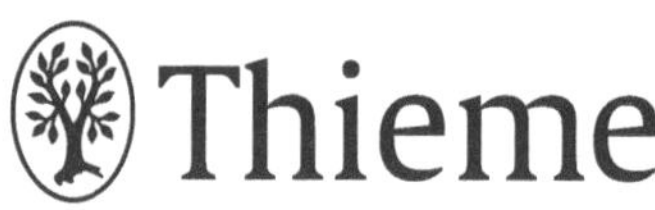

Clinical Anatomy, Histology, Embryology, and Neuroanatomy

An Integrated Textbook

Jamie C. Wikenheiser, PhD
Professor;
Director of Medical Gross Anatomy and Surgical Anatomy;
Program Director, Summer Gross Anatomy Academy;
Professor of Neuroscience and Clinical Foundations
Department of Anatomy and Neurobiology
University of California, Irvine School of Medicine
Irvine, California, USA

1952 Illustrations

Thieme
New York • Stuttgart • Delhi • Rio de Janeiro

Library of Congress Cataloging-in-Publication Data
is available with the publisher.

Important note: Medicine is an ever-changing science undergoing continual development. Research and clinical experience are continually expanding our knowledge, in particular our knowledge of proper treatment and drug therapy. Insofar as this book mentions any dosage or application, readers may rest assured that the authors, editors, and publishers have made every effort to ensure that such references are in accordance with **the state of knowledge at the time of production of the book.**

Nevertheless, this does not involve, imply, or express any guarantee or responsibility on the part of the publishers in respect to any dosage instructions and forms of applications stated in the book. **Every user is requested to examine carefully** the manufacturers' leaflets accompanying each drug and to check, if necessary in consultation with a physician or specialist, whether the dosage schedules mentioned therein or the contraindications stated by the manufacturers differ from the statements made in the present book. Such examination is particularly important with drugs that are either rarely used or have been newly released on the market. Every dosage schedule or every form of application used is entirely at the user's own risk and responsibility. The authors and publishers request every user to report to the publishers any discrepancies or inaccuracies noticed. If errors in this work are found after publication, errata will be posted at www.thieme. com on the product description page.

Some of the product names, patents, and registered designs referred to in this book are in fact registered trademarks or proprietary names even though specific reference to this fact is not always made in the text. Therefore, the appearance of a name without designation as proprietary is not to be construed as a representation by the publisher that it is in the public domain.

Thieme addresses people of all gender identities equally. We encourage our authors to use gender neutral or gender-equal expressions wherever the context allows.

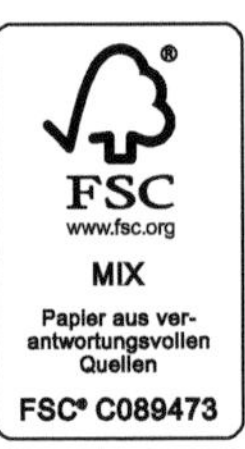

Thieme Medical Publishers, Inc.
333 Seventh Avenue, 18th Floor
New York, NY 10001, USA
www.thieme.com
+1 800 782 3488, customerservice@thieme.com

Illustrations by Markus Voll and Karl Wesker. From: Schuenke M, Schulte E, Schumacher U, *THIEME Atlas of Anatomy*.
Cover design: © Thieme
Cover images source: © Thieme
Typesetting by Thomson Digital, India

Printed in Germany by Beltz Grafische Betriebe 5 4 3 2 1

ISBN 978-1-62623-411-6
Also available as an e-book:
eISBN (PDF): 978-1-62623-412-3
eISBN (epub): 978-1-63853-427-3

My success would have not been possible without my wife Jen and my son Quinn. The two people who make my life complete. My parents, who along with my brother and closest friends encouraged me to be the best I can be.

I've had the good fortune to have worked with some of the brightest and knowledgeable in our field. My teaching career began in 1997 at the University of Minnesota, Twin Cities under the guidance of Anthony "Tony" Weinhaus. Tony to me was an encyclopedia of anatomical knowledge so I pushed myself to be just like him and model much of how I teach after him. He has always been there to give advice or talk shop.

At Case Western Reserve University, I had the privilege to have Michiko Watanabe as a mentor and research advisor focusing on pediatric cardiology and developmental biology. I can't say enough about how influential she was for myself and everyone in her laboratory. Nicole Ward for also sharpening my skills as a researcher. Individuals I taught alongside with included Charles Maier, Scott Simpson, Barbara Freeman, and John Fredieu.

At the David Geffen School of Medicine at UCLA, I had the opportunity to work with one of the greats in the field of human anatomy, the late Carmine Clemente. I thank him for his feedback and warmness as an individual. Joseph Miller and Robert Trelease for their advice. Warwick Peacock for sharpening my surgical skills and for advocating for more anatomy teaching. Individuals I taught alongside with included Elena Stark, Stephen Schettler, Jonathan Wisco, and Michael Zucker.

Here at the University of California, Irvine School of Medicine, I thank my former chair Ivan Soltesz and current chair Chris Gall for their support and confidence in how I approach medical training. My former colleague Justin Schaefer and postdoctoral scholars Zachary Gallaher and Rosie Santos for all their help and hard work. Michael Stamos, Dean of the Medical School; Khanh-Van Le-Bucklin, Vice Dean for Medical Education; Warren Weichman, Associate Dean of Clinical Science Education and Educational Technology; and Jeffery Suchard, Associate Dean of Basic Science Education for their leadership.

To all my past, current, and future students, thank you for your hard work and dedication to being the best medical professionals you can be. Your future patients will appreciate it.

To the donors and their families who graciously donate their bodies to the Willed Body programs across the country, because without you I cannot do my job the proper way.

Contents

Preface

For the past couple of decades, the anatomical sciences taught in North American professional schools have seen a steep decline in contact hours devoted to student training. With courses such as embryology and histology being hit the hardest, I set out to produce a text that would integrate the four anatomical sciences with an emphasis on clinical context. A text that could serve as a primary source for multiple courses, board-review preparation, or a reference book.

The introductory chapter will provide explanations to clarify anatomic terminology and an overview describing all systems of the body. The material is then organized by regions to not only better align with how most professional schools organize their curriculums, but also afford the flexibility to fit any other curriculum. The Back, Thorax, Abdomen, Pelvis and Perineum, Lower Extremity, Upper Extremity, and Head and Neck chapters are followed up by multiple chapters focused on neuroanatomy. There are over 350 up-to-date clinical correlates and nearly 250 board review-style multiple-choice questions.

The region-based chapters first introduce the gross anatomy of the structure, followed by descriptions of the neurovasculature and lymphatic drainage of that structure. Histology of the organ is then addressed, and after all structures that complement the particular system are described, the embryology of the larger system is depicted. Medical imaging focuses primarily on normal anatomy but select clinical cases are also presented. Examples include plain and contrast radiographs, CT, MRI, and ultrasonography studies. Radiology of the organs is generally addressed near the end of the chapter in order for future professionals to correlate information presented in the chapter with the reality in the professional setting. My hope is that this integration of the four anatomical sciences will further enhance a student's understanding of the subject matter, and better prepare them for national exams and most importantly enable them to deliver optimal care of their patients.

This textbook has over 1,100 exceptional images from the award-winning, three-volume *Thieme Atlas of Anatomy* by Michael Schuenke, Erik Schulte, and Udo Schumacher, with illustrations done by Markus Voll and Karl Wesker. In addition, there are images from the 4th edition of *Atlas of Anatomy*, published by Thieme, and co-edited by Anne Gilroy, Brian MacPherson, and me. I'm grateful for their advice and for the privilege to work alongside them on the *Atlas of Anatomy*. The histological images are from *Histology: An Essential Textbook* by D.J. Lowrie, also published by Thieme.

My former colleague at the David Geffen School of Medicine at UCLA, the late Carmine Clemente, looked over the early drafts I had written. His blessing and enthusiasm to move forward with the project meant the world to me. From a production standpoint, I'm in debt to the individuals at Thieme. Special thanks to Cathrin Weinstein (Managing Director) for continuing to believe in this project. Torsten Scheihagen (Senior Content Service Manager) for controlling the flow of this project. Calla Heald who produced exceptional new artwork and formally Delia DeTurris (Acquisitions Editor) and Nikole Conner (Managing Editor) for setting the pace and making things happen.

Jamie C. Wikenheiser, PhD
Irvine, California
July 2022

Acknowledgments

Mark Ajalat, MD
Division of Vascular Surgery; Department of Surgery
Ronald Reagan UCLA Medical Center
Los Angeles, California, USA

Kyle Barbour, MD
Emergency Medicine
Rochester General Hospital
Rochester, New York, USA

Roger A. Dashner, MS, PhD
Advanced Anatomical Services
Columbus, Ohio, USA

Rob Edwards, MD, PhD
Professor, Department of Pathology
University of California, Irvine, School of Medicine
Irvine, California, USA

Adachukwu Ezenekwe, MD
Primary Care
University of California, Irvine Medical Center
Irvine, California, USA

Ganga Karunamuni, PhD
Research Associate, Pediatrics
Case Western Reserve University, School of Medicine
Cleveland, Ohio, USA

Ismail Kasimoglu, MD
Internal Medicine
University of California, Irvine Medical Center
Irvine, California, USA

Kevin Labadie, MD
Department of Surgery
University of Washington, School of Medicine
Seattle, Washington, USA

Daniel Lama, MD
Division of Urology; Department of Surgery
University of Cincinnati, School of Medicine
Cincinnati, Ohio, USA

Joseph M. Miller, PhD
Department of Pathology and Laboratory Medicine
David Geffen School of Medicine at UCLA
Los Angeles, California, USA

Nathan Molina, MD
Plastic and Reconstructive Surgery; Department of Surgery
Icahn School of Medicine at Mount Sinai
New York, New York, USA

S. Carter Pace, MD, MS, FCAP, FASCP
Cleveland Clinic Union Hospital
Dover, Ohio, USA

Amanda Purdy, MD
General Surgery
Harbor UCLA Medical Center
Los Angeles, California, USA

Bob Trelease, PhD
Professor, Pathology and Laboratory Medicine
David Geffen School of Medicine at UCLA
Los Angeles, California, USA

Anthony J. Weinhaus, PhD
Department of Integrative Biology and Physiology
University of Minnesota, Twin Cities
Minneapolis, Minnesota, USA

Introductory Concepts and Imaging Techniques

LEARNING OBJECTIVES

- To understand the difference between systematic, regional, and clinical anatomy.
- Have a thorough knowledge of proper anatomical terminology. This will include terms that are associated with location and direction.
- Have a thorough knowledge of anatomical planes and axes in order to interpret radiological images.
- Have an understanding of the integumentary system that includes its functions and the five layers of the epidermis. Associated structures such as the dermis, nails, and glands will also be looked at along with clinical correlates such as surgical incisions and types of burns.
- Have an understanding of the skeletal system that involves bones, cartilage, and articulating joints. Types of bones, cartilage, and joints will be presented along with formation of bones and clinical correlates related to this system such as osteoporosis and bone fracture healing.
- Have an understanding of the muscular system and the three different types of muscles. This section examines the micro- and macrostructure of muscles along with contraction and movements produced by them. Clinical correlates would include muscular dystrophy and fibromyalgia.
- Have an understanding of the circulatory system that includes its functions, tunic layers, and types of blood vessels. This would also include a look at the lymphatic system and the specific structures associated with it. Clinical correlates will include a look at peripheral arterial disease, varicose veins, and the possible routes or pathways of cancer spreading.
- Have an understanding of the nervous system and the multiple parts of it. This would include the difference between the central and peripheral nervous systems as well as the difference between somatic and visceral innervation. A look at the micro- and macrostructure of neurons will be preceded by a look at the specific type of nerve fibers that pass through larger peripheral nerves. A closer look at the autonomic nervous system and its paired visceral sensory fibers will conclude this section.
- Introduce a brief synopsis of all other systems located in the body. These details will be presented during later chapters.
- Have a general understanding of the clinical imaging techniques used in today's medical field.

I.1 Studying Human Anatomy

There are three different approaches to studying human anatomy. These include a systematic, regional, or clinical (applied) anatomy approach. This text will focus on the clinical or applied anatomy approach that encompasses both regional and systematic approaches to studying human anatomy. The anatomical sciences are divided and studied as gross, microscopic (histology), development (embryology), and neuroanatomy with all aspects being touched upon in this text.

I.1.1 Systematic Anatomy

When organizing the body into organ systems that work together and carry out complex functions, this is known as the systematic approach to studying anatomy. For example, when the muscular system is active during exercise, it is not only the muscles that are functioning in this complex system. The heart and vessels of the cardiovascular system supply blood to the muscles. Within this blood, oxygen derived from the lungs of the respiratory system and glucose derived from the digestion of food from the digestive system supply the muscles with energy. Nerves of the nervous system are responsible for activating and turning off opposing muscles so that we have fluid movements. The basis of most of the systematic anatomy will be mentioned in this chapter but are relatable to almost all other chapters.

I.1.2 Regional Anatomy

When organizing the body into parts or regions, such as thorax or pelvis, this is the regional approach to studying anatomy. The body is divided into parts: head, neck, back, thorax, abdomen, pelvis/perineum, paired upper limbs, and paired lower limbs. The term "trunk" refers to the back, thorax, abdomen, and pelvis/perineum. The one thing to remember is that regions cannot only be thought of as just an isolated part of the body. The region is continuous or adjacent to other parts of the body being studied; thus, major neurovasculature bridging adjacent regions must be understood.

When a physician investigates the body for possible trauma or pathology, surface anatomy will be essential in understanding specific regional anatomy. **Surface anatomy** provides the treating physician landmarks of structures that are palpable under the skin and gives them a baseline of information to begin their diagnosis or further exploration (**Fig. I.1**). When a patient arrives to the emergency room with a gunshot to the upper left quadrant of the abdomen, the ER physician must know what organs were at risk of damage due to the bullet traveling through that region of the abdomen.

I.1.3 Clinical Anatomy

When systematic and regional anatomy is applied together and emphasis is on both structure and function, this is known as clinical anatomy. This is important in health care practice covering all fields such as medicine and the allied health sciences. Emphasis is placed on clinical application. This text emphasizes and bridges the four major areas of the anatomical sciences (gross anatomy, histology, embryology, and neuroanatomy) to better understand clinical practice. Gross, histology, and embryology will be the focus until near the end of the text when neuroanatomy is isolated and focus is on components of both the central and peripheral nervous systems.

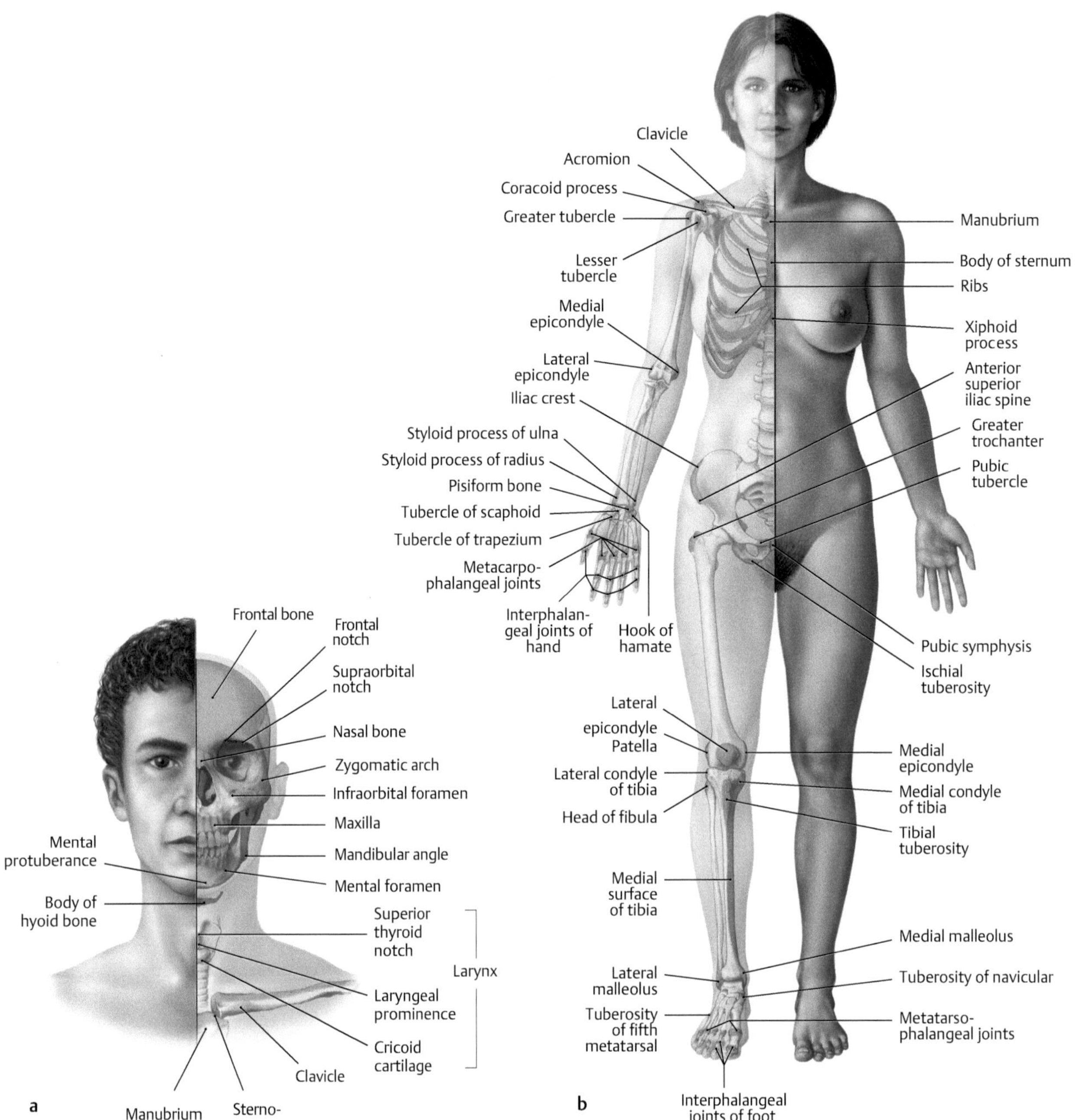

Fig. I.1 **(a)** Surface contours and palpable bony prominences of the face and neck, anterior view. **(b)** Surface contours and palpable bony prominences of the trunk and upper and lower limbs in the female, anterior view. (From Schuenke M, Schulte E, Schumacher U. THIEME Atlas of Anatomy. General Anatomy and Musculoskeletal System. Illustrations by Voll M and Wesker K. 3rd ed. New York: Thieme Medical Publishers; 2020.)

I.2 Anatomical Terminology and Position

In anatomy there is no need for translation because it has an international vocabulary that is the foundation of all medical terminology or nomenclature. All health professionals are able to communicate whether they are from clinical practice or basic sciences. Anatomical terms are mainly derived from Latin or Greek but many of these terms can provide a structure's location, size, shape, or function. **Eponyms** are the names of structures derived from the people who generally discovered them and are no longer listed as official anatomical terminology but are still seen in clinical practice. This text will mention the more common eponyms when appropriate. This standard was established during the *Terminologia Anatomica: International Anatomical Terminology* (Federative Committee on Anatomical Terminology or FCAT). It was released in 1998 and supersedes the previous standard, *Nomina Anatomica*.

All descriptions of the human body are expressed in terms of **anatomical position**. This is to ensure all clinical or scientific descriptions of the human body are not ambiguous. Anatomical position is a reference posture in which the human body is:

- Standing erect with the legs slightly spread apart.
- Upper limbs by the sides.
- Palms of the hands, toes of the feet, and head are facing forward.

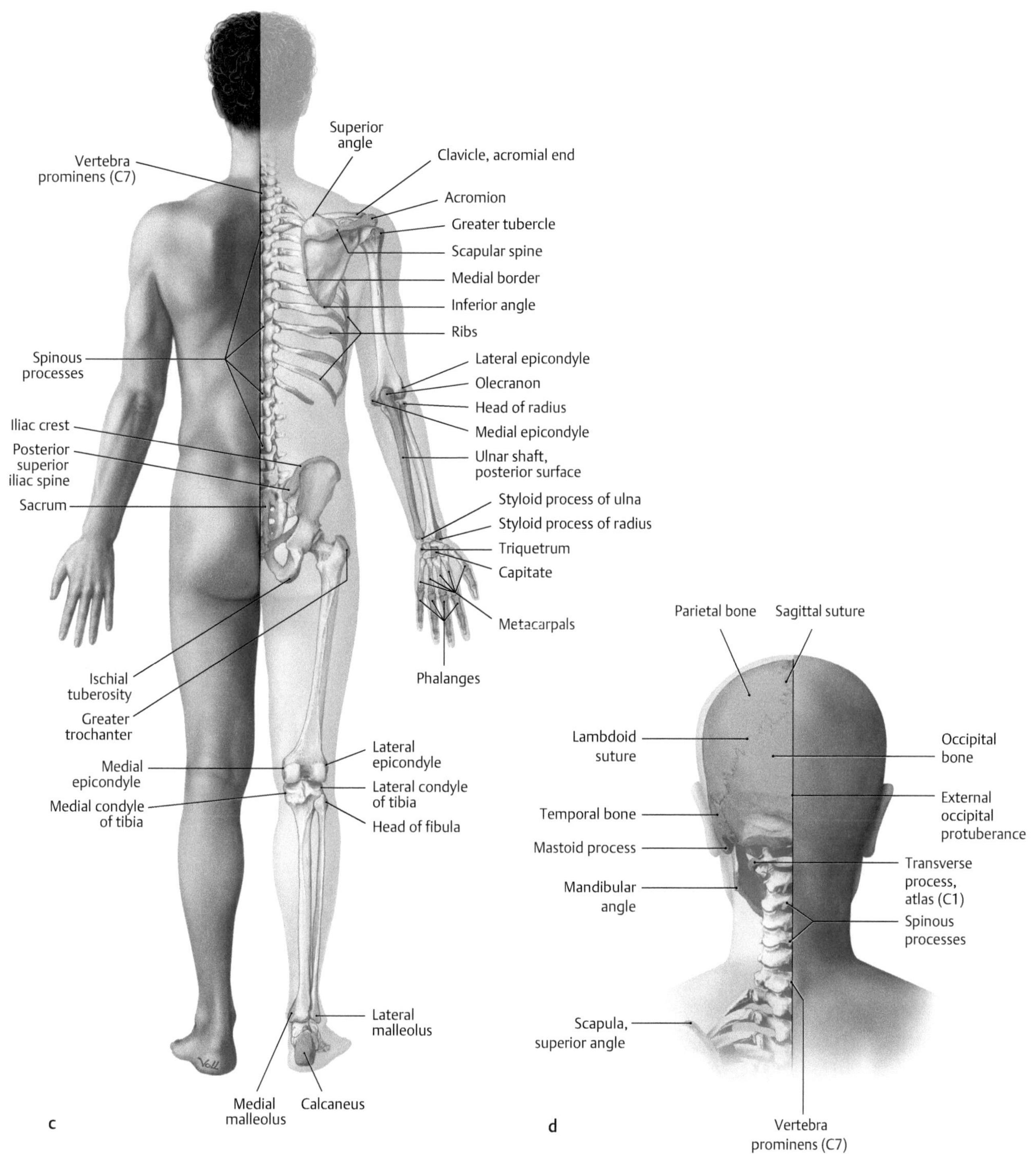

Fig. I.1 (*continued*) **(c)** Surface contours and palpable bony prominences of the trunk and upper and lower limbs in the male, posterior view. **(d)** Surface contours and palpable bony prominences of the face and neck, posterior view. (From Schuenke M, Schulte E, Schumacher U. THIEME Atlas of Anatomy. General Anatomy and Musculoskeletal System. Illustrations by Voll M and Wesker K. 3rd ed. New York: Thieme Medical Publishers; 2020.)

I.3 Anatomical Variation

The anatomy described in written texts and atlases is the observation of what is seen in most individuals. The most common pattern of structures is generally what is reported in these texts. Anatomical variation must be expected when a student is dissecting. Neurovasculature has a general theme with smaller veins varying the most, followed by arteries and then finally nerves.

I.4 Terms of Location and Direction

Location and directional terms used in the medical field will refer to the body in anatomical position. A list of terms describing the head, neck, trunk, and limb location and directions are listed in **Table I.1** (**Fig. I.2**).

Table I.1 **Terms of location and direction**

Head, neck, and trunk	
Superior (cranial)	Pertaining to, or located toward the head
Inferior (caudal)	Pertaining to, or located toward the feet
Anterior (ventral)	Located toward the front
Posterior (dorsal)	Located toward the back
Medial	Toward the median plane
Lateral	Away from the median plane or toward the side
Superficial	Near the surface
Intermediate	Between the superficial and deep surface
Deep	Further from the surface
Frontal	Pertaining to the forehead
Temporal	Pertaining to the lateral region of head (temple)
Occipital	Pertaining to the back of the head
Basilar	Pertaining to the base of the skull
Upper and lower limbs	
Proximal	Closer to the trunk or point of origin
Distal	Further from the trunk or point of origin
Ulnar	Pertaining to the ulna or medial forearm
Radial	Pertaining to the radius or lateral forearm
Tibial	Pertaining to the tibia or medial leg
Fibular	Pertaining to the fibula or lateral leg
Palmar (volar)	Pertaining to the palm or anterior surface of the hand
Plantar	Pertaining to the sole or inferior surface of the foot
Dorsum	Pertaining to the back of the hand or top of the foot

I.5 Anatomical Planes and Axes

Descriptions of the body are based on four imaginary planes that intersect the body in anatomical position. Each plane is perpendicular to the next and when movement occurs in a particular plane, it must rotate about an axis that has a 90-degree relationship to the other (**Fig. I.3**).

- The **coronal (frontal) plane** is a vertical plane passing through the body and is parallel to the coronal suture of the skull. This divides the body into an anterior and a posterior part.
- The **transverse (axial) plane** is any cross-sectional plane that divides the body into an upper (superior) and a lower (inferior) portion. A radiologist may refer to a transverse plane as a *transaxial plane* or just an *axial plane*. Axial anatomy is viewed as though the physician is looking from the feet toward the head.
- The **sagittal (parasagittal) plane** is a vertical plane that is parallel to the sagittal suture of the skull. The **midsagittal (median) plane** is the vertical plane passing longitudinally through the center of the body dividing it into left and right halves.
- The **longitudinal (vertical) axis**, while standing, runs through the body craniocaudally and is perpendicular to the ground. It lies at the intersection of the coronal and sagittal planes.
- The **transverse (horizontal) axis** runs from side to side and lies at the intersection of the coronal and transverse planes.
- The **sagittal axis** runs anteroposteriorly from the anterior to posterior surface of the body and lies at the intersection of the sagittal and transverse planes.

Anatomical planes may also be used to create a mental reconstruction of a two-dimensional section into a three-dimensional image, which is very helpful in describing a histological sample or section for example. These include transverse, longitudinal, and oblique sections (**Fig. I.4**).

- **Transverse (cross) sections** are slices of the body or its parts that are at right angles to the longitudinal axis of the body or any of its parts.
- **Longitudinal sections** run lengthwise or parallel to the long axis of the body or of any of its parts.
- **Oblique sections** are slices of the body or any of its parts that are not cut along any of the previously listed anatomical planes. Oblique sections are very common in radiographs because many of these sections do not lie perfectly in a frontal, transverse, or sagittal plane.

I.6 Center of Gravity

The *whole-body center of gravity* is located at the level of the second sacral vertebra (**Fig. I.5**). The *line of gravity* is an imaginary line that passes vertically along the midsagittal plane from the

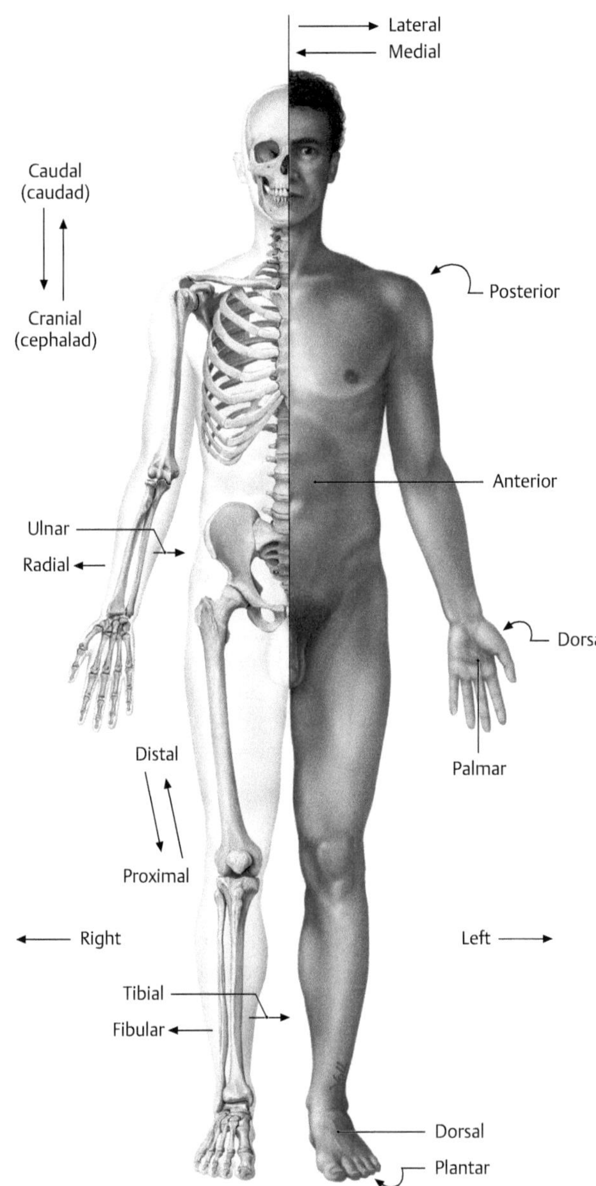

Fig. I.2 The anatomical body position. (From Schuenke M, Schulte E, Schumacher U. THIEME Atlas of Anatomy. General Anatomy and Musculoskeletal System. Illustrations by Voll M and Wesker K. 3rd ed. New York: Thieme Medical Publishers; 2020.)

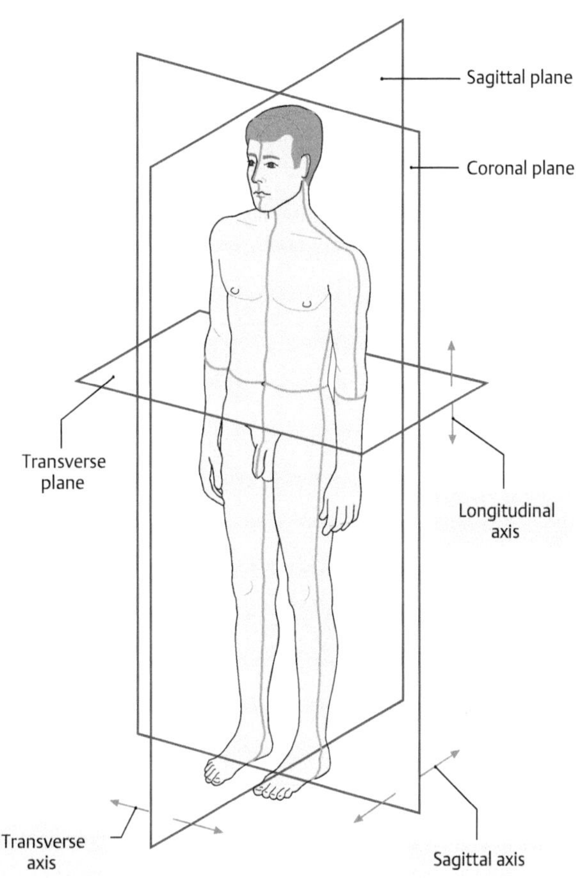

Fig. I.3 Cardinal planes and axes in the human body (neutral position, left anterolateral view). (From Schuenke M, Schulte E, Schumacher U. THIEME Atlas of Anatomy. General Anatomy and Musculoskeletal System. Illustrations by Voll M and Wesker K. 3rd ed. New York: Thieme Medical Publishers; 2020.)

anterior view. Laterally, the *line of gravity* passes through the external auditory meatus, dens of the C2 vertebra, anatomical and functional junctions of the spinal column, whole-body center of gravity, and finally through the hip, knee, and ankle joints.

I.7 Integumentary System

The skin and its appendages (hair, nails, oil glands, and sweat glands) are considered the **integumentary system**. The skin is considered the largest organ of the human body and it has five major functions:

1. **Protection** or barrier against environmental effects such as physical abrasions, chemical or biological insults, ultraviolet radiation, and fluid loss.

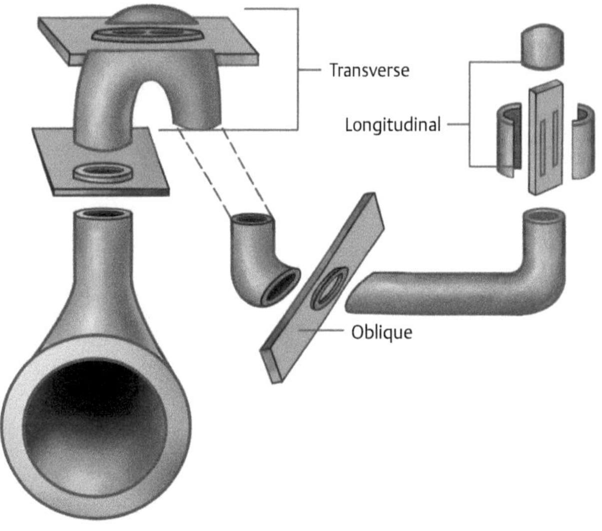

Fig. I.4 Histological sections in a transverse (cross), longitudinal, or oblique plane. Illustration by Calla Heald.

2. **Containment** of organs and extracellular fluids.
3. **Thermoregulation** by varying blood flow to superficial vessels and the evaporation of sweat.
4. **Storage and synthesis** of vitamin D by exposing bare skin to the sunlight and ultraviolet B rays.
5. **Sensory input** from the endings of superficial nerves and they transmit thermal, tactile, and painful stimuli.

The skin has a superficial cellular layer called the *epidermis* and a deep connective tissue layer known as the *dermis*. The **epidermis** is a *stratified squamous epithelium* consisting primarily of *keratinocytes*, divided into thick versus thin skin, avascular, and is organized into five layers (**Fig. I.6**).

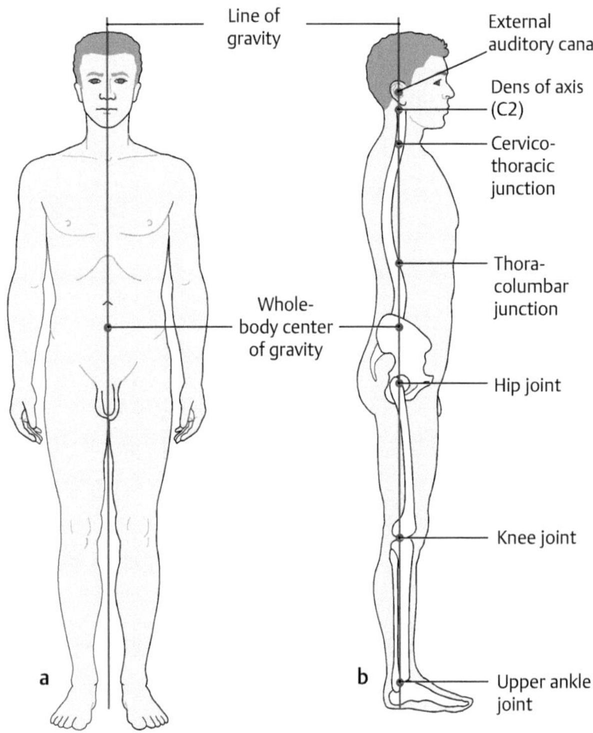

Fig. I.5 The whole-body center of gravity and the line of gravity: **(a)** anterior view, **(b)** lateral view. (From Schuenke M, Schulte E, Schumacher U. THIEME Atlas of Anatomy. General Anatomy and Musculoskeletal System. Illustrations by Voll M and Wesker K. 3rd ed. New York: Thieme Medical Publishers; 2020.)

1. **Stratum basale**: the deep, single layer of closely spaced cuboidal cells that anchors the epidermis to the dermis and contains the stem cells that produce new keratinocytes.
2. **Stratum spinosum**: contains several layers of keratinocytes that resemble spines. **Langerhans cells** are antigen-presenting dendritic cells found throughout the epidermis but mainly in the spinosum layer. These cells are distinguishable from melanocytes by the presence of *Birbeck granules* which have no known function.
3. **Stratum granulosum**: contains diamond-shaped keratinocytes that contain keratohyalin granules that appear to bind keratin filaments together. Cells begin to lose their nuclei closest to the stratum corneum layer. **Melanocytes** that produce the pigment **melanin** are scattered in this layer, the stratum spinosum layer, and within hair follicles. The amount of melanocytes is equivalent but their rate of melanin production and degradation differs between different races.
4. **Stratum lucidum**: seen only in thick skin such as the palms of the hands and soles of the feet. The anucleate keratinocytes form a translucent band directly next to the stratum corneum layer.
5. **Stratum corneum**: contains the anucleate, cornified, and stratified (15–20 layers) keratinocytes that also yield a continuous layer of lipids creating the barrier to help repel water.

The layer of dense interlacing collagen and elastic fibers just deep to the epidermis is called the **dermis**. The dermis is responsible for the strength, toughness, and tone of the skin. The dermis is divided into two parts: the *papillary* and *reticular layers*. The **papillary dermis** is the closest to the epidermis and includes the fingerlike projections called dermal papillae. The **dermal papillae** project into the epidermis between the **epidermal (rete) ridges**. They are most prominent near areas of high mechanical shearing stress such as the fingertips, palms of the hand, or soles of the feet and serve to increase the surface contact between the epidermis and dermis minimizing separation of the two layers. The papillary layer is relatively thin and contains type I and III collagen fibers, elastic fibers, capillaries, encapsulated nerve processes (Meissner corpuscles), and sweat glands.

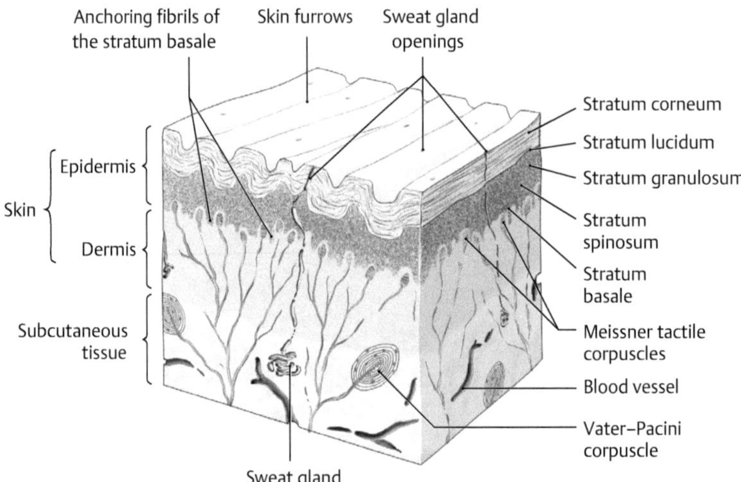

Fig. I.6 Structure of the skin and subcutaneous tissue and the five layers of the epidermis. (From Schuenke M, Schulte E, Schumacher U. THIEME Atlas of Anatomy. General Anatomy and Musculoskeletal System. Illustrations by Voll M and Wesker K. 3rd ed. New York: Thieme Medical Publishers; 2020.)

The **reticular dermis** is deeper and adjacent to the superficial fascia and contains thick type I collagen and elastic fibers that help dictate the *tension lines* of the skin. The **tension (Langer) lines** run in a longitudinal fashion in the limbs but more transversely in the neck and trunk regions (**Fig. I.7**). The predominant pattern of the collagen fibers will determine the characteristic tension line in the skin. Wrinkling of the skin in older individuals is the result of the weakening and loss of elastic fibers. The reticular layer also contains the base of the hair follicles, sweat glands, and mechanoreceptors (Ruffini and Pacinian corpuscles).

Other features of the skin include the *pilosebaceous units, nails,* and multiple types of *glands*. The **pilosebaceous unit** is primarily found in thin skin and is composed of the hair follicle and an attached sebaceous gland and arrector pili muscle. A single hair consists of keratinized cells that develop in hair follicles located in the deepest parts of the dermis and superficial fascia before reaching the epidermal surface. The expanded terminus of the hair follicle is called the **hair root** and along with the dermal papilla, they are known as the *hair bulb*. The base or **hair bulb** of the follicle contains the proliferating keratinocytes receiving nutrients from the dermal papillae and melanin from melanocytes. The majority of cells making up the hair root are called the **matrix**. They will account for the growth of the hair and produce keratin, which forms hard keratin. The **external root sheath** represents a tubular invagination of epidermis with a thickened basal lamina called the *glassy membrane*. The **glassy membrane** separates the dermis from the epithelium of the hair follicle. The **internal root sheath** consists of cells that immediately surround the *hair shaft* and produce a soft keratin. It ends where the duct of the sebaceous gland attaches to the hair follicle. The **hair shaft** is a long slender filament that consists of three regions known as the *medulla, cortex,* and *cuticle* of the hair. Hair growth averages about 1 cm per month but this growth is not continuous. The life span of a single hair can range from months to years and can be region specific. The **sebaceous glands** that attach to the follicle secrete a waxy sebum. The **arrector pili muscles** are smooth muscles that run obliquely from the hair follicle in the upper part of the dermis; elevate the hair in a vertical fashion; and are innervated by sympathetic postganglionic fibers (**Fig. I.8**).

The **nails** are located on the distal phalanx of each finger and toe and are composed of **nail plates** that are keratinized epithelial cells containing hard keratin resting on the epithelial cells of the **nail bed**. The epidermis will invade the dermis on a transverse line resulting in the formation of the **nail groove**. The nail matrix will form from proliferating cells in the **nail root** located in the nail groove. After the cells keratinize, the nail plate will advance pass the distal portion of the digit and over the nail bed. Fingernails grow continuously unlike hair at a rate of about 0.5 mm per week. Toenails grow slightly slower than fingernails. The **lunula** is the white, crescent-shaped junction of the nail root with the nail plate. The stratum corneum of the proximal nail fold forms the **eponychium (cuticle)** and it extends distally about 0.5 to 1.0 mm. The **hyponychium** represents the epidermis under the free distal end of the nail (**Fig. I.9**).

Glands of the integumentary system include the sebaceous, eccrine, and apocrine glands.

- **Sebaceous glands**: these are alveolar (saccular) type glands that secrete into a duct near the hair shaft. They are located in the dermis except at the glans penis, labia minora, and eyelids. They are prevalent in the skin of the forehead, face, and scalp and secrete sebum (oily secretions) to coat the hair and skin.
- **Eccrine sweat glands**: These are simple coiled tubular glands located in the dermis and superficial fascia throughout the skin of the body and can be quite numerous in the palms of the hands and soles of the feet. They secrete sweat onto the skin surface and are important for thermoregulation. They can excrete as much as 10 L of sweat in very active individuals and respond to sympathetic postganglionic stimulation.
- **Apocrine sweat glands**: These are sweat glands that are specifically located in areas such as the axilla, areola of the nipple, external genitalia, and anus. Modified versions of these glands are located in the eyelid (glands of Moll) and external auditory meatus (ceruminous wax glands). These are much longer than the eccrine sweat glands and their ducts drain into canals of the hair follicles just superficial to the insertion of the sebaceous gland ducts. They do not begin to secrete until puberty and under the influence of hormones but are also stimulated by sympathetic postganglionic fibers. These glands may have evolved from other glands that secreted sex attractants or pheromones seen in lower animals.

The **superficial fascia** located just deep to the dermis is composed primarily of loose connective tissue and stored fat along with

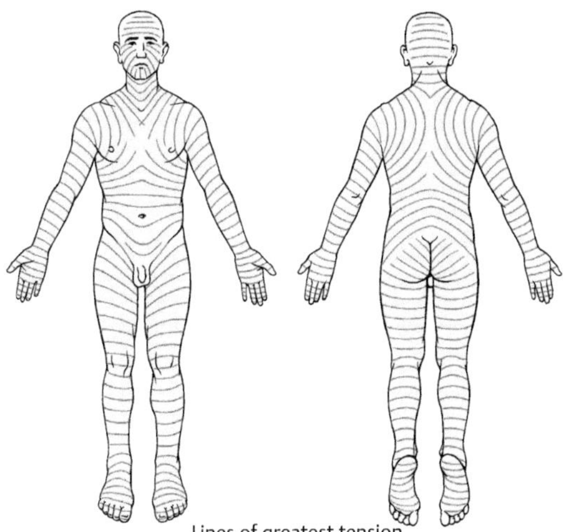

Fig. I.7 Tension lines of the skin. (Modified from Fritsch H, Kühnel W, ed. Color Atlas of Human Anatomy, Vol. 2: Internal Organs. 6th ed. Stuttgart: Thieme; 2014.)

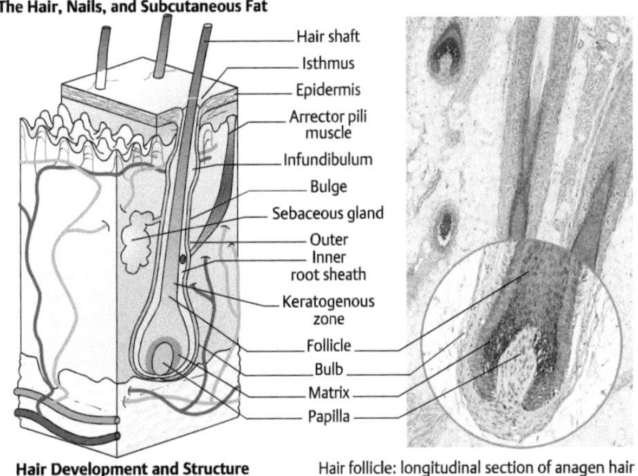

Fig. I.8 Structure of a hair follicle. (Modified from Rocken M, Schaller M, Sattler E, Burgdorf W. Color Atlas of Dermatology. 1st ed. Stuttgart: Thieme; 2012.)

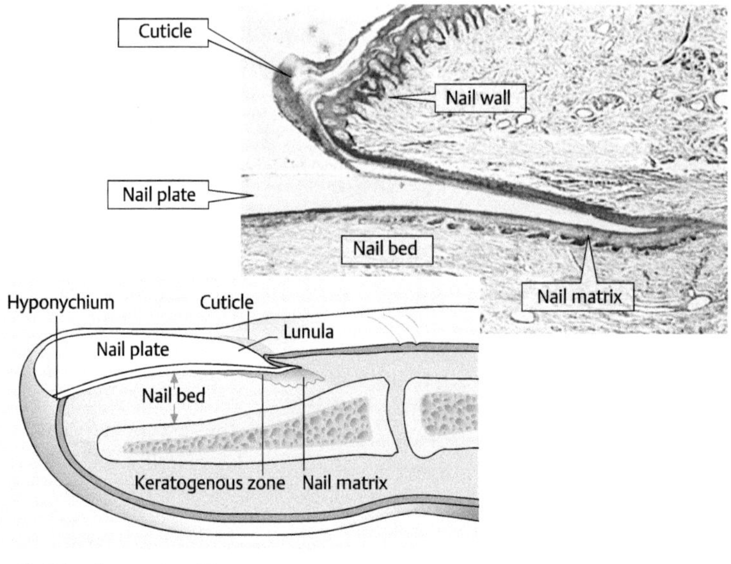

Fig. I.9 Structure of the thumbnail. (Modified from Rocken M, Schaller M, Sattler E, Burgdorf W. Color Atlas of Dermatology. 1st ed. Stuttgart: Thieme; 2012.)

cutaneous nerves and superficial blood and lymphatic vessels. The amount of subcutaneous tissue varies depending on the location of the body and nutritional state of the individual. It functions in thermoregulation and serves as padding to protect the skin from deeper bony projections. **Skin ligaments** are small but numerous bands that extend from the deeper aspect of the dermis back to the *deep fascia*. Mobility of the skin is determined by the density and length of these skin ligaments. **Deep fascia** is devoid of fat and can invest skeletal muscle, the periosteum of bone, and neurovascular bundles. This deep fascia will contribute to the **intermuscular septa** and the formation of **fascial compartments** that will be a focus during the lower and upper extremity chapters of this text (**Fig. I.10**).

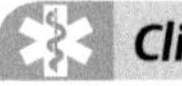

Clinical Correlate I.1

Skin Incisions, Lacerations, and Scarring

When an incision or laceration runs parallel to the tension lines there is generally good healing because there was minimal damage to the underlying fibers **(Fig. I.7)**. Certain surgical incisions such as the Pfannenstiel incision done during a Caesarean section or abdominal hysterectomy or even a McBurney incision during an open appendectomy are done in accordance with the tension lines. An incision made parallel with the tension lines results in less gaping to facilitate better healing and reduced scar tissue versus an incision perpendicular to the tension lines that creates more gaping, slower healing, and more scarring. Scarring is a natural part of healing and is composed of the same collagen it replaces; however, instead of the collagen fibers having a normal random formation, the fibers become aligned in a single direction and more pronounced. Scars are devoid of hair follicles and sweat glands and are less resistant to ultraviolet rays.

Clinical Correlate I.2

Types of Burns

Burns can be caused by thermal, chemical, electrical, or ionizing radiation sources and are classified depending on how deep and severe they penetrate the skin. Classification is set as first-, second-, third-, and fourth-degree burns.

- *First-degree (superficial) burns*: affect only the epidermis and the burn site will be red and hot (*erythema*), low-to-moderate pain level, and dry with no blisters present. Peeling of the skin may occur a few days after the initial exposure. Long-term damage is rare and sunburn would be an example. It will take typically 5 to 10 days to heal.
- *Second-degree (partial thickness) burns*: the epidermis and part of the dermis are affected with possible blistering. These burns are painful and highly sensitive to touch, have the sensation of being hot or cold, and feel moist. It will take anywhere from 2 to 3 weeks or a month or so to heal, and leave scarring.
- *Third-degree (full thickness) burns*: the epidermis and dermis are affected and possibly the superficial fascia. The burn site will appear charred or white with swelling. The site will be numb as most nerve endings will have been destroyed. Skin grafting will probably be needed to close the wound and it may take several months with special burn treatment to heal but full function may not be restored in some cases.
- *Fourth-degree burns*: underlying tendons, muscles, bones, and neurovasculatures are damaged. There is no pain due to all nerve endings being destroyed. Medical treatment will always be required with no healing occurring, thus possibly leading to amputation.

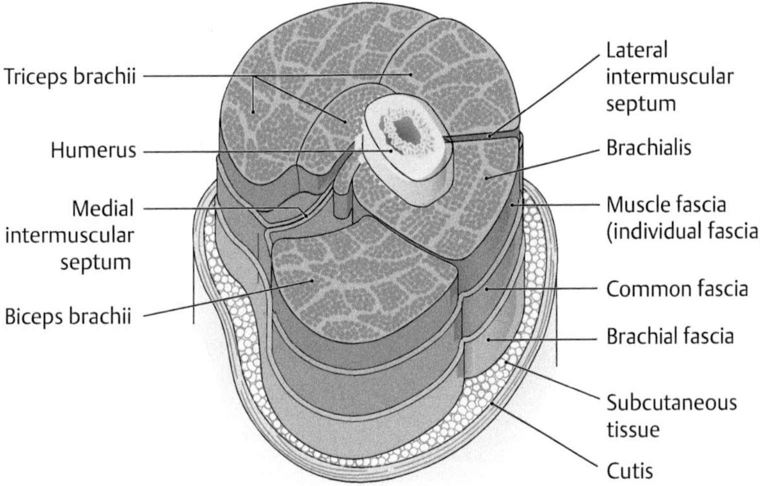

Fig. I.10 Muscle fasciae. (From Schuenke M, Schulte E, Schumacher U. THIEME Atlas of Anatomy. General Anatomy and Musculoskeletal System. Illustrations by Voll M and Wesker K. 3rd ed. New York: Thieme Medical Publishers; 2020.)

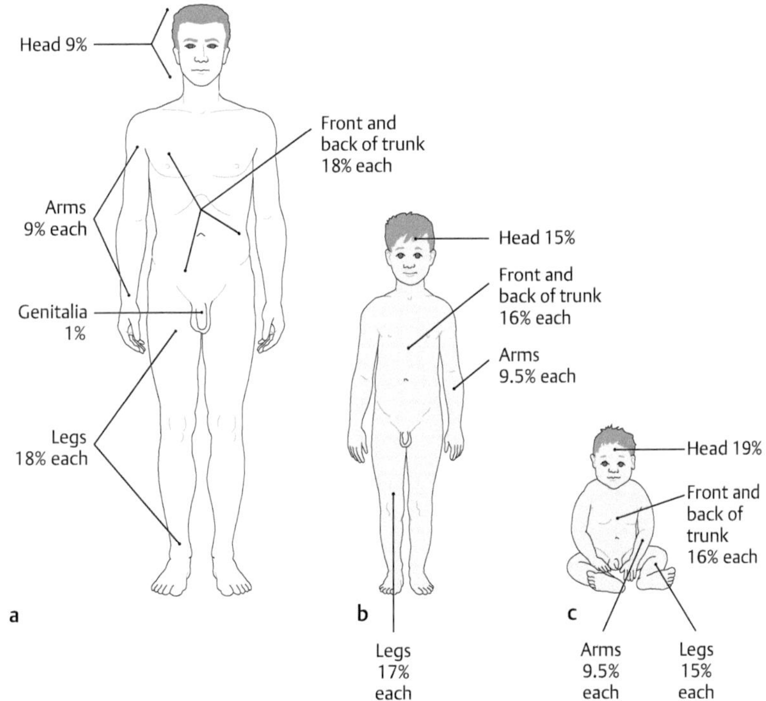

Fig. I.11 Distribution of body surface area in adults, children, and infants. (From Schuenke M, Schulte E, Schumacher U. THIEME Atlas of Anatomy. General Anatomy and Musculoskeletal System. Illustrations by Voll M and Wesker K. 3rd ed. New York: Thieme Medical Publishers; 2020.)

The percent of the total surface area of the body affected or extent of an individual burn is more significant than the degree of the initial burn. This will better predict the future prognosis of the victim. The **rule of nines** is a standardized method to assess how much surface area of the body has been burned on a patient and only applies to second- and third-degree burns. The body is divided into areas that account for approximately 9% of the total surface area compared to all the other surfaces or are measured in multiples of 9%. The rules of nine pertain to adults and are adjusted for children and infants (**Fig. I.11**).

I.8 Skeletal System

The **skeletal system** is made up of the bones and cartilage that provide support for the body and the protection of vital internal organs. Associated with the skeletal system is the **articular system**. This system involves the joints and associated ligaments that lie between two articulating bones. Certain movements, as dictated by the attachments of muscles, occur at these joints. The skeletal system is divided into two parts (**Fig. I.12**):

- **Axial skeleton**: consists of the skull, hyoid, vertebrae, sacrum, coccyx, sternum, and ribs.

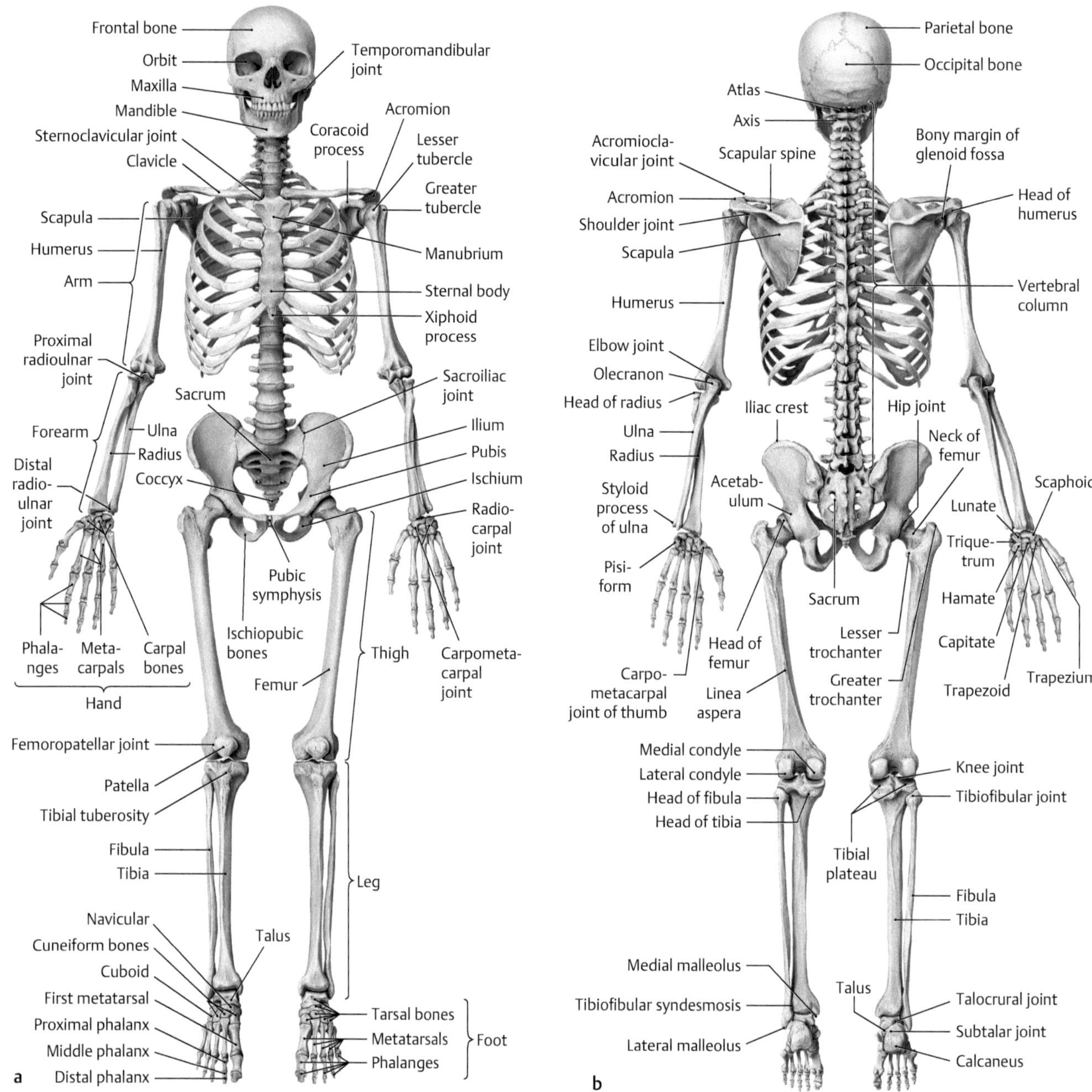

Fig. I.12 Human skeleton. **(a)** Anterior view. **(b)** Posterior view. (From Schuenke M, Schulte E, Schumacher U. THIEME Atlas of Anatomy. General Anatomy and Musculoskeletal System. Illustrations by Voll M and Wesker K. 3rd ed. New York: Thieme Medical Publishers; 2020.)

- **Appendicular skeleton**: consists of the bones of the upper limb that include the pectoral girdle (scapula and clavicle) and the bones of the lower limb that include the hip bones (made of the ilium, ischium, and pubis).

Cartilage is the flexible but semirigid form of connective tissue that adds flexibility to certain parts of the skeleton. Cartilage is avascular but receives nutrients by diffusion which limits its capacity for repair. There are three main types:

1. **Hyaline**: it is the most prevalent cartilage in the body and is made up mostly of type II collagen and may or may not have a perichondrium. It makes up most of the respiratory tract including the nose, larynx, trachea, and bronchi and the skeleton where it is located at the anterior ends of the ribs and articulating surfaces of weight-bearing bones. It also makes up the fetal skeleton before ossifying to become bone. The weight-bearing surfaces are associated with synovial joints and are capped by an **articular (hyaline) cartilage**. This articulating surface is responsible for a near frictionless and smooth surface allowing for free movement of these bones at their joints.
2. **Fibrocartilage**: it has both type I and II collagen but has no perichondrium. It is found in areas of high stress where tensile strength is necessary such as the intervertebral disks (annulus

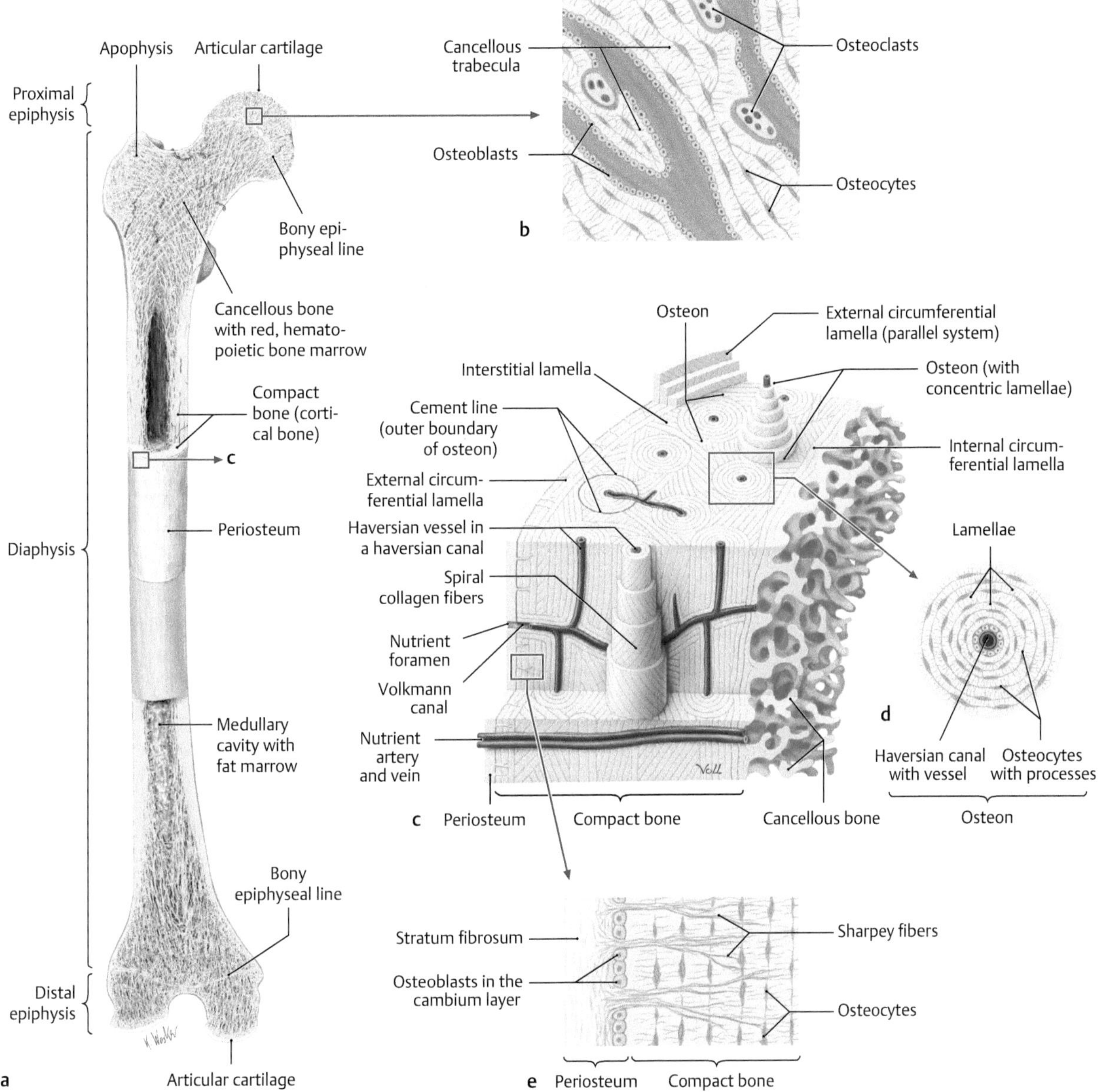

Fig. I.13 Structure of a typical tubular bone, illustrated for the femur. **(a)** Coronal sections of femur. **(b)** Detail from **a**: the sectioned areas display the lamellar architecture of the cancellous trabeculae. **(c)** Detail from **a**: three-dimensional representation of compact bone, whose structural units consist of osteons. **(d)** Detail from **c**: the microstructure of the osteon. **(e)** Detail from c: structure of the periosteum. (From Schuenke M, Schulte E, Schumacher U. THIEME Atlas of Anatomy. General Anatomy and Musculoskeletal System. Illustrations by Voll M and Wesker K. 3rd ed. New York: Thieme Medical Publishers; 2020.)

fibrosus), pubic symphysis, articulating surface of the temporomandibular joint, and the menisci for example.

3. **Elastic**: in addition to type II collagen there are elastic fibers that permit more flexibility than hyaline cartilage. It has a perichondrium and is located in the external ear, epiglottis of the larynx, and pharyngotympanic (auditory or Eustachian) tube.

Bone is a highly specialized living tissue and forms most of the skeleton. It consists of cells called **osteocytes** living in **lacunae** (gap or space) surrounded by an extracellular matrix that they themselves produce. The matrix is infiltrated with inorganic salts, making it rigid and somewhat inflexible. Bone is made up of both organic and inorganic material. About 95% of the organic portion or **osteoid** is made of type I collagen, while the inorganic portion is mostly calcium and phosphate ions that make up *hydroxyapatite crystals* and it also contains carbonate, magnesium, fluoride, and sulfate. There is an outer fibrous connective tissue called the **periosteum**, and unlike cartilage, it is highly vascular. Bone is constantly being remodeled in response to physical stresses being placed on it and the mineral needs of the body. The functions include supporting the body and its cavities; attachment sites for muscle tendons and ligaments; the basis of movement or leverage; mineral storage (calcium); the production of new blood cells and the protection of these hematopoietic tissues in medullary (marrow) cavity of most bones (**Fig. I.13**).

Table I.2 **Common bony surface markings and spaces**

General description	Structure	Definition	Example
Processes formed for articulation with adjacent bones	Head	A large, round articular end separated by the shaft by a neck	Head of femur
	Neck	The connection between the head and shaft	Anatomical neck of humerus
	Condyle	A smooth, rounded articular process	Lateral femoral condyle
	Epicondyle	A process superior or adjacent to a condyle	Medial epicondyle of humerus
	Trochlea	Smooth, grooved, or spool-like articular process that acts like a pulley	Trochlea of humerus
	Capitulum	A small, rounded articular head	Capitulum of humerus
	Facet	A small, flat articular surface	Superior articular facet of vertebrae
Processes formed by tendon or ligament attachments	Trochanter	A large, rough projection	Greater trochanter of femur
	Tuberosity	A small, rough projection	Ischial tuberosity of ischium
	Tubercle	A small, raised projection	Greater tubercle of humerus
	Crest	A prominent ridge of bone	Iliac crest of ilium
	Spine	A pointed process	Spine of the scapula
	Line	A low linear ridge	Soleal line of tibia
Elevation or projections	Protuberance	A projection of bone	External occipital protuberance
	Ramus	An extension of bone making an angle with the rest of the bone	Mandibular ramus of mandible
Depressions	Fossa	A shallow depressed area	Supraspinous fossa of scapula
	Sulcus	A narrow groove	Intertubercular sulcus
	Notch	A V-like depression in the margin of a flat area	Suprascapular notch of scapula
Openings	Foramen	A rounded passageway	Intervertebral foramen
	Fissure	An elongated cleft or crack	Superior orbital fissure
	Meatus	A tubelike opening or channel	External acoustic meatus
	Canal	A passageway through bone	Optic canal
	Sinus	A chamber within bone	Frontal sinus of the frontal bone

The two types of bones are *compact* and *spongy (trabecular) bone*. **Compact bone** is primarily calcified bone with small spaces containing vasculature and osteocytes. **Spongy bone** consists of thin plates of bony trabeculae (*spicules*) with relatively large medullary cavities. Spongy bone is covered by compact bone externally and by *endosteum* on the medullary cavity side. The **medullary** or **marrow cavity** is a soft connective tissue that fills the central cavities of long bones and all the spaces between the bony trabeculae. Bone marrow is classified as either red or yellow. The **red marrow** is mostly hematopoietic and responsible for producing blood cells while the **yellow marrow** is primarily adipose but can be converted back to red marrow in cases of severe blood loss (**Fig. I.13a**).

Bones are classified based on their shape and these will include the long, short, flat, irregular, and sesamoid bones (**Fig. I.12**).

- **Long bones**: are tubular and can include the femur of the thigh and humerus of the arm.
- **Short bones**: are cuboidal and are only found as tarsal (ankle) and carpal (wrist) bones.
- **Flat bones**: are just that, flat, and generally serve to protect. They can include multiple cranial bones, scapula of the shoulder, or the sternum and ribs of the thorax.
- **Irregular bones**: have odd shapes. These include bones of the face such as the sphenoid and the vertebrae.
- **Sesamoid bones**: develop in tendons and are located where tendons cross the ends of long bones or in areas that need to protect tendons from excessive wear. They can include the patella of the knee, pisiform of the wrist, or the paired sesamoid bones of the thumb and big toe.

Bone surface markings are located wherever tendons, ligaments, or fascia attaches to bone. They can also be identified as spaces or openings that allow certain neurovasculature to pass to and from other bones. A list of these markings or spaces is listed in **Table I.2.**

I.9 Bone Development

All bones are derived initially from embryonic mesenchyme but differentiate through two different processes known as *intramembranous* or *endochondral ossification*. Bones may take years to fully develop and mature.

- **Intramembranous ossification**: involves mesenchymal models of bone generally beginning to form during the second month of embryonic life and the direct ossification of this mesenchyme will not begin until the fetal period. This process involves mesenchymal migrating and aggregating forming

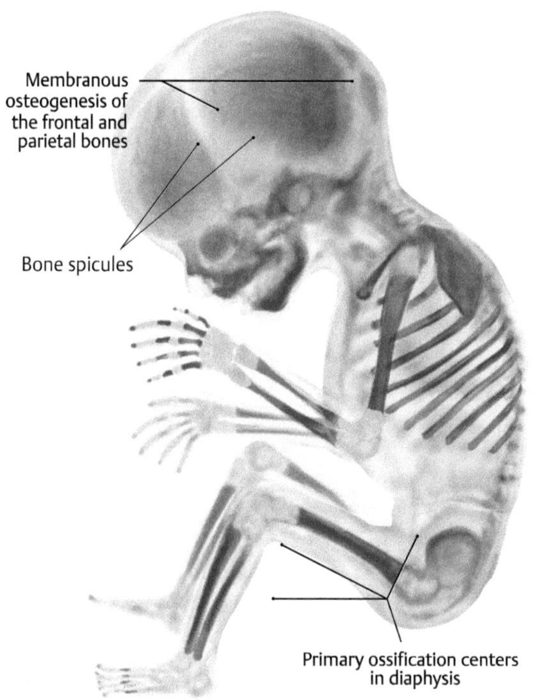

Fig. I.14 Bone spicule formation from primary ossification centers to the periphery. (From Schuenke M, Schulte E, Schumacher U. THIEME Atlas of Anatomy. General Anatomy and Musculoskeletal System. Illustrations by Voll M and Wesker K. 3rd ed. New York: Thieme Medical Publishers; 2020.)

specific areas called **ossification centers**. The mesenchymal cells differentiate into osteoblasts and they will produce bone matrix that undergoes calcification. As the osteoblasts become enclosed by bone matrix they become osteocytes. Bone growing from the ossification center forms linear extensions called **spicules** and blood vessels grow around them to support the bone tissue. Continued growth at multiple ossification leads to the eventual development of both spongy and compact bone along with the marrow cavities. This form of ossification involves many of the bones of the skull (**Fig. I.14**).

- **Endochondral ossification**: includes most bones of the body and form from a hyaline cartilage model that approximates the shape of the future bone. Growth occurs by both *interstitial* (from multiple centers) and *appositional* (addition of new layers to previous layers) growth. Multiple steps are involved (**Fig. I.15 a,b**):

1. **Formation of a primary ossification center**: osteoprogenitor cells around the center of the cartilage differentiate into osteoblasts and they produce the **diaphysis**. The perichondrium will become a periosteum. Chondrocytes within the cartilage degenerate and resorb their matrix causing an enlargement of the lacunae. Calcium deposits cause the cartilage to become calcified. The blood vessels and osteogenic cells from the periosteum invade the center of the cartilage and create larger lacunar spaces that lead to the creation of primary marrow cavities. The osteogenic cells will become the osteoblasts that line the calcified cartilage around these lacunar spaces and lead to the formation of the endosteum.
2. **Formation of a secondary ossification center**: once the primary ossification center is established, osteogenic vascular beds break into the distal ends of the hyaline cartilage model forming the **epiphyses**. The chondrocytes in the middle of the epiphyses will hypertrophy and the bone matrix between them will calcify. The **epiphyseal arteries** will migrate into this developing cavity. The flared portion between the diaphysis and epiphysis is called the **metaphysis**.
3. **Endochondral bone growth**: The primary and secondary ossification centers formed in the epiphyses and diaphysis are separated by a zone of cartilage and it is called the **epiphyseal plate** until growth of the long bones reach adult length. The epiphyseal plate maintains itself by interstitial growth and is vital for the bone to reach its final length. There are five zones exhibited within this cartilaginous plate, and proceeding from the epiphyseal to the diaphyseal side they are (**Fig. I.15c**):

    a. *Zone of resting cartilage:* chondrocytes exhibit no division or active matrix production.
    b. *Zone of proliferation*: chondrocytes undergo cell division and arrange themselves in distinct columns that are parallel to the direction of growth.
    c. *Zone of hypertrophy*: chondrocytes enlarge and compress the cartilage matrix surrounding them.
    d. *Zone of calcification*: these enlarged cells begin to degenerate as the matrix becomes calcified. Osteoblasts begin secreting matrix and calcification limits diffusion leading to chondrocyte death.
    e. *Zone of ossification*: osteoblasts align the spicules of remaining calicified cartilage and then lay down osteoid.

After reaching maturity at around 20 years of age, bone will constantly turn over and adapt to new mechanical stresses. It is a dynamic tissue and the compensatory deposition or resorption of compact bone or the realignment of the bony trabeculae is considered normal processes. Compact bone is always being resorbed and replaced in the following manner. **Osteoclasts** from the marrow will move into the area of compact bone being replaced and absorb the bone in what are called **resorption tunnels**. These are distinguishable from Haversian canals by their irregular outlines and the presence of osteoclasts lining their borders. These tunnels contain blood vessels along with **osteoprogenitor cells** and **osteoblasts** that proceed to produce concentric lamellae from the outside and back toward the inside of the tunnel before a central canal is left (**Fig. I.16**). Ultimately, these osteons develop through the progressive filling in of a tunnel with successive lamellae of bone. Osteoprogenitor cells are capable of differentiating into osteoblasts in highly vascular regions or chondroblasts in avascular regions. **Calcitonin** secreted by the thyroid gland lowers blood calcium levels by decreasing osteoclast activity and **parathyroid hormone** from the parathyroid glands raises blood calcium by increasing osteoclast activity.

I.9.1 Neurovasculature of the Bones

The **periosteal nerves** that originate from the nearby somatic nerves supply innervation to the bone periosteum. The periosteum is most sensitive to tension or tearing and thus the reason why breaking a bone is quite painful. The sympathetic postganglionic fibers coursing through these periosteal nerves are vasoconstrictive to the blood vessels associated with the bone marrow. A rich supply of blood reaches bones. Most of this comes from a single or multiple **nutrient arteries**. These nutrient arteries originate from nearby arteries located outside the periosteum and pass through a **nutrient foramen** in the compact bone before

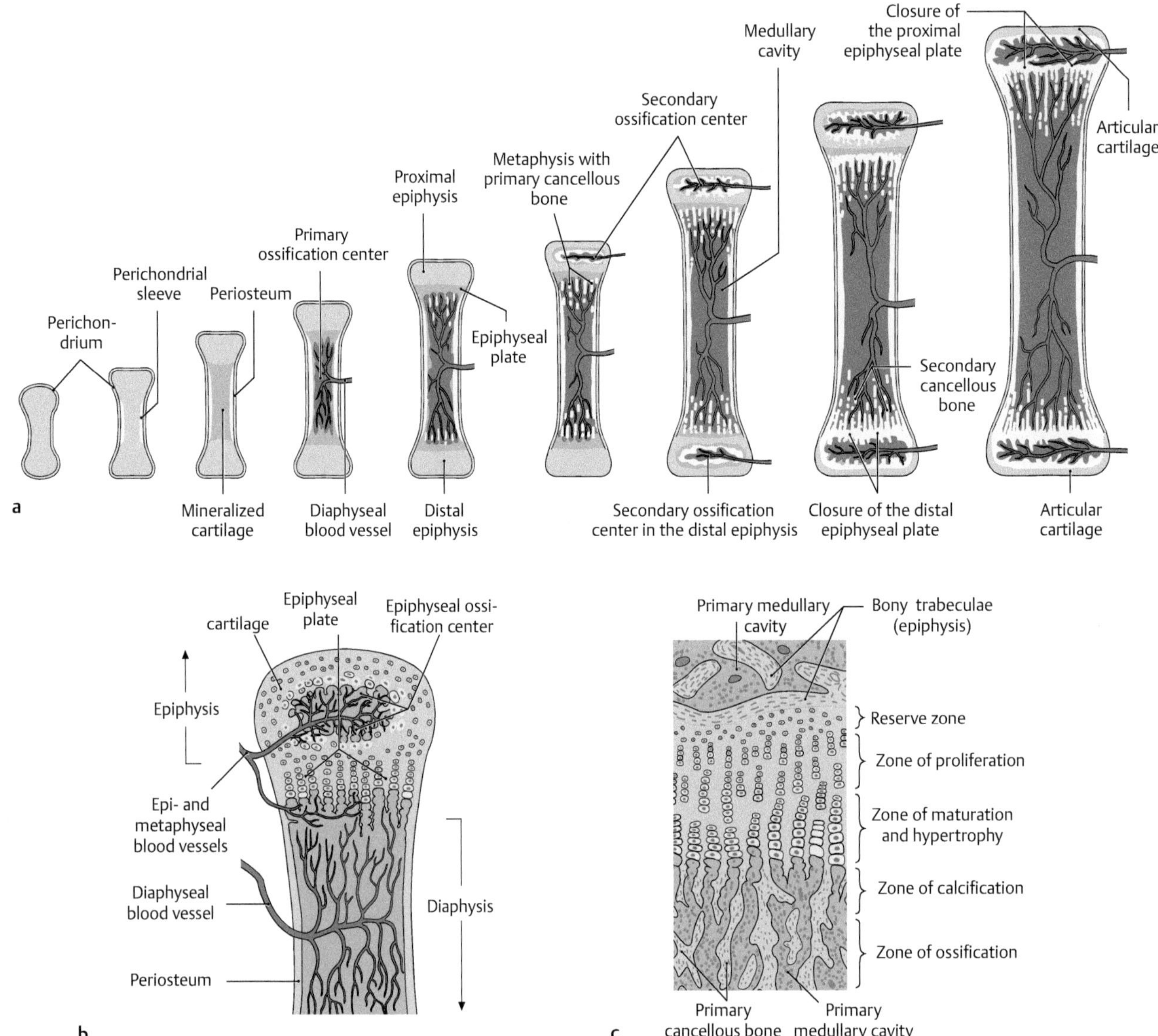

Fig. I.15 **(a)** Development of a long bone. **(b)** Structure of the epiphyseal plate and its blood supply. **(c)** Zones of the epiphyseal plate. (From Schuenke M, Schulte E, Schumacher U. THIEME Atlas of Anatomy. General Anatomy and Musculoskeletal System. Illustrations by Voll M and Wesker K. 3rd ed. New York: Thieme Medical Publishers; 2020.)

eventually reaching the medullary cavity of the bone. While in the medullary cavity, the nutrient artery divides into more longitudinal branches that extend to each end of the bone and will supply the spongy bone, compact bone, and bone marrow. Periosteal arteries supply most of the compact bone along with the periosteum and they themselves originate from the nutrient artery or other nearby systematic arteries. If the periosteum was to be removed the bone could not survive. Equivalent veins are paired with the arteries and there is an abundant supply of lymphatic vessels near the periosteum (**Fig. I.15b**).

The eventual vasculature reaches and drains at the level of the osteocytes by passing through the **haversian (osteon) system**. Osteocytes are arranged radially around their vascular supply. This cylindrical, lamellar arrangement of osteocytes is evident in compact bone. The osteocytes in their lacunae are arranged into progressively larger concentric circles around a central canal containing the blood vessels. In cross-section, the Haversian system has a central **Haversian canal** that will be surrounded by 4 to 20 **concentric lamellae** of matrix. Small **canaliculi** will be seen traversing the lamellae forming connections with the lacunae and central canals. Interstitial fluid from capillaries and within the canals percolates around osteocyte processes inside the canaliculi. Nutrients are thus able to be transported out to the most peripheral cells of the system. A **cement line** surrounds each Haversian system. Blood vessels will also traverse larger transverse channels known

Clinical Correlate I.3

Osteoporosis

Osteoporosis is the condition of fragile bones due to aging, a decrease in both the organic and inorganic composition of bone making an individual more susceptible to fractures. Bone density will begin to naturally decrease after 35 years of age and more rapidly in women after menopause. The risk factors can include the genetic predisposition of the individual, lack of calcium and vitamin D, reduced exercise levels, excessive alcohol consumption and cigarette smoking. A diagnosis can be made by taking an X-ray or by using tests to measure bone density but symptoms may not appear until after a bone fracture. Treatments may include using calcium and vitamin D supplements, prescription medications, increasing exercise activity, reducing alcohol consumption, and quitting smoking.

Clinical Correlate I.4

Stages of Bone Fracture Healing

Weakness of a bone when an individual is older or after trauma could be a reason for a bone fracture. Bones are strong but also susceptible to fractures. A **simple fracture** is when a bone fracture remains covered by the overlying skin. A **compound fracture** is when the broken bone penetrates the skin. Specific types can include *spiral, impacted, comminuted, epiphyseal, depressed,* and *greenstick fractures.* When a fracture occurs and a physician realigns the bone, this is known as **reduction. Open reduction** is when pins, rods, or wires surgically join the two broken ends together. A **closed reduction** is setting a broken bone into place without surgery. After reduction, the broken bones are immobilized by placing in a cast or traction unit and allowed to begin the healing process. The four phases of fracture healing:

1. *Hematoma formation*: blood vessels are broken in the periosteum and inside the bone, resulting in the formation of a hematoma. Inflammation occurs and the site is very painful. The bone cells are deprived of nutrients and die.
2. *Formation of a fibrocartilaginous callus*: within a few days new capillaries and blood vessels begin to grow into the hematoma and the dead cells begin to be cleared away by phagocytic cells. Osteoblasts and fibroblasts near the periosteum and endosteum of the fracture site begin to reform bone and this site is referred to as the **fibrocartilaginous callus.**
3. *Formation of a bony callus*: within a week, the fibrocartilaginous callus will be converted into a **bony callus** of spongy bone primarily by endochondral ossification. Approximately 2 months after the original fracture, the two ends will become firmly attached.
4. *Bone remodeling*: the bony callus will continue to be remodeled by osteoblasts and osteoclasts and any excess bony material will be removed from the exterior of the bone shaft and the interior of the medullary cavity. Compact bone is then added and displays the characteristics of the original unbroken bone.

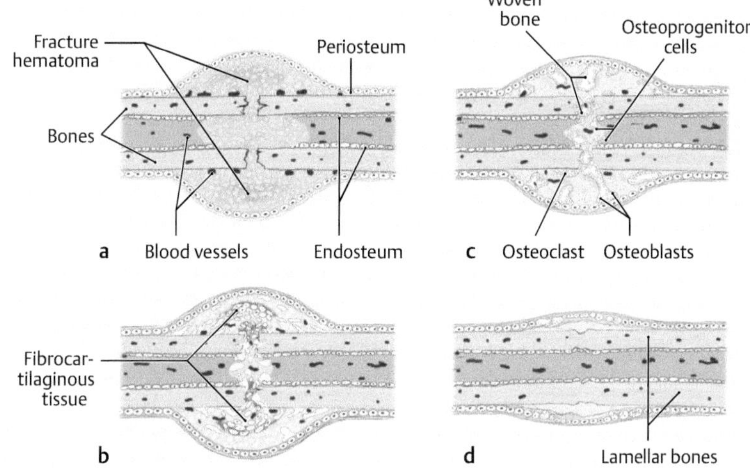

(a) Hematoma formation. **(b)** Formation of a fibrocartilaginous callus. **(c)** Formation of a bony callus. **(d)** Bone remodeling. (Modified from Schuenke M, Schulte E, Schumacher U. THIEME Atlas of Anatomy. General Anatomy and Musculoskeletal System. Illustrations by Voll M and Wesker K. 3rd ed. New York: Thieme Medical Publishers; 2020.)

as **Volkmann canals** and these will connect to adjacent Haversian canals. Structures called the **interstitial lamellae** are interspersed between complete Haversian systems and represent the remnants of concentric lamellae previously made of osteons that were partially removed in the remodeling process. **Circumferential lamellae** are the several layers of bone orientated parallel to the free surface of the outer periphery of compact bone **(Fig. I.13)**.

I.9.2 Joints

The articulations or junctions between two or more bones of the skeleton would constitute a **joint.** Joints can involve no movement at all or display a large range of motion (ROM). There are three classifications of joints and they include the fibrous, cartilaginous, and synovial joints.

- **Fibrous joints**: the bones are united by fibrous tissue. ROM at these joints is dependent on the length of the fibrous tissue but generally these joints are only partially moveable. Examples include the *sutures* between bones of the cranium; the presence of a fibrous membrane or ligament spanning two bones such as the *interosseous membrane* between the radius and ulna of the forearm and are also known as a **syndesmosis**; the socket articulation between the root of the tooth and alveolar process of the jaw is also a fibrous joint but is commonly referred to as a **dentoalveolar syndesmosis** (gomphosis) (**Fig. I.17**).
- **Cartilaginous joints**: are connected entirely by cartilage (hyaline or fibrocartilage) and consist of two types:
  1. *Primary cartilaginous* (synchondroses): are temporary articulations as with the development of the long bones at the epiphyseal plates and are united by hyaline cartilage. Slight bending may be allowed at these joints (**Fig. I.18**).
  2. *Secondary cartilaginous* (symphyses): these are strong and slightly movable joints united by fibrocartilage. Examples include the pubic symphysis and the intervertebral (IV)

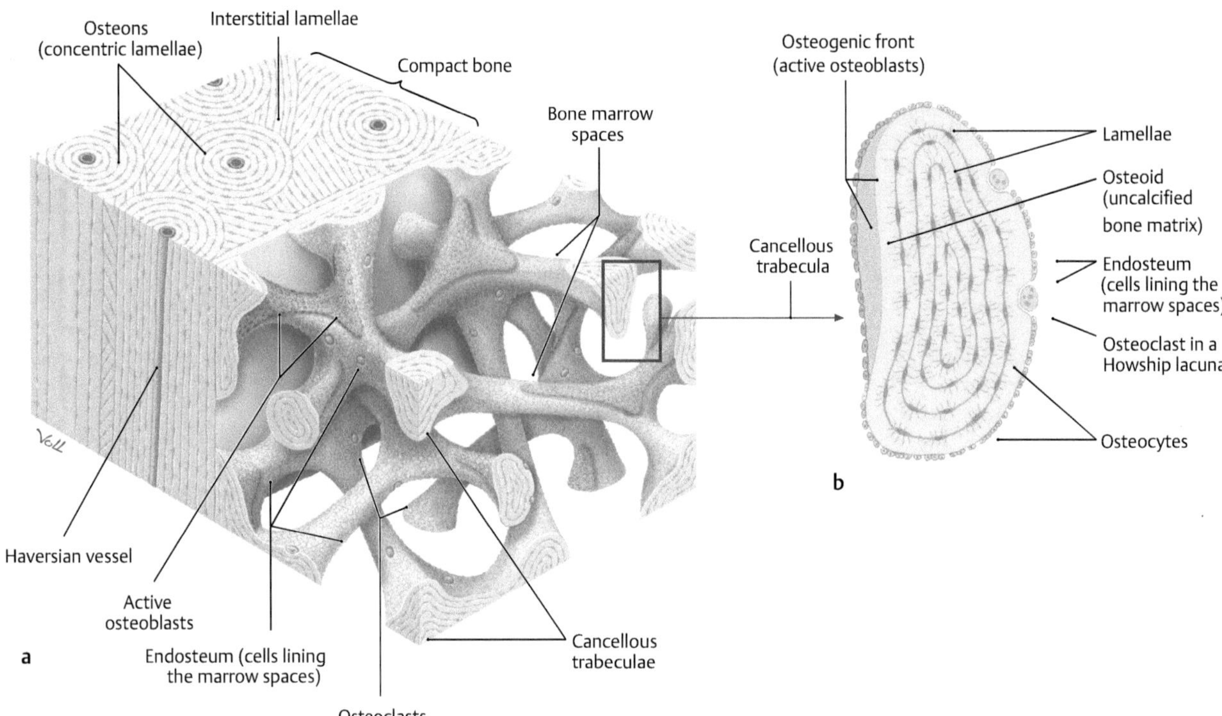

Fig. I.16 Growth and remodeling processes within the cancellous portion of a lamellar bone. **(a)** Three-dimensional representation of cancellous bone tissue. **(b)** Remodeling of a cancellous trabecula. (From Schuenke M, Schulte E, Schumacher U. THIEME Atlas of Anatomy. General Anatomy and Musculoskeletal System. Illustrations by Voll M and Wesker K. 3rd ed. New York: Thieme Medical Publishers; 2020.)

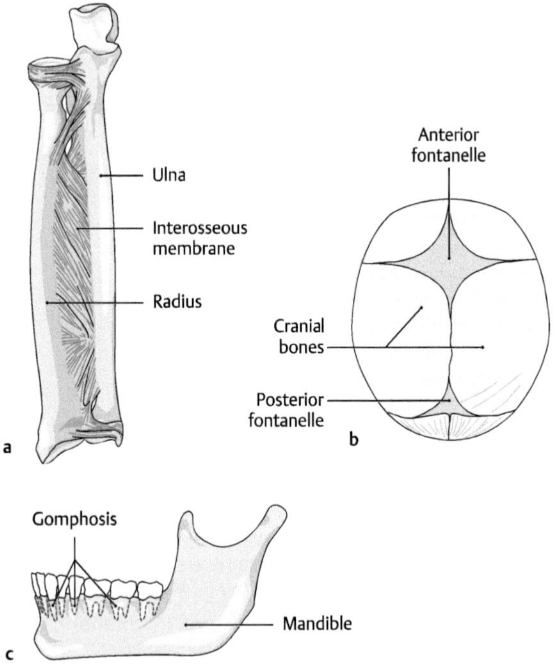

Fig. I.17 Syndesmoses (fibrous joints). **(a)** Interosseous membrane. **(b)** Fontanelles. **(c)** Gomphosis. (From Schuenke M, Schulte E, Schumacher U. THIEME Atlas of Anatomy. General Anatomy and Musculoskeletal System. Illustrations by Voll M and Wesker K. 3rd ed. New York: Thieme Medical Publishers; 2020.)

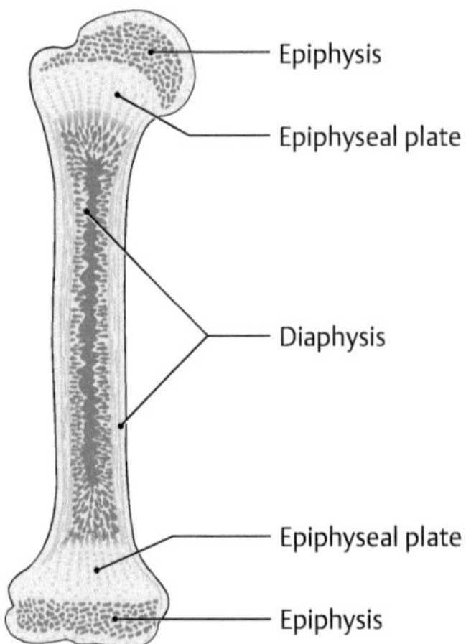

Fig. I.18 Epiphyseal plates prior to closure. (From Schuenke M, Schulte E, Schumacher U. THIEME Atlas of Anatomy. General Anatomy and Musculoskeletal System. Illustrations by Voll M and Wesker K. 3rd ed. New York: Thieme Medical Publishers; 2020.)

joints. The IV disks located between most adjacent vertebrae are made of fibrocartilage and act as their own IV joint and provide mobility, shock absorption, and strength to the vertebral column **(Fig. I.19)**.

- **Synovial joints**: are defined as consisting of four parts: (1) a **joint capsule** that has an outer fibrous layer and inner layer lined by a **synovial membrane**; (2) **synovial fluid** produced by the synovial membrane; (3) a **joint cavity** filled with the synovial fluid; and (4) an **articular cartilage** mostly made of hyaline cartilage (**Fig. I.20**). The synovial membrane will not pass over the articulating cartilage. For some of these joints, the larger the ROM, the less stable the overall integrity of the joint may be. There are six types of synovial joints (**Fig. I.21**):

1. *Ball and socket*: examples include the *glenohumeral* and *hip joints*. Movements occur in multiple axes and planes

and can include flexion, extension, abduction, adduction, lateral and medial rotations, and circumduction, making them *multiaxial joints.*

2. *Condyloid*: examples include *radiocarpal (wrist)* and *metacarpophalangeal (knuckle) joints.* Movements occur around two axes and in the sagittal or frontal plane and include flexion, extension, abduction, and adduction, making them *biaxial joints.*
3. *Saddle*: examples include the *sternoclavicular* and *carpometacarpal joint of the thumb.* Movements occur around two axes at right angles to one other in a sagittal and frontal plane and include flexion, extension, abduction, and adduction, making them *biaxial joints.*

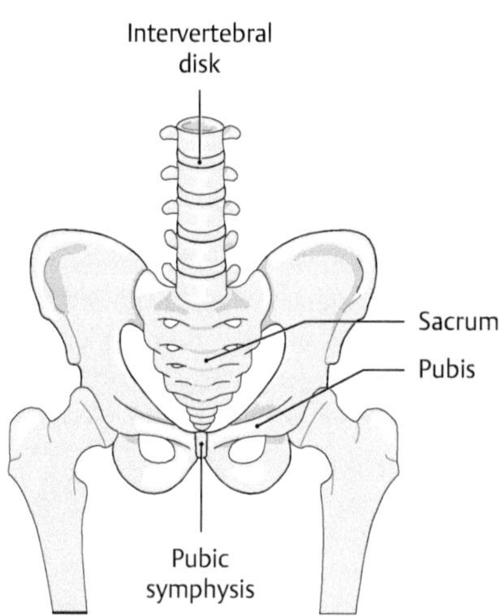

Fig. I.19 Pubic symphysis and intervertebral disks (intervertebral symphysis). (From Schuenke M, Schulte E, Schumacher U. THIEME Atlas of Anatomy. General Anatomy and Musculoskeletal System. Illustrations by Voll M and Wesker K. 3rd ed. New York: Thieme Medical Publishers; 2020.)

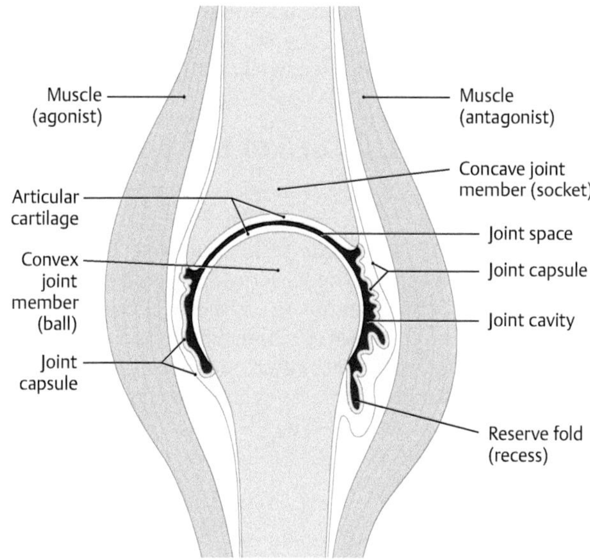

Fig. I.20 Structure of a true synovial joint. (From Schuenke M, Schulte E, Schumacher U. THIEME Atlas of Anatomy. General Anatomy and Musculoskeletal System. Illustrations by Voll M and Wesker K. 3rd ed. New York: Thieme Medical Publishers; 2020.)

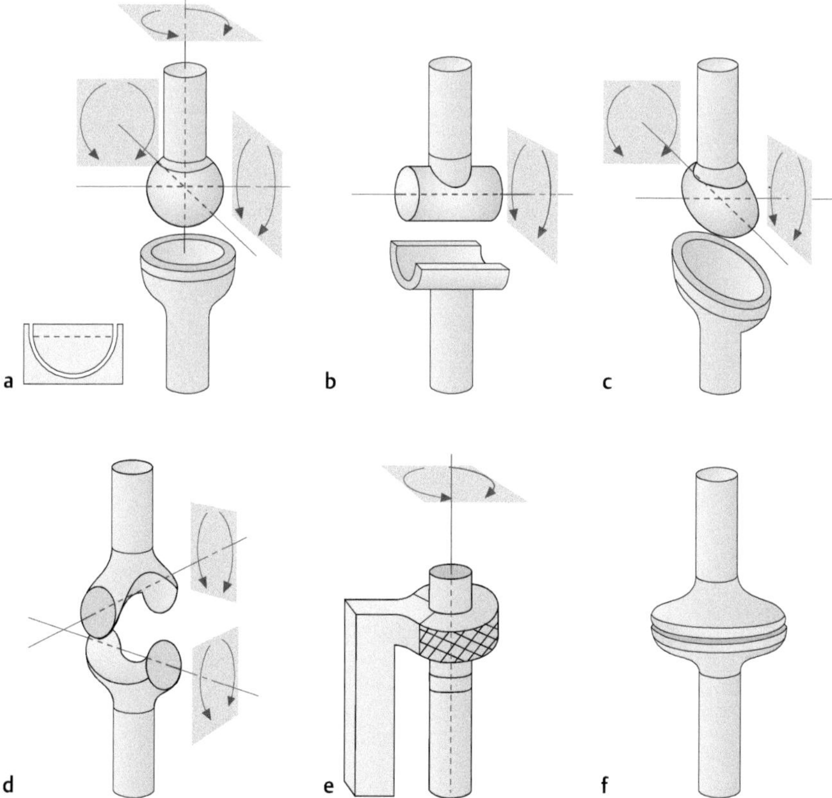

Fig. I.21 The classification of joints by shape. **(a)** Ball-and-socket joint. **(b)** Hinge joint. **(c)** Condyloid joint. **(d)** Saddle joint. **(e)** Pivot joint. **(f)** Plane joint. (From Schuenke M, Schulte E, Schumacher U. THIEME Atlas of Anatomy. General Anatomy and Musculoskeletal System. Illustrations by Voll M and Wesker K. 3rd ed. New York: Thieme Medical Publishers; 2020.)

4. *Hinge*: examples include the *elbow* and *ankle joints*. Movements occur in one axes and the sagittal plane and only include flexion and extension, making them *uniaxial joints*.
5. *Pivot*: examples include the *median atlantoaxial* and *proximal radioulnar joints*. Movement includes just rotation around a central axis, thus making them a *uniaxial joint*.
6. *Plane*: examples include *acromioclavicular* and *subtalar (talocalcaneal) joints*. Gliding and sliding movements occur at these joints but are considered *nonaxial joints*.

I.9.3 Neurovasculature of the Joints

The innervation to joints comes from the **articular nerves** that mostly originate from the nerves supplying the muscles but they also branch from the cutaneous nerves supplying the overlying skin of that particular joint. The sensory nerve endings are located in the joint capsule and transmit an awareness of movement and position sensation also known as *proprioception* back to the brain. When an injury occurs, the *pain* information comes from the joint capsule and surrounding ligaments. In general terms, it is **Hilton's law** that states the nerves supplying the muscles acting on or the skin overlying that particular joint will also be responsible for the innervation of the joint.

The **articular arteries** and **articular veins** that supply or drain the joint originate or form a tributary with the larger surrounding vessels near that same joint. The arteries are generally part of a larger anastomosis contributed to by other arteries surrounding the joint. This ensures a proper and redundant source of blood in the case of trauma, occlusion, or surgical ligation. These vessels can be located in both the joint capsule and synovial membrane.

I.10 Muscular System

All muscles of the body belong to the **muscular system** and its functions are movement, maintenance of posture, joint stabilization, and heat production and they are composed of three types of muscle tissue. Muscle tissue can also be found forming or part of the visceral organs. Muscle cells are specialized contractile cells and are most often referred to as muscle fibers. They have characteristics that describe whether or not they are striated (striped) or nonstriated due to sarcomeres; whether the contractions are voluntary or involuntary; and whether they are located on the body wall and limbs (somatic) or the internal organs and blood vessels (visceral). The three types of muscle tissue are as follows (**Fig. I.22**):

1. **Skeletal:** is striated and mostly voluntary. Most named muscles in the body are skeletal muscles with the biceps brachii

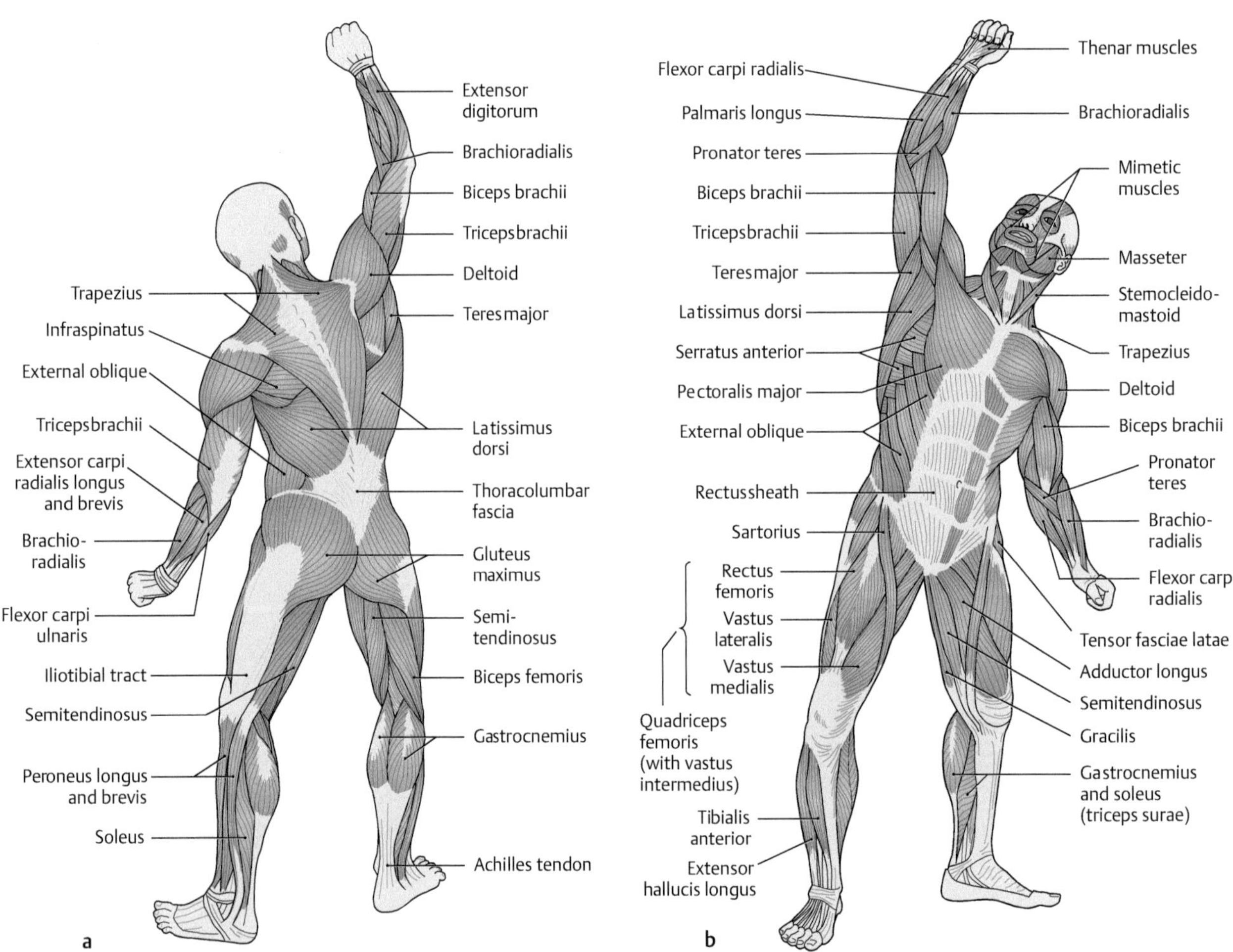

Fig. I.22 Postural muscles and muscles of movement. **(a)** Posterolateral view. **(b)** Anterolateral view. (From Schuenke M, Schulte E, Schumacher U. THIEME Atlas of Anatomy. General Anatomy and Musculoskeletal System. Illustrations by Voll M and Wesker K. 3rd ed. New York: Thieme Medical Publishers; 2020.)

being an example of a voluntary muscle and the diaphragm an involuntary muscle. These make up the bulk of gross skeletal muscles and about 40% of the total body weight, and their cells contract along the orientation of parallel fibers. Their strength, endurance, and fine motor control are dependent on the number, size, innervation, and fiber type. These muscles contain a rich supply of neurovasculature and it is the tendons or aponeuroses that transfer contractile force to the bone or other muscles. Skeletal muscle fibers themselves cannot divide but can hypertrophy or atrophy. When damaged, so-called satellite cells are stimulated to divide and will fuse with existing muscle fibers to regenerate and repair the damaged fibers.

A. *Basic structure:* (1) the **muscle fiber** (muscle cell) approximately 10 to 100 μm in diameter and up to 30 cm long is made up of numerous rodlike contractile elements called **myofibrils** that are composed of **sarcomeres**. The muscle fibers are surrounded by the **endomysium**. (2) The **fascicle** (muscle fiber bundles) is surrounded by the **perimysium**. (3) The named **muscle** is made up of large numbers of fascicles surrounded by the **epimysium (Fig. I.23; Fig. I.31)**.
B. *Sarcomere:* the myofibril is a long row of repeating segments called the **sarcomere** and it is the basic unit of contraction in skeletal muscle. It extends from Z-disk to Z-disk and it is the Z-disks that move closer to one another during muscle contraction. Attached to each **Z-disk** and extending toward the center of a sarcomere are **thin filaments** composed mainly of the protein *actin*. From the center of the sarcomere and extending just past the innermost borders of the thin filaments are the **thick filaments**. These filaments are made of the protein *myosin*, contain ATPase enzymes that split ATP in order to release energy required for muscle contraction, and have *myosin heads* that are key to the attachment-detachment cycle in contraction. Other features include the **I-band** that contains only thin filaments. The **A-band** stretches from I-band to I-band, contains both thin and thick filaments, and remains a constant size during contraction. The **H-band** contains only thick filaments and its width decreases during contraction. The **M-line** is located in the middle of the H-band and contains tiny rods that connect the adjacent thick filaments together (**Fig. I.24**).

Every skeletal muscle fiber contains two sets of tubules that will participate in the regulation of muscle contraction and these include the **sarcoplasmic reticulum (SR)** and **T-tubules**. The SR is an extensive smooth endoplasmic reticulum whose interconnecting tubules surround each myofibril. Most will run longitudinally along the myofibril while others called the **terminal cisterns** run perpendicular over

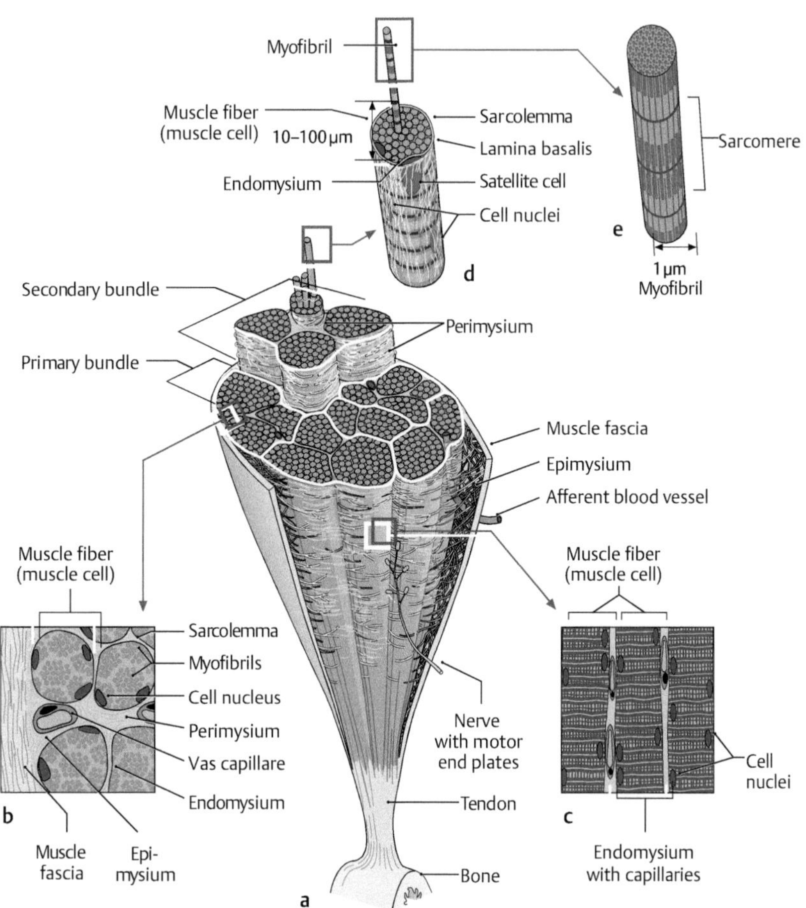

Fig. I.23 Structure of a skeletal muscle. **(a)** Cross section of a skeletal muscle. **(b)** Detail from **a** (cross section). **(c)** Detail from **a** (longitudinal section). **(d)** Structure of a muscle fiber (= muscle cell). **(e)** Structure of a myofibril. (From Schuenke M, Schulte E, Schumacher U. THIEME Atlas of Anatomy. General Anatomy and Musculoskeletal System. Illustrations by Voll M and Wesker K. 3rd ed. New York: Thieme Medical Publishers; 2020.)

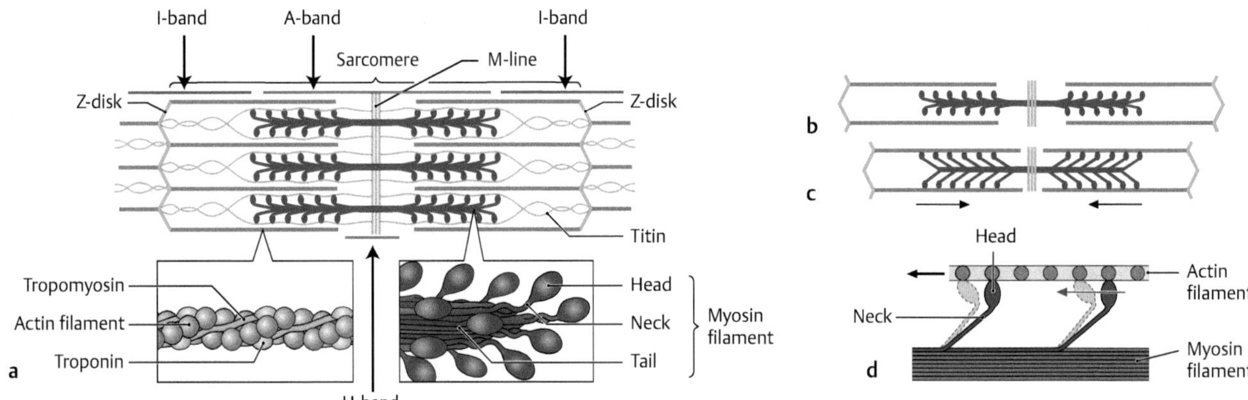

Fig. I.24 Histology of the sarcomere and the sliding filament mechanism. **(a)** Schematic representation of a sarcomere. **(b)** Myosin heads at rest. **(c)** Myosin heads during contraction. **(d)** Interaction between myosin heads and actin. (Modified from Schuenke M, Schulte E, Schumacher U. THIEME Atlas of Anatomy. General Anatomy and Musculoskeletal System. Illustrations by Voll M and Wesker K. 3rd ed. New York: Thieme Medical Publishers; 2020.)

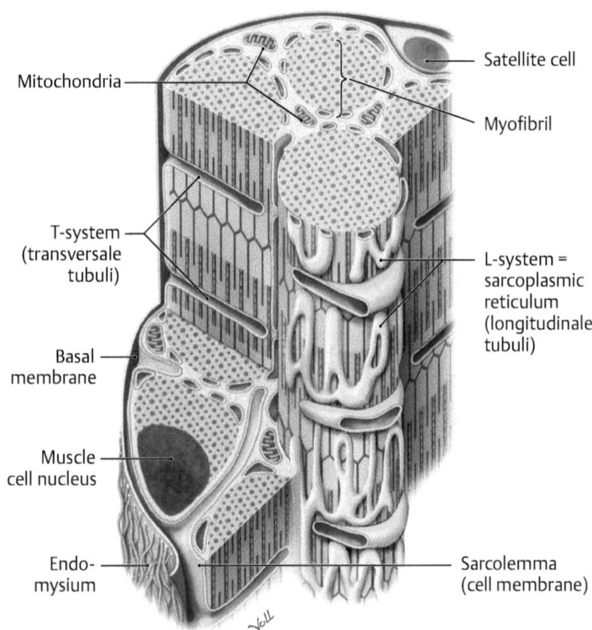

Fig. I.25 The sarcoplasmic reticulum and T-tubules of a skeletal muscle fiber. (From Schuenke M, Schulte E, Schumacher U. THIEME Atlas of Anatomy. General Anatomy and Musculoskeletal System. Illustrations by Voll M and Wesker K. 3rd ed. New York: Thieme Medical Publishers; 2020.)

the junctions between the A and I-bands. The SR and terminal cisterns store large amounts of calcium (Ca^{2+}) ions and these are released when the muscle contracts. The **T-tubules** are invaginations of the sarcolemma that run between each pair of terminal cistern and together are known as the **triad.** The T-tubules allow for conduction of impulses to the deepest parts of the muscle fibers creating an equal contraction between both the more superficial and deep myofibrils. The impulses traveling through T-tubules stimulate the release of calcium from the terminal cisterns. After the contraction, calcium is reabsorbed back into the SR **(Fig. I.25)**.

The **sliding filament mechanism** involves **concentric contraction**, or when a muscle shortens when innervated, and this is the result of the myosin heads of the thick filaments attaching to the thin filaments at both ends of the sarcomere and pulling the thin filaments toward the center of the sarcomere by swiveling inward. After the myosin head pivots at what is called its *hinge*, it will release itself and return to its original position. It will then bind to the thin filament further along its length before pivoting again. Contraction centers on the thin filaments sliding over the thick filaments. The thin and thick filaments do not shorten themselves.

C. *Three types of skeletal muscle:*

1. **Slow Oxidative (SO)** or red, slow twitch because these fibers have a large content of *myoglobin* and their energy comes from aerobic metabolism and have numerous mitochondria and capillaries. They contract slowly and are resistant to fatigue in the presence of oxygen. These fibers are fairly thin and would include postural muscles.
2. **Fast Glycolytic (FG)** or white, fast twitch because these fibers contain little myoglobin and their energy comes from anaerobic metabolism and have few mitochondria or capillaries. These fibers contract and fatigue quickly. These fibers have a diameter about twice as large as the SO fibers. Examples include upper limb muscles.
3. **Fast Oxidative (FO)** or the intermediate fibers because their contraction speeds and time before fatiguing are between that of the SO and FG fibers. Examples include muscles of the lower limbs. All muscles contain a mixture of these three types with the total amount being determined by genetics. It is possible through training or exercise to transform these fibers, but after stopping the training, a person's specific muscle fiber configuration will revert back to its original composition.

D. *Neuromuscular junction:* The nerve cells that innervate each skeletal muscle fiber are called **motor neurons** and where the nerve ending meets the fiber this is called the **neuromuscular junction** (motor end plate). Each skeletal muscle is innervated by one motor neuron. A nerve impulse will stimulate the release of the neurotransmitter acetylcholine (ACh) from the **axon terminal** and into the **synaptic cleft.** The synaptic cleft serves as a separation between the axon terminal and **sarcolemma** (plasma membrane of muscle cells) **(Fig. I.26)**.

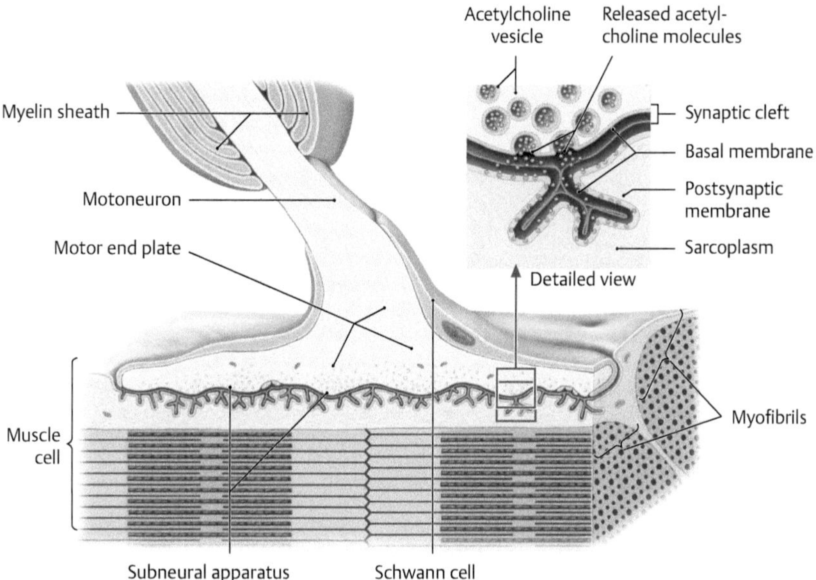

Fig. I.26 The neuromuscular junction (motor end plate). (From Schuenke M, Schulte E, Schumacher U. THIEME Atlas of Anatomy. General Anatomy and Musculoskeletal System. Illustrations by Voll M and Wesker K. 3rd ed. New York: Thieme Medical Publishers; 2020.)

Motor neuron axons branches numerous times to innervate a number of skeletal muscle fibers. The motor neuron and all of the muscle fibers it will innervate are called the **motor unit**. The number of muscle fibers associated with one motor unit can range from the single digits to several hundred. Larger weight-bearing muscles (i.e., gluteus maximus) have many muscle fibers per motor unit whereas a muscle involved in fine motor movements (i.e., muscles controlling the fingers) has very few muscle fibers per motor unit.

Sensory organs known as **proprioceptors** are located in each muscle as well as the tendons and joints, and they will provide feedback on the muscles' contractile state, tension on the tendon, and position of the joint. The **muscle spindle** consists of approximately seven **intrafusal muscle fibers** (two types technically) that are specialized muscle cells within a collagen sheath anchored to the endomysium and perimysium. They are innervated by both motor and sensory neurons but the sensory (afferent) nerves are a combination of fast-acting primary (***length***) and slow-acting secondary (***rate***) sensors. When the muscle stretches, the sensory nerves will feed back to the alpha motor neurons that innervate the **extrafusal muscle fibers**, of which most of the muscle is made of. The *simple reflex arc reaction* is the result of muscle spindles being suddenly stretched. The **Golgi tendon organ** is responsible for protecting the tendons from excessive muscle contraction and they specifically sense tension, not length or rate. This is an encapsulated receptor found at the junction between the tendon and muscle. The sensory nerves are responsible for inhibiting muscle contraction via a negative feedback loop (**Fig. I.27**).

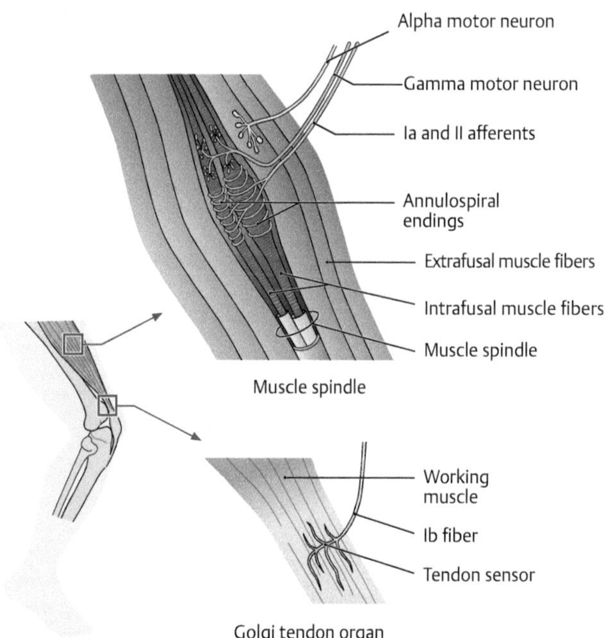

Fig. I.27 Receptors in the muscles and tendons. (From Schuenke M, Schulte E, Schumacher U. THIEME Atlas of Anatomy. General Anatomy and Musculoskeletal System. Illustrations by Voll M and Wesker K. 3rd ed. New York: Thieme Medical Publishers; 2020.)

E. <u>*Features of skeletal muscles:*</u> Muscles are the organs of locomotion and their more central, fleshy, and contractile portion that generally has a dark red appearance is known as the belly or head portion. The total length of a muscle includes the central contractile portion and the *tendons* or flat *aponeuroses* (flat tendonlike sheets) attached to them. Most skeletal muscles will attach to bones either directly or indirectly but also to cartilage, ligaments, or fascia mainly through tendons. They may also attach to skin, mucous membranes, or organs. **Tendons** consist of dense regular connective tissue primarily made of type I collagen fibers (>95%) and these fibers run as parallel bundles attaching muscle to bone. Tendons mainly, but also to an extent aponeuroses, will function by transmitting, absorbing, and modulating forces of the muscles during locomotion.

Most of the muscles are named based on their function or the bones they attach to while others are named according

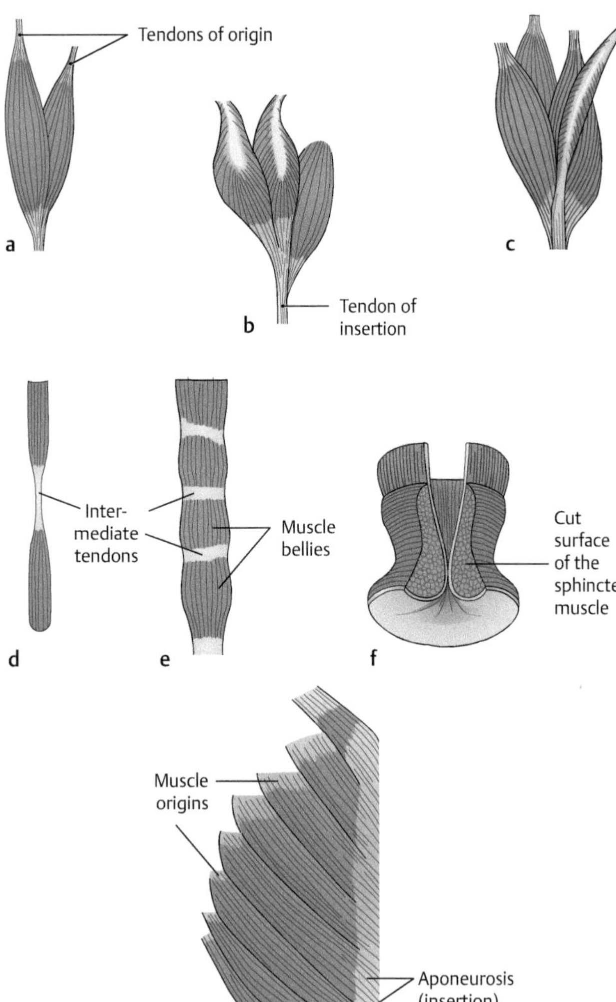

Fig. I.28 Morphological forms of muscles. **(a)** Two heads. **(b)** Three heads. **(c)** Four heads. **(d)** Two bellies = digastric. **(e)** Multiple bellies = multigastric. **(f)** Circular/sphincter. **(g)** Flat. (From Schuenke M, Schulte E, Schumacher U. THIEME Atlas of Anatomy. General Anatomy and Musculoskeletal System. Illustrations by Voll M and Wesker K. 3rd ed. New York: Thieme Medical Publishers; 2020.)

to their position. Muscles described based on shape are as follows **(Fig. I.28):**

- **Pennate**: feather-like based on their fascicle arrangement and may be *unipennate* (i.e., palmar interossei), *bipennate* (rectus femoris), or *multipennate* (deltoid).
- **Fusiform/parallel**: spindle-shaped with a round and thick belly (or bellies) are more fusiform (i.e., biceps brachii) or more straplike and parallel (i.e., sartorius).
- **Convergent**: will arise from a broad region and converge to form a single tendon. The pectoralis major is an example.
- **Circular/sphincter**: are located around a body opening or orifice. Examples include orbicularis oris or external anal sphincter.
- **Flat**: these muscles have parallel fibers often aligned with an aponeurosis. Examples include the external and internal obliques.
- **Multiheaded/bellied**: can include muscles from other classifications and may have more than one head of attachment (i.e., biceps and triceps brachii) or more than one contracting belly (i.e., rectus abdominis and digastric muscles).

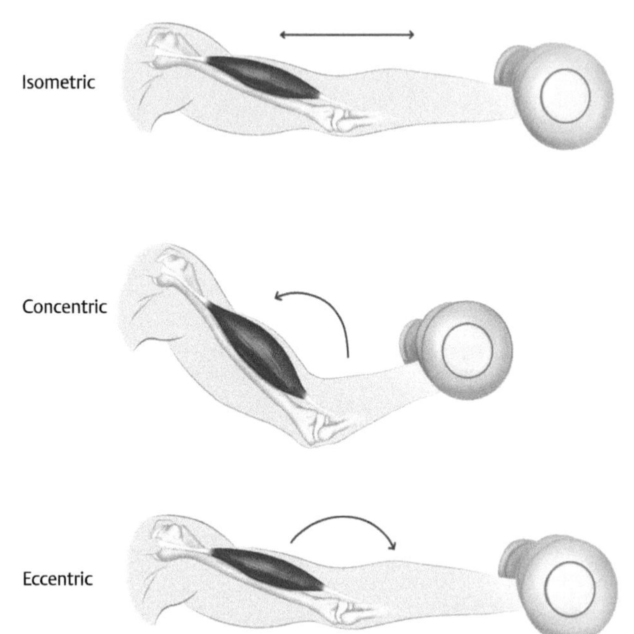

Fig. I.29 Isometric versus isotonic contractions. Illustration by Calla Heald.

F. <u>*Contraction and function of muscles*</u> **(Fig. I.29):**
Skeletal muscles function by contracting which results in pulling and never pushing. Fibers can shorten to a much as 70% of their resting length with the long parallel fascicle arranged muscles shortening the most. Muscle power increases as the total number of muscle cells increase. Thus, the short and wide pennate muscles are the most powerful. When contracting, usually the proximal end (origin) remains fixed while the distal attachment (insertion) is pulled toward the other. Contraction occurs in three ways:

1. ***Tonic contraction***: is a slight contraction that maintains muscle tone but does not produce movement or active resistance. This would be seen in maintaining posture or assisting with joint stability.
2. ***Phasic contraction***: there are two types of this type of contraction.
   - **Isometric contraction**: the muscle length will remain the same but force (muscle tension) is increased.
   - **Isotonic contraction**: the muscle changes length in order to produce movement. There are two forms of isotonic contraction:
     - **Concentric contraction**: movement occurs due to the muscle shortening (i.e., deltoid muscle shortens to abduct or elevate the arm).
     - **Eccentric contraction**: movement occurs due to the muscle lengthening (i.e., deltoid muscle lengthens to adduct or lower the arm).
3. ***Reflexive contraction***: is the automatic and not voluntarily controlled contraction. Respiratory movements involving the diaphragm and intercostal muscles are mostly reflexive. A *myotactic reflex*, the result of

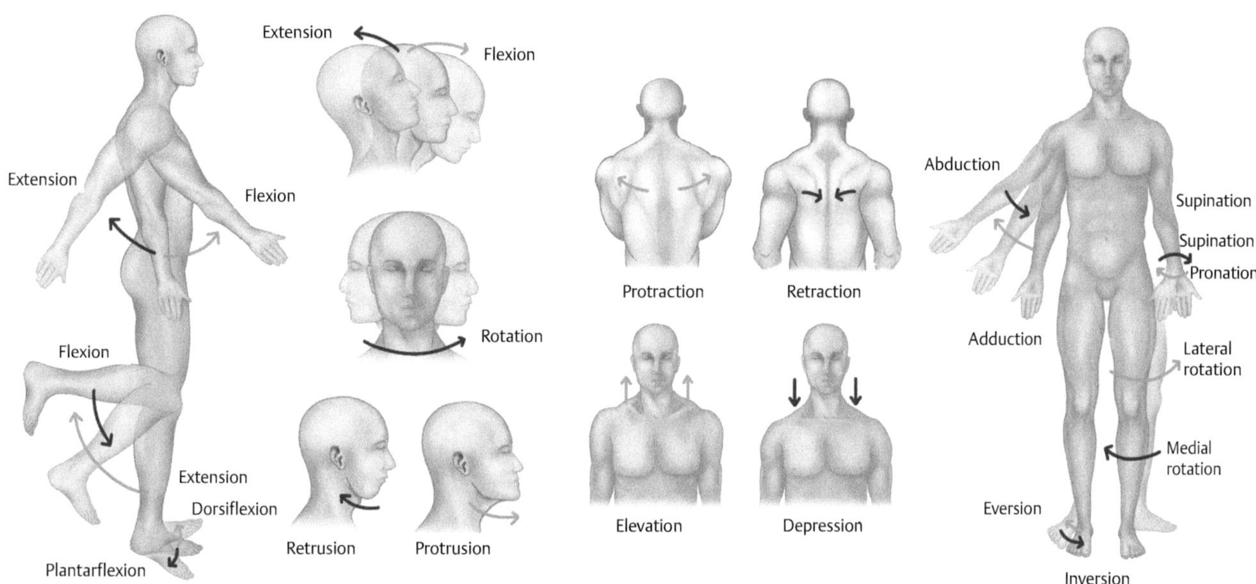

Fig. I.30 Terms for movement. Illustration by Calla Heald.

tapping a tendon with a reflex hammer, falls under this category.

The muscles will serve specific functions in moving and positioning the body and these functions include:

- **Agonist (prime mover)**: the main muscle for producing a specific movement of the body.
- **Synergist**: a muscle that complements the action of the agonist. This may mean directly assisting the agonist by providing a less mechanically advantaged component for the same movement. Or it may assist indirectly by serving as a *fixator* of an intervening joint when the agonist passes over more than one joint. Generally, several synergists assist the agonist in a particular movement.
- **Fixator**: will steady the proximal end of a limb while movements occur at the distal end.
- **Antagonist**: the muscle that opposes the action of the agonist. As the agonist contracts, the antagonist will progressively relax allowing for a more smooth and coordinated movement.

G. *Terms for movement:* Most movements occur at joints where two or more bones or cartilage articulate with one another. The movements that occur at joints are described relative to the axes around which the part of the body moves and the plane in which the movement takes place (**Fig. I.30**).

- **Elevation**: raising or moving a part of the body superiorly as in elevating the shoulders.
- **Depression**: lowering or moving a part of the body as in depressing the shoulders.
- **Flexion**: is the bending or decreasing of the angle between the bones or parts of the body. For most joints, flexion moves in an anterior direction. *Lateral flexion* or bending involves the neck flexing to the left or right.
- **Extension**: is the straightening or increasing of the angle between the bones or parts of the body. For most joints, extension moves in a posterior direction.
- **Plantarflexion**: is flexion of the foot at the ankle joint as in standing on one's toes.
- **Dorsiflexion**: is truly *extension* of the foot at the ankle joint. It refers to the notion that the foot is flexing toward the anterior or dorsal surface of the leg.
- **Abduction**: moving away from the median plane.
- **Adduction**: moving toward the median plane.
- **Circumduction**: the circular movement that involves the combination of flexion, abduction, extension, and adduction in that order (or in the opposite direction) such that the distal portion of the limb is moving in a circular fashion.
- **Rotation**: is the turning of the body around its longitudinal axis. **Medial (internal) rotation** moves the anterior surface of a limb closer to the median plane. **Lateral (external) rotation** moves the anterior surface away from the median plane.
- **Pronation**: rotation of the radius medially toward the ulna, resulting in the palm of the hand facing posteriorly.
- **Supination**: rotation of the radius laterally and away from the ulna (uncrossing), resulting in the palm of the hand and facing anteriorly and back in anatomical position.
- **Protraction**: the anterolateral movement of the scapula at the thoracic wall causing the scapula to move anteriorly.
- **Retraction**: the posteromedial movement of the scapula at the thoracic wall causing the scapula to move posteriorly.
- **Protrusion**: anterior or forward movement of the tongue, mandible, or lips.
- **Retrusion**: posterior or backward movement of the tongue, mandible, or lips.
- **Eversion**: the sole of the foot moves away from the median plane, turning the sole laterally. When fully everted, the foot is also dorsiflexed.
- **Inversion**: the sole of the foot moves toward the median plane, turning the sole medially. When fully inverted, the foot is also plantarflexed.

- **Opposition**: the ability of the first digit of the hand (thumb) to move into contact with other fingers across the palm. This is for the purpose of grasping objects between the thumb and fingers.
- **Reposition**: the ability of the first digit of the hand (thumb) to move back from opposition and back into its anatomical position.

2. **Cardiac:** is striated and involuntary and associated primarily with the myocardium of the heart. The individual cells are joined by electromechanical junctions called **intercalated disks** and these are important for supporting the synchronized contraction of cardiac muscle. There are no organized bundles but more of a branching appearance interspersed with connective tissue. There is no direct innervation but the autonomic nervous system fibers travel through the myocardium and affect the heart rate, force of contraction, and the constriction and dilation of the coronary arteries. Cardiac muscle cells are capable of hypertrophy and atrophy but do not have an equivalent to the satellite cell found in skeletal muscle and it was generally thought that they do not regenerate. However, recent work has shown that cardiomyocytes may renew themselves, albeit at a limited level but it occurs throughout the individual's life. Connective tissue will still replace the dead cardiac cells if there was an infarct leading to a fibrotic scar (**Fig. I.31**).

   T-tubules in cardiac muscle are larger and wider and located at the Z-disk. There are fewer T-tubules in comparison with skeletal muscle. The SR and T-tubule junction is not a triad but a diad, resulting in there being a single T-tubule paired with a terminal cisterna of the SR. This diad will play an important role in excitation-contraction coupling by juxtaposing an inlet for the action potential near a source of calcium. This is so that the wave of depolarization can be coupled to calcium-mediated cardiac muscle contraction via the sliding filament mechanism.
3. **Smooth:** is nonstriated and involuntary. They can be arranged in bundles or sheets and orientated either circularly or longitudinally. They are located in areas such as the blood vessels and gastrointestinal (GI) tract. They have no striations, sarcomeres, or T-tubules. Gap junctions between the cells help spread the depolarization signal, and the autonomic nervous system innervates these types of cells. Smooth muscle cells are capable of hypertrophy, hyperplasia, and maintain the capacity to divide; thus, they can regenerate (**Fig. I.31**).

Clinical Correlate I.5

Muscular Dystrophy

Muscular dystrophies (MD) are a group of more than 30 genetic diseases characterized by progressive weakness and degeneration of the skeletal muscles. Some forms are seen as early as infancy while others may not appear until middle age or later. MD can differ in terms of age of onset, the extent of the muscle weakness, the rate of progression, or the pattern of inheritance. The most common form is **Duchenne MD** and it primarily affects boys. The absence of a protein called dystrophin, which is involved in maintaining the integrity of muscle is the cause. The onset is generally between 3 and 5 years of age and it progresses rapidly. Most will be unable to walk before their teenage years and will later need a respirator to breathe. The most common adult form is **myotonic MD** and it presets with prolonged muscle spasms, cardiac abnormalities, endocrine disturbances, and cataracts. Individuals have long, thin faces with a swan-like neck and drooping eyelids.

Prognosis for individuals with MD will vary according to their type and the progression of the disorder. Cases can be mild and progress very slowly over a normal lifespan or others will produce severe muscle weakness and functional disability. Early onset during infancy can lead to death while others can reach adulthood with only moderate disability. No specific treatment can stop or reverse any form of MD. Physical, speech, occupational, and respiratory therapies are used for treatment but corrective orthopaedic surgery may also be needed. Corticosteroids along with immunosuppressants can slow muscle degeneration; anticonvulsants would control seizures; assisted ventilation to treat respiratory muscle weakness and a pacemaker for cardiac issues can all be utilized if needed.

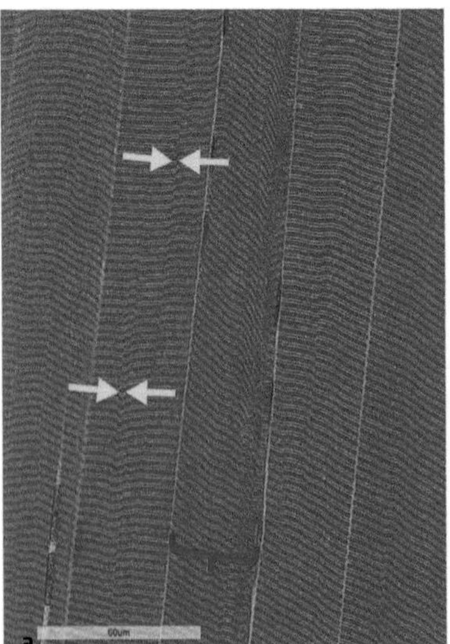

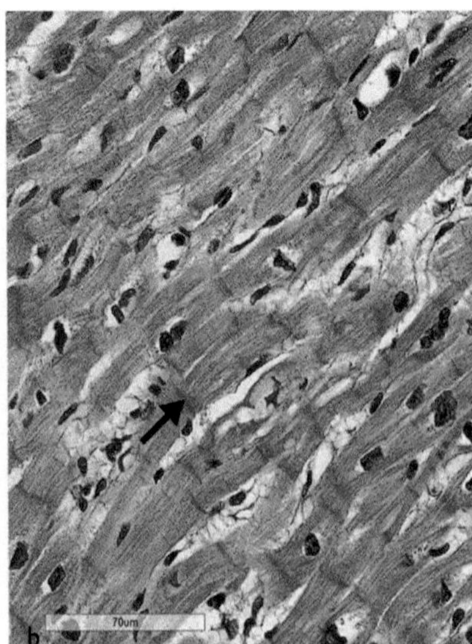

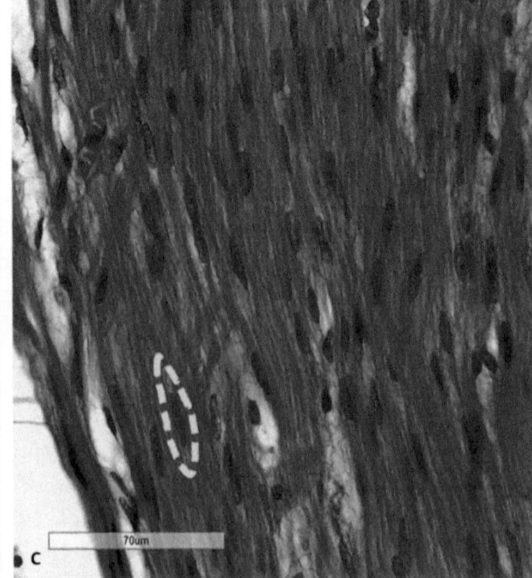

Fig. I.31 Types of muscle. **(a)** Skeletal muscle in longitudinal section showing myofibrils; muscle fiber or cell (*green bracket*), width of one or possibly two myofibrils (*yellow arrows*). **(b)** Cardiac muscle in longitudinal section; intercalated disks (*black arrows*). **(c)** Smooth muscle in longitudinal section with a single smooth muscle cell highlighted (*yellow outline*). (Modified from Lowrie Jr. D, ed. Histology: An Essential Textbook. 1st Edition. New York: Thieme; 2020.)

Clinical Correlate I.6

Fibromyalgia

Fibromyalgia (FM) is a disorder characterized by chronic and widespread pain that is heightened and painful in response to touch. There is no known cause but symptoms can include joint stiffness, tingling, numbness, difficulty swallowing, and feeling tired which could be due to sleep disturbances. It is frequently associated with anxiety, depression, and cognitive dysfunction. The widespread pain appears to be due to neurochemical imbalances and the activation of inflammatory pathways in the brain. There are 18 designated tender points but in the past few years it was decided that diagnosis is not dependent on the number of present tender points.

I.11 Circulatory System

The **circulatory system** is divided into the **cardiovascular system** (heart, blood, and blood vessels) that is responsible for propelling blood throughout the body and the **lymphatic system** (vessels that carry lymph), which is responsible for filtering excess interstitial (intercellular) fluid (or lymph) through the lymph nodes and finally back to the bloodstream **(Fig. I.32)**.

The heart is made up of two muscular pumps that act in series to pump blood to both the pulmonary and systematic circulations. The right ventricle of the heart pumps low-oxygen blood originating from the right atrium to the pulmonary circulation that centers on the lungs, which are responsible for exchanging carbon dioxide for more oxygen. The left atrium receives the now oxygen-rich blood from the lungs and via the left ventricle; this blood will be pumped throughout the systematic circulation to the rest of the body.

There are three different types of blood vessels and these consist of the arteries, capillaries, and veins. The general concept revolves around the high-pressure blood leaving the heart and traveling through thick-walled arteries before it is distributed to other parts of the body by the thinner arterioles before reaching the capillaries where there is an exchange of oxygen and nutrients. From the capillaries, waste products and carbon dioxide travel through the venules, small, medium, and large veins before reaching the heart. The veins are more abundant than the arteries and make up around 70 to 80% of all blood vessels in the body. Veins also have thinner walls and that allows them to expand. This can occur if any blood should be impeded on its way back to the heart, such as when a person takes a deep breath and holds it (*Valsalva maneuver*). In most regions of the body, there will be at least two smaller veins paired up with a slightly larger artery. This is quite evident in the vasculature of the limbs. When this occurs, there is a thin **vascular sheath** that wraps around all of the vessels and this creates the **arteriovenous pump** (**Fig. I.33**). This pump is created as the pulsating arteries stretch and flatten the surrounding veins aiding in return of blood back to the heart. The close proximity of the warmer artery to the colder veins allows for a *heat exchanger effect* and the venous drainage warms up as it travels back to the heart. Muscular contractions of the lower limbs function alongside the venous valves to move blood back toward the heart. With the outward expansion of contracting muscle bellies limited by the deep fascia, this creates a compressive force and propels blood against gravity. This is called the **musculovenous pump** (**Fig. I.34**).

An **anastomosis** between multiple branches of an artery will provide a potential route for blood in case of an occlusion or trauma involving the artery. Understanding anastomoses is important in surgical ligations because there may only be one route to a particular structure and some ligations are not feasible. A **collateral circulation** can form when a main blood supply is occluded leading the smaller channels to increase in size and now allow sufficient blood supply to a structure distal to the blockage. An **end (terminal) artery** is an artery that has no anastomosis with another artery and is the only artery responsible for blood supply to that particular structure. An example would include the central artery of the retina, and if an occlusion were to occur in this vessel, death to the retinal tissue would lead to blindness. Arteries that have ineffective anastomoses and are similar to end arteries are known as *functional terminal arteries* and they include central branches of the cerebral arteries, splenic, renal, and vasa recta of the mesenteric arteries.

Blood vessels have three layers or coats called tunics (**Fig. I.35**):

1. **Tunica intima**: the innermost layer or endothelium consists of a *simple squamous epithelium* and this is surrounded by a *basal lamina*. This layer plays an important role in many vascular diseases such as atherosclerosis that could lead to a myocardial infarction (heart attack) and cerebral ischemia. *Atheromas* are an accumulation of degenerative materials that include macrophages and lipids among other things and form a swelling in the artery. The *internal elastic lamina* is its outer border.
2. **Tunica media**: the middle layer made mostly of varying layers of smooth muscle cells. There is also collagen and elastic fibers produced by and interspersed between the smooth muscle layers. It has an *external elastic lamina* but it is less distinct than the internal layer.
3. **Tunica adventitia**: the outermost layer that blends with the connective tissue surrounding vessels. It has type I collagen and elastic fibers along with fibroblasts and some smooth muscle cells and is generally the thickest layer of venules and veins. The vessels supplying the vessels with blood (*vasa varosum*) and the autonomic fibers are located in this layer.

A summary of all blood vessels (**Fig. I.36**):

- **Elastic arteries**: a large artery that conducts blood from the heart and these include the aorta (~2.5 cm), brachiocephalic, common carotids, subclavian, vertebral, and common iliac arteries. They have a relatively thick tunica intima with a multilayered internal elastic lamina. The many elastic fibers in the tunica media stretch in response to high blood pressure and they do not contain as many smooth muscle cell layers as the muscular arteries. They passively contract during diastole to maintain systematic pressure.
- **Muscular arteries**: have a diameter between 0.3 mm and 1.0 cm. These arteries distribute the blood to various parts of the body and include arteries such as the coronary, femoral, tibial, popliteal, axillary, radial, splenic, and hepatic arteries. There can be up to 40 layers of smooth muscle and they have a prominent internal elastic lamina. The tunica media and adventitia layers are equal in thickness.
- **Small arteries** and **arterioles**: have a diameter including all three layers of less than 0.5 mm. The arterioles have a lumen less than 100 to 300 µm in diameter. The internal elastic lamina is present in small arteries but not arterioles and the tunica media is very thin and layers in the single digits. The arterioles are important in determining a person's blood pressure as their narrow diameter resists blood flow; thus, the back pressure helps to stretch the walls of the arteries during heart contractions.

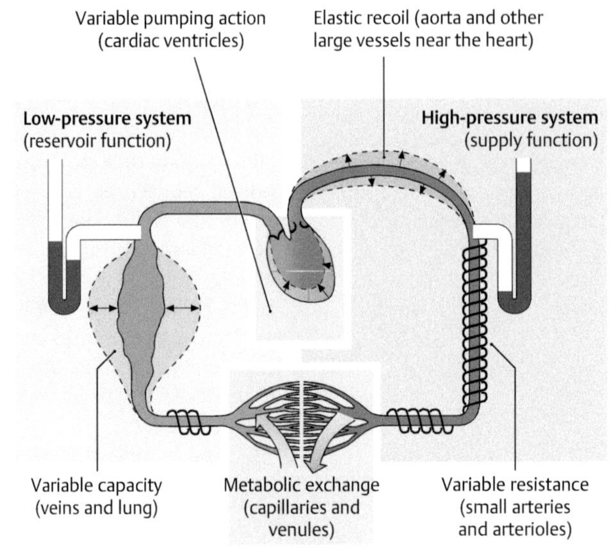

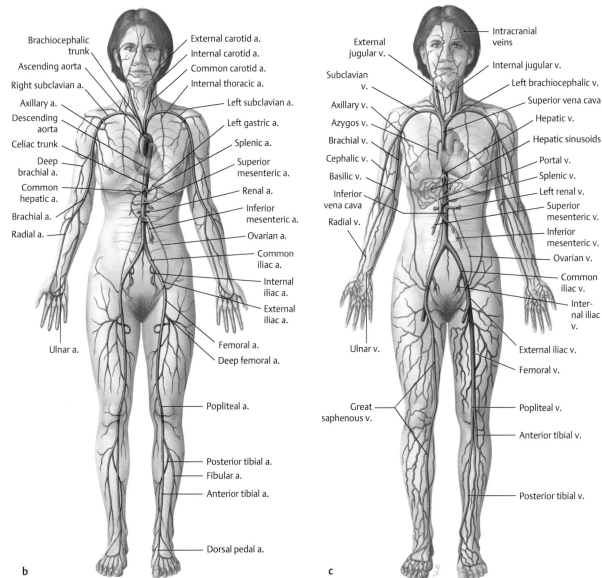

Fig. I.32 (a) Basic functional diagram of the circulatory system. **(b)** Overview of the principal arteries in the systemic circulation. **(c)** Overview of the principal veins in the systemic circulation. (From Schuenke M, Schulte E, Schumacher U. THIEME Atlas of Anatomy. General Anatomy and Musculoskeletal System. Illustrations by Voll M and Wesker K. 3rd ed. New York: Thieme Medical Publishers; 2020.)

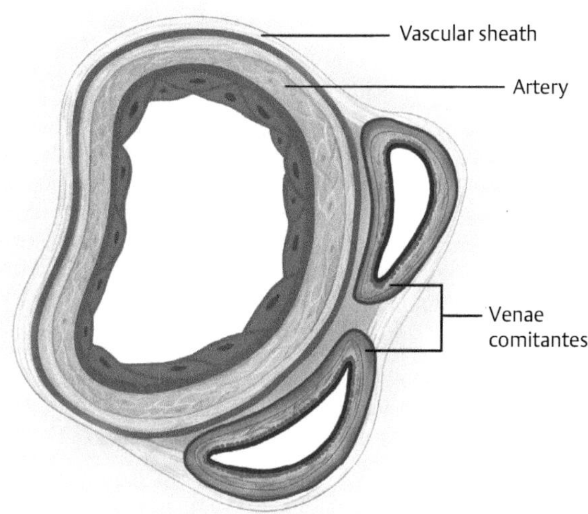

Fig. I.33 Vascular sheath creating the arteriovenous pump. Illustration by Calla Heald.

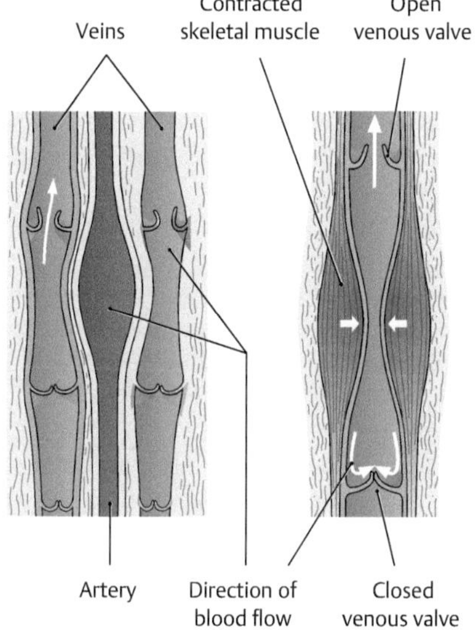

Fig. I.34 Musculovenous pump. (From Schuenke M, Schulte E, Schumacher U. THIEME Atlas of Anatomy. General Anatomy and Musculoskeletal System. Illustrations by Voll M and Wesker K. 3rd ed. New York: Thieme Medical Publishers; 2020.)

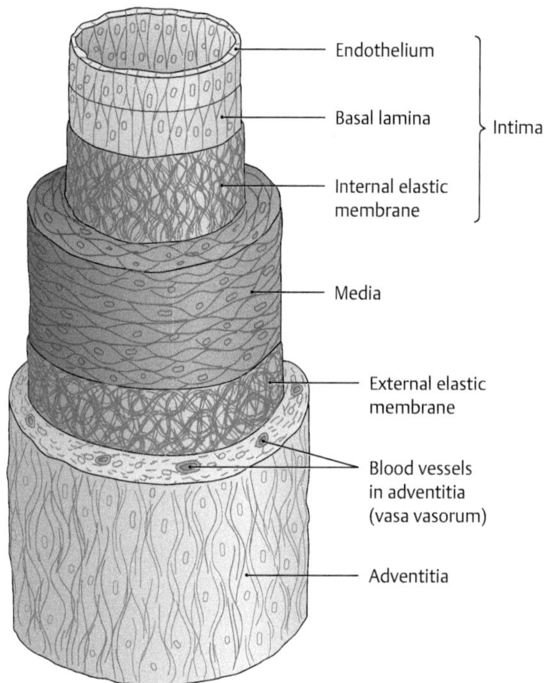

Fig. I.35 Wall structure of a blood vessel illustrated for a muscular-type artery. (From Schuenke M, Schulte E, Schumacher U. THIEME Atlas of Anatomy. General Anatomy and Musculoskeletal System. Illustrations by Voll M and Wesker K. 3rd ed. New York: Thieme Medical Publishers; 2020.)

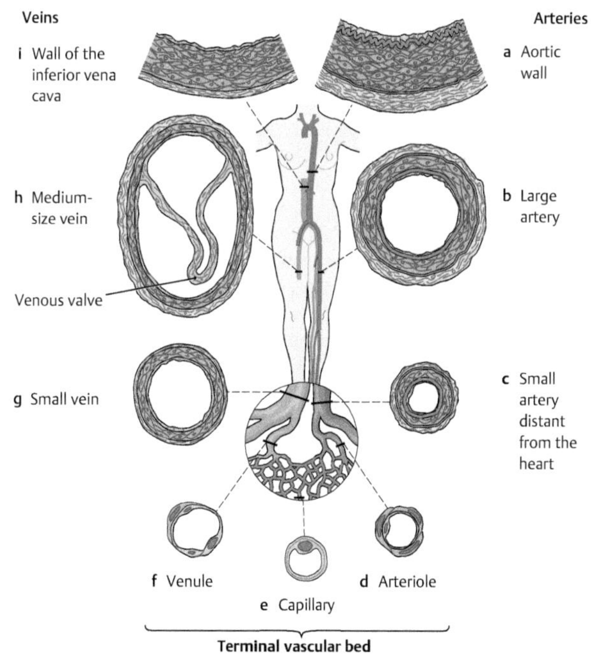

Fig. I.36 Structure of the blood vessels in different regions of the systemic circulation. (From Schuenke M, Schulte E, Schumacher U. THIEME Atlas of Anatomy. General Anatomy and Musculoskeletal System. Illustrations by Voll M and Wesker K. 3rd ed. New York: Thieme Medical Publishers; 2020.)

- **Capillaries**: they are responsible for connecting the arterioles and venules. Their diameter can range from 5 to 10 µm to as thin as 0.2 µm. Their permeability depends on the structural characteristics of endothelial cells and basal lamina because they lack muscular and adventitial layers. The density of capillaries is dependent on an organ's metabolic activity; thus, skeletal muscle and myocardium have high densities. There are three types:

  1. **Continuous**: the endothelium is uninterrupted due to tight junctions and there is a continuous basal lamina. Transport of nutrients is through pinocytosis and there are often *pericytes* associated with them, a source of new fibroblasts, which are seen in many tissues such as in muscle, lung, and the blood-brain barrier of the central nervous system.
  2. **Fenestrated**: the endothelium is fenestrated (having pores) but there is still a continuous basal lamina. They allow for the passage of small molecules and limited amounts of protein and are present in tissues of the intestines, endocrine glands, kidney, and pancreas.
  3. **Discontinuous (sinusoidal)**: the endothelium have large fenestrations that slow the flow of blood and there is an incomplete or absent basal lamina. This allows for a direct

exchange of molecules between the blood and cells. They exhibit irregular and torturous paths and they can be found in organs such as the liver, spleen, bone marrow, lymphoid tissue, and endocrine glands.

- **Venules**: are the smallest veins, have a diameter of around 10 to 50 µm and contain approximately 25% of the total blood volume. They have a tunica intima without any elastic fibers and a tunica media layer with only a couple of smooth muscle cell layers. The tunica adventitia is fused with the surrounding tissue.
- **Small** and **medium-sized veins**: small veins range from 0.2 to 1 mm and medium veins range from 1 to 9 mm in diameter. One-way valves that are folds in the tunica intima and are covered with endothelium will be first seen in medium-sized veins. The tunica media consist of two to four layers of smooth muscle cells and the vasa vasorum penetrate deep into this layer. The tunica adventitia is thicker than the tunica media. Small veins are unnamed but are the tributaries of medium-sized veins and help form **venous plexuses**. Examples of medium-sized veins would be the great saphenous, cephalic, and any other vein paired with an artery.
- **Large veins**: have a diameter of more than 9 mm and can include the venae cavae, internal jugular, portal, splenic, superior mesenteric, femoral, and external iliac veins. The valves are located in the tunica intima, and the tunica media is similar in size to the small and medium veins. The tunica adventitia layer is the thickest of the three layers in a large vein.
- **Perforating veins**: these veins connect the deeper veins to the more superficial veins in the leg and also contain valves. These valves prevent regurgitation of blood back to the superficial veins.

The **lymphatic system** runs parallel with the venous circulation of the body. It is the equivalent of an overflow system that provides for (1) the drainage or removal of interstitial fluid **(lymph)**, a component of extracellular fluid which also includes plasma from around the extracellular spaces of most tissues; (2) the absorption and transport of fatty acids and fats as *chyle* from the digestive system through lacteals; and (3) the defense against foreign microorganisms and disease. Fluid and electrolytes enter the extracellular spaces by way of the capillaries, but these same capillaries will reabsorb 90% of that fluid. The remaining 10% or approximately 3 L of this fluid each day must be picked up by the lymphatic system. It is similar to the venous system, in that it has a one-way flow due to its valves. Additional parts of this system include **(Fig. I.37)**:

- **Lymphatic capillaries**: originate in the extracellular spaces of most tissues and they consist of endothelium made of a single layer of *simple squamous epithelium* and are blind-ended vessels. They have no fenestrae or tight junctions and little to no basal lamina.
- **Lymphatic vessels**: lymph from the capillaries leads first to the lymphatic vessels. They have thin, veinlike walls. They have an endothelium, a thin layer of smooth muscle cells, an adventitia that helps bind it to surrounding tissue and numerous valves. The *afferent vessels* carry lymph toward the lymph node while *efferent vessels* lead lymph away from the lymph node **(Fig. I.38)**.
- **Lymph nodes**: are small, oval masses of lymphatic tissue where lymph is filtered. This is also a site where lymphocytes can be activated **(Fig. I.39)**.
- **Lymphocytes**: a subset of white blood cells that include B cells, T cells, and natural killer (NK) cells. These circulating cells react to foreign materials.
- **Lymphoid organs**: are broken down into primary versus secondary lymphoid organs. Primary lymphoid organs are where lymphocytes are *produced* and *mature* and these include the thymus and red bone marrow. Secondary lymphoid organs are where lymphocytes are *activated* and they include the lymph nodes, spleen, MALT in the tonsils, Peyer's patches, and vermiform appendix.
- **Lymphatic ducts**: after leaving lymph nodes, lymph will travel through efferent vessels before they soon become trunks and finally lymphatic ducts. The **right lymphatic duct** drains lymph from the right half of the head, neck, thorax, and right upper limb. It enters near the *right venous angle* or junction between the right internal jugular and subclavian veins. Lymph from the remaining parts of the body passes through the **thoracic duct**. Lymph from the lower limbs, pelvis, and abdomen will reach the **cisterna chyli** before it becomes the thoracic duct. Along with lymph from the left head, neck, and thorax, the thoracic duct drains into the venous circulation at the *left venous angle* located at the junction of the left internal jugular and subclavian veins.

Clinical Correlate I.7

Peripheral Arterial Disease

Peripheral artery disease (PAD) is when plaque builds up in the arteries that carry blood to the head, limbs, or organs. The plaque is related to the tunica intima and can be made up of cholesterol, calcium, fibrous tissue, and macrophages. When plaque builds up in the arteries, it is referred to as atherosclerosis. Over time, these arteries will become narrow and stiff, limiting the flow of oxygen-rich blood to parts of the body and may result in claudication most notably in the legs. PAD is generally thought of to be associated with the lower limbs but it can also affect arteries of the head, upper limbs, stomach, or kidneys.

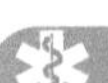

Clinical Correlate I.8

Varicose Veins

Varicose veins are twisted and swollen veins located just beneath the skin. They are most commonly associated with veins of the leg but they can also include *hemorrhoids* of the lower rectum and anal regions. They are caused when the valves of these veins responsible for the one-way flow of blood back toward the heart becomes weak or damaged. Blood may back up or pool causing the characteristic swelling or twisting. Risk factors include being female, older, obese, and a lack of exercise. They can be surgically removed but adding exercise and losing weight, avoid standing for long periods and elevating the legs when resting can help prevent or reduce the pain associated with varicose veins.

I.12 Nervous System

The major details associated with the nervous system will be discussed in Chapters 8–12 of this text. However, a general understanding of how it controls and coordinates somatic or visceral movements and sensation of the body must be addressed to make sense of the general architecture of our body. The cells (neurons) of this system communicate by way of electrical signals that produce almost immediate responses. This system is divided into a structural versus functional component.

- The **central nervous system (CNS)** and **peripheral nervous system (PNS)** make up the structural portion of this system. The CNS is made up of the brain and spinal cord. The PNS

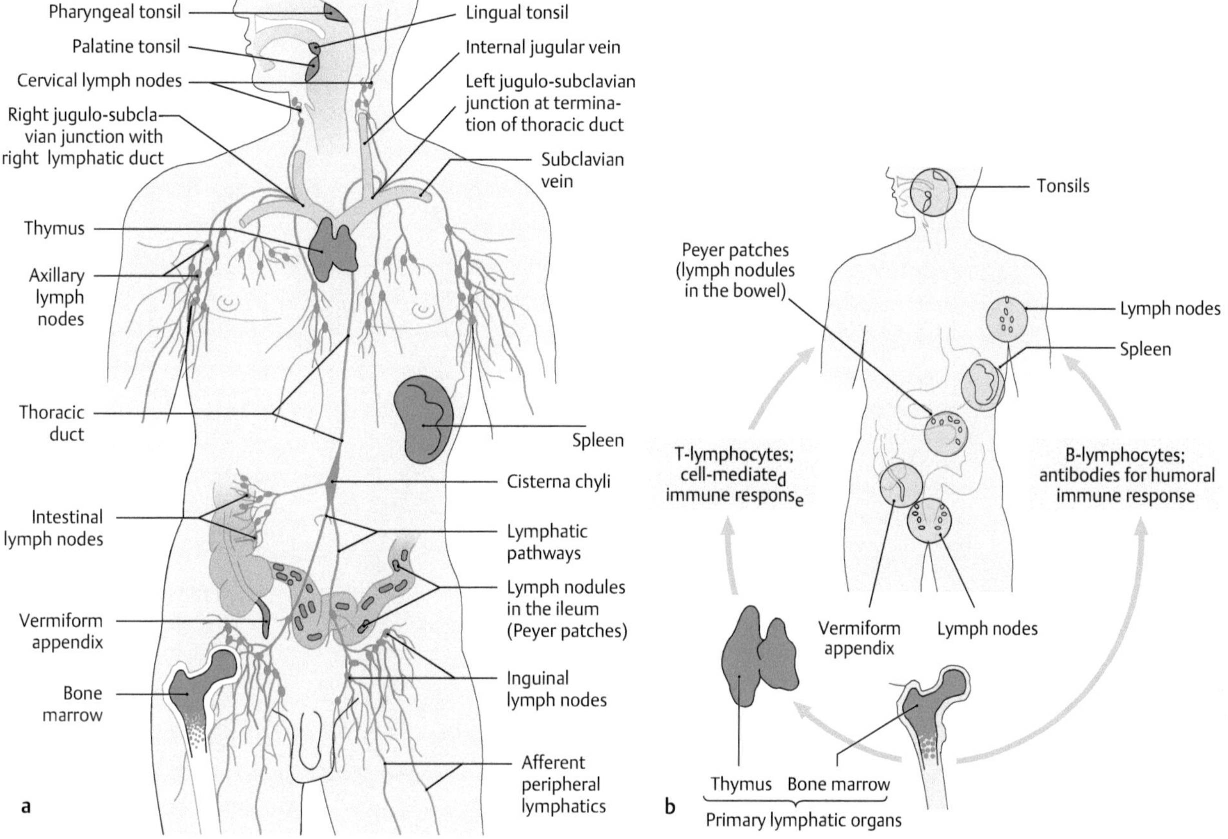

Fig. I.37 **(a)** The human lymphatic system. **(b)** Primary and secondary lymphatic organs. (From Schuenke M, Schulte E, Schumacher U. THIEME Atlas of Anatomy. General Anatomy and Musculoskeletal System. Illustrations by Voll M and Wesker K. 3rd ed. New York: Thieme Medical Publishers; 2020.)

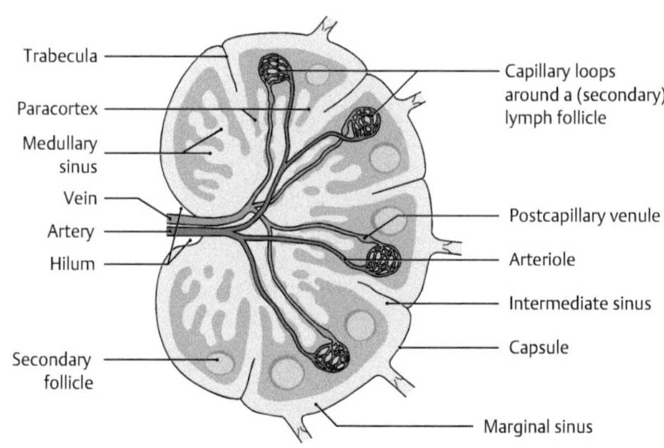

Fig. I.38 Blood supply to the lymph node. (From Schuenke M, Schulte E, Schumacher U. THIEME Atlas of Anatomy. General Anatomy and Musculoskeletal System. Illustrations by Voll M and Wesker K. 3rd ed. New York: Thieme Medical Publishers; 2020.)

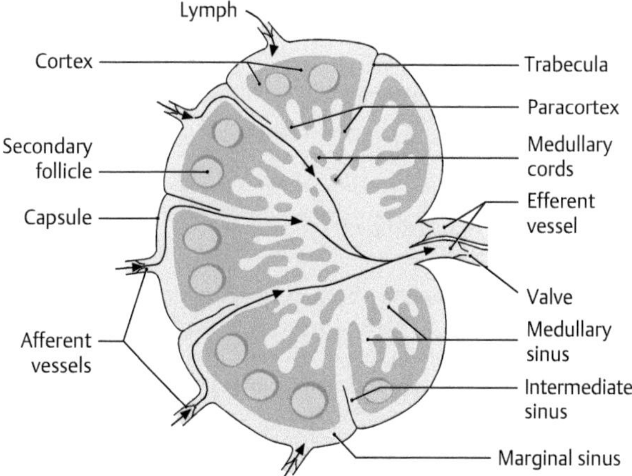

Fig. I.39 Lymph circulation. (From Schuenke M, Schulte E, Schumacher U. THIEME Atlas of Anatomy. General Anatomy and Musculoskeletal System. Illustrations by Voll M and Wesker K. 3rd ed. New York: Thieme Medical Publishers; 2020.)

consists of most cranial nerves, all the spinal nerves and their associated motor fibers, sensory fibers and their cell bodies or ganglia, and the autonomic nervous system (ANS) (**Fig. I.40**).

- The **somatic nervous system (SNS)** and the **autonomic nervous system (ANS)** make up the functional portion of this system. Somatic motor and sensory fibers supply the skeletal muscles and the sensation from the skin and joints. The ANS is motor only to visceral organs, smooth muscle, and glands and consists of *parasympathetic* and *sympathetic* fibers. Visceral sensory fibers can pair with the visceral motor fibers but then by definition are not part of the ANS (**Fig. I.41**).

There are two cell types in nervous tissue. The parenchymal cell is known as the **neuron** while the supportive/stromal cells are called **neuroglia (Fig. I.42)**.

- The structural and functional components of the nervous system are the **neurons**. These are nonmitotic in the adult meaning cell death is permanent. A neuron is a cell that processes and transmits information through electrical and chemical signals via *synapses*. All neurons have a **cell body** (soma) and a variable

Clinical Correlate I.9

Pathways of Cancer Spreading

Cancer is able to invade the body by successively growing into surrounding tissue (*contiguity*) or by *metastasis*. Metastatic cancer is the spreading of cancer from the original site it first began to develop at, to another place in the body. A metastatic cancer will be named according to where it originated from (*primary cancer*) and not where it has metastasized. Lung cancer that has metastasized to the brain is still referred to as lung cancer. The most common sites of cancer metastasis are to the liver, lungs, and bone. Metastatic tumors can originate from any form of cancer and the metastasis of them will occur in three different ways:

1. By **lymphogenesis spreading** through lymphatic vessels: the most common route for *carcinomas*. Carcinomas develop from epithelial cells, or the cells that line the cavities and surfaces of an organ or blood vessel, of which they are the most common type of cancer. The affected epithelial cells from the primary cancer will loosen and pass through the lymphatic vessels to travel to other places in the body. The staging of cancer is done by removing and examining the lymph nodes associated with the normal lymphatic drainage pattern of the organ currently the site of a primary tumor. Generally when a lymph node becomes swollen due to an illness it will become painful when palpated or compressed. In the case of an enlarged cancerous node, there generally is no pain associated with it.
2. By **hematogenous spreading** through blood vessels: spreading through the venous drainage is more common than arterial supply spreading because veins have thinner walls offering less resistance and are the most abundant vessels in the body. Connective tissue cancers or *sarcomas* are less common but generally spread by this route.
3. By the **direct seeding** of body cavities: the malignant tumors that arise in organs adjacent to body cavities can shed malignant cells into body cavities such as the pleural and peritoneal cavities. Tumor cells that reach a body cavity can spread by the associated fluid of that cavity to new locations on the serous membrane. An example would include certain ovarian cancers seeding the peritoneal cavity.

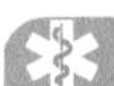

Clinical Correlate I.10

Lymphedema, Lymphangitis, and Lymphadenitis

After the removal of cancerous lymph nodes as part of a cancer treatment, or even with parasitic infections, a blockage of the lymphatic drainage can occur resulting in localized fluid retention or lymphedema. Most frequently this condition is the result of cancer and radiation treatment (secondary lymphedema) but it can also be inherited. The cause of inherited (primary) lymphedema is still not understood but it is common in newborns with Turner syndrome. Conditions that may be related to or involve bacterial transport after an infection, for instance, could result in inflammation of the lymphatic vessels (lymphangitis) or lymph nodes (lymphadenitis). Lymphatic vessels are not normally seen but if they display a red streak under the skin and have sore or painful lymph nodes associated with them this could be a sign of blood poisoning (septicemia).

number of processes including at least one **axon** and one or more **dendrites**. Axons transmit impulses away from the cell body and these signals can be amplified or increased when **myelin** or the **myelin sheath** is present around these axons.

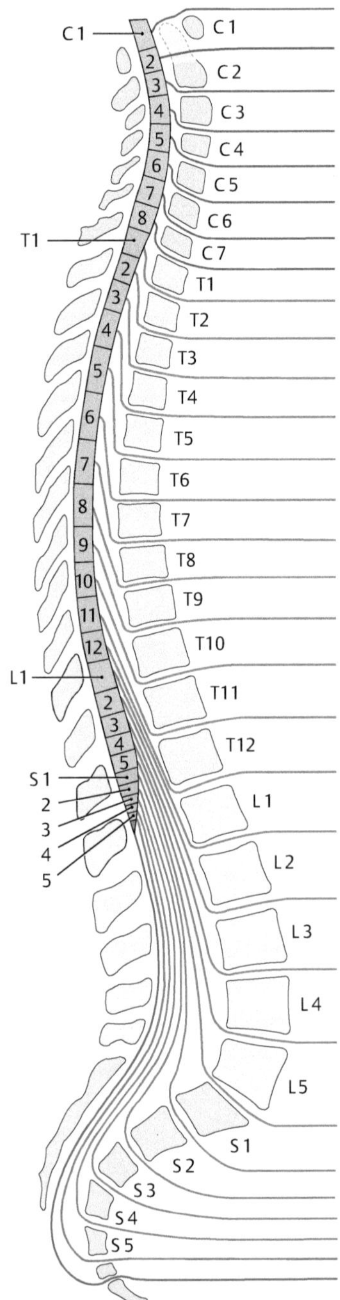

Fig. I.40 Location and designation of spinal cord segments in relation to the spinal canal. (From Schuenke M, Schulte E, Schumacher U. THIEME Atlas of Anatomy. General Anatomy and Musculoskeletal System. Illustrations by Voll M and Wesker K. 3rd ed. New York: Thieme Medical Publishers; 2020.)

Myelin does not form a continuous layer because it is interrupted at regular intervals called **nodes of Ranvier**. The distance between two nodes is called an **internode** and represents the distance covered by a single *oligodendroglia* or *Schwann cell*. Depolarization occurs at the nodes and demonstrates a salutatory (or leaping) conduction; thus, the myelin serves to increase the velocity of conduction of the nerve impulse. Dendrites propagate or spread the incoming signal from other neurons to the cell body and are found with all neurons except in pseudounipolar neurons. There are three types of neurons (**Fig. I.43**):

1. **Multipolar**: have one axon and multiple dendrites. They make up the majority of all neurons and include all motor (somatic and autonomic) neurons and interneurons.
2. **Pseudounipolar**: has one axon extending from the cell body that splits into two branches. They are the *peripheral* (impulses from the receptor organ to cell body) and *central* (cell body to CNS) *branches*. These make up the sensory neurons of the PNS and select cranial nerves. Incoming impulses do not have to route through the cell body but instead pass directly from the incoming to outgoing process.
3. **Bipolar**: have a single axon and dendrite that arise at opposite ends of the cell body and both of them have many distal branches. They are associated with special senses that include sensory pathways for *smell, sight, hearing, vestibulation (balance)*, and *taste*.

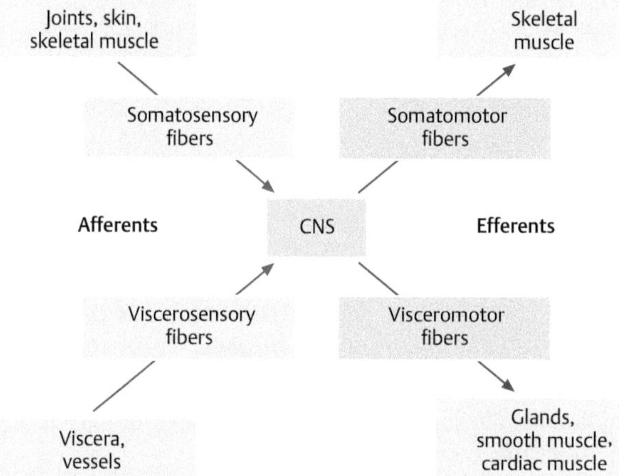

Fig. I.41 Schematic representation of information flow in the nervous system. (From Schuenke M, Schulte E, Schumacher U. THIEME Atlas of Anatomy. General Anatomy and Musculoskeletal System. Illustrations by Voll M and Wesker K. 3rd ed. New York: Thieme Medical Publishers; 2020.)

- Communications between the neurons occurs at **synapses**. These are the contact points between axons, dendrites, cell bodies, and rarely other axons that allow the neuron to pass an electrical or chemical signal to another neuron. The axon terminates as a rounded structure called the **synaptic bouton**. A thickened presynaptic and postsynaptic membrane forms the actual synapse with a **synaptic cleft** located between them. Numerous vesicles containing neurotransmitters are located in each synaptic bouton, and they are released with the arrival of an action potential, then they diffuse across the synapse and bind to receptors on the postsynaptic membrane **(Fig. I.44)**.
- The **neuroglia (glial) cells** provide structural and metabolic support and can outnumber neurons as much as 50:1. They are non-neuronal and nonexcitable and vary depending on if they are found in the CNS or PNS. Details of individual neuroglia and their functions are discussed in the relevant CNS and PNS chapters.

I.13 Structure of the Central Nervous System

Made up of the brain and spinal cord, the CNS has the role of integrating and coordinating incoming and outgoing neuron signals. It is also involved in carrying out higher mental functions such as learning and memory. The brain and spinal cord are made up of **gray matter** and **white matter**. The gray matter contains numerous collections of cell bodies (or a **nucleus**), supporting neuroglia, and relatively few myelinated axons. The spinal cord in cross-section has an H-shaped region of gray matter embedded in the surrounding white matter. The H-shaped structure has a **ventral horn** associated with *efferent (motor) neurons*; a **dorsal horn** associated with *afferent (sensory) neurons*; and in specific regions, a **lateral (intermediolateral) horn** that is associated with

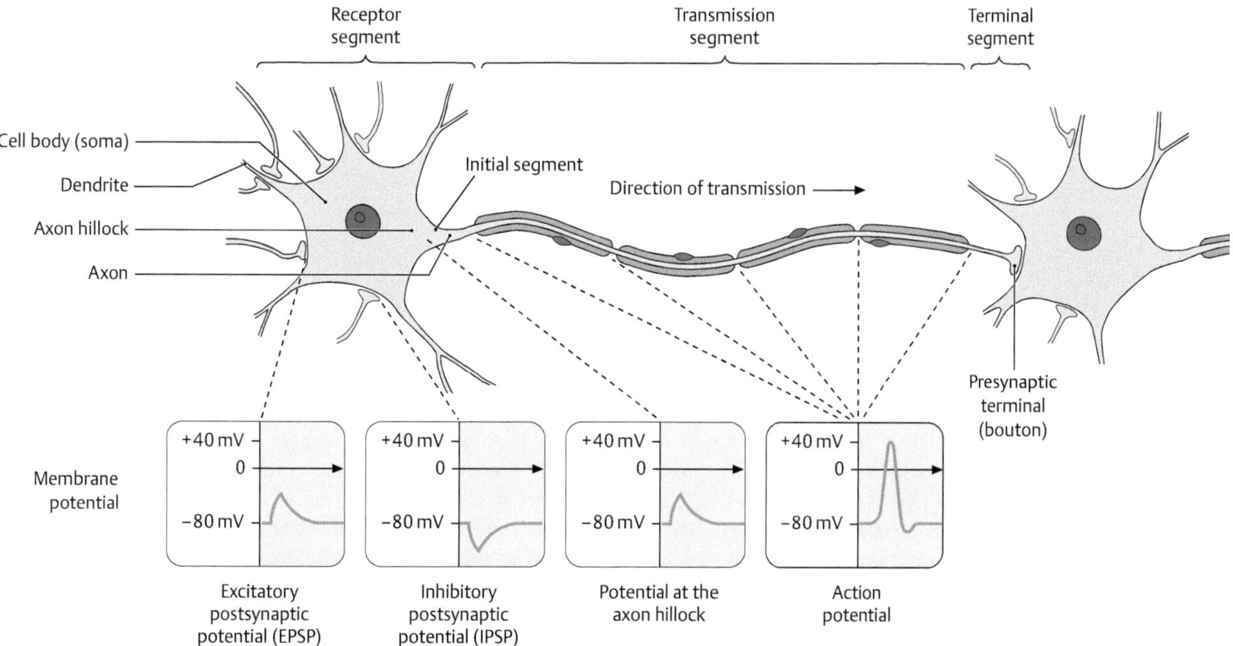

Fig. I.42 The neuron (nerve cell). (From Schuenke M, Schulte E, Schumacher U. THIEME Atlas of Anatomy. General Anatomy and Musculoskeletal System. Illustrations by Voll M and Wesker K. 3rd ed. New York: Thieme Medical Publishers; 2020.)

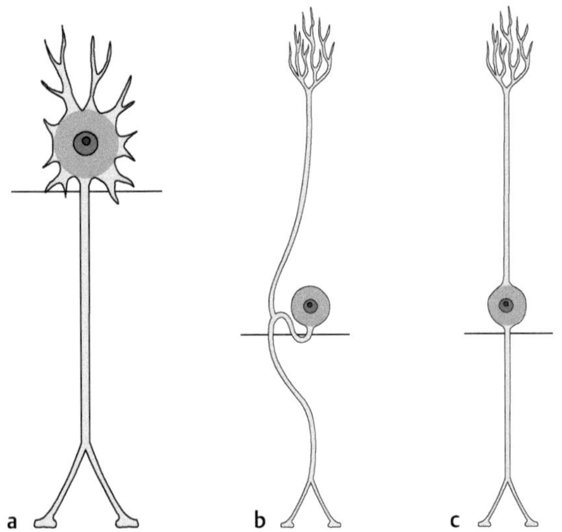

Fig. I.43 Types of neurons. **(a)** Multipolar neuron. **(b)** Pseudounipolar neuron. **(c)** Bipolar neuron. (Modified from Schuenke M, Schulte E, Schumacher U. THIEME Atlas of Anatomy. General Anatomy and Musculoskeletal System. Illustrations by Voll M and Wesker K. 3rd ed. New York: Thieme Medical Publishers; 2020.)

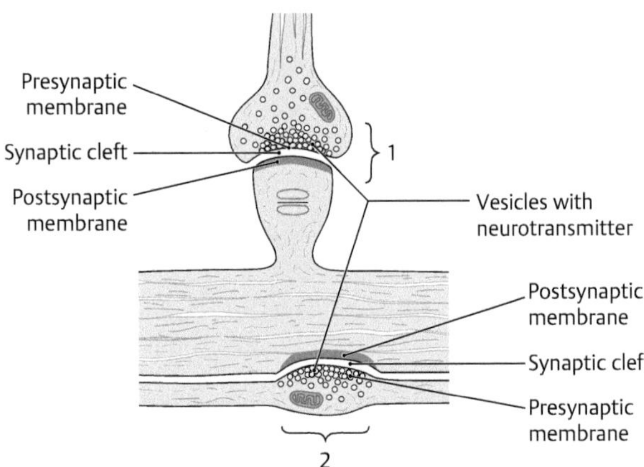

Fig. I.44 Electron microscopy of synapses in the central nervous system (CNS). A synapse with a dendritic spine (1). A side-by-side synapse called a parallel contact or *bouton en passage* (2). (From Schuenke M, Schulte E, Schumacher U. THIEME Atlas of Anatomy. General Anatomy and Musculoskeletal System. Illustrations by Voll M and Wesker K. 3rd ed. New York: Thieme Medical Publishers; 2020.)

preganglionic autonomic neurons. The white matter is composed of bundles of myelinated axons that connect to various gray matter locations along with supporting neuroglia. A bundle of axons (nerve fibers) within the CNS that connects nuclei of the cerebral cortex are known as **tracts** (**Fig. I.45**).

The external surface of the CNS is covered by the meninges and there are three of these membranes. They are called the dura mater, arachnoid mater, and pia mater. The layer adjacent to the CNS tissue is the **pia mater**. The space located between the pia and the next layer or arachnoid mater is called the **subarachnoid space** and it is occupied by a delicate connective tissue or trabeculae and intercommunicating channels that contain the **cerebrospinal fluid (CSF)**. The CSF serves as a cushion and shock absorber for the CNS; circulates nutrients and chemicals filtered from the blood; and removes waste products from the brain. It is produced by ependymal cells of the choroid plexuses and reabsorbed by the *arachnoid granulations*. Adjacent to the arachnoid is the dura mater. The dura is the furthest from the brain but closest to the surrounding bone (**Fig. I.46**).

I.14 Structure of the Peripheral Nervous System

All of the nerve fibers and cell bodies located outside of the CNS that conduct impulses to or away from the CNS are part of the PNS. It is organized into nerves that connect the CNS with peripheral structures. A **nerve fiber** is defined as consisting of an *axon*, a *neurolemma*, and its surrounding *endoneurium*. The **neurolemma** is the outermost nucleated cytoplasmic layer of the Schwann cells that surround the axon of the neuron and separates it from other axons. It takes two forms in the PNS: (1) with myelinated nerve fibers, the neurolemma consists of Schwann cells specific to an individual axon, and it is organized into a *continuous series* or enwrapping cells that form myelin; and (2) with unmyelinated nerve fibers, the neurolemma composed of Schwann cells do not produce myelin with these types of nerve fibers; thus, they will not form a continuous series of wrapped myelin sheets. Multiple axons will be embedded separately within the cytoplasm of each cell.

A **nerve** will consist of the following characteristics: (1) a bundle of nerve fibers outside the CNS or have fascicles that are a bundle of bundled fibers; (2) connective tissue that surrounds and binds nerve fibers and fascicles together; and (3) nourished by blood vessels known as *vasa nervorum*. The connective tissues of the nerve fibers are as follows (**Fig. I.47**):

- **Endoneurium**: surrounds the neurolemma of myelinated and unmyelinated nerve fibers.
- **Perineurium**: a dense connective tissue layer that encloses a fascicle and prevents penetration of most foreign substances.
- **Epineurium**: the outermost layer of a nerve and is a thick, dense connective tissue sheath that wraps around multiple bundles of fascicles. Blood vessel and lymphatics can also be found near this layer.

Types of nerves associated with the PNS include the cranial and spinal nerves. The 12 pairs of **cranial nerves** are discussed extensively in Chapter 7 and exclusively in Chapter 12 but they are peripheral nerves that arise from the brain with the exception of one that originates from the spinal cord (spinal accessory nerve or CN XI). Originating from the spinal cord are 31 pairs of spinal nerves that all correspond to a particular spinal segment of the spinal cord. There are 8 cervical, 12 thoracic, 5 lumbar, 5 sacral, and 1 coccygeal set of spinal nerves.

The architecture extending out from the spinal cord is as such **ventral/dorsal rootlets**, **ventral/dorsal roots**, and the spinal nerve that will bifurcate into a ventral or dorsal ramus branch just distal to the intervertebral foramen. The dorsal root contains a **dorsal root ganglion**. The dorsal rami branches of spinal nerves target the deep muscles of the back, the overlying skin of the back, and the synovial joints of the vertebral column. The ventral rami branches of spinal nerves make up the majority of named nerves, can form plexuses, and innervate the anterior and lateral body walls along with the upper and lower limbs, thus becoming a bigger contributor than the dorsal rami (**Fig. I.48**).

The **ventral rootlet** and **roots** contain **efferent (motor) fibers**. These are always somatic motor in nature but there are visceral motor fibers traveling through the T1–L2 and S2–S4 ventral rootlets and roots. The visceral motor fibers are part of the autonomic

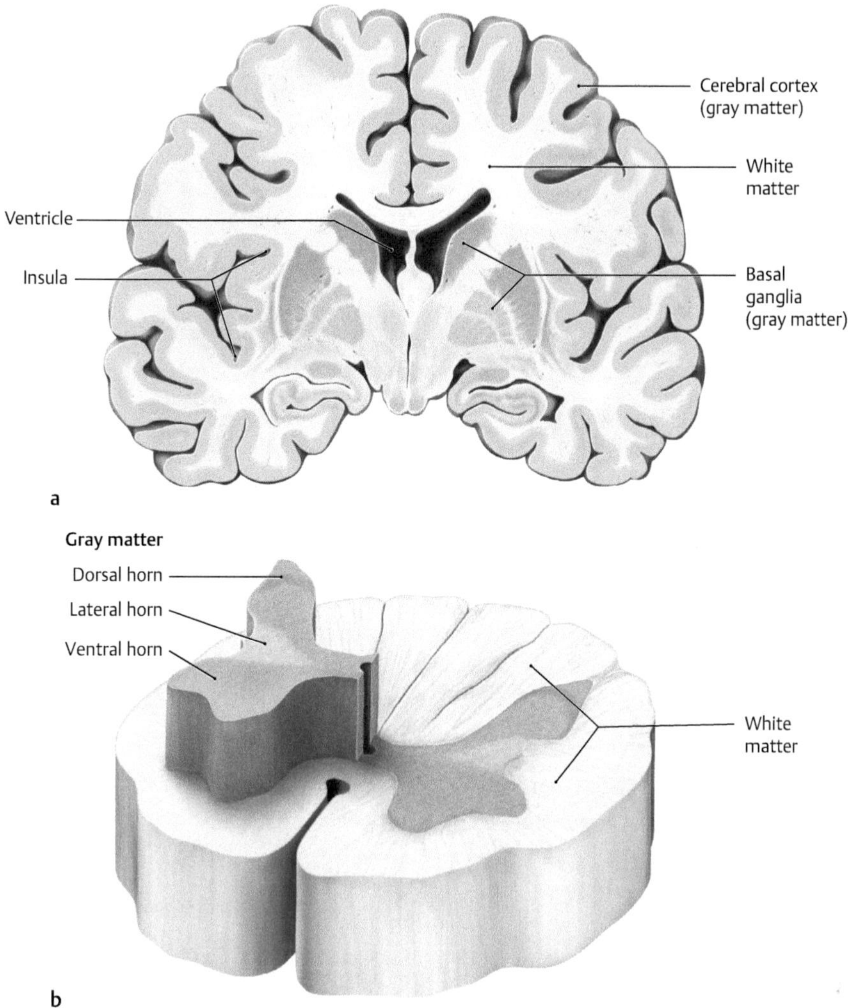

Fig. I.45 **(a)** Distribution of white and gray matter in the central nervous system (CNS). **(b)** Gray and white matter of the spinal cord. (Modified from Schuenke M, Schulte E, Schumacher U. THIEME Atlas of Anatomy. General Anatomy and Musculoskeletal System. Illustrations by Voll M and Wesker K. 3rd ed. New York: Thieme Medical Publishers; 2020.)

nervous system, which in itself is divided into a sympathetic and parasympathetic division. The fibers passing through T1–L2 are sympathetic while those through S2–S4 are parasympathetic. The **dorsal rootlets** and **roots** contain only **afferent (sensory) fibers**. They will include both somatic and visceral sensory fibers with their cell bodies both located in the **dorsal root ganglion**.

Motor and sensory fibers will not mix until reaching the **spinal nerve**. The **ventral** and **dorsal rami** branches of the spinal nerve are both considered mixed nerves. Each contains a combination of somatic motor (GSE), somatic sensory (GSA), visceral motor (GVE-sym/post), and in some locations visceral sensory (GVA) fibers that briefly pass back through with a ventral rami branch (**Fig. I.49**).

I.15 Dermatomes and Myotomes

The area of skin that is mainly supplied by the sensory neurons of a single spinal nerve of the ipsilateral (same) side is called a **dermatome**. There is overlap from one dermatome to the next, and therefore if a lesion of a specific spinal nerve was to occur, there is still some sensory input to the affected dermatome. For example, if there was compression or a lesion of the fourth spinal nerve which corresponds to the dermatome the nipple is located in, fibers of the adjacent third and fifth spinal nerves overlap the fourth dermatome and thus provide a double or redundant coverage. Consecutive or adjacent spinal nerves would have to be affected in order to eliminate the sensation to a particular dermatome. It is important to distinguish the fibers carried by an individual spinal nerve that contributes to a segmental innervation such as a dermatome and the fibers carried by a named cutaneous nerve that can originate from a plexus of peripheral nerves and thus innervates a peripheral region not defined by dermatomes (**Fig. I.50**).

A cutaneous nerve supplies an area of the skin that is related to a peripheral nerve. This cutaneous nerve may contain fibers from several individual spinal nerves, and therefore the peripheral cutaneous nerve and dermatome-mapped regions will show much overlapping. A cutaneous nerve area is generally broader and wider than an area or segment defined as a single dermatome. Overlap is seen with individual cutaneous nerves much like that of an individual spinal nerve overlapping another defined dermatome. The details listed above are the reason a dermatome map differs from that of a peripheral cutaneous nerve map (**Fig. I.51**).

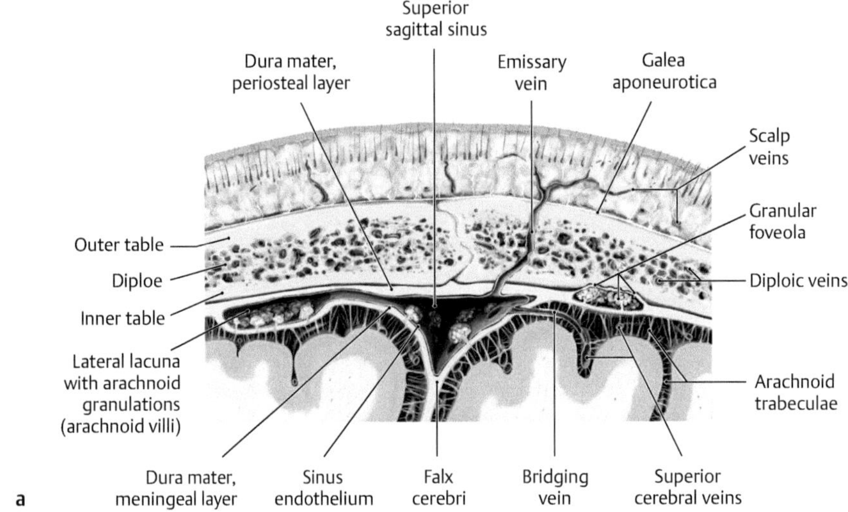

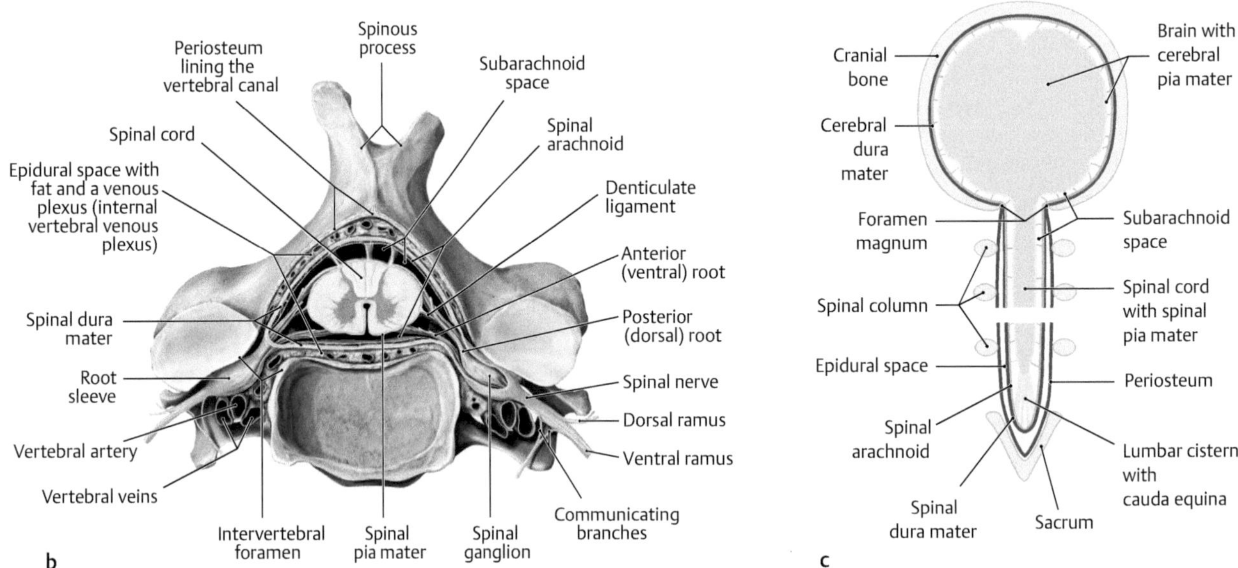

Fig. I.46 (a) Relationship of the meninges to the cavarium. **(b)** Transverse section through a cervical vertebra demostrating the menigeal layers. **(c)** Relationship of the meninges within the cranial cavity and spinal canal. Formation of the naturally occuring epidural space of the spinal canal is shown in **b** and **c**. (Modified from Schuenke M, Schulte E, Schumacher U. THIEME Atlas of Anatomy. Head, Neck, and Neuroanatomy. Illustrations by Voll M and Wesker K. 3rd ed. New York: Thieme Medical Publishers; 2020.)

The concept of **referred pain** is the perception of somatic pain at a particular location but in reality it is pain from a visceral organ and travels back with the *visceral sensory fibers* associated with the sympathetic nervous system. It may be located in an area corresponding to multiple dermatomes but referred pain in itself is not associated with a specific dermatome.

A **myotome** represents a group of muscles that a single spinal nerve innervates. Most of the muscles located in the upper and lower limbs receive innervation from one or more spinal nerves that collectively form a "nerve" and are therefore comprised of multiple myotomes. When spinal nerves become compressed or irritated by trauma, disk herniation, bone spurs, or even reduced blood supply due to diabetes, for example, it leads to what is known as radiculopathy. The result could be pain, numbness, or even muscle weakness, with it generally occurring at the level of the cervical and lumbar regions **(Fig. I.52)**.

I.16 Somatic Nervous System

The **somatic nervous system (SNS)** is the part of the PNS that provides both motor and sensory innervation to the outer body wall **(Fig. I.53)**. This will include innervation of the striated, voluntary skeletal muscle and skin but not visceral structures such as vital internal organs, glandular tissue, and smooth muscle. The SNS is broken down as such.

- **General somatic motor (GSE)**: these fibers transmit impulses from the CNS to striated, skeletal muscles for voluntary movement or for movements associated with involuntary reflex arcs.
- **General somatic sensory (GSA)**: these fibers transmit impulses back to the CNS. They include *proprioceptive* information about tension from muscles and tendons and positioning of the joints. There is also exteroceptive information that includes pain, temperature, pressure, and touch passing back to the CNS through these fibers.

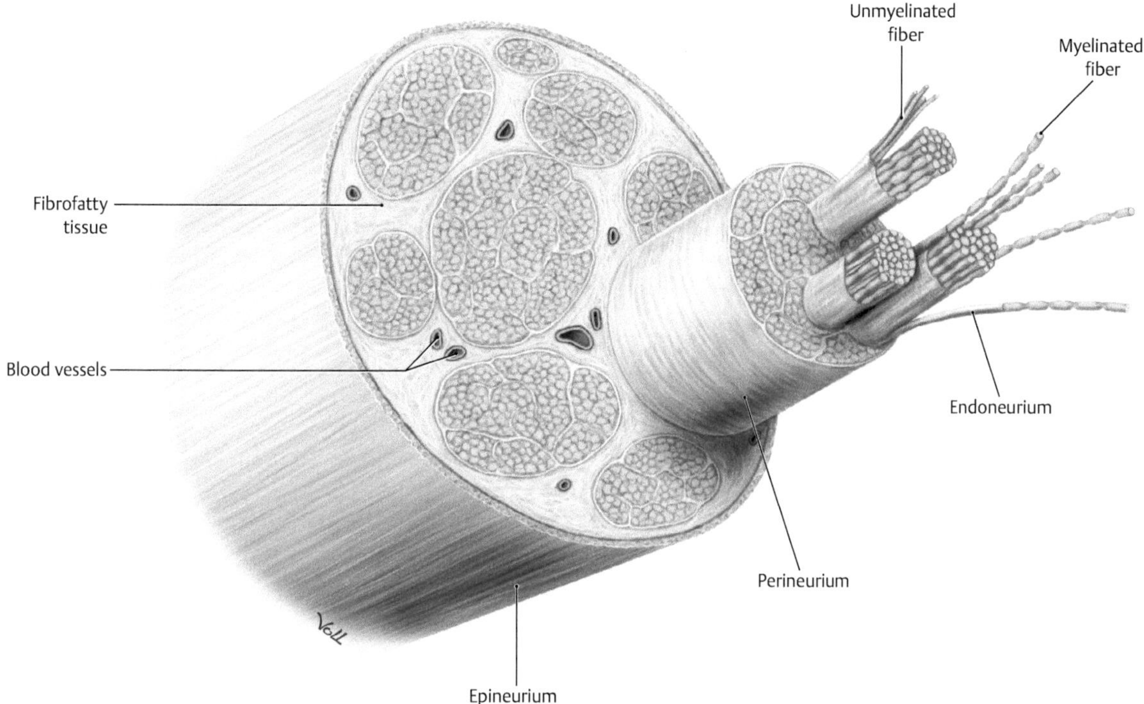

Fig. I.47 Peripheral nerve. (From Schuenke M, Schulte E, Schumacher U. THIEME Atlas of Anatomy. General Anatomy and Musculoskeletal System. Illustrations by Voll M and Wesker K. 3rd ed. New York: Thieme Medical Publishers; 2020.)

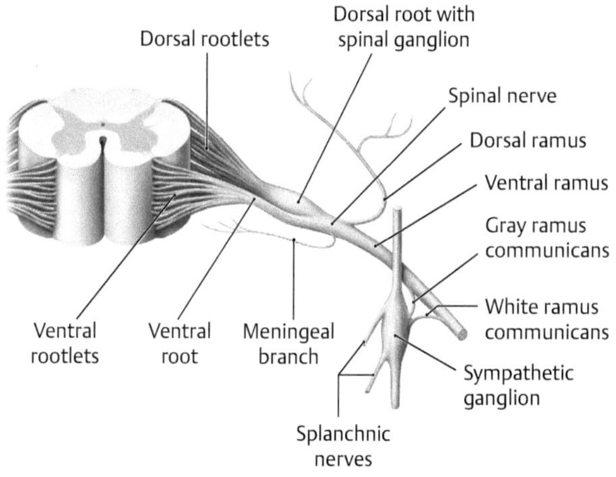

Fig. I.48 Structure of a spinal cord segment. (From Schuenke M, Schulte E, Schumacher U. THIEME Atlas of Anatomy. Head, Neck, and Neuroanatomy. Illustrations by Voll M and Wesker K. 3rd ed. New York: Thieme Medical Publishers; 2020.)

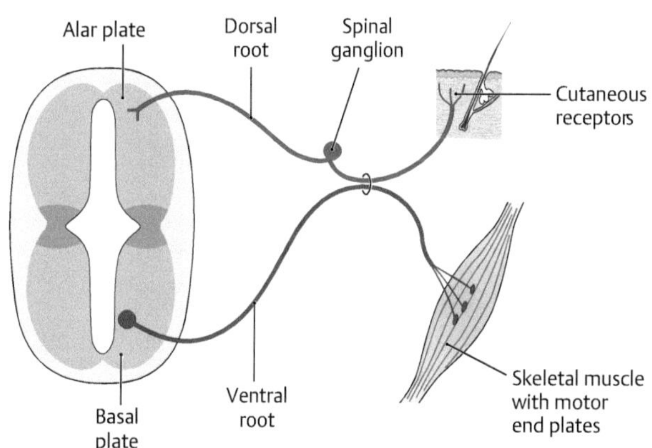

Fig. I.49 Topographical and functional organization of a spinal cord segment. (From Schuenke M, Schulte E, Schumacher U. THIEME Atlas of Anatomy. General Anatomy and Musculoskeletal System. Illustrations by Voll M and Wesker K. 3rd ed. New York: Thieme Medical Publishers; 2020.)

I.17 Autonomic Nervous System

The **autonomic nervous system (ANS)** is defined as the visceral motor fibers that innervate visceral organs, and these can include vital organs, smooth muscle, or glandular tissues (**Fig. I.54**). The fibers are labeled as **general visceral motor (GVE)** and it consists of a two-neuron motor system that differs from the entire SNS that only has one neuron involved. The cell body of the first **preganglionic (presynaptic) neuron** is located in the gray matter of the CNS. After traveling through the nerve fiber, a synapse will occur on the cell body of the **postganglionic (postsynaptic) neuron** that is located in *autonomic ganglion* outside the CNS. The postganglionic fibers will then terminate on a target organ that could include cardiac muscle, smooth muscle, or glandular tissue. The ANS has a *parasympathetic* and *sympathetic division.*

- **Parasympathetic division**: is a *homeostatic system* or energy conserving system concerned with the calming, resting, or digestive actions of the body. Functions are described in **Table I.3.**
  - This division is also known as the *craniosacral division* because it originates from the brainstem or sacral regions of the spinal cord. The fibers of the cranial portion will travel initially through cranial nerves III, VII, IX, and X. The fibers of the sacral region originate from the S2–S4 spinal segments in a region of the spinal cord gray matter similar in location to the lateral (intermediolateral) horns that will be discussed with the sympathetic division.

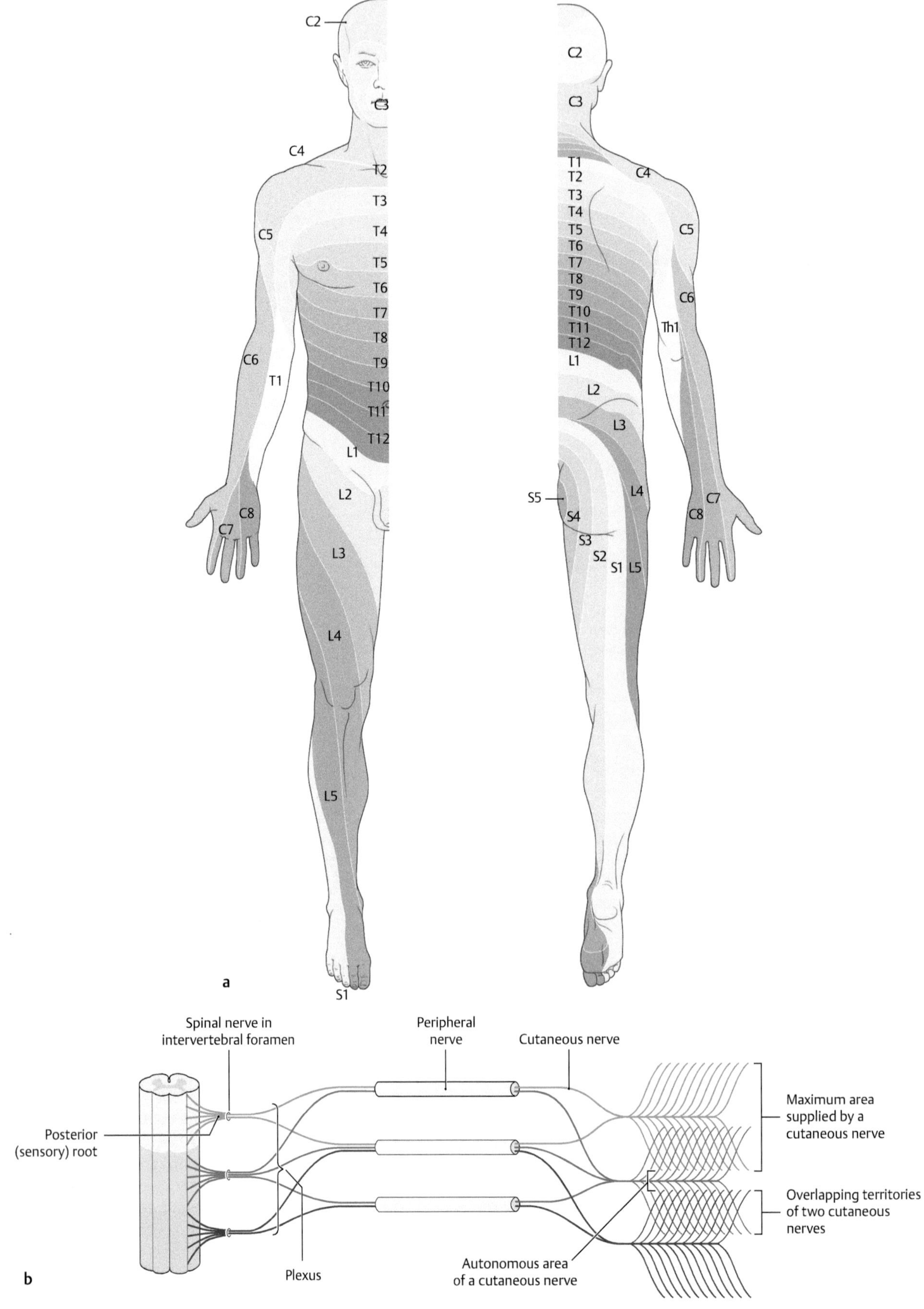

Fig. I.50 (a) Pattern of radicular (segmental) sensory innervation. **(b)** Course of sensory fibers from the dorsal root to the dermatome. (From Schuenke M, Schulte E, Schumacher U. THIEME Atlas of Anatomy. General Anatomy and Musculoskeletal System. Illustrations by Voll M and Wesker K. 3rd ed. New York: Thieme Medical Publishers; 2020.)

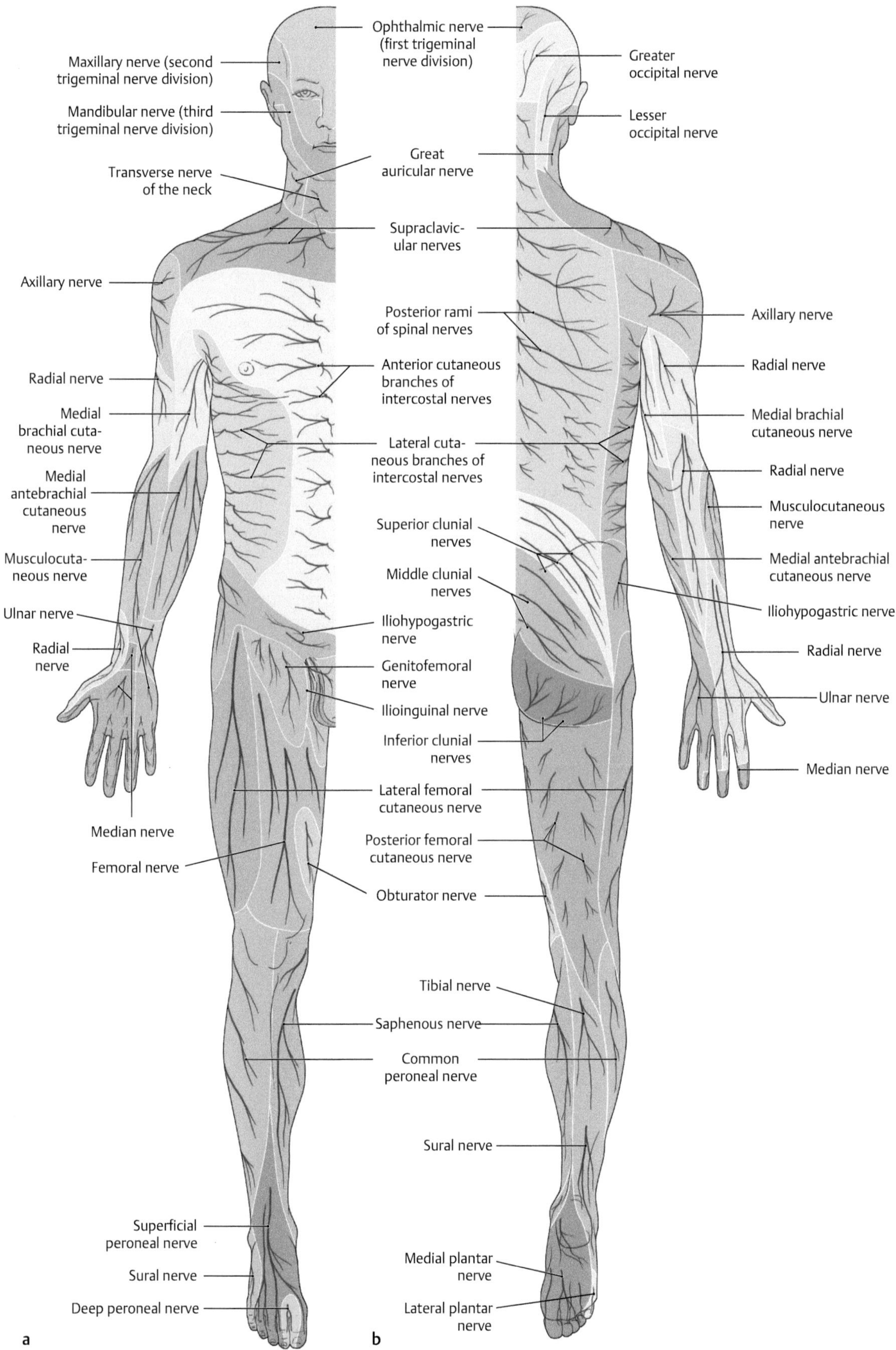

Fig. I.51 Pattern of peripheral sensory innervation. **(a)** Anterior view. **(b)** Posterior view. (From Schuenke M, Schulte E, Schumacher U. THIEME Atlas of Anatomy. General Anatomy and Musculoskeletal System. Illustrations by Voll M and Wesker K. 3rd ed. New York: Thieme Medical Publishers; 2020.)

Parasympathetics are never located on the outer body wall.

- *Preganglionics (para/pre)*: the para/pre fibers associated with cranial nerves III, VII, IX, and X originate from brainstem nuclei called **Edinger-Westphal**, **superior salivatory**, **inferior salivatory**, and the **dorsal motor nucleus of vagus**, respectively. The para/pre fibers from the sacral region originate from the S2–S4 spinal segments in a region of the spinal cord gray matter similar in location to the lateral (intermediolateral) horns that will be discussed with the sympathetic division. They then travel through the ventral roots of spinal nerves S2–S4, ventral rami of S2–S4, and the pelvic splanchnic nerves that arise from the S2–S4 ventral rami. From the pelvic splanchnic nerves, para/pre fibers travel to hindgut and pelvic structures before synapsing on para/post cell bodies (**Fig. 1.55**).
- *Postganglionic (para/post)*: the para/post cell bodies are located in the **ciliary**, **pterygopalatine**, **submandibular**, and **otic ganglion** of the head or the **submucosal ganglion** of a target organ such as the heart, lungs, esophagus, and most of the GI tract. The para/post fibers extending out from the four-head ganglion will normally travel on one of the three branches of the trigeminal nerve (CN V) before reaching its target organ. Submucosal ganglion lies adjacent to the target organ already, so the para/post fibers have a very short course (**Fig. I.55**).

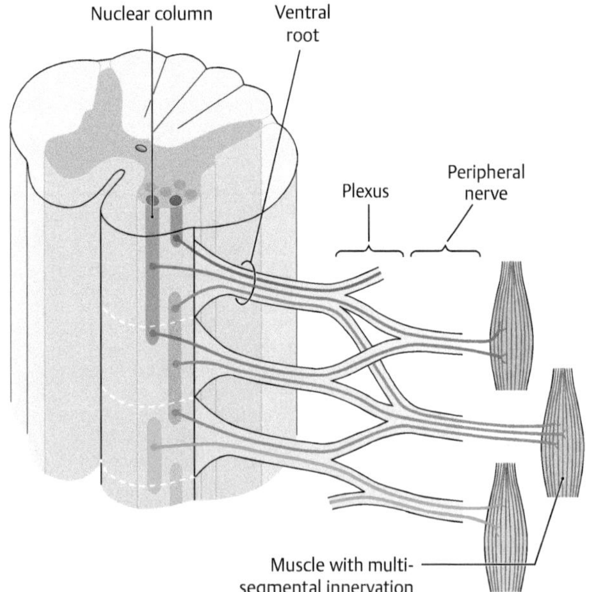

Fig. I.52 Organizational principles of the anterior column of the spinal cord. (From Schuenke M, Schulte E, Schumacher U. THIEME Atlas of Anatomy. General Anatomy and Musculoskeletal System. Illustrations by Voll M and Wesker K. 3rd ed. New York: Thieme Medical Publishers; 2020.)

- **Sympathetic division**: is a *catabolic system* or energy expending system concerned with the "fight or flight" response. This division is also known as the *thoracolumbar division* because it originates from the thoracic and upper lumbar regions of the spinal cord, and its functions are described in **Table I.3.**
  - *Preganglionic (sym/pre)*: the sym/pre cell bodies are located in the lateral horns of gray matter of the T1–L2 spinal segments. The sym/pre fibers leave the spinal cord by coursing through the ventral rootlets, ventral root, spinal nerve, and very briefly through the ventral rami before entering the sympathetic trunk (or chain) by passing through the **white rami communicantes**. White rami communicantes are only located between T1 and L2.

Once in the sympathetic trunk, these sym/pre fibers can (1) *synapse immediately* at a sympathetic chain (paravertebral)

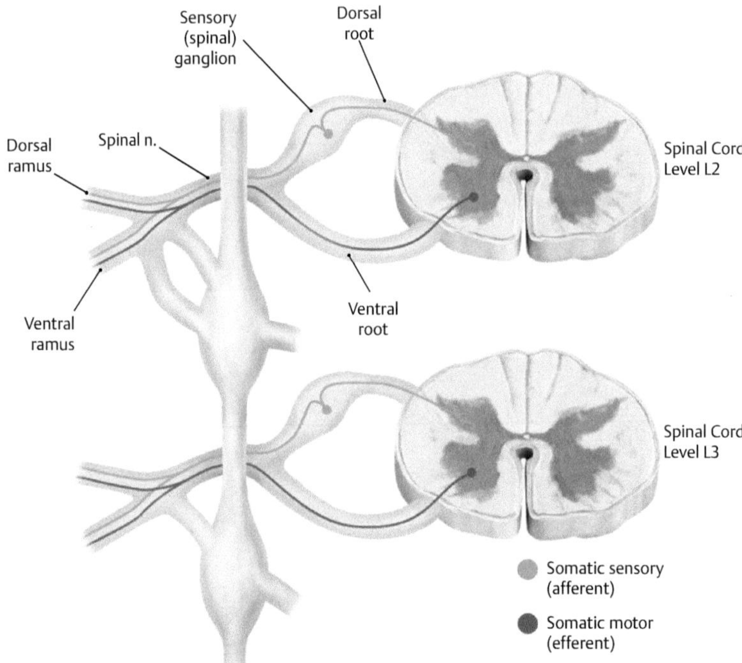

Fig. I.53 Typical spinal nerve. (From Schuenke M, Schulte E, Schumacher U. THIEME Atlas of Anatomy. Head, Neck, and Neuroanatomy. Illustrations by Voll M and Wesker K. 3rd ed. New York: Thieme Medical Publishers; 2020.)

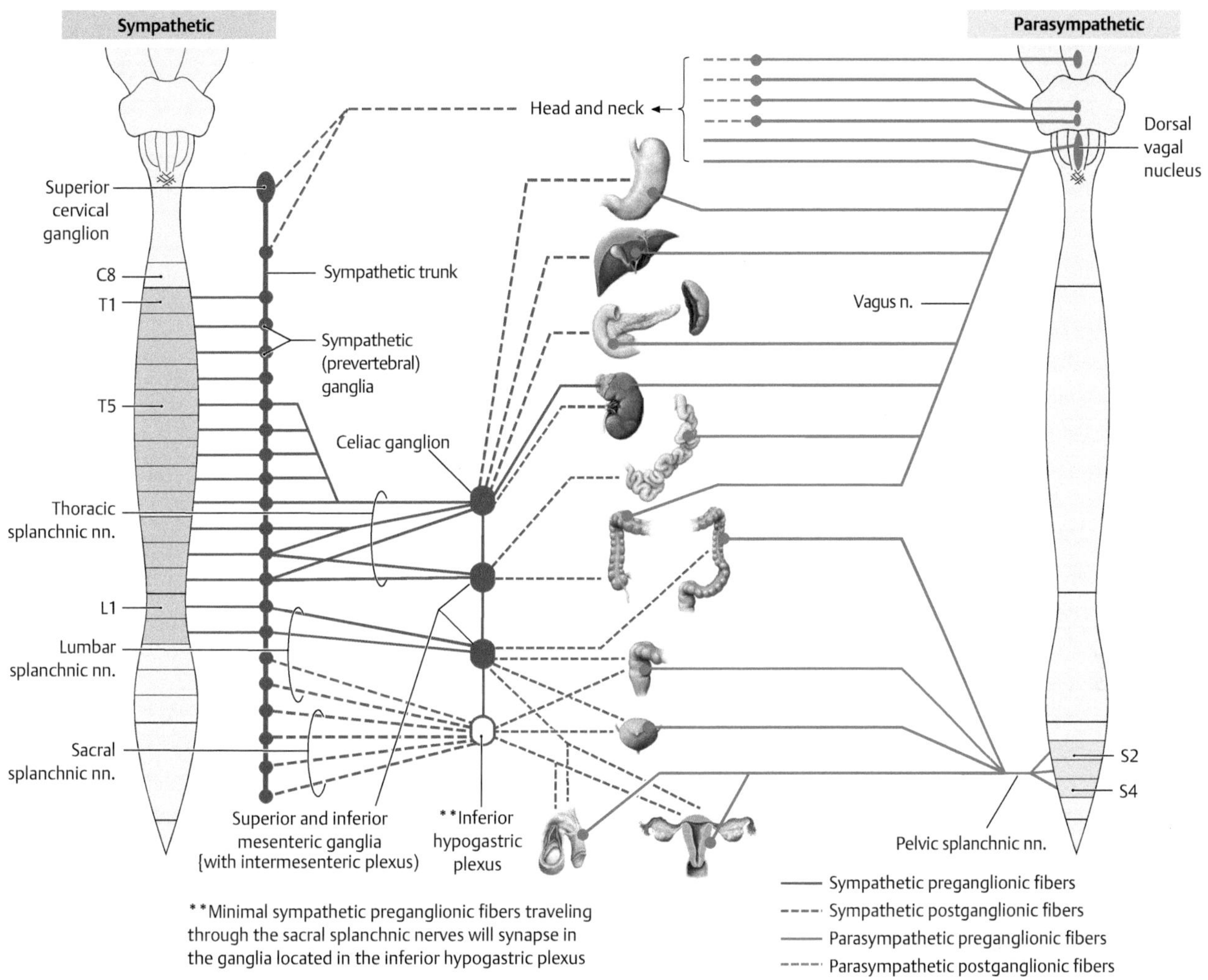

Fig. I.54 Overview of the autonomic nervous system. (From Schuenke M, Schulte E, Schumacher U. THIEME Atlas of Anatomy. Internal Organs. Illustrations by Voll M and Wesker K. 3rd ed. New York: Thieme Medical Publishers; 2020.)

ganglion; (2) *ascend* or *descend* through the trunk before finally synapsing at a sympathetic chain ganglion; (3) *continue through a splanchnic nerve* before synapsing at a preaortic (prevertebral) ganglion of the aortic plexus; or (4) *innervate the suprarenal gland* by first passing through a splanchnic nerve and then bypassing the preaortic ganglion of the aortic plexus before synapsing on chromaffin cells of the suprarenal gland medulla.

- *Postganglionic (sym/post)*: after the sym/pre fibers have synapsed at a **sympathetic chain (paravertebral) ganglion,** the sym/post fibers must pass through **gray rami communicantes** attached to one of the 31 spinal nerves before continuing through either a ventral or dorsal rami branch. Sym/post fibers traveling through this route are destined to innervate the blood vessels, arrector pili muscles, and sweat glands of the head, neck, trunk, or limb regions. The sym/pre fibers that passed through splanchnic nerves synapse on the sym/post cell bodies primarily at the **preaortic ganglion** and these include the **celiac, aorticorenal, superior mesenteric,** and **inferior mesenteric ganglion**. The sym/post fibers then pass through the aortic plexus and onto a blood vessel (periarterial plexus) or down into the pelvic region and innervate blood vessels or certain sphincters of the abdominal and pelvic organs (**Fig. I.56**).

Some splanchnic nerves originating from the neck region (cardiopulmonary splanchnics) are already carrying sym/post fibers and deliver them to the cardiopulmonary plexus. The esophageal plexus may receive its sym/post fibers directly from the sympathetic chain by way of splanchnic nervelike branches. **Chromaffin cells** located in the medulla of the suprarenal gland are structurally similar to sympathetic postganglionic neurons, and when stimulated by the sym/pre fibers, they release epinephrine and norepinephrine into the systematic circulation.

I.18 Visceral Sensory

The **general visceral sensory (GVA)** fibers transmit reflex or pain impulses from the blood vessels or visceral organs such as the heart, lungs, and GI tract back to the CNS. These fibers are not considered part of the ANS but the information that passes through them can help alter blood pressure and chemistry and digestion activity. If visceral sensation reaches a conscious level it is generally perceived as poorly localized pain related possibly to hunger, cramps, or nausea. Visceral reflex arcs can be associated with urination (micturition), defecation, baroreceptors, chemoreceptors, and the enteric nervous system.

Table I.3 **Effects of the ANS on various organs**

Organ		Parasympathetic effects	Sympathetic effects
Systematic arteries			
	Skin		Constricts
	Skeletal		Dilates (β_2); constricts (α_1)
	Abdominal		Constricts
Arrector pili muscles			Contracts
Adipose			Lipolysis
Glands			
	Sweat		Stimulates sweating
	Lacrimal, parotid, submandibular, sublingual and nasal	Stimulates secretion	Reduces secretion
Eye			
	Pupil	Constrict	Dilate
	Ciliary muscle	Contract	
Heart			
	Cardiac muscle	Decrease force of contraction	Increases force of contraction
	Coronary arteries (mainly effected by metabolic factors)	Constrict	Dilate
Lungs		Constrict bronchioles; dilate arteries; increased secretions	Dilate bronchioles; constrict arteries; decreased secretions
GI tract			
	Peristalsis activity	Increase	Decrease
	Sphincters	Relax	Contract
	Glands	Increases secretions	Decreases secretions
	Liver		Glycogenolysis
	Gallbladder	Contract	Relax
Adrenal gland			
	Cortex		Stimulates release of cortex hormones
	Medulla		Stimulates release of epinephrine and norepinephrine
Kidney			Constricts arteries to reduce urine output
Urinary bladder		Contracts detrusor muscle; relaxes urethral sphincter	Relaxes detrusor muscle; contracts urethral sphincter
Male genitalia		Causes an erection	Ejaculation
Uterus (mainly under hormonal control)		Relaxes smooth muscle; dilates arteries	Contracts smooth muscle; constricts arteries
Vagina			Contracts smooth muscle

- **GVA pain fibers** from all locations will travel back primarily with sympathetic fibers and their cell bodies are located in a dorsal root ganglion. Visceral pain fibers have a strong correlation with ***referred pain*** **(Fig. I.57)**.
- **GVA reflex fibers** from the thorax, foregut, and midgut travel back through the vagus nerve (CN X) and their cell bodies are located in the inferior sensory ganglion of CN X. The GVA reflex fibers originating from the hindgut or pelvis travel back through the pelvis splanchnic nerves and their cell bodies are located in the S2–S4 dorsal root ganglions.

I.18.1 Visceral Nerve Plexus

A **visceral nerve plexus** is located near a visceral organ and are generally named according to that specific organ or region they lie near. Examples include the cardiopulmonary, aortic, or

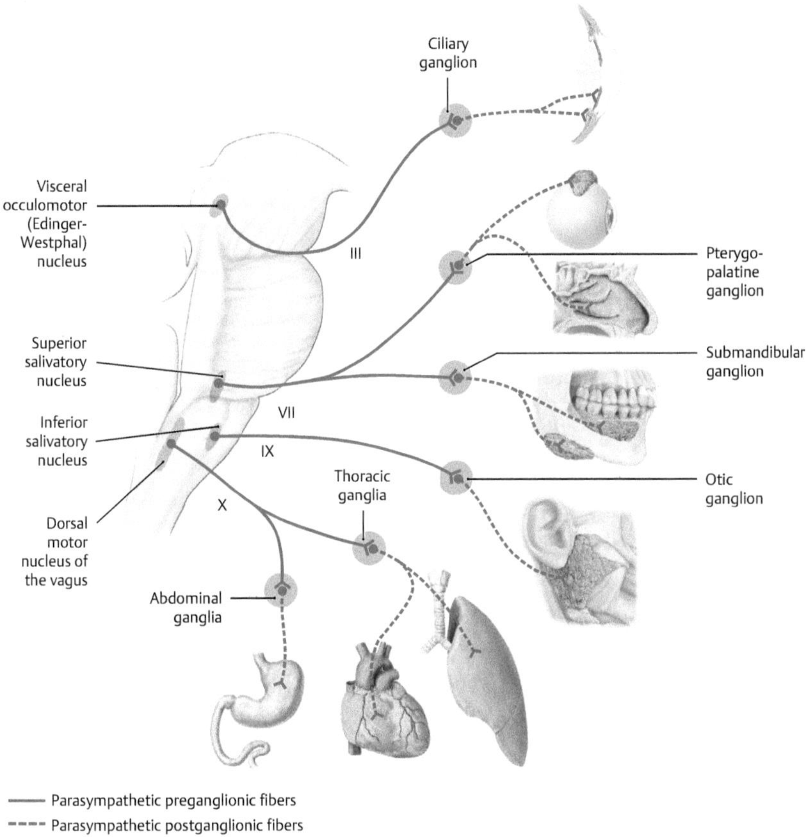

Fig. I.55 Parasympathetic nervous system (cranial part): overview. (From Schuenke M, Schulte E, Schumacher U. THIEME Atlas of Anatomy. Head, Neck, and Neuroanatomy. Illustrations by Voll M and Wesker K. 3rd ed. New York: Thieme Medical Publishers; 2020.)

inferior hypogastric plexuses. The plexuses will be composed of both visceral efferent (GVE) and visceral afferent (GVA) fibers. The GVE fibers that pass through these plexuses consist of sympathetic postganglionic (sym/post) and parasympathetic preganglionic (para/pre) fibers and they are accompanied by either visceral pain or reflex fibers. There is generally no ganglion located in a visceral nerve plexus except for that of the aortic plexus. The inferior hypogastric (pelvic) plexuses have a minimal amount of ganglion-like cells that involve sympathetic synapses.

I.19 Respiratory System

The structures related to this system include the air passages (trachea, bronchi, etc.) and the lungs that are responsible for supplying oxygen and eliminating carbon dioxide from the body. The majority of these structures will be found in Chapter 2 but will also be discussed in Chapter 7.

I.20 Digestive (Alimentary) System

The organs associated with this system are responsible for taking in food, breaking it down into smaller nutrients, absorbing the nutrients, and then eliminating excess or indigestible wastes. The digestive process involves the processes of ingestion, propulsion, mechanical and chemical digestion, absorption, and finally defection. The alimentary canal or GI tract extends from the mouth to the anus. This system is detailed in both Chapters 3 and 7.

I.21 Endocrine System

This system includes a series of ductless glands, cells of the intestine and blood vessel walls, as well as specialized nerve endings that secrete messenger molecules known as hormones. These hormones will be transported by the cardiovascular system in order to reach receptors on cells and influence characteristic physiological responses in those cells. Major endocrine glands include the thymus (Chapter 2); testes, pancreas, kidneys, and suprarenal glands (Chapter 3); ovaries (Chapter 4); thyroid and parathyroid glands (Chapter 7); and the pituitary and pineal glands (Chapter 9).

I.22 Reproductive System

The reproductive system is made up of the gonads (testes in males, ovaries in females) that are responsible for the production of sperm in males and oocytes or eggs in females. Internal structures that include the ductus deferens, seminal vesicles, and prostate gland in the male; the uterine tubes, uterus, and vagina in the female along with the external genitalia of both sexes are

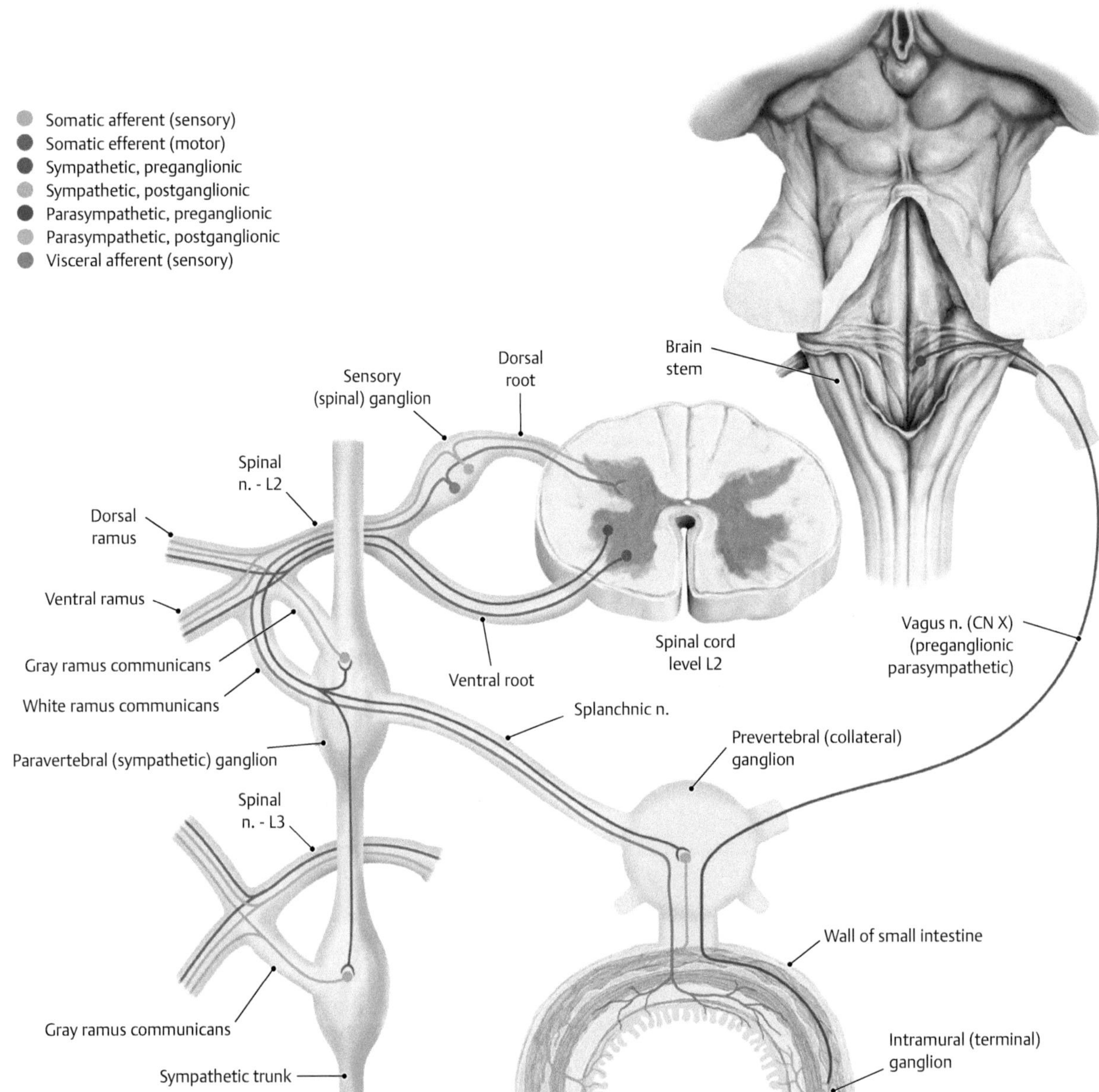

Fig. I.56 Incorporation of both the somatic and autonomic nervous system. (From Schuenke M, Schulte E, Schumacher U. THIEME Atlas of Anatomy. Head, Neck, and Neuroanatomy. Illustrations by Voll M and Wesker K. 3rd ed. New York: Thieme Medical Publishers; 2020.)

considered part of the reproductive system. Most of the structures related to this system are discussed in Chapter 4.

I.23 Urinary System

The urinary system is made up of the kidneys, ureters, urinary bladder, and urethra. This system is responsible for filtering blood of waste and will ultimately produce, transport, store, and excrete urine. These structures are detailed in both Chapters 3 and 4.

I.24 Imaging Techniques

The principles of anatomical structure and function are fundamental to one being able to understand imaging techniques of the human body. These techniques are used in order to recognize abnormalities such as tumors, fractures, and congenital abnormalities. This section describes the principles behind commonly used diagnostic imaging techniques: conventional radiography (CR), ultrasonography (US), computerized tomography (CT), magnetic resonance imaging (MRI), and positron emission tomography (PET).

I.24.1 Conventional Radiography (CR)

Conventional radiography known as a simple X-ray image to most is considered the foundation of diagnostic imaging, and it works by having highly penetrating beams of X-rays transilluminate a patient and display tissues of different densities of mass within the body. These images are then displayed on an X-ray film or more recently in clinical practice with digital acquisition. The tissue or organ that is relatively dense in mass will absorb more X-rays than does a less dense structure. A very dense structure

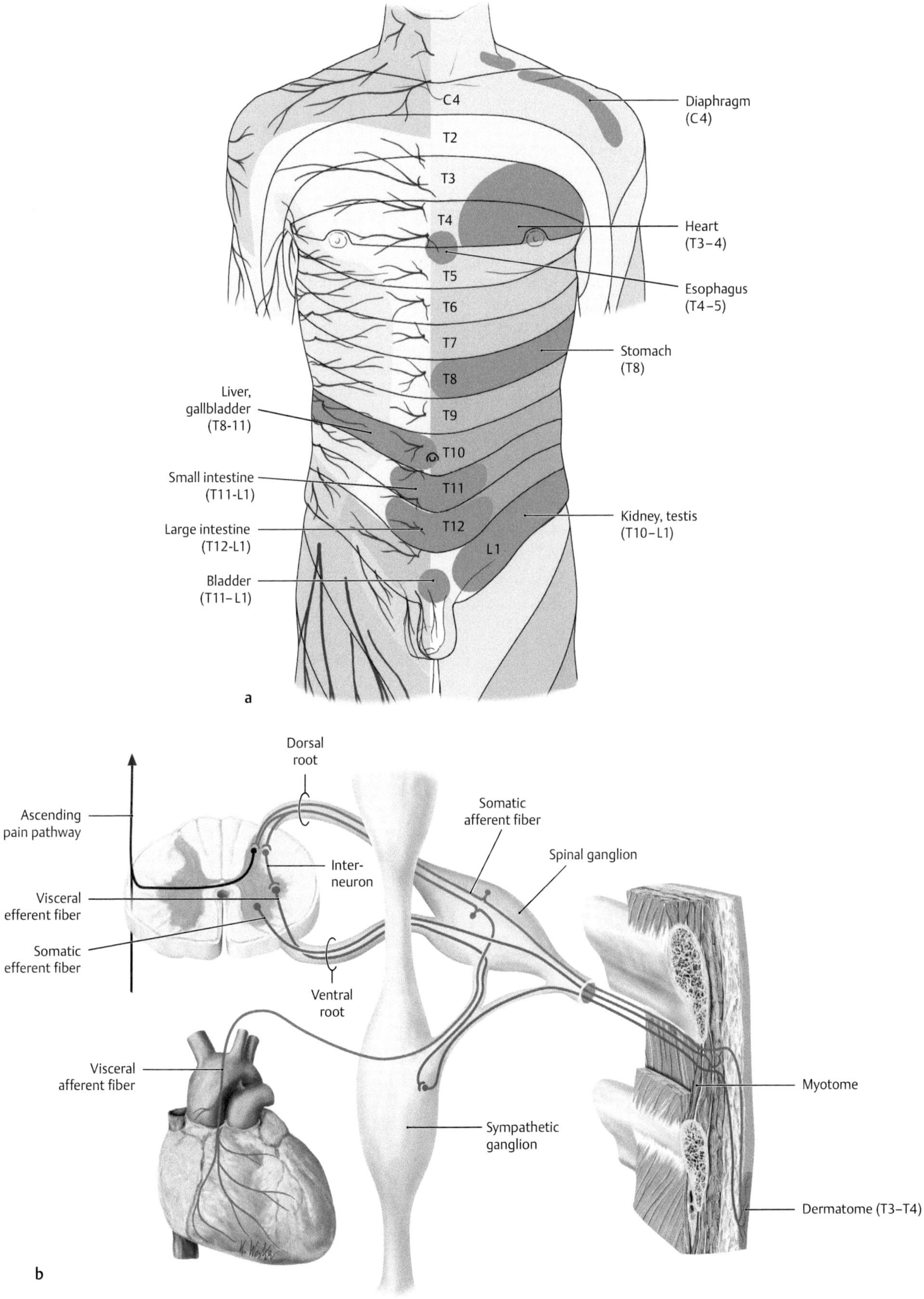

Fig. I.57 Referred pain. **(a)** Pain impulses from a particular internal organ are consistently projected to the same well-defined skin area. **(b)** The convergence of somatic and visceral afferent pain. (From Schuenke M, Schulte E, Schumacher U. THIEME Atlas of Anatomy. Internal Organs. Illustrations by Voll M and Wesker K. 3rd ed. New York: Thieme Medical Publishers; 2020.)

(compact bone) is known as *radiopaque* because it absorbs more X-rays while a less dense structure (lungs) is known as *radiolucent* because it absorbs less X-rays. Radiographs are generally done with the patient's body resting near the X-ray film or detector to maximize magnification artifacts.

The depiction of anatomic features may be limited by the overlap of structures along the path of an X-ray beam. However, in the case of orthopaedic imaging, the anatomy involved in these images tend to be simple with intrinsic tissue contrast high enough so that a fracture or break in the leg for instance can be visualized quite easily. Radiography provides a very high spatial resolution of the internal structure. Ingestion of a radiopaque substance or injection of an iodinated contrast media will enhance the resolution of radiographs. A *noninvasive study* would involve the injection of contrast medium into a peripheral intravenous line while an arteriogram procedure involving an arterial puncture and injection of contrast medium would be considered an *invasive study*.

I.24.2 Computerized Tomography (CT)

Computerized tomography or CT uses X-ray tubes and detector arrays that rotate around a stationary patient and displays images resembling transverse sections of the body. It is a procedure that can be done in as little as five to ten minutes. Radiation absorbed by different tissues varies with a computer then compiling and generating two-dimensional slices but also have the ability to create three-dimensional reconstructions.

I.24.3 Magnetic Resonance Imaging (MRI)

A procedure similar to CT but not exposing the patient to radiation, **magnetic resonance imaging**, is considered better than CT for soft tissue differentiation. An MRI scan usually takes longer to run than a CT scan (approximately 30 minutes). Tissues can be reconstructed from any plane, even arbitrary oblique planes. While a person lies in a scanner much like CT, a strong magnetic field is applied to the individual and pulsed with radio waves. Patient tissues emit signals that are stored in a computer and reconstructed images can be reproduced in either two or three dimensions. These MRI scanners can be gated or paced to visualize moving structures such as the heart in real time but the tissue appearance will vary depending on the amount of radiofrequency pulses applied to the patient.

I.24.4 Positron Emission Tomography (PET)

Positron emission tomography is a form of *nuclear medicine* used to measure and evaluate physiological functions of an organ such as brain or the metabolic activity of a tumor. PET scans expose a patient to radiation by way of injecting a radioactive tracer such as cyclotron-produced isotopes that have extremely short half-life emitting positrons. The areas of increased physiological activity display selective uptake of the injected isotopes.

I.24.5 Fluoroscopy and Angiography

Fluoroscopy is an imaging technique that uses X-rays to obtain real-time images of many areas of the body including the digestive, respiratory, urinary, and reproductive systems. A continuous X-ray is passed through the body part being examined and the information is transmitted to a nearby monitor so that the body part and its motion can be seen in detail. Fluoroscopy as an imaging tool is similar to both conventional radiography and computerized tomography. It may be used simply for diagnostic procedures in conjunction with other diagnostic or therapeutic procedures. An example would include a ***barium swallow evaluation*** that uses a barium sulfate suspension as a radiocontrast agent to diagnose the underlying issues associated with difficulty swallowing (dysphagia), hiatal hernias, gastroesophageal reflux disease, or possible pharynx cancers.

Angiography is a form of fluoroscopy that focuses on real-time blood flow in an artery in order to assess any blockage, narrowing, or widening as in the case of an aneurysm with a contrast agent that is generally iodine based. Angiography may also be used to guide procedures dealing with vessel abnormalities as with coronary artery blockages that require a stent to be inserted. Angiography using CT and MRI is only able to demonstrate the appearance of a vessel and cannot be used for treatment procedures.

I.24.6 Ultrasonography (US)

Ultrasonography or just ultrasound involves exposing a portion of the body to high-frequency pulses of sound waves that originate from a transducer and produce images of the inside of the body. There is no ionizing radiation used and the frame rate of images captured is rapid enough to be in real-time showing structure and movements of internal structures. Very high spatial resolution can be obtained; however, ultrasound images are generally not as visually comparable to images obtained using imaging techniques such as CT or MRI. Ultrasound planes are not as restricted as CT or MRI because an individual can move the transducer in an almost infinite number of angles to produce an image. When blood flow through a vessel for instance needs to be evaluated, ***Doppler ultrasound*** may be used to determine if a blockage or narrowing of the vessel exists.

PRACTICE QUESTIONS

1. Anatomical position is defined as a medical reference posture or standard in which the human body is positioned in such a way to eliminate any ambiguous classifications. What particular position is not considered anatomical position?
   A. Upper limbs rest by ones side.
   B. An individual stands erect.
   C. Feet face anteriorly.
   D. Palms face posteriorly.
   E. Head faces anteriorly.
2. The epidermis of the palms and feet are organized into five layers and are referred to as the thick skin. All other areas of the body have an epidermis that only has four layers and it is generally referred to as thin skin. What stratum layer is not seen in thin skin?
   A. Stratum granulosum.
   B. Stratum lucidum.
   C. Stratum spinosum.
   D. Stratum corneum.
   E. Stratum basale.
3. A 23-year-old man presents in the emergency room after burning himself with fireworks in his backyard. The burns affect his left forearm and there is blistering demonstrating damage to the epidermis and a part of the dermis. The burns are painful and highly sensitive to touch and the patient describes the

sensation of being hot and cold with the injury site looking moist. This type of burn is known to take up to a month to heal and leaves a scar. What type of burn has this man obtained?
A. First-degree.
B. Second-degree.
C. Third-degree.
D. Fourth-degree.
E. This type of burn could represent multiple degrees.

4. A patient is brought into the emergency department after a motor vehicle accident with multiple bone fractures. After an X-ray is performed, it is discovered that the individual has fractures of the L5 vertebral body, sacrum, pubic bone, sternum, and the lower three ribs on the left side. Which listed bone is considered part of the appendicular skeleton?
A. L5 vertebral body.
B. Sacrum.
C. Pubic bone.
D. Sternum.
E. Ribs.

5. Of the listed joints, which one is a synovial joint?
A. Pubic symphysis.
B. Cranial sutures.
C. Epiphyseal plate.
D. Intervertebral joints.
E. Condyloid joint.

6. The basic unit of contraction in skeletal muscle is called the sarcomere. Which statement regarding the sarcomere and its mechanism of contraction are FALSE?
A. Muscle contraction is dependent on thick filaments sliding over the thin filaments.
B. T-tubules allow for conduction of impulses to the deepest muscle fibers.
C. The Z-disks move closer to one another during muscle contraction.
D. The H-band contains only thick filaments.
E. Thin filaments are made of the actin protein.

7. What statement regarding the muscular system is INCORRECT?
A. A nerve impulse stimulates the release of acetylcholine from the axon terminal.
B. Eccentric contraction is movement occurring due to the muscle lengthening.
C. If a limb moves toward the median plane this is called adduction.
D. Large numbers of fascicles in skeletal muscle are surrounded by perimysium.
E. A muscle that complements the action of an agonist is called a synergist.

8. What type of vessel is best described by the following description? The tunic media is thin and is made up of only a few layers but these vessels generally do not have an internal elastic lamina. These vessels have a total diameter including all three tunic layers of about 0.5 mm. The lumen is less than 100 to 300 μm in diameter and these vessels are important in determining the blood pressure of an individual.
A. Large veins.
B. Muscular arteries.
C. Arterioles.
D. Venules.
E. Discontinuous capillaries.

9. The lymphatic drainage of what particular part of the body or region will ultimately drain to the right lymphatic duct before reaching the venous circulation?
A. Spleen.
B. Left gluteal region.
C. Right thigh region.
D. Left ear.
E. Right axillary region.

10. Which statement about the nervous system is INCORRECT?
A. The ventral roots of S2–S4 consist of sympathetic preganglionic autonomic fibers.
B. The area of skin supplied primarily by one spinal nerve is called a dermatome.
C. The majority of neurons are multipolar.
D. Gray matter of the CNS contains numerous collections of cell bodies.
E. The dorsal rami contain GSE, GSA, and GVE-sympathetic postganglionic fibers.

ANSWERS

1. D. All other answers are correct and associated with the correct anatomical position. An individual stands erect with the upper limbs resting to the side. The head, palms, and feet must face forward or anteriorly.

2. B. The stratum lucidum is a layer of the epidermis only found in thick skin or the skin of the palms and feet.

3. B. Second-degree burns affect the epidermis and part of the dermis and can demonstrate possible blistering. These types of burns are painful and highly sensitive to touch and there is a sensation of being hot or cold and these injuries feel moist. These types of burns take approximately 2 to 4 weeks to heal and leave behind scarring.
A. First-degree burns only affect the epidermis and are red and hot, have a low-to-moderate pain level, and have no blistering. The skin will begin to peel in a few days and typically take 5 to 10 days to fully heel.
C. Third-degree burns affect the epidermis and all of the dermis and possibly the superficial fascia. The burn site is white and charred and swelling is evident. The nerve endings will have been destroyed and the area will feel numb. It will take several months to heal and generally a skin graft is needed as part of an individual's treatment.
D. Fourth-degree burns damage underlying muscles, tendons, bones, and the surrounding neurovasculature. No pain is present because all nerve endings have been destroyed. Medical treatment will always be needed and because of limited healing this could lead to a possible amputation.
E. Degrees of burn severity are defined clearly and thus do not generally overlap.

4. C. The lower limb bones along with the ilium, ischium, and pubis of the hip bone are all considered part of the appendicular skeleton. The scapula and clavicle and all other upper limb ones are also part of the appendicular skeleton.
A. All vertebrae are part of the axial skeleton.
B. The sacrum and coccyx are part of the axial skeleton.
D. The sternum is part of the axial skeleton.
E. All of the ribs are part of the axial skeleton.

5. **E**. A condyloid joint is a synovial joint.
   A. The pubic symphysis is a secondary cartilaginous joint.
   B. Cranial sutures are fibrous joints.
   C. Epiphyseal or growth plates are primary cartilaginous joints.
   D. Intervertebral joints are a secondary cartilaginous joint.
6. **A**. All answers are true except for A. During the sliding filament mechanism or when a muscle contracts and shortens, the myosin heads of the thick filaments attach to the actin of the thin filaments and pull the thin filaments toward the center of the sarcomere. After the myosin head pivots, at what is called the hinge, it will release itself and return to its original position. It will then bind to the thin filament further along its length before pivoting again but contraction centers on the thin filaments sliding over the thick filaments.
7. **D**. All answers are correct except for D. A named muscle is made up of large numbers of fascicles that are surrounded by the epimysium.
8. **C**. The arterioles have the listed diameters, have few layers of smooth muscle, have no internal elastic lamina, and are the blood vessels that determine an individual's blood pressure.
   A. Large veins have diameters that are more than 9 mm and have valves located in the tunica intima. These veins connect to perforating veins.
   B. Muscular arteries have diameters between 0.3 and 1.0 cm and they are responsible for distributing blood to various parts of the body. They can have up to 40 layers of smooth muscle and have a prominent internal elastic lamina.
   D. Venules are the smallest veins, have a 10 to 50 μm diameter, and contain about 25% of the total blood volume.
   E. Discontinuous capillaries have an endothelium with large fenestrations, incomplete or absent basal lamina, and a slow blood flow. These capillaries are important in allowing direct exchange of molecules between the blood and cells.
9. **E**. The right half of the thorax, upper limb, and head and neck regions drain to the right lymphatic duct before entering the venous circulation. All other areas and structures of the body eventually drain to the thoracic duct.
10. **A**. All answers are correct except A. The ventral roots of S2–S4 consist of parasympathetic preganglionic autonomic fibers. They would also contain somatic motor, somatic sensory, and visceral sensory fibers.

Reference

1. Bergmann, et al. Evidence for cardiomyocyte renewal in humans. Science 324, 98; 2009

1 Back

LEARNING OBJECTIVES

- To understand the regions of the back
- To understand the fascia and surface anatomy of the back.
- To distinguish the different regions, curvatures and structures associated with specific regions of the vertebral column.
- To understand the major ligaments that add to the structural stability of the vertebral column.
- To understand the individual joints and how they add to the overall mobility of the vertebral column.
- To understand the clinical correlates that relate to the overall architecture of the vertebral column including osteoporosis, Jefferson fractures, hangman fractures, flexion and extension teardrop fractures, spondylolysis, spondylolisthesis, spinal stenosis, herniation of intervertebral discs, low back pain and the laminectomy procedure.
- To understand the vertebral column neurovasculature and the metastasis of cancer.
- To understand the structure of the spinal cord and the meninges that surround it. The clinical correlates will include a look at myelography and lumbar puncture procedures.
- To understand the functions and innervations of both extrinsic and intrinsic muscles of the back.
- To understand how the vertebral column and back muscles develop, and the types of spina bifida.

1.1 Overview of the Back

In this chapter, "the back" will include the vertebral column, spinal cord (detailed in Chapter 9), spinal meninges, extrinsic and intrinsic back muscles, suboccipital triangle, and the overlying fascia and skin. It encompasses the posterior aspect of the trunk and is located between the inferior neck and the region just superior to the buttocks. The skin is generally thick and highly protective and is described as having low discriminatory nervous sensation. The skin tension lines form segments of two adjacent circles in the thoracic region but run horizontally in the cervical and lumbosacral regions. The superficial fascia can be thick and fatty, especially in the lower back region.

The deep fascia of the muscles of the back and trunk are covered by **thoracolumbar fascia**. This fascia extends laterally from the spinous processes, forming a thick covering over muscles originating from the lumbar region as well as a thin covering over the intrinsic back muscles such as the erector spinae muscle group. The thoracolumbar fascia contributes to the deep fascia of the *external oblique, internal oblique, transversus abdominis, quadratus lumborum, latissimus dorsi* and *serratus posterior inferior* muscles. It is divided into *anterior, middle* and *posterior layers.* The anterior layer lies on the anterior surface of the quadratus lumborum muscle while the middle layer is located between the quadratus lumborum and intrinsic back muscles. The posterior layer is posterior to the intrinsic back muscles. A lateral raphe of thoracolumbar fascia extends laterally near the anterior surface of the latissimus dorsi muscle before contributing to the oblique muscles (**Fig. 1.1**).

The dorsal (posterior) rami cutaneous branches of spinal nerves innervate the bulk of the overall back region, including the posterior neck (**Fig. 1.2**). Cutaneous artery branches that supply the skin originate from the occipital, deep cervical, transverse cervical, dorsal scapular, suprascapular, subscapular, posterior intercostal, lumbar and lateral sacral arteries. Cutaneous veins drain primarily back to the azygos vein by way of the posterior intercostal and lumbar veins. Drainage also includes the occipital and deep cervical veins. Lymphatic drainage includes the *occipital, deep cervical, axillary* and *superficial inguinal lymph nodes.*

1.2 Surface Anatomy

Near the level of the suboccipital region of the neck, the prominent projection on the back of one's skull is called the **external occipital protuberance**. Extending down the midline of the back near the inferior neck, the **nuchal groove** representing the site of the *nuchal ligament* can be located a few centimeters superior to the **vertebra prominens** or *spinous process of the C7 vertebra* (**Fig. 1.3**). The groove that extends inferiorly from the nuchal groove down near the level of the iliac crests is known as the **posterior median furrow**. This furrow splits the *trapezius* and *erector spinae muscles* into a left and right half and overlies the spinous processes of the vertebral column. The superior half of the back displays the superior, middle and inferior bellies of trapezius muscle. Near the juncture of the middle and inferior bellies of the trapezius muscle, the **medial border of the scapula** along with the beginning of the **spine of the scapula** can be palpated. The spine of the scapula is primarily at the T3 vertebral level and extends laterally to the shoulder region before ending as the **acromion**. The **superior border of the scapula** is near T1 while the **inferior border** is located at T7. The *teres major muscle* can be located near the inferior angle of the scapula and extends laterally toward the humerus. Each numbered rib will correlate with the same numbered thoracic spinous process (**Fig. 1.3**).

Adjacent to the posterior median furrow in the lower back region, two prominent and thicker portions of the erector spinae muscles can be seen. Just lateral to these erector spinae muscles, a thinner muscular sheet extending toward the superior portion of the humerus represents the *latissimus dorsi muscle.* A dimple inferior and just lateral to each of the erector spinae muscle bellies indicates the **posterior superior iliac spines**. The two ridges extending laterally from the L4 vertebral level represent the **iliac crest** of the hip. The **sacral triangle**, which is defined by the lines that join the posterior superior iliac spines (generally represented by dimples) and the superior part of the **intergluteal (anal) cleft** is a common site associated with low back sprains (**Fig. 1.3**).

When a patient is asked to bend forward and fold their arms across the chest, the scapula expose the **triangle of auscultation.** This position is used for listening to respiratory sounds with a stethoscope. The borders of this triangle include a medial (lateral border of inferior trapezius), lateral (medial border of scapula) and inferior border (superior border of latissimus dorsi). The **lumbar triangle** near the iliac crest can be further subdivided into an **inferior lumbar** (***Petit***) and **superior lumbar** (***Grynfeltt-Lesshaft***)

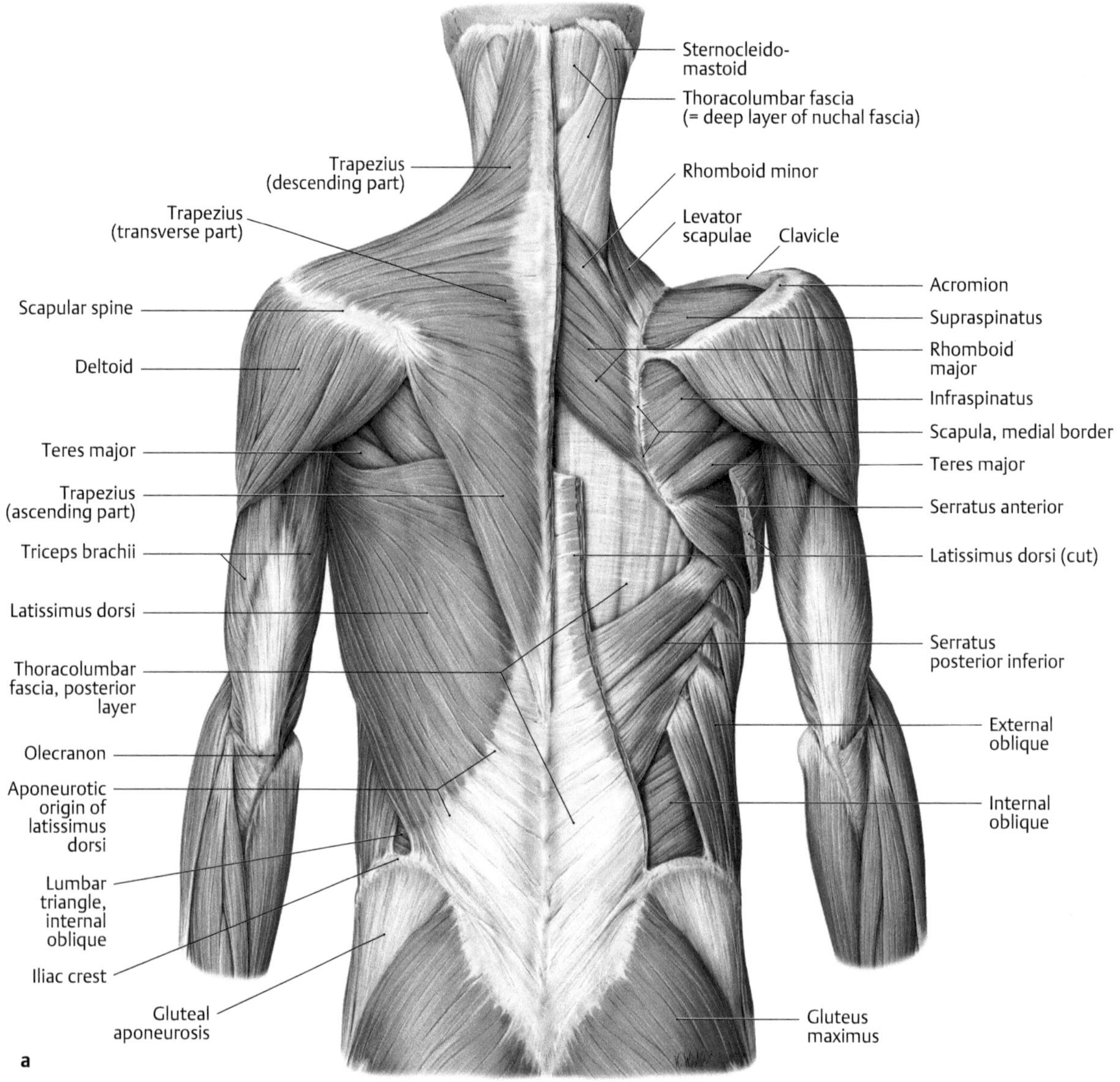

Sternocleido-
mastoid
Thoracolumbar fascia
(= deep layer of nuchal fascia)
Trapezius
(descending part)
Rhomboid minor
Trapezius
(transverse part)
Levator
scapulae
Clavicle
Acromion
Scapular spine
Supraspinatus
Rhomboid
major
Deltoid
Infraspinatus
Scapula, medial border
Teres major
Teres major
Trapezius
(ascending part)
Serratus anterior
Triceps brachii
Latissimus dorsi (cut)
Latissimus dorsi
Serratus
posterior inferior
Thoracolumbar
fascia, posterior
layer
External
oblique
Olecranon
Aponeurotic
origin of
latissimus
dorsi
Internal
oblique
Lumbar
triangle,
internal
oblique
Iliac crest
Gluteal
aponeurosis
Gluteus
maximus
a

Psoas fascia
Abdominal
aorta
Inferior
vena cava
Parietal
peritoneum
Kidney
Renal fascia,
anterior layer
Lateral
abdominal
wall muscles
Transversalis
fascia
L2 vertebra
Fibrous capsule
Psoas major
Renal fascia,
posterior layer
Vertebral arch
Latissimus dorsi
Transverse process
of L2
Serratus
posterior inferior
Spinous process
of L1
Quadratus lumborum
Intrinsic
back muscles
Anterior layer
(quadratus lumborum fascia)
Middle layer
Posterior
layer
Thoracolumbar
fascia
b

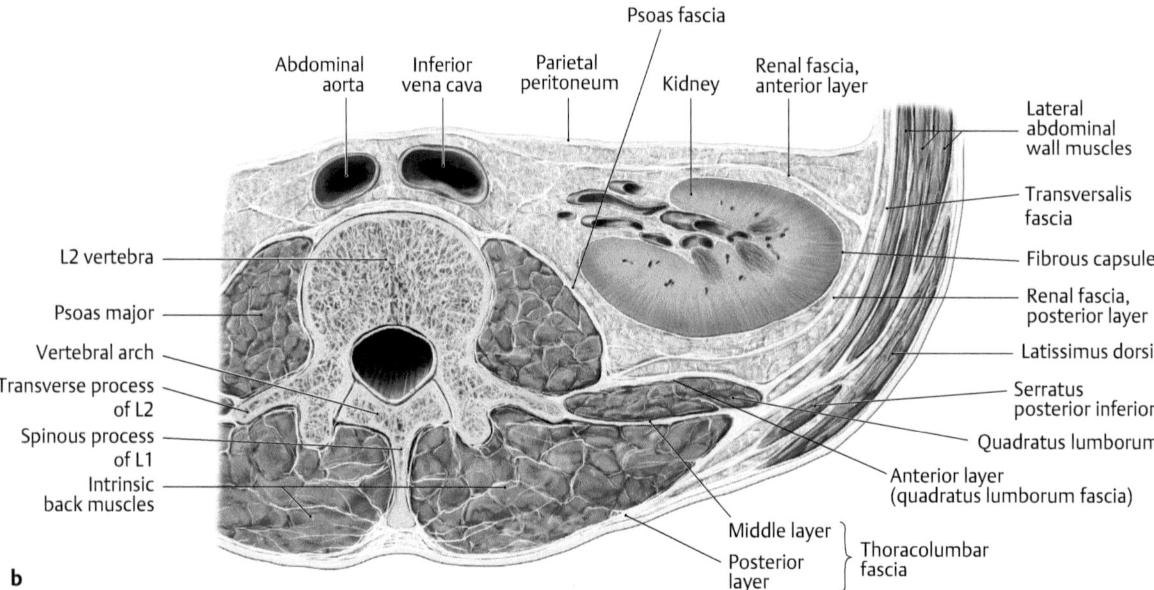

Fig. 1.1 **(a)** Superficial extrinsic muscles of the back, posterior view; **(b)** thoracolumbar fascia; transverse section at vertebral level L2, superior view. (From Schuenke M, Schulte E, Schumacher U. THIEME Atlas of Anatomy. General Anatomy and Musculoskeletal System. Illustrations by Voll M and Wesker K. 3rd ed. New York: Thieme Medical Publishers; 2020.)

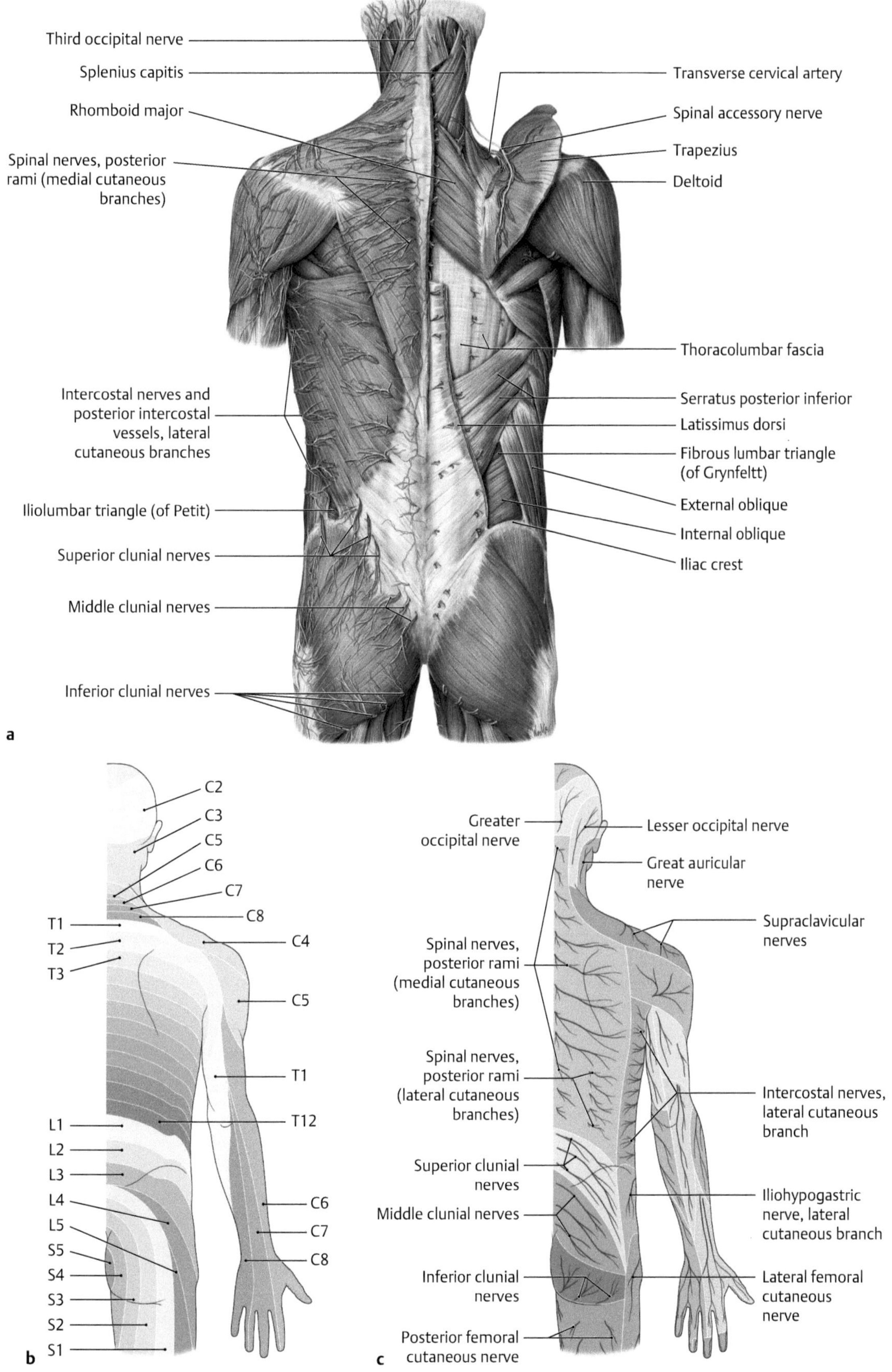

Fig. 1.2 (a) Neurovascular structures of the posterior trunk wall and nuchal region, posterior view. **(b, c)** Neurovascular structures of the posterior trunk wall and nuchal region, posterior view. (From Schuenke M, Schulte E, Schumacher U. THIEME Atlas of Anatomy. General Anatomy and Musculoskeletal System. Illustrations by Voll M and Wesker K. 3rd ed. New York: Thieme Medical Publishers; 2020.)

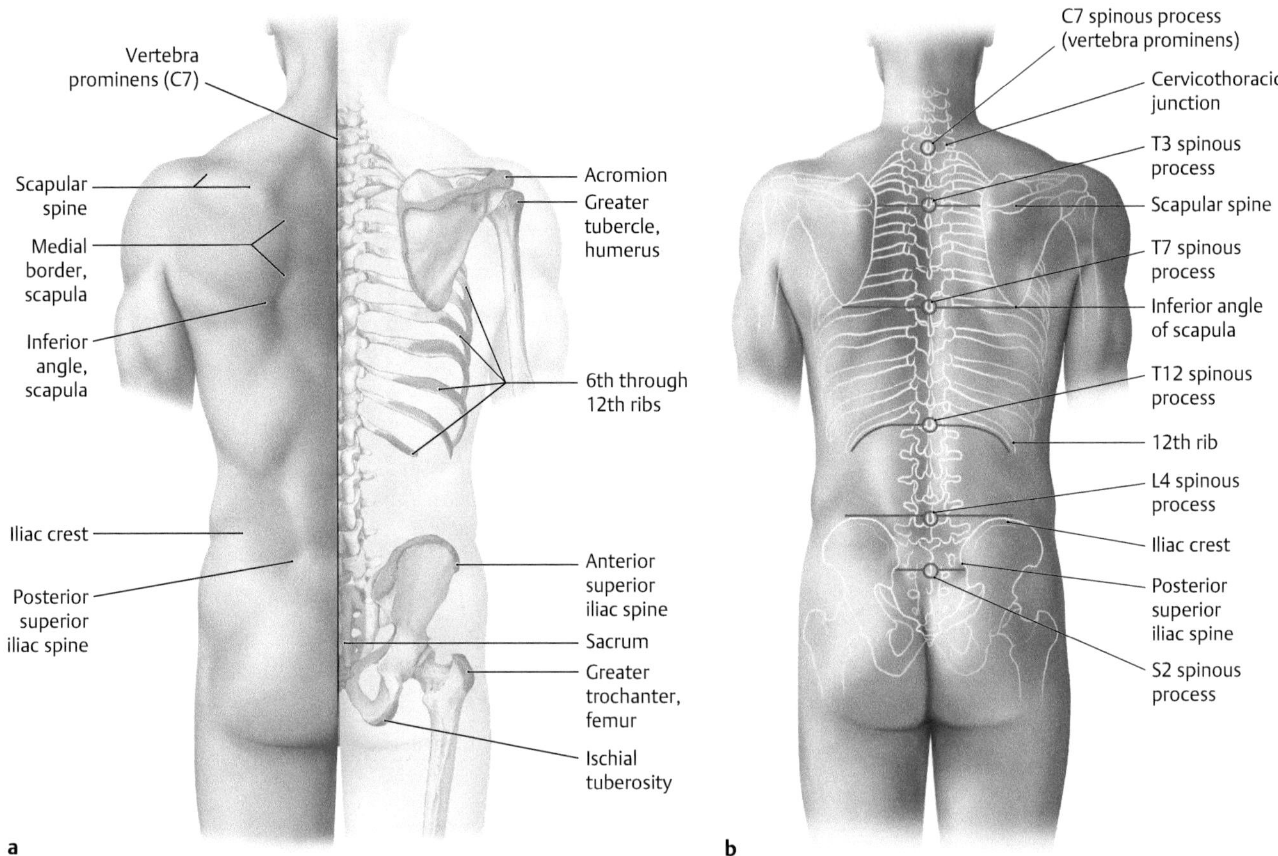

Fig. 1.3 **(a)** Palpable structures of the back, posterior view. **(b)** Spinous processes and landmarks of the back, posterior view. (From Schuenke M, Schulte E, Schumacher U. THIEME Atlas of Anatomy. Illustrations by Voll M and Wesker K.)

triangles. The inferior lumbar triangle is superficial while the superior lumbar triangle is deeper. The lumbar triangle is of clinical significance because it is the site of a possible herniation. These herniations are rare compared to inguinal hernias and are mostly acquired due to trauma or unrelated surgical intervention. The lumbar triangle can also serve as a surgical approach to the kidney or ureter. The *inferior lumbar triangle* is bordered by the iliac crest (inferiorly), external oblique (laterally), latissimus dorsi (medially) and internal oblique (floor). The *superior lumbar triangle* is bordered by the 12th rib (superiorly), internal oblique (laterally), quadratus lumborum (medially), external oblique (roof) and transversalis fascia (floor) **(Fig. 1.2)**.

1.3 Vertebral Column

The **vertebral column** consists of 33 vertebrae arranged into five regions. There are 7 cervical, 12 thoracic, 5 lumbar, 5 fused sacral and 3-5 fused coccygeal vertebrae (**Fig. 1.4**). Most individuals have 4 coccygeal vertebrae so this number of vertebrae is assumed and they are generally not completely fused until the third decade of life. The functions of the vertebral column include:

- Body weight support superior to the level of the pelvis
- Provide in part a rigid but flexible axis for body and head movements
- Provide a role for both posture and locomotion
- Protect the spinal meninges, cord, roots, and nerves

The vertebrae become progressively larger until reaching their maximum size just above the sacrum, which transfers the weight to the pelvic girdle at the sacro-iliac joints. Size differences are related to successive vertebrae bearing more weight than the previous. From the sacrum, the vertebrae become progressively smaller until reaching the apex of the coccyx. Flexibility of the vertebral column is due to *intervertebral (IV) discs* located between most of the individual vertebrae.

The vertebral column has four curvatures in adults. These curvatures provide additional flexibility and shock absorption. Curvatures tend to increase when a load is carried because this causes an increase in compression of the curvatures themselves and IV discs. If additional weight is placed anterior to the body's gravitational axis, as in late pregnancy or in patients with an extensive lower abdominal region, this too can increase the curvatures.

The **thoracic** and **sacral curvatures** (kyphoses) are the **primary curvatures** that develop during the fetal period and are concave anteriorly. The primary curvatures are retained throughout life due to the differences in height between the anterior and posterior vertebral parts. Clinically, an excessive amount of kyphosis, especially at the thoracic vertebrae, is called "humpback." The **cervical** and **lumbar curvatures** (lordoses) are the **secondary curvatures** that are the result of extension from the flexed fetal position **(Fig. 1.5)**. The curvatures are concave posteriorly and do not become evident until late infancy, when the child begins to stand and take their first steps. Maintaining these curvatures is primarily due to the thickness between anterior and posterior parts of

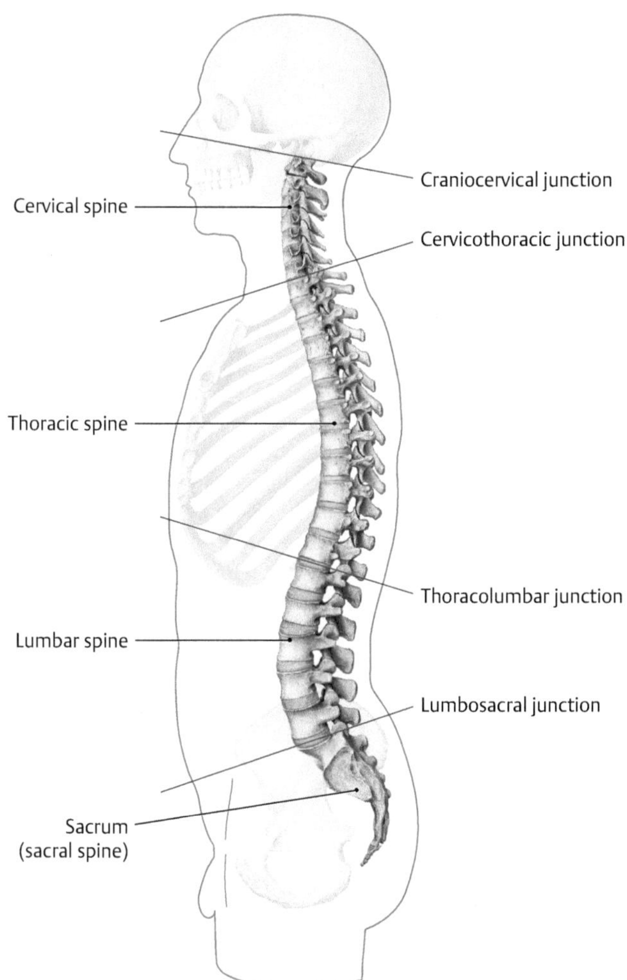

Fig. 1.4 Vertebral column, left lateral view. (From Schuenke M, Schulte E, Schumacher U. THIEME Atlas of Anatomy. General Anatomy and Musculoskeletal System. Illustrations by Voll M and Wesker K. 3rd ed. New York: Thieme Medical Publishers; 2020.)

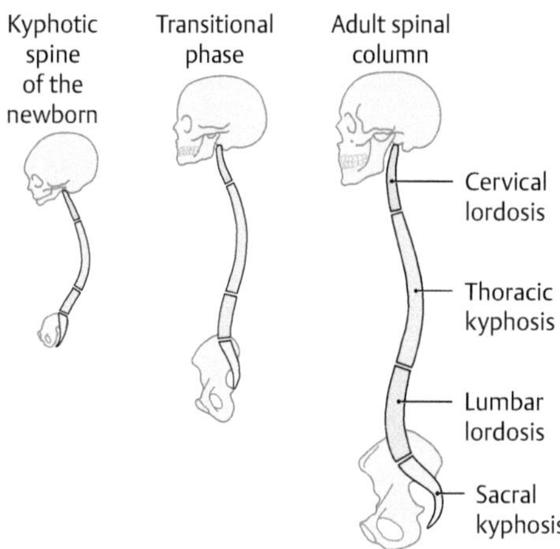

Fig. 1.5 Spinal development. (From Schuenke M, Schulte E, Schumacher U. THIEME Atlas of Anatomy. General Anatomy and Musculoskeletal System. Illustrations by Voll M and Wesker K. 3rd ed. New York: Thieme Medical Publishers; 2020.)

the IV discs. *Cervical lordosis* is clearly visible once an infant begins to extend or raise the head while prone or hold the head erect when sitting. *Lumbar lordosis* is visible once late infants and early toddlers assume an upright posture while standing or walking. This curvature ends at the *lumbosacral angle* located at the junction of the L5 vertebra and the sacrum and is more pronounced in females. Excessive lordosis is called "hollow back" **(Fig. 1.6)**.

An abnormal lateral curvature of the vertebrae that is accompanied by rotation is known as **scoliosis**. Scoliosis can be seen in as many as 2-3% of adolescents but very few will have spinal curvatures over 40°. Most scoliosis cases have one of three causes: they can be *idiopathic* (no specific cause), potentiallydue to *neuromuscular* issues resulting in asymmetric weakness of intrinsic back muscles, *degenerative* because of trauma or early onset of osteoporosis, or *congenital* because a portion of a vertebra fails to develop correctly (as in *hemivertebra*). Treatment includes braces for individuals still maturing with spinal curves between 25-40°. However, the spinal curve may return to its original form when the brace is removed. Surgery is generally recommended for individuals who have spinal curvatures over 40°, but this alone does not completely straighten the vertebral column. Spinal fusion is generally involved. This procedurepermanently joins the vertebrae together using a combination of bone grafts and metal implants **(Fig. 1.6)**.

1.4 Structure of the Vertebrae

The vertebrae vary in size and shape and display certain characteristics that distinguish the regions of the vertebral column from one another. The typical vertebra consists of a vertebral body, a vertebral arch and seven processes that arise from the vertebral arch. The **vertebral body** is anterior to all the other structures and gives strength to the vertebral column to support the body weight. They are the more extensive portion of the vertebra and increase in size as the vertebral column descends. The central portion of the vertebral body originates from its primary ossification center called the **centrum**. The outer edges of both the superior and inferior surfaces of a vertebral body are called the **epiphyseal rim** and are derived from an **anular epiphysis**. Located posterior to the vertebral body is the **vertebral arch**, which is made up of two pedicles and laminae. The short and cylindrical left and right **pedicles** extend posteriorly to meet the left and right **laminae**. The vertebral arch is the structure that gives rise to all seven **processes (Fig. 1.7)**.

- **Transverse processes**: there are two that project posterolaterally from the junction of the pedicles and laminae. They serve as attachment sites for deep back muscles.
  - **Articular processes**: there are two **superior articular** and two **inferior articular processes** that arise near the junctions of the pedicles and laminae. They all have an **articular surface** (or **facet**) that lies in apposition with the corresponding processes of adjacent vertebrae and establishes the **zygapophysial (facet) joints.** These processes generally only bear limited weight but primarily function in aligning the adjacent vertebrae.
  - **Spinous processes**: these processes project posteriorly and mostly inferiorly from the midline of the vertebral arch and fused laminae.

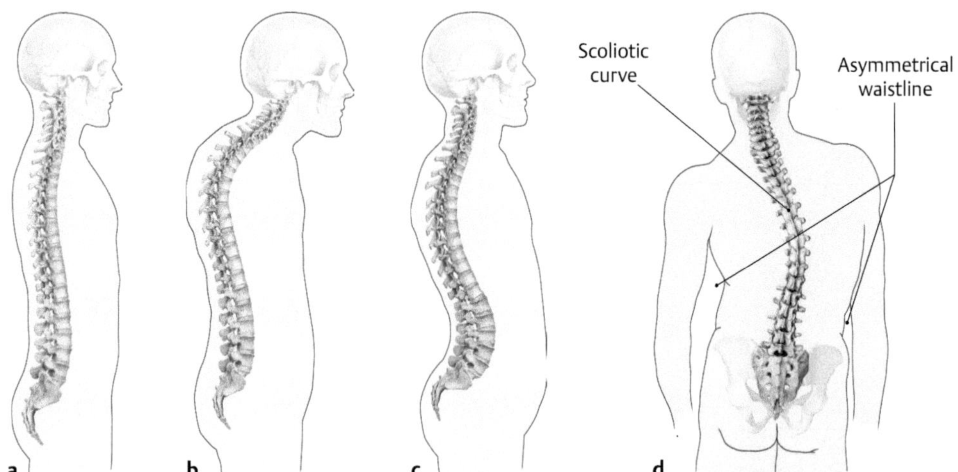

Fig. 1.6 Vertebral column curvatures. **(a)** Normal. **(b)** Excessive kyphosis. **(c)** Excessive lordosis. **(d)** Scoliosis. (From Gilroy AM et al. Atlas of Anatomy. 4th ed. 2020. Based on: Schuenke M, Schulte E, Schumacher U. THIEME Atlas of Anatomy. General Anatomy and Musculoskeletal System. Illustrations by Voll M and Wesker K. 3rd ed. New York: Thieme Medical Publishers; 2020.)

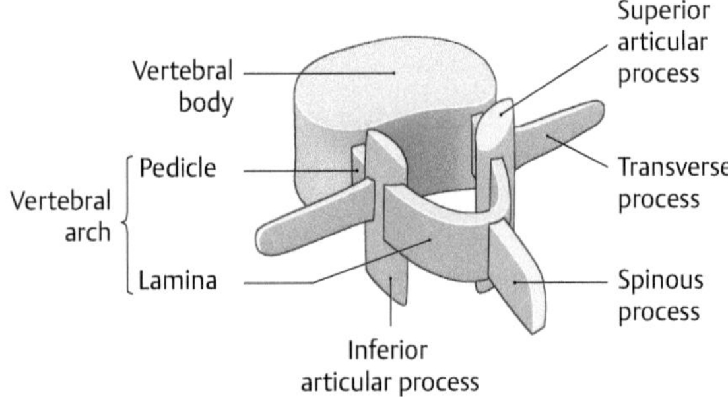

Fig. 1.7 Structural elements of a vertebra, left posterosuperior view. (From Schuenke M, Schulte E, Schumacher U. THIEME Atlas of Anatomy. General Anatomy and Musculoskeletal System. Illustrations by Voll M and Wesker K. 3rd ed. New York: Thieme Medical Publishers; 2020.)

Other features include the **vertebral foramen** that is defined as the space located between the posterior border of the vertebral body and the vertebral arch. Successive vertebral foramina form the **vertebral canal**, which contains the spinal cord, roots of the spinal nerves, meninges, blood vessels and fat. Viewed from the lateral side of the vertebral column are the **superior** and **inferior vertebral notches** located superior or inferior to the pedicles. The space between both notches and a portion of the IV disc is called the **intervertebral foramen** and it is the location of the emerging spinal nerves and dorsal root ganglion. The **pars interarticularis** (or just **pars**) is the part of the vertebra located between the superior and inferior articular processes that help form the zygapophysial (facet) joints.

1.5 Region Specifics of the Vertebrae

1.5.1 Cervical Vertebrae

There are seven **cervical vertebrae (Fig. 1.8)**. They are the smallest of all vertebrae and are located between the cranium and thoracic vertebrae. These vertebrae have the largest range of motion of all vertebrae and this is owed to the fact the IV discs are relatively thick compared to the connecting vertebral bodies, the articular facets are nearly horizontal in their orientation, and there is a minimal amount of body mass near these vertebrae.

All cervical vertebrae have an oval hole called a **transverse foramen** passing through the transverse processes. These foramina allow passage of the vertebral artery and the corresponding veins. The vertebral artery in most individuals bypasses the C7 transverse foramen and will first enter at C6. The transverse processes also have an **anterior tubercle** and **posterior tubercle**, which provide attachment sites for cervical muscles such as the scalenes. The C6 anterior tubercles are also known as the **carotid tubercles**. They are a common site for compressing the common carotid artery and serve as an insertion site for a procedure called a *stellate ganglion block*. A groove exists between the two tubercles and allows for the ventral rami of spinal nerves to extend past them. The spinous processes of C2-C6 are generally bifid with the C7 spinous process being non-bifid. C2 and C7 tend to have longer spinous processes. A hook-shaped **uncinate process** is located on the superolateral margin of the body of the C3-C7 vertebrae and limits lateral flexion. The cervical vertebrae are described as being *atypical* (C1, C2, and C7) or *typical* (C3-C6) in nature.

The **C1 vertebra (atlas)** articulates with the *occipital condyles* of the cranium at the **superior articular surface** of the **lateral masses**. This vertebra is unique because it does not contain a body or spinous process and is the widest of all cervical vertebrae. The transverse processes extend out from the lateral masses and are more laterally placed than all the others inferior to it. Extending between the lateral masses and forming a complete ring are the **anterior** and **posterior arches**. The posterior arch is the equivalent of the laminae of typical vertebrae. On its superior surface there is a **groove for the 3rd part of the vertebral artery**. Both the anterior and posterior arches contain an **anterior** or **posterior tubercle** respectively located in the center of its external aspect.

The **C2 vertebra (axis)** is the strongest of all cervical vertebrae and contains two **superior articular facets** that the C1 vertebra rotates on. The distinguishing feature of C2 is the **dens (odontoid process)** that projects superiorly from the C2 body. The dens is part of the *median atlanto-axial joint* that serves as a pivot joint.

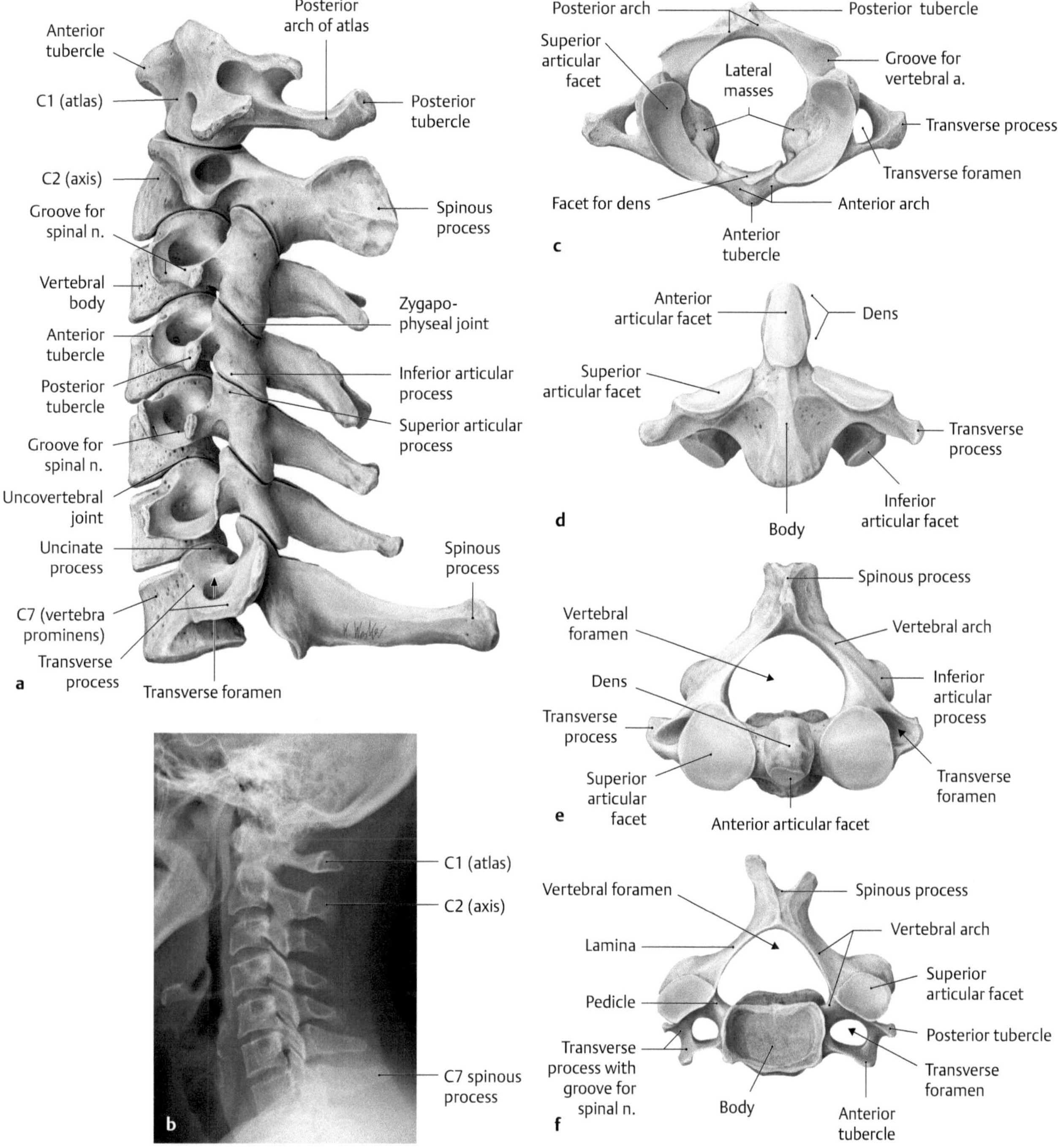

Fig. 1.8 **(a)** Cervical spine, left lateral view. **(b)** Radiograph of cervical spine, left lateral view. **(c)** Atlas (C1), superior view. **(d)** Axis (C2), anterior view. **(e)** Axis (C2), superior view. **(f)** Typical cervical vertebra (C4), superior view. (From Schuenke M, Schulte E, Schumacher U. THIEME Atlas of Anatomy. General Anatomy and Musculoskeletal System. Illustrations by Voll M and Wesker K. 3rd ed. New York: Thieme Medical Publishers; 2020.)

The dens is located anterior to the spinal cord and is held in position against the posterior aspect of the C1 anterior arch by the **transverse ligament of the atlas**. This ligament prevents anterior displacement of the atlas and posterior displacement of the dens. The atlas encircles the dens, spinal cord and its surrounding meninges.

The **C7 vertebra** is characterized by a long, non-bifid spinous process and it is generally the most prominent spinous process. It can be felt by running a finger down the central portion of the vertebral column. Thus C7 is also called the **vertebra prominens**. The anterior tubercle is fairly small and the transverse foramina may be absent in C7.

The typical (C3-C6) vertebrae have larger vertebral foramina in order to accommodate the cervical enlargement of the spinal cord, even though the cervical enlargement is made up of the C5-T1 spinal segments of the spinal cord. These typical vertebrae have a superior border of the vertebral bodies that is elevated both posteriorly and especially laterally while the anterior border is depressed. These elevations on the superolateral aspects were earlier referred to as the uncinate processes. The inferior borders are in an opposite orientation in order to articulate with the superior borders of adjacent vertebrae. The articulation pattern of cervical vertebrae allow for free flexion and extension, limited lateral flexion and restricted rotational movements.

1.5.2 Thoracic Vertebrae

There are twelve **thoracic vertebrae** located between the cervical and lumbar vertebrae (**Fig. 1.9**). Features include vertebral foramina with smaller diameters, transverse processes that articulate with most ribs and spinous processes that are long and mostly slope postero-inferiorly.

The most prevalent feature of these vertebrae is the **costal facets** that are involved in the articulation of both the heads and transverse processes of the ribs. For most thoracic vertebrae and specifically those of T2-T9, there is a **superior** and **inferior costal (demifacet) facet**. For these vertebrae, the head of a rib would articulate with both superior and inferior demifacets. The superior costal facet on the T1 vertebral body is not considered a demifacet because there is no corresponding demifacet on the C7 vertebra. The head of the 2nd rib articulates with both the 1st and 2nd thoracic vertebrae, the head of the 3rd rib articulates with both the 2nd and 3rd thoracic vertebrae, and so on until T10. T10 has only a superior demifacet that corresponds with the 10th rib. The 1st, 11th and 12th head of the ribs do not articulate with two vertebrae but with only an isolated costal facet. The **costal facets of the transverse**

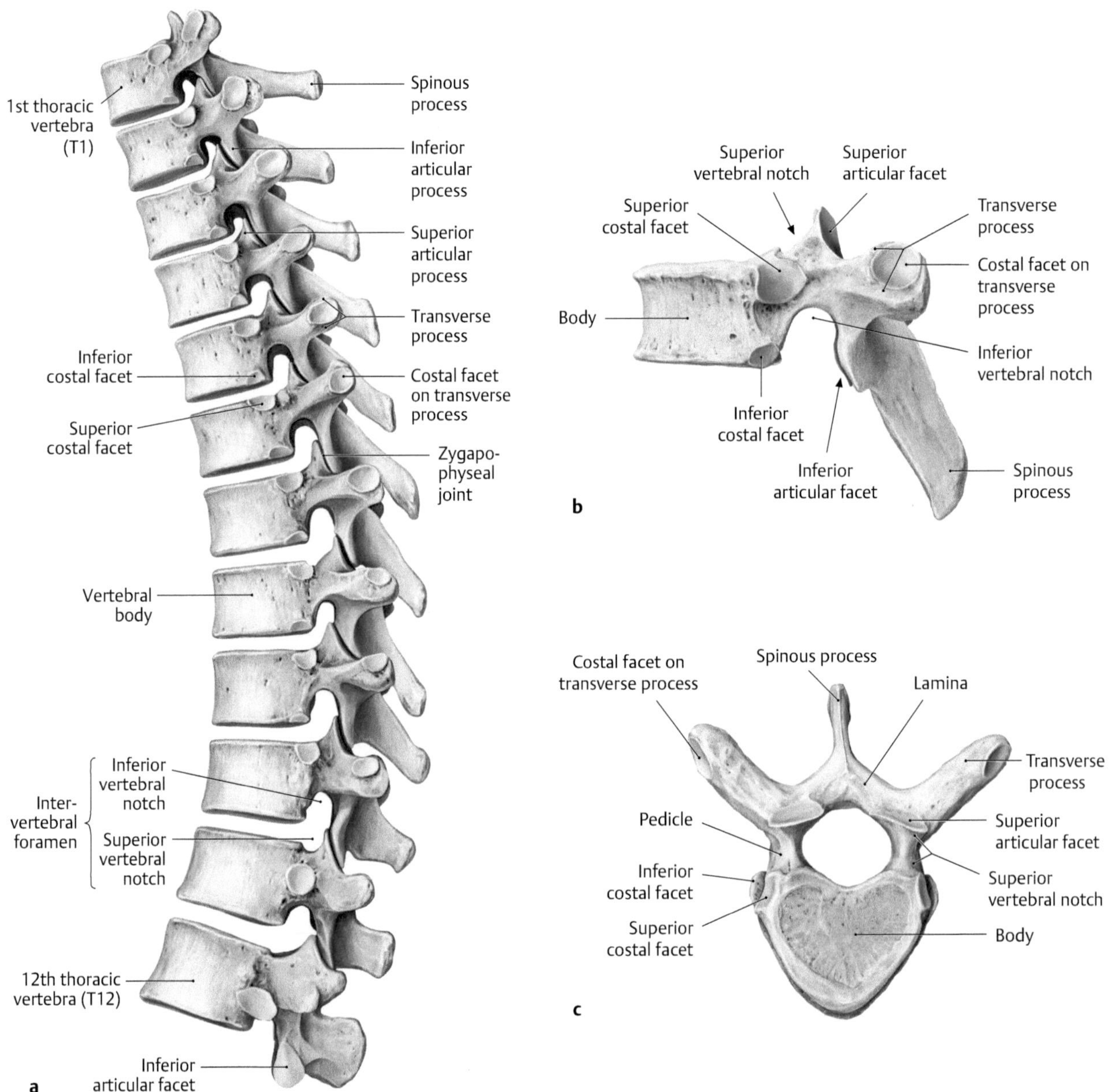

Fig. 1.9 **(a)** Thoracic spine, left lateral view. Typical thoracic vertebra (T6), left lateral view **(b)** and superior view **(c)**. (From Schuenke M, Schulte E, Schumacher U. THIEME Atlas of Anatomy. General Anatomy and Musculoskeletal System. Illustrations by Voll M and Wesker K. 3rd ed. New York: Thieme Medical Publishers; 2020.)

process articulate with the corresponding rib, except at T11 and T12, where there is no facet located on the transverse process.

The T1-T4 vertebrae have features in common with the cervical vertebrae. The T1 spinous process, for example, is prominent like C7 but is more horizontal than C7 in its orientation. The T5-T8 vertebrae have the greatest degree of rotation, but flexion, extension and lateral flexion are limited due to the overlapping spinous processes, vertical orientation of the articular facets, and attachment of the rib cage. The T12 vertebra has the greatest degree of change from thoracic to lumbar vertebrae with its hatchet-like spinous process and no costal facts on the transverse processes. T12 is the most commonly fractured vertebra and this is because it is the site of extensive transitional forces. The upper half of T12 is the site of primarily rotational movements while the inferior half is associated with flexion and extension.

1.5.3 Lumbar Vertebrae

There are five **lumbar vertebrae** and they possess large vertebral bodies, a vertebral foramen with a slightly smaller diameter than the cervical region but a more triangular shape, spinous processes that are thick, broad and hatchet shaped, and articular processes with nearly vertical facets (**Fig. 1.10**). The superior articular process contains smaller **mammillary processes** that allow attachment of the multifidus and intertransversarii muscles. The **accessory processes** are located on the posterior surface of the transverse processes and also provide attachments for the intertransversarii muscles.

The L5 vertebra is the largest mobile vertebra and it carries the weight of the entire upper body. Due to its height on the anterior side, it is largely responsible for the **lumbosacral angle** located between the long axis of the lumbar region of the vertebral column and the sacrum. This angle varies between 130-160° (avg. 143°). Body weight is transferred from L5 to the base of the sacrum located at the superior portion of the S1 vertebra. The L5-S1 facets are orientated coronally and this allows for flexion, extension and lateral flexion but no rotational movement (**Fig. 1.11**).

1.5.4 Sacrum

The **sacrum** is composed of five fused vertebrae, is wedge-shaped and has a pelvic (ventral), dorsal and lateral surface along with a base and an apex (**Fig. 1.12**). It is located inferior to the lumbar vertebrae, superior to the coccyx, and medial to the hip bones. The sacrum provides strength and stability to the pelvis and transmits body weight through the pelvic girdle or the combination of the sacrum and hip bones. Only the superior half is weight-bearing while the inferior half is not.

The **pelvic surface** is concave and smooth. The four transverse lines on this surface represent where fusion of the sacral vertebrae occurrs. Fusion of the sacral vertebrae does not begin until after

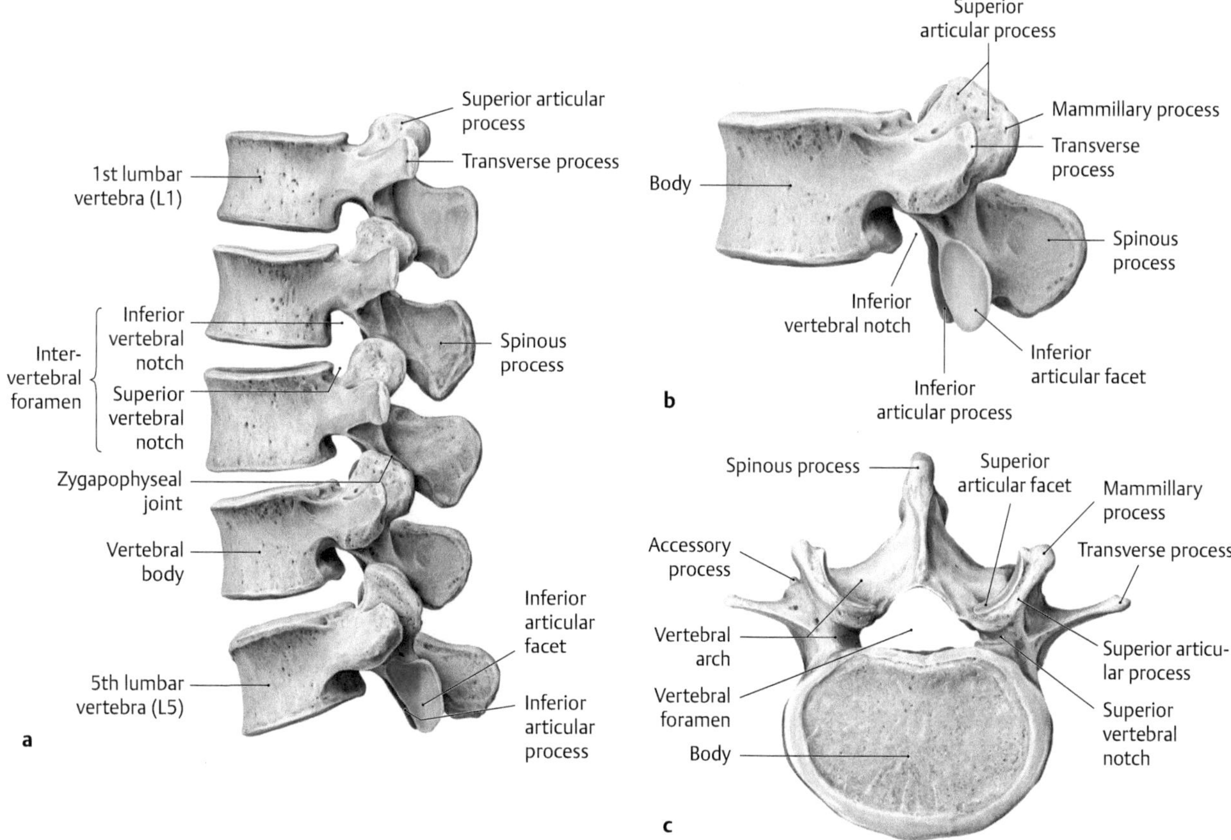

Fig. 1.10 **(a)** Lumbar spine, left lateral view. Typical lumbar vertebra (L4), left lateral view **(b)** and superior view **(c)**. (From Schuenke M, Schulte E, Schumacher U. THIEME Atlas of Anatomy. General Anatomy and Musculoskeletal System. Illustrations by Voll M and Wesker K. 3rd ed. New York: Thieme Medical Publishers; 2020.)

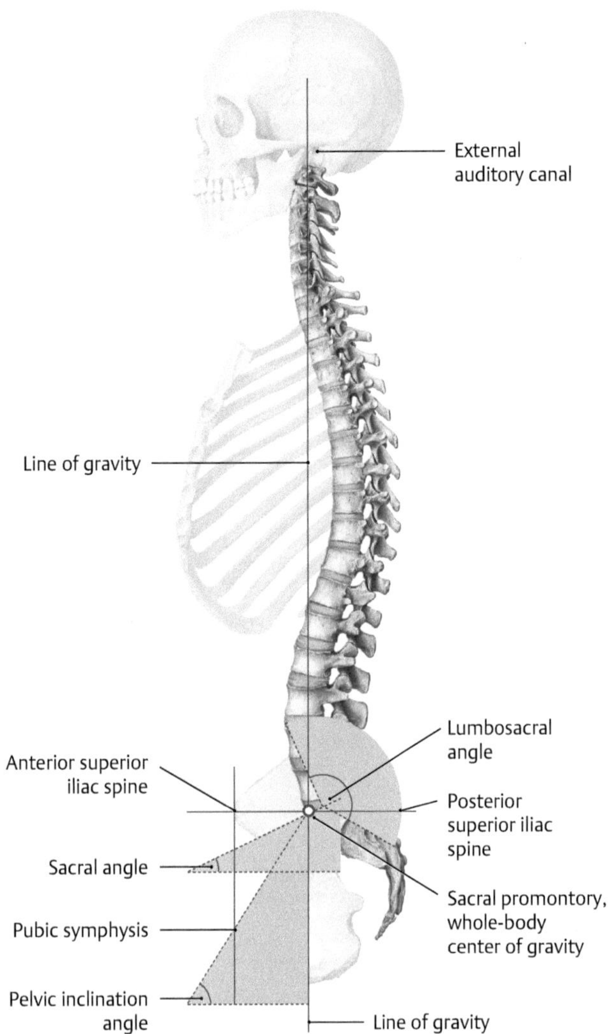

Fig. 1.11 Location of the lumbosacral angle. The sacral angle is the angle between the horizontal plane and superior surface of the sacrum (~30 degrees). The pelvic inclination angle is formed by the plane of the pelvic inlet and the horizontal plane and is approximately 60 degrees when standing upright. The line of gravity passes through the external auditory canal, the dens of C2, and the whole-body center of gravity just anterior to the sacral promontory. (From Schuenke M, Schulte E, Schumacher U. THIEME Atlas of Anatomy. General Anatomy and Musculoskeletal System. Illustrations by Voll M and Wesker K. 3rd ed. New York: Thieme Medical Publishers; 2020.).

age 20, but during childhood, the individual sacral vertebrae are connected by hyaline cartilage and separated by IV discs. These IV discs remain unossified until or even after middle age.

The **dorsal surface** is convex, rough and displays five longitudinal crests. The **median sacral crest** lies in the midline and represents the fused primitive spinous processes of the upper 3-4 sacral vertebrae. S5 is devoid of a spinous process. Located just lateral on both sides of the median sacral crest are the **medial sacral crests** and they represent fused articular processes. The **lateral sacral crests** are located just lateral to the medial sacral crests and are the tips of the transverse processes of the fused sacral vertebrae.

The **lateral surface** has a superior portion called the **auricular surface** (ear-shaped) and it is the site of the synovial part of the sacro-iliac joint between the sacrum and ilium. Posterior to the auricular surface is a rough surface called the **sacral tuberosity** that allows for the attachment of the posterior sacro-iliac ligaments, which form the syndesmotic portion of the sacro-iliac joint.

The **base** is formed by the superior surface of the S1 vertebra. Its superior articular processes will articulate with the inferior articular processes of L5. The anterior projection from the superior portion of the S1 body is called the **sacral promontory**. The **apex** is the portion that tapers off and articulates with the coccyx.

The continuation of the vertebral canal into the sacrum is called the **sacral canal**. It contains a bundle of spinal nerves associated with the cauda equina and they pass through the intervertebral foramen before their anterior and posterior rami branches course through the **anterior** or **posterior sacral foramina**, respectively. The **sacral hiatus** is a U-shaped space and continuation of the sacral canal that is created due to the absence of the S5 spinous process and laminae. The hiatus has lateral margins formed by the **sacral cornua** and they represent the inferior articular processes of the S5 vertebra. The paired coccygeal (Co1) nerves along with the *filum terminale* pass through the sacral hiatus.

1.5.5 Coccyx

The **coccyx** is the most distal and inferior portion of the vertebral column (**Fig. 1.12**). It is made up of four primitive coccygeal vertebrae. Coccygeal vertebra 1 is the largest of the group but may remain separate from the fused group. It is the remnant of the embryonic tail-like caudal eminence present during development. The coccyx has no weight-bearing function but when sitting it will flex forward. It provides an attachment site for the anococcygeal ligament and gluteus maximus and coccygeus muscles. The coccyx and sacrum attach at the sacrum at the **sacrococcygeal joint**.

1.6 Ligaments of the Vertebral Column

- **Anterior longitudinal ligament**: a strong, wide and flat band that is continuous from the occipital bone anterior to the foramen magnum and extends inferiorly on the anterior surface of the vertebral column onto the pelvic surface of the sacrum. It connects the anterolateral surface of the vertebral bodies and IV discs together and primarily functions to prevent hyperextension of the vertebral column. Due to its width, it also makes it difficult for a herniated disc to pass anteriorly.
- **Posterior longitudinal ligament**: a narrow ligament that extends from the posterior edge of C2 and inferiorly to the sacrum. It primarily functions in preventing hyperflexion of the vertebral column. A herniated disc passes posteriorly on either side of this ligament and can compress nerve roots.
- **Nuchal ligament**: a strong and broad midline ligament that extends from the external occipital protuberance and posterior border of the foramen magnum to the spinous processes of the cervical vertebrae. It is composed of a thickened fibroelastic tissue and provides for muscle attachments (**Fig. 1.13**).
- **Supraspinous ligament**: a cord-like ligament that extends from the C7 spinous process down to the sacrum. It fuses with the nuchal ligament of the cervical region and helps to stabilize the vertebral column.
- **Interspinous ligaments**: thin ligaments that connect adjacent spinous processes from the root to the apex of each spinous process. They are weak stabilizers of the vertebral column.
- **Intertransverse ligaments**: thin ligaments that connect adjacent transverse processes.

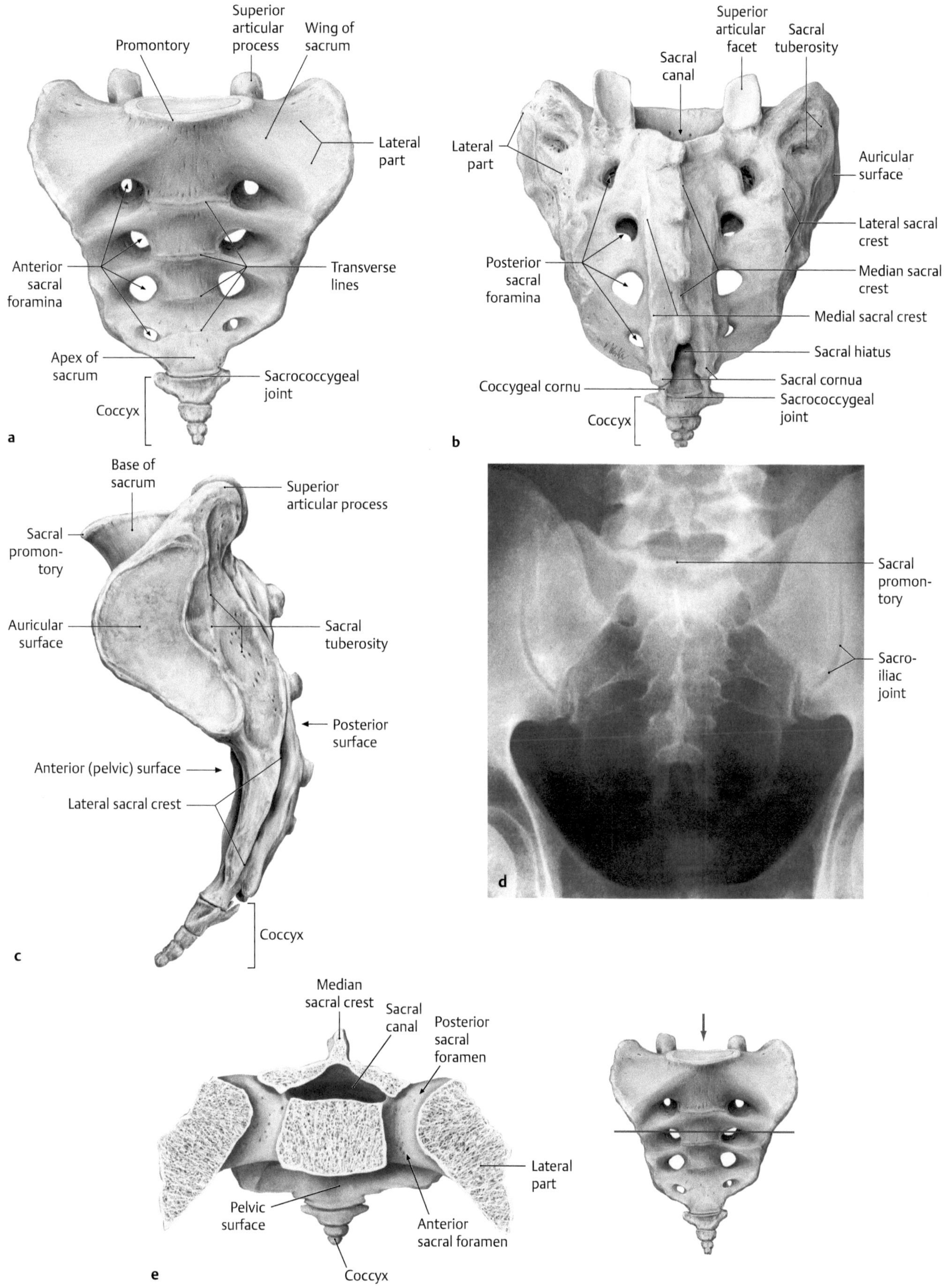

Fig. 1.12 Sacrum and coccyx. **(a)** Anterior view. **(b)** Posterior view. **(c)** Left lateral view. **(d)** Radiograph of sacrum, anteroposterior view. **(e)** Transverse section through second sacral vertebra. (**a, b, c, e** from Schuenke M, Schulte E, Schumacher U. THIEME Atlas of Anatomy. General Anatomy and Musculoskeletal System. Illustrations by Voll M and Wesker K. 3rd ed. New York: Thieme Medical Publishers; 2020. **d** from Moeller TB, Reif E. Pocket Atlas of Radiographic Anatomy, 3rd ed. New York, NY: Thieme; 2010.)

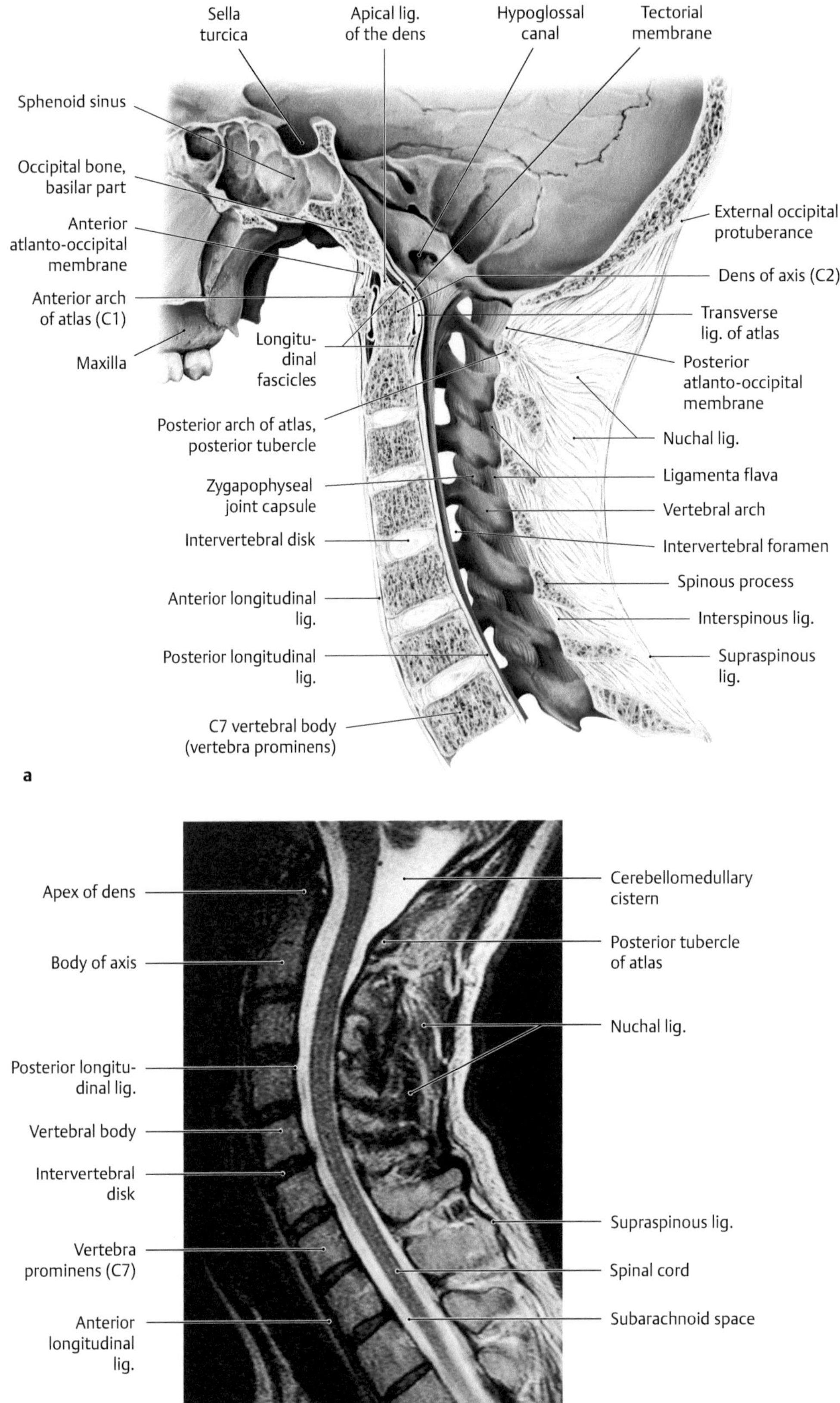

Fig. 1.13 Ligaments of the cervical spine. **(a)** Midsagittal section, left lateral view. **(b)** Midsagittal T2-weighted MRI, left lateral view. (From Schuenke M, Schulte E, Schumacher U. THIEME Atlas of Anatomy. General Anatomy and Musculoskeletal System. Illustrations by Voll M and Wesker K. 3rd ed. New York: Thieme Medical Publishers; 2020.)

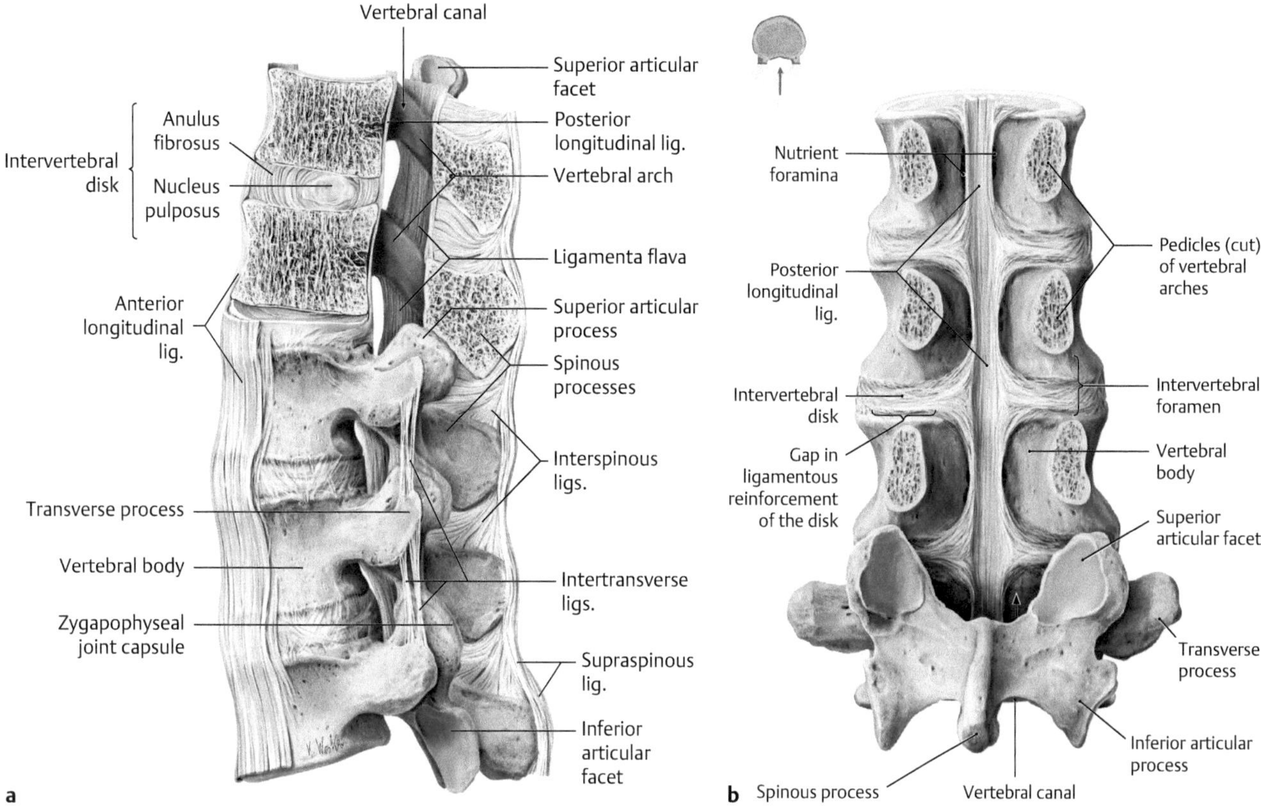

Fig. 1.14 Ligaments of the vertebral column. **(a)** Left lateral view of T11-L3, with T11-T12 sectioned in the midsagittal section. **(b)** Posterior view of opened vertebral canal at level L2-L5. (From Schuenke M, Schulte E, Schumacher U. THIEME Atlas of Anatomy. General Anatomy and Musculoskeletal System. Illustrations by Voll M and Wesker K. 3rd ed. New York: Thieme Medical Publishers; 2020.)

- **Ligamentum flava**: broad and pale yellow ligaments made of elastic tissue that connect adjacent laminae. They resist the separation of the vertebral lamina by limiting abrupt flexion of the vertebral column. They help preserve the curvatures of the vertebral column (**Fig. 1.14**).

1.7 Joints of the Vertebral Column

1.7.1 Intervertebral (IV) Joints

The **intervertebral (IV) joints** are located between non-fused, adjacent vertebral bodies and are secondary cartilaginous (symphyses) joints connected by **intervertebral (IV) discs** and ligaments (**Fig. 1.13; Fig. 1.14; Fig. 1.15; Fig. 1.16**). The IV discs provide strong attachments between the vertebral bodies and are designed for weight bearing and shock absorption. The IV discs are not located between the C1 and C2 vertebrae but extend to the position between the L5 and S1 vertebrae. Thickness correlates with range of movement. The cervical and lumbar regions are thicker, specifically along their anterior edges with uniformity in size seen in the thoracic region. The IV disc has an outer *anulus fibrous* and inner gelatinous central mass called the *nucleus pulposus*.

The **anulus fibrosus** is the bulging fibrous outer ring of the IV disc made of concentric lamellae (layers) of fibrocartilage that are made up of type I and II collagen. The anuli insert into the smooth and rounded *epiphyseal rims* on the articular surfaces of the vertebral bodies that are formed by the fused *anular epiphyses*. Rotation is limited between adjacent vertebrae because the fibers forming each lamella run obliquely from one vertebra to the next at about 30° from vertical axis and the fibers of adjacent lamellae cross each other obliquely in opposite directions at angles of greater than 60°. Only the outer one-third is innervated and this is by way of the *recurrent meningeal nerves of spinal nerves*. It receives less blood as it moves closer to the nucleus pulposus (**Fig. 1.16**).

The **nucleus pulposus** is the core of the IV disc and is made up of approximately 90% water and type II collagen fibers at birth. As one ages, the type II collagen will be replaced with type I collagen. In general, the semifluid nature of the nucleus allows for the great flexibility and resilience seen with the IV disc and vertebral column as a combined structure. The nucleus is not in the center of the IV disc but more between the center and posterior aspect of the disc. This is due to the lamellae of the anulus fibrosus being thinner and less numerous posteriorly. When vertical forces compress the IV discs, the nuclei become broader, but when the IV disc is stretched, the nuclei become thinner. When the vertebral column is undergoing anterior flexion, lateral flexion or extension, compression and stretching occur simultaneously. During these movements the nucleus acts much like a fulcrum. There is no innervation to the nucleus pulposus and it only receives nourishment through diffusion from blood vessels supplying the vertebral body and peripheral anulus fibrosus (**Fig. 1.16**).

1.7.2 Zygapophyseal (Facet) Joints

The **zygapophyseal (facet) joints** are considered the joints of the vertebral arches and are plane-type synovial joints located

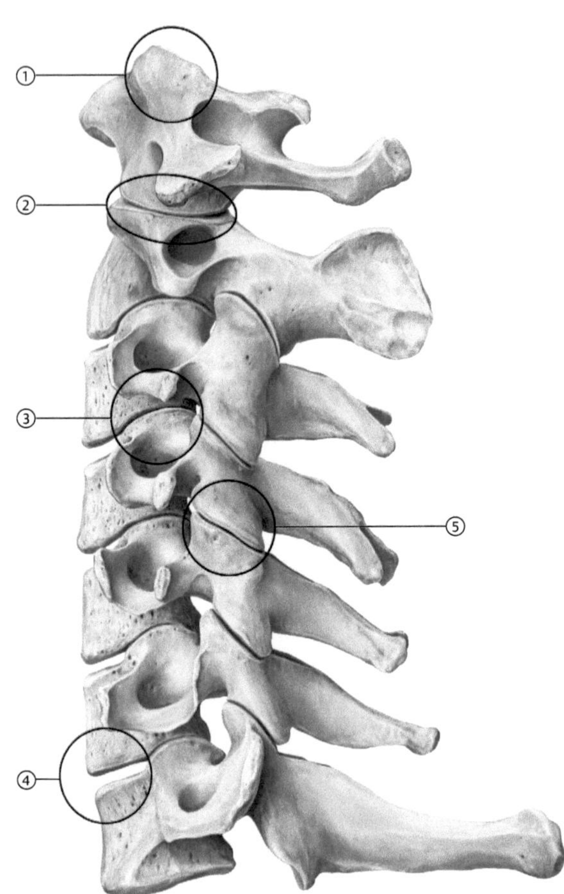

Fig. 1.15 Joints of the vertebral column: (1) atlanto-occipital joint; (2) atlanto-axial joint; (3) uncovertebral joint; (4) intervertebral (IV) joint; and (5) zygapophysial (facet) joint. (From Schuenke M, Schulte E, Schumacher U. THIEME Atlas of Anatomy. General Anatomy and Musculoskeletal System. Illustrations by Voll M and Wesker K. 3rd ed. New York: Thieme Medical Publishers; 2020.)

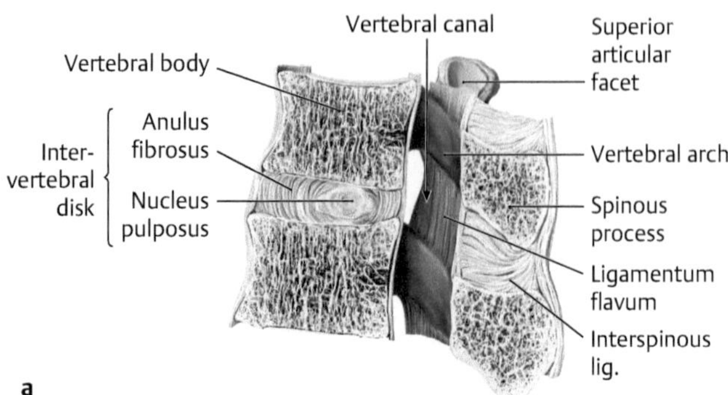

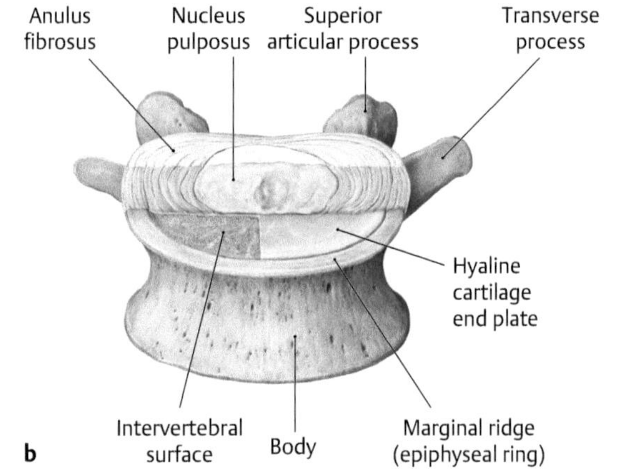

Fig. 1.16 Intervertebral joint. **(a)** Sagittal section of T11-T12, left lateral view. **(b)** Structure of the intervertebral disk. (From Schuenke M, Schulte E, Schumacher U. THIEME Atlas of Anatomy. General Anatomy and Musculoskeletal System. Illustrations by Voll M and Wesker K. 3rd ed. New York: Thieme Medical Publishers; 2020.)

between the superior and inferior articular processes of adjacent vertebrae that allow for gliding movements (**Fig. 1.17**). They naturally have a joint capsule because they are synovial joints but their elasticity in the cervical region allows for a wider range of movement. Their range of motion is determined by the size of the IV disc relative to that of the vertebral body. These joints, found in the cervical and lumbar regions, share some of the weight-bearing functions normally seen with the IV discs, especially during lateral flexion. The articular branches that originate from the medial branches of the dorsal rami branches innervate these joints. Each articular branch supplies two adjacent joints because they lie in grooves on the posterior surface of the medial parts of the transverse processes. Thus two nerves supply each joint (**Fig. 1.18**).

1.7.3 Atlanto-occipital Joints

The articulations between the occipital condyles of the occipital bone and the superior articular surfaces of the lateral masses of the C1 (atlas) vertebra are called the **atlanto-occipital joints** (**Fig. 1.19**). They are condyloid-type synovial joints that allow mainly flexion but also extension and minimal rotation or lateral flexion. The characteristic nodding "yes" movement of the head is

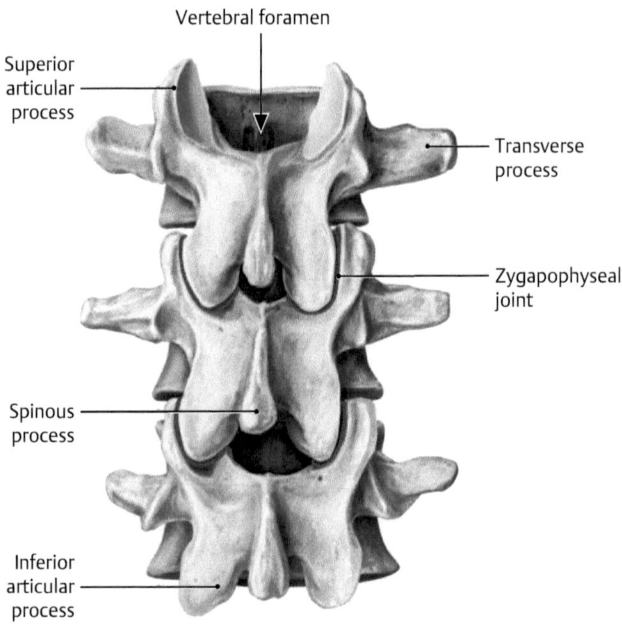

Fig. 1.17 Zygapophysial (facet) joint, posterior view. (From Schuenke M, Schulte E, Schumacher U. THIEME Atlas of Anatomy. General Anatomy and Musculoskeletal System. Illustrations by Voll M and Wesker K. 3rd ed. New York: Thieme Medical Publishers; 2020.)

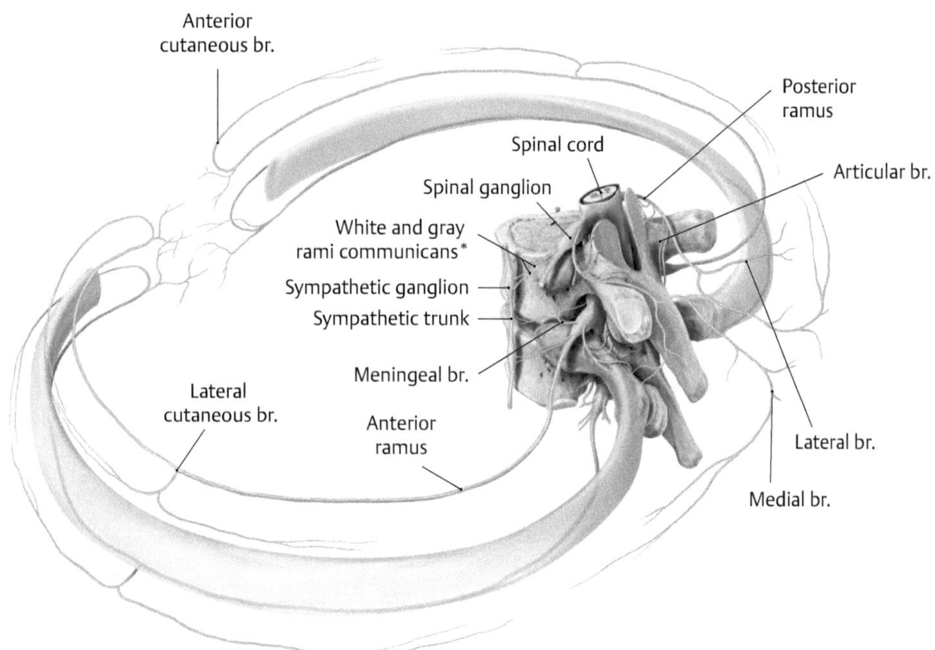

Fig. 1.18 Spinal nerve branches. (From Schuenke M, Schulte E, Schumacher U. THIEME Atlas of Anatomy. General Anatomy and Musculoskeletal System. Illustrations by Voll M and Wesker K. 3rd ed. New York: Thieme Medical Publishers; 2020.)

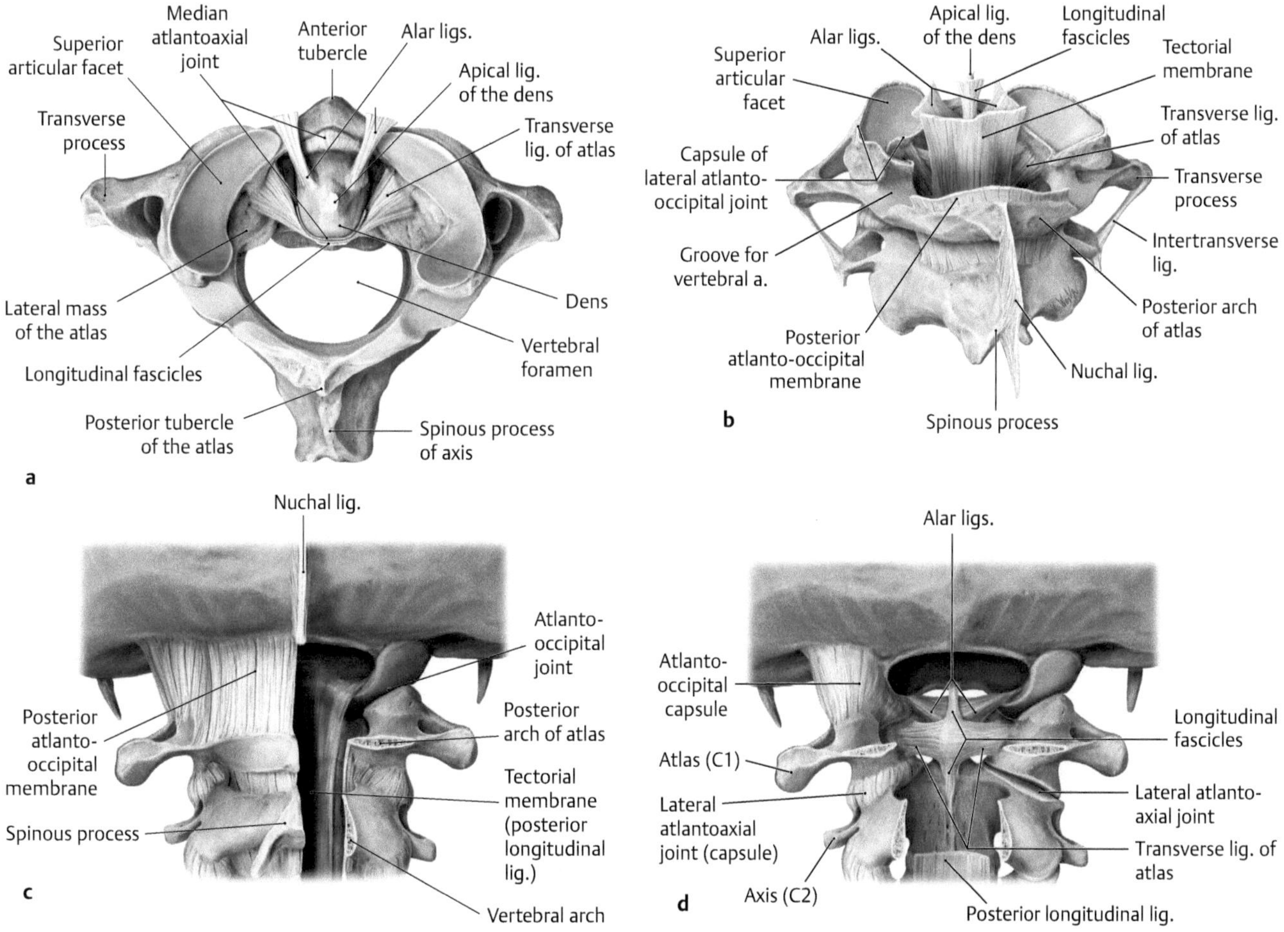

Fig. 1.19 Joints and ligaments related to the atlas (C1) and axis (C2). (**a**) Ligaments of the median atlanto-axial joint, superior view. (**b**) Posterosuperior view with the dens hidden by the tectorial membrane. (**c**) Posterior view with the vertebral canal windowed. (**d**) Posterior view with the tectorial membrane, posterior atlanto-occipital membrane, and vertebral arches removed. (From Schuenke M, Schulte E, Schumacher U. THIEME Atlas of Anatomy. General Anatomy and Musculoskeletal System. Illustrations by Voll M and Wesker K. 3rd ed. New York: Thieme Medical Publishers; 2020.)

facilitated by this joint. The **anterior** and **posterior atlanto-occipital membranes** extend from the anterior and posterior arches of C1 to the anterior and posterior margins of the foramen magnum. The membranes help prevent excessive movements of these joints (**Fig. 1.13; Fig. 1.19**).

1.7.4 Atlanto-axial Joints

There are three articulations associated with the **atlanto-axial joints** (**Fig. 1.19**). The **lateral atlanto-axial joints** are the articulations between the inferior facets of the lateral masses of the C1 vertebra and the superior facets of C2. They are gliding-type synovial joints. The **median atlanto-axial joint** is the articulation between the anterior arch of C1 and the dens of C2. This is a pivot-type synovial joint. The characteristic shaking "no" movement of the head involves all three of these joints and during this movement the cranium and C1 rotate as a unit on C2.

During rotation, the dens of C2 is the pivot that is held in a socket formed anteriorly by the anterior arch of C1 and posteriorly by the **transverse ligament** of C1, which spans between the tubercles on the medial aspects of the lateral masses of C1. Vertical **superior** and **inferior longitudinal bands** extend from the *transverse ligament* to attach to the occipital bone and C2 respectively. Extending from the dens of C2 to the lateral margins of the foramen magnum are the **alar ligaments**. These act as check ligaments to prevent excessive rotation at the joints. The superior continuation of the posterior longitudinal ligament from the body of C2 up through the foramen magnum is called the **tectorial membrane**. This membrane passes posteriorly over the median atlanto-axial joint and its ligaments.

1.7.5 Uncovertebral Joints (*of Luschka*)

Located between the hook-shaped uncinate processes of the C3-C6 (C7) vertebrae and the angled inferolateral surfaces of the vertebral bodies superior to them are the **uncovertebral joints** (**Fig. 1.20**). These so-called joints are also located at the posterolateral margins of the IV discs. The articulating surfaces are covered by cartilage and contain a capsule filled with fluid. Whether this is a true joint or not is debated as some consider it a synovial joint while others believe it to be more of a degenerative space in the discs filled with extracellular fluid. Bone spur formation (osteophytes) is frequent at these locations and can lead to compression of the vertebral artery or nearby spinal nerves that result in chronic neck pain.

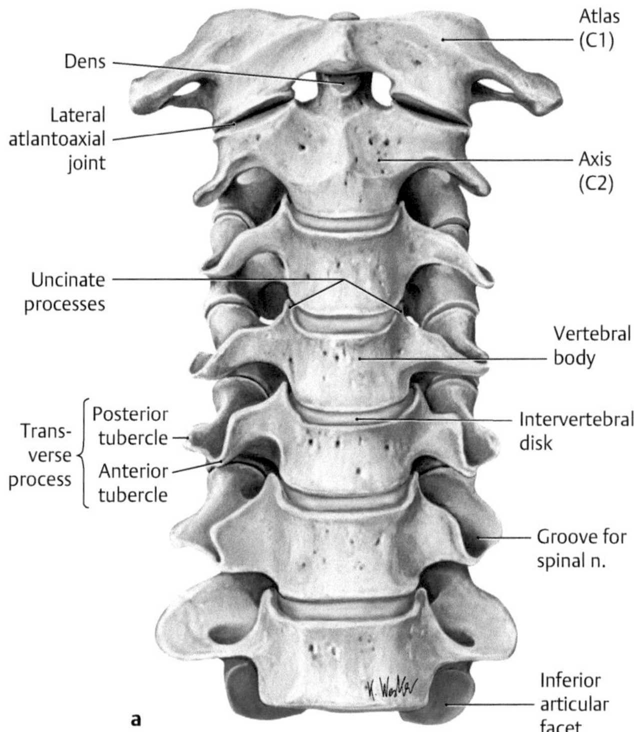

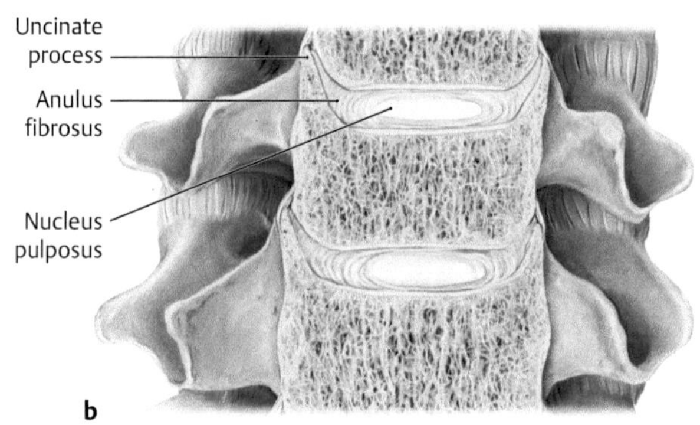

Fig. 1.20 Uncovertebral joints. (**a**) Anterior view of cervical vertebrae. (**b**) Uncovertebral joints enlarged, anterior view of coronal section. (From Schuenke M, Schulte E, Schumacher U. THIEME Atlas of Anatomy. General Anatomy and Musculoskeletal System. Illustrations by Voll M and Wesker K. 3rd ed. New York: Thieme Medical Publishers; 2020.)

1.8 Mobility of the Vertebral Column

Mobility of the vertebral column varies according to the specific region and even the age of an individual (**Fig. 1.21**). Vertebral column mobility primarily originates from the compressibility and elasticity of the IV discs. Movements between adjacent vertebrae occur at both the strong but flexible nuclei pulposi of the IV discs and at the zygapophysial joints. The movements between adjacent vertebrae are small but it is the multiplying effect of these smaller movements that create a larger range of motion. This never occurs at a single segment of the vertebral column except for between C1-C2. These movements seen with the vertebral column include flexion, extension, rotation and lateral flexion and extension. Movements and mobility of the vertebral column are limited by:

- Compressibility, thickness and elasticity of IV discs.
- Tension, shape and orientation of the zygapophysial (facet) joints.
- Resistance of vertebral column ligaments and the back muscles that act on it.
- Surrounding tissue of an individual (i.e., being overweight).
- Thoracic wall attachments.

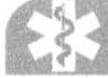

Clinical Correlate 1.1

Osteoporosis of the Vertebral Column

Osteoporosis is a thinning of the bones and is the result of demineralization of these bones due to the rate of reabsorption by osteoclasts exceeding that of bone formation by osteoblasts. Risk factors can include natural aging, being female, menopause, smoking, and having a low body weight. One of the areas most affected by osteoporosis is the vertebral column, especially the vertebral bodies, and osteoporosis is the most common cause of vertebral compression fractures. The spongy bone of the vertebral body can begin to demineralize and a common pattern of vertical striations can be seen fairly early in a radiograph if an individual has osteoporosis. Further progression of the osteoporosis will demonstrate near radiolucent (more transparent) vertebral bodies in later radiographs. In late osteoporosis, a patient may display increased thoracic kyphosis on examination and possible vertebral collapses in an X-ray. The thoracic vertebrae are the most commonly affected by osteoporosis, although all vertebrae are subject to it.

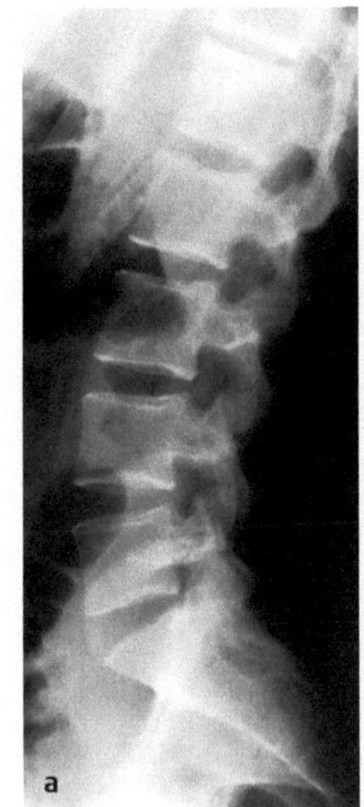

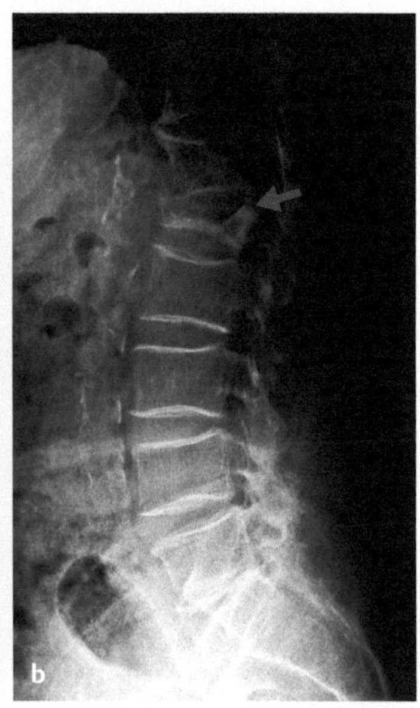

(**a**) Radiograph of a normal lumbar spine, left lateral view. (Reproduced from Moeller TB, Reif E. Pocket Atlas of Radiographic Anatomy, 3rd ed. New York, NY: Thieme; 2010.) (**b**) Radiograph of an osteoporotic lumbar spine with a compression fracture at L1 (*arrow*). Note that the vertebral bodies are decreased in density, and the internal trabecular structure is coarse. (Reproduced from Jallo J, Vaccaro AR. Neurotrauma and Critical Care of the Spine, 1st ed. New York, NY: Thieme; 2009.)

Clinical Correlate 1.2

Laminectomy

The surgical removal of a spinous process and a portion of each lamina adjacent to it is called a **laminectomy**. The laminae are generally excised in succession from a particular region of the vertebral column in order to provide access to the vertebral canal and the posterior aspect of the spinal cord. This access allows for direct targeting of the nerve roots as in a rhizotomy or repair of a herniated disc. This procedure is generally performed in order to relieve pressure on the spinal cord or its nerve roots brought on by stenosis of the vertebral canal, a herniated disc, or a tumor. In the case of a herniated disc, an outpatient *microdiscectomy* may be performed by removing a small portion of the bone over the nerve root and/or disc material from under the nerve root to relieve impingement and may replace the need for a more extensive laminectomy.

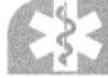

Clinical Correlate 1.3

Spinal Stenosis

Any form of abnormal narrowing of the vertebral canal is called **spinal stenosis**. The most common areas for this to occur are in the lumbar region followed by the cervical region of the vertebral column. Stenosis can lead to symptoms of paresthesia, numbness, pain or even loss of motor innervation. Lumbar stenosis is much more common but cervical stenosis could involve spinal cord compression and is considered more serious. Lumbar stenosis will center on portions of the cauda equina because the spinal cord ends at vertebral level L1. The lumbar spinal nerves increase in size as they travel down through the vertebral canal and the intervertebral foramina decrease in size. Any narrowing tends to be maximal at the level of the IV discs and may involve one or more spinal nerve roots. Causes can include a thickening of nearby ligaments such as the ligamentum flavum, bone spurs, osteoarthritis, herniated discs, tumors or hereditary in nature.

The cervical and lumbar regions of the vertebral column have the greatest range of motion. All movements are quite free to act in the cervical region due to the neck being thinner compared to the trunk, it has loose and nearly horizontal zygapophysial joints, and it has thick IV discs relative to the size of their vertebral bodies. The cervical region has the greatest range of flexion. The lumbar region allows for a great deal of both flexion and extension but no rotation. The largest range of extension comes from the lumbar region. The thoracic region has limited flexion but considerable rotation.

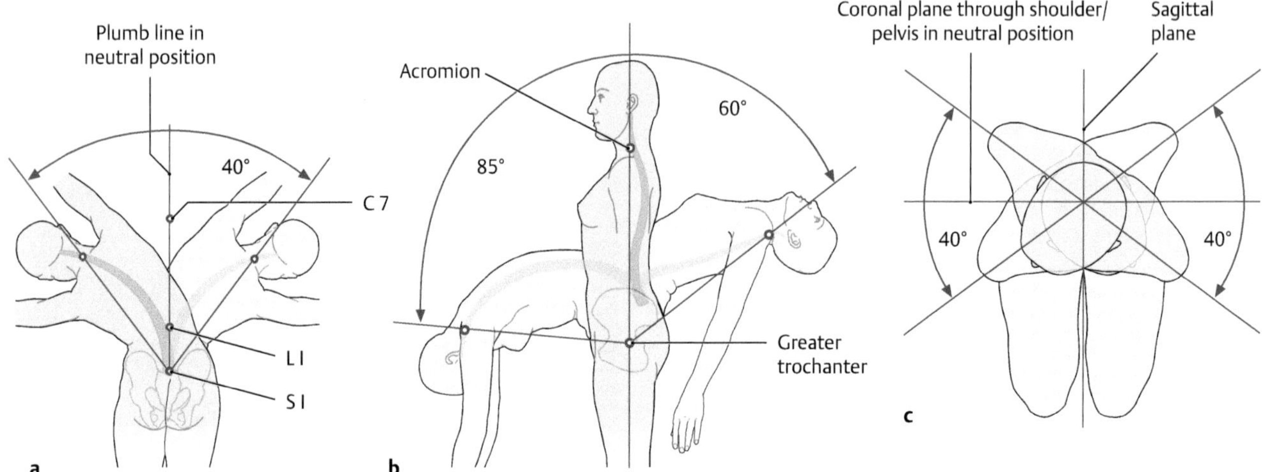

Fig 1.21 Mobility of the vertebral column. **(a)** Lateral flexion. **(b)** Flexion/extension. **(c)** Rotation. (From Schuenke M, Schulte E, Schumacher U. THIEME Atlas of Anatomy. General Anatomy and Musculoskeletal System. Illustrations by Voll M and Wesker K. 3rd ed. New York: Thieme Medical Publishers; 2020.)

1.9 Neurovasculature of the Vertebral Column

The **meningeal branches of the spinal nerves** innervate the vertebral column and generally originate from the spinal nerve prior to the bifurcation of ventral and dorsal rami branches. These nerves will carry somatic sensory and sympathetic postganglionic fibers. There are two to four of these branches that originate from each side of every vertebral level. They receive communicating branches from gray rami communicantes near their origin **(Fig. 1.23)**.

Most of these branches pass back through the intervertebral foramen and into the vertebral canal, while others remain external to the canal and distribute themselves to the anterolateral aspect of the IV discs and vertebral bodies. These more external branches supply the anterior longitudinal ligament, periosteum and annuli fibrosi. The true recurrent branches pass back into the vertebral canal and branch further. They innervate the periosteum and anuli fibrosi, and also the posterior longitudinal ligament, dura mater, ligamenta flava and blood vessels passing through the vertebral canal.

Blood supply to the vertebrae comes from *periosteal* and *equatorial* branches of the major cervical and segmental arteries and *spinal* branches. The cervical vertebrae receive blood originating

Clinical Correlate 1.4

Fractures and Dislocations of Vertebrae

When the occipital condyles are driven into the lateral masses of the C1 vertebra, a **Jefferson or burst fracture** occurs resulting in the lateral masses moving away from each other and causing the anterior and posterior arches to fracture in as many as four places (**Fig. 1.22 a,b**). Up to two fractures can occur in each arch. These can be seen in diving accidents but because the vertebral canal is enlarging with the lateral masses moving laterally themselves, the spinal cord may be spared of any damage.

When the pars interarticularis of the C2 vertebra fractures, which is generally due to trauma involving hyperextension of the neck as in motor vehicular accidents, it is called a Hangman's fracture (**Fig. 1.22 c,d**). It is also known as a **traumatic spondylolysis of C2**. Although it is commonly known as Hangman's fracture, the fracture itself is rarely seen in judicial or suicidal hangings. Instead, asphyxiation is generally the mode of actual death and not the fracture. Fracture of the dens (odontoid process) is a common fracture of C2 and generally occurs near the base of the dens or where it meets the body of C2. These fractures generally result in avascular necrosis because the blood supply is cut off. If the fracture occurs below the level of the base, the blood supply is generally still good enough to allow for proper healing.

Flexion teardrop fractures are the most severe fracture of the cervical spine and typically occur from hyperflexion and compression. There is an anteroinferior vertebral fragment (teardrop), anterior longitudinal ligament tearing, posterior vertebral body displacement (subluxation) into the vertebral canal resulting in spinal cord compression, and fracture of the spinous process. This could also be due to a diving accident or even a motor vehicular accident. **Extension teardrop fractures** typically occur due to hyperextension of the neck and are not as severe as flexion teardrop fractures because there is no displacement of the vertebral body. They are similar in that they both involve a fracture of the anteroinferior corner of the vertebral body and that the anterior longitudinal ligament is disrupted.

A fracture of the pars interarticularis or bony region located between the superior and inferior articulating processes of a vertebra is called **spondylolysis**. This is most commonly seen in in the lower lumbar region of the vertebrae. When there is a shift or dislocation between adjacent vertebrae, most commonly between L5 and S1, it is now known as **spondylolisthesis**. When an oblique view radiograph is taken of the vertebral column, the appearance of a "*Scotty dog*" is seen (**Fig. 1.22 e,f**). The superior articular process represents the ear, the pedicle is the eye, the transverse process marks the nose, the pars interarticularis represents the neck, the inferior articular process is the front leg, the lamina is the body; the spinous process is the tail, and the contralateral inferior articular process is the back leg. When the neck of "*Scotty dog*" is broken this represents spondylolysis.

Clinical Correlate 1.5

Herniation of Intervertebral Discs and Lower Back Pain

Flexion of the vertebral column produces compression anteriorly but stretching or tension posteriorly. If there is any degeneration of the anulus fibrosus, the nucleus pulposus may be able to protrude toward the thinnest portion of the anulus fibrosus. This protrusion or herniation of the nucleus pulposus into or through the annulus fibrosus may lead to compression of the spinal cord or nerve roots. Most herniations occur between the L4-L5 or L5-S1 levels and pass posterolaterally (*posterolateral disc herniation*) to the posterior longitudinal ligament. A general rule applies in that when a disc herniation occurs, the nerve root compressed is the one numbered one inferior to the location of the herniated disc. For example, if the herniation involves the disc between L5 and S1, the S1 nerve root would be compressed. Recall that this is due to the intervertebral disc forming the inferior half of the anterior border of the intervertebral foramen and that the superior half is formed by the bone of the body of the superior vertebra in the thoracic and lumbar regions.

The protrusion of the nucleus pulposus could push the posterior longitudinal ligament to the side or pass directly through it (*posteromedial disc herniation*) and generally results in the compression of multiple lower spinal nerves. For example, a posteromedial protrusion at the IV disc between L4-L5 affects the L5 and possibly multiple sacral spinal nerves associated with the cauda equina.

In the cervical region, the cervical spinal nerves exit superior to the vertebra of the same number, thus the relationship of the herniated disc to the affected spinal nerve is the same. For example, a protrusion between C5-C6 would affect the C6 spinal nerve.

A localized back pain, which is usually acute pain, is generally the result of pressure on the longitudinal ligament and the periphery of the anulus fibrosus. When there is compression of the spinal nerve, the pain becomes more chronic and results in referred pain that is perceived in certain dermatomes associated with that particular spinal nerve.

Lower back pain affects most individuals at some time in their lifetime. Pain from this specific region of the back will generally involve the muscles, joints or fibroskeletal structures that include the periosteum, anuli fibrosi and ligaments. Tension, stress, cramping or overuse could bring on muscular pain while normal aging of the zygapophysial joints could be the cause of joint pain. Any referred pain would most likely be the result of a herniated disc.

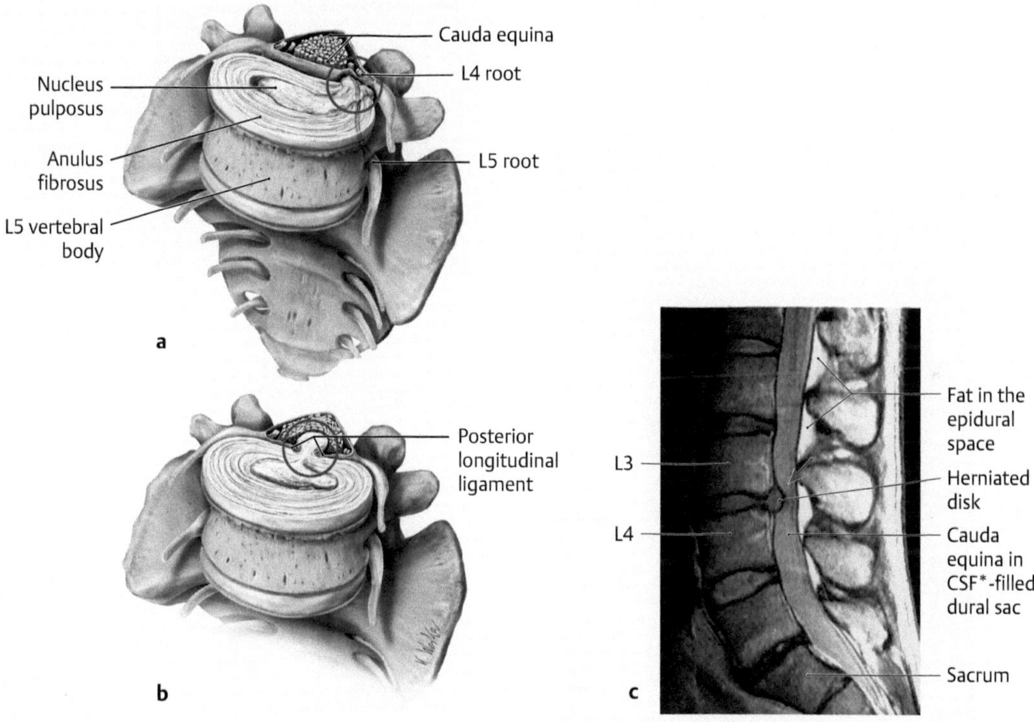

(**a**) Posterolateral disk herniation at the L4/L5 level. (**b**) Posteromedial disk herniation at the L4/L5 level. (**c**) Midsagittal T2-weighted MRI (magnetic resonance image). (**a**, **b** from Schuenke M, Schulte E, Schumacher U. THIEME Atlas of Anatomy. Head, Neck, and Neuroanatomy. Illustrations by Voll M and Wesker K. 3rd ed. New York: Thieme Medical Publishers; 2020. **c** from Schuenke M, Schulte E, Schumacher U. THIEME Atlas of Anatomy. General Anatomy and Musculoskeletal System. Illustrations by Voll M and Wesker K. 3rd ed. New York: Thieme Medical Publishers; 2020.)

from the **vertebral** and *ascending cervical arteries*. The thoracic vertebrae receive blood originating from the **posterior intercostal arteries**. The lumbar vertebrae receive blood originating from the **subcostal** and **lumbar arteries**. The sacrum and coccyx receive blood originating from the **median sacral**, **lateral sacral**, and *iliolumbar arteries* (**Fig. 1.24**).

A typical blood supply would involve this pattern. The posterior intercostal arteries that originate from the thoracic aorta themselves pass along both anterolateral sides of the vertebra and branch off the **periosteal** and **equatorial arteries**. This occurs before the posterior intercostal artery reaches the intervertebral foramen, where it gives off the spinal artery branch or continues

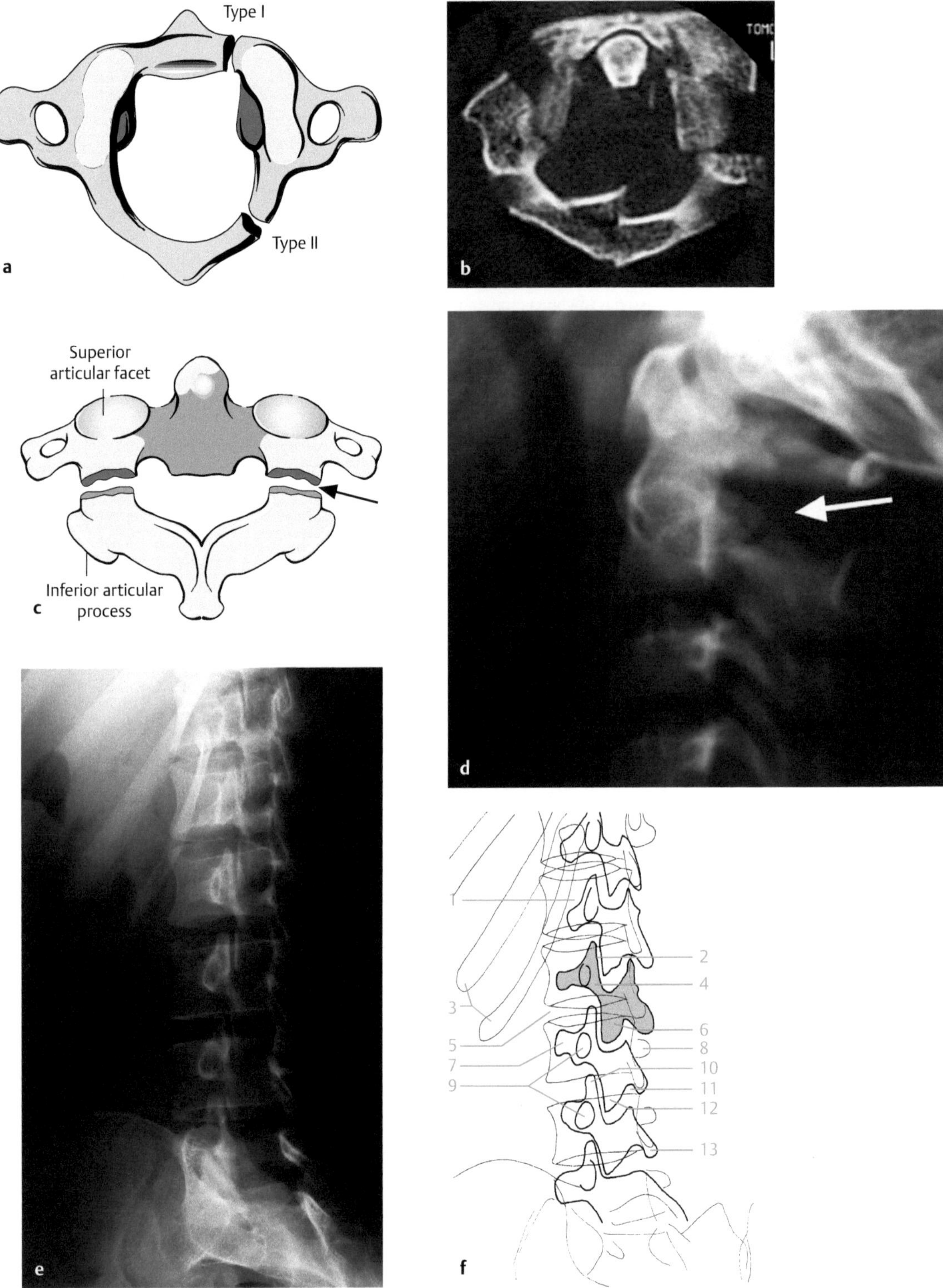

Fig 1.22 Fractures and dislocations of vertebrae. **(a)** Schematic of Jefferson fracture. **(b)** Jefferson fracture. **(c)** Schematic of Hangman's fracture. **(d)** Hangman's fracture. **(e)** Scotty dog. **(f)** Schematic of lumbar vertebrae and Scotty dog. 1, body of vertebra; 2, intervertebral disk space; 3, ribs; 4, interarticular part; 5, intervertebral disk space; 6, lamina; 7, ipsilateral transverse process; 8, contralateral transverse process; 9, pedicle; 10, superior articular process; 11, intervertebral foramen; 12, inferior articular process; 13, spinous process. (**a-d** reproduced from Imhof H. Direct Diagnosis in Radiology: Spinal Imaging. New York, NY: Thieme; 2008. **e, f** reproduced from Moeller TB, Reif E. Pocket Atlas of Radiographic Anatomy, 3rd ed. New York, NY: Thieme; 2010.)

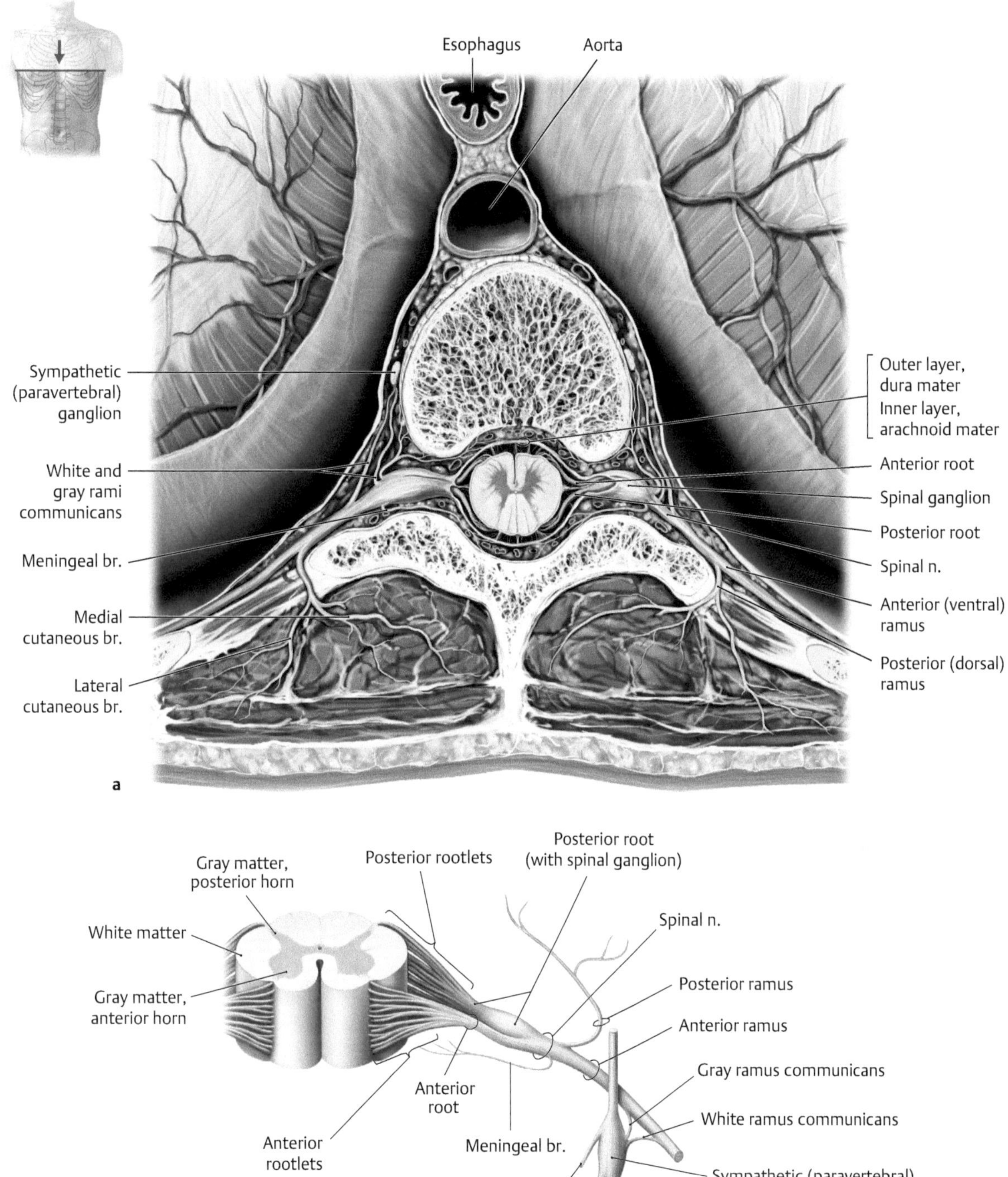

Fig. 1.23 **(a)** Cross section of the vertebral column and spinal cord, superior view. **(b)** A spinal cord segment. (**a** from Schuenke M, Schulte E, Schumacher U. THIEME Atlas of Anatomy. Illustrations by Voll M and Wesker K. **b** from Schuenke M, Schulte E, Schumacher U. THIEME Atlas of Anatomy. Head, Neck, and Neuroanatomy. Illustrations by Voll M and Wesker K. 3rd ed. New York: Thieme Medical Publishers; 2020.)

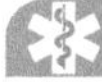

Clinical Correlate 1.6

Metastasis of Cancer

The venous drainage of the brain along with that of the thorax, abdomen and pelvic viscera, all have a connection with the vertebral venous plexuses. Due to these connections and the lack of valves in the vertebral venous plexuses, metastasis of cancer from one region to another is common and should be considered when an individual is being treated for specific cancers. For example, prostate cancer is known to metastasize to the brain and the route it could take to reach the brain would be through the vertebral venous plexuses. The vertebral column is the most common site of bone metastasis.

If there has been no initial diagnosis of cancer, constant pain in the neck or back regions could be due to metastases of a particular cancer to the bones of the vertebral column and this is now leading to compression of the spinal cord.

Clinical Correlate 1.7

Myelography

Myelography is a fluoroscopic imaging technique that involves the introduction of a spinal needle into the spinal canal and the injection of contrast material into the subarachnoid space. Nowadays, myelography is slowly being replaced with high resolution MRI, but it is still needed in the event an individual has a medical device such as a cardiac pacemaker. The procedure involves CSF being withdrawn by lumbar puncture and then replaced with contrast material. This is most commonly used to detect abnormalities of the spinal cord, vertebral canal, spinal nerve roots or even the blood vessels that supply the spinal cord.

toward the more posterior aspects of the vertebral arch. The **spinal artery** enters the intervertebral foramen and divides into the *anterior* and *posterior vertebral canal branches.* The anterior vertebral canal branch gives off a *nutrient artery* that supplies the bulk of the vertebral body and the posterior vertebral canal artery supplies blood to the more anterior aspect of the vertebral arch. Both vertebral canal arteries have branches that anastomose with other arteries that supply the meninges and spinal cord. The posterior intercostal artery that continues past the intervertebral foramen gives off *posterior branches* that supply the remainder of the vertebral arch and they have their own periosteal and nutrient artery branches. The spinal arteries may also branch off *segmental medullary* and *radicular arteries* that supply blood to specific portions of the spinal cord or ventral and dorsal roots of spinal nerves (**Fig. 1.24**).

There are valve-less venous plexuses found both internally and externally to the vertebral column that communicate with one another. The plexuses help equalize pressure in adjacent veins and due to the lack of valves allow for metastasis of cancer. The **external vertebral venous plexus** has both an anterior and posterior plexus associated with it. The *anterior portion* is adjacent to the vertebral body while the *posterior portion* is adjacent to the vertebral arch. The **internal vertebral (epidural or *Batson's*) venous plexus** is also divided into an anterior and posterior plexus. Both of these lie in the epidural space between the vertebral column and dura mater surrounding the spinal cord. **Basivertebral veins** originate from the vertebral bodies

Clinical Correlate 1.8

Lumbar Spinal Puncture (Spinal Tap)

A lumbar spinal puncture or *spinal tap* is used to obtain a sample of cerebrospinal fluid. Under aseptic conditions, a lumbar puncture needle (with stylet) is inserted in the midline between the spinous processes of L3 and L4 (or L4 and L5) vertebrae and into the lumbar cistern. The patient is lying down or sitting in a flexed position. This will facilitate the stretching of the ligamenta flava, spinous processes and laminae making it easier to insert the needle. This procedure can help diagnose infections such as meningitis or encephalitis, central nervous system conditions such as multiple sclerosis and Guillain-Barre syndrome, and it can determine if there is a subarachnoid hemorrhage or certain cancers involving the brain or spinal cord.

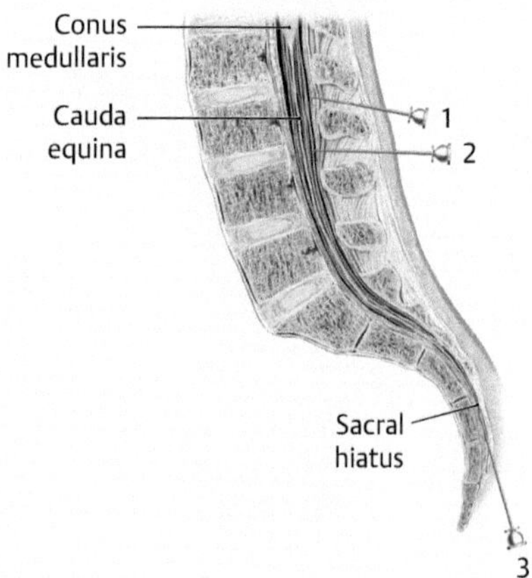

Anesthesia

Lumbar anesthesia may be administered in a similar fashion (2). Epidural anesthesia is administered by placing a catheter in the epidural space without penetrating the dural sac (1). This may also be done by passing a needle through the sacral hiatus (3). (From Schuenke M, Schulte E, Schumacher U. THIEME Atlas of Anatomy. Head, Neck, and Neuroanatomy. Illustrations by Voll M and Wesker K. 3rd ed. New York: Thieme Medical Publishers; 2020.)

and primarily drain through a canal or foramina into the anterior portion of the intervertebral venous plexus. The **intervertebral veins** are located in the intervertebral foramen and receive venous drainage from the vertebral venous plexuses and spinal cord. They will drain into the cervical and segmental veins that pair up with the equivalent arteries (**Fig. 1.25**).

1.10 Spinal Cord and Meninges

Located in the vertebral canal is the spinal cord, spinal nerve roots, spinal meningeal layers and the neurovasculature related to these structures. The majority of the details related to these structures are discussed in Chapter 9 of this text, thus only a brief description of these structures will be given here.

1.10.1 Spinal Cord

The major bundle of nervous tissue that begins at the *medulla oblongata* at the level of the foramen magnum and terminates

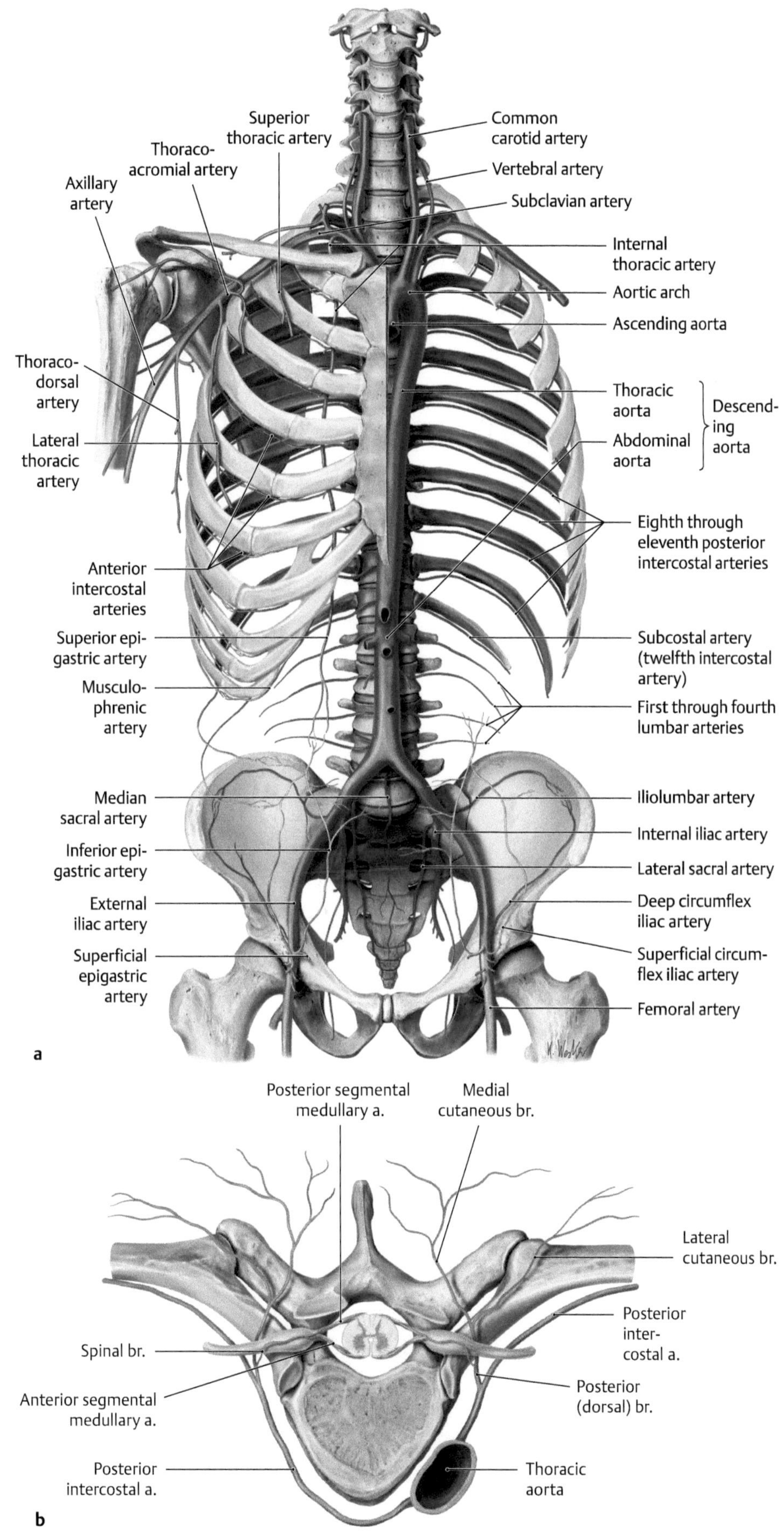

Fig. 1.24 (**a**) Arteries of the trunk wall. (**b**) Branches of the posterior intercostal arteries, superior view. (From Schuenke M, Schulte E, Schumacher U. THIEME Atlas of Anatomy. General Anatomy and Musculoskeletal System. Illustrations by Voll M and Wesker K. 3rd ed. New York: Thieme Medical Publishers; 2020.)

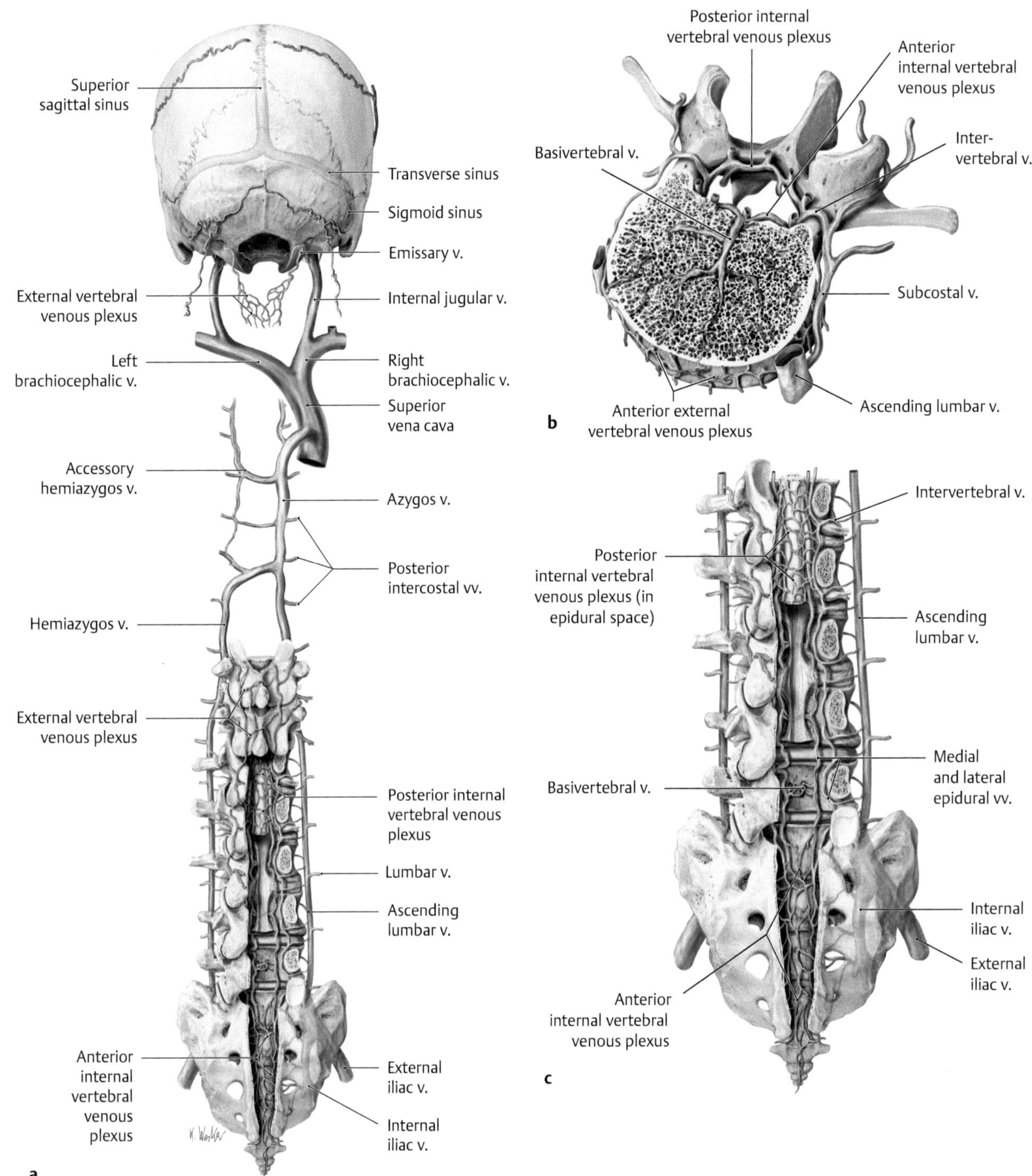

Fig. 1.25 **(a)** Intercostal veins and anterior vertebral venous plexus, anterosuperior view. **(b)** Vertebral venous plexuses. **(c)** Veins in the sacral and lumbar canals. (From Schuenke M, Schulte E, Schumacher U. THIEME Atlas of Anatomy. Head, Neck, and Neuroanatomy. Illustrations by Voll M and Wesker K. 3rd ed. New York: Thieme Medical Publishers; 2020.)

Clinical Correlate 1.9

Spina Bifida

Spina bifida is a neural tube defect that occurs when the spine and spinal cord do not form properly. In the United States, it affects about one out of every 1,500 newborns. There are three main types.

- **Spina bifida occulta (a)** is the most common congenital anomaly of the vertebral column in which the laminae of L5 and/or S1 fail to develop. The defect is often hidden and most individuals are unaware they have the condition because there is only a small defect in the vertebrae. There is generally no disturbance of spinal function.
- **Spina bifida (meningocele) (b)** occurs when one or more vertebral arches fail to develop and presents with a herniation or sac of only the meninges. The spinal cord and nerves are normal and not severely affected.
- **Spina bifida (myelomeningocele) (c)** occurs when multiple vertebral arches fail to develop resulting in a herniation of both the meninges and spinal nerves. This is the most severe form exposing the newborn to life threatening infections, bowel and bladder dysfunction, and total paralysis of the lower extremities.

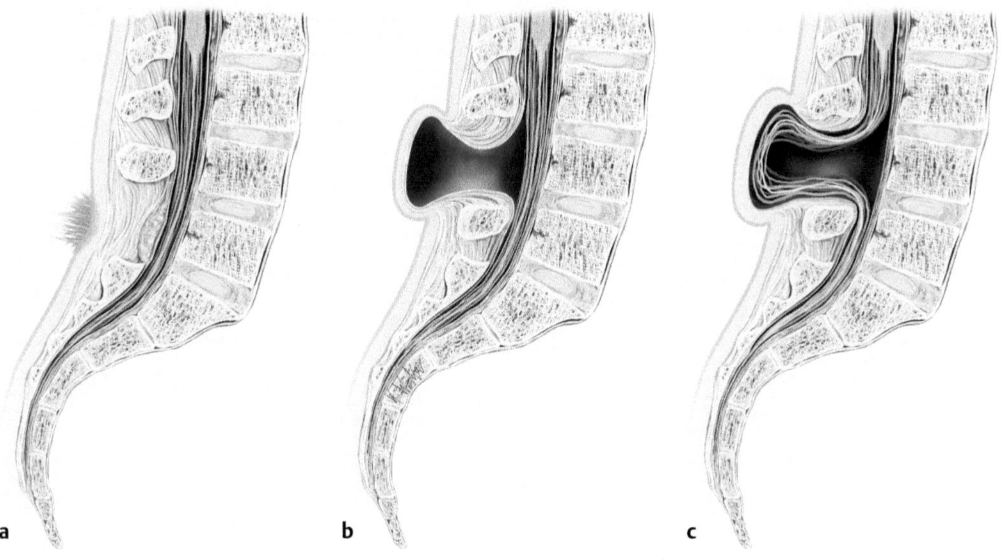

inferiorly at the L1 vertebral level represents the **spinal cord**. The tapering off end of the spinal cord is called the **conus medullaris** and in newborns may extend down to the L3 vertebral level or even lower. The spinal cord is made up of **spinal segments**, of which each has a paired ventral and dorsal root that will fuse to become a spinal nerve. There are 31 total and specifically 8 cervical, 12 thoracic, 5 lumbar, 5 sacral and 1 coccygeal spinal segments **(Fig. 1.26)**.

There are two enlargements of the spinal cord that are associated with the innervation to the limbs. The **cervical enlargement** is made up of the C4-T1 spinal segments and the ventral rami that are associated with these spinal segments form the *brachial plexuses* that are responsible for innervating the upper limbs. The **lumbosacral enlargement** is made up of the L1-S3 spinal segments (between the T9-T12 vertebral levels) and the ventral rami that are associated with them form the *lumbar* and *sacral plexuses* that are responsible for innervating the lower limbs **(Fig. 1.26)**.

As described in the introductory chapter, the spinal cord has a set of ventral and dorsal rootlets and roots, of which the dorsal root contains a ganglion (DRG), before fusing to become the spinal nerve. In approximately 50% of the population, the C1 nerves do not contain a dorsal root. The T1-C1 nerves bear the same alphanumeric name as the vertebra forming the superior margin of their intervertebral foramen thus the T6 spinal nerve passes between the T6 and T7 vertebrae. Due to the cervical nerves having eight pairs and there only being seven pairs of cervical vertebrae, the C1-C7 spinal nerves pass above their same alphanumeric vertebra but the C8 spinal nerve passes between the C7 and T1 vertebrae.

The spinal cord in adults is shorter than the vertebral column so there will be a progressive increase in length of both the ventral and dorsal rootlets and roots before they reach the corresponding intervertebral foramen and become a spinal nerve. The lumbar and sacral rootlets and roots are the longest and any of these located inferior to the conus medullaris are known collectively as the **cauda equina**. The cauda equina is located in a particular portion of the subarachnoid space called the **lumbar cistern** and is a clinically relevant location when doing *spinal taps*. Also passing through this region is an isolated extension from the conus medullaris called the **filum terminale** and it acts as an anchor for the spinal cord and spinal meninges **(Fig. 1.27)**.

1.10.2 Spinal Meninges

Dura Mater

The dura mater at the level of the spinal cord consists of only one layer, unlike the dura mater of the cranium that consists of two layers (**Fig. 1.28**). It is the outermost meningeal layer of the spinal cord and it is composed of a tough, fibrous and elastic tissue. The dura mater forms the **dural sac** (**Fig. 1.27**), a long tubular sheath

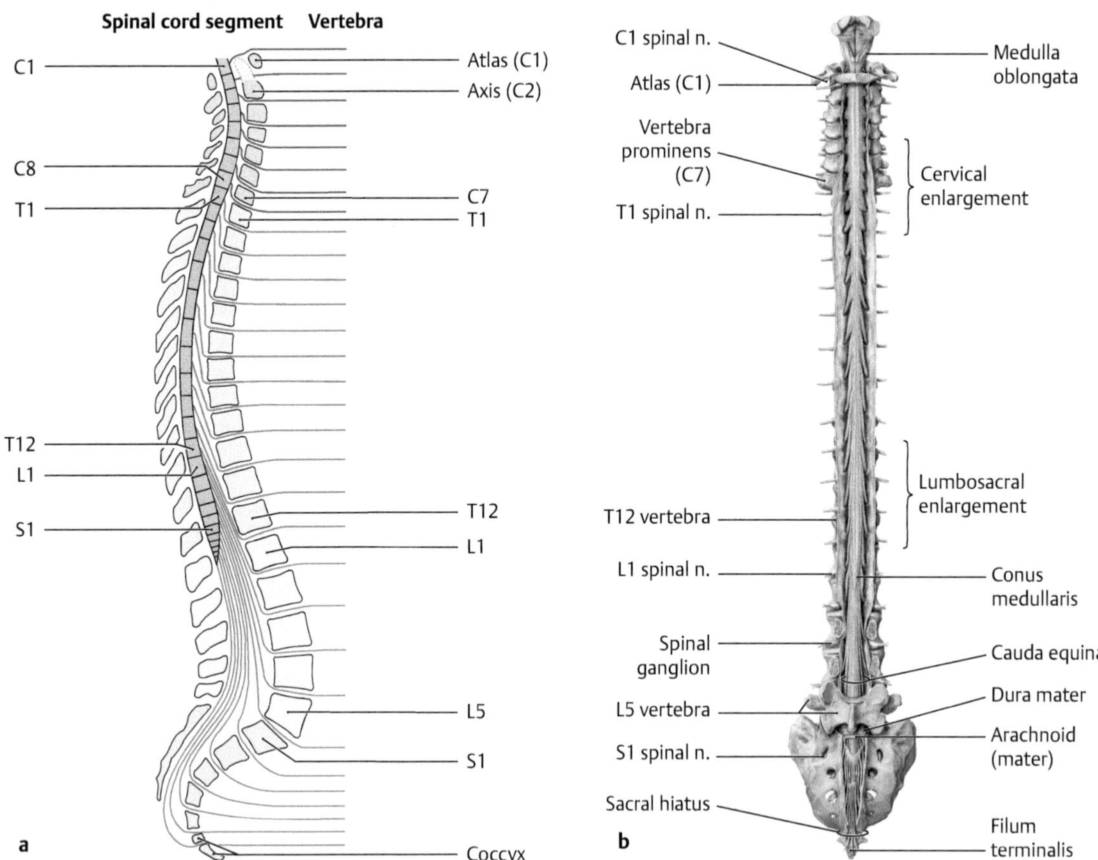

Fig. 1.26 (a) Spinal cord segments. (b) Spinal cord in situ, posterior view with vertebral canal windowed. (From Schuenke M, Schulte E, Schumacher U. THIEME Atlas of Anatomy. Head, Neck, and Neuroanatomy. Illustrations by Voll M and Wesker K. 3rd ed. New York: Thieme Medical Publishers; 2020.)

within the vertebral canal structure that extends from the junction of the cranial dura mater located at the foramen magnum and inferiorly to about the S2 vertebral level. The spinal nerves will ultimately pierce the dural sac as well as the filum terminale that helps to anchor it. The dural sac will extend into the intervertebral foramina and along the ventral and dorsal nerve roots distal to the dorsal root ganglia to form the **dural root sheaths**. The dural root sheaths are continuous with the outer epineurium of the spinal nerves.

The space located between the vertebrae and the dura mater is called the **epidural space**. This space runs the entire length of the vertebral canal beginning at the level of the foramen magnum and inferiorly to the level of the sacral hiatus being sealed off by the *sacrococcygeal ligament*. It also extends laterally at the intervertebral foramina just as the dura mater adheres to the periosteum surrounding each opening. In addition to a thin layer of **epidural fat** the *internal vertebral venous plexus* fills the epidural space.

Arachnoid Mater

The arachnoid mater is the thin, avascular intermediate meningeal layer that is composed of fibrous and elastic tissue (**Fig. 1.28**; **Fig. 1.29**). It lines the internal surface of the dural sac and dural root sheaths but is not technically attached to them. Instead it is held up against the dura mater by the pressure of the **cerebrospinal fluid (CSF)**. CSF is located in the **subarachnoid space** located between the arachnoid and pia mater. The subarachnoid space matches the location of the dural sac but also extends into the cranium. Spanning the subarachnoid space are very delicate strands of connective tissue called the **arachnoid trabeculae** and they connect the arachnoid to the pia mater (**Fig. 1.29**).

There is a potential space between arachnoid and dura mater layers and it is called the *subdural space*. It is generally a trauma situation involving bleeding that results in the creation of this space. The lack of CSF passing through the subarachnoid space in a cadaver opens the *subdural space* that normally is not present in living individuals.

Pia Mater

The innermost layer of the meninges is the pia mater (**Fig. 1.28**; **Fig. 1.29**). It is made of flattened cells with long and equally flattened processes that follow the surface of the spinal cord, spinal blood vessels and roots of the spinal cord. The filum terminale, while passing through the lumbar cistern of the subarachnoid space, is made of condensed pia mater. The filum terminale, along with the structures called denticulate ligaments, help to suspend the spinal cord within the dural sac, but both have a limited role in preventing unwanted motion of the spinal cord.

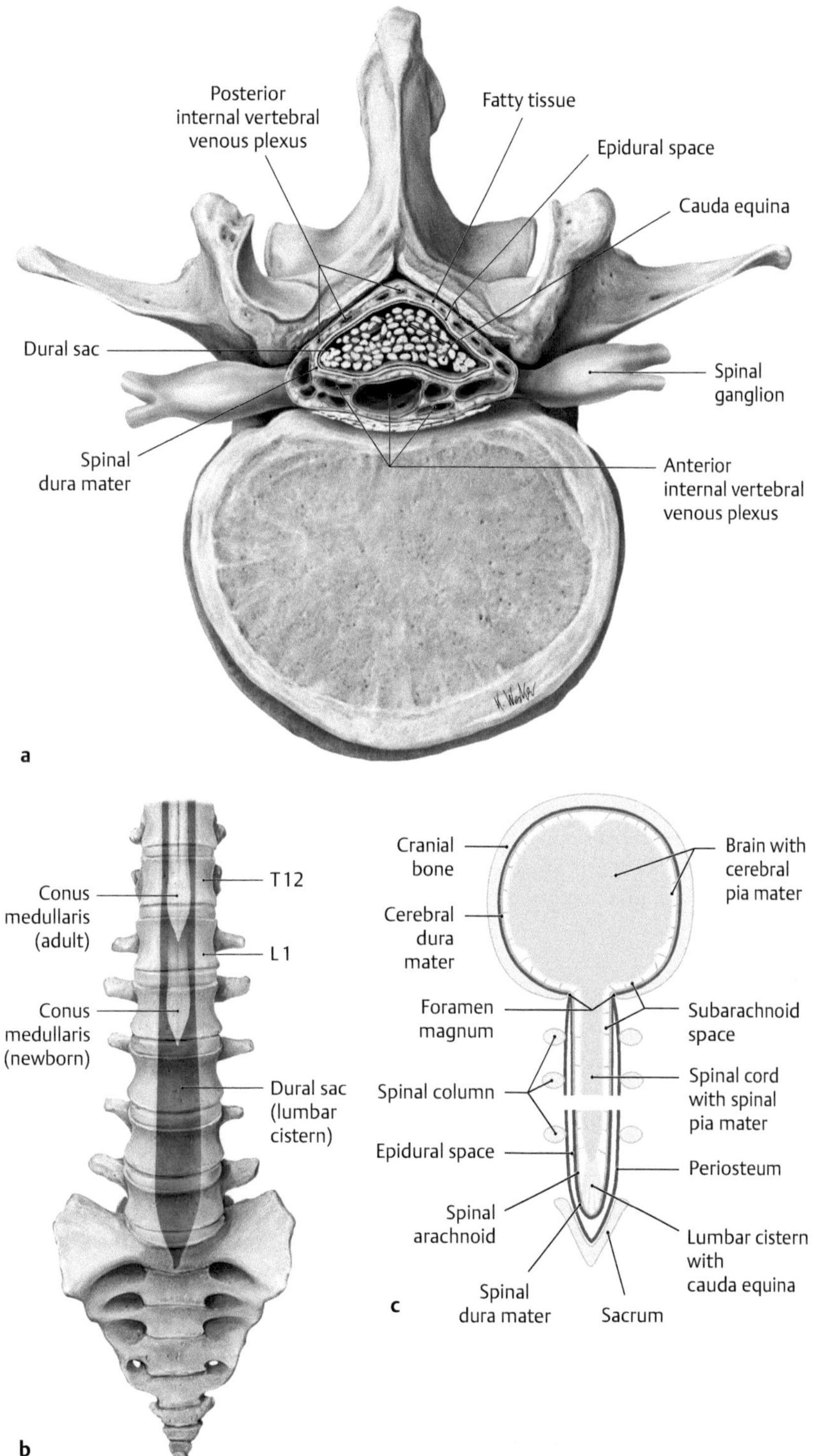

Fig. 1.27 **(a)** Cauda equina in situ, transverse section at L2, superior view. **(b)** The spinal cord, dural sac, and vertebral column at different stages, anterior view. **(c)** Meninges in the cranial cavity and spinal canal. (From Schuenke M, Schulte E, Schumacher U. THIEME Atlas of Anatomy. Head, Neck, and Neuroanatomy. Illustrations by Voll M and Wesker K. 3rd ed. New York: Thieme Medical Publishers; 2020.)

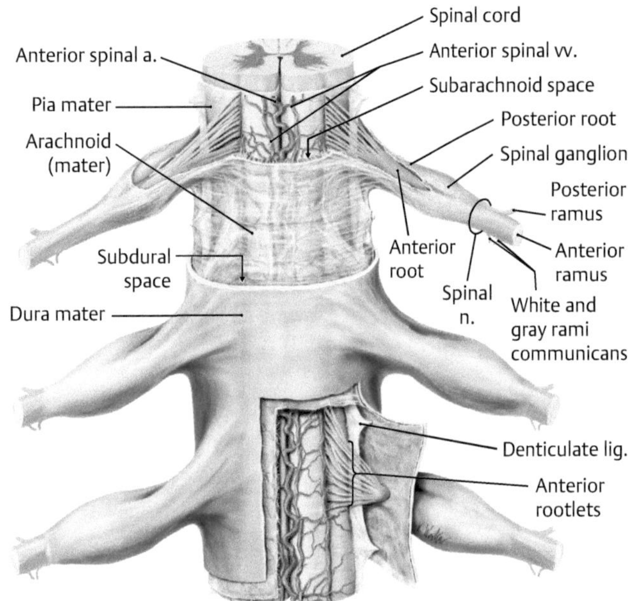

Fig. 1.28 Spinal cord and its meningeal layers, anterior view. (From Schuenke M, Schulte E, Schumacher U. THIEME Atlas of Anatomy. Head, Neck, and Neuroanatomy. Illustrations by Voll M and Wesker K. 3rd ed. New York: Thieme Medical Publishers; 2020.)

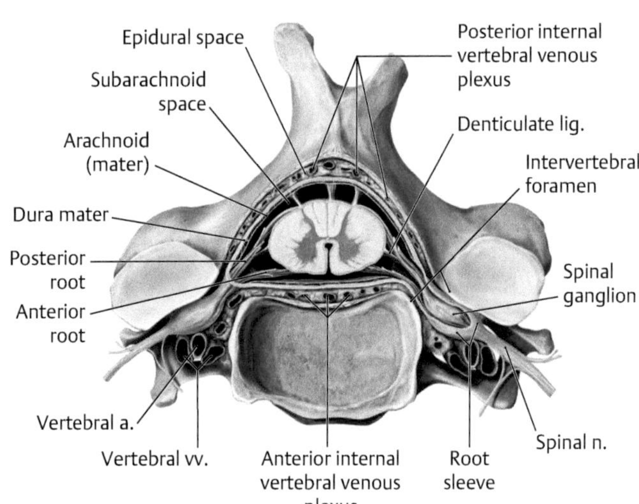

Fig. 1.29 Cervical spinal cord in situ, transverse section at C4. (From Schuenke M, Schulte E, Schumacher U. THIEME Atlas of Anatomy. Head, Neck, and Neuroanatomy. Illustrations by Voll M and Wesker K. 3rd ed. New York: Thieme Medical Publishers; 2020.)

Denticulate ligaments are tooth-like extensions or sheets of pia mater passing between a ventral and dorsal nerve root before anchoring into the dura mater. There are approximately 20-22 of them located from the craniovertebral junction down to T12-L1 nerve root (**Fig. 1.28**).

1.11 Muscles of the Back

There are two major groups of muscles associated with the back, the extrinsic and intrinsic muscles. The extrinsic back muscles are further subdivided into superficial and intermediate muscle groups. They control the upper limbs and respiratory muscles. The intrinsic back muscles are subdivided into superficial, intermediate and deep muscle groups and act specifically on the vertebral column in order to control its movements and maintain normal posture.

Most muscles acting on the cervical portion of the vertebral column are known as the prevertebral muscles and they are described in detail in Chapter 7. When a person is standing erect, the back muscles are fairly inactive. They are primarily acting in this situation as postural muscles, maintaining the stability of the vertebral column by providing constant tension. Most movements of the vertebral column, except for extension, will involve the anterolateral abdominal wall muscles. It is the abdominal wall muscles that create the concentric contraction and the intrinsic back muscles that provide the eccentric contraction creating a smooth and controlled movement.

1.11.1 Extrinsic Back Muscles

The **superficial extrinsic back muscles** make up the posterior axio-appendicular muscles that attach the vertebral column of the axial skeleton to the pectoral girdle and humerus of the superior appendicular skeleton (**Fig. 1.30**). These muscles include the *trapezius, latissimus dorsi, levator scapulae* and *rhomboids* and they are responsible for producing and controlling upper limb movements. Nerves originating from the ventral rami and a cranial nerve are responsible for innervating extrinsic back muscles. Descriptions of these muscles are found in **Table 1.1**.

The **intermediate extrinsic back muscles** consist of two very thin muscles known as the *serratus posterior superior* and *serratus posterior inferior*. These two muscles are also considered muscles of the thoracic wall and have been known in the past as accessory respiratory muscles but probably have more of a proprioceptive function. Details of these are presented in Chapter 2 (**Fig. 1.30**).

1.11.2 Intrinsic Back Muscles

The **intrinsic "true" back muscles** (deep back) have the primary function of maintaining posture and exerting control of vertebral column movements directly. These muscles can be found between the base of the skull and the pelvic region. There are three layers of intrinsic back muscles: superficial, intermediate and deep. All intrinsic back muscles are innervated by dorsal rami of spinal nerves.

The *superficial layer* consists of the **splenius muscles** (**splenius capitis** and **splenius cervicis**) that are thick and flat and located on the posterior neck and are described in **Table 1.2**. The *intermediate layer* is made up of the **erector spinae**, which is located over large portions of the back and divided into three parts or columns. These columns are arranged from medial to lateral as the **spinalis**, **longissimus** and **iliocostalis** of the larger erector spinae. Each of these columns is divided into three parts and named based on the region of its superior attachment. They function as lateral flexors and as the chief extensors of the vertebral column. Descriptions of these muscles are found in **Table 1.3** (**Fig. 1.31**).

The *deep layer* is made up of a group of muscles known as the **transversospinalis muscles**. These muscles are located in an area known as the "gutter" region between the spinous and transverse processes of the vertebrae and just deep to the erector spinae. They are arranged from superficial to deep as the **semispinalis**,

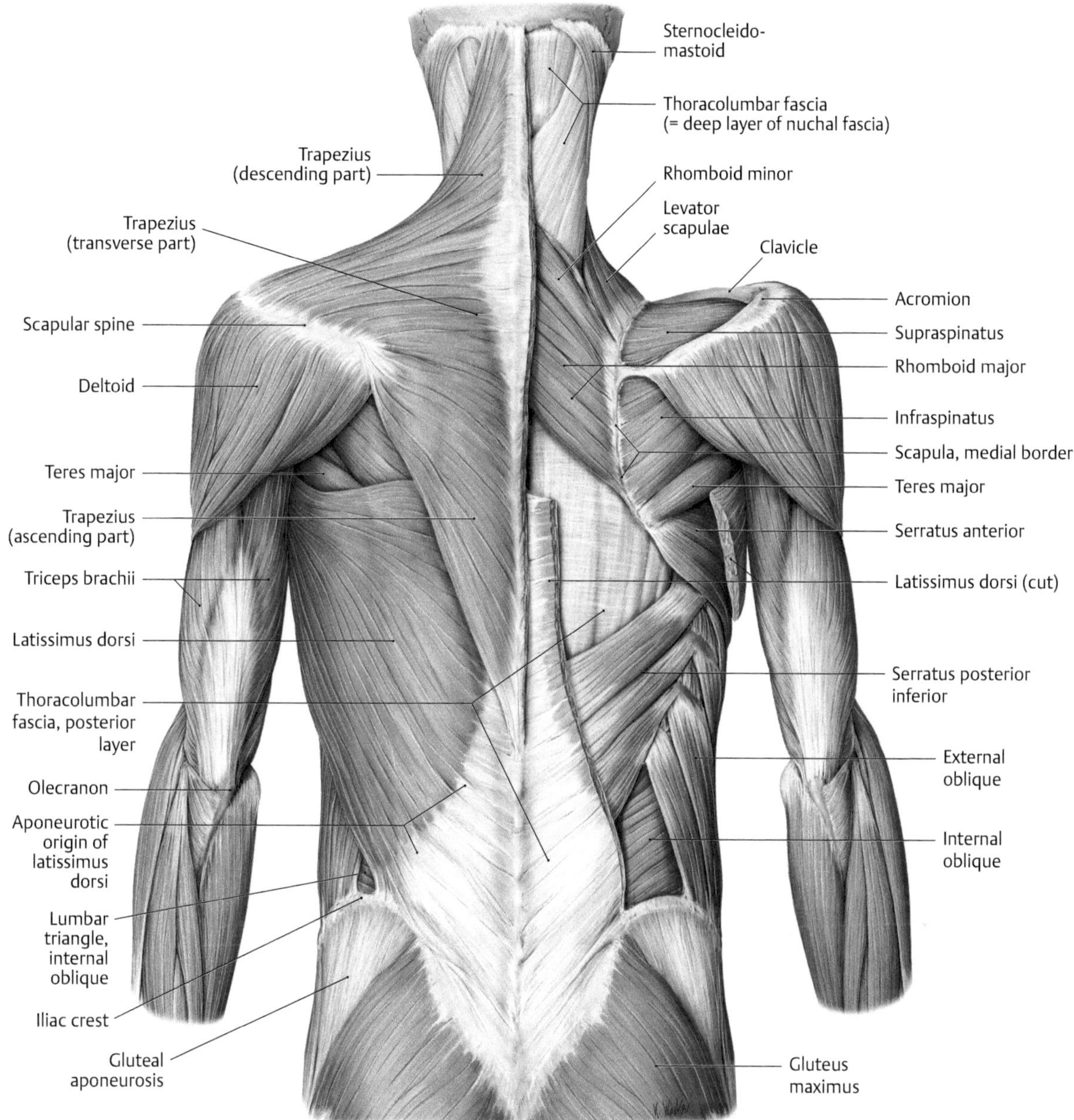

Fig. 1.30 Extrinsic back muscles. (From Schuenke M, Schulte E, Schumacher U. THIEME Atlas of Anatomy. General Anatomy and Musculoskeletal System. Illustrations by Voll M and Wesker K. 3rd ed. New York: Thieme Medical Publishers; 2020.)

Table 1.1 **Superficial extrinsic back muscles**

Muscle	Innervation	Function(s)	Origin	Insertion
Trapezius	Spinal accessory nerve (CN XI) and ventral rami of C2–C4 for pain and proprioception	*Superior fibers*: elevate scapula; *Middle fibers*: retract scapula; *Inferior fibers*: depress scapula; *superior and inferior fibers* together superiorly rotate the scapula	Medial 1/3 of superior nuchal line; external occipital protuberance; nuchal ligament; C7-T12 spinous processes	Lateral 1/3 of clavicle; acromion and spine of scapula
Latissimus dorsi	Thoracodorsal nerve	Adducts, extends and medially rotates humerus	T7-T12 spinous processes; thoracolumbar fascia; iliac crest; inferior 3-4 ribs	Intertubercular sulcus (bicipital groove) of humerus (floor of)
Levator scapulae	Dorsal scapular nerve	Elevates and inferiorly rotates scapula	C1-C4 transverse processes	Superior angle and superomedial border of scapula
Rhomboids (major and minor)	Dorsal scapular nerve	Retracts and inferiorly rotates scapula	*Minor*: nuchal ligament, C7-T1 spinous processes; *Major*: T2-T5 spinous processes	*Minor*: medial border of scapula (above scapular spine); *Major*: medial border of scapula (below scapular spine)

Table 1.2 **Superficial layer of intrinsic back muscles**

Muscle	Innervation	Function(s)	Origin	Insertion
Splenius (*capitis* and *cervicis*)	Dorsal rami of spinal nerves	*As an individual muscle*: lateral flexion of neck; rotate head to side of active muscles *As a group*: extension of head and neck	Nuchal ligament and spinous processes of C7-T4	*Splenius capitis*: mastoid process of temporal bone and lateral 1/3 of superior nuchal line of occipital bone *Splenius cervicis*: tubercles of transverse processes of C1-C4 vertebrae

Table 1.3 **Intermediate layer of intrinsic back muscles**

Muscle	Innervation	Function(s)	Origin	Insertion
Erector spinae (*spinalis*, *longissimus* and *iliocostalis*)	Dorsal rami of spinal nerves	*Acting unilaterally the erector spinae*: laterally flexes vertebral column; *Acting bilaterally the erector spinae*: extends vertebral column and head; control flexion of back by gradually lengthening their fibers	The erector spinae arises as a broad tendon from the posterior part of the iliac crest, posterior surface of sacrum, spinous processes of sacrum and lower lumbar vertebrae, and supraspinous ligament	*Spinalis* (thoracis, cervicis, capitis): spinous processes in upper thoracic region and to cranium *Longissimus* (thoracis, cervicis, capitis): between tubercles and angles of ribs; transverse processes in thoracic and cervical regions; mastoid process of temporal bone *Iliocostalis* (lumborum, thoracis, cervicis): angles of lower ribs; cervical transverse processes

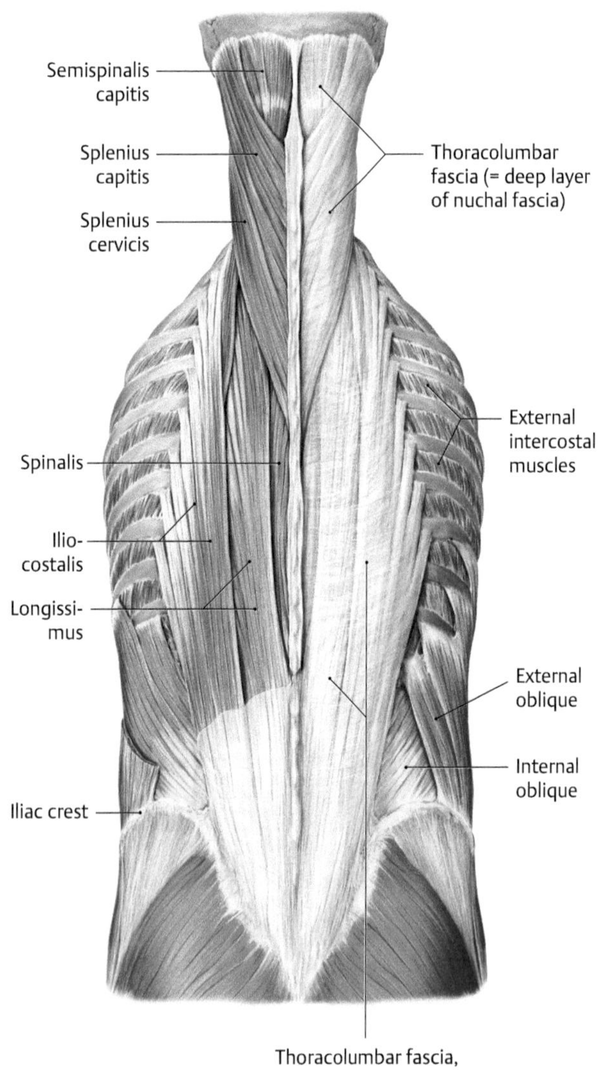

Fig. 1.31 Superficial and intermediate intrinsic back muscles. (From Schuenke M, Schulte E, Schumacher U. THIEME Atlas of Anatomy. General Anatomy and Musculoskeletal System. Illustrations by Voll M and Wesker K. 3rd ed. New York: Thieme Medical Publishers; 2020.)

multifidus and **rotatores** muscles. The semispinalis is further divided into three parts and named based on their locations: the **semispinalis capitis**, **semispinalis cervicis** and **semispinalis thoracis**. Descriptions of these muscles are found in **Table 1.4 (Fig. 1.32)**.

There is a group of *minor muscles* located in the deep layer. They are, from medial to lateral, the **interspinales**, **intertransversarii** and **levator costarum**. They are initially named based on the attachment points that include the spinous process, transverse process and ribs. The interspinales and intertransversarii muscles can also be classified based on their location. Descriptions of these muscles are found in **Table 1.5 (Fig. 1.33)**.

1.11.3 Suboccipital Triangle

The **suboccipital triangle** is a bilateral region deep to the superior part of the posterior cervical region and it underlies the sternocleidomastoid, trapezius, splenius and semispinalis muscles. There are four muscles specifically located in this region and they are the **obliquus capitis superior**, **obliquus capitis inferior**, **rectus capitis posterior major** and **rectus capitis posterior minor**. Only the rectus capitis posterior minor does not help define a border of the suboccipital triangle. These muscles serve as postural muscles. Descriptions of these muscles are found in **Table 1.6 (Fig. 1.34)**.

The obliquus capitis superior forms the superolateral border; the obliquus capitis inferior forms the inferolateral border; and the rectus capitis posterior major forms the superomedial border. The posterior atlanto-occipital membrane along with the posterior arch of the C1 vertebra defines the floor while the roof of the triangle is considered the semispinalis capitis muscle.

The contents of this triangle include the **suboccipital nerve**, the dorsal rami nerve branch of C1 that innervates all four muscles of this region. The **3rd (suboccipital) part of the vertebral artery** courses along an arterial groove of the C1 vertebrae before passing through the *posterior atlanto-occipital membrane*. This defect allows for the passage of the suboccipital nerve as well. The **suboccipital venous plexus** collects blood from this region and drains into the vertebral veins **(Fig. 1.35)**.

Table 1.4 **Deep layer of intrinsic back muscles (transversospinalis)**

Muscle	Innervation	Function(s)	Origin	Insertion
Semispinalis (*capitis*, *cervicis* and *thoracis*)	Dorsal rami of spinal nerves	Extends head and cervical and thoracic regions of vertebral column; and rotates these regions contralaterally	Transverse processes of C4-T10 vertebrae	Fibers run superomedially to the occipital bone and spinous processes of cervical and upper thoracic regions spanning 4-6 segments
Multifidus	Dorsal rami of spinal nerves	Unilateral contraction rotates vertebral column to contralateral side; stabilizes vertebrae during local vertebral column movements	Posterior sacrum, posterior superior iliac spine of ilium, aponeurosis of erector spinae, sacro-iliac ligaments, mammillary processes of lumbar vertebrae, transverse processes of T1-T3, and articular processes of C4-C7.	Fibers run superomedially to spinous processes 2-4 segments above the origin throughout the entire vertebral column
Rotatores (*longus* and *brevis*)	Dorsal rami of spinal nerves	Possible proprioception function; stabilize vertebrae and assist with local extension and rotary movements of vertebral column	Transverse processes of primarily the thoracic vertebrae	Fibers run superomedially to attach to junction of lamina and transverse or spinous process of vertebra 2 segments above (longus) or immediately (brevis) of origin

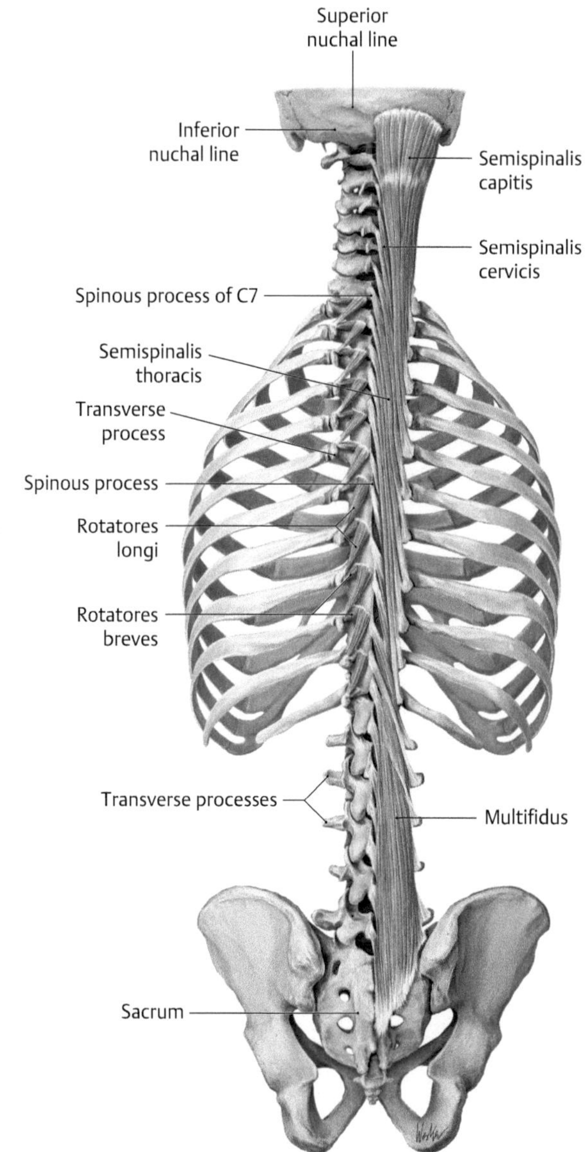

Fig. 1.32 Transverosospinalis muscles: rotatores, multifidus, and semispinalis. (From Schuenke M, Schulte E, Schumacher U. THIEME Atlas of Anatomy. General Anatomy and Musculoskeletal System. Illustrations by Voll M and Wesker K. 3rd ed. New York: Thieme Medical Publishers; 2020.)

1.12 Development of the Vertebral Column and Back Region

The vertebrae originate from the sclerotome portion of the somites (**Fig. 1.36**). During the fourth week of development, the sclerotome cells migrate around the notochord and spinal cord and eventually blend with cells from the opposing somite located on the other side of the neural tube. The sclerotomes consist of loosely arranged cells cranially and densely packed cells caudally. Some of the densely packed cells move cranially and opposite the center of the myotome where they contribute to the development of the IV disc. The remaining densely packed cells fuse with the loosely arranged cells of the immediately caudal sclerotomes to form the **centrum**, or early vertebral body. The mesenchymal cells that surround the neural tube form the **neural arch**, the future vertebral arches.

With continued growth, the sclerotome portion of each somite undergoes a process called **resegmentation**, by which the caudal half of each sclerotome expands into and fuses with the cranial half of each underlying sclerotome. Thus the vertebrae are formed by a combination of the caudal half of one somite and the cranial half of an adjacent somite.

The mesenchymal cells located between the cranial and caudal portions of the original sclerotome segment do not proliferate but instead fill the space between two precartilaginous vertebral bodies and contribute to the formation of the IV disc. The notochord regresses completely in the areas of the vertebral bodies but persists and enlarges in the region of the intervertebral disc to become the *nucleus pulposus*. This is then surrounded by the circular fibers of the *anulus fibrosus* and can be considered a complete intervertebral disc.

Resegmentation also causes the myotomes to bridge the intervertebral discs, giving them the ability to move the spine. For similar reasons, the **intersegmental arteries** at first lie between the sclerotomes but later pass midway over the vertebral bodies. These would become the *intercostal arteries* or *nutrient arteries* supplying the vertebral bodies, for example. The spinal nerves will come to lie adjacent to the intervertebral discs and exit through the intervertebral foramen.

Ossification begins at around the 8th week of development and there are three **primary ossification centers**: the *centrum* and an

Table 1.5 **(Minor) deep layer of intrinsic back muscles**

Muscle	Innervation	Function(s)	Origin	Insertion
Interspinales (*cervicis* and *lumbora*)	Dorsal rami of spinal nerves	*Cervicis*: extend cervical region; *Lumborum*: extend lumbar region	Superior surface of cervical or lumbar spinous processes	Inferior surface of cervical or lumbar spinous processes
Intertransversarii (*anterior cervices, posterior cervices, medial lumbora,* and *lateral lumbora*)	Dorsal rami of spinal nerves (*posterior cervices* and *medial lumbora*) and ventral rami of spinal nerves (*anterior cervices* and *lateral lumbora*)	*Acting unilaterally*: lateral flexion of the cervical or lumbar vertebral column to ipsilateral side; *Acting bilaterally*: extends and stabilizes the cervical or lumbar vertebral column	Transverse processes of cervical or lumbar vertebrae	Transverse processes of adjacent cervical or lumbar vertebrae
Levatores costarum (*longi* and *breves*)	Dorsal rami of C7-T11 spinal nerves	Elevate ribs; *Acting unilaterally*: lateral flexion of thoracic vertebral column to ipsilateral side and rotates to contralateral side; *Acting bilaterally*: extends thoracic vertebral column	Transverse processes of C7-T11	Near costal angles of T1-T12

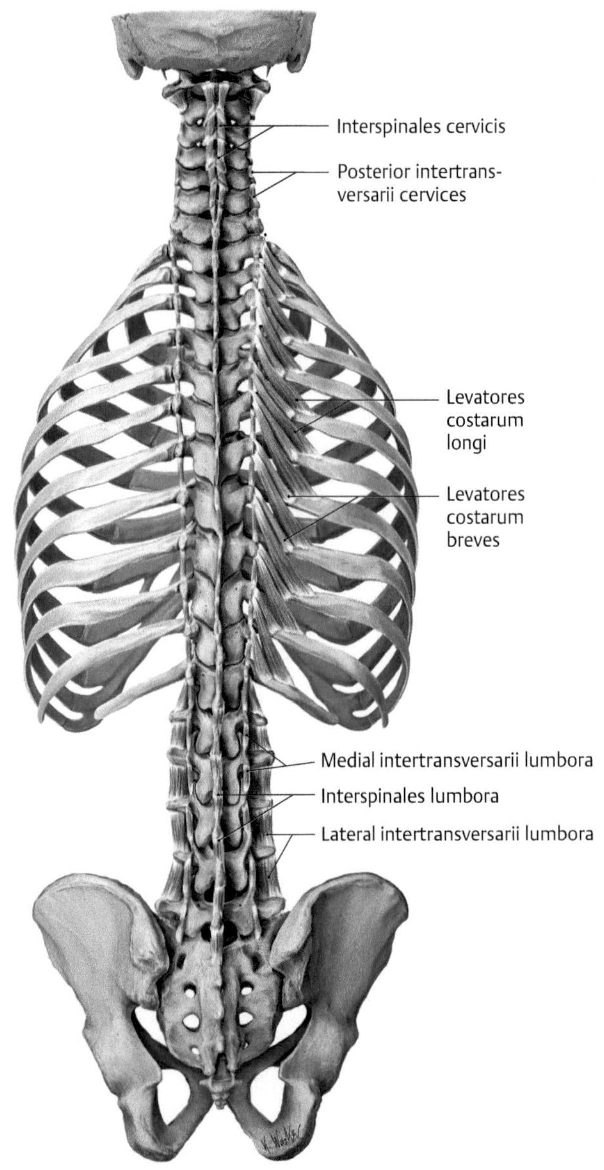

Fig. 1.33 Deep segmental muscles: interspinales, intertransversarii, and levatores costarum. (From Schuenke M, Schulte E, Schumacher U. THIEME Atlas of Anatomy. General Anatomy and Musculoskeletal System. Illustrations by Voll M and Wesker K. 3rd ed. New York: Thieme Medical Publishers; 2020.)

isolated portion on *each side of the neural arch*. At birth, each vertebra will consist of three bony portions connected by cartilage. The bony halves of the vertebral arch usually fuse between 3-5 years of age. The arches of the lumbar region are the first to unite and extend cranially. Where the vertebral arches articulate with the centrum is called the **neurocentral joints** and these joints allow the vertebral arches to grow while the spinal cord enlarges and they themselves will disappear by 3-6 years of age. There are five **secondary ossification centers** that appear after puberty and they are located at the *tip of the spinous process*, the *tip of each transverse process*, and at the *anular epiphyses* of both the superior and inferior edges of the vertebral body.

The C1 and C2 vertebrae develop slightly differently in that the centrum of C1 fuses with that of C2 and becomes the dens (odontoid process). This will leave only the neural arch, which grows anteriorly before finally fusing in the midline to form the characteristic ring shape of C1.

Skeletal muscle development originates from the myotome. The myotomes will divide into a dorsal **epaxial** and ventral **hypaxial** set of muscles. The epaxial muscles will develop into muscles associated with the vertebral column, the ribs and the base of the skull and are all innervated by dorsal rami spinal nerve branches. This includes the splenius, erector spinae and transversospinalis muscle groups along with the suboccipital region muscles. The hypaxial muscles include all the remaining muscles such as the diaphragm, abdominal wall and both of the limbs muscles. These muscles are innervated by ventral rami branches of the spinal nerves and would include the extrinsic muscles of the back region (**Fig. 1.36**).

Table 1.6 **Suboccipital muscles**

Muscle	Innervation	Function(s)	Origin	Insertion
Obliquus capitis superior	Suboccipital nerve	*Acting unilaterally*: lateral flexion of head to ipsilateral side; rotates head to contralateral side *Acting bilaterally*: extends head	Transverse process of C1 vertebra	Occipital bone between superior and inferior nuchal lines just above rectus capitis posterior major
Obliquus capitis inferior	Suboccipital nerve	*Acting unilaterally*: rotates head to ipsilateral side *Acting bilaterally*: extends head	Posterior tubercle of posterior arch of C2 vertebra	Transverse process of C1 vertebra
Rectus capitis posterior major	Suboccipital nerve	*Acting unilaterally*: rotates head to ipsilateral side *Acting bilaterally*: extends head	Spinous process of C2 vertebra	Lateral portion of inferior nuchal line
Rectus capitis posterior minor	Suboccipital nerve	*Acting unilaterally*: rotates head to ipsilateral side *Acting bilaterally*: extends head	Posterior tubercle of posterior arch of C1 vertebra	Medial portion of inferior nuchal line

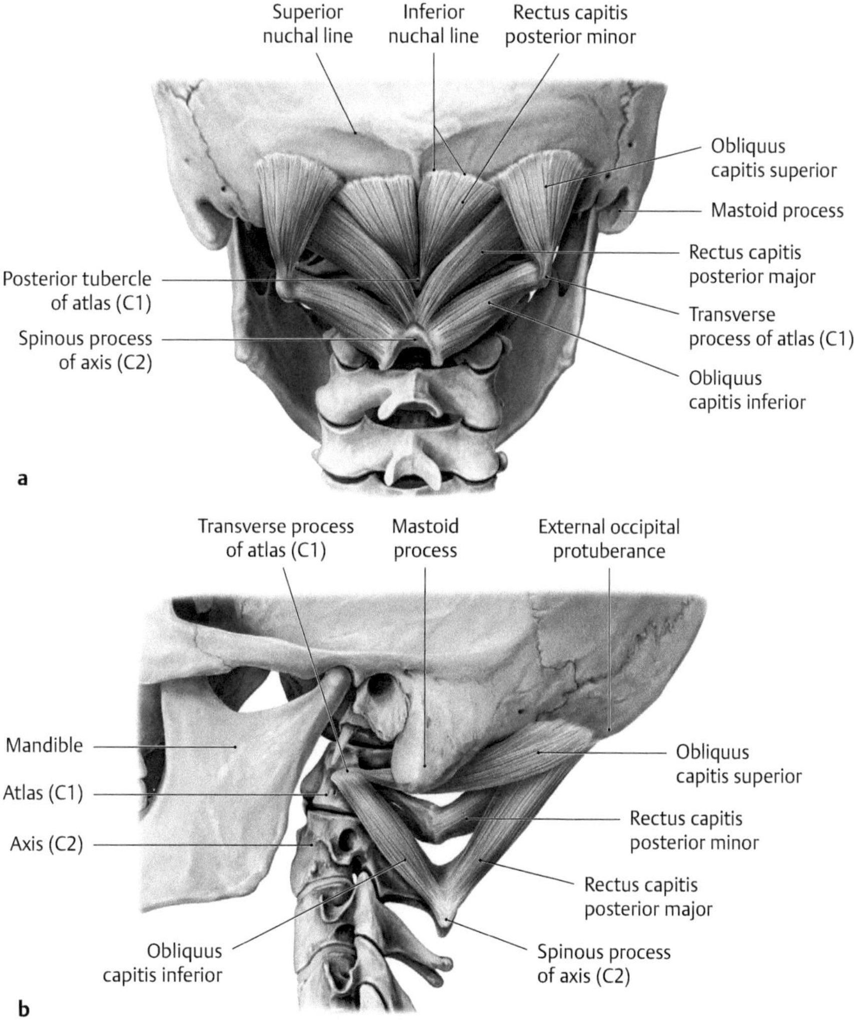

Fig. 1.34 Suboccipital muscle. **(a)** Posterior view. **(b)** Left lateral view. (From Schuenke M, Schulte E, Schumacher U. THIEME Atlas of Anatomy. General Anatomy and Musculoskeletal System. Illustrations by Voll M and Wesker K. 3rd ed. New York: Thieme Medical Publishers; 2020.)

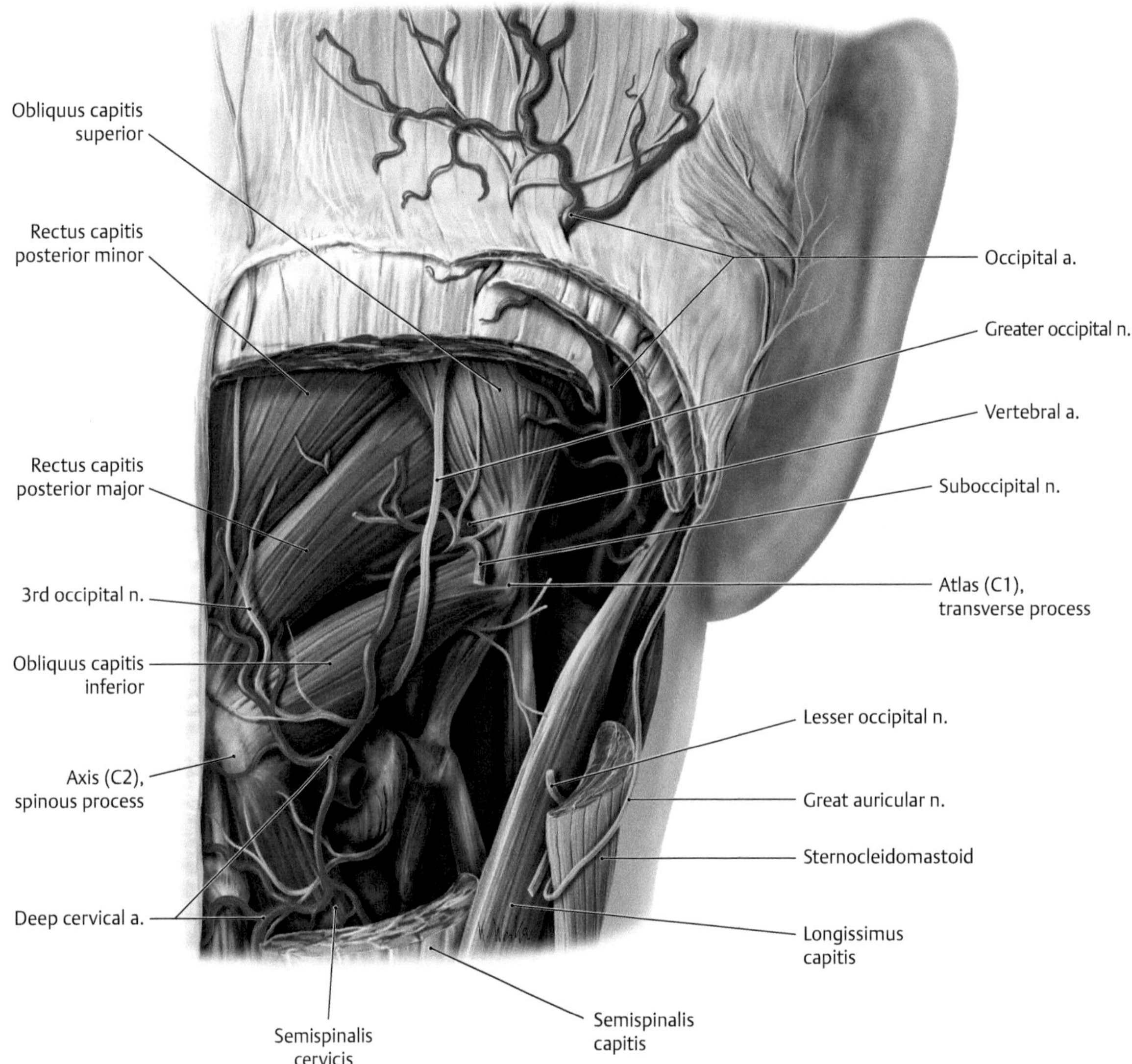

Fig. 1.35 Neurovasculature of the suboccipital region, posterior view. (From Schuenke M, Schulte E, Schumacher U. THIEME Atlas of Anatomy. General Anatomy and Musculoskeletal System. Illustrations by Voll M and Wesker K. 3rd ed. New York: Thieme Medical Publishers; 2020.)

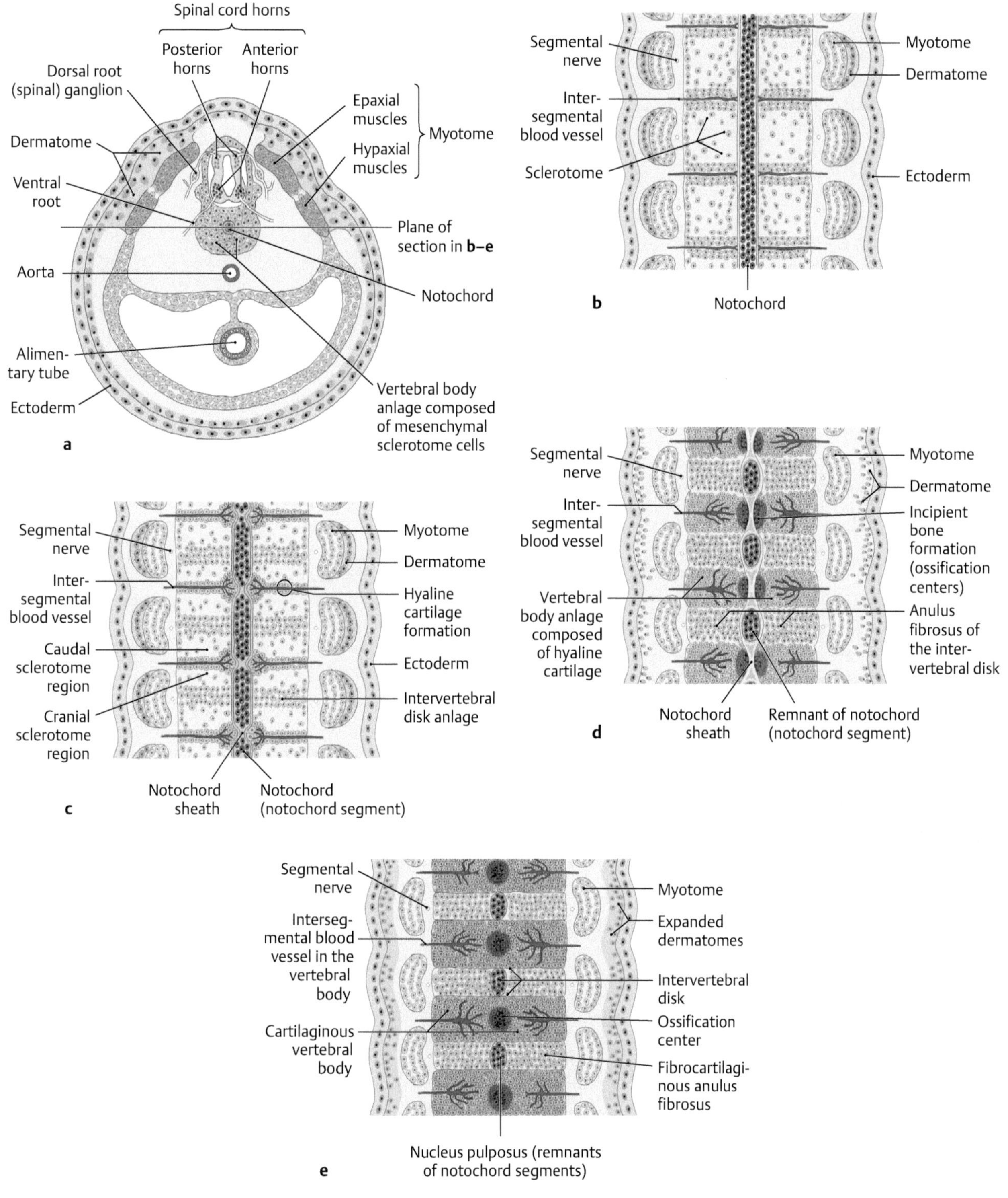

Fig. 1.36 Development of the spinal column (weeks 4-10). **(a)** Schematic cross section. **(b-e)** Schematic coronal sections as identified in **a**. **(a,b)** The somites have differentiated into the dermatome, myotome, and sclerotome. The sclerotome cells separate and migrate toward the notochord and form a cluster of mesenechymal cells around the notochord. **(c)** The adjacent cranial and caudal sclerotome segments above and below the intersegmental vessels join together and begin to chondrify in the sixth week, displacing notochordal material. **(d)** The IV disks with their nucleus pulposus and anulus fibrosus develop between the rudimentary vertebral bodies. Ossification begins at the center of the vertebral bodies in the eighth week. **(e)** By fusion of the cranial and caudal sclerotome segments, the segmentally arranged myotomes interconnect the processes of two adjacent vertebral horns (a), bridging the gap across the intervertebral disks. The segmental spinal nerve courses at the level of the future intervertebral foramen, and the intersegmental vessels become the nutrient vessels of the vertebral bodies. (From Schuenke M, Schulte E, Schumacher U. THIEME Atlas of Anatomy. General Anatomy and Musculoskeletal System. Illustrations by Voll M and Wesker K. 3rd ed. New York: Thieme Medical Publishers; 2020.)

PRACTICE QUESTIONS

1. A patient is admitted to the hospital after dropping a large box onto their lower neck and upper shoulder regions. The patient is having difficulty elevating and depressing their scapula and they are unable to inferiorly rotate their shoulder. Which nerve is most likely to be compressed if these functions are unable to occur?
   A. Suboccipital.
   B. Dorsal scapular.
   C. Thoracodorsal.
   D. Spinal accessory.
   E. Multiple dorsal rami branches.
2. Which statement related to the spinal cord is CORRECT?
   A. The cervical enlargement is made up of C1-C4 spinal segments.
   B. The adult spinal cord terminates at vertebral level L3.
   C. Cerebrospinal fluid flows through the subdural space.
   D. The spinal cord consists of 31 spinal segments.
   E. The lumbar cistern is the part of the dorsal sac that extends from the base of the skull to vertebral level L1.
3. Which statement related to the back region is CORRECT?
   A. The ventral rami of C1 is called the suboccipital nerve.
   B. The most common congenital anomaly of the vertebral column is spina bifida cystica.
   C. The nucleus pulposus of the IV disc is situated on the anterior aspect of the disc.
   D. Excessive lordosis would affect the thoracic or sacral curvatures and is called "humpback."
   E. A posterolateral herniation of the nucleus pulposus of the IV disk between L3 and L4, would result in compression of the L4 spinal nerve.
4. A brawl breaks out and an individual is stabbed in the suboccipital triangle, damaging the suboccipital nerve. Which muscle would NOT be affected by injury to the suboccipital nerve?
   A. Rectus capitis posterior minor.
   B. Obliquus capitis superior.
   C. Obliquus capitis inferior.
   D. Splenius capitis.
   E. Rectus capitis posterior major.
5. Which statement about the trapezius muscle is INCORRECT?
   A. Superior fibers elevate the scapula.
   B. Inferior fibers depress the scapula.
   C. Superior and inferior fibers inferiorly rotate the scapula.
   D. Superior and inferior fibers superiorly rotate the scapula.
   E. It is innervated by the spinal accessory nerve (CN XI).
6. When palpating the spinous processes of the vertebral column during a physical examination, which spinous process matches the CORRECT corresponding anatomical structure?
   A. T7 – inferior angle of the scapula.
   B. T3 – vertebra prominens.
   C. T5 – superior angle of the scapula.
   D. C7 – spine of the scapula.
   E. T12 – iliac crest.
7. A 22-year-old college student is brought to the emergency department after complaining of a constant and severe headache along with a fever and chills. There has been a recent outbreak of meningitis on campus, so the physician would like to perform a spinal tap to confirm or rule out a meningitis infection. In what order would a needle pierce certain structures before it reached the cerebrospinal fluid (CSF)?
   A. Skin, ligamentum flavum, posterior longitudinal ligament, epidural space, dura mater, arachnoid mater, then subarachnoid space.
   B. Skin, ligamentum flavum, epidural space, dura mater, arachnoid mater, then subarachnoid space.
   C. Skin, posterior longitudinal ligament, ligamentum flavum, epidural space, dura mater, arachnoid mater, then subarachnoid space.
   D. Skin, ligamentum flavum, dura mater, arachnoid mater, pia mater, then subarachnoid space.
   E. Skin, epidural space, ligamentum flavum, dura mater, arachnoid mater, then subarachnoid space.
8. Which statement about the spinal meninges is CORRECT?
   A. The subdural space is between the arachnoid and pia mater.
   B. The dural sac extends inferiorly to vertebral level L5.
   C. Denticulate ligaments originate from pia mater.
   D. Arachnoid trabeculae connect the dura to the arachnoid mater.
   E. The pia mater is the outermost meningeal layer.
9. What is the function of the posterior longitudinal ligament?
   A. Prevents excessive rotation of the spine.
   B. Prevents hyperflexion of the spine.
   C. Preserve the curvatures of the spine.
   D. Prevents hyperextension of the spine.
   E. Weak stabilizer of the vertebral column.
10. A 71-year-old woman with a history of osteoporosis has recently fallen. She complains of pain in the lower back region, so her doctor orders an oblique view X-ray to examine the appearance of "Scotty Dog" as he suspects that there is a fracture leading to spondylolysis. On the X-ray, if a fracture is present, what structure on Scotty Dog would be broken?
    A. Ear.
    B. Nose.
    C. Front leg.
    D. Neck.
    E. Eye.
11. A 51-year-old woman has been brought into the emergency department due to an apparent diving accident. After a CT scan, there was no apparent damage to the spinal cord, but she was diagnosed with a Jefferson fracture. Which vertebra has been fractured?
    A. C1.
    B. C2.
    C. C7.
    D. L5.
    E. S1.
12. Which muscle of the back listed below is NOT innervated by a dorsal rami nerve branch?
    A. Splenius capitis.
    B. Multifidis.
    C. Rhomboids.
    D. Semispinalis.
    E. Longissimus of erector spinae.
13. There are certain characteristic structures seen on specific types of vertebrae. Of the ones listed below, which structure is correctly paired with the vertebral region?
    A. Demifacet/cervical vertebrae.
    B. Hatchet-shaped spinous process/lumbar vertebrae.
    C. Promontory/thoracic vertebrae.
    D. Transverse foramen/lumbar vertebrae.
    E. Costal facet/sacrum.
14. A 61 year-old obese female presents to her physician initially complaining of low back pain. The pain has gradually become

worse over the past few years. A bone mineral density scan is performed and osteoporosis has been diagnosed at the L2 and L3 vertebrae. The normal curvature of the lumbar vertebrae now is much more exaggerated and it was noted the gap between the exam table and her lower back was quite pronounced. What would your diagnosis be?
A. Lordosis.
B. Scoliosis.
C. Spondylolysis.
D. Kyphosis.
E. Spinal stenosis.

15. An individual presents with bone spurs or osteophytes at multiple uncovertebral joints of the vertebral column. The bone spurs are already leading to compression of the nearby spinal nerves but what artery would be at risk to damage?
A. Posterior intercostal artery.
B. Lumbar artery.
C. Vertebral artery.
D. Median sacral.
E. Lateral sacral.

ANSWERS

1. **B.** The functional deficits displayed are consistent with the functions of both the levator scapulae and rhomboid muscles and these muscles are innervated by the dorsal scapular nerve.
2. **D.** There 8 cervical, 12 thoracic, 5 lumbar, 5 sacral and 1 coccygeal spinal segments for a total of 31.
A. The cervical enlargement includes spinal segments C4-T1.
B. The adult spinal cord terminates at vertebral level L1.
C. Cerebrospinal fluid flows through the subarachnoid space.
E. The lumbar cistern is the part of the dorsal sac that extends from vertebral levels L1-S2.
3. **E.** A posterolateral herniation resulting in compression between L3 and L4 would only affect the L4 nerve roots.
A. The dorsal rami of C1 is called the suboccipital nerve.
B. The most common congenital anomaly of the vertebral column is spina bifida occulta.
C. The nucleus pulposus of the IV disc is situated on the posterior aspect of the disc.
D. Excessive lordosis would affect the cervical and lumbar curvatures of the vertebral column and is known as "hollow back."
4. **D.** All of the muscles listed are innervated by the suboccipital nerve except for the splenius capitis.
5. **C.** All answers are incorrect except for C. The superior and inferior fibers of the trapezius when working in concert with one another inferiorly rotate the scapula.
6. **A.** The inferior angle of the scapula is located at T7.
B. The vertebra prominens is located at C7.
C. The superior angle of the scapula is located at about T1.
D. The spine of the scapula is located at T3.
E. The iliac crest is located at L4.
7. **B.** The correct order a needle would pass through before reaching CSF would be skin, ligamentum flavum, epidural space, dura mater, arachnoid mater, then subarachnoid space.
8. **C.** Denticulate ligaments originate from the pia before passing toward the dura mater.
A. The subdural space is a potential space located between the dura and arachnoid maters.
B. The dural sac extends inferiorly to vertebral level S2.
D. The arachnoid trabeculae connect the arachnoid to the pia mater.
E. The pia mater is the innermost meningeal layer.
9. **B.** The posterior longitudinal ligament prevents hyperflexion.
A. The alar ligament prevents excessive rotation between the C1 and C2 vertebrae.
C. The ligamentum flavum help preserve the curvatures of the vertebral column.
D. The anterior longitudinal ligament prevents hyperextension.
E. The interspinous ligaments are a weak stabilizer of the vertebral column.
10. **D.** If spondylolysis is present, a fracture of Scotty Dog's neck is present and this represents a fracture of the pars interarticularis.
A. The ear represents the superior articular process.
B. The nose represents the transverse process.
C. The front leg represents the inferior articular process.
E. The eye represents the pedicle.
11. **A.** Jefferson fractures involve the C1 vertebrae.
12. **C.** All the muscles listed are intrinsic or true back muscles and are thus innervated by dorsal rami nerve branches. The rhomboids are an extrinsic back muscle and they are innervated by ventral rami nerve, specifically the dorsal scapular nerve.
13. **B.** Hatched-shaped spinous processes are located in the lumbar vertebrae.
A. Demifacets are related to the thoracic vertebrae and are the sites for articulation of the 2nd to 9th or 10th heads of the ribs.
C. The promontory is an anterior projection from the superior portion of the S1 body of the sacrum.
D. The transverse foramina are located in the cervical vertebrae and allow passage of the vertebral vessels.
E. Costal facets are located on the transverse processes of the thoracic vertebrae and are the sites of rib articulations specifically at the tubercle.
14. **A.** The lumbar region of the vertebral column is naturally in a lordotic state but an excessive amount is known as lordosis or "hollow back". Lordosis is often seen with pregnant women.
B. Scoliosis presents as a lateral deviation of the spine.
C. Spondylolysis would refer to a fracture located at the pars interarticularis of a vertebra.
D. Kyphosis is an abnormal curvature of the thoracic vertebrae.
E. Spinal stenosis would refer to the abnormal narrowing of the vertebral canal.
15. **C.** The uncovertebral joints are specific to the cervical vertebrae and are located adjacent to the transverse foramen that allows for passage of the vertebral artery.

2 Thorax

LEARNING OBJECTIVES

- To understand the surface anatomy and structures that make up the thoracic wall.
- To describe how the ribs and sternum develop.
- To distinguish the fascia, neurovasculature, muscles, joints, and different movements of the thoracic wall.
- A look at the clinical correlates that relate to the thoracic wall will include supernumerary ribs, rib fractures, separations and dislocations, flail chest, thoracotomies, video-assisted thoracoscopic surgery (VATS), thoracic outlet syndrome (TOS) and intercostal nerve blocks.
- To understand the structure, neurovasculature and specific lymphatic drainage of the breast.
- Clinical correlates that relate to the breast will include mammography, breast carcinoma and mastectomies, and supernumerary breasts and nipples.
- To understand the structures located in the superior, anterior, and posterior mediastinum. The clinical correlates will include a look at the variations and anomalies of the arch of the aorta, double aortic arch, retro-esophageal right subclavian artery and coarctation of aorta.
- To understand the pericardium and structures of the heart along with their neurovasculature and development.
- Clinical correlates that relate to the pericardium and heart will include cardiac tamponade, pericardial effusion, pericarditis, pericardial friction rub, pericardiocentesis, valvular heart disease, tricuspid, aortic and pulmonary valve stenosis/insufficiency, mitral/bicuspid valve prolapse, echocardiogram, coronary atherosclerosis, (acute) myocardial infarction, coronary angiography, coronary angioplasty, coronary artery bypass surgery, electrocardiogram, artificial pacemaker, fibrillation of the Heart, cardiopulmonary resuscitation (CPR), referred pain of the heart, septal defects, tetralogy of Fallot, and persistent truncus arteriosus.
- To understand prenatal and postnatal circulation.
- To understand the pleurae and structures associated with the lungs, tracheobronchial tree, and histology of the alveoli.
- To describe the neurovasculature, lymphatic drainage, and development of the pleurae and parts of the lungs.
- Clinical correlates that relate to the pleurae and lungs will include pulmonary (lung) collapse, pleuritis, pulmonary embolism, carcinoma of the lungs, thoracentesis, chest tube placement, and bronchoscopy.
- To understand auscultatory areas of the heart and lungs and radiology of the thorax region.

The part of the body between the neck and abdomen is known as the **thorax**. When the term "chest" is used, it commonly refers to the thorax and the pectoral (shoulder) girdle together. The specifics of the pectoral girdle will be discussed in Chapter 6. The term thorax will refer to the region located between the diaphragm and the superior thoracic aperture. The thorax contains and protects the central mediastinum and pleural cavities, all of which are found within a larger **thoracic cavity (Fig. 2.1)**.

The thoracic cavity walls are formed by the **thoracic cage** (rib cage) which is made up of the ribs and costal cartilage primarily. Due to the coverage of the thoracic cage, the thoracic cavity and upper abdomen are protected by the bony structures making up the thoracic cage. The diaphragm and important structures located within the thorax tend to always be in motion, hence the thorax is one of the most dynamic regions of the body.

2.1 Thoracic Wall

The thoracic wall includes the thoracic cage and the skin, subcutaneous tissue, fascia, and muscles located anterolaterally to the wall, within intercostal spaces of the ribs and posteriorly in the back region. Breasts are found within the subcutaneous tissue of the thoracic wall. The functions of the thoracic wall include:

- Resistance to the negative internal pressures generated by elastic recoil of the lungs and inspiratory movements.
- Protection of vital thoracic and abdominal structures.
- Provide attachment sites for muscles that maintain the position and move the upper limbs relative to the trunk.
- Provide attachment sites for abdominal, neck and back muscles important in respiration.

In short, with every breath, the diaphragm and muscles of the thoracic and abdominal walls help change the volume of the thoracic cavity. This causes the lungs to expand and draw air in and then, because of lung elasticity and muscle relaxation, cavity volume decreases, causing the lung to eject air.

2.2 Surface Anatomy of the Thoracic Wall

The clavicles form a bony ridge just below the skin at the junction of the neck and thorax. The sternum lies in the midline and can be palpated from the jugular notch down to the tip of the xiphoid process. The ribs and the intercostal spaces between them can be palpated and used to determine the correct insertion points for a chest tube or needle in the case of a thoracentesis.

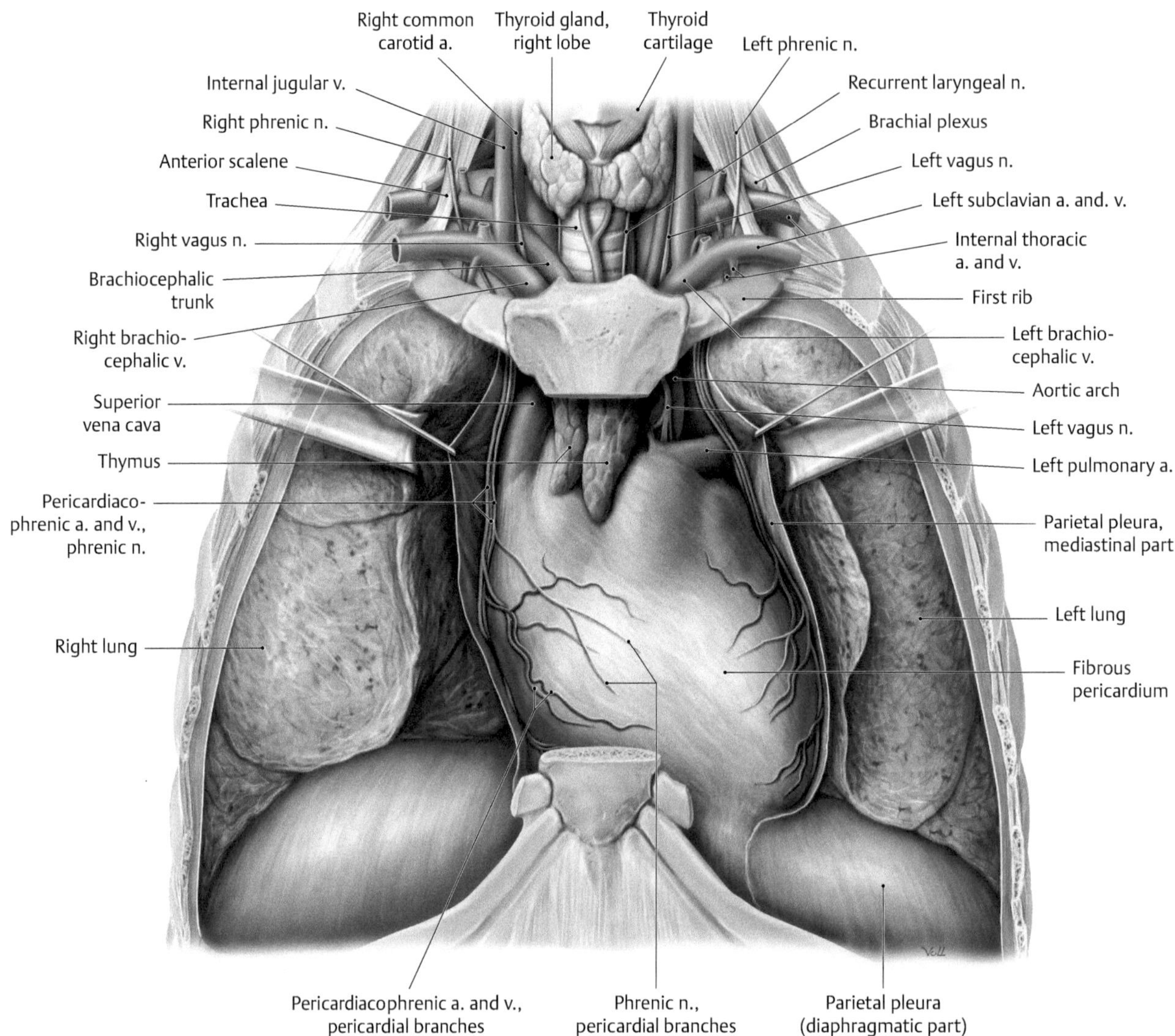

Fig. 2.1 Opened thoracic cavity. The anterior portion of the chest plate has been removed. (From Schuenke M, Schulte E, Schumacher U. THIEME Atlas of Anatomy. Internal Organs. Illustrations by Voll M and Wesker K. 3rd ed. New York: Thieme Medical Publishers; 2020.)

A few imaginary lines are used for anatomical positioning of the thorax (**Fig. 2.2**).

- Anteriorly:
  - The **anterior median (midsternal) line** is a vertical line in the median plane that divides the thorax into left and right halves from the anterior aspect.
  - The **midclavicular lines** pass through the middle of both clavicles and are parallel to the anterior median line.
- Posteriorly:
  - **Posterior median (midvertebral) line** is a vertical line in the median plane passing along the spinous processes of vertebrae that also divides the body into left and right halves.
  - The **scapular lines** intersect the inferior angles of the scapula and run parallel to the posterior median line.
- Laterally:
  - The **anterior axillary line** is a vertical line passing along the anterior axillary fold that is formed by the lateral border of the pectoralis major.
  - The **midaxillary line** is a vertical line parallel to the anterior and posterior axillary lines extending down from the apex of the axillary fossa.
  - The **posterior axillary line** is a vertical line passing along the posterior axillary fold that is formed by the lateral borders of the latissimus dorsi and teres major muscles.

2.3 Skeleton of the Thoracic Wall

The thoracic skeleton forms the larger osteocartilaginous thoracic cage, which includes a sternum, 12 pairs of ribs, costal cartilages of the ribs, 12 thoracic vertebrae and the intervertebral (IV) disks located between the thoracic vertebrae. Most of the thoracic wall is formed by the ribs and costal cartilage (**Fig. 2.3**).

2.3.1 Sternum

The **sternum** is a flat and stretched out bone that forms the middle of the anterior thoracic cage. It directly overlies mediastinal viscera and much of the heart. The sternum consists of three parts: manubrium, sternal body and xiphoid process (**Fig. 2.4**).

The **manubrium** is the superior portion of the larger sternum. It is located between vertebral levels T3-T4/T5. A small depression or groove is located on the superior border and is called

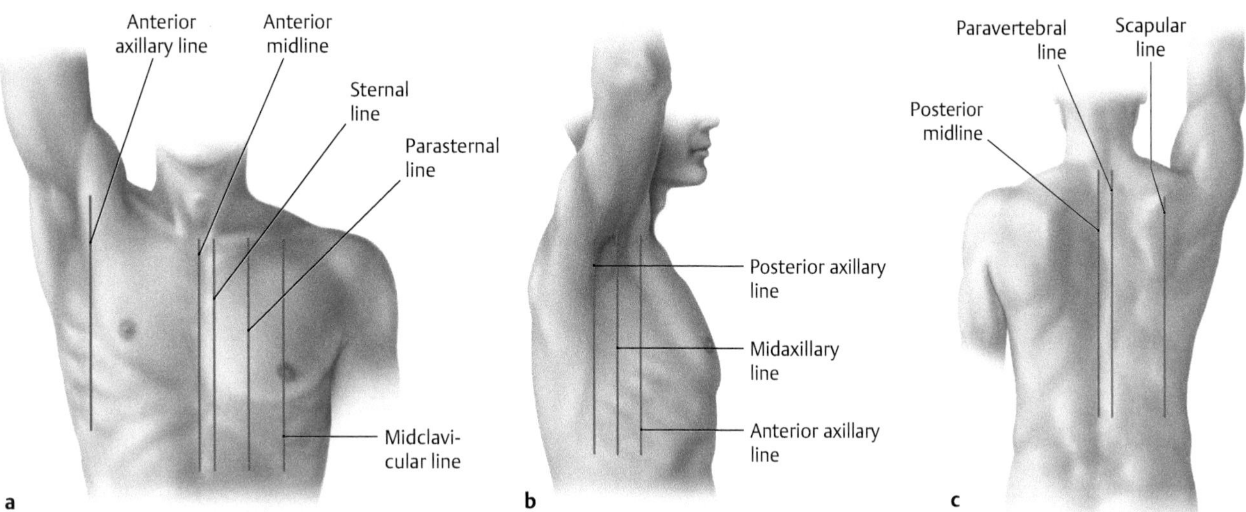

Fig. 2.2 Vertical reference lines of the thorax. **(a)** Anterior view. **(b)** Right lateral view. **(c)** Posterior view. (From Schuenke M, Schulte E, Schumacher U. THIEME Atlas of Anatomy. General Anatomy and Musculoskeletal System. Illustrations by Voll M and Wesker K. 3rd ed. New York: Thieme Medical Publishers; 2020.)

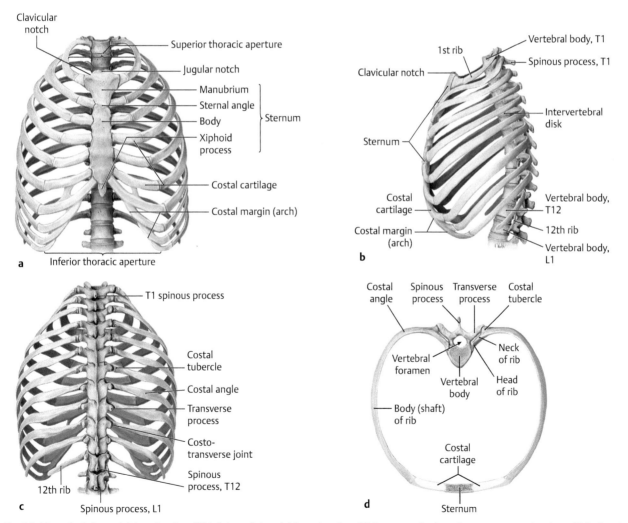

Fig. 2.3 Thoracic skeleton. **(a)** Anterior view. **(b)** Left lateral view. **(c)** Posterior view. **(d)** Structure of a thoracic segment, superior view of 6th rib pair. (From Schuenke M, Schulte E, Schumacher U. THIEME Atlas of Anatomy. General Anatomy and Musculoskeletal System. Illustrations by Voll M and Wesker K. 3rd ed. New York: Thieme Medical Publishers; 2020.)

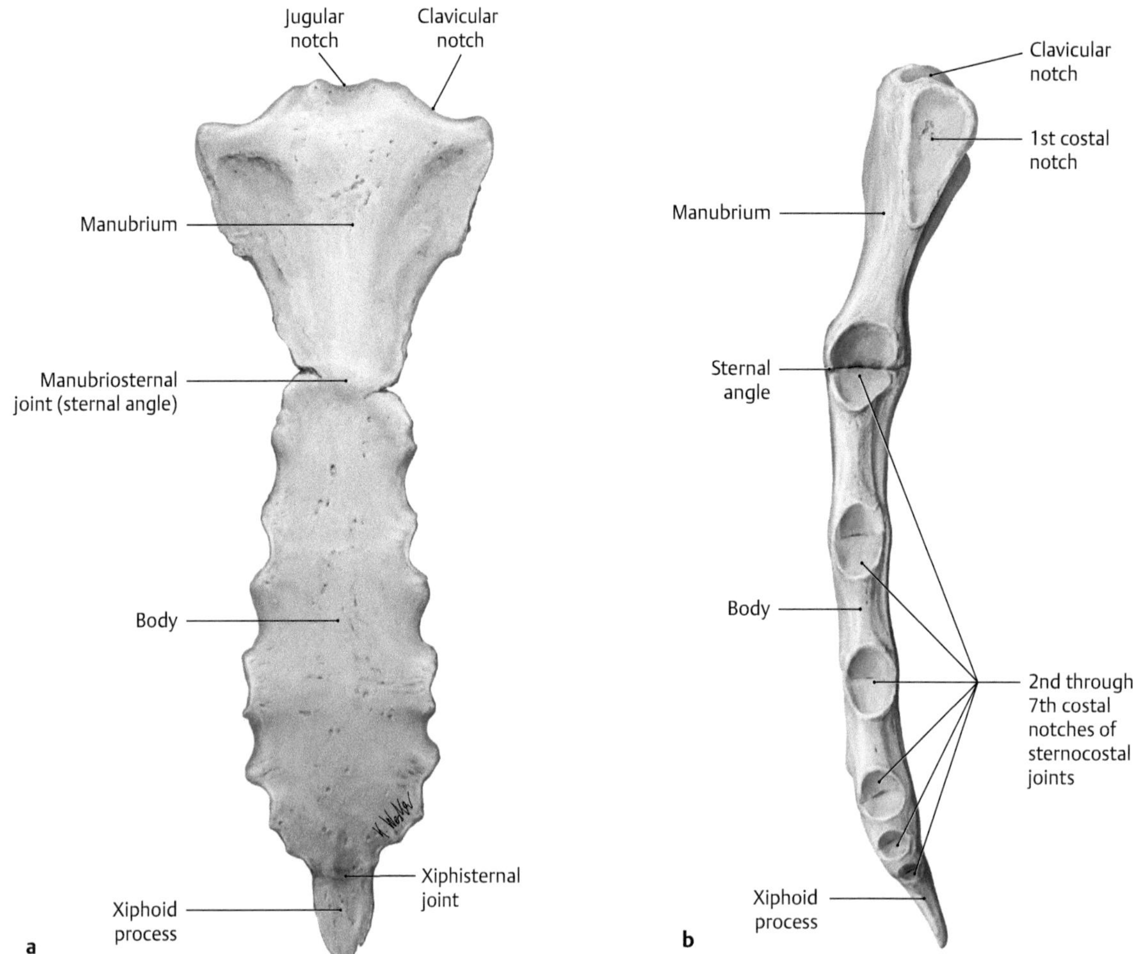

Fig. 2.4 Sternum. **(a)** Anterior view. **(b)** Left lateral view. (From Schuenke M, Schulte E, Schumacher U. THIEME Atlas of Anatomy. General Anatomy and Musculoskeletal System. Illustrations by Voll M and Wesker K. 3rd ed. New York: Thieme Medical Publishers; 2020.)

the **jugular notch** (suprasternal notch). The clavicle articulates with the manubrium at the **sternoclavicular (SC) joint** and this is a saddle-type synovial joint. Just inferior to the sternoclavicular joint, the first rib articulates to the manubrium, forming the first of seven sternocostal joints. This particular joint is a primary cartilaginous (synchondrosis) joint. The articulation between the manubrium and sternal body is known as the **manubriosternal joint** and it is a secondary cartilaginous (symphysis) joint. Due to the articulation between the manubrium and sternal body, a small projection known as the **sternal angle** (of Louis) forms and serves as a good landmark for identifying the T4/T5 vertebral level. The second set of ribs and their costal cartilages are found attached to the sternum at the level of the sternal angle **(Fig. 2.4)**.

The **sternal body** is the middle portion of the larger sternum and is located between vertebral levels T4/T5-T9. It is longer, thinner and narrower than the manubrium. **Costal notches** are located on the lateral borders of the sternum and will be the site of the 2nd-7th costal cartilage attachments. These articulations are also known as **sternocostal joints** but they are plane type synovial joints. The adult sternal body has three slight elevations known as the **transverse ridges** and they represent the fusion lines of the original four separate sternebrae **(Fig. 2.4)**.

The **xiphoid process** is located at approximately the level of the T10 vertebra and is the smallest part of the sternum. This process is quite variable and it articulates with the sternal body at the **xiphisternal joint**. The xiphisternal joint is the site of the **infrasternal angle** that is formed by the left and right costal margins. It will also serve as a marker demarcating the inferior border of the heart, superior limit of the liver and central tendon of the diaphragm **(Fig. 2.4)**.

2.3.2 Ribs and Costal Cartilage

Ribs are flat and curved bones that form the majority of the thoracic cage. They are highly resilient and light in weight. There are three types of ribs but they can be classified as either typical or atypical ribs **(Fig. 2.5)**:

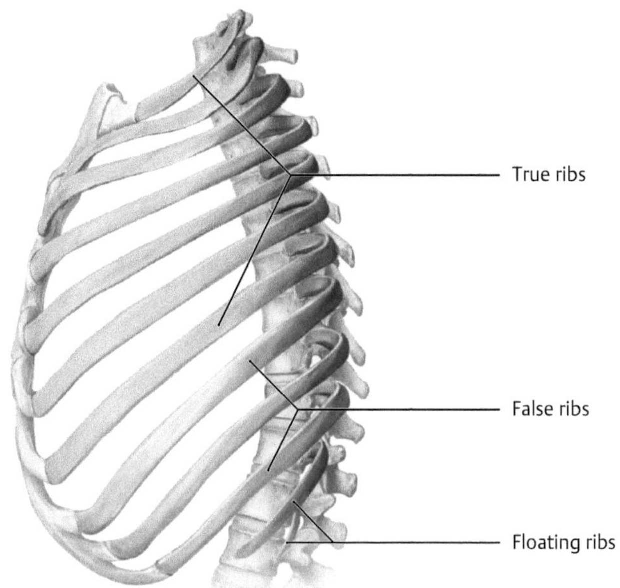

Fig. 2.5 Types of ribs. (From Schuenke M, Schulte E, Schumacher U. THIEME Atlas of Anatomy. General Anatomy and Musculoskeletal System. Illustrations by Voll M and Wesker K. 3rd ed. New York: Thieme Medical Publishers; 2020.)

- **True ribs** are the 1st-7th ribs and they attach directly to the sternum by costal cartilages.
- **False ribs** are the 8th-10th ribs and they attach indirectly to the sternum by costal cartilages.
- **Floating ribs** are the 11th and 12th ribs and they have no attachment to the sternum.

Typical ribs include the 3rd-9th ribs and they have a head, neck, tubercle and body **(Fig. 2.6)**.

- The **head** is wedge-shaped and has two facets that articulate with corresponding vertebral bodies. These two facets are separated by a small projection known as the **crest**.
- The **neck** connects the head with the body near the tubercle.
- The **tubercle** is the smooth articular portion that articulates with the transverse process of the corresponding vertebra. This articulation helps form the *costotransverse joint*.
- The **body** or *shaft* of the rib is flat, thin and curved. The curved portion is most evident at the **costal angle**. The weakest point of the rib is just anterior to the costal angle and this serves as the most common site for *rib fractures*.
- The **costal groove** is located on the inferior border of the rib and it is where the intercostal neurovasculature courses.

Atypical ribs include the 1st, 2nd, 10th-12th ribs **(Fig. 2.6)**.

- The 1st rib is the shortest, broadest and has the sharpest curve of the true ribs. It has a groove on its superior surface for both the subclavian vein and artery. The grooves are separated by the **scalene tubercle**, which is the attachment site for the anterior scalene muscle. From anterior to posterior on the 1st rib you would find the subclavian vein, anterior scalene muscle and then the subclavian artery.
- The 2nd rib is thinner and less curved but much longer than the 1st rib. The **tuberosity of the serratus anterior muscle** is located approximately in the middle of the body region and acts as an attachment site for this muscle.
- The 11th and 12th ribs only have one facet at the head region and thus only articulate with the 11th and 12th vertebrae individually and respectively. The 11th and 12th ribs are also short and have no neck or tubercles.

Costal cartilages are the anterior extensions of the ribs and will contribute to the elasticity of the thoracic wall **(Fig. 2.3)**. The lengths of these cartilages increase through the first 7 ribs but then gradually decrease with ribs 8-10. The fusion of the 8-10th costal cartilages forms a continuous cartilage that results in the formation of the **costal margin**. The costal cartilages of the 11th and 12th ribs form only a cap over the distal end of the rib.

The gaps between ribs are known as **intercostal spaces** and are the widest anterolaterally. There are a total of 11 spaces and are named according to the rib forming the superior border of the space. For example, the 6th intercostal space is located between the 6th and 7th ribs. The space below the 12th rib is known as the subcostal space. These spaces are filled with the external, internal and innermost intercostal muscles. However, between the internal and innermost intercostal muscles, lies a *neurovascular plane* that permits the passage of the intercostal neurovasculature and their collateral branches **(Fig. 2.7)**. The subcostal neurovasculature is located in the subcostal space just below the 12th rib.

2.3.3 Thoracic Vertebrae

As discussed in Chapter 1, **thoracic vertebrae** are so-called standard vertebrae consisting of bodies, vertebral arches and seven processes. Thoracic vertebrae have spinous processes that are long and project posteroinferiorly. They cover the intervals between the laminae of adjacent vertebrae. The head of the rib will articulate directly with the first, eleventh, and twelfth thoracic vertebrae. For the remainder, the head of the rib articulates at costal (demifacets) facets, which is an articulation bridging two adjacent vertebrae. These articulations are known as the **superior** and **inferior demifacets**. They occur as bilateral pairs on the superior and inferior posterolateral margins of the bodies of thoracic vertebrae T2-T9 **(Fig. 2.8)**.

The inferior demifacet is found on the superior vertebra while the superior demifacet is located on the inferior vertebra of the articulation with the head of the rib. This articulation also includes the IV disk located between the corresponding demifacets. The **costal facets of the transverse processes** articulate with the tubercles of the upper 9-10 ribs. The last two ribs generally do not attach to the transverse processes. For example, most rib articulations are as follows: the 6th rib tubercle would articulate with the 6th transverse process while the inferior articular facet of the head of the rib articulates with the superior demifacet of the 6th vertebrae. The superior articular facet of the head of the rib would articulate with the inferior demifacet of the 5th vertebrae **(Fig. 2.8)**.

2.4 Development of the Ribs and Sternum

Costal processes are small lateral mesenchymal condensations that develop in association with the vertebral arches of the neck and thoracic region. However, only in the thoracic region do these

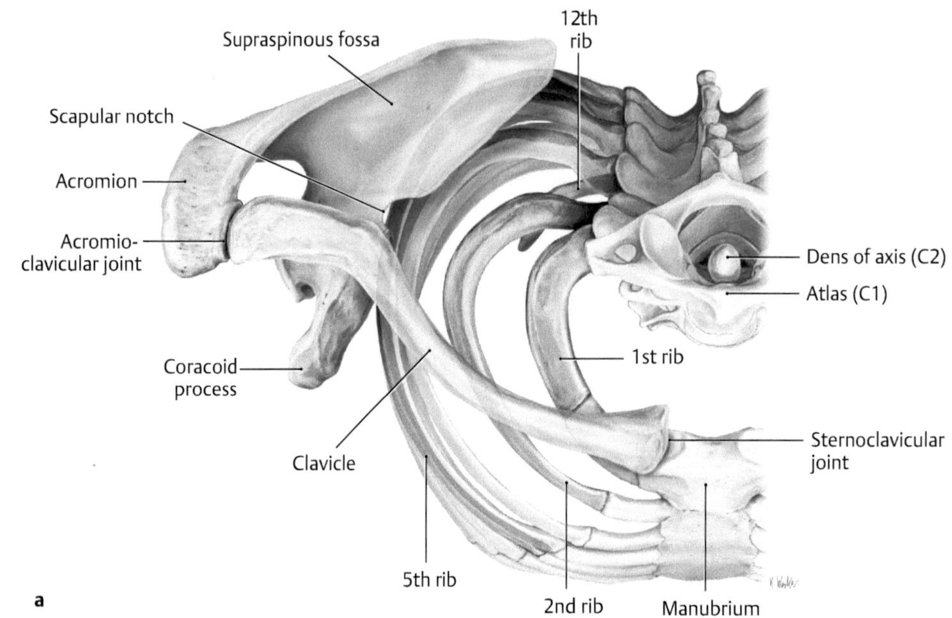

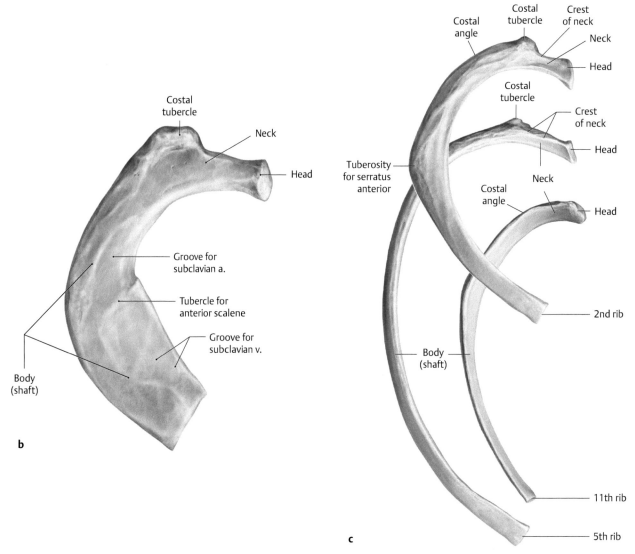

Fig. 2.6 Ribs. **(a)** Superior view of right ribs. **(b)** 1st rib. **(c)** 2nd, 5th, and 11th ribs, superior view. (From Schuenke M, Schulte E, Schumacher U. THIEME Atlas of Anatomy. General Anatomy and Musculoskeletal System. Illustrations by Voll M and Wesker K. 3rd ed. New York: Thieme Medical Publishers; 2020.)

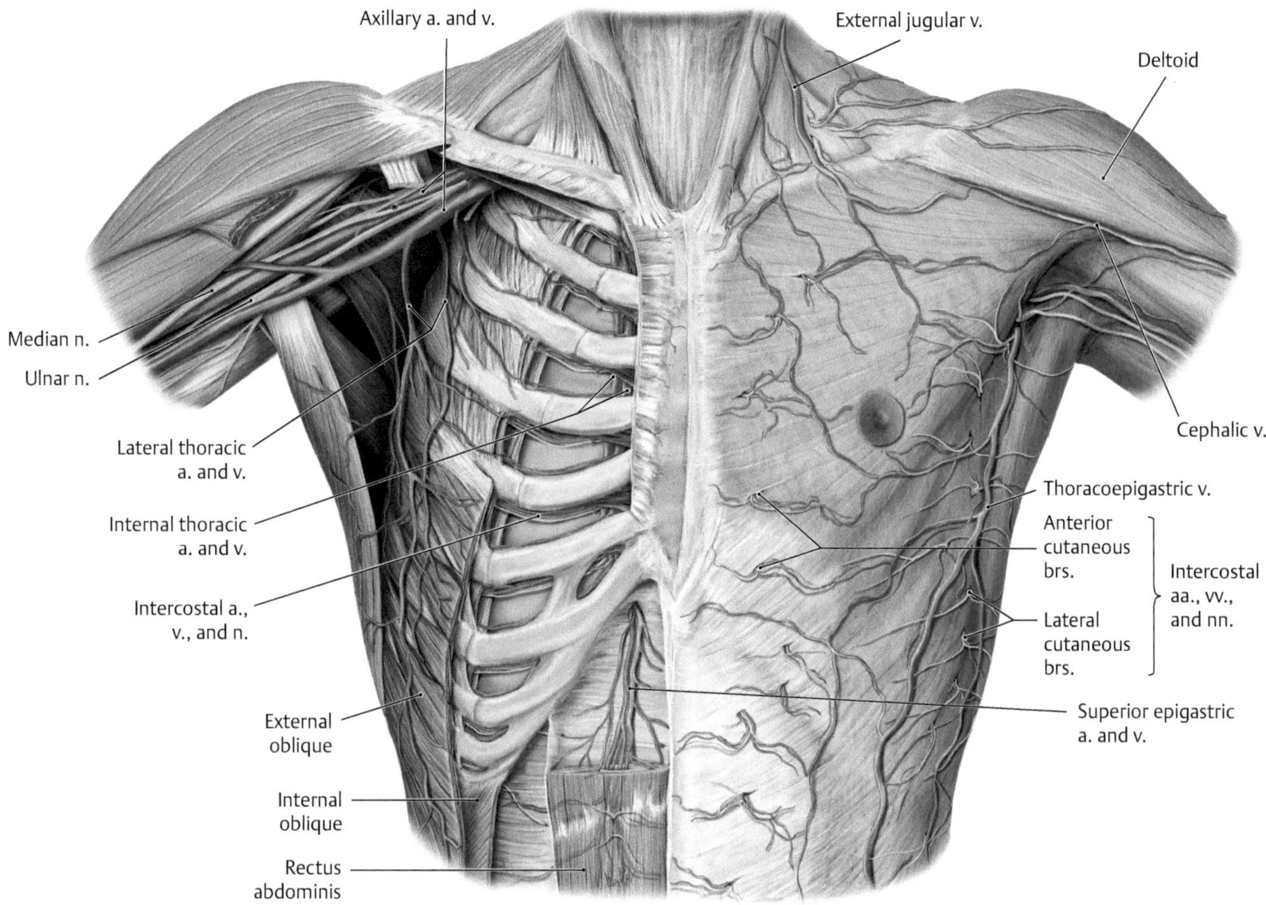

Fig. 2.7 Intercostal neurovasculature. (From Schuenke M, Schulte E, Schumacher U. THIEME Atlas of Anatomy. General Anatomy and Musculoskeletal System. Illustrations by Voll M and Wesker K. 3rd ed. New York: Thieme Medical Publishers; 2020.)

costal processes elongate to form ribs. The ribs begin to lengthen and form on the 35th day of development. The ribs develop as cartilaginous precursors that later ossify in a process known as **endochondral ossification (Fig. 2.9)**.

The sternum develops from a pair of longitudinal mesenchymal condensations known as **sternal bars**. The sternal bars begin to fuse at the midline just as the most cranial ribs begin to make contact with them at approximately day 45 of development. Fusion occurs in a cranial to caudal fashion with the xiphoid process finally forming in the 9th week of development. Ossification centers appear in the sternum by the 60th day of development and ossification progresses in a cranial to caudal direction until shortly after birth. This results in the formation of the manubrium, sternal body and xiphoid process (**Fig. 2.9**).

2.5 Apertures of the Thorax

The thorax is open both superiorly and inferiorly. These openings are known as the superior thoracic and inferior thoracic apertures (**Fig. 2.3a**).

- The **superior thoracic aperture** allows for the passage of structures such as the esophagus, trachea, and neurovasculature to and from the head, neck and upper limbs. This aperture is formed as follows:
  - Anteriorly by the superior border of the manubrium.
  - Laterally by the 1st pair of costal cartilages and their attached ribs.
  - Posteriorly by the T1 vertebra.
- The **inferior thoracic aperture** is much larger than the superior thoracic aperture but the diaphragm closes it separating the thoracic and abdominal cavities. Openings found penetrating the diaphragm allow structures to pass to and from the thorax and abdomen. The diaphragm can extend as high as the 4th intercostal space on the right side of the body. This aperture is formed as follows:
  - Anteriorly by the xiphisternal joint.
  - Anterolaterally by the costal margins, which are the combination of 7-10th costal cartilages.
  - Posterolaterally by the 11th and 12th pairs of ribs.
  - Posteriorly by the 12th thoracic vertebra.

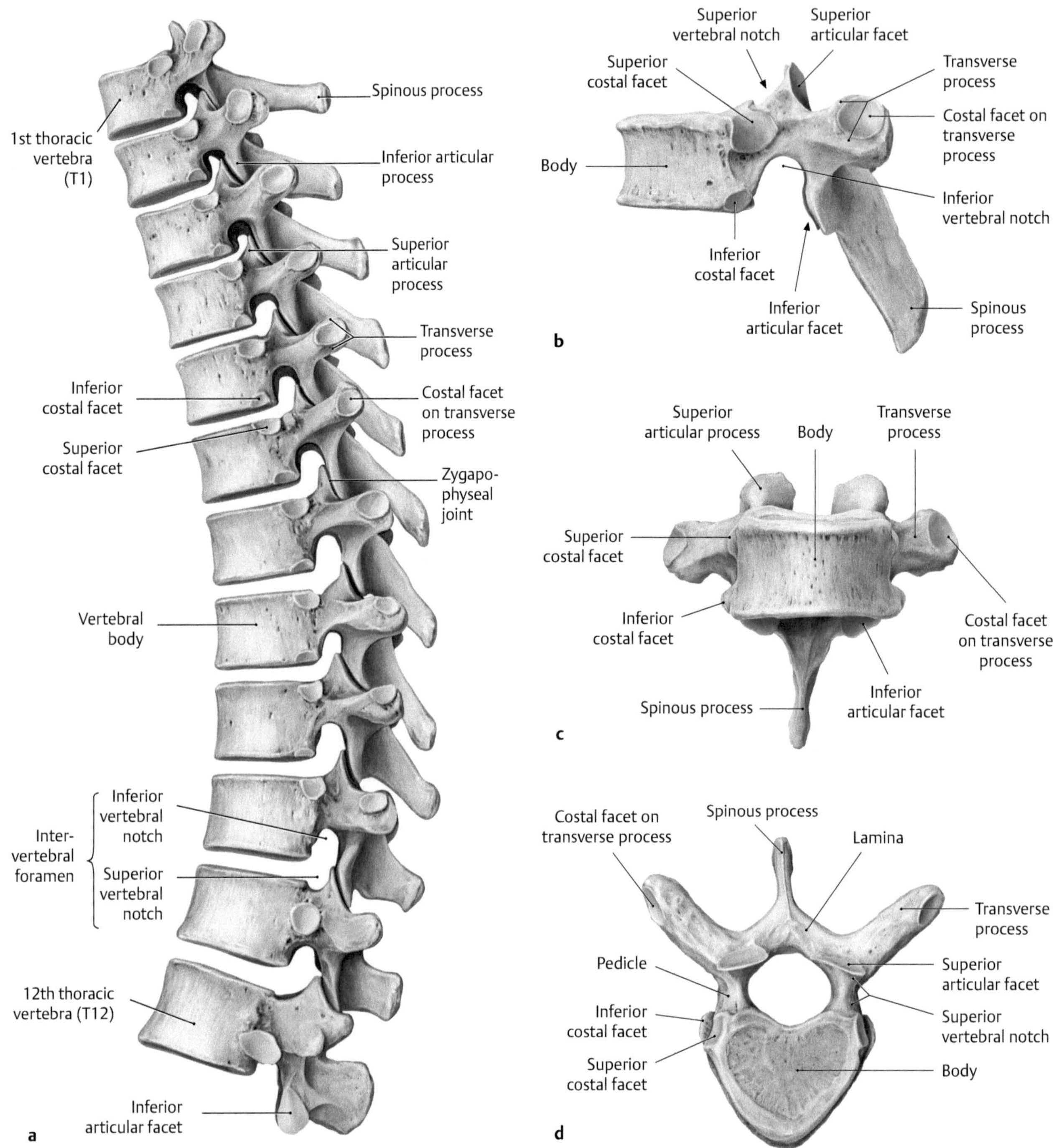

Fig. 2.8 (a) Thoracic spine. Typical thoracic vertebra (T6). **(b)** Left lateral view. **(c)** Anterior view. **(d)** Superior view. (From Schuenke M, Schulte E, Schumacher U. THIEME Atlas of Anatomy. General Anatomy and Musculoskeletal System. Illustrations by Voll M and Wesker K. 3rd ed. New York: Thieme Medical Publishers; 2020.)

2.6 Thoracic Wall Joints

Movements at the joints of the thoracic wall are frequent during normal respiration. Range of motion at these same joints is limited, however. Any alteration of the mobility of these joints can cause difficulty breathing. A couple of joints related to the thorax, the intervertebral (IV) joints (Chapter 1) and sternoclavicular joints (Chapter 6), are discussed in detail elsewhere.

Costovertebral joints are the articulations of ribs with their corresponding vertebrae **(Fig. 2.10bc)**. The articulation of the vertebra with the head of the rib occurs at two different locations for ribs 2-10. Ribs 1, 11, and 12 attach only with the vertebral body

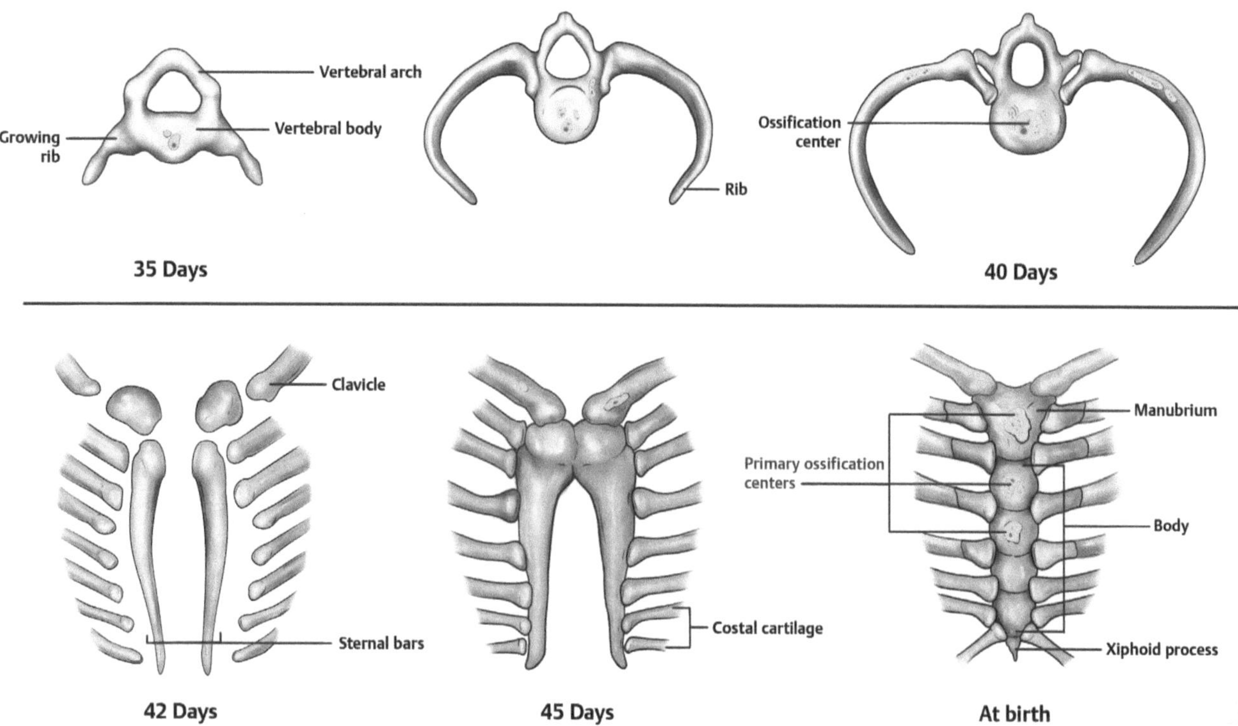

Fig. 2.9 Development of the ribs and sternum. Illustration by Calla Heald.

of the same number. As described in the thoracic vertebrae section, the *inferior articular facet* of the head of the rib articulates with the *superior demifacet* of the corresponding same-numbered vertebra. The *superior articular facet* of the head of the rib articulates with the *inferior demifacet* of the vertebra above it. The *crest* of the head of the rib will attach to the IV disk by way of the **intra-articular ligament** within the joint. This essentially divides the enclosed space into two smaller synovial joints. The **radiate ligament** forms a strong, anterior attachment from the rib to the bodies of the two corresponding vertebrae and IV disk between them.

The articulation between a tubercle of a rib with the costal facet of the transverse process of the same numbered vertebrae is known as a **costotransverse joint (Fig. 2.10b,c)**. These joints are plane type synovial joints strengthened by a **costotransverse, lateral** and **superior costotransverse ligament**. The superior costotransverse ligament can be further divided into individual *anterior costotransverse* and *posterior costotransverse ligaments*. The 1st-7th ribs and their costotransverse joints allow for rotational movements around a transverse axis. This results in elevation and depression of the sternal ends of the ribs and sternum in a sagittal plane depicting the look of a pump handle movement. The 8th-10th ribs and their costotransverse joints allow for more gliding movements. This results in elevation and depression of the lateral-most aspects of the ribs in a transverse plane and depicts a bucket handle movement.

The **sternocostal joints** are the articulations between the costal cartilages of ribs 1-7 and the sternum **(Fig. 2.4b; Fig. 2.10a)**. The 1st sternocostal joint is a primary cartilaginous (synchondrosis) joint while the 2nd through 7th sternocostal joints are plane type synovial joints. **Anterior** and **posterior radiate sternocostal ligaments** add additional strength to these weak joint capsules. *Rib dislocations* occur at the sternocostal joints.

Additional joints of this region include the **costochondral joints** located between the sternal ends of ribs 1-10 and the lateral ends of costal cartilage. These are primary cartilaginous joints and the site of rib separations. The **interchondral joints** are the anterior articulations between costal cartilages of the 6th-10th ribs **(Fig. 2.10a)**. They are plane type synovial joints and have interchondral ligaments that add support to these joints. The **manubriosternal joint** is the articulation between the manubrium and sternal body while the **xiphisternal joint** is the articulation between the sternal body and xiphoid process **(Fig. 2.4a)**. The manubriosternal joint is a secondary cartilaginous (symphysis) joint while the xiphisternal joint is a primary cartilaginous (synchondrosis) joint.

2.7 Thoracic Wall Fascia

Deep to the skin there is a thin layer of superficial fascia which is primarily made of loose areolar connective tissue and adipose. Deep fascia in this region attaches to the clavicle and sternum and is known as **pectoral fascia** because it adheres to the pectoralis major muscle. It is continuous with the fascia of the anterior abdominal wall and helps form the **axillary fascia (Fig. 2.11)**. The pectoral fascia also forms much of the *bed of the breast* which is the area the posterior surface of the breast lies against.

Just deep to the pectoralis major is the pectoralis minor muscle. The pectoralis minor along with parts of the subclavius muscle and clavicle are covered with deep fascia known as **clavipectoral fascia**. This fascia forms the *costocoracoid membrane* and *suspensory*

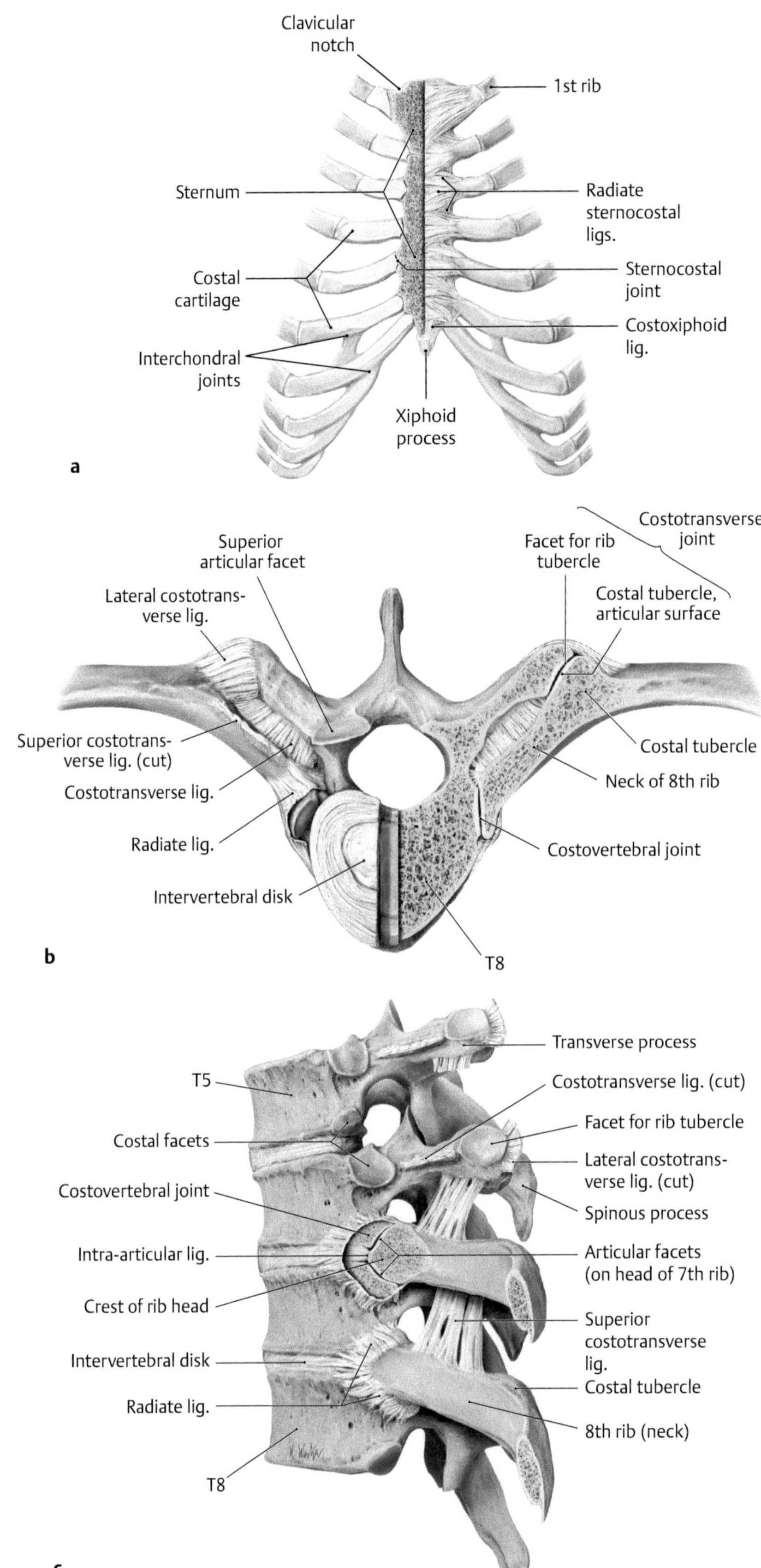

Fig. 2.10 **(a)** Sternocostal joints. **(b)** Costotransverse joint. **(c)** Costovertebral joints. (From Schuenke M, Schulte E, Schumacher U. THIEME Atlas of Anatomy. General Anatomy and Musculoskeletal System. Illustrations by Voll M and Wesker K. 3rd ed. New York: Thieme Medical Publishers; 2020.)

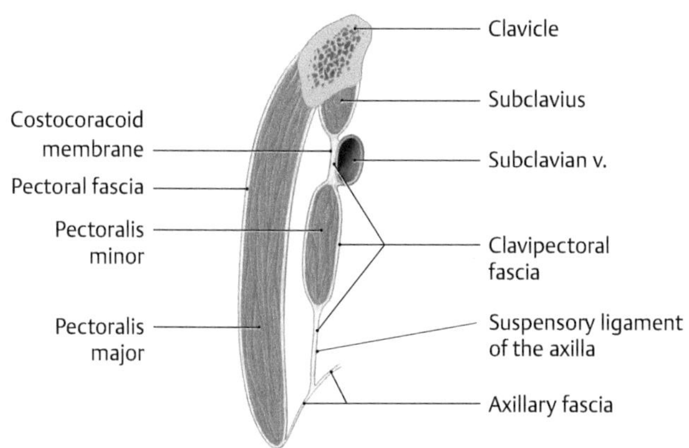

Fig. 2.11 Axillary fascia. (From Gilroy AM et al. Atlas of Anatomy. 4th ed. 2020. Based on: Schuenke M, Schulte E, Schumacher U. THIEME Atlas of Anatomy. General Anatomy and Musculoskeletal System. Illustrations by Voll M and Wesker K. 3rd ed. New York: Thieme Medical Publishers; 2020.)

ligament of the axilla (**Fig. 2.11**). Further details of these fascias will be discussed in Chapter 6. Generally, the deep fascia of a particular muscle is given the name of the muscle in which it adheres to except for the pectoralis minor. For example, deep fascia of the serratus anterior.

2.8 Thoracic Wall Muscles

The thoracic wall has muscles that extend to and from the upper limb, anterolateral abdominal wall, neck, and back (**Fig. 2.12**). Although the pectoralis major, pectoralis minor, serratus anterior and scalene muscles are attached to the thoracic wall, they act more as accessory respiratory muscles outside of their normal functions. The primary muscle of inspiration is the ***diaphragm***, which is discussed in detail in Chapter 3. Muscles of the thoracic wall that assist in respiration but on a smaller scale include the ***intercostals***, ***transversus thoracis***, ***subcostal***, ***serratus posteriors*** and ***levatores costarum***.

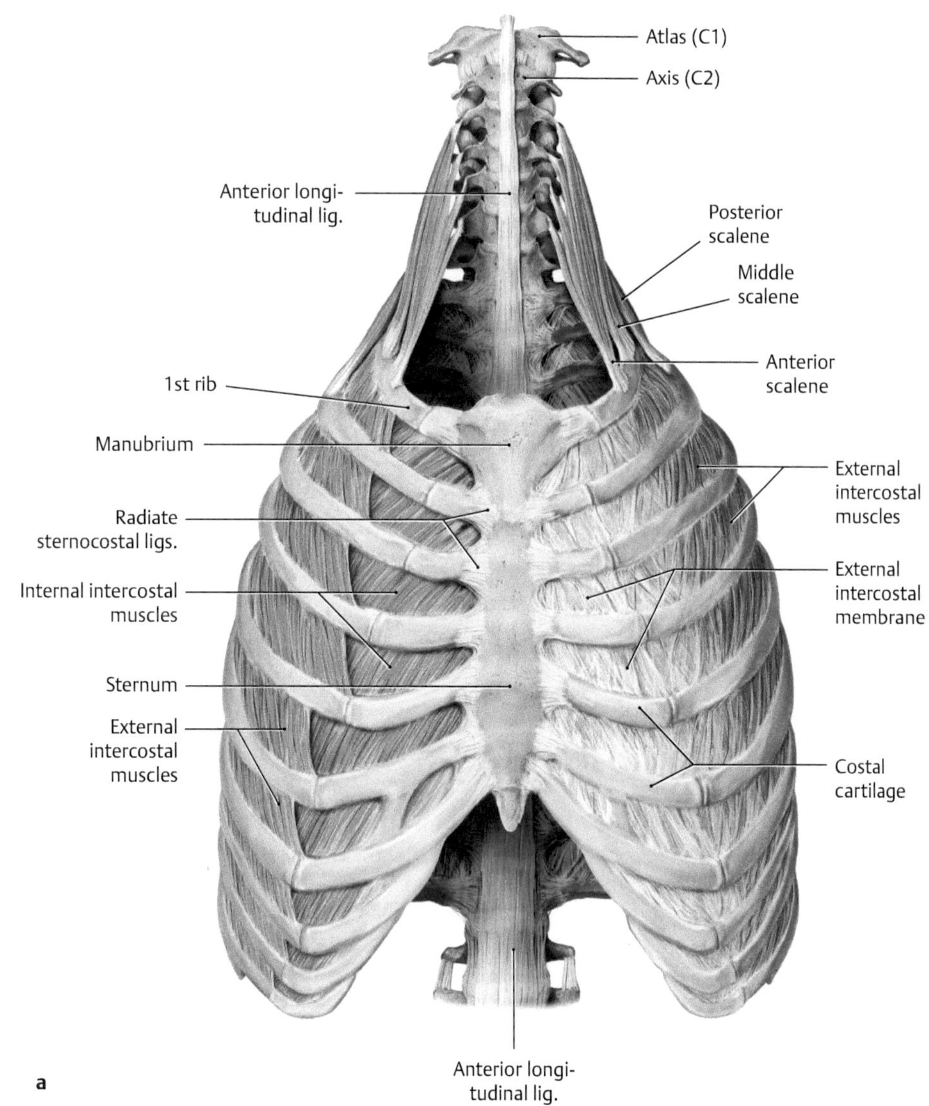

Fig. 2.12 Thoracic wall muscles. (a) Anterior view. (*continued*) (From Schuenke M, Schulte E, Schumacher U. THIEME Atlas of Anatomy. General Anatomy and Musculoskeletal System. Illustrations by Voll M and Wesker K. 3rd ed. New York: Thieme Medical Publishers; 2020.)

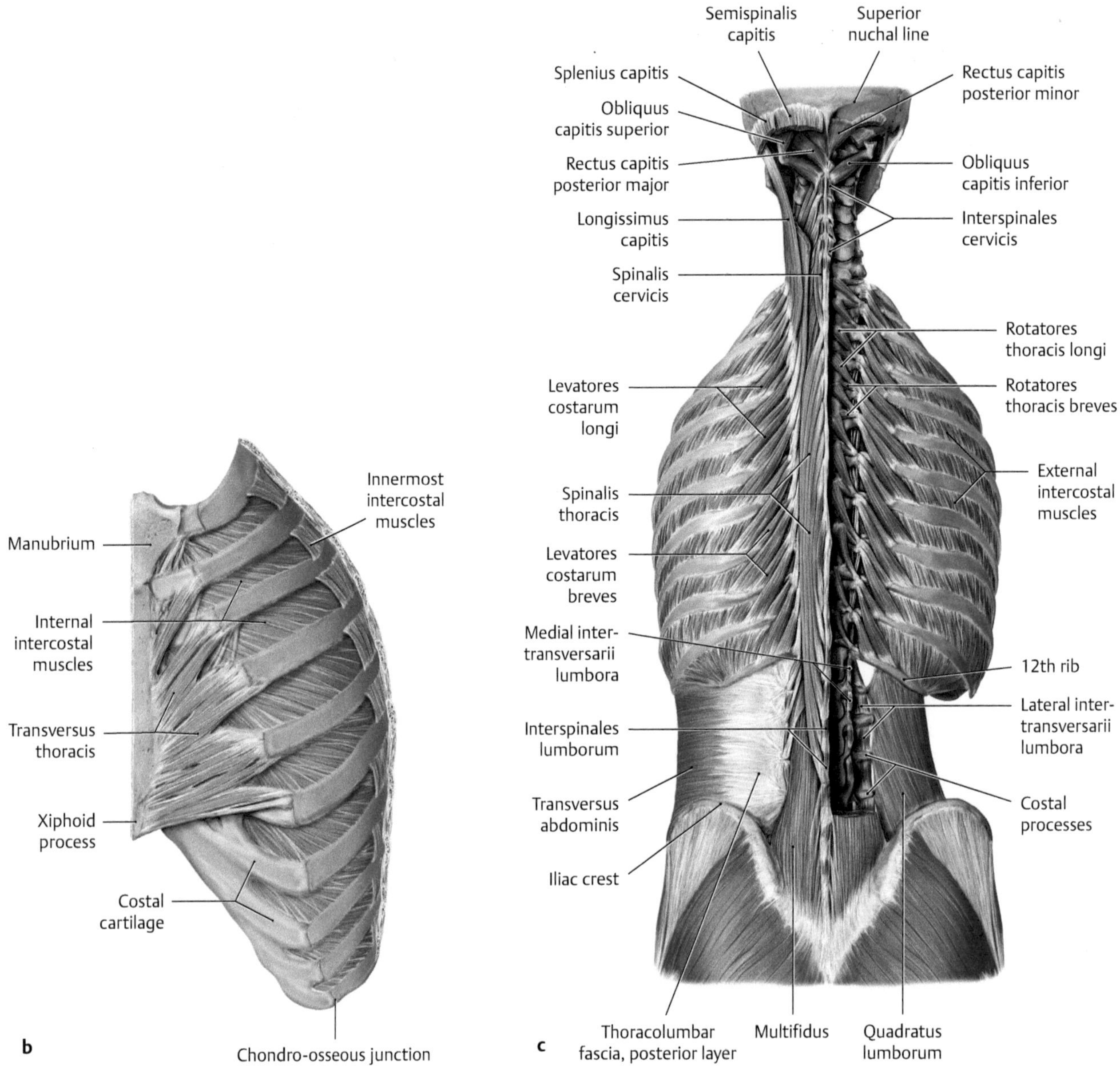

Fig. 2.12 (*continued*) Thoracic wall muscles. **(b)** Anterior view with thoracic cage opened to expose posterior surface of anterior wall. **(c)** Posterior view along with the deep intrinsic back muscles. (From Schuenke M, Schulte E, Schumacher U. THIEME Atlas of Anatomy. General Anatomy and Musculoskeletal System. Illustrations by Voll M and Wesker K. 3rd ed. New York: Thieme Medical Publishers; 2020.)

These muscles are all innervated by the intercostal nerves except for the levatores costarum muscles. The intercostal muscles are located within the intercostal spaces between the ribs. The most superficial muscle is the external intercostal with the internal intercostal just deep to it. There is a neurovascular plane where the intercostal neurovasculature passes between the internal intercostal and the deepest muscle filling the intercostal space, the innermost intercostal.

The **external intercostals** are found in all 11 intercostal spaces and are responsible for elevation of the ribs and are most active during forced inspiration. They begin near the tubercles of the ribs and extend anteriorly to about the costochondral joints before forming the **external intercostal membrane**. These muscles are continuous inferiorly with the external oblique muscles of the anterolateral abdominal wall. The **internal intercostals** are found in all 11 intercostal spaces and are responsible for depression of the ribs and are most active during forced expiration. They begin near the lateral walls of the sternum and extend posteriorly to about the angles of the ribs before forming the **internal intercostal membrane**. These muscles are continuous inferiorly with the internal oblique muscles of the anterolateral abdominal wall. The **innermost intercostals** are the deepest of all intercostal muscles. They act similar to the internal intercostals as weak depressors of the ribs.

The **transversus thoracis** consist of 4-5 slips of muscle extending superiorly from the inferior internal sternum on both sides. This muscle is continuous inferiorly with the transversus abdominis muscles of the anterolateral wall. They generally act as weak depressors of the ribs and may have a proprioception function. The **subcostals** are variable in size and shape but are generally found only in the lower thoracic wall internally closest to the endothoracic fascia. Most often they will span at least two ribs and act as depressors of the ribs.

The **serratus posterior superior** was once said to elevate the ribs while the **serratus posterior inferior** depressed the ribs. Most people agree that both of these muscles have more of a proprioception function and the elevation versus depression functions is minor at best. The **levatores costarums** are 12 fan-shaped muscles extending down from transverse processes and are responsible for weakly elevating the ribs. They are the only ones within this group of thoracic wall muscles innervated by dorsal rami nerves. Refer to **Table 2.1** for descriptions of these muscles.

2.9 Thoracic Wall Movements

Movements of the thoracic wall and diaphragm produce changes in the diameters and intrathoracic volume of the thorax. Pressure changes result in air passing through the nose, mouth, larynx, down through the trachea and finally into the lungs (inspiration). Air will be expelled from the lungs and back through these same passages (expiration). Expiration for the most part is passive and results from the diaphragm and intercostal muscles relaxing. This decreases *intrathoracic volume* but increases *intrathoracic pressure*. In parallel, *intra-abdominal pressure decreases* and the abdominal viscera are no longer being compressed. There are three different thorax dimensions to consider when discussing movements of the thoracic wall: the *anteroposterior, vertical* and *transverse dimensions* (**Fig. 2.13**).

The **anteroposterior (AP) dimension** increases when the intercostal muscles contract and movement of the ribs (especially the 2nd-6th ribs) at the costovertebral joints around an axis passing through the necks of the ribs causes the anterior aspects of the ribs to rise. This gives the illusion of a *pump handle-like movement*. This dimension increases during inspiration and decreases during expiration.

The **vertical dimension** of the thorax increases during inspiration due to the contraction of the diaphragm. When the diaphragm contracts it will descend inferiorly toward the abdomen. During expiration, the diaphragm relaxes and the vertical dimension decreases.

The **transverse dimension** of the thorax increases when the intercostal muscles contract during inspiration and results in the raising of the lateral most parts of the ribs especially the inferior ones. This produces a *bucket handle-like movement* that increases during inspiration but decreases during expiration. In summary, the AP, vertical and transverse dimensions increase during inspiration but decrease during expiration.

2.10 Thoracic Wall Neurovasculature

There are 11 pairs of **intercostal nerves** followed by one pair of **subcostal nerves**, all of which are ventral rami nerves and the focus of this section. These intercostal nerves are divided into either a typical or atypical nerve. Dorsal rami nerves are present but pass posteriorly just lateral to the intervertebral foramen and supply deep back muscles, joints and skin of the posterior 1/3 of the back adjacent to the thorax region (**Fig. 2.14**).

Typical intercostal nerves are considered the 3rd-6th intercostal nerves and they enter the medial most parts of the posterior intercostal spaces initially running within the endothoracic fascia between the parietal fascia and internal intercostal membrane. Near the angle of the rib, the nerve passes between the internal and innermost intercostal muscles to enter the neurovascular plane and is located near the costal groove of the rib. It is paired with intercostal vessels in a vein,

Table 2.1 **Thoracic wall muscles**

Muscle	Innervation	Function(s)	Origin	Insertion
External intercostal	Intercostal nerves	Elevate ribs (mainly during forced inspiration)	Inferior border of ribs	Superior border of ribs one below the origin
Internal intercostal	Intercostal nerves	Depress ribs (mainly during forced expiration)	Inferior border of ribs	Superior border of ribs one below the origin
Innermost intercostal	Intercostal nerves	Depress ribs (mainly during forced expiration)	Inferior border of ribs	Superior border of ribs one below the origin
Transversus thoracis	Intercostal nerves	Weakly depresses ribs	Inner surface of sternum and xiphoid process	Inner surface of 2-6 ribs
Subcostal	Intercostal nerves	Depress ribs	Inner surface of lower half of ribs	Superior border of 2-3 ribs below the origin
Serratus posterior superior	2-5th intercostal nerves	Proprioception (elevate ribs)	Nuchal ligament; C7-T3 spinous processes	Superior borders of 2-4th ribs
Serratus posterior inferior	9-12th intercostal nerves	Proprioception (depress ribs)	T11-L2 spinous processes	Inferior borders of 8-12th ribs
Levatores costarum	Dorsal rami of C8-T11	Elevate ribs; extend and rotates thoracic spine	C7-T11 transverse processes	Adjacent tubercle and angle of rib below origin

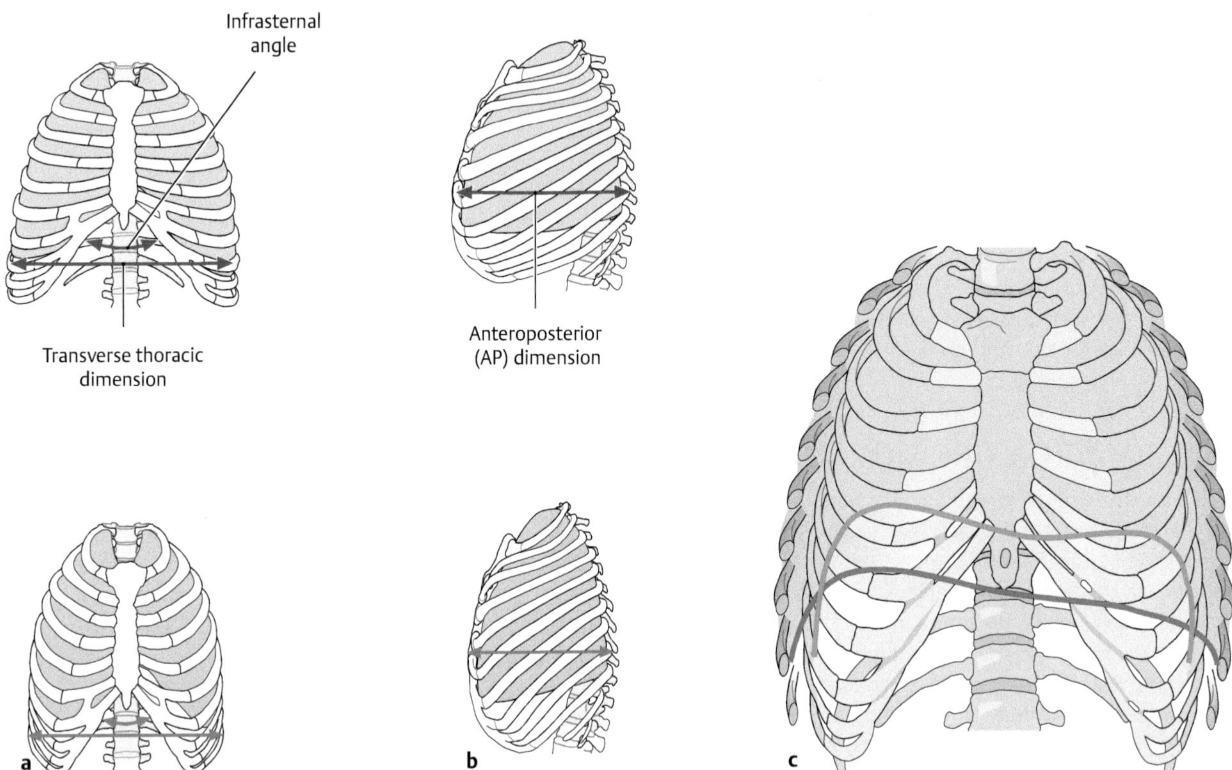

Fig. 2.13 Rib cage movements; full inspiration (red) and full expiration (blue). **(a)** Transverse dimension. **(b)** Anteroposterior dimension. **(c)** Vertical dimension. (From Schuenke M, Schulte E, Schumacher U. THIEME Atlas of Anatomy. General Anatomy and Musculoskeletal System. Illustrations by Voll M and Wesker K. 3rd ed. New York: Thieme Medical Publishers; 2020.)

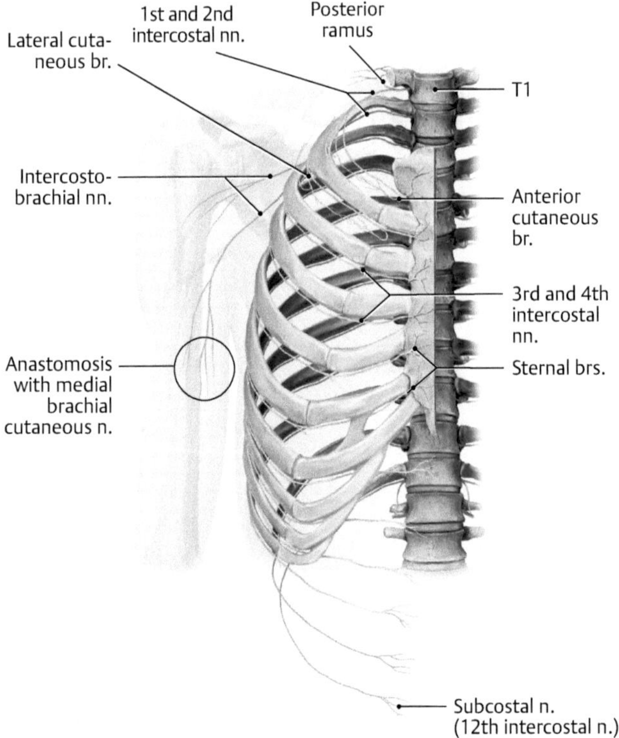

Fig. 2.14 Thoracic wall nerves. Anterior view demonstrating the 12 right sided intercostal nerves with the 1st rib removed. (From Schuenke M, Schulte E, Schumacher U. THIEME Atlas of Anatomy. General Anatomy and Musculoskeletal System. Illustrations by Voll M and Wesker K. 3rd ed. New York: Thieme Medical Publishers; 2020.)

artery and nerve (VAN) orientation within the costal groove **(Fig. 2.15)**.

The anterior, lateral and dorsal cutaneous branches (T2-T12) are represented in a segmental pattern or *dermatome* from the anterior to the posterior median lines **(Fig. 2.16)**. A group of muscles supplied by the ventral ramus (intercostal) and dorsal ramus of each pair of thoracic spinal nerves would constitute a *myotome*.

2.10.1 Branches of a Typical Intercostal Nerve

- **Rami communicantes** are the branches that connect the ipsilateral sympathetic trunk to each of the corresponding intercostal and subcostal nerves **(Fig. 2.17)**. The white rami communicantes are located lateral to the gray rami communicantes but are only found attached to all the thoracic intercostals, subcostal and upper two lumbar ventral rami branches. The white rami contain GVE-sym/pre fibers entering the sympathetic trunk. The gray rami are attached to all of the ventral rami from C1 to Co1 (if present). However, GVE-sym/pre fibers passing through the gray rami will continue on a ventral or dorsal rami branch. This means sym/post fibers will be distributed through all branches of the spinal nerves in order to reach smooth muscle of the blood vessels and arrector pili and sweat glands.
- **Collateral branches** that are generally smaller than the intercostals originate near the angle of the rib but run along the superior border with collateral vessels. The collateral

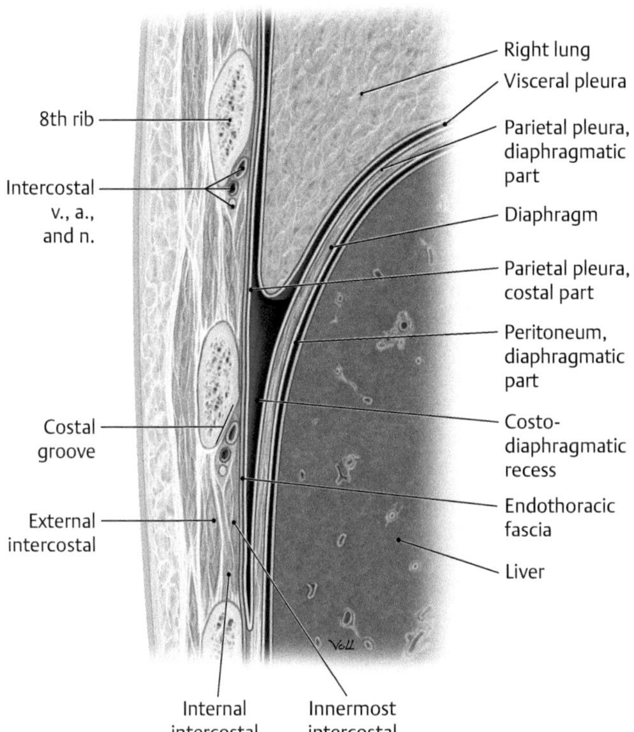

Fig. 2.15 Thoracic wall neurovasculature. Coronal section, anterior view. (From Schuenke M, Schulte E, Schumacher U. THIEME Atlas of Anatomy. Internal Organs. Illustrations by Voll M and Wesker K. 3rd ed. New York: Thieme Medical Publishers; 2020.)

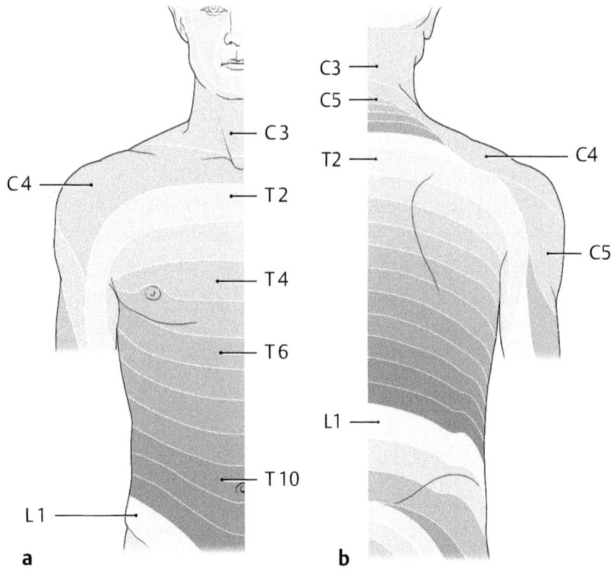

Fig. 2.16 Dermatomes of the thoracic wall. **(a)** Anterior view. **(b)** Posterior view. (From Schuenke M, Schulte E, Schumacher U. THIEME Atlas of Anatomy. General Anatomy and Musculoskeletal System. Illustrations by Voll M and Wesker K. 3rd ed. New York: Thieme Medical Publishers; 2020.)

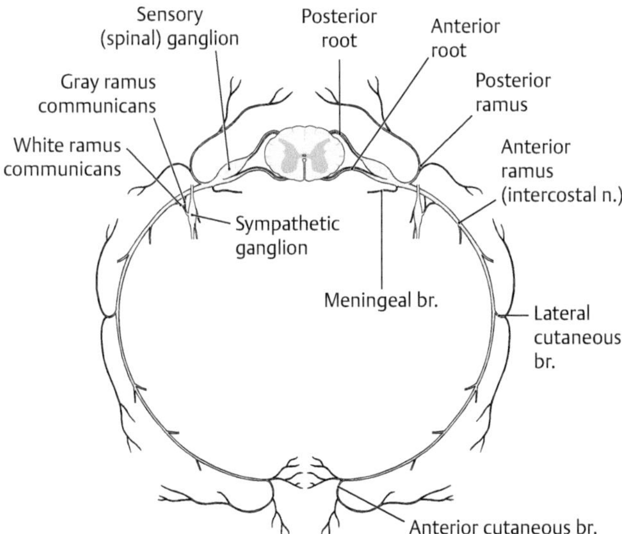

Fig. 2.17 Branches of a spinal nerve and typical intercostal nerve, superior view. (From Schuenke M, Schulte E, Schumacher U. THIEME Atlas of Anatomy. General Anatomy and Musculoskeletal System. Illustrations by Voll M and Wesker K. 3rd ed. New York: Thieme Medical Publishers; 2020.)

neurovasculature on the superior border of a rib is in a nerve, artery and vein (NAV) orientation. They help supply intercostal muscles and the parietal pleura.

- **Lateral cutaneous branches** leave the larger intercostal nerve at the midaxillary line, pierce the internal then external intercostal muscles, and then divide into an ***anterior*** and ***posterior branch***. These nerve branches supply the skin of the lateral thorax and abdominal walls.
- **Anterior cutaneous branches** are the terminal branches of an intercostal nerve and pierce the muscles and membranes of the intercostal space near the lateral sternum. Here it bifurcates into a lateral and medial branch that supplies the skin of the anterior thorax and abdomen.
- **Muscular branches** supply the intercostal, serratus posterior, transverse thoracis, subcostal and levator costarum muscles.
- The functional components of the intercostal nerves are GSE, GSA and GVE-sym/post. Any cutaneous branch would have GSA and GVE-sym/post fibers.

2.10.2 Characteristics of Atypical Intercostal Nerves

The above lists of branches that originate from a typical nerve are also associated, for the most part, with atypical intercostal nerves. Most of the characteristics of an atypical nerve are related to position or extra branching patterns. The ventral ramus of T1 actually has a larger superior and a smaller inferior portion. The superior portion becomes associated with the *brachial plexus* of the arm while the inferior portion actually becomes the 1st intercostal nerve.

- The 1st intercostal nerve has no anterior cutaneous branch and on occasion no lateral cutaneous branch. If the lateral cutaneous branch is present, it helps supply the skin of the axilla.
- The 1st and 2nd intercostal nerves course alongside the internal surface of the 1st and 2nd ribs respectively instead of in the costal groove.

- The 2nd intercostal nerve gives rise to the **intercostobrachial nerve** which is a larger cutaneous nerve supplying the skin of the axillary floor and superomedial posterior arm. It passes through the 2nd intercostal space near the midaxillary line and may communicate with the *medial cutaneous nerve of the arm*. A second intercostobrachial nerve may originate from the lateral cutaneous branch of the 3rd intercostal nerve.
- After giving rise to their lateral cutaneous branches, the 7th-11th intercostal nerves cross the costal margin posteriorly and continue on to supply abdominal muscles and skin. They are no longer intercostal at this point and have become the *thoraco-abdominal nerves*. The anterior cutaneous branches of these nerves supply the midline of the abdomen.

2.11 Thoracic Wall Blood Supply

Arterial supply to the thoracic wall originates from branches off the thoracic aorta, subclavian and axillary arteries. Each intercostal space (except for the 10th and 11th) is supplied by a posterior intercostal and its collateral branch, as well as a superior and inferior anterior intercostal artery (**Fig. 2.18**). Near the midaxillary line, the posterior intercostal forms an anastomosis with the *superior* anterior intercostal artery and the collateral branch will anastomose with the *inferior* anterior intercostal artery. Below are the characteristics of these thoracic wall arteries.

- **Posterior Intercostal Arteries**:
  - The ones located in the 1st and 2nd intercostal spaces originated from the **superior intercostal artery**, which is a branch off the **costocervical trunk** of the 2nd part of the subclavian artery.
  - The 3rd-11th posterior intercostal and **subcostal** (*12th posterior intercostal*) branches originate from the thoracic aorta.
  - All of them give off spinal branches that help supply the vertebral column, back muscles, spinal cord and skin.
  - Found in the neurovascular plane between the internal and innermost intercostal muscles.
  - Form an anastomosis with the *superior* anterior intercostal arteries.
  - Collateral branches near the angle of the rib are given off which then anastomose with the *inferior* anterior intercostal artery. Along with its collateral branch they are the only arteries to supply the 10th and 11th intercostal spaces.
- **Internal Thoracic (Internal Mammary) Arteries**:
  - Originate from the 1st part of the subclavian artery.
  - Terminate near the 6th intercostal space as the **superior epigastric** and **musculophrenic arteries**.
  - Pass posterior to the clavicle and 1st costal cartilage on their way to the anterior thorax just posterior to the sternum.
  - They are crossed near their origins by the phrenic nerves.
  - Give rise directly to the upper six sets of superior/inferior anterior intercostal arteries.
- **Anterior intercostal arteries**:
  - The upper six sets of anterior intercostals originate from the internal thoracic arteries.
  - The next three sets of anterior intercostal arteries originate from the musculophrenic arteries.
  - Are not located in the 10th or 11th intercostal spaces.

2.12 Thoracic Wall Venous Drainage

There are 11 **posterior intercostal**, a **subcostal** and 9 superior/inferior **anterior intercostal veins** on each side of the thorax (**Fig. 2.19**). Just like with the arteries, there is an anastomosis between the posterior intercostal, its collateral branch and the anterior intercostal veins. The posterior intercostal vein, along with its spinal tributary draining the vertebral column and spinal cord, and subcostal vein on the right side of the thorax drain primarily to the azygos vein. Blood from the azygos vein drains into the superior vena cava.

The right 1st posterior intercostal vein drains into the right brachiocephalic vein. The right 2nd and 3rd posterior intercostal veins drain first into the **right superior intercostal vein** before it drains near the arch of the azygos vein. The remaining posterior intercostals and the subcostal vein on the right drain directly into the azygos vein.

The left 1st posterior intercostal vein drains into the left brachiocephalic vein. The left 2nd-4th posterior intercostal veins drain first into the **left superior intercostal vein** before they drain into the left brachiocephalic vein as well. The left superior intercostal vein may also drain into the **accessory hemiazygos vein**. The 5th-8th posterior intercostal veins generally drain first into the accessory hemiazygos vein and blood from here will drain into the larger azygos vein. The left 9th-11th posterior intercostals and subcostal vein drain into the **hemiazygos vein** and blood from here will also drain to the azygos vein.

The superior 6 sets of **anterior intercostal veins** drain directly into the internal thoracic veins. The inferior 3 sets of anterior intercostal veins drain first into the **musculophrenic veins** prior to reaching the internal thoracic veins. The **internal thoracic veins** drain into the brachiocephalic veins.

2.13 Breasts

2.13.1 Structure of the Breast

Breasts are the most prominent feature of the anterior thoracic wall in women (**Fig. 2.20**). Breast size and shape are determined in part by genetic, ethnic and dietary factors. Breasts in men are generally due to an overabundance of subcutaneous tissue. For females, the breast size, shape and symmetry can even vary on the same individual. The breasts are separated medially by the **intermammary cleft** and divided clinically into superolateral, superomedial, inferolateral and inferomedial quadrants. The quadrants are important to understand when discussing lymphatic drainage and cancer metastasis of the breast.

The breasts consist of glandular and supporting fibrous tissue that is embedded within a fatty matrix mixed in with nerves, vessels and lymphatics. The amount of fat surrounding the glandular tissue will determine the size of a non-lactating breast. The breast is generally located vertically from the 2nd-6th ribs and transversely from the sternum's lateral border to the midaxillary line. The mostly circular, posterior surface of the breast rests on the **bed of the breast**. The pectoral fascia or deep fascia of the pectoralis major muscle forms two-thirds of the bed while the other one-third is formed by the deep fascia of the serratus anterior muscle. A potential space does exist between the breast and pectoral fascia known as the **retromammary space**.

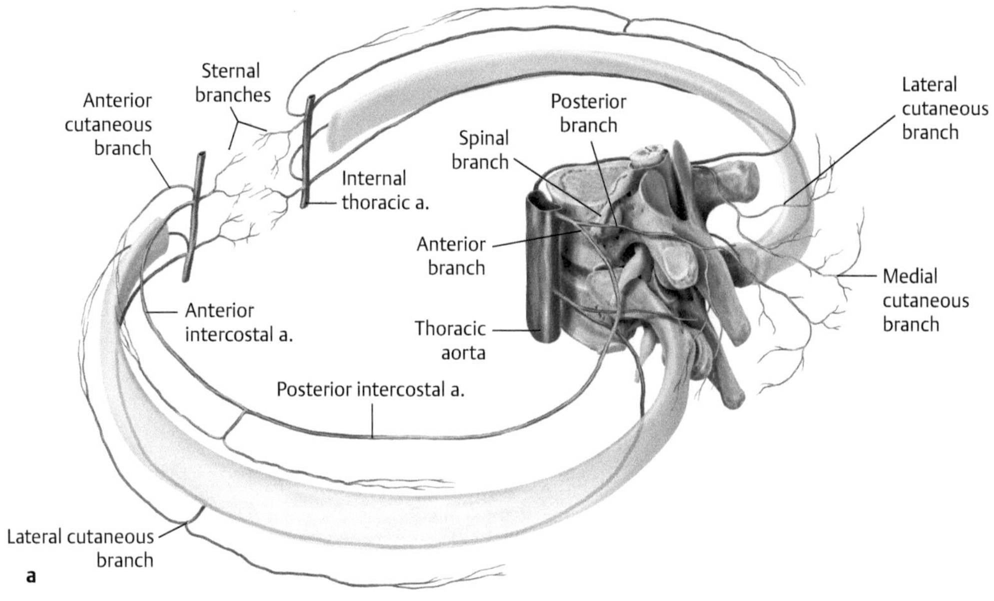

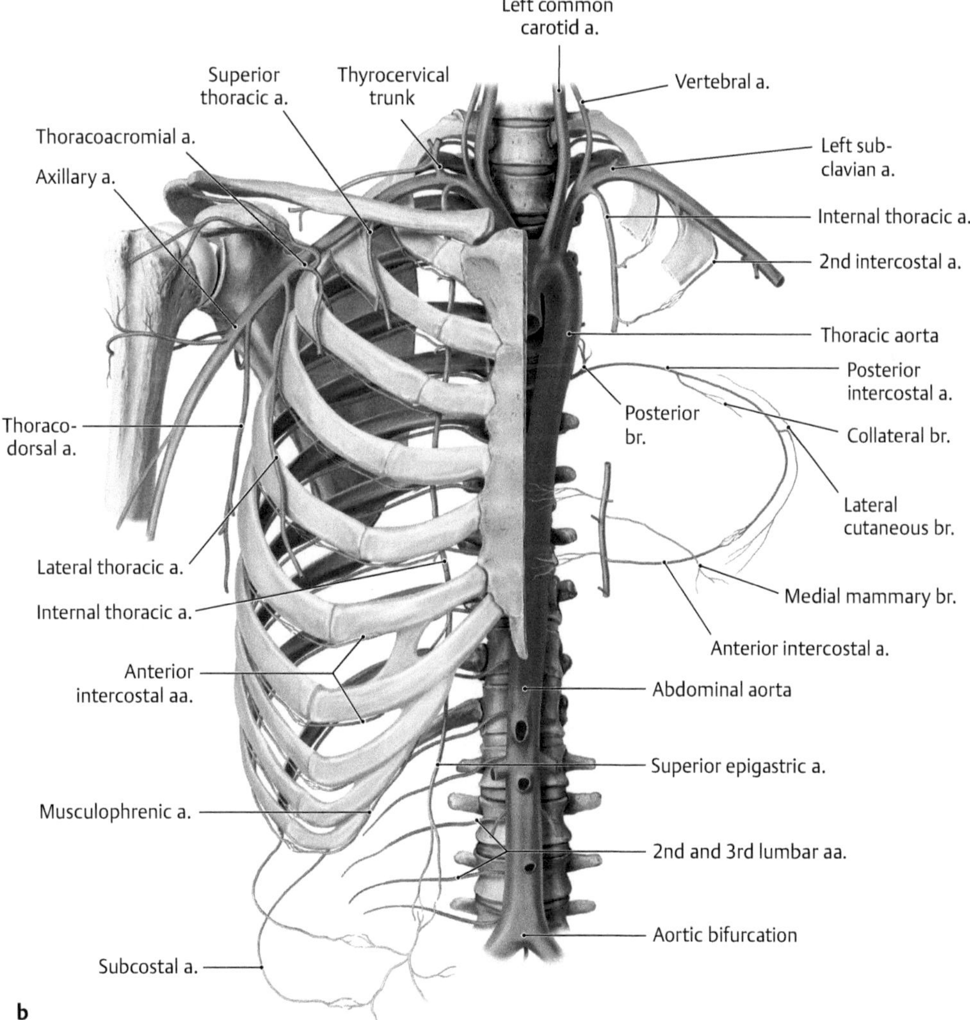

Fig. 2.18 Intercostal arteries. **(a)** Oblique posterosuperior view. **(b)** Anterior view. (From Schuenke M, Schulte E, Schumacher U. THIEME Atlas of Anatomy. General Anatomy and Musculoskeletal System. Illustrations by Voll M and Wesker K. 3rd ed. New York: Thieme Medical Publishers; 2020.)

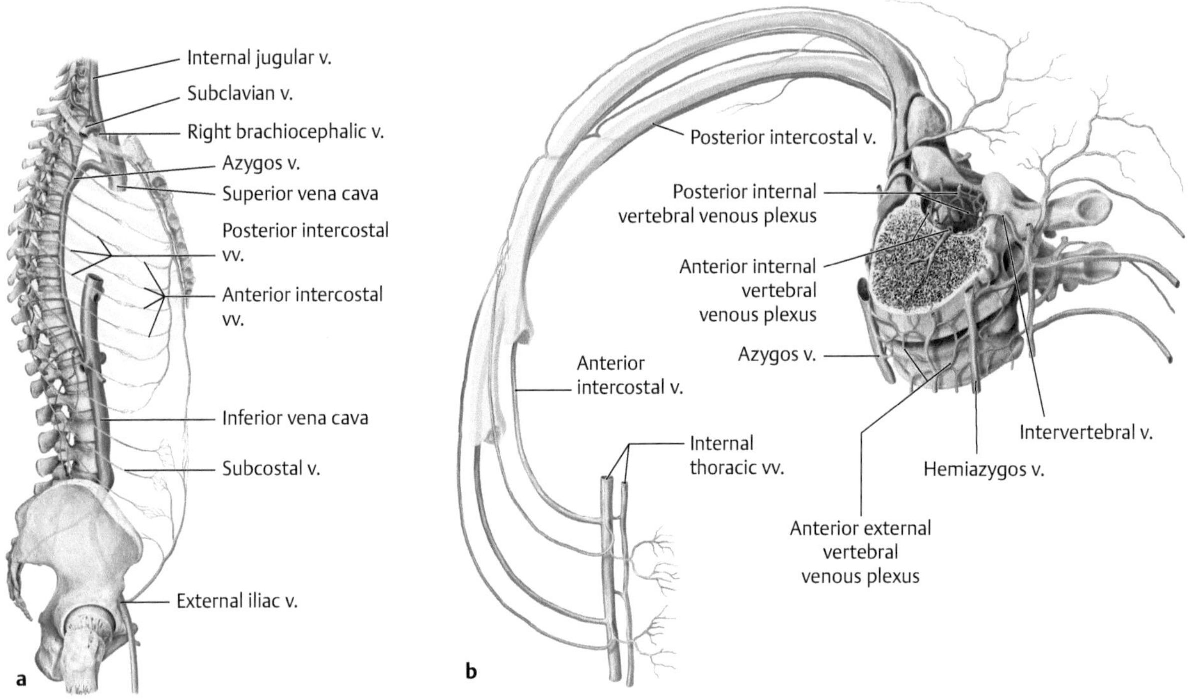

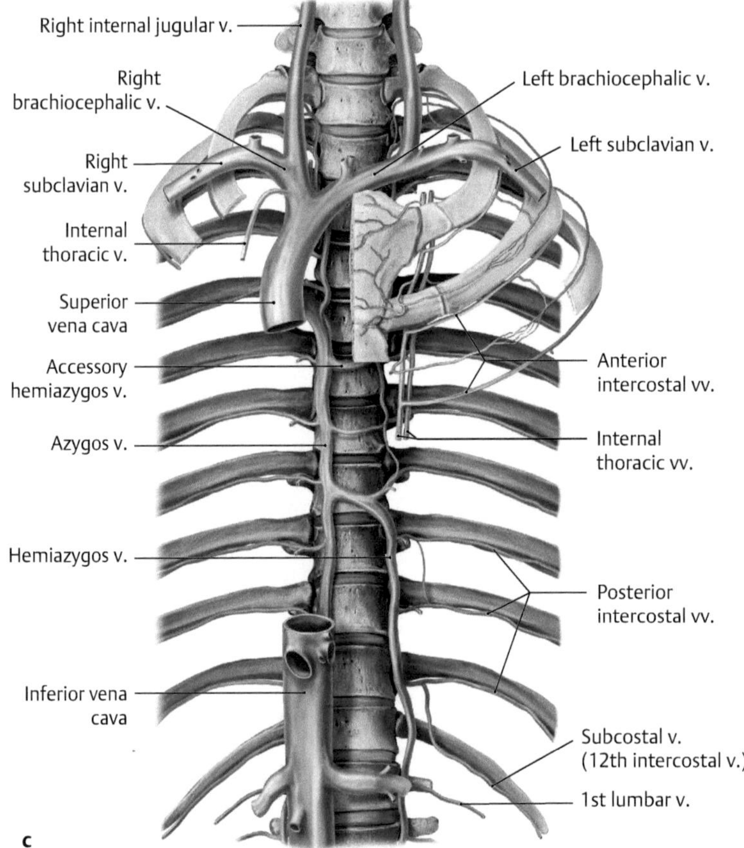

Fig. 2.19 Veins of the thoracic wall. **(a)** Right lateral view. **(b)** Anterosuperior view. **(c)** Anterior view with rib cage opened. (From Schuenke M, Schulte E, Schumacher U. THIEME Atlas of Anatomy. General Anatomy and Musculoskeletal System. Illustrations by Voll M and Wesker K. 3rd ed. New York: Thieme Medical Publishers; 2020.)

Clinical Correlate 2.1

Supernumerary Ribs

An individual normally has 24 total ribs, 12 on each side. A small percentage of people (0.5%) have a cervical rib articulating with the C7 vertebra. This extra cervical rib could be the reason an individual is experiencing thoracic outlet syndrome. A less common supernumerary rib would be a lumbar rib articulating with the L1 vertebra.

Clinical Correlate 2.2

Rib Fractures

Blunt trauma generally exerts direct pressure on the ribs and is the most common mechanism for causing rib fractures. Rib fractures are easily identified using a standard chest x-ray. A CT scan could be useful in determining if a contusion was present or to identify air that may have escaped the lung as a pneumothorax after the fracture. The weakest part of the rib is just anterior to the angle of the rib but fractures can occur anywhere on the rib. The 7th-10th ribs are the most common ribs fractured and this may result in the tearing of the diaphragm or puncturing of the spleen and liver. Fractures of the 1st and 2nd ribs are rare but when the 1st rib is involved the subclavian vessels and the brachial (nerve) plexus are at risk for damage. Pain may be felt for some time after the initial fracture because of the constant movement of the ribs during normal breathing.

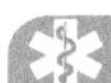

Clinical Correlate 2.3

Rib Dislocations

A rib dislocation involves the *sternocostal joints* or the displacement of the *interchondral joints*. "Slipping rib syndrome" is another term used to describe these dislocations. They are common in contact sports and may result in damage of the nearby intercostal neurovasculature. Interchondral joints are the synovial joints between costal cartilages of the 6th-10th ribs but generally the dislocation involves ribs 8-10.

Clinical Correlate 2.4

Rib Separations

Rib separations generally involve one or more of the 3rd-10th costochondral joints and results in tearing of the perichondrium and periosteum. Ribs may separate superiorly and override the rib above it causing great pain.

Clinical Correlate 2.5

Flail Chest

Flail chest involves multiple but mostly adjacent rib fractures allowing a large segment of the anterior or lateral thoracic wall to move freely. In all cases, a flail chest is accompanied by a pulmonary contusion and may result in a clinical entity called acute lung injury. In the most severe form, acute lung injury can lead to adult respiratory distress syndrome (ARDS) which is life threatening. Respiratory failure is usually caused by the underlying pulmonary contusion but not by the anatomic flail chest itself. In addition, the flail segment moves in the opposite direction as the rest of the chest wall because of the ambient pressure in comparison to the pressure inside the lungs. This paradoxical motion can increase the pain and work involved with breathing.

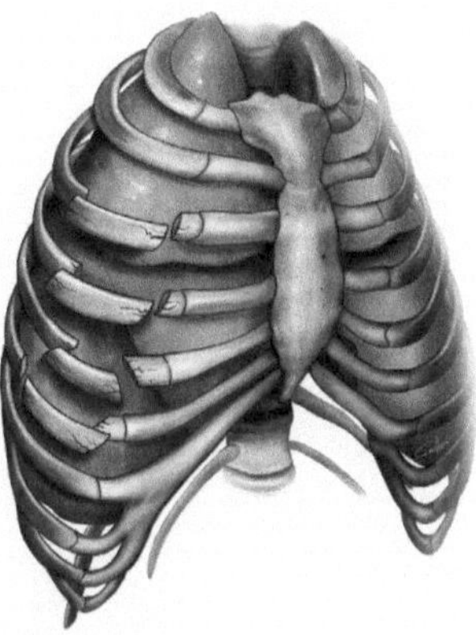

Illustration by Calla Heald.

Mammary glands are located in the subcutaneous tissue overlying mainly the pectoralis major. Mammary glands are considered by most to be modified sweat glands while others believe they are modified sebaceous glands. They are accessory to reproduction in females and are responsible for producing milk in order to feed newborns. A small portion of the mammary gland extends up near the axilla and is known as the **axillary tail (of Spence)**. It is often mistaken as a cancerous lump during the menstrual cycle.

The mammary glands are attached to the dermis of overlying skin by fibrous connective tissue known as the **suspensory ligaments (of Cooper)**. They help support the lobes and lobules of the mammary gland and are well developed in the superior part of the gland. Normal enlargement of the breasts occurs during puberty and is the result primarily of increased fat deposits and glandular development. The milk-producing part of the gland is known as the parenchyma. This parenchyma consists of lobes that are divided into 15-20 **lobules of the mammary gland**. The lobules contain grape-like clusters of milk-secreting **alveoli**. A **lactiferous duct** drains each lobule, and it has a dilated portion known as the **lactiferous sinus**. However, recent studies have shown that there may not be a lactiferous sinus.

The **nipple** is a conical structure located in the middle of the areola and contains the merging lactiferous ducts (assuming no sinus is present). In males and young women, the nipple is located at the level of the 4th intercostal space; however, in multiparous women the nipples may be located at a different intercostal space and vary considerably. Smooth muscle fibers of the nipple wrap around the lactiferous ducts and compress them during lactation. These smooth muscle fibers are also responsible for erecting the nipple during arousal or infant suckling. Nipples contain no hair, sweat glands or fat.

The **areola** is the circular pigmented area of skin surrounding the nipple. The areolae contain numerous sebaceous glands that enlarge during pregnancy and secrete an oily substance that provides a protective lubricant for both the nipple and areola. Compression of the areola during infant suckling results in milk being secreted into the mouth of the infant and not sucked from the gland. The *let-down reflex*, which is influenced by the infant suckling and the hormone oxytocin, causes milk to freely flow during breastfeeding.

Clinical Correlate 2.6

Thoracotomy

A surgical opening into an individual's pleural space of the chest and performed in either a controlled or emergency situation, is known as a thoracotomy. A thoracotomy may be used in many thoracic surgeries some of which include heart and lung transplants; open heart bypass surgeries; segmentectomy, lobectomy or pneumonectomy of the lungs; or an esophagectomy. Types of thoracotomies include median sternotomy and anterolateral or posterolateral thoractomies. These surgical incisions will require the use of a rib retractor to maintain patency of the intercostal space. In addition, the latissmus dorsi and serratus anterior muscles are commonly divided unless a modified thoracotomy is performed. Complications include heart, lung or vessel damage, persistent pain, pneumothorax, and consistent numbness near the incision and surrounding area.

- *Median sternotomy*: an incision through the center of the sternum and the choice for most open heart surgeries. This incision also allows access to the lungs.
- *Anterolateral thoracotomy*: generally a smaller incision through the intercostal space to allow access to the heart for open chest/heart massage, for example.
- *Posterolateral thoracotomy*: generally a larger incision near the 5th-7th intercostal spaces allowing greater access to the lungs, heart, aorta and esophagus. This is the approach most likely taken for a lobe or pneumoectomy of the lung.

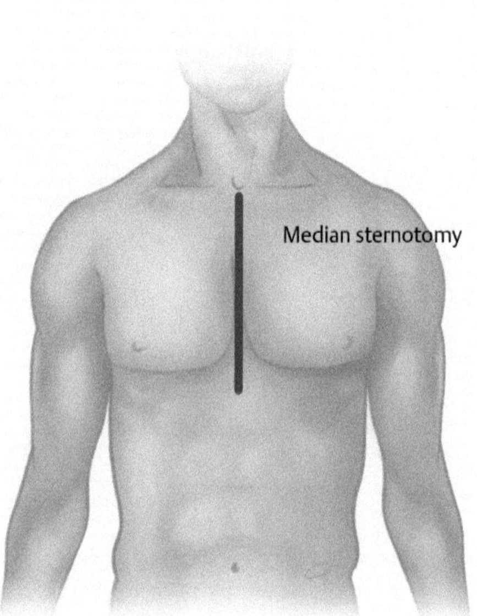

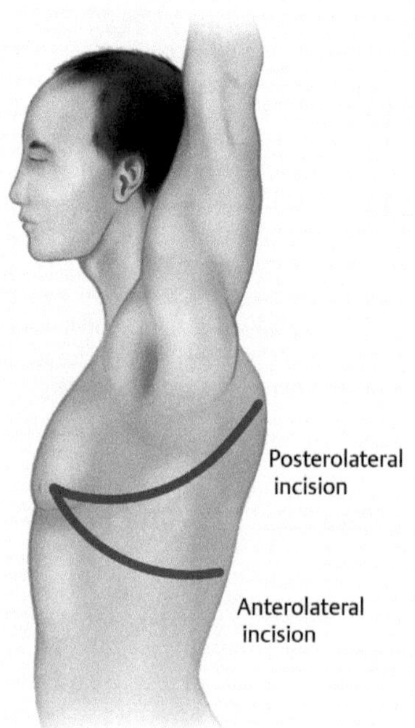

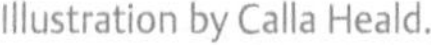
Illustration by Calla Heald.

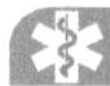

Clinical Correlate 2.7

Video-Assisted Thoracoscopic Surgery (VATS)

To reduce the need for thoracotomies, a type of thoracic surgery known as video-assisted thoracoscopic surgery (or VATS) was developed and involves a camera and laparoscopic instruments being inserted into the chest wall through small ports. This type of surgery became popular in the early 1990s to replace the traditional thoracotomy to do common procedures such as pulmonary biopsies and decortication (pleural layer removal), pleurodesis (adhesion of pleurae), lymphadenectomy for lung cancer and segmentectomy of the lung, thoracic sympathectomy to control hyperhidrosis (excessive sweating), esophageal resections, and the repair of diaphragmatic hernias.

Clinical Correlate 2.8

Thoracic Outlet Syndrome (TOS)

There are various types of TOS but it is generally due to the compression of nerves and vessels passing near the clavicle. This neurovasculature originates from between the anterior and middle scalene muscles of the neck and passes through to the upper limbs. These structures include the brachial plexus and subclavian artery (the subclavian vein is rarely involved). It may present initially with pain in the shoulder and neck regions or more than normal paresthesia and motor deficits of the upper limb. The *superior thoracic aperture* that anatomists refer to is the same as the *thoracic outlet* that clinicians refer to. Compression of these structures actually occurs in the root of the neck and not the thoracic region as the name implies. Treatment may include resection of the extra cervical rib, abnormal fascial band release, physical therapy or even a bypass of an abnormally placed blood vessel. Complications could include pneumothorax or damage to the nearby muscles, nerves and blood vessels.

Clinical Correlate 2.9

Intercostal Nerve Blocks

An **intercostal nerve block** is an injection of a steroid or local anesthetic near the location of an intercostal nerve or one of its collateral branches adjacent to the rib. This procedure is typically ordered by a physician for pain near the ribs following surgery in that area (i.e., after a thoracotomy), a rib fracture or for an individual suffering from herpes zoster (shingles). Due to the overlapping nature of dermatomes, injections of two or more consecutive intercostal nerves must be done in order to completely knock out sensation from that region.

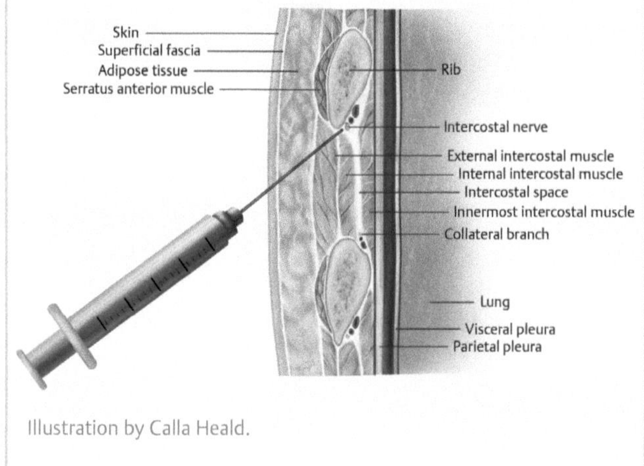

Illustration by Calla Heald.

2.13.2 Neurovasculature of the Breasts

- Cutaneous innervation of the breast comes from the **anterior and lateral cutaneous nerve branches of the 4th-6th intercostal nerves (Fig. 2.21a)**.
- Arterial supply originates mainly from the **lateral thoracic artery** (axillary artery branch) and the **internal thoracic artery** (subclavian artery branch) **(Fig. 2.21b)**.
  - **Lateral mammary arteries** from both the lateral thoracic and lateral cutaneous branches of the posterior intercostal arteries.
  - **Medial mammary arteries** from the perforating branches of the internal thoracic artery.
- Venous drainage follows the arteries to either the **lateral thoracic** or **internal thoracic veins**. Venous drainage leads back to either the axillary or brachiocephalic veins and to a lesser degree the azygos venous system **(Fig. 2.21b)**.

2.13.3 Lymphatic Drainage of the Breasts

Breast cancer will typically spread by way of the lymphatic vessels, which carry these cancer cells from the breast primarily to the lymph nodes of the axilla. Due to the abundant lymphatic vessels in the breast, a thorough understanding of all lymphatic drainage patterns is warranted because breast cancer can spread to multiple areas.

Lymph will first pass through the **subareolar lymphatic plexus** from the nipple, areola gland lobules. From here lymph drainage can follow multiple routes **(Fig. 2.22)**:

- Most lymph (>75%), mainly from the superolateral and inferolateral quadrants, drains to the **pectoral (anterior) lymph nodes** of the larger collection of **axillary lymph nodes.** The axillary lymph nodes are made up of the **pectoral (anterior)**, **humeral (lateral)**, **subscapular (posterior)**, **central** and **apical lymph nodes**. Lymph from the axillary lymph nodes will drain superiorly to the **infraclavicular** and **supraclavicular lymph nodes** before reaching the **subclavian lymphatic trunk**. Form here lymph will drain into the **right lymphatic duct** on the right side or **thoracic duct** on the left side, before finally draining into the venous circulation near the **venous angles** marked by the junction of the internal jugular and subclavian veins.
- Cancer metastasis from the superior quadrants can sometimes pass from the subareolar lymphatic plexus to the **interpectoral (Rotter's) lymph nodes** located between the pectoralis major and minor muscles before reaching the axillary nodes.
- Lymph from the medial quadrants can drain to the ipsilateral **parasternal lymph nodes** or even to the contralateral breast. From the parasternal lymph nodes, lymph will travel to the **bronchomediastinal lymphatic trunk**, followed by the drainage into either the right lymphatic duct of thoracic duct.
- Lymph from the inferior quadrants may pass to the *abdominal (subdiaphragmatic) lymph nodes* specifically the **inferior phrenic lymph nodes**.

2.14 Overview of the Mediastinum

The mediastinum is the region and central component of the thorax that contains structures located between the two pulmonary cavities **(Fig. 2.24)**. The mediastinum is located from the superior thoracic aperture down to the diaphragm, from the sternum and costal cartilages to the thoracic vertebrae, and is covered on each side by mediastinal pleura. The mediastinum is quite mobile due to the hollow nature of the heart and lungs as well as the loose connective tissue, nerves, vessels and lymph nodes that surround these visceral structures.

The mediastinum is initially divided into a superior and inferior mediastinum. The **superior mediastinum** will extend from the superior thoracic aperture down to the **transverse thoracic plane** located at the level of the sternal angle and vertebral level T4/T5. The **inferior mediastinum** extends down from the transverse thoracic plane to the level of the diaphragm, which varies depending on the specific location of the diaphragm but can reach as low as the T12 vertebral level. The inferior mediastinum is further divided into an *anterior*, *middle* and *posterior mediastinum* and will be examined in that order.

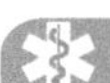

Clinical Correlate 2.10

Mammography

A mammogram is the radiographic examination of the breasts using low-energy x-rays **(Fig. 2.23a)**. The exam is used for early detection of breast cancer and the results are reported by way of a Breast Imaging-Reporting and Data System (BI-RADS™) score.

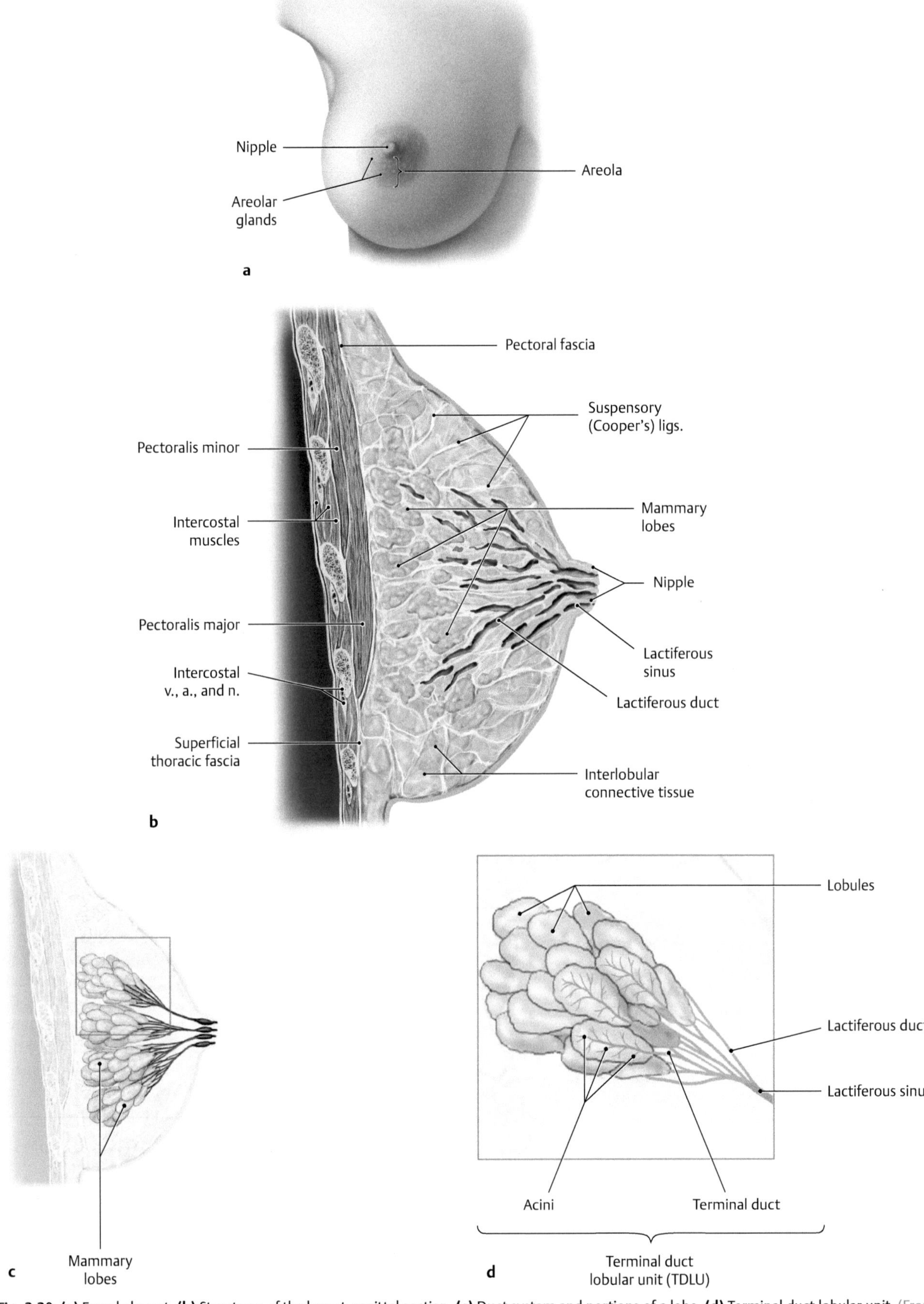

Fig. 2.20 **(a)** Female breast. **(b)** Structures of the breast, sagittal section. **(c)** Duct system and portions of a lobe. **(d)** Terminal duct lobular unit. (From Schuenke M, Schulte E, Schumacher U. THIEME Atlas of Anatomy. General Anatomy and Musculoskeletal System. Illustrations by Voll M and Wesker K. 3rd ed. New York: Thieme Medical Publishers; 2020.)

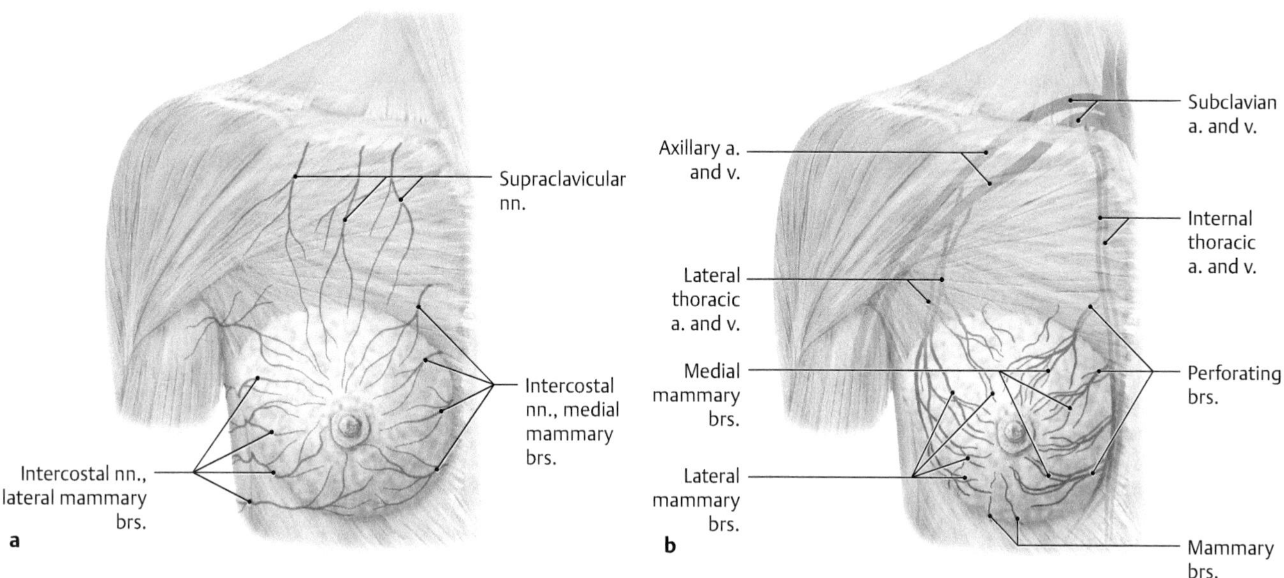

Fig. 2.21 **(a)** Sensory innervation of the breast. **(b)** Vasculature of the breast. (From Schuenke M, Schulte E, Schumacher U. THIEME Atlas of Anatomy. General Anatomy and Musculoskeletal System. Illustrations by Voll M and Wesker K. 3rd ed. New York: Thieme Medical Publishers; 2020.)

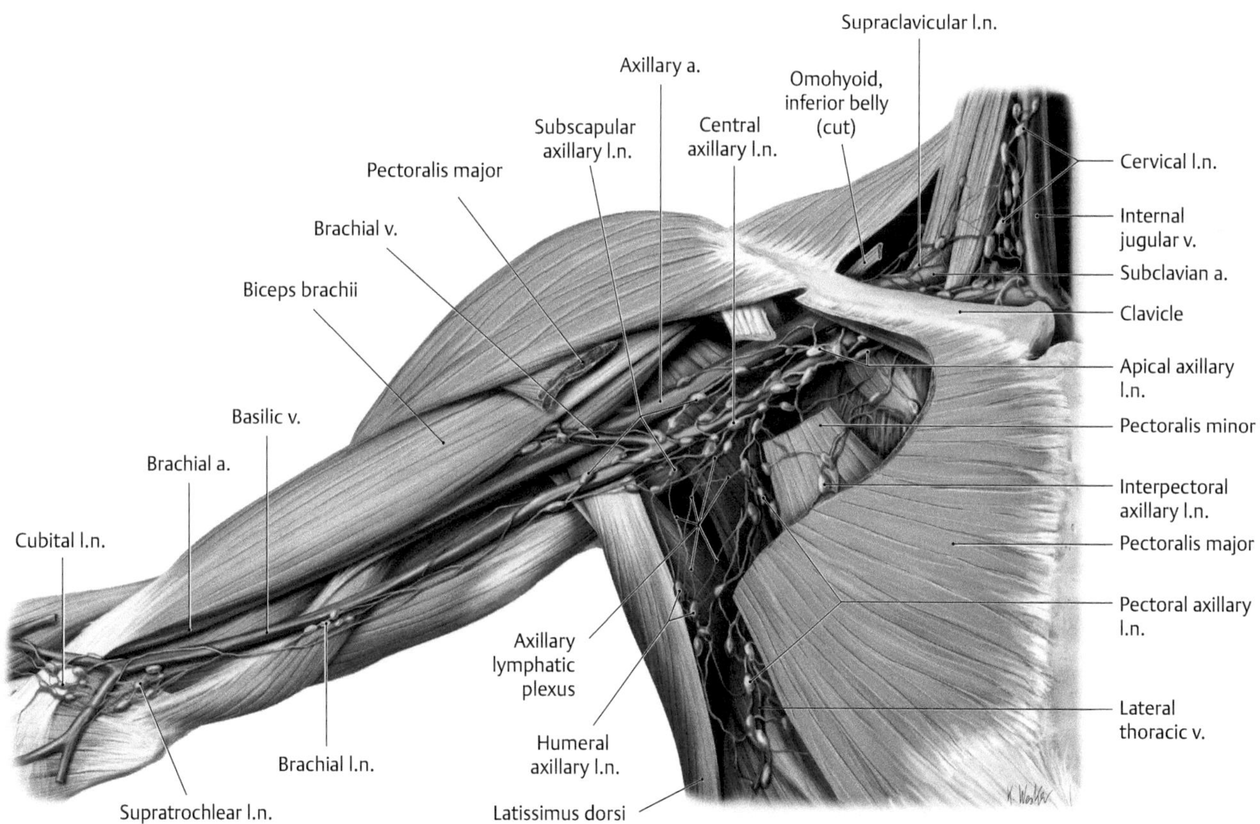

Fig. 2.22 Lymphatic drainage of the breasts. (From Schuenke M, Schulte E, Schumacher U. THIEME Atlas of Anatomy. General Anatomy and Musculoskeletal System. Illustrations by Voll M and Wesker K. 3rd ed. New York: Thieme Medical Publishers; 2020.)

Clinical Correlate 2.11

Carcinoma of the Breast and Mastectomies

Breast cancers are usually adenocarcinomas (glandular in nature) developing from epithelial cells of the lactiferous ducts in the mammary gland lobules. They also generally present as malignant tumors **(Fig. 2.23b)**. Most breast cancers spread through lymphatic vessels to the axillary lymph nodes. There is however a number of lymphatic communications between the axillary, cervical, parasternal and abdominal regions, meaning metastasis can occur to more than just the axillary lymph nodes.

With breast cancer, abnormal breast contours may be visible externally. If lymphatic drainage is impeded by cancer, this may result in edema that causes swelling and in turn causes the nipple to deviate. A leather-like appearance of the skin and prominent puffiness between dimpled pores makes the surface much like an orange peel. This is called *peau d'orange*. Cancerous invasion of the glandular tissue and fibrosis add traction and shorten the suspensory ligaments (of Cooper) creating larger skin dimpling. Cancerous invasion affecting the lactiferous ducts, as in *subareolar breast cancer*, can result in nipple retraction.

Five-year survival rates can be established by dividing the axillary lymph nodes into three levels. **Level I (lower axillary group)** is located lateral to the pectoralis minor and consists of the *humeral (lateral)*, *pectoral (anterior)* and *subscapular (posterior)* lymph nodes. **Level II (middle axillary group)** is located at the level of the pectoralis minor and consists of the *central* and *interpectoral* lymph nodes. **Level III (upper infraclavicular group)** is located medial to the pectoralis minor and consists of the *apical* lymph nodes. The 5-year survival rate if malignancy has reached level I, II, and III is about 65%, 31% and nearly 0% respectively **(Fig. 2.23c)**.

The distribution of malignant tumors can be described as originating from one of four breast quadrants. The breast is divided into a superolateral, inferolateral, superomedial and inferomedial quadrant. Most malignancies originate from the superolateral quadrant and account for approximately 60% of all malignant tumors of the breast. Although part of all four quadrants, malignancies originating from the areola account for approximately 10% of malignant tumors of the breast **(Fig. 2.23d)**.

The removal of the breast is known as a **mastectomy**. A **simple mastectomy** (or *total mastectomy*) involves the entire breast tissue down to the retromammary space being removed but the axillary tissue and lymph nodes are left intact. A **radial mastectomy** involves the removal of the entire breast tissue along with the axillary lymph nodes, surrounding fat, pectoralis major and minor muscles. The **modified radical mastectomy** is similar to the radical mastectomy but the pectoral muscles are left intact.

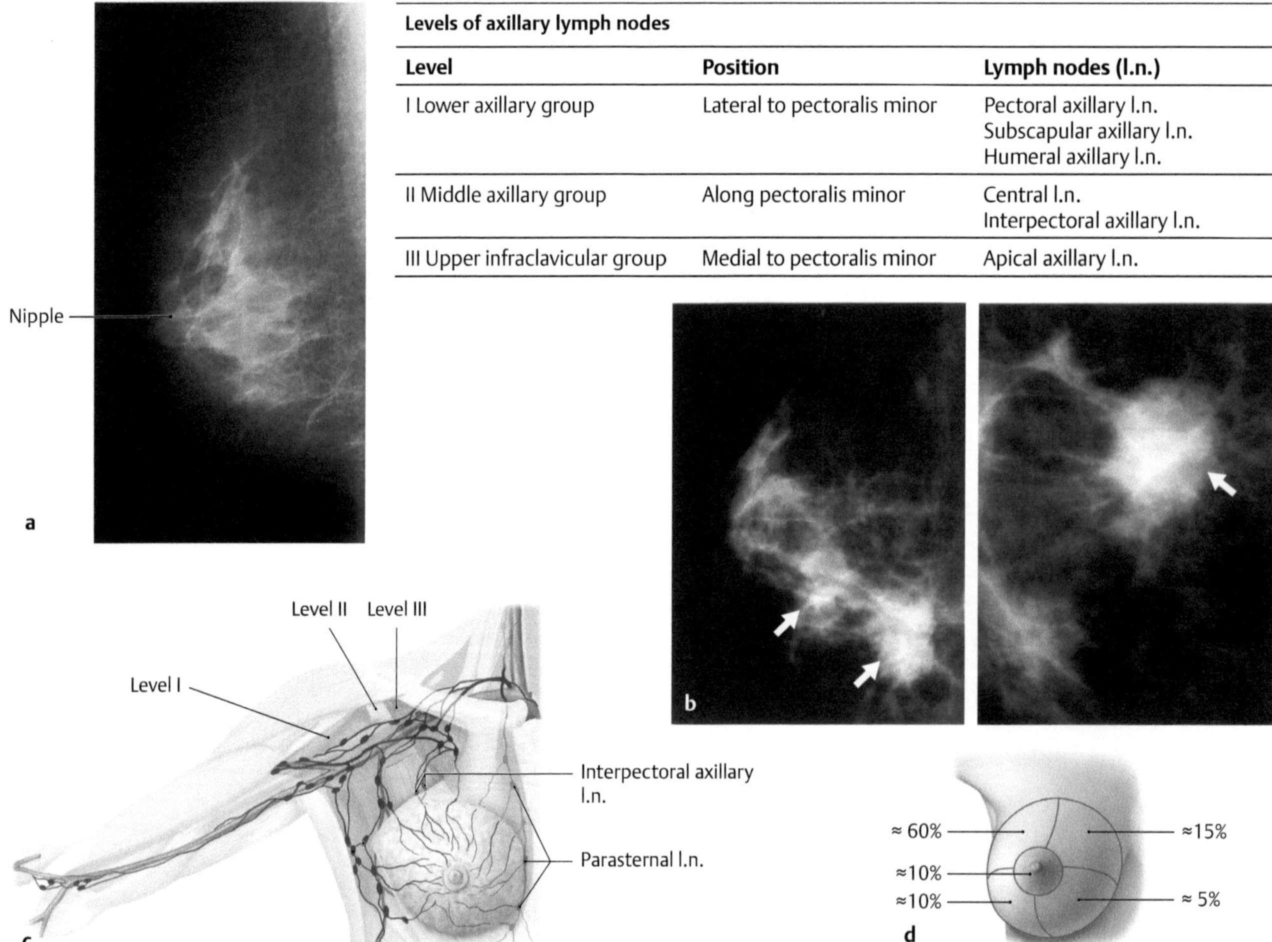

Levels of axillary lymph nodes

Level	Position	Lymph nodes (l.n.)
I Lower axillary group	Lateral to pectoralis minor	Pectoral axillary l.n. Subscapular axillary l.n. Humeral axillary l.n.
II Middle axillary group	Along pectoralis minor	Central l.n. Interpectoral axillary l.n.
III Upper infraclavicular group	Medial to pectoralis minor	Apical axillary l.n.

Fig. 2.23 **(a)** Normal mammogram. **(b)** Mammogram of invasive ductal carcinoma (irregular white areas, *arrows*). **(c)** Lymphatic drainage of the breast. **(d)** Origin of malignant tumors by quadrant. (From Schuenke M, Schulte E, Schumacher U. THIEME Atlas of Anatomy. General Anatomy and Musculoskeletal System. Illustrations by Voll M and Wesker K. 3rd ed. New York: Thieme Medical Publishers; 2020.)

Clinical Correlate 2.12

Supernumerary Breasts and Nipples

Supernumerary breasts (*polymastia*) or nipples (*polythelia*) are relatively common and can affect both men and women. Most supernumerary breasts do not contain any glandular tissue and only have a rudimentary areola and nipple. However, if there is extra glandular tissue it may not be noticeable until a woman becomes pregnant. Supernumerary breasts and nipples will be noticed along the embryonic mammary ridges or "milk lines" that extend from the axilla down to the groin. The two most common sites are in the axilla and just beneath a normal breast. It is rare to encounter a patient with the absence of breast tissue, areola and nipple (*amastia*) or no breast tissue but the areola and nipple are still present (*amazia*). Both conditions can be treated with breast augmentation.

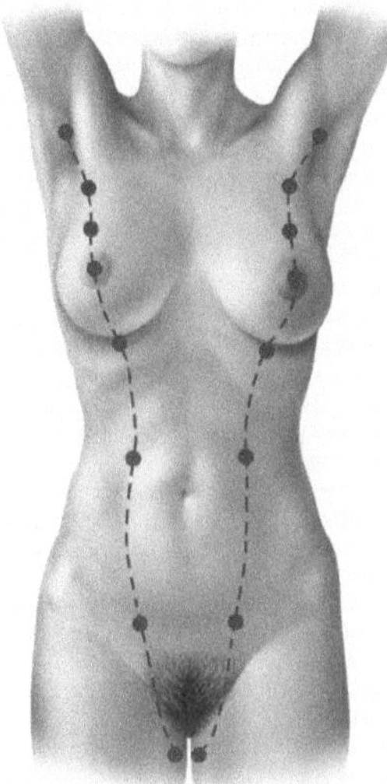

(From Schuenke M, Schulte E, Schumacher U. THIEME Atlas of Anatomy. Internal Organs. Illustrations by Voll M and Wesker K. 3rd ed. New York: Thieme Medical Publishers; 2020.)

2.14.1 Superior Mediastinum

As previously mentioned, the **superior mediastinum** extends from the superior thoracic aperture down to the transverse thoracic plane located at the level of the sternal angle and vertebral level T4/T5 (**Fig. 2.25**). The orientation of structures located within the superior mediastinum from anterior to posterior includes:

- Thymus.
- Brachiocephalic veins.
- Superior vena cava and the location of where the arch of the azygos drains into it.
- Great vessels including the arch of the aorta, its branches and the closely adjacent nerves
  - Brachiocephalic trunk
  - Left common carotid artery
  - Left subclavian artery
- Phrenic nerve, vagus nerve, and cardiac and pulmonary plexuses.
- Trachea (limited) (**Fig. 2.26**).
- Esophagus (limited) (**Fig. 2.26**).
- Thoracic duct (limited) (**Fig. 2.26**).

The **thymus** is a flat gland with two flask-shaped lobes located in the inferior part of the neck and the anterior part of the superior mediastinum. It is a primary lymphoid organ (along with bone marrow) important in the maturation of T-lymphocytes. During puberty, the thymus will undergo a gradual involution and will be replaced with fat. However, residual T-cell lymphopoiesis will continue even after atrophy of the organ (**Fig. 2.25**).

- Blood supply originates mainly from branches of the *internal thoracic* and the *inferior thyroid arteries*.
- Venous drainage is to either the *brachiocephalic, internal thoracic* and *inferior thyroid veins* or occasionally it may drain directly to the *superior vena cava*.
- Lymphatic drainage is to the *brachiocephalic, parasternal* and *tracheobronchial lymph nodes*.

The thymus has a dual embryonic origin with its lymphocytes arising from bone marrow (mesoderm in origin) and the thymus epithelium developing from endoderm of the 3rd pharyngeal pouch (**Fig. 2.27**).

Histologically, the thymus is made up of lobes surrounded by an *outer capsule*, peripheral *cortex* and central *medulla*. The connective tissue **outer capsule** penetrates the parenchyma and divides the thymus into incomplete lobules. This results in continuity between the cortex and medulla of adjoining lobules. The **cortex** is made up of an extensive population of T-cell precursors (thymocytes) mixed in with macrophages and epithelial reticular cells. The **medulla** contains *thymic (Hassall) corpuscles* that are characteristic of this region however the function of these corpuscles is unknown. The medulla also consists of differentiated T-lymphocytes and epithelial reticular cells (**Fig. 2.28**).

The union of the internal jugular and subclavian veins forms the **left and right brachiocephalic veins**. This occurs just posterior to the sternoclavicular joints. These veins drain blood originating from the head, neck and upper limbs. Near the level of the right 1st costal cartilage, the brachiocephalic veins will unite and form the superior vena cava (SVC). The left brachiocephalic vein is longer because it must pass from the left to the right side before helping to form the SVC (**Fig. 2.29**).

The **superior vena cava** drains the blood from the brachiocephalic veins and the arch of the azygos vein into the right atrium of the heart. It essentially drains all the blood superior to the diaphragm except for that of the heart and lungs. The terminal half of the SVC ends at the level of the right 3rd costal cartilage and within the middle mediastinum where it also forms the posterior border of the *transverse pericardial sinus*. The upper half is found in the superior mediastinum. The SVC lies anterolateral to the to the trachea and posterolateral to the ascending aorta. The right phrenic nerve is situated between the SVC and mediastinal pleura. The **arch of the azygos vein** loops over the right root of the lung prior to draining into the SVC (**Fig. 2.29**).

The **arch of the aorta** (or aortic arch) is the continuation of the **ascending aorta** which itself originates from within the pericardium of the middle mediastinum. It is clearly shown at vertebral level T3 on an axial or transverse plane of a CT scan. The arch begins to descend posterior to the left root of the lung just beside the T4 vertebra and ends as the **thoracic (descending) aorta**. This is approximately at the left 2nd sternocostal joint. The arch generally gives off three branches: the brachiocephalic (innominate) trunk, left common carotid artery and the left subclavian artery (**Fig. 2.30**).

The **brachiocephalic trunk** is the first and largest branch off the aortic arch and divides into a *right common carotid* and *right*

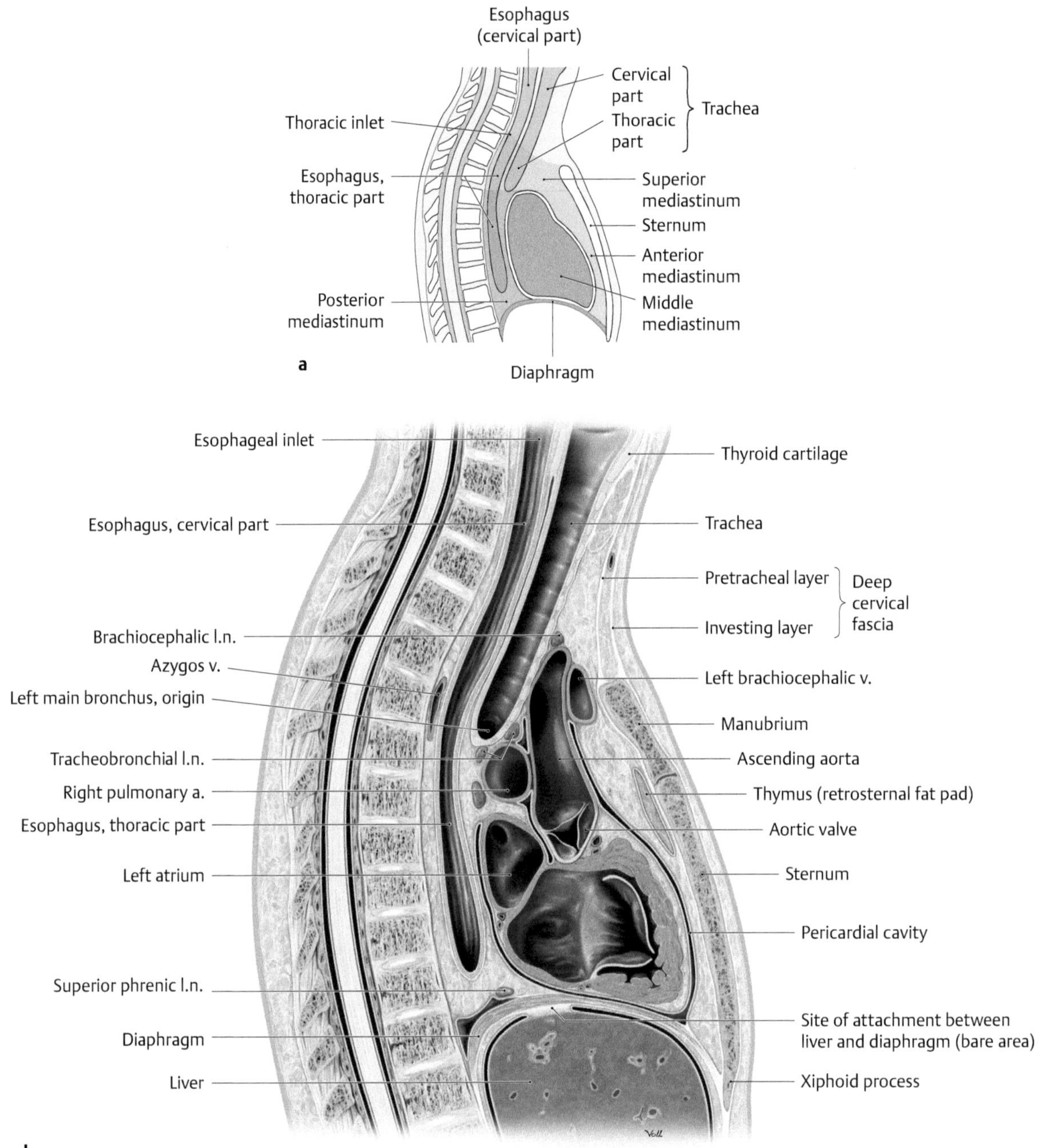

Fig. 2.24 Divisions of the mediastinum. **(a)** Schematic. **(b)** Midsagittal section, right lateral view. (From Schuenke M, Schulte E, Schumacher U. THIEME Atlas of Anatomy. Internal Organs. Illustrations by Voll M and Wesker K. 2nd ed. New York: Thieme Medical Publishers; 2016.)

subclavian artery. It is anterior to the trachea and posterior to the left brachiocephalic vein. The **left common carotid artery** is the second branch off the aortic arch and is slightly posterior and to the left of the brachiocephalic trunk. It then passes anterior and then to the left of the trachea before extending into the neck. The **left subclavian artery** is the third branch off the aortic arch and courses lateral to the trachea. On their way out of the thorax, the left common carotid and left subclavian arteries can be found posterior to the sternocostal joint **(Fig. 2.31)**.

The **phrenic nerves** originate from the ventral rami of the cervical nerves C3-C5 and are seen initially resting on the anterior surface of the anterior scalene muscles. The phrenic nerves are located lateral to the vagus nerves and they course along the fibrous pericardium on their way to the diaphragm. Most phrenic nerve branching does not occur until reaching the inferior surface of the diaphragm. They supply the diaphragm with both motor and sensory fibers. The phrenic nerves supply the sensory innervation of the pericardium and mediastinal pleura. The functional components of these nerves are GSE, GSA, GVE-sym/post and GVA **(Fig. 2.32)**.

The **left phrenic nerve** descends between the anterior scalene muscle and distal left brachiocephalic vein, above the anterior surface of the aortic arch, anterior to the root of the left lung and along the fibrous pericardium before reaching and then innervating the diaphragm. The **right phrenic nerve** descends initially between the anterior scalene muscle and right subclavian vein, lateral to the right brachiocephalic vein and SVC, anterior to the root of the right lung and along the fibrous pericardium before

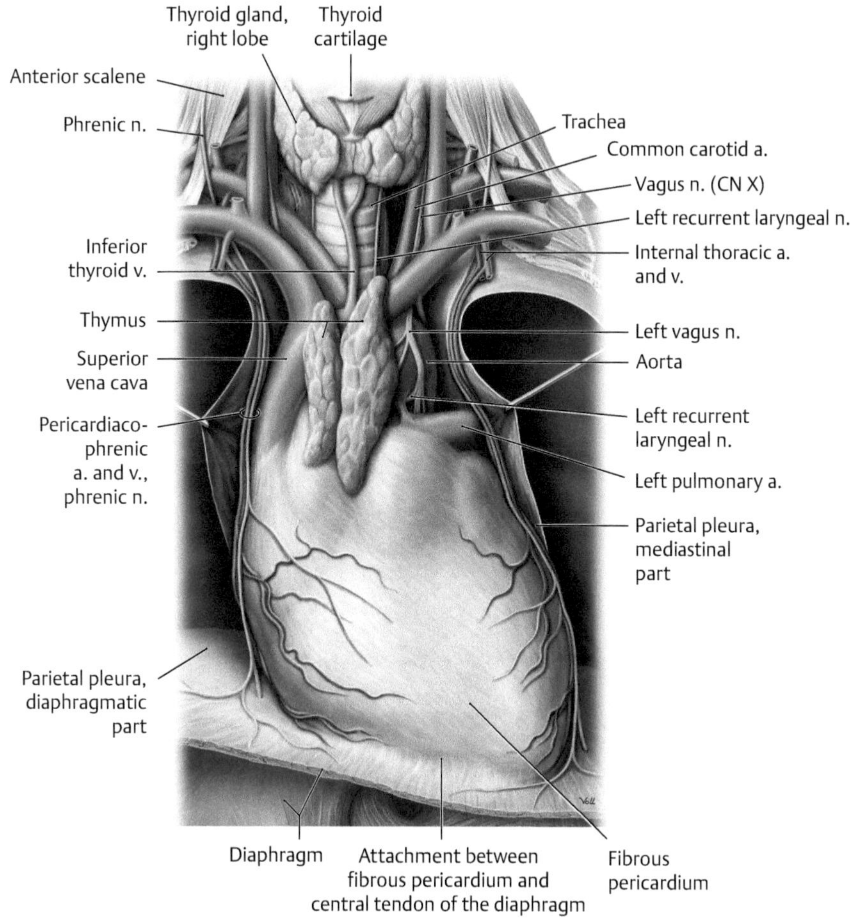

Fig. 2.25 Superior and middle mediastinum, anterior view. (From Schuenke M, Schulte E, Schumacher U. THIEME Atlas of Anatomy. Internal Organs. Illustrations by Voll M and Wesker K. 3rd ed. New York: Thieme Medical Publishers; 2016.)

piercing through the diaphragm just lateral to the caval opening for the inferior vena cava.

The **vagus nerves** are also known as the tenth cranial nerve (CN X) and exit the cranium through the jugular foramen. These nerves descend through the neck posterior to both the internal jugular vein and common carotid arteries within the carotid sheath before reaching the thorax. The **left vagus nerve** descends initially posterior to the left common carotid artery but enters the superior mediastinum between the left common carotid and left subclavian arteries. It will then cross the anterior surface of the aortic arch before giving off the **left recurrent laryngeal nerve** that hooks around the arch of the aorta just posterior to the *ligamentum arteriosum*. The left recurrent laryngeal nerve extends back up straight towards the larynx within the neck. The left vagus continues posterior to the root of the left lung at which point it gives off many branches that contribute to the **left pulmonary plexus**. After these branches are given off, the left vagus becomes the **anterior vagal trunk** and contributes to the *esophageal plexus* (**Fig. 2.31**).

The **right vagus nerve** enters the superior mediastinum anterior to the right subclavian artery where it immediately gives rise the **right recurrent laryngeal nerve** that hooks around the right subclavian artery. The right recurrent laryngeal nerve extends back up towards the larynx within the neck at an angle that has clinical significance (Chapter 7). The right vagus continues on the right side of the trachea and then passes posterior to the right brachiocephalic vein, SVC and root of the right lung, where it gives off branches to contribute to the *right pulmonary plexus*. Once these branches are given off, the right vagus becomes the **posterior vagal trunk** and contributes to the *esophageal plexus.*

Functional components of the vagus nerves in the superior mediastinum proximal to the recurrent laryngeal nerve branches are SVE (or BM), GSA, GVE-para/pre, and GVA and these fibers continue through the recurrent laryngeal nerves. Branchiomotor (BM) fibers are responsible for innervating laryngeal muscles and are discussed in more detail in Chapter 7. Vagus nerves and vagal trunks distal to the recurrent laryngeal nerve branches have GVE-para/pre and GVA fibers. The **cardiac** and **pulmonary plexuses** contain the typical GVE-sym/post, GVE-para/pre and GVA fibers seen in most visceral nerve plexuses. Details of these plexuses are discussed during their respective heart and lung sections.

The **trachea** is located anterior to the esophagus and enters the superior mediastinum slightly to the right of the median plane. It is a semi-circular, fibrocartilaginous tube surrounded by C-shaped **tracheal (cartilaginous) rings**. It originates at vertebral level C6 and ends when it bifurcates at vertebral level T4/T5 (**Fig. 2.26**).

The **esophagus** is a fibromuscular tube that connects the pharynx to the stomach. Similar to the trachea, it originates from vertebral level C6 but terminates at vertebral level T11. While in the superior mediastinum, it lies just to the left of the trachea and anterior to the thoracic vertebrae but by the time it reaches the level of the *transverse thoracic plane*, it is pushed to the right and closer to the median plane by the arch of the aorta. Further details of the esophagus are discussed in the *Posterior Mediastinum* section (**Fig. 2.65**).

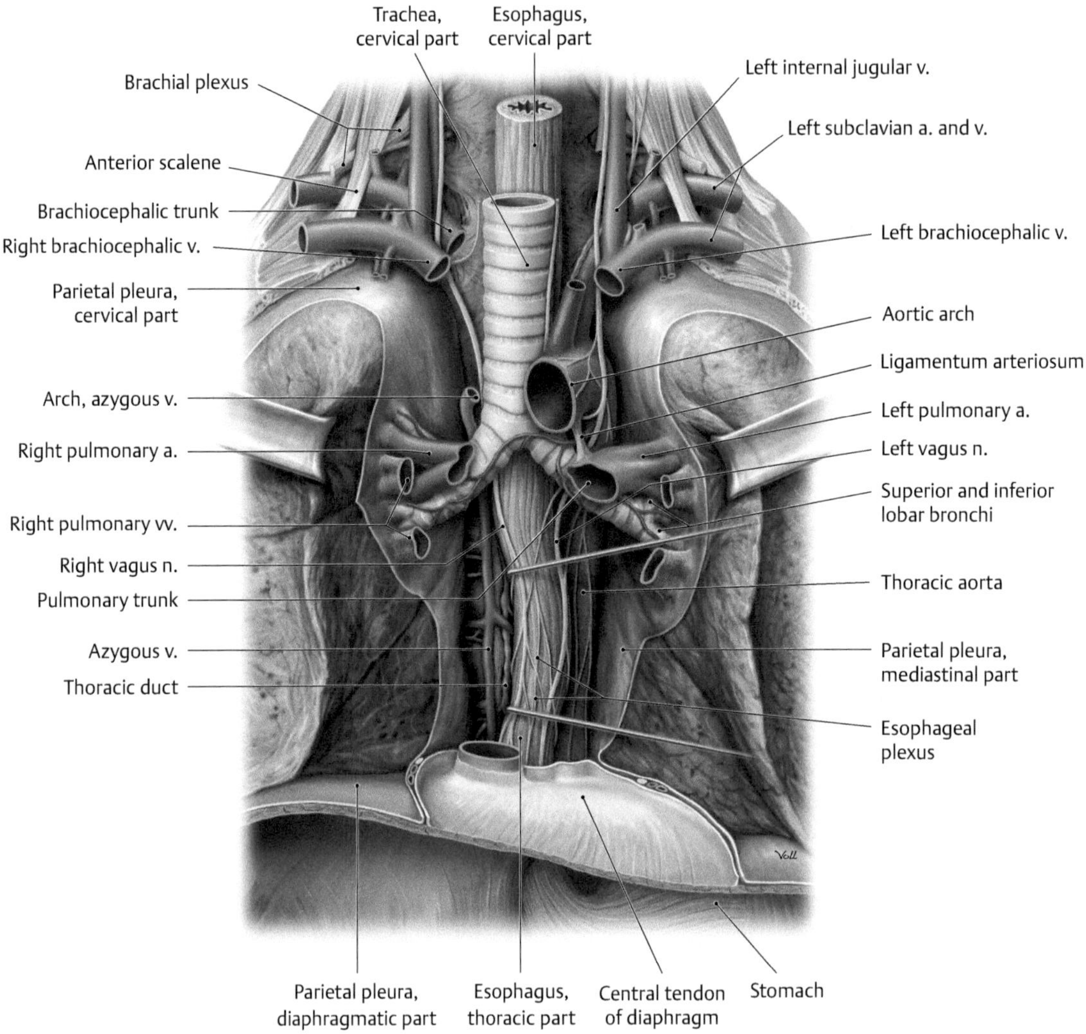

Fig. 2.26 Structures passing through multiple mediastinums. (From Schuenke M, Schulte E, Schumacher U. THIEME Atlas of Anatomy. Internal Organs. Illustrations by Voll M and Wesker K. 3rd ed. New York: Thieme Medical Publishers; 2016.)

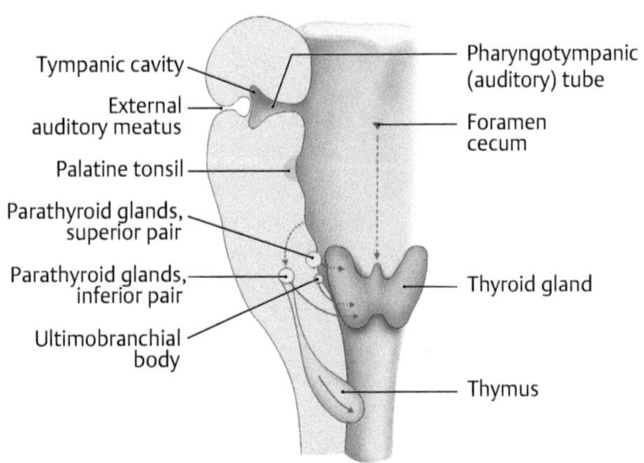

Fig. 2.27 Migration movements of the pharyngeal pouch tissues. (After Sadler. From Schuenke M, Schulte E, Schumacher U. THIEME Atlas of Anatomy. Head, Neck, and Neuroanatomy. Illustrations by Voll M and Wesker K. 3rd ed. New York: Thieme Medical Publishers; 2020.)

The **thoracic duct** has a long course but while it is in the superior mediastinum, it lies just left of the esophagus before terminating at the junction of the left internal jugular and subclavian veins of the lower neck. Further details involving the thoracic duct are discussed in the *Posterior Mediastinum* section (**Fig. 2.67**).

2.14.2 Anterior Mediastinum

The **anterior mediastinum** is a small portion of the overall mediastinum and is located from the body of the sternum anteriorly, to the pericardium posteriorly (**Fig. 2.33**). It is continuous with the superior mediastinum at the sternal angle but is limited inferiorly by the diaphragm. During infancy and in young children the inferior portion of the thymus lies within the anterior mediastinum. Structures are limited but include the *internal thoracic vessels, transversus thoracic muscles, sternopericardial ligaments, lymphatic vessels*, and *fat*.

2.14.3 Middle Mediastinum

The middle mediastinum contains the pericardium, roots of the great vessels and the heart (**Fig. 2.32**). It is the part of the larger inferior mediastinum located between the anterior and posterior

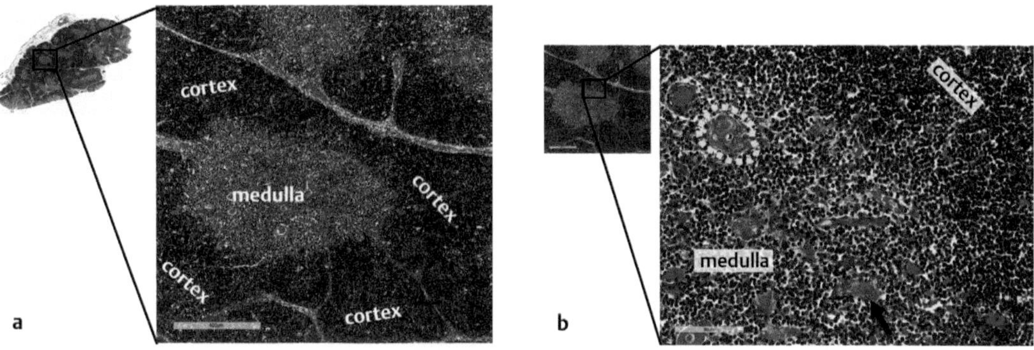

Fig. 2.28 **(a)** Thymus of an infant at medium magnification showing medulla and cortex. **(b)** Thymus of an infant at medium to high magnification showing an epithelial reticular cell (*arrow*) and Hassal's corpuscle (*outlined*). (From Lowrie DJ. Histology: An Essential Textbook. New York: Thieme Medical Publishers; 2020.)

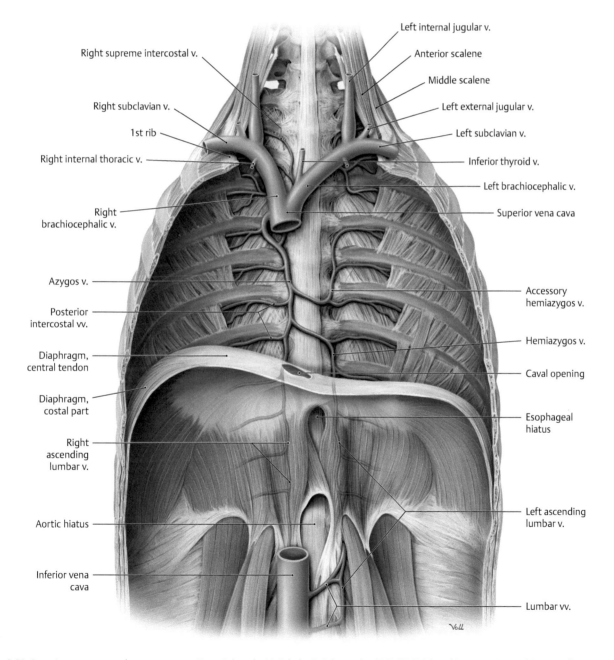

Fig. 2.29 Superior vena cava and azygos system. (From Schuenke M, Schulte E, Schumacher U. THIEME Atlas of Anatomy. Internal Organs. Illustrations by Voll M and Wesker K. 3rd ed. New York: Thieme Medical Publishers; 2020.)

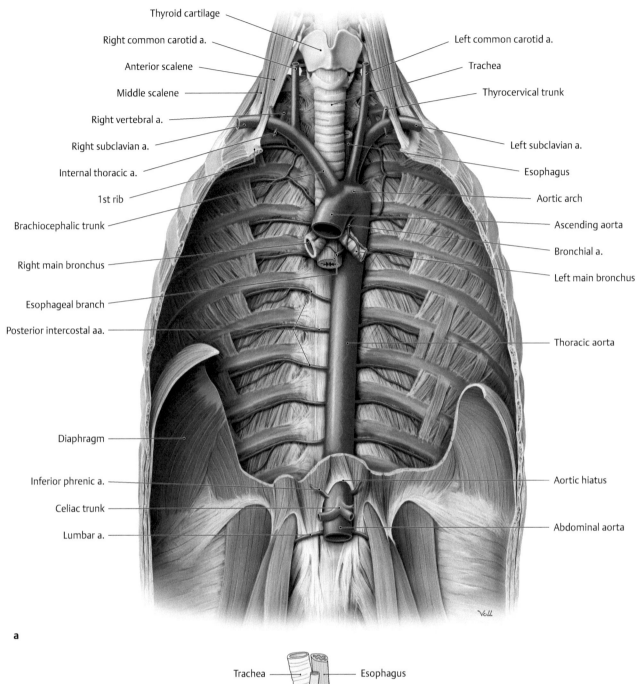

Thyroid cartilage
Right common carotid a.
Anterior scalene
Middle scalene
Right vertebral a.
Right subclavian a.
Internal thoracic a.
1st rib
Brachiocephalic trunk
Right main bronchus
Esophageal branch
Posterior intercostal aa.
Diaphragm
Inferior phrenic a.
Celiac trunk
Lumbar a.
Left common carotid a.
Trachea
Thyrocervical trunk
Left subclavian a.
Esophagus
Aortic arch
Ascending aorta
Bronchial a.
Left main bronchus
Thoracic aorta
Aortic hiatus
Abdominal aorta
Voll

a

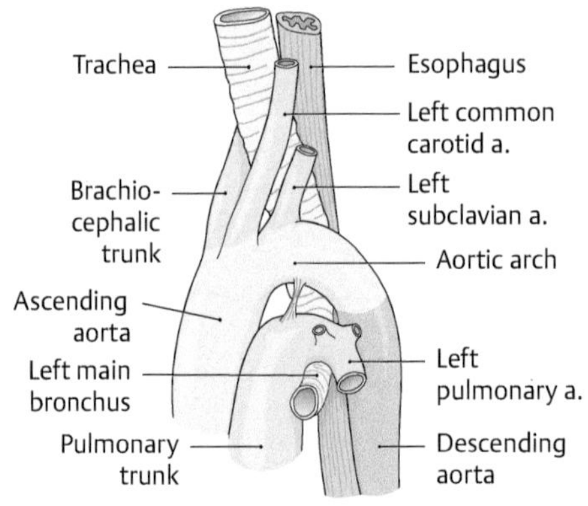

b

Fig. 2.30 **(a)** Thoracic aorta in situ. **(b)** Parts of the aorta, left lateral view. (From Schuenke M, Schulte E, Schumacher U. THIEME Atlas of Anatomy. Internal Organs. Illustrations by Voll M and Wesker K. 3rd ed. New York: Thieme Medical Publishers; 2020.)

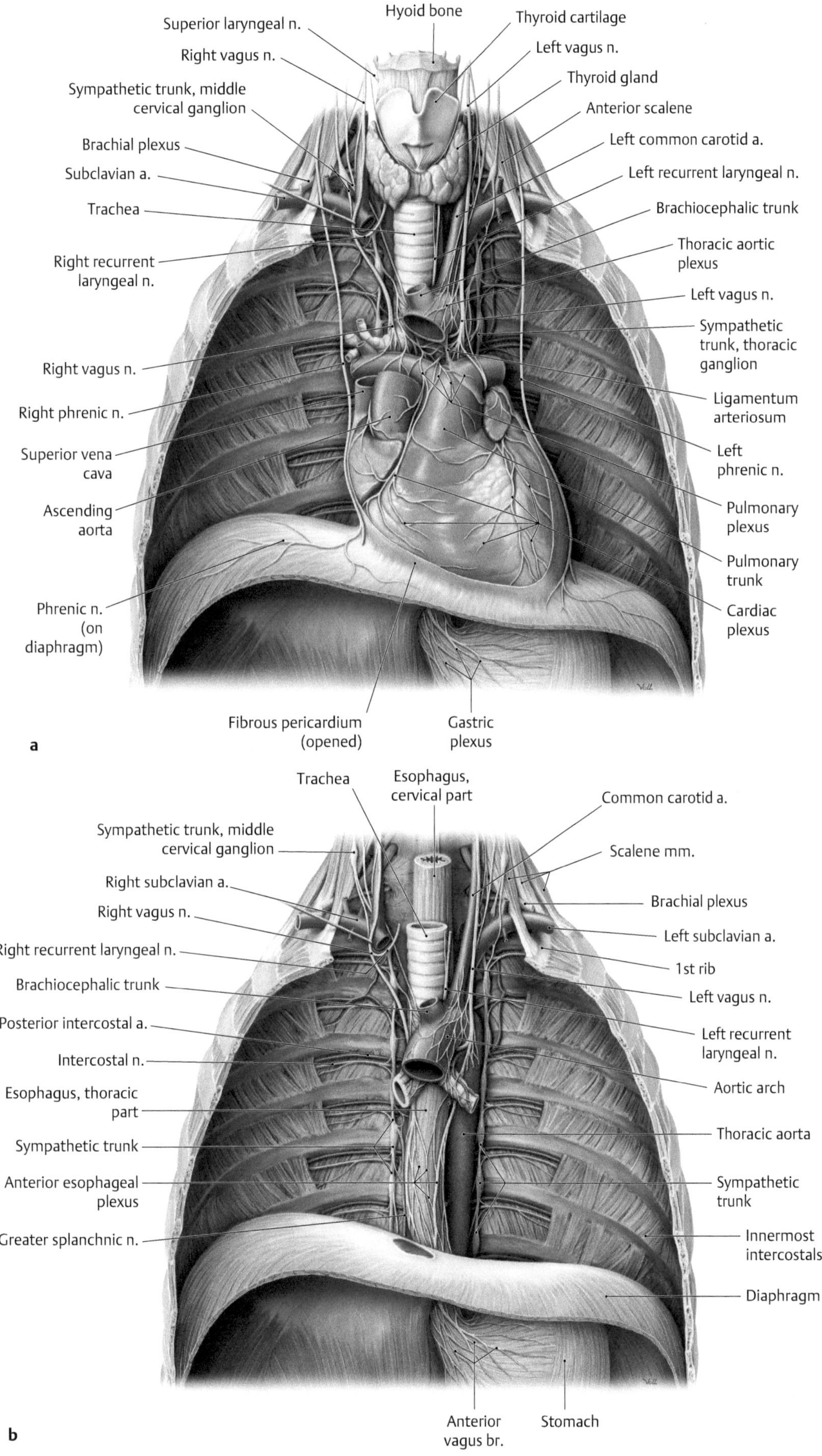

Fig. 2.31 Nerves of the thorax. **(a)** Anterior view with the heart in situ. **(b)** Anterior view with the heart removed. (From Schuenke M, Schulte E, Schumacher U. THIEME Atlas of Anatomy. Internal Organs. Illustrations by Voll M and Wesker K. 3rd ed. New York: Thieme Medical Publishers; 2020.)

Clinical Correlate 2.13

Variations and Anomalies of the Arch of the Aorta

The normal pattern of aortic arch artery branches seen in anatomical texts and atlases accounts for approximately 70% of all individuals meaning variation is quite common in the general population. Additional variations are demonstrated in **b-f**.

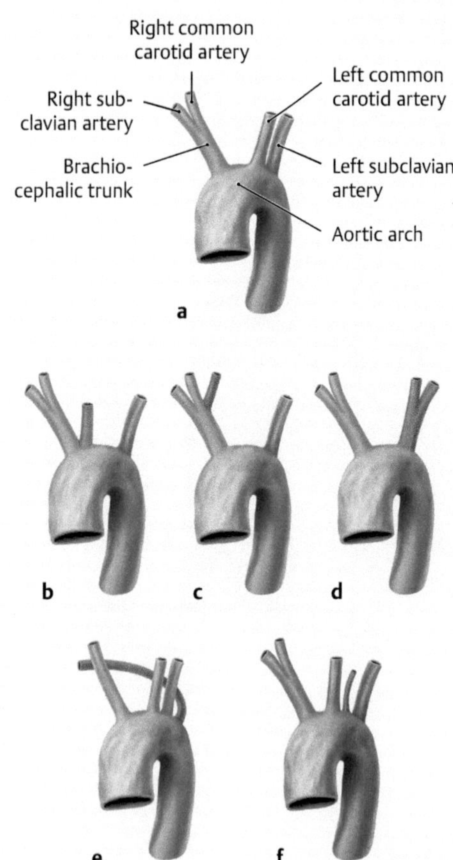

(a) Common pattern (~70%). **(b)** The left common carotid arises from the aortic arch next to the brachiocephalic trunk (~13%). **(c)** The left common carotid artery arises from the brachiocephalic trunk (~9%). **(d)** There are two brachiocephalic trunks (~1%). **(e)** Retro-esophageal right subclavian artery (~1%). **(f)** The left vertebral artery arises from the aortic arch (~1%). (From Schuenke M, Schulte E, Schumacher U. THIEME Atlas of Anatomy. Internal Organs. Illustrations by Voll M and Wesker K. 3rd ed. New York: Thieme Medical Publishers; 2020.)

Clinical Correlate 2.14

Double Aortic Arch

The **double aortic arch** involves a complete *vascular ring* surrounding the trachea and esophagus. This leads to compression of these structures causing difficulty breathing and swallowing. It is the result of a persistent right dorsal aorta between its junction with the left dorsal aorta and the origin of the 7th intersegmental artery. The distal portion of the right dorsal aorta is normally obliterated during development.

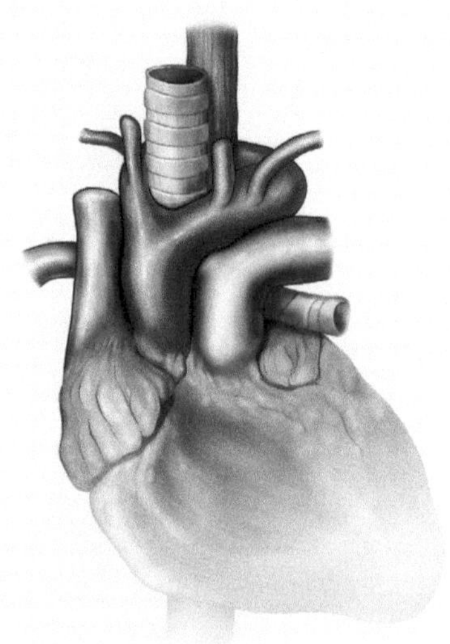

Illustration by Calla Heald.

Clinical Correlate 2.15

Retro-Esophageal Right Subclavian Artery

The **retro-esophageal right subclavian artery** forms an incomplete vascular ring around the trachea and esophagus. Obliteration of the right 4th aortic arch and proximal portion of the right dorsal aorta forms this anomaly. The right subclavian artery is thus formed by the 7th intersegmental artery and distal portion of the right aortic arch.

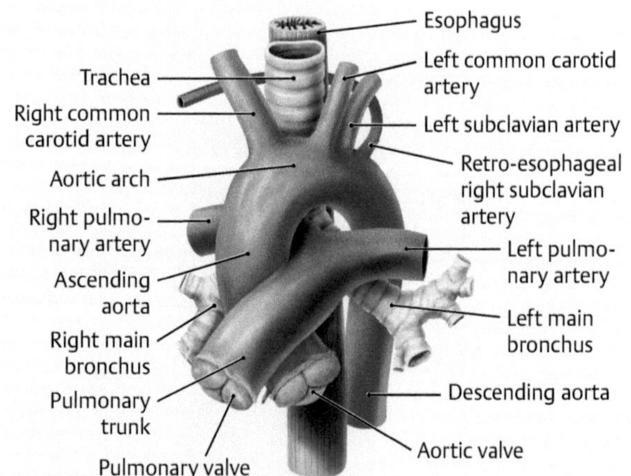

(From Schuenke M, Schulte E, Schumacher U. THIEME Atlas of Anatomy. Internal Organs. Illustrations by Voll M and Wesker K. 3rd ed. New York: Thieme Medical Publishers; 2020.)

mediastinums. It also constitutes the cardiac silhouette in a conventional radiograph or x-ray.

Pericardium

A fibroserous membrane known as the **pericardium** covers the root of the great vessels and heart (**Fig. 2.33**). It is influenced by movements of the heart, great vessels, diaphragm and sternum. It is a closed sac composed of two layers the first being an outer and tough **fibrous pericardium.** Just on the opposite side of the outer fibrous pericardium is the **parietal layer of the serous pericardium.** This layer will be reflected onto the heart near the aorta, SVC, pulmonary trunk and pulmonary veins. This reflected layer and resting on the heart itself is known as the **visceral**

Clinical Correlate 2.16

Coarctation of the Aorta

Coarctation of the aorta (~3/10,000 live births) is described as an abnormal stenosis or narrowing of the aorta most commonly identified near the ductus arteriosus. It consists of two types, a **preductal (a)** and **postductal (b)** version. Coarctation reduces the size of the aortic lumen thus impeding normal blood flow to the systematic circulation. It is caused primarily by an abnormality involving the media of the aorta and followed by intima proliferations. Generally it is present at birth alongside additional heart defects but may range from mild to severe and may not be detected until adulthood. If the *preductal* version is present, the ductus arteriosus still persists. In the more common *postductal* version, the ligamentum arteriosum is present and collateral circulation may involve the intercostal and internal thoracic arteries.

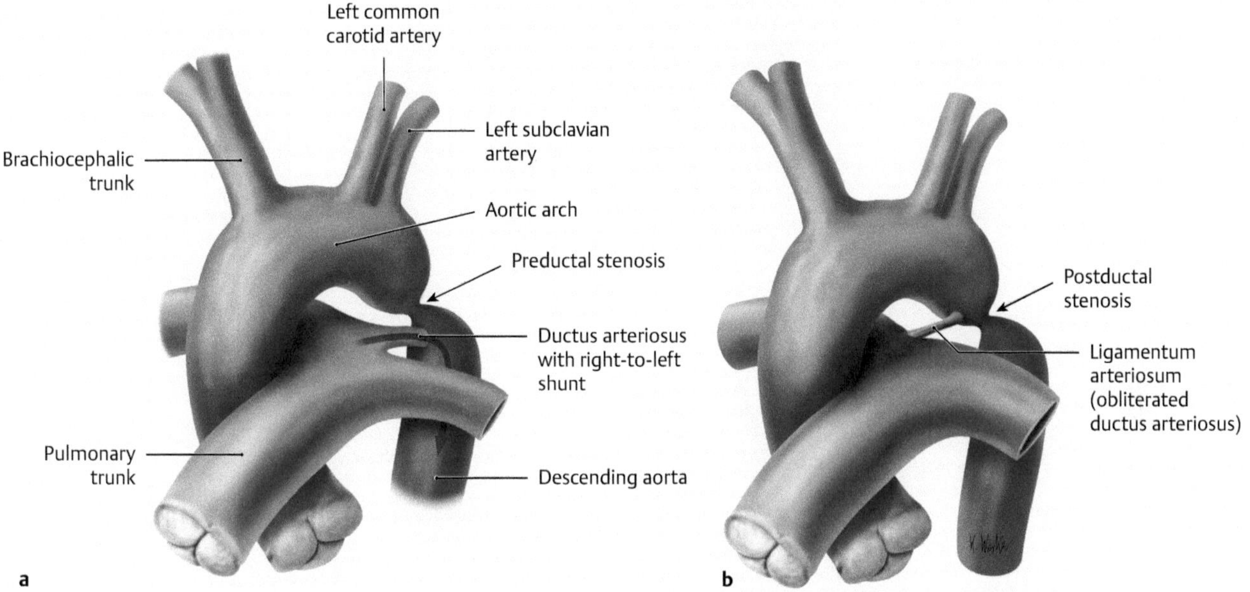

(From Schuenke M, Schulte E, Schumacher U. THIEME Atlas of Anatomy. Internal Organs. Illustrations by Voll M and Wesker K. 3rd ed. New York: Thieme Medical Publishers; 2020.)

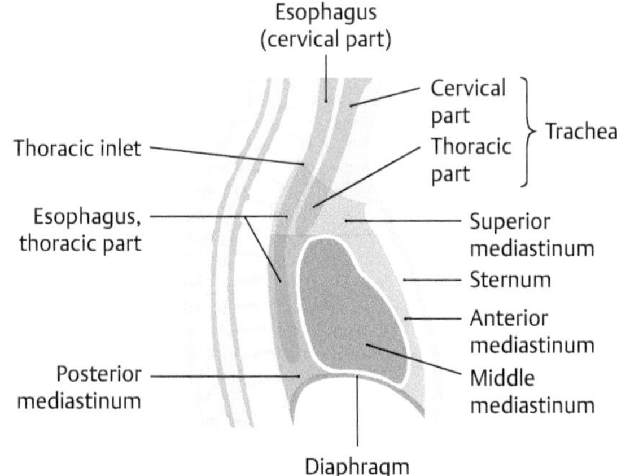

Fig. 2.32 Divisions of the mediastinum. (From Schuenke M, Schulte E, Schumacher U. THIEME Atlas of Anatomy. Internal Organs. Illustrations by Voll M and Wesker K. 3rd ed. New York: Thieme Medical Publishers; 2020.)

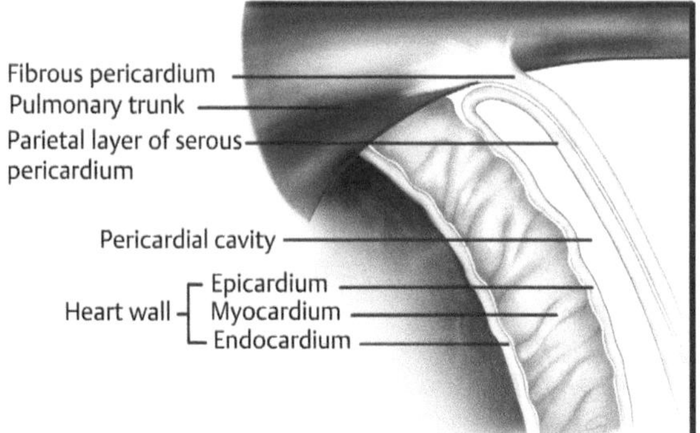

Fig. 2.33 Layers of the pericardium. Illustration by Calla Heald.

layer of serous pericardium (or epicardium). The epicardium is considered the outermost layer of the overall three layers of the heart.

The serous pericardium is composed of mesothelium which is a single layer of flattened cells forming an epithelium. It secretes a thin film of serous fluid and is found lining the internal surface of the fibrous pericardium (parietal layer) and external surface of the heart (visceral layer). The thin film of serous fluid is secreted into a potential space located between the parietal and visceral layers of serous pericardium known as the **pericardial cavity**. The serous fluid located in this cavity enables the heart to beat in a frictionless environment.

Locations where there is a reflection of the parietal and visceral layers of the serous pericardium can be found near the aorta, SVC

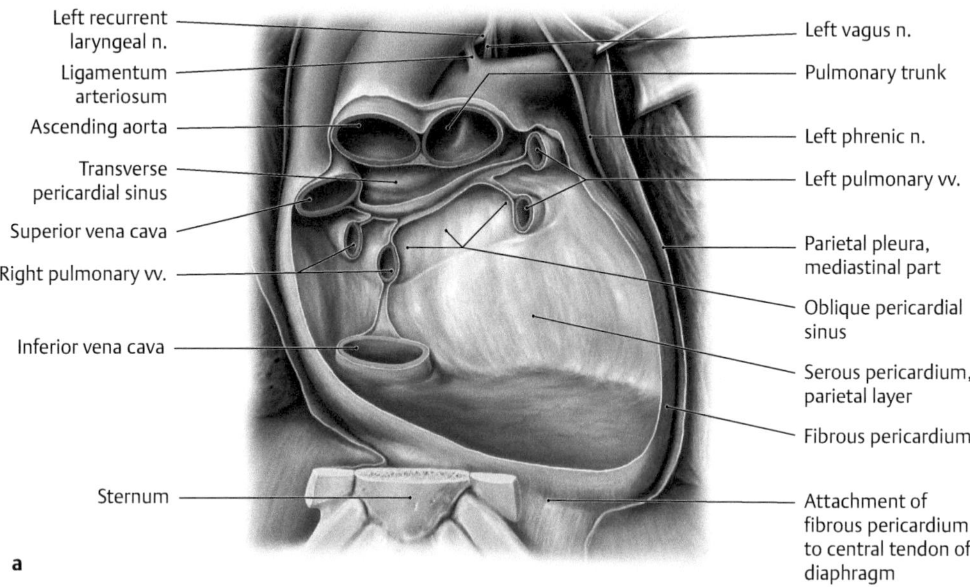

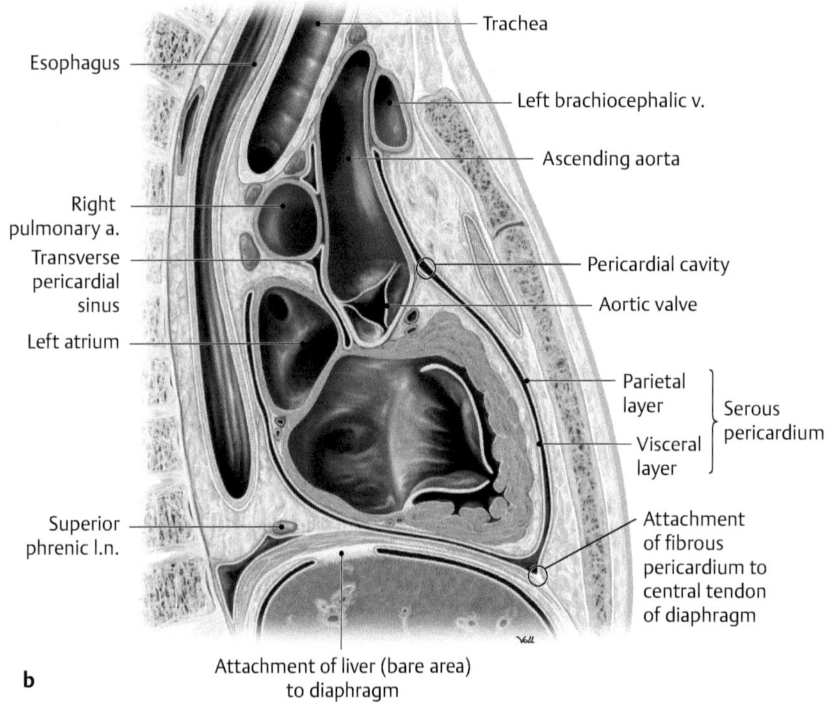

Fig. 2.34 **(a)** View of the posterior pericardium and oblique pericardial sinus. **(b)** Midsagittal view demonstrating the pericardium, pericardial cavity, and transverse pericardial sinus. (From Schuenke M, Schulte E, Schumacher U. THIEME Atlas of Anatomy. Internal Organs. Illustrations by Voll M and Wesker K. 3rd ed. New York: Thieme Medical Publishers; 2020.)

and pulmonary vessels. Two recesses form within the pericardial cavity due to these reflections and can be accessed after opening the anterior wall of the pericardium. Thoracic surgeons can access these recesses so that they may manipulate, clamp or ligate these proximal vessels during a surgical procedure such as coronary artery bypass. The **transverse pericardial sinus** is located posterior to the pulmonary trunk and ascending aorta but anterior to the SVC. The **oblique pericardial sinus** is located posterior to the heart and between the left and right pulmonary veins (**Fig. 2.34**).

The *fibrous pericardium* is unyielding and protects the heart against sudden overfilling. If extensive pericardial effusion was to occur, it could lead to unwanted heart compression or *cardiac tamponade*. It is also capable of attaching to surrounding areas in order to keep the pericardium and heart located in a central location. It is continuous:

- Superiorly with the tunica adventitia of the great vessels near the heart and the pretracheal layer of deep cervical fascia.
- Inferiorly with the central tendon of the diaphragm. This connection is really continuity between the fibrous pericardium and central tendon of the diaphragm and it is called the **pericardiacophrenic ligament**.

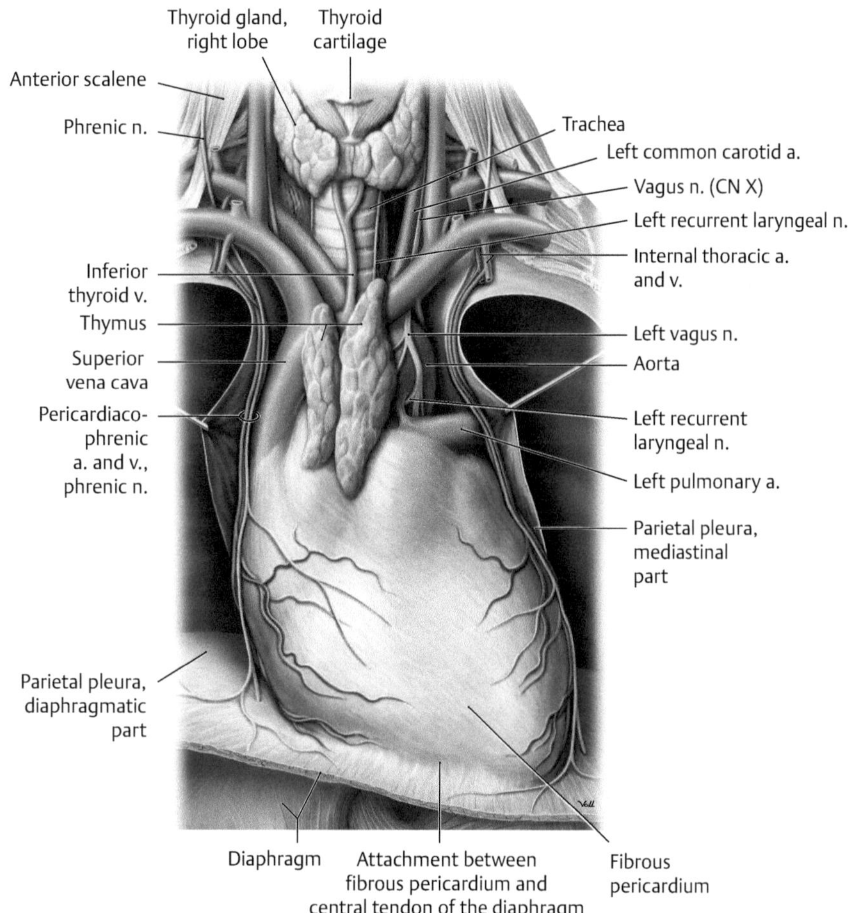

Fig. 2.35 Neurovasculature of the pericardium. (From Schuenke M, Schulte E, Schumacher U. THIEME Atlas of Anatomy. Internal Organs. Illustrations by Voll M and Wesker K. 3rd ed. New York: Thieme Medical Publishers; 2020.)

- Anteriorly with the posterior sternum by way of the **sterno-pericardial ligaments**.
- Posteriorly with posterior mediastinum structures by way of loose connective tissue.

Neurovasculature of the Pericardium

- Innervation is from multiple sources **(Fig. 2.35)**:
  - **Phrenic nerves** (ventral rami of C3-C5) are the primary source of sensory fibers. Referred pain from this region would correspond to the C3-C5 dermatomes of the ipsilateral supraclavicular and shoulder regions.
  - **Sympathetics** are vasomotor to the vessels supplying the pericardium.
  - **Parasympathetics** (vagus nerve) have an uncertain function.
- Arterial supply originates mainly from the **pericardiacophrenic arteries** which are branches from the internal thoracic arteries. Additional blood supply comes from:
  - **Coronary arteries** (visceral layer only).
  - **Musculophrenic** (internal thoracic), **esophageal** (thoracic aorta), **bronchial** (thoracic aorta) and **superior phrenic arteries** (thoracic aorta).
- Venous drainage is primarily from the **pericardiacophrenic veins** which drain to the internal thoracic or brachiocephalic veins. To a lesser degree venous drainage can lead back to the *azygos venous system*.

Development of the Pericardium

Extensive growth of the lungs into the early pleural cavities, or **pleuroperitoneal canals**, results in the extension of the **pleuropericardial folds** from the body wall and this creates the **pleuropericardial membranes**. The pleuropericardial membranes will fuse and separate the pericardial and pleural cavities from one another as well as become the fibrous pericardium **(Fig. 2.36)**. These membranes contain the phrenic nerves and this is why the nerves are in close relationship with the adult fibrous pericardium. They will go on to primarily innervate the diaphragm.

Heart

The **heart** is the structure that makes up most of the middle mediastinum. It is found between the T5-T8/T9 vertebral levels and is the approximate size of a loosely clenched fist. It has four chambers of which the right side is associated with deoxygenated blood while the left side is associated with oxygenated blood. The left and right atria receive blood but the left and right ventricles pump blood to the systematic and pulmonary circulations respectively **(Fig. 2.37)**.

Tissue Layers and Fibrous Skeleton

The heart chambers consist of three layers with the middle myocardial layer varying the most in thickness. They are in order from external to internal **(Fig. 2.33)**.

Fig. 2.36 (a-d) Separation of the pericardial cavity from the pleural cavities beginning at about 5 weeks of development. (From Schuenke M, Schulte E, Schumacher U. THIEME Atlas of Anatomy. Internal Organs. Illustrations by Voll M and Wesker K. 3rd ed. New York: Thieme Medical Publishers; 2020.)

1. **Epicardium**: the thin external layer formed of mesothelium and also known as the visceral layer of serous pericardium.
2. **Myocardium**: the thick layer composed of involuntary striated cardiac muscle.
3. **Endocardium**: the thin internal layer made of endothelium and subendothelial connective tissue that also lies over individual valves. Purkinje branches of the hearts conduction system course through the *subendocardial* connective tissue layer located between the endocardium and myocardium.

The walls of the heart are made up of primarily myocardium and this is most evident with the ventricles. Ventricular contraction produces a wringing or twisting motion because of the double helical orientation of the cardiac muscle fibers. This process results in blood initially being ejected from the ventricles as the outer (basal) spiral region, first narrowing and then shortening the heart, reduces ventricular volume. The continued and sequential

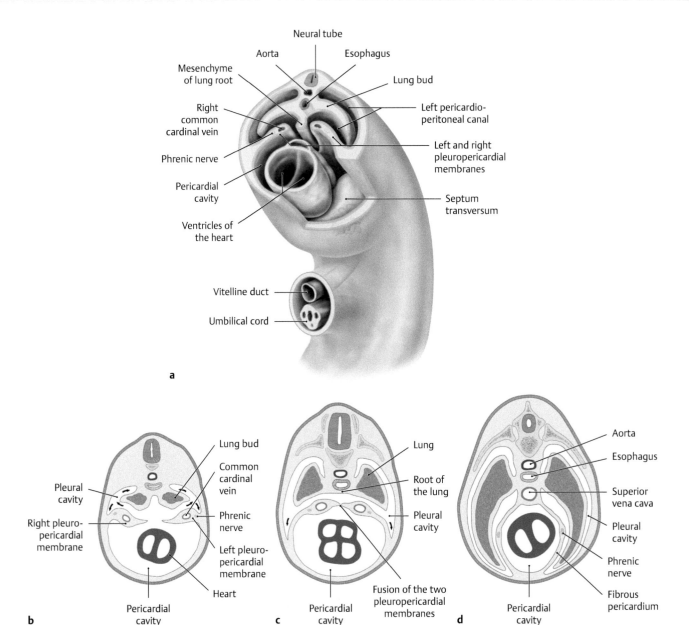

Clinical Correlate 2.17

Cardiac Tamponade, Pericardial Effusion, Pericarditis & Pericardial Friction Rub

The pericardium does not normally allow for expansion mainly due to its outer fibrous layer. Air or blood that enters the pericardial cavity (*pneumopericardium* or *hemopericardium* respectively) creates a potentially lethal situation where the heart becomes compressed and this is known as **cardiac tamponade**. Cardiac tamponade limits the amount of blood the heart can receive thus reducing cardiac output. **Pericardial effusion** also produces compression of the heart but is the result of an imbalance between the production and re-absorption of pericardial fluid at the level of the pericardial capillaries. Inflammation of the pericardium is known as **pericarditis** and generally causes chest pain. Inflammation also causes the serous pericardial layers to become rough and rub up against each other creating an audible friction called **pericardial friction rub**.

Clinical Correlate 2.18

Pericardiocentesis

A **pericardiocentesis** (pericardial tap) is an invasive procedure in which a needle and catheter aspirate fluid from the pericardial space surrounding the heart. The pericardial fluid may be tested for the presence of blood, inflammation or infection. In an emergency situation, a pericardiocentesis may need to be performed to treat cardiac tamponade and relieve the pressure on the heart affecting its pumping ability. The patient can be in a semi-recumbent (~30-45 degrees) or supine position but the semi-recumbent position brings the heart closer to the anterior chest wall. The needle is inserted near the subxiphoid or left sternocostal margin.

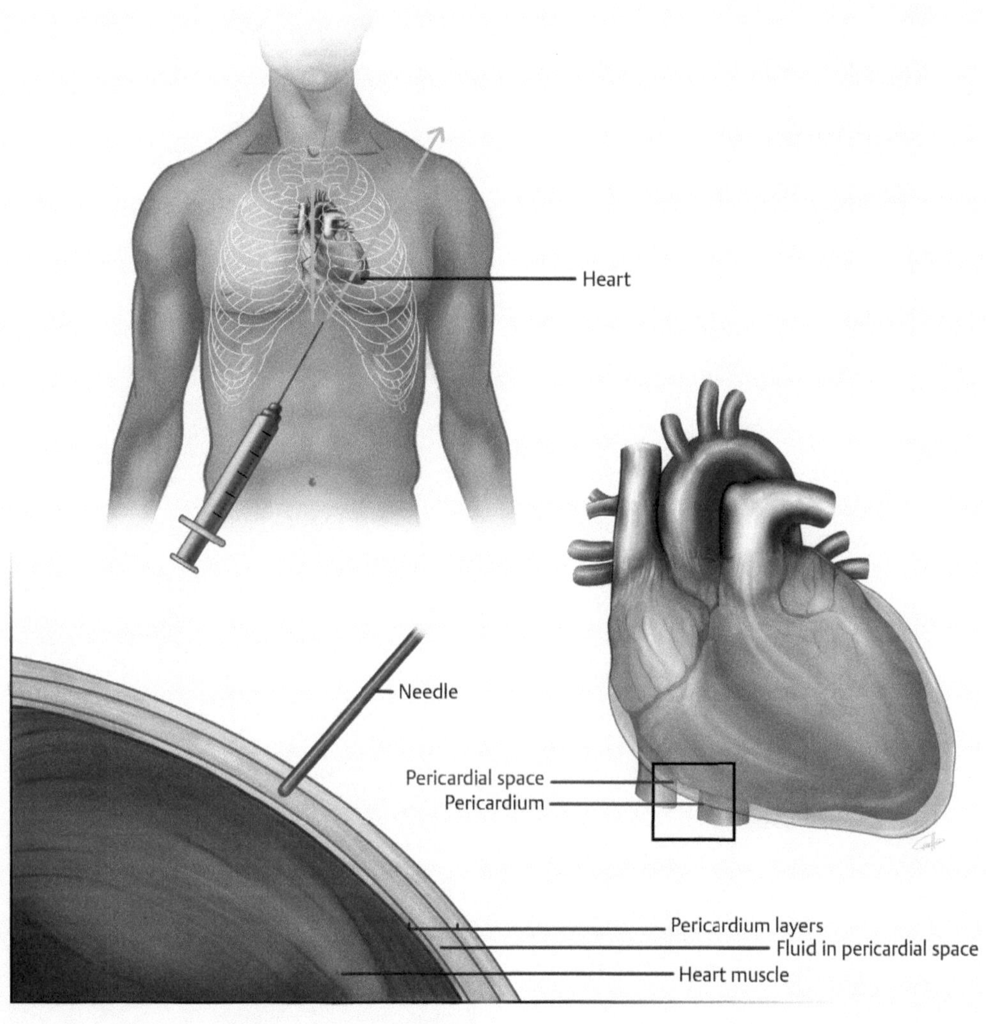

Illustration by Calla Heald.

contraction of the inner (apical) spiral region will first elongate then widen the heart. This is due to the myocardium briefly relaxing, which increases the volume of the chambers to draw blood from the atria.[1]

The **cardiac skeleton of the heart** is a complex framework of dense fibrous collagen forming four **fibrous rings**, two **fibrous trigones**, and the **membranous portion of the interatrial, interventricular** and **atrioventricular septa**. The *fibrous rings* surround the orifices of the aortic and pulmonary semilunar valves as well as the bicuspid and tricuspid valves. The *fibrous trigones* are formed at the regions of fibrous ring connections. The membranous portions of certain septa are in intimate contact with the parts of the *conducting system* of the heart. The fibrous skeleton has four major functions **(Fig. 2.38)**:

1. It anchors the valve cusps.
2. It prevents the over dilation of the valve openings.
3. It provides the attachment points for the cusps and leaflets of valves and the myocardium.
4. It forms an electrical insulator by blocking the direct spread of electrical impulses from atrial to ventricular muscles. This provides a passage for the initial part of the AV bundle of the conducting system.

Histology of the Myocardium

As previously mentioned, the myocardial layer of the heart is composed of involuntary striated cardiac muscle. A **cardiac muscle cell** is a short, branching cell with one or two large centrally localized

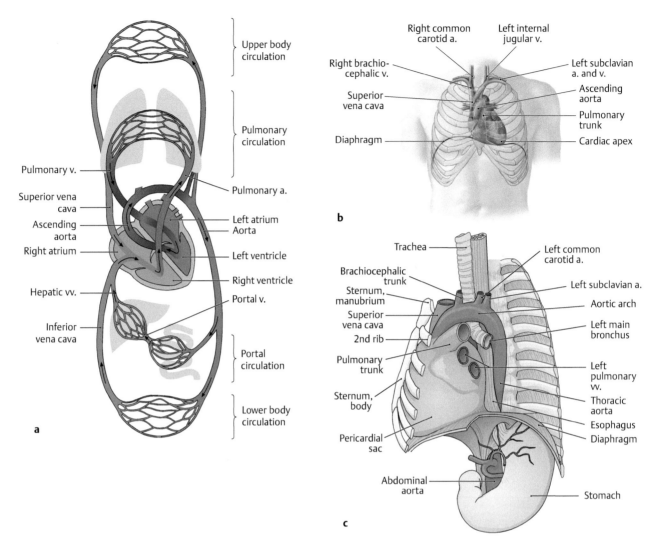

Fig. 2.37 **(a)** Circulation of blood. **(b)** Projection of the heart and great vessels onto chest, anterior view. **(c)** Left lateral view with the left lung removed. (From Schuenke M, Schulte E, Schumacher U. THIEME Atlas of Anatomy. Internal Organs. Illustrations by Voll M and Wesker K. 3rd ed. New York: Thieme Medical Publishers; 2020.)

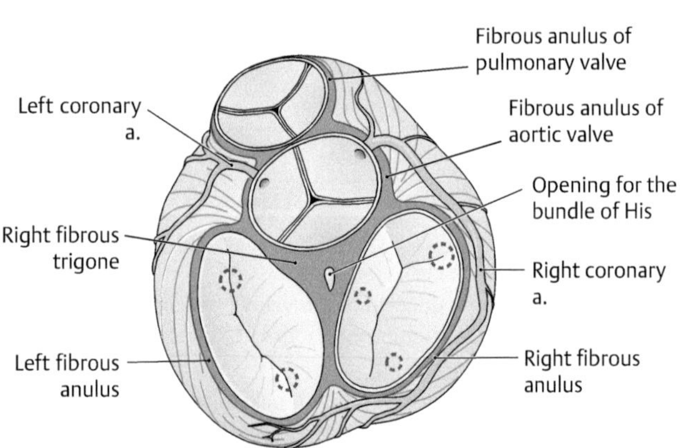

Fig. 2.38 Cardiac skeleton of the heart. (From Schuenke M, Schulte E, Schumacher U. THIEME Atlas of Anatomy. Internal Organs. Illustrations by Voll M and Wesker K. 3rd ed. New York: Thieme Medical Publishers; 2020.)

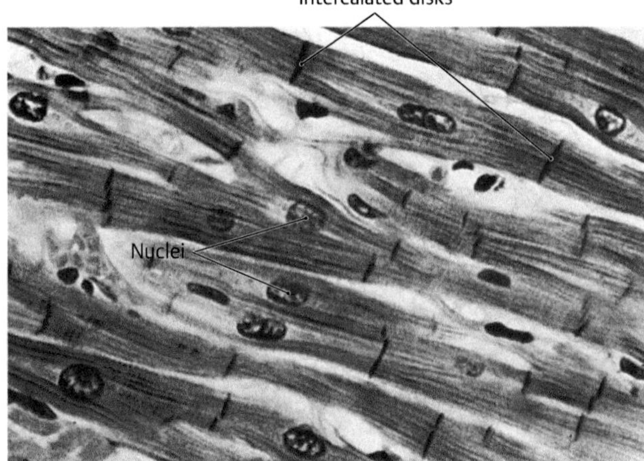

Fig. 2.39 Histology of the myocardium. (From Kuehnel, Taschenatlas Histologie, 13th ed. Stuttgart: Thieme; 2014.)

nuclei compared to skeletal muscle cells, which are long, multinucleated and cylindrical in nature. Branching networks of cardiac cells are called cardiac fibers. The atria myocardium is thinner with fewer t-tubules, more gap junctions, more elastic tissue and a faster conduction rate than the ventricular myocardium. Due to the high demands of cardiac muscle, dense vascularization is also present (**Fig. 2.39**).

The specialized and complex electro-mechanical junctions that join cardiac muscle cells are called **intercalated disks.** They connect cardiac muscles cells at the membranes of their longitudinal ends by way of three distinct types of membrane specialization.

- **Fascia adherens**: are located at the transverse "end" region and connect the closest sarcomere. They also act as the anchoring site for actin filaments.
- **Macula adherens** (desmosomes): are located at the transverse "end" region and stop separation during contractions by binding intermediate filaments. There are no actin filaments.
- **Gap junctions**: are located on the lateral "side" regions and allow action potentials or low resistance electrical coupling between two cardiac cells which are individually innervated. The wave of depolarization is transmitted from cell to cell.

Borders, Surfaces and External Sulci

- **Apex of the heart**
  - Formed by the inferolateral portion of the heart.
  - Located in the left 5th intercostal space.
  - Projects anteriorly, inferiorly and to the left.
  - Is motionless throughout the cardiac cycle.
  - The best location for auscultation of the bicuspid (mitral) valve.
- **Base of the heart**
  - Posterior aspect of the heart and opposite the apex.
  - Formed primarily by the left atrium with a smaller contribution from the right atrium.
  - Located approximately between the T6-T8 vertebral bodies and in between the bifurcation of the pulmonary trunk down to the coronary sulcus.
  - Receives all four pulmonary veins at the left atrial portion.
  - Receives the SVC and IVC at the right atrial portion.
- There are four borders of the heart
  1. **Superior border**: formed by the left and right atria and their auricles from the anterior aspect. The pulmonary trunk and ascending aorta leave from this border but the SVC joins it. This border also forms the inferior boundary of the transverse pericardial sinus.
  2. **Left border**: formed by the left ventricle.
  3. **Inferior border**: primarily formed by the right ventricle and partially by the left ventricle.
  4. **Right border**: formed by the right atrium.
- There are 4 four surfaces of the heart **(Fig. 2.40)**
  1. **Anterior (sternocostal) surface**: primarily formed by the right ventricle.
  2. **Diaphragmatic surface**: related to the central tendon of the diaphragm. Primarily formed by the left ventricle and partially by the right ventricle.
  3. **Left pulmonary surface**: related to the cardiac impression of the left lung. Formed by the left ventricle.
  4. **Right pulmonary surface**: formed by the right atrium.
- There are **three sulci of the external surface of the heart**:
  1. **Anterior interventricular sulcus**: a groove that forms between the left and right ventricles on the anterior aspect of the heart. This is the sulcus that contains the *anterior interventricular (left anterior descending) artery* and the *great cardiac vein.*
  2. **Posterior interventricular sulcus**: a groove that forms between the left and right ventricles on the posterior aspect of the heart. This is the sulcus that contains the *posterior interventricular (posterior descending) artery* and the *middle cardiac vein.*
  3. **Coronary sulcus (atrioventricular groove)**: a groove that extends around the heart separating the atria from the ventricles. On the left half, it contains the circumflex artery and continuation of the great cardiac vein along with the coronary sinus. On the right half, it contains the right coronary artery and a portion of the small cardiac vein.

Chambers

Right atrium: the right atrium receives blood from the SVC, IVC and coronary sinus and forms the right border of the heart. Smaller anterior cardiac veins located on the anterior surface can also drain into the right atrium but they are of minor significance. An ear-like projection extends out from the right atrium and over the ascending aorta is known as the **right auricle** (appendage). The auricle functions simply to increase the capacity of the atrium **(Fig. 2.41)**.

The interior of the right atrium is both rough and smooth. The anterior and rough portion is due to the presence of **pectinate muscle** and resembles the teeth of a comb. The right auricle is lined with pectinate muscle as well. The posterior, smooth and thin walled portion is specifically known as the **sinus venarum.** A small, thumbprint impression is located on the interatrial septum known as the **oval fossa**, which is the remnant of the **oval foramen**. The smooth portion of the right atrium receives deoxygenated blood from the SVC, IVC and coronary sinus. The SVC is located at the level of the right 3rd costal cartilage while the IVC is located at approximately the right 5th costal cartilage. The rough and smooth portions are separated externally by the **sulcus terminalis** and internally by the **crista terminalis (Fig. 2.41)**.

There are several valves located in the right atrium and they include the **valve of the IVC (Eustachian)** and the **valve of the coronary sinus (Thebesian)**. The *right atrioventricular orifice* is where the right atrium delivers blood to the right ventricle and it is also the location of the **tricuspid valve**. Being able to identify these valves is important because they help define the *Triangle of Koch*. The apex of this triangle represents the location of the *atrioventricular (AV) node* of the conducting system and the following structures form its borders **(Fig. 2.41)**:

- The *tendon of Todaro*, which is a tendinous structure connecting the valve of the IVC to the right fibrous (central body) trigone.
- The origination of the septal leaflet of the tricuspid valve.
- The level of the opening of the coronary sinus.

Right ventricle: the right ventricle makes up most of the anterior surface of the heart and receives blood from the right atrium. The interior of this chamber is filled with meaty ridges that are almost web-like called **trabeculae carneae.** The right ventricle begins to taper off as it heads towards the **pulmonary semilunar valve** and this portion of it is called the **conus arteriosus**. Separating the smooth conus region from the rough meaty ridges is the **supraventricular crest**. This crest is important in deflecting the incoming flow of blood from the right atrium from that of the outgoing blood heading towards the pulmonary trunk **(Fig. 2.42)**.

The **tricuspid valve** is located in the right atrioventricular orifice and it consists of an **anterior**, **posterior** and **septal cusp**. **Tendinous cords** (*chordae tendineae*) attach to the free edges of these cusps. The tendinous cords then attach to an anterior, posterior or septal **papillary muscle**. These papillary muscles look

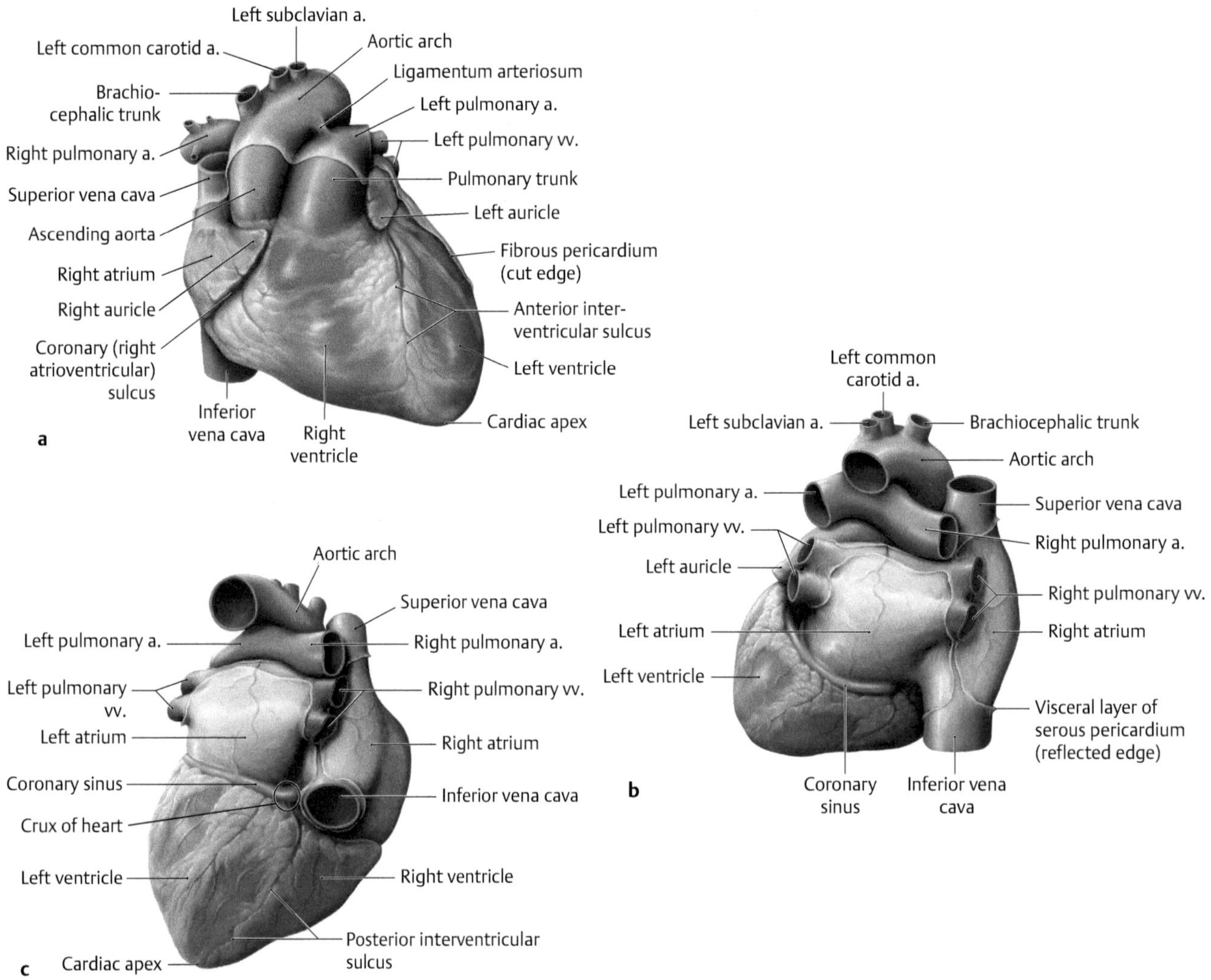

Left subclavian a.
Left common carotid a.
Aortic arch
Ligamentum arteriosum
Brachio-cephalic trunk
Left pulmonary a.
Right pulmonary a.
Left pulmonary vv.
Superior vena cava
Pulmonary trunk
Left auricle
Ascending aorta
Fibrous pericardium (cut edge)
Right atrium
Right auricle
Anterior inter-ventricular sulcus
Coronary (right atrioventricular) sulcus
Left ventricle
Inferior vena cava
Right ventricle
Cardiac apex
a
Left common carotid a.
Left subclavian a.
Brachiocephalic trunk
Aortic arch
Left pulmonary a.
Superior vena cava
Left pulmonary vv.
Right pulmonary a.
Left auricle
Right pulmonary vv.
Left atrium
Right atrium
Left ventricle
Visceral layer of serous pericardium (reflected edge)
b
Coronary sinus
Inferior vena cava
Aortic arch
Superior vena cava
Left pulmonary a.
Right pulmonary a.
Left pulmonary vv.
Right pulmonary vv.
Left atrium
Right atrium
Coronary sinus
Inferior vena cava
Crux of heart
Left ventricle
Right ventricle
Posterior interventricular sulcus
c
Cardiac apex

Fig. 2.40 Surfaces of the heart. **(a)** Anterior (sternocostal). **(b)** Posterior. **(c)** Inferior (diaphragmatic). (From Schuenke M, Schulte E, Schumacher U. THIEME Atlas of Anatomy. Internal Organs. Illustrations by Voll M and Wesker K. 3rd ed. New York: Thieme Medical Publishers; 2020.)

Ascending aorta
Pulmonary trunk
Superior vena cava
Right auricle
Right pulmonary a.
Terminal crest
Left atrium
Pectinate mm.
Right pulmonary vv.
Right ventricle
Interatrial septum
Limbus of oval fossa
Right atrioventricular orifice with atrioventricular valve
Oval fossa
Inferior vena cava
Valve of inferior vena cava
Valve of coronary sinus

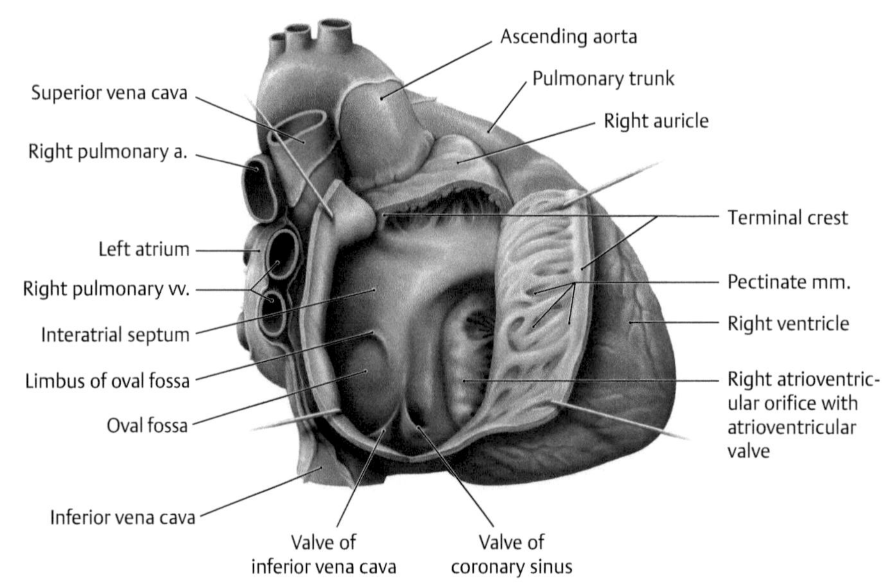

Fig. 2.41 Right atrium, right lateral view. (From Schuenke M, Schulte E, Schumacher U. THIEME Atlas of Anatomy. Internal Organs. Illustrations by Voll M and Wesker K. 3rd ed. New York: Thieme Medical Publishers; 2020.)

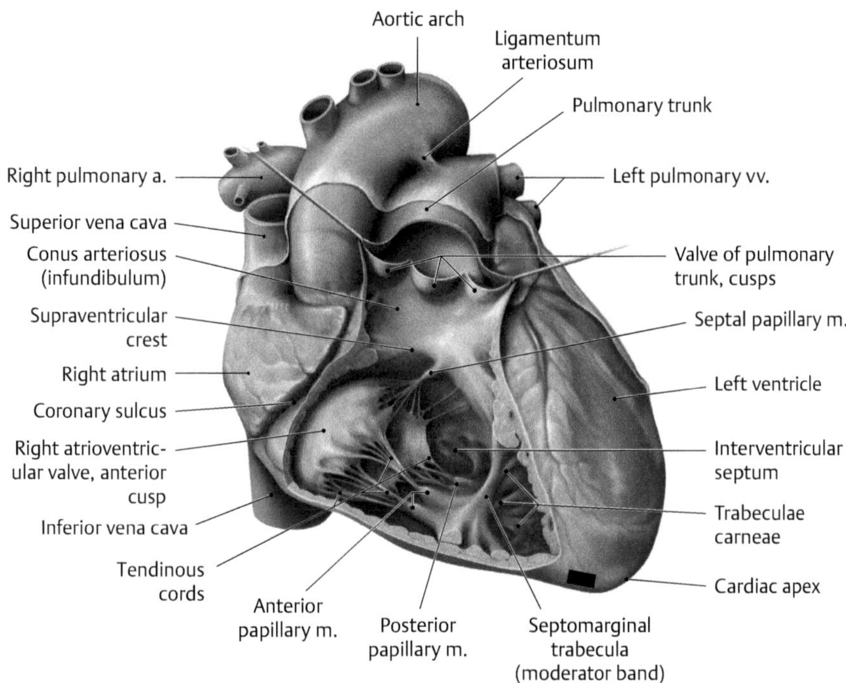

Fig. 2.42 Right ventricle, anterior view. (From Schuenke M, Schulte E, Schumacher U. THIEME Atlas of Anatomy. Internal Organs. Illustrations by Voll M and Wesker K. 3rd ed. New York: Thieme Medical Publishers; 2020.)

like muscular projections or pillars from the ventricular wall. The **anterior papillary muscle** is the largest and its tendinous cords attach to both the *anterior and posterior cusps*. The **posterior papillary muscle** and its tendinous cords attach to the *posterior and septal cusps*. The **septal papillary muscle** originates from the interventricular septum and its tendinous cords attach to the *septal and anterior cusps*. They function by contracting just before the right ventricle contracts and thus prevents prolapse of the tricuspid valve back into the right atrium. The valve cusps essentially block regurgitation of blood from the right ventricle back into the right atrium during ventricular systole (**Fig. 2.43**).

The **septomarginal trabecula (moderator band)** is an extra muscular bundle found only in the right ventricle and resembles a smaller papillary muscle that traverses the chamber from the inferior aspect of the interventricular septum to the base of the anterior papillary muscle. It carries within it the **right bundle branch of the AV bundle** which is associated with the conducting system of the heart. It is a shortcut of the conducting system fibers to facilitate the conduction time, thus allowing for a coordinated contraction of the anterior papillary muscle.

Left atrium: the left atrium receives all four of the valveless pairs of pulmonary veins that deliver oxygenated blood from the lungs and it forms the majority of the base or posterior aspect of the heart. The walls of the left atrium are smooth and are derived from the embryonic pulmonary vein. It has a larger smooth-walled portion and slightly thicker wall than the right atrium. The *left atrioventricular orifice* is where the left atrium delivers blood to the left ventricle and it is also the location of the **bicuspid (mitral) valve**. The **left auricle** (appendage) overlaps the pulmonary trunk and increases the capacity of the atrium. It contains pectinate muscle just like the right auricle (**Fig. 2.44**).

Left ventricle: the left ventricle forms the left pulmonary and diaphragmatic surfaces as well as the apex of the heart. The left ventricle pumps harder than the right ventricle and is thus 2-3 times thicker than the right side. *Trabeculae carneae, papillary muscles* and *tendinous cords* are found in the left ventricle just like in the right ventricle. The major differences being that the **trabeculae carneae** are finer and more numerous than those found in the right ventricle; there are only the **anterior** and **posterior papillary muscles** (multiple bellies) and the **tendinous cords** are fewer in numbers but tend to be stronger and thicker (**Fig. 2.44**). The cords have overlapping attachments on the cusps similar to how they attach to the tricuspid valve. The **bicuspid (mitral) valve** is located in the left atrioventricular orifice and it consists of an **anterior** and **posterior cusp**. The **aortic vestibule** is the non-muscular, smooth-walled outflow portion of the left ventricle that leads to the **aortic orifice** that contains the **aortic semilunar valve** (**Fig. 2.43**).

Chamber Septum

The **interatrial septum (IAS)** separates the right and left atria from one another. In the adult, an **oval fossa** (*fossa ovalis*) about the size of a thumbprint is present and was formed by the closing of the **valve of the oval foramen**, part of the *septum primum* of the septating atria. During development, an **oval foramen** (*foramen ovale*) between the right and left atria is present and acts to divert blood away from the lungs and pulmonary arteries. The pulmonary arteries still receive some blood but because there is no major exchange of oxygen and carbon dioxide taking place during this time, not as much blood is needed. Instead the majority of the blood is allowed to enter the left atrium, followed by the left ventricle, and then through the aorta to the systematic circulation (**Fig. 2.41**).

The **interventricular septum (IVS)** is made up of a membranous and muscular portion and is responsible for separating the left and right ventricles. The **muscular portion** that forms the majority of this septum has the thickness consistent with the rest of the left ventricle. This is because the blood pressure is higher in the left ventricle due to it needing to pump blood

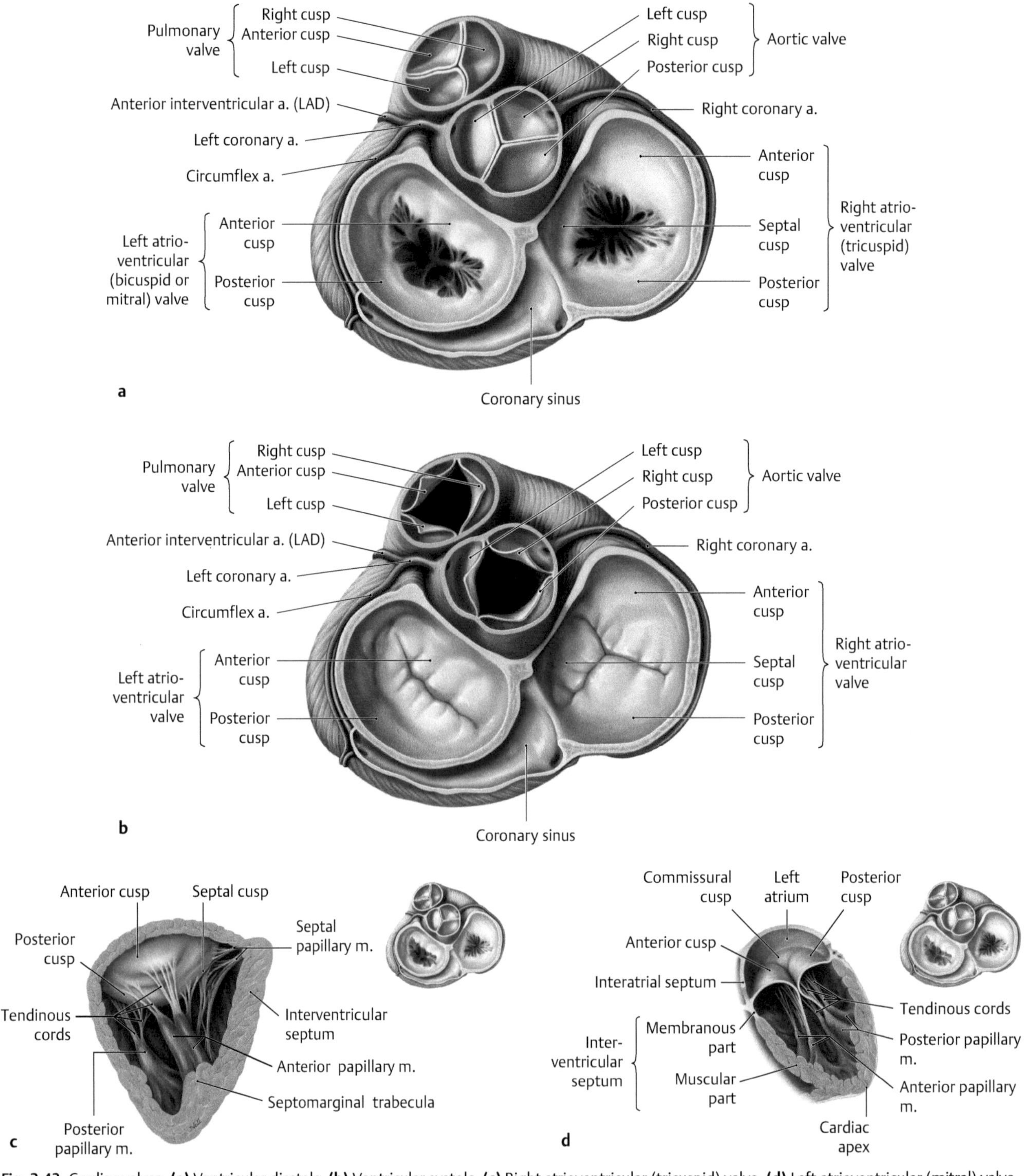

Fig. 2.43 Cardiac valves. **(a)** Ventricular diastole. **(b)** Ventricular systole. **(c)** Right atrioventricular (tricuspid) valve. **(d)** Left atrioventricular (mitral) valve. (From Schuenke M, Schulte E, Schumacher U. THIEME Atlas of Anatomy. Internal Organs. Illustrations by Voll M and Wesker K. 3rd ed. New York: Thieme Medical Publishers; 2020.)

throughout the body versus just to the lungs. The **membranous portion** is superior to the muscular portion and much smaller. This portion is also a part of the fibrous skeleton, develops from multiple sources, and is the site of most *ventricular septal defects* (**Fig. 2.42**).

Semilunar Valve Components

Blood passing from the right ventricle to the pulmonary trunk must pass through the **pulmonary semilunar valve** while blood passing from the left ventricle to the ascending aorta must pass through **aortic semilunar valve.** Both semilunar valves have three cusps each (**Fig. 2.45**). The pulmonary semilunar valve has an anterior, left and right cusp and the aortic semilunar valve has a left, right and posterior cusp. The names of these cusps originate from their embryological origin and not their adult position.

The thickened edge of each cusp is the **lunule** and in the middle or apex of the lunule, there is an additional thickening known as the **nodule**. The **aortic sinuses** and **pulmonary sinuses** are the spaces between the superior aspect of the cusps and the dilated

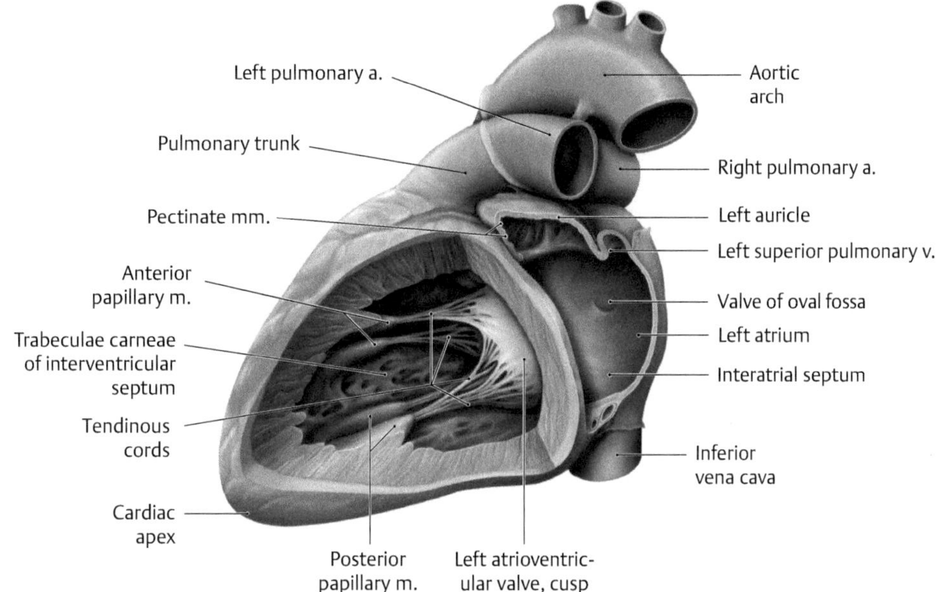

Fig. 2.44 Left atrium and ventricle, left lateral view. (From Schuenke M, Schulte E, Schumacher U. THIEME Atlas of Anatomy. Internal Organs. Illustrations by Voll M and Wesker K. 3rd ed. New York: Thieme Medical Publishers; 2020.)

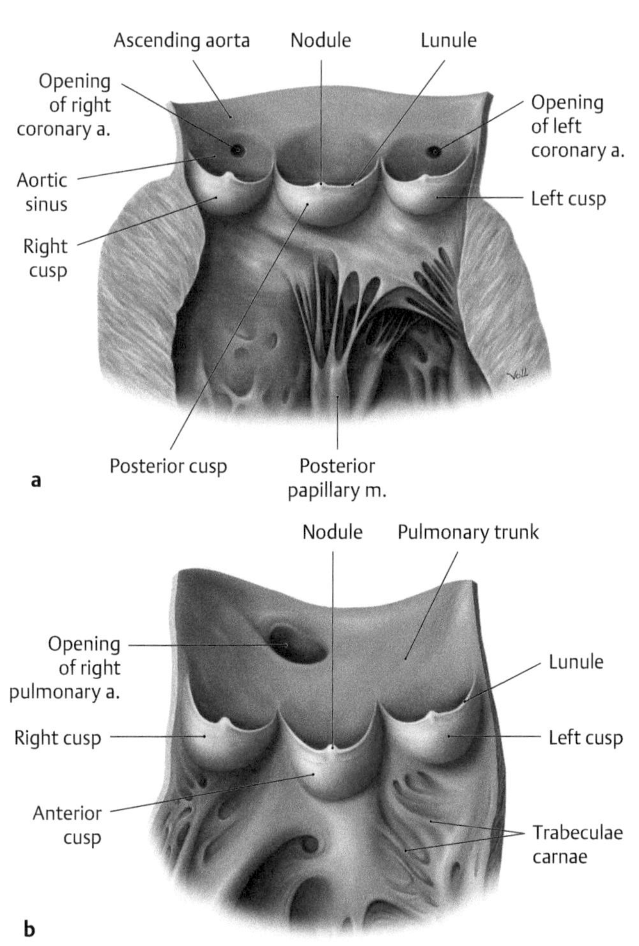

Fig. 2.45 **(a)** Aortic semilunar valve. **(b)** Pulmonary semilunar valve. (From Schuenke M, Schulte E, Schumacher U. THIEME Atlas of Anatomy. Internal Organs. Illustrations by Voll M and Wesker K. 3rd ed. New York: Thieme Medical Publishers; 2020.)

Clinical Correlate 2.19

Valvular Heart Disease

Valvular heart disease is a group of disorders that involve either the tricuspid, bicuspid (mitral) or semilunar valves and can be classified as either acquired or congenital. If not congenital, examples of the causes of valvular disease could include radiation therapy, rheumatic fever, endocarditis, high blood pressure, atherosclerosis, rheumatoid arthritis, systematic lupus, or simply the age of an individual's valve. Clinical significance can range from minor to a severe functional deficit but the acquired valvular abnormalities develop over a longer period of time.

Valvular heart disease can lead to valvular stenois or insufficiency conditions. **Valvular stenosis** involves the valve leaflets becoming stiff which narrows the valve opening thus reducing blood flow passing through it. **Valvular insufficiency** (or "leaky valve") occurs when the leaflets do not close completely, allowing for regurgitation of blood to occur. Both valvular stenosis and insufficiency result in a greater workload for the heart. As blood passes through these stenotic or insufficient valves, turbulence is produced leading to the development of small whirlpools (or *eddies*). These *eddies* produce vibrations that are audible as *murmurs*. On the skin over an area of turbulence, vibratory sensations known as *thrills* can be felt. Due to the mechanical nature of valvular disease, heart valves can be replaced surgically in a procedure known as valvuloplasty.

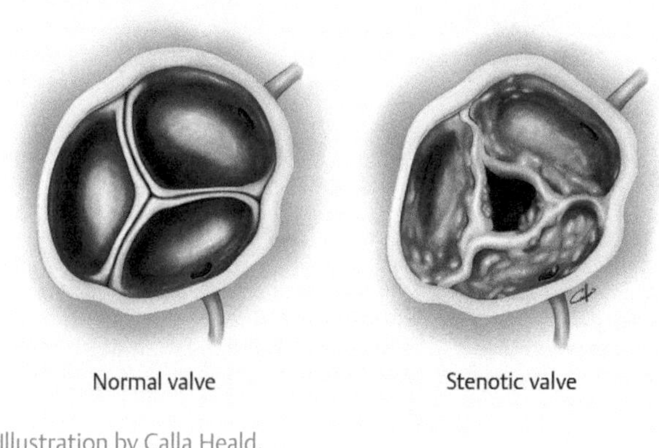

Illustration by Calla Heald.

Clinical Correlate 2.20

Tricuspid Valve Stenosis/Insufficiency

Tricuspid stenosis/insufficiency of the tricuspid valve is associated with rheumatic fever. Generally individuals with **tricuspid stenosis** also have mitral valve stenosis. Tricuspid stenosis leads to a reduction of blood filling the right ventricle and the right atrium will enlarge. **Tricuspid insufficiency** is the regurgitation of blood from the right ventricle back into the right atrium. The main cause of this form of insufficiency is an enlarged right ventricle.

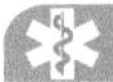

Clinical Correlate 2.21

Mitral/Bicuspid Valve Prolapse (MVP)

Mitral valve prolapse is among the most common heart conditions and is described as an insufficient or incompetent mitral valve that prolapses back into the left atrium during left ventricular contraction, the cause of which is unknown. The regurgitation of blood back into the left atrium produces a characteristic *murmur* or "clicking" sound. For most people, MVP is generally not a serious problem and they can still lead active lives. For others, surgery may be warranted to repair or replace the defective valves.

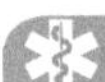

Clinical Correlate 2.22

Aortic Valve Stenosis/Insufficiency

Aortic valve stenosis of the aortic semilunar valve is primarily associated with degenerative calcification. The extra workload the heart is under due to this stenosis results in left ventricular hypertrophy. **Aortic valve insufficiency** can be caused by an acute endocarditis or chronic exposure to rheumatic fever or the presence of a bicuspid aortic semilunar valve when normally there are three valves. It is described as a regurgitation of blood back into the left ventricle during diastole producing a heart murmur and *collapsing pulse* (pulse with rapid upstrokes and downstrokes).

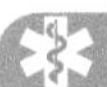

Clinical Correlate 2.23

Pulmonary Stenosis/Insufficiency

Pulmonary valve stenosis of the pulmonary semilunar valve is usually congenital and the valve cusps are fused forming a dome with a narrow opening. Most cases are considered mild presenting no symptoms but right ventricular hypertrophy can occur. **Pulmonary valve insufficiency** can be caused by pulmonary hypertension or most often in patients who had corrective surgery for *Tetralogy of Fallot* as a child. It is described as a regurgitation of blood back into the right ventricle during diastole producing a heart murmur (*Graham Steell murmur*).

outer walls of the ascending aorta or pulmonary trunk. The abnormal closure of these cusps is prevented by blood that fills these sinuses and the dilated portions of the ascending aorta and pulmonary trunk.

When the ventricles relax during diastole, this results in the elastic recoil of the wall of the aorta and pulmonary trunk which forces blood back toward the heart. The cusps then quickly close and seal as they catch the backflow of blood thus preventing regurgitation of blood back into the ventricles.

Clinical Correlate 2.24

Echocardiogram

An **echocardiogram** (or *echo*) is a type of ultrasound that uses high-pitched sound waves sent through a device called a transducer and picks up echoes of the sound waves as they bounce off different structures of the heart. The echoes are then turned into moving pictures that can be seen on a screen. This test can be used to check for heart wall thickness, heart valve function, size of the heart chambers, or to detect heart diseases such as cardiomyopathy. The different types include the transthoracic (most common), Doppler, stress and transesophageal echocardiograms.

Blood Supply and Venous Drainage of the Heart

The blood supply and venous drainage of the myocardium and epicardium of the heart are by way of the **coronary vessels** (**Fig. 2.46; Fig. 2.47**). The left and right coronary arteries originate from the left and right aortic sinuses (of Valsalva) of the aortic semilunar valve respectively. Coronary artery dominance is defined by which artery gives rise to the posterior interventricular artery. The right coronary artery gives rise to the posterior interventricular in approximately 70% of the population while the left coronary (via the circumflex) gives rise to it in only 15% of the population. The left and right coronaries both contribute to the posterior interventricular artery in approximately 15-20% of the population. Coronary dominance does not describe the artery and its branches that supply most of the cardiac tissue. Though the right coronary gives rise to the posterior interventricular artery a larger percentage of the time, it is almost always the left coronary and its branches that supply a greater volume of the myocardium (**Fig. 2.47; Fig. 2.48**).

Branches of the coronary arteries supply both the atria and ventricles but are considered **functional end arteries**. Functional end arteries lack sufficient anastomoses from larger branches if an occlusion of the vessel occurs. Some anastomoses do occur between branches of the coronary arteries, subepicardial or myocardial, and between these arteries and extracardiac vessels such as the thoracic vessels.[2] A very low percentage of normal hearts display anastomoses near the terminations of the interventricular branches near the apex and the left and right coronary arteries in the coronary sulcus.

After arising from the left aortic sinus, the **left coronary artery (LCA)** passes between the left auricle and the left side of the pulmonary trunk and for a very brief moment in the coronary sinus. Immediately after entering the coronary sulcus and at the superior end of the *anterior interventricular sulcus*, the LCA bifurcates into the circumflex and anterior interventricular (left anterior descending) arteries (**Fig. 2.46; Fig. 2.47**).

The **anterior interventricular** (or **left anterior descending**) **artery** courses along the anterior interventricular sulcus and within 2-2.5 cm the **lateral (diagonal) artery** is given off to help supply the left ventricle. The anterior interventricular artery will continue until it reaches the apex and possibly anastomose with the *posterior interventricular artery*. **Septal artery** branches of the anterior interventricular supply the adjacent sides of both ventricles and the anterior two thirds of the IVS, which includes the AV bundle branches of the conducting system. The anterior interventricular artery is paired with the **great cardiac vein**.

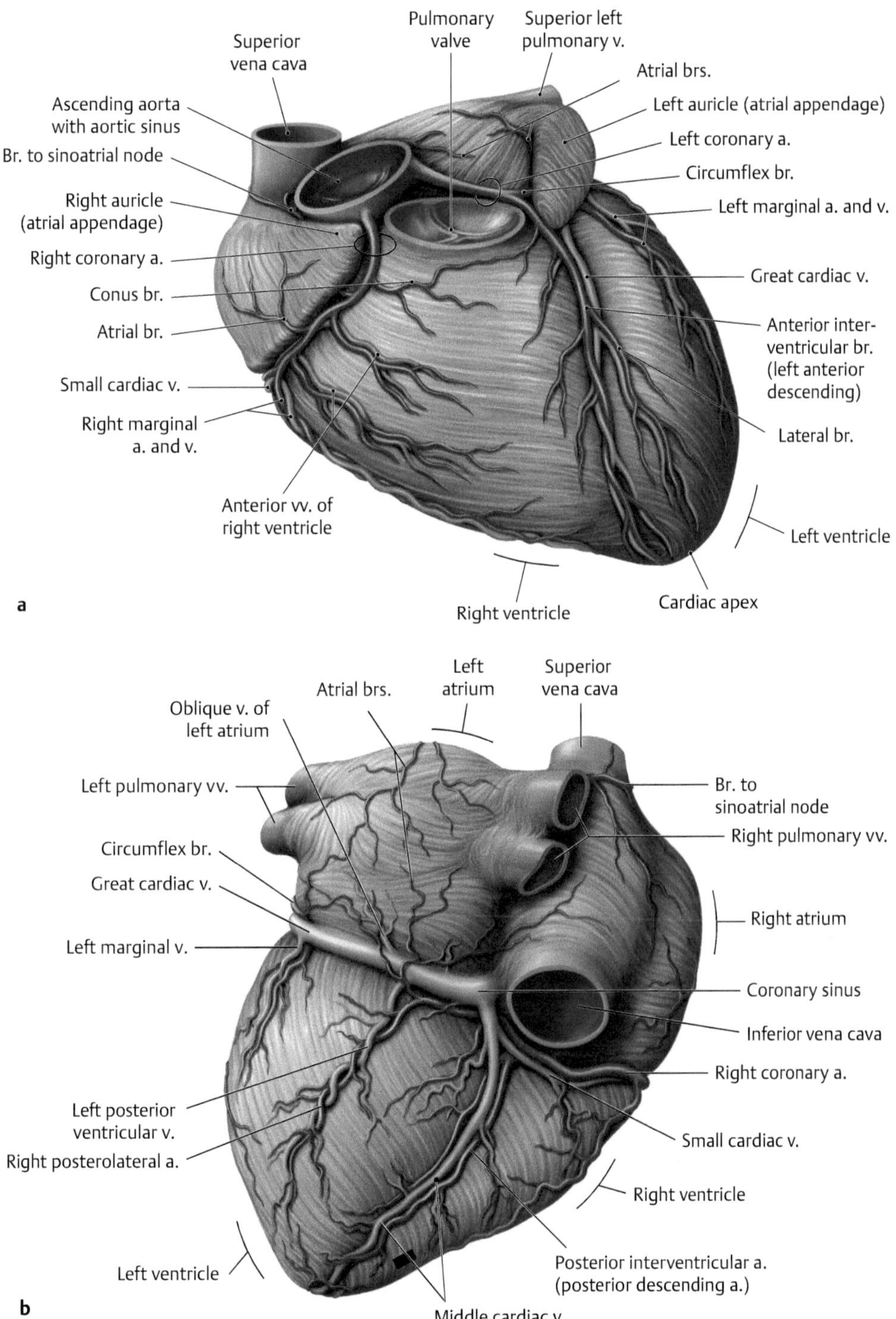

Fig. 2.46 (a) Coronary vessels as seen from the sterncostal surface of the heart. **(b)** Posteroinferior view of the coronary vessels on the diaphragmatic surface of the heart. (From Schuenke M, Schulte E, Schumacher U. THIEME Atlas of Anatomy. Internal Organs. Illustrations by Voll M and Wesker K. 3rd ed. New York: Thieme Medical Publishers; 2020.)

The **circumflex artery** follows the coronary sulcus around the left border and to the posterior surface of the heart where it generally terminates near the *coronary sinus* (**Fig. 2.46; Fig. 2.47; Fig. 2.48**). The circumflex may continue directly as the *posterior interventricular artery* but this only occurs in about 15% of the population. The **left marginal artery** branches off the circumflex near the left margin of the heart. In approximately 40% of the population the **sinoatrial (SA) nodal artery** originates off the circumflex artery while the **atrioventricular (AV) nodal artery** only arises from the terminal circumflex about 20% of the time. These arteries supply the SA node and AV nodes of the cardiac conducting system respectively. The **great cardiac vein** originally was paired with the anterior interventricular artery but after reaching the coronary sulcus region it will continue with the circumflex artery in the coronary sulcus. The circumflex contributes to both the left ventricle and left atrium blood supply.

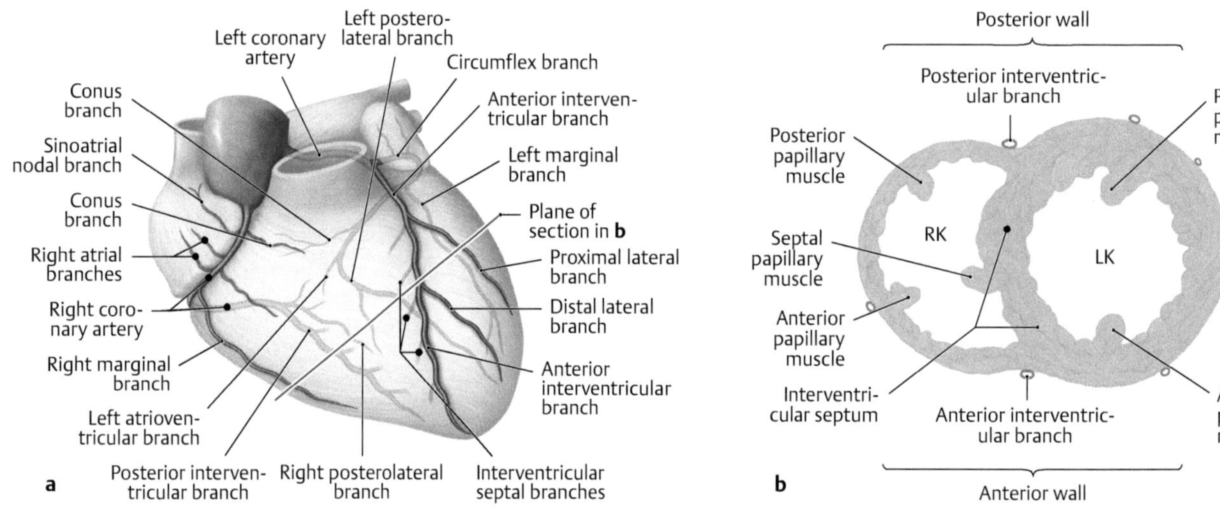

Fig. 2.47 Balanced (normal) coronary supply. **(a)** Course of the left and right coronary arteries, anterior view. **(b)** Cross-section of both ventricles: area supplied by left coronary (colored red); area supplied by right coronary (colored green). (From Schuenke M, Schulte E, Schumacher U. THIEME Atlas of Anatomy. Internal Organs. Illustrations by Voll M and Wesker K. 3rd ed. New York: Thieme Medical Publishers; 2020.)

- The left coronary and its branches will supply blood to **(Fig. 2.47)**:
  - Majority of the left ventricle.
  - Majority of the left atrium.
  - Small portion of the right ventricle.
  - Anterior two thirds of the interventricular septum.
  - AV bundle branches of the conducting system.
  - SA node (~40%) and AV node (~20%).

After arising from the right aortic sinus, the **right coronary artery (RCA)** passes between the right side of the pulmonary trunk and within the coronary sinus **(Fig. 2.46)**. Just after leaving the ascending aorta, the **SA nodal artery** (~60%) is generally given off. It passes posteriorly and in between the right auricle and ascending aorta before reaching the SA node situated near the superior portion of the sulcus terminalis. While the RCA is still in the coronary sulcus, it gives off a smaller **conus arteriosus branch**, along with multiple **anterior cardiac branches** as well as a possible **atrial branch**. The LCA is also known to branch off a conus arteriosus branch. Near the right border of the heart, the **right marginal artery** branches off the RCA. This artery is paired with the **right marginal vein** and is a tributary of the **small cardiac vein**.

After giving off the right marginal branch, the RCA will wrap around the right border of the heart and continue within the posterior aspect of the coronary sulcus with the small cardiac vein before reaching the *posterior interventricular sulcus*. At the superior part of the sulcus, the RCA terminates as the **posterior interventricular artery**. Quite common as well, this is the location of the **AV nodal branch** (~80%) which supplies the AV node.

The **posterior interventricular** (or **posterior descending**) **artery** courses along the *posterior interventricular sulcus* paired with the **middle cardiac vein** and will continue until it reaches the apex before possibly forming anastomoses with the *anterior interventricular artery*. **Septal artery** branches of the posterior interventricular supply the posterior one third of the IVS. A **right posterolateral artery** is commonly seen as a branch of the posterior interventricular or it may serve as the termination of the RCA. This artery crosses the sulcus and helps supply blood to the diaphragmatic surface of the left ventricle. A *left posterolateral artery* may exist but it is generally a branch of the circumflex artery.

- The right coronary and its branches supply blood to **(Fig. 2.47)**:
  - Majority of the right ventricle.
  - Majority of the right atrium.
  - Small portion of the left ventricle.
  - Posterior one third of the interventricular septum.
  - AV bundle branches of the conducting system.
  - SA node (~60%) and AV node (~80%).

Most venous drainage of the heart will eventually make it to the **coronary sinus** before finally draining into the right atrium. The *great cardiac, middle cardiac, small cardiac* and the *posterior vein of left ventricle* drain directly into the coronary sinus. The **great cardiac vein** begins near the apex on the anterior side of the heart and travels alongside the *anterior interventricular* and *circumflex arteries* before fusing with the **oblique vein of the left atrium** (of Marshall) to form the coronary sinus. The great cardiac vein is the largest tributary of the coronary sinus and is responsible for draining most of the blood originally supplied by the LCA.

The **middle cardiac vein** begins near the apex on the posterior side of the heart and is paired with the posterior interventricular artery. The **small cardiac vein** first receives blood from the **right marginal vein** and then courses along with the last half of the RCA in the coronary sulcus before reaching the coronary sinus. The **posterior vein of left ventricle** is located somewhere between the left marginal and middle cardiac veins and it can pair with the *posterolateral artery* (left or right). Multiple veins can be located on the diaphragmatic surface of the left ventricle thus veins in this region are highly variable **(Fig. 2.46b)**.

The **anterior cardiac veins** are located over the anterior surface of the right ventricle and generally drain directly into the right atrium. Occasionally they may drain into the small cardiac vein. Originating from the capillary beds of myocardium, miniature veins called the *smallest cardiac veins* can open directly into all chambers of the heart and bypass the coronary sinus.

Coronary Artery Variations and Anomalies

The location of the left and right coronary arteries has a stereotypical architecture that is conserved across individuals within a species and across species. The transcription factor HIF-1α plays a

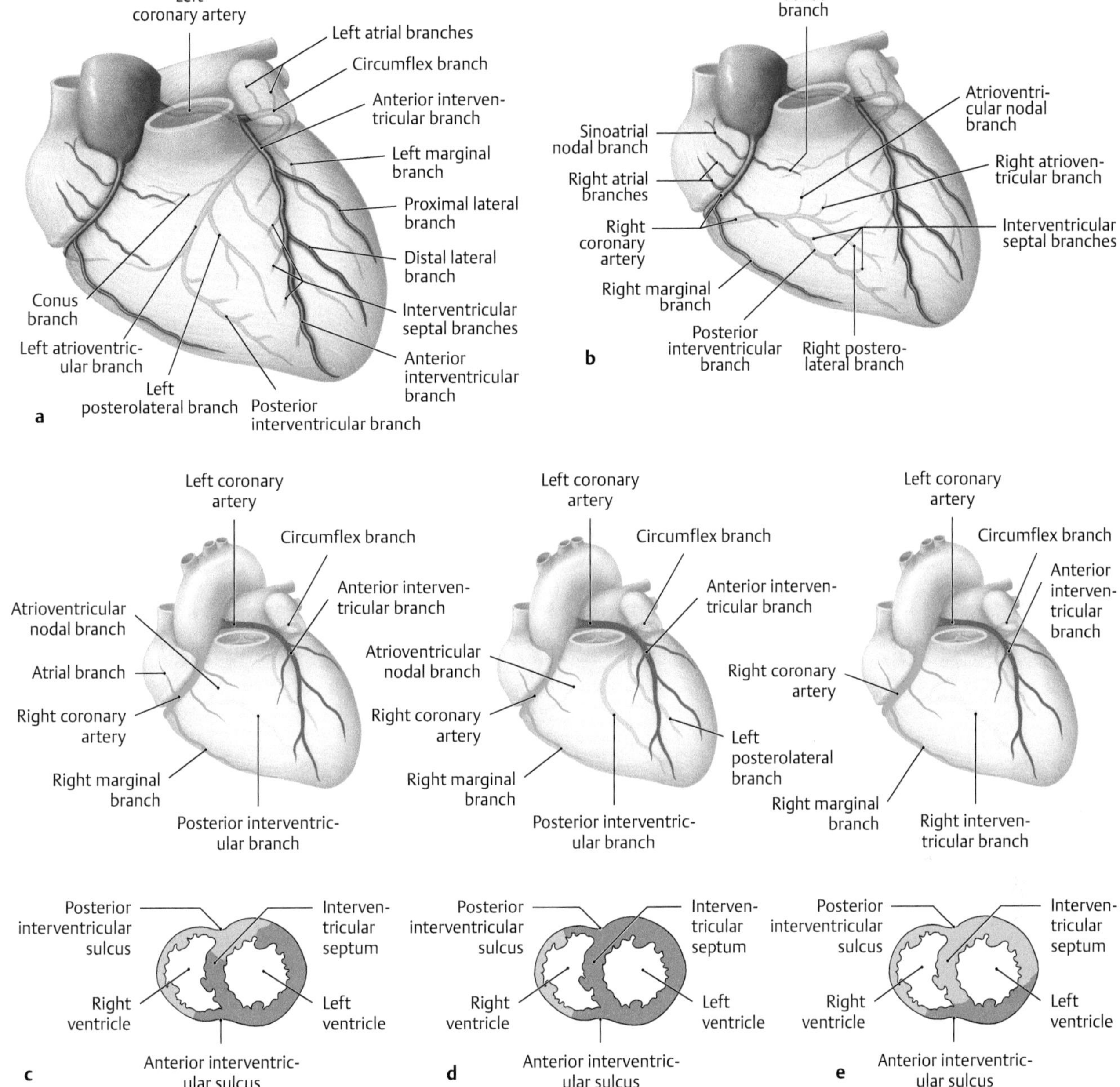

Fig. 2.48 (a) Left dominant circulation. **(b)** Right dominant circulation. **(c)** Balanced circulation (~70% of population). **(d)** Left dominant circulation (~15% of population). **(e)** Right dominant circulation (~15% of population). (From Schuenke M, Schulte E, Schumacher U. THIEME Atlas of Anatomy. Internal Organs. Illustrations by Voll M and Wesker K. 3rd ed. New York: Thieme Medical Publishers; 2020.)

large role in coronary artery development and depending on the condition, alteration of HIF-1α results in a 75-90% rate in coronary artery anomalies. The proximal attachment of coronary arteries is of greater clinical significance versus the more distal branching patterns.[3,4] Listed are some of the more common or clinically significant coronary artery anomalies **(Fig. 2.49)**.

- The **circumflex artery arising from the right main coronary artery** and passing posterior to the aorta (retro-aortic) is the most common anomaly accounting for about 35% of all anomaly cases. Major clinical complications are not seen with this anomaly.
- The **left coronary artery arising from the (opposite) right aortic sinus (Left-ACAOS)** that passes between the aorta and the pulmonary trunk is rare (3% of anomaly cases), but has been associated with sudden death. The presumption is that during exercise the abnormal coronary artery running between the aorta and pulmonary trunk is compressed by the dilated vessels thus reducing blood flow to a large portion of the heart.
- The **right coronary artery arising from the (opposite) left aortic sinus (Right-ACAOS)** occurs in approximately 30% of all coronary anomalies. In this condition, the right coronary artery runs between the aorta and the pulmonary trunk similar to left-ACAOS. It has an increased risk for sudden death, as does certain cases of left-ACAOS, and surgical re-implantation is recommended.
- The **left coronary artery arising from the pulmonary artery/trunk (ALCAPA)** results in left ventricular

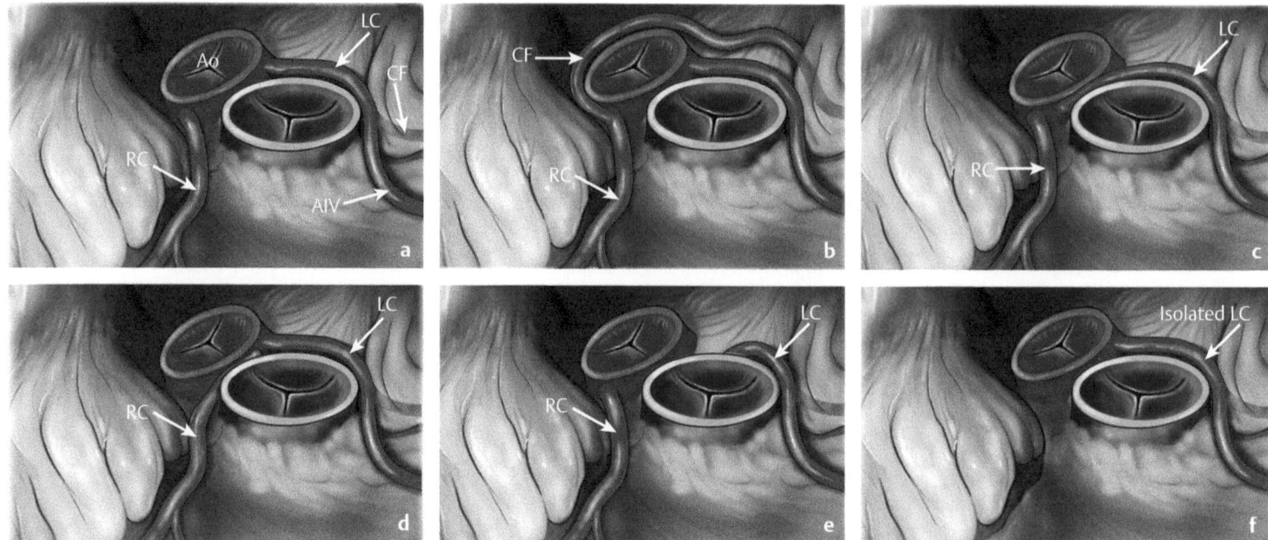

Fig. 2.49 Coronary artery variations and anomalies. **(a)** Normal orientation. **(b)** Retro-aortic circumflex artery originating from the proximal right coronary. **(c)** Left coronary artery originating from the right aortic sinus. **(d)** Right coronary artery originating from the left aortic sinus. **(e)** Left coronary artery originating from the pulmonary trunk. **(f)** A single coronary artery which can be either from the left or right side. LA, left atrium; RA, right atrium; Ao, aorta; Pt, pulmonary trunk; LC, left coronary; RC, right coronary; AIV, anterior interventricular; CF, circumflex. Illustration by Calla Heald.

insufficiency or infarction and infants with this condition have a high mortality rate with 65-90% dying before age 1 from congestive heart failure. This anomaly is usually isolated but can be associated with other congenital heart defects such as Tetralogy of Fallot or coarctation of the aorta. It usually presents at birth or shortly thereafter with an increase in myocardial ischemia followed by exhaustion of the coronary vascular reserve.

- A **single coronary artery** originates from the aorta and then branches to give rise to the left and right coronaries and make up around 5-20% of coronary anomalies. Approximately 40% of single coronary artery cases are associated with other congenital cardiac defects such as Tetralogy of Fallot. This anomaly has a mildly increased risk of sudden death but with only one initial main coronary, there is a greater vulnerability to future plaque buildup.

Lymphatic Drainage of the Heart

Lymphatic drainage of the heart displays a crossed drainage pattern and it divides the heart into a left versus right region (**Fig. 2.50**). The *left region* consists of the left ventricle, left atrium, and a small strip of the right ventricle and lymph from these regions is conveyed through the **"left coronary trunk."** Lymph would originate from either of the locations listed above and travel to the **bronchopulmonary lymph nodes**, followed by the **inferior tracheobronchial (carinal) lymph nodes** located deep to the ascending aorta but adjacent to the tracheal bifurcation. From the inferior tracheobronchial lymph nodes, lymph will travel through the **right bronchomediastinal trunk** before reaching the **right lymphatic duct** and from here lymph enters the venous circulation at the *right venous angle.*

The *right region* consists of the majority of the right ventricle and all of the right atrium. Lymph from these regions is conveyed through the **"right coronary trunk."** Lymph would originate from either of the locations listed above and travel to the **anterior mediastinal lymph nodes** located on the ascending aorta, followed by the **brachiocephalic lymph nodes** located near the left brachiocephalic vein. From the brachiocephalic lymph nodes, lymph will meet and then travel through the **left bronchomediastinal trunk** before reaching the **thoracic duct** and from here lymph enters the venous circulation at the *left venous angle.* Lymph from the right atrium can also drain directly to the **bronchopulmonary lymph nodes** before reaching the left bronchomediastinal trunk.

The Conducting System and Cardiac Cycle

The **conducting system of the heart** is responsible for coordinating the *cardiac cycle* of the heart. It is a series of specialized cardiac muscle cells that carry impulses throughout the heart musculature and signal the heart chambers to contract in their proper sequence. The **sinoatrial (SA) node** is made from specialized cardiomyocytes and serves as the heart's *pacemaker.* It initiates and regulates an impulse that averages about 70 beats per minute in most people. *Bradycardia* is the term to describe a resting heart rate that is slower than normal whereas *tachycardia* is the term to indicate a resting heart rate that is faster than normal. The SA node is located just deep to the epicardium near the superior end of the sulcus terminalis and at the junction of the SVC and right atrium. From the SA node, impulses spread along cardiac muscle fibers of the atria causing them to contract, but some impulses travel along an *internodal pathway* that targets the atrioventricular node. The **atrioventricular (AV) node** is located in the interatrial septum near the opening of the coronary sinus and is slightly smaller in size compared to the SA node. Its purpose is to delay ventricular contraction until after both of the atria have contracted (**Fig. 2.51**).

After a fraction of a second delay, impulses travel from the AV node, through the **AV bundle** (*bundle of His*) that serves as the only bridge of conduction between the atria and ventricular myocardium. From the AV node, the AV bundle passes through the right fibrous trigone of the cardiac skeleton and after reaching the border of the membranous and muscular interventricular septum, it bifurcates into a **left** and **right bundle branch**. The left bundle branch is associated with the left ventricle and the right bundle branch gives off a trunk that enters the **septomarginal trabeculae** (moderator band) and targets the anterior papillary muscle of the right ventricle. Impulses continue through the left and right

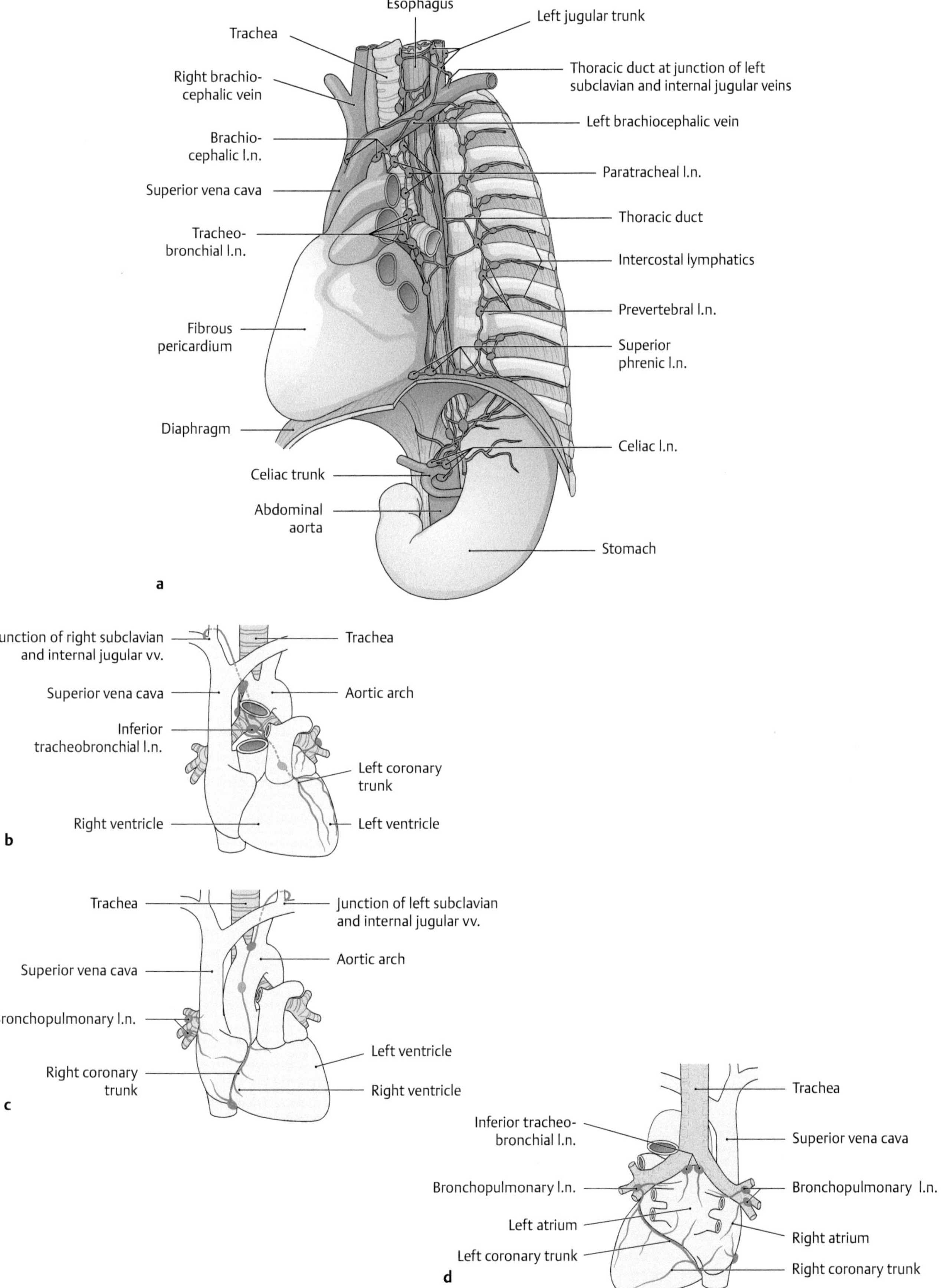

Fig. 2.50 **(a)** Lymph nodes of the mediastinum and thoracic cavity. **(b)** Lymph drainage of the left chambers, anterior view. **(c)** Lymph drainage of the right chambers, anterior view. **(d)** Posterior view. (From Schuenke M, Schulte E, Schumacher U. THIEME Atlas of Anatomy. Internal Organs. Illustrations by Voll M and Wesker K. 3rd ed. New York: Thieme Medical Publishers; 2020.)

Clinical Correlate 2.25

Coronary Atherosclerosis

Coronary artery disease (CAD) is the leading cause of death in the world and **coronary atherosclerosis** is the principal cause of CAD, which can create life-threatening blockages within the walls of the coronary arteries. Plaques that develop on the intima (internal lining) of the coronary arteries can obstruct blood flow and are caused by the buildup of low-density lipoprotein (LDL) cholesterol. These plaques may grow slowly, never blocking the artery or cause symptoms, or may expand and significantly block the blood flow in a coronary artery that may or may not lead to a myocardial infarction (MI). High blood pressure, cigarette smoking, and diabetes can also have an effect on plaque development.

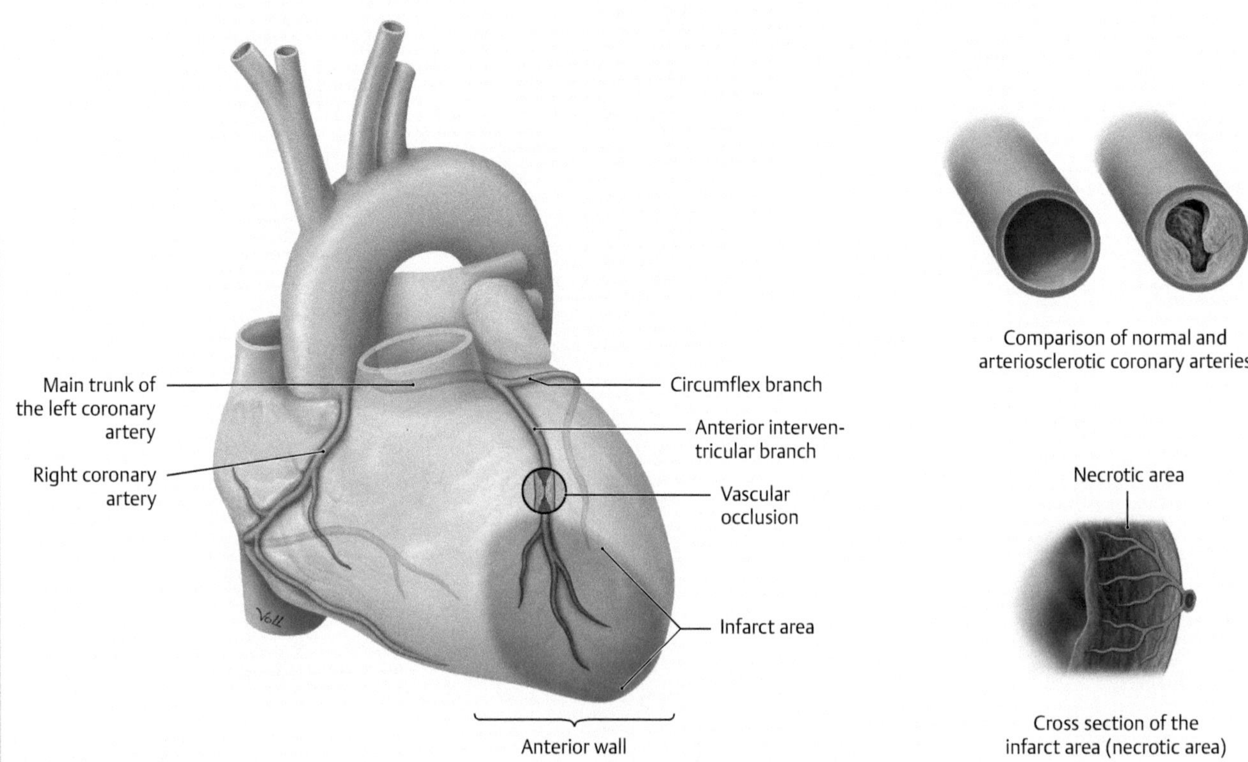

(From Schuenke M, Schulte E, Schumacher U. THIEME Atlas of Anatomy. Internal Organs. Illustrations by Voll M and Wesker K. 2nd ed. New York: Thieme Medical Publishers; 2016.)

Clinical Correlate 2.26

(Acute) Myocardial Infarction (AMI or "Heart Attack")

Refer to the image seen in Clinical Correlate 2.25. When a coronary artery suddenly becomes occluded resulting in an imbalance between the myocardial blood flow and the metabolic demand of the myocardium, the myocardium being supplied by that artery becomes infarcted and necrotic. *Angina pectoris* (constricting pain of the chest) pain is the result of ischemia of the myocardium that just falls short of inducing cellular necrosis that defines infarction. Angina pectoris is hence the result of narrowed coronary arteries supplying that region of myocardium. This angina pain is commonly felt radiating from the sternum, left pectoral and medial portion of the left upper limb regions. Myocardial infarction (MI) is the area of myocardium that has undergone necrosis.

There are six common sites of coronary artery occlusions that may lead to a MI. The first three sites listed account for 80–85% of all coronary artery occlusions.

1. Proximal anterior interventricular (AIV or LAD) near the LCA bifurcation.
2. Proximal RCA near its attachment to the ascending aorta.
3. Proximal circumflex artery near the LCA bifurcation.
4. Distal LCA near its bifurcation.
5. Proximal posterior interventricular (PIV or PDA) near where it branches off the RCA.
6. RCA approximately equal distances from both the ascending aorta and its PIV branch.

bundle branches located in the subendocardium. About midway down the septum, bundle branches become **Purkinje fibers**. These fibers stimulate the ventricular walls from the apex of the heart towards the atria thus resulting in the apex being pulled toward the plane of the valves. Direct stimulation of the papillary muscles prior to ventricular contraction ensures that the atrioventricular valves remain closed during ventricular systole (**Fig. 2.51**).

The **cardiac plexus** is a visceral nerve plexus responsible for the innervation of the heart. It consists of a *superficial portion* located on the inferior aspect of the aortic arch and anterior to the right

Clinical Correlate 2.27

Coronary Angiography

Coronary angiography is a test that employs the use of a dye and x-ray to visualize the lumen shape of a coronary artery. If there is suspected coronary artery blockage, a procedure known as *cardiac catheterization* involves inserting a thin, flexible catheter initially through an artery found in the groin, arm or neck until it reaches the openings of either the left or right coronary arteries. At this point, a special dye is released into the bloodstream and makes the coronary arteries visible on x-ray allowing physicians to view any blockages within the arteries.

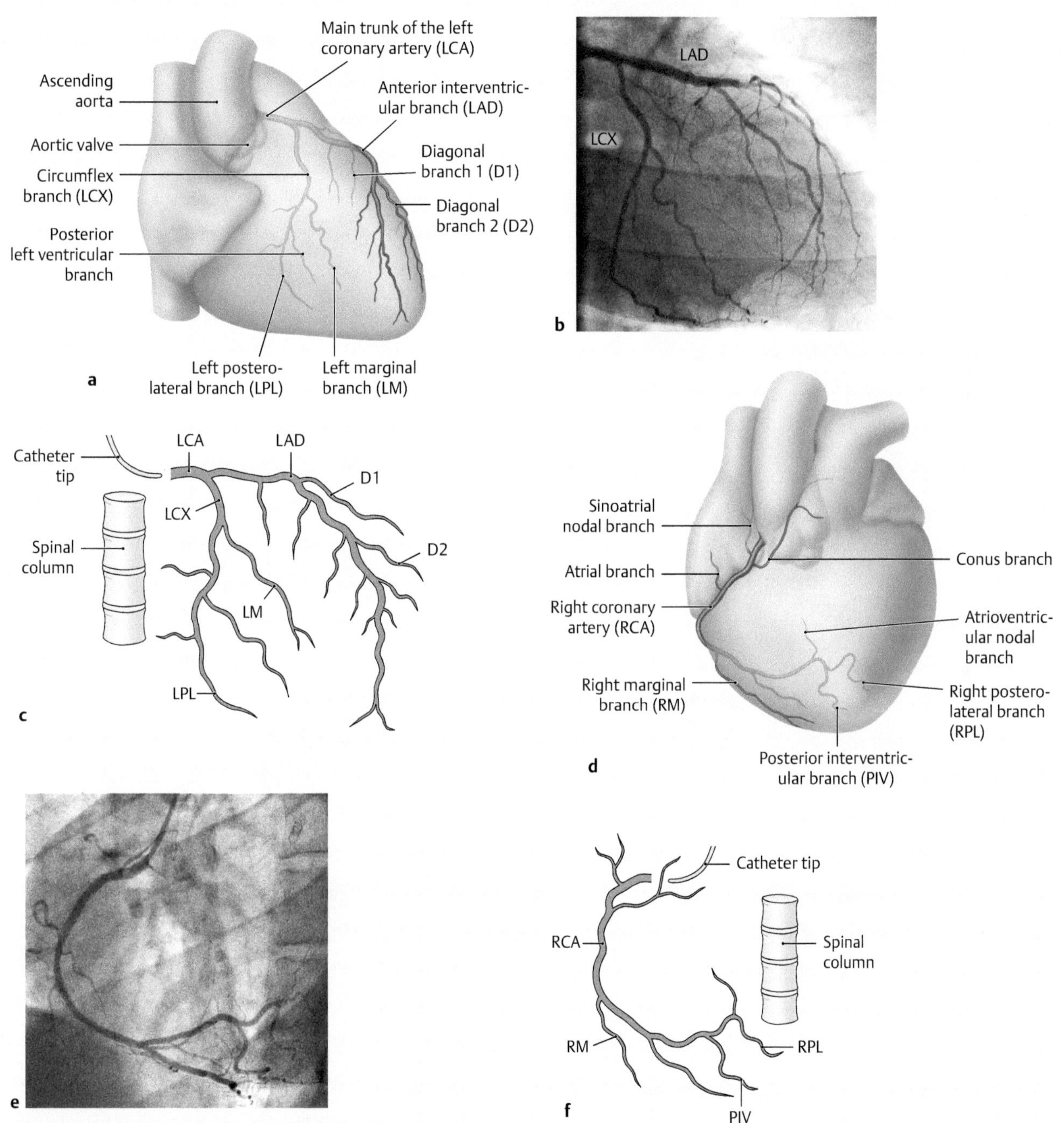

(a) Course of the left coronary artery (LCA) in a right anterior oblique (RAO) view. **(b)** Selective coronary angiography of the LCA. **(c)** Schematic representation of the individual branches. **(d)** Course of the right coronary artery (RCA) in a left anterior oblique (LAO) view. **(e)** Selective coronary angiography of the RCA. **(f)** Schematic representation of the individual branches. Note: In RAO projections, the spinal column is always projected to the left side. (**a, c, d, f** from Schuenke M, Schulte E, Schumacher U. THIEME Atlas of Anatomy. Internal Organs. Illustrations by Voll M and Wesker K. 2nd ed. New York: Thieme Medical Publishers; 2016. **b, e** from Thelen. M. et al.: Bildgebende Kardiodiagnostik/Cardiac Imaging. Stuttgart: Thieme; 2007.)

Clinical Correlate 2.28

Coronary Angioplasty

Coronary angioplasty is a procedure used to open a narrow or occluded coronary artery. During the procedure, a thin, flexible catheter with a balloon at its tip is threaded through the groin or an arm artery (*cardiac catheterization*), until it reaches the affected coronary artery. Once in place, the balloon is inflated to compress the plaque against the inner wall restoring blood flow through the artery. The balloon can also be used to place a stent in the artery to maintain patency. Some stents, called drug-eluting stents, are coated with medicine that can prevent re-stenosis of the vessel. Stents can also help prevent small pieces of plaque from breaking off and causing a heart attack or stroke.

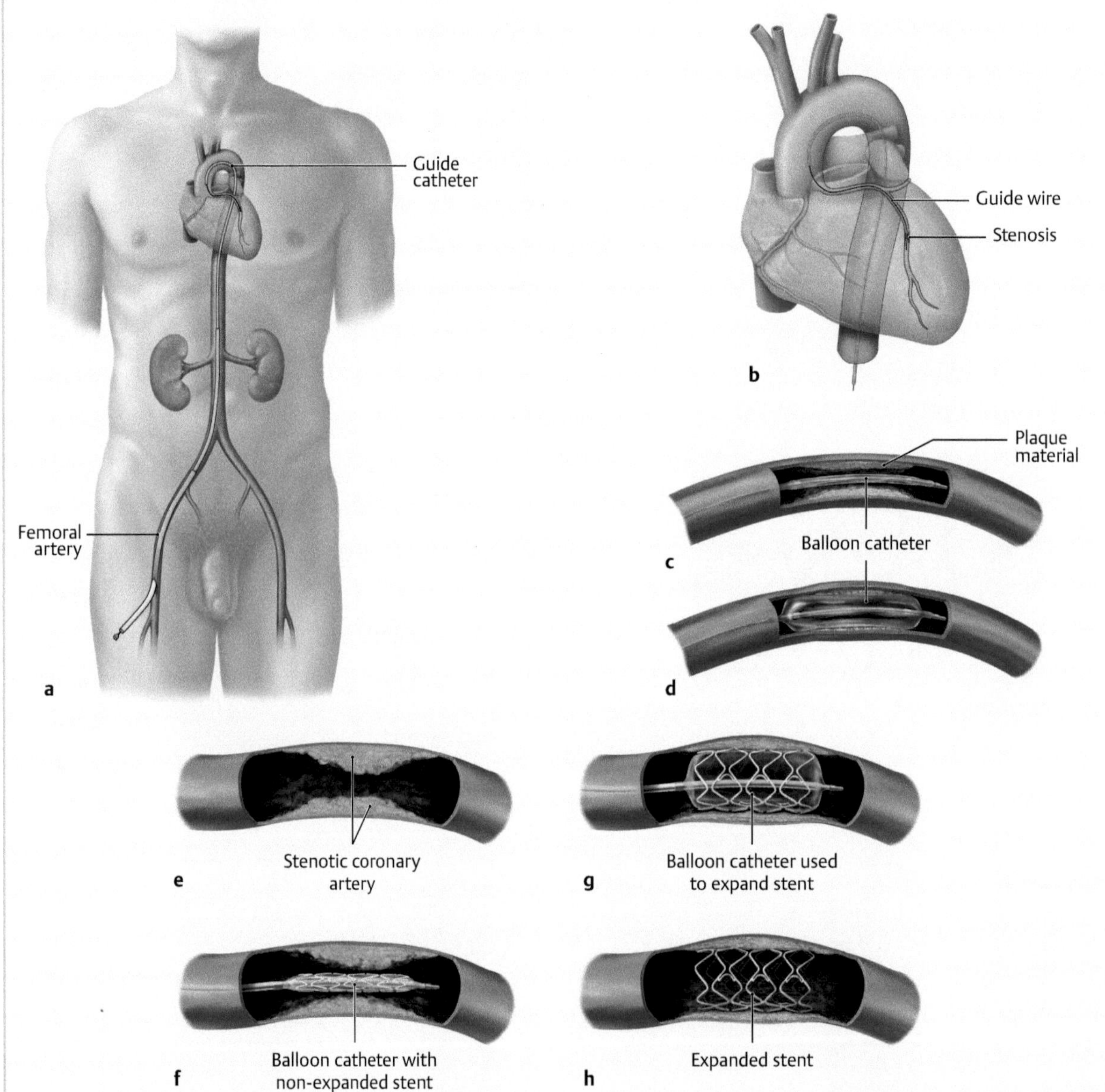

Percutaneous transluminal coronary angioplasty (PTCA) and stent placement. **(a)** Probing the coronary artery using a guide catheter to insert a guide wire. **(b)** Passing the stenosis with a guide wire. **(c,d)** Placement of a balloon catheter over the guide wire and dilatation of the stenosis. **(e–h)** The placement of wire mesh stents. (From Schuenke M, Schulte E, Schumacher U. THIEME Atlas of Anatomy. Internal Organs. Illustrations by Voll M and Wesker K. 2nd ed. New York: Thieme Medical Publishers; 2016.)

pulmonary artery. The *deep portion* is located posterior to the aortic arch but anterior to the tracheal bifurcation. Extensions of the superficial and deep portions include the *left and right coronary plexuses* and the *atrial plexus*. The majority of visceral nerve plexuses have no ganglion associated with the plexus. The cardiac plexus does contain limited amounts of isolated ganglion that consist of para/post cell bodies. The majority of ganglions that para/pre fibers synapse on in the thorax region are intrinsic to the organ they act upon. The functional components of this plexus are mostly GVE-sym/post, GVE-para/pre, and GVA with a limited amount of GVE-para/post fibers. The autonomic fibers of this plexus are motor to nodal, coronary vessel smooth muscle and cardiac musculature and contain visceral afferent fibers that convey nociceptive and reflexive fibers from the heart (**Fig. 2.52**).

The sympathetic fibers originate as sym/pre cell bodies from the **intermediolateral cell columns** (or **lateral horns**) of the

Clinical Correlate 2.29

Coronary Artery Bypass Surgery

When the coronary arteries become obstructed over time with plaque buildup, a patient may undergo a **coronary artery bypass surgery** to improve the blood flow to the heart. The surgery involves sewing a section of vein (great saphenous) from the leg and/or artery (internal thoracic) from the chest to bypass a part of the occluded coronary artery. This creates a new route for blood to flow, so that the heart muscle will get the oxygen-rich blood it needs to work properly. The surgery generally involves performing a median sternotomy, stopping the heart and sending blood through a heart-lung machine; however, variations of this procedure exist. The results of coronary bypass are usually excellent but individuals may still need to have blockages removed from the grafted vessels or arteries that were not originally occluded prior to the first operation.

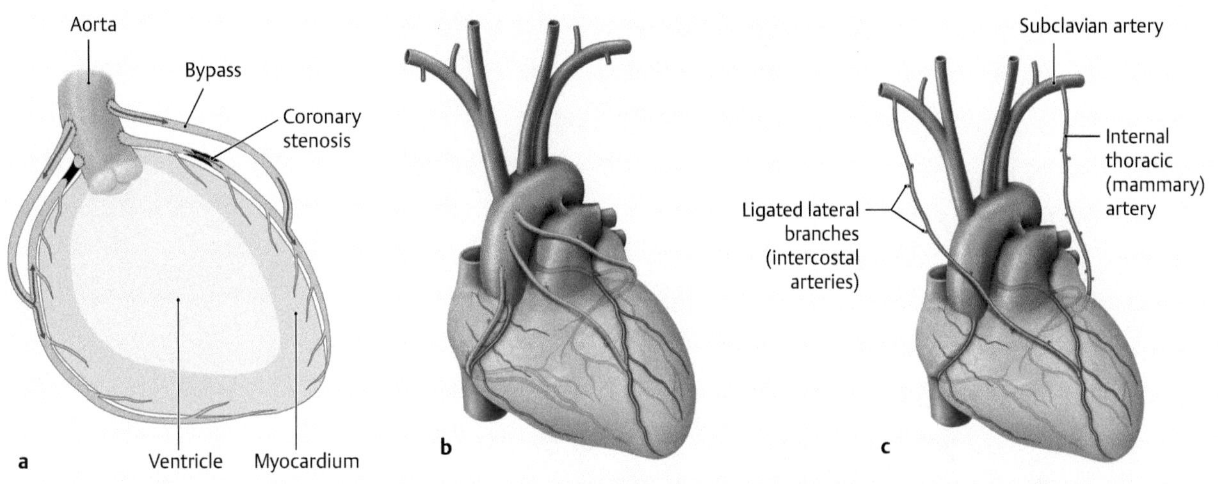

(a) Aortocoronary venous bypass (ACVB). **(b)** Aortocoronary venous bypass in a patient with three vessel disease. **(c)** Arterial internal thoracic (mammary) artery bypass. (From Schuenke M, Schulte E, Schumacher U. THIEME Atlas of Anatomy. Internal Organs. Illustrations by Voll M and Wesker K. 2nd ed. New York: Thieme Medical Publishers; 2016.)

T1-T5/T6 spinal cord segments. The **cardiopulmonary splanchnic nerves** originating from the neck deliver sym/post fibers to the cardiac plexus. Both pathways have their sym/post cell bodies located in the cervical and upper thoracic sympathetic chain ganglion. The sympathetic fibers are responsible for increasing heart rate and the force of contraction, as well as dilating (indirectly) the coronary vessels. Visceral afferent fibers that pass back with the sympathetics convey nociceptive information from the heart **(Fig. 2.53)**.

The parasympathetic fibers targeting the heart originate from para/pre cell bodies located in the medulla of the brainstem and they course through the vagus nerves (CN X) on their way to the cardiac plexus. The para/pre fibers synapse mostly on intrinsic ganglion of the cardiac plexus located in the atrial wall and adjacent to the interatrial septum near the SA and AV nodes as well as along the coronary arteries. The parasympathetic fibers are responsible for decreasing heart rate and the force of contraction and also for constricting the coronary vessels. Both autonomic divisions innervate the SA and AV nodes and the atrial muscle cells but ventricular muscle cells are predominately innervated by sympathetic fibers. Visceral afferent fibers that pass back with the parasympathetics convey reflexive fibers back from the heart **(Fig. 2.53)**.

The reticular formation of the medulla oblongata contains *cardiac centers* that are responsible for cardiac control. The **cardioacceleratory center** controls sympathetic neurons that increase the heart rate and the adjacent **cardioinhibitory center** controls the parasympathetic neurons that slow the heart rate. The activities of the *cardiac centers* are influenced by reflex pathways and through higher brain regions such as the anterior (parasympathetic) and posterior (sympathetic) nuclei of the hypothalamus, periaqueductal gray matter, amygdala and the insular cortex.

The **cardiac cycle** represents the period from the beginning of one heartbeat to the beginning of the next heartbeat. The cycle involves two major periods known as diastole and systole. **Diastole** is when the ventricles elongate/relax and fill while **systole** is when the ventricles contract/shorten and empty. Two heart sounds are normally heard while using a stethoscope. They are described as a *lub* and *dub* sound and are the result of the heart valves closing. The "lub" (S_1) sound is created by the closure of the AV valves while the "dub" (S_2) sound is due to the semilunar valves closing. A third and fourth sound may also be heard and are clinically described as S_3 and S_4. S_3 or the ventricular gallop ("Kentucky" gallop) is thought to be caused by the back and forth oscillation of blood between the walls of the ventricles initiated by blood rushing in from the atria. It could be the sign of a failing left ventricle, indicative of congestive heart failure. If present, it occurs at the beginning of diastole right after S_2. S_4 or atrial gallop ("Tennessee" gallop) is produced by the sound of blood being forced into a hypertrophic ventricle. It could be a sign of aortic stenosis, hypertrophic cardiomyopathy or a hypertrophic left ventricle as is seen in systemic hypertension. If present, the sound will be heard just after atrial contraction at the end of diastole and immediately before the S_1 sound.

The cardiac cycle can be divided into seven different phases:

- **Phase 1: Atrial systole** is preceded by the P wave of an ECG and represents the electrical activation of the atria. It contributes to ventricular filling and causes the S_4 heart sound that is generally not heard in normal adult hearts.

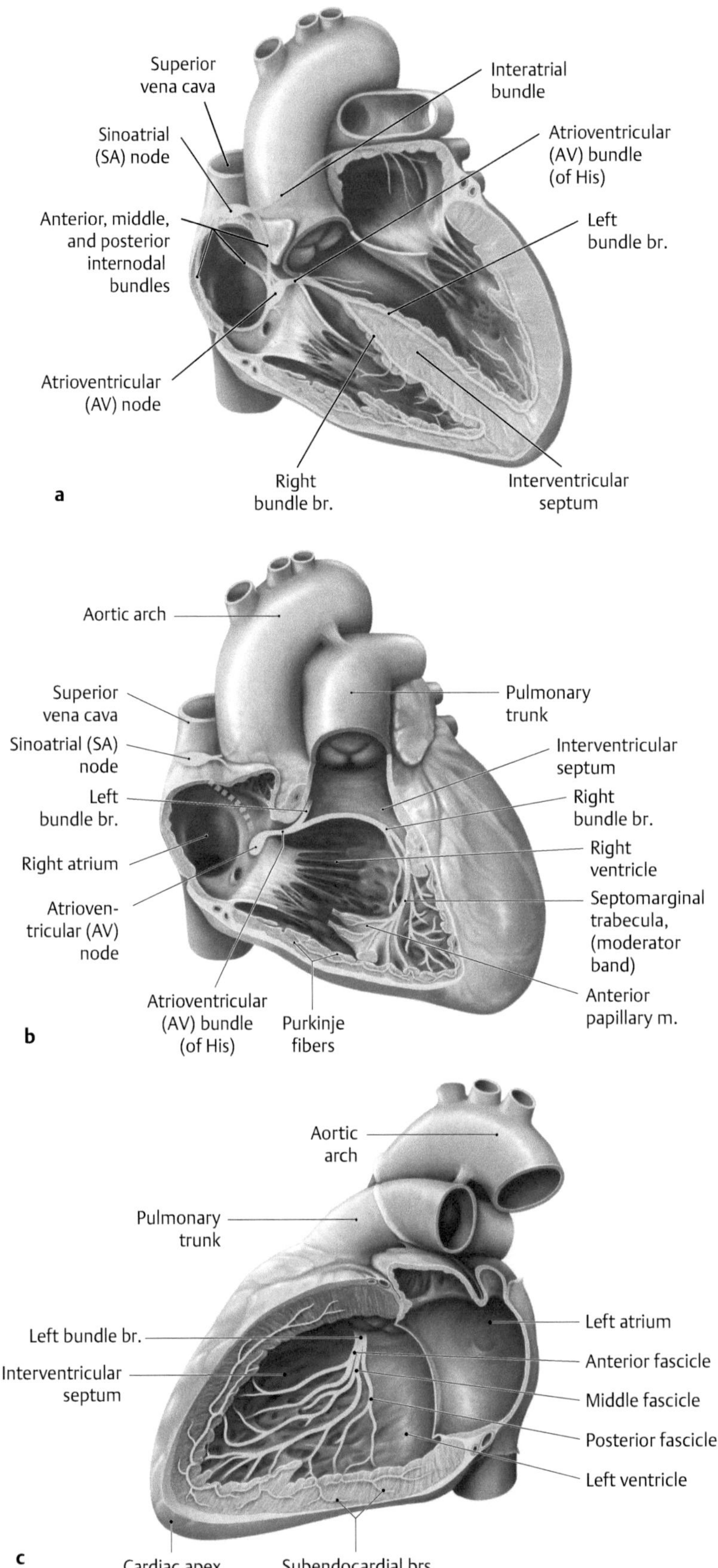

Fig. 2.51 Cardiac conduction system. **(a)** Anterior view. **(b)** Right lateral view. **(c)** Left lateral view. (From Schuenke M, Schulte E, Schumacher U. THIEME Atlas of Anatomy. Internal Organs. Illustrations by Voll M and Wesker K. 3rd ed. New York: Thieme Medical Publishers; 2020.)

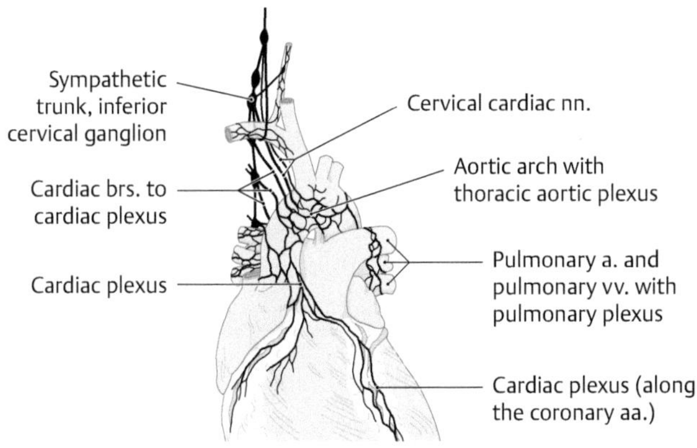

Fig. 2.52 Automatic plexuses of the heart, right lateral view. (From Schuenke M, Schulte E, Schumacher U. THIEME Atlas of Anatomy. Internal Organs. Illustrations by Voll M and Wesker K. 3rd ed. New York: Thieme Medical Publishers; 2020.)

- **Phase 2: Isovolumetric ventricular contraction** occurs after the onset of the QRS complex and represents the electrical activation of the ventricles. The AV valves close when the ventricular pressure becomes greater than the atrial pressure. The AV valves closing represent the first or S_1 heart sound. Ventricular pressure increases but the volume remains constant during this phase. Blood will not exit the ventricle at this time due to the aortic semilunar valves being closed.
- **Phase 3: Ventricular ejection** occurs rapidly after the ventricular pressure has peaked and is greater than aortic pressure resulting in the opening of the aortic semilunar valves. Most of the stroke volume is ejected reducing ventricular volume. The onset of the T wave is seen on an ECG and the atria begin to fill.
- **Phase 4: Reduced ventricular ejection** occurs when ventricular and aortic pressures begin to decease while the atria continue to fill.
- **Phase 5: Isovolumetric ventricular relaxation** occurs at the end of the T wave and represents a complete repolarization of the ventricles. The aortic then pulmonary semilunar valves close, creating the second or S_2 heart sound. Ventricular pressure decreases but the ventricular volume remains constant during this phase. The mitral valve opens when ventricular pressure is less than atrial pressure.
- **Phase 6: Ventricular filling** occurs rapidly when blood from the atria flows into the ventricles. This causes a third or S_3 heart sound that normally can only be heard in children or as an adult with heart pathology.
- **Phase 7: Reduced ventricular filling** is the longest cardiac cycle phase. The ventricles continue to fill but at a slower rate. Heart rate plays a role in the time required for ventricular filling. A higher heart rate will decrease the time for ventricular refilling.

2.15 Development of the Heart

2.15.1 Primary vs. Secondary Heart Fields

The cardiovascular system begins to form during the middle of the third week of development, when the embryo can no longer rely on diffusion for nutrition. The **progenitor heart cells** come from the epiblast and are immediately adjacent to the cranial end of the primitive streak. After migrating through the primitive streak and reaching the splanchnic (visceral) layer of lateral plate mesoderm, these cells form a horseshoe-shaped cluster of cells known as the **primary heart field (PHF)** during days 16-18 of development. The PHF is specified on both sides of the horseshoe-shaped structure to become, from lateral to medial, the *atria*, *left ventricle* and *most of the right ventricle* (**Fig. 2.54**).

The most medial portion of this heart field is known as the **secondary heart field (SHF)** and doesn't appear until about the 20th or 21st day of development. The SHF does not differentiate as myocardium until the looping stage of heart development. The SHF contributes to the *remainder of the right ventricle* and the *conus cordis* and *truncus arteriosus* of the outflow tract (OFT). All three regions together are referred to as the *bulbus cordis*. The SHF constitutes the source of cells that gives rise to both the most distal outflow tract myocardium and the most proximal smooth muscle that forms the tunica media of the arterial trunks. OFT defects are the result of reduced migration or abnormal proliferation of cells from the SHF.

Normal patterning of progenitor heart cells in both heart fields occurs at the same time that laterality (left-right sidedness) is being established for the entire embryo and is essential for normal heart development. Cells from the SHF on the left will contribute to the right while the right contributes to the left and this helps explain the spiraling effect of the aorta and pulmonary trunk so that they match up with the left ventricle and right ventricle respectively.

2.15.2 Primary Heart Tube Formation

During the fourth week of development, embryonic folding of the head, tail and lateral regions converts the flat trilaminar embryonic disk into a more cylindrical embryo. Mainly the lateral and head (cephalic) folding of the trilaminar disc brings the endocardial tubes together and tucks them along with the rest of the pericardial cavity ventral in the thoracic region anterior to the foregut and caudal to the oropharyngeal membrane.

With the fusion of the endocardial tubes, a **primary heart tube** forms and through which blood eventually flows in a cranial direction. The splanchnic (visceral) mesoderm surrounding the endocardial tube condenses to form the myocardium. The myocardium will then thicken and secrete a thick layer of extracellular matrix rich in hyaluronic acid called **cardiac jelly**. The cardiac jelly separates the myocardium from the endothelial layer (future **endocardium**) of the heart tube. Mesothelial cells originating from the **septum transversum** will form the **proepicardium** located near the sinus venosus. These mesothelial cells will continue to migrate over the heart and form most of the **epicardium** (visceral pericardium). The epicardium is responsible for the formation of smooth muscle and endothelium of the coronary arteries. Originally the primary heart tube is suspended in the pericardial cavity by the dorsal mesocardium. Shortly thereafter, the connection ruptures and the dorsal mesocardium becomes the **transverse pericardial sinus (Fig. 2.55)**.

A series of constrictions and dilations divide the heart tube into 4-5 sections (depending on the anatomist). The cranial portion begins as the **bulbus cordis** and is divided into three sections. The most distal portion is the **truncus arteriosus** and this portion is continuous with the **aortic sac**. It forms the roots and proximal portions of the aorta and pulmonary trunk. The middle portion is the **conus cordis** and becomes the OFT portions of the left and right ventricles. The proximal portion develops into the **trabeculated portion of the right ventricle**. The second dilation is known as the **primitive ventricle** and becomes the left ventricle after it becomes trabeculated. The third dilation is the **primitive atrium** and becomes both the left and right atria. The last dilation is the

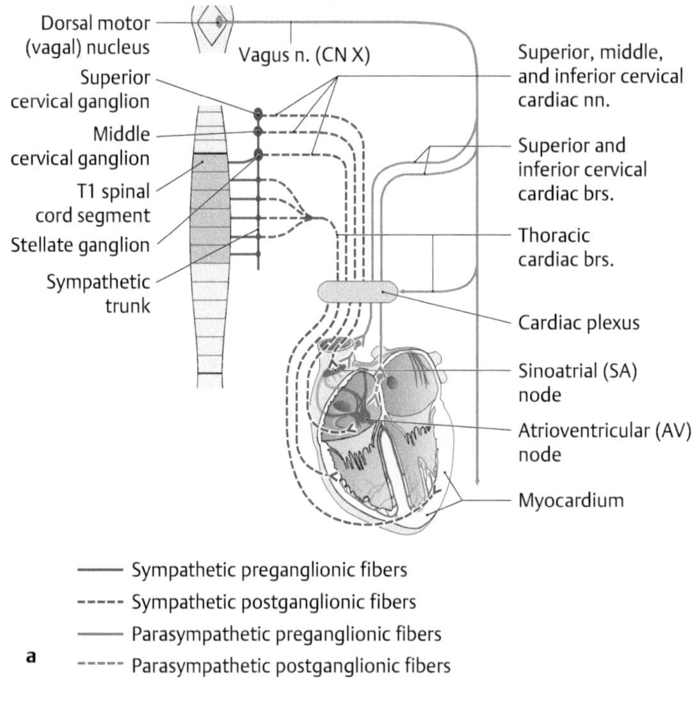

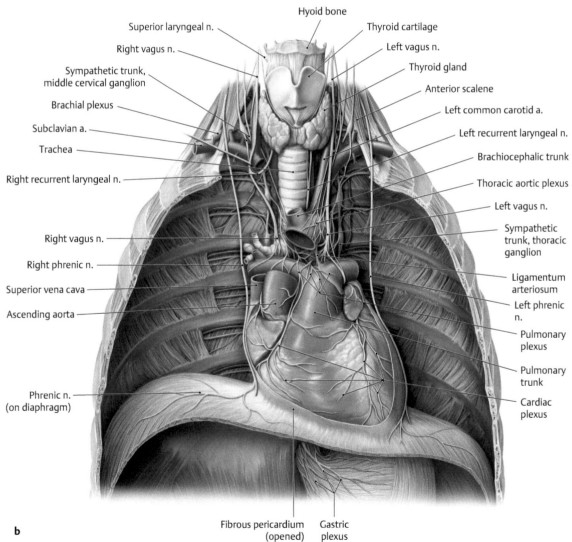

Hyoid bone
Superior laryngeal n.
Thyroid cartilage
Right vagus n.
Left vagus n.
Sympathetic trunk, middle cervical ganglion
Thyroid gland
Anterior scalene
Brachial plexus
Left common carotid a.
Subclavian a.
Left recurrent laryngeal n.
Trachea
Brachiocephalic trunk
Right recurrent laryngeal n.
Thoracic aortic plexus
Left vagus n.
Right vagus n.
Sympathetic trunk, thoracic ganglion
Right phrenic n.
Ligamentum arteriosum
Superior vena cava
Left phrenic n.
Ascending aorta
Pulmonary plexus
Pulmonary trunk
Phrenic n. (on diaphragm)
Cardiac plexus
b
Fibrous pericardium (opened)
Gastric plexus

Fig. 2.53 (a) Schematic of the autonomic innervation of the heart. **(b)** Autonomic nerves of the heart, anterior view. (From Schuenke M, Schulte E, Schumacher U. THIEME Atlas of Anatomy. Internal Organs. Illustrations by Voll M and Wesker K. 3rd ed. New York: Thieme Medical Publishers; 2020.)

Clinical Correlate 2.30

Electrocardiogram

An **electrocardiogram** (ECG or EKG) is a noninvasive interpretation of the electrical activity of the heart over a period of time. Ten electrodes are attached to the surface of the skin and an external device displays the recorded activity. The electrical impulses recorded by the ECG are generated by the polarization and depolarization of cardiac tissue and are displayed by waves. These waves can be used to measure the rate and regularity of heartbeats, the presence of any heart damage, the size and position of the chambers, and the effects of devices (i.e., pacemaker) or drugs used to regulate the heart. It may also give information regarding the balance of electrolytes in the blood or reveal problems with sodium channels within the heart muscle cells.

An ECG has multiple waves, intervals and segments. The **P wave** represents *atrial depolarization*. The **PR interval** is the time from the beginning of the P wave to the beginning of the Q wave. The **QRS (waves) complex** represents *ventricular depolarization*. Atrial repolarization is not heard but is “lost” within the QRS complex. The **T wave** demonstrates *ventricular repolarization*. The **QT interval** is the time from the beginning of the Q wave until the end of the T wave and represents the entire period of depolarization and repolarization of the ventricles. The **ST segment** is the time from the end of the S wave until the beginning of the T wave and it represents the period when the ventricles are depolarized.

Name	Definition
P wave	Atrial depolarization (< 0.1 s)
Q, R, and S wave (the QRS complex)	Beginning of ventricular excitation (< 0,1 s)
T wave	End of ventricular excitation
PQ interval	Onset of atrial excitation until the onset of ventricular excitation = conduction time = 0.1–0.2 s
QT interval	Q spike until the end of the T wave = time needed for both ventricles for de- and repolarization = 0.32–0.39 s. Varies based on the heart rate of the individual
Cardiac cycle	Interval between two R spikes
Heart rate	60 s/distance between R spikes (s) = beats/minute; e.g., 60/0.8 = 75

a

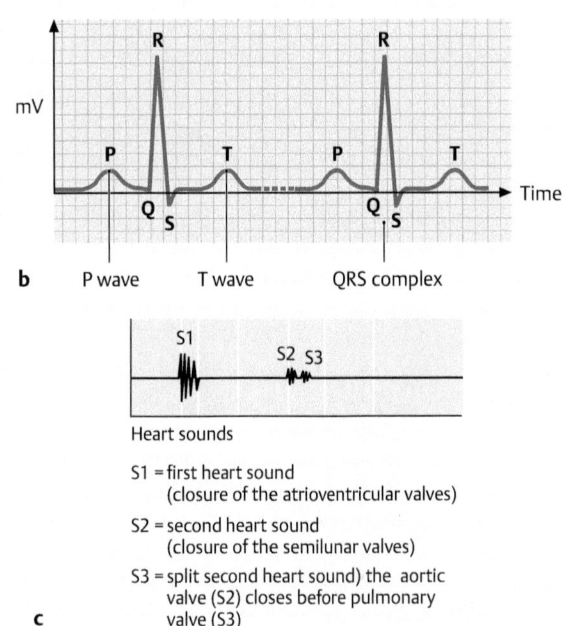

(a) Names and definitions of waves, spikes, and intervals in the ECG. **(b)** ECG curve: excitation cycle (recording of two heartbeats). **(c)** Heart sounds in relation to the ECG. (From Schuenke M, Schulte E, Schumacher U. THIEME Atlas of Anatomy. Internal Organs. Illustrations by Voll M and Wesker K. 2nd ed. New York: Thieme Medical Publishers; 2016.)

sinus venosus, which receives blood from the left and right sinus horns that consequently receive blood from the common cardinal, umbilical and vitelline veins. The sinus venosus does not contribute to any adult heart structure (**Fig. 2.56**).

2.15.3 Cardiac Looping

The heart begins to beat at day 22 of development, but these contractions are likened to peristalsis. Just a day later, the heart tube and its dilations must undergo cardiac (dextral) looping. The heart tube continues to elongate and is forced into looping due to the addition of these cells originating from the SHF, a process regulated by neural crest cells. Lengthening of the heart tube is considered essential for the looping process and normal formation of the outflow tract region and right ventricle.

Cardiac looping begins at day 23 of development. The cranial portion of the tube bends ventrally, caudally and to the right. The caudal portion of the tube bends dorsally, cranially and to the left. Cardiac looping is complete by day 28 (**Fig. 2.56**).

2.15.4 Chamber Formation and Septation

The **interatrial septum** that creates a separation between the left and right atria is formed by the combination of two embryonic septa. These are the septum primum and the septum secundum. The **septum primum** grows near the midsagittal plane as a crescent-shaped structure toward the atrioventricular canal. This septum separates the two atria, except for a temporary space at the inferior edge of the septum primum near the atrioventricular cushions called the **foramen primum**. Before the septum primum is able to completely close, apoptosis at the center of the septum primum (near the superior edge) begins to form a second opening, the **foramen secundum**. This foramen provides an alternate right-to-left shunt (**Fig. 2.57**).

Clinical Correlate 2.31

Artificial Cardiac Pacemaker

An **artificial pacemaker** is a small device that is put just underneath the skin of the chest to help the heart pump blood more efficiently. It uses small electrical currents to stimulate the heart muscle and will not be rejected by the body. Pacemakers contain a pulse generator with one or more leads. The pulse generator is a tiny computer powered by a battery that lasts many years. The leads connect the pulse generator to the inner wall of the heart (occasionally the outer wall). Each lead consists of a metal coil covered by a soft plastic insulating material with small metal electrodes. There are three types of artificial pacemakers:

- *Single chamber pacemakers*: set the pace of only one heart chamber (generally the left ventricle) and have just one lead.
- *Dual chamber pacemakers*: set the pace of two heart chambers and have two leads. These are more sophisticated and use information about the atrial electrical activity to set the pumping rate for the ventricles. Dual chamber pacemakers are ideal if an individual has heart block (electrical signals are slow or disrupted).
- *Biventricular pacemakers*: use three leads, one in the right atrium and one in each ventricle. These are a newer type of pacemaker and are more complex.

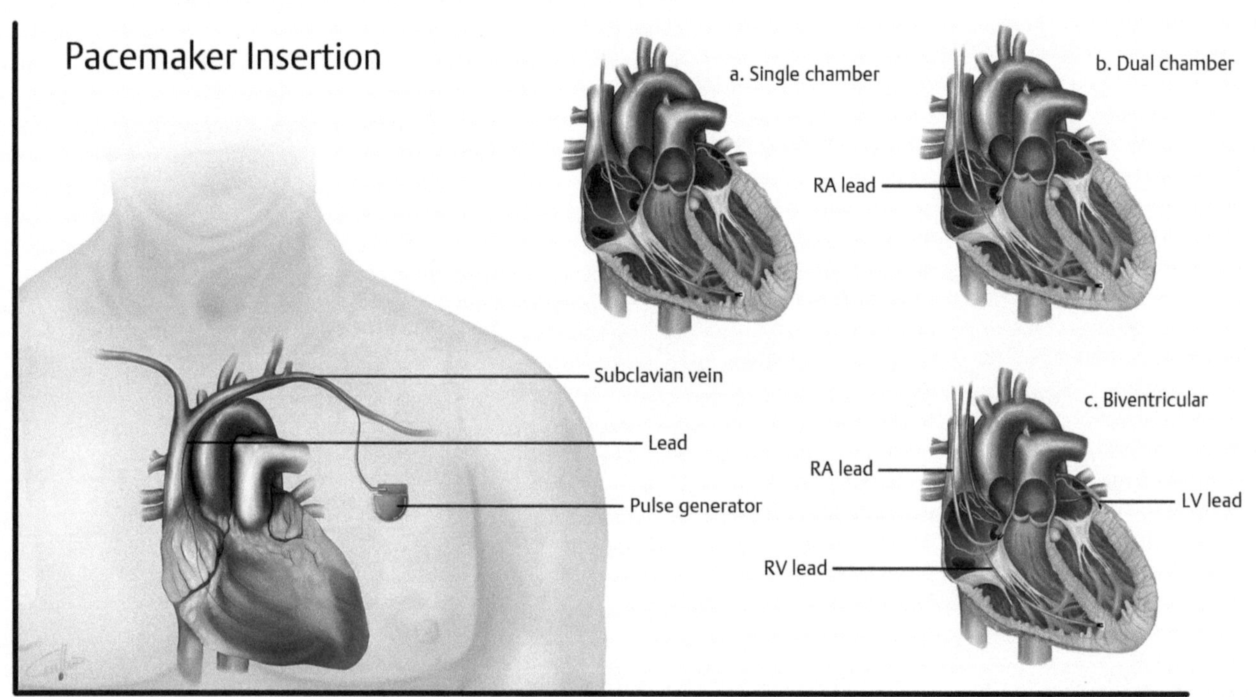

(a) Names and definitions of waves, spikes, and intervals in the ECG. **(b)** ECG curve: excitation cycle (recording of two heartbeats). **(c)** Heart sounds in relation to the ECG. Illustration by Calla Heald.

Clinical Correlate 2.32

Fibrillation of the Heart

Fibrillation is defined as the irregular rapid, unsynchronized contractions of the atrial or ventricular cardiac muscle. **Atrial fibrillation** is the most common type of cardiac arrhythmia and can be confirmed with the absence of the P wave in an ECG. Normal atrial contractions are replaced with irregular and rapid contractions from different locations within the atria and hence compete to stimulate the AV node. The risk of stroke increases if an individual has atrial fibrillation. Anticoagulants along with medications to restore normal heart rhythm may be prescribed.

Ventricular fibrillation is a sudden and lethal arrhythmia where normal ventricular contractions are replaced with irregular and rapid contractions that are not efficient to pump any blood. Ventricular fibrillation is an emergency situation and requires immediate medical attention. Patients who are at high risk of ventricular fibrillation may have an implantable cardioverter defibrillator (ICD) implanted that delivers a high-energy electrical pulse to correct dangerous arrhythmias. A pacemaker is implanted in a similar fashion but only delivers a low-energy electrical pulse.

Clinical Correlate 2.33

Cardiopulmonary Resuscitation (CPR)

Cardiopulmonary resuscitation (CPR) is performed in an emergency situation on a person who is in cardiac arrest with the objective to restore cardiac output and pulmonary ventilation. CPR is generally not enough to restart the heart but delays tissue death until an electric shock from a defibrillator can be used to restore a heart rhythm. Defibrillation provides a therapeutic dose of electrical energy to help establish normal contraction rhythms in the heart. CPR involves firm pressure being applied over multiple compressions (or "pumps") of the thorax over the inferior portion of the sternal body or center of the chest. Giving breaths in between the sets of multiple pumps provides artificial respiration consisting of approximately 16% oxygen. CPR is generally continued until there is a return of spontaneous circulation or a person is declared deceased.

Clinical Correlate 2.34

Referred Pain of the Heart

The heart is a visceral organ so it is insensitive to heat, cold and touch but ischemia can stimulate visceral pain sensory endings in the myocardium. Visceral afferent fibers travel back through the cardiopulmonary splanchnic (cervical cardiac) nerves and especially through the thoracic cardiac branches of the sympathetic trunk. The axons of these visceral afferent fibers generally enter the left T1-T5/T6 spinal segments. The phenomenon known as referred pain is when a person perceives pain in a superficial part of the body. Cardiac pain (angina) is referred in most individuals from the regions of the sternum, left pectoral and the medial portion of the left upper limb. Other areas of referred pain may include the left neck, left epigastric and the mid-back regions.

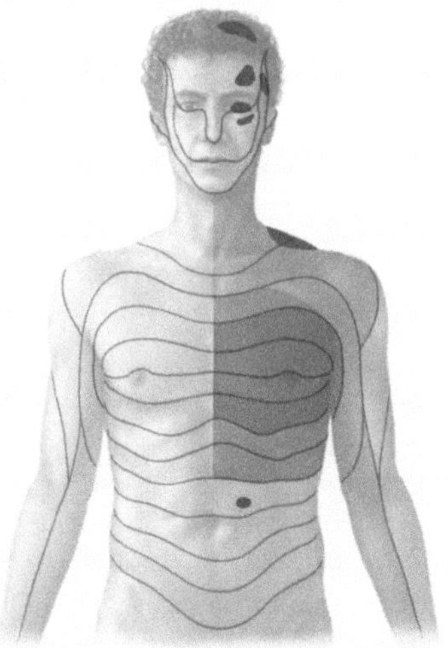

(From Schuenke M, Schulte E, Schumacher U. THIEME Atlas of Anatomy. Internal Organs. Illustrations by Voll M and Wesker K. 2nd ed. New York: Thieme Medical Publishers; 2016.)

During this process and after the incorporation of the right sinus horn, a second crescent-shaped septum known as the **septum secundum** begins to grow down from the roof of the right atrium just to right of the septum primum. This septum never forms a complete partition but permits the right-to-left shunt of blood through a space called the **oval foramen** (*foramen ovale*). The septum secundum eventually fuses inferiorly, but the oval foramen remains patent. Essentially, fetal blood is shunted from the right atrium to the left atrium through two staggered openings, the foramen ovale and the foramen secundum. After birth, when pulmonary circulation increases blood pressure in the left atrium, the septum primum is pressed against the septum secundum and becomes the **valve of the oval foramen** and this closure creates the **oval fossa** (*fossa ovalis*) (**Fig. 2.57**).

The primitive right atrium is pushed anteriorly and to the right, eventually becoming the right auricle. This portion of the atrial wall and the right auricle are lined with trabeculated pectinate muscle. The smooth portion of the right atrium or **sinus venarum** is derived from the **right sinus horn** that was originally connected to the sinus venosus, a structure that represents nothing seen in the adult. The *crista terminalis* (internally) and the *sulcus terminalis* (externally) delineate the smooth from the pectinate (rough) lined right atrium.

The primitive left atrium sprouts a single primitive pulmonary vein that promptly bifurcates into a left and right pulmonary vein and this is followed by another bifurcation resulting in a total of two left and right pulmonary veins that grow toward the developing lungs. The smooth walled portion of the left atrium is formed by the invagination of the primitive pulmonary vein and its main tributaries leaving behind four smaller pulmonary veins. The trabeculated left side of the primitive atrium is pushed anteriorly and to the left and is lined with pectinate muscle.

Endocardial cushions (or swellings) are masses of tissue involved in the formation of a septum by active growth that eventually reaches the opposite side. Neural crest cells contribute to the endocardial cushion formation. Cushions develop in the atrioventricular and OFT regions and assist in the formation of the *atrioventricular canals and valves, aorta (ascending) and pulmonary trunk*, and finally the *membranous portions of the atrial and ventricular septa*.

By the end of the 4th week of development, endocardial cushions form on the anterior and posterior walls of the common **atrioventricular (AV) canal**. The *anterior* and *posterior cushions* then migrate towards each other and eventually fuse forming and **AV septum** and an individual **left and right AV canal**. There are two *lateral cushions* located on the left and right borders of the canal (**Fig. 2.58**).

During the 5th week of development, a **left inferior** and **right superior truncus ridge/cushions** appear on the internal wall of the truncus arteriosus. The left cushion grows cranially and to the right while the right cushion also grows cranially but to the left. This leads to the development of the **aorticopulmonary septum** that divides the truncus arteriosus into the aorta (ascending portion) and pulmonary trunk. This spiraling motion the aorticopulmonary septum undertakes results in the pulmonary trunk lying anterior to the ascending portion of the aorta (**Fig. 2.59**).

The conus cordis has a **left** and **right cushion** that appears when the truncus arteriosus cushions develop. Both cushions move toward each other to form a conus septum while currently extending distally to meet and fuse with the aorticopulmonary septum of the truncus arteriosus. With fusion of the conus septum and aorticopulmonary septum, this will connect the left ventricular OFT with the ascending aorta and the right ventricular OFT with the pulmonary trunk (**Fig. 2.59**).

The primitive ventricles begin to expand near the end of the 4th week of development. The left ventricle is formed primarily from the primitive ventricle while the right ventricle is formed primarily from the inferior 1/3 of the bulbus cordis. The **muscular interventricular septum** begins to develop by the medial walls of the

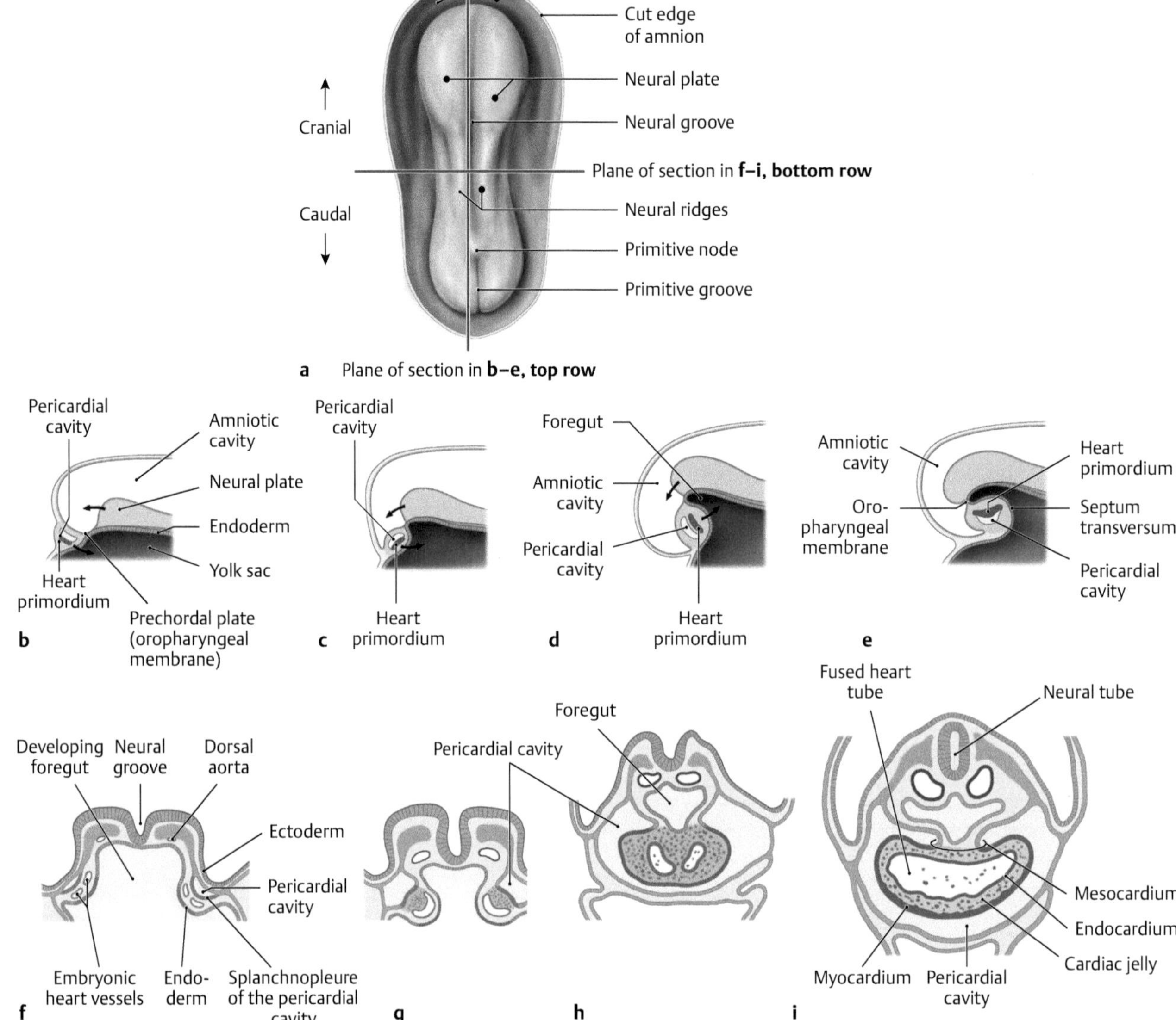

Fig. 2.54 Formation of the heart. **(a)** Origin of the cardiac tissue (cardiogenic area). **(b–e)** Sagittal sections. **(f–i)** Cross-sections (21-23 days/4-12 somites). Lateral **(b–e)** and rostral **(f–i)** views. For location of the respective plane of section see **a.** (From Schuenke M, Schulte E, Schumacher U. THIEME Atlas of Anatomy. Internal Organs. Illustrations by Voll M and Wesker K. 2nd ed. New York: Thieme Medical Publishers; 2016.)

expanding ventricles gradually merging and extending superiorly from the ventricular floor between the presumptive right and left ventricles. This septum stops short of the AV septum, leaving a space called the **interventricular foramen**. The **membranous portion of the interventricular septum** is complete after the anterior AV cushion fuses with the complete conus septum of the former conus cordis region effectively sealing off the interventricular foramen (**Fig. 2.60**).

2.15.5 Atrioventricular Valves

After the formation of the left and right AV canals by the fusion of the AV endocardial cushions, the borders of the canals will be surrounded by proliferations of dense mesenchymal tissue. Blood flow passing by the ventricular surface of these proliferations hollows out and thins this tissue forming valves. Three valves (tricuspid) will form at the right atrioventricular canal while only two (bicuspid/mitral) valves form at the left AV canal.

The valves remain attached to the ventricular walls by muscular cords. The cords' muscular tissue degenerates and is replaced by dense connective tissue eventually becoming *tendinous cords*. Tendinous cords attach to valves consisting of dense connective tissue covered by endocardium. The tendinous cords attach to the outer ventricular walls by way of the *papillary muscles* (**Fig. 2.60**).

2.15.6 Semilunar Valves

Before the truncus arteriosus completes its septation, additional but smaller swellings (tubercles) appear on the larger main truncus swellings. There will be one assigned to either the aortic or pulmonary trunk. A third tubercle will appear in both channels opposite the fused truncus swellings. From the 6-8th weeks of development, these tubercles will hollow out on their superior surface and form defined semilunar valves. Neural crest cells have been shown to contribute to the formation of these valves.

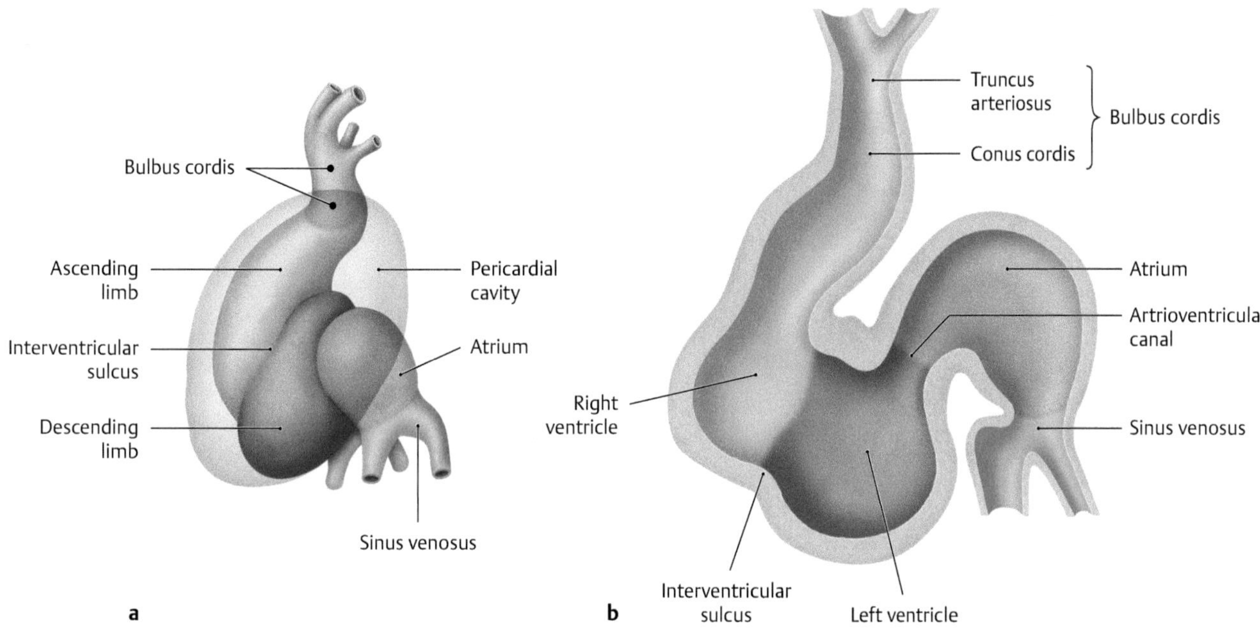

Fig. 2.55 Formation of the heart tube. **(a)** Cardiac loop, left lateral view. **(b)** Sagittal section of the cardiac loop. By the end of the 3rd or beginning of the 4th week, the precursors of the definitive parts of the heart are clearly visible. (From Schuenke M, Schulte E, Schumacher U. THIEME Atlas of Anatomy. Internal Organs. Illustrations by Voll M and Wesker K. 2nd ed. New York: Thieme Medical Publishers; 2016.)

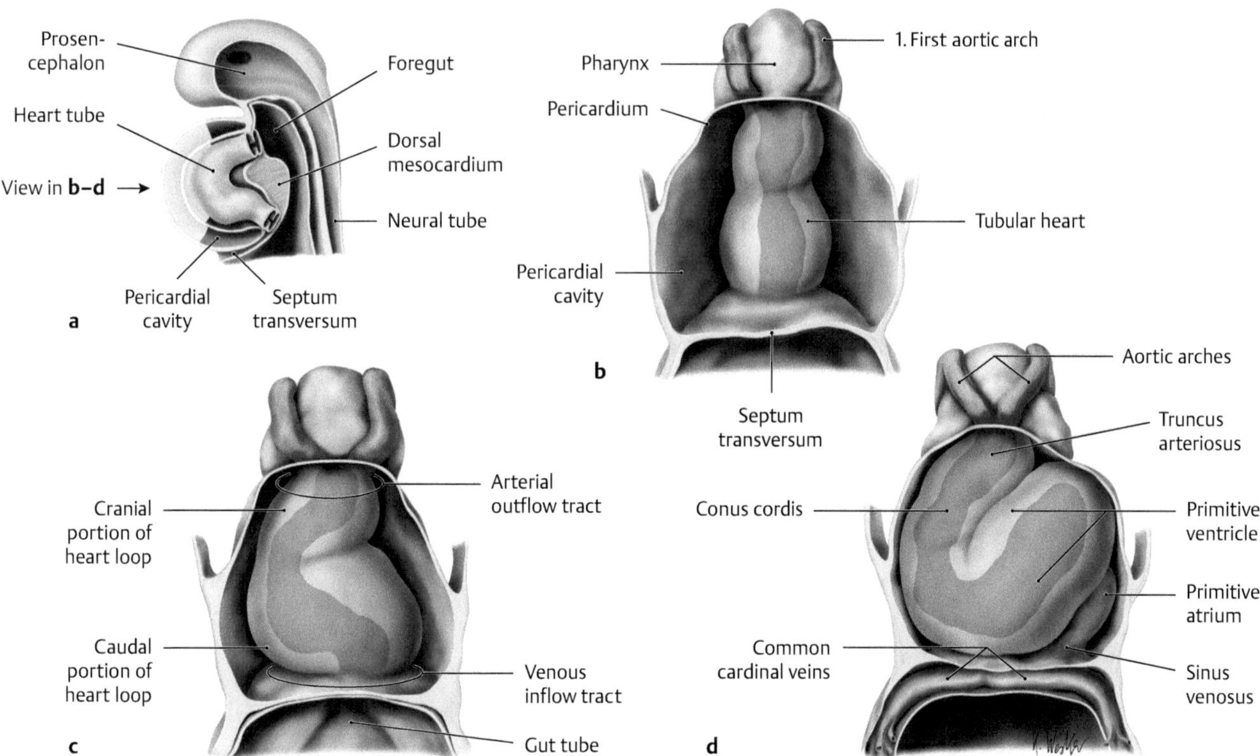

Fig. 2.56 Formation of the cardiac loop. **(a)** Left lateral view. **(b–d)** Anterior view (with the pericardial cavity opened). (From Schuenke M, Schulte E, Schumacher U. THIEME Atlas of Anatomy. Internal Organs. Illustrations by Voll M and Wesker K. 2nd ed. New York: Thieme Medical Publishers; 2016.)

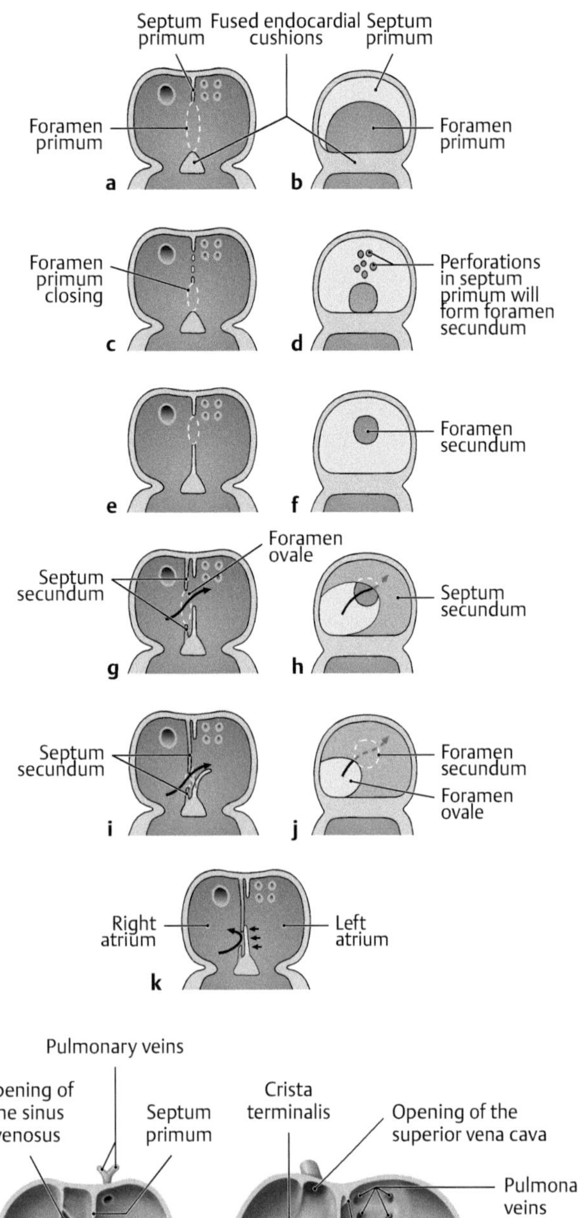

Fig. 2.57 Formation of the atrial septum. **(a,c,e,g,i,k)** Frontal sections, ventral view. **(b,d,f,h,j)** Sagittal sections, viewed from the right side. **(l)** Transformation of the atria. (From Schuenke M, Schulte E, Schumacher U. THIEME Atlas of Anatomy. Internal Organs. Illustrations by Voll M and Wesker K. 2nd ed. New York: Thieme Medical Publishers; 2016.)

2.15.7 Conducting System

During the 5th week of development, cardiac myocytes within the sinus venosus of the early heart tube begin to undergo spontaneous electrical depolarizations that are at a faster rate than that of the cardiac myocytes anywhere else. During the process of cardiac looping, these isolated and faster-rate depolarizing cells cardiomyocytes become the SA node and AV node. The AV node will become the only pathway for depolarizations after the formation of the fibrous skeleton. The AV bundle will develop from a ring-like cluster of cells found at the AV junction while Purkinje fibers develop from currently contractile cardiomyocytes within the myocardium.

2.16 Prenatal and Postnatal Circulation

Before birth, the blood that originates from the placenta and passes to the fetus by way of the one remaining **umbilical vein** has an O_2 saturation of 80%. As blood courses through the fetus, there are five particular areas where mixing of different O_2 saturated blood mixes, those are the (1) liver, (2) IVC, (3) right atrium, (4) left atrium and the (5) descending aorta near the site of the ductus arteriosus (**Fig. 2.61**).

As much as 50% of the blood originating from the umbilical vein bypasses the liver via the **ductus venosus** and enter the IVC. The remaining blood enters the **portal vein** and supplies the liver with oxygen and nutrients. The blood continues superiorly through the IVC before reaching the right atrium. This blood mixes with blood returning from the SVC and blood from the right atrium either passes through the **oval foramen** (*foramen ovale*) to enter the left atrium or continue into the right ventricle. The left atrium sends blood to the left ventricle where it is pumped into the ascending aorta before continuing through the arch of the aorta. The blood that was in the right ventricle is pumped through the pulmonary trunk and pulmonary arteries. Since there is not any gas exchange occurring in the lungs, this blood passes through the **ductus arteriosus** where it mixes with the blood of the descending aorta. Blood continuing through the descending aorta eventually passes back through the two **umbilical arteries** and returns blood that has circulated through the fetus back to the placenta. The O_2 saturation of this particular blood is approximately 58%.

After birth, the closure of the *oval foramen* is caused by an increase in the pressure of the left atrium, combined with decreased pressure in the right atrium. The first breath presses the septum primum against the septum secundum and it may take up to one year to completely close this foramen now known as the **oval fossa** (*fossa ovalis*). Up to as many as 20% of the population may still have a **patent foramen ovale** as adults. Closure of the *ductus arteriosus* is accomplished by contraction of the smooth muscles in its walls and this occurs almost immediately after birth. It is mediated by *bradykinin*, which originates from the lungs during the initial inflation of them. It can take 1-3 months to become obliterated but it is now known as the **ligamentum arteriosum**. Failure of the ductus arteriosus to close is known as patent ductus arteriosus (PDA). This is frequently seen in premature infants and is the result of increased backflow of aortic blood into the pulmonary trunk, which leads to volume overload on the pulmonary circulation.

When the infant is being separated from the placenta during delivery, closure of the *umbilical arteries* occur and these become the **medial umbilical ligaments**. The most proximal portion remains patent and is involved in some blood supply in the pelvis. Closure of the *umbilical vein* and *ductus venosus* occurs just after the umbilical arteries and they become the **round ligament of the liver (ligamentum teres)** and the **ligamentum venosum** respectively.

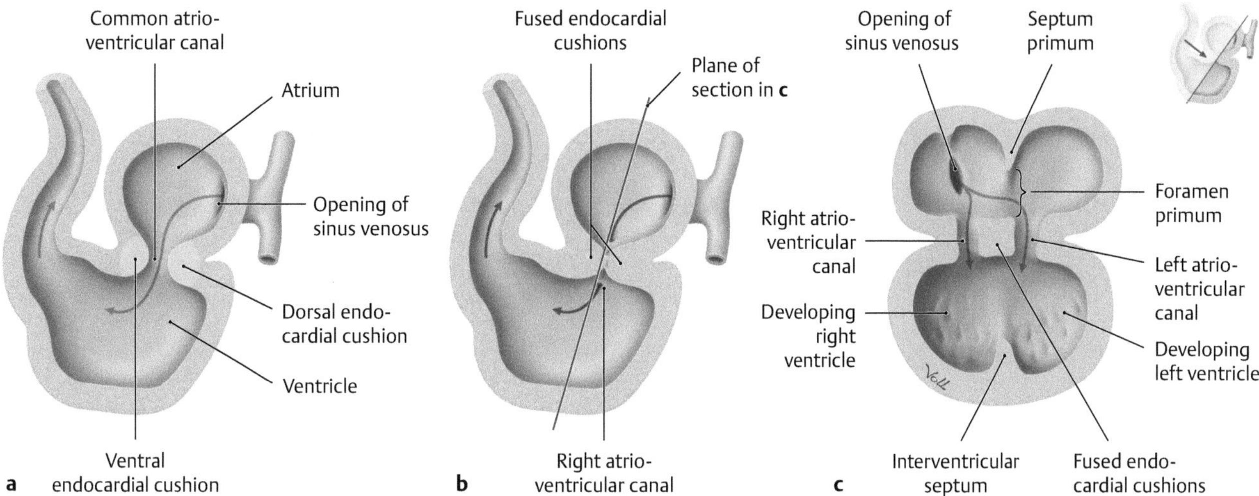

Fig. 2.58 Formation of the atrioventricular septum and canals. **(a,b)** Sagittal section of the cardiac loop. **(c)** Anterior view at the level of the endocardial cushions (for plane of section see **b**). (From Schuenke M, Schulte E, Schumacher U. THIEME Atlas of Anatomy. Internal Organs. Illustrations by Voll M and Wesker K. 2nd ed. New York: Thieme Medical Publishers; 2016.)

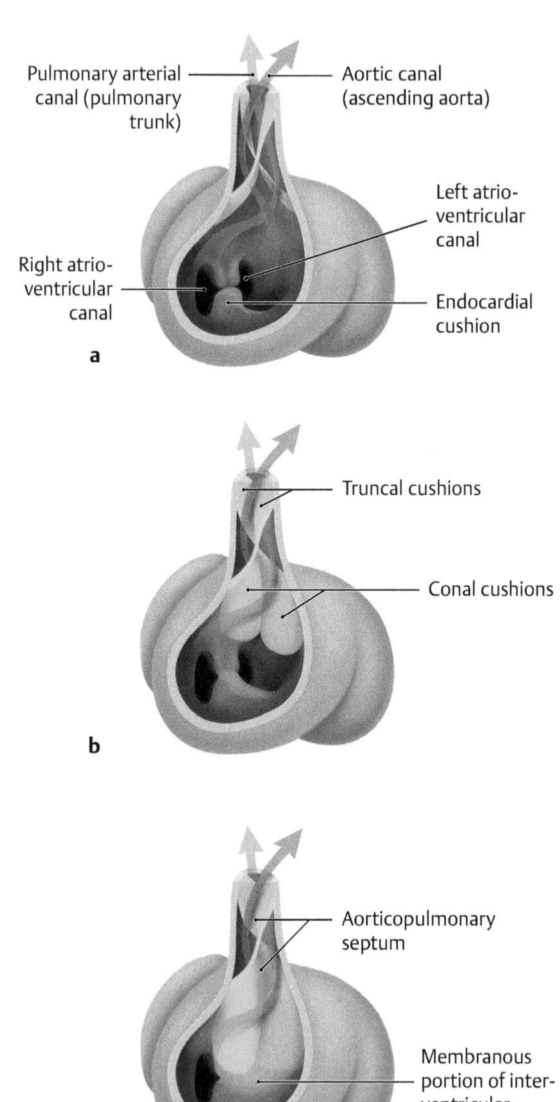

Fig. 2.59 (a–c) Septation of the outflow tract. (From Schuenke M, Schulte E, Schumacher U. THIEME Atlas of Anatomy. Internal Organs. Illustrations by Voll M and Wesker K. 2nd ed. New York: Thieme Medical Publishers; 2016.)

2.17 Posterior Mediastinum

The **posterior mediastinum** is located inferior to the transverse thoracic plane, posterior to the pericardium but anterior to the T5-T12 thoracic vertebrae and in between the parietal pleura of both lungs (**Fig. 2.62**). Structures located within the posterior mediastinum include:

- Thoracic aorta.
- Azygos, accessory hemiazygos and hemiazygos veins.
- Esophagus and esophageal (visceral) nerve plexus.
- Thoracic duct.
- Posterior mediastinal lymph nodes.
- Sympathetic trunk and splanchnic nerves.

The **thoracic aorta** is the continuation of the arch of the aorta and begins on the left side of the inferior border of the T4 vertebral body (**Fig. 2.63**). It will descend along the left borders of the upper eight thoracic vertebrae before reaching the aortic hiatus of the diaphragm at vertebral level T12. At this point the thoracic aorta continues as the abdominal aorta. The azygos vein and thoracic duct also pass through the aortic hiatus. Within this mediastinum, the thoracic aorta will be located posterior to the root of the left lung, esophagus and pericardium. A lesser-defined visceral nerve plexus known as the **thoracic aortic plexus** is found wrapped around this portion of the aorta.

The larger descending aorta that includes both the thoracic and abdominal aortas displays arterial branches coursing through one of three vascular planes and they are described as such:

- (1) anterior/midline plane with unpaired visceral branches.
- (2) lateral plane with paired visceral branches.
- (3) posterolateral plane with paired parietal branches.

In the thorax, the planes are represented by these arteries:

- (1) anterior/midline plane: 2-5 **esophageal arteries.**
- (2) lateral plane: **bronchial arteries.**
- (3) posterolateral plane: 9 lower **posterior intercostal** and **subcostal arteries**. Exceptions to this pattern include the paired **superior phrenic arteries** that course anterolaterally and the unpaired **pericardial** and **mediastinal arteries** that course anteriorly.

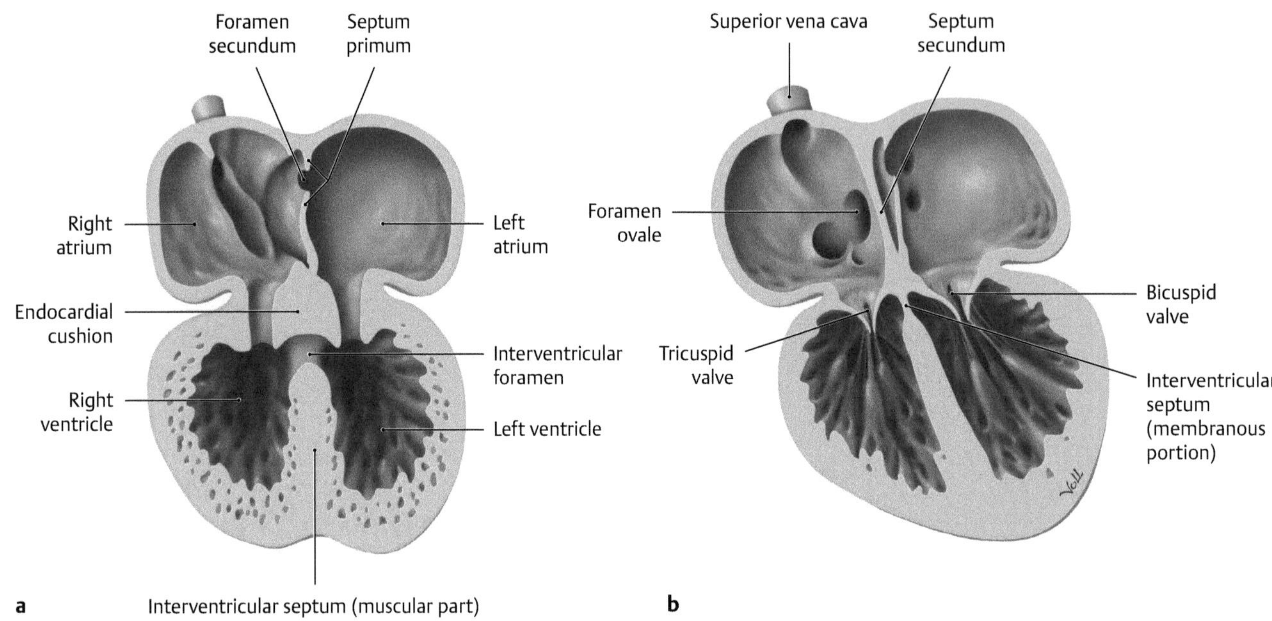

Fig. 2.60 Ventricular septation. **(a)** The medial walls of the expanding ventricles will become apposed and gradually merge, forming the muscular interventricular septum. **(b)** Complete closure of the interventricular foramen forms the membranous portion of the interventricular septum. (From Schuenke M, Schulte E, Schumacher U. THIEME Atlas of Anatomy. Internal Organs. Illustrations by Voll M and Wesker K. 2nd ed. New York: Thieme Medical Publishers; 2016.)

Clinical Correlate 2.35

Septal Defects

Atrial septal defects (ASD) are congenital and located within the interatrial septum. ASDs are usually due to an incomplete closure of the oval foramen (*foramen ovale*). They allow oxygenated blood to pass from the left to the right atrium. Large shunts cause hypertrophy of the right atrium and ventricle as well as the pulmonary trunk.

Ventricular septal defects (VSD) are the most common of all cardiac defects and account for about 25% of all congenital heart defects. They are described mostly as the failure of the membranous portion of the interventricular septum to develop. Defects within the muscular portion of the interventricular septum are less common and tend to close naturally on their own during childhood. The size of the defect varies considerably and can be as big as 25 mm. VSD's cause a left-to-right ventricular shunting of blood with the larger defects increasing pulmonary blood flow leading to pulmonary hypertension.

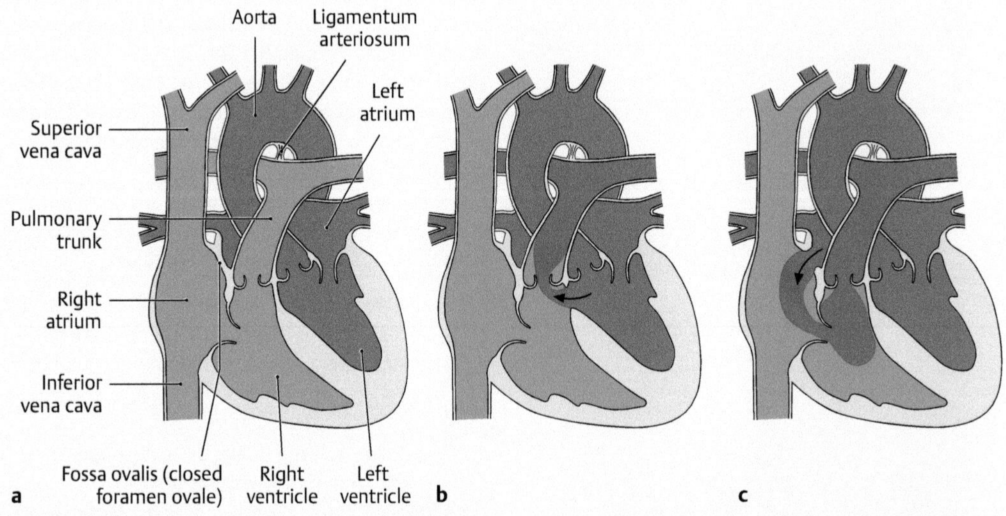

Congenital heart defects. **(a)** Normal postnatal heart. **(b)** Ventricular septal defect (VSD). **(c)** Atrial septal defect (ASD). (From Schuenke M, Schulte E, Schumacher U. THIEME Atlas of Anatomy. Internal Organs. Illustrations by Voll M and Wesker K. 2nd ed. New York: Thieme Medical Publishers; 2016.)

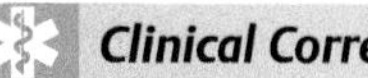

Clinical Correlate 2.36

Tetralogy of Fallot

Tetralogy of Fallot (~1/1,000 live births) is the most common of all conotruncal region abnormalities. It is due to the unequal division of the conus resulting from the anterior displacement of the larger conotruncal (conus cordis and truncus arteriosus) septum. This produces four alterations to the heart: (1) overriding aorta; (2) pulmonary stenosis; (3) interventricular septal defect; and (4) right ventricular hypertrophy.

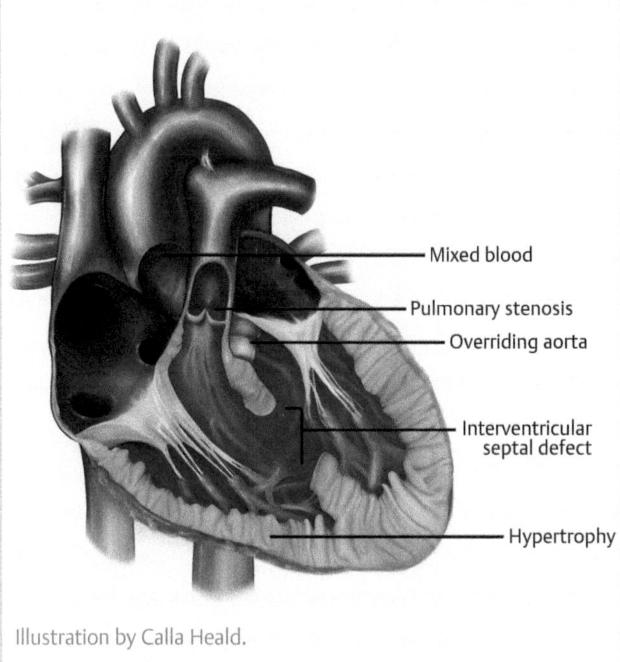

Illustration by Calla Heald.

Clinical Correlate 2.37

Persistent Truncus Arteriosus

Persistent truncus arteriosus (~1/10,000 live births) is the result of the conotruncal cushions failing to form and thus not forming a divided outflow tract. The pulmonary trunk is forced to originate above the origin of the undivided truncus region. The undivided truncus will override both ventricles and receive blood from both. An interventricular septal defect is always present because the cushions that normally contribute to development of the interventricular septum are not present.

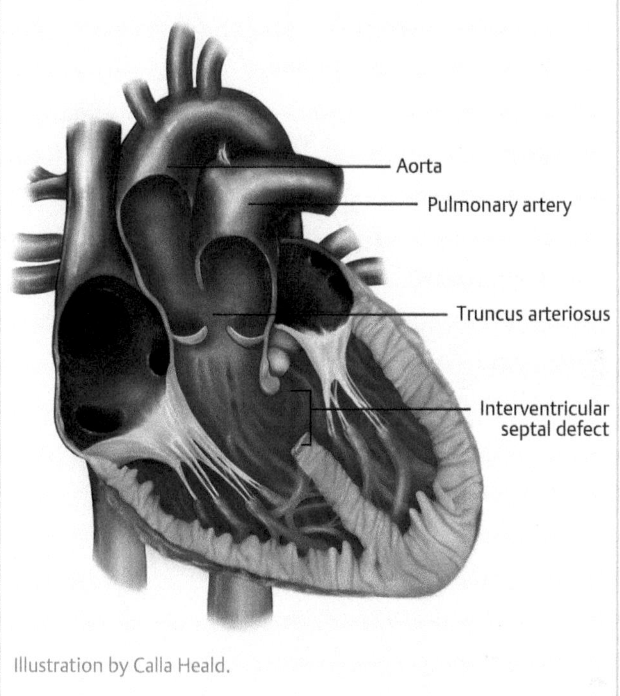

Illustration by Calla Heald.

The *azygos system of veins* was briefly described with the venous drainage of the thoracic wall. This system is located on each side of the vertebral column and is responsible for draining blood originating from the back, vertebral canal, mediastinal viscera and the thoracoabdominal walls. This system includes the azygos, accessory hemiazygos and hemiazygos veins and it must be noted that it is highly variable. The azygos and hemiazygos veins originate in a large part from the **ascending lumbar veins** but also from smaller root tributaries that come from the IVC and/or renal veins.

The **azygos vein** will form a collateral pathway between the SVC and IVC and receives blood directly from the lower right 8 posterior intercostals and subcostal vein (**Fig. 2.64**). The hemiazygos and accessory hemiazygos veins after receiving blood from most of the left posterior intercostals and subcostal vein will also drain into the larger azygos vein. The azygos vein passes superiorly near the right sides of the lower 7-8 thoracic vertebrae before arching over the root of the right lung and draining into the SVC. The right 1st posterior intercostal vein generally drains directly into the right brachiocephalic vein but the right 2nd and 3rd posterior intercostals drain into the **right superior intercostal vein** before reaching the azygos vein.

The **accessory hemiazygos** is located on the left side of the thoracic vertebrae and deep to the thoracic aorta. It receives blood from the left 5th-8th posterior intercostal veins and the **left superior intercostal vein** frequently drains into it. Recall that the left superior intercostal vein receives the left 2nd-4th posterior intercostals while the left 1st posterior intercostal vein generally drains directly into the left brachiocephalic vein. The accessory hemiazygos occasionally merges with the hemiazygos or it can drain straight to the azygos vein at approximately the level of the T7 or T8 vertebrae (**Fig. 2.64**).

The **hemiazygos vein** is located on the left side of the thoracic vertebrae and hidden by the thoracic aorta. It receives blood from the left 9th-11th posterior intercostals and subcostal vein before draining into the azygos vein. At approximately the T9 vertebra, the hemiazygos crosses over the anterior surface of this vertebra and drains into the azygos vein (**Fig. 2.64**).

The **esophagus** descends down from the superior mediastinum and into the posterior mediastinum where it will be anterior to the thoracic vertebrae and thoracic duct. The thoracic aorta is to the left while the azygos vein is to the right of it. The esophagus passes through the esophageal hiatus of the diaphragm at vertebral level T10. At T11 it will join the stomach within the abdomen. There are three main constrictions of the esophagus (**Fig. 2.65**):

- In the neck at vertebral level C6 due to the cricopharyngeus muscle.
- At approximately the vertebral level T4/T5 due to the combination of the arch of the aorta and left primary bronchus.
- At vertebral level T10 due to the diaphragm.

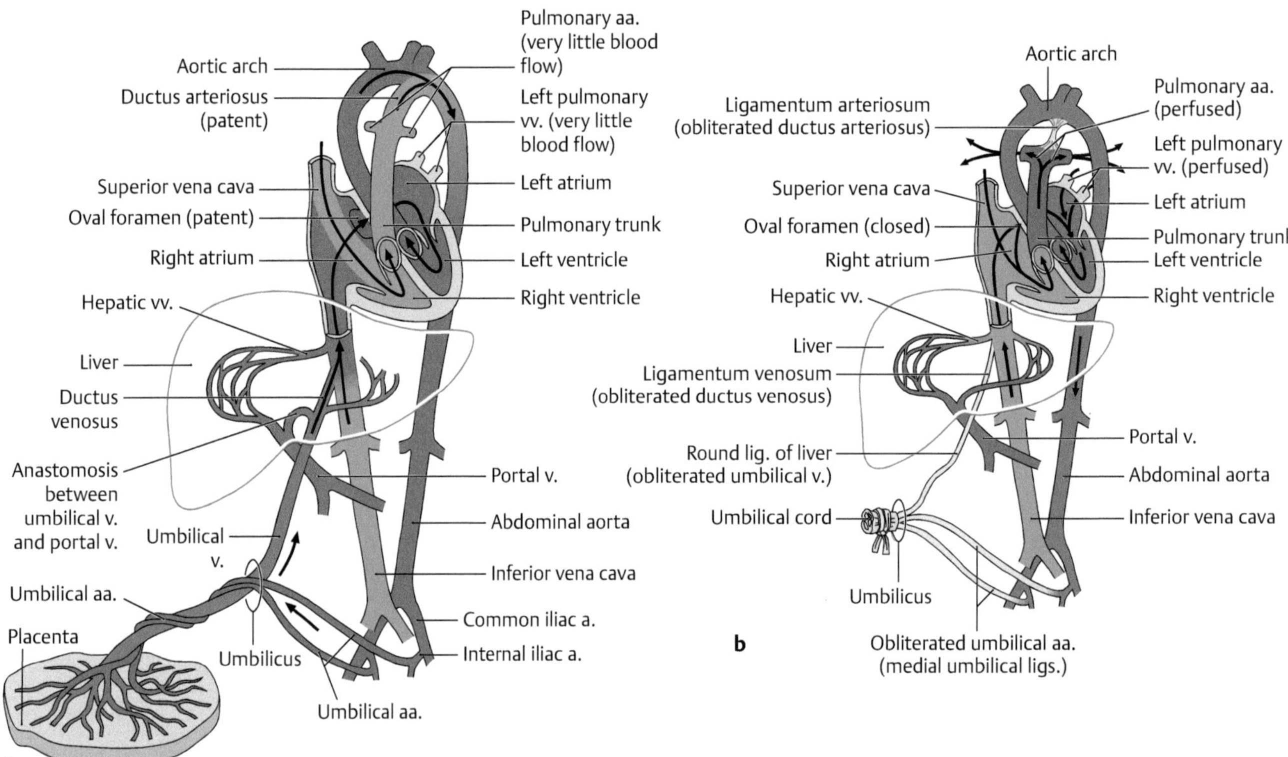

Fig. 2.61 (a) Prenatal circulation. **(b)** Postnatal circulation. (From Schuenke M, Schulte E, Schumacher U. THIEME Atlas of Anatomy. Internal Organs. Illustrations by Voll M and Wesker K. 3rd ed. New York: Thieme Medical Publishers; 2020.)

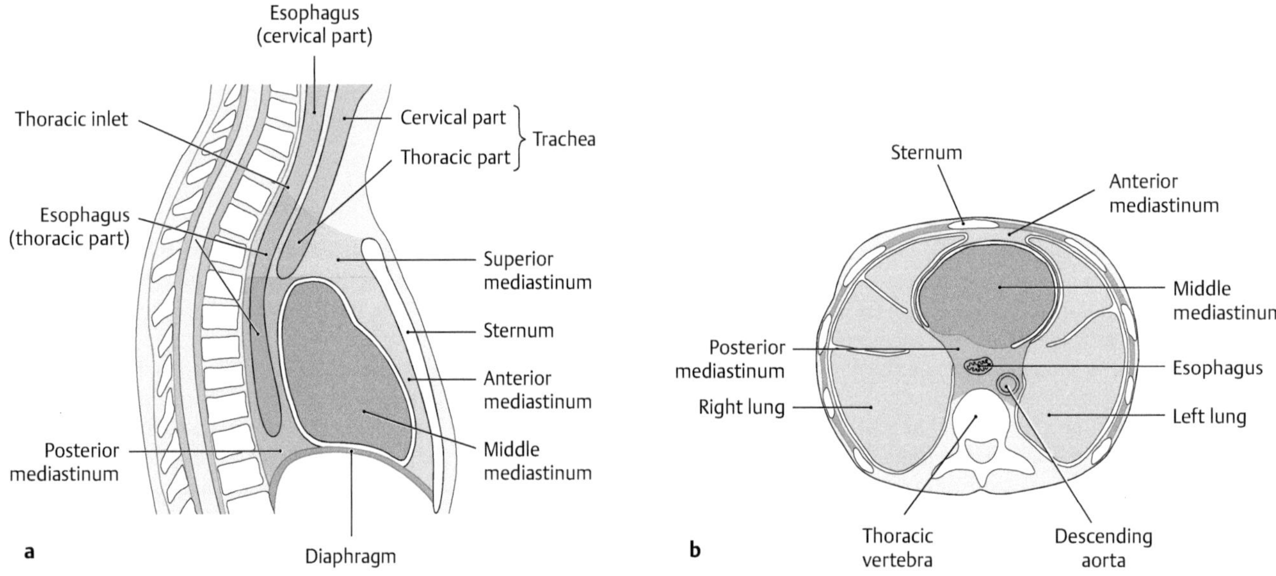

Fig. 2.62 Divisions of the mediastinum. **(a)** Lateral view. **(b)** Inferior view. (From Schuenke M, Schulte E, Schumacher U. THIEME Atlas of Anatomy. Internal Organs. Illustrations by Voll M and Wesker K. 3rd ed. New York: Thieme Medical Publishers; 2020.)

Most of the blood supply to this portion of the esophagus comes from the esophageal arteries with a minor amount from the bronchial arteries. The **esophageal nerve plexus** is a visceral nerve plexus that wraps around both the anterior and posterior aspects of the esophagus. It contains the functional components GVE-sym/post, GVE-para/pre, and GVA fibers. Sympathetics can act as blood vessel and sphincter constrictors while the parasympathetics increase motility (peristalsis), sphincter relaxation and mucosal glands secretions **(Fig. 2.66; Fig. 2.68)**.

The **thoracic duct** is the largest lymphatic channel in the body and it has many valves to prevent any backflow of lymph. It drains all the lymph from the body except for the right upper quadrant that is drained by the right lymphatic duct. Its long course first originates in the abdomen from the cisterna chyli before coursing through the posterior mediastinum between the azygos vein and thoracic aorta. It enters the superior mediastinum just left of the esophagus, and then terminates at the junction between the left internal jugular and subclavian veins or **left venous angle** found

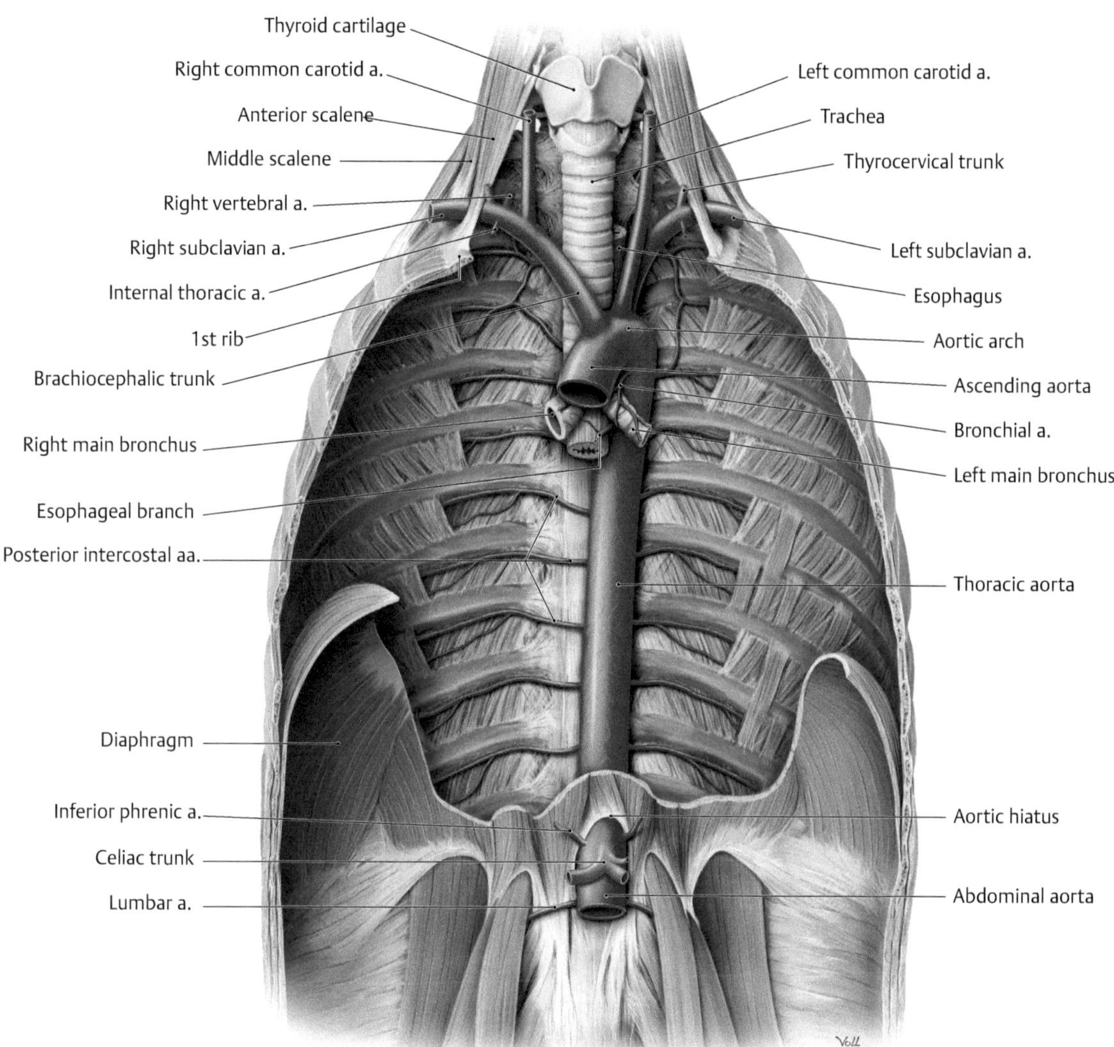

Fig. 2.63 Thoracic aorta. (From Schuenke M, Schulte E, Schumacher U. THIEME Atlas of Anatomy. Internal Organs. Illustrations by Voll M and Wesker K. 3rd ed. New York: Thieme Medical Publishers; 2020.)

near the lower neck. Near the termination, the *bronchomediastinal, jugular* and *subclavian lymphatic trunks* join the thoracic duct prior to it draining adjacent to the left venous angle. These additional lymphatic trunks do not always join the thoracic duct but instead terminate independently into nearby veins. The *collecting trunks* from intercostal spaces drain into the thoracic duct (**Fig. 2.67**).

The **posterior mediastinal lymph nodes** are located posterior to the pericardium and are closely associated with the esophagus and thoracic aorta. They consist of several nodes posterior to the inferior esophagus and up to eight more anterior and lateral to the esophagus. They receive lymph not only from the esophagus but from the diaphragm, posterior pericardium and mid-level posterior intercostal spaces. This lymph may pass superiorly through the bronchomediastinal trunks or the thoracic duct.

The **sympathetic trunks and ganglion** are located on the lateral walls of the entire vertebral column. Some may or may not consider the sympathetic trunk, its ganglion and the splanchnic nerves heading to the gut as part of the posterior mediastinum but here we will. The sympathetic trunk in the thoracic region is initially near the head of the ribs (upper portion), followed by the costovertebral joint (middle portion), and finally the vertebral bodies (lower portion). The **thoracic splanchnic nerves** known as the greater, lesser and least splanchnic nerves are responsible for innervating gut structures below the diaphragm and are all carrying autonomic sympathetic preganglionic (GVE-sym/pre) as well as visceral afferent (GVA) fibers. The splanchnic nerves will generally originate directly off of the sympathetic chain ganglion. Multiple contributions lead to the formation of a more defined splanchnic nerve before it passes through the crura region of the diaphragm to reach the abdomen (**Fig. 2.68**).

- **Greater splanchnic nerve** originates from the T5-T9 ganglions of the sympathetic trunk.
- **Lesser splanchnic nerve** originates from the T10-T11 ganglions of the sympathetic trunk.
- **Least splanchnic nerve** originates from the T12 ganglion of the sympathetic trunk.

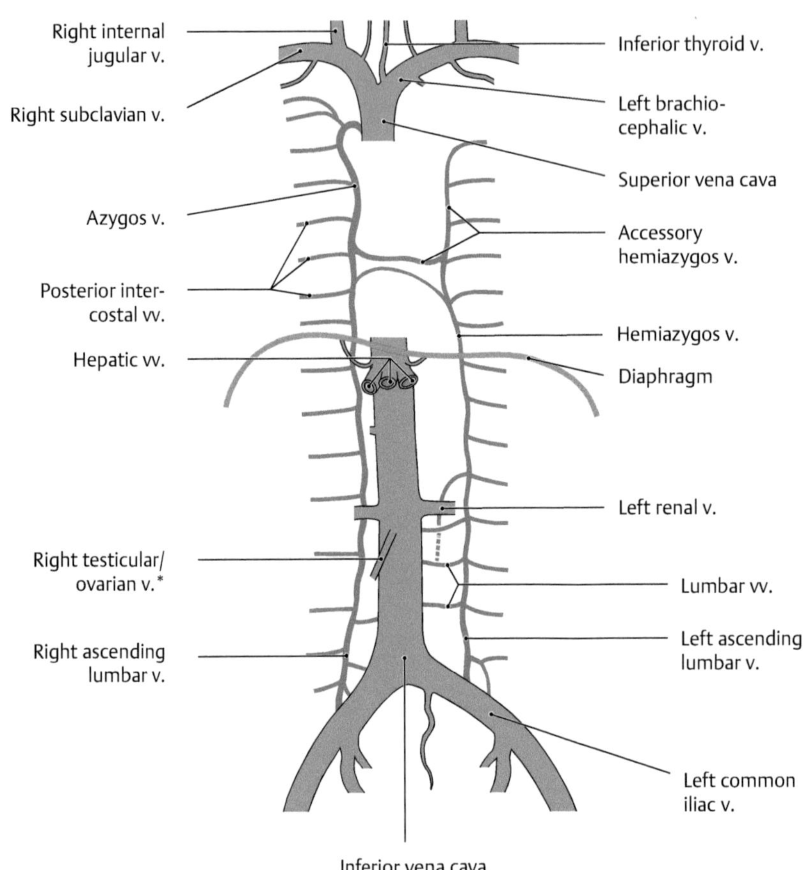

Fig. 2.64 Superior and inferior venae cavae, and the azygos system. (From Schuenke M, Schulte E, Schumacher U. THIEME Atlas of Anatomy. Internal Organs. Illustrations by Voll M and Wesker K. 3rd ed. New York: Thieme Medical Publishers; 2020.)

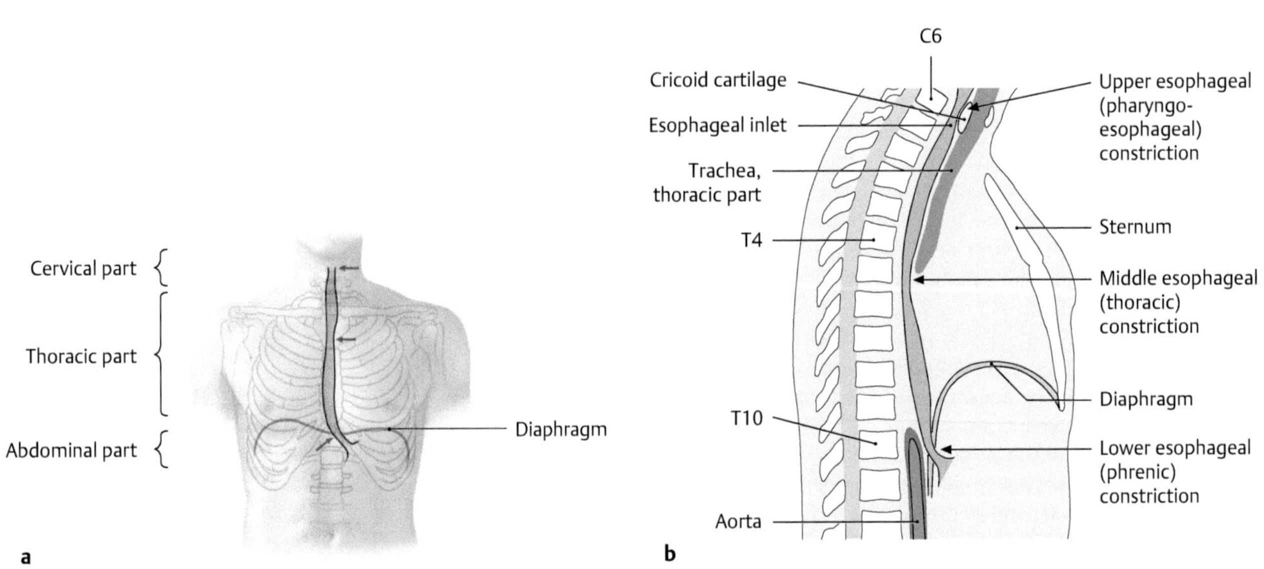

Fig. 2.65 (a) Projection of esophagus onto chest wall. Esophageal constrictions are indicated with arrows. **(b)** Esophageal constrictions, right lateral view. (From Schuenke M, Schulte E, Schumacher U. THIEME Atlas of Anatomy. Internal Organs. Illustrations by Voll M and Wesker K. 3rd ed. New York: Thieme Medical Publishers; 2020.)

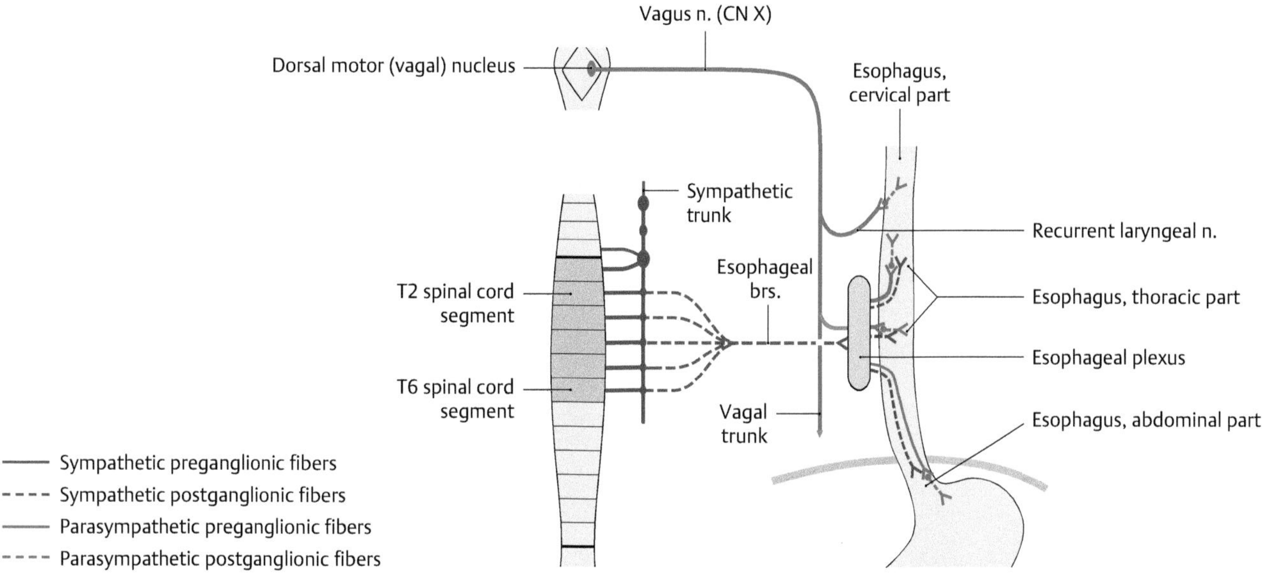

Fig. 2.66 Autonomic innervation of the esophagus. (From Schuenke M, Schulte E, Schumacher U. THIEME Atlas of Anatomy. Internal Organs. Illustrations by Voll M and Wesker K. 3rd ed. New York: Thieme Medical Publishers; 2020.)

- **Note**: there are on occasion only 11 thoracic sympathetic chain ganglion in which the lesser and least splanchnic nerves may act as a combined nerve.

2.18 Pulmonary Cavities

The majority of the thoracic cavity is occupied by the **left** and **right pulmonary cavities** which contain the lungs and pleurae (**Fig. 2.69**). The pulmonary cavities are separate from one another with the mediastinum between the two cavities. **Endothoracic fascia** is a thin fibroareolar layer located between the internal aspect of the thoracic cage and the lining of the parietal pleura of the pleural cavity. The innermost and internal intercostals, subcostal and transversus thoracis muscles are invested by this fascia. It will also blend in with the periosteum of the sternum and ribs as well as the perichondrium of the costal cartilages. The endothoracic fascia is important clinically because it provides a cleavage plane for a surgeon to separate the parietal pleura from the thoracic wall giving access to the intrathoracic structures.

2.19 Pleurae

Both lungs are invested by and enclosed in a serous pleural sac consisting of two continuous membranes much like the pericardial cavity surrounding the heart. There is a **parietal pleura** which lines the pulmonary cavities and is adjacent to the **endothoracic fascia** and a **visceral pleura** which invests all surfaces of the lungs including the oblique and horizontal fissures and forms their outer slippery surface. The parietal and visceral pleura are continuous with each other at the hilum of the lung. A potential space lies between the two pleural layers and is called the **pleural cavity.** The pleura are serous membranes and thus secrete a thin layer of serous fluid into the pleural cavity allowing the pleura to slide smoothly against each other during respiration. Surface tension allows the pleura to remain in contact with one another; however, if this surface contact is lost, a "collapsed lung" results (**Fig. 2.70**).

The **parietal pleura** lines the pulmonary cavities and thus adheres to the thoracic wall, diaphragm and mediastinum. The parietal pleura consists of four parts; the *cervical, costal, diaphragmatic* and *mediastinal* (**Fig. 2.71**).

- The **cervical part** extends through the superior thoracic aperture into the root of the neck about 2-3 cm superior to the medial 1/3 of the clavicle at the level of the first rib. It forms a cup-shaped dome (cupula) over the apex portion of the lung and is reinforced by the **suprapleural membrane (Sibson fascia)** which is an extension of the endothoracic fascia. It attaches to the internal border of the 1st rib and transverse process of the C7 vertebra. The cervical part is an extension of both the costal and mediastinal parietal pleura.
- The **costal part** covers the internal surfaces of the thoracic wall but is technically separated from the wall by endothoracic fascia.
- The **diaphragmatic part** covers the superior surface of the diaphragm on each side of the mediastinum except near its costal attachments and where the diaphragm is fused with the pericardium. The diaphragmatic part is connected to the muscular fibers of the diaphragm by another extension of endothoracic fascia known as the **phrenicopleural fascia**.
- The **mediastinal part** covers the lateral portion of the mediastinum and is a continuous sheet passing anteroposteriorly between the sternum and vertebral column superior to the root of the lung. It reflects laterally onto the root of the lung to become continuous with the visceral pleura at the hilum of the lung.

The parietal pleura abruptly changes direction as it reflects from one wall of the pleural cavity to the next. These are known as the **lines of pleural reflection** and there are five reference lines used to identify the inferior-most extent to which the parietal pleura can extend. These *reference lines* are known from anterior to posterior as the **sternal**, **midclavicular**, **midaxillary**, **scapular** and **paravertebral lines.** Refer to the images and table to understand the inferior-most aspect of the parietal pleura versus the inferior most part of the lungs while at rest at these same reference lines (**Fig. 2.72, Table 2.2**).

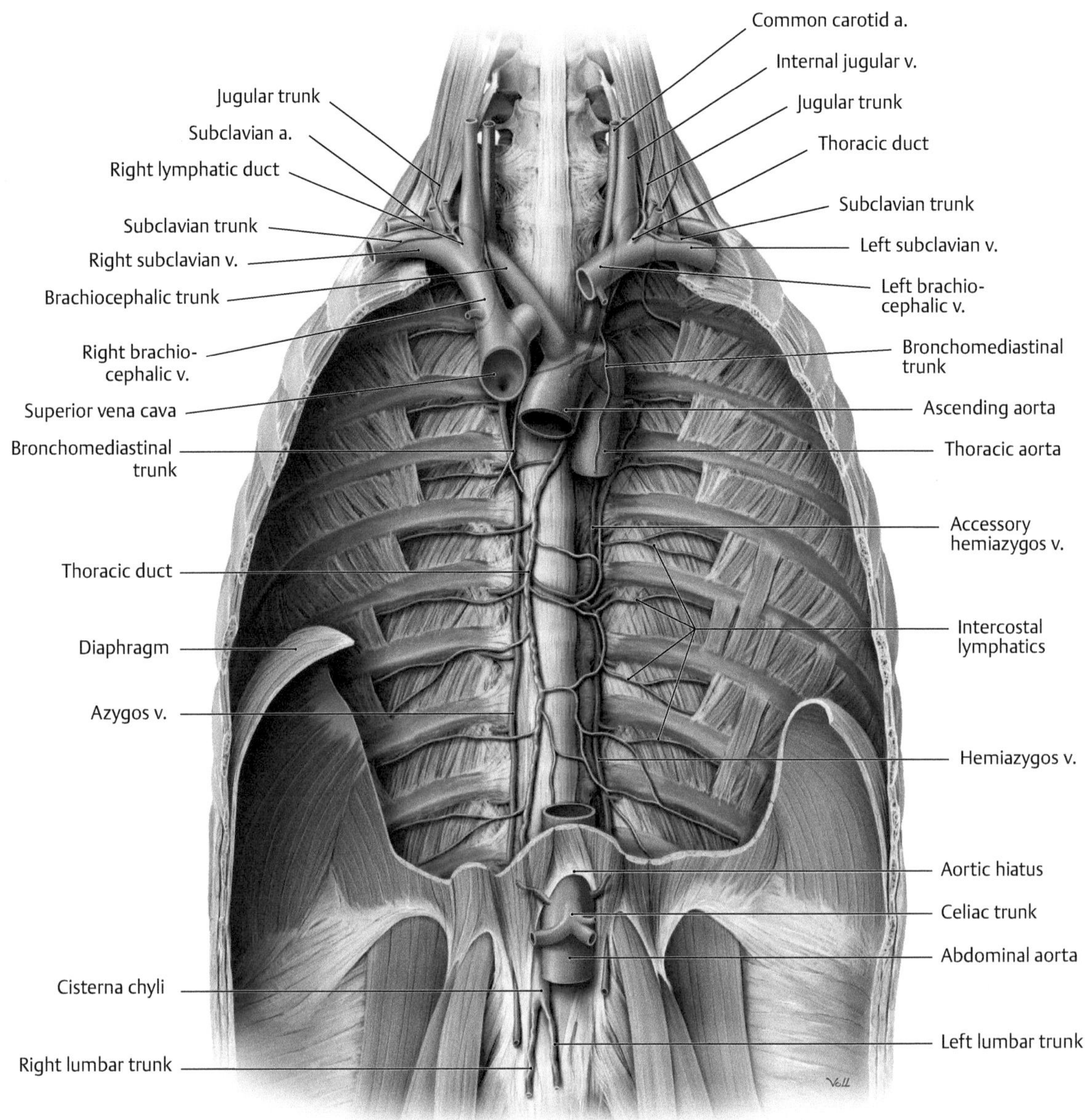

Fig. 2.67 (a) Lymphatic trunks in the thorax. (*continued*) (From Schuenke M, Schulte E, Schumacher U. THIEME Atlas of Anatomy. Internal Organs. Illustrations by Voll M and Wesker K. 3rd ed. New York: Thieme Medical Publishers; 2020.)

On the right side, the line of pleural reflection runs inferiorly down the sternum from the cupula to near the xiphoid process in a fairly straight line. It then deviates from about the 6th costal cartilage to the 8th rib, 10th rib and finally the 12th rib near the neck in a fairly uniform fashion. On the left side, the reflection descends similarly to the right side, but after reaching the 4th costal cartilage, it deviates to the 6th costal cartilage to accommodate the pericardium and cardiac notch. From the 6th costal cartilage, the pleural reflection begins to resemble that of the right side and deviates to the 8th rib near the midclavicular line, crosses the 10th rib at the midaxillary line and finishes near the neck of the 12th rib.

During regular respiration, the inferior borders of both lungs do not come in contact with the edges of the parietal pleura, resulting in the formation of two pleural spaces. The **costomediastinal recesses** are small and located posterior to the sternum where the costal pleura is in contact with the mediastinal pleura. The left costomediastinal recess is larger because of the pronounced *cardiac notch* of the left lung. The **costodiaphragmatic recesses** are larger "gutters" that surround the upward convexity of the diaphragm within the thoracic wall and it is a common site for a *thoracentesis*. At rest, the inferior borders of both lungs are located respectively from anterior, lateral and posterior at approximately the T6, T8 and T10 vertebral levels. During heavy breathing and again from anterior, lateral and posteriorly, the inferior borders fill the recesses by extending down to the T8, T10 and T12 vertebral levels respectively (**Fig. 2.70; Fig. 2.71; Fig. 2.72**).

2.20 Lungs

The **lungs** are the main organs of respiration and their main function is to oxygenate the blood and release carbon dioxide from the bloodstream into the atmosphere (**Fig. 2.73**). There is a left and right lung. The left lung is smaller and lighter than the right

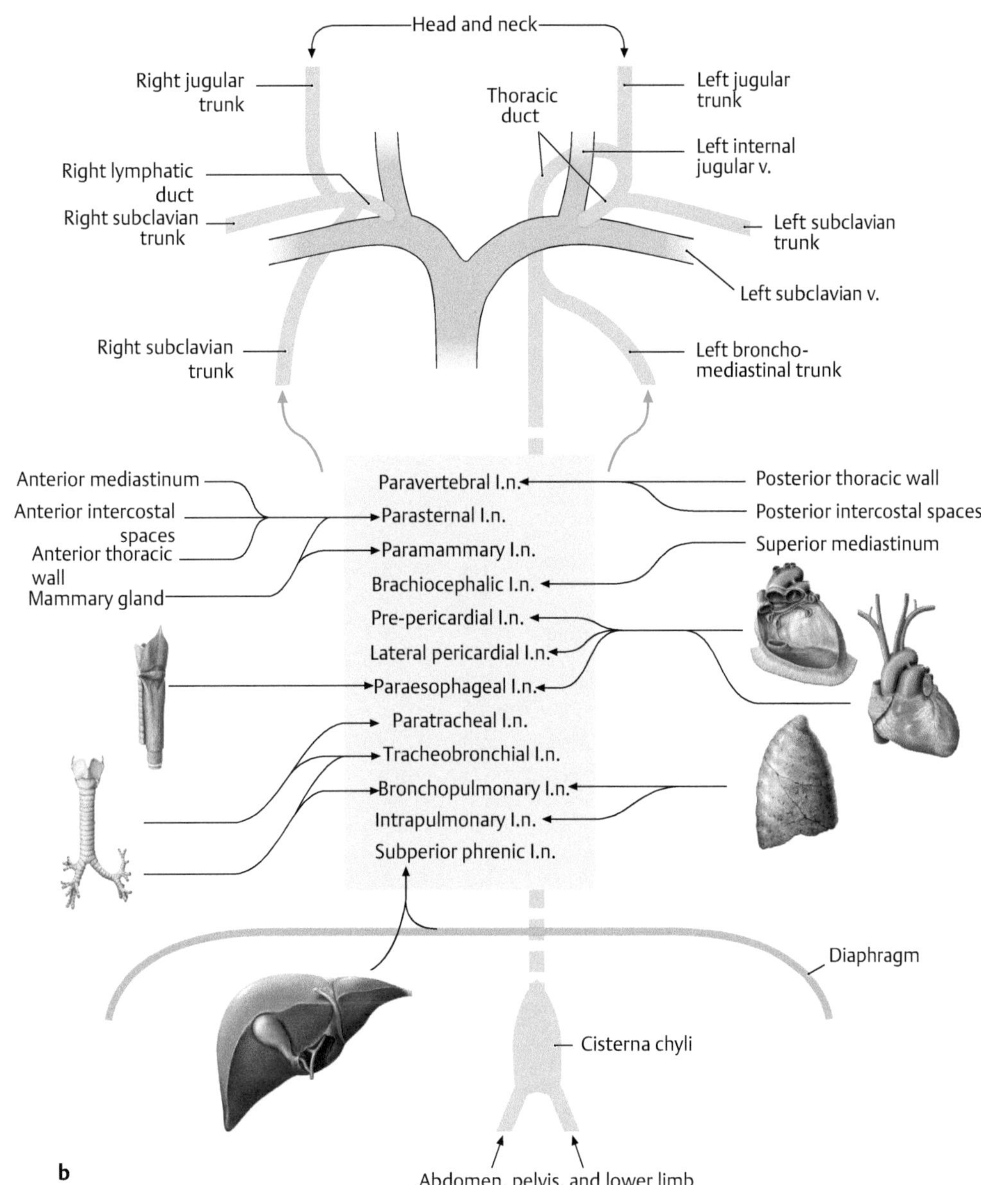

Fig. 2.67 *(continued)* **(b)** Lymphatic pathways in the thorax. (From Schuenke M, Schulte E, Schumacher U. THIEME Atlas of Anatomy. Internal Organs. Illustrations by Voll M and Wesker K. 3rd ed. New York: Thieme Medical Publishers; 2020.)

lung because the pericardium and heart bulge towards the left. The right lung is higher because the diaphragm and liver extend farther superiorly. The left lung is made up of two lobes (superior and inferior) separated by an **oblique fissure** while the right lung is made up of three lobes (superior, middle and inferior) which are separated from one another by an **oblique** and **horizontal fissure**. On the posterior border of both lungs, the oblique fissures are located at vertebral level T4/T5. Each lung has certain features and they are listed below.

- **Apex**: the blunt superior end of the lung that passes above the level of the first rib and into the root of the neck. It is covered by cervical parietal pleura.
- **Base**: the inferior border and diaphragmatic surfaces of the lungs opposite the apex.
- **3 surfaces**:
  - **Costal surface** is related to the costal parietal pleura and adjacent to the sternum, costal cartilages and ribs.
  - **Mediastinal surface** is related to the middle mediastinum and includes the *hilum of the lung*.
  - **Diaphragmatic surface** is related to the diaphragm and helps form the base of the lung.
- **3 borders**:
  - **Anterior border** is where the costal and mediastinal surfaces meet anteriorly and rest over the heart.
  - **Posterior border** is where the costal and mediasinal surfaces meet posteriorly.
  - **Inferior border** is the outer border of the diaphragmatic surface separating it from the costal and mediastinal surfaces.

The **hilum of the lung** is the area located on the mediastinal surface of each lung and its border is formed by the pleural sleeve. The **pleural sleeve** is the area of continuity between the parietal and visceral layers of pleura. On both lungs, there is an inferior extension from the pleural sleeve known as the **pulmonary ligament**.

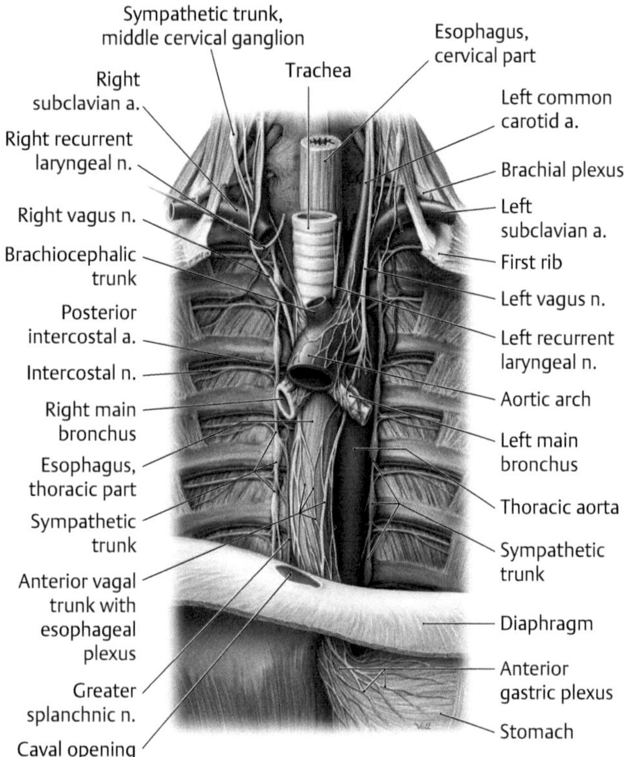

Fig. 2.68 Esophageal plexus and sympathetic trunk. (From Schuenke M, Schulte E, Schumacher U. THIEME Atlas of Anatomy. Internal Organs. Illustrations by Voll M and Wesker K. 3rd ed. New York: Thieme Medical Publishers; 2020.)

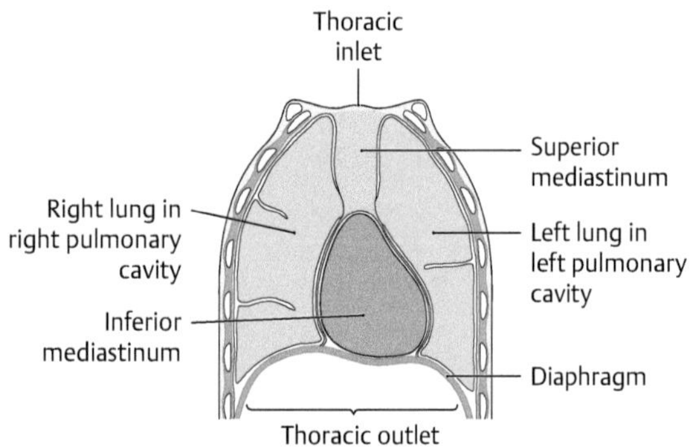

Fig. 2.69 Divisions of the thoracic cavity. (From Schuenke M, Schulte E, Schumacher U. THIEME Atlas of Anatomy. Internal Organs. Illustrations by Voll M and Wesker K. 3rd ed. New York: Thieme Medical Publishers; 2020.)

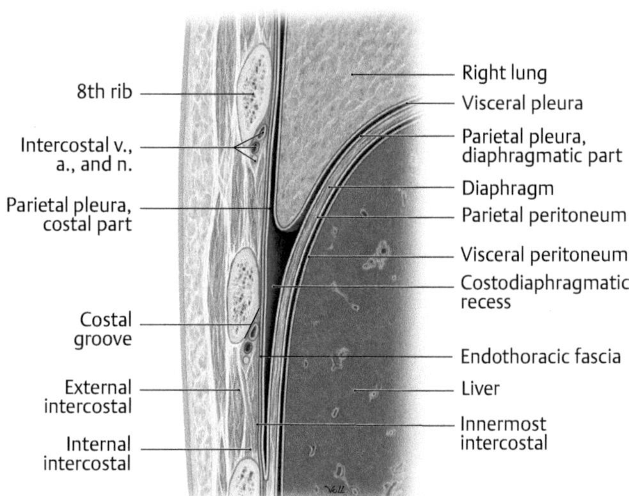

Fig. 2.70 Costodiaphragmatic recess, coronal section, anterior view. (From Schuenke M, Schulte E, Schumacher U. THIEME Atlas of Anatomy. Internal Organs. Illustrations by Voll M and Wesker K. 3rd ed. New York: Thieme Medical Publishers; 2020.)

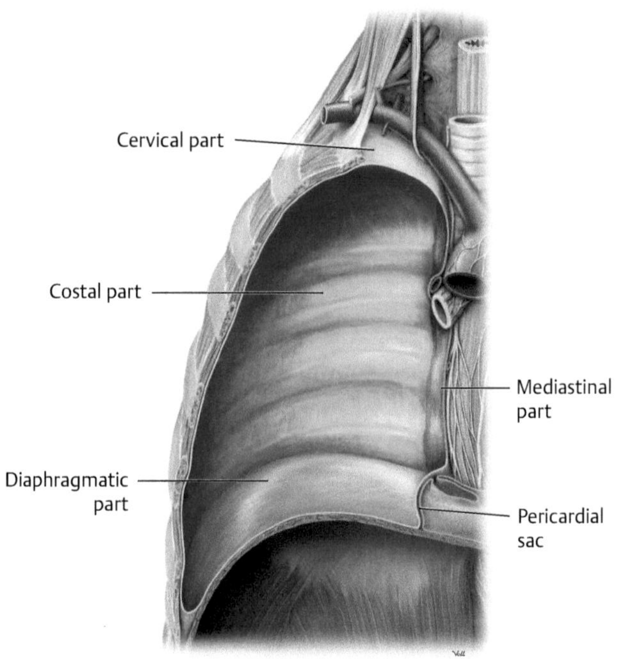

Fig. 2.71 Parts of the parietal pleura. (From Schuenke M, Schulte E, Schumacher U. THIEME Atlas of Anatomy. Internal Organs. Illustrations by Voll M and Wesker K. 3rd ed. New York: Thieme Medical Publishers; 2020.)

This ligament actually consists of a double layer of pleura separated by a very small amount of connective tissue (**Fig. 2.73**).

The **root of the lung** is formed by structures entering and exiting from the lung at the hilum. The root connects each lung with both the heart and trachea. A general arrangement can be viewed if the root is sectioned before the branching of the main (primary) bronchus and pulmonary vessels.

- The **main (primary) bronchus** is inferior to the pulmonary artery on the left lung but posterior to the pulmonary artery on the right lung.
- The **pulmonary artery** is superior to the main bronchus on the left lung but anterior to the main bronchus on the right lung.
- The **pulmonary veins** on both lungs are located anterior and inferior to any other structures.

The surface anatomy of the lungs' mediastinal surfaces can present grooves or impressions from additional nearby structures, especially on an embalmed cadaver. On the left lung, the *cardiac impression, cardiac notch, lingula,* and *grooves for the arch of the aorta* and *thoracic/descending aorta* are quite evident. On the right lung, *grooves of the arch of the azygos* and *azygos vein* as well as the *impression of the esophagus* could be evident.

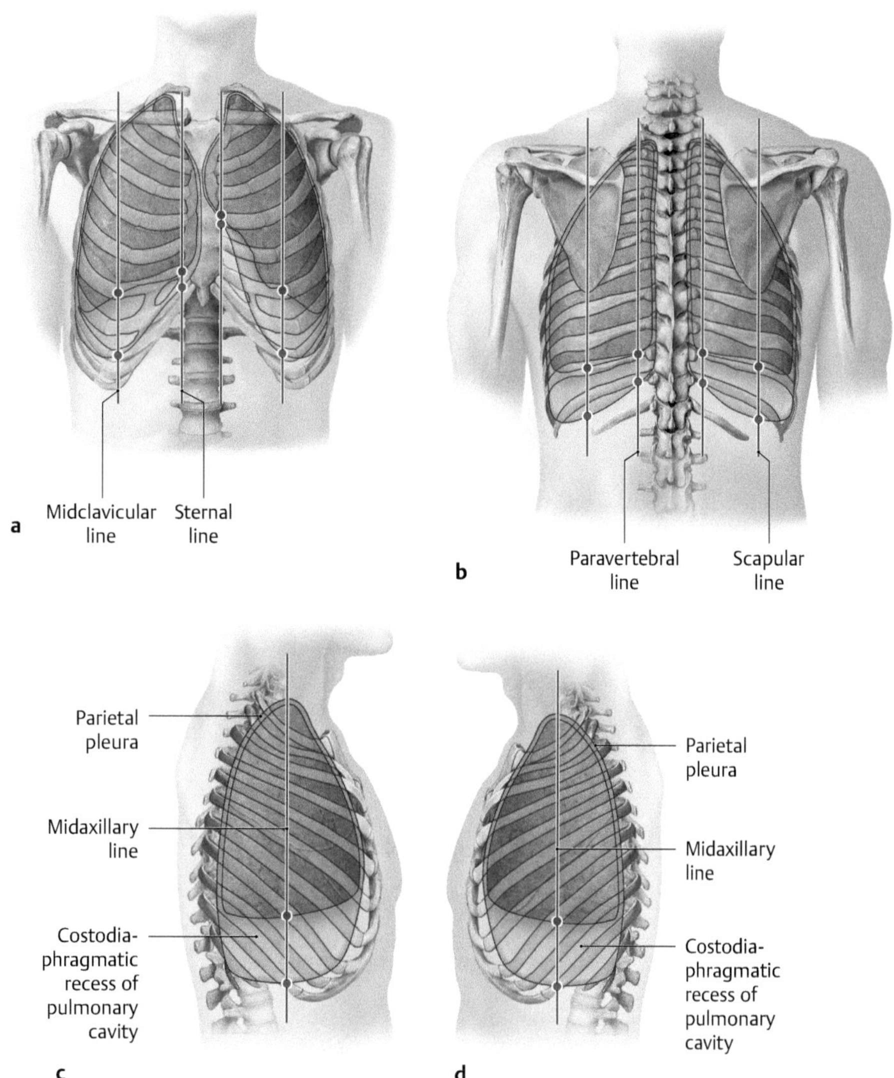

Fig. 2.72 Boundaries of the lungs and pleural cavities. **(a)** Anterior view. **(b)** Posterior view. **(c)** Right lateral view. **(d)** left lateral view. The red dot represents the inferior boundary of the lung and the blue dot represents the inferior boundary of the pulmonary cavity. (From Schuenke M, Schulte E, Schumacher U. THIEME Atlas of Anatomy. Internal Organs. Illustrations by Voll M and Wesker K. 3rd ed. New York: Thieme Medical Publishers; 2020.)

Table 2.2 **Pleural cavity boundaries and reference points**

Reference line	Right lung	Right parietal pleura	Left lung	Left parietal pleura
Sternal line (STL)	6th rib	7th rib	4th rib	4th rib
Midclavicular line (MCL)	6th rib	8th costal cartilage	6th rib	8th rib
Midaxillary line (MAL)	8th rib	10th rib	8th rib	10th rib
Scapular line (SL)	10th rib	11th rib	10th rib	11th rib
Paravertebral line (PV)	10th rib	T12 vertebra	10th rib	T12 vertebra

2.20.1 Tracheobronchial Tree

The **tracheobronchial tree** is the trachea and bronchi located within the mediastinum as well as the bronchial tree located within the lungs. It consists of a *conducting* and *respiratory component.* At vertebral level C6, the larynx ends and the trachea begins (**Fig. 2.74**). The **trachea** is located anterior to the esophagus until it bifurcates into the main (primary) bronchi at vertebral level T4/T5. It is a semi-circular, fibrocartilaginous tube with approximately 15 incomplete C-shaped **tracheal (cartilaginous-hyaline) rings** with a flat, non-cartilaginous posterior surface adjacent to the esophagus. These posterior gaps in the tracheal rings are filled in with smooth muscle known as the **trachealis muscle.**

At vertebral level T4/T5, the trachea bifurcates into the left and right main (primary) bronchi. The **left main bronchus** passes

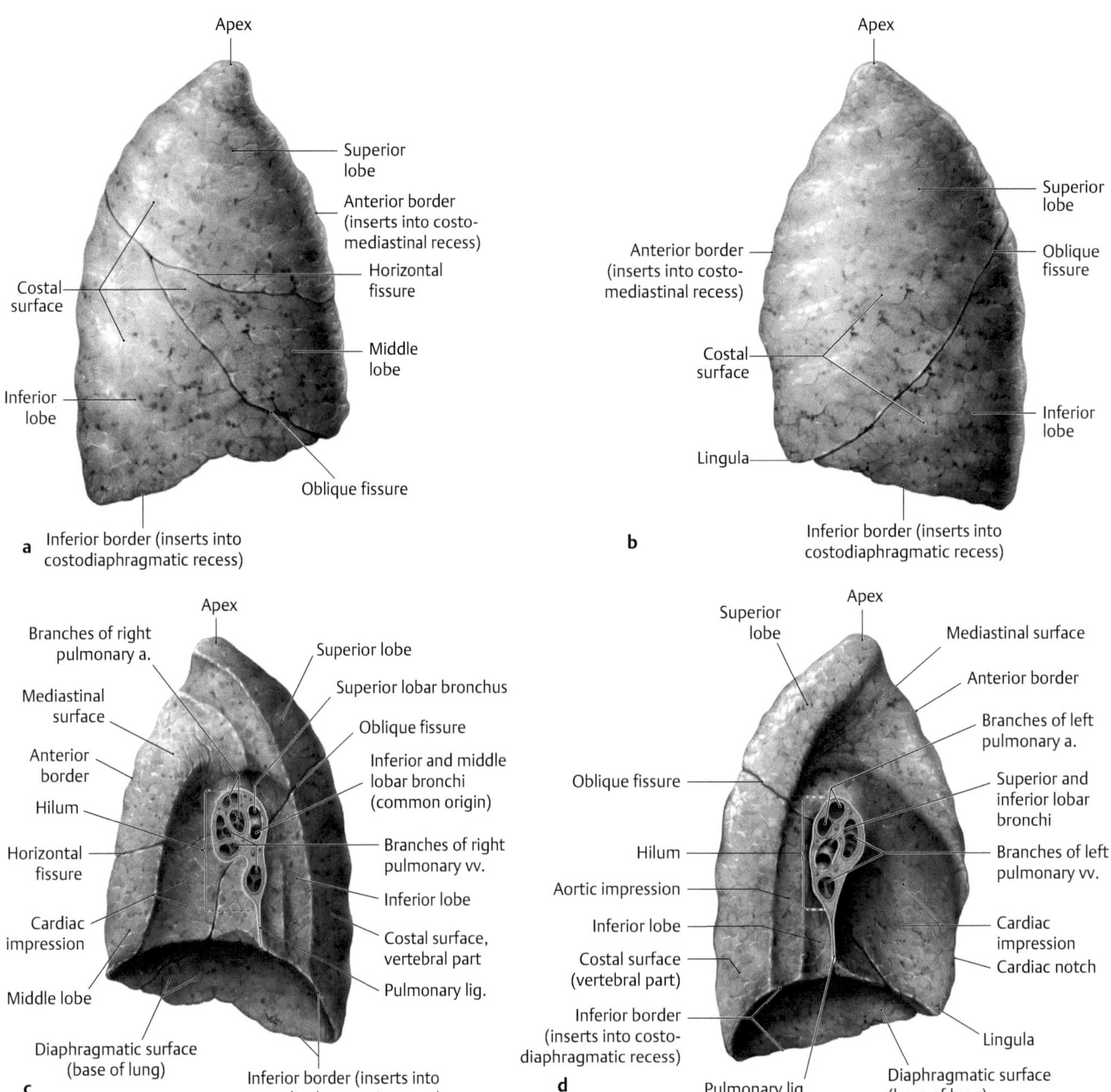

Fig. 2.73 Gross anatomy of the lungs. **(a)** Right lung, lateral view. **(b)** Left lung, lateral view. **(c)** Right lung, medial view. **(d)** Left lung, medial view. (From Schuenke M, Schulte E, Schumacher U. THIEME Atlas of Anatomy. Internal Organs. Illustrations by Voll M and Wesker K. 3rd ed. New York: Thieme Medical Publishers; 2020.)

inferolaterally at approximately a 45 degree angle to reach the hilum of the lung. It is longer than but not as wide as the right main bronchus. It passes inferior to the arch of the aorta but anterior to the thoracic aorta and esophagus. The **right main bronchus** is more vertical on its way to the hilum. It is also wider and shorter than the left main bronchus. The bronchi branch while in the lungs to form additional branches of the tracheobronchial tree. All tracheobronchial tree branches are components of the root of the lung and consist of their own pulmonary artery and vein branches. Internally and at the bifurcation of the trachea, there is a cartilaginous ridge known as the **carina**. The carina leans to the left of the midline, and if any foreign bodies fall down the trachea, they tend to enter the right main bronchus **(Fig. 2.74)**.

Each main bronchus divides into multiple **lobar (secondary) bronchi** and they supply each lobe of the lung. The left lung has a **superior** and **inferior lobar bronchus** while the right lung has a **superior**, **middle** and **inferior lobar bronchus**. The superior lobar bronchus is also known as the *eparterial bronchus* because it arises above the level of the pulmonary artery. All other lobar bronchi branching are *hyparterial* because they are below the level of the pulmonary artery. The right main bronchus gives off the superior lobar bronchus prior to entering the hilum of the lung **(Fig. 2.74)**.

All secondary lobar bronchi divide into **segmental (tertiary) bronchi** which are responsible for supplying the bronchopulmonary segments of the lung. A **bronchopulmonary segment** is a

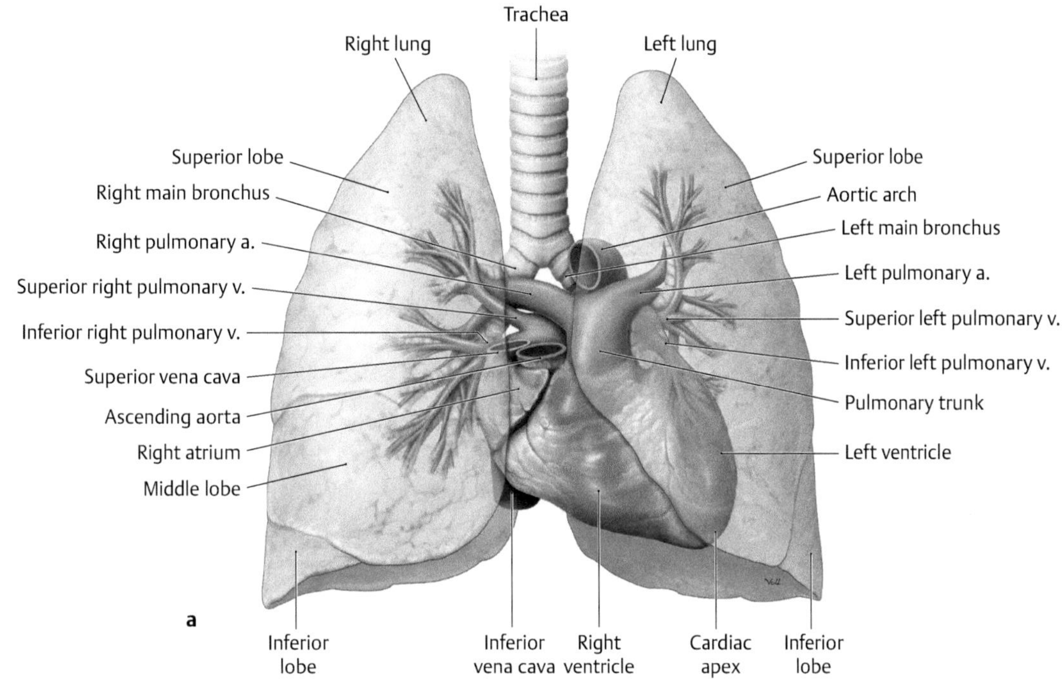

Thyroid cartilage
Cricoid cartilage
Median cricothyroid lig.
Tracheal cartilages
Anular ligs.
Right main bronchus
Right superior lobar bronchus
Right middle lobar bronchus
Left main bronchus
Left superior lobar bronchus
Tracheal bifurcation
Right/left inferior lobar bronchi
I II III IV V VI VII VIII IX X
b

Thyroid cartilage
Arytenoid cartilage
Cricoid cartilage
Membranous posterior wall (with tracheal glands)
Tracheal cartilages
Mucosa
Position of carina (at tracheal bifurcation)
Right main bronchus
Left main bronchus
I II III IV V VI VII VIII IX X
c

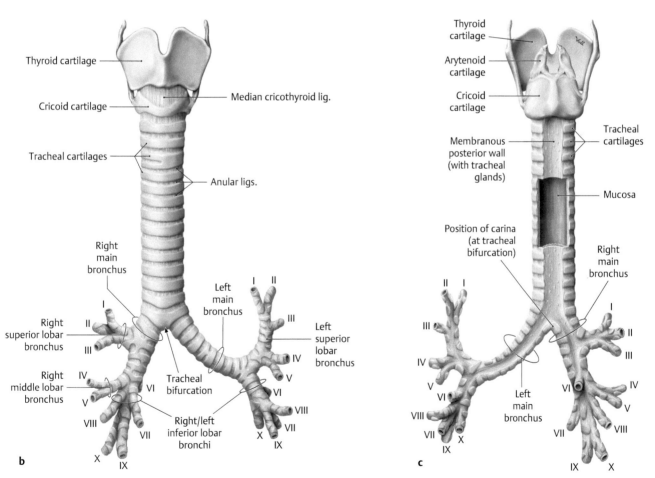

Fig. 2.74 **(a)** Distribution of the pulmonary arteries and veins, anterior view. **(b)** Trachea, anterior view. **(c)** Trachea, posterior view with opened posterior wall. (From Schuenke M, Schulte E, Schumacher U. THIEME Atlas of Anatomy. Internal Organs. Illustrations by Voll M and Wesker K. 3rd ed. New York: Thieme Medical Publishers; 2020.)

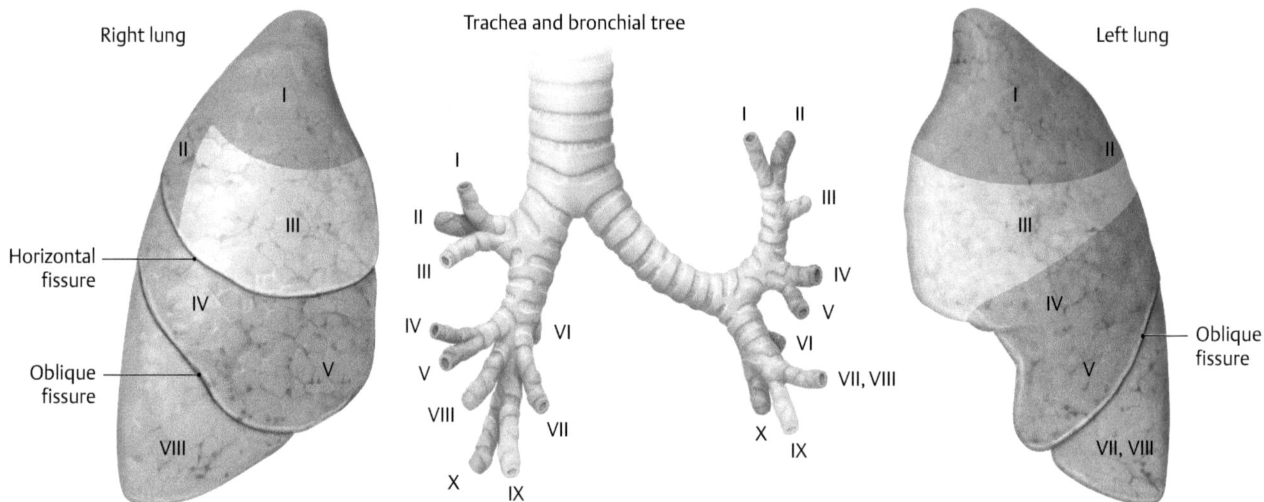

Fig. 2.75 Segmentation of the lung, anterior view. (From Schuenke M, Schulte E, Schumacher U. THIEME Atlas of Anatomy. Internal Organs. Illustrations by Voll M and Wesker K. 3rd ed. New York: Thieme Medical Publishers; 2020.)

division of the lung that is separated from the rest of the lung by a connective tissue septum. This allows for a particular segment to be surgically removed without affecting another segment. Characteristics of the bronchopulmonary segments include:

- They are the largest subdivisions of a lobe.
- They are named according to the segmental bronchi supplying it.
- The left lung has 8-10 and the right lung has 10.
- The segment is shaped similar to a pyramid with the apex facing the root of the lung and the base facing the pleural surface.
- They are supplied independently by a segmental bronchus and a tertiary branch of the pulmonary artery.
- They are drained by intersegmental portions of the pulmonary veins that are found in the connective tissue in between adjacent segments. This can result in drainage of two separate segments.

The segmental bronchi of each lobe of a lung are listed below **(Fig. 2.75; Fig. 2.76; Fig. 2.77)**:

- Left superior lobe: **apical**, **anterior**, **posterior**, **superior lingular** and **inferior lingular.**
- Left inferior lobe: **superior**, **anterior basal**, **medial basal**, **lateral basal** and **posterior basal.**
- Right superior lobe: **apical**, **anterior** and **posterior.**
- Right middle lobe: **lateral** and **medial.**
- Right inferior lobe: **superior**, **anterior basal**, **medial basal**, **lateral basal** and **posterior basal.**

The apical and posterior segmental bronchi of the left superior lobe often fuse to form the **apicoposterior segmental bronchi**. The anterior basal and medial basal segmental bronchi of the left inferior lobe often fuse to form the **anteromedial basal segmental bronchi**.

After the segmental (tertiary) bronchi there will be 20-25 generations of **conducting bronchioles** that end as **terminal bronchioles**. The terminal bronchioles represent the end of the *conducting component* of the tracheobronchial tree. The conducting and terminal bronchioles lack any cartilage, glands or alveoli. They simply "conduct" or transport air to the *respiratory component* of the tracheobronchial tree (**Fig. 2.78**).

The terminal bronchioles give rise to several generations of **respiratory bronchioles** that have scattered, thin-walled evaginations extending from their lumens and are known as alveoli. Because alveoli are already present on respiratory bronchioles, this means these bronchioles are both transporting air and involve in gas exchange. The respiratory bronchioles give rise to 2-10 ill-defined **alveolar ducts** which are elongated airways densely lined with alveoli. The alveolar ducts give rise to 3-6 **alveolar sacs** into which clusters of **alveoli** open and it is the alveoli that represent the end of the respiratory component of the tracheobronchial tree.

2.20.2 Histology of the Alveoli

The **pulmonary alveoli** represent the basic structural unit for gas exchange in the lungs. The functional unit of the lung could be defined as the entire *pulmonary acinus* which includes the entire portion of the lung distal to the terminal bronchioles. Not including the *endothelial cells* of pulmonary capillaries or the *interstitial cells* such as fibroblasts and mast cells, there are three main cell types of the alveolus (**Fig. 2.79**).

- **Type I pneumocytes**: a simple squamous epithelium representing more than 90% of the alveolar surface area. Also contribute to the blood-air barrier.
- **Type II pneumocytes**: a cuboidal shaped cell intermixed with type I cells that produces and secretes surfactant and is thought to be stem cells for both type I and type II cells. This is important in reducing the surface tension of the fluid lining the alveoli subsequently preventing collapse of the alveoli. Lack of surfactant, especially in a preterm baby prior to seven months' gestation, is central to *respiratory distress syndrome*.
- **Pulmonary macrophages**: phagocytize particulate matter and form the primary defense mechanism of the alveoli.

The **blood-air barrier** is formed by the type I pneumocyte, endothelium of the capillary and a simple basement membrane. The **pores of Kohn** allow collateral air flow and macrophage migration by forming passages between adjacent alveoli.

2.20.3 Blood Supply and Venous Drainage of the Lungs

Each lung has a pulmonary artery and two pulmonary veins assigned to it. The pulmonary trunk that diverts blood away from the right ventricle of the heart, divides into a left and right

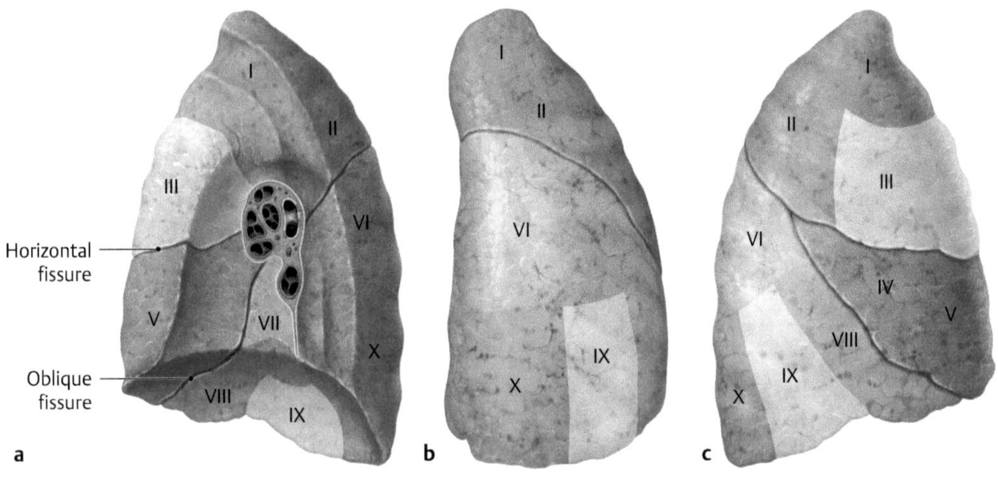

Fig. 2.76 Bronchopulmonary segments of the right lung. **(a)** Medial view. **(b)** Posterior view. **(c)** Lateral view. (From Schuenke M, Schulte E, Schumacher U. THIEME Atlas of Anatomy. Internal Organs. Illustrations by Voll M and Wesker K. 3rd ed. New York: Thieme Medical Publishers; 2020.)

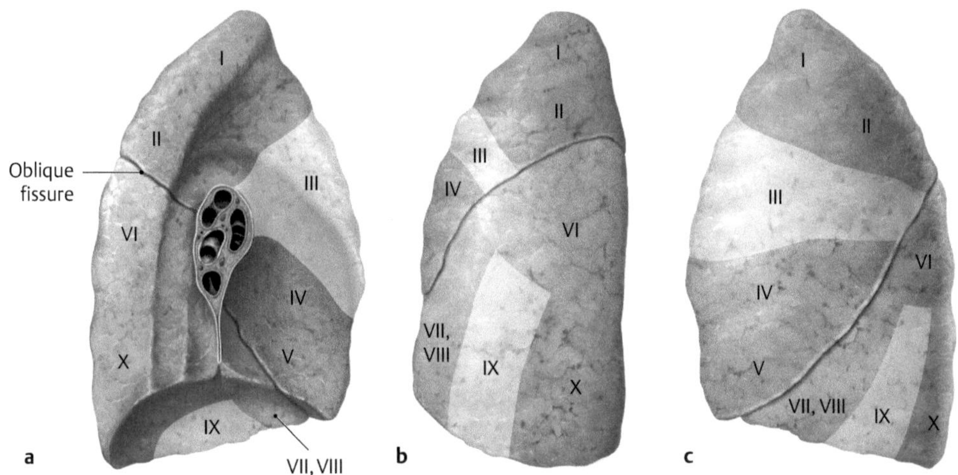

Fig. 2.77 Bronchopulmonary segments of the left lung. **(a)** Medial view. **(b)** Posterior view. **(c)** Lateral view. (From Schuenke M, Schulte E, Schumacher U. THIEME Atlas of Anatomy. Internal Organs. Illustrations by Voll M and Wesker K. 3rd ed. New York: Thieme Medical Publishers; 2020.)

pulmonary artery near the level of the T4/T5 vertebral level. The left pulmonary artery is located anterior to the arch of the aorta while the right pulmonary artery slides underneath the aortic arch before reaching the hilum of the right lung.

The **pulmonary arteries** transport deoxygenated blood to the capillaries surrounding the alveoli. Each pulmonary artery becomes part of the root of the lung. With the exception of the left and right superior lobar arteries, while within the lungs, the pulmonary arteries divide into **lobar (secondary) arteries** followed by **segmental (tertiary) arteries**. The lobar and segmental arteries are paired with their corresponding bronchi and bronchopulmonary segment. The artery is generally located on the anterior aspect of these bronchi. The parietal pleura is supplied by outer systematic arteries such as the posterior and anterior intercostal arteries (**Fig. 2.80**).

The **pulmonary veins** transport oxygenated blood back towards the heart and originate from the capillary beds surrounding the alveoli. They begin first as small veins that leave the alveoli capillary beds and travel within the intersegmental septa to receive veins from the adjacent bronchopulmonary segments as well as the visceral pleura. These veins follow the **segmental** and **lobar** patterns seen with the arteries however the veins run independently of the arteries and bronchi in each lung. The lobar veins eventually form a superior and inferior pulmonary vein within each lung. These veins pass through the hilum of the lung to reach the left atrium of the heart. It should be noted that veins from the visceral pleura and the bronchial veins can drain into the pulmonary veins. This results in a minimal amount of deoxygenated blood entering an area of highly oxygenated blood. The parietal pleura is drained by systematic veins such as the posterior and anterior intercostal veins (**Fig. 2.80**).

The **bronchial arteries** are responsible for supplying blood to structures of the root of the lungs, visceral pleura and supporting tissues of the lungs. Bronchial arteries are generally located posterior to the bronchi and supply blood down to the respiratory bronchioles. At that point they anastomose with the pulmonary arteries in the walls of the bronchioles and visceral pleura. There are two **left (superior/inferior) bronchial arteries** and one **right bronchial artery**. Both of the left bronchial arteries originate from

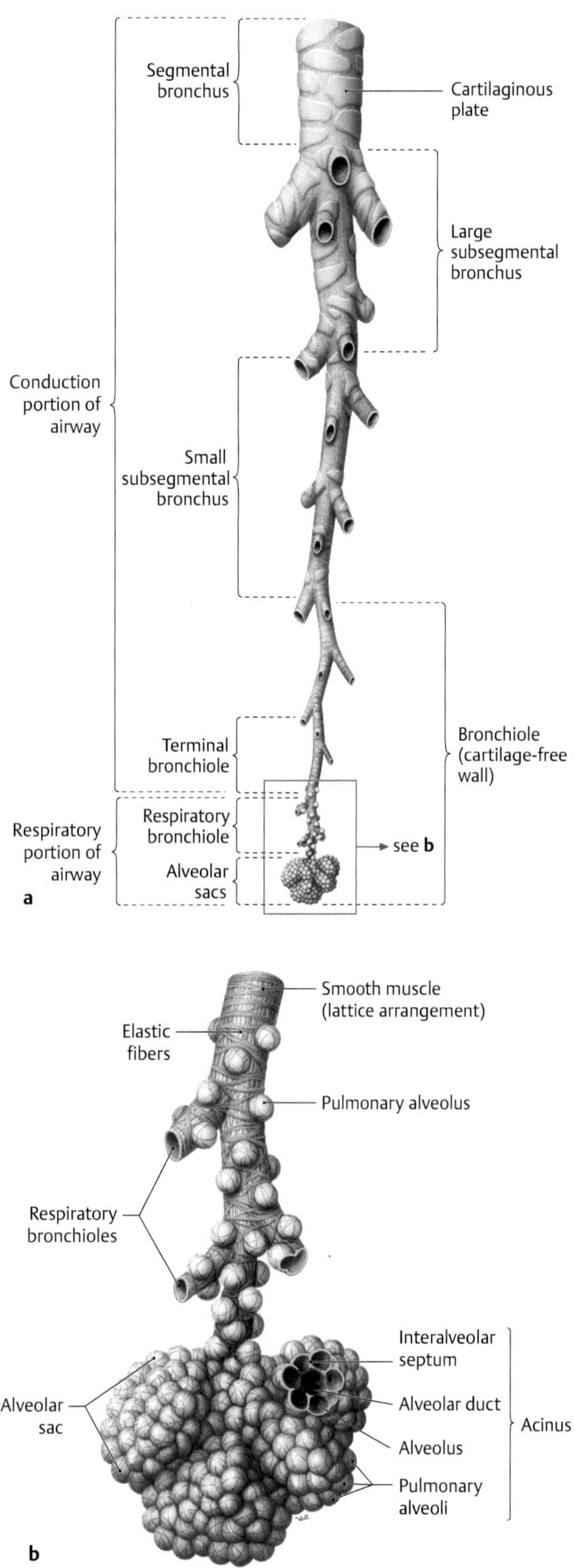

Fig. 2.78 Bronchial tree. **(a)** Divisions of the bronchial tree. **(b)** Respiratory portion of the bronchial tree. (From Schuenke M, Schulte E, Schumacher U. THIEME Atlas of Anatomy. Internal Organs. Illustrations by Voll M and Wesker K. 3rd ed. New York: Thieme Medical Publishers; 2020.)

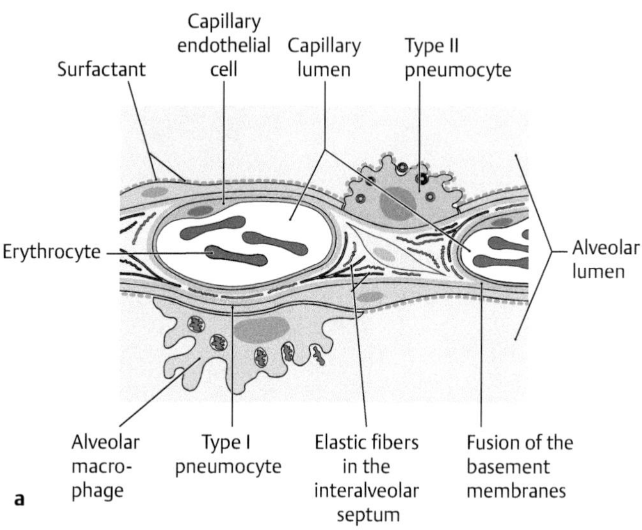

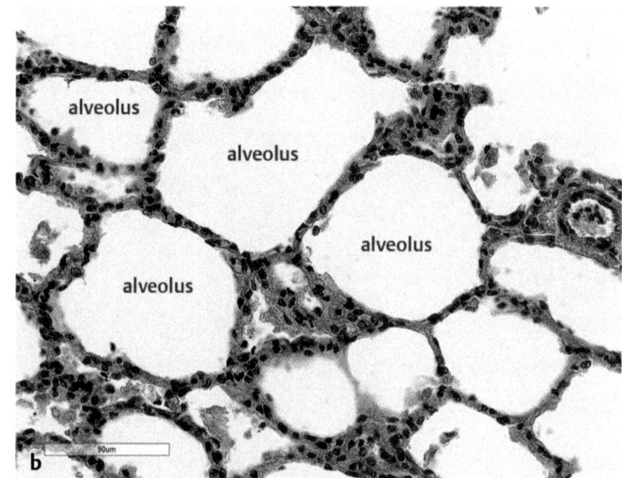

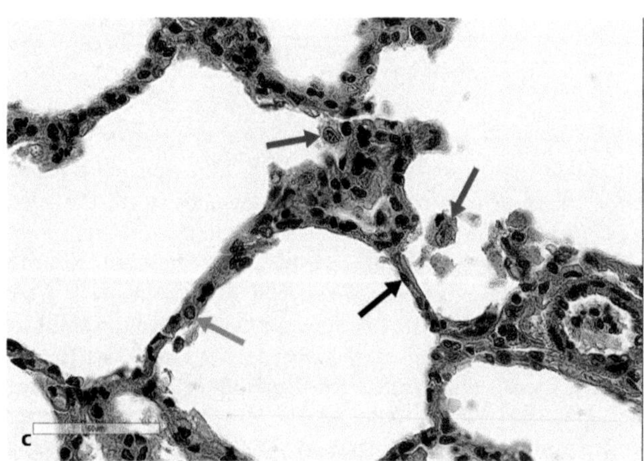

Fig. 2.79 Histology of the alveoli. **(a)** Epithelial lining of the alveoli. **(b)** Alveoli, light micrograph, medium magnification. **(c)** Alveoli, light micrograph, high magnification, showing type I alveolar cell *(black arrow)*, type II alveolar cell *(blue arrow)*, and alveolar macrophages *(green arrows)*. (**a** from Schuenke M, Schulte E, Schumacher U. THIEME Atlas of Anatomy. Internal Organs. Illustrations by Voll M and Wesker K. 3rd ed. New York: Thieme Medical Publishers; 2020. **b** and **c** from Lowrie DJ. Histology: An Essential Textbook. New York: Thieme Medical Publishers; 2020.)

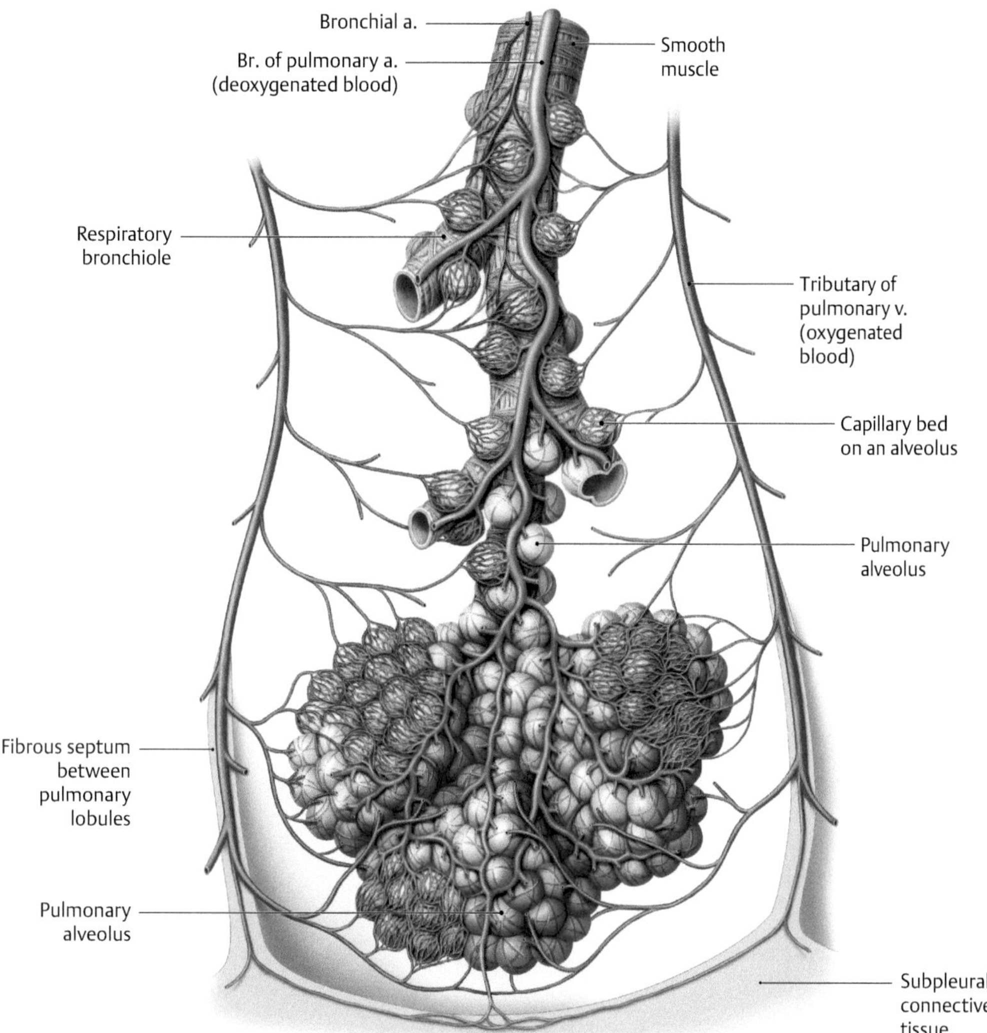

Fig. 2.80 Pulmonary vasculature. (From Schuenke M, Schulte E, Schumacher U. THIEME Atlas of Anatomy. Internal Organs. Illustrations by Voll M and Wesker K. 3rd ed. New York: Thieme Medical Publishers; 2020.)

the *thoracic aorta* but the right bronchial artery can originate from one of three locations **(Fig. 2.81)**:

- From the proximal *right 3rd posterior intercostal artery.*
- From a common trunk with the *left superior bronchial artery.*
- Directly from the *thoracic aorta* (rare).

The **bronchial veins** drain a limited amount of blood with it coming from near the proximal portion of the root of the lungs. The *pulmonary veins* are responsible for draining the rest including the peripheral regions of the lung, the distal portions of the root of the lungs and the visceral pleura. The **left bronchial veins** drain into either the *left superior intercostal* or *accessory hemiazygos veins.* The right bronchial veins (1 or 2 total) drain into the *azygos vein* **(Fig. 2.82)**.

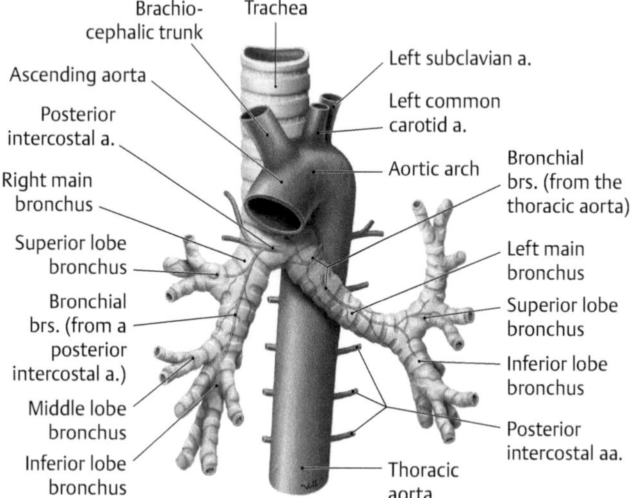

Fig. 2.81 Arteries of the tracheobronchial tree. (From Schuenke M, Schulte E, Schumacher U. THIEME Atlas of Anatomy. Internal Organs. Illustrations by Voll M and Wesker K. 3rd ed. New York: Thieme Medical Publishers; 2020.)

2.20.4 Lymphatic Drainage of the Lungs

With the *parietal pleura* being closely associated with the thoracic wall and diaphragm, lymph drains to the **intercostal, mediastinal, parasternal** and **phrenic lymph nodes.** Lymph drainage from the visceral pleura and lung parenchyma is a little more extensive. The **subpleural (superficial) lymphatic plexus** is just deep to the

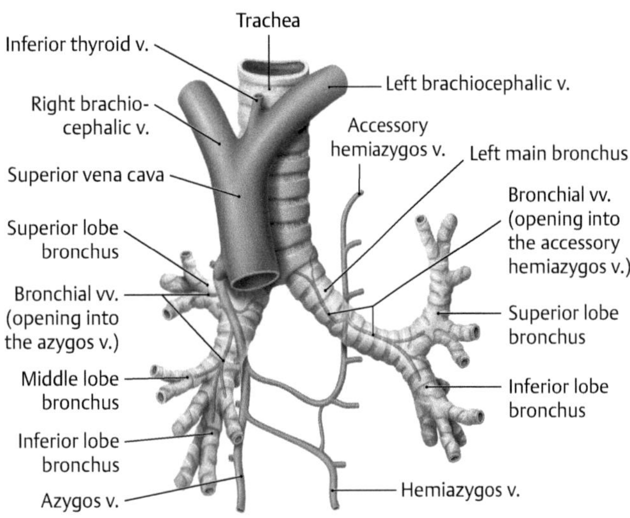

Fig. 2.82 Veins of the tracheobronchial tree. (From Schuenke M, Schulte E, Schumacher U. THIEME Atlas of Anatomy. Internal Organs. Illustrations by Voll M and Wesker K. 3rd ed. New York: Thieme Medical Publishers; 2020.)

visceral pleura and drains both the visceral pleura and lung parenchyma. Lymph from this plexus drains to the **bronchopulmonary (hilar) lymph nodes** located at the hilum of the lung. The **bronchopulmonary (deep) lymphatic plexus** is found in the submucosa of the bronchi and peribronchial connective tissue and it is responsible for draining structures that form the root of the lung. Lymph from this deep plexus first drains near the lobar bronchi to the **pulmonary lymph nodes**, followed by the bronchopulmonary (hilar) lymph nodes that also drain the subpleural plexus (**Fig. 2.83**).

The bronchopulmonary (hilar) lymph nodes drain to the **superior** or **inferior tracheobronchial lymph nodes** near the bifurcation of the trachea. Lymph from the tracheobronchial lymph nodes drains to either the **left** or **right bronchomediastinal lymph trunks**. The left bronchomediastinal lymph terminates in the **thoracic duct** while the right bronchomediastinal lymph trunk helps form the **right lymphatic duct**.

2.20.5 Innervation of the Pleura and Lungs

The *intercostal nerves* innervate the parietal pleura, specifically the *costal* and *peripheral portions of the diaphragmatic parietal*

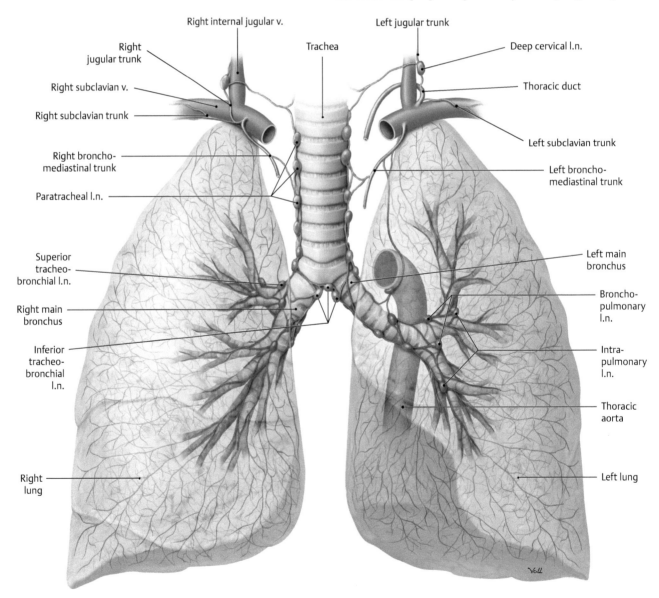

Fig. 2.83 Lymph nodes of the pleural cavity. (From Schuenke M, Schulte E, Schumacher U. THIEME Atlas of Anatomy. Internal Organs. Illustrations by Voll M and Wesker K. 3rd ed. New York: Thieme Medical Publishers; 2020.)

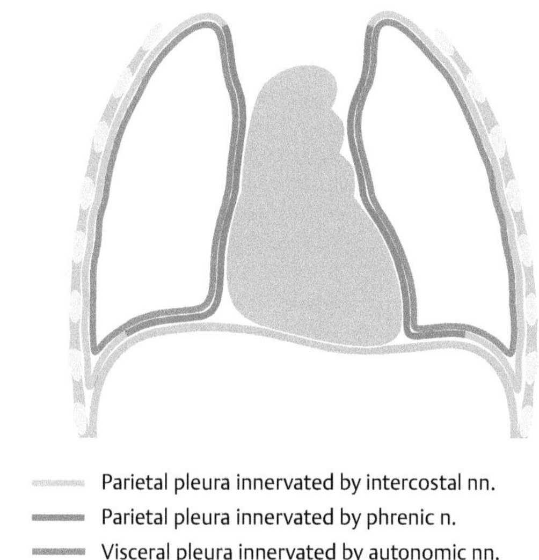

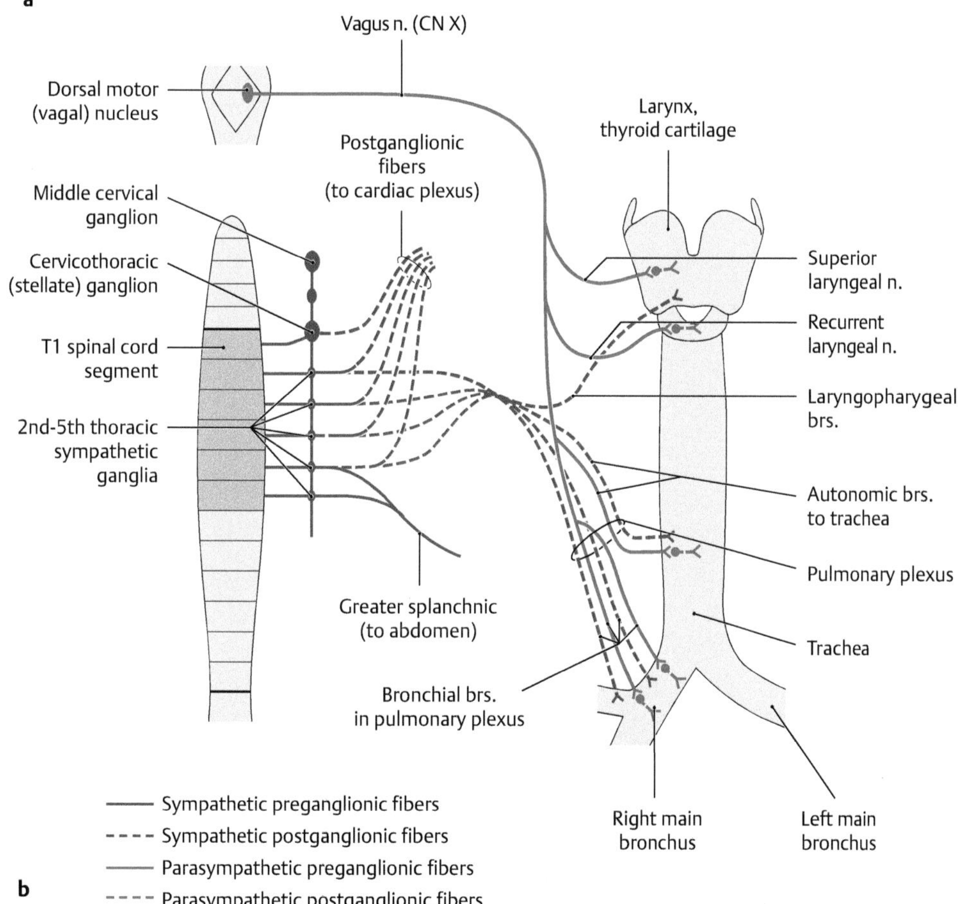

Fig. 2.84 (a) Innervation of the pleura. **(b)** Autonomic innervation of the tracheobronchial tree. (From Schuenke M, Schulte E, Schumacher U. THIEME Atlas of Anatomy. Internal Organs. Illustrations by Voll M and Wesker K. 3rd ed. New York: Thieme Medical Publishers; 2020.)

pleura. The *mediastinal* and *central portion of the diaphragmatic parietal pleura* are innervated by the *phrenic nerve*. The **left** and **right pulmonary plexuses** are visceral nerve plexuses important in the innervation of the lungs and visceral pleura. Like the majority of other visceral nerve plexuses there is no ganglion associated with this plexus. The functional components are GVE-sym/post, GVE-para/pre, and GVA. The pulmonary plexus receives sympathetic fibers originating directly from the sympathetic trunk in the thorax and from the cardiopulmonary splanchnic nerves that originate from the sympathetic trunk in the neck. The parasympathetic fibers originate from the vagus nerve (CN X) (**Fig. 2.84**).

- Sympathetics are responsible for:
  - Dilating the bronchioles (bronchodilator).
  - Constricting the pulmonary vessels (vasoconstrictor).
  - Inhibiting gland secretion (secretoinhibitory).

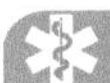

Clinical Correlate 2.38

Pulmonary (Lung) Collapse

Surface tension exists between the parietal and visceral layers of pleura. If the surface tension were broken due to trauma from a broken rib or a penetrating wound for instance, this would allow air to enter the pleural cavity that is generally a potential space. The expansion of the pleural cavity causes the inherent elasticity of the lung to be lost resulting in a collapsed lung. The pleural cavities are separate from one another meaning if one lung collapses the other lung remains functional. Air (*pneumothorax*), blood (*hemothorax*), lymph (*chylothorax*), pus (*pyothorax*) or general serous fluid (*hydrothorax*) is known to enter the pleural cavity. A *tension pneumothorax* occurs when a detached or displaced piece of tissue covers the site of trauma from the inside and allows air to enter but not escape. This will create pressure to build up within the pleural cavity. **Pleural effusion** is the clinical term when an excessive amount of fluid accumulates between the parietal and visceral layers of pleura. With this extra fluid present, the effectiveness of the lungs during normal breathing is reduced and an individual may complain of a shortness of breath.

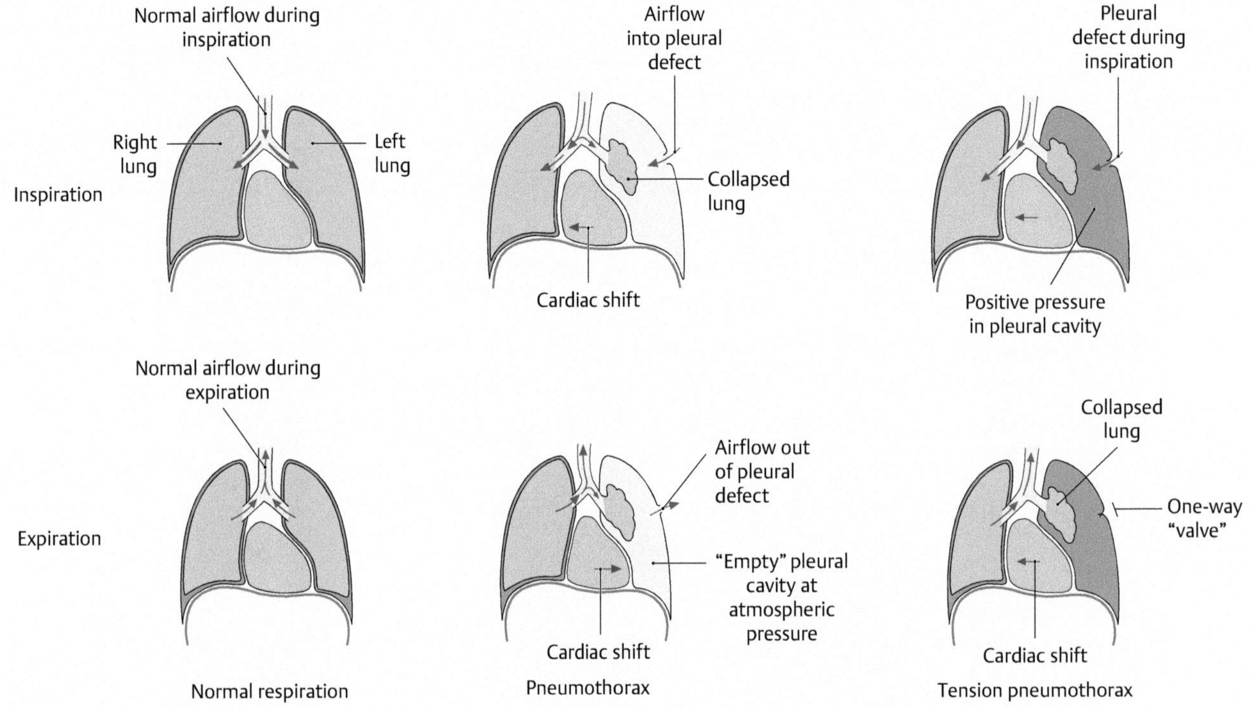

(From Schuenke M, Schulte E, Schumacher U. THIEME Atlas of Anatomy. Internal Organs. Illustrations by Voll M and Wesker K. 3rd ed. New York: Thieme Medical Publishers; 2020.)

Clinical Correlate 2.39

Pleuritis

During normal auscultation of the lungs, no sound is normally heard because the pleural layers slide smoothly against each other. Inflammation of the pleura or **pleuritis**, causes friction (*pleural rub*) and can now be heard during auscultation.

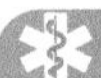

Clinical Correlate 2.40

Pulmonary Embolism

A **pulmonary embolism** is a life-threatening situation when one or more pulmonary arteries in your lungs become blocked. In most cases, blood clots that traveled to the lungs from the legs (*deep vein thrombosis* or *DVT*) are the cause of the block. A high percentage of pulmonary embolisms occur in conjunction with a DVT leading some physicians to refer to the two conditions together as *venous thromboembolism* (*VTE*). A recent surgery, cancer or immobility can increase the odds of having a pulmonary embolism.

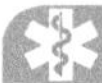

Clinical Correlate 2.41

Carcinoma of the Lungs

There are two major forms of lung cancer, the non-small cell lung cancer (NSCLC) or small cell lung cancer (SCLC). Non-small cell lung cancer is measured by stages I-IV and accounts for approximately 85% of all cases. Staging of lung cancer is determined by whether the cancer is local or has spread from the lungs to additional lymph nodes or other organs. Stage I and II (early-stage) are difficult to detect due to the size of the lungs. Tumors can grow in the lungs for a long period of time before they cause any symptoms beyond coughing and fatigue which individuals may feel are due to other causes. By the time a diagnosis is made, most individuals are generally at stage III or IV meaning the cancer has spread. Small cell lung cancers are referred to as being in a *limited* or *extensive stage* and account for the remaining 15% of lung cancers. During the treatment of lung cancer, portions of the lung may have to be removed. This includes the removal of a bronchopulmonary segment (*segmentectomy*), a lung lobe (*lobectomy*), or even the entire lung (*pneumonectomy*).

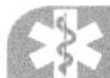

Clinical Correlate 2.42

Thoracentesis

A **thoracentesis** is a procedure that involves inserting a needle into the pleural cavity to remove air or fluid for diagnostic or therapeutic purposes. Location of where the procedure is done can vary but the most common location is in the 8th or 9th intercostal space near the midaxillary line. This would target the costodiaphragmatic recess of the pleural cavity. Complications could include a pneumothorax or hemothorax.

Clinical Correlate 2.43

Chest Tube

A **chest tube** is used to drain air, blood or fluid from around the lungs. The chest tube is inserted into an area known as the *"triangle of safety"* located between the level of 4th and 5th intercostal spaces near the anterior axillary line. The borders of this triangle are formed anteriorly by the pectoralis major muscle, posteriorly by latissimus dorsi muscle, and inferiorly by a horizontal line at the level of the nipple. The level of the nipple may differ in women. After an incision near the location of the 5th rib, the chest tube is inserted and guided into the pleural cavity.

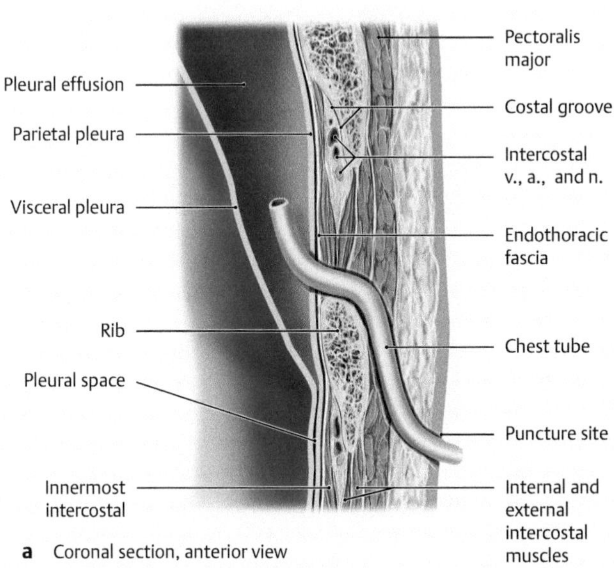

a Coronal section, anterior view

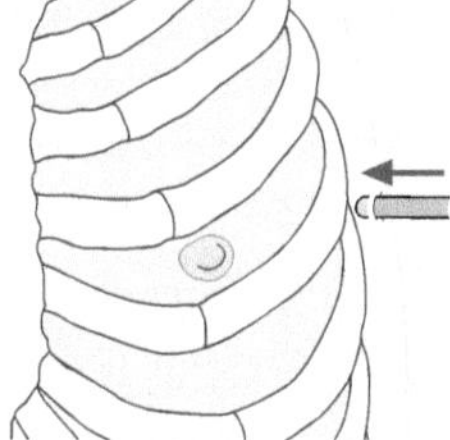

b Drainage tube is inserted perpendicular to chest wall.

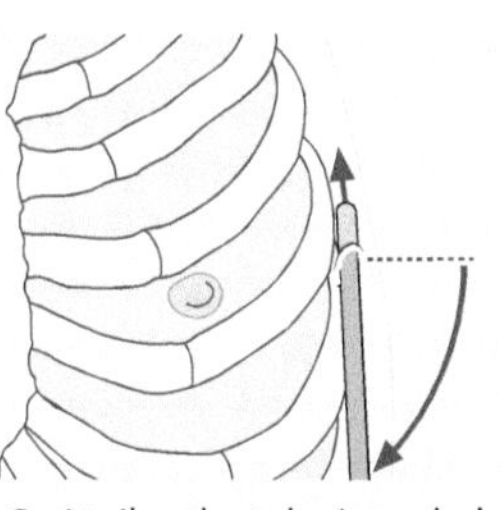

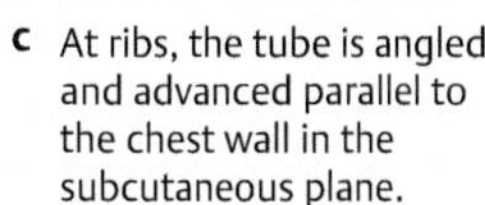

c At ribs, the tube is angled and advanced parallel to the chest wall in the subcutaneous plane.

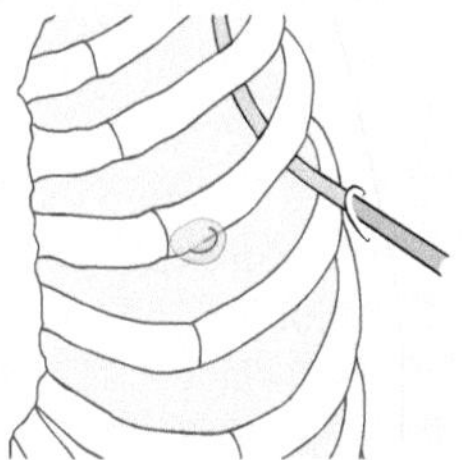

d At the superior margin of the rib, the tube is passed through the intercostal muscles and advanced into the pleural cavity.

(a-d) Insertion of a chest tube. (From Schuenke M, Schulte E, Schumacher U. THIEME Atlas of Anatomy. Internal Organs. Illustrations by Voll M and Wesker K. 3rd ed. New York: Thieme Medical Publishers; 2020.)

Clinical Correlate 2.44

Bronchoscopy

Bronchoscopy is a procedure that utilizes a bronchoscope to allow for visualization of the airway. Bronchoscopy can also be used to remove objects that are blocking the airway, collect tissue biopsies, and diagnose lung cancer and other lung diseases. The carina, which is a superior projection of the last tracheal ring, is used as a diagnostic tool to determine if an individual has some form of a bronchogenic carcinoma. It becomes distorted and posteriorly widened if the tracheobronchial lymph nodes are enlarged. The mucous membrane overlying the carina is also a very sensitive area of the tracheobronchial tree and is associated with the cough reflex.

Clinical Correlate 2.45

Opacity in Lung Diseases

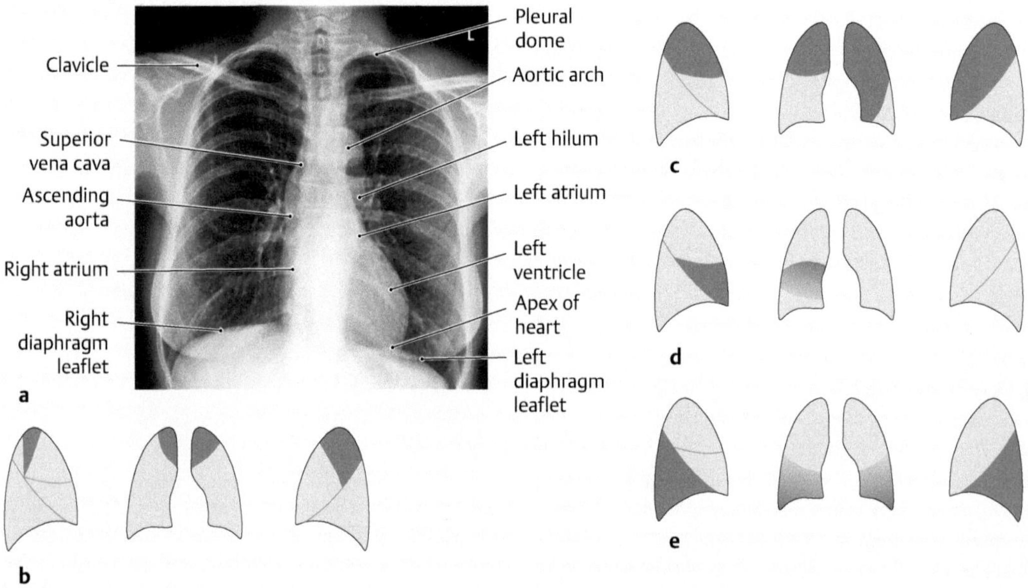

Lateral and anterior views of the right and left lungs. **(a)** Normal posteroanterior chest radiograph. **(b)** Apical segment opacity. **(c)** Upper lobe opacity. **(d)** Middle lobe opacity found only in the right lung. **(e)** Lower lobe opacity. (From Schuenke M, Schulte E, Schumacher U. THIEME Atlas of Anatomy. Internal Organs. Illustrations by Voll M and Wesker K. 1st ed. New York: Thieme Medical Publishers; 2010.)

- Visceral afferent fibers passing back with the *sympathetics* are nociceptive in nature and convey pain impulses due to excessive stretch or chemical irritation.
- Parasympathetics are responsible for:
  - Constricting the bronchioles (bronchoconstrictor).
  - Dilating the pulmonary vessels (vasodilator).
  - Exciting gland secretion (secretomotor).
- Visceral afferent fibers passing back with the *parasympathetics* are reflexive in nature and convey impulses back from:
  - Bronchial mucosa (cough reflexes) and muscles (stretch reception).
  - Interalveolar connective tissue (Hering-Breuer reflexes limiting respiratory excursions).
  - Pulmonary arteries (baroreceptors) and pulmonary veins (chemoreceptors).

2.21 Development of the Lungs

During the 4th week of development and on the anterior wall of the primitive foregut, the **respiratory diverticulum** begins to form (**Fig. 2.85**). The opening of the respiratory diverticulum is known as the **laryngeal orifice** and will lead to further development of the larynx. These details will be discussed during Chapter 7. The most distal end of the respiratory diverticulum enlarges and forms the **lung bud**. The lung bud will form the **trachea** and split into two **bronchial buds**. A definite separation between the trachea and foregut does not form until the **tracheoesophageal folds** begin to form between the respiratory diverticulum and early foregut. The tracheoesophageal folds fuse in the center to form the **tracheoesophageal septum** officially separating the primitive trachea and foregut. The epithelium and glands of the trachea and bronchioles originate from the endoderm. All other tissues of the trachea and bronchioles that include the C-shaped tracheal cartilaginous rings, bronchial cartilage, smooth muscle and surrounding connective tissue are all derived from visceral mesoderm.

At the beginning of the fifth week of development, both of the bronchial buds enlarge and split into the **left** and **right main (primary) bronchi** with the right main bronchus lying more vertical. The left main bronchus further divides into two **lobar (secondary) bronchi** while the right main bronchus divides into three lobar bronchi. The two left lobar bronchi divide into 8-10 **segmental (tertiary) bronchi** while the right lobar bronchi always divide into 10 segmental bronchi. Segmental bronchi are the early

Clinical Correlate 2.46

Diseases of the Lung

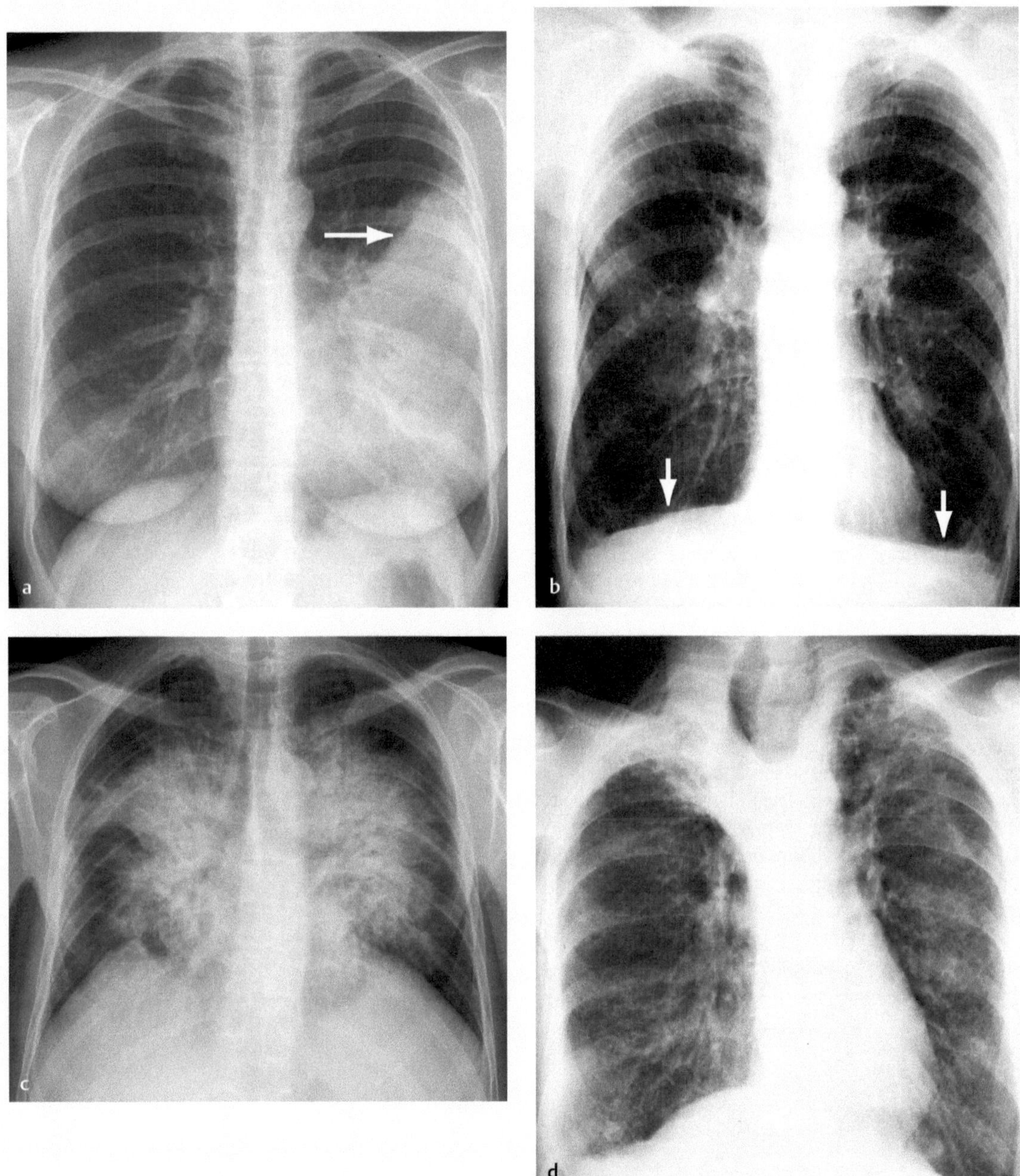

(a) Lingular pneumonia. The arrow shows the boundary between bronchopulmonary segments III and IV. **(b)** Pulmonary pneumonia. Arrows show diaphragmatic dome depression. **(c)** Pulmonary edema complicating acute myocardial infarction. This image shows a butterfly pattern of edema and bilateral pleural effusion. **(d)** Tuberculosis. Note the thickening of the pleura and the radiating fibrous bands. This image does not contain the small pulmonary nodules (tuberculomas) often found in the upper zones of the lung. (From Schuenke M, Schulte E, Schumacher U. THIEME Atlas of Anatomy. Internal Organs. Illustrations by Voll M and Wesker K. 1st ed. New York: Thieme Medical Publishers; 2010.)

bronchopulmonary segments of the lungs that are morphologically and functionally individual respiratory units.

The lung buds expand in the caudal and lateral directions resulting in growth and expansion into the body cavity. The initial spaces for the lungs are the pericardioperitoneal canals and they are narrow and located on each side of the foregut. The pleuropericardial and pleuroperitoneal folds eventually separate the pericardioperitoneal canals from the pericardial and peritoneal cavities respectively. The somatic mesoderm covering the inside of the body wall forms the **parietal pleura** while the visceral mesoderm adjacent to the developing bronchi becomes the **visceral pleura**. The space located between the visceral and parietal pleura is the **pleural cavity**.

The maturation of the lungs occurs in a proximal to distal direction meaning proximal tissue is in a more advanced stage of development versus distal tissue. Bronchioles continuously divide until the seventh prenatal month. From the seventh month, there are sufficient numbers of mature alveolar sacs and capillaries to provide adequate gas exchange in the event the infant is born prematurely. For the remaining two months of prenatal life and extending for several years after birth, the terminal sacs continue to increase at a steady pace as well as the type 1 pneumocytes that surround these sacs become thinner and become more intimate with capillaries thus providing a more efficient blood-air barrier. Lung maturation progresses through four different periods: the **pseudoglandular**, **canalicular**, **terminal sac** and **alveolar periods (Fig. 2.86)**.

- **Pseudoglandular period**: occurs during prenatal weeks 5-16. This period involves numerous *simple columnar epithelial-lined* **endodermal tubules** branching into 15-25 **terminal bronchioles**. No respiratory bronchioles or alveoli are present during this period.
- **Canalicular period**: occurs during prenatal weeks 16-26. This period involves the terminal bronchioles branching into three or more **respiratory bronchioles**. The respiratory bronchioles subsequently divide into as low as 2 or as high as 10 **alveolar ducts**. The terminal bronchioles, respiratory bronchioles and alveolar ducts are now lined with *simple cuboidal epithelium*.
- **Terminal sac period**: occurs from the prenatal week 26 until birth. This period is described as the time when **terminal sacs (primitive alveoli)** sprout from the alveolar ducts and then expand into surrounding mesoderm. **Primary septae** separate the terminal sacs from one another. The simple cuboidal epithelium located here differentiates into type 1 and type 2 pneumocytes. Capillaries within the surrounding mesoderm are in close contact with the terminal sacs and specifically the type 1 pneumocytes and now establish the blood-air barrier.
- **Alveolar period**: occurs from the prenatal week 32 until 8 years of age. This period is when terminal sacs are further separated by **secondary septae** to form mature **alveoli**. The formation of additional secondary septae between the alveoli is what is responsible for the millions of additional alveoli seen in the adult lung. There are approximately 20-70 million alveoi present at birth but by 8 years of age there can be as many as 300-400 million alveoli. The increase in the size of the lung after birth is due to the increase in the number of respiratory bronchioles and not alveoli.

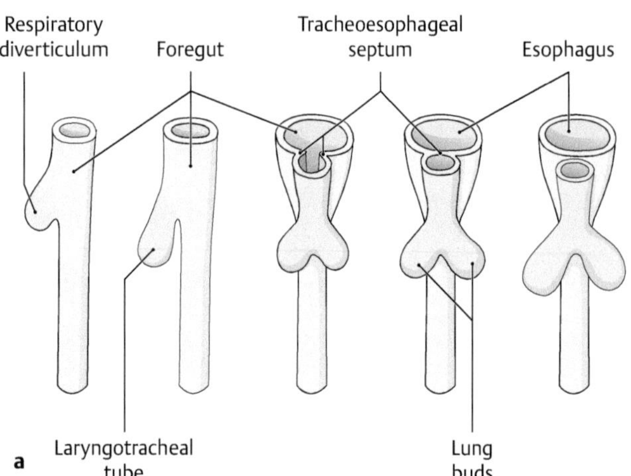

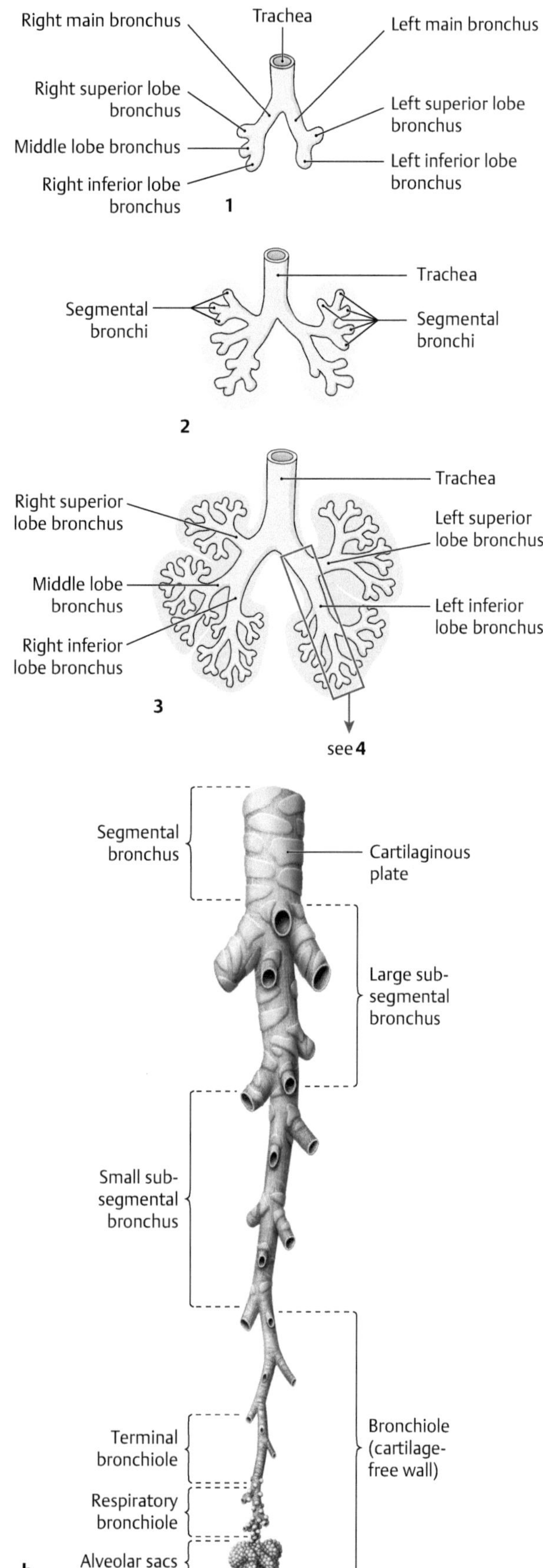

Fig. 2.85 Development of the lungs. **(a)** Development of the trachea and lungs: laryngotracheal tube and lung buds. **(b)** Development of the trachea and lungs: bronchial tree at (1) 5 weeks, (2) 6 weeks, (3) 8 weeks, (4) fully developed. (*continued*) (From Schuenke M, Schulte E, Schumacher U. THIEME Atlas of Anatomy. Internal Organs. Illustrations by Voll M and Wesker K. 3rd ed. New York: Thieme Medical Publishers; 2020.)

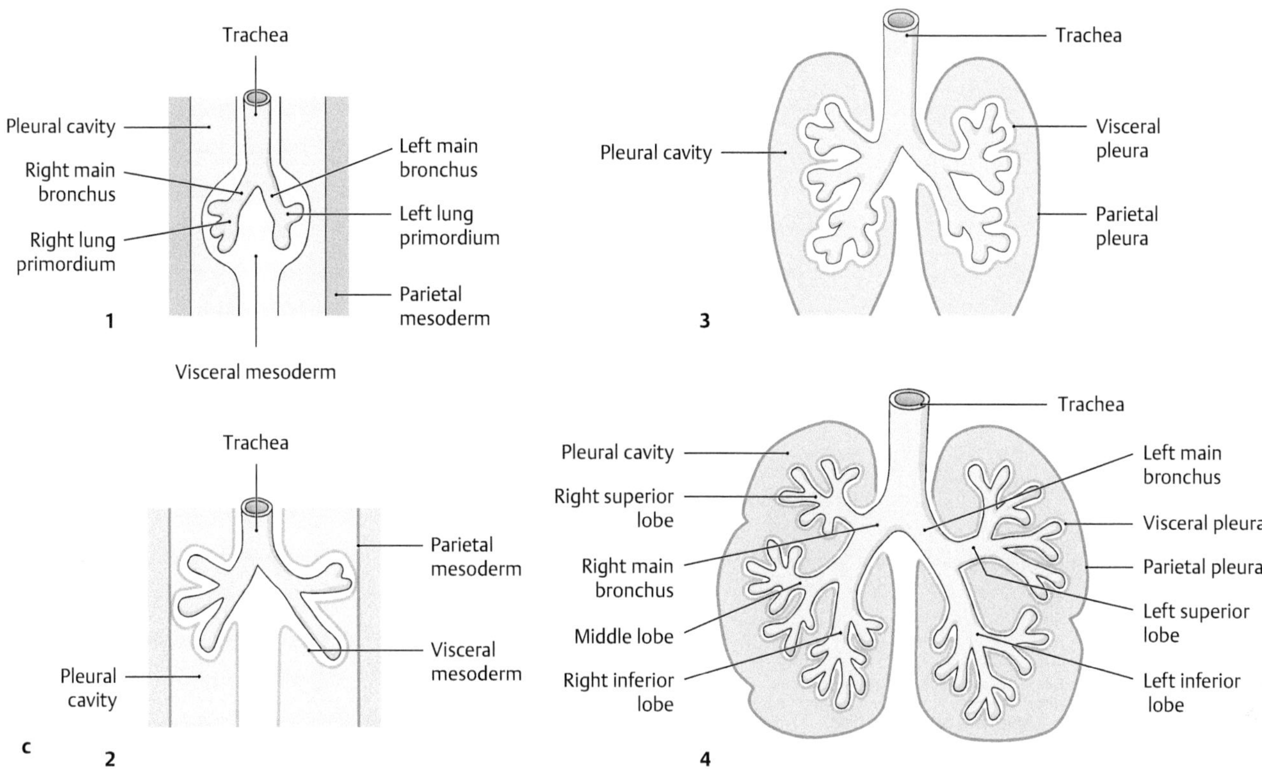

Fig. 2.85 (*continued*) Development of the lungs. **(c)** Development of the trachea and lungs: the pleural cavities. Pleural cavities at 5 weeks (1) and 6 weeks (2). Expanding lung tissue, covered by visceral pleura, progressively filling the parietal pleura lined body cavity (3,4). (From Schuenke M, Schulte E, Schumacher U. THIEME Atlas of Anatomy. Internal Organs. Illustrations by Voll M and Wesker K. 3rd ed. New York: Thieme Medical Publishers; 2020.)

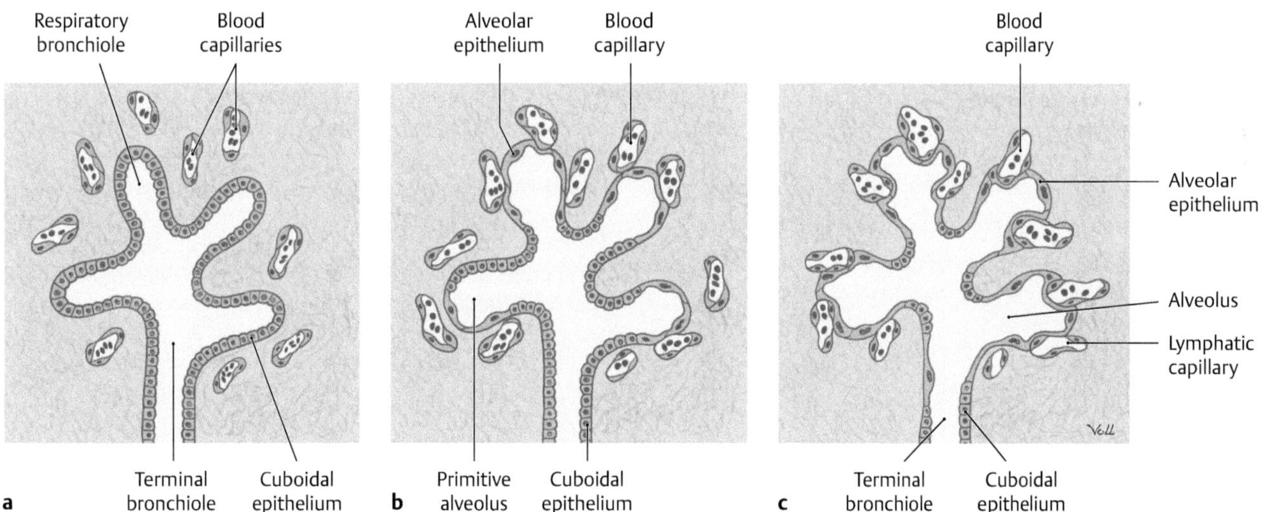

Fig. 2.86 Development of the lungs: alveolar formation and lung maturation. **(a)** Pseudoglandular. **(b)** Canalicular. **(c)** Terminal sac. Note: These phases can overlap. (From Schuenke M, Schulte E, Schumacher U. THIEME Atlas of Anatomy. Internal Organs. Illustrations by Voll M and Wesker K. 3rd ed. New York: Thieme Medical Publishers; 2020.)

2.22 Auscultatory Areas of the Heart and Lungs

Understanding the surface anatomy of the thorax during a physical examination is important for a health care professional so they know where to put their stethoscope in order to hear heart valves and specific lobes of the lung. For the heart valves, there are five specific areas that are used to distinguish valve sounds. The blood carries the sound in the direction of its flow and each auscultatory area is situated superficial to the chamber or vessel into which the blood passes and in a direct line with the valve orifices. Two of these can be used for the pulmonary semilunar valves (or pulmonic areas). Most are located to the left of the sternum (**Fig. 2.87** and **Table 2.3**).

- The **aortic semilunar valve** (or aortic area) is located in the right 2nd intercostal space near the sternum (parasternal).
- The **pulmonary semilunar valve** (or pulmonic area) is located in the left 2nd intercostal space near the sternum.

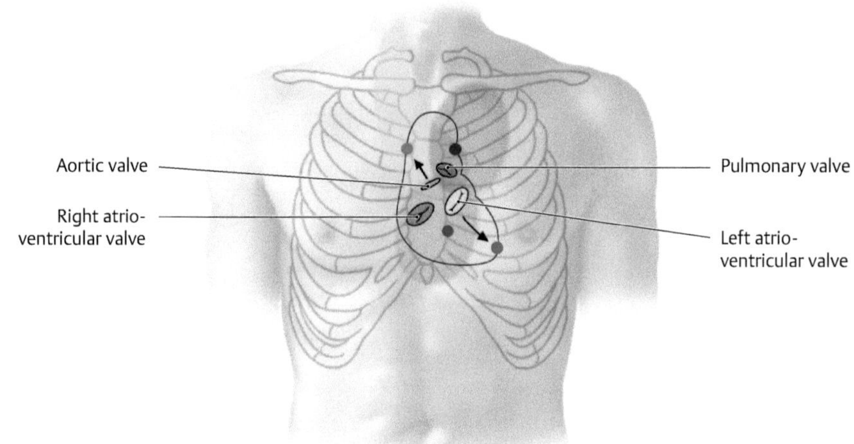

Fig. 2.87 Auscultation of the cardiac valves. (From Schuenke M, Schulte E, Schumacher U. THIEME Atlas of Anatomy. Internal Organs. Illustrations by Voll M and Wesker K. 3rd ed. New York: Thieme Medical Publishers; 2020.)

Table 2.3 **Position and auscultation sites of cardiac valves**

Valve	Anatomical projection	Auscultation site
Aortic valve	Left sternal border (at level of 3rd rib)	Right 2nd intercostal space (at sternal margin)
Pulmonary valve	Left sternal border (at level of 3rd costal cartilage)	Left 2nd intercostal space (at sternal margin)
Bicuspid (mitral) valve	Left 4th/5th costal cartilage	Left 5th intercostal space (at midclavicular line) or cardiac apex
Tricuspid valve	Sternum (at level of 5th costal cartilage)	Left 5th intercostal space (at sternal margin)

- A **second pulmonic area** is located in the left 3rd intercostal space near the sternum.
- The **tricuspid valve** (or tricuspid area) is located at either the left 4th or 5th intercostal spaces near the sternum.
- The **bicuspid (mitral) valve** (or mitral area) is located at the left 5th intercostal space near the midclavicular line just below the nipple.

Recall that the left lung has two lobes while the right lung has three lobes. This is important when trying to listen for sounds within individual lobes. In addition, an individual wants to stay lateral to where they normally would have auscultated for the heart valves.

- The **apex** of each lung, from an anterior or posterior approach, can be heard from within the posterior triangle of the neck.
- The left and right **superior lobes anteriorly**, can be heard at the 2nd intercostal space near the midclavicular line.
- The left and right **superior lobes posteriorly**, can be heard well at the 2nd intercostal space somewhere between the posterior median and scapular lines. Interference from the scapula and vertebral column should be limited.
- The left and right **inferior lobes anteriorly**, can be heard at the 6th intercostal spaces near the anterior axillary line.
- The left and right **inferior lobes posteriorly**, can be heard well somewhere between the 6th and 7th intercostal spaces somewhere between the posterior median and scapular lines similar to the superior lobes.
- The **middle lobe** of the right lung can only be approached from the anterior aspect. It is heard best at the right 4th intercostal space near the midclavicular line adjacent to the nipple.

2.23 Radiology of the Thorax

Most chest x-rays are done as a posteroanterior (PA) projection meaning that the x-rays pass through the patient's thorax from the vertebrae to the sternum. However, when the standard chest x-ray (film) is read it will be from the anteroposterior (AP) view. This remains true for a chest x-ray done as an AP projection. If a lateral projection is done, generally a L or R are placed on the film to indicate the side closest to the film or detector. While viewing in the clinic, it is best to place the lateral projection film pointing towards the patients AP view. If a lesion or some form of pathology is suspected, the side the lesion is located on should point toward the AP view film.

2.23.1 Conventional Radiograph (CR) of the Chest

The *radiodense* structures that absorb or reflect more x-rays on a normal CR include the cardiac silhouette, vertebrae and ribs. By 35 years of age, the costal cartilages should have ossified enough to look more *radiodense*. The **cardiac silhouette** includes the heart and pericardium. Lungs would be considered *radiolucent* because the x-ray beams pass through structures that are less dense.

The **cardiothoracic ratio** is the width of the cardiac silhouette divided by the width of the thoracic cavity in the same plane as the cardiac silhouette being measured. This ratio is approximately 0.5 in normal patients. Useful landmarks on a CR include the **costodiaphragmatic** and **cardiophrenic angles**. These angles should be sharp. If dull, there could be pathology or trauma involved (**Fig. 2.88**).

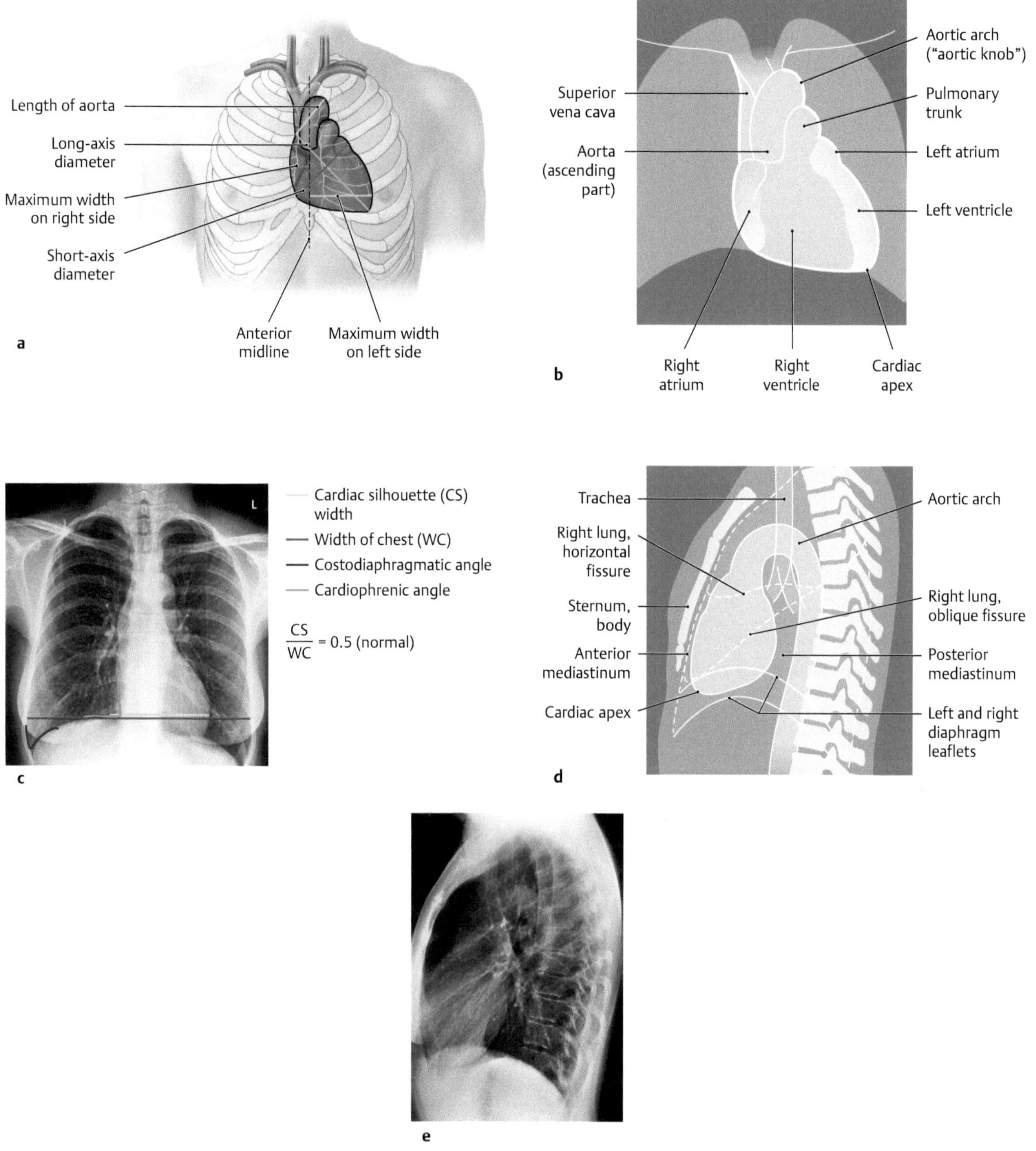

Fig. 2.88 **(a)** Cardiac borders and configurations. **(b)** Radiographic appearance of the heart, anterior view. **(c)** Posteroanterior chest radiograph. **(d)** Lateral view. **(e)** Left lateral chest radiograph. (From Schuenke M, Schulte E, Schumacher U. THIEME Atlas of Anatomy. Internal Organs. Illustrations by Voll M and Wesker K. 2nd ed. New York: Thieme Medical Publishers; 2016.)

2.23.2 CT and MRI of the Thorax

When looking at serial transverse/axial sections of CT or MRI scans, it is important to take note of the vertebral levels to better identify possible pathology. Whether a person is tall or short, vertebral level locations of structures are very consistent. Below are serial sections of a CT scan through the thorax at multiple vertebral levels. Anatomical position refers to an individual standing which means gravity will pull the viscera downward. However, an individual is lying down or in the supine position when they are having a CT scan or MRI done. Vertebral levels will thus correlate with the superior shift of the viscera while the person is supine (**Fig. 2.89; Fig. 2.90**).

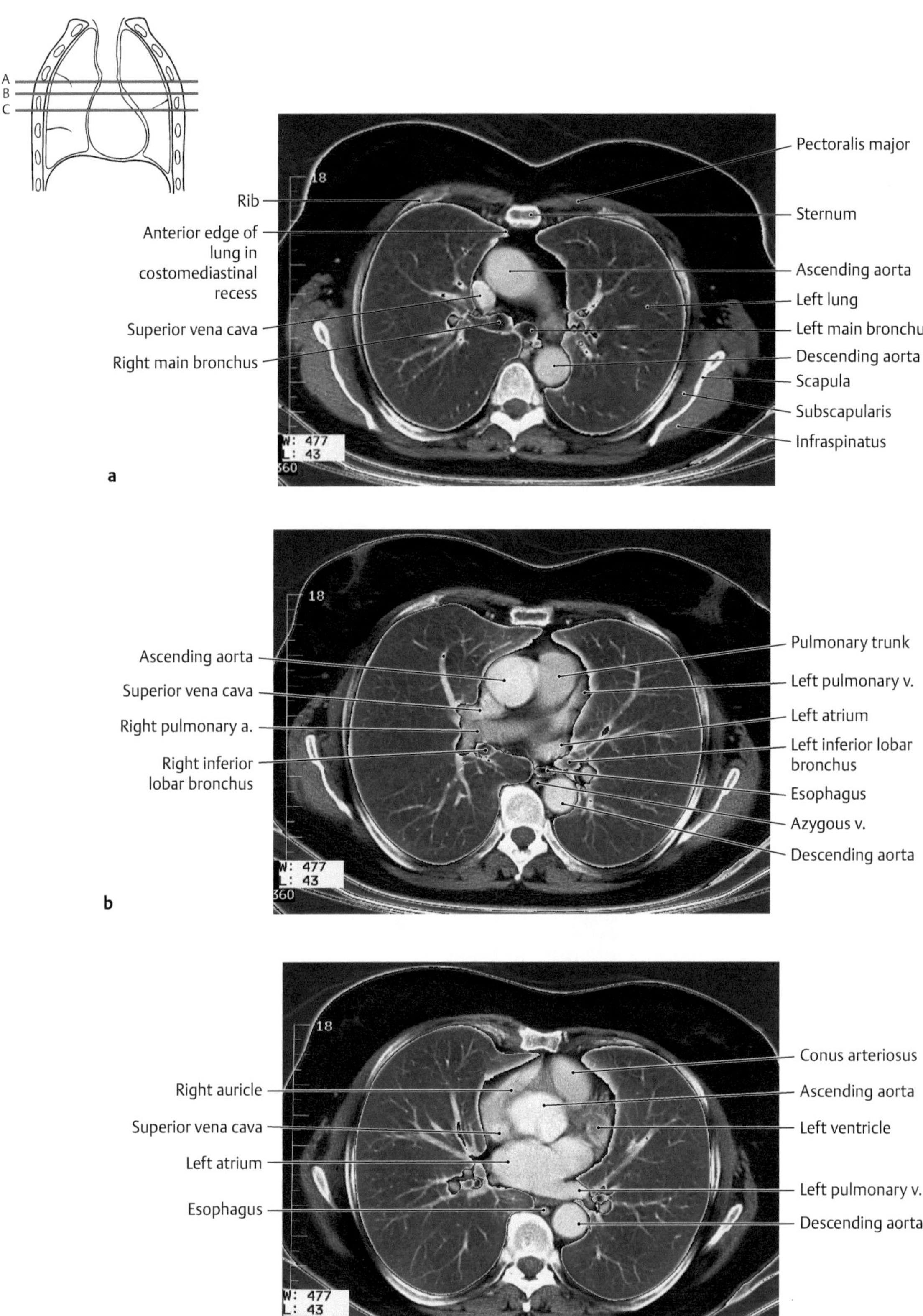

Fig. 2.89 (a-c) CT of the thorax. (*continued*) (From Moeller TB, Reif E. Pocket Atlas of Sectional Anatomy, Vol 2, 4th ed. New York, NY: Thieme; 2014.)

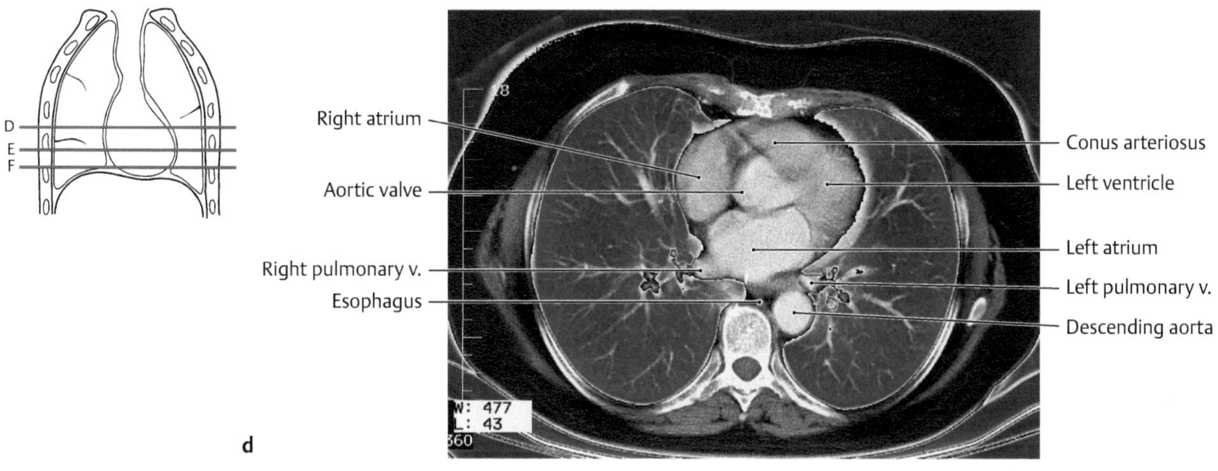

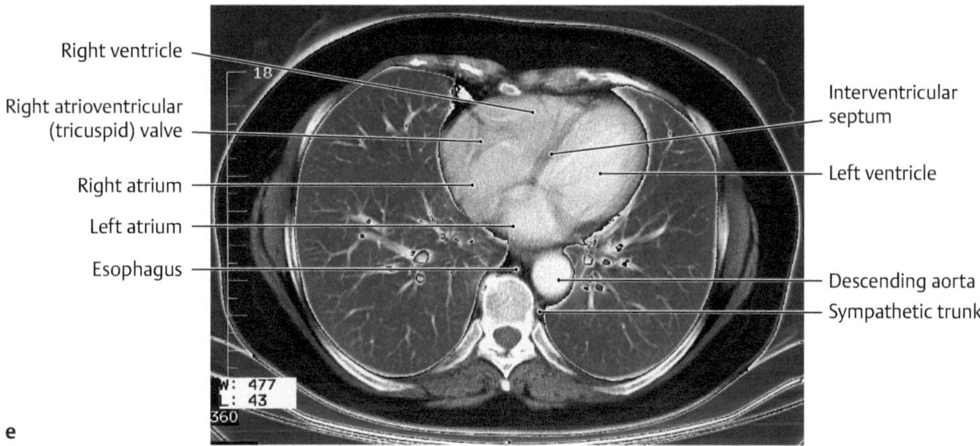

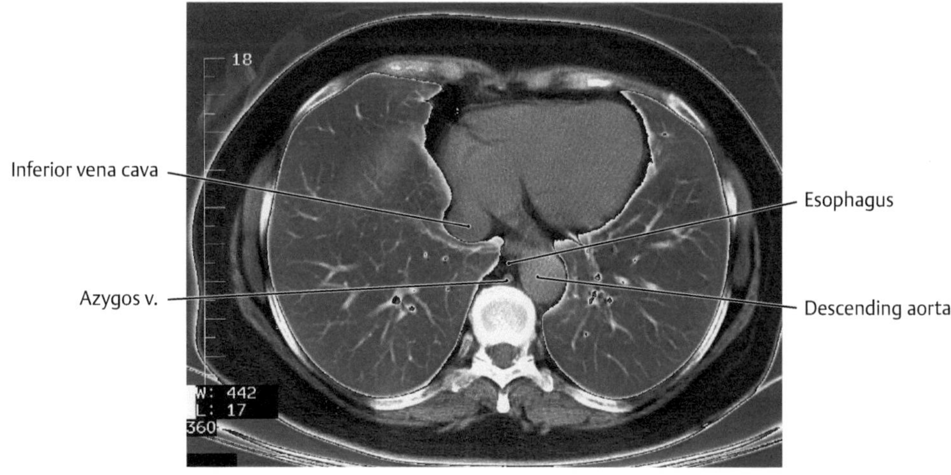

Fig. 2.89 (*continued*) **(d-f)** CT of the thorax. (From Moeller TB, Reif E. Pocket Atlas of Sectional Anatomy, Vol 2, 4th ed. New York, NY: Thieme; 2014.)

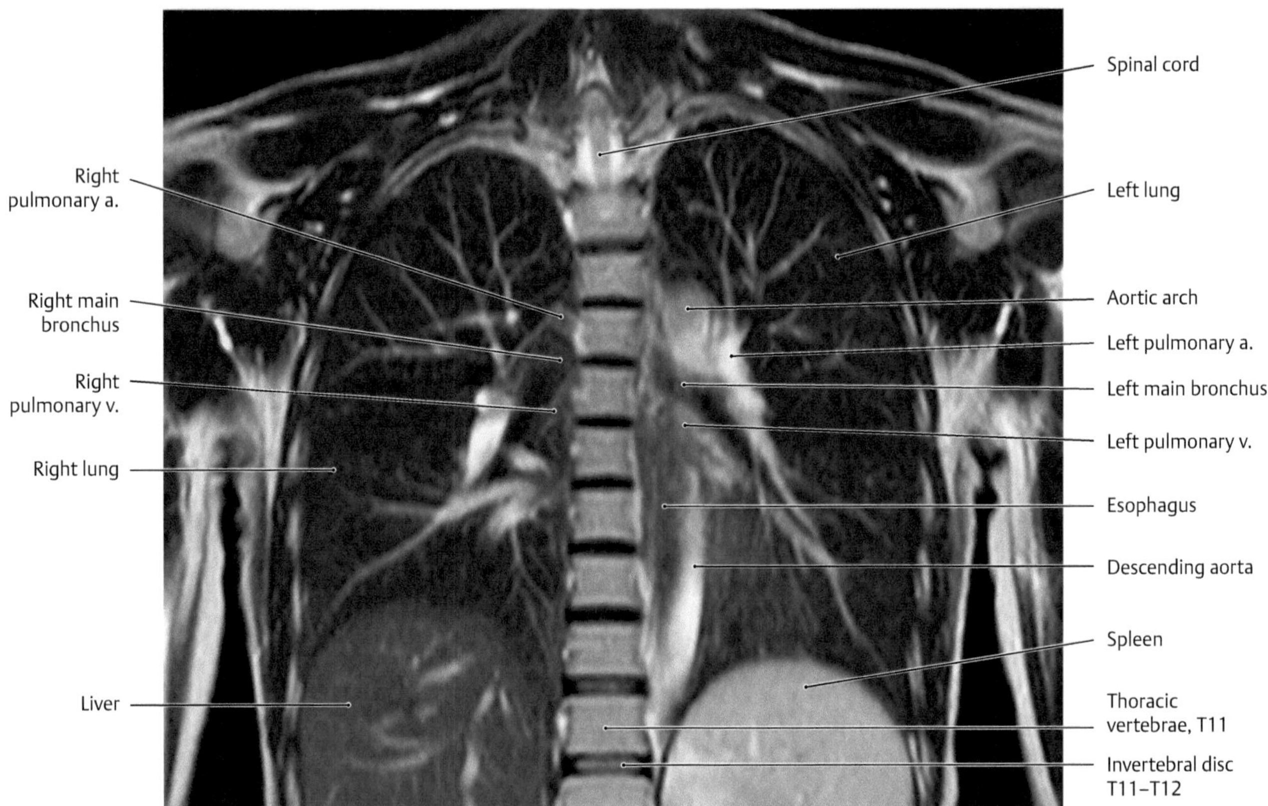

Fig. 2.90 MRI of the thorax. (Moeller TB, Reif E. Pocket Atlas of Sectional Anatomy, Vol 2, 3rd ed. New York, NY: Thieme; 2007.)

2.23.3 Additional Radiology of the Thorax

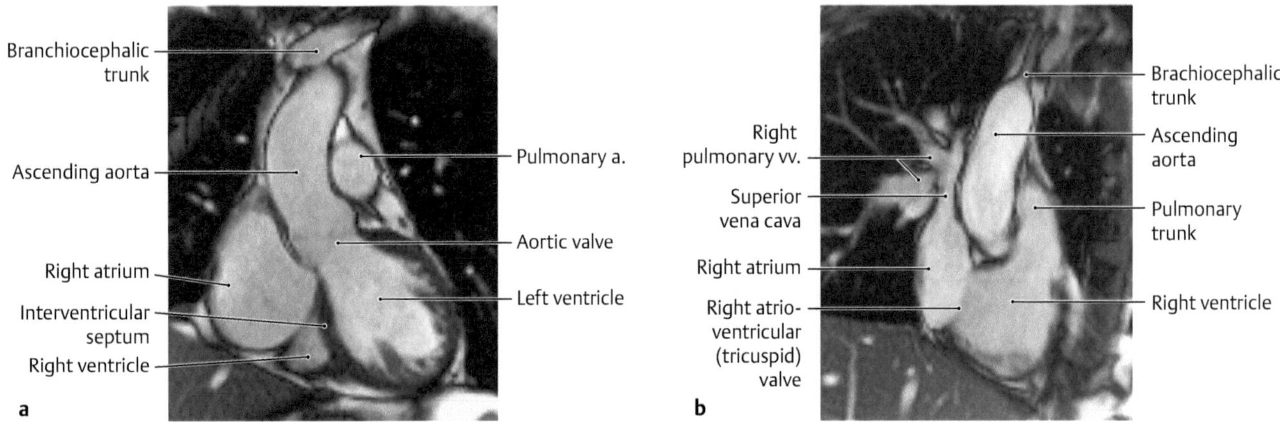

Fig. 2.91 MRI of the heart. **(a)** Left ventricular outflow tract. **(b)** Two chambers of right ventricle. (From Moeller TB, Reif E. Pocket Atlas of Sectional Anatomy, Vol 2, 4th ed. New York, NY: Thieme; 2014.)

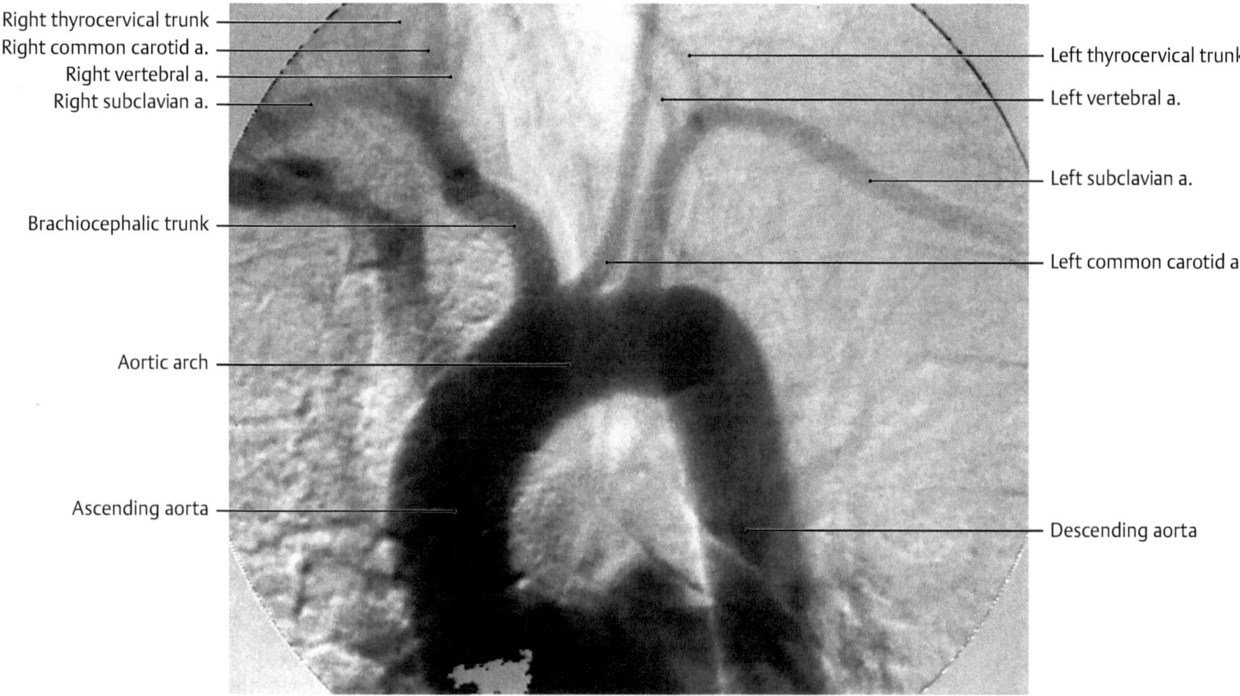

Fig. 2.92 Aortic arch angiogram, left lateral view. (From Moeller TB, Reif E. Pocket Atlas of Sectional Anatomy, Vol 2, 4th ed. New York, NY: Thieme; 2014.)

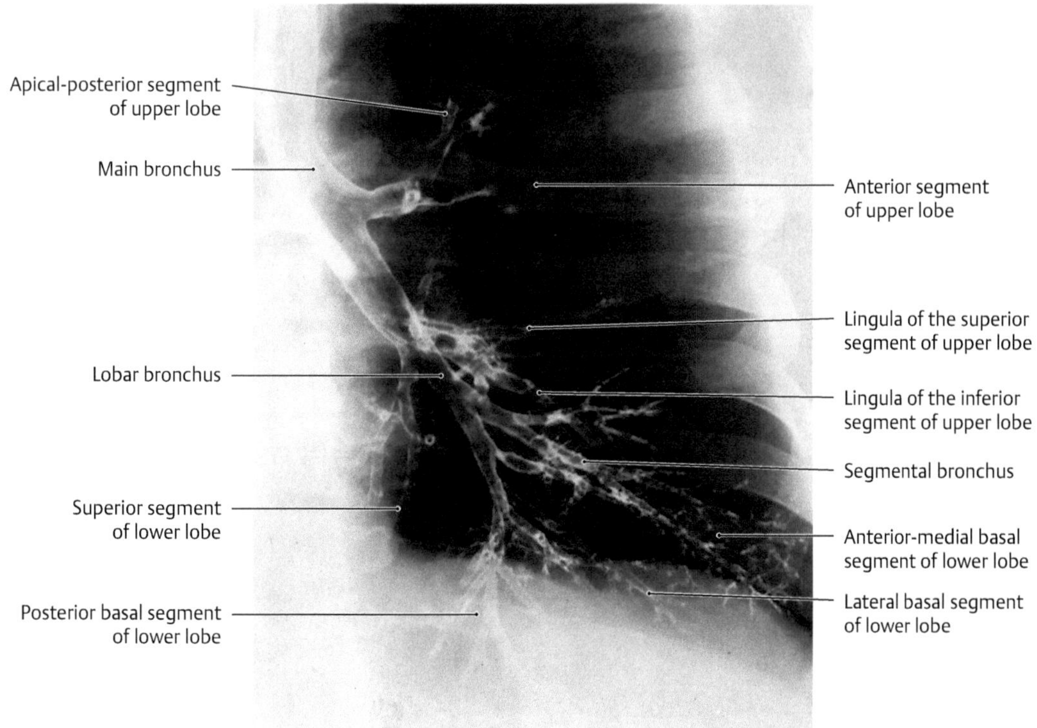

Fig. 2.93 Left bronchogram, anteroposterior view. (From Moeller TB, Reif E. Pocket Atlas of Radiographic Anatomy, 3rd ed. New York, NY: Thieme; 2010.)

QUESTIONS

1. Which statement about the thoracic wall is CORRECT?
   A. Rib fractures most frequently occur just anterior to the angle of the rib.
   B. Ribs 8-10 are considered true ribs.
   C. Demifacets articulate with the tubercle of a rib.
   D. Transverse costal facets articulate with the angle of a rib.
   E. Only the first 3 costal cartilages directly attach to the sternum.
2. During expiration, the vertical, anteroposterior and transverse dimensions will:
   A. Vertical (increase), anteroposterior (decrease), transverse (decrease).
   B. Vertical (increase), anteroposterior (increase), transverse (decrease).
   C. Vertical (increase), anteroposterior (increase), transverse (increase).
   D. Vertical (decrease), anteroposterior (increase), transverse (increase).
   E. Vertical (decrease), anteroposterior (decrease), transverse (decrease).
3. Which statement about the neurovasculature of the thoracic wall is CORRECT?
   A. The NAV orientated neurovasculature is found near the costal groove of the rib.
   B. The lateral thoracic artery is a branch of the 1st part of the axillary artery.
   C. The posterior intercostal and subcostal arteries are branches of the internal thoracic.
   D. The VAN orientated neurovasculature passes between the innermost and internal intercostals.
   E. The internal thoracic artery is a branch of the pericardiacophrenic artery.
4. Of the thoracic wall joints listed, which joint is considered a secondary cartilaginous joint?
   A. Costochondral joints.
   B. 2nd-7th sternocostal joints.
   C. Manubriosternal joint.
   D. Costotransverse joints.
   E. Xiphisternal joint.
5. A 23-year-old male is involved in motor vehicular accident and a few weeks after his discharge from the hospital he is assessed by a physician. The patient prefers to take breaths similar to that of respiration at rest. He is still recovering from his broken ribs but which muscle would function in elevating the ribs and thus possibly increase the patient's pain when he ties to take a deep breath?
   A. Innermost intercostals.
   B. Transversus thoracis.
   C. Internal intercostals.
   D. Subcostals.
   E. External intercostals.
6. Most lymph, especially from the lateral quadrants of the breast, drains to the ________ of the axillary lymph nodes.
   A. Central lymph nodes.
   B. Pectoral (anterior) lymph nodes.
   C. Humeral (lateral) lymph nodes.
   D. Subscapular (posterior) lymph nodes.
   E. Apical lymph nodes.
7. Which statement about the pericardium is INCORRECT?
   A. The phrenic nerves are the primary source of sensory fibers.
   B. The pericardial cavity is found between the parietal & visceral serous pericardium.
   C. The parietal and visceral serous pericardium adhere to the epicardium of the heart.
   D. The fibrous pericardium is the tough external layer that is unyielding and firm.
   E. The transverse pericardial sinus is found posterior to the pulmonary trunk and aorta but anterior to the superior vena cava.
8. A 45-year-old patient has come in for his yearly checkup. During his physical examination the physician listens to the valves of his heart with a stethoscope. In what location would the aortic semilunar valve be heard?
   A. Right 2nd intercostal space near the sternum.
   B. Left 2nd intercostal space near the sternum.
   C. Left 3rd intercostal space near the sternum.
   D. Left 4th or 5th intercostal spaces near the sternum.
   E. Left 5th intercostal space near the midclavicular line.
9. Which statement about the heart chambers is CORRECT?
   A. The tendinous cords attach to the semilunar valves.
   B. Trabeculae carneae are located in both left and right ventricles.
   C. The tricuspid valve is found between the left atrium and left ventricle.
   D. The septomarginal trabecula (moderator band) carries the left bundle branches of the conducting system to the anterior papillary muscle of the left ventricle.
   E. The SA is located in the interatrial septum near the opening of the coronary sinus.
10. Which statement about the coronary vessels is CORRECT?
   A. The left coronary is the dominant coronary artery 85% of the time.
   B. The posterior interventricular (PDA) artery is paired with the small cardiac vein.
   C. The right coronary and its branches supply the anterior 2/3 of the interventricular septum, AV bundle branches, and the SA node 40% of the time.
   D. The anterior interventricular (LAD) artery is paired with the great cardiac vein.
   E. The left coronary bifurcates into a circumflex and posterior interventricular (PDA) artery.
11. A 66-year-old male is scheduled to have triple bypass surgery. One of the bypasses will pass over the proximal circumflex artery near the bifurcation of the left coronary artery. Of all the major sites for a coronary occlusion to occur, how common is it to be seen at the proximal circumflex artery?
   A. The most.
   B. 2nd most.
   C. 3rd most.
   D. 4th most.
   E. 5th most.
12. A newborn appears to have cyanosis or a bluish discoloration of the skin due to inadequate oxygenation of the blood. Although there are many causes of being born with cyanosis that are related to the heart specifically, what is the most common congenital heart defect?
   A. Patent ductus arteriosus.
   B. Atrial septal defect.
   C. Tetralogy of Fallot.
   D. Ventricular septal defect.
   E. Transposition of the great arteries.

13. What is the main function of the ductus venous during fetal life?
    A. Provides a bypass for blood from the right atrium to the left atrium.
    B. Diverts blood away from the liver.
    C. Allows blood to bypass the lungs.
    D. Diverts blood into the liver.
    E. Returns blood back to the fetus.

14. A newborn has cyanosis or a bluish tint to the skin for some time after being born. A heart murmur is first detected and an echocardiogram is then ordered to identify any problem with the way the heart is formed or functioning. The newborn is diagnosed with tetralogy of Fallot. Which defect is NOT seen in tetralogy of Fallot?
    A. Pulmonary stenosis.
    B. Interventricular septal defect.
    C. Hypertrophy of the right ventricle.
    D. Overriding aorta.
    E. Aortic stenosis.

15. During development, fetal circulation is known to have 5 areas where mixing of the oxygenated and poorly oxygenated blood occur. Which area is known to be the 2nd site for which mixing of the blood would occur?
    A. Inferior vena cava.
    B. Liver.
    C. Left atrium.
    D. Near the ductus arteriosus.
    E. Right atrium.

16. Which statement about the surface anatomy of the lung is CORRECT?
    A. The left lung has the groove for the arch of the azygos vein.
    B. The right lung has the groove for the arch of the aorta.
    C. The pulmonary artery is superior to the main bronchus on the left lung.
    D. The horizontal fissure is located on the left lung.
    E. The pulmonary artery is posterior to the main bronchus on the right lung.

17. A 62-year-old female who has smoked most of her life comes into the clinic and describes that she has had difficulty breathing after long walks for the past few months. A CT scan is performed and it is confirmed that she has stage 3 lung cancer and the cancerous lesions are located on the ipsilateral side near the periphery next to the ribs and adjacent to the root of the lung. If the masses have spread from both superficial and deep structures, at what set of lymph nodes do the superficial and deep lymphatic plexuses draining the lung meet before continuing superiorly toward the neck?
    A. Pulmonary lymph nodes.
    B. Bronchopulmonary (hilar) lymph nodes.
    C. Inferior tracheobronchial lymph nodes.
    D. Superior tracheobronchial lymph nodes.
    E. Bronchomediastinal trunks.

18. A 55-year-old male has been diagnosed with lung cancer. A CT scan confirms that multiple masses are located in both the superior and inferior lingular bronchopulmonary segments. If surgery was performed, which specific lung lobe would the surgeon need to focus on?
    A. Superior lobe of left lung.
    B. Inferior lobe of left lung.
    C. Superior lobe of right lung.
    D. Middle lobe of right lung.
    E. Inferior lobe of right lung.

19. A 31-year-old male has received a deep penetrating wound while working in a factory. The wound is so deep it has severed the white rami communicantes at the T8 location. What combination of the following nerve fibers would have been damaged?
    A. Sympathetic/postganglionic, parasympathetic/preganglionic, visceral sensory.
    B. Parasympathetic/postganglionic, visceral sensory.
    C. Visceral sensory only.
    D. Sympathetic/preganglionic, parasympathetic/preganglionic.
    E. Sympathetic/preganglionic, visceral sensory.

20. A 44-year-old had a chest X-ray performed after the individual presents with shortness of breath. It is discovered that they have pleural effusion or an abnormal amount of fluid in the pleural cavity surrounding the lung. The physician would like to do a thoracentesis for analysis of this fluid. If remaining on the midaxillary line, what intercostal space would be the best space to target for aspirating a sample of this fluid?
    A. 1st.
    B. 3rd.
    C. 4th.
    D. 6th.
    E. 8th.

21. A medical student is learning how to properly use a stethoscope by listening to heart sounds. She recognizes the continuous and characteristic "lub" and "dub" sounds. What two valves close almost simultaneously to create the second or "dub" sound?
    A. Tricuspid and pulmonary valves.
    B. Aortic and tricuspid valves.
    C. Aortic and pulmonary valves.
    D. Tricuspid and bicuspid/mitral valves.
    E. Pulmonary and bicuspid/mitral valves.

22. Which statement about the posterior mediastinum is CORRECT?
    A. The greater splanchnic nerve contains parasympathetic preganglionic fibers.
    B. The first esophageal constriction occurs at T10 near the diaphragm.
    C. The hemiazygos vein receives blood from the right 9-11th posterior intercostal and subcostal veins.
    D. The azygos vein drains into the superior vena cava.
    E. The thoracic aorta passes posterior to the diaphragm at vertebral level T8 to become the abdominal aorta.

23. Which statement involving the lungs and pleura is CORRECT?
    A. The carina of the trachea is located at the C6 vertebral level.
    B. Parasympathetic innervation constricts the bronchioles.
    C. Type I pneumocytes produce and secrete surfactant.
    D. Bronchial arteries are located on the anterior surface of the bronchi.
    E. Type II pneumocytes contribute to the blood-air barrier.

24. A 2-month-old baby is initially brought into her pediatrician's office because she seems very lethargic, has a poor appetite, and the baby's skin and nails have cyanosis or a bluish discoloration. She is referred to a pediatric cardiologist and a chest X-ray demonstrates an enlarged heart, in addition to cardiac catheterization identifying a coronary artery anomaly. Which is the most consistent coronary artery anomaly to present in this situation?
    A. A single right coronary arising from the aorta.
    B. Left coronary artery arising from the (opposite) right aortic sinus.
    C. Circumflex artery arising from the right main coronary artery.

D. Right coronary artery arising from the (opposite) left aortic sinus.
E. Left coronary artery arising from the pulmonary trunk.

25. A 24-year-old college football player collides with an opponent and takes most of the blunt force near the sternum. The player complains of a deep pain and leaves the game to have an X-ray taken at the nearby hospital. The player does not have any rib fractures but is diagnosed with a rib dislocation. At what joint do rib dislocations occur?
A. Costochondral joint.
B. Costotransverse joint.
C. Sternocostal joint.
D. Xiphisternal joint.
E. Manubriosternal joint.

ANSWERS

1. **A.** The most common location for a rib fracture to occur is just anterior to the angle of the rib.
B. Ribs 8-10 are false ribs.
C. Demifacets articulate with the heads of ribs.
D. Transverse costal facets articulate with the tubercle of a rib.
E. The first 7 costal cartilages directly attach to the sternum.

2. **E.** During expiration, all three different dimensions of the thoracic wall decrease as a combined unit. During inspiration, all three dimensions increase together.

3. **D.** The VAN orientated neurovasculature passes between the innermost and internal intercostals.
A. The NAV orientated neurovasculature is located on the superior border of the rib.
B. The lateral thoracic artery is a branch of the 2nd part of the axillary artery.
C. The posterior intercostal and subcostal arteries are branches thoracic aorta. The 1st and 2nd posterior intercostals originate from the superior intercostal, a branch of the costocervical trunk.
E. The internal thoracic artery is a branch of the 1st part of the subclavian artery.

4. **C.** The manubriosternal joint is a secondary cartilaginous joint.
A. The costochondral joints are primary cartilaginous joints.
B. The 2nd-7th sternocostal joints are plane type synovial joints. The 1st sternocostal joint is a primary cartilaginous joint.
D. The costotransverse joints are plane type synovial joints.
E. The xiphisternal joint is a primary cartilaginous joint.

5. **E.** The external intercostals elevate the ribs while all of the other muscles listed are depressors of the ribs.

6. **B.** Most lymph from the lateral quadrants of the breast drains to the pectoral (anterior) lymph nodes.

7. **C.** All statements are correct except for C. The visceral pericardium is also known as the epicardium. The parietal and visceral serous pericardiums are separated from one another by the pericardial cavity and the serous fluid that fills it. These two layers are only connected at sites of reflections found near the aorta, superior vena cava and pulmonary vessels.

8. **A.** The aortic semilunar valve is located at the right 2nd intercostal space near the sternum.
B. (Pulmonary semilunar valve) right 2nd intercostal space near the midclavicular line.
C. (Second pulmonic area) left 3rd intercostal space near the sternum.
D. (Tricuspid valve) left 4th or 5th intercostal spaces near the sternum.
E. (Bicuspid/mitral valve) left 5th intercostal space near the midclavicular line.

9. **B.** The trabeculae carneae are located in both the left and right ventricles.
A. The tendinous cords attach to the either the tricuspid or bicuspid/mitral valves located at the atrioventricular junctions and not the semilunar valves.
C. The tricuspid valve is found between the right atrium and right ventricle.
D. The septomarginal trabecula (moderator band) carries the right bundle branches of the conducting system to the anterior papillary muscle of the left ventricle.
E. The SA node is located just deep to the epicardium near the superior end of the sulcus terminalis and at the junction of the SVC and right atrium. The AV node is located in the interatrial septum near the opening of the coronary sinus.

10. **D.** The anterior interventricular (Left Anterior Descending) artery is paired with the great cardiac vein.
A. The right coronary is the dominant coronary artery 85% of the time.
B. The posterior interventricular (PDA) artery is paired with the middle cardiac vein.
C. The left coronary and its branches supply the anterior 2/3 of the interventricular septum, AV bundle branches, and the SA node 40% of the time.
E. The left coronary bifurcates into a circumflex and anterior interventricular (LDA) artery.

11. **C.** The proximal circumflex is the 3rd most common site of coronary occlusion.
A. Most common site of occlusion is the proximal anterior interventricular (LAD) near the left coronary artery bifurcation.
B. The 2nd most common site is the proximal right coronary artery near its attachment to the ascending aorta.
D. The 4th most common site is the distal left coronary artery just prior to it bifurcating into the anterior interventricular (LAD) and circumflex arteries.
E. The 5th most common site is the proximal posterior interventricular (PDA) near the termination of the right coronary artery.

12. **D.** The most common congenital heart defect is a ventricular septal defect.

13. **B.** The ductus venous diverts blood away from the liver.
A. The oval foramen (*foramen ovale*) provides a bypass for blood from the right atrium to the left atrium.
C. The ductus arteriosus allows blood to bypass the lungs.
D. The portal vein diverts blood into the liver.
E. The umbilical arteries returns blood back to the fetus.

14. **E.** All listed defects are seen with tetralogy of Fallot except for aortic stenosis.

15. **A.** The inferior vena cava is the 2nd site of mixing of the blood.
B. Liver (1st).
C. Left atrium (4th).
D. Near the ductus arteriosus (5th).
E. Right atrium (3rd).

16. **C.** The pulmonary artery is superior to the main bronchus on the left lung.
A. The right lung has the groove for the arch of the azygos vein.
B. The left lung has the groove for the arch of the aorta.

D. The horizontal fissure is located on the right lung.
E. The pulmonary artery is anterior to the main bronchus on the right lung.

17. **B.** The superficial (directly) and deep lymphatic (via the pulmonary lymph nodes) plexuses both drain lymph to bronchopulmonary (hilar) lymph nodes and hence the spread of cancer could continue superiorly from this point and up into the neck.

18. **A.** The superior lobe of the left lung is the only lobe of the lungs that contains a superior and inferior lingular bronchopulmonary segment.

19. **E.** The nerve fibers that pass through a white rami communicantes, located between T1-L2 levels of the sympathetic trunk, would always be sympathetic preganglionic (sym/pre) and visceral sensory (GVA). The GVA fibers are visceral pain in nature since they are paired with sympathetic fibers. These visceral pain fibers are associated with referred pain.

20. **E.** The most common location to aspirate fluid with a thoracentesis is the 8th or 9th intercostal space near the midaxillary line. The needle enters the costodiaphragmatic recess of the pleural cavity.

21. **C.** The second or "dub" sound is created by the aortic and pulmonary semilunar valves closing. The first or "lub" sound would have been caused by the tricuspid and bicuspid/mitral valves closing together.

22. **D.** The azygos vein drains into the superior vena cava.
A. The greater splanchnic nerve contains sympathetic preganglionic and visceral sensory fibers.
B. The first esophageal constriction occurs at vertebral level C6.
C. The hemiazygos vein receives blood from the left 9-11th posterior intercostal and subcostal veins.
E. The thoracic aorta passes posterior to the diaphragm at vertebral level T12 to become the abdominal aorta.

23. **B.** Parasympathetic innervation constricts the bronchioles.
A. The carina of the trachea is located at the T4/T5 vertebral level.
C. Type II pneumocytes are the cells that produce and secrete surfactant.
D. Bronchial arteries are generally located on the posterior surface of the bronchi.
E. Type II pneumocytes do not contribute to the blood-air barrier but Type I does.

24. **E.** Most coronary anomalies do not present any clinical complications until adulthood and may not be diagnosed until after a coronary angiogram has been performed or after a sudden death autopsy. A left coronary artery arising from the pulmonary trunk will usually present at birth after the patient begins showing signs of left ventricular insufficiency. This anomaly is usually isolated and can be surgically fixed, but it can be associated with other congenital heart defects, such as Tetralogy of Fallot.

25. **C.** The sternocostal joints are the sites of rib dislocations but they may also involve the interchondral joints located between costal cartilages of the 6-10th ribs. Rib dislocations are also known as *slipping rib syndrome*. Alternatively, rib separations generally involve one or more of the 3rd-10th costochondral joints.

References

1. Torrent-Guasp et al. The structure and function of the helical heart and its buttress wrapping. I. The normal macroscopic structure of the heart, Semin Thorac Cardiovasc Surg. 2001. 13:301–19.
2. Standring S, ed., Gray's Anatomy: The Anatomical Basis of Clinical Practice, 40th ed. 2008.
3. Wikenheiser et al. Altered hypoxia-inducible factor-1 alpha levels correlate with coronary artery anomalies, Dev Dynam. 2009. 238:2688-2700.
4. Angelini P. Coronary Artery Anomalies: An Entity in Search of an Identity. Circulation. 2007. 115: 1296-1305.

3 Abdomen

LEARNING OBJECTIVES

- To understand how to identify underlying structures through abdominal quadrants or regions. Know the different planes that help define a quadrant versus regions.
- To understand the muscles, rectus sheathes, and neurovasculature of the anterior abdominal wall.
- To understand the inguinal region and the structures that contirbute to the spermatic cord. Clinical correlates that relate to the inguinal region and spermatic cord will include a hematocele, hydrocele, and the difference between direct and indirect hernias.
- To understand the neurovasculature and histology of the testes and the process of spermatogenesis versus spermiogenesis. Clinical correlates include a look at testicular cancer and the vasectomy procedure.
- To understand the relationship between peritoneum and the viscera and why these organs are referred to as intraperitoneal, primarily retroperitoneal, secondarily retroperitoneal or subperitoneal. There will be an understanding of the different types of double layered peritoneum and how they are connected to the viscera.
- To understand the digestive system and the five different processes involved in digestion. Be able to describe the difference between segmentation and peristalsis and the general histology of the gastrointestinal tract.
- To describe the gross structure, histology and neurovasculature associated with structures of the foregut. Clinical correlates include a look at esophageal varices, helicobacter pylori, gastric and duodenal ulcers, cirrhosis of the liver, portal hypertension, gallstones, pancreatitis and splenomegaly.
- To describe the gross structure, histology and neurovasculature associated with structures of the midgut. Clinical correlates include a look at appendicitis.
- To describe the gross structure, histology and neurovasculature associated with structures of the hindgut. Clinical correlates include a look at constipation, colorectal cancer, diverticulosis and hemorrhoids.
- To understand how the foregut, midgut and hindgut all develop and related clinical correlates such as esophageal atresia, gastroschisis, omphalocele and Hirschsprung's disease.
- To describe the diaphragm and all other muscles of the posterior abdominal wall. Have an understanding of the lumbar plexus and the specific nerves associated with it.
- To describe the gross structure, histology and development of the viscera found on the posterior abdominal wall, including the suprarenal gland, kidney and ureter. Clinical correlates include Addison disease, polycystic kidney disease, renal and ureteric calculi.
- To understand the autonomic innervation to the abdominal viscera and the pathway of individual sympathetic and parasympathetic fibers through the aortic plexus. Describe the individual splanchnic nerves and their target sections of the abdominal viscera and understand the connection with the enteric nervous system.

The anatomical trunk consists of the thorax, abdomen and pelvis with the **abdomen** located between the other two. It contains the majority of the **gastrointestional (GI) tract** and a portion of the urogenital system. All GI tract organs are contained within the larger and continuous *abdominopelvic cavity* by an anterolateral musculo-aponeurotic wall, the diaphragm and pelvic muscles. Voluntary or reflexive contractions of the anterolateral wall, diaphragm and pelvic floor muscles can increase the internal intra-abdominal pressure thus aiding in the removal of urine, feces and even air through the thoracic cavity (**Fig. 3.1**).

The abdominopelvic cavity is made up of a larger and superiorly placed abdominal cavity and a smaller and inferiorly placed pelvic cavity thus extending from the thoracic diaphragm to the pelvic diaphragm. An arbitrary plane called the pelvic inlet separates the abdominal and pelvic cavities from one another. The abdominal cavity is located as high as the 4th intercostal space with a good portion of the upper GI tract and spleen being protected by the thoracic cage.

3.1 Abdominal Planes, Quadrants, and Regions

While viewing the surface anatomy of the anterolateral abdominal wall, it is important to understand that this region can be divided into quadrants or regions. The *quadrants* are formed by two planes and are more general if pain is being described. The *regions* are formed by four planes and are more specific in describing pain or surgical manipulation. Understanding clinically which organs can be palpated and auscultated in a particular quadrant or region helps during a physical examination.

The median and transumbilical planes form **abdominal quadrants (Fig. 3.2)**. The **median plane** is vertical and extends from the xiphoid process down to the pubic symphysis and will divide it into a left and right half. The **transumbilical plane** passes through the area of the umbilicus that is located at the IV disk between the L3 and L4 vertebrae and creates an upper versus lower quadrant. Collectively theses planes create a left upper (LUQ), right upper (RUQ), left lower (LLQ) and right lower (RLQ) quadrant. Organs located in these individual quadrants are listed in **Table 3.1**.

Four planes, of which two are vertical and two are horizontal, form a total of nine **abdominal regions**. The vertical planes include a left and right **midclavicular plane** that extends from the *mid-clavicle* down to the *midinguinal point* located between a line connecting the *anterior superior iliac spine (ASIS)* and *pubic tubercle*. The horizontal planes include the subcostal plane and transtubercular plane. The **subcostal plane** passes across and connects the inferior borders of the 10th costal cartilages of the thoracic cage. The **transtubercular plane** passes through the body of the L5 vertebra and connects the iliac tubercles. Additional terminology used by clinicians to describe these horizontal planes includes the transpyloric and interspinous planes. The **transpyloric plane** is located at the level of the 9th costal cartilages and 1st lumbar vertebra. This plane is also approximately located between the jugular notch and pubic symphysis. The 1st lumbar vertebra represents the termination of the adult spinal cord, locations of the pyloric region of the stomach, 1st part of the duodenum, origin of portal vein and the superior mesenteric artery off of the aorta, hilum of the kidneys, neck of the pancreas, and the fundus of the gallbladder, among some other additional structures. The **interspinous plane** connects the anterior superior iliac spines. The regions are named accordingly: epigastric, left and right hypochondriac, umbilical, left and right lumbar, pubic (hypogastric), left and right inguinal (**Fig. 3.2**).

3.2 Anterolateral Abdominal Wall

The abdominal wall is continuous from anterior to posterior. It is divided into an anterolateral and posterior abdominal wall for descriptive purposes. The anterolateral wall is musculo-aponeurotic and is bounded by the xiphoid process and cartilages of the 7th – 10th ribs superiorly and the anterolateral aspects of the pelvic girdle and inguinal ligament inferiorly. Contents of this wall include skin, subcutaneous (superficial) fascia, three musculotendinous layers, deep fascia, extraperitoneal fat and parietal

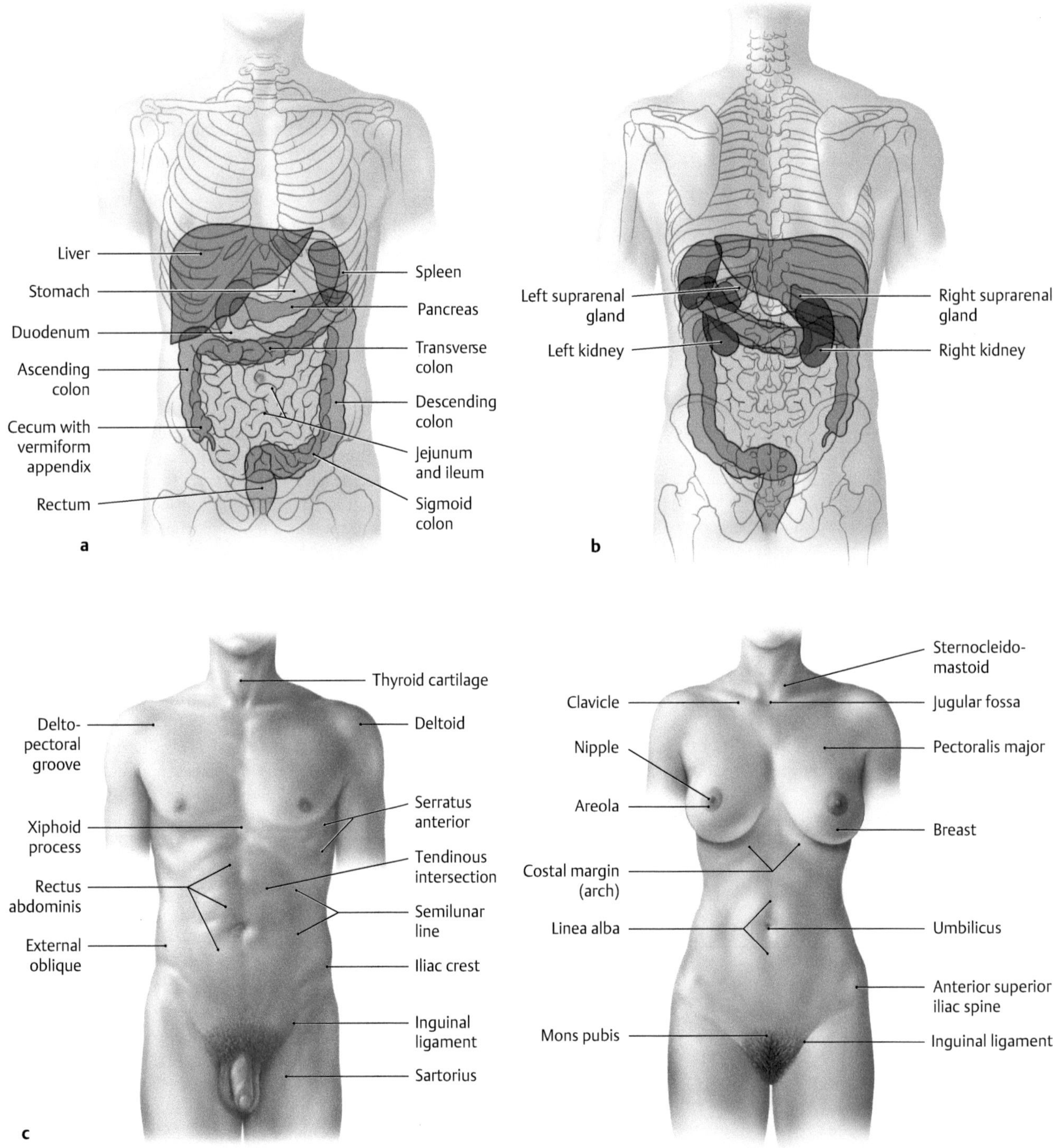

Fig. 3.1 Projection of the abdominal and pelvic organs onto the **(a)** anterior trunk wall and **(b)** posterior trunk wall. **(c)** Surface anatomy of the anterior trunk wall. (*continued*) (From Schuenke M, Schulte E, Schumacher U. THIEME Atlas of Anatomy. Internal Organs. Illustrations by Voll M and Wesker K. 3rd ed. New York: Thieme Medical Publishers; 2020, and General Anatomy and Musculoskeletal System. Illustrations by Voll M and Wesker K. 3rd ed. New York: Thieme Medical Publishers; 2020.)

Fig. 3.1 (*continued*) **(d)** Criteria for dividing the abdomen into regions. **(e)** Projection of the abdominal organs onto the four quadrants of the anterior abdominal wall. (From Schuenke M, Schulte E, Schumacher U. THIEME Atlas of Anatomy. General Anatomy and Musculoskeletal System. Illustrations by Voll M and Wesker K. 3rd ed. New York: Thieme Medical Publishers; 2020.)

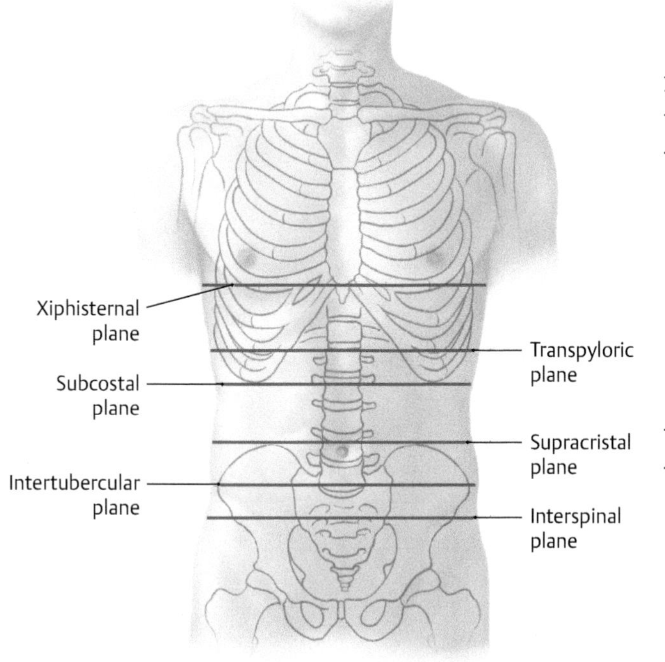

Fig. 3.2 Horizontal (transverse) planes in the anterior trunk wall. (From Schuenke M, Schulte E, Schumacher U. THIEME Atlas of Anatomy. Internal Organs. Illustrations by Voll M and Wesker K. 3rd ed. New York: Thieme Medical Publishers; 2020.)

Table 3.1 **Abdominal quadrant contents**

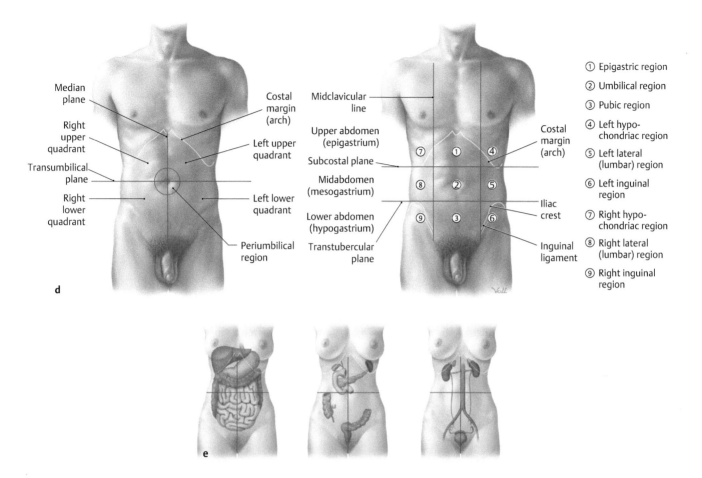

Right Upper Quadrant (RUQ)	Left Upper Quadrant (LUQ)
• Pyloric region of stomach • Parts 1-3 of duodenum • Head and uncinate process of pancreas • Right lobe of liver • Gallbladder • Right kidney • Right suprarenal gland • Superior part of ascending colon • Right half of transverse colon	• Majority of stomach • Left lobe of liver • Spleen • Body and tail of pancreas • Jejunum and proximal ileum • Left kidney • Left suprarenal gland • Left half of transverse colon • Superior part of descending colon
Right Lower Quadrant (RLQ)	**Left Lower Quadrant (LLQ)**
• Majority of ileum • Cecum • Appendix • Inferior part of ascending colon • Right abdominal part of ureter • Right abdominal part of spermatic cord • Right uterine tube • Right ovary • If enlarged the uterus and urinary bladder	• Inferior part of descending colon • Sigmoid colon • Left abdominal part of ureter • Left abdominal part of spermatic cord • Left uterine tube • Left ovary • If enlarged, the uterus and urinary bladder

peritoneum. Fiber orientation of the muscle layers is similar to that of the intercostal muscles.

Fascia characteristics can vary based on location relative to the umbilicus. Above the umbilicus, superficial fascia is consistent with fascia located elsewhere on the body. However, below the level of the umbilicus, there is a superficial fatty layer (*Camper's fascia*) and a deep membranous layer (*Scarpa's fascia*). Aponeuroses extend distally from the deep fascia investing the three muscle layers and contribute to the rectus sheaths that envelop the rectus abdominis muscles. The innermost layer of the aponeurosis and closest to the transversus abdominis muscle is lined with **transversalis fascia**. A thin layer of **extraperitoneal fat** follows and the layer closest to the abdominal viscera is the **parietal peritoneum**. The transversalis fascia, extraperitoneal fat and the parietal peritoneum extend posteriorly to contribute to the posterior abdominal wall.

3.2.1 Muscles of the Anterolateral Wall

There are three paired lateral muscles and a pair of vertical muscles just lateral to the midline on the anterior wall. The lateral most muscles include the **external oblique**, **internal oblique** and **transversus abdominis** and the vertical muscles include the **rectus abdominis** and **pyramidalis (Fig. 3.3; Fig. 3.4)**. Orientation of the muscle fibers in different directions adds to the overall strength of the anterolateral wall. The external oblique muscles run in a down-and-in ("hands in the pocket") orientation while the internal oblique muscles travel perpendicular to the externals. The transversus abdominis muscles run perpendicular to the rectus abdominis muscles. The rectus abdominis muscle is not continuous from superior to inferior but is interrupted by 3-4 **tendinous intersections**. These intersections are what give the appearance of a "six pack". All muscles of the anterolateral wall are innervated by a combination of nerves known as the thoraco-abdominal nerves. These include the ventral rami of T7-T12 and L1 spinal nerves. The pyramidalis only receives innervation from the subcostal nerve (T12) due to its size. Approximately 80% of the population has a pyramidalis muscle. These muscles as a group can compress and support the anterior trunk. Flexion, rotation of the trunk and maintenance of posture are the primary functions of these muscles. Descriptions of these muscles are found in **Table 3.2**.

3.2.2 Rectus Sheath

The aponeuroses of the external oblique, internal oblique and transversus abdominis muscles terminate anteriorly to help form the **rectus sheath (Fig. 3.5)**. The aponeuroses of these muscles interweave and cross from one side to the other and encase the majority of the rectus abdominis and pyramidalis muscles. The

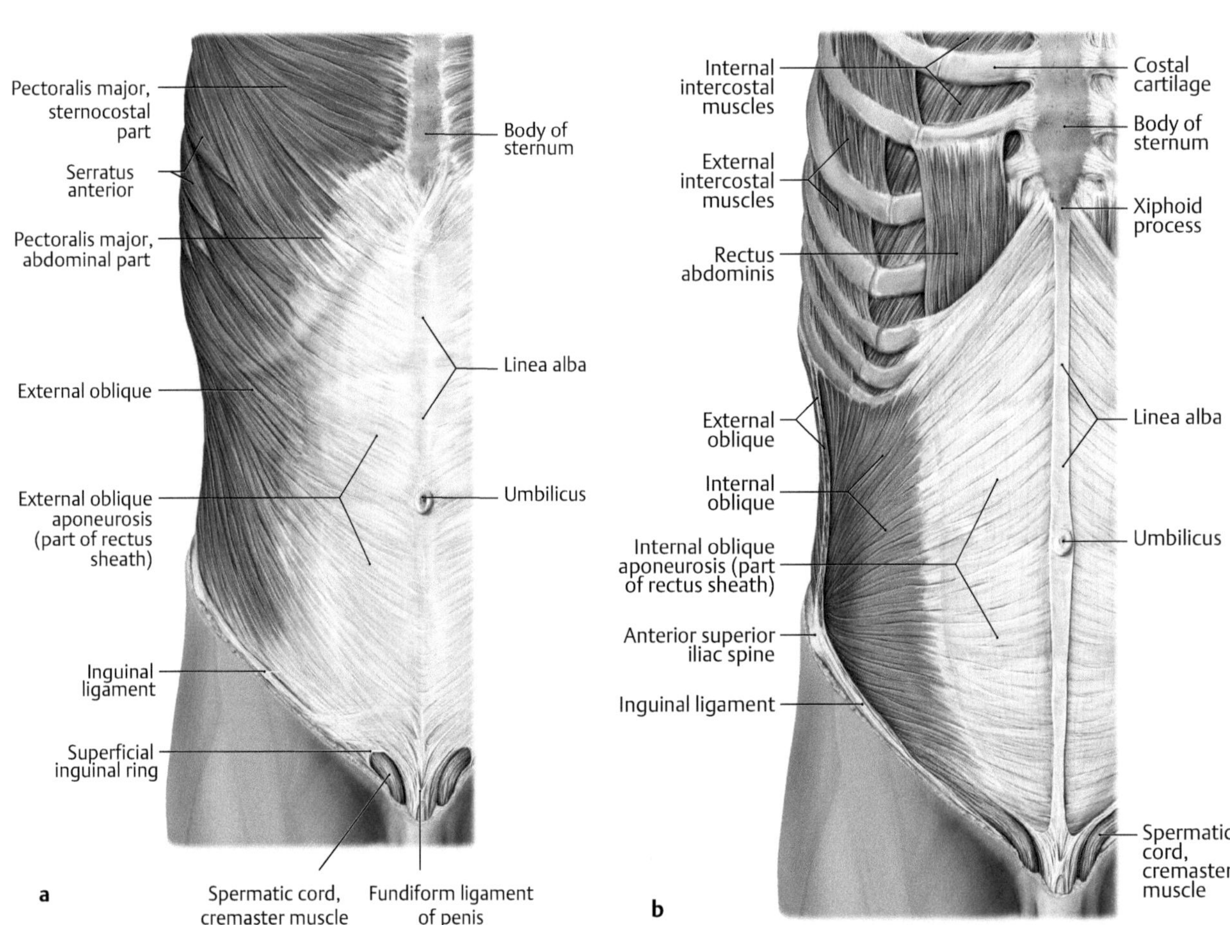

Fig. 3.3 Muscles of the abdominal wall. Right side, anterior view. **(a)** Superficial abdominal wall muscles. **(b)** Removed: external oblique, pectoralis major, and serratus anterior. (From Schuenke M, Schulte E, Schumacher U. THIEME Atlas of Anatomy. General Anatomy and Musculoskeletal System. Illustrations by Voll M and Wesker K. 3rd ed. New York: Thieme Medical Publishers; 2020.)

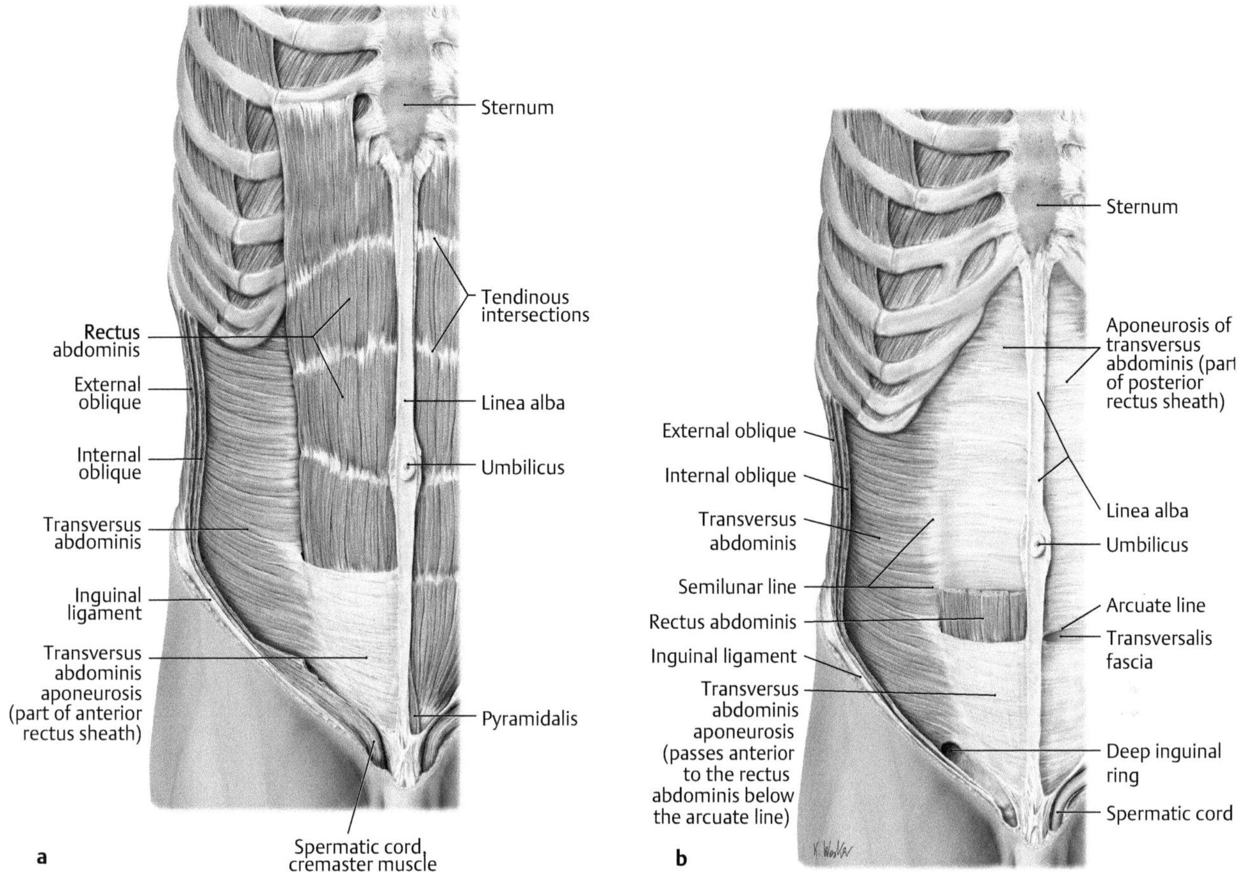

Fig. 3.4 Muscles of the abdominal wall. Right side, anterior view. **(a)** Removed: external and internal obliques. **(b)** Removed: rectus abdominis. Muscles of the anterolateral wall. (From Schuenke M, Schulte E, Schumacher U. THIEME Atlas of Anatomy. General Anatomy and Musculoskeletal System. Illustrations by Voll M and Wesker K. 3rd ed. New York: Thieme Medical Publishers; 2020.)

Table 3.2 **Anterior abdominal wall muscles**

Muscle	Innervation	Function(s)	Origin	Insertion
External oblique	Thoraco-abdominal nerves (T7-T12, L1)	Lateral flexion and rotation of trunk; maintains abdominal tone; compresses viscera increasing intra-abdominal pressure	External surface of the 5th – 12th ribs	Anterior half of iliac crest, pubic tubercle, and linea alba
Internal oblique	Thoraco-abdominal nerves (T7-T12, L1)	Lateral flexion and rotation of trunk; maintains abdominal tone; compresses viscera increasing intra-abdominal pressure	Thoracolumbar fascia, lateral two-thirds of inguinal ligament, and anterior two-thirds of iliac crest	Inferior borders of 10th – 12th ribs, pectineal line (pecten pubis) of pubic bone, and linea alba
Transversus abdominis	Thoraco-abdominal nerves (T7-T12, L1)	Maintains abdominal tone; compresses viscera increasing intra-abdominal pressure	Thoracolumbar fascia, internal surface of 7th – 12th ribs and their costal cartilage, and lateral one-third of inguinal ligament	Pubic crest, pectineal line (pecten pubis) and linea alba
Rectus abdominis	Thoraco-abdominal nerves (T7-T12, L1)	Flexes trunk and maintains abdominal tone	Pubic crest and pubic symphysis	Xiphoid process and 5th – 7th costal cartilages
Pyramidalis	Subcostal nerve (T12)	Tenses the lower part of linea alba	Body of pubic bone and pubic symphysis	Linea alba

superior epigastric and **inferior epigastric blood vessels** along with the distal portions of the T7-L1 ventral rami branches also reside within the rectus sheath.

The rectus sheath is divided into an anterior versus posterior layer (lamina) and the **arcuate line** seen only from the internal surface of the anterolateral abdominal wall defines the aponeuroses that contribute to each specific layer. The arcuate line is located approximately one-third of the way between the umbilicus and pubic crest and is the site of where the inferior epigastric vessels enter the rectus sheath.

- *Above the arcuate line*, the external oblique and anterior half of the internal oblique aponeuroses form the *anterior layer* of

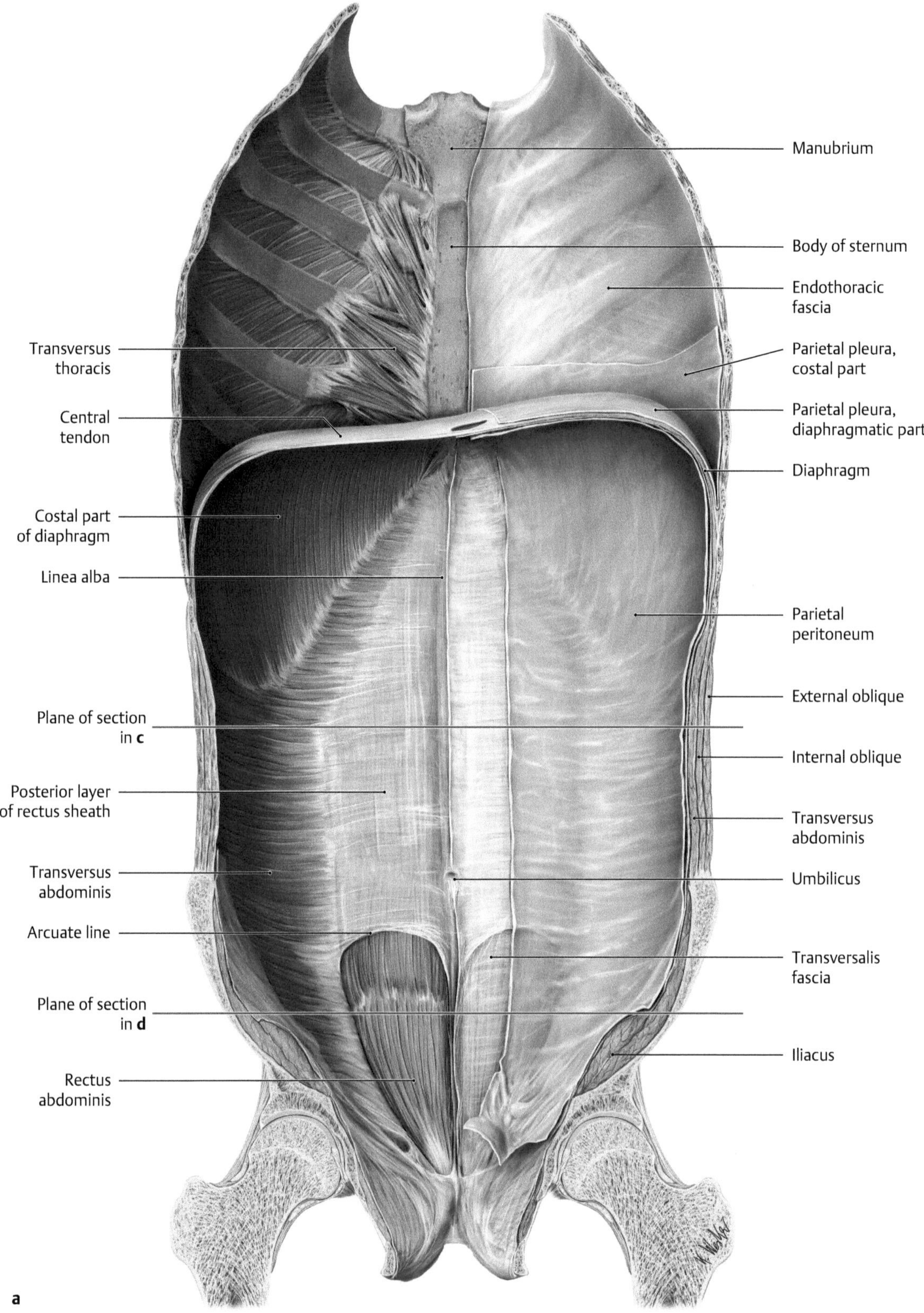

Fig. 3.5 Rectus sheath. **(a)** Posterior (inferior) view of the anterior wall. Peritoneum and transversalis fascia have been removed on the left side to reveal the rectus sheath. (*continued*) (From Schuenke M, Schulte E, Schumacher U. THIEME Atlas of Anatomy. General Anatomy and Musculoskeletal System. Illustrations by Voll M and Wesker K. 3rd ed. New York: Thieme Medical Publishers; 2020.)

the rectus sheath. The posterior half of the internal oblique and transversus abdominis aponeuroses contribute to the *posterior layer*.
- *Below the arcuate line*, the aponeurosis of the external oblique, internal oblique and transversus abdominis form the *anterior layer* of the rectus sheath. There is *no posterior layer* of the rectus sheath below the arcuate line because the arcuate line demarcates the inferior edge of the posterior rectus sheath.

Only the transversalis fascia directly covers the rectus abdominis muscle at this point.

The **linea alba** is located on the midline and extends from the xiphoid process down to the pubic symphysis. It is formed by the aponeuroses that contribute to the anterior and posterior layers of the rectus sheath. The linea alba forms the medial borders of the rectus abdominis muscles while the **semilunar lines** form

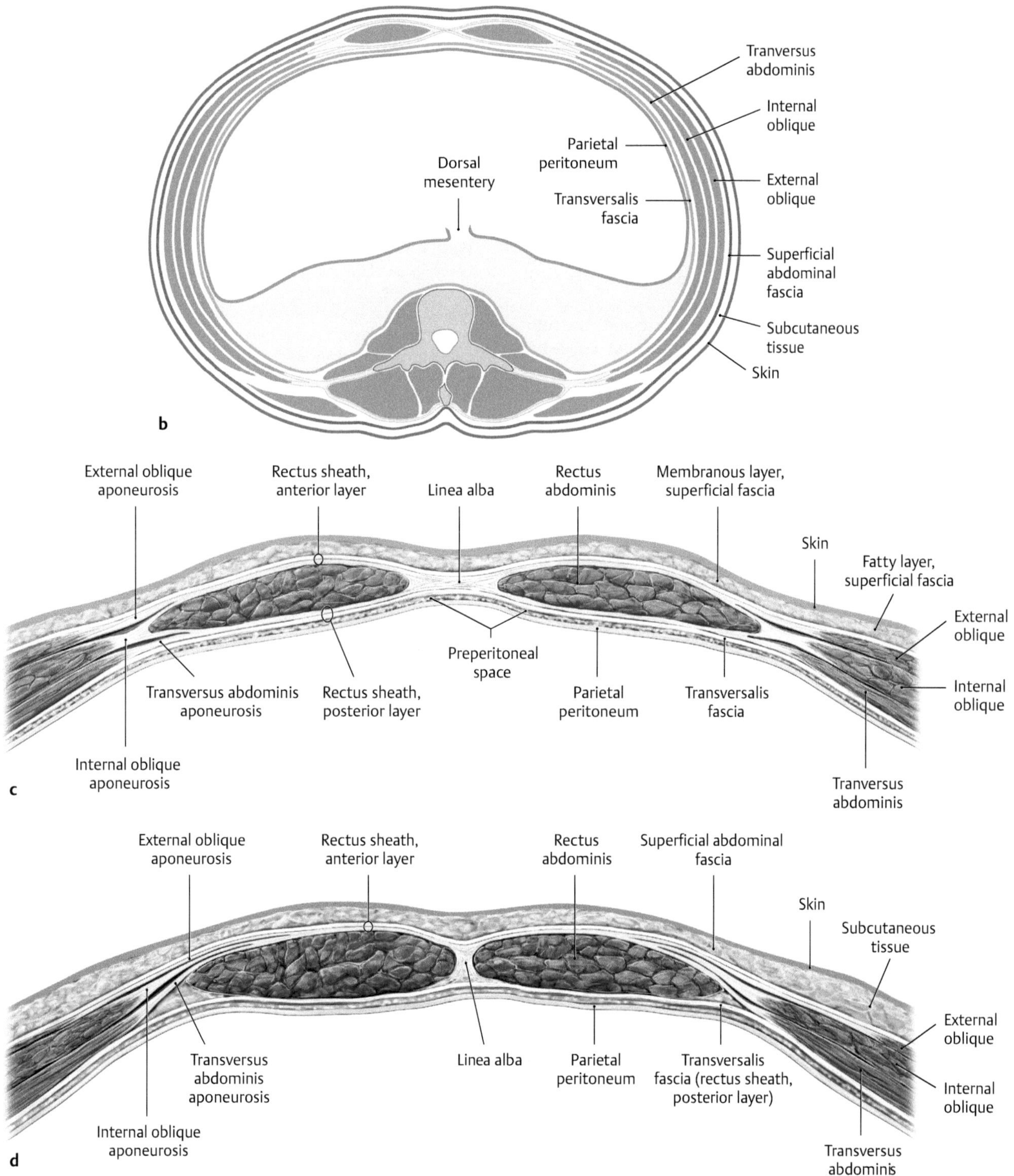

Fig. 3.5 (*continued*) **(b)** Relationship between rectus sheath and the parietal peritoneum and transversalis fascia. **(c)** Section through the abdominal wall superior to the arcuate line. **(d)** Section through the abdominal wall inferior to the arcuate line. (From Schuenke M, Schulte E, Schumacher U. THIEME Atlas of Anatomy. General Anatomy and Musculoskeletal System. Illustrations by Voll M and Wesker K. 3rd ed. New York: Thieme Medical Publishers; 2020.)

the lateral borders. The linea alba also contains a defect called the **umbilical ring** that during development allowed the fetal umbilical vessels to pass from umbilical cord to the placenta.

3.2.3 Neurovasculature of the Anterolateral Abdominal Wall

As mentioned previously, the **thoraco-abdominal nerves** are a combination of ventral rami spinal nerves originating from T7-L1 and are responsible for innervating the muscles of this region. T12 is also known as the **subcostal nerve** while L1 is a combination of two nerves known as the **iliohypogastric** and **ilioinguinal nerves** (**Fig. 3.6**). All of the thoraco-abdominal nerves contain the functional components GSE, GSA, and GVE-sym/post while the anterior and lateral cutaneous branches originating from these same nerves are like all typical cutaneous nerves and contain the functional components GSA and GVE-sym/post. These nerves are responsible for the characteristic dermatome map located on the anterolateral abdominal wall. If a lesion were to occur on an individual intercostal nerve, there would not be any major clinical effect. This is due to the anterolateral wall muscles receiving innervation from multiple nerves. If a lesion of the ilioinguinal nerve occurs, paresthesia may be felt over the anterior scrotum or labia majora because this nerve continues as the anterior scrotal/labial nerve.

Blood supply is from the **superior epigastric** and **musculophrenic arteries** (brs. of internal thoracic); **inferior epigastric** and **deep circumflex iliac arteries** (brs. of external iliac); **posterior intercostal**, **subcostal** and upper **lumbar arteries** (brs. of the thoracic/abdominal aorta); and finally the **superficial epigastric** and **superficial circumflex iliac arteries** (brs. of the femoral). The superior epigastric and inferior epigastric arteries form an anastomosis near the umbilicus.

Venous drainage includes the veins paired with the above listed arteries as well as the **thoracoepigastric vein** that drains blood from the superficial portion of the anterolateral abdominal wall above the level of the umbilicus before reaching the axillary vein. Smaller cutaneous veins near the umbilicus anastomose with the **para-umbilical veins** (tributaries of the hepatic portal vein).

Lymphatic drainage will be based on a superficial or deep drainage pattern. Above the umbilicus and superficial, lymph drains toward the **parasternal** and **axillary lymph nodes**. Below the umbilicus and still superficial, lymph drains to the **superficial inguinal lymph nodes**. Deeper lymphatic vessels from the majority of the anterolateral abdominal wall drain to the **external iliac**, **common iliac** and **lumbar lymph nodes**.

A neurovascular plane located between the internal oblique and transversus abdominis muscles serves as the passage for the neurovasculature responsible for supplying the majority of the anterolateral abdominal wall. Anterior and lateral cutaneous nerve branches originating from the nerves originally passing through the neurovascular plane along with smaller vessels such as the superficial epigastric and superficial circumflex iliac supply the subcutaneous tissue layer.

 *Clinical Correlate 3.1*

Palpation of the Abdominal Wall

To avoid the anterolateral abdominal muscles from contracting involuntarily, warm hands must be used instead of cold because this will cause the muscles to tense up and become **guarded**. These involuntary muscle contractions protect the viscera from outside pressure that can lead to painful stimulation if an abdominal infection is present. A patient is generally lying down and supine with their thighs and knees partially flexed to relax the abdominal wall muscles. If not properly done, the deep fascia of the thighs can pull on the membranous layer of the abdominal subcutaneous tissue and end up tensing the abdominal wall. By placing a pillow underneath the persons knees while resting the upper limbs to the side can also relax the abdominal wall muscles.

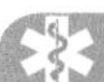 *Clinical Correlate 3.2*

Umbilical Hernia

An umbilical hernia may be due to the protrusion of the bowel through a natural weak defect at the umbilicus or occur because of the failure of the midgut to return to the abdomen during fetal development. They are most common in infants and occur equally between males and females but can also occur in adults. When present in an infant, an umbilical hernia generally doesn't cause pain and will close on its own with surgery only needed in a small percentage of cases. If present in an adult, and generally brought on by obesity or multiple pregnancies, surgery is generally the first choice of action and this can involve inserting a mesh product at the level of the defect in order to add strength to the abdominal wall. The defect can also be simply sutured closed.

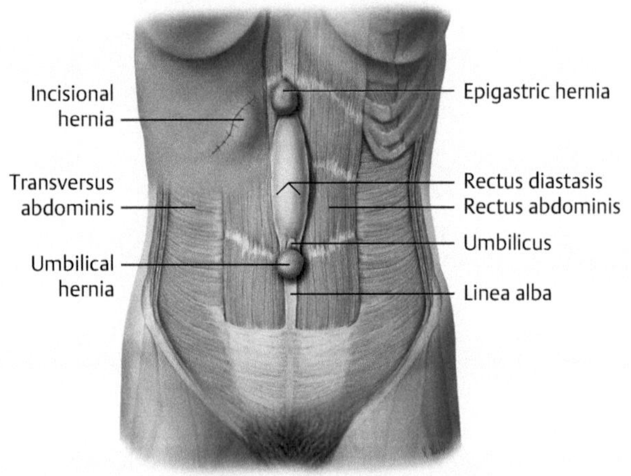

(From Schuenke M, Schulte E, Schumacher U. THIEME Atlas of Anatomy. General Anatomy and Musculoskeletal System. Illustrations by Voll M and Wesker K. 3rd ed. New York: Thieme Medical Publishers; 2020.)

3.3 Inguinal Region

The **inguinal region** (or groin) extends from between the anterior superior iliac spine and the pubic tubercle. It serves as a region for structures passing to and from the abdominal cavity. This region is reinforced by multiple ligaments of which originate mostly from the aponeurosis of the external oblique muscle and transversalis fascia (**Fig. 3.7; Fig. 3.8**).

The dense band-like structure called the **inguinal ligament** originates from the aponeurosis of the external oblique muscle and connects the anterior superior iliac spine to the pubic tubercle. Fibers of this ligament pass superiorly to the pubic tubercle and form the **reflected inguinal ligament** that helps form the posterior wall of the *inguinal canal* and may contribute to the *conjoint tendon.* Additional fibers will pass posteriorly and lateral to the pubic tubercle before attaching to the *superior pubic ramus* becoming the **lacunar** (*Gimbernat*) **ligament.** This ligament contributes to the floor of the inguinal canal. A lateral extension of the lacunar ligament that attaches to the *pectineal line (pecten pubis)* becomes the **pectineal** (*Cooper*) **ligament.** The transversalis fascia thickens on the posterior surface of the inguinal ligament to become the **iliopubic tract.** This structure is important for adding strength to the floor and posterior wall of the inguinal canal as it passes over the *retroinguinal space.*

The **retroinguinal** (*Bogro's*) **space** is located below the level of the inguinal ligament and allows for the passage of neurovasculature and muscles related to the anterior thigh region of the lower limb (**Fig 3.9**). The **myopectineal orifice** is a natural weakness of the inguinal region spanned by the inguinal ligament and iliopubic tract and that includes a portion of the retroinguinal space. It will serve as the site for femoral, direct and indirect hernias.

The **inguinal canal** runs parallel and superior to the distal one-half of the inguinal ligament. It is present in both sexes but more prominent males. It allows for the passage of the spermatic cord in the male and the round ligament in the female along with the ilioinguinal nerve, genital branch of the genitofemoral nerve, and relevant blood vessels and lymphatics of both sexes. This canal is open at both ends by a deep inguinal ring and superficial inguinal ring. The **deep inguinal ring** serves as the entrance of the inguinal canal and is located superior to the inguinal ligament near its midpoint and just lateral to the inferior epigastric vessels. The deep inguinal ring is formed by the transversalis fascia that begins to evaginate and thus creates this opening. The **superficial inguinal ring** represents the exit for the inguinal canal and is formed by the aponeurosis of the external oblique muscle and is located just superior and lateral to the pubic crest. This ring is bounded on either side by crura and intercrural fibers. The **medial crus** attaches to the pubic crest while the **lateral crus** connects to the pubic tubercle. The lateral crura are much stronger with both of them originating from the aponeurosis of the external oblique muscle. The **intercrural fibers** help prevent the crura from splitting but originate from the superficial layer of the deep fascia surrounding the external oblique muscle and aponeurosis.

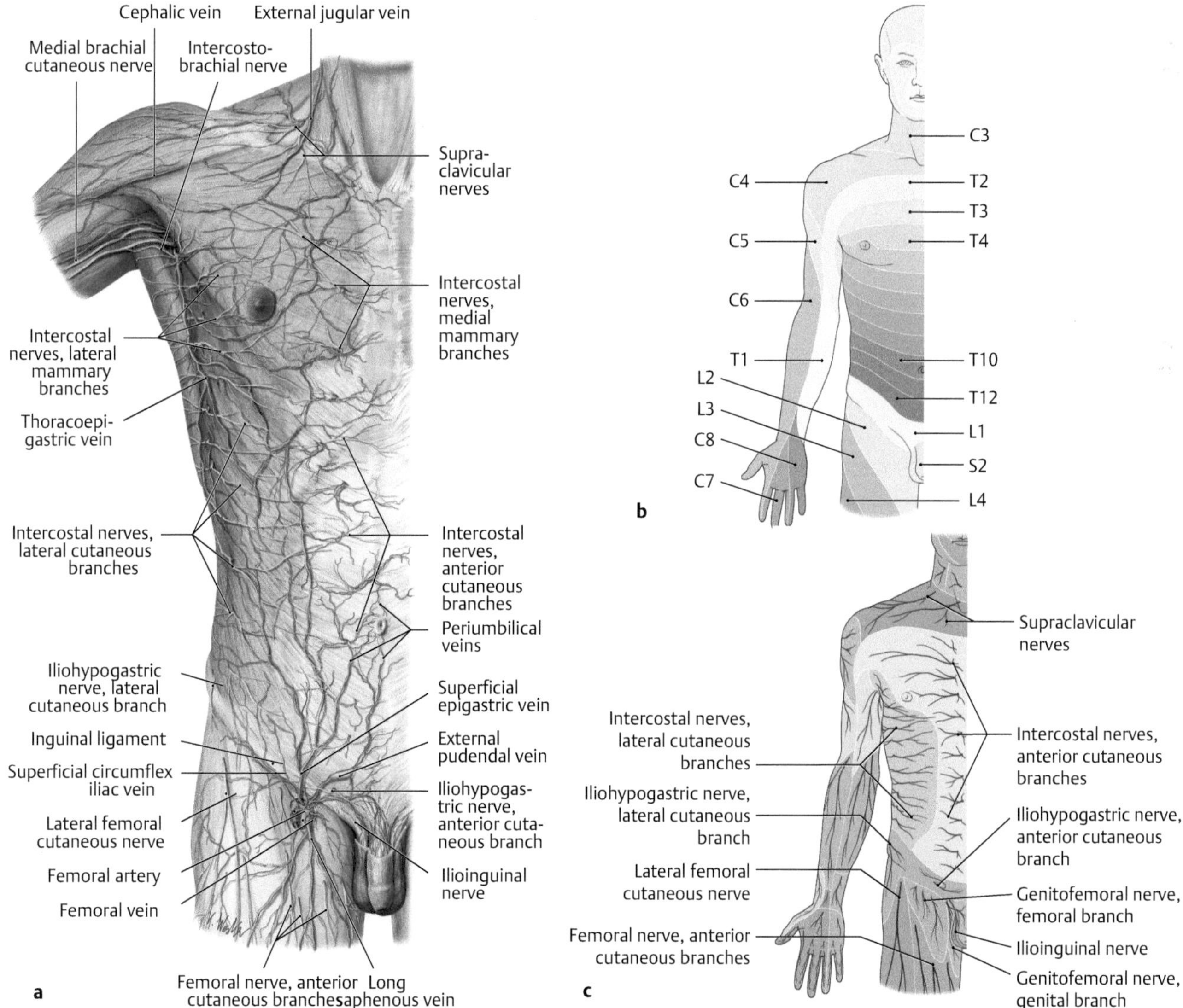

Fig. 3.6 Neurovasculature of the anterior trunk wall. **(a)** Superficial surface neurovasculature. **(b)** Dermatomes of the anterior trunk. **(c)** Cutaneous innervation of the anterior trunk. (From Schuenke M, Schulte E, Schumacher U. THIEME Atlas of Anatomy. General Anatomy and Musculoskeletal System. Illustrations by Voll M and Wesker K. 3rd ed. New York: Thieme Medical Publishers; 2020.)

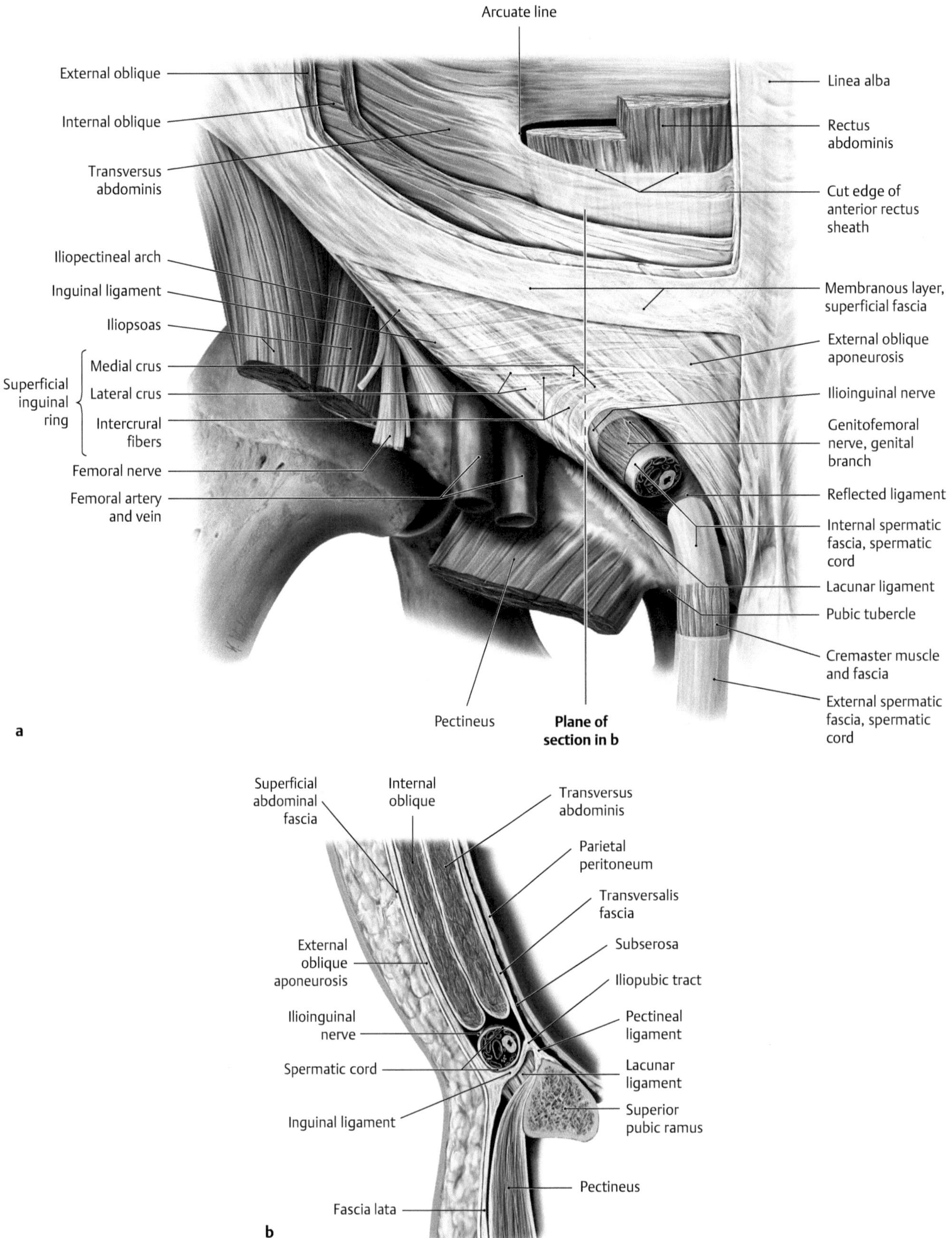

Fig. 3.7 Inguinal canal. **(a)** Location of the inguinal canal in the male. **(b)** Sagittal section through the inguinal canal in the male. (From Schuenke M, Schulte E, Schumacher U. THIEME Atlas of Anatomy. General Anatomy and Musculoskeletal System. Illustrations by Voll M and Wesker K. 3rd ed. New York: Thieme Medical Publishers; 2020.)

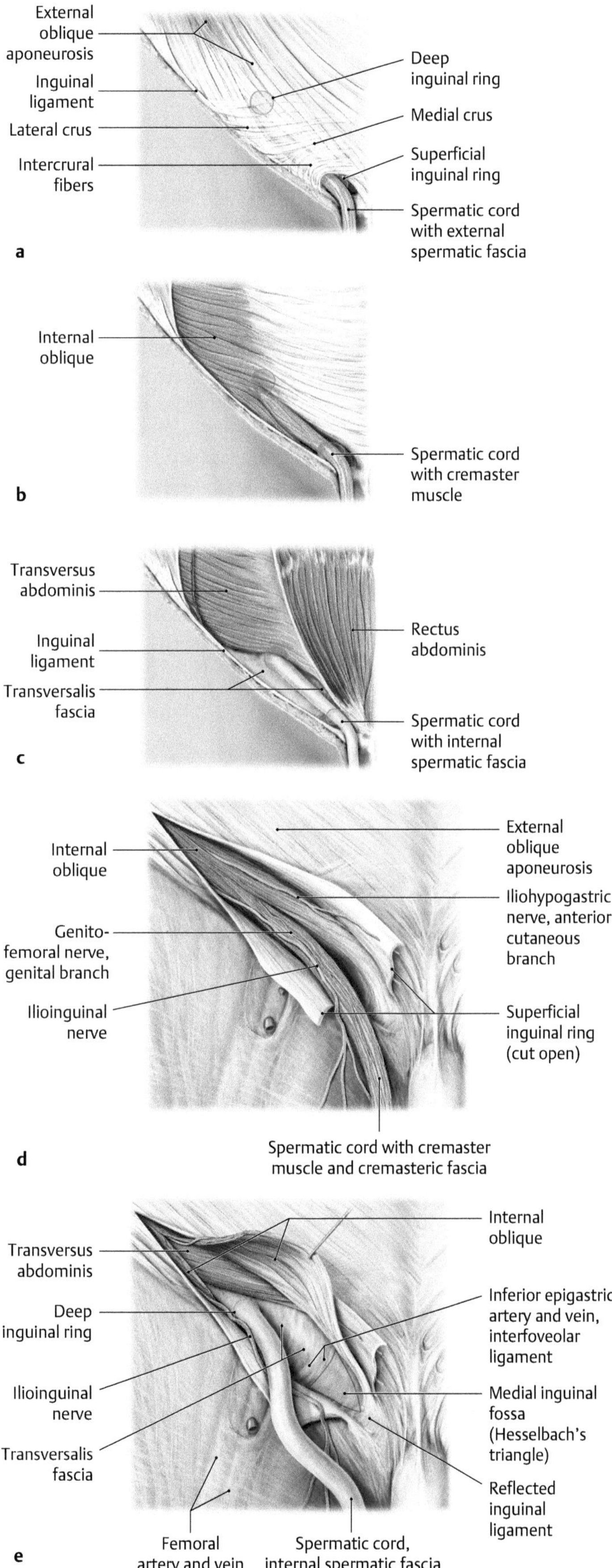

Fig. 3.8 Right inguinal region, anterior view. **(a-c)** Progressive removal of the abdominal wall muscles. **(d,e)** Progressive opening of the inguinal canal to expose the spermatic cord. (From Schuenke M, Schulte E, Schumacher U. THIEME Atlas of Anatomy. General Anatomy and Musculoskeletal System. Illustrations by Voll M and Wesker K. 3rd ed. New York: Thieme Medical Publishers; 2020.)

The inguinal canal is described as having an anterior and posterior wall, roof and floor but generally has the appearance of being collapsed (**Fig. 3.7**).

- Anterior wall: formed by the aponeurosis of the external oblique with its lateral portion reinforced by internal oblique muscle fibers.
- Posterior wall: formed by the transversalis fascia. The medial portion is reinforced by the **inguinal falx (or conjoint tendon)**; a structure formed by the inferior fibers of the internal oblique and transversus abdominis aponeuroses. The reflected inguinal ligament also adds support to this wall.
- Roof: formed by the transversalis fascia (laterally); musculo-aponeurotic arches of the internal oblique and transversus abdominis (centrally); and the medial crus of the external oblique aponeurosis (medially).
- Floor: formed by the iliopubic tract (laterally); the gutter formed by the infolded inguinal ligament (centrally); and lacunar ligament (medially).

3.4 Spermatic Cord and Scrotum

Structures that help define the anterolateral abdominal wall and inguinal canal contribute to the layers of the spermatic cord and scrotum for males. The spermatic cord serves as the conduit for the structures that pass to and from the testes (**Fig. 3.10; Fig. 3.11**). It begins at the deep inguinal ring and courses through the inguinal canal before passing through the superficial inguinal ring. It extends inferiorly to engulf the testes and assists in suspending them. Fascial layers of the spermatic cord include an external spermatic, cremasteric and internal spermatic fascia all of which are derived from the anterolateral abdominal wall.

The **external spermatic fascia** originates from the *external oblique aponeurosis* and its deep fascia; the **cremasteric fascia** comes from the deep fascia of the *internal oblique muscle*; the **internal spermatic fascia** originates from the *transversalis fascia*. The **cremaster muscle** is skeletal in nature and is found in the cremasteric fascia (**Fig. 3.10; Fig. 3.11**). This muscle is formed by the inferior fascicles of the *internal oblique muscle* and reflexively elevates the testis in the scrotum toward the body generally in response to a cold environment. A constant temperature is needed in the formation of sperm (spermatogenesis) thus the cremaster muscle serves that purpose. The genital branch of the genitofemoral nerve innervates the cremaster muscle.

Contents of the spermatic cord enveloped by the internal spermatic fascia include: **testicular nervous (autonomic) plexus**; **testicular artery** (abdominal aorta br.); **testicular veins** and the **pampiniform venous plexus** that develops from them; **lymphatic vessels** draining testes back to the lumbar lymph nodes; **ductus (vas) deferens** that transports sperm from the epididymis to the ejaculatory duct; and **artery/vein of ductus deferens** (artery br. of both superior/inferior vesical); and the **obliterated processus**

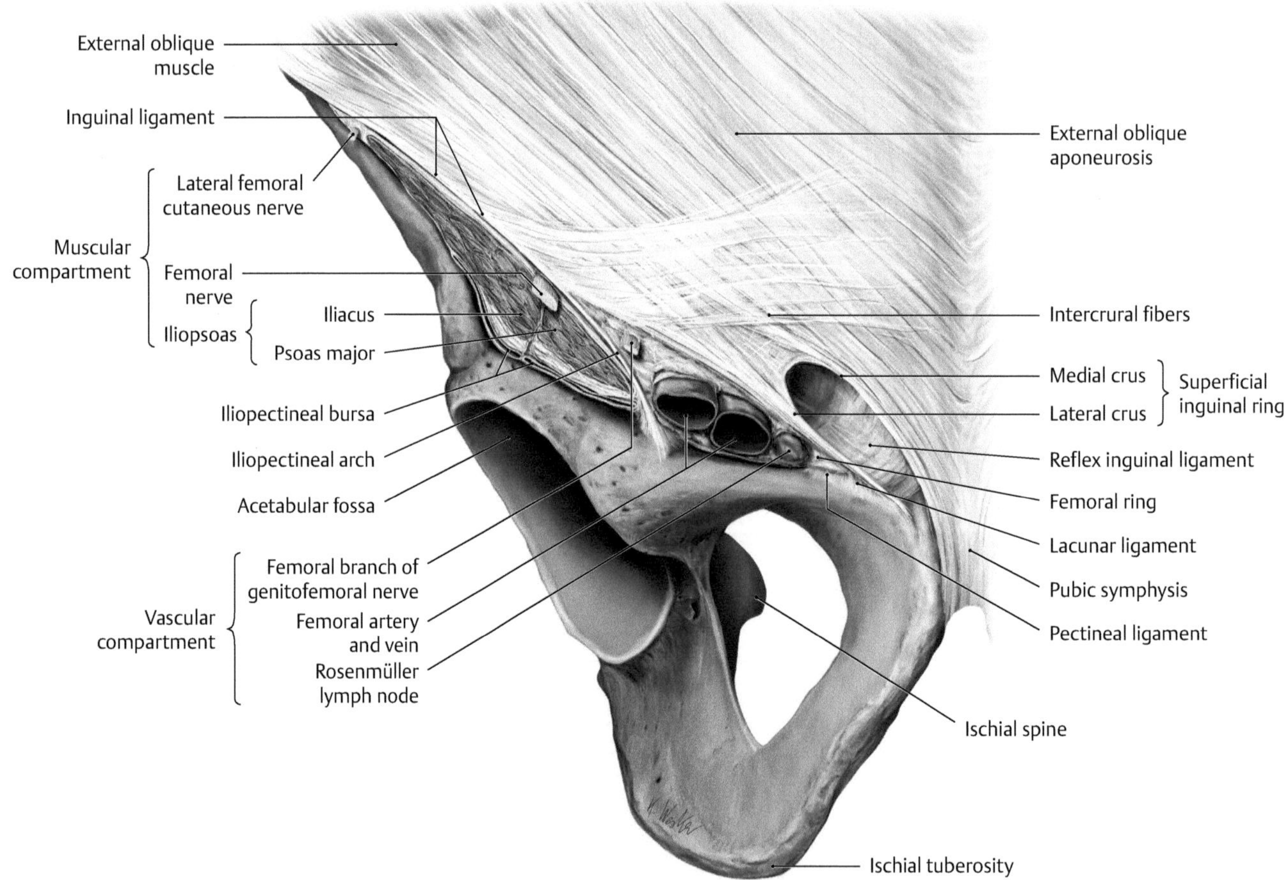

Fig. 3.9 Inguinal region and the division of the retroinguinal space into a muscular compartment (lacuna musculorm) and a vascular compartment (lacuna vasorum). (From Schuenke M, Schulte E, Schumacher U. THIEME Atlas of Anatomy. General Anatomy and Musculoskeletal System. Illustrations by Voll M and Wesker K. 1st ed. New York: Thieme Medical Publishers; 2010.)

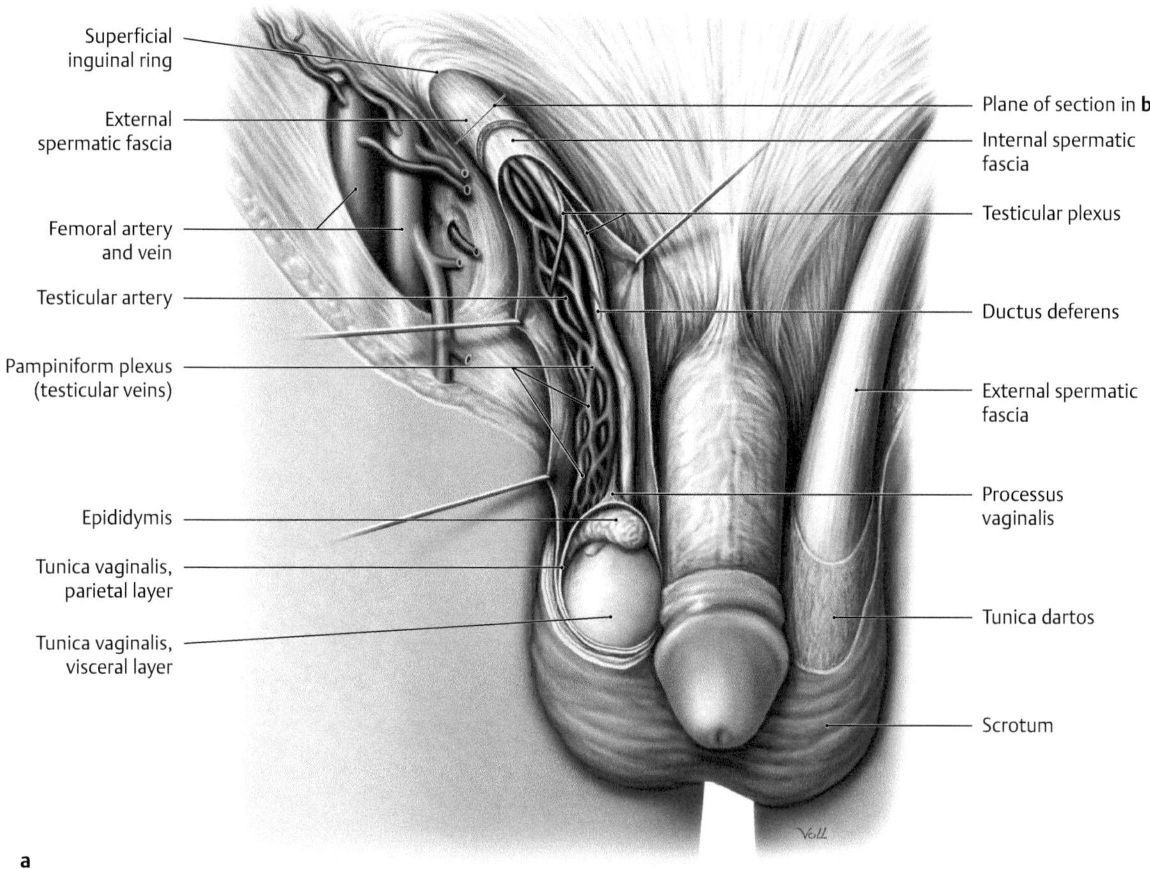

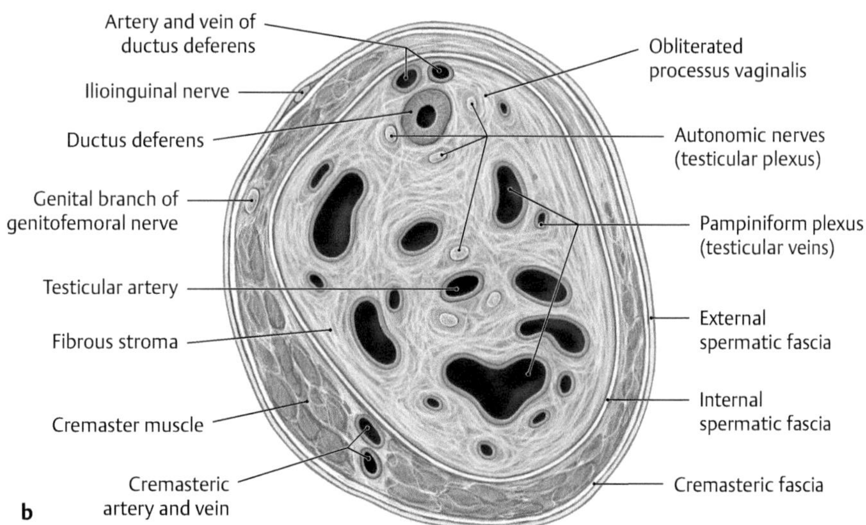

Fig. 3.10 **(a)** Fascial and muscular layers of the spermatic cord opened. **(b)** Contents of the spermatic cord. (From Schuenke M, Schulte E, Schumacher U. THIEME Atlas of Anatomy. General Anatomy and Musculoskeletal System. Illustrations by Voll M and Wesker K. 3rd ed. New York: Thieme Medical Publishers; 2020.)

vaginalis, a fibrous remnant of the formally opened process vaginalis, an extension of peritoneum. Structures located superficial to the internal spermatic fascia include: **genital branch of the genitofemoral nerve** and the **cremasteric artery/vein** (artery br. of inferior epigastric br.). The **ilioinguinal nerve** is generally located on the superficial surface of the external spermatic fascia. The round ligament in the female is not considered a homolog of the spermatic cord.

The testicular nerve plexus originates from the periarterial autonomic fibers wrapped around the testicular arteries. These same testicular arteries originate as a pair from the abdominal aorta just below the renal arteries at approximately the L2 vertebral level. They descend to the deep inguinal ring and pass through the spermatic cord before reaching the ipsilateral testicle. The pampiniform venous plexus condenses to form a testicular vein that eventually pairs with the artery. The veins ascend from the left

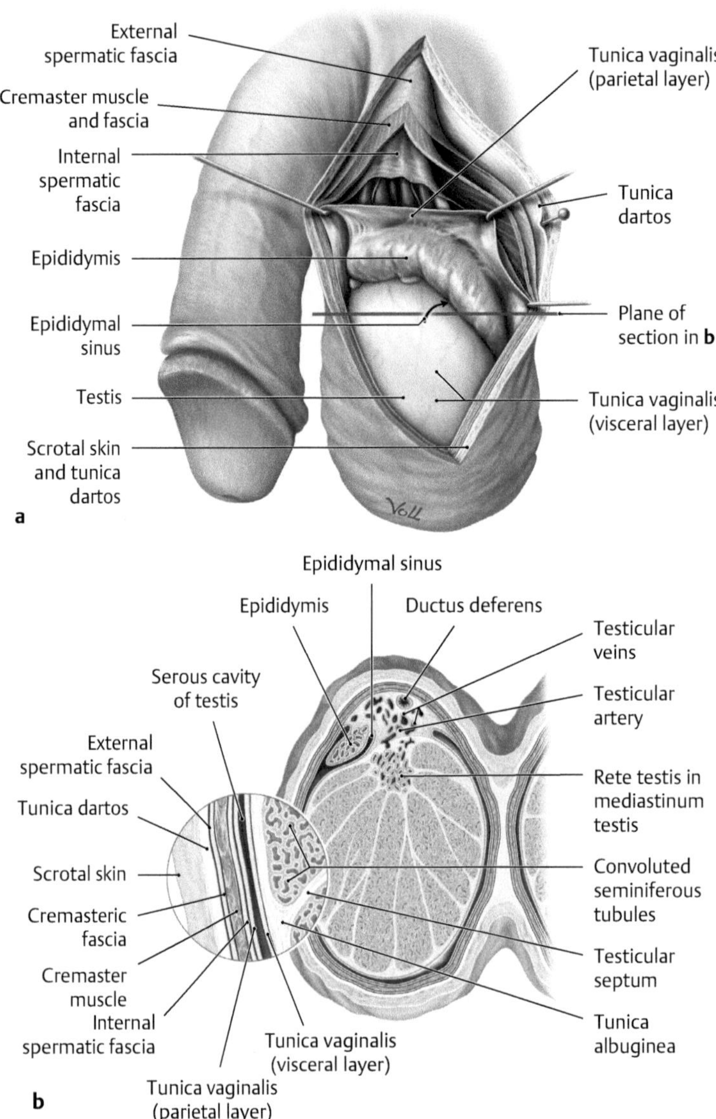

Fig. 3.11 **(a)** Testis and epididymis, left lateral view. **(b)** Coverings of the testis. Transverse section through the right testis, superior view. (From Schuenke M, Schulte E, Schumacher U. THIEME Atlas of Anatomy. General Anatomy and Musculoskeletal System. Illustrations by Voll M and Wesker K. 3rd ed. New York: Thieme Medical Publishers; 2020.)

testicle to the *left renal vein* while from the right testicle venous drainage ascends back to the *IVC*.

The **scrotum** is a double chambered, suspended sac made up of an outer-pigmented skin layer and an internal fat-free **dartos fascia** with **dartos muscle** layer. Dartos fascia is continuous with the *membranous layer of subcutaneous tissue of the perineum (Colles' fascia)* and the *membranous layer of subcutaneous tissue of the abdomen (Scarpa's fascia)*. A left and right chamber are formed by the **septum of the scrotum**, a central continuation of the dartos fascia. The external demarcation of the septum is displayed by the **scrotal raphe**, a fusion of the embryonic *labioscrotal swellings*. Dartos muscle is smooth muscle that is located deep to the skin and continuous with the septum of the scrotum. When it contracts, the attachment to the skin gives the scrotum a wrinkled appearance along with assisting the cremaster muscle in elevation of the testes.

At the level of the testes the order of layers from skin of the scrotum to the testes is: skin, subcutaneous tissue (dartos fascia/muscle), external spermatic fascia, cremasteric fascia/muscle, internal spermatic fascia, parietal layer of tunic vaginalis, visceral layer of tunica vaginalis and tunica albuginea of the testes.

3.4.1 Neurovasculature of the Scrotum

The **anterior scrotal nerve** (ilioinguinal br.) supplies the anterior surface and the **posterior scrotal nerve** (pudendal br.) supplies the posterior surface of the scrotum. The **genital branch of the genitofemoral nerve** not only innervates the cremaster muscle but it can also supply the anterolateral surface of the skin. The **perineal nerves** (posterior femoral cutaneous br.) supply the posteroinferior surface of the skin. The functional components of these nerves are GSA and GVE-sym/post. The dartos muscle is innervated by GVE-sym/post fibers that originate from the nerves listed above (**Fig. 3.12**).

Blood supply to the scrotum includes the **anterior scrotal** (external pudendal br.), **posterior scrotal** (perineal br.), and the

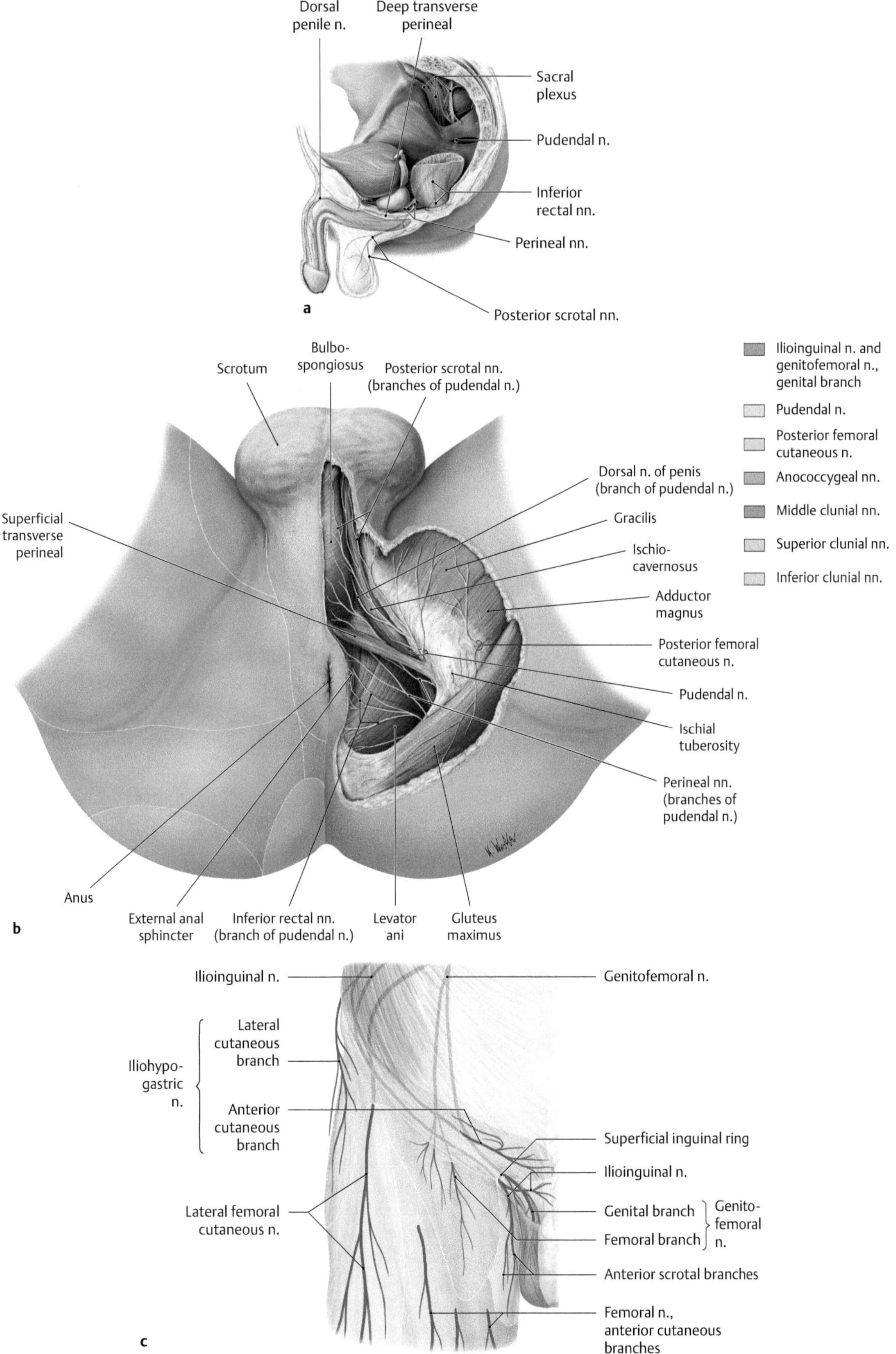

Fig. 3.12 Nerve supply of the male genitalia. **(a)** Neurovasculature of the scrotum. **(b)** Lithotomy position. **(c)** Cutaneous innervation of the inguinal region. Right male inguinal region, anterior view. (From Schuenke M, Schulte E, Schumacher U. Thieme Atlas of Anatomy, General Anatomy and Musculoskeletal System. Illustrations by Voll M and Wesker K. 1st ed. New York: Thieme Medical Publishers; 2010.)

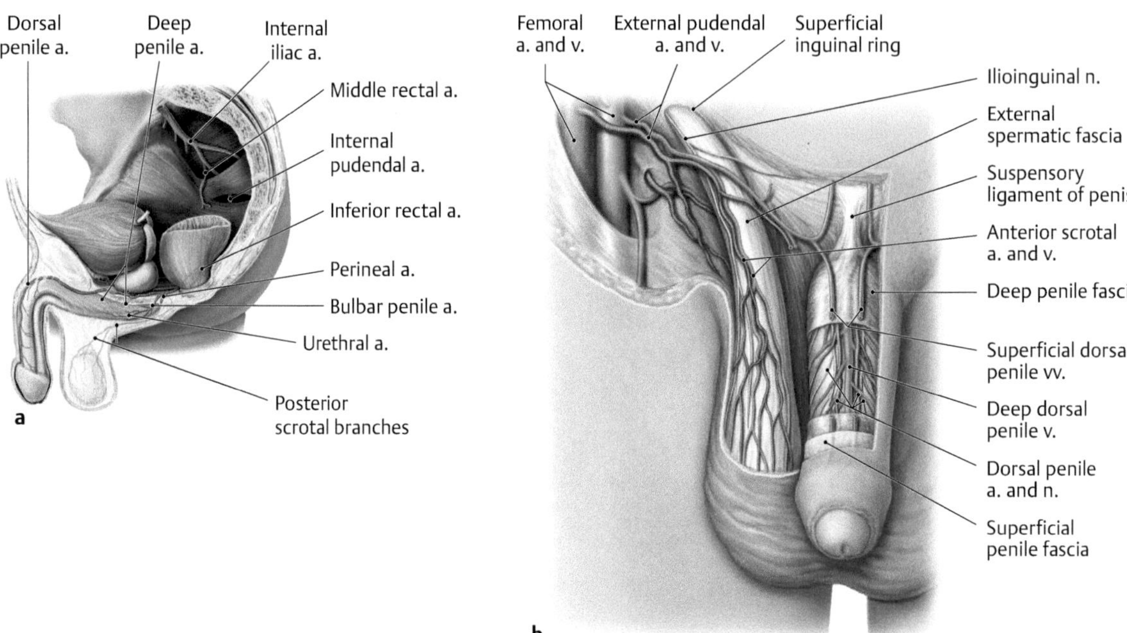

Fig. 3.13 (a) Blood supply of the male genitalia. **(b)** Neurovasculature of the penis and scrotum. (From Schuenke M, Schulte E, Schumacher U. Thieme Atlas of Anatomy, General Anatomy and Musculoskeletal System. Illustrations by Voll M and Wesker K. 1st ed. New York: Thieme Medical Publishers; 2010.)

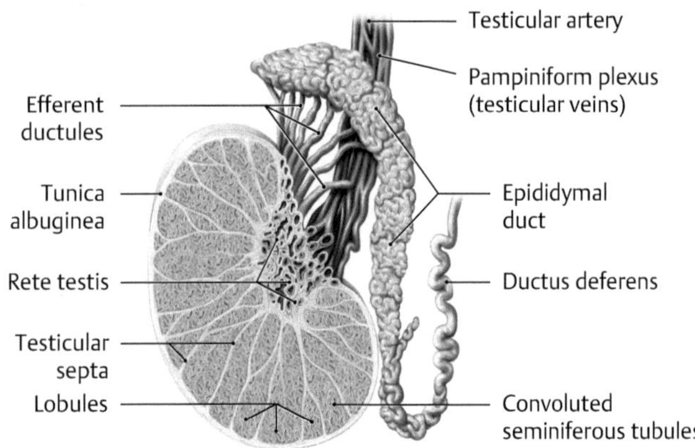

Fig. 3.14 Sagittal section of the testes and epididymis. (From Schuenke M, Schulte E, Schumacher U. THIEME Atlas of Anatomy. General Anatomy and Musculoskeletal System. Illustrations by Voll M and Wesker K. 3rd ed. New York: Thieme Medical Publishers; 2020.).

cremasteric (inferior epigastric br.) **arteries (Fig. 3.13)**. These vessels all have paired venous drainage and its lymphatic drainage is to the **superficial inguinal lymph nodes**.

3.5 Testes

The **testes** are the paired male gonads suspended by the spermatic cords that produce *sperm* and the male hormone *testosterone* **(Fig. 3.14)**. The left testicle generally rests more inferiorly than the right. The **tunica vaginalis** is the closed peritoneal sac that surrounds the majority of the testis and contains very little fluid allowing limited internal movement of the testis. It represents the closed distal portion of the of the embryonic processus vaginalis. It consists of an outer parietal and inner visceral layer.

The **parietal layer of tunica vaginalis** is adjacent to the internal spermatic fascia and it folds back on itself to form the **visceral layer of tunica vaginalis**. The visceral layer rests up against the *tunica albuginea* of the testis, epididymis and inferior portion of the ductus deferens. Between the body of the epididymis and posterolateral surface of the testis, a small recess of the tunica vaginalis can be found and is called the **sinus of the epididymis**.

3.5.1 Vasculature and Lymphatic Drainage of the Testes

The **testicular plexus** is an autonomic nervous plexus that contains sympathetic, parasympathetic and visceral afferent fibers. The sympathetics are important in blood vessel constriction while the parasympathetics are more associated with smooth muscle contraction. The paired testicular arteries supply the testes and originate from the abdominal aorta at approximately the L2 vertebral level.

Venous drainage of the testes (and epididymis) begins as a network of veins called the **pampiniform venous plexus.** This plexus along with the cremasteric and dartos muscles is part of a thermoregulatory system that regulates the temperature of the testes. The plexus coalesces to form more individualized veins as it progresses superiorly through the spermatic cord. The result is the formation of a **left testicular vein** that drains into the left renal vein while the **right testicular vein** drains directly into the IVC. Lymphatic drainage of the testes follows the testicular vessels back to the **lumbar** and **pre-aortic lymph nodes (Fig. 3.15)**.

3.5.2 Histology of the Testes

The tough outer surface of the testes is known as the **tunica albuginea (Fig. 3.16)** and it thickens into a highly vascularized

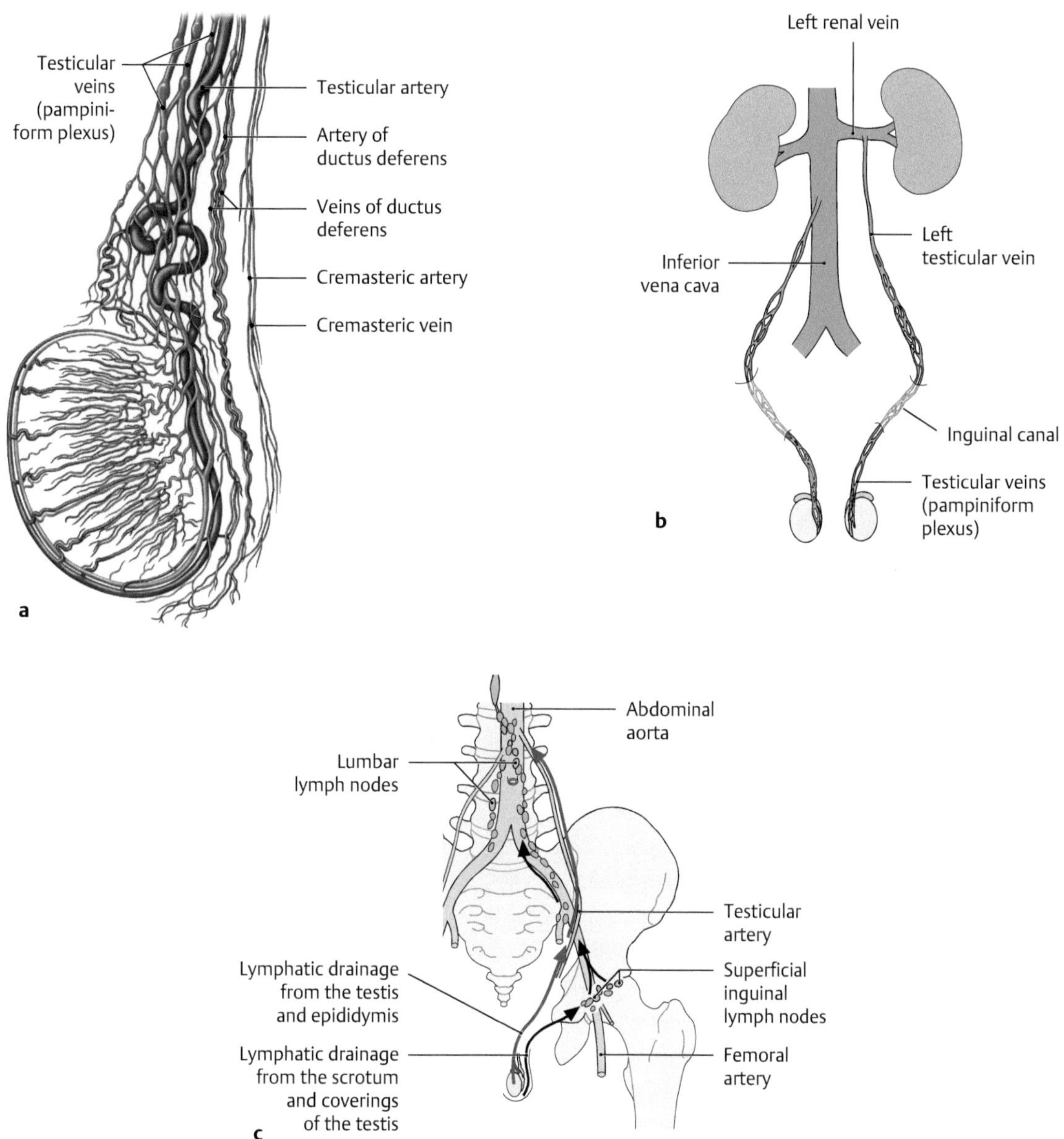

Fig. 3.15 (a-c) Vasculature and lymphatic drainage of the testes. (From Schuenke M, Schulte E, Schumacher U. THIEME Atlas of Anatomy. General Anatomy and Musculoskeletal System. Illustrations by Voll M and Wesker K. 3rd ed. New York: Thieme Medical Publishers; 2020.)

ridge on its internal and posterior surface becoming the **mediastinum testis (Fig. 3.17)**. From this internal ridge there are fibrous septa that extend inward and between lobules of long, highly coiled **seminiferous tubules (Fig. 3.16)**. The seminiferous tubules are the site of sperm production. The spermatogenic (germ) cells within the seminiferous epithelium are surrounded by the processes of Sertoli cells. The **Sertoli cells** are elongated cells that: provide physical and nutritional support to differentiating spermatogenic cells; form the *blood-testis barrier*; facilitate phagocytosis of excess spermatid cytoplasmic fragments during spermiogenesis; secrete *androgen binding protein* which concentrates testosterone; secrete *anti-Müllerian factor* during embryogenesis to produce a male fetus; and secrete inhibin, a substance that suppresses *follicle stimulating hormone (FSH)*. Within the stroma located between the seminiferous tubules, **Leydig cells** are responsible for producing testosterone. This process is regulated by *luteinizing hormone (LH)* released by the pituitary gland **(Fig. 3.16)**.

The **straight tubules** have a simple cuboidal/columnar epithelium comprised of Sertoli cells and drain the seminiferous tubules into the rete testis. The **rete testis (Fig. 3.16)** is an anastomosing network of channels lined by simple cuboidal cells with microvilli and a single cilium that carries sperm to the efferent ductules **(Fig. 3.16)**. The **efferent ductules** are lined by a pseudostratified epithelium of either a ciliated columnar cell or non-ciliated cuboidal cell **(Fig. 3.16a)**. The cuboidal cells are believed to absorb most of the fluid produced by Sertoli cells of the seminiferous tubules. A thin layer of smooth muscle that surrounds these ductules aids in the transport of non-motile sperm toward the epididymis.

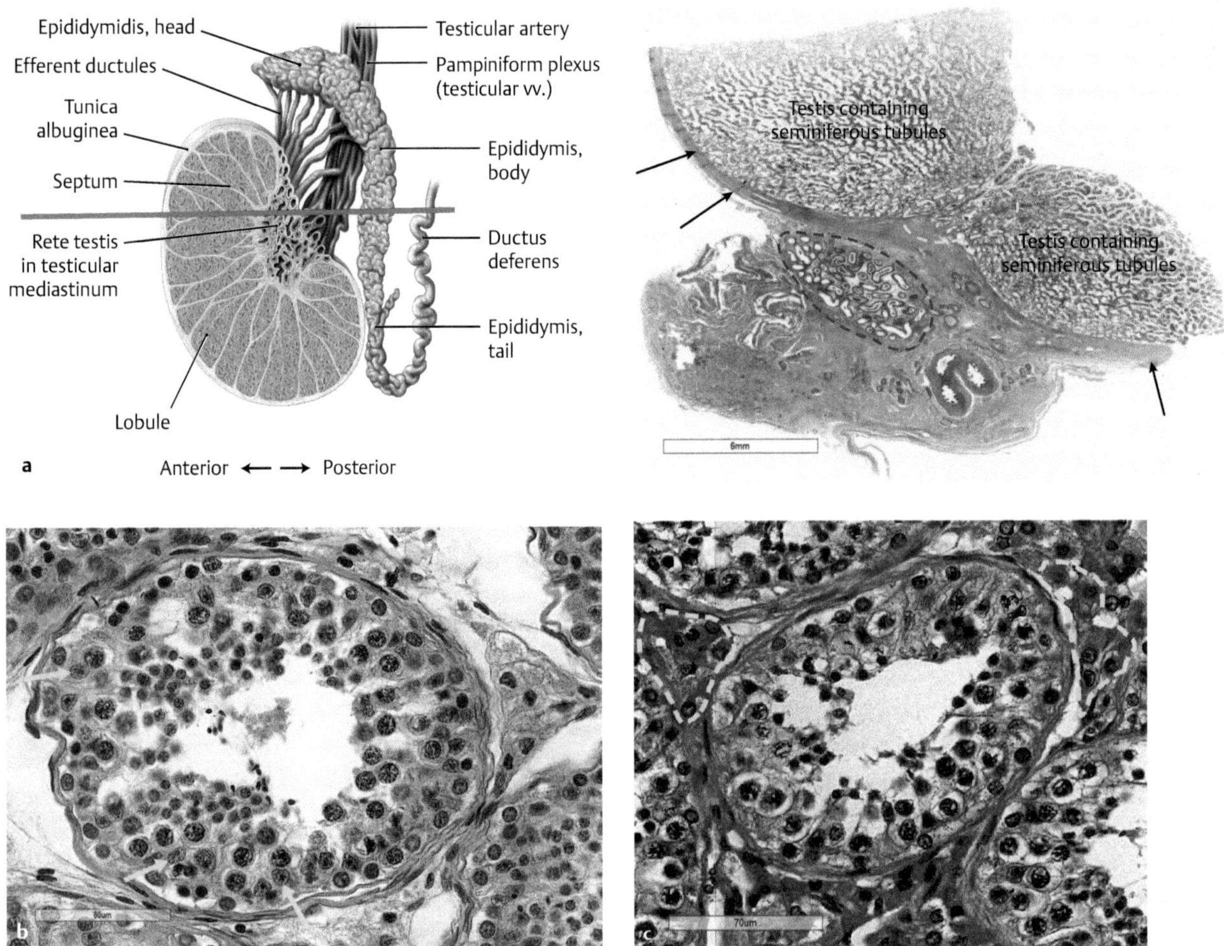

Fig. 3.16 Histology of the testes. **(a)** Scanning view of a horizontal section through the testis. The mediastinum (*yellow outline*), epididymis (*blue outline*), ductus deferens (*green outline*), and tunica albuginea (*black arrows*). **(b)** Seminiferous tubule, high magnification, showing Sertoli cells (*arrows*). **(c)** Seminiferous tubule, medium-high magnification, showing Leydig cells (*yellow outline*). (From Lowrie DJ. Histology: An Essential Textbook. New York: Thieme Medical Publishers; 2020.)

3.6 Epididymis

The **epididymis (Fig. 3.17)** is located on the posterior surface of each testis and is formed by minute convolutions of the **duct of the epididymis**. It is 4-6 meters in total length but tightly convoluted and compact with subdivisions called the head, body and tail region. It serves as a storage site for sperm as they become motile. The *head* is the portion formed by the coiled ends of 12-14 efferent ductules. The *body* is the major part consisting of the tightly convoluted duct of the epididymis. The *tail* represents the smallest portion of the duct and becomes continuous with the ductus deferens. It has a pseudostratified epithelium with stereocilia responsible for absorbing the remainder of fluid from the seminiferous tubules. The peristaltic contraction of circular smooth muscle aids in the propulsion of sperm during ejaculation. Neurovasculture of the epididymis mirrors that of the testes.

3.7 Spermatogenesis and Spermiogenesis

Sperm are specialized gametes that contain half the normal required chromosomes (haploid 23 versus diploid 46). **Meiosis** includes two meiotic cell divisions (meiosis I and II) and is the process by which the chromosome number is reduced by one half.

Spermatogonia begin the transformation into mature sperm at puberty during the process of **spermatogenesis**. Spermatogonia are dormant in the seminiferous tubules of the testes from the late fetal period until puberty. After passing through several mitotic cell divisions and progressing through the type A and type B spermatogonia, it is the type B spermatogonia that divide and form a **primary spermatocyte** containing a diploid number of chromosomes. After the first meiotic division, two **secondary spermatocytes** remain and have a haploid number of chromosomes. After a second meiotic division, four haploid **spermatids** are produced **(Fig. 3.18)**.

Spermatids are transformed into mature sperms by a process known as **spermiogenesis**. This is a metamorphosis in which the nucleus condenses, an acrosome forms, and the shedding of most of the cytoplasm takes place. The mature sperm consists of a *head*, *neck* and *tail*. The **head** contains the nucleus and forms the bulk of the sperm. The **acrosome** is located on the anterior two thirds of the head and it contains enzymes that facilitate sperm penetration during fertilization. The **neck** is simply the junction between the head and tail. The **tail** consists of three parts: the **middle**, **principal**, and **end piece**. The **middle piece**

Clinical Correlate 3.3

Indirect (Congenital) Inguinal Hernia

An **indirect inguinal hernia** makes up 70-75% of all inguinal hernias and is much more prevalent in males. Generally the processus vaginalis is obliterated prior to birth except for the portion that forms the tunica vaginalis. The peritoneal portion of the hernial sac is formed by the lingering patent processus vaginalis. This type of hernia has the possibility of traveling all the way to the top of the testes in the scrotum thus traversing the entire inguinal canal. The hernia passes lateral to the inferior epigastric vessels and through the deep inguinal ring. The hernial sac is located in the spermatic cord (assuming male) and consists of the periosteum of the persistent processus vaginalis and all three of the spermatic cord fascial layers **(a)**.

To test, the examiner should follow the course of the spermatic cord until reaching the superficial inguinal ring. If a hernia exists, a sudden impulse will be felt against the examiner's finger when the patient is asked to cough. If no hernia exists, the superficial inguinal ring will admit the tip of the finger. The distinction between an indirect and direct hernia is tough to isolate at the superficial ring. However, if the examiner's finger is pressed near the area of the deep inguinal ring (located about 3-4 cm superolateral from the pubic tubercle) and a mass is felt, coupled with an impulse at the superficial inguinal ring, the individual has an indirect inguinal hernia **(b, c)**.

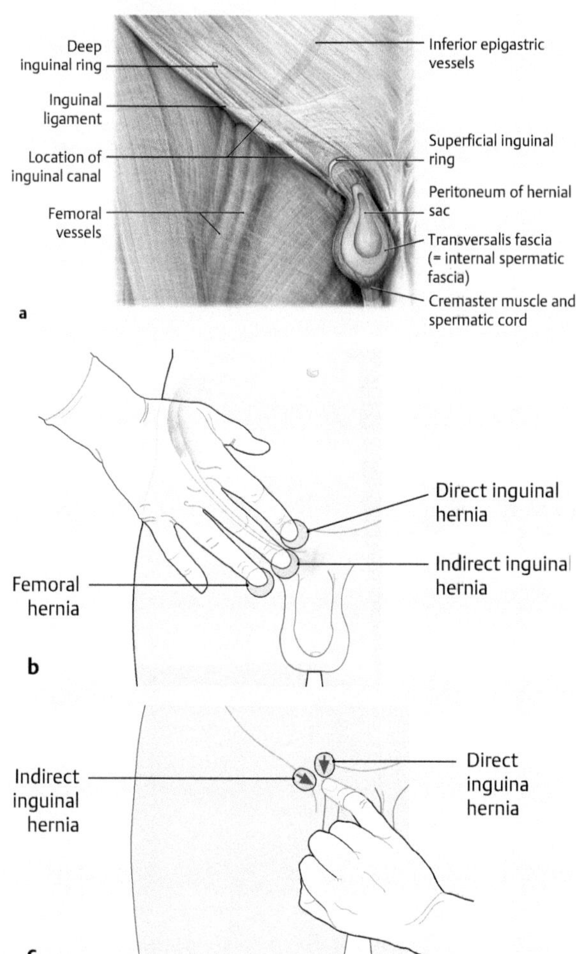

(From Schuenke M, Schulte E, Schumacher U. THIEME Atlas of Anatomy. General Anatomy and Musculoskeletal System. Illustrations by Voll M and Wesker K. 3rd ed. New York: Thieme Medical Publishers; 2020.)

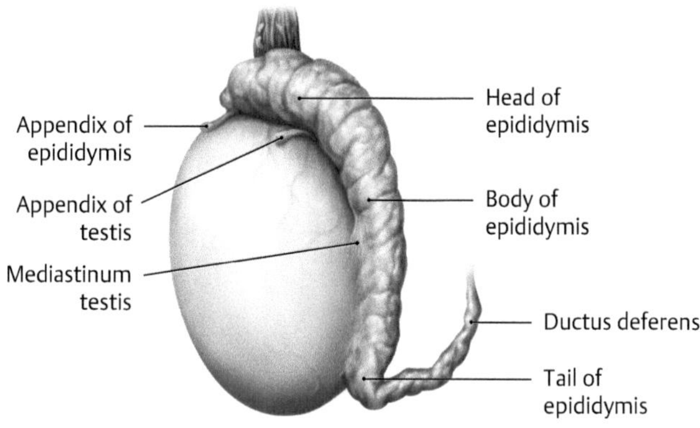

Fig. 3.17 Surface anatomy of the testis and epididymis. (From Schuenke M, Schulte E, Schumacher U. THIEME Atlas of Anatomy. General Anatomy and Musculoskeletal System. Illustrations by Voll M and Wesker K. 3rd ed. New York: Thieme Medical Publishers; 2020.)

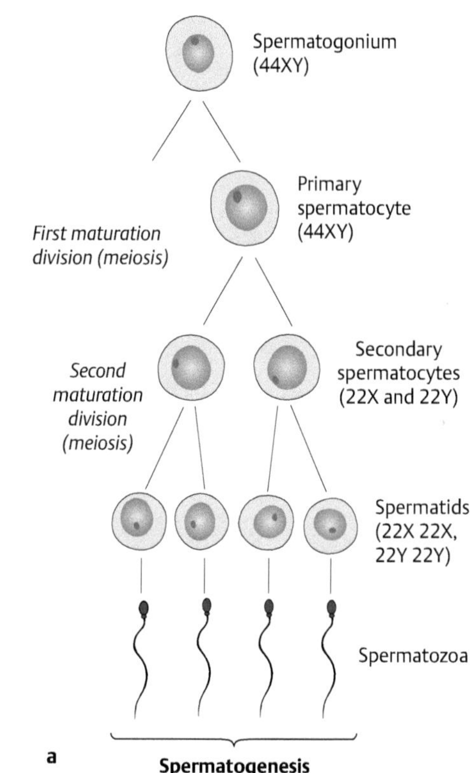

Fig. 3.18 (a) Spermatogenesis and spermiogenesis. (*continued*) (From Schuenke M, Schulte E, Schumacher U. THIEME Atlas of Anatomy. General Anatomy and Musculoskeletal System. Illustrations by Voll M and Wesker K. 3rd ed. New York: Thieme Medical Publishers; 2020.)

is the part that contains the mitochondria and provides motility for the sperm.

During ejaculation, there are normally 200-300 million spermatozoa (mature sperm) deposited. Only 200-500 actually reach the site of fertilization (generally the ampulla of the uterine tube). The process from spermatogenesis through spermiogenesis takes approximately two months to complete and continues throughout the lifetime of a male.

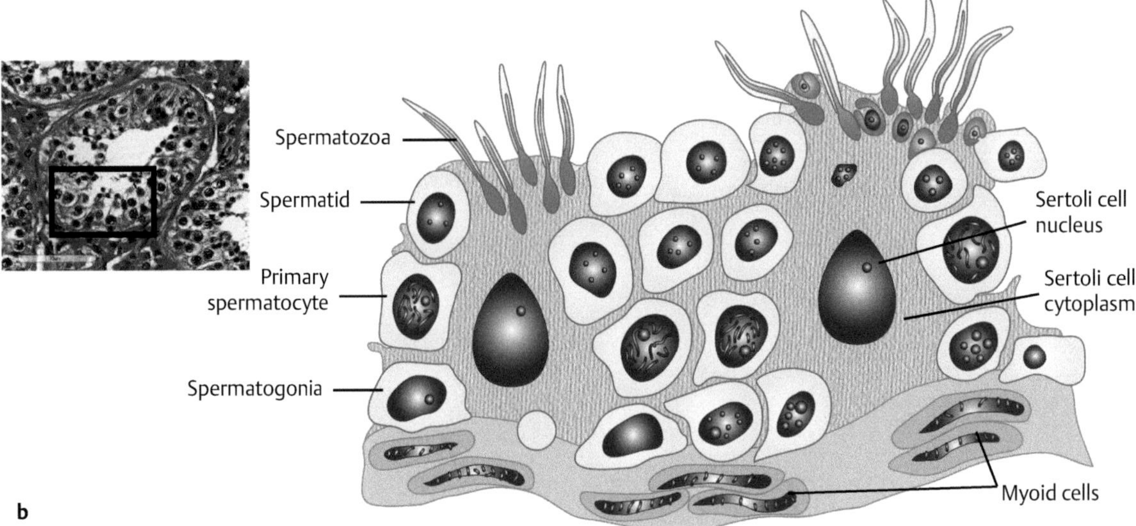

Fig. 3.18 *(continued)* **(b)** Drawing of a portion of the wall of a seminiferous tubule. (From Lowrie DJ. Histology: An Essential Textbook. New York: Thieme Medical Publishers; 2020.)

Clinical Correlate 3.4

Direct (Acquired) Inguinal Hernia

The other type of inguinal hernia is a **direct inguinal hernia**. Weakness of the abdominal wall at the level of the inguinal (*Hesselbach's*) triangle is a predisposing factor, but these only make up about 25-30% of all inguinal hernias. The hernia passes medial to the inferior epigastric vessels adjacent to the deep inguinal ring and is unable to traverse the entire inguinal canal. The hernial sac consists of the periosteum covered by the transversalis fascia. To test, the examiner should press their finger against the superficial inguinal ring and an area in between the superficial and deep inguinal rings, ask the patient to cough, and if pressure is felt against both locations, the individual has a direct inguinal hernia.

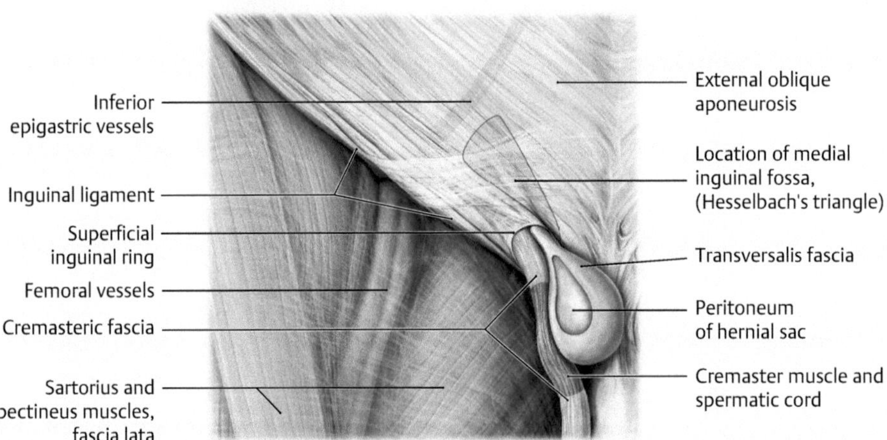

(From Schuenke M, Schulte E, Schumacher U. THIEME Atlas of Anatomy. General Anatomy and Musculoskeletal System. Illustrations by Voll M and Wesker K. 3rd ed. New York: Thieme Medical Publishers; 2020.)

Clinical Correlate 3.5

Appendicular (Amyand's) Hernia

When the appendix is trapped within the hernia sac of an inguinal hernia it is referred to as an Amyand's hernia. The incidence of this type of hernia is rare (1% of inguinal hernias) and clinical presentation generally mimics a typical inguinal hernia. The appendix may or may not be inflamed. Adhesions may ultimately be the reason the appendix is unable to retract from within the hernia sac. An appendectomy is generally performed and the hernia is fixed much like any other inguinal hernia repair (Ivanschuk et al., 2014).

 Clinical Correlate 3.6

Hematocele and Hydrocele

Trauma to the testis can result in the damaged testicular vessels passing blood into the tunica vaginalis, resulting in a **testis hematocele.** If the surrounding scrotal tissue has received the blood from the damaged testicular vessels, then a **scrotal hematocele** could be present. If a hematocele is relatively small and not much pain is associated with it, foot elevation and bed rest may be sufficient to fix the problem. In extreme situations, surgical intervention is done to drain the accumulated blood from the scrotum. If the cause of bleeding is due to a testicular tumor, the entire testicle is generally removed to prevent the cancer from spreading.

A **hydrocele** may be found in a few locations. A **congenital hydrocele** may be associated with an indirect inguinal hernia with excess fluid being found in a *persistent processus vaginalis*. If a **testis hydrocele** is present, the fluid is confined to the scrotum but it distends the tunica vaginalis. A **spermatic cord hydrocele** is isolated in the spermatic cord but it distends the persistent part of the stalk. Blood does not transluminate, so a physician can differentiate between a hematocele and hydrocele.

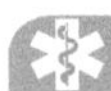 Clinical Correlate 3.7

Cremasteric Reflex

The cremaster reflex is elicited by lightly stroking the superior and medial portions of the thigh. The normal response would be an immediate contraction of the cremaster muscle resulting in elevation of the ipsilateral testes. The afferent limb involves the femoral branch of the genitofemoral (L1-L2) and ilioinguinal nerves (L1). The efferent limb involves the genital branch of the genitofemoral nerve, which in turn innervates the cremaster muscle causing the elevation of the testis.

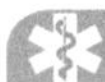 Clinical Correlate 3.8

Vasectomy

A procedure that can sterilize a man and prevent pregnancy involves the ligation of the ductus (vas) deferens while in the scrotum and bilaterally, sealing both ends. This is called a **vasectomy.** Sperm can no longer pass through the male genital duct system but the testicle is unaffected and still functioning normally. A vasectomy is 99.9% effective in preventing pregnancy. If a pregnancy occurs it most likely occurs soon after the procedure, before the man had a sperm count taken. There is a fairly low rate of complications, but a small percentage of men may develop *post-vasectomy pain syndrome* that is chronic and possibly debilitating with very little but pain management to comfort the patient.

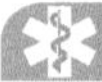 Clinical Correlate 3.9

Varicocele

When the pampiniform plexus, located within the spermatic cord, becomes **varicose** (dilated), it produces a varicocele. These are generally visible when a man is standing or straining, but when they are palpated they are described as feeling like a bag of worms. They are generally found on the left side, presumably because there is a more direct venous drainage on the right side. They can be the result of renal vein drainage problems or defective valves of the testicular veins.

Clinical Correlate 3.10

Testicular Cancer

Testicular cancer is rare but it is the most common cancer in males between 15-35 years of age. Even if the cancer has spread beyond the testicle, this cancer is highly treatable. Regular testicular self-examinations can help identify any growths early. Symptoms can include a lump on either testicle, consistent back pain, the feeling of a heavy scrotum, and dull aches or pain in the abdomen. Treatment can be as simple as surgically removing the diseased testicle.

3.8 Development of the Inguinal Canal

On the superior portion of the posterior abdominal wall, the **urogenital ridge** (formed of **intermediate mesoderm**) proliferates and forms a **gonadal ridge** in both sexes. With the development of primary sex cords and incorporation of primordial germ cells from the yolk sac, the gonad will take on characteristics of either a primordial testis or an ovary.

The **primordial testes** are connected at their caudal end by a band of fibrous tissue known as a **gubernaculum**. This structure extends into the scrotum. The peritoneum evaginates alongside the gubernaculum forming the **processus vaginalis** and this open space passes through the inguinal canal into the **primordial scrotum**. Possibly due to disproportionate growth of the upper abdomen and other factors not completely understood, the testes descend, and by the 12th week they are located in the pelvic region. Around the 28th week, the testes are located near the deep inguinal ring and over the course of approximately three days pass through the inguinal canal. Four weeks later, the testes completely enter the scrotum. The left testes generally descend before the right, and in over 95% of full-term neonates, the testes are completely descended. The **scrotal ligament** is the remnant of the male gubernaculum **(Fig. 3.19)**.

The **primordial ovaries** originate from the superior portion of the posterior abdominal wall, much like the primordial testes. By the 15th week of development, the ovaries have reached the pelvis. The gubernaculum of the female is originally one longer fibrous structure; however, early descent of the ovaries splits this gubernaculum into an upper and lower portion. The upper portion connects the ovary to the primordial uterus near the junction of the uterine tubes while the lower portion connects near this same primordial uterus/uterine tube junction but extends into the labia majora. The **ovarian ligament** is a remnant of the upper portion and the **round ligament of the uterus** is a remnant of the lower portion. The **processus vaginalis** generally disintegrates in the female, but if it persists and extends down into the labia majora, this is known as the *canal of Nuck*. If the *canal of Nuck* is present an individual may show signs of a hydrocele or cyst near or in the labia majora.

The deep and superficial inguinal rings are nearly superimposed and the inguinal canal is very short in a newborn. With growth, the anterior abdominal wall muscles rapidly increase in size and this causes a lengthening of the canal and the separation of the inguinal rings.

3.9 Internal Surface of the Anterolateral Abdominal Wall

After the anterolateral abdominal wall is opened and reflected thus allowing for a view of the posterior surface of the anterolateral wall, a number of folds and fossae can be identified. These structures represent past embryological structures and allow a clinician to distinguish between different inguinal hernia types. An inguinal hernia is a protrusion of parietal peritoneum and viscera through a normal or abnormal opening from the cavity in which they belong and generally involves the small intestine. This internal wall is covered by transversalis fascia and is closest to the muscle layer, an extraperitoneal fat layer that varies in thickness and allows for the passage of embryological remnants, and finally the parietal peritoneum that lies closest to the abdominal viscera.

The **median umbilical fold** extends between the umbilicus and apex of the urinary bladder. It covers the **median umbilical ligament**, which is the fibrous remnant of the *urachus*. The **medial umbilical folds** are located lateral to the median umbilical fold and cover the **medial umbilical ligaments**, the fibrous remnants of the *occluded umbilical arteries*. The **lateral umbilical folds** are located lateral to the medial umbilical folds and cover the patent *inferior epigastric vessels* (**Fig. 3.20**).

The **supravesical fossae** rest on the bladder and are located between the median and medial umbilical folds. These fossae rise and fall due to the filling and emptying of the bladder. The **medial inguinal fossae** are located between the medial and lateral umbilical folds. Within this larger fossae is a more defined **inguinal/Hesselbach's triangle**. The borders of this triangle include the lateral border of the rectus abdominis muscle (medial); inferior epigastric vessels (lateral); and the inguinal ligament (inferiorly). This triangle is filled mostly by the conjoint tendon but contains a small depression near the inferior epigastric vessels. This depression is the location of the less common *direct inguinal hernia*. The **lateral inguinal fossae** are located lateral to the lateral umbilical folds. They are the location of the deep inguinal ring which itself is located near the inferior portion of the inferior epigastric vessels. Passage of bowels through the deep inguinal ring would represent an *indirect inguinal hernia* (**Fig. 3.20**).

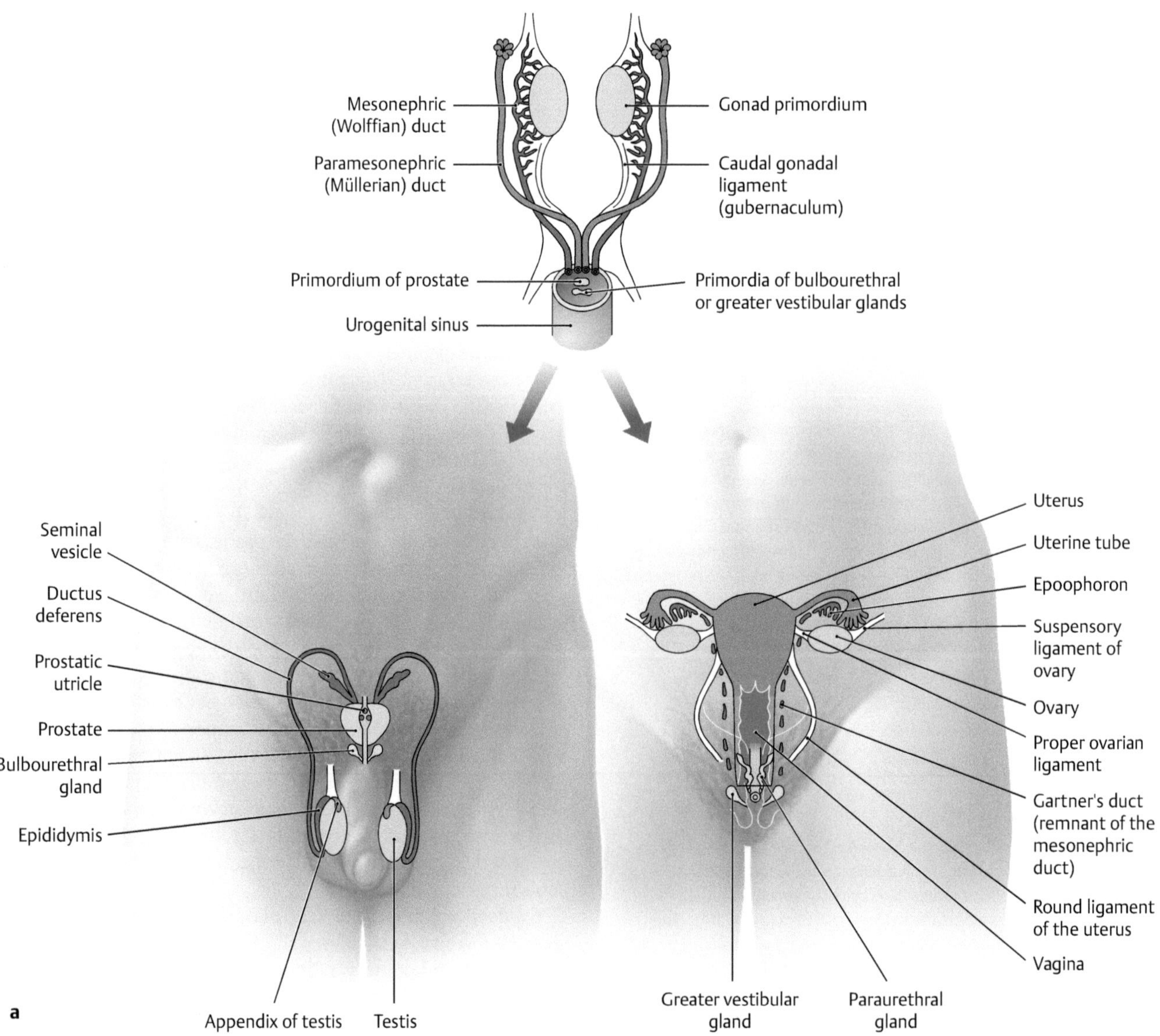

Fig. 3.19 (a) Development of the internal genitalia. (*continued*) (From Schuenke M, Schulte E, Schumacher U. THIEME Atlas of Anatomy. Internal Organs. Illustrations by Voll M and Wesker K. 3rd ed. New York: Thieme Medical Publishers; 2020.)

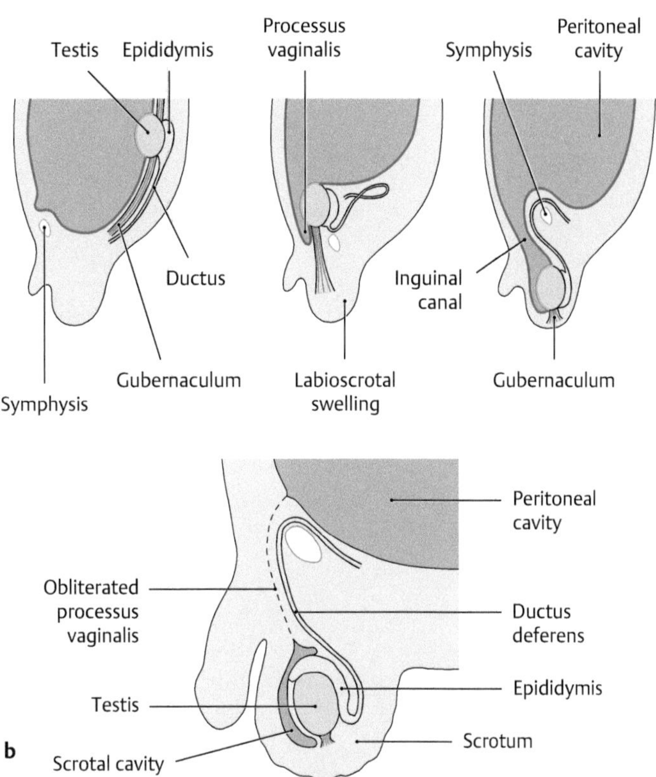

Fig. 3.19 *(continued)* **(b)** Development of the inguinal canal. (From Schuenke M, Schulte E, Schumacher U. THIEME Atlas of Anatomy. General Anatomy and Musculoskeletal System. Illustrations by Voll M and Wesker K. 3rd ed. New York: Thieme Medical Publishers; 2020.)

The listed folds and fossae above correspond with the area below the level of the umbilicus. However, extending from the umbilicus to the liver is a peritoneal reflection called the **falciform ligament**. It contains the *round ligament of the liver (ligamentum teres)* and this is the fibrous remnant of the *umbilical vein.*

3.10 Peritoneal Cavity

After entering through the abdominal wall a continuous, thin and wet serous membrane (a simple squamous mesothelium) known as the **peritoneum** can be seen lining the abdominopelvic wall and infesting the majority of the internal viscera. There is an outer *parietal layer of peritoneum* attached to the internal surface of the abdominopelvic wall and there is the inner *visceral layer* of peritoneum that invests the viscera. The parietal peritoneum is supplied by all the same neurovasculature of the outer abdominal wall thus it is somatically innervated and sensitive to heat, cold, pressure and pain (possibly due to a laceration). Visceral peritoneum and the organs it is associated with are supplied by the same neurovasculature. This layer is stimulated for the most part by stretching and chemical irritation and it is insensitive to such factors as heat, cold and touch. Pain related to this layer of peritoneum is poorly localized and may present according to the principal of referred pain **(Fig. 3.21)**.

The **peritoneal cavity** is the potential space between the parietal and visceral layers of peritoneum **(Table 3.1)**. In males this cavity is completely closed off. In females, however, there is a communication from this cavity to the outer body by way of the uterine tubes, uterus and vagina and constitutes the potential for an infection. The peritoneal cavity does not contain any organs, just peritoneal fluid, which is derived from interstitial fluid and is made mainly of water, but also consists of electrolytes, antibodies and leukocytes. Peritoneal fluid functions mainly to lubricate adjacent viscera so they do not adhere to one another but it also can fight off infections.

The peritoneal cavity is divided into a greater and lesser sac. The **greater sac** is located between the anterolateral abdominal wall and the internal organs and it extends from the diaphragm down to the pelvis. It is a remnant of the embryonic left pleuroperitoneal space. The *transverse mesocolon* divides the greater sac into a **supracolic compartment** that contains the stomach, liver and spleen and an **infracolic compartment** that contains the small intestine, ascending colon and descending colon. The infracolic compartment is further subdivided into a left and right **infracolic space** by *"the mesentery."* The **lesser sac (omental bursa)** is located mainly posterior to the stomach and anterior to the pancreas. This sac is continuous superiorly up to the diaphragm and coronary ligaments of the liver. In an infant, the lesser sac continues inferiorly between the layers of the greater omentum. The lesser sac opens into the greater sac at the **epiploic (omental) foramen** or *foramen of Winslow* **(Fig. 3.22)**. This foramen can be located with a finger posterior to the hepatoduodenal ligament. This is the same location of the *portal triad*, or the combination of the hepatic portal vein, hepatic arteries and (common) bile duct.

There is a relationship between the peritoneum and viscera, with these organs being referred to as intraperitoneal, primarily retroperitoneal, secondarily retroperitoneal or subperitoneal. The retroperitoneal and subperitoneal structures are also grouped together as extraperitoneal structures **(Fig. 3.21)**.

- **Intraperitoneal**: the structures that are almost completely enveloped by visceral peritoneum and attach to the abdominal

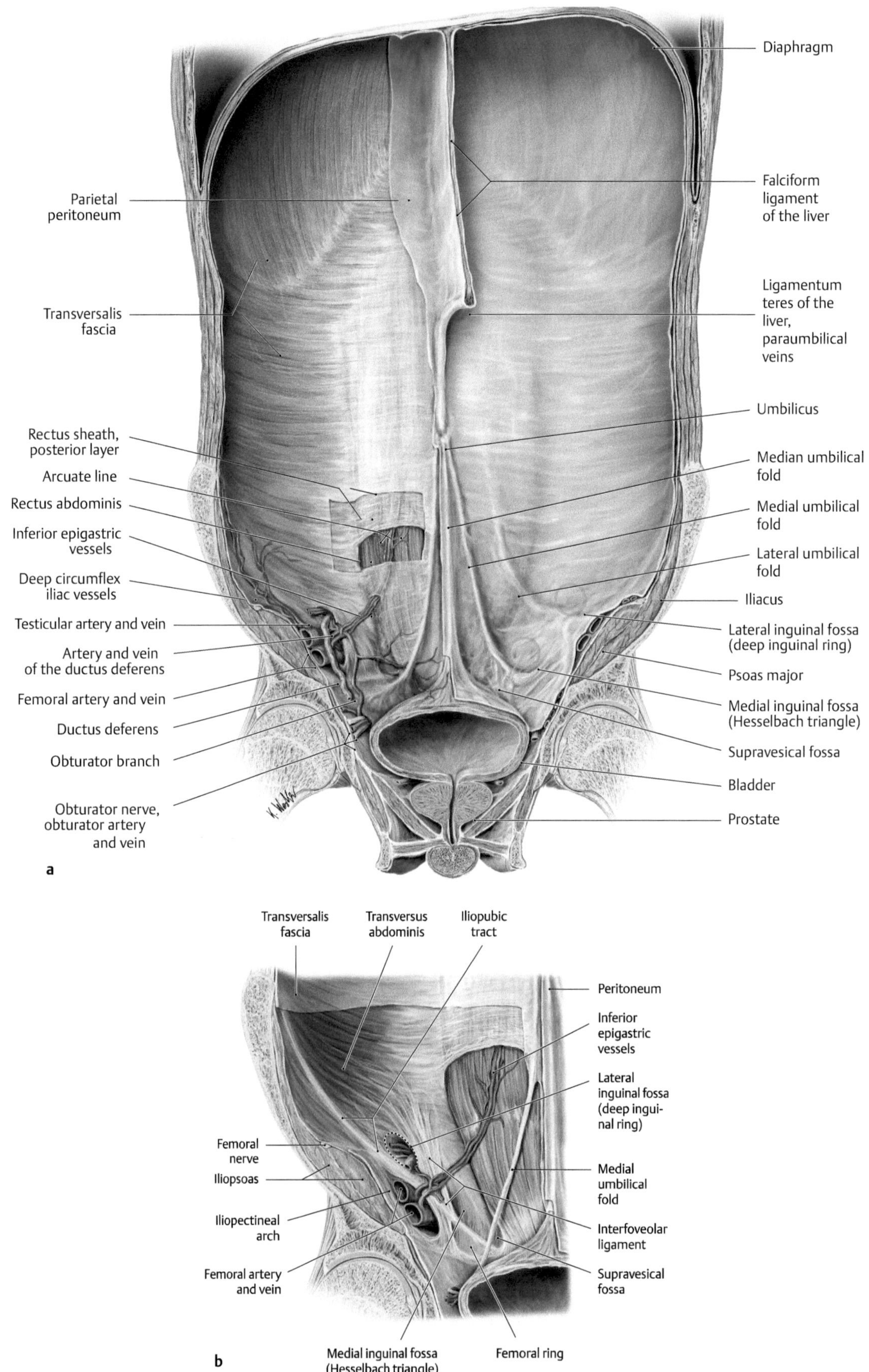

Fig. 3.20 (a) Coronal section, posterior (internal) view of anterior abdominal wall. The three fossae (circled) are potential sites of herniation. **(b)** Inferior anterior abdominal wall. (From Schuenke M, Schulte E, Schumacher U. THIEME Atlas of Anatomy. General Anatomy and Musculoskeletal System. Illustrations by Voll M and Wesker K. 1st ed. New York: Thieme Medical Publishers; 2010.)

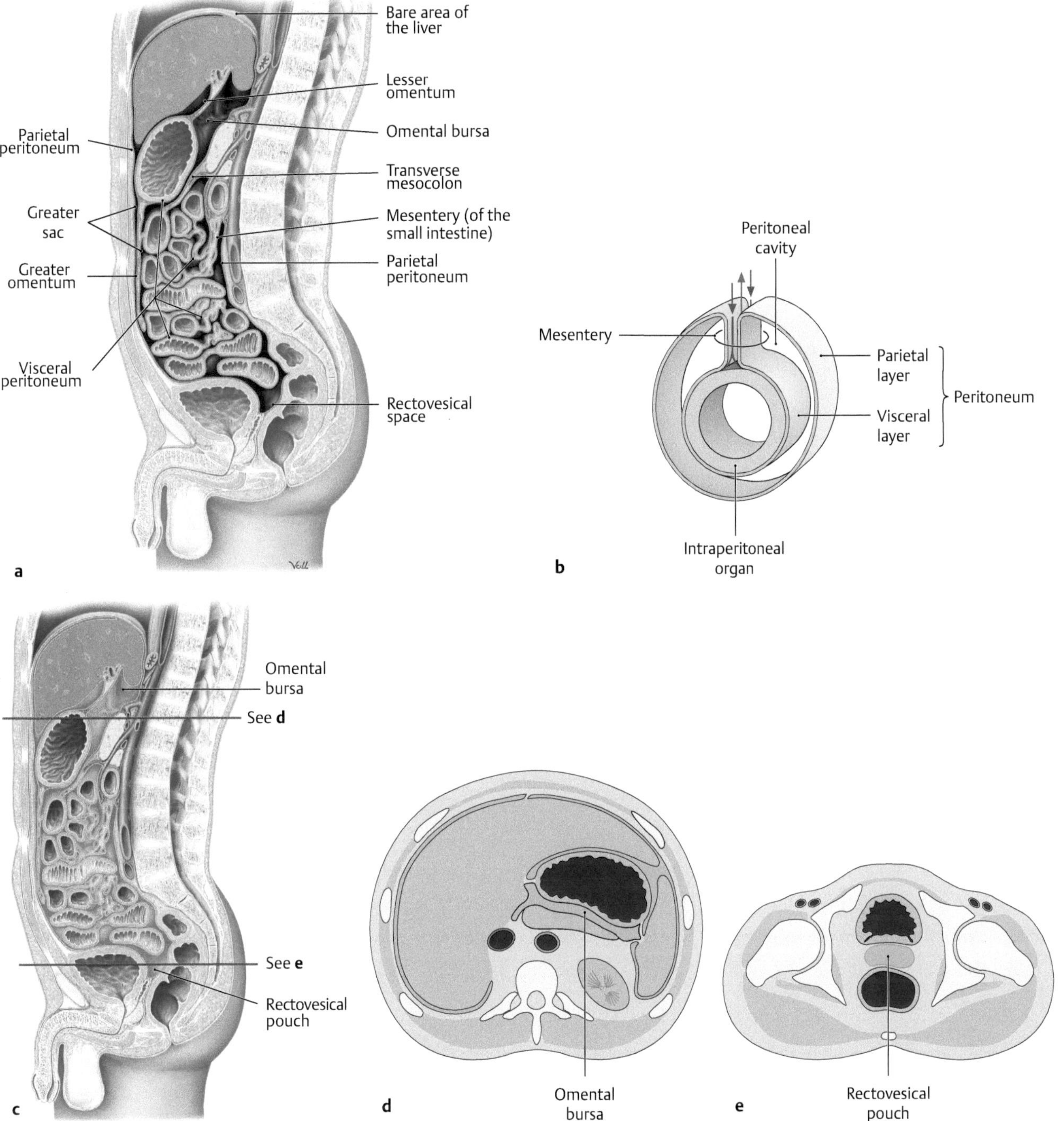

Fig. 3.21 (a) Midsagittal section through the male abdominopelvic cavity, viewed from the left. The peritoneum is shown in red. **(b)** Relationship of the intraperitoneal organ to the mesentery and peritoneum, *arrows* indicate blood vessels in the mesentery. **(c-e)** Serous cavities (peritoneal spaces): abdominal peritoneal cavity and pelvic peritoneal cavity. (From Schuenke M, Schulte E, Schumacher U. Thieme Atlas of Anatomy, Internal Organs. Illustrations by Voll M and Wesker K. 3rd ed. New York: Thieme Medical Publishers; 2020.)

walls by a mesentery. There is always a portion of an intraperitoneal visceral organ that is not covered with peritoneum and this serves as the location of passing neurovasculature. These organs include the liver (except at the *bare area*), spleen, stomach, the first part of the duodenum, jejunum, ileum, cecum (occasionally retroperitoneal), appendix, transverse colon and sigmoid colon.

- **Primarily retroperitoneal**: these structures lie between the parietal peritoneum and posterior abdominal wall and are not supported by a mesentery but are surrounded by large amounts of fat. These organs include the suprarenal (adrenal) glands, kidneys, ureters, upper rectum, aorta and IVC.
- **Secondary retroperitoneal**: these structures are originally intraperitoneal but during development become fixed to the posterior abdominal wall and have a layer of parietal peritoneum resting on their anterior surface. These organs include the 2nd, 3rd, and 4th parts of the duodenum, pancreas (except tail), ascending colon and descending colon.

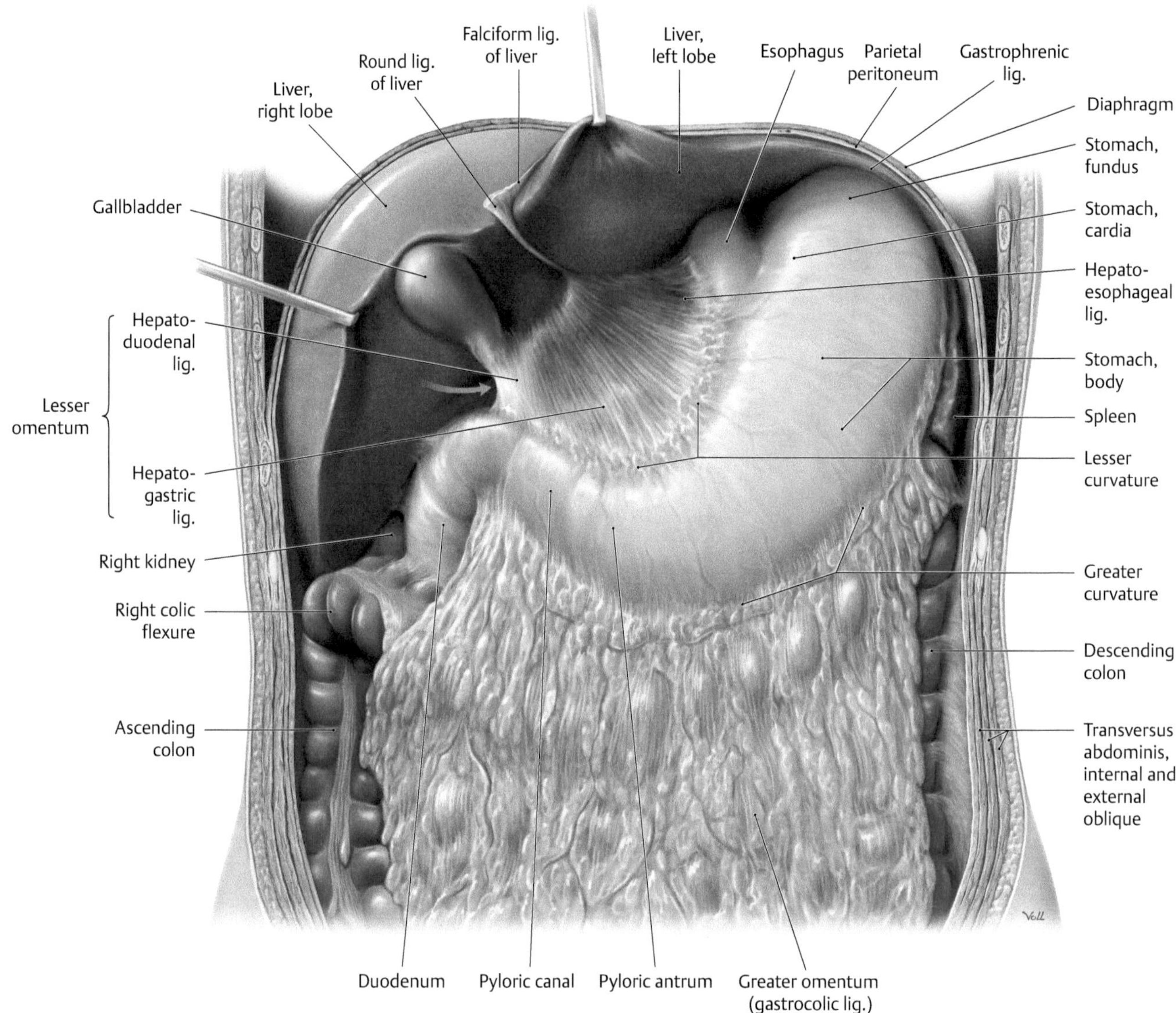

Fig. 3.22 Stomach in situ, great and lesser omentums, and epiploic (omental) foramen (*arrow*). (From Schuenke M, Schulte E, Schumacher U. Thieme Atlas of Anatomy, Internal Organs. Illustrations by Voll M and Wesker K. 3rd ed. New York: Thieme Medical Publishers; 2020.)

- **Subperitoneal**: these organs are located below the inferior margin of peritoneum and include the bladder, lower rectum, anal canal and organs associated with sexual reproduction.

A double layer of peritoneum can also form reflections that attach to viscera and these are known as an *omentum, mesentery* or *peritoneal ligament.* Peritoneal ligaments are also known to help contribute to the formation of an omentum.

An **omentum** connects the stomach to the transverse colon (greater omentum) as well as the liver to the stomach and first part of the duodenum (lesser omentum). The majority of the **greater omentum** begins at the greater curvature of the stomach and descends anterior to the small intestine and parts of the large intestine before ascending back towards the transverse colon to form an apron-like structure. It also attaches to the diaphragm and spleen. It functions as a site for fat to be deposited and responds to intraperitoneal infections and internal wounds by physically containing the area of trauma or infection. It is quite common to find the greater omentum wrapped around an organ in a cadaver.

The greater omentum is made up of three peritoneal ligaments (**Fig. 3.22; Fig. 3.23**).

- **Gastrocolic ligament**: connects the greater curvature of the stomach to the inferior border of the transverse colon. This portion of the greater omentum has an apron-like appearance.
- **Gastrophrenic ligament**: connects the fundus of the stomach to the diaphragm.
- **Gastrosplenic ligament**: connects the greater curvature of the stomach to the hilum of the spleen. Allows for the passage of the short gastric and left gastro-omental vessels.

The **lesser omentum** connects the liver to both the lesser curvature of the stomach and first part of the duodenum. It is made up of two peritoneal ligaments that are connected to one another (**Fig. 3.22**).

- **Hepatogastric ligament**: the thinner portion of the lesser omentum that connects the liver to the lesser curvature of the stomach.

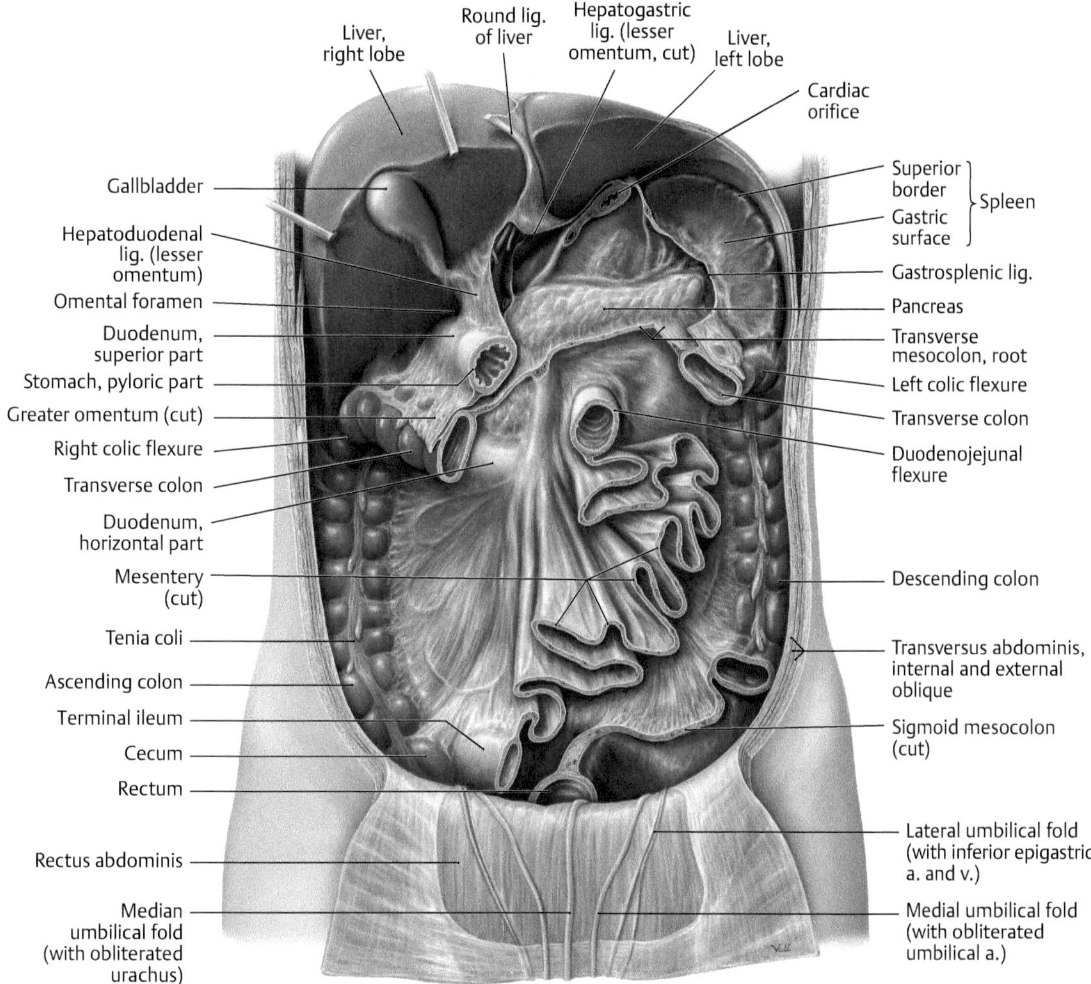

Fig. 3.23 Mesenteries and organs of the peritoneal cavity. (From Schuenke M, Schulte E, Schumacher U. Thieme Atlas of Anatomy, Internal Organs. Illustrations by Voll M and Wesker K. 3rd ed. New York: Thieme Medical Publishers; 2020.)

Clinical Correlate 3.11

Peritonitis

If a bacterial contamination occurs after trauma or an open incision (laparotomy) that could result in fecal matter entering the peritoneal cavity, the result is an inflammation of the surrounding peritoneum called **peritonitis**. Peritonitis can be lethal and quite painful because the peritoneal surface is semipermeable and can rapidly absorb different fluid compositions in which bacterial toxins could be present. Any excess fluid in the peritoneal cavity is called ascitic fluid or **ascities**. If large amounts of fluid are present in the peritoneal cavity, this can alter the general movements of the GI tract. Ascites can be the result of portal hypertension or metastasis of cancer cells, among other things. The *paracolic gutters* can provide a pathway for ascitic fluid to pass thus causing an infection to spread.

- **Hepatoduodenal ligament**: the thicker portion of the lesser omentum that allows for the passage of the ***portal triad***. The triad includes the hepatic arteries, portal vein and (common) bile duct.

A **mesentery** represents a continuation between the visceral and parietal layers of peritoneum. A mesentery serves as the connection between an intraperitoneal organ and the body wall and allows for the passage of neurovasculature and lymph drainage associated with that portion of the gut. The mesentery associated with the jejunum and ileum is sometimes referred to as *"the mesentery (proper)"* and the portion closest to the vertebral column and extending toward the ileocecal junction is known as the "*root of the mesentery*." The superior mesenteric neurovasculature and lymph drainage is associated with "the mesentery." Other mesenteries include **(Fig. 3.24)**:

- **Transverse mesocolon**: connects the posterior surface of the transverse colon to the posterior abdominal wall. The layers of this mesentery are continuous with that of the gastrocolic ligament. It allows for the passage of the middle colic vessels, autonomics and lymphatics.
- **Sigmoid mesocolon**: connects the sigmoid colon to the posterior abdominal and pelvic walls. The sigmoid and superior rectal vessels, autonomics and lymphatics pass through this mesentery.
- **Mesoappendix**: connects the appendix to the mesentery of the ileum. It allows for passage of the appendicular vessels, autonomics and lymphatics.

A **peritoneal ligament** connects two organs to one another or an organ to the abdominal wall. The individual peritoneal ligaments

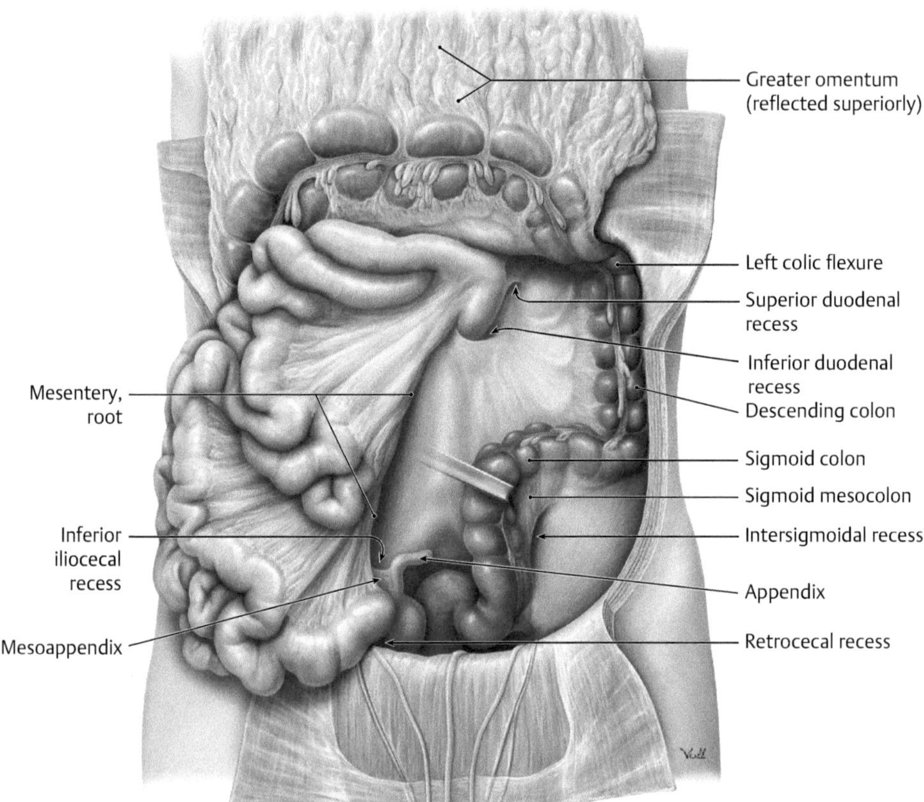

Fig. 3.24 Mesenteries of the peritoneal cavity. (From Schuenke M, Schulte E, Schumacher U. Thieme Atlas of Anatomy, Internal Organs. Illustrations by Voll M and Wesker K. 3rd ed. New York: Thieme Medical Publishers; 2020.)

that help form the omentum have already been discussed but a number of others exist (**Fig. 3.37**):

- **Falciform ligament**: connects the liver to the anterior abdominal wall. The falciform ligament creates a left and right **subphrenic space** on the anterior surface of the liver. These spaces extend as far superiorly as the coronary ligaments of the liver. Passing through it are the *paraumbilical veins* and *round ligament of the liver* (**Fig. 3.37**).
- **Round ligament of the liver (ligamentum teres)**, which is the remnant of the *umbilical vein*, is enclosed by the falciform ligament (**Fig. 3.37**).
- **Ligamentum venosum**: a remnant of the *ductus venosus*, a structure that shunts blood from the *umbilical vein* to the IVC in order to bypass the liver during embryonic development (**Fig. 3.37**).
- **Coronary ligament of liver**: the peritoneal reflection from mostly the posterior aspect of the liver back onto the diaphragm. The lateral extensions of the coronary ligaments are known as the left and right **triangular ligaments**. These ligaments define the **bare area of the liver**, a region devoid of a visceral layer of peritoneum resting on the liver's surface (**Fig. 3.37**).
- **Splenorenal ligament**: serves as the attachment between the hilum of the spleen and left kidney and allows passage of the splenic vessels and possibly the tail of the pancreas (**Fig. 3.23**).
- **Splenocolic ligament**: connects the splenic capsule to the left colic/splenic flexure, the sharp bend at the border of the transverse and descending colons. It is generally avascular (**Fig. 3.23**).
- **Pancreaticocolic ligament**: connects the body and proximal tail region of the pancreas to the transverse colon near the left colic/splenic flexure. It is generally avascular (**Fig. 3.23**).
- **Phrenicocolic ligament**: connects the left colic/splenic flexure to the diaphragm opposite the tenth and eleventh ribs and it functions by supporting the spleen.

With the framework created by the peritoneum, spaces evolve and allow peritoneal fluid to flow from one space to another. As mentioned earlier, the transverse colon divides the greater sac into a supracolic and infracolic compartment. The infracolic compartment is further subdivided into a left versus right infracolic space by *the mesentery*. The space just lateral to both the ascending and descending colons are known as **paracolic gutters**. These gutters serve as a communication between themselves and the supra/infracolic compartments. The **hepatorenal recess** (*Morison's pouch*) continuous with the **subhepatic space** is found on the right side of the liver adjacent to the right suprarenal gland and kidney. It is a gravity-dependent recess that receives drainage from the lesser sac and supracolic compartments and must be considered when patients are bed ridden for extended periods of time (**Fig. 3.25**).

3.11 Viscera of the Abdomen

The **gastrointestinal (GI) tract** or **alimentary canal** is the muscular tube that passes through the body and is responsible for digestion and absorption of nutrients. The food first inserted into the oral cavity will travel through the GI tract before its undigested

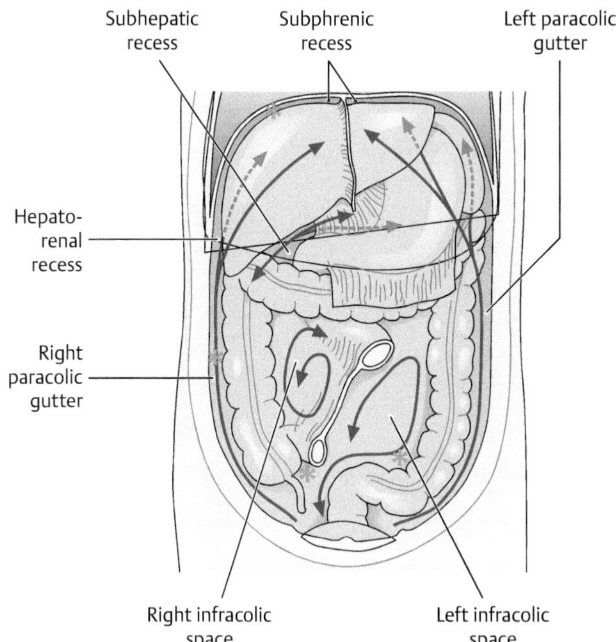

Fig. 3.25 Drainage spaces within the peritoneal cavity. (From Schuenke M, Schulte E, Schumacher U. Thieme Atlas of Anatomy, Internal Organs. Illustrations by Voll M and Wesker K. 3rd ed. New York: Thieme Medical Publishers; 2020.)

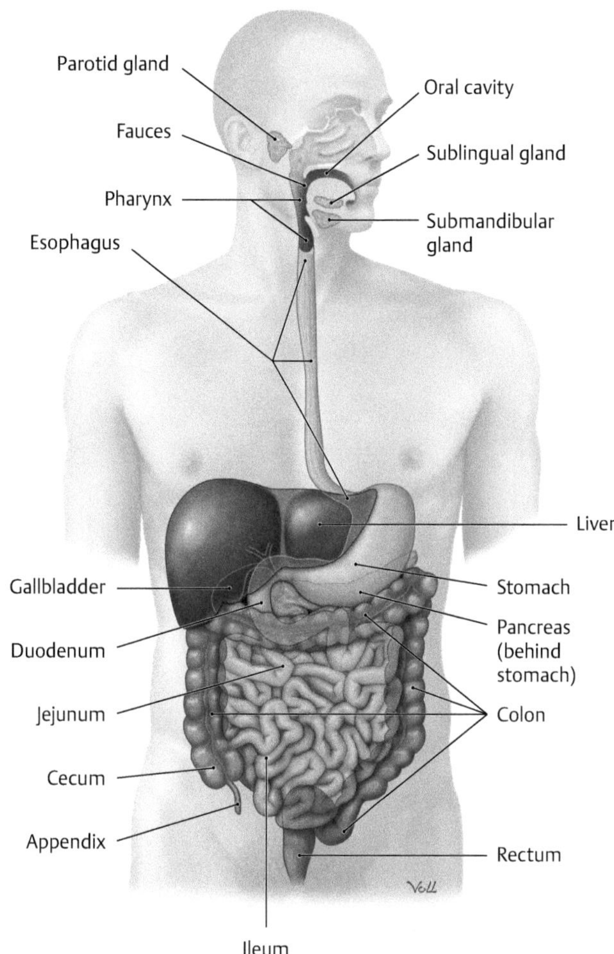

Fig. 3.26 The gastrointestional tract. (From Schuenke M, Schulte E, Schumacher U. Thieme Atlas of Anatomy, Internal Organs. Illustrations by Voll M and Wesker K. 3rd ed. New York: Thieme Medical Publishers; 2020.)

bolus exits the anal canal by defecation. The majority of digestion occurs in the stomach and the first part of the small intestine known as the duodenum. The absorption of chemical compounds primarily occurs in the small intestine while most water absorption takes place in the large intestine and this helps contribute to the formation of solid feces.

The organs of the GI tract include the mouth/oral cavity, pharynx, esophagus, stomach, small intestine, large intestine and anus (**Fig. 3.26**). The total length can reach as much as 30 feet in a cadaver due to the loss of muscle tone. The food that enters this muscular tube can technically be considered to be outside the body because the GI tract is open to the outside environment from mouth to anus.

Accessory digestive organs are found external but connected to the GI tract by ducts. These organs include the teeth, tongue, salivary glands, liver, gallbladder and pancreas. These structures can help break down larger pieces of food or can be involved in chemical digestion.

The process of digestion involves five steps and these steps may be out of order or repeated. These steps include: *ingestion*, *mechanical breakdown*, *chemical breakdown*, *absorption* and *defecation*.

1. **Ingestion**: putting food into one's mouth.
2. **Mechanical breakdown**: physically breaking down food by chewing, churning in the stomach, and segmentation (mainly through the small intestines). This type of breakdown creates smaller pieces of food thus making chemical digestion more efficient.
3. **Chemical breakdown**: reducing food from larger molecules such as carbohydrates, proteins and lipids into smaller nutrients capable of being taken up by cells such as glucose, amino acids and fatty acids. The accessory organs of the GI tract carry out chemical digestion by producing enzymes along with other substances that are secreted into the lumen in order to make contact with the mechanically broken down food.
4. **Absorption**: the passing of most small nutrients from the epithelial cells lining the lumen of the GI tract to blood capillaries. Fat absorption involves the formation of chylomicrons in the cell, which then pass through the lacteals of the lymphatic system before finally reaching the bloodstream. Over 90% of all nutrition is absorbed through the small intestine.
5. **Defecation**: the elimination of feces, the indigestible food that cannot be absorbed.

3.12 Segmentation versus Peristalsis

The movement of a food bolus is mitigated through the processes of segmentation and peristalsis. **Segmentation** involves the rhythmic and localized constrictions of nonadjacent segments of the intestine. The process repeats itself by moving chyme (partially digested food) back and forth within the same area of the segment. This increases the efficiency of the mechanical breakdown of food, allows for more exposure to the digestive juices

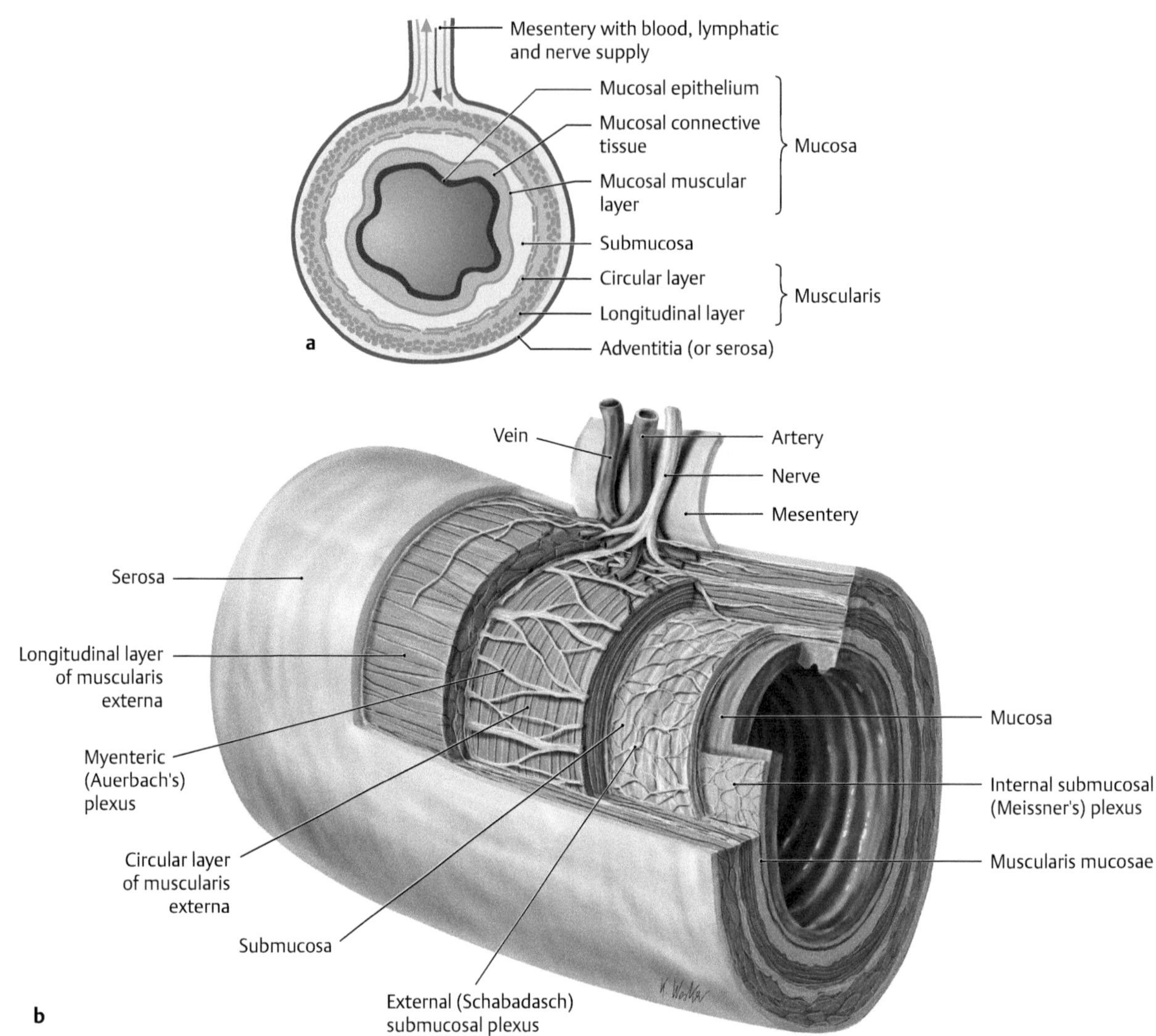

Fig. 3.27 **(a)** Schematic cross-section illustrating the histology of the gastrointestinal tract. **(b)** The enteric nervous system in the small intestine. (From Schuenke M, Schulte E, Schumacher U. Thieme Atlas of Anatomy, Internal Organs. Illustrations by Voll M and Wesker K. 3rd ed. New York: Thieme Medical Publishers; 2020.)

important in chemical breakdown, and increases nutrient absorption. Segmentation is most prominent in the small intestine but also occurs in the large intestine. **Peristalsis** is a more continuous and slow propulsion of food that involves alternate waves of contraction and relaxation of adjacent segments. There is not as much mixing of the food bolus with digestive juices, but peristalsis complements the mechanical process of segmentation. Most peristalsis takes place from the esophagus through the end of the small intestine.

Presentation of the GI tract will be based on the structures area of embryonic development. The GI tract during development is divided into a foregut, midgut and hindgut. The foregut is made up of the esophagus, stomach, first two parts of the duodenum, liver, gallbladder and pancreas. The spleen is associated with the foregut because of its neurovasculature but it does not develop as a foregut structure. The midgut consists of the final two parts of the duodenum, jejunum, ileum, cecum, appendix, ascending colon and the proximal two-thirds of the transverse colon. Finally, the hindgut is made up of the distal one-third of the transverse colon, descending colon, sigmoid colon, rectum and upper one-half of the anal canal.

The function of the GI tract is controlled by the enteric nervous system (ENS) and it is associated with *Meissner's submucosal plexus* and *Auerbach's myenteric plexus.* It can be found continuously from the esophagus down to the anus. It receives considerable input from the autonomic nervous system (ANS) but can operate autonomously. Due to its own independent reflex activities the ENS can be considered separate from the ANS. The ENS communicates with the central nervous system through the ANS (**Fig. 3.27**).

The abdominal aorta has three main branches that supply blood to the GI tract. The celiac trunk and its branches supply the foregut. The superior mesenteric artery and its branches supply the midgut. Finally the inferior mesenteric artery and its branches supply the hindgut. Nutrients that are absorbed through the lumen of the GI tract will enter the portal venous system before reaching the liver to be processed. It is the union of the superior mesenteric and splenic veins that form the hepatic portal vein, the major blood supply to the liver.

3.13 Overview of GI Tract Histology

The tubular wall of the GI tract is subdivided into four different layers. These include the mucosa, submucosa, muscularis externa and the serosa/adventitia (**Fig. 3.27**). The *Meissner* and *Auerbach* nervous plexuses help form the enteric nervous system, a nervous system that compares in size to the central nervous system and drives the innervation of the GI tract (**Fig. 3.27**). Although all four of these layers are found in each organ of the digestive tract, it is the organization and composition of these layers that distinguish one organ from the next.

The **muscosa** is the innermost layer and is broken down into an epithelium, lamina propria and muscularis mucosa. The surface area of this layer can increase depending on features such as *rugae, crypts, pits* and *villi* (**Fig. 3.27**).

- Epithelium: the mucosa is either stratified squamous or simple columnar.
- Lamina propria: a loose connective tissue underlying the epithelium and containing neurovasculature, lymphatic vessels and in specific regions intestinal glands.
- Muscularis mucosa: a thin layer of multiple smooth muscle layers underlying the lamina propria. Smooth muscle is usually situated in an inner circular and outer longitudinal orientation.

The **submucosa** is a connective tissue layer that underlies the mucosa and contains larger neurovasculature including the *Meissner's submucosal plexus* of the enteric nervous system. Specific regions such as the duodenum have submucosal glands (*Brunner's glands*) that have their acini (secreting cells) located in the submucosa layer but their ducts must pass back towards the epithelium (**Fig. 3.27**).

The **muscularis externa** underlies the submucosa and contains at least an inner circular and outer longitudinal layer of smooth muscle. Skeletal muscle can be located in the upper and middle portions of the esophagus as well as the anal sphincter. When the inner circular layer contracts, it narrows the lumen of the GI tract. The inner layer may also thicken in specific regions and form sphincters that regulate the flow of a food bolus. Contraction of the outer longitudinal layer is associated with peristalsis and propels food through the lumen. The part of the enteric nervous system known as the *Auerbach's myenteric plexus* is located between the inner circular and outer longitudinal muscle layers (**Fig. 3.27**).

The **serosa/adventitia** serves as the outermost layer of connective tissue and consists of neurovasculature and lymphatics. Major structures or contributors of these layers will be discussed with each visceral organ or group.

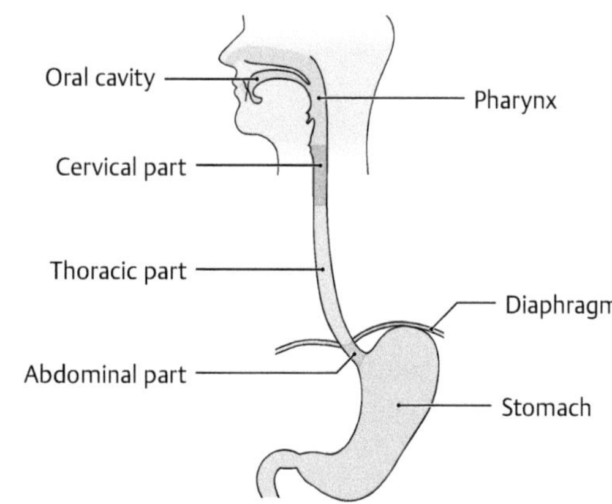

Fig. 3.28 Divisions of the esophagus. (From Schuenke M, Schulte E, Schumacher U. Thieme Atlas of Anatomy, Internal Organs. Illustrations by Voll M and Wesker K. 3rd ed. New York: Thieme Medical Publishers; 2020.)

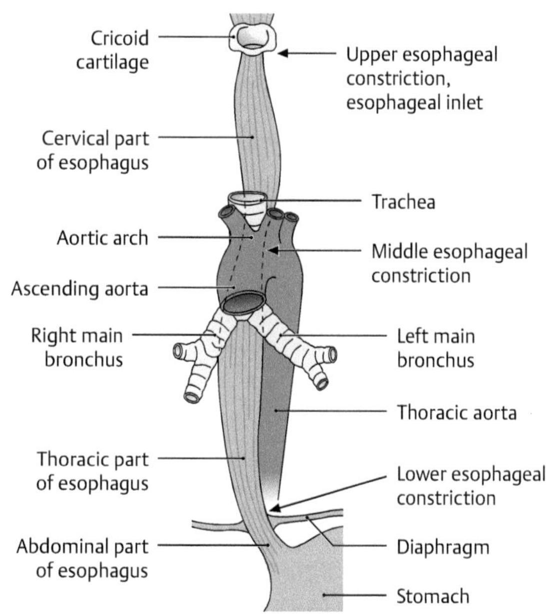

Fig. 3.29 Constrictions of the esophagus. (From Schuenke M, Schulte E, Schumacher U. Thieme Atlas of Anatomy, Internal Organs. Illustrations by Voll M and Wesker K. 3rd ed. New York: Thieme Medical Publishers; 2020.)

3.14 Esophagus

The muscular tube that extends from the end of the laryngopharynx (hypopharynx) at vertebral level C6 down through the neck, thorax and finally through the diaphragm before reaching the stomach at vertebral level T11 is known as the **esophagus** (**Fig. 3.28**). The junction between the esophagus and stomach is known as the *esophagogastric junction* and is clinically known as the **Z-line**. This is the region where an abrupt change from the esophageal *stratified squamous* to the stomachs *simple columnar epithelium* takes place. It is approximately 20-25 cm in total length and subdivided into three unequal parts, the *cervical, thoracic*, and *abdominal*. The esophagus has varying degrees of skeletal versus smooth muscle contributions. The upper one third is primarily skeletal; the middle one third is a combination of skeletal and smooth; and the lower one third is primarily smooth muscle.

There are three constrictions associated with the esophagus. The cricopharyngeus muscle serves as the upper esophageal sphincter (UES) and relaxes during swallowing but contracts when swallowing is not taking place. The middle constriction is due to the left main bronchus and aortic arch pressing against the esophagus at approximately the T4/T5 vertebral level. The lower constriction is formed as the esophagus passes through the diaphragm at vertebral level T10 (**Fig. 3.29**).

3.14.1 Neurovasculature of the Esophagus

Branchiomotor fibers from the recurrent laryngeal nerve (of CN X) innervate the skeletal muscle while the smooth muscle is innervated by parasympathetic fibers coursing through the vagus nerve (CN X) and the **esophageal plexus**, an autonomic plexus wrapped around the abdominal portion of the esophagus. Sympathetic fibers mostly from the esophageal plexus innervate the blood vessels (**Fig. 3.30a**).

The *cervical region* is supplied by branches of the **inferior thyroid artery** (subclavian br.). The *thoracic region* receives blood from the **esophageal** and **bronchial arteries** (thoracic aorta brs.). The *abdominal region* is supplied by the **left gastric** (celiac trunk br.) and **left inferior phrenic** (abdominal aorta br.) **arteries** (**Fig. 3.30b**).

Venous drainage of the *cervical region* is through tributaries of the **inferior thyroid veins**. The *thoracic region* is drained by numerous **esophageal veins** before they reach the azygos, hemiazygos or accessory hemiazygos veins. The *submucosal veins* of the *abdominal region* drain to either the **left gastric** or **esophageal veins**. The left gastric vein is part of the *portal venous drainage* and eventually reaches the portal vein while the esophageal veins are part of the *systematic venous drainage* and drain to the azygos vein. The anastomosis between submucosal veins between the portal and systematic venous drainage in the abdominal esophagus can lead to esophageal varices during portal hypertension (**Fig. 3.30c**).

Lymphatic drainage of the *cervical region* is to the **paratracheal** and **deep cervical lymph nodes**. The *thoracic region* drains to the **superior diaphragmatic**, **posterior mediastinal** and **tracheobronchial lymph nodes** along with the **bronchomediastinal trunk**. The *abdominal region* drains to the **left gastric lymph nodes** (**Fig. 3.30d**).

3.14.2 Histology of the Esophagus

The esophagus has a *stratified squamous epithelium*, the lamina propria contains esophageal "cardiac" glands near the junction of the esophagus and stomach. The muscularis mucosa has a longitudinal smooth muscle that is thin and discontinuous. The submucosa has mucous secreting esophageal glands and contains a large venous plexus near the junction of the stomach. The esophagus and duodenum are the only areas of the GI tract that have submucosal glands. The muscularis externa layer is the layer that varies in skeletal versus smooth muscle composition. The circular layer of the muscularis externa near the pharynx/esophagus junction forms the cricopharyngeus or UES. At the esophagus/cardiac region of stomach junction this layer becomes the lower esophageal sphincter (LES). Adventitia covers the majority of the esophagus except after it passes the diaphragm where it is then surrounded by serosa (**Fig. 3.31**).

3.15 Stomach

The most dilated portion of the GI tract is the **stomach**. The stomach is generally located in the LUQ and RUQ or left hypochondriac, epigastric and umbilical regions. It functions as a reservoir (up to 2-3 liters of food) for accumulated food waiting to be broken down further both mechanically and chemically before being passed to the duodenum. Gastric juices convert the food bolus into a semi-liquid mixture called **chyme**.

The stomach has four parts and two curvatures: the cardia, fundus, body and pyloric region (**Fig. 3.32**).

- **Cardia**: surrounds the cardial orifice and is connected to the esophagus.
- **Fundus**: the dilated superior portion that extends as high as T10 and rests against the left dome of the diaphragm. Located between the junction of the esophagus, cardia and fundus is the **cardiac notch**. On a radiograph, gas is commonly present in the fundus.
- **Body**: the largest portion of the stomach, located between the fundus and pyloric region.
- **Pyloric region**: made up of multiple parts and shaped like a funnel with the wider portion represented by the **pyloric antrum** which leads into a narrower **pyloric canal**. The **pyloric sphincter** is the most distal portion of the pyloric region and is marked by a thickening of the circular layer of smooth muscle. The sphincter controls discharge of chyme through the pyloric orifice. The pyloric region crosses the transpyloric plane located at vertebral level L1.
- **Lesser curvature**: the smaller, concave, right border of the stomach. It is associated with the lesser omentum and the **angular notch**, the junction of the body and pyloric regions.
- **Greater curvature**: the larger, convex, left border of the stomach. It is associated with the greater omentum.

3.15.1 Vasculature and Lymphatic Drainage of the Stomach

Blood supply related to the *lesser curvature* is by way of the **left gastric** (celiac trunk br.) and **right gastric** (hepatic proper br.) **arteries**. The *fundus* and *upper portion of the body* are supplied by the **short gastric** and **posterior gastric** (splenic brs.) **arteries**. The region of the greater curvature is supplied by the **left** and **right gastro-omental (or gastroepiploic) arteries**. The left gastro-omental is a branch of the splenic artery while the right gastro-omental is a branch of the gastroduodenal artery (**Fig. 3.33a**).

Venous drainage mirrors the arteries. The **left** and **right gastric veins** drain into the hepatic portal vein. The left gastric on occasion will drain into the splenic vein. The right gastric vein receives the **prepyloric vein** (*of Mayo*), a landmark for surgeons when they are identifying the pyloric sphincter. The **short gastric**, **middle gastric**, **posterior gastric** and **left gastro-omental veins** drain into the splenic vein. The **right gastro-omental vein** drains into the superior mesenteric vein (**Fig. 3.33b**).

Lymphatic drainage of the *superoposterior 2/3 of the stomach* drains to the **pancreaticosplenic lymph nodes**. Areas near the *lesser curvature* drain to the **gastric** and **superior pyloric lymph nodes**. Areas near the greater curvature drain to the **gastro-omental** and **inferior pyloric lymph nodes**. Lymph will continue to drain towards the **celiac** or **superior mesenteric lymph nodes** after initially draining to the above lymph nodes (**Fig. 3.33c**).

3.15.2 Histology of the Stomach

The stomach has an internal surface or mucosa consisting of prominent longitudinal folds called **rugae** that serve to increase the surface area of the stomach. The rugae are most prominent near the greater curvature and pyloric regions and are directed

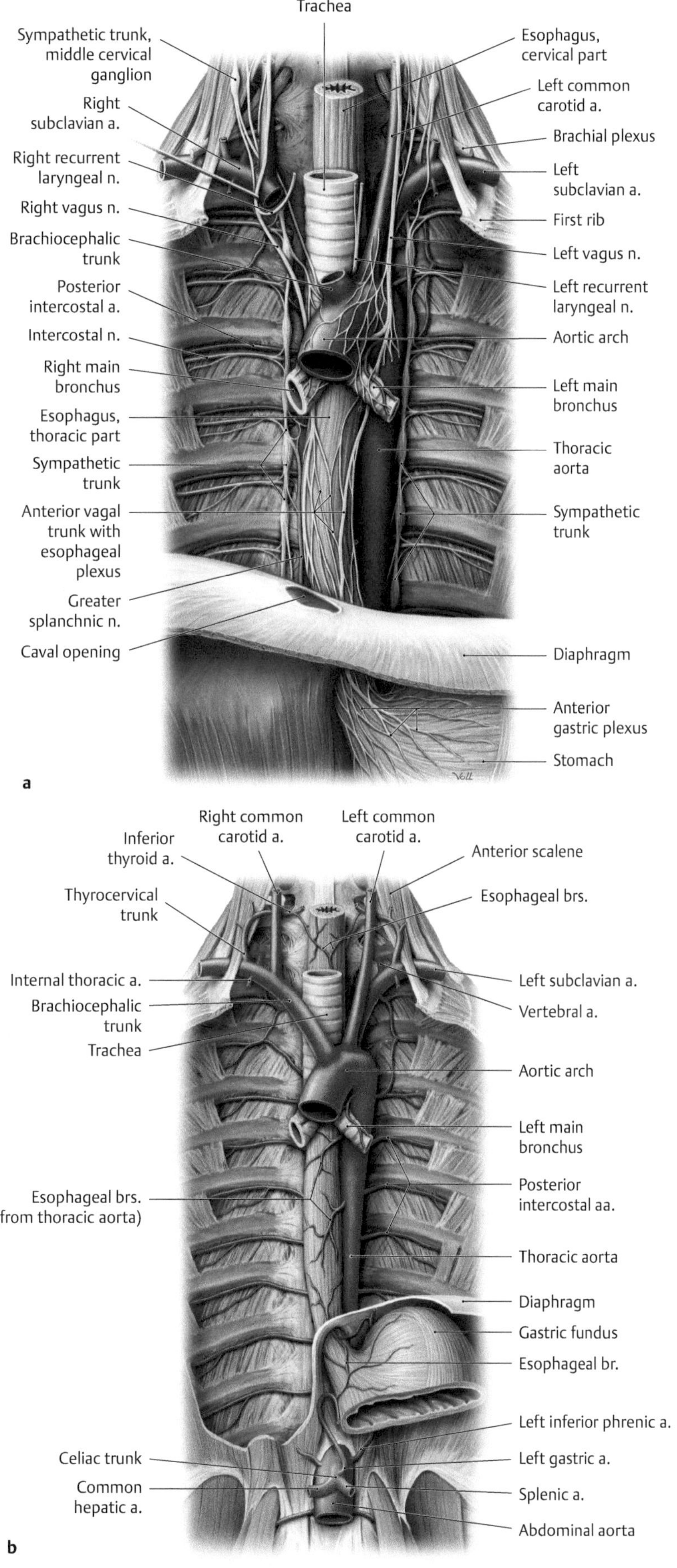

Fig. 3.30 **(a)** Innervation of the esophagus. **(b)** Blood supply of the esophagus. (*continued*) (From Schuenke M, Schulte E, Schumacher U. Thieme Atlas of Anatomy, Internal Organs. Illustrations by Voll M and Wesker K. 3rd ed. New York: Thieme Medical Publishers; 2020.)

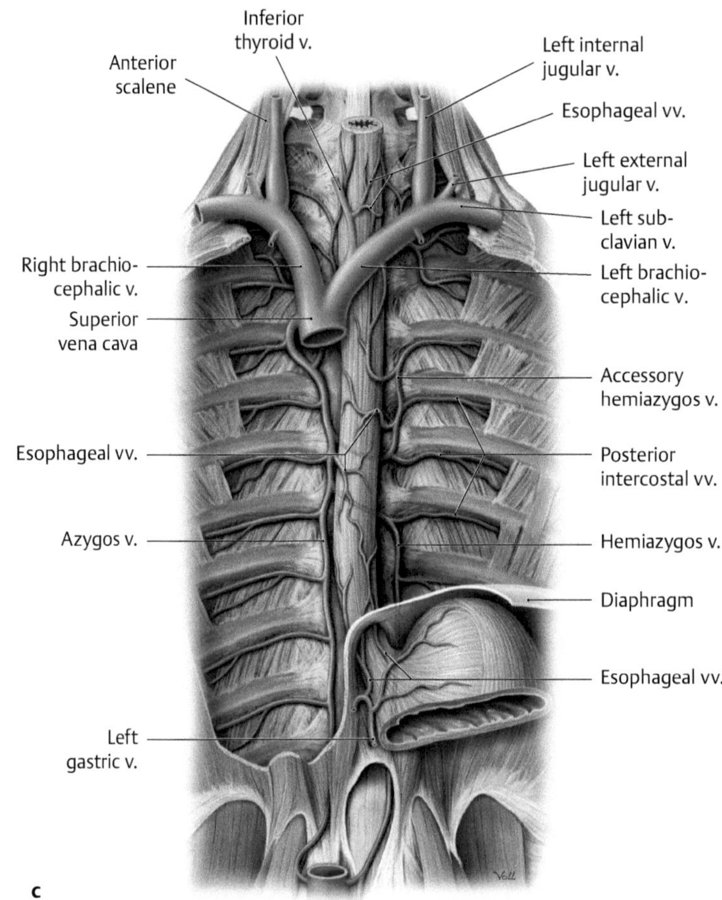

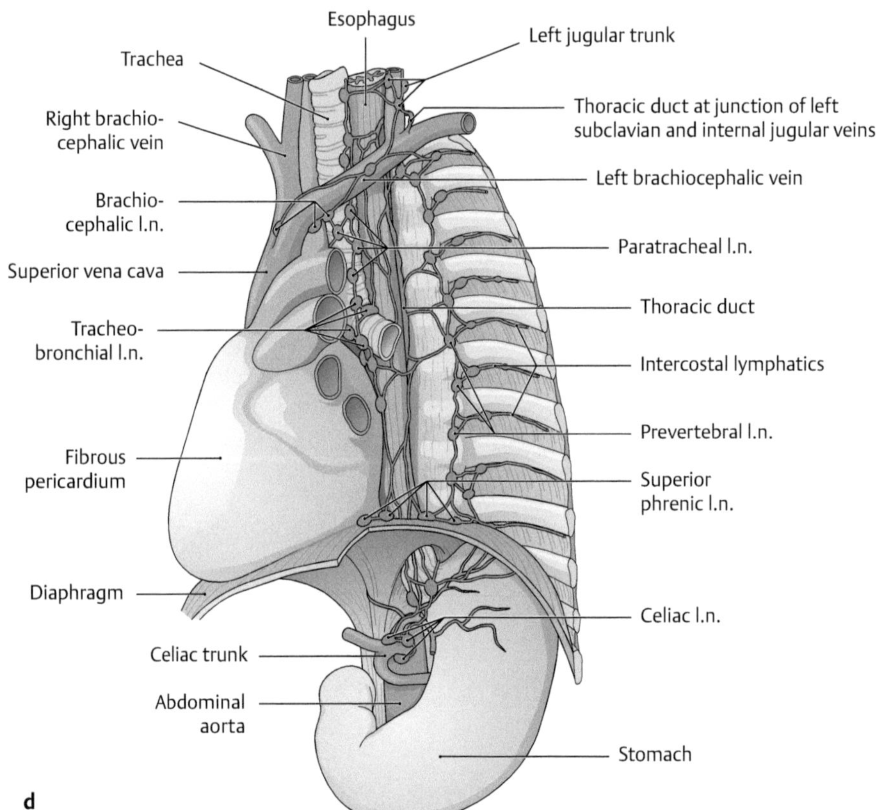

Fig. 3.30 (*continued*) **(c)** Venous drainage of the esophagus. **(d)** Lymphatic drainage of the esophagus. (From Schuenke M, Schulte E, Schumacher U. Thieme Atlas of Anatomy, Internal Organs. Illustrations by Voll M and Wesker K. 3rd ed. New York: Thieme Medical Publishers; 2020.)

Clinical Correlate 3.12

Zenker's Diverticulum

A **Zenker's diverticulum** is a diverticulum of the pharynx just superior to the cricopharyngeus muscle or UES. It is considered a pseudo-diverticulum because it only involves a herniation of mucosa and submucosa in the laryngopharynx (or hypopharynx) between the fibers of the inferior pharyngeal constrictor and cricopharyngeus muscles. This can lead to the development of a sac capable of trapping food or liquids. Confirmation may be done with a barium swallow evaluation and can be fixed endoscopically.

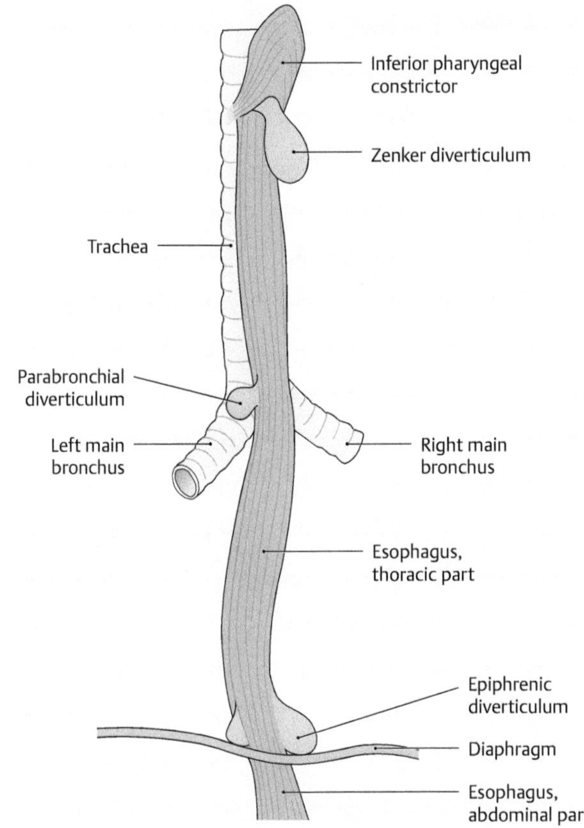

(From Schuenke M, Schulte E, Schumacher U. Thieme Atlas of Anatomy, Internal Organs. Illustrations by Voll M and Wesker K. 3rd ed. New York: Thieme Medical Publishers; 2020.)

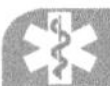

Clinical Correlate 3.13

Gastroesophageal Reflux Disease (GERD)

GERD is due to stomach acid of stomach contents passing back up through the esophagus because there has been an abnormal relaxation of the lower esophageal sphincter (LES). This reflux of stomach contents irritates the esophageal lining and results in GERD. Symptoms generally include consistent heartburn occurring multiple times a week. Regurgitation back into the esophagus is possible with sliding hiatal hernias because the right crus of the diaphragm is weak resulting in no natural LES constriction. Complications due to GERD can include Barrett's esophagus or ulcers.

Clinical Correlate 3.14

Barrett's Esophagus

A **Barrett's esophagus** is the abnormal change or metaplasia of the cells located in the distal esophagus. It is characterized by replacing the normal stratified squamous epithelium lining the esophagus with a simple columnar epithelium that contains goblet cells, but this is normally seen in the lower parts of the GI tract. There is a strong correlation between Barrett's esophagus and esophageal adenocarcinoma.

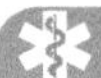

Clinical Correlate 3.15

Esophageal Varices

A consequence of portal hypertension and cirrhosis of the liver is the dilation of submucosal veins located in the distal esophagus. These are known as **esophageal varices** and they can lead to bleeding. Symptoms generally involve a patient coughing up blood or having tar–like, bloody stools, but varices may be suspected if an individual is jaundiced or has a swollen spleen. The primary goal is to prevent bleeding because varices are life-threatening. Treatments include tying off the veins using elastic bands with endoscopy or prescribing beta-blocker medications to reduce portal vein pressure.

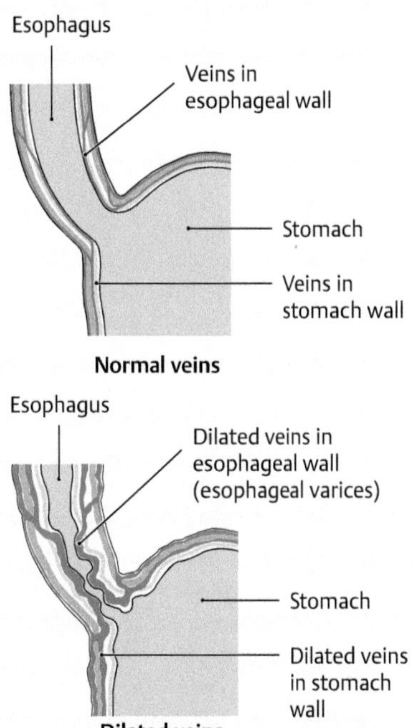

(From Schuenke M, Schulte E, Schumacher U. Thieme Atlas of Anatomy, Internal Organs. Illustrations by Voll M and Wesker K. 3rd ed. New York: Thieme Medical Publishers; 2020.)

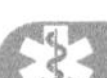

Clinical Correlate 3.16

Dysphagia and Achalasia

Having a persistent difficulty swallowing or **dysphagia** could be the result of a serious medical condition. Symptoms may include the inability to swallow, frequent heartburn, coughing or gagging and having the sensation that food is stuck in the throat. Causes could include esophageal tumors, GERD, diffuse spasms of the esophageal smooth muscle, current radiation therapy or a rare disorder called achalasia. **Achalasia** is the result of the esophagus losing the ability to pass food into the stomach because the LES remains closed during swallowing forcing food back up towards the mouth.

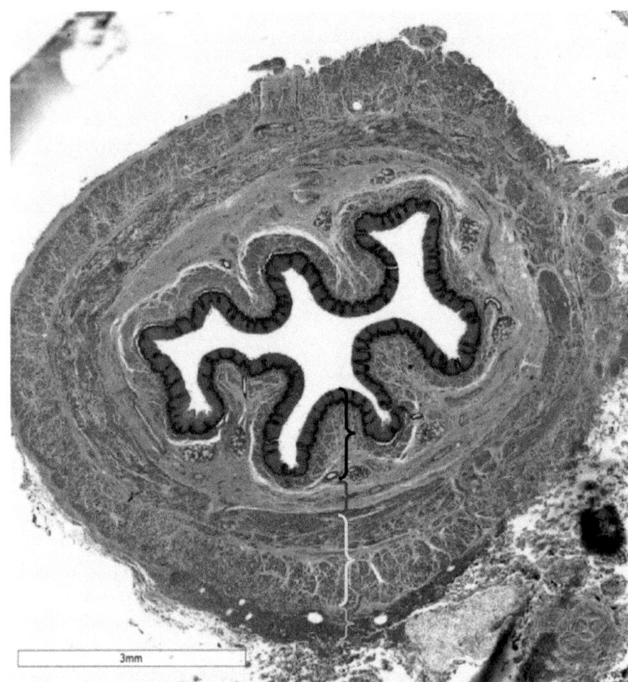

Fig. 3.31 Histology of the esophagus. Mucosa (*black bracket*), submucosa (*blue bracket*), muscularis externa (yellow bracket), adventitia (*green bracket*). (From Lowrie DJ. Histology: An Essential Textbook. New York: Thieme Medical Publishers; 2020.)

toward this same pyloric region. They become reduced or flat when the stomach is full and distended. The mucosa also displays **gastric pits** lined with a simple columnar epithelium of surface mucous cells neighboring with the adjacent **gastric glands (Fig. 3.34)**.

There are five major cell types that are found in the gastric pit/gland assembly and these include the *surface mucous*, *neck mucous*, *parietal*, *chief* and *enteroendocrine cells*. Undifferentiated stem cells are found throughout the internal surface. Due to the harsh conditions within the stomach, the entire epithelial lining is replaced every 3-7 days. Gastric pits consist only of surface mucous cells while the gastric glands contain the remaining four types. The cardiac and pyloric regions have primarily mucous cells with the pyloric region also containing enteroendocrine cells. The fundus and body regions contain the mucous cells in addition to the parietal, chief and enteroendocrine cells.

- **Surface mucous cells**: located in the gastric pits and secrete a neutral barrier mucous.
- **Neck mucous cells**: located in the neck of the gastric glands and secrete a slightly acidic mucous.
- **Parietal (oxyntic) cells**: abundant in the gastric glands and secrete **hydrochloric acid (HCl)** and **gastric intrinsic factor**. HCl is used to break down food while gastric intrinsic factor is required for later absorption of vitamin B_{12} in the ileum. Vitamin B_{12} is required for normal erythropoiesis.
- **Chief cells**: abundant near the base of the gastric glands and secrete **pepsinogen**. Pepsinogen is converted to **pepsin** in the presence of an acidic environment. Pepsin is responsible for breaking down proteins.

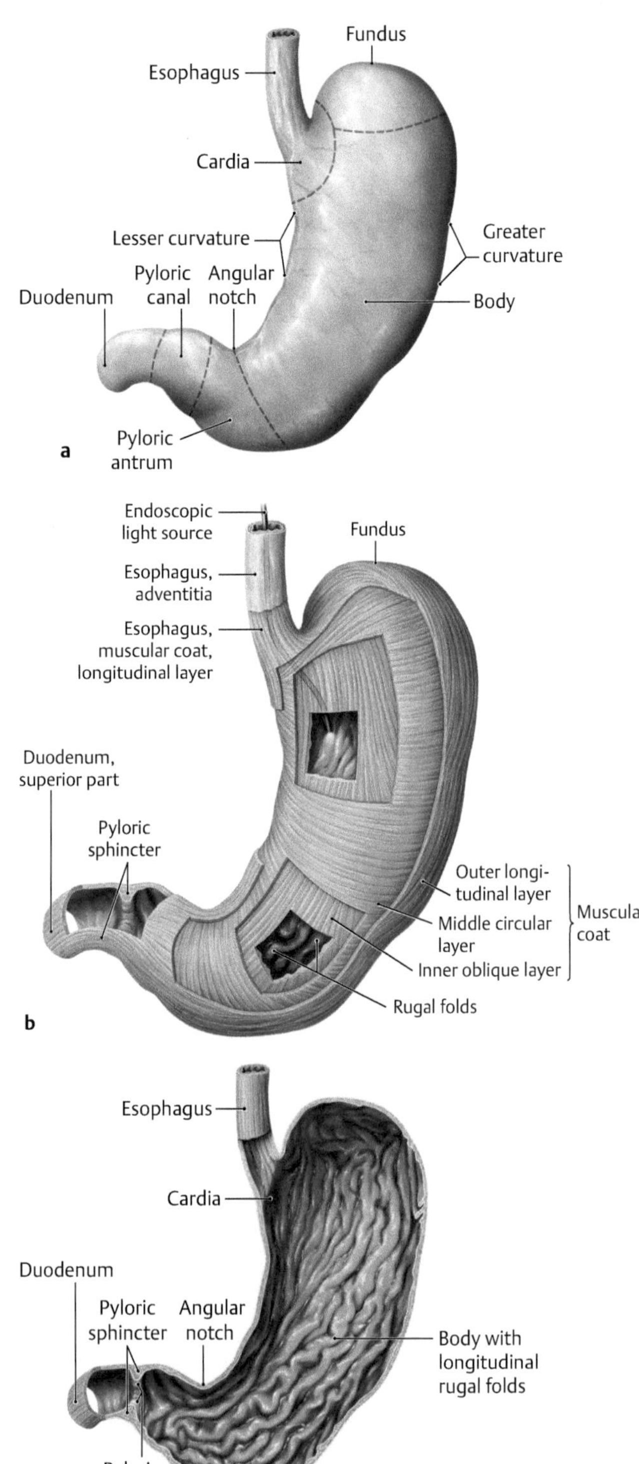

Fig. 3.32 Stomach. **(a)** Anterior wall. **(b)** Muscular layers. Removed: serosa and subserosa. Windowed: muscular coat. **(c)** Interior. Removed: anterior wall. (From Schuenke M, Schulte E, Schumacher U. Thieme Atlas of Anatomy, Internal Organs. Illustrations by M. Voll, and K. Wesker. 3rd ed. New York: Thieme Medical Publishers; 2020.)

- **Enteroendocrine cells**: located at the base of the gastric glands and help regulate GI tract activity. They can release gastrin, somatostatin and serotonin. **Gastrin** triggers the parietal cells to produce HCl; **somatostatin** inhibits gastrin release; and **serotonin** helps stimulate peristalsis.

Clinical Correlate 3.17

Stomach Cancer

Almost all gastric cancers are adenocarcinomas (beginning with cells that make and secrete mucus and other fluids) while other types include lymphoma, gastrointestinal carcinoid tumors and gastrointestinal stromal tumors. Gastric cancer is often diagnosed at an advanced stage because there are no early signs or symptoms and the 5 year survival rate is less than 5% if found this late. Infection with bacteria called *H. pylori* is a major cause of gastric cancer. Additional risk factors include being male, over 50, a diet high in smoked foods, salted meat or fish and being a smoker. After confirming gastric cancer using endoscopy, a mix of chemotherapy, radiation or surgery may be used to treat the patient. Surgical intervention may involve removing a portion of the stomach but rarely the entire stomach. However, additional surrounding tissue and lymph nodes may be removed.

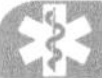

Clinical Correlate 3.18

Helicobacter Pylori

Helicobacter Pylori or *H. pylori*, is a Gram-negative, microaerophilic bacterium that colonizes the stomach and can induce a long-lasting inflammation of the stomach or *chronic gastritis*. The *H. pylori* bacterium can persist for decades and most individuals infected will never experience clinical symptoms despite having the chronic gastritis. Gastric and duodenal ulcers will ultimately develop in about 10–20% of those colonized by *H. pylori* but this infection is only associated with a 1–2% chance of developing stomach cancer. Once established, it is widely believed the infection persists for life. In the elderly, the stomach becomes increasingly atrophic and inhospitable to colonization and an infection will likely disappear. *H. pylori* infection is thought to play an important role in the natural stomach ecology.

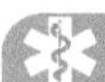

Clinical Correlate 3.19

Vagatomy

A **vagatomy** is a surgical procedure that targets the anterior or posterior vagal trunks as they descend onto the surface of the stomach. The vagus nerve and its trunks deliver the bulk of the parasympathetic fibers that innervate the GI tract (all but the hindgut). Parasympathetic innervation is responsible for parietal cell secretion of HCl, thus if the parasympathetic fibers were not allowed to function, there would be very little acid secretion. Clinicians must be very selective about where they choose to perform a vagatomy. The more distal a branch of vagal trunk is severed, the smaller the effect it will have on the function of the foregut and midgut. This also allows for a more targeted reduction in parietal cell secretion.

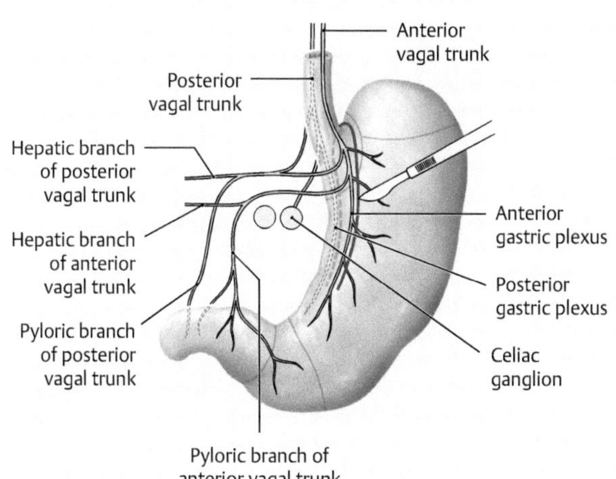

(From Schuenke M, Schulte E, Schumacher U. THIEME Atlas of Anatomy. Neck and Internal Organs. Illustrations by Voll M and Wesker K. 3rd ed. New York: Thieme Medical Publishers; 2010.)

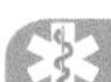

Clinical Correlate 3.20

Gastric Bypass Surgery and Lap Band Procedures

Gastric bypass surgery is intended to reduce the amount of food an individual is able to consume. With less food to absorb, a patient will reduce their body weight. The operation is intended for the morbidly obese with body mass indexes over 40. The most common form of gastric bypass surgery is known as the *Roux-en-Y procedure*. The surgeon first staples the stomach in such a way that a small (useable) and large (unused) pouch is created. The surgeon then attaches a Y-shaped section of the small intestine generally from the jejunum to the small stomach pouch. The reminder of the stomach still attached to the duodenum and proximal jejunum will be attached to the new bypass tube. The bypass creates an environment where less absorption of nutrients and calories will take place.

The **lap-band procedure** also known as gastric banding is a procedure that wraps an inflatable silicone device around the upper portions of the stomach. This band can be filled with saline in order to reduce the size of the stomach and hence limit the amount of food a person is able to consume. A physician is able to inflate or deflate the band because a thin tube connects the band to the access port seen just under the skin.

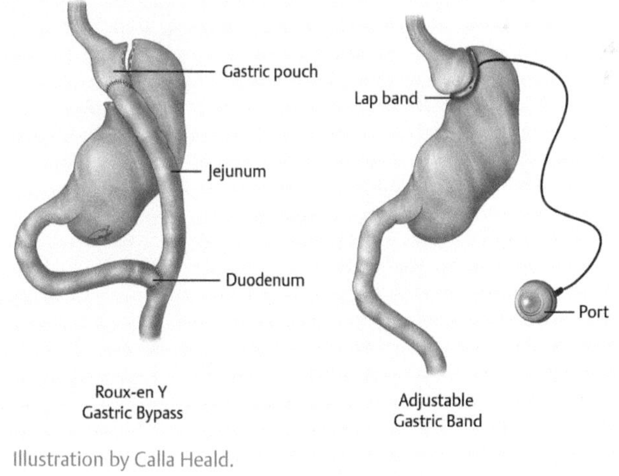

Illustration by Calla Heald.

The lamina propria, muscularis mucosa, submucosa and serosa demonstrate no remarkable structures. The muscularis externa has an inner oblique, middle circular and outer longitudinal layer. It is the middle circular layer that contributes the thickness seen with the cardiac and pyloric sphincter.

3.16 Duodenum (First and Second Parts)

The first of three parts of the small intestine is the duodenum. The duodenum itself is divided into four parts but is only about 30 cm (~12 in) in total length and is by far the shortest portion of the small intestine. The first two parts are considered part of the foregut while the last two parts are considered midgut. The duodenum has a C-shaped course and is adjacent to the pancreas **(Fig. 3.35)**.

The **1st (superior) part of the duodenum** begins on the right side of the pyloric sphincter, adjacent to the neck of the pancreas. It is short and located at vertebral level L1. The first couple centimeters of the 1st part are known as the *duodenal cap* and are dilated forming an ampulla. The proximal portion of this part of the duodenum is attached to the *hepatoduodenal ligament* thus making it mobile and intraperitoneal. The *gastroduodenal artery* passes posterior to this portion of the duodenum and is at risk of being damaged if there were a duodenal ulcer.

The **2nd (descending) part of the duodenum** lies to the right of the head of the pancreas and is located between vertebral levels L2-L3. The (common) bile duct and main pancreatic duct fuse to form the **hepatopancreatic ampulla** (*of Vater*) and it opens into this portion of the duodenum as the **major duodenal papilla**. If

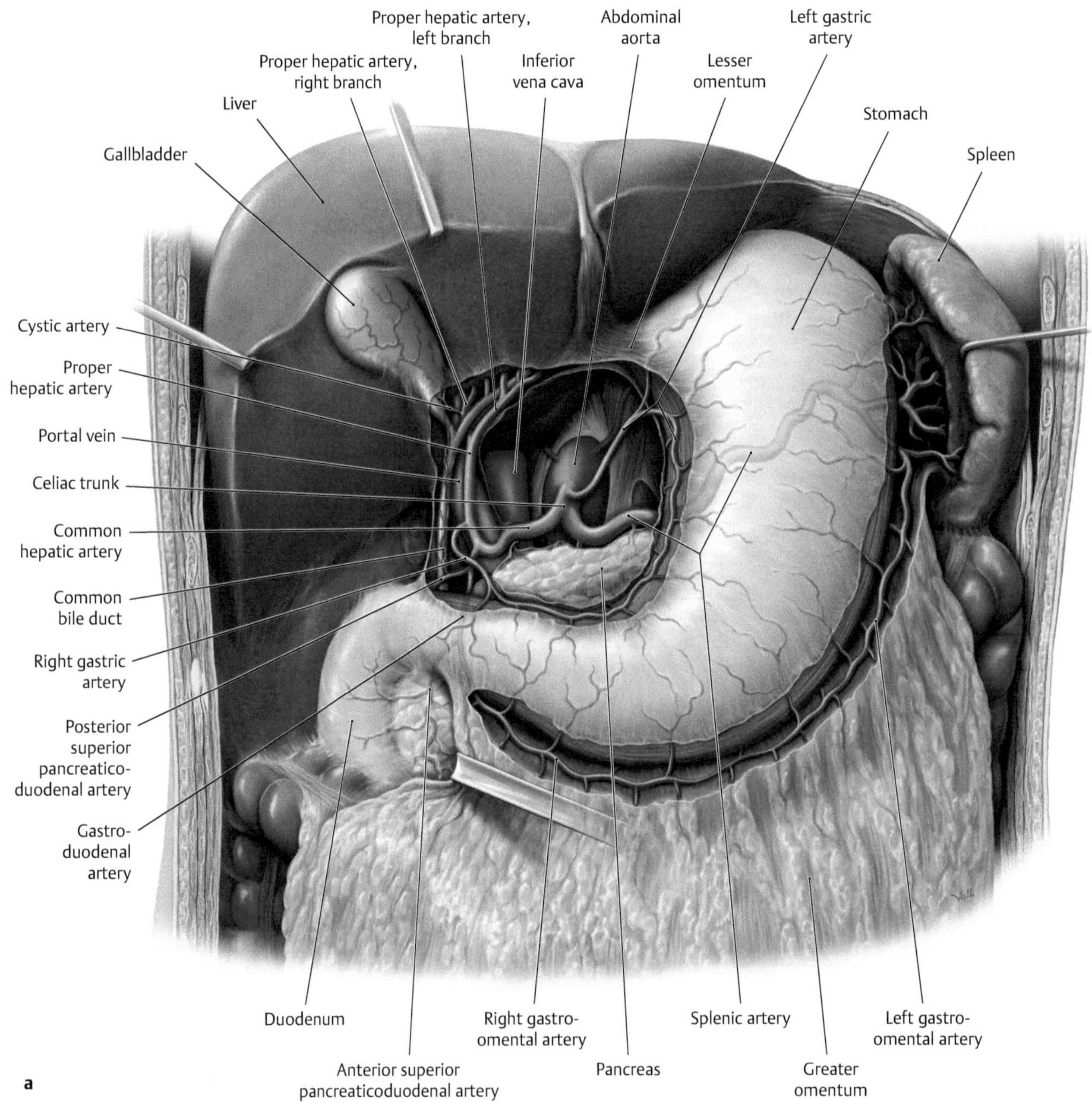

Fig. 3.33 **(a)** Celiac trunk: blood supply to the stomach, liver, and gallbladder. (*continued*) (From Schuenke M, Schulte E, Schumacher U. Thieme Atlas of Anatomy, Internal Organs. Illustrations by Voll M and Wesker K. 3rd ed. New York: Thieme Medical Publishers; 2020.)

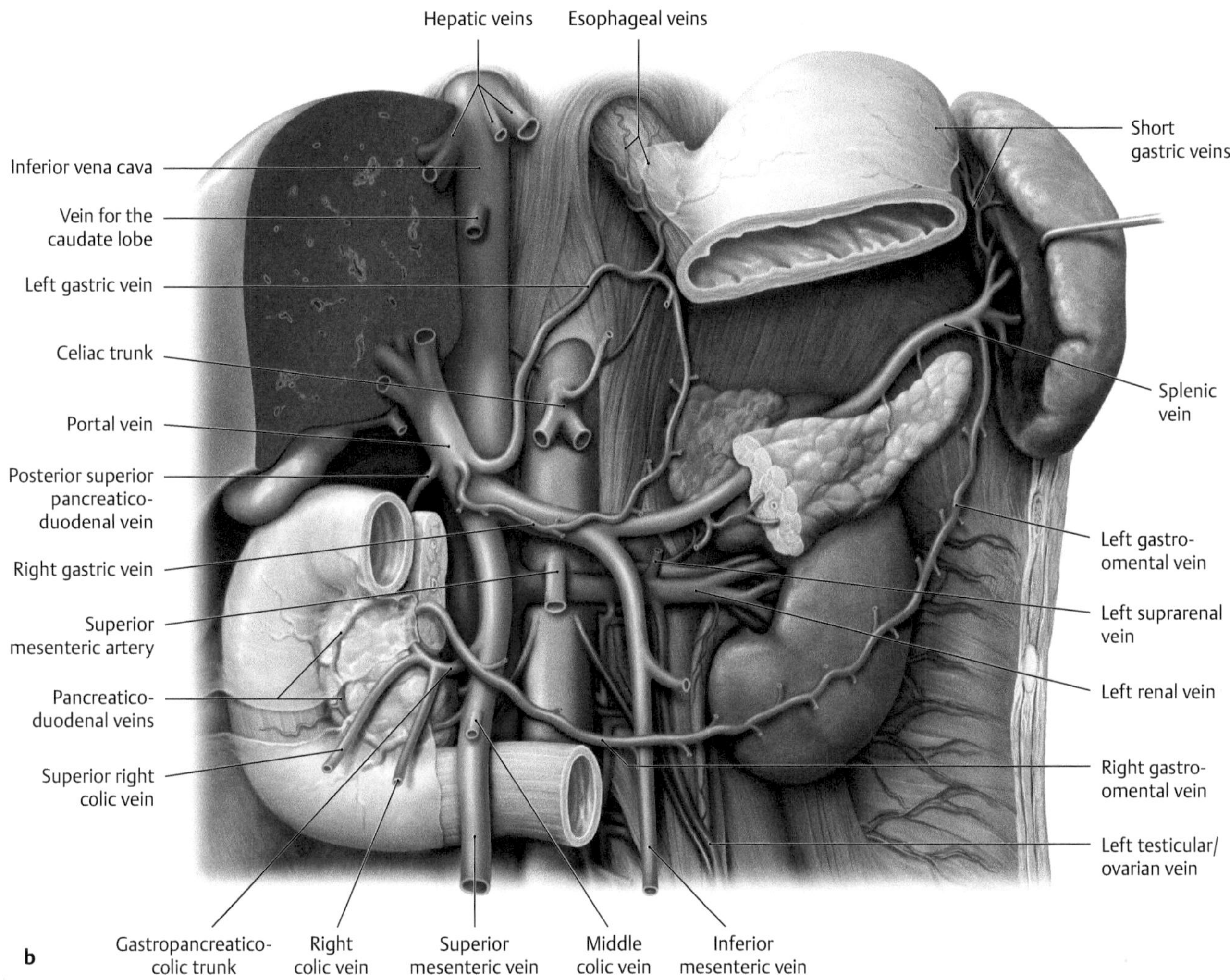

Fig. 3.33 (*continued*) **(b)** Tributaries of the portal vein. (*continued*) (From Schuenke M, Schulte E, Schumacher U. Thieme Atlas of Anatomy, Internal Organs. Illustrations by Voll M and Wesker K. 3rd ed. New York: Thieme Medical Publishers; 2020.)

an accessory duct originating from the pancreas exists, a **minor duodenal papilla** will be present superiorly to the major duodenal papilla. This portion of the duodenum is retroperitoneal.

Clinical Correlate 3.21

Gastric and Duodenal Ulcers

Open lesions or ulcers involving the stomach and duodenum are generally associated with a *H. pylori* infection. Gastric acid production is generally well above normal even if a meal is not being consumed and digested. The general thinking is that the higher than normal acid levels overwhelm the bicarbonate produced in the duodenum, leaving the mucosa vulnerable to *H. pylori*. *H. pylori* then erodes the mucosal lining, making it susceptible to any acid levels or digestive enzymes secreted by the stomach. Posterior gastric ulcers can erode and damage the *splenic artery* lying on the superior border of the pancreas while a duodenal ulcer is common in the 1st part (or cap) of the duodenum. An ulcer located here has the ability to erode the *gastroduodenal artery*. Any damage to an artery would lead to hemorrhaging and subsequent leaking of chyme could lead to peritonitis.

3.16.1 Vasculature and Lymphatic Drainage of the Duodenum (Foregut Portion)

Blood supply to this portion of the duodenum is originally derived from the **celiac trunk**. The **supraduodenal**, **anterior superior pancreaticoduodenal**, and **posterior superior pancreaticoduodenal arteries** originate from the **gastroduodenal artery** (common hepatic br.). The supraduodenal artery targets the 1st part of the duodenum while the anterior/posterior superior pancreaticoduodenal arteries lie in a groove between the pancreas and duodenum and supply both structures. They form an anastomosis with the anterior/posterior inferior pancreaticoduodenal arteries **(Fig. 3.36a)**.

Venous drainage mirrors the arteries and drains either directly or indirectly back into the **hepatic portal vein (Fig. 3.33b)**. Lymphatic drainage from this portion of the anterior duodenum is to the **pancreaticoduodenal lymph nodes**, followed by the **pyloric lymph nodes** before reaching the **celiac lymph nodes**. Lymphatic drainage from this portion of the posterior duodenum is generally straight to the **celiac lymph nodes (Fig. 3.36b)**.

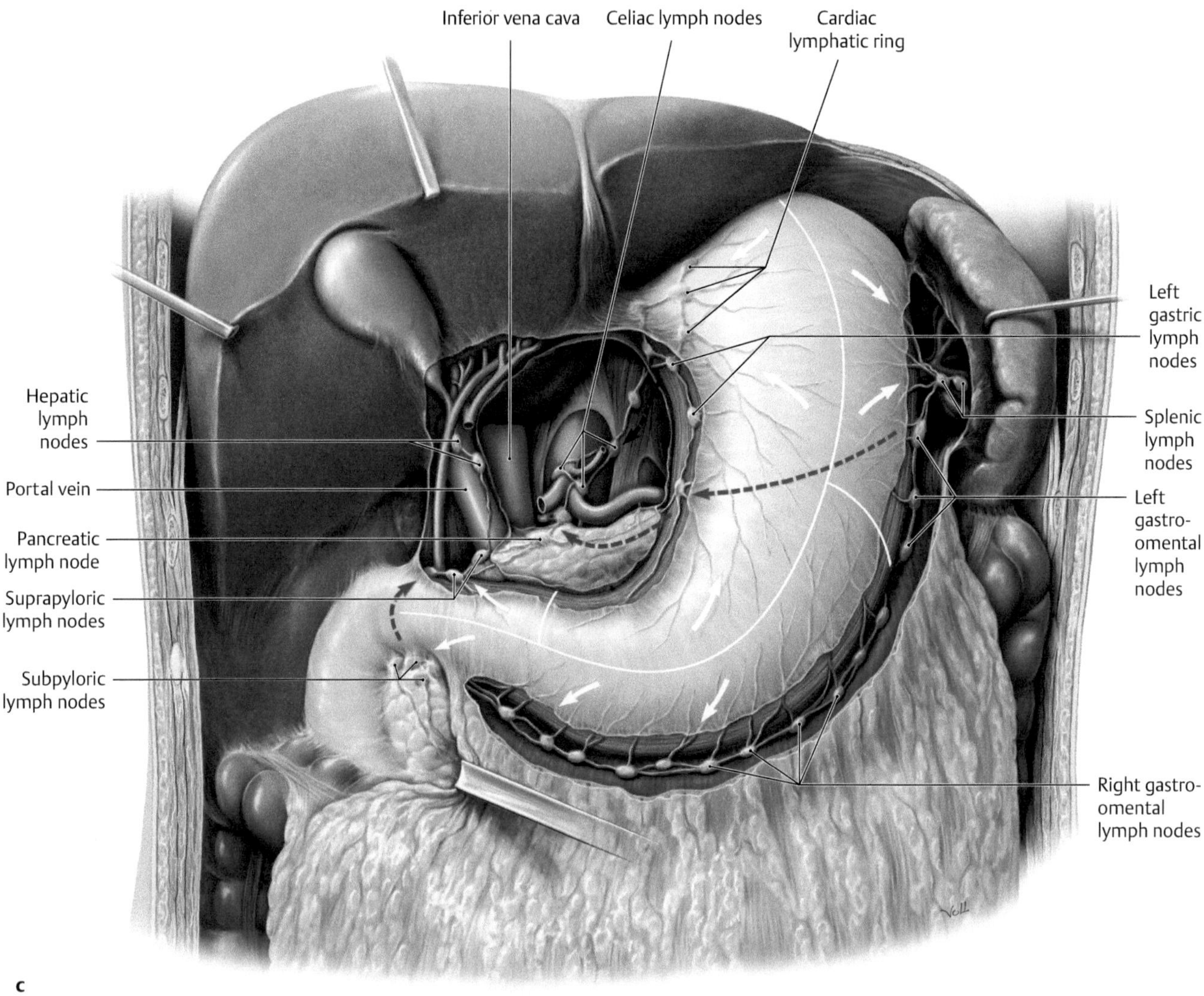

Inferior vena cava
Celiac lymph nodes
Cardiac lymphatic ring
Left gastric lymph nodes
Hepatic lymph nodes
Splenic lymph nodes
Portal vein
Left gastro-omental lymph nodes
Pancreatic lymph node
Suprapyloric lymph nodes
Subpyloric lymph nodes
Right gastro-omental lymph nodes
c

Fig. 3.33 *(continued)* **(c)** Lymphatic drainage of the stomach and liver. (From Schuenke M, Schulte E, Schumacher U. Thieme Atlas of Anatomy, Internal Organs. Illustrations by Voll M and Wesker K. 3rd ed. New York: Thieme Medical Publishers; 2020.)

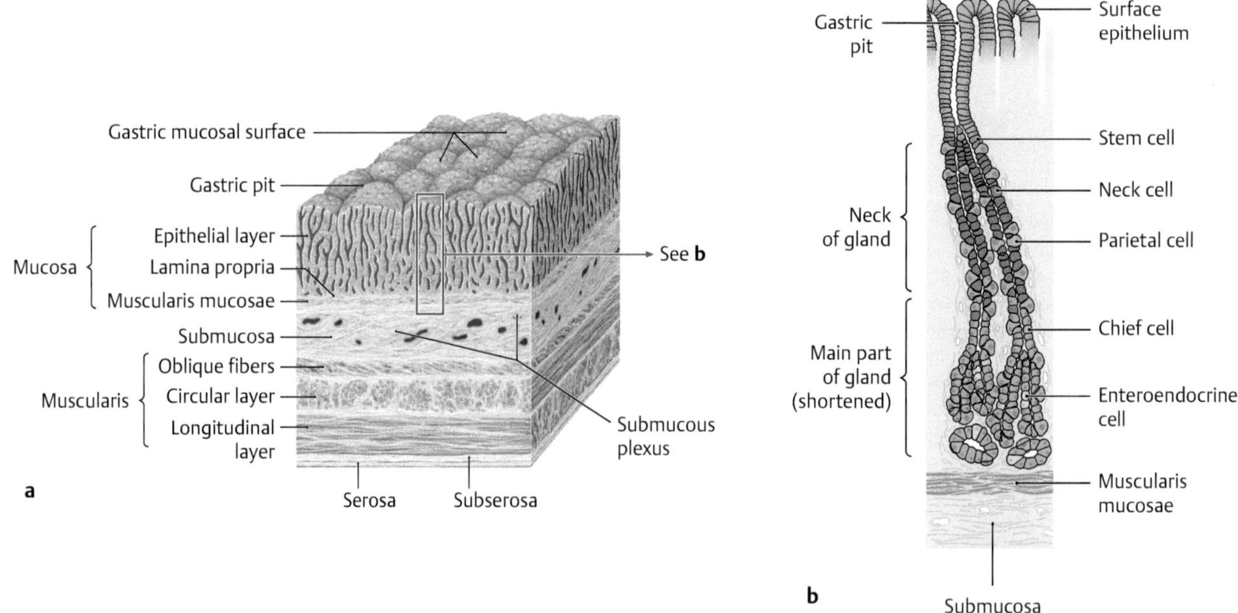

Fig. 3.34 Histology of the stomach. **(a)** Structure of the stomach wall. **(b)** Structure of the gastric glands. (From Schuenke M, Schulte E, Schumacher U. Thieme Atlas of Anatomy, Internal Organs. Illustrations by Voll M and Wesker K. 3rd ed. New York: Thieme Medical Publishers; 2020.)

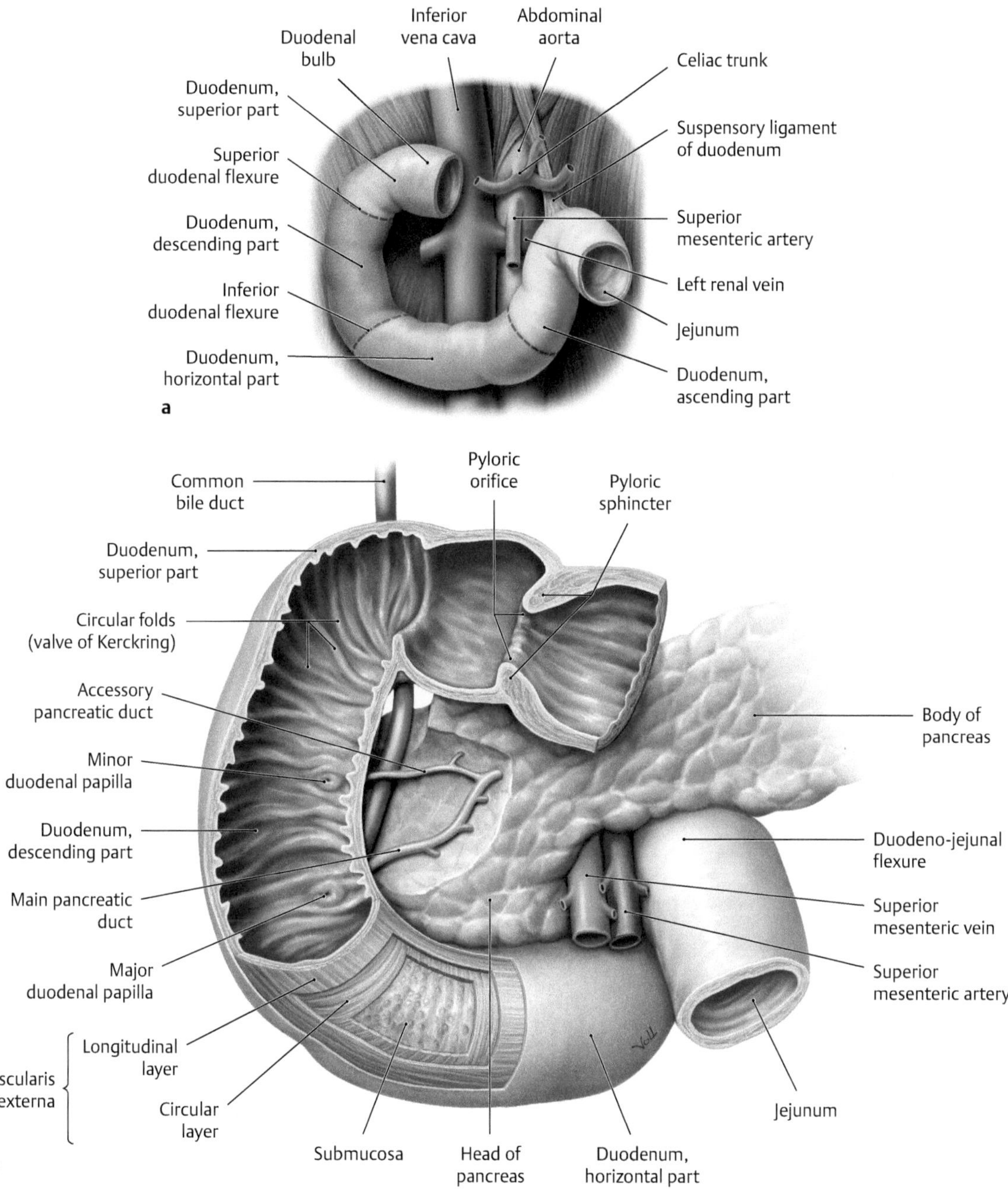

Fig. 3.35 **(a)** Parts of the duodenum, anterior view. **(b)** Anterior wall of the first two parts of the duodenum opened. (From Schuenke M, Schulte E, Schumacher U. Thieme Atlas of Anatomy, Internal Organs. Illustrations by Voll M and Wesker K. 3rd ed. New York: Thieme Medical Publishers; 2020.)

3.17 Liver

The largest internal organ and gland in the body and weighing approximately 1.5 kg (~3.3 lbs) is the **liver**. It is located in the RUQ between vertebral levels T7-L2/L3 and has been estimated to have 500 different functions **(Fig. 3.37)**. These can include the processing of every substance absorbed by the GI tract except for lipids; storing glycogen and numerous vitamins, secreting bile; synthesizing angiotensinogen; and producing albumin among many other functions. It is the only human internal organ capable of natural regeneration of lost tissue. However, this regrowth of the tissue does not lead to the original anatomical form.

The liver has two different surfaces: a convex diaphragmatic and a flat concave visceral surface. The **diaphragmatic surface** is intimately related to the inferior surface of the diaphragm. The **subphrenic recesses** that were divided into a left and right side by the *falciform ligament* are related to this surface. The **subhepatic space** represents the portion of the supracolic compartment immediately inferior to the liver. The subhepatic space extends back toward the **hepatorenal recess** (*Morison's pouch*). All but the **bare area** that is demarcated by the **coronary ligaments** is covered by visceral peritoneum on the diaphragmatic surface. The lateral extensions of the coronary ligaments are called the **left** and **right triangular ligaments**. The IVC passes through the bare area of the liver.

The liver is intraperitoneal and its **visceral surface** is covered with visceral peritoneum except at the porta hepatis and gallbladder fossa. The **porta hepatis** is the passage for structures to pass to and from the liver. These structures include the hepatic portal vein, hepatic arteries, hepatic ducts, autonomic fibers and lymphatics. The **gallbladder fossa** is where the gallbladder rests against the liver. A couple of fissures can be located on this surface. The **left sagittal fissure (umbilical fissure)** is a continuous groove formed by the anteriorly orientated **fissure of the round ligament** and the posteriorly orientated **fissure of the ligamentum venosum**. The structures located in these fissures are the round ligament and ligamentum venosum respectively. The **round ligament (ligamentum teres)** is the remnant of the *umbilical vein* that was responsible for delivering nutrient-rich oxygenated blood to the fetus from the placenta. The **ligamentum venosum** is the remnant of the *ductus venosus* that was responsible for shunting blood from the umbilical vein to the IVC, thus bypassing the liver. This fissure separates the left lobe from the quadrate and caudate lobes. The **right sagittal fissure** is the continuous groove between the anteriorly placed **gallbladder fossa** and the posteriorly placed **vena cava groove** containing the IVC. This fissure appears to separate the right lobe from the quadrate and caudate lobes, however the quadrate and caudate lobes are not true lobes but accessory lobes that are actually part of the anatomical right lobe. These two fissures are linked centrally by the porta hepatis.

The **hepatoduodenal ligament** of the lesser omentum extends from the porta hepatis to the 1st part of the duodenum and encloses

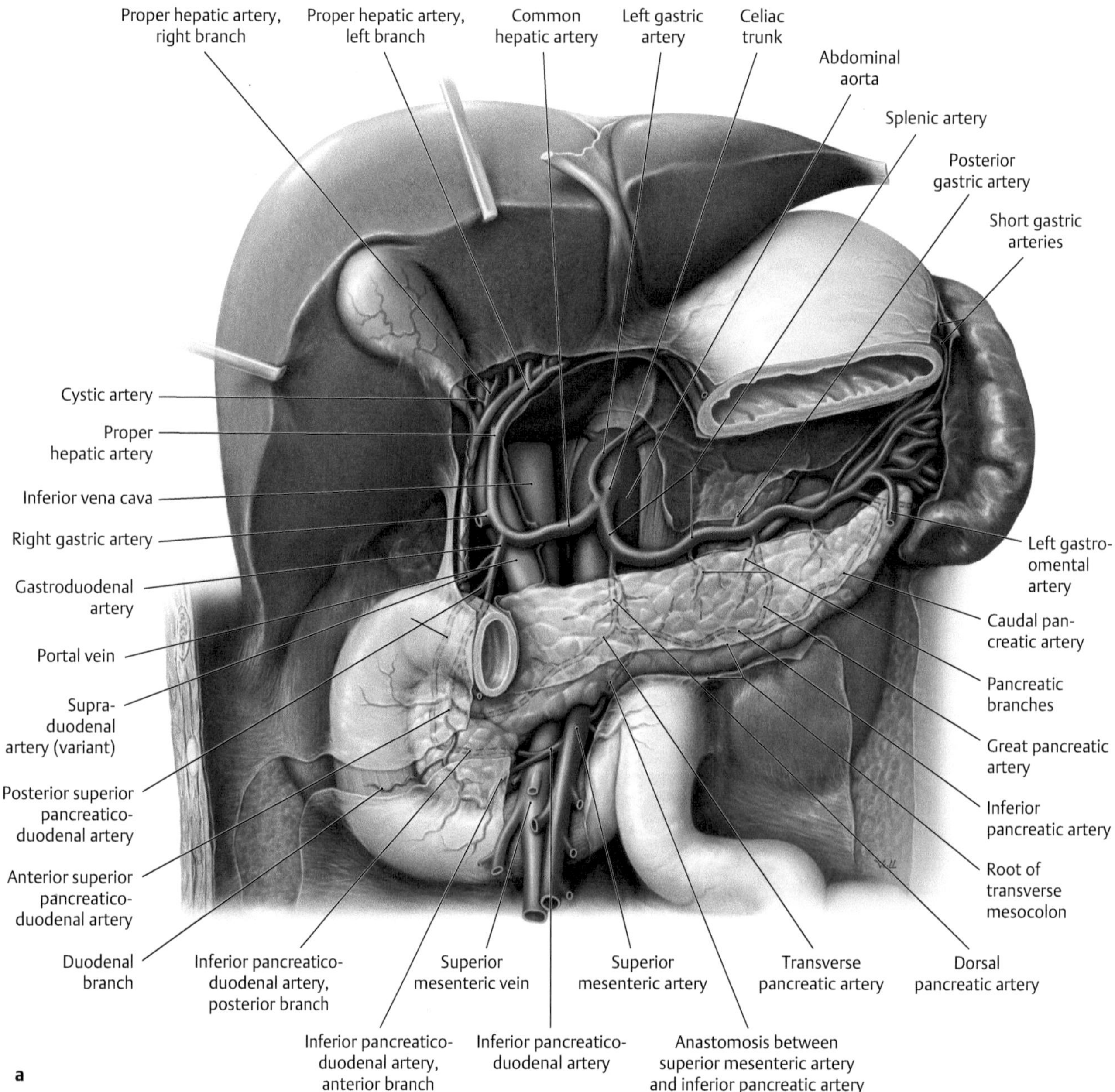

Fig. 3.36 (a) Celiac trunk: blood supply to the duodenum, pancreas, and spleen. *(continued)* (From Schuenke M, Schulte E, Schumacher U. Thieme Atlas of Anatomy, Internal Organs. Illustrations by Voll M and Wesker K. 3rd ed. New York: Thieme Medical Publishers; 2020.)

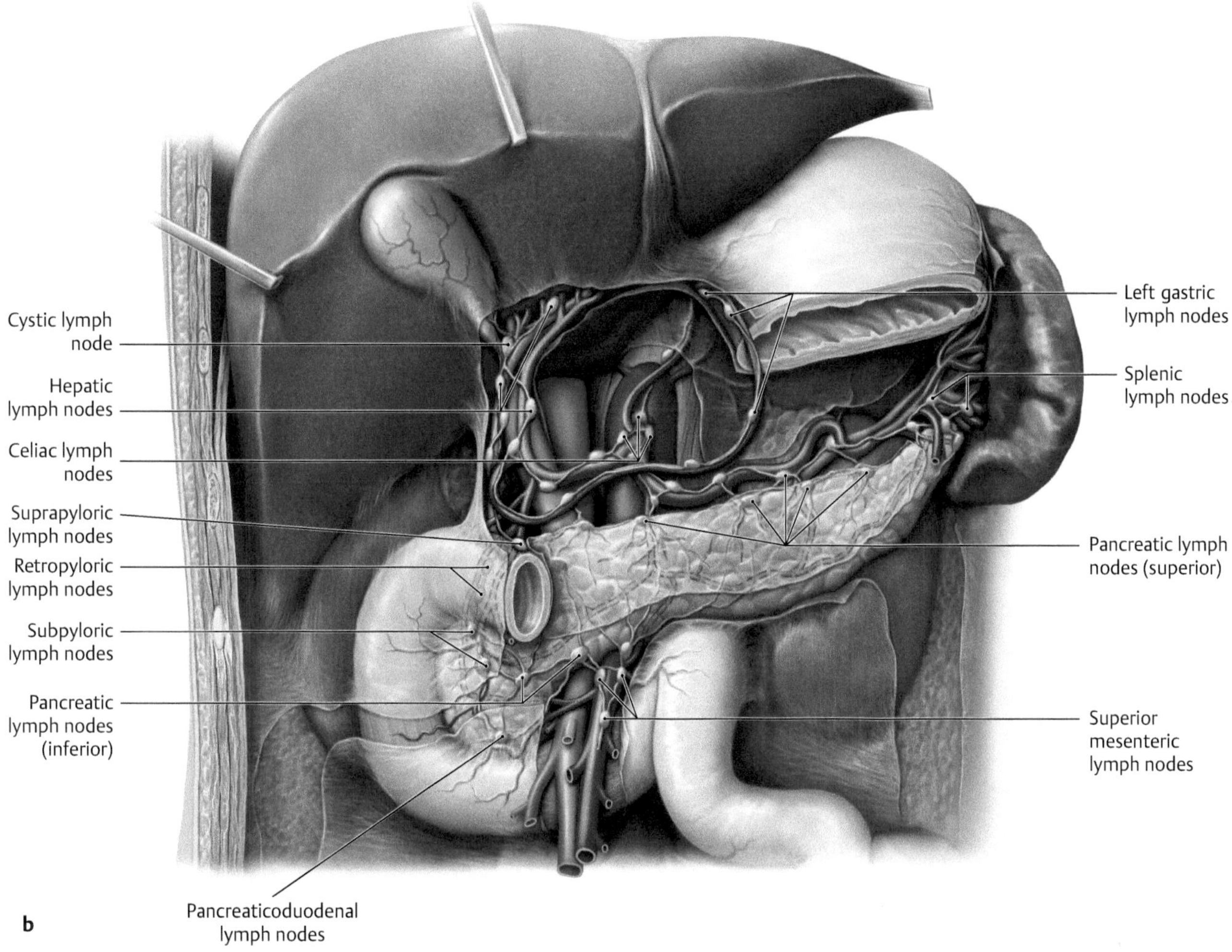

Fig. 3.36 *(continued)* (b) Lymphatic drainage of the duodenum, pancreas, and spleen. (From Schuenke M, Schulte E, Schumacher U. Thieme Atlas of Anatomy, Internal Organs. Illustrations by Voll M and Wesker K. 3rd ed. New York: Thieme Medical Publishers; 2020.)

the structures of the **portal triad**, the **hepatic portal vein**, **hepatic arteries** and **(common) bile duct**. The **hepatogastric ligament** of the lesser omentum connects the fissure of the ligamentum venosum and the lesser curvature of the stomach.

The liver is divided into two anatomical lobes and two accessory lobes. It is the attachment of the falciform ligament and the left sagittal fissure that are responsible for dividing the liver into a small **left lobe** and large **right lobe**. As previously mentioned, the quadrate and caudate lobes are accessory lobes and part of the anatomical right lobe.

From a functional standpoint, the liver has an independent **left** and **right liver**, which are fairly equal in size. There are no clearly defined internal demarcations because the liver parenchyma is continuous in nature. The liver may also be divided into **four divisions** or **eight hepatic (surgical) segments** that can be surgically removed (**Fig. 3.38**).

The liver is divided into a left and right liver based on the primary division of the portal triad into left and right branches except for the caudate lobe (segment I). The **main portal fissure** is the plane between the left and right livers and represents the location for the **middle hepatic vein**. This plane is defined on the diaphragmatic surface by the *Cantlie line*, an imaginary line that runs from the notch of the gallbladder fossa back to the IVC. On the visceral surface, the right sagittal fissure represents this same plane. Each portion receives its own *primary branch* of the hepatic artery and hepatic portal vein as well as its own hepatic duct.

The *left sagittal (umbilical) fissure* along with the **right portal fissure** vertically divides each left and right liver into its own *medial* and *lateral division*, thus creating four total divisions that receive independent *secondary branches* of portal triad structures. The fissures represent the locations of the **left** and **right hepatic veins** respectively. The right portal fissure is difficult to isolate because it has no visible external markings to help identify it.

While following the horizontal orientated left and right portal vein branches, a **transverse hepatic plane** divides three of the four divisions into smaller segments (segments II-VIII). This plane does not divide the left medial division of the liver (*Couinaud classification*), which includes the quadrate lobe and is known as segment IV. It is on occasion divided into an IV_A and IV_B segment by the left hepatic portal vein branch (*Bismuth classification*). The caudate lobe (segment I) is located posteriorly and is not visible from the anterior view. It could be considered a third part of the liver because it has a vascularization pattern independent of the bifurcation of the portal triad and smaller hepatic veins that drain

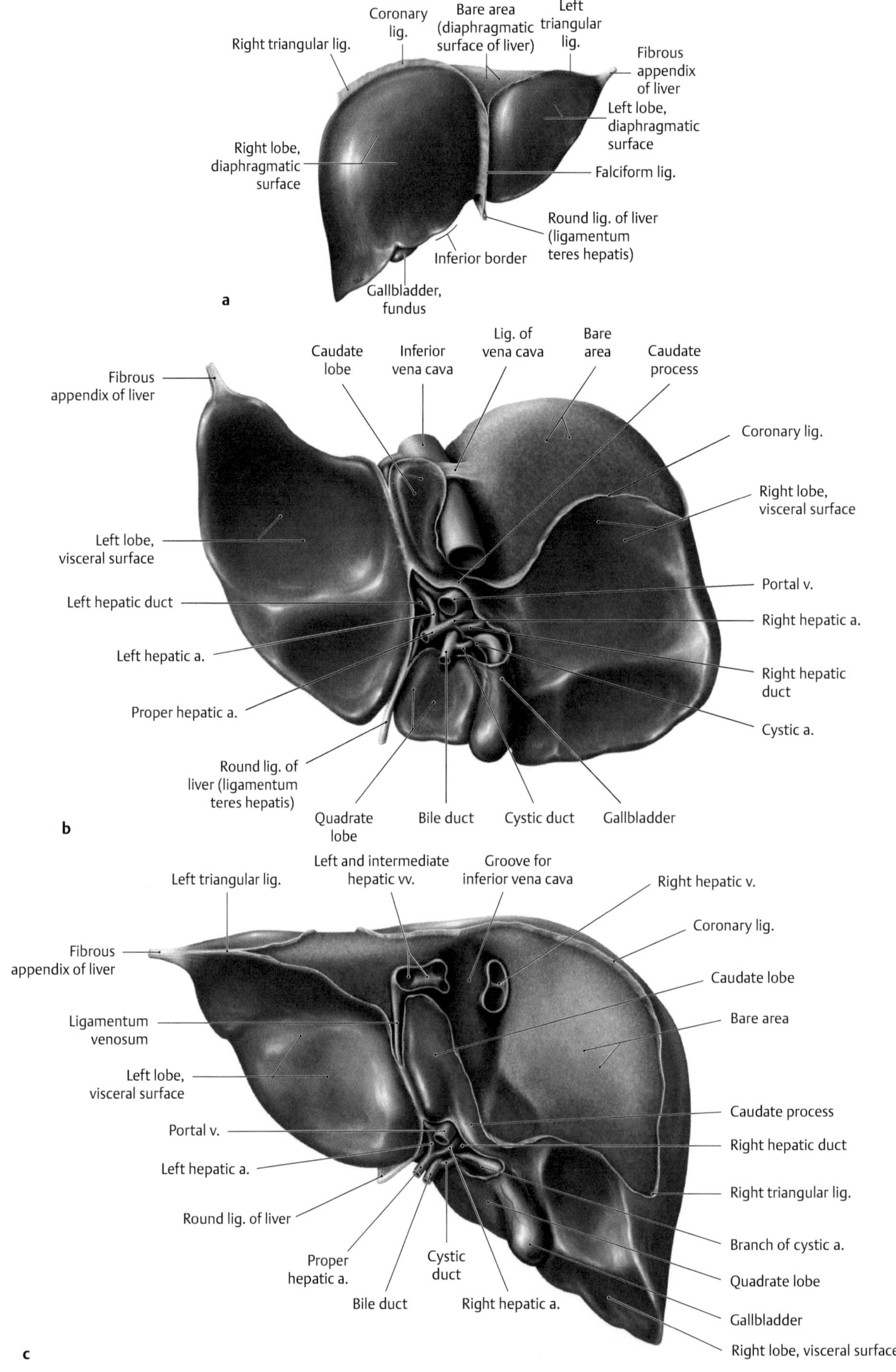

Fig. 3.37 Liver. **(a)** Anterior view. **(b)** Inferior view. **(c)** Posterior view. (From Schuenke M, Schulte E, Schumacher U. THIEME Atlas of Anatomy. Internal Organs. Illustrations by Voll M and Wesker K. 3rd ed. New York: Thieme Medical Publishers; 2020.)

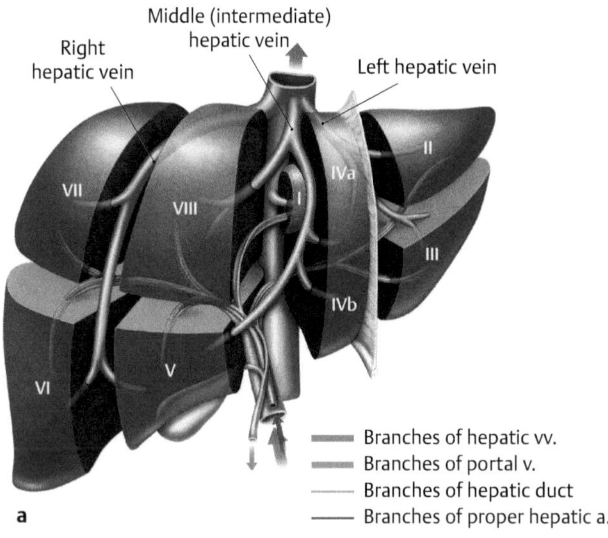

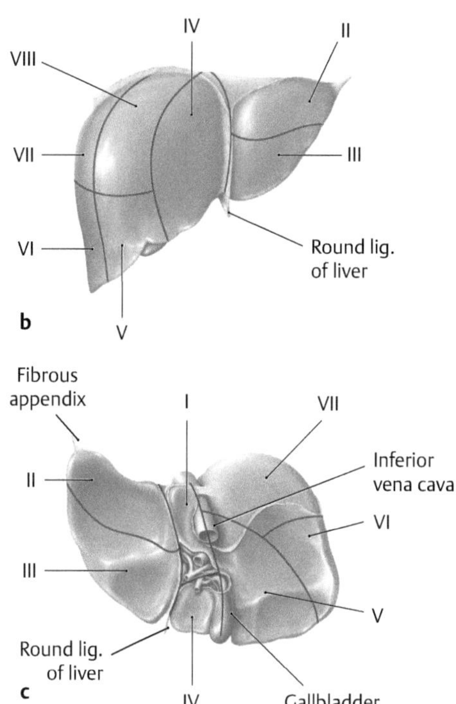

Fig. 3.38 (a) Segmentation of the liver. **(b)** Diaphragmatic surface, anterior view. **(c)** Visceral surface, inferior view. (From Schuenke M, Schulte E, Schumacher U. THIEME Atlas of Anatomy. Internal Organs. Illustrations by Voll M and Wesker K. 3rd ed. New York: Thieme Medical Publishers; 2020.)

directly into the IVC. Thus seven of the eight segments receive independent *tertiary branches* of portal triad structures.

3.17.1 Vasculature and Lymphatic Drainage of the Liver

The liver has a dual blood supply with the dominant source being venous in nature. The **hepatic portal vein**, which is formed by the *superior mesenteric* (SMV) and *splenic veins* and is located anterior to the IVC, delivers approximately 75-80% of the blood to the liver. In about 30% of the population the *inferior mesenteric vein* will join the SMV and splenic vein to form the hepatic portal vein. This blood contains nutrients (except lipids) absorbed by the GI tract and is then sent to the sinusoids. The parenchyma (hepatocytes) is supplied by this portal blood, of which it has a 40% higher oxygen content than what passes through the IVC **(Fig. 3.33b)**.

The **hepatic arteries** supply 20-25% of the blood to the liver and primarily support non-parenchymal structures such as the intrahepatic bile ducts. The **common hepatic artery** (celiac trunk br.) bifurcates into the *hepatic proper* and *gastroduodenal arteries*. The **hepatic proper artery** bifurcates into a **left** and **right hepatic artery** and they are responsible for supplying the left and right liver respectively **(Fig. 3.33a)**.

After blood has been processed in the liver, the central veins send blood through the interlobular veins that drain themselves into the **left**, **middle (intermediate)** or **right hepatic veins** located between specific divisions of the liver. The hepatic veins then drain into the IVC just inferior to the diaphragm.

The major lymph-producing organ is the liver and between one-quarter and one-half of all lymph passing through the thoracic duct originates from the liver. Lymphatic drainage of the liver consists of a superficial versus deep drainage pattern. The *superficial lymphatics* located within the **fibrous** (*Glisson*) **capsule** drain the *anterior surfaces* of the liver toward the **hepatic lymph nodes.** They also drain the *posterior surfaces* toward the **phrenic** and **posterior mediastinal lymph nodes** or to the *lymph nodes adjacent to the IVC*. The majority of the liver is drained by *deep lymphatics* that are found accompanying vessels in an *interlobular portal triad*. The deep lymphatics receive lymph from the **perisinusoidal spaces** (*of Disse*) and they drain mainly to the **hepatic lymph nodes** while the rest will reach *lymph nodes adjacent to the IVC* above the diaphragm **(Fig. 3.39)**.

3.17.2 Histology of the Liver

The majority of the liver is covered by visceral peritoneum along with a thin, dense, irregular connective tissue that becomes thicker near the hilum known as **Glisson's capsule**. The parenchyma of the liver is made of **hepatocytes** and they are normally arranged in interconnected plates and constitute about two-thirds of the liver's total mass. Liver (hepatic) tissue is described as having a hexagonal-shaped pattern of *liver lobules*.

These **liver lobules** are polygonal masses of tissue with **portal triads** (or tracks) at the periphery and a **central vein** located in the center **(Fig. 3.40a,b)**. The portal triads are located in the corners of the lobules and contain connective tissue, neurovasculature, bile ducts and lymphatics. There are three to six portal spaces per lobule with each containing an arteriole (hepatic artery br.), venule (portal vein br.), duct (bile duct br.) and lymphatics. Lymphocytes and macrophages could also be present along with inflammatory cells that may increase with age or certain liver diseases.

Hepatocytes in the liver lobule are radially orientated and arranged like plates or bricks on a wall. These plates are separated by **sinusoids** that have blood passing through them. These sinusoids are lined by

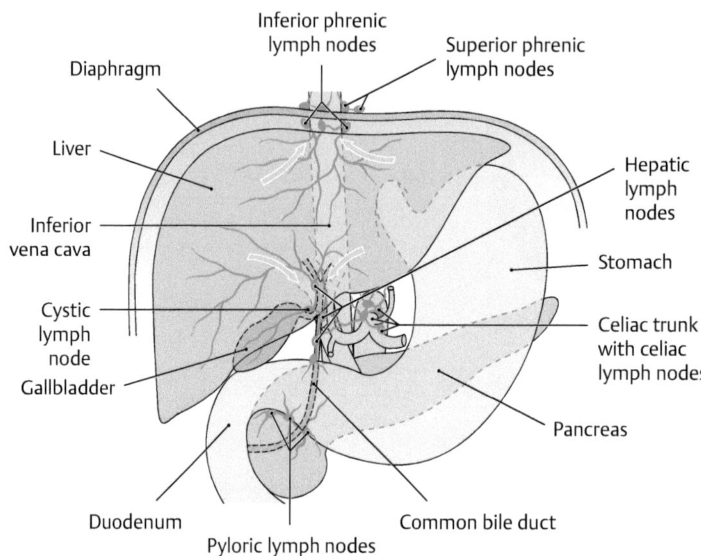

Fig. 3.39 Lymphatic drainage of the liver and gallbladder. (From Schuenke M, Schulte E, Schumacher U. Thieme Atlas of Anatomy, Internal Organs. Illustrations by Voll M and Wesker K. 3rd ed. New York: Thieme Medical Publishers; 2020.)

a discontinuous fenestrated endothelium making them highly permeable and allowing for free flow of plasma but not of any cellular elements. Located on the luminal surfaces of the sinusoids, macrophages known as **Kupffer cells**, are responsible for digesting hemoglobin, metabolizing aged erythrocytes, destroying bacteria and secreting proteins related to immunological processes (**Fig. 3.40c**).

Located between the endothelium of the sinusoid and the hepatocyte is the **perisinusoidal space** (*space of Disse*), the space that accepts the free flowing plasma from the sinusoid thus allowing for an easy exchange of molecules from the lumen of the sinusoids to the hepatocytes and vice versa (**Fig. 3.40d**). This exchange is important physiologically because of the large number of macromolecules secreted in the blood by hepatocytes but also because the liver takes up and catabolizes many of these large molecules. **Ito cells** are also located in the perisinusoidal space and they are important in storing fat-soluble vitamins such as vitamin A.

The architecture of the liver is established in such a way to allow: (1) a mix of hepatic venous (mainly) and arterial blood originating from the portal triads to flow through the sinusoids and toward the central veins and (2) hepatic bile to flow from the hepatocytes, to the bile canaliculi, through the *canals of Hering* before reaching the interlobular bile ducts located in the portal triads. The entire pathway of bile secretion and drainage is discussed fully in the "Biliary System" section of this chapter.

3.18 Gallbladder

The **gallbladder** is a pear-shaped structure that lies in the *gallbladder fossa* on the visceral surface of the livers right lobe. It concentrates bile and stores between 30-50 ml of it. The liver produces about 250 ml – 1 L of bile per day, much of that passing to and from the gallbladder. The gallbladder is made up of three parts: the *fundus*, *body* and *neck* (**Fig. 3.41**).

- **Fundus**: the widest portion projecting from the inferior border of the liver. The fundus and body are located at about the L1 vertebral level near the midclavicular line.
- **Body**: lies in contact with the visceral surface of the liver, 1st part of the duodenum and transverse colon.
- **Neck**: the narrow portion that has an S-shaped curve that connects to the **cystic duct**, which itself connects to the **common hepatic duct** to form the **(common) bile duct**. The mucosa of the neck internally forms the **spiral valve** and this keeps the cystic duct open so that bile can easily pass into the gallbladder when the *hepatopancreatic sphincter* is closed.

3.18.1 Vasculature and Lymphatic Drainage of the Gallbladder

Blood supply to the gallbladder is from the **cystic artery**, and over 90% of the time it is a branch of the **right hepatic artery** (**Fig. 3.36a**). The cystic artery travels through a surgically important site called the **cystohepatic** (*Calot's*) **triangle** defined by the cystic duct (laterally), common hepatic duct (medially) and the inferior border of the liver (superiorly). The **cystic veins** drain the neck of the gallbladder and the biliary ducts to the **hepatic portal vein**. The body and fundus of the gallbladder drain directly through the visceral surface of the liver and into the **hepatic sinusoids**.

Lymphatic drainage of the gallbladder is to the **cystic lymph nodes** before reaching the **hepatic lymph nodes** (**Fig. 3.36b; Fig. 3.39**). From here lymph will travel to the **celiac lymph nodes**. Within the cystohepatic triangle, the sentinel lymph node corresponding to pathology related to the gallbladder is known as the *Lund* **(or** *Mascagni*) **lymph node**.

3.18.2 Histology of the Gallbladder

The gallbladder has only three layers: a mucosa, muscularis externa and an adventitia/serosa. It lacks a muscularis mucosae and submucosa layer. The mucosa consists of a *simple columnar epithelium* that can be highly folded unless it is distended and filled with bile. The epithelium has microvilli that help absorb water and this results in more concentrated bile.

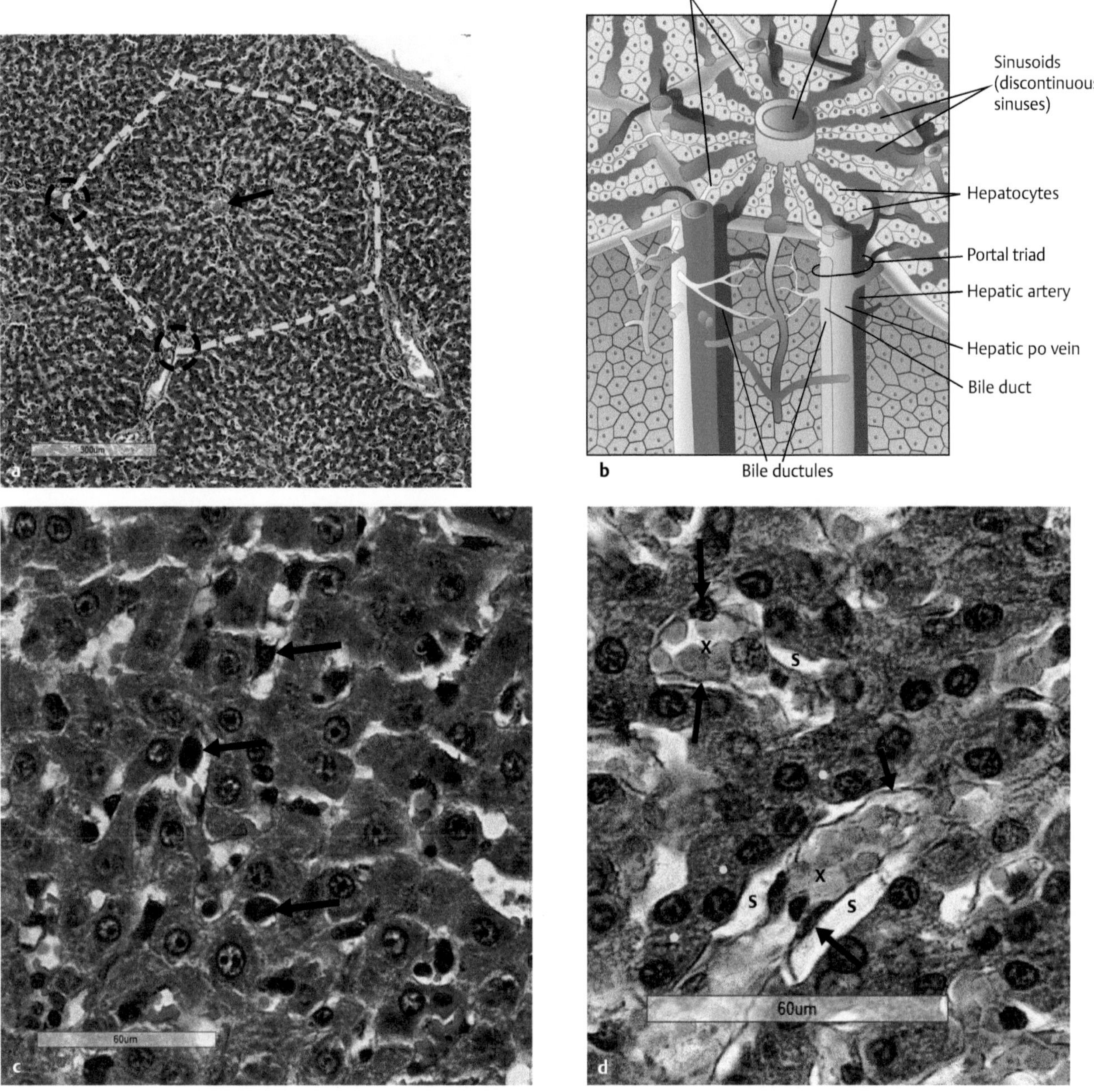

Fig. 3.40 Histology of the liver. **(a)** Low magnification showing a classic liver lobule (*yellow outline*), portal triads/canals (*black outlines*), and central vein (*black arrow*). **(b)** Detailed drawing of the liver histology. **(c)** Liver macrophages or Kupffer cells (*black arrows*). **(d)** Liver sinusoids (x) at high magnification, lined by endothelial cells (nuclei and cytoplasm marked with black arrows). Perisinusoidal spaces of Disse (S) are visible. The approximate size and location of canaliculi are indicated by the yellow dots. (From Lowrie DJ. Histology: An Essential Textbook. New York: Thieme Medical Publishers; 2020.)

The muscularis externa contains circular and longitudinal layers of smooth muscle but they are inconsistent. This layer lies up against the lamina propria. The adventitia is continuous with *Glisson's capsule* of the liver and peritoneum is found lining the portions of the gallbladder not directly attached to the liver (**Fig. 3.42**).

3.19 Biliary System

The **biliary system** is the combination of bile ducts associated with the liver and gallbladder. Bile is continuously produced in the liver by the hepatocytes but it is stored and concentrated in the gallbladder. Bile emulsifies fat so that it is able to be absorbed through the intestinal wall.

The pathway begins with the hepatocytes secreting bile into the **bile canaliculi** located between them. From the bile canaliculi, bile continues through the *canals of Hering* and then the **interlobular bile ducts** before reaching either the **left** or **right hepatic ducts**. The left and right hepatic ducts unite to form the **common hepatic duct**. Where the common hepatic duct and cystic duct of the gallbladder merge represents the formation of the **(common) bile duct**. The bile duct descends posterior to the 1st part of the duodenum before lying in a groove located on the posterior surface of the pancreas. It then penetrates the head of the pancreas

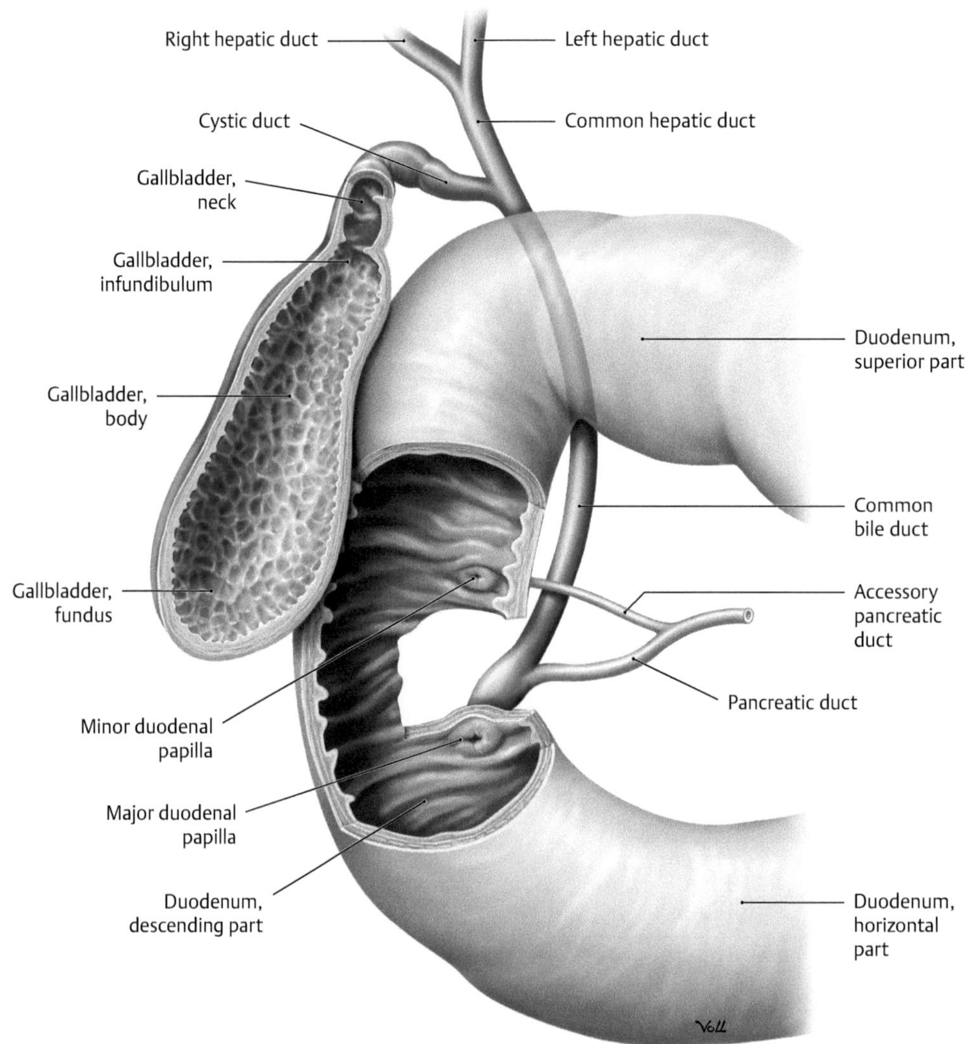

Fig. 3.41 Gallbladder and duodenum opened and extrahepatic bile ducts, anterior view. (From Schuenke M, Schulte E, Schumacher U. THIEME Atlas of Anatomy. Internal Organs. Illustrations by Voll M and Wesker K. 3rd ed. New York: Thieme Medical Publishers; 2020.)

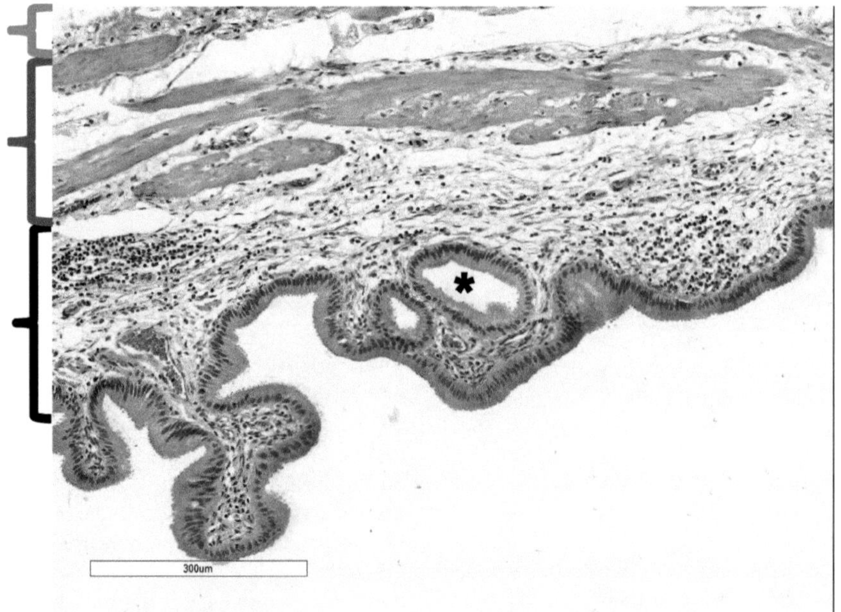

Fig. 3.42 Histology of the gallbladder showing the mucosa (*black bracket*), muscularis externa (*red bracket*), and adventitia/serosa (*green bracket*). Asterisk (*) indicates a mucosal fold that has the appearance of a gland. (From Lowrie DJ. Histology: An Essential Textbook. New York: Thieme Medical Publishers; 2020.)

for only a short distance near the left border of the 2nd part of the duodenum. The bile duct then meets the *main pancreatic duct* to form the **hepatopancreatic ampulla** (*of Vater*) and this is where bile mixes with pancreatic digestive juices. The distal portion of the ampulla projects out into the 2nd part of the duodenum and constitutes the **major duodenal papilla (Fig. 3.41; Fig. 3.43)**.

When the sphincters surrounding both the hepatopancreatic ampulla (the *sphincter of Oddi*) and the distal bile duct contract, bile is forced to backflow through the bile and cystic ducts before filling the gallbladder.

3.20 Pancreas

The **pancreas** is a mixed exocrine (~80%) and endocrine (~20%) organ located at vertebral levels L1 and L2. The exocrine portion secretes digestive pancreatic juices that originate from acinar cells and enter the 2nd part of the duodenum while the endocrine secretions originate from pancreatic islets (*of Langerhans*) and enter the bloodstream. It is about 12-15 cm in length and located primarily up against the duodenum, to the right of the spleen and posterior to the stomach. It consists of a *head, neck, body* and *tail region*. The head, neck and body regions are retroperitoneal while the tail is intraperitoneal and lies up against the hilum of the spleen **(Fig. 3.44)**.

The **head** is the expanded portion of the pancreas and lies up against the C-shaped duodenum firmly attaching to its 2nd and 3rd parts. The distal bile duct is embedded in the head of the pancreas prior to fusing with the main pancreatic duct. The SMV

Clinical Correlate 3.24

Portal Hypertension

Cirrhosis leads to scarring and fibrosis of the liver and these compress and obstruct the hepatic portal vein that delivers most of the blood to the liver. When the pressure increases in the hepatic portal vein and all of its tributaries, this is known as **portal hypertension**. Compression or blockage leading to portal hypertension can be located at different locations near or in the liver. Liver cirrhosis is an *intrahepatic* cause of blockage while thrombosis of the hepatic portal vein is a *pre-hepatic* cause and hepatic vein thrombosis is a *post-hepatic* cause of portal hypertension. Blood is essentially forced through alternate channels that include the portosystematic anastomoses and a greater pressure located here can lead to *esophageal* and *anorectal varices* or *caput medusae*.

The former way to treat or reduce portal hypertension was by performing a **portosystematic shunt** in order to divert blood from the portal venous system to the systematic venous system. This created a communication between the hepatic portal vein and the inferior vena cava. An example would include connecting the splenic vein to the left renal vein. The development of **transjugular intrahepatic portosystematic shunt (TIPS)** procedure has drastically reduced the need for a traditional portosystematic shunt. TIPS involves entering the internal jugular vein with a guidewire and catheter and passing it inferiorly through both venae cavae before reaching the hepatic veins. A passage is formed using a *Colapinto needle* through the parenchyma of the liver to bridge a hepatic vein with the hepatic portal vein. After the opening is created, a stent is placed to keep this passageway open, thus creating a new blood shunt.

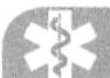

Clinical Correlate 3.22

Cirrhosis of the Liver

Cirrhosis of the liver is a condition where the liver is not functioning properly and is most commonly caused by of alcohol abuse, chronic hepatitis B and C, or non-alcoholic fatty liver disease. The disease itself progresses slowly over many years and symptoms such as jaundice, ascites, hepatomegaly, spider angiomata, and many others are the direct consequence of improper hepatocyte functioning. Portal hypertension due to cirrhosis increases blood flow resistance and this alone can lead to other effects such as esophageal varices and splenomegaly. The hepatitis B vaccination can prevent cirrhosis but generally preventing a worsening of the complications is the only course of treatment because cirrhosis cannot be reversed.

Clinical Correlate 3.23

Lobectomies and Segmentectomy of the Liver

With the separation of hepatic vasculature and duct branches that supply individual sections of the liver, it is possible to have portions of the liver removed if a disease state is diagnosed. A hepatic left or right lobe can be removed (lobectomy) and excessive bleeding can be avoided. With cauterizing scalpels and laser surgery, along with a combination of dye injection, balloon catheter occlusion and ultrasound imaging, segmentectomies of the liver are a possibility and more detailed than a lobectomy. Because of the potential of major bleeding during the procedure, vascular patterns based on the left, intermediate and right hepatic veins help distinguish the fissures of the liver for better guidance to remove a segment.

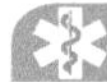

Clinical Correlate 3.25

Gallstones

Gallstones (or *cholelithiasis* if located in the actual gallbladder) which can also be found in the cystic or bile ducts (*choledocholithiasis*), develop when the concentration of cholesterol in bile is high but bile salts are low. An incomplete or infrequent emptying of the gallbladder could lead to the bile becoming overconcentrated and contribute to gallstone formation. Gallstones are more prevalent in women due increased estrogen levels that result from pregnancy or hormone supplement therapy. Diagnosis can be made easily with ultrasound. Most individuals are asymptomatic, but if a blockage occurs and causes a "gallstone attack", a cholecystectomy may need to be performed.

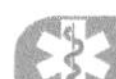

Clinical Correlate 3.26

Cholecystectomy

The surgical removal of the gallbladder is called a cholecystectomy and is the recommended treatment the first time a patient is admitted to a hospital for inflammation of the gallbladder (*cholecystitis*). This procedure is also performed if *gall bladder cancer*, *biliary colic* (spastic pain from the cystic duct) or *pancreatitis* is diagnosed. The laparoscopic cholecystectomy is the most common approach to removing the gallbladder with the most serious complication being damage to the bile duct (<1% of cases).

and occasionally the SMA pass over the projection from the inferior part of the head called the **uncinate process**. A tumor of this structure does not cause any obstruction of the bile duct. The **neck** overlies the superior mesenteric vessels and its anterior surface lies adjacent to the pylorus of the stomach. On the posterosuperior portion of the neck is where the SMV joins the splenic vein to form the hepatic portal vein. The **body** lies between the neck and tail of the pancreas. It is left of the superior mesenteric vessels, passes over the aorta, and also forms the floor of the lesser sac. The **tail** is closely associated with the hilum of the spleen and anterior to the left kidney. It is generally intraperitoneal and relatively mobile.

The tail region is also where the **main pancreatic duct** (*of Wirsung*) originates before continuing through the parenchyma of the pancreas and terminating at the hepatopancreatic ampulla. The sphincter on the distal portion of this duct contributes to the flow of digestive juices. An **accessory pancreatic duct** (*of Santorini*) is present in approximately 70-80% of individuals and mostly connects to the main pancreatic duct. It passes through the head region before forming the **minor duodenal papilla** and draining into the 2nd part of the duodenum **(Fig. 3.41)**.

3.20.1 Vasculature and Lymphatic Drainage of the Pancreas

Blood supply to the pancreas originates from multiple sources associated with the celiac trunk and SMA. The **anterior/posterior superior pancreaticoduodenal arteries** originate from the **gastroduodenal artery** (common hepatic br.). There is a direct **inferior pancreaticoduodenal artery** (SMA br.) before it bifurcates into **anterior/posterior inferior pancreaticoduodenal arteries.** These arteries form an anastomosis with each other and lie in a groove between the pancreas and duodenum to supply both structures. They supply specifically the uncinate process, head and tail of the pancreas. The **splenic artery** has a highly torturous course on the superior border of the pancreas and it gives off the *dorsal pancreatic, great pancreatic, caudal pancreatic* and many minute *unnamed pancreatic arteries.* The **dorsal (superior) pancreatic artery** mostly originates from the proximal portion of the splenic artery and supplies mainly the head and neck region. The **great pancreatic (pancreatic magna) artery** originates from about the midportion of the splenic artery and supplies the body and tail regions. The **caudal pancreatic artery** originates from the distal splenic artery and targets mainly the tail region. The **transverse pancreatic artery** forms an anastomosis between the dorsal pancreatic, greater pancreatic and caudal pancreatic arteries and provides a redundant blood supply to the body and tail regions **(Fig. 3.36a)**.

Venous drainage follows the arteries and they drain either to the **hepatic portal vein** (superior pancreaticoduodenal tributaries), **SMV** (inferior pancreaticoduodenal tributaries) or the **splenic vein.** The splenic vein is located on the posterosuperior edge of the pancreas and does not have a torturous course and is fairly straight. It does receive the **inferior mesenteric vein** posterior

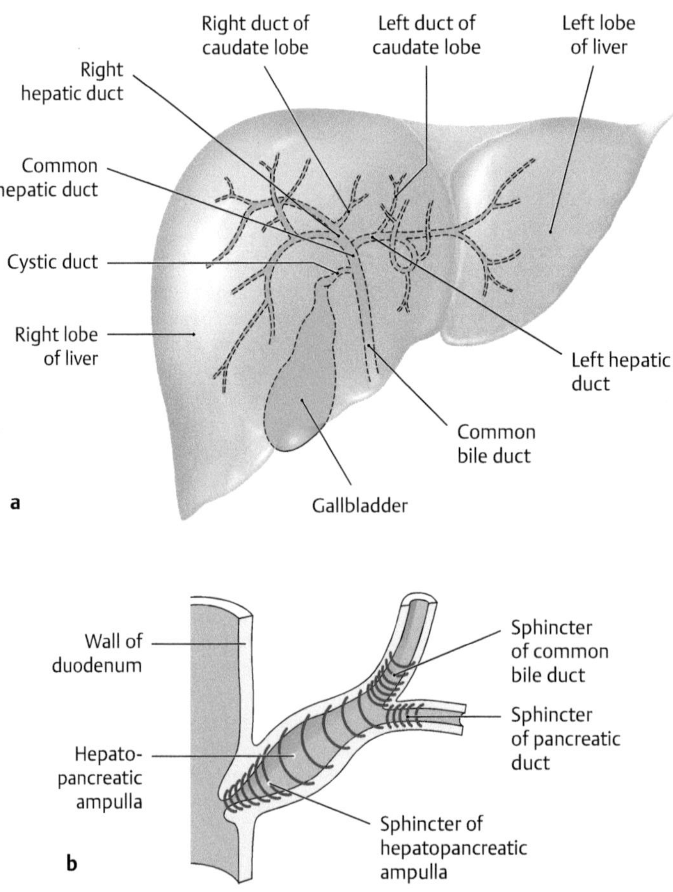

Fig. 3.43 Biliary system. **(a)** Projection onto surface of the liver, anterior view. **(b)** Sphincters of the pancreatic and bile ducts. (From Schuenke M, Schulte E, Schumacher U. THIEME Atlas of Anatomy. Internal Organs. Illustrations by Voll M and Wesker K. 3rd ed. New York: Thieme Medical Publishers; 2020.)

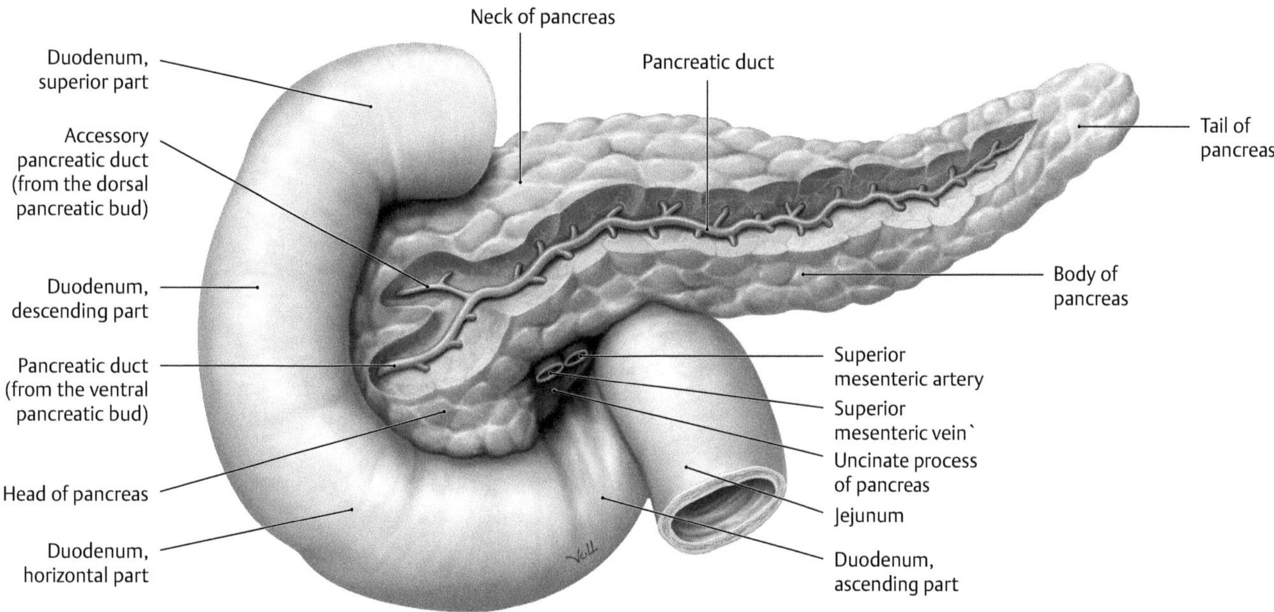

Fig. 3.44 Pancreas. (From Schuenke M, Schulte E, Schumacher U. THIEME Atlas of Anatomy. Internal Organs. Illustrations by Voll M and Wesker K. 3rd ed. New York: Thieme Medical Publishers; 2020.)

to the body region in most individuals. Lymphatic drainage from the uncinate process, head and neck regions primarily drain to the **pyloric** and **pancreaticoduodenal lymph nodes**. Lymphatic drainage from the body and tail regions is to the **pancreaticosplenic lymph nodes (Fig. 3.36b)**.

3.20.2 Histology of the Pancreas

The exocrine portion of the pancreas makes up approximately 98% of this organ's mass and consists of numerous grape-like clusters of acini segregated into lobules that secrete an enzyme-rich fluid that aids in digestion **(Fig. 3.45)**. The parenchyma has the appearance of mostly exocrine acini with ducts mixed in with isolated endocrine cells known as *pancreatic islets.*

The normally large **acinar cells** have the appearance of a truncated pyramid with the apex facing toward the lumen of the acinus. Secretions of the acinar cells drain through a duct system that begins within the center of the acinus as an **intercalated duct** lined with *simple cuboidal* **centroacinar cells**. Intercalated ducts drain into slightly larger *simple cuboidal* lined **intralobular ducts** before several of these ducts converge to form an even larger *simple columnar* lined **interlobular duct** located between adjacent lobules. It is the interlobular ducts that drain directly into the *simple columnar* lined *main pancreatic duct* **(Fig. 3.45)**.

The exocrine secretions of digestive enzymes originate from the zymogen granules of an acinar cell and include enzymes or inactive enzyme precursors known as proenzymes that are activated in the intestinal lumen. These digestive enzymes can include but are not limited to *amylase* (for carbohydrate breakdown); *trypsinogen*, *chymotrypsin* and *carboxypeptidase* (for protein breakdown); *lipase* and *phospholipase* (for lipid breakdown); and finally *deoxyribonuclease* and *ribonuclease* (for nucleic acid breakdown). The release of these enzymes is stimulated by the hormones *cholecystokinin*, *gastrin* and *secretin*. The epithelial cells in pancreatic ducts are the source of the *bicarbonate* and water secreted by the pancreas. Bicarbonate is a base and it is critical for neutralizing the acidic chyme entering the small intestine from the stomach and its secretion is dependent on enzyme *carbonic anhydrase*. The total amount of pancreatic digestive juices produced per day is around 2 liters. The endocrine portion is approximately 2% of the pancreas's mass and its secretions originate from cells of the **pancreatic islets** (*of Langerhans*). These islets are made of **(Fig. 3.45)**:

- **Alpha cells**: ~20% of the islets and positioned mostly on the periphery; secretes *glucagon* which elevates blood glucose levels.
- **Beta cells**: ~70% of the islets and concentrated mainly in the central regions but present throughout; secretes *insulin* which decreases blood glucose levels.
- **Delta cells**: < 5% of the islets and positioned mostly on the periphery; secretes somatostatin and gastrin. *Somatostatin* inhibits hormone release of nearby secretory cells and reduces the contractions and motility of GI tract and gallbladder. *Gastrin* stimulates HCl secretion by the parietal cells and aids in stomach motility.
- **F cells**: rare but positioned mostly on the periphery; secrete *pancreatic polypeptide* that regulates pancreatic secretion activities.

3.21 Spleen

The **spleen** is a left-sided organ similar in shape to an oval, purplish with a pulpy texture, close to the size of a person's fist. It is located in the LUQ between vertebral levels T10 and L1 (9th–11th ribs) and it rests up against the lower parts of the thoracic cage providing it protection **(Fig. 3.46)**. It is the largest lymphatic organ and participates in the production of immunological responses against blood-borne antigens and the removal of defective erythrocytes or particulate matter. It serves as a blood reservoir storing

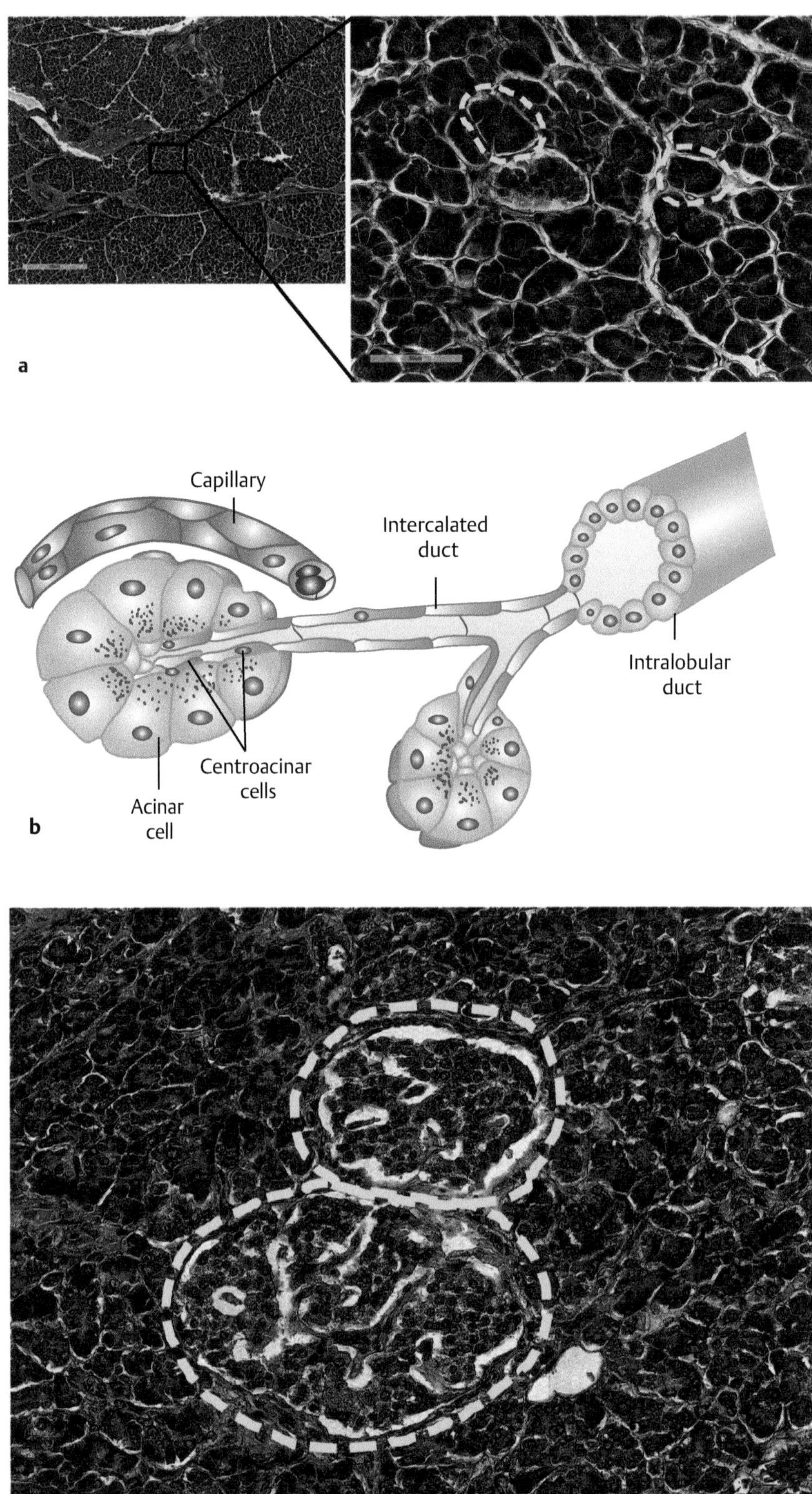

Fig. 3.45 Histology of the pancreas. **(a)** Exocrine pancreas, showing acini (*yellow outlines*). **(b)** Schematic showing the cells and ducts of the exocrine pancreas. **(c)** Pancreatic islets of Langerhans (*yellow outlines*). (From Lowrie DJ. Histology: An Essential Textbook. New York: Thieme Medical Publishers; 2020.)

Clinical Correlate 3.27

Pancreatitis

Inflammation of the pancreas is known as **pancreatitis** and it can present as either acute or chronic. The presence of gallstones in the *hepatopancreatic ampulla* is the most common cause for acute pancreatitis while heavy alcohol use or alcoholism is the most common cause for chronic pancreatitis. Smoking increases the risk for both the acute and chronic pancreatitis. Pain presentation in the upper abdomen and/or back, nausea and vomiting may occur. Weight loss, diarrhea and fatty stools may be an indicator of a more chronic pancreatitis. Treatment can include pain medication, intravenous fluids, abstinence from alcohol and antibiotics. An *endoscopic retrograde cholangiopancreatography* (ERCP) may be performed to open the pancreatic duct if it has become blocked with stones. The gallbladder may also be removed to prevent further development of stones. Nutrition provided through a tube or pancreatic enzyme replacement may need to be provided in chronic cases.

Clinical Correlate 3.28

Pancreatic Cancer

One of the most devastating forms of cancer is **pancreatic cancer** because it is generally found in an advanced stage of development and has a poor prognosis. A loss of appetite followed by weight loss, upper abdominal pain that can radiate to the back and jaundice are all possible symptoms. Having chronic pancreatitis, diabetes, certain gene mutations, or being overweight and a smoker can all increase the risk of developing pancreatic cancer. The most common form is pancreatic adenocarcinoma and this affects the exocrine portion of the gland. The only cure for this type of cancer is surgical removal but this is only possible in a low percentage of patients because the cancer is generally aggressive and has passed to other parts of the pancreas or surrounding tissue. Chemotherapy is generally used in the case of pancreatic cancer to prolong or improve quality of life.

red blood cells and platelets and can increase blood volume in case of a hemorrhage, although this response is limited. Prenatally, the spleen plays a role in hematopoiesis.

The stomach lies anterior to the spleen and the diaphragm lies posterior to it. It is entirely surrounded by peritoneum except at its hilum where the splenic vessels pass to and from the organ. The *splenocolic ligament* that attaches the spleens capsule to the left colic/splenic flexure must be considered when working in this area. If the capsule is damaged, this could result in the rupture of the spleen and an emergency *splenectomy* may have to be performed. Removal of the spleen during childhood will make the individual more susceptible to infection by certain bacteria but in adults this is not as much of a concern.

The presence of an **accessory spleen** is fairly common, relatively small, and they are mostly found near the splenic hilum. Other possible locations include adjacent to the splenic vessels; between the layers of the splenocolic or gastrosplenic ligaments; embedded in the tail of the pancreas, mesentery of the small intestine; and even near the uterus, ovary or testicle.

Clinical Correlate 3.29

Diabetes

Diabetes mellitus type 1 (type 1 diabetes, insulin-dependent or juvenile diabetes) is the result of an autoimmune destruction of the insulin-producing beta cells located in the pancreas. The subsequent lack of insulin leads to an increase in blood and urine glucose levels. The classical symptoms include increased thirst (polydipsia) and hunger (polyphagia), weight loss and frequent urination (polyuria). Although the cause of type 1 diabetes is unknown it can be distinguished from type 2 diabetes by the C-peptide assay that measures endogenous insulin production. Insulin is essential for survival and must be administrated continuously throughout the day. Complications due to non-compliance or the inability to inject insulin when needed can lead to long-term conditions such as kidney failure, retinal damage, heart disease, stroke, neuropathy and foot ulcers. A more acute complication would include *diabetic ketoacidosis*. This is a shortage of insulin that forces the body to begin breaking down fatty acids creating acidic ketone bodies.

Diabetes mellitus type 2 (type 2 diabetes, noninsulin-dependent or adult-onset diabetes) is a metabolic disorder characterized by high blood sugar (hyperglycemia) due to insulin resistance. In this case, insulin is present but cells fail to respond or have become resistant to its action hence the reason for continuously high blood sugar levels. The symptoms are similar to type 1 and include excess thirst and hunger with frequent urination. About 90% of all diabetes cases are of the type 2 nature. The primary cause of type 2 diabetes seems to center on obesity and this has reached epidemic proportions in the western world. Making changes to a person's diet and increasing the amount of exercise per day can help manage type 2 diabetes. Medications can also be prescribed if a person's blood sugar levels cannot be adequately lowered with diet and exercise alone. *Ketoacidosis* is uncommon in type 2 diabetics but a person may be at more risk for *hyperosmolar hyperglycemic state* where high blood sugar levels cause severe dehydration increasing the osmolarity of the blood possibly leading to a coma or even death. Long-term complications are similar to type 1 diabetics and include diabetic retinopathy, kidney failure, heart disease and stroke.

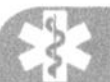

Clinical Correlate 3.30

Splenomegaly

An enlargement of the spleen is known as **splenomegaly**. There are generally no symptoms but abdominal pain, frequent infections, anemia, fatigue or even feeling full after eating a small meal could be a sign of splenomegaly. Infectious mononucleosis, portal hypertension or cancers from a hematological malignancy are the most common causes of splenomegaly. Treatment may involve doing a splenectomy.

3.21.1 Vasculature and Lymphatic Drainage of the Spleen

Blood supply to the spleen is from the **splenic artery**, the largest branch of the celiac trunk. It follows a very tortuous course on the superior border of the pancreas and is found within the *splenorenal ligament* (**Fig. 3.36a**).

The **splenic vein** receives tributaries from the *short gastric, left gastro-omental* and numerous *pancreatic veins* before merging

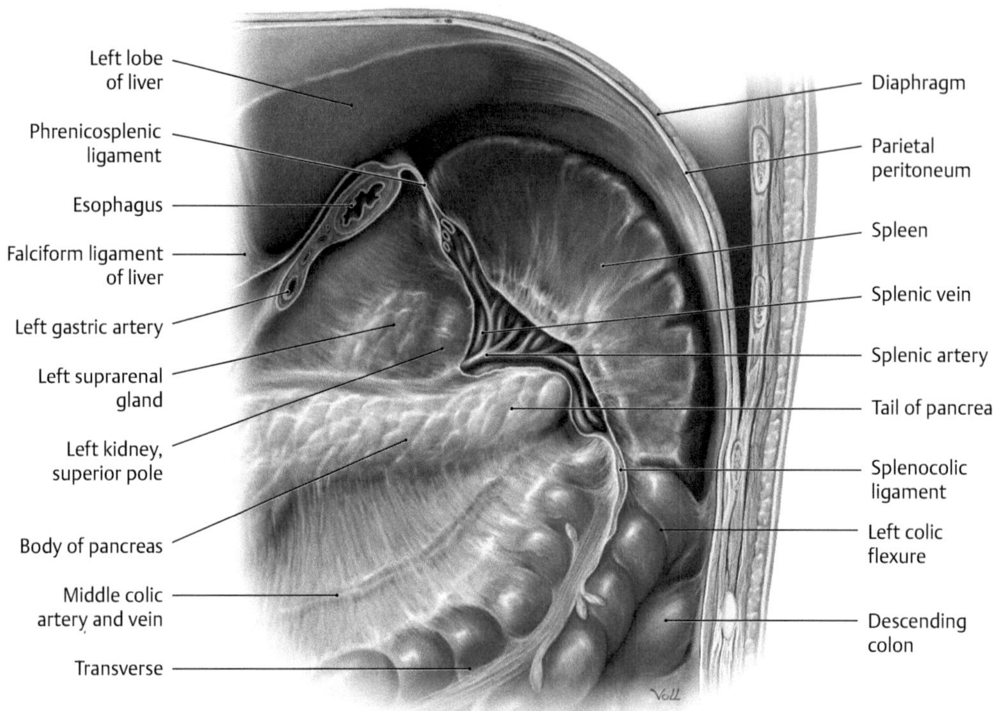

Fig. 3.46 Spleen. (From Schuenke M, Schulte E, Schumacher U. THIEME Atlas of Anatomy. Internal Organs. Illustrations by Voll M and Wesker K. 3rd ed. New York: Thieme Medical Publishers; 2020.)

with the *superior mesenteric vein* to form the *hepatic portal vein* **(Fig. 3.33b)**. Lymphatic drainage passes to the **pancreaticosplenic lymph nodes (Fig. 3.33c; Fig. 3.36b)**.

3.21.2 Histology of the Spleen

The spleen is made up primarily of **red pulp** (~75% of total volume) which is embedded with **white pulp**. Red pulp is analogous to the medulla of a lymph node while the white pulp is analogous to the cortex of a lymph node. The spleen has a thin outer capsule from which short trabeculae extend into the parenchyma and the capsule is thickest near the hilum.

The red pulp is a highly vascular tissue traversed by thin walled venous sinusoids lined by *littoral cells*, a type of endothelial cell that allows the passing of red blood cells between the sinus and cords (*of Billroth*). The sinuses are separated by these cords, which contain a labyrinth of splenic macrophages responsible for filtering red blood cells **(Fig. 3.47)**.

The white pulp functions by trapping antigens for processing. It forms a wrapping of lymphoid cells around arteries called **periarteriolar lymphoid sheaths (PALS)** that are composed of T cells and lymphoid follicles (or B cells). The follicles have a surrounding mantle zone (proliferating B cells) and an outer marginal zone (memory B cells).

3.22 Duodenum (Third and Fourth Part)

The continuation of the duodenum at the junction of the 2nd and 3rd parts represents the end of the foregut and the beginning of the midgut. The **3rd (horizontal) part of the duodenum** lies adjacent to the head and uncinate process of the pancreas and is located at vertebral level L3. The superior mesenteric vessels course superficial to this portion of the duodenum. This portion of the duodenum is retroperitoneal.

The **4th (ascending) part of the duodenum** lies posterior to the root of the mesentery and inferior to the body of the pancreas. It ascends back from vertebral level L3 to L2. This portion of the duodenum is retroperitoneal. At its distal end it curves anteriorly to become the jejunum, the second of three parts of the small intestine. This is also known as the **duodenojejunal flexure**. This junction is supported by the **suspensory muscle of the duodenum** (*ligament of Treitz*) a thin slip of skeletal muscle that mostly originates from the right crus of the diaphragm. In addition, there are some smooth muscle fibers that originate from the 3rd and 4th parts of the duodenum and contribute to this structure. The duodenojejunal flexure is widened by contraction of this muscle.

3.22.1 Vasculature and Lymphatic Drainage of the Duodenum (Midgut Portion)

Blood supply to this portion of the duodenum is originally derived from the **superior mesenteric artery (SMA)**. There is a direct **inferior pancreaticoduodenal artery** that branches off the SMA before bifurcating into **anterior/posterior inferior pancreaticoduodenal arteries**. These arteries lie in a groove between the pancreas and duodenum and supply both structures. They form an anastomosis with the anterior/posterior superior pancreaticoduodenal arteries **(Fig. 3.36a)**.

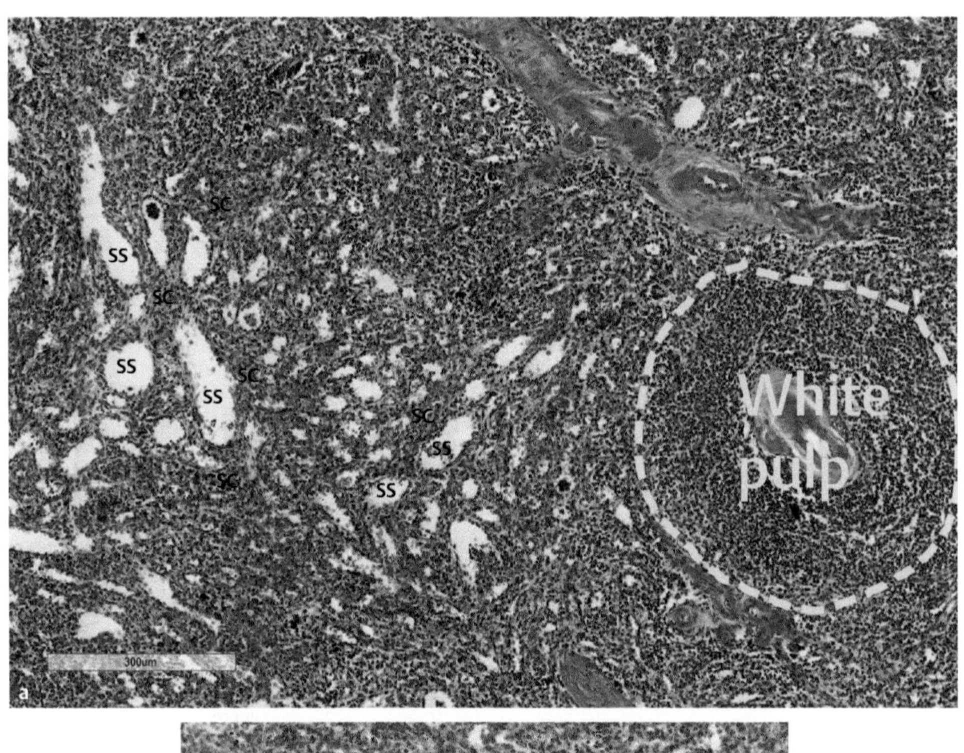

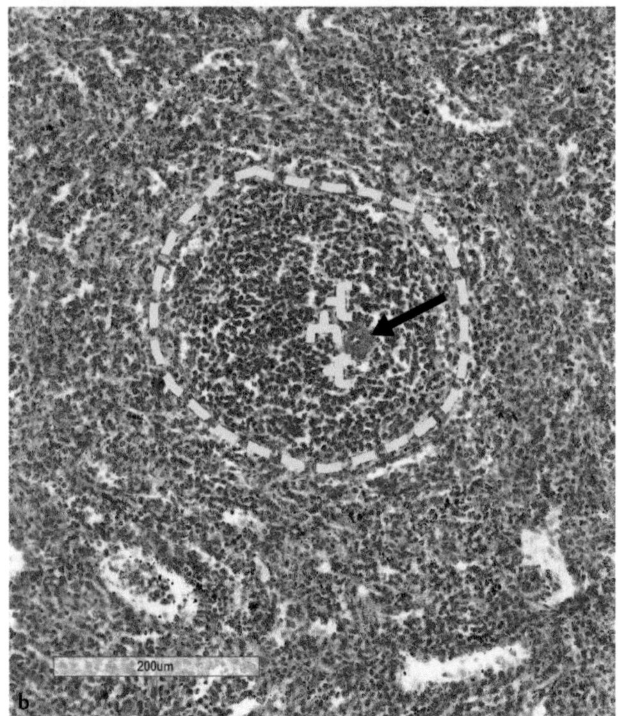

Fig. 3.47 Histology of the spleen. **(a)** Red pulp of the spleen, low-medium magnification. Splenic sinusoids (*SS*) are the predominant vessels in this region; the pulp tissue here consists of splenic cords (of Billroth, *SC*). A nodule of white pulp is indicated. **(b)** White pulp (*yellow outline*) showing a central arteriole (*black arrow*). T lymphocytes immediately surrounding the central arteriole make up the periarterial lymphatic sheath (PALS, *yellow brackets*). The remainder of the outlined area is a lymphoid nodule rich in B lymphocytes. (From Lowrie DJ. Histology: An Essential Textbook. New York: Thieme Medical Publishers; 2020.)

Venous drainage follows the arteries and drains back to the **superior mesenteric vein** before ultimately making it to the **hepatic portal vein**. Lymphatic drainage from this portion of the anterior and posterior duodenum is to the **pancreaticoduodenal lymph nodes** followed by the **superior mesenteric lymph nodes** (**Fig. 3.36b**).

3.23 Jejunum and Ileum

The second and third parts of the small intestine are the **jejunum** and **ileum** respectively (**Fig. 3.26; Fig. 3.48**). The jejunum rests mainly in the LUQ and the ileum is found mostly in the RLQ. The jejunum has a larger lumen, is heavier and tends to be a brighter

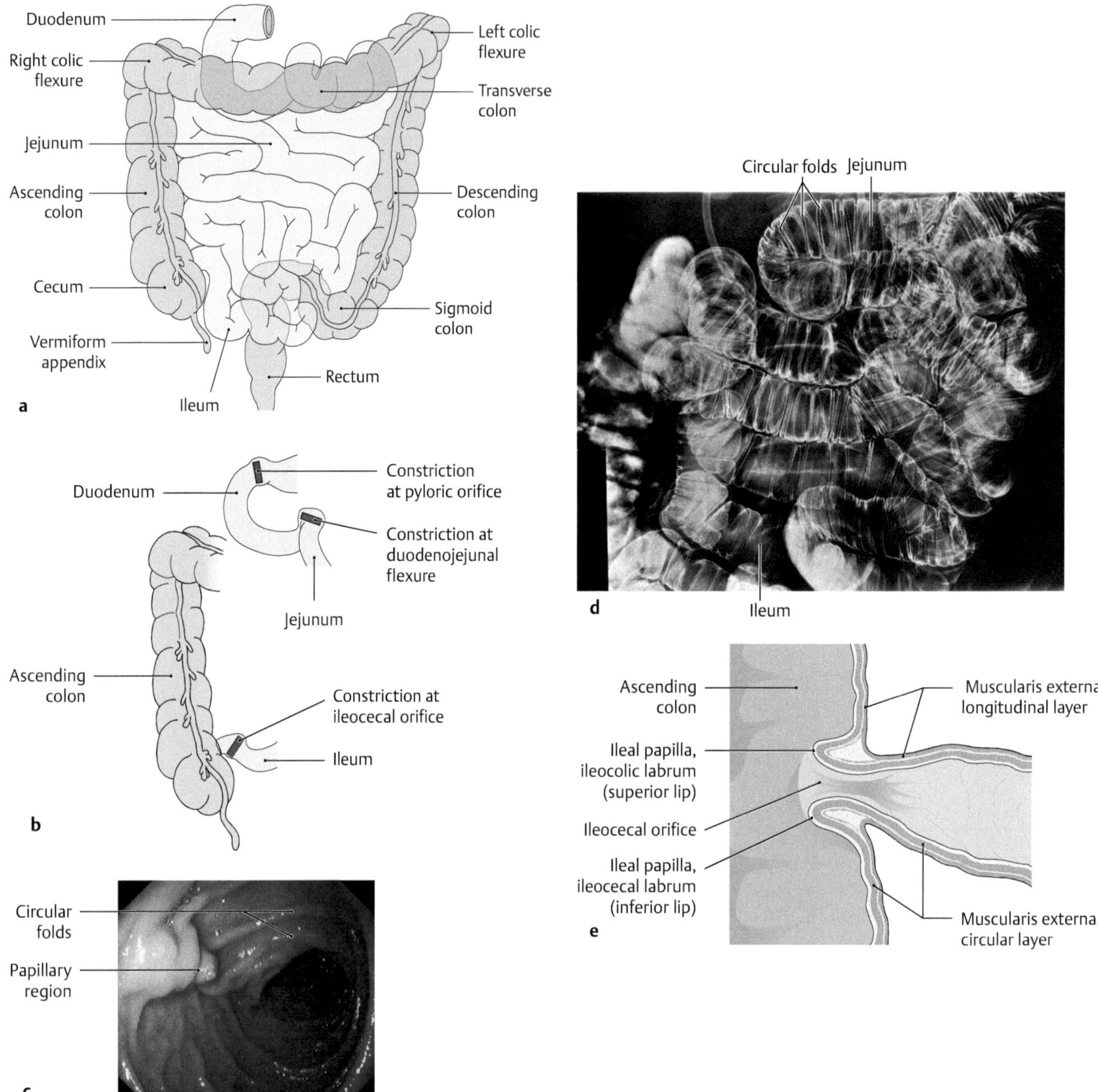

Fig. 3.48 (a) Location of small intestine. **(b)** Anatomical constrictions of the small intestine. **(c)** Endoscopic appearance of the descending portion of the duodenum near the major duodenal papilla. **(d)** Double contrast barium enema of the small intestine, anterior view. **(e)** Structure of the ileocecal valve. (**a**, **b**, **d**, **e** from Schuenke M, Schulte E, Schumacher U. THIEME Atlas of Anatomy. Neck and Internal Organs. Illustrations by Voll M and Wesker K. 1st ed. New York: Thieme Medical Publishers; 2010. **c** from Block, Schachschal and Schmidt. Endoscopy of the Upper G I Tract. Stuttgart: Thieme; 2004.)

red in color compared to the ileum. It also has less fat located in its adjacent mesentery versus the ileum that has more fat and displays encroaching fat, the appearance of fat extending over the outer wall. The jejunum begins at the duodenojejunal flexure and the ileum ends at the **ileocecal junction**. There is no clear demarcation separating the two structures but the characteristics listed above from a surgical perspective are useful.

The combined length of these structures is 6-7 meters with the jejunum accounting for two fifths and the ileum three fifths of the total length. The *mesentery* attaches to the entire jejunum and ileum to the posterior abdominal wall thus making it mobile and intraperitoneal. The *root of the mesentery* extends from the duodenojejunal flexure to the ileocecal junction.

3.23.1 Vasculature and Lymphatic Drainage of the Small Intestine

Blood supply to the jejunum and ileum is from the 15-18 **jejunal** and **ileal artery** branches of the **superior mesenteric artery (SMA) (Fig. 3.49)**. The arterial supply and patterns differ between these two parts of the small intestine. The jejunum has a greater

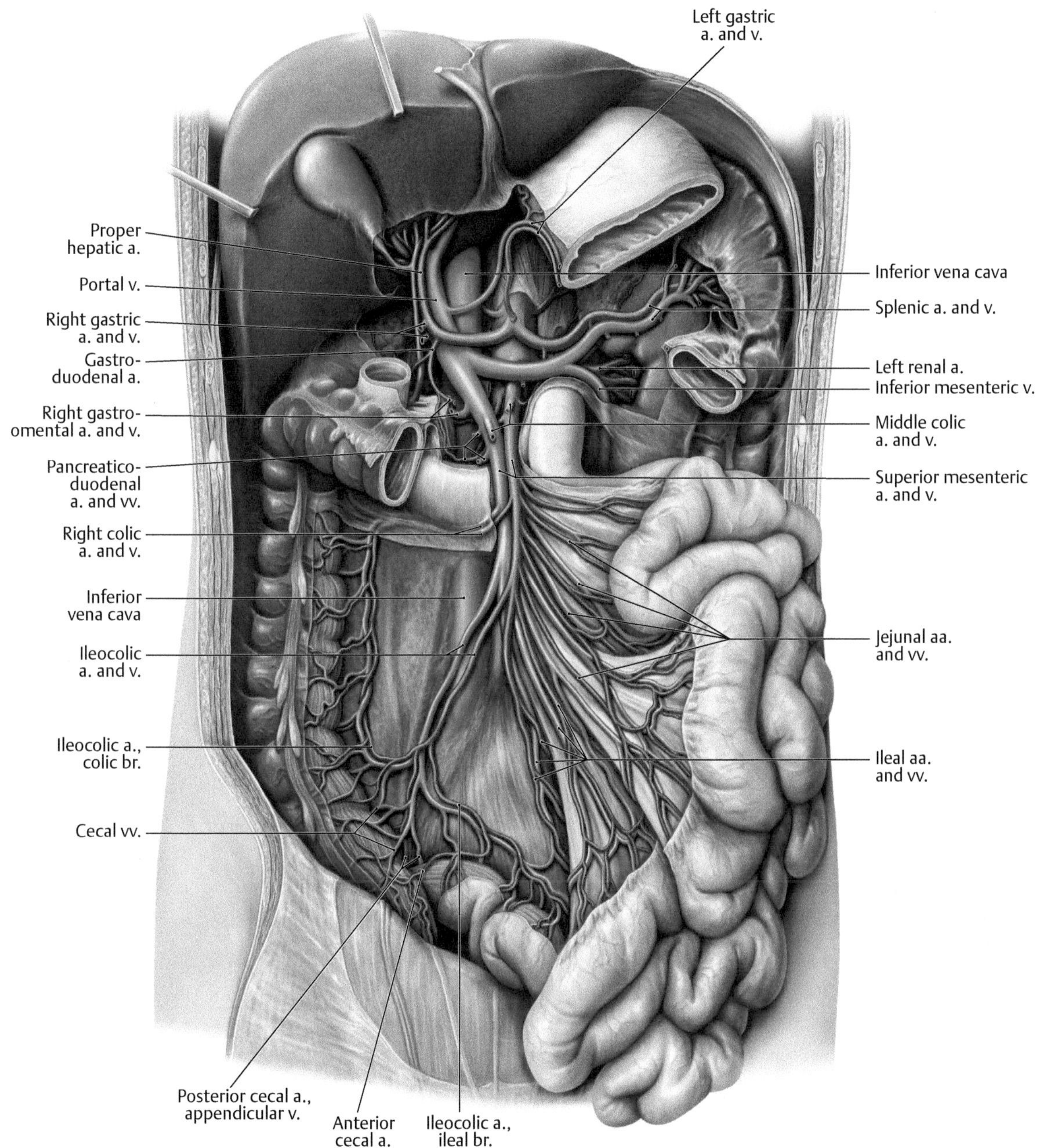

Fig. 3.49 Superior mesenteric vessels. (From Schuenke M, Schulte E, Schumacher U. THIEME Atlas of Anatomy. Internal Organs. Illustrations by Voll M and Wesker K. 3rd ed. New York: Thieme Medical Publishers; 2020.)

amount of vascularity attributed to **vasa recta** that are *long* and **arterial arcades** having *large but few loops*. The ileum presents with **vasa recta** that are *short* and **arterial arcades** that are *numerous but very short* (**Fig. 3.50**).

Venous drainage follows the arterial supply and eventually drains into the **superior mesenteric vein (SMV)**. The absorption of fat is through **lacteals**, specialized lymphatic vessels located in the intestinal villi. A milk-like fluid drains into the lymphatic plexuses located in the walls of the jejunum and ileum. Between the layers of the mesentery, the lymph passes in order through three groups of lymph nodes. The first being **juxta-intestinal lymph nodes** located near the intestinal wall. Drainage is then to the **intermediate (mesenteric) lymph nodes** scattered along the arterial arcades. Lymph will pass through the **central (superior) lymph nodes** before ultimately reaching the **superior mesenteric lymph nodes (Fig. 3.51)**. **Lymphoid nodules** (*Peyer patches*) are present in larger numbers within the ileum but are less prevalent in the jejunum. These lymphoid nodules are involved in the immune surveillance of pathogenic microorganisms. Hypertrophy of these lymphoid nodules could lead to *intussusception*, this is when a part of the intestine invaginates into another section of the intestine creating an obstruction.

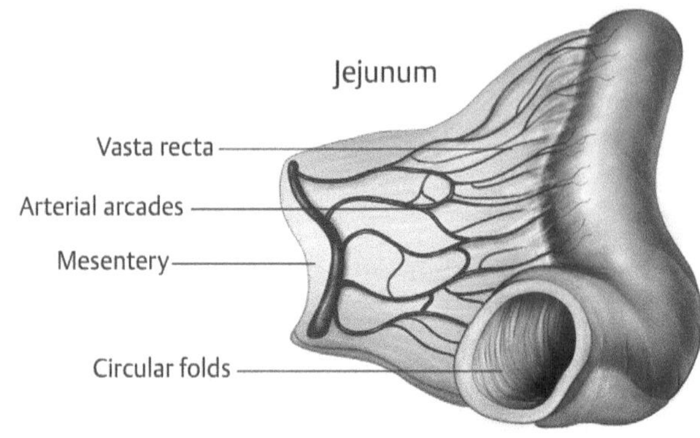

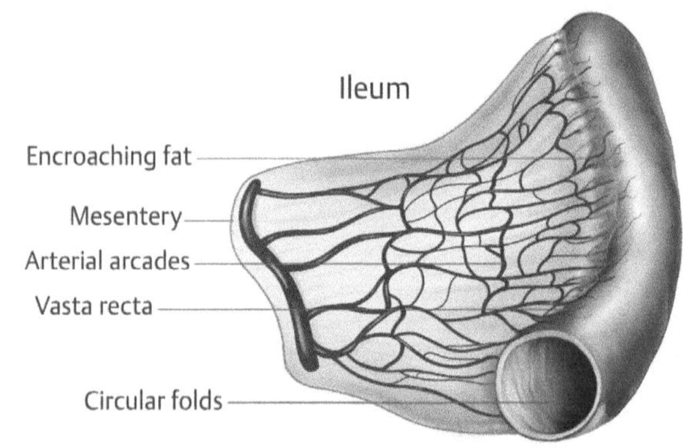

Fig. 3.50 Blood supply pattern of the jejunum and ileum. Illustration by Calla Heald.

3.23.2 Histology of the Small Intestine

The majority of the small intestines mucosa consists of *plicae circulares, villi* and *microvilli* in order to increase to total surface area (600 fold) and maximize the efficient digestive and absorptive functions.

The mucosa is made up of a *simple columnar epithelium*. The lamina propria contains much immunocompetent *gut-associated lymphatic tissue* (GALT) that may be solitary or confluent in nature. Lymphocytes that secrete IgA predominate in this layer as well. The **plicae circulares (circular folds** or *valves of Kerckring*) are permanent folds that consist of epithelium, lamina propria and muscularis mucosa along with a submucosa. They are located from the distal duodenum to the proximal ileum and are the most pronounced in the jejunum. Mucosal evaginations called **villi** are characteristic of the small intestine and vary in appearance such as a leaf-like structure in the duodenum or a short and simple version in the ileum. A villus contains an arteriole, venule, capillaries, autonomics, smooth muscle and a lacteal. They are primarily made of absorptive cells. The **microvilli** are located on the apical surface of the epithelial cells. Besides amplifying the surface area, these structures secrete enzymes that help complete the breakdown of nutrients. Between the villi deep invaginations that extend to the muscularis mucosa form the **intestinal glands** (*crypts of Lieberkuhn*). These glands secrete *intestinal juice* a watery solution that mixes with chyme and can contain mucus, digestive enzymes, hormones and substances to neutralize HCl from the stomach. There are several epithelial cell types that are known to cover the villi or line the glands and they include (**Fig. 3.52**):

- **Enterocyte (absorptive) cells**: located on the villi and upper intestinal glands. They absorb digested nutrients and contain many mitochondria because this is an energy-dependent process. They also assemble absorbed lipid molecules into lipid-protein complexes known as chylomicrons so that they may enter the lacteals.
- **Goblet cells**: located on the villi and secrete mucus to lubricate the chyme and form a protective barrier from any enzymatic digestion of the intestinal wall.
- **Enteroendocrine cells**: scattered on the villi and intestinal glands. They secrete *gastrin* (influences gastric secretions), *cholecystokinin* (stimulate gallbladder contraction), *secretin* (signal pancreas to secrete a bicarbonate juice to neutralize the acidic chyme) and *motilin* (stimulate the production of pepsin and improve peristalsis) as well as others.
- **Paneth cells**: located in the lower intestinal gland. They secrete enzymes that destroy certain bacteria. There is a permanent intestinal bacterial presence called the *intestinal flora* that manufactures certain vitamins one of which is vitamin K. This vitamin is important in blood coagulation.
- **Undifferentiated cells**: found in the lower regions of the intestinal glands. They renew the mucosal epithelium continuously and rapidly onto the villi. A complete renewal of the intestinal lining of the small intestine occurs every 3-6 days.

The submucosa is fairly common in all areas of the small intestine except in the duodenum where special **duodenal glands** (*Brunner's glands*) exist. These glands secrete a mucus-rich alkaline substance that is important for neutralizing the acidic chyme, lubricating the intestinal wall, and providing a more alkaline environment that helps intestinal enzymes become more active, thus stimulating more absorption. The lamina propria and submucosa of the ileum contain numerous **lymphoid nodules** (*Peyer's patches*). All other layers have no unusual features.

3.24 Large Intestine

The large intestine consists of the cecum, appendix, ascending colon, transverse colon, descending colon, sigmoid colon, rectum and upper anal canal. These structures are part of both the midgut and hindgut. The function of the large intestine as a whole is to absorb water from the indigestible food bolus in order to solidify a stool or feces and act as a temporary storage site before defecation occurs. The large intestine has characteristics that distinguish it from the small intestine and these include (**Fig. 3.53**):

- **Lumen size**: has a larger diameter than the small intestine.
- **Haustra**: the appearance of small pouches caused by sacculation.
- **Teniae coli**: three separate longitudinal bands (*free, mesocolic* and *omental*) of smooth muscle that contract and produce haustra. The three bands begin at the base of the appendix and end at the *rectosigmoid junction*. The **free taenia** is devoid of both omental appendices and any mesentery attachments. The **mesocolic taenia** attaches to both the transverse and sigmoid mesocolons. The **omental taenia** attaches to both the greater omentum and numerous omental appendices (**Fig. 3.54**).
- **Omental appendices**: small, omentum-like projections attached to most of the tenia. These can be larger depending on body fat percentage.
- **Semilunar folds**: internal features corresponding to external constrictions that separate the haustra (**Fig. 3.55**).
- **Marginal artery** (*of Drummond*): forms an anastomosis between the distal branches of the superior mesenteric and

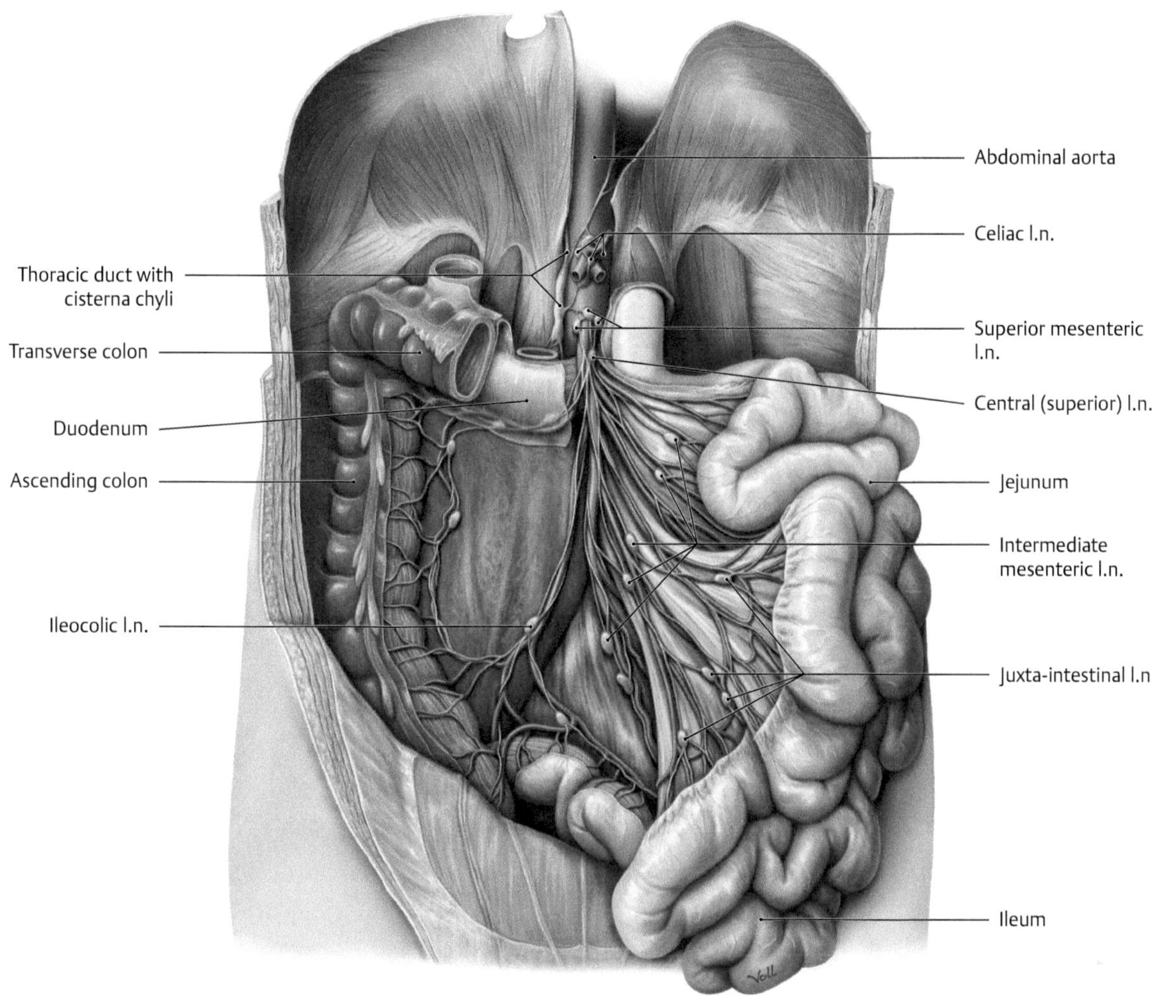

Fig. 3.51 Lymph nodes of the jejunum and ileum. (From Schuenke M, Schulte E, Schumacher U. THIEME Atlas of Anatomy. Internal Organs. Illustrations by Voll M and Wesker K. 3rd ed. New York: Thieme Medical Publishers; 2020.)

inferior mesenteric arteries. In the case of an abdominal aortic aneurysm surgical repair, the inferior mesenteric artery does not have to be reattached because of this anastomosis.

3.25 Cecum

The first part of the large intestine is a blind intestinal pouch called the **cecum**. It is located in the RLQ and iliac fossa and it is enveloped by peritoneum. It has no mesentery but is still considered an intraperitoneal structure (**Fig. 3.53; Fig. 3.56**). It is generally bound to the lateral abdominal wall by a couple of **cecal folds** made of peritoneum and this helps create a **retrocecal space**, a common location for the appendix. The cecum has a variable peritoneal covering at times making the cecum a retroperitoneal structure. The ileum terminates as an invagination into the cecum. The **ileal orifice**, surrounded by the **ileal papilla**, can be located just deep to the **frenula of the ileal orifice**. The ileal papilla is thought to prevent the reflux of cecal contents back into the ileum.

3.26 Appendix

The **appendix** (vermiform appendix) is a blind intestinal diverticulum in the RLQ and ranges from 6 to 10 cm (**Fig. 3.53; Fig. 3.56**). It originates from the posteromedial aspect of the cecum but rests nearly 70% of the time in a retrocecal position within the retrocecal space. It is attached to a mesentery called the mesoappendix thus making it an intraperitoneal structure. It contains masses of lymphoid tissue and it used to be generally regarded as a vestigial organ with no significant function. Recently a study has shown that the appendix may serve to re-inoculate the colon with beneficial bacteria after a bout of dysentery (Bollinger et al., 2007).

3.26.1 Vasculature and Lymphatic Drainage of the Cecum and Appendix

The blood supply to the cecum is from the **anterior** and **posterior cecal arteries** (ileocolic brs.) while the appendix receives blood from the **appendicular artery** (ileocolic br.) (**Fig. 3.49**).

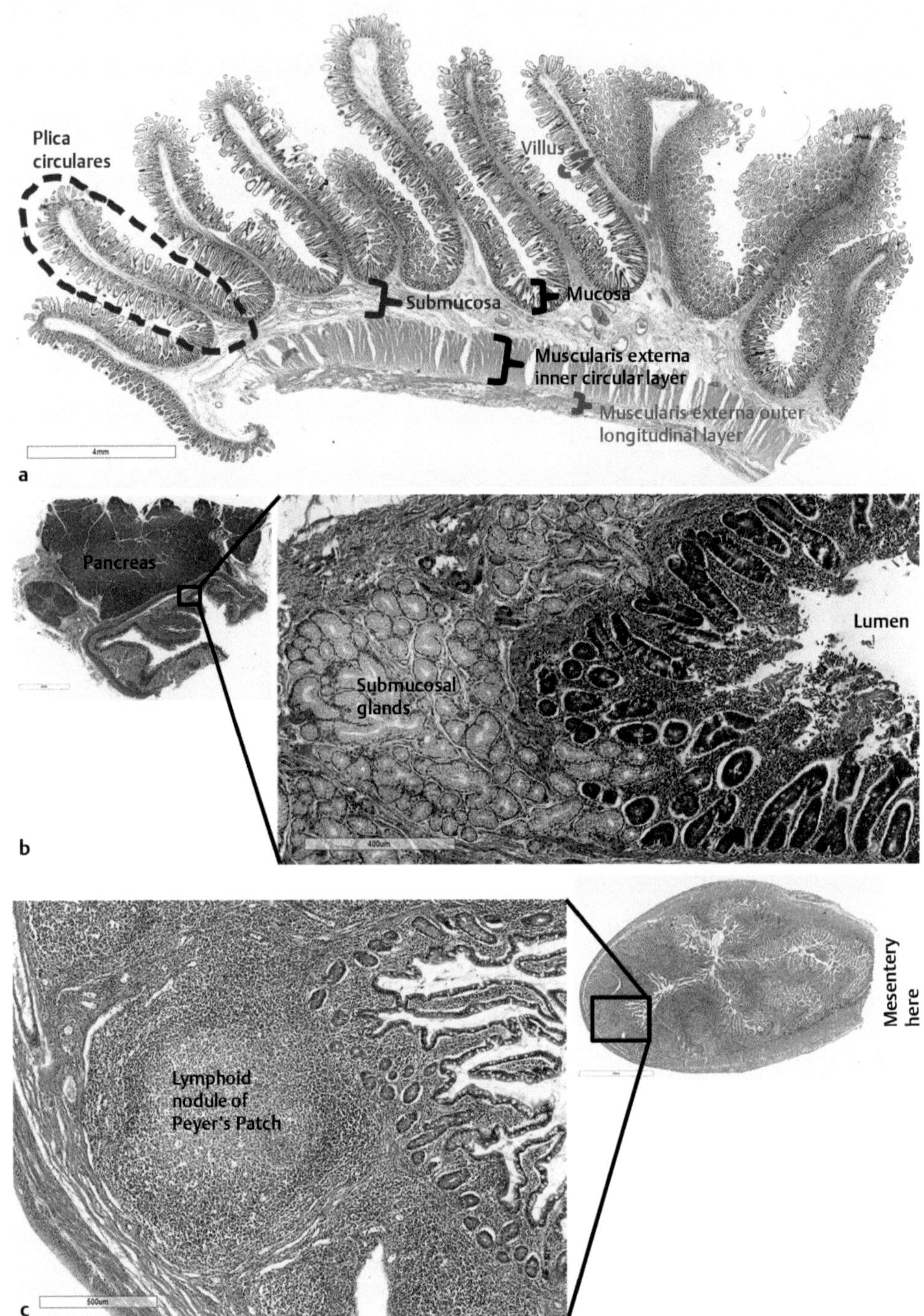

Fig. 3.52 Histology of the small intestine. **(a)** Jejunum in longitudinal section, showing the four-layered structure typical of the GI tract. A plicae circularis (*black outline*) and a villus (*red outline*) are also shown. **(b)** Duodenum showing mucus (Brunner's) glands in the submucosa. **(c)** Ileum showing lymphoid nodules (Peyer's patches). (From Lowrie DJ. Histology: An Essential Textbook. New York: Thieme Medical Publishers; 2020.)

Venous drainage matches the arteries before reaching the **SMV**. Lymphatic drainage of the cecum generally passes to the **ileocolic lymph nodes** before reaching the **superior mesenteric lymph nodes**. The appendix drains first to the **appendicular lymph nodes** before following the course of the cecum's drainage (**Fig. 3.51**).

3.27 Ascending Colon

The **ascending colon** passes superiorly from the cecum toward the right lobe of the liver (**Fig. 3.53**). At this point it turns to the left to become the transverse colon at the *right colic/hepatic flexure.* The flexure lies deep to the 9th and 10th ribs and is overlapped by the inferior aspect of the liver. The ascending colon is retroperitoneal and narrower that the cecum. The *right paracolic gutter* rests between the abdominal wall and the ascending colon.

3.27.1 Vasculature and Lymphatic Drainage of the Ascending Colon

The blood supply to the ascending colon is from the **right colic** and **ileocolic arteries** both branches of the **SMA**. The right colic

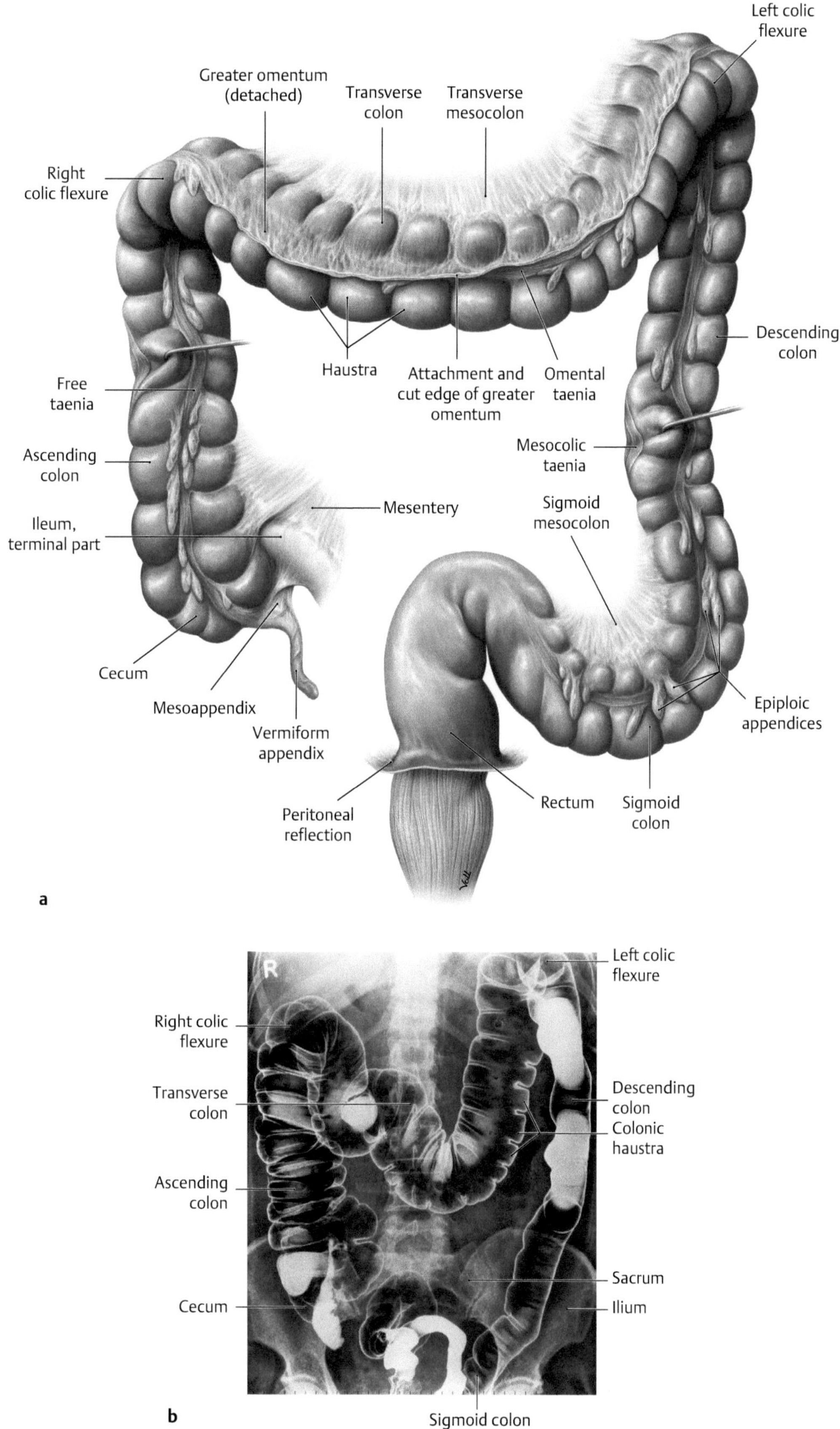

Fig. 3.53 (a) Large intestine, anterior view. **(b)** Double contrast barium enema of the large intestine, anterior view. (**a** from Schuenke M, Schulte E, Schumacher U. THIEME Atlas of Anatomy. Internal Organs. Illustrations by Voll M and Wesker K. 3rd ed. New York: Thieme Medical Publishers; 2020. **b** from Reiser, M. et al.: Radiologie [Duale Reihe], 2nd ed. Stuttgart: Thieme Medical Publishers; 2006.)

Clinical Correlate 3.31

Appendicitis and Appendectomy

Sudden pain in the right lower quadrant at within the T10 dermatome has a high correlation to inflammation of the appendix or **appendicitis.** In younger individuals it is usually hyperplasia of lymphatic follicles in the appendix that results in occlusion of the lumen that leads to appendicitis. Obstruction by way of a fecalith (coprolith), a core of fecal matter surrounded by surrounding tissue is generally the cause of appendicitis in older individuals. If there was not a full rotation of the gut during development, appendicitis has been localized to the RUQ. An **appendectomy** has now become routinely performed using laparoscopic surgery. The location for the appendix is generally located at the McBurney point.

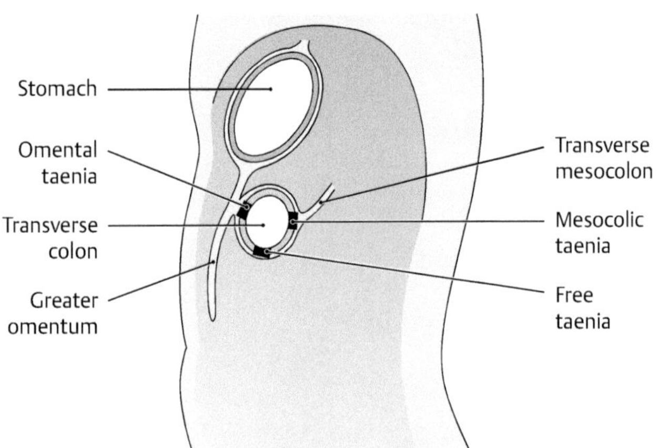

Fig. 3.54 The three taeniae of the colon. (From Schuenke M, Schulte E, Schumacher U. THIEME Atlas of Anatomy. Internal Organs. Illustrations by Voll M and Wesker K. 3rd ed. New York: Thieme Medical Publishers; 2020.)

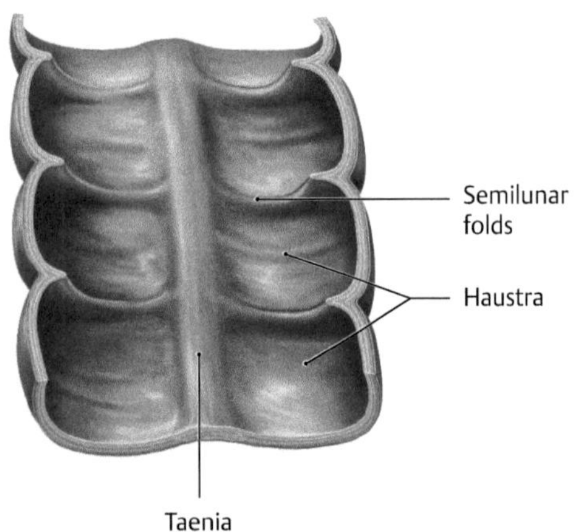

Fig. 3.55 Interior of the colon. (From Schuenke M, Schulte E, Schumacher U. THIEME Atlas of Anatomy. Internal Organs. Illustrations by Voll M and Wesker K. 3rd ed. New York: Thieme Medical Publishers; 2020.)

will anastomose with the ileocolic and the *right branch of the middle colic* arteries. If the right colic artery is highly variable and if it does not originate directly from the SMA, it may arise from a common trunk with the ileocolic or middle colic arteries (**Fig. 3.49**).

Venous drainage is by way of the **right colic** and **ileocolic veins** to the **SMV**. Lymphatic drainage is first to the **epiploic** and **paracolic lymph nodes.** Lymph will then travel to the **right colic** and **ileocolic lymph nodes** before finally reaching the **superior mesenteric lymph nodes** (**Fig. 3.51**).

3.28 Transverse Colon

The **transverse colon** is the longest and most mobile portion of the large intestine (**Fig. 3.53**). It extends from the *right colic/hepatic flexure* to the more superiorly and more acute *left colic/splenic flexure* before becoming the descending colon. The proximal two-thirds is part of the *midgut* while the distal one-third is associated with the *hindgut*. The transverse colon does have a mesentery attached to it called the **transverse mesocolon** and its *root* lies along the inferior border of the pancreas.

3.28.1 Vasculature and Lymphatic Drainage of the Transverse Colon

The blood supply to the transverse colon is from the **middle colic artery**, a branch of the **SMA**. The middle colic has both a *left* and *right branch* that help distribute blood throughout the length of the transverse colon (**Fig. 3.49; Fig. 3.57b**).

Venous drainage is by way of the **middle colic vein** to the **SMV**. Lymphatic drainage is first to the **epiploic** and **paracolic lymph nodes**, followed by the **middle colic lymph nodes** before finally reaching the **superior mesenteric lymph nodes** (**Fig. 3.57c**).

3.29 Descending Colon

The **descending colon** begins at the *left colic/splenic flexure* where the transverse colon ends and extends inferiorly before becoming the sigmoid colon (**Fig. 3.53**). It is a retroperitoneal structure and the *left paracolic gutter* rests between it and the abdominal wall. It functions by continuing to solidify the feces and storing it before it progresses through the rest of the large intestine.

3.29.1 Vasculature and Lymphatic Drainage of the Descending Colon

The blood supply to the descending colon is from the **left colic artery**, a branch of the **inferior mesenteric artery** (**IMA**). The left colic has both an *ascending* and *descending branch* that helps distribute blood throughout the length of the descending colon (**Fig. 3.57**).

Venous drainage flows from the **left colic veins** to the **inferior mesenteric vein (IMV)**. Lymphatic drainage is first to the **epiploic** and **paracolic lymph nodes**, followed by the **left colic (intermediate colic) lymph nodes** before reaching the **inferior mesenteric lymph nodes** (**Fig. 3.57**).

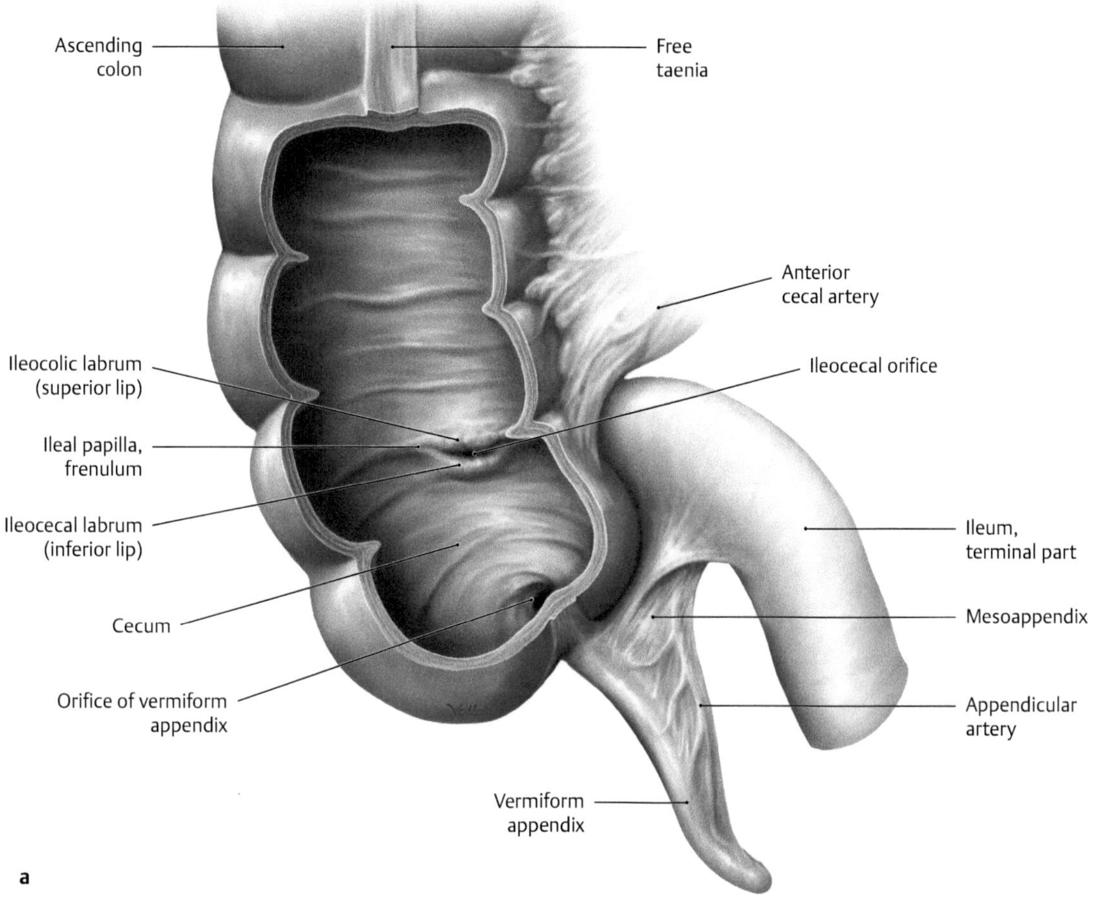

Ascending colon
Free taenia
Anterior cecal artery
Ileocolic labrum (superior lip)
Ileocecal orifice
Ileal papilla, frenulum
Ileocecal labrum (inferior lip)
Ileum, terminal part
Cecum
Mesoappendix
Orifice of vermiform appendix
Appendicular artery
Vermiform appendix
a

Location of umbilicus
L 4 vertebra
McBurney point
Right anterior superior iliac spine
Left anterior superior iliac spine
Lanz point
b

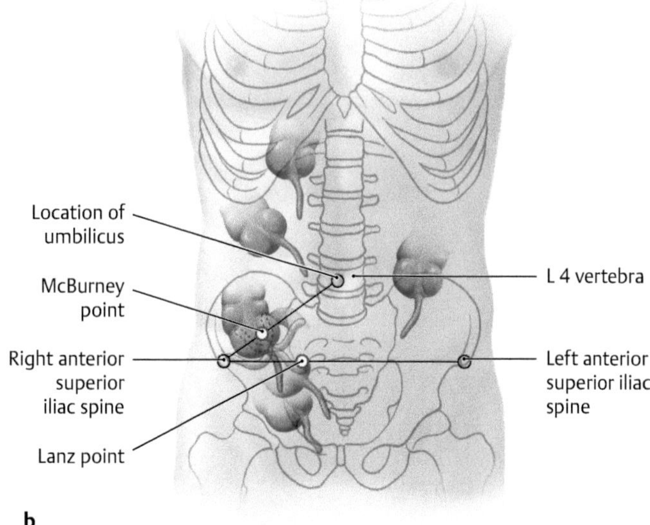

Fig. 3.56 **(a)** Windowed cecum and terminal ileum, anterior view. **(b)** Variants in the position of the vermiform appendix. (From Schuenke M, Schulte E, Schumacher U. THIEME Atlas of Anatomy. Internal Organs. Illustrations by Voll M and Wesker K. 3rd ed. New York: Thieme Medical Publishers; 2020.)

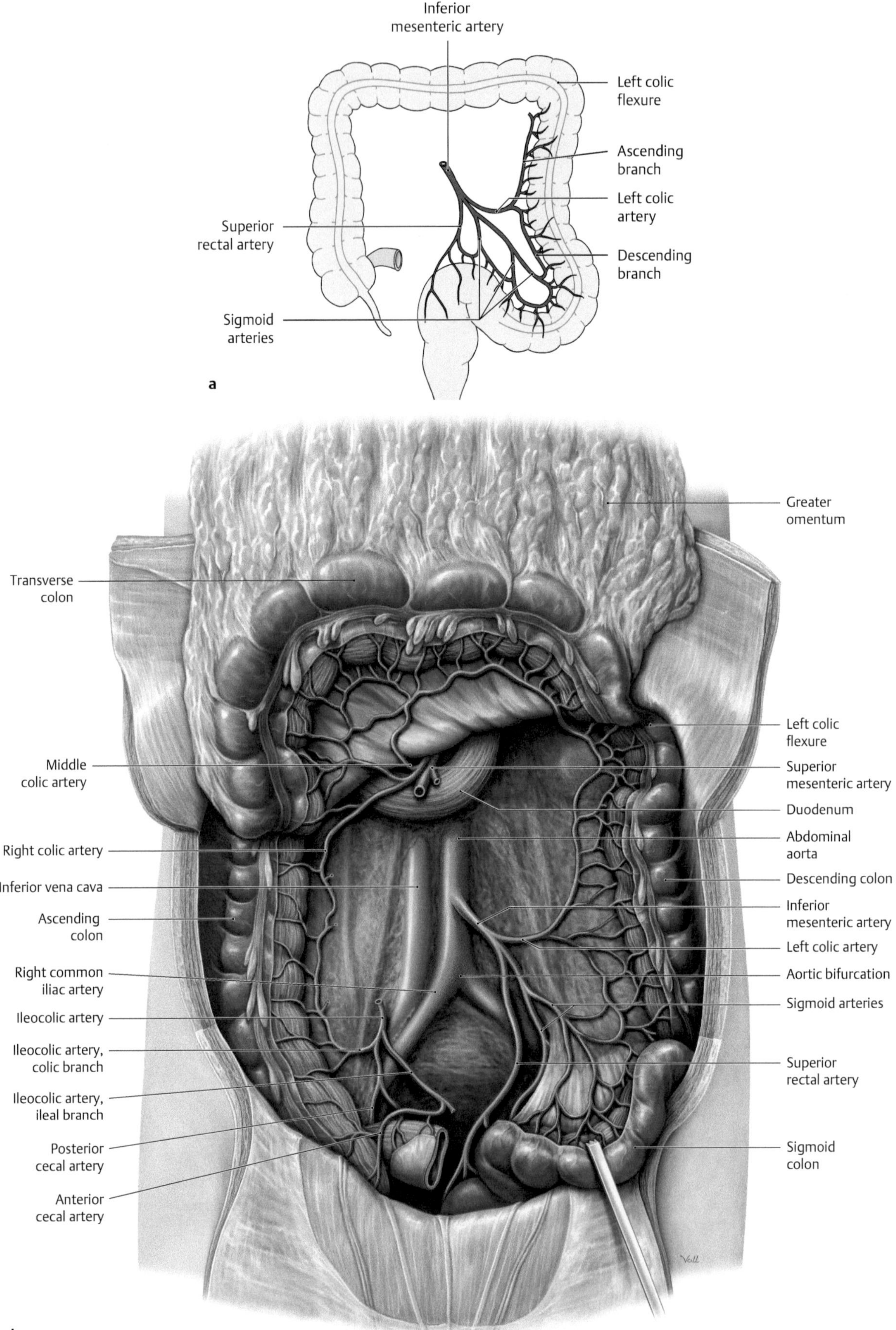

Fig. 3.57 (a) Sequence of branches from the inferior mesenteric artery. **(b)** Branches of the inferior mesenteric artery. (*continued*) (From Schuenke M, Schulte E, Schumacher U. THIEME Atlas of Anatomy. Internal Organs. Illustrations by Voll M and Wesker K. 3rd ed. New York: Thieme Medical Publishers; 2020.)

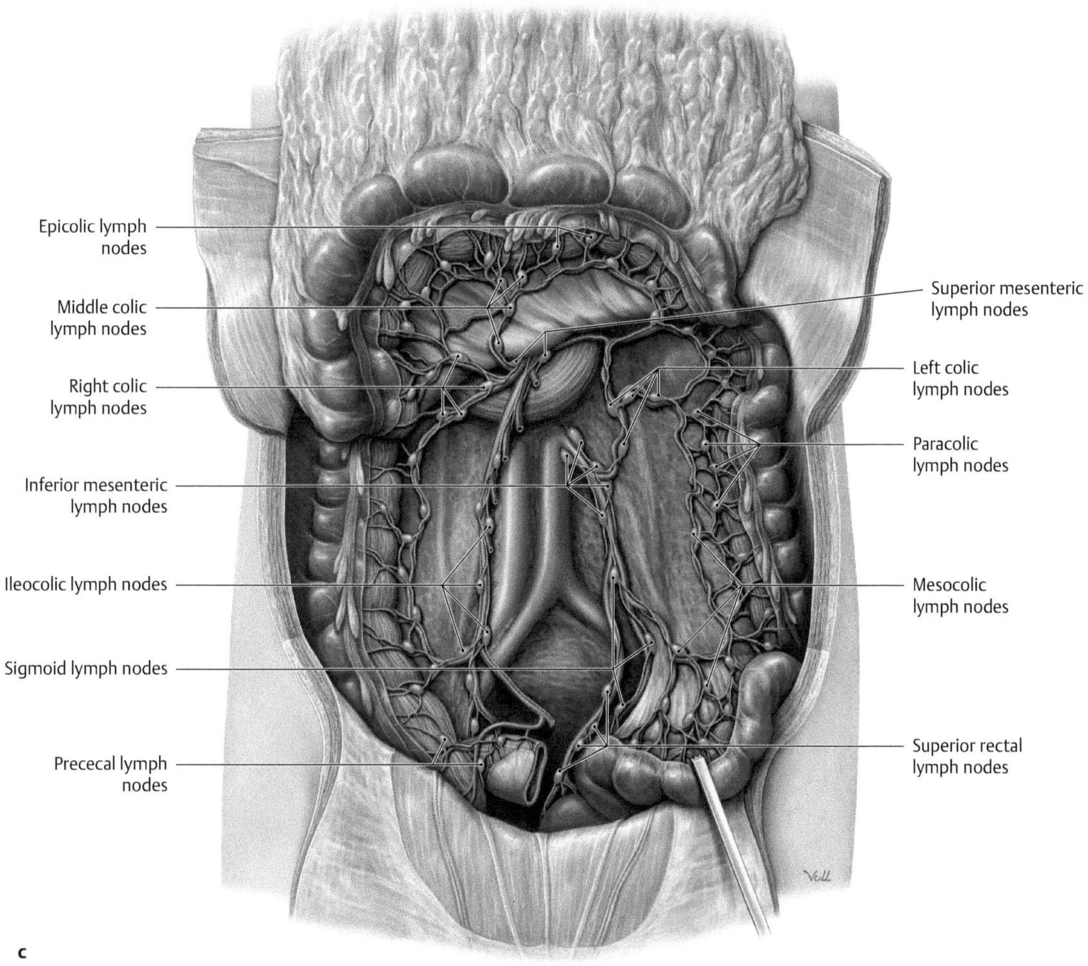

Fig. 3.57 *(continued)* **(c)** Lymphatic drainage of the large intestine. (From Schuenke M, Schulte E, Schumacher U. THIEME Atlas of Anatomy. Internal Organs. Illustrations by Voll M and Wesker K. 3rd ed. New York: Thieme Medical Publishers; 2020.)

3.30 Sigmoid Colon

The **sigmoid colon** is located between the descending colon and the rectum and has a characteristic S-shaped loop to it **(Fig. 3.53)**. It is located in the iliac fossa and LLQ and extends to the S3 vertebra where it becomes the rectum. There is a mesentery associated with it known as the **sigmoid mesocolon** thus making it mobile and intraperitoneal. The *root* of this sigmoid mesocolon extends from the external iliac vessels, back to the bifurcation of the common iliac vessels before reaching the anterior sacrum. An **intersigmoid recess (fossa)** is formed and the left ureter passes through this fossa just deep to the peritoneum. The sigmoid colon is the most common site for *diverticulosis*, a disorder in which multiple external evaginations called diverticula are present and susceptible to infection and rupture.

3.30.1 Vasculature and Lymphatic Drainage of the Sigmoid Colon

The blood supply to the sigmoid colon is from multiple **sigmoid arteries** that branch from the **IMA (Fig. 3.57)**. Venous drainage is by way of the **sigmoid veins**, a tributary of the **inferior mesenteric vein (IMV)**. Lymphatic drainage is first to the **epiploic** and **paracolic lymph nodes**, followed by the **sigmoid (intermediate colic) lymph nodes** before finally reaching the **inferior mesenteric lymph nodes**.

3.31 Rectum

The rectum is the pelvic portion of the GI tract and it is connected to the sigmoid colon and begins at the **rectosigmoid junction** at vertebral level S3 **(Fig. 3.53; Fig. 3.58)**. The upper portion of the rectum is primary retroperitoneal while the lower portion is subperitoneal. The lumen is similar to that of the sigmoid colon initially but it becomes progressively more dilated near its termination known as the **rectal ampulla**. The definition of the rectal ampulla is the region between the *middle transverse rectal fold* and *anorectal junction*. The rectum follows the curve of the sacrum resulting in the **sacral flexure** of the rectum. There are three **lateral flexures** that can be seen externally and are known as the **superior**, **middle**, and **inferior flexures**. They are formed in relationship to the three internal rectal folds. These are known as the **superior**, **middle**, and **inferior transverse rectal folds**. The superior and inferior lateral flexures along with their corresponding

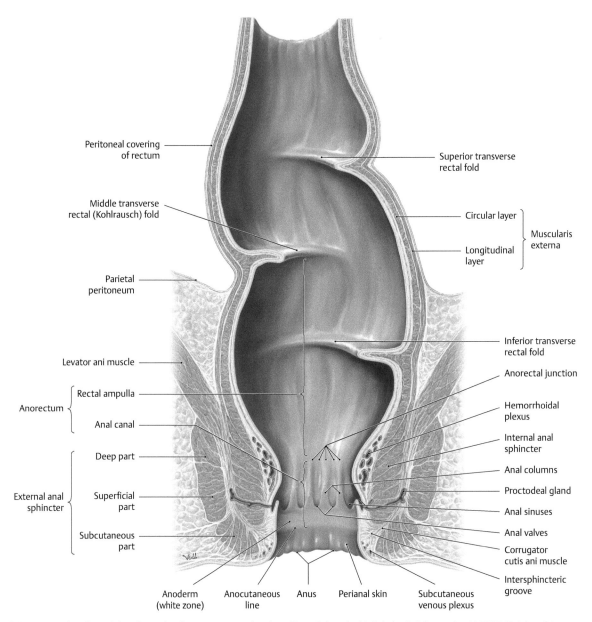

Fig. 3.58 Rectum and anal canal: interior and wall structure, anterior view. (From Schuenke M, Schulte E, Schumacher U. THIEME Atlas of Anatomy. Internal Organs. Illustrations by Voll M and Wesker K. 3rd ed. New York: Thieme Medical Publishers; 2020.)

superior and inferior transverse rectal folds are located on the left side of the rectum while the middle flexure and transverse rectal fold are located on the right side of the rectum.

The rectum terminates anteroinferior to the tip of the coccyx and just before a sharp posteroinferior angle called the **anorectal flexure** occurs or when the rectum passes through the pelvic diaphragm to become the anal canal. The anorectal flexure and its ~80° angle is an important mechanism associated with fecal continence and it is maintained during the resting state by the strength of the puborectalis muscle, and by its active contraction during peristaltic contractions if defecation is not to occur or is to be delayed **(Fig. 3.59)**.

The rectum functions as a temporary storage site for feces. The urge to defecate comes from the continued filling of the rectum that stimulates stretch receptors found along the rectal wall. The length of the rectum shortens as peristalsis propels feces out of the rectum and into the anal canal before exiting the body.

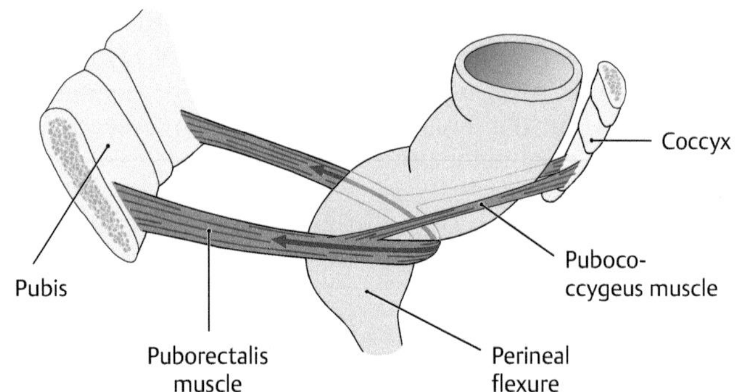

Fig. 3.59 Continence organ: closure by the puborectalis muscle. (From Schuenke M, Schulte E, Schumacher U. THIEME Atlas of Anatomy. Neck and Internal Organs. Illustrations by Voll M and Wesker K. 1st ed. New York: Thieme Medical Publishers; 2010.)

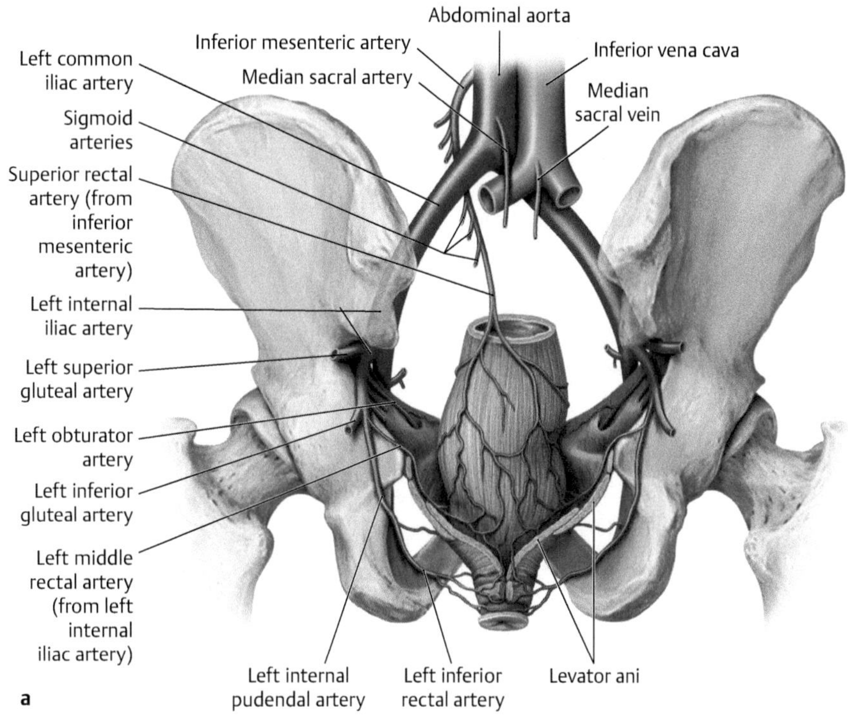

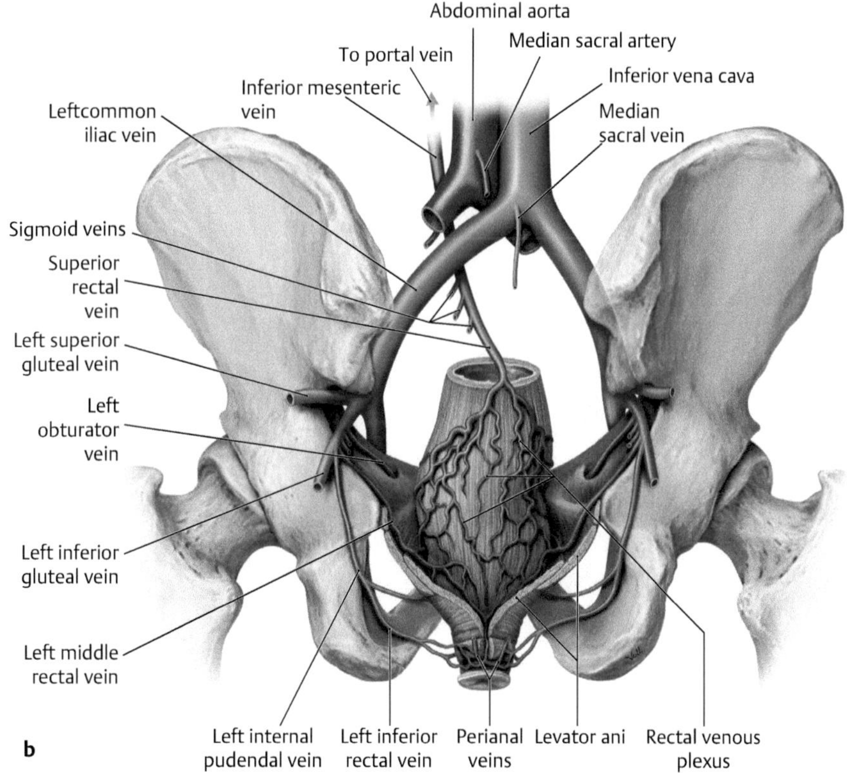

Fig. 3.60 Posterior view. **(a)** Arterial supply of the rectum and anal canal. **(b)** Venous drainage of the rectum and anal canal. (From Schuenke M, Schulte E, Schumacher U. THIEME Atlas of Anatomy. Internal Organs. Illustrations by Voll M and Wesker K. 3rd ed. New York: Thieme Medical Publishers; 2020.)

3.31.1 Vasculature and Lymphatic Drainage of the Rectum

The blood supply to the rectum is from the **superior rectal** (IMA br.), **middle rectal** (anterior division of internal iliac br.) and **inferior rectal arteries** (internal pudendal br.). The inferior rectal arteries generally supply more of the anal canal and only the rectum near the anorectal junction. A potential collateral circulation occurs with the anastomosis of the superior and inferior rectal arteries. However, the middle rectal arteries are only minor contributors to this anastomosis (**Fig. 3.57; Fig. 3.60a**).

Venous drainage parallels the arterial supply and thus there is a *superior, middle* and *inferior rectal vein.* The **superior rectal vein** is a tributary of the **IMV** and is part of the *portal venous circulation.*

The **middle rectal** and **inferior rectal veins** are tributaries of the **internal iliac** and **internal pudendal veins** respectively **(Fig. 3.60b)**. These veins together belong to the *systematic venous circulation*. The anastomosis between the superior rectal (portal) and the middle rectal and inferior rectal veins (systematic) are of clinical importance and are associated with the larger portocaval anastomosis.

Lymphatic drainage of the *superior portion of the rectum* drains to the **pararectal**, **sacral** and then the **inferior mesenteric lymph nodes**. The *inferior portion of the rectum* can drain to the **sacral lymph nodes** before ascending to the **inferior mesenteric lymph nodes** or if it is more near the ampulla, lymph may travel first **internal iliac** followed by the **common iliac** and **lumbar lymph nodes (Fig. 3.57c)**.

3.32 Anal Canal

The terminal portion of the GI tract is the **anal canal** and is separate from the rectum at the **anorectal junction**. It is divided embryologically into an upper two-thirds and a lower one-third anal canal by the **pectinate (dentate) line**. This is also the delineation of columnar versus squamous epithelium. The mucosa of the upper anal canal has **anal columns** (*of Morgagni*) that help define and form the **anal valves** and **anal sinuses**. When fecal matter compresses the anal sinuses, mucus is secreted to assist in the passage of the feces **(Fig. 3.58)**.

The inner circular smooth muscle layer of the muscularis externa that is associated with the superior two-thirds of the anal canal forms the **internal anal sphincter**. This structure is under autonomic control with sympathetic fibers providing a tonic or continuous contraction of the muscle while parasympathetic fibers would be responsible for inhibiting this contraction. This is generally in response to distension detected within the rectal ampulla and the progression of fecal movement by peristalsis.

The circular bands of skeletal muscle wrapped around the inferior two-thirds of the anal canal form the **external anal sphincter** and this is under conscious control. The sphincter is divided into **subcutaneous**, **superficial** and **deep zones** that are often indistinct from one another and not exactly individual muscle bellies. It blends in with the puborectalis muscle superiorly. It is also attached to the *perineal body* anteriorly and to the coccyx by the *anococcygeal ligament* posteriorly.

3.32.1 Vasculature and Lymphatic Drainage of the Anal Canal

The blood supply to the anal canal *above the pectinate line* is from the **superior rectal artery** (IMA br.). *Below the pectinate line*, the **inferior rectal arteries** (internal pudendal br.) supply the anal canal in addition to the surrounding skin and musculature **(Fig. 3.60)**.

There is a **submucosal rectal venous plexus** that consists of two parts: an **external rectal venous plexus** just external to the muscular wall of the rectum; and an **internal rectal venous plexus** located just deep to the mucosa at the anorectal junction. These plexuses are named rectal but are associated more with venous drainage of the anal canal and not so much with the rectum. These venous plexuses are associated with hemorrhoids.

Lymphatic drainage above the pectinate line is to the **internal iliac lymph nodes** while below the pectinate line lymph travels to the **superficial inguinal lymph nodes**.

3.33 Histology of the Large Intestine

The mucosa of the large intestine consists of a *simple columnar epithelium* and as a whole is fairly smooth and does not contain plicae circulares or villi. Similar to the small intestine, **intestinal glands** (*crypts of Lieberkuhn*) extend down to the muscularis mucosa. Isolated lymphatic nodules can be found in the lamina propria and the number of goblet cells in the rectum increases. The appendix displays a nearly identical surface epithelium and intestinal glands set up as the rest of the colon however there are no villi or teniae coli. The epithelium is mostly goblet cells and the lamina propria contains numerous lymphoid nodules **(Fig. 3.61)**.

The *simple columnar epithelium* of the upper anal canal abruptly changes to a *stratified squamous epithelium* at the *pectinate (dentate) line*, and this serves as the delineation between

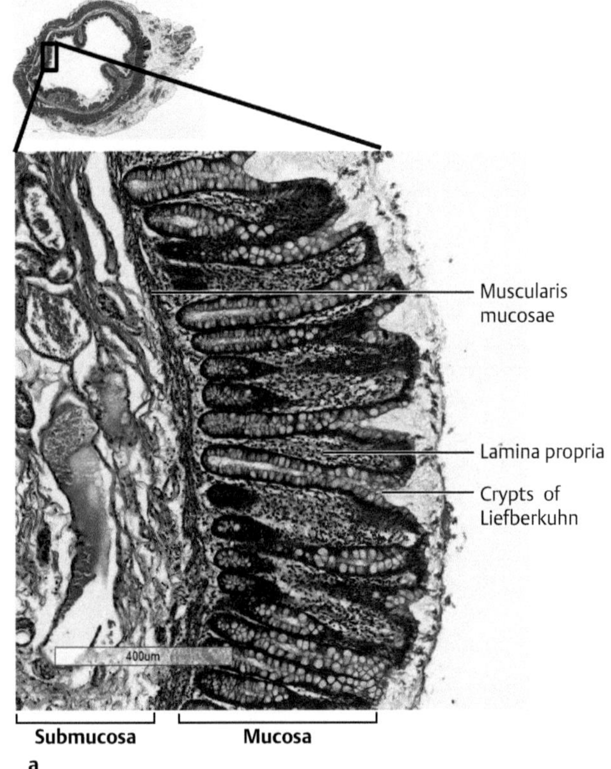

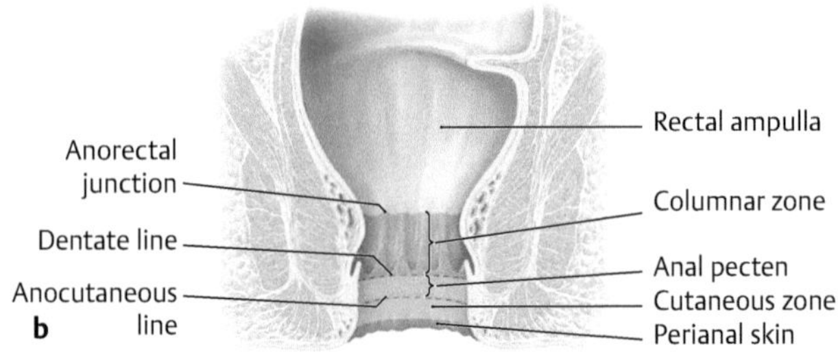

Fig. 3.61 **(a)** Histology of the large intestine showing mucosa and submucosa. **(b)** Epithelial regions of the anal canal. (**a** from Lowrie DJ. Histology: An Essential Textbook. New York: Thieme Medical Publishers; 2020. **b** from Schuenke M, Schulte E, Schumacher U. THIEME Atlas of Anatomy. Neck and Internal Organs. Illustrations by Voll M and Wesker K. 1st ed. New York: Thieme Medical Publishers; 2010.)

the upper and lower anal canals. The lower anal canal, which does not derive itself from the embryonic hindgut but the proctodeum, can be divided in half by *Hilton's white line* (*anocutaneous line*). Above this line the lower anal canal has a *stratified squamous non-keratinized* epithelium and it is considered to be located within the **anal pecten** (white zone). Below this line it becomes a *stratified squamous keratinized epithelium* that blends with the skin of the anus.

3.34 Portal-Systematic Anastomoses

The communication between the veins of notable structures involving the portal venous system and the systematic venous system is commonly referred to as the **portal-systematic anastomoses (Fig. 3.62)**. Portal drainage is related to the hepatic portal vein while systematic drainage is related to the IVC. An anastomosis can be located in the submucosa of the inferior esophagus or anal canal, the posterior aspects (or bare areas) of secondarily retroperitoneal viscera and the liver, and finally the peri-umbilical region. The anastomosis provides a collateral circulation if an obstruction is present in the liver or hepatic portal vein. These collateral routes are allowed to function because there are no valves in the hepatic portal vein or its tributaries thus blood from the GI tract is capable of traveling back towards the IVC. There are four major areas where these anastomoses can be located and the most common clinically relevant areas tend to involve the esophagus and anal canal/rectal regions:

1. At the junction of the **left gastric** (portal) and **esophageal veins** (caval). The important clinical issue at this location involves the formation of *esophageal varices* that form because of portal hypertension commonly due to liver cirrhosis.
2. At the junction of the **superior rectal** (portal) and the **middle rectal** and **inferior rectal veins** (caval). Varices involving the anorectal region are again generally due to portal hypertension and as high as 80% of individuals with portal hypertension have some form of anorectal varix. When the mucosa containing these submucosal veins collapses this is known as *hemorrhoids*.
3. At the junction of the **para-umbilical veins** (portal) near the umbilicus and the **superior and inferior epigastric veins** (caval) of the anterior abdominal wall. Engorgement of these veins near the umbilicus is known as *caput medusae*. The initially closed and obliterated umbilical vein may re-canalize

Clinical Correlate 3.32

Constipation
Infrequent or difficult bowel movements are a symptom called **constipation**. This is quite common in the general population and can present randomly depending on certain factors. There are many causes of constipation with the minor effect based on diet, hypothyroidism or medication side effects that can be easily managed through the use of laxatives, enemas or simply changing one's diet to include more dietary fiber. If severe constipation has become an issue, this could be due to a more serious condition such as colon cancer. Complications that can arise due to constipation include hemorrhoids, rectal prolapse or anal fissures, so it is advised not to strain when passing a bowel movement.

Clinical Correlate 3.33

Inflammatory Bowel Disease
A group of inflammatory conditions generally involving the small and large intestine is known as **inflammatory bowel disease (IBD)**. Symptoms for both major forms of IBD include diarrhea, abdominal discomfort due to muscle cramps, vomiting, rectal bleeding and anemia. Causes are related to environmental and genetic factors but alterations in the normally present beneficial bacteria contribute to IBD. There is an increased risk for colorectal cancer if an individual has IBD. The most common types of IBD are *Crohn's disease* and *ulcerative colitis*. Crohn's targets both the small and large intestine but can also affect the esophagus, stomach or anus. Ulcerative colitis is associated mainly with just the colon and rectum. Rarely fatal, but the quality of life can be largely affected as the individual has to deal with consistent loose fecal movements and abdominal pain. Surgery can eliminate ulcerative colitis if most of the large intestine is removed but *Crohn's disease* involves too many other organs.

Clinical Correlate 3.34

Colorectal Cancer
The development of cancer in the colon or rectum or both is known as the broad **colorectal cancer**. Symptoms can include chronic constipation, bloody stools and weight loss. Risk factors can include smoking, obesity, alcoholism, eating red and processed meat or having IBS. Treatment can involve a combination of surgery, chemotherapy and/or radiation. Diagnosis is generally made after a colonoscopy.

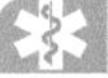

Clinical Correlate 3.35

Diverticulosis
A disorder where numerous diverticula (out-pocketings of mucosa) develop primarily in the sigmoid colon is called **diverticulosis**. They are mostly found on the mesenteric side of the two non-mesenteric teniae coli where nutrient arteries are found penetrating the muscular coat in order to reach the submucosa. When these diverticula become infected this is known as **diverticulitis** and these diverticula still have a chance to rupture spilling fecal matter into the peritoneal cavity.

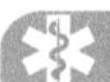

Clinical Correlate 3.36

Colonoscopy
In order to observe and take pictures of a potential problem with the colon, a procedure called a **colonoscopy** is performed. This procedure makes use of a long but flexible fiberoptic endoscope that is first sent through the anal canal before reaching its target location. There are smaller instruments that can be passed through a colonoscope to facilitate minor procedures and operations including biopsies and polyp removal.

Clinical Correlate 3.37

Volvulus of the Sigmoid Colon

The sigmoid colon is movable and has some range of movement because of the sigmoid mesocolon attached to it. Large bowel obstructions that present after initial complaints of constant constipation involve the sigmoid colon nearly 80% of the time. They have a high rate of returning and a surgical resection of the sigmoid colon may be needed. A volvulus involving a portion of the large bowel is much more common than one involving the small bowel.

Clinical Correlate 3.38

Importance of Rectal Exams

Although embarrassing and an inconvenience for most patients, rectal exams are able to provide much valuable information to the treating physician. The anterior borders of the rectum lie against the prostate and seminal vesicles in males and the vagina and cervix region of the uterus in females. More laterally, the ischial spine and tuberosity, any enlargement of the ureters as in an *ureterocele*, or swollen internal iliac lymph nodes can be palpated with this exam.

Clinical Correlate 3.39

Hemorrhoids

Hemorrhoids are normal and tortuous vascular structures located at the level of the anal canal and these vessels are in relationship to the rectal venous plexuses. There is no real cause but numerous factors can lead to their formation. These include constipation, low fiber diets, sedentary lifestyle, straining during bowel movements and even pregnancy. Simple treatments include eating more dietary fiber or using topical agents but in situations where they keep developing, rubber band ligation and cauterization procedures may be employed. Hemorrhoids are classified as being either *internal* or *external*.

- **Internal hemorrhoids** are prolapses resulting from the breakdown of the muscularis mucosae of the rectal mucosa containing the *internal rectal venous plexus*. As they continue to prolapse inferiorly after enlargement, internal hemorrhoids will end up resting near the level of the sphincters and are subject to their blood flow being impeded and becoming ulcerated. Any bleeding from this type of hemorrhoid is bright red and tends to cover the stool. Visceral afferents supply the area above the pectinate line so there is no pain associated with internal hemorrhoids.
- **External hemorrhoids** are thromboses of the veins involving the external rectal venous plexus and are located near the skin and become irritated and itchy near the anus.

Clinical Correlate 3.40

Esophageal Atresia

Esophageal atresia is the result of the tracheoesophageal septum deviating too far dorsally, resulting in the esophagus ending as a blind tube. The most common esophageal atresia is one presenting with a **trachoeoesophageal fistula** or TEF (~1 in 4,000 live births). The esophageal atresia presents with its typical upper esophagus blind sac appearance but the TEF represents the lower portion of the esophagus inserting near the bifurcation of the trachea. Esophageal atresia is generally present with other congenital defects and this is part of the **VACTERL** association. These children can have a combination of either a **v**ertebral, **a**nal, **c**ardiac, **t**racheoesophageal fistula, **e**sophageal atresia, **r**enal or **l**imb defects.

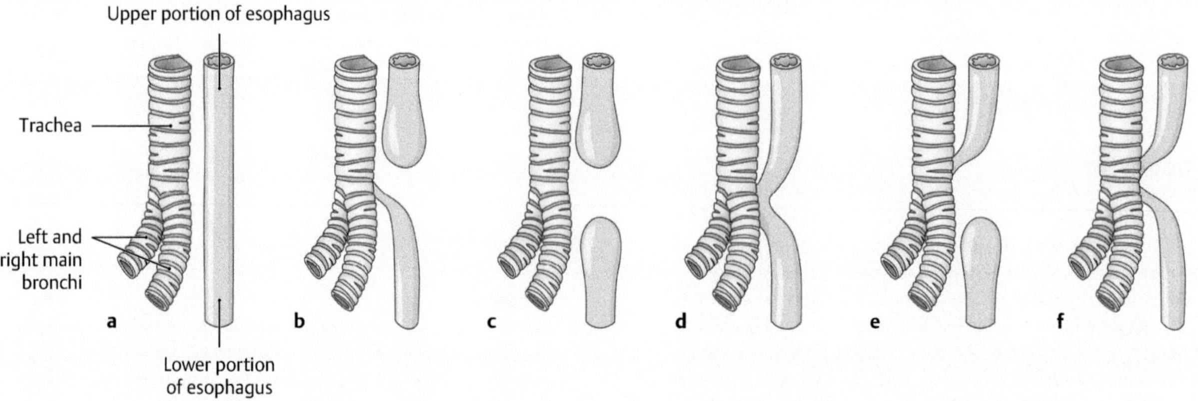

(a) Normal anatomy. **(b-f)** Abnormalities with **(b)** being the most common type of esophageal atresia (~90%) and it presents with a tracheoesophageal fistula (TEF). (From Schuenke M, Schulte E, Schumacher U. THIEME Atlas of Anatomy. Internal Organs. Illustrations by Voll M and Wesker K. 2nd ed. New York: Thieme Medical Publishers; 2016.)

Clinical Correlate 3.41

Volvulus of the Superior Mesenteric Artery

A midgut volvulus involves the superior mesenteric vessels of a malrotated small bowel and this can occur at any age but almost 90% of them happen within the first year of life. They are rare but the neonate or infant is acting normal before a sudden presentation of bilious vomiting and perceived pain occur. This represents a medical emergency and if the volvulus does not spontaneously reduce or is released surgically in a timely matter, then the obstruction of the superior mesenteric vessels will result in the gradual onset of ischemia and eventual necrosis could occur. The abdomen becomes swollen as fluid accumulates in the lumen of the bowel becoming tender and the child could go into shock. The superior mesenteric vessels supply much of the GI tract associated with absorption of nutrients thus any substantial ischemic death to this tissue would result in the inability of the body to absorb meaningful nutrition and may not be able to sustain life.

and become patent again and form a connection with para-umbilical veins.

4. At the junction of smaller **colic veins** (portal) connected to the SMV and **retroperitoneal veins** (caval) connecting to the lumbar or ascending lumbar veins.

Clinical Correlate 3.42

Ileal Diverticulum

A congenital anomaly of the proximal portion of the **omphaloenteric (vitelline) duct** on the non-mesenteric border of ileum located about 50 cm (~2 ft) from the ileocecal junction and occurring in 1-2% of the population is known as an **ileal** (*Meckel*) **diverticulum**. When it becomes inflamed, it may mimic the pain similar to appendicitis. It has been shown to contain not only ileal tissue but also gastric, jejunal or colonic tissues.

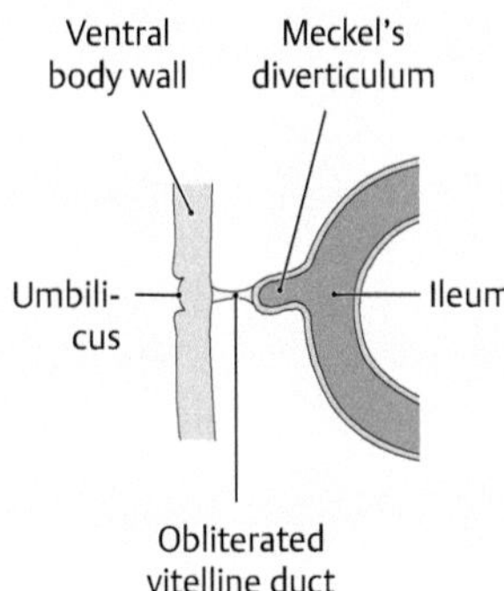

(From Schuenke M, Schulte E, Schumacher U. THIEME Atlas of Anatomy. Internal Organs. Illustrations by Voll M and Wesker K. 2nd ed. New York: Thieme Medical Publishers; 2016.)

3.35 Development of the GI Tract

The **primitive gut tube** begins to develop at the beginning of the fourth week and is formed initially after the fusion of the dorsal part of the yolk sac into the embryo during the processes of head and tail (craniocaudal) and lateral folding. This primitive gut tube will extend from the **buccopharyngeal (oropharyngeal) membrane** to the **cloacal membrane** and is divided into the foregut, midgut and hindgut. The mucosa's epithelial lining and the associated glands all derive from **endoderm**. All other layers from the lamina propria of the mucosa to the adventitia/serosa develop from **visceral mesoderm**. The lumen is initially closed because of the rapid proliferation of the epithelium but it later recanalizes, forming a continuous tube.

3.35.1 Foregut Development

During the fourth week, the cranial portion of the gut tube develops **tracheoesophageal folds** internally and as this happens, a ventral diverticulum extends from the initial tube. After these folds fuse, a **tracheoesophageal septum** will form. The dorsal portion is the early **esophagus**, short at first but which lengthens later while the ventral diverticulum represents the **respiratory bud**, which is a combination of both the early *trachea* and *lungs*.

A dilation of the gut tube distal to the esophagus represents the early **stomach**. The dorsal portion of the dilation grows quicker than the ventral part and this is what gives the stomach the greater versus lesser curvature orientation. The early stomach rotates 90° *clockwise* on its longitudinal access which affects the whole developing foregut. This rotation is the reason the left and right vagus nerves become the anterior and posterior vagal trunks respectively. This also forces the dorsal mesentery to rotate to the left to eventually form the *greater omentum* (**Fig. 3.63**).

The early **duodenum** elongates and forms a C-shaped loop that initially extends ventrally but with early stomach rotation the duodenum along with the pancreas are forced against the posterior abdominal wall. The 1st part remains free and intraperitoneal while the 2nd-4th parts along with the pancreas become retroperitoneal. The first two parts are considered foregut and the last two parts are midgut (**Fig. 3.64**).

An outgrowth of endoderm from the foregut called the **hepatic diverticulum (liver bud)** extends into the surrounding mesoderm of the **septum transversum**. This interaction is induced by the release of fibroblast growth factors (FGF's) released by the cardiac mesoderm. The **hepatic cords (hepatoblasts)** that originate from the hepatic diverticulum grow into the septum transversum and form a crucial interaction with the mesoderm. **Hepatic sinusoids** are created after the hepatic cords arrange themselves around the *umbilical* and *vitelline veins* while in the septum transversum. Rapid growth of the liver stretches the septum transversum and forms the **ventral mesentery**, the precursor to multiple peritoneal ligaments. The endothelium of the sinusoids, *Kupffer cells*, connective tissue and hematopoietic cells are derived from mesoderm whereas everything else originates from endoderm including the lining of the biliary system. The narrowing of the connection between the hepatic diverticulum and the foregut forms the **bile duct**. The outgrowth of endoderm from the early bile duct forms the **cystic duct** and **gallbladder bud**. With further development, the lumen of the cystic duct and gallbladder canalizes creating an open space for each structure (**Fig. 3.64**).

The larger **dorsal pancreatic bud** is a direct outgrowth of endoderm near the location of the liver bud. The much smaller **ventral pancreatic bud** is an endodermal outgrowth near the distal bile duct near its insertion into the duodenum. The ventral pancreatic bud rotates dorsally and fuses with the dorsal pancreatic bud after the 90° clockwise rotation of the duodenum and this leads to the definitive (adult) pancreas appearance. Abnormal rotation of the ventral bud may result in an **anular pancreas** and this may cause an obstruction of the duodenum (duodenal stenosis). The dorsal

Clinical Correlate 3.43

Gastroschisis and Omphalocele

Gastroschisis is defined by when the bowel loops herniate through the abdominal wall but without a sac. They occur in about 1/2,000 births and could be associated with an umbilical vein rupture and are considered a surgical emergency. An **omphalocele** is a persistent herniation of bowel loops through an enlarged umbilical ring. These are generally small bowel loops that are enclosed in the amniotic sac around the base of the umbilical cord. They occur in about 1/5,000 births and have approximately a 25% mortality rate. These are also fixed with surgery.

Gastroschisis

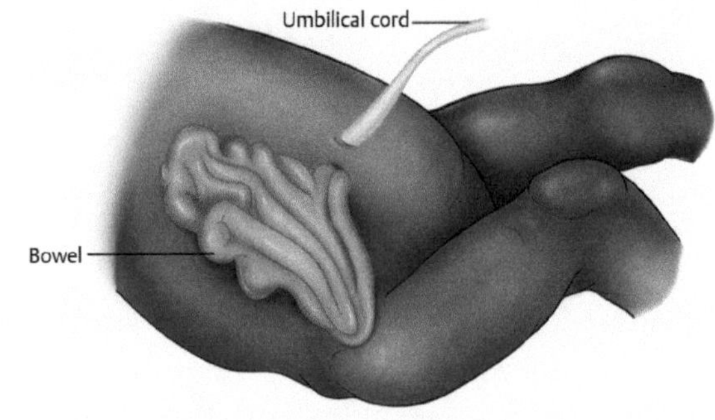

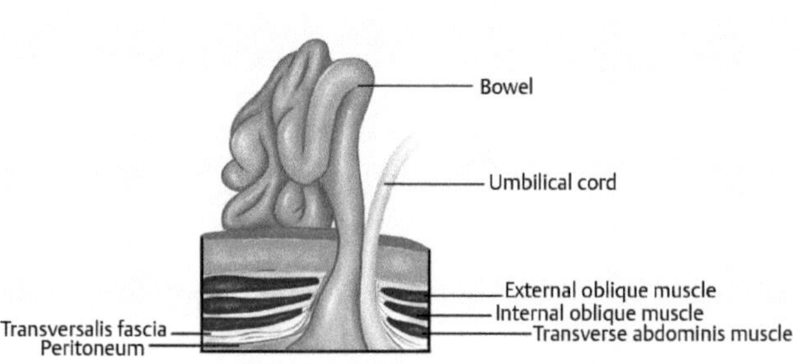

Omphalocele

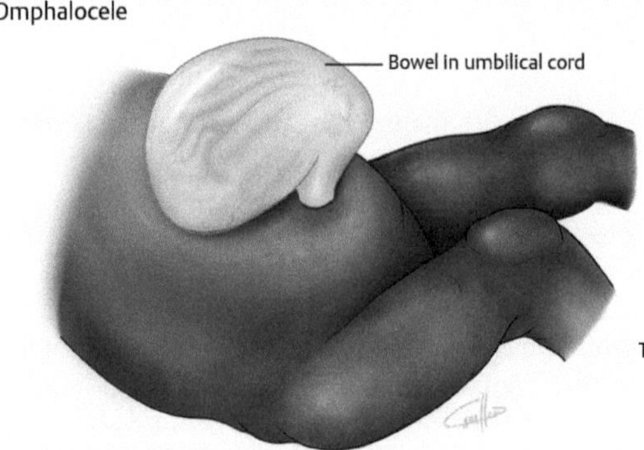

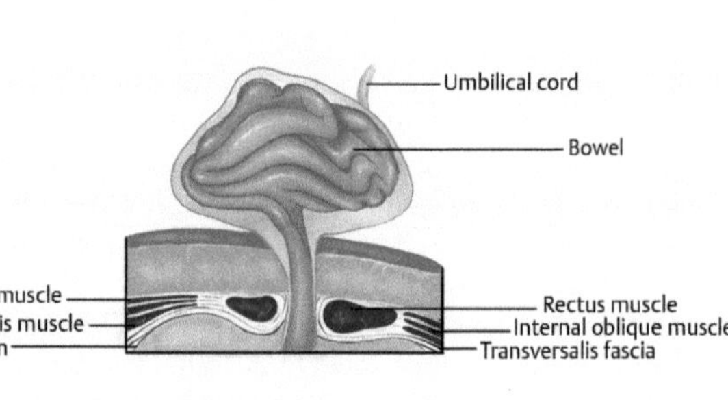

Illustration by Calla Heald.

Clinical Correlate 3.44

Hirschsprung's Disease or Congenital Megacolon

A disorder affecting the large intestine and the nerve plexuses associated with the enteric nervous system primarily in the hindgut portion is called *Hirschsprung's disease*. It occurs in approximately 1/5000 live births and affects males more than females. The failure to pass a bowel movement within the first couple of days after birth, or the presence of a large bowel, are signs a newborn may have this condition. The cause can be traced back to the lack of neural crest cells migrating to that portion of the gut and not forming the *Meissner's* and *Auerbach's nervous plexuses* of the enteric nervous system. Treatment consists of the surgical removal of the abnormal section of the colon and a later reattachment. A reversible colostomy is done and after the child has aged a few years the bowel is then attached to the lower rectum or upper anus.

pancreatic bud forms most of the *head*, *neck*, *body* and *tail* while the ventral pancreatic bud forms a small portion of the *head* and the *uncinate process*. The endodermal tubules of both buds branch multiple times to form **acinar cells** and ducts. Isolated clumps of endoderm that bud off of the tubules and accumulate within the surrounding mesoderm form the **pancreatic islets**. The order that the islets cells develop in is *alpha*, *beta*, *delta* and finally the *F cells*. The **main pancreatic duct** is formed when the distal two-thirds of the dorsal pancreatic duct and the entire ventral pancreatic duct fuse. If the **accessory pancreatic duct** is present, it was formed when the proximal one-third of the main pancreatic duct failed to regress like it normally does.

The **spleen** begins to develop during the fifth week and is derived from a mass of *mesoderm* located between the layers of the **dorsal mesentery**. It is attached to the dorsal wall by the *splenorenal ligament* and to the stomach by the *gastrosplenic ligament*. Although the vasculature of the spleen is associated with the foregut, the spleen is not considered a part of the foregut because it

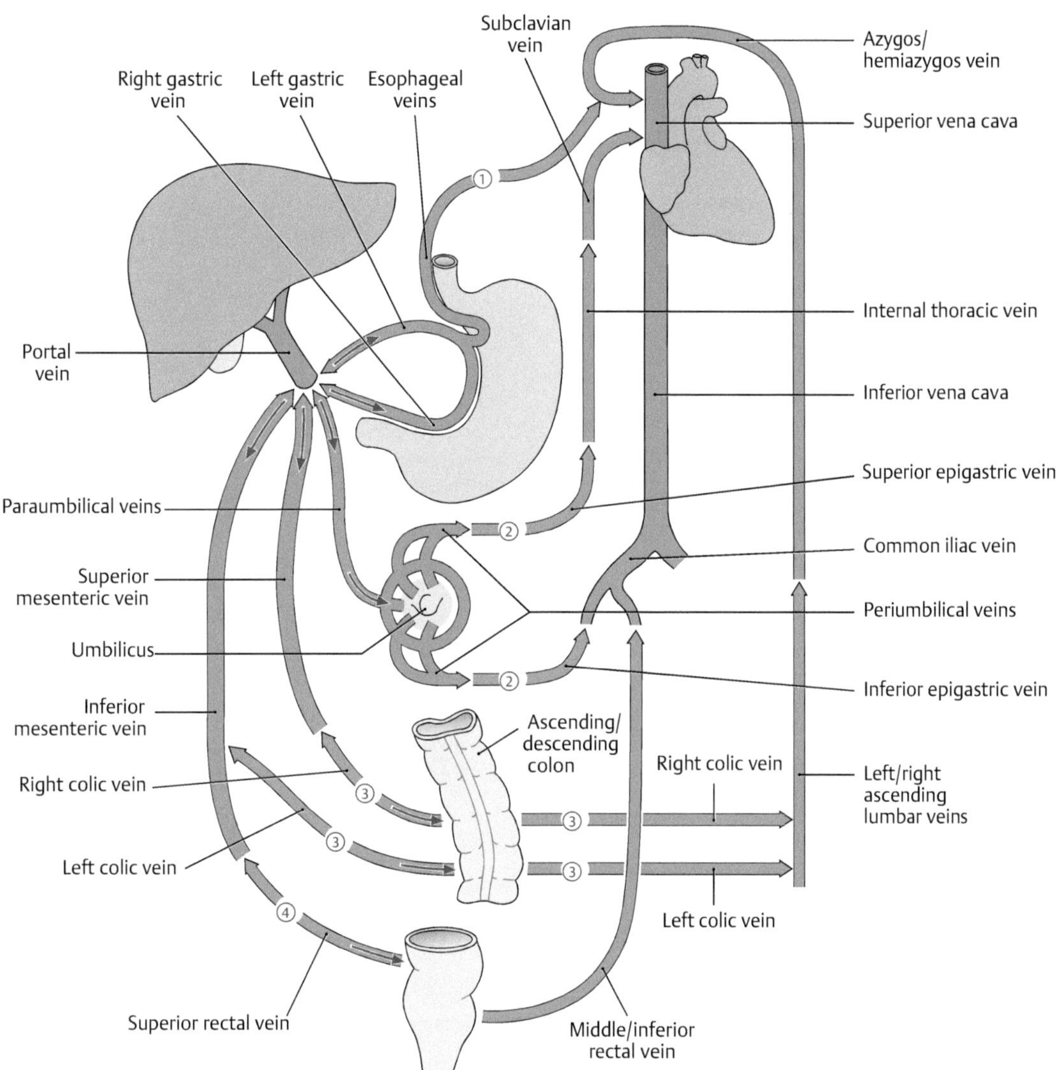

Fig. 3.62 Portal-systematic anastomoses. (From Schuenke M, Schulte E, Schumacher U. THIEME Atlas of Anatomy. Internal Organs. Illustrations by Voll M and Wesker K. 3rd ed. New York: Thieme Medical Publishers; 2020.)

develops from mesoderm and not endoderm like the rest of the gut viscera (**Fig. 3.63**).

3.35.2 Midgut Development

The midgut includes the GI tract from the 3rd part of the duodenum all the way to the border between the proximal two-thirds and distal one-third of the transverse colon. As the midgut rapidly elongates it initially forms a U-shaped loop, also known as the **midgut loop**, which herniates into the umbilical cord and extraembryonic coelom. This naturally occurring herniation is known as the *physiological umbilical herniation* and is seen during the sixth week of development. The basis of this occurring is due to the fact the abdomen is occupied already by the massive liver and kidneys and with the midgut outpacing their growth an additional space is needed to accommodate this rapid growth. The midgut loop consists of a proximal limb and distal limb.

The **proximal (cranial) limb** gives rise to the distal parts of the duodenum, jejunum and upper portion of the ileum and the **distal (caudal) limb** forms the lower portion of the ileum, cecum, appendix, ascending colon and the proximal two-thirds of the transverse colon. While in the umbilical cord, the midgut loop will rotate 90° counterclockwise around the axis of the SMA and this brings the proximal limb of the loop to the right and the distal limb to the left. During the tenth week the small intestines (of proximal limb) return first to occupy the central portion of the abdomen (reduction of physiological hernia) and as the large intestine (of distal limb) returns, the midgut undergoes an additional 180° counterclockwise rotation. This places the cecum and appendix near the right lobe of the liver and they descend into the right iliac fossa at a later date. Hence the midgut rotates a total of 270° counterclockwise and the GI tract is back in the abdomen by the eleventh week (**Fig. 3.65**).

3.35.3 Hindgut Development

The hindgut follows the midgut back into the abdomen and does not rotate. It gives rise to the distal one-third of the transverse

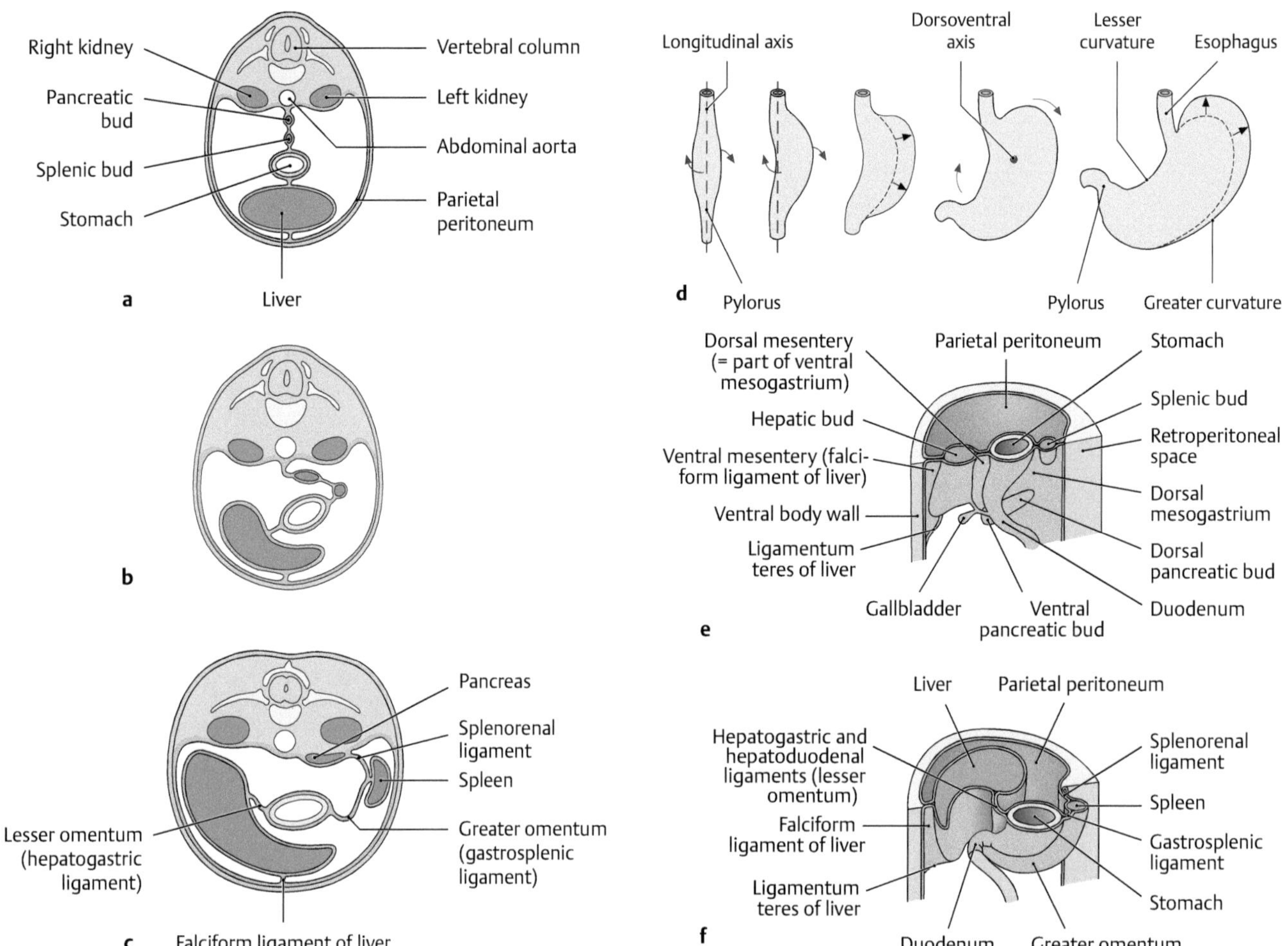

Fig. 3.63 **(a-c)** Rotation of organs in the upper abdomen; transverse sections and viewed from above. **(d)** Stomach rotation viewed from the anterior side. **(e-f)** Formation of the omentums from the mesogastriums; transverse section, left superior view. (From Schuenke M, Schulte E, Schumacher U. THIEME Atlas of Anatomy. Neck and Internal Organs. Illustrations by Voll M and Wesker K. 1st ed. New York: Thieme Medical Publishers; 2010.)

colon, descending colon and sigmoid colon and finally terminates as a pouch called the **cloaca** **(Fig. 3.66)**. The cloaca is lined with endoderm and lies in contact with the surface ectoderm of the **proctodeum** to form the **cloacal membrane**. The **urorectal septum** subdivides the cloaca into a dorsally placed **rectum** and the *upper two-thirds* of the **anal canal** and a ventrally placed **urogenital sinus**. After the urorectal septum fuses with the cloacal membrane, it divides it into a ventral *urogenital membrane* and dorsal **anal membrane**. The invagination of surface ectoderm caused by the proliferation of mesoderm around the anal membrane is the proctodeum and the *lower one-third* of the **anal canal** develops from it. The anal membrane ruptures at the end of the eighth week of development and is represented in the adult as the **pectinate line**, located at the inferior border of the anal columns. The pectinate line serves as the border between the upper and lower anal canals.

3.35.4 The Mesenteries

After the embryo has folded, the caudal portions of the foregut, midgut and hindgut are suspended from the dorsal abdominal wall by the **dorsal mesentery**. It gives rise to the *mesentery (proper)*, *transverse mesocolon*, *sigmoid mesocolon* and *mesoappendix*. As the stomach rotates clockwise, a specific portion of the dorsal mesentery called the **dorsal mesogastrium** rotates and drapes itself over the transverse colon to become the *greater omentum*. The space formed posterior to the stomach becomes the *lesser sac (omental bursa)* **(Fig. 3.67)**.

The **ventral mesogastrium** originates from the septum transversum and it attaches the anterior abdominal wall to the liver as well as the stomach and duodenum to the liver. It gives rise to the *falciform ligament, lesser omentum, coronary* and *triangular ligaments of the liver* **(Fig. 3.67)**.

3.36 Posterior Abdominal Wall

The posterior abdominal wall is a combination of multiple structures consisting of muscles, neurovasculature and fascia. This section also includes viscera such as the suprarenal glands, kidneys and ureters.

The five lumbar vertebrae extend out anteriorly in such a way that two laterally placed deep depressions are created. The

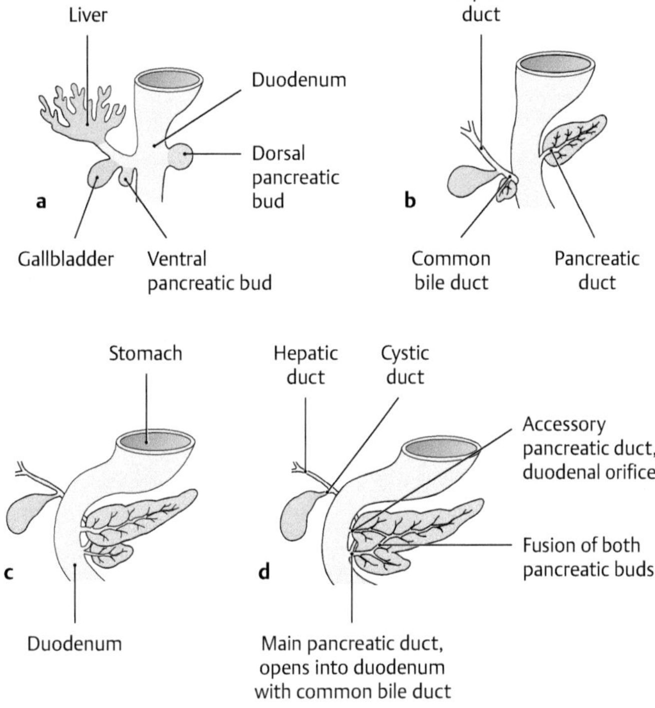

Fig. 3.64 Development of the pancreas: dorsal and ventral pancreatic buds. (From Schuenke M, Schulte E, Schumacher U. THIEME Atlas of Anatomy. Neck and Internal Organs. Illustrations by Voll M and Wesker K. 1st ed. New York: Thieme Medical Publishers; 2010.)

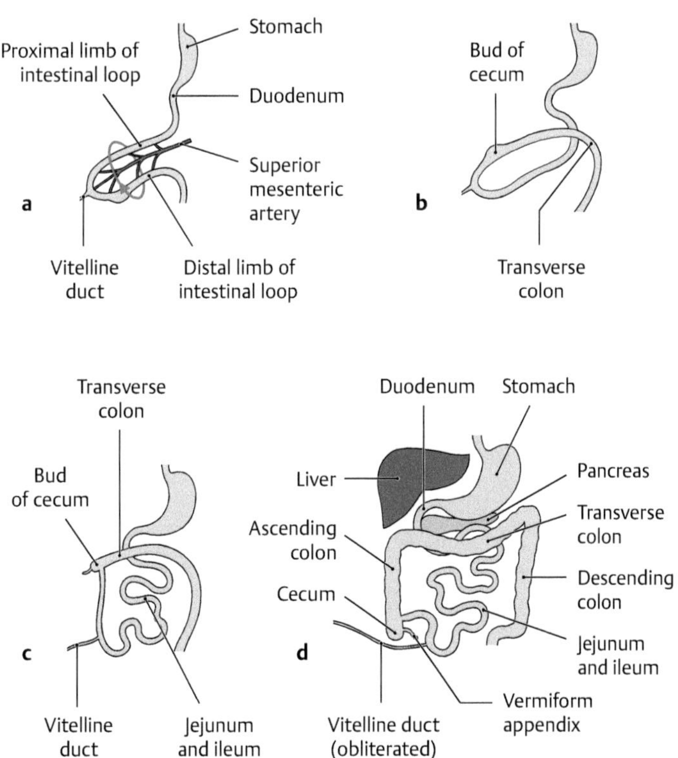

Fig. 3.65 Development of the embryonic intestine and its rotation around the intestinal loop. **(a)** Proximal and distal limbs of the intestinal loop rotate 90 degrees counterclockwise. **(b-c)** Rotated loops shift the the right upper quadrant and rotate an additional 180 degrees counterclockwise. **(d)** The region of the ileocecal junction and ascending colon descends into the right lower quadrant. (From Schuenke M, Schulte E, Schumacher U. THIEME Atlas of Anatomy. Neck and Internal Organs. Illustrations by Voll M and Wesker K. 1st ed. New York: Thieme Medical Publishers; 2010.)

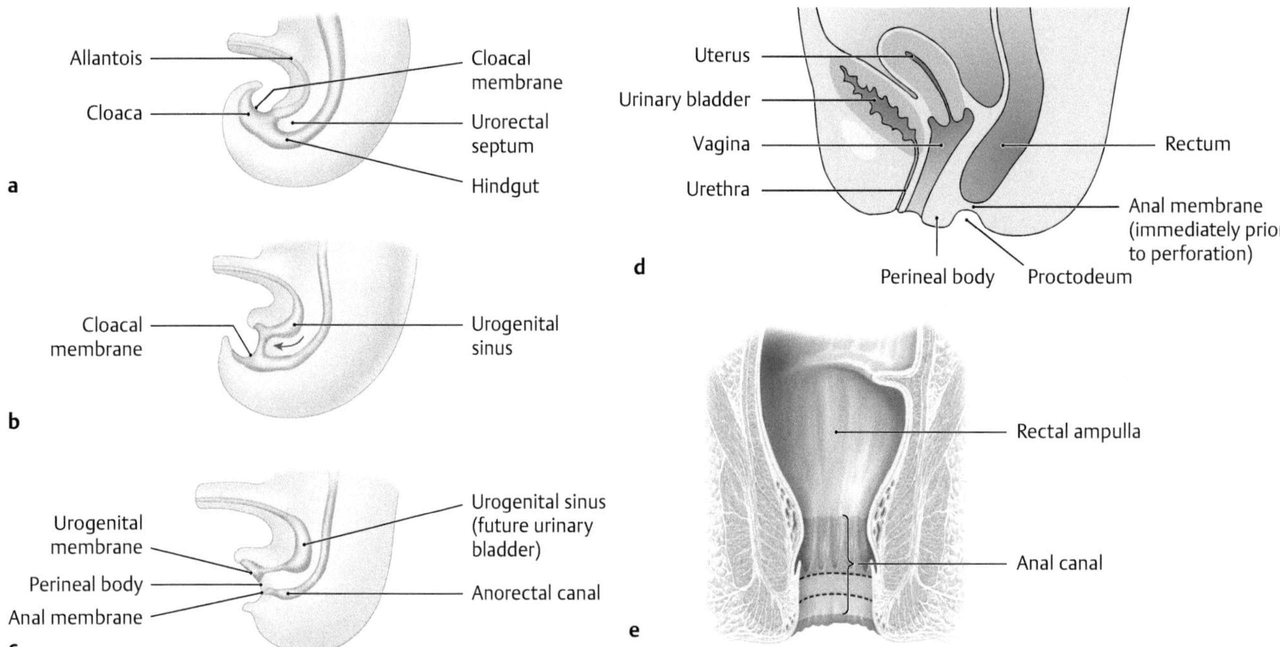

Fig. 3.66 Hindgut development: the division of the cloaca into the rectum and urogenital septum. **(a)** 4 weeks. **(b)** 5 weeks. **(c)** 7 weeks. **(d)** Mesenchymal swellings form at the margins of the anal membrane and as a result, the anal membrane lies in a depression called the proctodeum (or anal pit). **(e)** By the 9th week, the anal membrane has ruptures and the rectum is an open communication with the body's exterior. (From Schuenke M, Schulte E, Schumacher U. THIEME Atlas of Anatomy. Internal Organs. Illustrations by Voll M and Wesker K. 3rd ed. New York: Thieme Medical Publishers; 2020.)

kidneys and the fascia that surrounds them mostly occupy these depressions. The abdominal aorta and IVC are located on the anterior surfaces of these same vertebrae with the aortic autonomic plexus being intimately associated with the aorta.

3.37 Diaphragm

The **diaphragm** is a double-domed musculotendinous structure that separates the superiorly located thoracic cavity from the inferiorly located abdomen. This is the primary muscle of inspiration but only its central portion and domes actually move due to the peripheral muscle fibers being fixed to the thoracic cage and upper lumbar vertebrae. The **central tendon** has no bony attachments but there is a **caval opening** located at about vertebral level T8 and this is where the inferior vena cava passes before reaching the right atrium of the heart. The distal *right phrenic nerve* and a few lymphatics from the liver also pass through this opening. The superior portion of the central tendon fuses with the inferior portion of the *fibrous pericardium*.

The right done is situated slightly higher than the left dome and with expiration of air can reach the height of approximately the 4th intercostal space or 5th rib. The level of either the left or right domes is dependent on if the individual is supine or standing; inspiring or expiring air; and the degree of distension involving the abdominal viscera. The peripherally located skeletal muscle fibers of the diaphragm radiate toward the centrally located aponeurotic portion of the central tendon. The muscular portion is divided into three parts the *costal, lumbar*, and *sternal parts* (**Fig. 3.68**).

- **Costal**: wide slips of muscle that attach to the internal surfaces of the last six costal cartilages and their adjoining ribs bilaterally. This part of the diaphragm establishes the *left* and *right domes*.
- **Lumbar**: forms the *left* and *right diaphragmatic crura* that ascend to the central tendon. It originates from the medial and lateral arcuate ligaments as well as the superior three lumbar vertebrae.
- **Sternal**: if present, the sternal part is made of just two slips of muscle that attach to the posterior aspect of the xiphoid process. The **sternocostal foramen** is the small opening located between the sternal and costal attachments of the diaphragm. The *superior epigastric vessels* and *lymphatics from the diaphragmatic surface of the liver* pass through this foramen.

The musculotendinous extensions that arise from the anterior surfaces of the L1, L2, and L3 vertebrae, anterior longitudinal ligament and the intervertebral disks are known as the **left** and **right diaphragmatic crura**. The **right crus** is much larger and ascends mostly from the upper three lumbar vertebrae to form the **esophageal hiatus** at vertebral level T10 while the **left crus** ascends from the upper two lumbar vertebrae. The **median arcuate ligament** unites the left and right crura and these structures together form the **aortic hiatus** located at vertebral level T12 (**Fig. 3.69**). The lumbar portion of the diaphragm is attached to the psoas major muscles by the **medial arcuate ligaments** and to the quadratus lumborum muscles by the **lateral arcuate ligaments**. The median, medial and lateral arcuate ligaments are more of a condensation of the deep fascia associated with the diaphragm and the adjacent skeletal muscle (**Fig. 3.68**).

Contraction of the diaphragm results in the central portion and domes being pulled inferiorly creating a somewhat flattened diaphragm. There is an increase in thoracic cavity volume and a decrease in intrathoracic pressure and this allows an individual to freely breathe in air. At the same time, the abdominal cavity volume decreases and the intra-abdominal pressure increases. A decrease in intrathoracic pressure and an increase in intra-abdominal pressure help return venous blood through the IVC back to the heart.

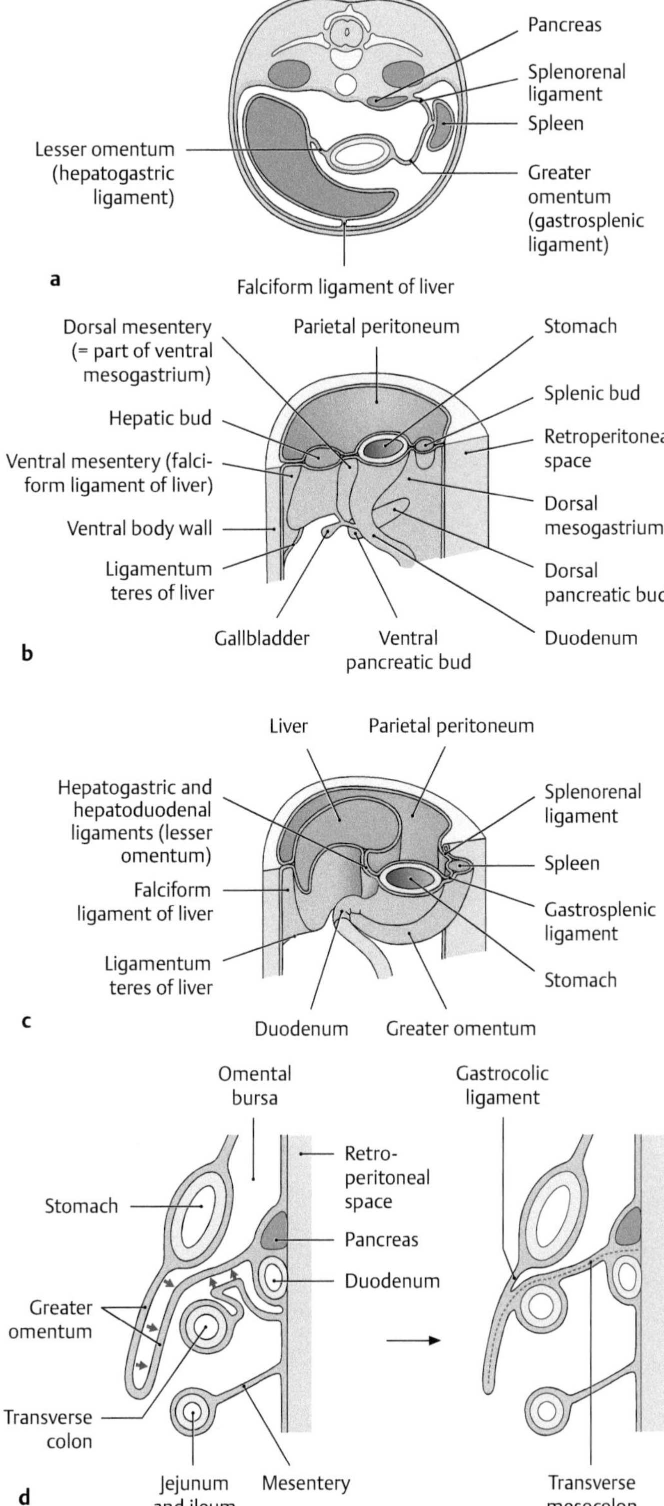

Fig. 3.67 **(a)** Transverse section of developing abdomen and viewed form above. This view would be seen after rotation demonstrated by the c image. Formation of the dorsal and ventral mesogastrium and migration of organs in the upper abdomen at: **(b)** 5th week and **(c)** 11th week. **(d)** Fusion of the greater omentum. (From Schuenke M, Schulte E, Schumacher U. THIEME Atlas of Anatomy. Internal Organs. Illustrations by Voll M and Wesker K. 3rd ed. New York: Thieme Medical Publishers; 2020.)

When an individual is in the *Trendelenburg position* (upper body is lowered while on a table 15-30 degrees), the diaphragm extends more superiorly into the thoracic cavity because of the abdominal contents putting pressure on it and the diaphragm is at its lowest point while standing. Individuals that have difficulty breathing (dyspnea) prefer to sit up versus lying down because non-tidal (reserve) lung volume is increased and the diaphragm is then working with gravity rather than against it.

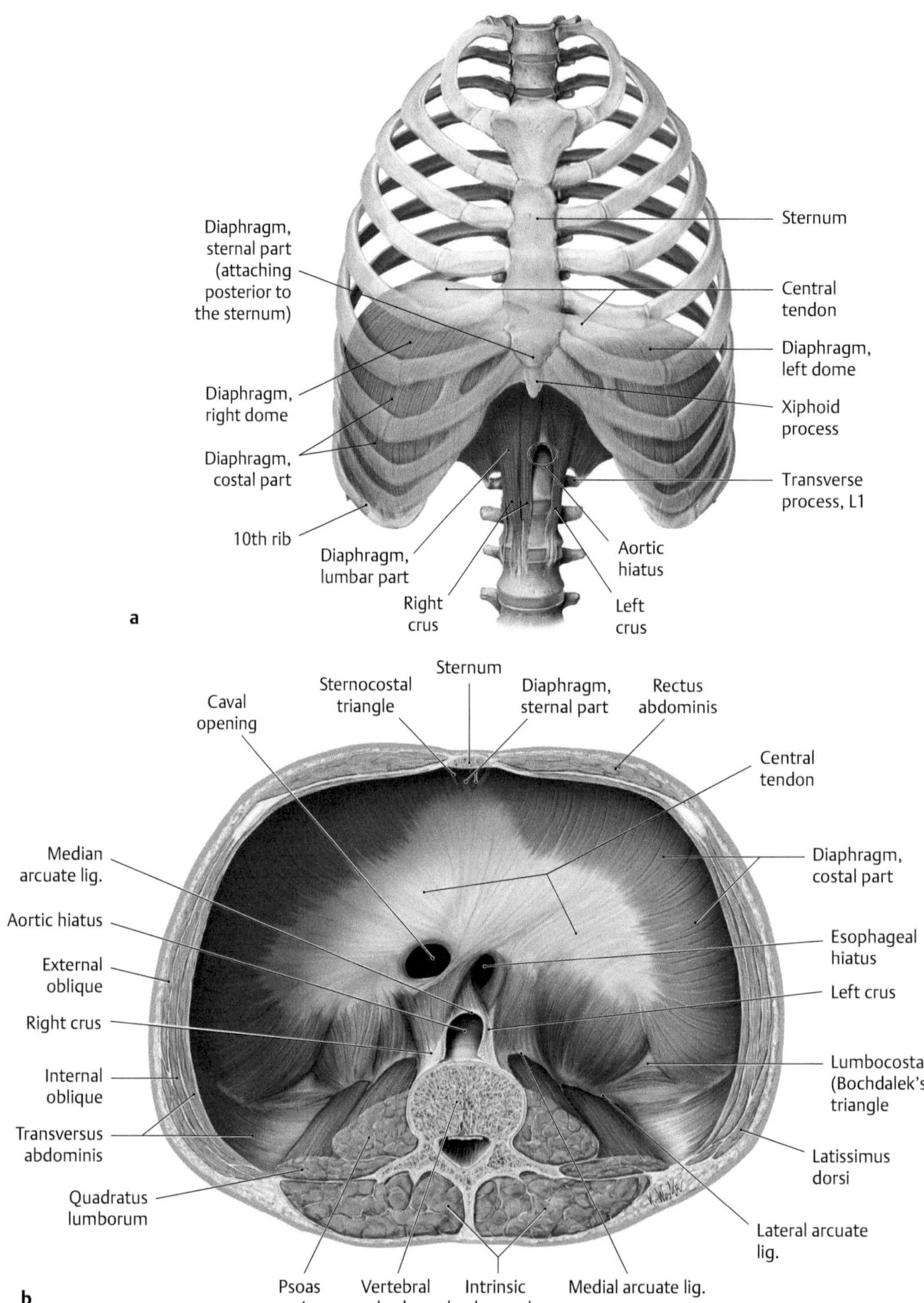

Fig. 3.68 (a) Anterior view of the diaphragm. **(b)** Inferior view of the diaphragm. (From Schuenke M, Schulte E, Schumacher U. THIEME Atlas of Anatomy. Internal Organs. Illustrations by Voll M and Wesker K. 3rd ed. New York: Thieme Medical Publishers; 2020.)

3.37.1 Neurovasculature of the Diaphragm

The **left** and **right phrenic nerves** supply motor innervation to the individual domes of the diaphragm. These nerves arise from the ventral rami of C3-C5 in the neck and have the functional components GSE, GSA, GVE-sym/post and GVA (**Fig. 3.70**). The phrenic nerves receive pain and proprioception information primarily for the central portion of the diaphragm. The sensory information from the peripheral portions of the diaphragm are supplied by the lower 6-7 **intercostal nerves** and the **subcostal nerve** (T12).

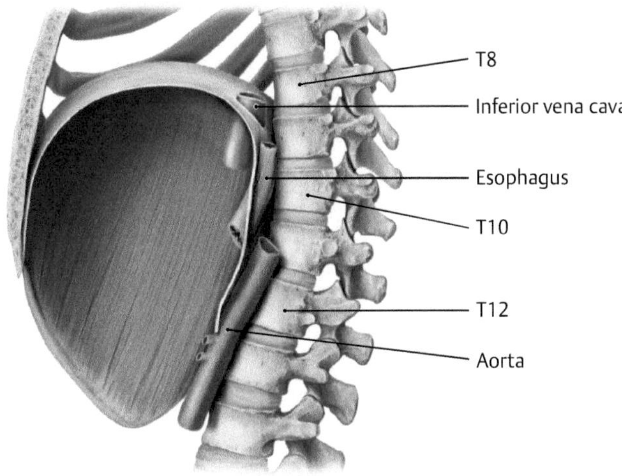

Fig. 3.69 Opened thorax viewed from the left side. Caval opening at T8; esophageal hiatus at T10; aortic hiatus at T12. (From Schuenke M, Schulte E, Schumacher U. THIEME Atlas of Anatomy. Internal Organs. Illustrations by Voll M and Wesker K. 3rd ed. New York: Thieme Medical Publishers; 2020.)

The *superior surface* of the diaphragm receives its blood supply from the **pericardiacophrenic** (internal thoracic br.), **musculophrenic** (internal thoracic br.) and the **superior phrenic arteries** (thoracic aorta br.). The *inferior surface* of the diaphragm is supplied by the **inferior phrenic arteries** (abdominal aorta br.).

Venous drainage of the *superior surface* is by the **pericardiacophrenic** and **musculophrenic veins**, both tributaries of the **internal thoracic vein** and specifically on the right side the **superior phrenic vein** drains into the IVC. The *inferior surface* is drained by the inferior phrenic veins. The **left inferior phrenic vein** is actually a double vein and is a tributary to both the left suprarenal vein and IVC. The **right inferior phrenic vein** drains into the IVC.

There is a free communication between the lymphatic plexuses of the thoracic and abdominal surfaces of the diaphragm. The *thoracic surface* is associated with the **anterior** and **posterior diaphragmatic lymph nodes** and drainage from these nodes travel to the **phrenic**, **parasternal** and **posterior mediastinal lymph nodes**. Lymph from the *abdominal surface* drains to the **phrenic**, **anterior diaphragmatic** and the more superior **lumbar lymph nodes**.

Inferior thyroid v.
Left common carotid a.
Left internal jugular v.
Left external jugular v.
Left subclavian a. and v.
Right phrenic n.
Superior vena cava
Internal thoracic a.
Azygos v.
Left brachiocephalic v.
Left phrenic n.
Posterior intercostal vv.
Accessory hemiazygous v.
Pericardiacophrenic a.
Hemiazygos v.
Musculophrenic a.
Superior phrenic aa.
Left phrenic n.
Inferior phrenic aa.
Celiac trunk
a
Inferior vena cava

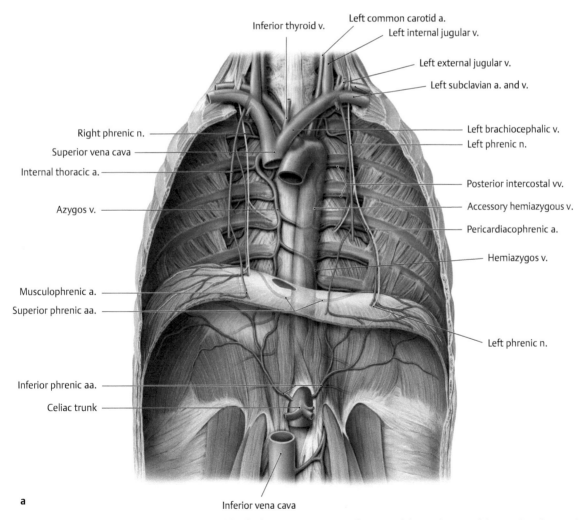

Fig. 3.70 Neurovasculature of the diaphragm. **(a)** Arteries of the diaphragm, anterior view of an opened thorax. (*continued*) (From Schuenke M, Schulte E, Schumacher U. THIEME Atlas of Anatomy. Internal Organs. Illustrations by Voll M and Wesker K. 3rd ed. New York: Thieme Medical Publishers; 2020.)

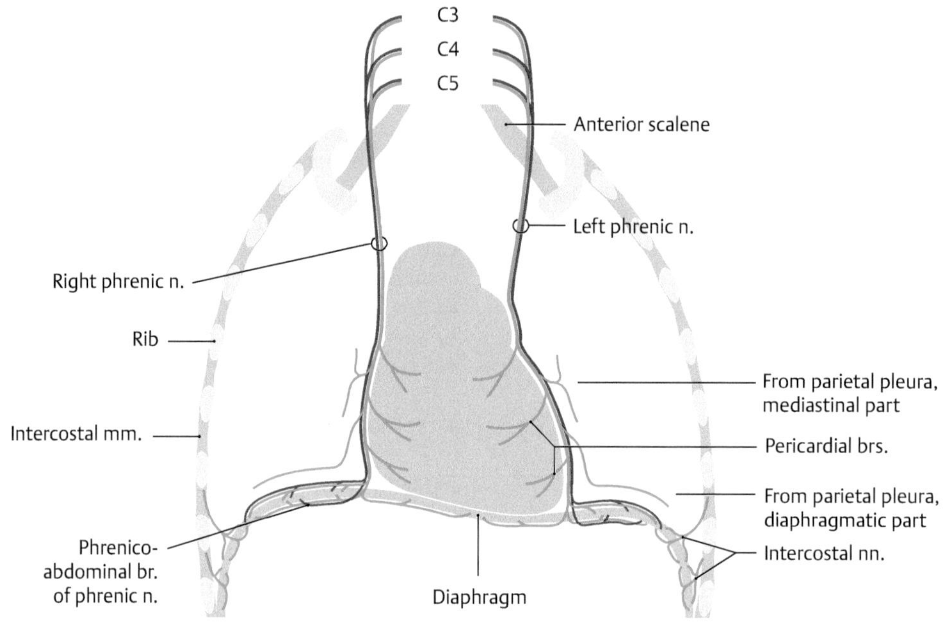

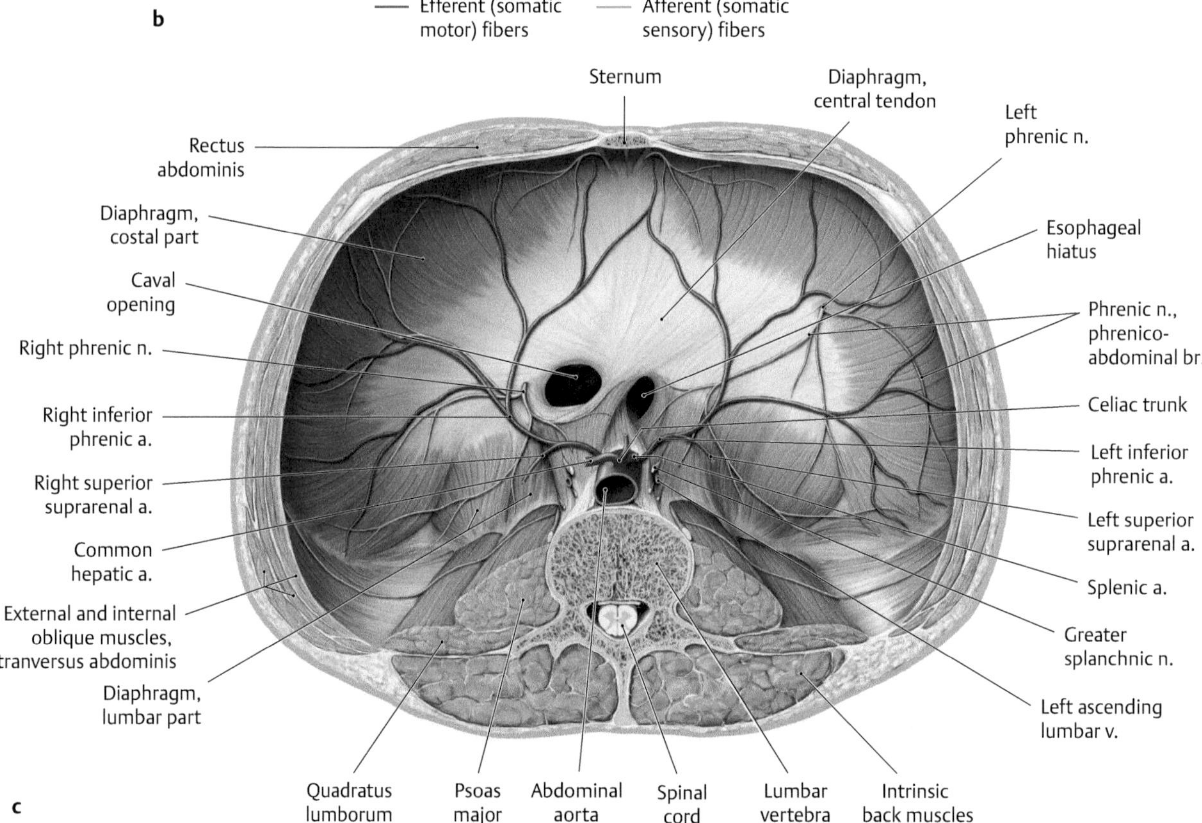

Fig. 3.70 (*continued*) Neurovasculature of the diaphragm. **(b)** Phrenic nerve branching patterns. **(c)** Arterial supply of inferior diaphragm. (From Schuenke M, Schulte E, Schumacher U. THIEME Atlas of Anatomy. Internal Organs. Illustrations by Voll M and Wesker K. 3rd ed. New York: Thieme Medical Publishers; 2020.)

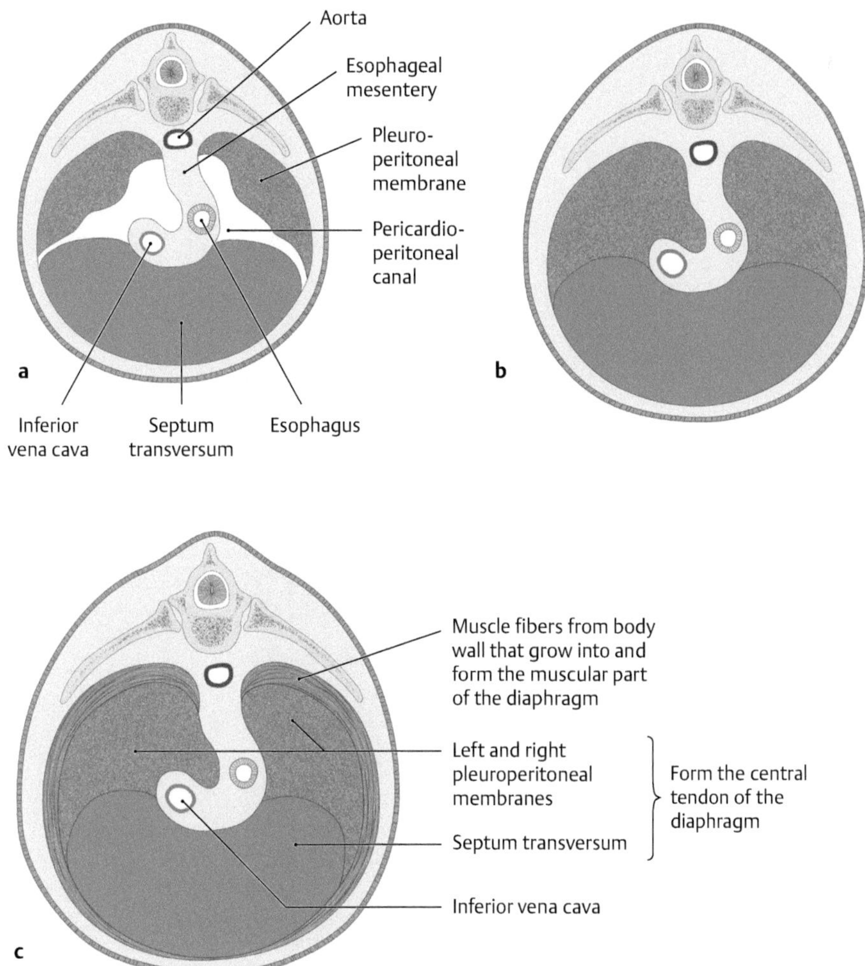

Fig. 3.71 Development of the diaphragm. **(a)** The septum transversum moving dorsally and the pleuroperitoneal membrane moving ventrally. **(b)** Fusion of the septum transversum and pleuroperitoneal membranes forming the future central tendon. **(c)** The dorsal mesentery of the esophagus and adjacent bod wall musculature give rise to the muscular part of the diaphragm. (From Schuenke M, Schulte E, Schumacher U. THIEME Atlas of Anatomy. Internal Organs. Illustrations by Voll M and Wesker K. 3rd ed. New York: Thieme Medical Publishers; 2020.)

3.37.2 Development of the Diaphragm

Early in the fourth week, the **intraembryonic coelom** appears as a horseshoe-shaped cavity in the cardiogenic and lateral plate mesoderms. It gives rise to the *pericardial cavity*, the *peritoneal cavity* and two *pericardioperitoneal canals* that connect these two cavities. However, there are two partitions needed to accomplish the separation of the early body cavity in to multiple regions. These include the paired *pleuropericardial membranes* and the *diaphragm*. The **pleuropericardial membranes** are made of somatic mesoderm and they fuse to separate the pericardial and pleural cavities.

The **diaphragm** must first develop from four different sources before it is capable of separating the thoracic cavity from the peritoneal cavity. Ultimately all of these sources fuse to close off the pericardioperitoneal canals and form the definitive diaphragm (**Fig. 3.71**).

1. The **septum transversum** is found between the primitive heart tube and developing liver and is made of mesoderm. It becomes the **central tendon of the diaphragm**.
2. The paired **pleuroperitoneal membranes** are derived from somatic mesoderm and fuse to form the early diaphragm.
3. The **outer body walls** provide muscular components from the 3rd, 4th, and 5th cervical somites that incorporate themselves into the pleuroperitoneal membranes and form the **peripheral muscular portion** of the diaphragm.
4. Myoblasts that grow into the **dorsal mesentery of the esophagus** contribute to the **crura of the diaphragm**.

3.38 Muscles of the Posterior Abdominal Wall

Muscles of the posterior abdominal wall are primarily made up of the **psoas major**, **iliacus**, and **quadratus lumborum**. The psoas major and iliacus muscles merge together to form the **iliopsoas muscle** and this is one of the strongest hip flexors (**Fig. 3.72**). The inconstant **psoas minor** is a muscle located on the superficial surface of the psoas major but it is only found in about 50% of the

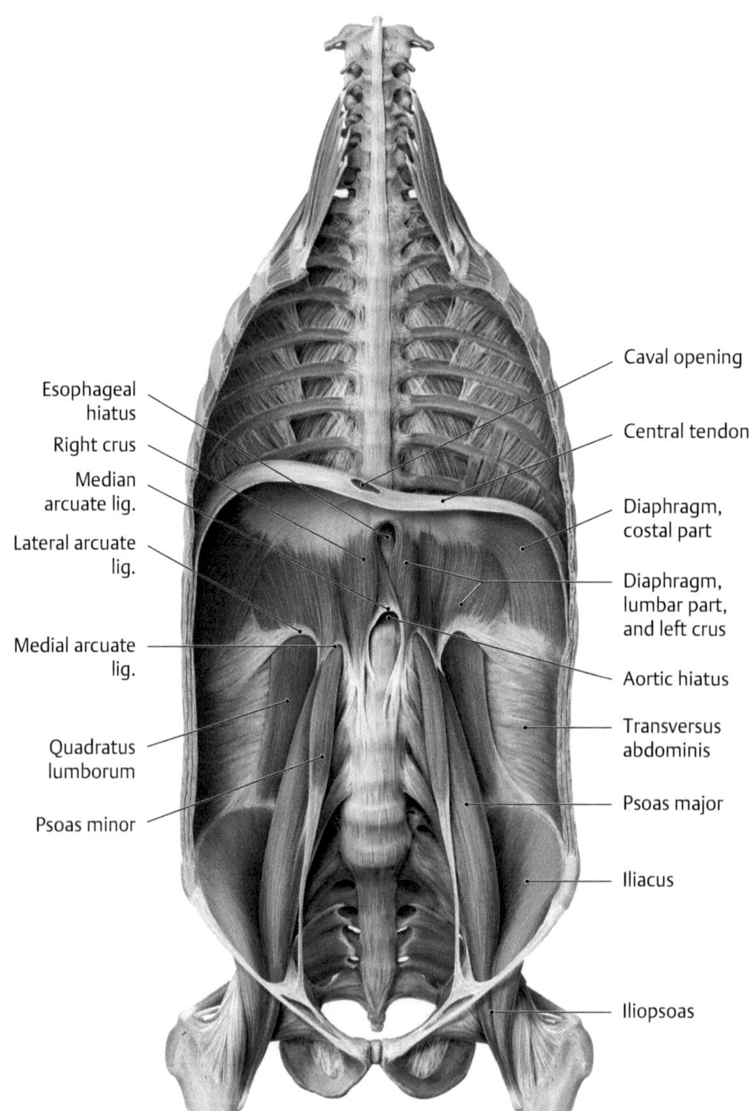

Fig. 3.72 Muscles of the posterior abdominal wall, coronal section through the trunk. (From Schuenke M, Schulte E, Schumacher U. THIEME Atlas of Anatomy. General Anatomy and Musculoskeletal System. Illustrations by Voll M and Wesker K. 3rd ed. New York: Thieme Medical Publishers; 2020.)

population, thus its importance is minimal. These muscles are described in **Table 3.3**.

3.39 Fascia of the Posterior Abdominal Wall

Structures related to the posterior abdominal wall are generally retroperitoneal which means a layer of parietal peritoneum forms what looks like a blanket over these structures. Fascia that was seen in the anterolateral abdominal wall is continuous with much of the posterior abdominal wall. The *parietal peritoneum, extraperitoneal fat* and *transversalis fascia* continue posteriorly with the parietal peritoneum forming the blanket or roof, transversalis fascia becoming continuous with *renal fascia* and in between these two layers a now thicker layer of extraperitoneal fat that also contributes to the *perinephric* and *paranephric fat* surrounding the kidneys. The **perinephric (perirenal) fat** is a layer of fat the directly contacts the kidney, suprarenal gland and the ureter. The **renal fascia** is a membranous layer of fascia continuous with the transversalis fascia that surrounds the perinephric fat. The **paranephric (pararenal) fat** is located outside the renal fascia and adjacent to the fascia along the posterior abdominal wall that was also a continuation of the transversalis fascia (**Fig. 3.73**).

The **thoracolumbar fascia** was first described on the superficial back but what could not be seen at that time is that it is quite extensive and is made of an *anterior, middle* and *posterior layers*. The **posterior** and **middle layers** enclose the erector spinae muscle group. The **middle** and **anterior layers** enclose the quadratus lumborum muscle. The **anterior layer** extends over a portion of the anterior surface of the latissimus dorsi muscle before continuing laterally with the aponeurosis of the transversus abdominis muscle. The anterior layer passes medially from the quadratus lumborum and becomes continuous with the **psoas fascia (Fig. 3.73)**.

Clinical Correlate 3.45

Hiatal Hernias

Diaphragmatic hernias are those that allow abdominal structures to enter the thoracic cavity by passing through the diaphragm. These hernias are described as either being hiatal or congenital but can also be due to trauma. **Hiatal hernias** are protrusions of a part of the stomach through the esophageal hiatus and are described as either being *sliding* or *paraesophageal* in nature. **Sliding hernias** involve the abdominal portion of the esophagus and the cardia and fundus of the stomach sliding superiorly through the esophageal hiatus and into the thoracic cavity. They account for about 90% of all hiatal hernias. When only the fundus of the stomach passes superiorly this is called a **paraesophageal hernia**.

A **congenital diaphragmatic hernia (CDH)** involves the presence of a posterolateral defect of the diaphragm that is generally caused by the failure of the left pleuroperitoneal membrane to close. The failure of both sides to close is possible. It is one of the most common congenital malformations of a newborn with an incidence rate of about 1 in 2,000 live births. It is the most common cause of pulmonary hypoplasia (incomplete lung development) due to the fact the GI tract filled portions of the thoracic cavity.

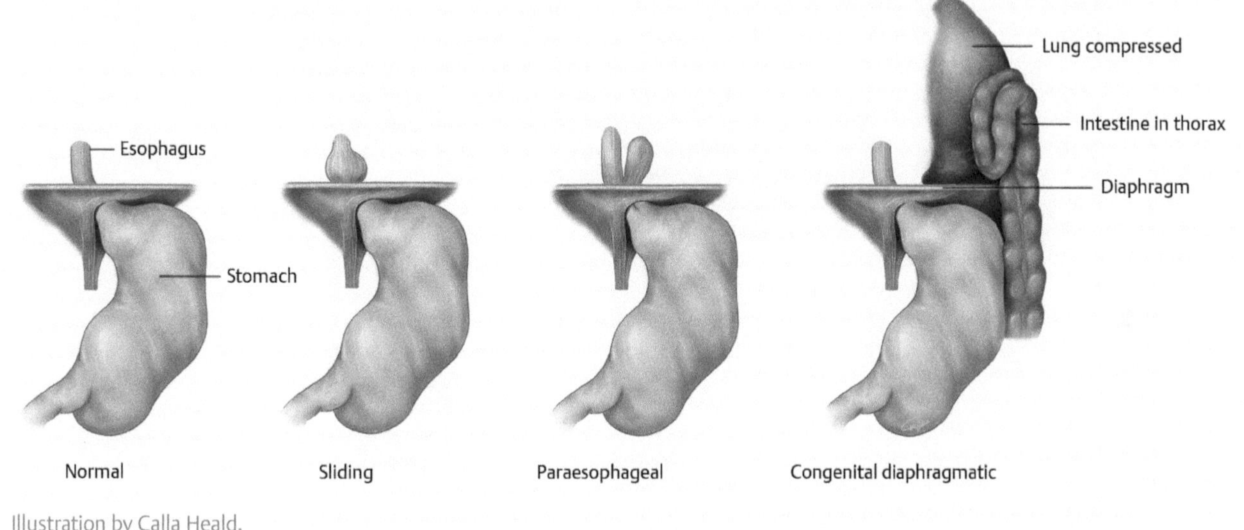

Illustration by Calla Heald.

Table 3.3 **Posterior abdominal wall muscles**

Muscle	Innervation	Function(s)	Origin	Insertion
Psoas major	Lumbar plexus via ventral rami of L1-L4	Flexes thigh and trunk with iliacus; flexes vertebral column laterally to balance trunk	Transverse process and body of T12, L1-L4 vertebrae; intervertebral disks between T12 and L5	Combines with iliacus to form the iliopsoas muscle and inserts on lesser trochanter of femur
Psoas minor	L1 of lumbar plexus	If present, very weak flexor of the thigh	Lateral surfaces of T12 and L1 vertebral bodies	Pectineal line, iliopectineal eminence and iliac fascia. Often fuses with tendon of psoas major
Iliacus	Femoral nerve	Acts with psoas major to flex thigh, flex trunk and stabilize hip joint	Superior two-thirds of the iliac fossa, ala of the sacrum and anterior sacro-iliac ligaments	Combines with psoas major to form the iliopsoas muscle and inserts on lesser trochanter of femur
Quadratus lumborum	Ventral rami of T12, L1-L4	Laterally flexes and extends vertebral column; fixes 12th rib during inspiration	Medial portion of the 12th rib and transverse processes (tips) of the L1-L4 vertebrae	Iliolumbar ligament and iliac crest

Viscera of the Posterior Abdominal Wall

3.40 Suprarenal (Adrenal) Glands

The **suprarenal glands** are retroperitoneal structures that lie adjacent to the superior poles of the kidneys (**Fig. 3.74**). They are surrounded by a significant amount of *perinephric fat* and the *renal fascia*, which attaches to the diaphragmatic crura and prevents excessive movement. Both suprarenal glands are made of two parts: a **cortex** that secretes androgens and corticosteroids and a **medulla** that secretes epinephrine and norepinephrine. The left suprarenal gland is more crescent-shaped and is located adjacent to the left crus of the diaphragm, stomach, pancreas and spleen. The right suprarenal gland is shaped more like a pyramid and makes contact with the IVC and liver.

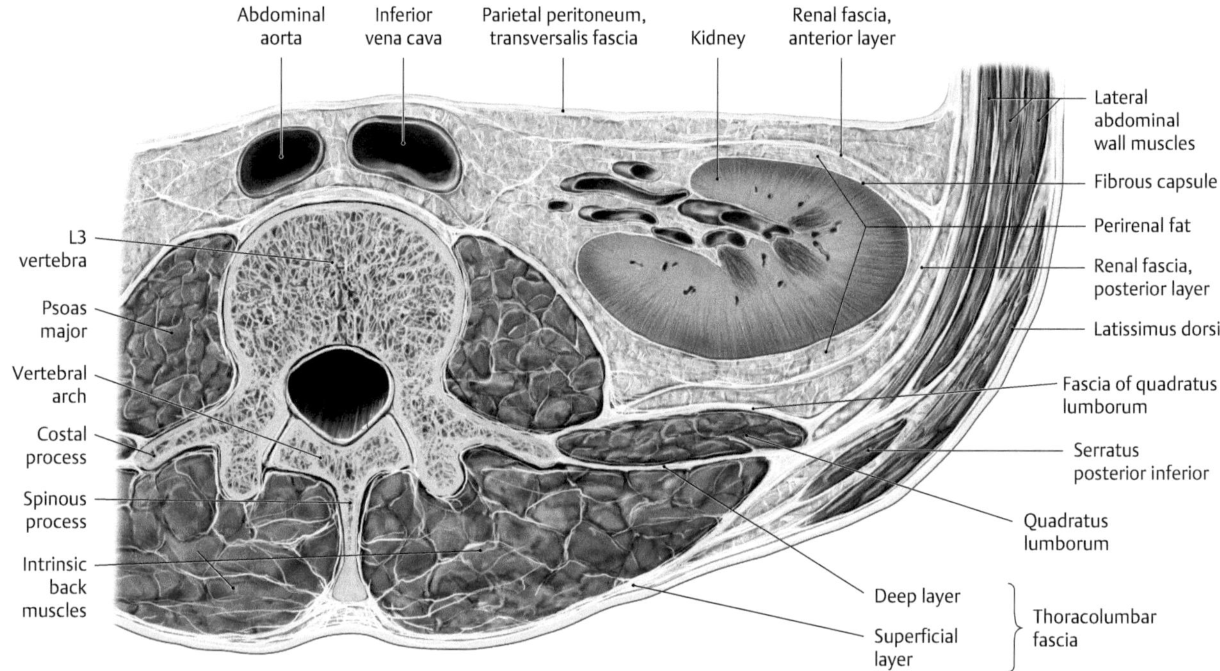

Fig. 3.73 Transverse section through the posterior trunk wall at the level of the L3 vertebra, superior view. (From Schuenke M, Schulte E, Schumacher U. THIEME Atlas of Anatomy. General Anatomy and Musculoskeletal System. Illustrations by Voll M and Wesker K. 3rd ed. New York: Thieme Medical Publishers; 2020.)

Clinical Correlate 3.46

Disorders of the Suprarenal Cortex and Medulla

- **Cushing Syndrome** (hypercortisolism) is uncommon and is caused by the overproduction of the hormone cortisol. Symptoms include high blood pressure, rapid weight gain around the trunk but a loss at the limbs, reddish stretch mark and round face and muscle weakness. It is generally caused by taking too much glucocorticosteroid medicine used to treat asthma, rheumatoid arthritis, bowel disease or skin inflammation.
- **Conn Syndrome** is a small tumor that produces an excessive amount of the hormone aldosterone and is generally related to a pituitary adenoma resulting in excessive production of ACTH. Excessive production of aldosterone by the tumor leads to high blood pressure and low potassium levels. The preferred treatment is a laparoscopic adrenalectomy that removes the entire gland and tumor.
- **Addison Disease** (hypocortisolism) is destruction of the cortex that leads to adrenocortical insufficiency. Tumors, tuberculosis, HIV or fungal infections infection, or an autoimmune disease targeting the suprarenal gland causes this type of cortex damage. Symptoms include dehydration, chronic diarrhea, mouth lesions, salt craving and dizziness when standing up. Treatment includes replacement corticosteroids to control the disease or injections of hydrocortisone.

Carcinomas of the suprarenal cortex are rare but a **phaeochromocytoma** is a tumor of the chromaffin cells within the medulla and it causes symptoms and signs of episodic catecholamine release, hyperglycemia and hypertension. Most are unilateral and solitary benign tumors found in adults. Only about 10% are malignant or seen in children. Medications involved in adrenergic alpha-blockades are given prior to surgical intervention that typically provides a cure.

3.40.1 Vasculature and Lymphatic Drainage of the Suprarenal Glands

There is an abundant amount of blood supply to the suprarenal glands and this involves multiple arteries. The blood supply pattern is bilateral. The **superior suprarenals** (inferior phrenic brs.) have multiple branches whereas the **middle suprarenal** (abdominal aorta br.) and the **inferior suprarenal arteries** (renal br.) are generally isolated arteries. On occasion there may be multiple branches associated with the latter two arteries (**Fig. 3.74**).

The above arteries enter through the capsule and form cortical and medullary arteries. The **cortical arterioles** become capillary beds that are fenestrated sinusoidal networks located between the cords of the parenchyma and essentially supply blood to the cortex. After supplying the cortex these vessels drain into the medullary capillary beds. The **medullary arterioles** penetrate the cortex, but they do not branch within it. They just continue to the medulla where they form capillary beds of the medulla. Hence the medulla has a dual blood supply that is both arterial (medullary) and venous (cortical). The blood returning from both cortical and medullary veins empties through a single central vein and drains the left adrenal gland to the left renal vein and the right adrenal gland to the IVC.

The venous drainage pattern is side-specific and these veins have a larger diameter than the arteries. The **left suprarenal vein** is short and drains into the **left renal vein**. The **right suprarenal vein** drains directly into the IVC. Lymphatic drainage of both suprarenal glands is to the **lumbar lymph nodes** (**Fig. 3.79**).

3.40.2 Histology of the Suprarenal Glands

The suprarenal glands have a *capsule*, *cortex* and *medulla*. The **cortex** of the adrenal gland is divided into three poorly anatomically defined layers but the functions of the layers are more discrete.

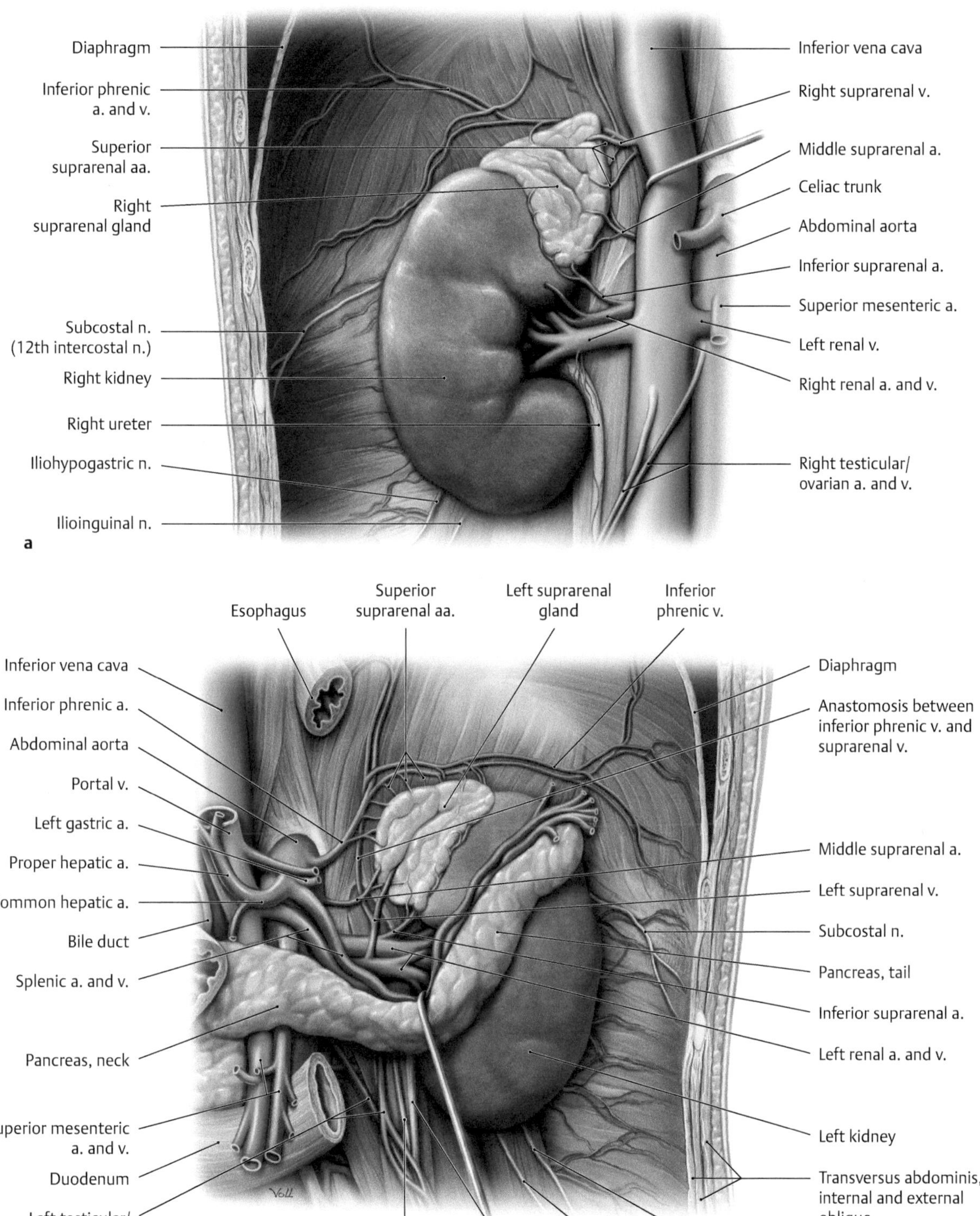

Fig. 3.74 (a) Right suprarenal (adrenal) gland and kidney, anterior view with perirenal fat removed. **(b)** Left suprarenal (adrenal) gland and kidney, anterior view with perirenal fat removed. (From Schuenke M, Schulte E, Schumacher U. THIEME Atlas of Anatomy. Internal Organs. Illustrations by Voll M and Wesker K. 3rd ed. New York: Thieme Medical Publishers; 2020.)

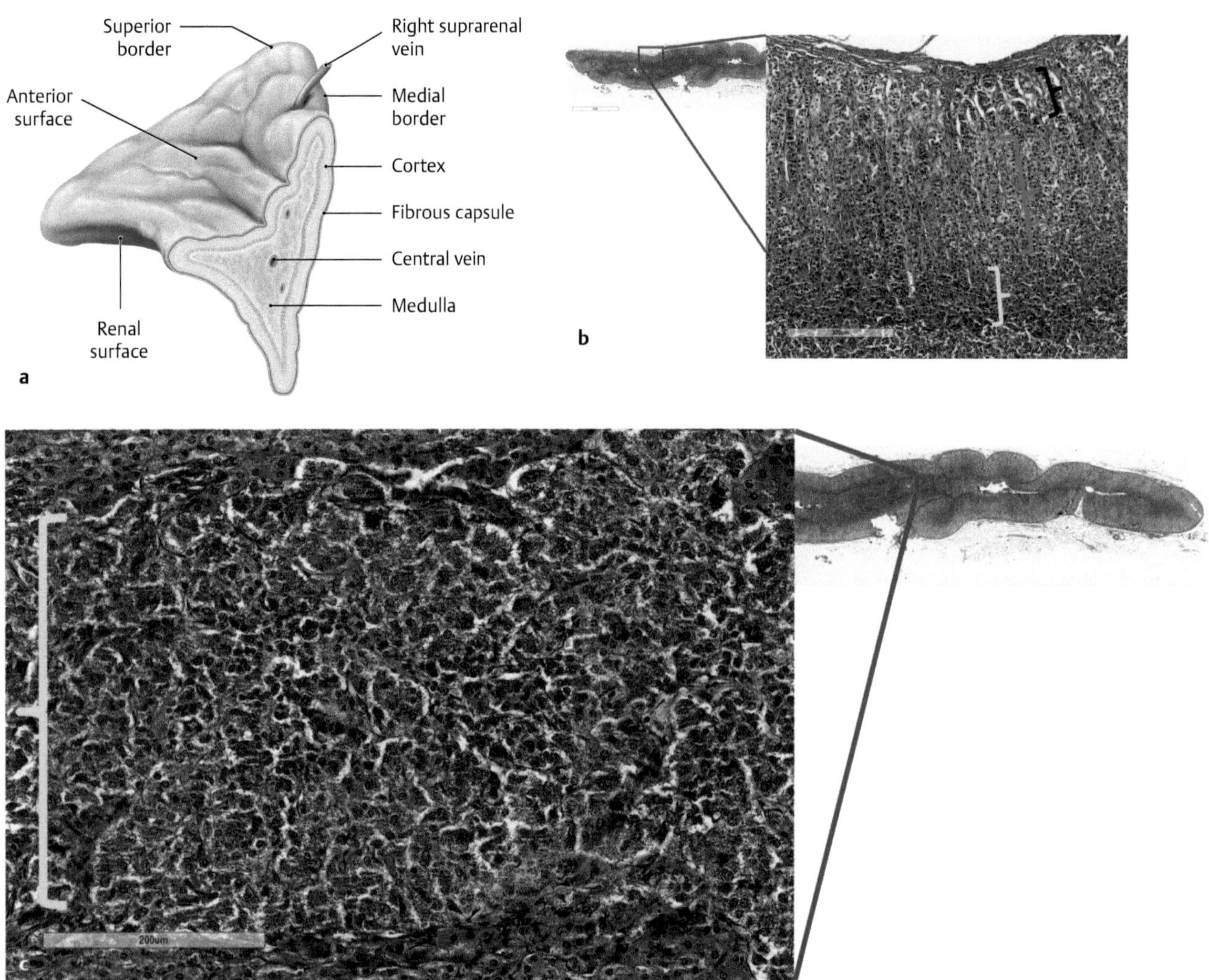

Fig. 3.75 Histology of the suprarenal gland. **(a)** Coronal section through the right suprarenal gland. **(b)** Suprarenal cortex. The three zones are indicated: zona glomerulosa (*black bracket*); zona fasciculata (*blue bracket*); zona reticularis (*yellow bracket*). **(c)** Suprarenal medulla (*yellow bracket*), medium magnification. (**a** from Schuenke M, Schulte E, Schumacher U. THIEME Atlas of Anatomy. Internal Organs. Illustrations by Voll M and Wesker K. 3rd ed. New York: Thieme Medical Publishers; 2020. **b** and **c** from Lowrie DJ. Histology: An Essential Textbook. New York: Thieme Medical Publishers; 2020.)

The cortex synthesizes and secretes steroid hormones only upon demand but does not store these secretory products. From superficial to deep, they are arranged as the *zona glomerulosa*, *zona fasciculata* and *zona reticularis* (**Fig. 3.75**).

- **Zona glomerulosa**: the most superficial layer and closest to the capsule. The columnar or pyramidal shaped cells of this layer are arranged like arched cords and account for approximately 15% of the suprarenal gland. The cells of this layer secrete steroid hormones called **mineralocorticoids** and they function by affecting the salt and water balances of the blood. The primary mineralocorticoid is called **aldosterone**, which acts on the distal tubules of the kidneys nephrons to maintain electrolyte levels and blood volume. More details involving aldosterone can be seen in the discussion about the juxtaglomerular apparatus in the histology of the kidney section.
- **Zona fasciculata**: the middle layer and also the largest of the cortex. The cells are arranged as columns or cords that are perpendicular to the capsule and account for 65% of the entire gland. These columns or cords are separated by sinusoidal capillaries as described in the blood supply section above. These cells also have a foamy appearance because they are filled with many lipid droplets and hence are referred to as **spongiocytes**. Steroid hormones called **glucocorticoids** are secreted by this layer and they function by increasing blood glucose levels (glucose metabolism), suppressing inflammatory and immunologic responses and can also affect arousal and cognition. The most important glucocorticoid and essential for life is **cortisol**. It is released in response to stress and low blood glucose levels and is essential for homeostasis maintenance. The glucocorticoids released are about 95% cortisol and the remaining 5% a combination of cortisone and corticosterone (precursor to aldosterone).
- **Zona reticularis**: the deepest layer of the cortex and closest to the medulla. The cells of this layer are arranged as a network of irregular anastomosing cords and account for only 7% of the suprarenal gland. Cells here produce precursor androgens with the primary product of this layer being *dehydroepiandrosterone*

(DHEA). These precursor androgens do not go through any conversion in the suprarenal cortex but instead are released into the blood stream and are taken up by the gonads to help produce testosterone in the male and estrogen in the female, for example.

The **medulla** of the suprarenal gland is characterized by **chromaffin cells** that are large, polyhedral and arranged as irregular cords and clumps. They are modified sympathetic postganglionic neurons that have lost their axons and dendrites during development. They have instead become secretory cells that are responsible for synthesizing and secreting catecholamines. The majority of the secreted product is **epinephrine** or *adrenaline* (~80%) and **norepinephrine** (~20%) and this is especially evident during a *fight-or-flight response*. The sympathetic preganglionic fibers of a **splanchnic** (*greater*, *lesser* or *least*) **nerve** innervate these chromaffin cells and they then release their product into the extensive capillary network found within the medulla (**Fig. 3.75**).

3.41 Kidneys

The **kidneys** are retroperitoneal structures located on the left from T12-L3 and on the right from L1-L4. The superior aspects of both kidneys are related to the diaphragm while inferiorly they are close to the quadratus lumborum muscles. The left kidney more specifically is found near the stomach, jejunum, pancreas, spleen and descending colon. The right kidney is located closer to the liver, duodenum and ascending colon.

The kidneys have a superior and inferior pole, an anterior and posterior surface, and a medial and lateral margin. The superior poles are where the suprarenal glands are located. The **renal hilum** is associated with the medial margin and this is where the *renal sinus* and *renal pelvis* of the ureter are located. The **renal sinus** contains the renal pelvis, renal calices, neurovasculature and fat. If viewing the kidney from the anterior aspect, the renal vein is the most anterior, the renal artery is in the middle, and the renal pelvis is the most posterior of these structures (**Fig. 3.76**).

The apex or **renal papilla** of the **renal pyramid** is where urine is excreted and it is the renal pyramids and their associated cortex that contribute to the lobes of the kidney. The lobes are most prevalent during fetal development (7-18 total lobes) however in the adult the lobes have been smoothed out. The pyramids drain through the papilla to the **minor calyx**, of which there are about three minor calices that drain into a **major calyx**. There are about two to three major calices that merge to form the renal pelvis. The **renal pelvis** represents the superior portion of the ureter.

The functions of the kidneys are to filter the blood and remove excess organic wastes of metabolism, maintain the acid-base balance by regulating pH in blood plasma, regulate electrolytes, regulate blood pressure by maintaining water and salt balance, and secrete hormones. The kidneys receive about 25% of the total cardiac output at rest thus blood is filtered through the kidneys numerous times per day and the final product of kidney filtration is urine. Approximately 180 L of filtrate is produced from the blood but about 99% of that is reabsorbed. The net amount of excreted urine is about 1 L.

3.41.1 Neurovasculature and Lymphatic Drainage of the Kidneys

The **renal plexus** is a mixed autonomic plexus originating from the intermesenteric plexus of the larger aortic plexus. Sympathetics from this plexus are vasoconstrictive to the arteries, increase renin release from juxtaglomerular cells, and increase sodium reabsorption of the renal tubules. These combined effects contribute to the development and maintenance of hypertension. Parasympathetics have little to no effect on the kidney (**Fig. 3.77**).

The **renal arteries** originate from the abdominal aorta at about the L1/L2 vertebral level. The right renal artery is naturally longer because it must pass posterior to the IVC before reaching the right kidney. Near the renal hilum, the renal arteries branch into five segmental arteries that are defined as *end arteries*. End arteries are those that do not anastomose significantly with other arteries and thus each segmental artery has its own independent and surgically resectable *renal segment*. These segmental arteries include: **superior (apical) segmental artery**, **anterosuperior segmental artery**, **anteroinferior segmental artery**, **inferior segmental artery** and the **posterior segmental artery**. The branching pattern displayed in most textbooks and atlases regarding these segmental branches is only consistent in approximately 9% of the population so there is much variation involving these arteries (**Fig. 3.78**).

The **renal veins** drain each kidney into the IVC. The left renal vein must pass over the abdominal aorta to reach the IVC. The left renal vein receives the left suprarenal vein and left gonadal veins. The right renal vein does not receive a suprarenal or a gonadal vein. Due to the close proximity of the SMA as it extends inferiorly over the left renal vein, compression of the left renal vein by the SMA is known as "*nutcracker syndrome*". Lymphatic drainage of the kidneys is to the **lumbar lymph nodes** (**Fig. 3.79**).

3.41.2 Histology of the Kidneys

A thin **renal capsule** encloses the parenchyma that consists of a *cortex* and *medulla* and it extends around to contain the renal hilum. The larger *arcuate blood vessels* demarcate the cortex from the medulla. Epithelial tubules occupy most of the total renal volume but some connective tissue surrounds each tubule. Numerous capillaries occupy the interstitium of the stroma. The **renal cortex** is located on the outermost portion of the kidney between the capsule and medulla and has a thickness of about 1 cm. The renal corpuscles are found within the cortex. The **renal medulla** is made up of numerous cone-shaped **renal pyramids** that are separated from one another by the **renal columns** (*of Bertin*). The renal columns are continuous with the cortex (**Fig. 3.76; Fig. 3.80**).

As the blood enters the kidney as a **segmental branch of the renal artery**, an **interlobar artery** branches off it and runs within the renal columns to supply each lobe. From the interlobar arteries, **arcuate arteries** branch off at right angles and run along the cortico-meduallry junction before branching into **interlobular arteries** that enter the cortex and radiate toward the renal surface. The **afferent glomerular arterioles** originate from the interlobular arteries and supply blood to the **glomerular capillaries** within the renal corpuscle. These glomerular capillaries converge into the **efferent glomerular arteriole** that drains in order from the **peritubular capillaries**, **interlobular veins**, **arcuate veins**, **interlobar veins**, and finally the **renal veins** (**Fig. 3.81**).

The **renal** (*uriniferous*) **tubule** is considered the functional unit of the kidney and it is comprised of a **nephron** and **collecting duct**. In some texts, the nephron is stated to be the functional unit of a kidney. Each nephron is composed of a *renal corpuscle* along with its *proximal convoluted tubule*, *thin and thick limbs of the loop of Henle*, and the *distal convoluted tubule*. There are approximately 1 million nephrons in each kidney and they are subdivided based on the location of the renal corpuscles in the cortex. They are

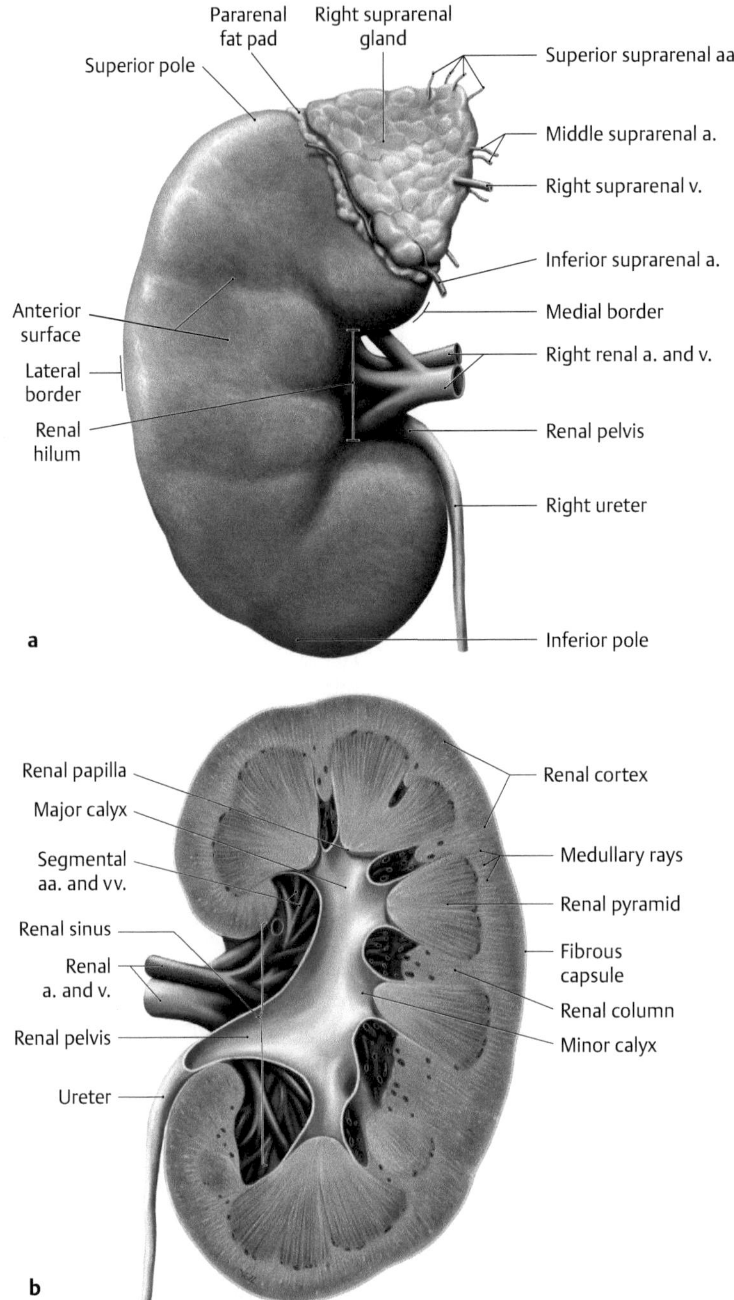

Fig. 3.76 (a) Right kidney with suprarenal gland, anterior view. **(b)** Right kidney, posterior view, midsagittal section. (From Schuenke M, Schulte E, Schumacher U. THIEME Atlas of Anatomy. Internal Organs. Illustrations by Voll M and Wesker K. 3rd ed. New York: Thieme Medical Publishers; 2020.)

either *superficial*, *midcortical*, or *juxtamedullary* (adjacent to the medulla).

The **renal corpuscle** is the complex filtration apparatus consisting of a capillary tuft or *glomerulus* enclosed by a double epithelial wall, the first of which includes a capillary endothelium next to a fused basal lamina and outer *podocytes* that make up the **visceral layer of Bowman's capsule**, followed by **Bowman's space**, and finally an outer border called the **parietal layer of Bowman's capsule (Fig. 3.80; Fig. 3.82)**.

The **glomerulus** receives blood from an **afferent arteriole** that subdivides into a convolution of capillaries that merge back into a single **efferent arteriole** rather than a venule. The high pressure within the glomerulus aids in the process of ultrafiltration where fluids and soluble materials in the blood are forced out of the capillaries and into Bowman's space. These capillaries are characterized by an inner *simple squamous fenestrated endothelium* with no diaphragms across the fenestrae (openings) thus making these capillaries very leaky and not much of a barrier to the movement of plasma. There are modified smooth muscle cells within the walls of the afferent (mainly) and efferent arterioles called **juxtaglomerular cells** and they contain *renin*. Renin is related to the *renin-angiotensin*

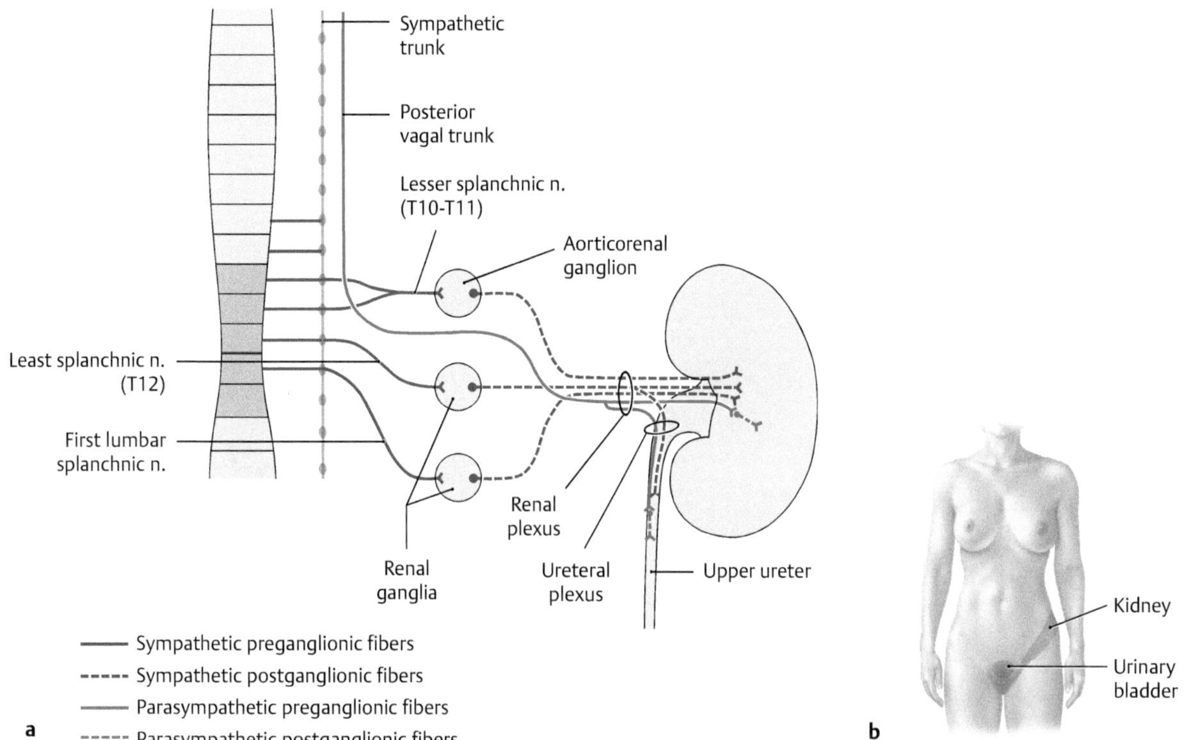

Fig. 3.77 **(a)** Autonomic innervation of the kidneys and upper ureters. **(b)** Referred pain from the left kidney and bladder. (From Schuenke M, Schulte E, Schumacher U. THIEME Atlas of Anatomy. Internal Organs. Illustrations by Voll M and Wesker K. 3rd ed. New York: Thieme Medical Publishers; 2020.)

system that is important in the reabsorption of water and sodium (**Fig. 3.82**).

The **basal lamina** is comprised of three layers and is the functional component of the renal filtration barrier. It is also referred to as the **glomerular basement membrane (GBM)**. The **visceral epithelium of Bowman's capsule** consists of podocytes that encircle the capillaries with foot-like processes known as **pedicels**. The pedicels rest directly against the GBM but have considerable spaces that provide little resistance to flow (**Fig. 3.82**).

The **parietal layer of Bowman's capsule** is lined by a *simple squamous epithelium* that is continuous with the visceral layer at the *vascular pole* of the renal corpuscle. The space that is located between the visceral and parietal layers of Bowman's capsule is called **Bowman's space** and is the location of plasma filtrate. The filtrate located in this space exits towards the proximal convoluted tubule at the *urinary pole* of the renal corpuscle. The tubular system, which begins with the PCT, modifies the glomerular filtrate by absorbing molecules like water, sodium, and glucose but also secreting substances such as creatine. These molecules are then removed from interstitium by post-glomerular capillaries closely associated with the renal tubules. Urine becomes more hypertonic after this process (**Fig. 3.80; Fig. 3.82**).

The **proximal convoluted tubule (PCT)** extends from the parietal layer of Bowman's capsule and consists of a *simple cuboidal to columnar epithelium* lined by a dense microvillous border that greatly increase surface area for filtrate absorption. Between 65-80% of all filtrate is absorbed by the PCT and this also includes reabsorption of glucose, amino acids, electrolytes and water (**Fig. 3.80; Fig. 3.82**).

The **loop of Henle** is located in the medulla and includes a *thick descending limb*, followed by a *thin descending and ascending limb*, and finally a *thick ascending limb*. The thick limbs are made of a *simple cuboidal epithelium* while the thin limbs consist of *simple squamous epithelium*. The descending and ascending loops lie next to each other, and there is an increasing osmotic gradient from the cortex to the tip. Urea, sodium and chloride ions are actively transported into the interstitial space of the medulla by the ascending limb, and these are taken up by the descending limb that has a lower osmotic concentration. This means that while moving from the cortex and into the medulla of the kidney, the salt concentration in the interstitial space increases becoming more and more hypertonic, relative to the fluid passing through the collecting ducts. This helps to extract water from the filtrate and produce more concentrated urine. The efficient modification of ultrafiltrate into urine based on the differential permeability between thick and thin limbs is known as *countercurrent exchange*.

The thin descending limbs are permeable to water (passes out) and electrolytes (passes in) allowing for an equilibration with the interstitium. Thin and thick ascending limbs are impermeable to water but will transport Cl^- into the medullary interstitium resulting in hypotonic fluid. Na^+ follows passively during the transport of Cl^- (**Fig. 3.80; Fig. 3.82**).

The **distal convoluted tubule (DCT)** is located in the cortex and consists of a *simple cuboidal epithelium*. Near the vascular pole of the glomerulus, the epithelium of the DCT becomes specialized and is called the macula densa. The **macula densa** are responsible for sensing changes in the NaCl levels, and they will trigger an autoregulatory response to increase or decrease reabsorption

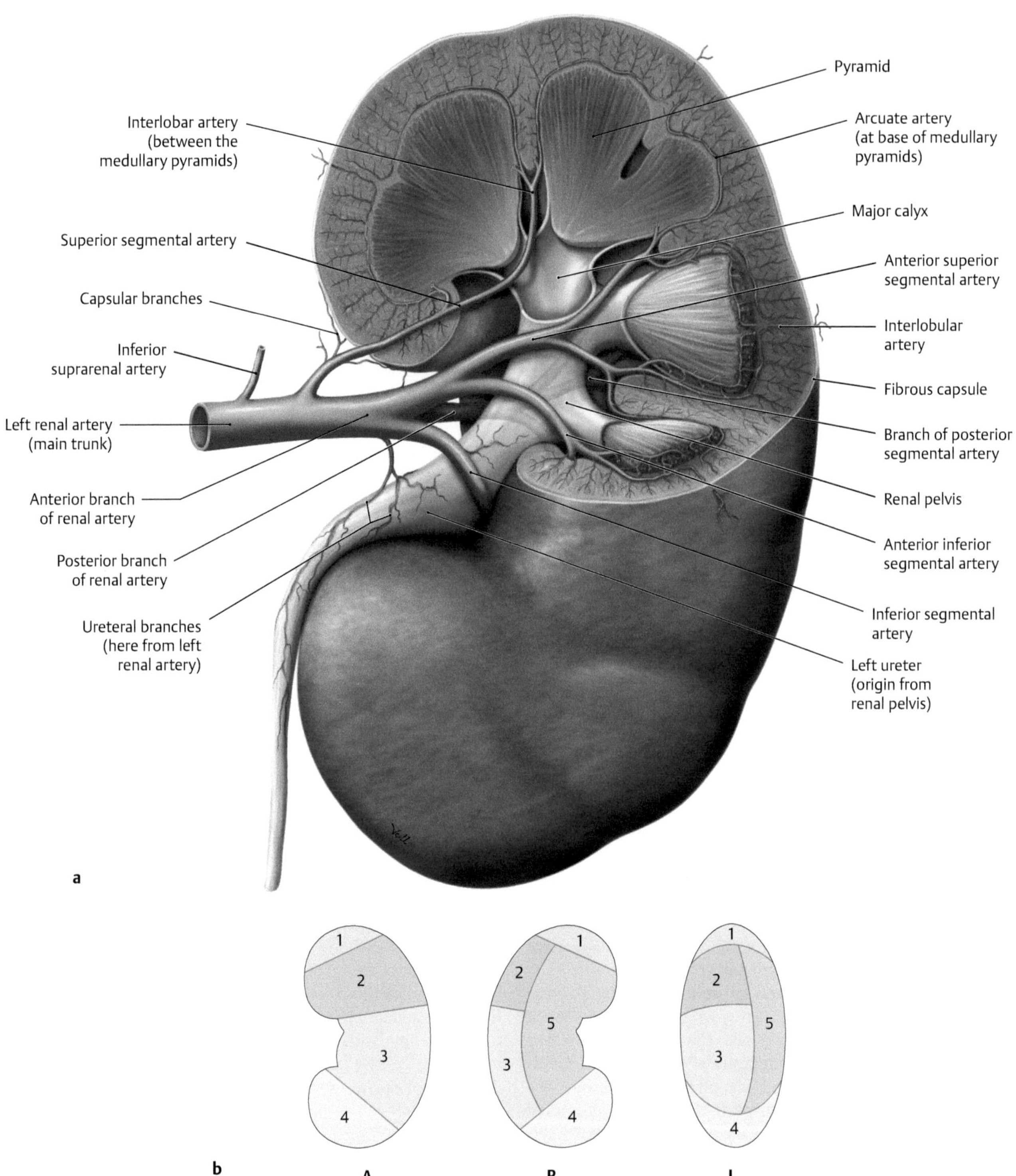

Fig. 3.78 (a) Division of the renal artery into segmental arteries. **(b)** Vascular segmentation of the kidney. A, anterior; P, posterior; and L, lateral side. (From Schuenke M, Schulte E, Schumacher U. THIEME Atlas of Anatomy. Internal Organs. Illustrations by Voll M and Wesker K. 3rd ed. New York: Thieme Medical Publishers; 2020.)

of ions and water to the blood in order to alter blood volume and return the blood pressure to normal. The DCT actively absorbs sodium and is involved in potassium and hydrogen ion secretion. Calcium absorption can also occur here but this is influenced by parathyroid hormone (PTH) **(Fig. 3.80; Fig. 3.82)**.

The **juxtaglomerular apparatus** is a small complex near the vascular pole composed of the **macula densa** (of the DCT), **extraglomerular mesangial cells** (connective tissue cells near afferent and efferent arterioles) and the **juxtaglomerular cells** mainly of the afferent arterioles. Decreased blood volume and/or

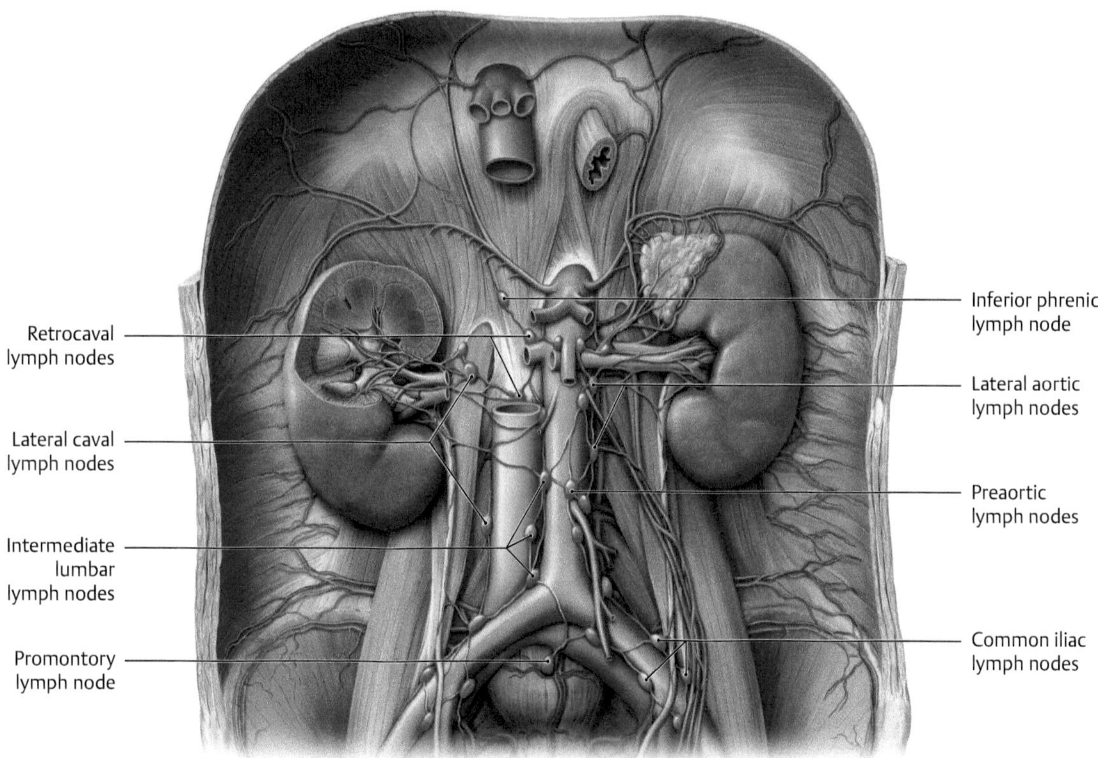

Fig. 3.79 Lymphatic drainage of the kidney, suprarenal gland, and ureter. (From Schuenke M, Schulte E, Schumacher U. THIEME Atlas of Anatomy. Internal Organs. Illustrations by Voll M and Wesker K. 3rd ed. New York: Thieme Medical Publishers; 2020.)

sodium concentration sensed by the macula densa, stimulates the juxtaglomerular cells to release the enzyme **renin**. Renin will activate the circulating angiotensinogen released by the liver to angiotensin I. Angiotensin I is then converted to angiotensin II by angiotensin-converting enzyme (ACE) while passing through the pulmonary vasculature of the lungs. Angiotensin II causes blood vessels to constrict, resulting in increased blood pressure and it also stimulates the secretion of the hormone *aldosterone* from the zona glomerulosa of the adrenal cortex. *Aldosterone* causes the tubules of the kidneys to increase the reabsorption of sodium and water into the blood, while at the same time causing the excretion of potassium thus maintaining the electrochemical balance. This increases the volume of extracellular fluid in the body, which then also increases blood pressure.

The DCT becomes the **connecting tubules** and they consist of a *simple cuboidal epithelium*. The collecting tubules are not part of the nephron but the first part of the **collecting duct system**, the final portion of the kidney that influences the electrolyte and fluid balance of the body. This system accounts for 4–5% of the kidney's reabsorption of sodium and water. The collecting tubules pass through the cortex and help form the collecting ducts at the medullary ray region of the cortex (**Fig. 3.82**).

The **collecting ducts** have a *simple cubodial epithelium* and consist of two different cell types: the principal and intercalated cells. The **principal cells** are found throughout the collecting duct and they mediate the collecting ducts' influence on sodium and potassium balance. The **intercalated cells** are located in between principal cells but most of these are located in the upper, cortical portions of the collecting duct. They actively transport and secrete hydrogen ions against high concentration gradients; this in turn modulates the acid-base balance of the body. The initial portion of the collecting duct is sensitive to aldosterone but the entire collecting duct is sensitive to antidiuretic hormone (ADH). When ADH is present, this allows for more reabsorption of water creating more concentrated urine instead of excessive amounts of diluted urine as in *diuresis*. After urine drains through the renal papilla connecting to a collecting duct, it passes through the minor calyx, major calyx and renal pelvis before reaching the ureter. All of these tissues have a *transitional epithelium* (**Fig. 3.80; Fig. 3.82**).

Clinical Correlate 3.47

Polycystic Kidney Disease

Polycystic kidney disease is an inherited disorder that is both autosomal dominant (ADPKD) and autosomal recessive (ARPKD). Bilaterally located, diffuse renal cysts that replace the normal kidney parenchyma characterize both of these disorders. There is a progressive renal insufficiency associated with the presence of these cysts of which there is no direct treatment to slow additional cyst formation. **ADPKD** is fairly common and occurs in 1 in4001,000 live births and cysts form from on all segments of the nephron but usually do not cause renal failure until adulthood. **ARPKD** is much rarer and may only be present in 1 in 20,000 live births. This progressive disorder involves cysts forming from the ascending limb and collecting ducts. The kidneys become very large and renal failure can occur during infancy or childhood.

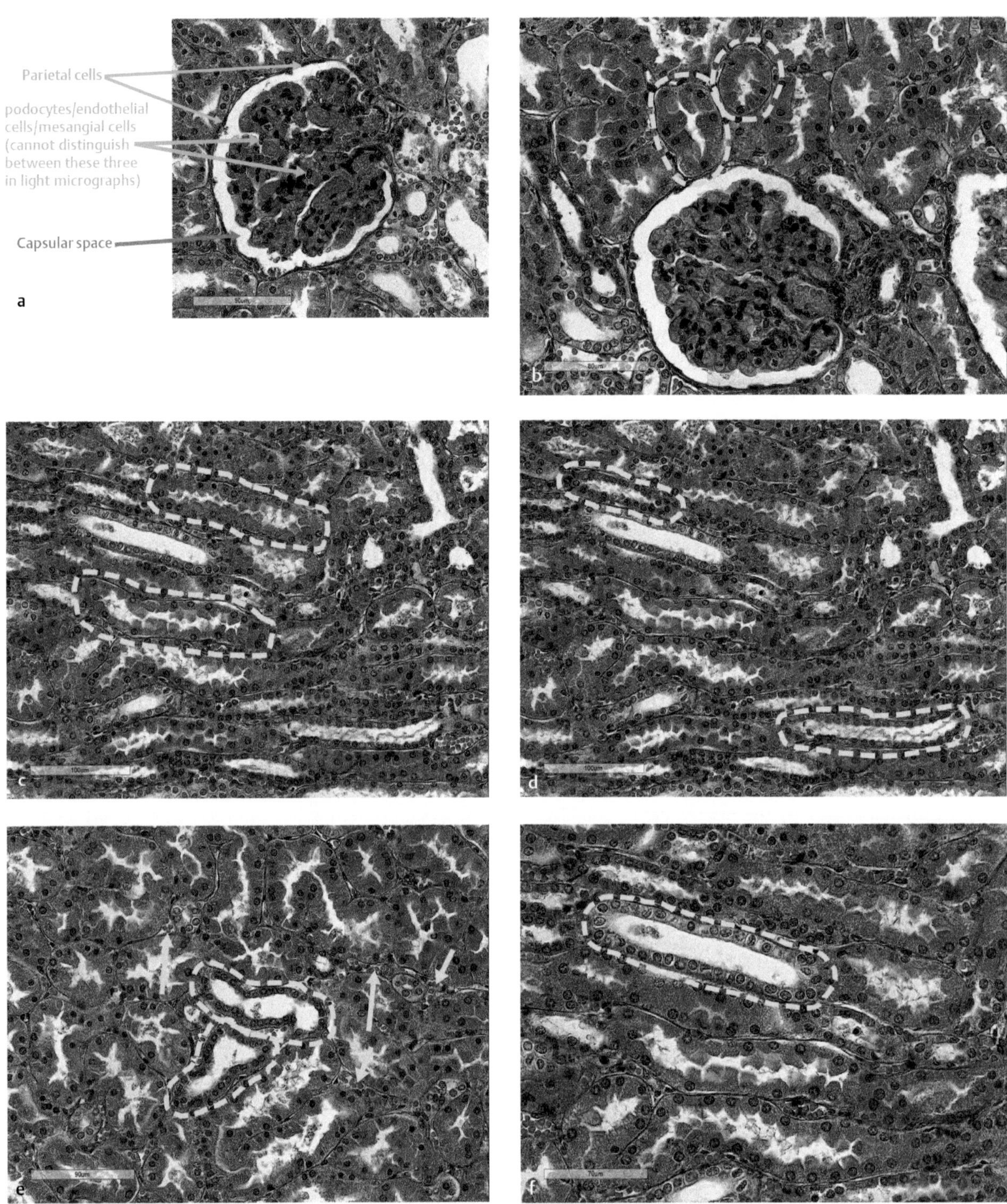

Fig. 3.80 Histology of the kidneys. **(a)** Renal corpuscle. **(b)** Proximal convoluted tubules (*outlined*). **(c)** Descending thick limbs of loop of Henle (*outlined*). **(d)** Ascending thick limbs of loops of Henle (*outlined*). **(e)** Distal convoluted tubules (*outlined*). Peritubular capillaries are indicated by the arrows. **(f)** Collecting duct (*outlined*). (From Lowrie DJ. Histology: An Essential Textbook. New York: Thieme Medical Publishers; 2020.)

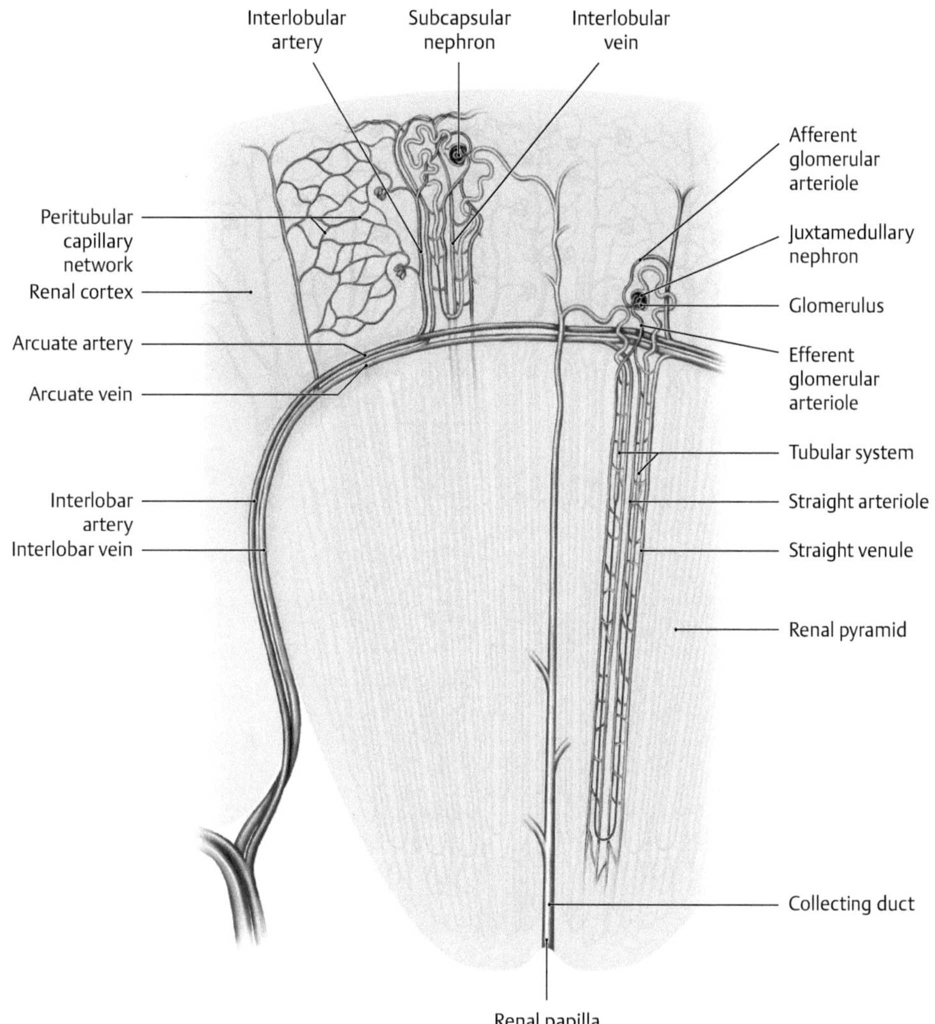

Fig. 3.81 Architecture of the renal vessels. (From Schuenke M, Schulte E, Schumacher U. THIEME Atlas of Anatomy. Internal Organs. Illustrations by Voll M and Wesker K. 3rd ed. New York: Thieme Medical Publishers; 2020.)

3.42 Ureter

The ureters are muscular ducts that transfer urine from the renal pelvis down to the urinary bladder (**Fig. 3.83**). They are approximately 25 cm (~10 in) in length and retroperitoneal. They are one of the most common structures damaged during general or gynecological surgery. The ureters run posterior to the gonadal vessels and anterior to the psoas muscle before reaching the pelvic brim. From here they cross over near the bifurcation of the common iliac into external iliac and internal iliac arteries. After entering the pelvis near its lateral wall, the ureters then curve anteromedially to enter the urinary bladder. There are three areas of constriction during the decent of the ureters (**Fig. 3.84**):

1. At the junction of the renal pelvis and ureter near the inferior renal pole.
2. As the ureters enter the pelvis near the bifurcation of the common iliac arteries.
3. As they traverse the urinary bladder.

3.42.1 Neurovasculature and Lymphatic Drainage of the Ureters

The **ureteric plexus**, which is distal from the renal plexus, contains autonomic fibers with the sympathetics acting primarily as vasoconstrictors. The autonomics in general have not been shown to have a large effect on peristaltic waves involving the ureter. Instead, peristaltic contractions are instigated by spontaneously depolarizing smooth muscles cells beginning at the renal pelvis (**Fig. 3.85**).

Blood supply to the ureters is segmental and from multiple smaller **ureter arteries**. The ureter artery branches originate from the *abdominal aorta, renal, ovarian* or *testicular arteries*. Venous drainage is by multiple and smaller **ureter veins** that drain to the renal, ovarian or testicular veins (**Fig. 3.86**).

Lymphatic drainage is also segmental. The *upper portion* of the ureter drains to the **lumbar lymph nodes**. The *middle portion* of the ureter drains mostly to the **common iliac lymph nodes** while the *lower portion* drains to the **external iliac** and **internal iliac lymph nodes** (**Fig. 3.87**).

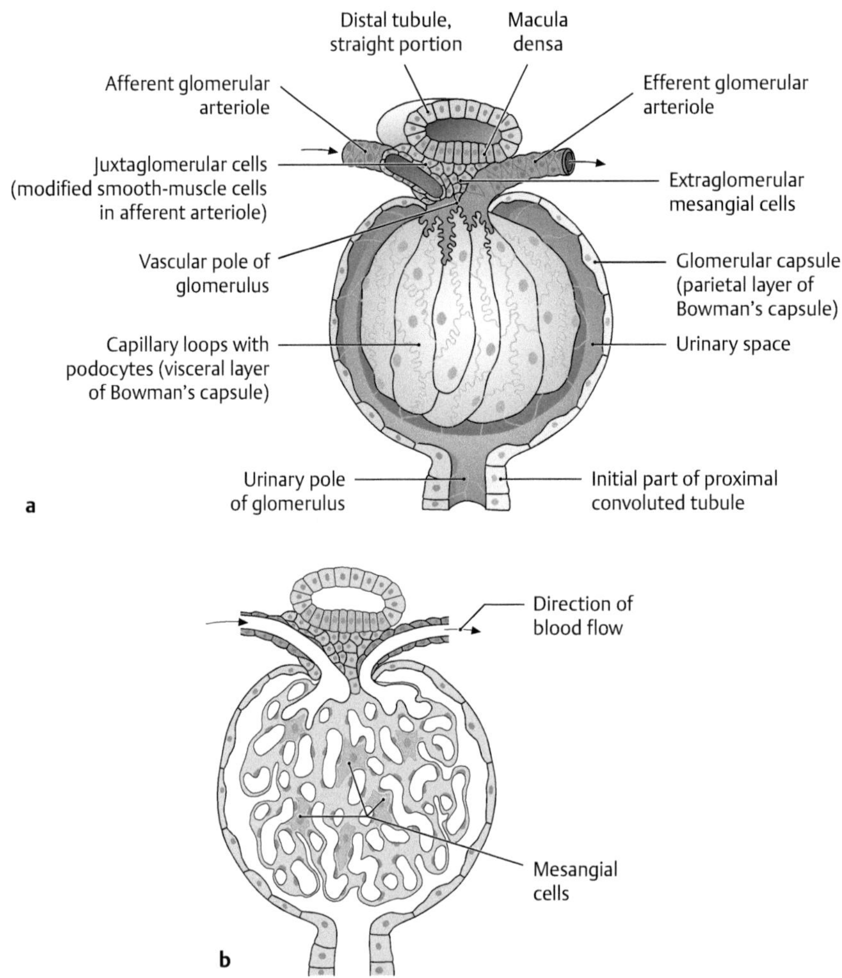

Fig. 3.82 Renal capsule **(a)** with the capsule opened **(b)** in section. (From Schuenke M, Schulte E, Schumacher U. THIEME Atlas of Anatomy. Internal Organs. Illustrations by Voll M and Wesker K. 3rd ed. New York: Thieme Medical Publishers; 2020.)

3.42.2 Histology of the Ureter

The mucosa has a stellate-shaped lumen lined with *transitional epithelium* and a lamina propria. The muscularis externa layer has an inner longitudinal and middle circular layer of smooth muscle. An outer longitudinal layer is present with the distal ureter near the bladder. The main function of the muscularis layer is to produce peristalsis and help propel the urine toward the urinary bladder. The mucosa creates a flap near the ureter/bladder junction and this helps prevent reflux of urine back into the ureter (**Fig. 3.88**).

3.43 Development of the Suprarenal Glands, Kidney, and Ureter

3.43.1 Suprarenal Gland Development

The cortex of the suprarenal gland develops from *mesoderm* while the medulla portion develops from *neuroectoderm*. The **cortex** develops from two different incidents of mesodermal proliferations. During the 5th week, mesothelial cells between the root of the dorsal mesentery and developing gonad begin to proliferate and penetrate the underlying mesenchyme. These cells differentiate into the **fetal (primitive) cortex**. Shortly after this, a second wave of cells from the mesothelium penetrates the mesenchyme and surrounds the fetal cortex. These cells will form the **adult (definitive) cortex** by the ninth week. The differentiation of the cortical zones begins during the late fetal period and first creates the *zona glomerulosa* and *zona fasciculata* layers. The *zona reticularis* will not be recognizable until approximately three years of age. This will also represent the same age that the fetal cortex will have completely disappeared by (**Fig. 3.89**).

As the fetal cortex is developing, neural crest cells cluster at the medial aspect of the fetal cortex and give rise to the **medulla**. The fetal and adult cortexes eventually surround the medulla. The neural crest cells differentiate into **chromaffin cells**, which are structurally similar to sympathetic postganglionic cell bodies. Chromaffin cells are scattered throughout the developing embryo but only persist in the medulla of the suprarenal gland as an adult.

3.43.2 Kidney Development

From an embryological standpoint, the urinary and genital systems are closely associated with one another. During the folding

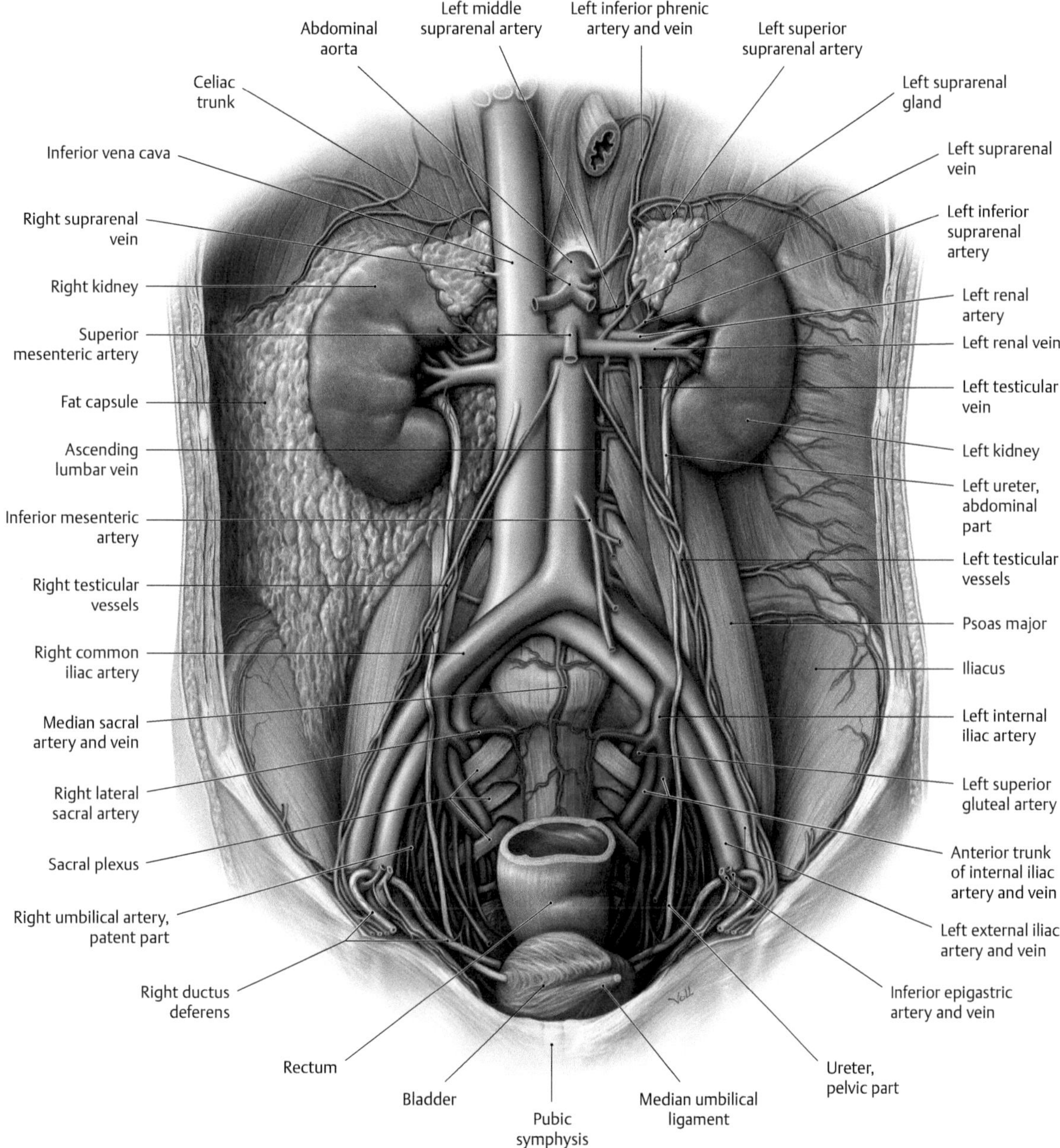

Fig. 3.83 Course of the ureter in the abdomen and pelvis. (From Schuenke M, Schulte E, Schumacher U. THIEME Atlas of Anatomy. Internal Organs. Illustrations by Voll M and Wesker K. 3rd ed. New York: Thieme Medical Publishers; 2020.)

Clinical Correlate 3.48

Renal and Ureteric Calculi

A **renal calculus** better known as a kidney stone distends the ureter and causes pain as it is forced through the ureter by peristaltic waves. A kidney stone is capable of partially or completely obstructing urinary flow and most are made of calcium while others are made from struvite, uric acid and cysteine. **Ureteric calculi** are the original kidney calculi that now lie in the ureter. If the stones are small enough they can generally just pass through without incidence. Risk factors include not staying properly hydrated and diets high in animal proteins, apple juice, grapefruit juice, high fructose corn syrup, refined sugars, oxalate and high sodium intake. The hallmark of this condition is the excruciating, intermittent pain radiating from the flank to the groin region known as **renal colic**.

Renal colic is commonly accompanied with the urgency to urinate, sweating, nausea, hematuria and restlessness. The pain comes in increments lasting 20-60 minutes and this corresponds to the peristaltic contractions of the ureter. Renal calculi are common in people suffering from Crohn's disease because it is associated with the malabsorption of magnesium and hyperoxaluria (excessive oxalate excretion while urinating).

Treatments begin with increasing water intake and taking a NSAID to curb the pain. **Extracorporeal shock wave lithotripsy (ESWL)** uses sound waves and the strong vibrations that come from them to break down larger stones into smaller stones. Larger stones may need to be surgically removed by way of **percutaneous nephrolithotomy** and this procedure uses small instruments through a posterior incision in order to remove the stones. An **ureteroscope** equipped with special tools can be passed through the urethra and bladder to reach the stone where they are then collected or broken up.

process of the embryo the intermediate mesoderm is carried ventrally and this results in it losing its connection with the somites. A longitudinal ridge of this mesoderm, known as the **urogenital ridge**, forms on each side of the dorsal aorta. This urogenital ridge has a **nephrogenic cord** region that gives rise to the urinary system along with a **gonadal ridge** that gives rise to the genital system (discussed in Chapter 4).

The **nephrogenic cord** develops into three sets of nephric structures/kidney systems that lie in a cranial-to-caudal sequence and in order: the **pronephros**, **mesonephros** and **metanephros** (**Fig. 3.90**).

- **Pronephros**: includes the *pronephric tubules* and a *pronephric duct.* They appear early during the fourth week and are located in the cervical region. The pronephros form **nephrotomes**, which are vestigial excretory units that regress before more caudal ones form. By the fifth week all signs of the pronephros have disappeared and thus are not functional in an adult.
- **Mesonephros**: includes the *mesonephric tubules* and a *mesonephric duct (Wolffian duct).* They appear during the 4th week and are located from the upper thoracic to upper

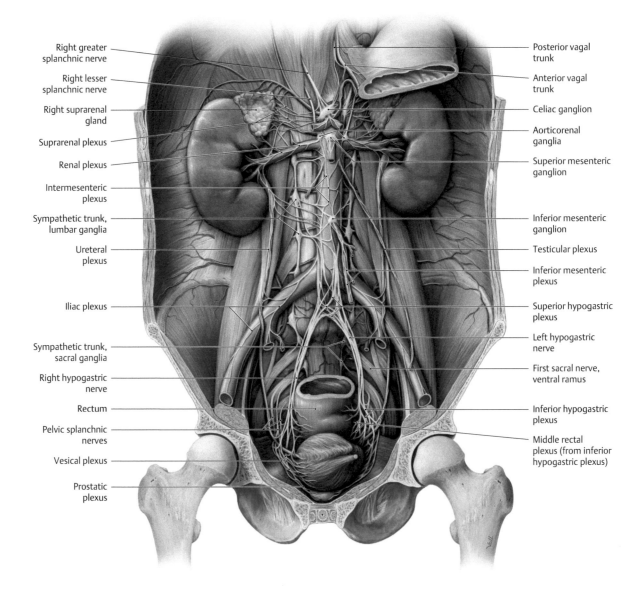

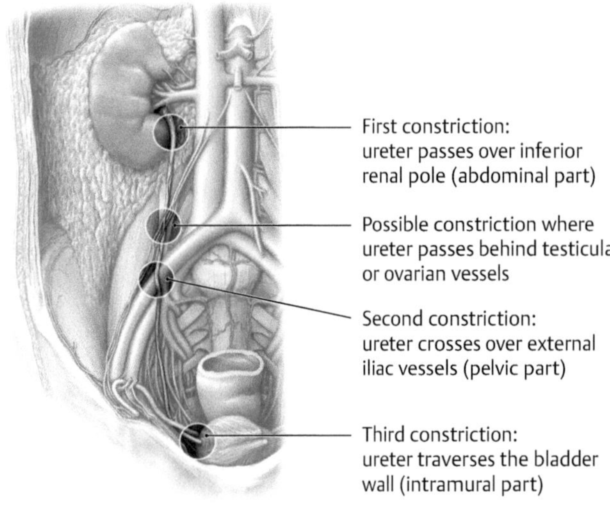

Fig. 3.84 Anatomical constructions of the ureter. (From Schuenke M, Schulte E, Schumacher U. THIEME Atlas of Anatomy. Internal Organs. Illustrations by Voll M and Wesker K. 3rd ed. New York: Thieme Medical Publishers; 2020.)

Fig. 3.85 Overview of the autonomic innervation of the urinary organs and suprarenal glands. (From Schuenke M, Schulte E, Schumacher U. THIEME Atlas of Anatomy. Internal Organs. Illustrations by Voll M and Wesker K. 3rd ed. New York: Thieme Medical Publishers; 2020.)

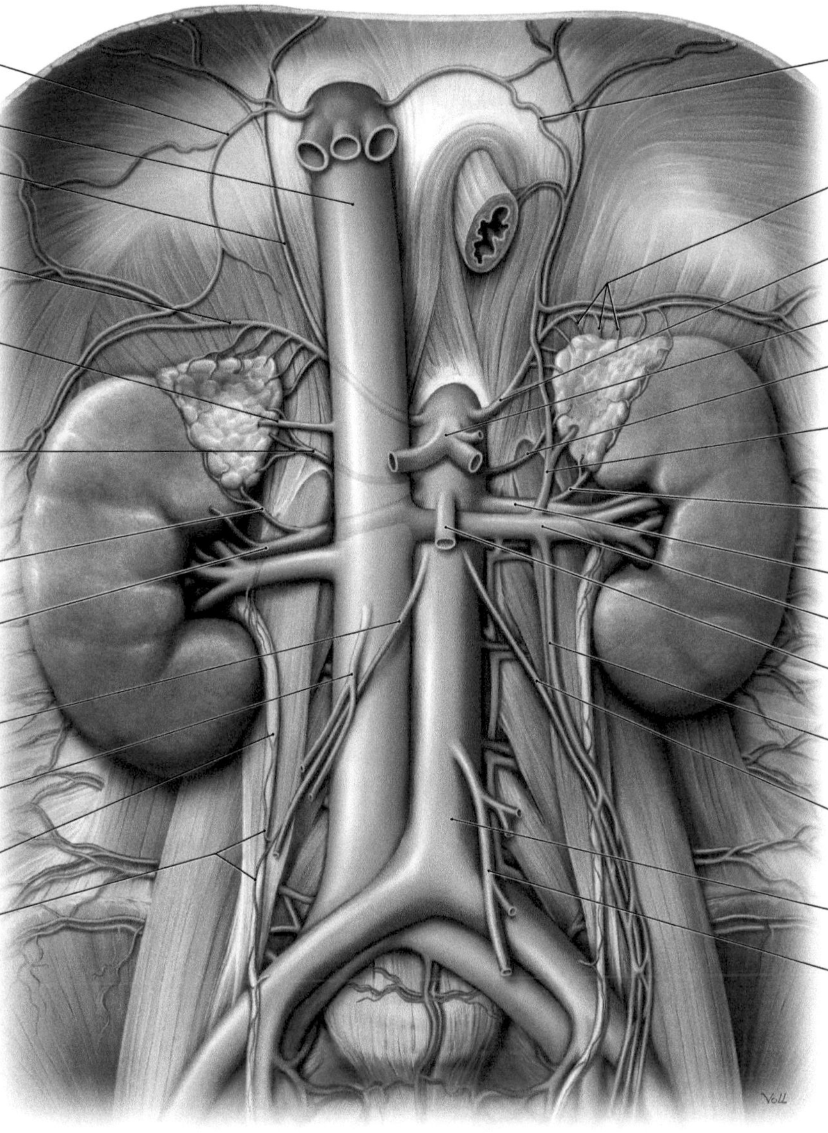

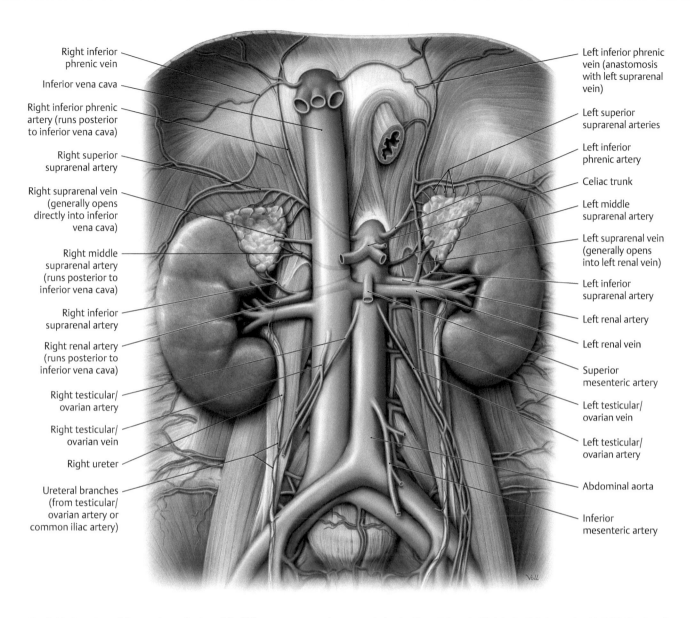

Right inferior phrenic vein
Inferior vena cava
Right inferior phrenic artery (runs posterior to inferior vena cava)
Right superior suprarenal artery
Right suprarenal vein (generally opens directly into inferior vena cava)
Right middle suprarenal artery (runs posterior to inferior vena cava)
Right inferior suprarenal artery
Right renal artery (runs posterior to inferior vena cava)
Right testicular/ ovarian artery
Right testicular/ ovarian vein
Right ureter
Ureteral branches (from testicular/ ovarian artery or common iliac artery)
Left inferior phrenic vein (anastomosis with left suprarenal vein)
Left superior suprarenal arteries
Left inferior phrenic artery
Celiac trunk
Left middle suprarenal artery
Left suprarenal vein (generally opens into left renal vein)
Left inferior suprarenal artery
Left renal artery
Left renal vein
Superior mesenteric artery
Left testicular/ ovarian vein
Left testicular/ ovarian artery
Abdominal aorta
Inferior mesenteric artery

Fig. 3.86 Overview of the arteries and veins of the kidneys, ureters, and suprarenal glands. (From Schuenke M, Schulte E, Schumacher U. THIEME Atlas of Anatomy. Internal Organs. Illustrations by Voll M and Wesker K. 3rd ed. New York: Thieme Medical Publishers; 2020.)

Abdominal aorta
Lateral lymph nodes
Inferior vena cava
Right ureter, abdominal part
Common iliac artery
External iliac lymph nodes
External iliac artery
Internal iliac lymph nodes
Internal iliac artery
Right ureter, pelvic part

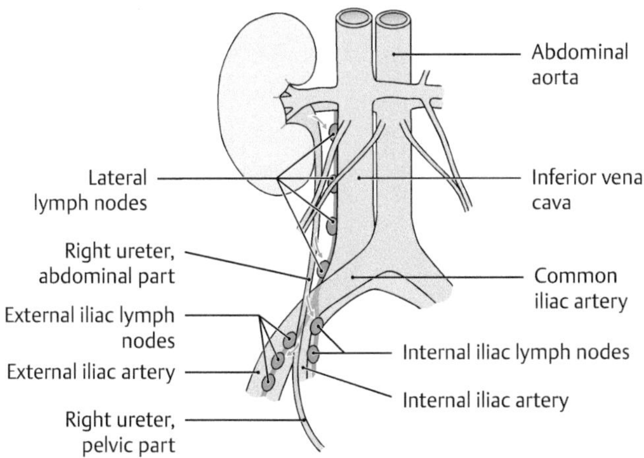

Fig. 3.87 Lymph nodes of the ureter. (From Schuenke M, Schulte E, Schumacher U. THIEME Atlas of Anatomy. Internal Organs. Illustrations by Voll M and Wesker K. 3rd ed. New York: Thieme Medical Publishers; 2020.)

lumbar regions. They lengthen rapidly and form an S-shaped loop, and acquire a tuft of capillaries that form a *glomerulus* at their medial end. Around the **glomerulus**, the tubules form **Bowman's capsule**, and together these structures constitute a **renal corpuscle**. Laterally, the tubules enter the longitudinal *mesonephric duct*. Most *mesonephric tubules* regress but the *mesonephric duct* persists and opens into the urogenital sinus. For a short period the mesonephros is functional. With the more caudal tubules still differentiating, the cranial most tubules and glomeruli disappear for the most part by the end of the second month.

- **Metanephros**, appears during the fifth week and develops from an outgrowth of the mesonephric duct called the **ureteric bud** and from a condensation of mesoderm within the nephrogenic cord called the **metanephric blastema.** This is the most caudal nephric structure and becomes functional at approximately the tenth week of development. The metanephros becomes the **permanent adult kidney**.

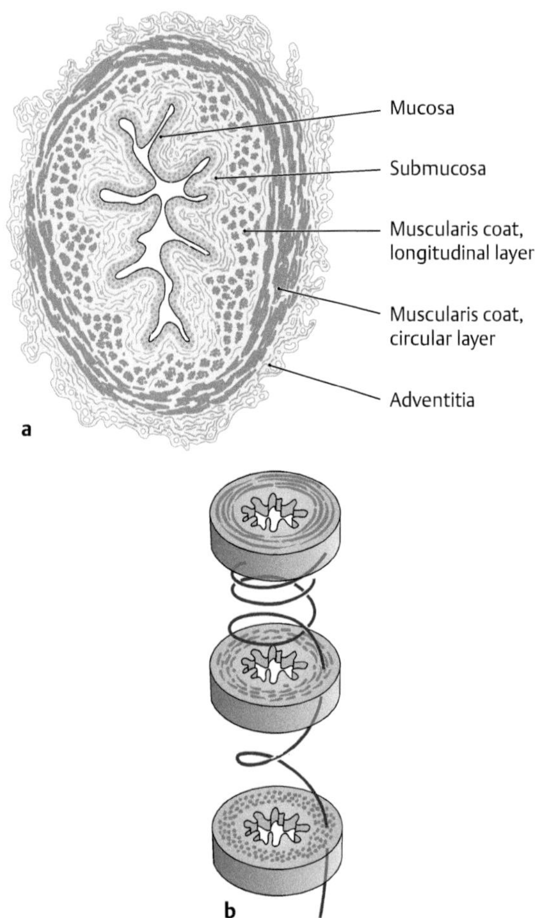

Fig. 3.88 (a) Wall structure of the ureter. **(b)** Arrangement of the ureter musculature. (From Schuenke M, Schulte E, Schumacher U. THIEME Atlas of Anatomy. Internal Organs. Illustrations by Voll M and Wesker K. 3rd ed. New York: Thieme Medical Publishers; 2020.)

The kidney is initially located in the pelvis at about the S1-S2 vertebral level. Hence, the kidneys must ascend because their final adult positions are in the upper lumbar region. The hilum of a kidney is initially facing anteriorly but after a *90° rotation inward*, they point toward the midline. As kidneys ascend their blood originates from arteries that continuously form and regress. If one of these arteries does not regress they persist as **supernumerary arteries**.

3.43.3 Collecting System

The **ureteric bud**, which is an outgrowth of the mesonephric duct near the cloaca, penetrates the **metanephric blastema** and subsequently dilates to form the **renal pelvis (Fig. 3.90; Fig. 3.91)**. The section of the ureteric bud extending from the mesonephric duct to the renal pelvis becomes the **ureters**. From the renal pelvis, the bud splits and undergoes repeated branching in order to develop into the **major calyces, minor calyces**, and the **collecting tubules/ ducts**. The ureteric bud thus gives rise to the ureters, renal pelvis, major and minor calyces and about 1-2 million collecting ducts.

3.43.4 Nephron/Excretory System

The newly formed collecting ducts are covered at their distal end by a **metanephric tissue cap**.

The collecting ducts induce these metanephric tissue caps to differentiate into **renal (metanephric) vesicles**, which later give rise to small **S-shaped renal tubules** that are critical to formation of the nephron. The S-shaped renal tubules differentiate into **Bowman's capsule, proximal convoluted tubule, loop of Henle, distal convoluted tubule** and the **connecting tubule (Fig. 3.92)**. Capillaries protrude into Bowman's capsule and differentiate into **glomeruli**. Together the glomeruli and Bowman's capsule constitute a **renal corpuscle**.

The **nephron** extends from the renal corpuscle to the distal convoluted tubule. The connecting tubule is generally considered part of the collecting system although it developed from the renal tubule. Structural formation of a nephron is complete at birth and there are 1-2 million of them. Functional maturation continues through infancy but the definitive kidney has been functional since the 12th week of development.

3.44 Lumbar Plexus and Vasculature of the Posterior Abdominal Wall

The somatic nerves located in the posterior abdominal wall are the subcostal nerve and nerves of the lumbar plexus. The

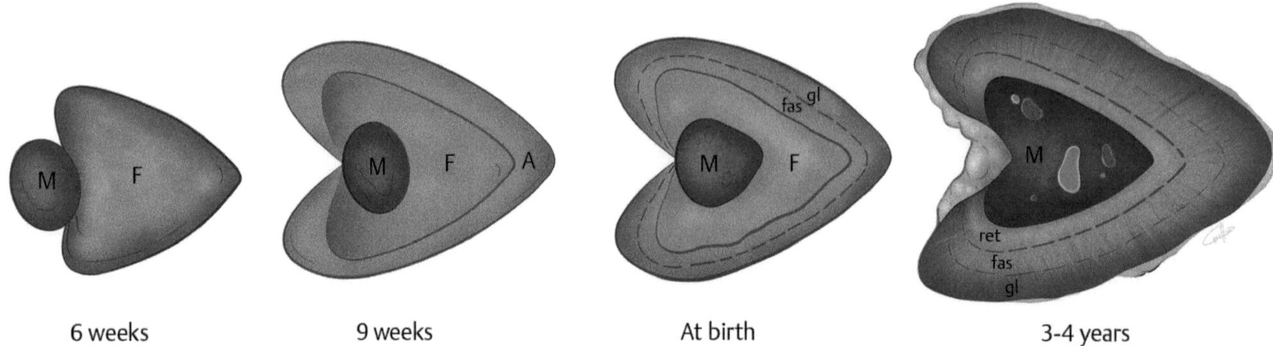

Fig. 3.89 Development of the suprarenal glands. Illustration by Calla Heald.

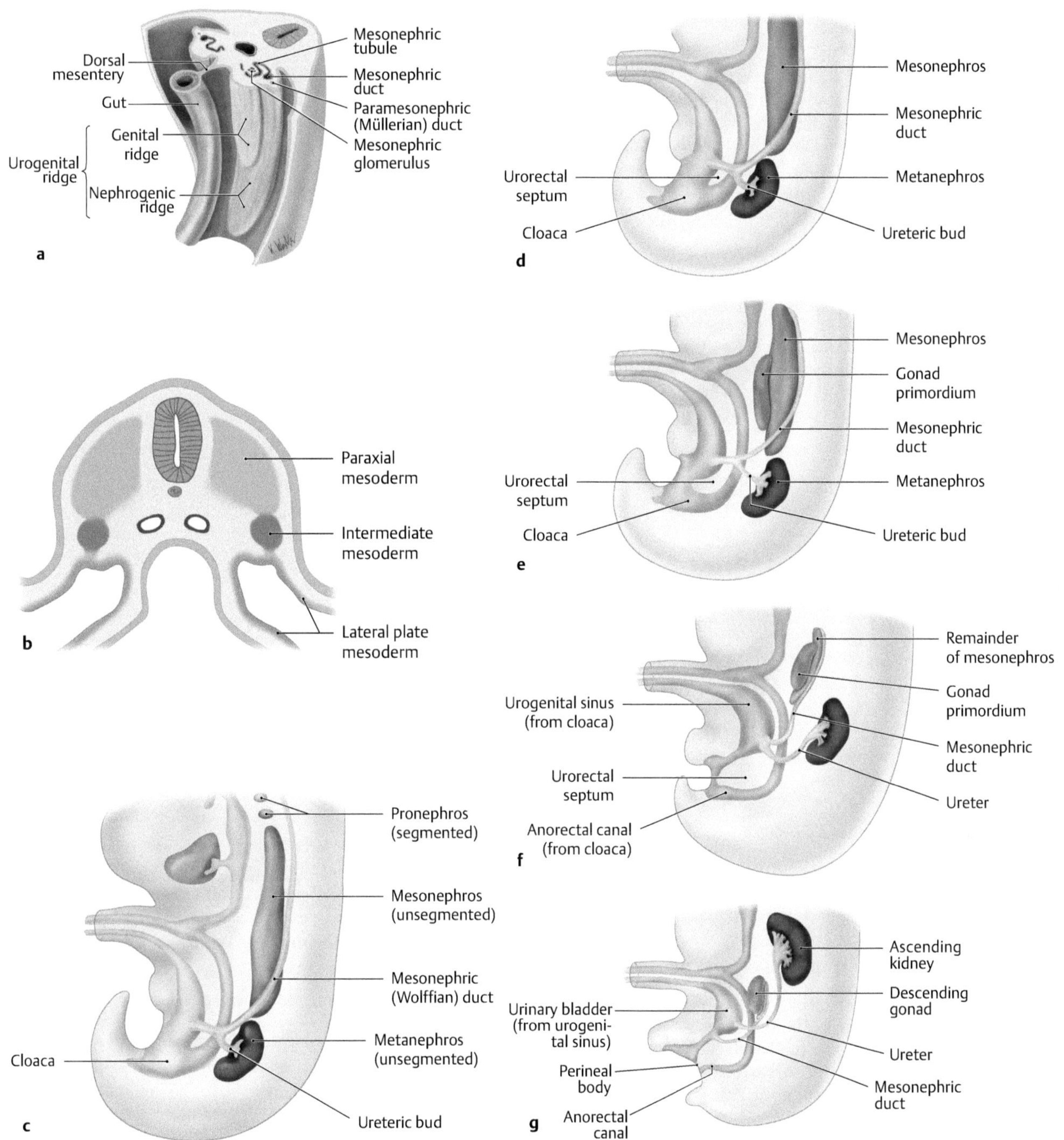

Fig. 3.90 Kidney development. **(a)** The urogenital ridge consists of the nephrogenic cord and gonadal ridge. **(b)** Cross-section of an embryo, approx. 21 days, cranial view. **(c)** Location of the developing renal primordia and what they would look like if they all existed in the embryo at the same time. **(d)** the metanephros appears during the fifth week in the most caudal portion of the intermediate mesoderm. The ureteric bud sprouts from the mesonephric duct and grows into the metanephros. **(e-g)** The metanephros and ureteric bud grow from the pelvic region in a cranila direction and later come to lie just below the diaphragm. This ascent is partially the result of a reduction of bending and increased growth of the sacro-lumbar region of the embryo. (From Schuenke M, Schulte E, Schumacher U. THIEME Atlas of Anatomy. Internal Organs. Illustrations by Voll M and Wesker K. 3rd ed. New York: Thieme Medical Publishers; 2020.)

subcostal nerve is the ventral rami branch of T12. It will pass posterior to the lateral arcuate ligament and on the anterior surface of the quadratus lumborum before entering a neurovascular plane between the transversus abdominis and internal oblique muscles.

The **lumbar plexus** is a network of ventral rami branches from L1-L4 (**Fig. 3.93**). It is first located anterior to the lumbar transverse processes and can be exposed by removing the psoas major muscle. It is further divided into a group of either anterior or posterior portions of ventral rami branches. Its branches contribute to the innervation of the anterolateral abdominal wall, scrotum, labia majora, and the anterior and medial thighs. Beginning from the superior most part of the plexus and extending down near the pelvis the lumbar plexus consists of:

Clinical Correlate 3.49

Congenital Anomalies of Kidney Placement

The most common form of renal ectopia is a **pelvic kidney**. With this birth defect, generally only one of the kidneys fails to ascend towards the posterior abdominal wall. It is estimated that this occurs in about 1 in 1000 live births, but pelvic kidneys have been associated with other abnormalities such as vascular and genital anomalies as well as agenesis of the contralateral kidney. An individual may remain asymptomatic their life but they do have a greater chance of having kidney stones or a urinary tract infection.

A **horseshoe kidney** occurs in about 1 in 500 live births and is characterized by fusion of the lower poles of the two kidneys during their initial ascent towards the posterior abdominal wall. The now fused kidney is prevented from reaching the posterior abdominal wall by the inferior mesenteric artery. Around one-third of these children also present with another anomaly related to the genitourinary, cardiovascular or central nervous systems.

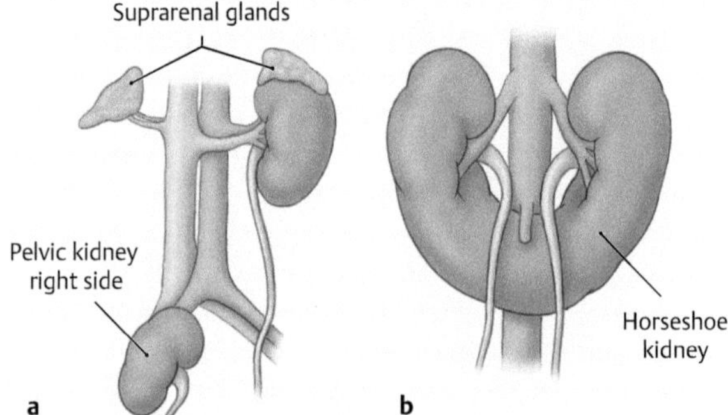

(a) Pelvic kidney. **(b)** Horseshoe kidney. (From Schuenke M, Schulte E, Schumacher U. THIEME Atlas of Anatomy. Internal Organs. Illustrations by Voll M and Wesker K. 3rd ed. New York: Thieme Medical Publishers; 2020.)

Clinical Correlate 3.50

Additional Renal Conditions

Wilm's tumor is a rare cancer (nephroblastoma) of the kidneys that generally affects children by 3-4 years of age but may also occur in the fetus. It is due to mutations in the WT1 gene on the 11p13 chromosome. It tends to recapitulate different stages of the embryological formation of the kidney thus displaying a metanephric blastema and portions of the stroma and epithelium.

Renal dysplasia is abnormal tissue development resulting in immature nephrons of the renal parenchyma that can be confined to a small section of one or both kidneys. There is an incidence rate of approximately 1 in 4,000 individuals. **Renal hypoplasia** is a congenitally small kidney containing normal levels of parenchyma but have smaller calyces, papillae and lobules. **Renal agenesis** is when the ureteric bud has failed to form thus eliminating the induction of the renal vesicles and nephron formation. Two forms exist:

- *Unilateral*: is relatively common (1 in 1,000) so a physician should not assume every patient has two kidneys. It is generally asymptomatic because the remaining kidney hypertrophies. These individuals do have a higher rate of developing hypertension.
- *Bilateral*: is relatively uncommon (1 in 3,000) and it causes oligohydramnios (amniotic fluid deficiency) that results in compression of the fetus leading to **Potter syndrome/ sequence**. These fetuses will display wrinkly skin, deformed limbs, abnormal facial appearances and are usually stillborn.

Clinical Correlate 3.51

Duplications of the Kidney and Ureter

If the ureteric bud divides prematurely before it penetrates the metanephric blastema this results in either a **double kidney** or a **duplicated ureter**. If there are two ureters draining a single kidney this is commonly called a *duplex kidney*. Most individuals are asymptomatic and are generally diagnosed by accident while the patient is in the clinic for another issue.

Clinical Correlate 3.52

Ureterocele

An **ureterocele** is a cyst-like protrusion of the ureter that is caused by a ureteral opening near the bladder being abnormally small resulting in the obstruction of urine flow. A **simple ureterocele** is located at the distal ureter and is a protrusion into the submucosal layer of the bladder. An **ectopic ureterocele** masks the simple version but is generally seen when there is a duplication of the ureters. An ureterocele predisposes individuals to kidney infections and *vesicoureteral reflux*, or the backward flow of urine from the bladder into the kidneys. The normal one-way valve that is seen at the junction between the ureter and bladder is quite distorted allowing for reflux to occur. Most ureteroceles are diagnosed before the age of two and present with flank, back or abdominal pain, excessive and painful urination, and possibly blood present in the urine.

- **Iliohypogastric** and **ilioinguinal nerves** (L1): the iliohypogastric nerve normally lies just superior to the ilioinguinal nerve. It may begin as an isolated L1 branch before bifurcating near the ASIS so its course is variable. Both pass through the same neurovascular plane as the subcostal nerve does and innervate anterolateral abdominal wall muscles as well as the skin of the inguinal and pubic regions.
- **Lateral femoral cutaneous** (L2-L3): this nerve lies against the iliacus muscle between the iliac crest and psoas major muscle, passes deep to the inguinal ligament just medial to the ASIS, and innervates the skin of the anterolateral thigh.
- **Femoral nerve** (L2-L4): located just lateral and deep to the psoas major muscle and presents as a fairly individual and bulky nerve. Just after passing deep to the inguinal ligament and entering the anterior thigh, the femoral nerve branches into many individual nerves that target muscles primarily involved in hip flexion and knee extension.
- **Genitofemoral nerve** (L1-L2): is found on the superficial surface of the psoas major muscle running towards the inguinal and femoral regions. The genital branch innervates the cremaster muscle and skin of the anterior scrotum in the male while in the female it is only sensory to the anterior labia majora. The femoral branch in both sexes innervates skin of the upper anterior thigh.
- **Obturator nerve** (L2-L4): is found on the medial border of the psoas major muscle and course into the lesser pelvis before passing through the *obturator foramen*. This nerve innervates muscles located in the medial thigh that function mainly in hip adduction. An **accessory obturator nerve** (L3-L4) is present in a small percentage of individuals and is located just lateral to the obturator nerve. It generally replaces the femoral nerve branch innervating the pectineus muscle with itself. This is the

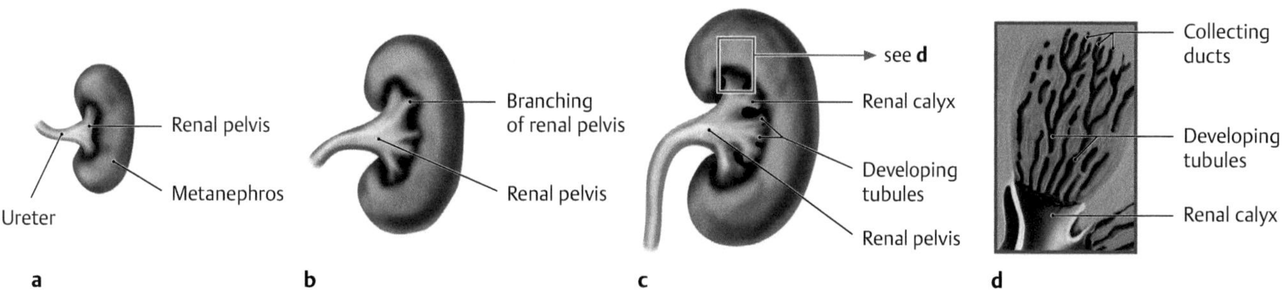

Fig. 3.91 (a-d) Development of the collecting system. The ureteric bud gives rise to the ureters, renal pelvis, major and minor calyces, and collecting **ducts.** (From Schuenke M, Schulte E, Schumacher U. THIEME Atlas of Anatomy. Internal Organs. Illustrations by Voll M and Wesker K. 3rd ed. New York: Thieme Medical Publishers; 2020.)

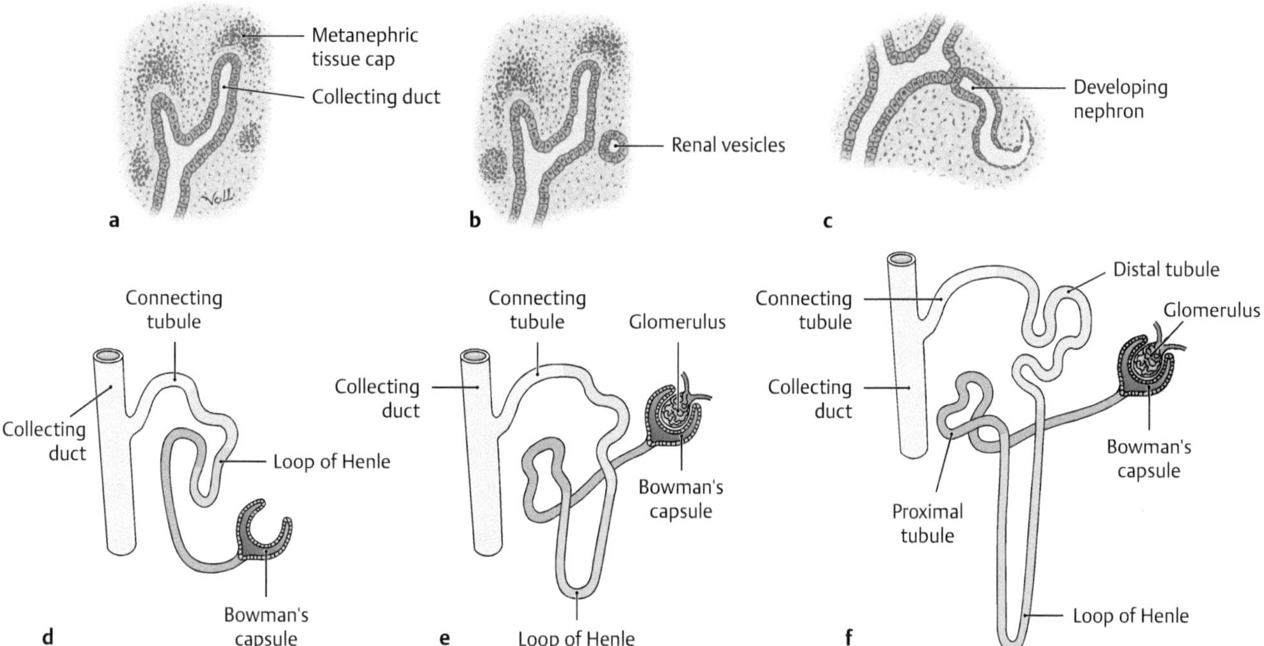

Fig. 3.92 Development of the nephron/excretory system. Nephron formation is induced by branching of the ureteric bud, with each terminal collecting duct being covered by a metanephric tissue cap **(a)**. Cells of the tissue cap move laterally and develop into renal vesicles **(b)**. Each vesicle gives rise to a small S-shaped tubule **(c)**. While segments of the tubule continue to differentiate and elongate, its distal end, the connecting tubule, connects it to a collecting duct **(d)**. Its proximal end (Bowman's capsule) becomes invaginated by a tuft of capillaries (the glomerulus), which is supplied by a branch of the renal artery **(e)**. Continuous lengthening and differentiation of the tubules result in the formation of the tubular system including the loop of Henle **(f)**. The loop of Henle helps to concentrate primary urine (approximately 170 liters every 24 hours) to 1% of its volume to produce the final urine. At the start of the 13th week, almost 20% of nephrons are functional and can form urine. (From Schuenke M, Schulte E, Schumacher U. THIEME Atlas of Anatomy. Internal Organs. Illustrations by Voll M and Wesker K. 3rd ed. New York: Thieme Medical Publishers; 2020.)

reason the pectineus muscle can be innervated by either the femoral or accessory obturator nerve.

The *sympathetic trunk* located near the lumbar vertebrae delivers sym/post fibers by way of the *gray rami communicantes*. Due to this, the functional components of these nerves are either true motor nerves or cutaneous sensory nerves with sym/post fibers. The functional components of a motor branch would contain GSE, GSA, GVE-sym/post while a cutaneous sensory branch has GSA and GVE-sym/post.

The **abdominal aorta** is the major artery located in this region and it lies to the left of the IVC. It has many branches that are responsible for supplying portions of the foregut, midgut and hindgut as well as the diaphragm and visceral structures of the posterior abdominal wall. It begins at the aortic hiatus (T12) and ends as a bifurcation into common iliac arteries (L4). Branches from the abdominal aorta are said to be associated with a particular vascular plane, these include the *anterior midline*, *lateral* and *posterolateral vascular planes*. The vertebral levels of the arteries associated with these planes are given in **(Fig. 3.94)**.

The **anterior midline vascular plane** is made up of three *unpaired visceral* arteries responsible for blood supply destined for the GI tract. These include the **celiac trunk** (T12), **superior mesenteric** (L1) and the **inferior mesenteric** (L3). These arteries and their related branches supply the foregut, midgut and hindgut, respectively.

The **lateral vascular plane** is made up of three *paired visceral* arteries responsible for the blood supply to urogenital and

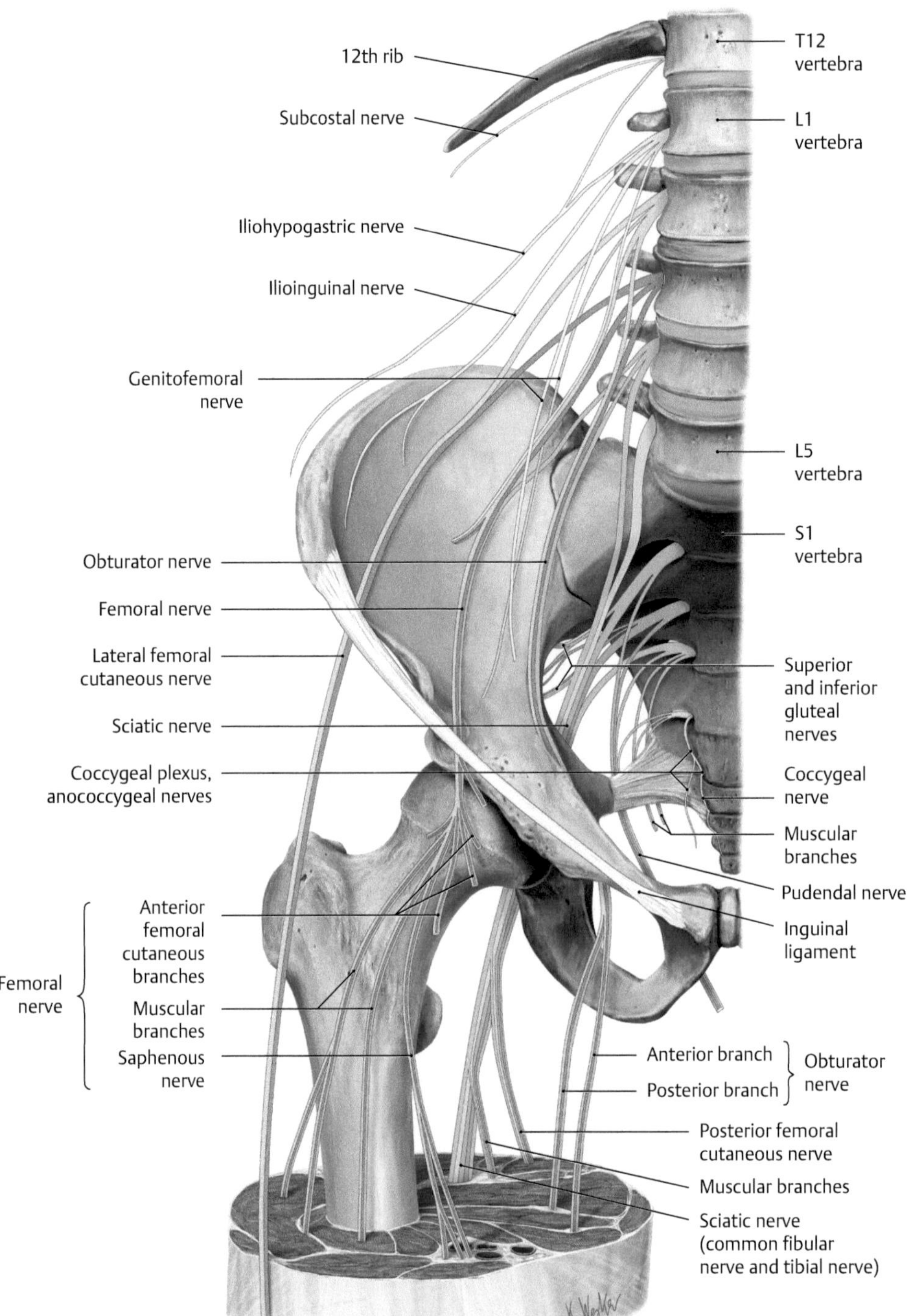

Fig. 3.93 Lumbar plexus of the posterior abdominal wall. (From Schuenke M, Schulte E, Schumacher U. THIEME Atlas of Anatomy. General Anatomy and Musculoskeletal System. Illustrations by Voll M and Wesker K. 3rd ed. New York: Thieme Medical Publishers; 2020.)

endocrine visceral organs. These include the **middle suprarenal** (L1), **renal** (L1/L2) and **gonadal arteries** (L2). These arteries are responsible for supplying the suprarenal glands, kidneys and gonads. The *superior suprarenals* (inferior phrenic br.) and *inferior suprarenals* (renal br.) are both bilateral and contribute to the suprarenal blood supply but come from arteries located somewhere between the T12 and L1 vertebral levels but are not considered part of this plane.

The **posterolateral vascular plane** is made up of three *paired parietal* or segmental arteries responsible for supplying blood to the diaphragm and outer body wall. These arteries include the **subcostal** (T12), **inferior phrenic** (T12) and **lumbar arteries** (L1-L4). The **median sacral artery** is an *unpaired parietal* branch off of the bifurcation of the abdominal aorta at L4. It branches off a pair of 5th lumbar arteries which are markedly small and do not supply much.

The **inferior vena cava** is formed by the left and right common iliac veins at vertebral level L5 and lies to the right of the abdominal aorta. It ascends through the abdomen and eventually passes through the caval opening of the diaphragm before terminating

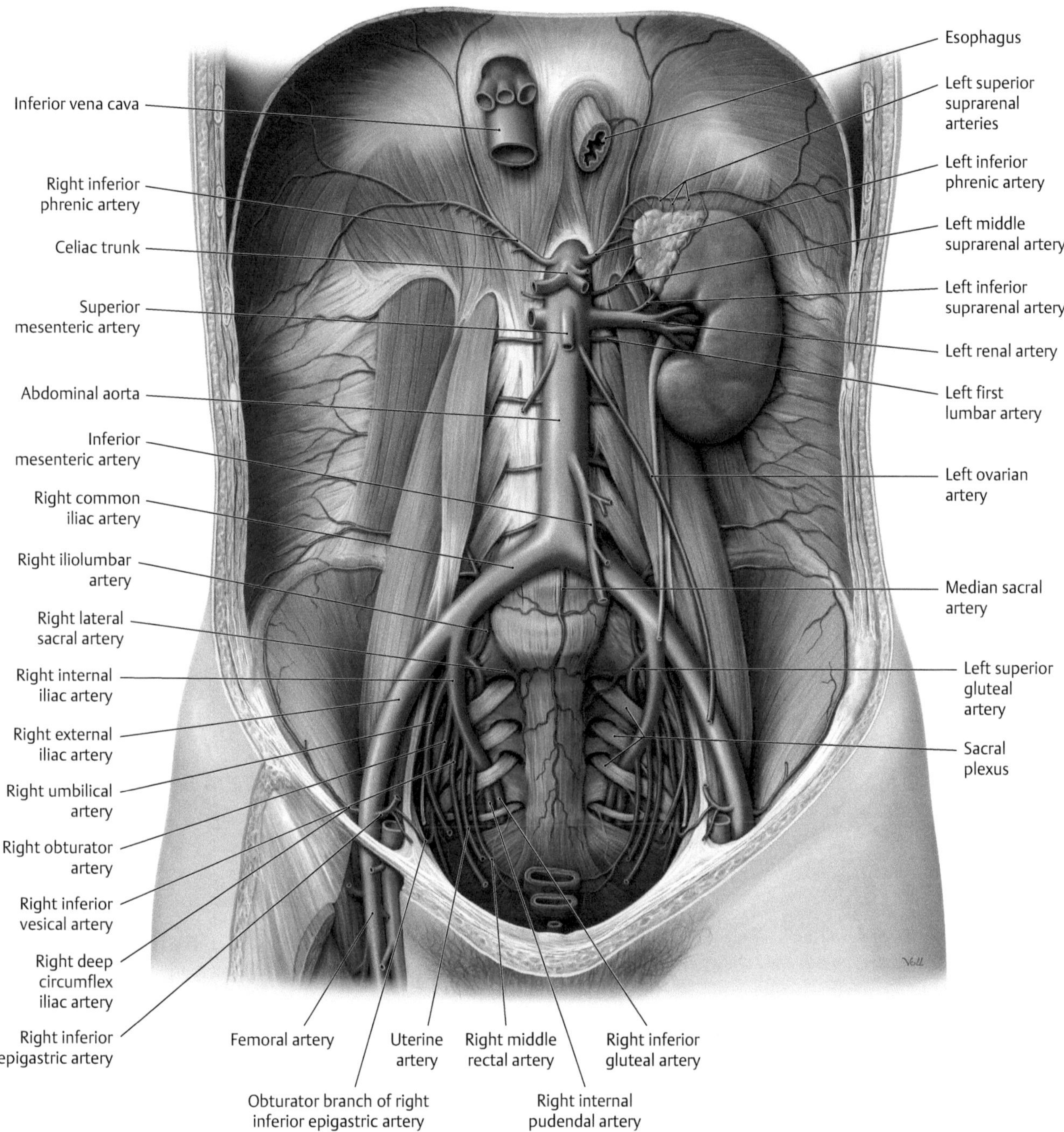

Fig. 3.94 Overview of the abdominal aorta and pelvic arteries (abdominal organs removed). (From Schuenke M, Schulte E, Schumacher U. THIEME Atlas of Anatomy. Internal Organs. Illustrations by Voll M and Wesker K. 3rd ed. New York: Thieme Medical Publishers; 2020.)

at the right atrium of the heart. The IVC receives blood from the following veins **(Fig. 3.95)**:

- **Left** and **right common iliac** (L5).
- **3**rd (L3) and **4**th **lumbar** (L4). The other lumbar veins tend to be tributaries of veins that eventually reach the IVC such as the ascending lumbar, renal and the L3 lumbar vein itself.
- **Ascending lumbar**: the precursor to the azygos and hemiazygos veins.
- **Right gonadal vein (testicular/ovarian)**: the left gonadal vein drains into the left renal vein, not the IVC.
- **Left** and **right renal veins** (L1): the veins drain the kidney with the left one passing over the abdominal aorta before draining into the IVC.
- **Right suprarenal vein**: the left suprarenal vein drains into the left renal vein. These veins drain the suprarenal gland.
- **Hepatic veins** (T8/T9): the left, middle and right hepatic veins drain the liver.
- **Left** and **right inferior phrenic veins**: drain the diaphragm.

Lymph nodes in the abdomen are predominately found near an artery. The general lymphatic drainage of this region begins at the

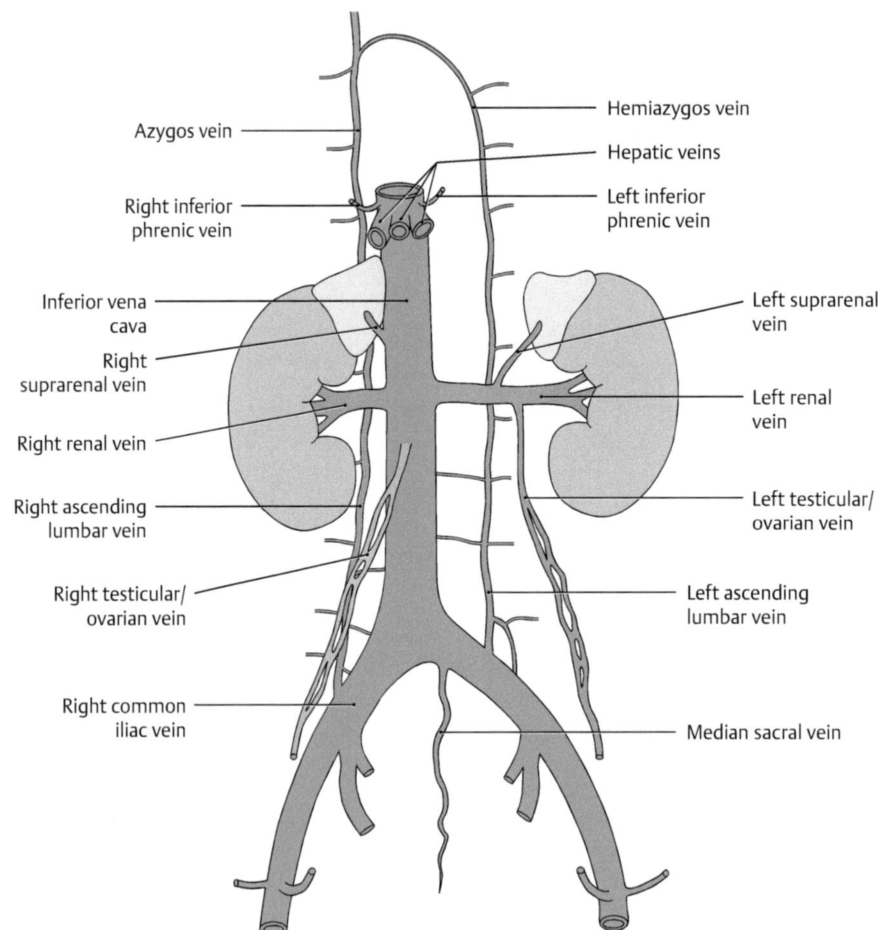

Fig. 3.95 Tributaries of the inferior vena cava. (From Schuenke M, Schulte E, Schumacher U. THIEME Atlas of Anatomy. Internal Organs. Illustrations by Voll M and Wesker K. 3rd ed. New York: Thieme Medical Publishers; 2020.)

common iliac lymph nodes of which they received lymph from both the *external iliac* and *internal iliac lymph nodes* that drained mostly the lower limbs and pelvic region. Lymph from the common iliacs ascends to the **lumbar lymph nodes** and these lymph nodes receive drainage from not only the posterior abdominal wall but also areas such as the gonads, pelvic viscera, and parts of the urinary system and GI tract.

Lymph continues superiorly towards a larger network of **preaortic lymph nodes** that include the **inferior mesenteric, superior mesenteric** and **celiac lymph nodes**. Lymph originating from the GI tract passes back with the main artery that supplies that part of the gut meaning structures of the foregut mostly drain to the celiac lymph nodes because it receives its arterial supply form branches of the celiac trunk. Lymph eventually reaches the **cisterna chyli**, a smaller sac-like structure located between the vertebral levels L1-L2 and at the inferior end of the **thoracic duct (Fig. 3.96)**.

The thoracic duct passes through the aortic hiatus and eventually terminates at the left venous angle between the left internal jugular and subclavian veins. Lymph from the lower limbs, pelvis, abdomen, left half of the thorax, left upper limb and left half of the head and neck drain to the thoracic duct. The right half of the thorax, head and neck and right upper limb all drain to the **right lymphatic duct** before reaching the right venous angle between the right internal jugular and subclavian veins.

3.45 Autonomic Innervation of the GI Tract and Posterior Abdominal Wall

The abdominal viscera are innervated by visceral efferent (GVE) parasympathetic (para) and sympathetic (sym) and visceral sensory (GVA) fibers. The parasympathetic fibers are delivered by way of the vagal trunks originally of the vagus nerve (CN X) and pelvic splanchnic nerves. They do not synapse at a ganglion until reaching the target organ. The sympathetic fibers are delivered initially by way of multiple splanchnic nerves, which after synapsing at a ganglion associated with the aortic plexus follow a peri-arterial plexus to their target organ. The only instance that a synapse does not occur at a ganglion associated with the aortic ganglion is in the case involving innervation to the medulla of the suprarenal gland **(Fig. 3.97)**.

3.45.1 Aortic Nerve Plexus

The major visceral nerve plexus associated with the innervation to the abdominal viscera and lying adjacent to the abdominal aorta is the **aortic plexus (Fig. 3.98)**. There are smaller plexuses that help define the larger aortic plexus and these include the **celiac, superior mesenteric**, **intermesenteric** and the **inferior mesenteric**

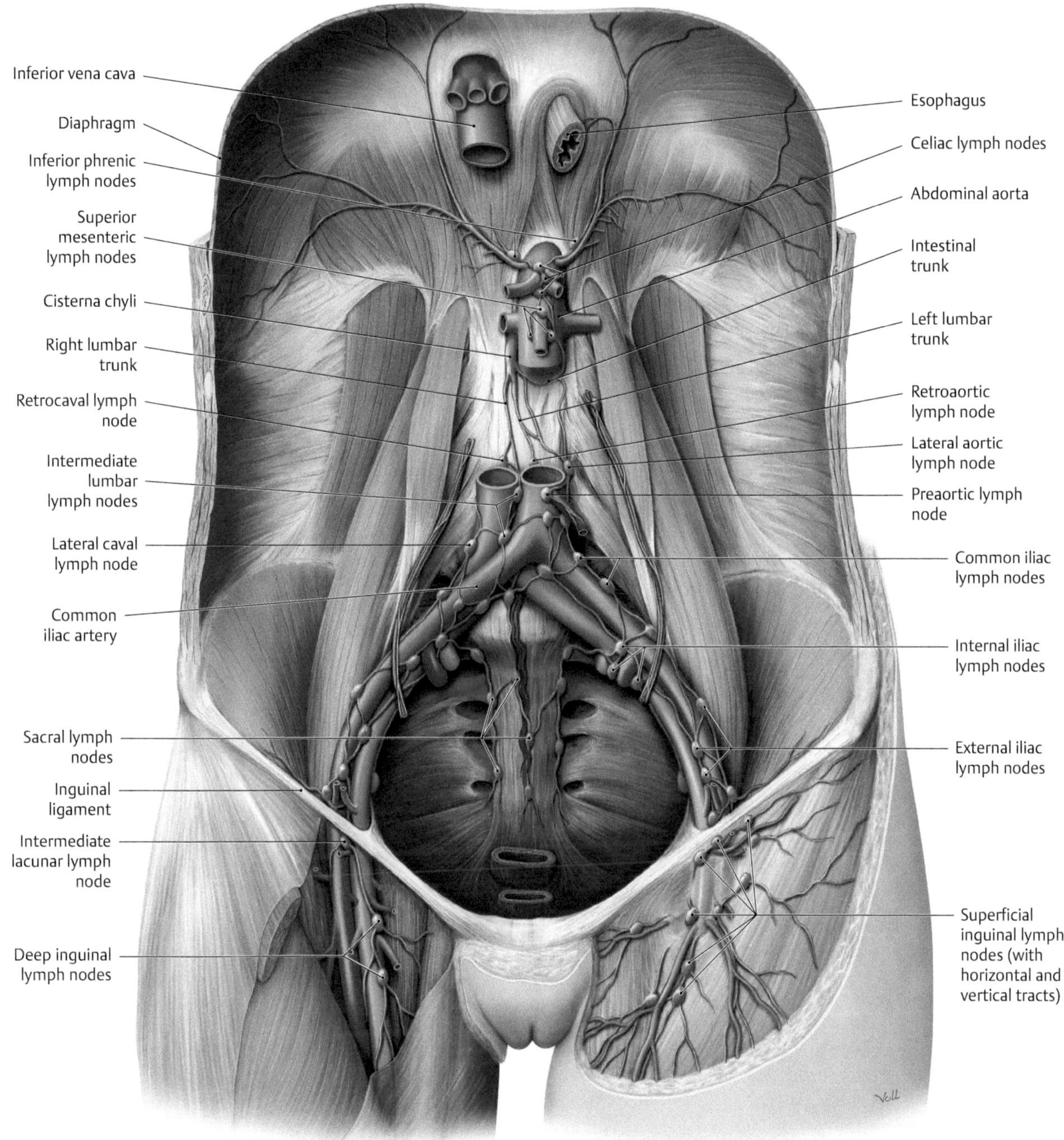

Fig. 3.96 Overview of lymph nodes in the abdomen and pelvis. (From Schuenke M, Schulte E, Schumacher U. THIEME Atlas of Anatomy. Internal Organs. Illustrations by Voll M and Wesker K. 3rd ed. New York: Thieme Medical Publishers; 2020.)

Clinical Correlate 3.53

Abdominal Aortic Aneurysm

The localized enlargement of the aorta, mostly found inferior to the level of the renal arteries, is known as an **abdominal aortic aneurysm (AAA)**. There are generally no symptoms unless it has ruptured and if this occurs the mortality rate is near 90%. Surgery is generally recommended for any aortic diameter greater than 5 cm. AAA's can be fixed with a procedure called endovascular aneurysm repair and this involves the placement of an expandable stent graft without actually operating directly on the aorta. Smoking is a big contributor to their development along with alcoholism and hypertension.

plexuses. The *intermesenteric plexus* is located between the superior and inferior mesenteric plexuses but gives rise to the **gonadal**, **renal** and **ureteric plexuses**. The aortic plexus is continuous with the *superior hypogastric plexus*, *hypogastric nerves* and the *inferior hypogastric plexus* of which the autonomic fibers passing through these structures center mostly on the pelvic viscera. However, parasympathetic fibers targeting the hindgut must pass back through these plexuses.

There are **pre-aortic ganglia** called the **celiac**, **superior mesenteric** and **inferior mesenteric ganglia** that are associated with the artery and plexus of the same name. In addition, **aorticorenal ganglia** are located near the border of the aorta and renal arteries

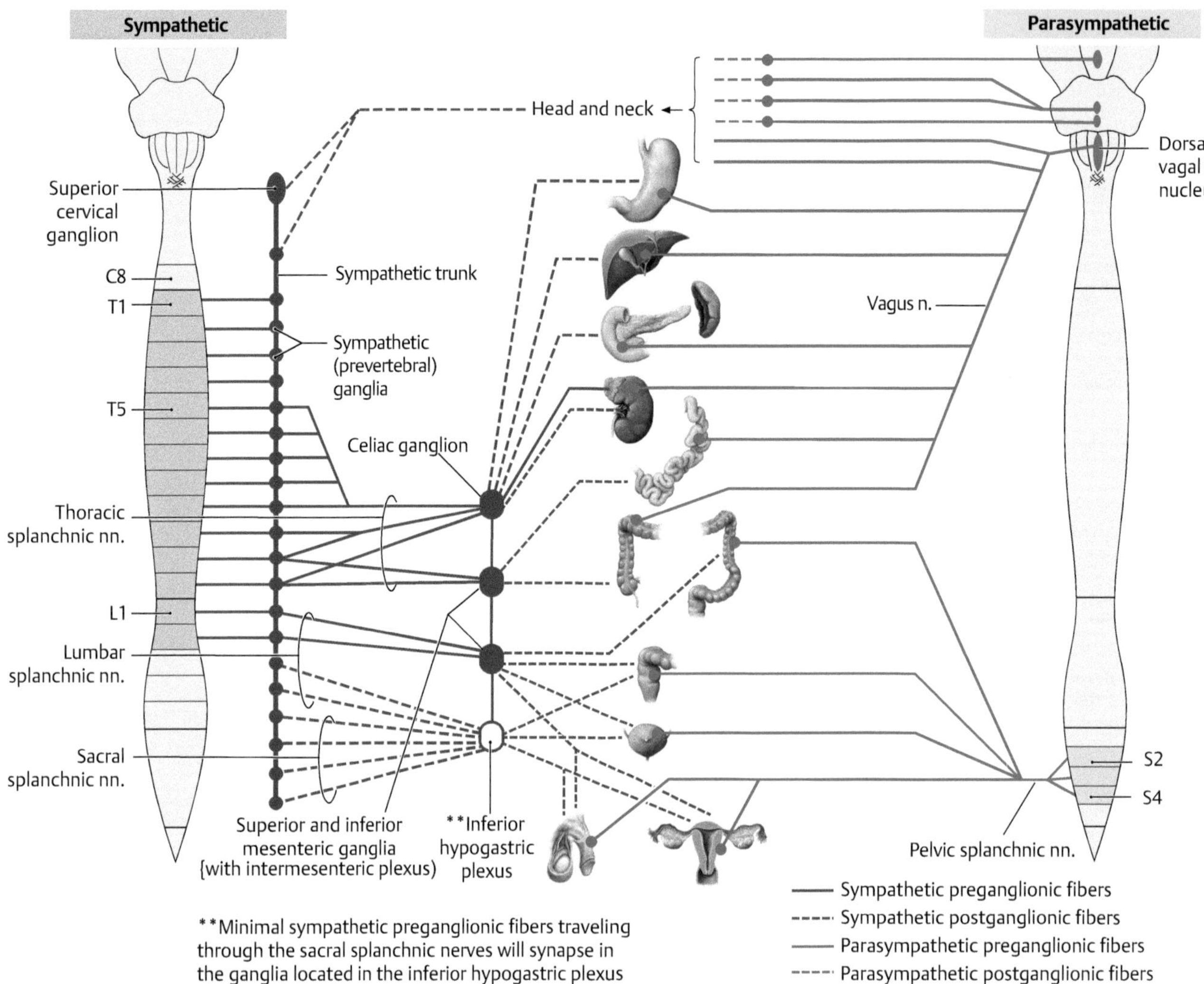

Fig. 3.97 Overview of the autonomic nervous system. (From Schuenke M, Schulte E, Schumacher U. THIEME Atlas of Anatomy. Internal Organs. Illustrations by Voll M and Wesker K. 3rd ed. New York: Thieme Medical Publishers; 2020.)

(Fig. 3.98). Only the sympathetic preganglionic fibers that traveled through the *greater, lesser, least* or *lumbar splanchnic nerves* may synapse at one of these pre-aortic ganglia.

The aortic plexus along with all of its connected plexuses contain GVE-sym/post, GVE-para/pre and GVA fibers. The aortic plexus receives its parasympathetic fibers from the *anterior vagal trunk, posterior vagal trunk* and *pelvic splanchnic nerves* (indirectly). The **peri-arterial plexuses** wrapped around the arteries that are direct or indirect branches of the abdominal aorta continue as GVE-sym/post, GVE-para/pre and GVA until they hit the target organ. The GVE-para/pre fibers finally synapse at the submucosal ganglion of the target organ and become postganglionic. Only in the special situation involving the innervation of the medulla of the suprarenal gland does GVE-sym/pre fibers bypass a pre-aortic ganglion to later synapse at a chromaffin cell. The sympathetics are responsible for inhibiting peristalsis, contracting sphincters and vasoconstriction. The parasympathetics are then responsible for promoting peristalsis and secretion of digestive juices as well as relaxing the sphincters.

Note that there is considerable overlap to where sympathetic splanchnic nerves deliver their GVE-sym/pre fibers to a pre-aortic ganglion. This is much the same case involving the anterior and posterior vagal trunks overlapping in their innervation of the foregut and midgut viscera. The pelvic splanchnic nerves are consistent as the source of GVE-para/pre fibers destined to innervate the hindgut and pelvic structures.

3.45.2 Sympathetic Pathway to GI Tract and Posterior Abdominal Wall Viscera

From the lateral horn between the T5-L2 portions of the spinal cord, a sym/pre fiber passes through the ventral root, then the spinal nerve, next the ventral rami for a short distance, and then through a white rami communicans to finally reach the sympathetic trunk. There is no synapse at a sympathetic trunk (paravertebral) ganglion but this sym/pre fiber continues through a splanchnic nerve (greater, lesser, least & lumbar) and synapses at a pre-aortic (prevertebral) ganglion located in the abdomen. The sym/post fiber then passes from the pre-aortic ganglion and continues through a peri-arterial plexus, an extension of the larger aortic plexus, in order to reach the target organ.

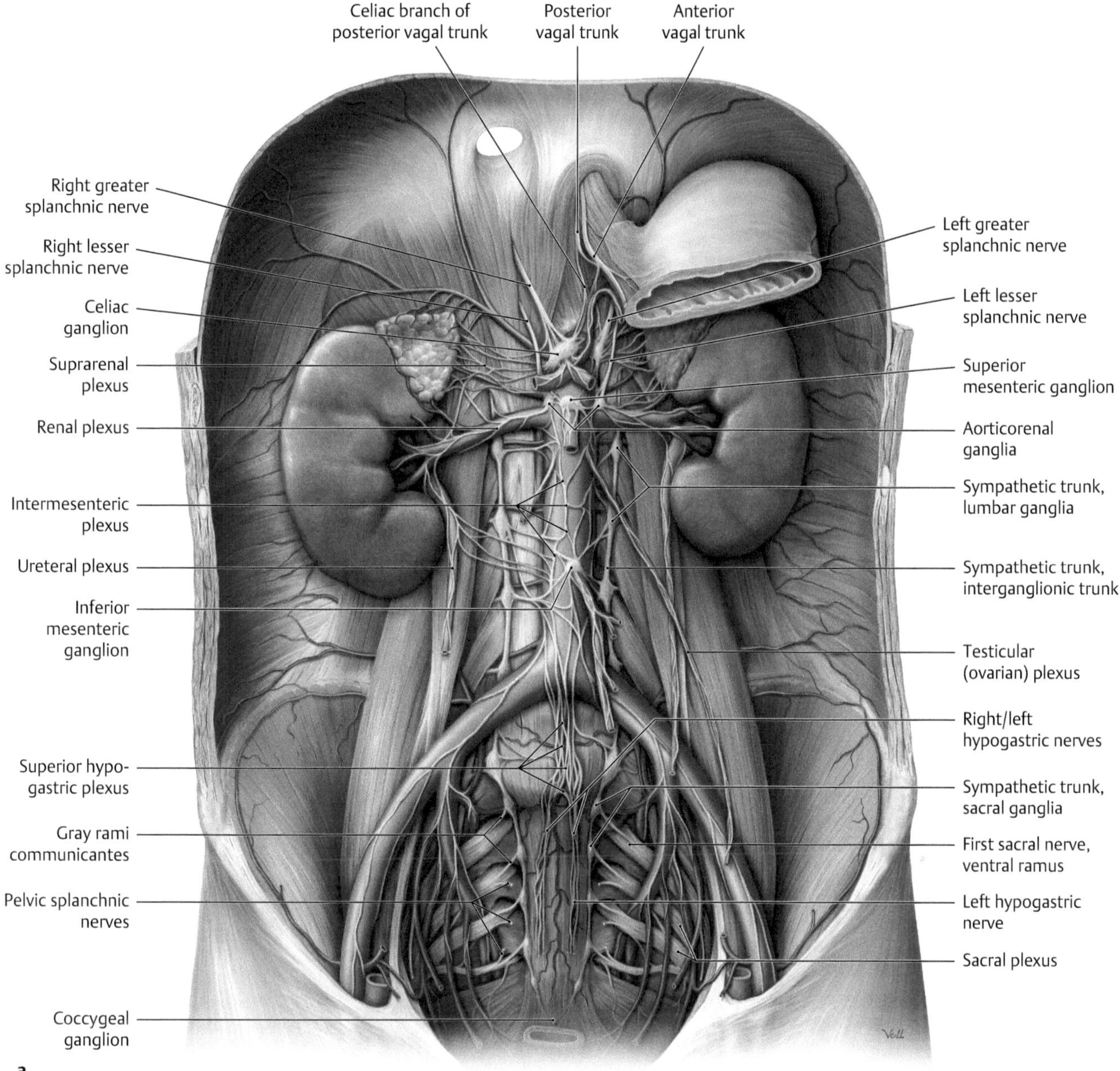

Fig. 3.98 (a) Overview of autonomic ganglia and plexuses in the abdomen and pelvis. (*continued*) (From Schuenke M, Schulte E, Schumacher U. THIEME Atlas of Anatomy. Internal Organs. Illustrations by Voll M and Wesker K. 3rd ed. New York: Thieme Medical Publishers; 2020.)

There are numerous splanchnic nerves that originate from the sympathetic trunk. The *upper thoracic splanchnic nerves* (first four) are small and less defined than the rest of the thoracic splanchnics. They are associated with a larger group known as the *cardiopulmonary splanchnic nerves* and they target the head, neck and thorax viscera. The **abdominopelvic splanchnic nerves** are a group consisting of the *lower thoracic* (greater, lesser and least) and *upper lumbar splanchnic nerves* and they innervate the GI tract and posterior abdominal wall viscera. The lower thoracic splanchnics must pierce the crus of the diaphragm before reaching the pre-aortic ganglion located on the aortic plexus. The splanchnic nerves originate for the most part off of a ganglion closely associated with the same vertebral level. For example, the T5 ganglion is near the T5 vertebral level. It is known however that the sympathetic trunk does not always have a **paravertebral (sympathetic trunk) ganglion** at every vertebral level but this is assumed for description purposes. The specific splanchnic nerves include:

- **Greater splanchnic nerve (T5-T9)**: their sym/pre fibers synapse primarily at the celiac ganglion but also the superior mesenteric ganglion. The sym/post fibers from these ganglions course along an artery targeting foregut viscera and the spleen **(Fig. 3.99; Fig. 3.100)**.
- **Lesser (T10-T11)** and **Least (T12) splanchnic nerves**: their sym/pre fibers synapse primarily at the superior mesenteric ganglion but also at the aorticorenal ganglions. The sym/post fibers from these ganglions course along an artery

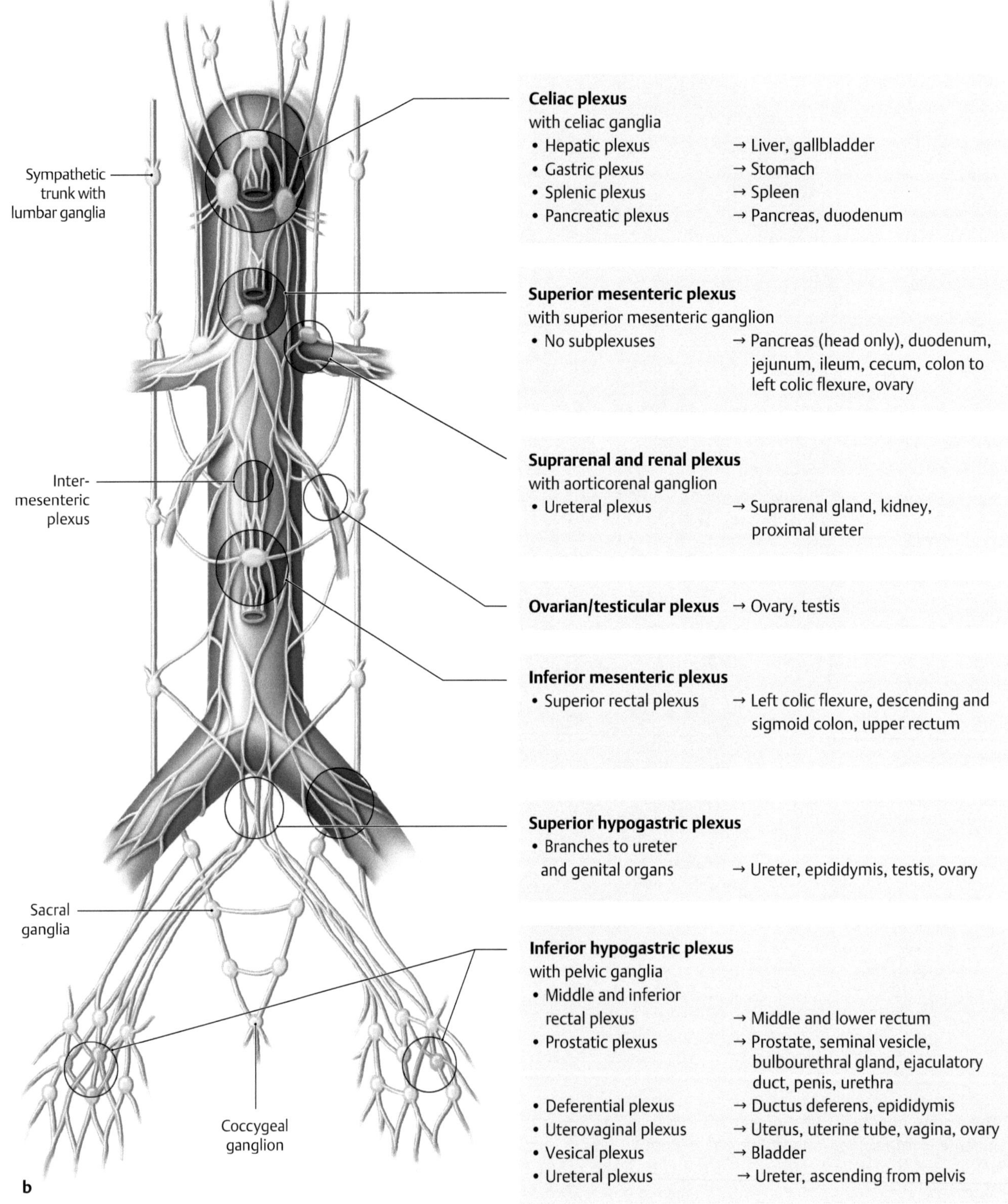

Fig. 3.98 (*continued*) **(b)** Organization of autonomic ganglia and plexuses. (From Schuenke M, Schulte E, Schumacher U. THIEME Atlas of Anatomy. Internal Organs. Illustrations by Voll M and Wesker K. 3rd ed. New York: Thieme Medical Publishers; 2020.)

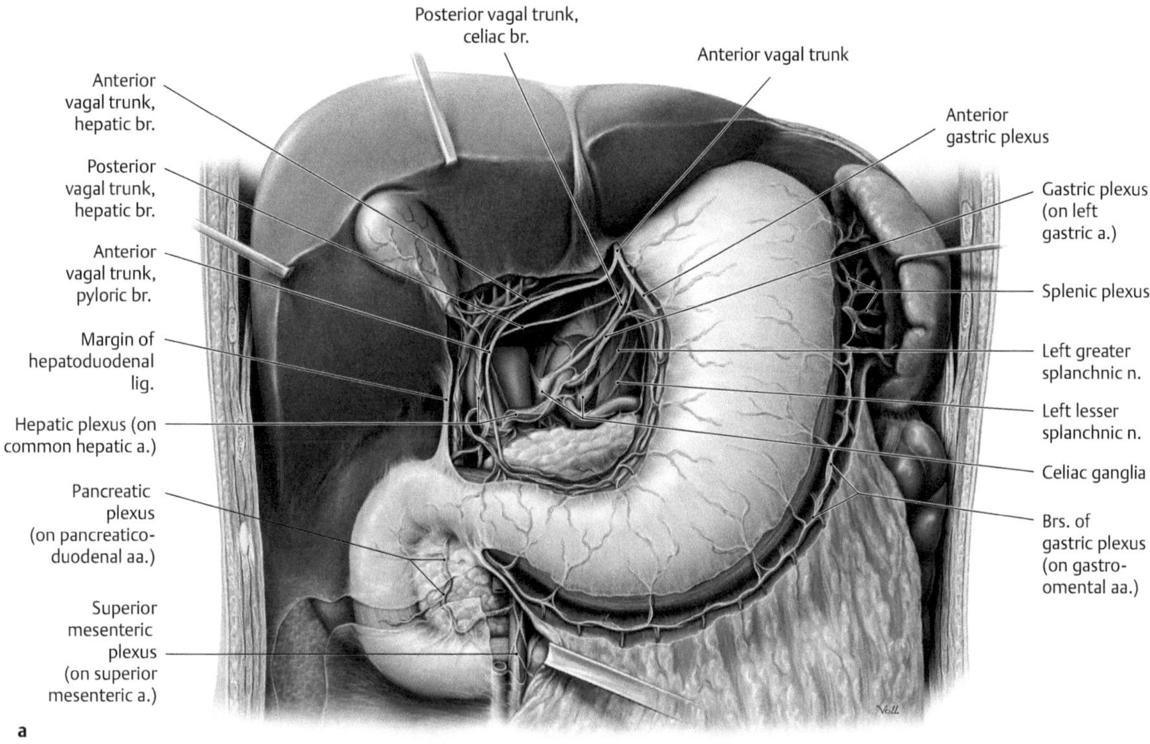

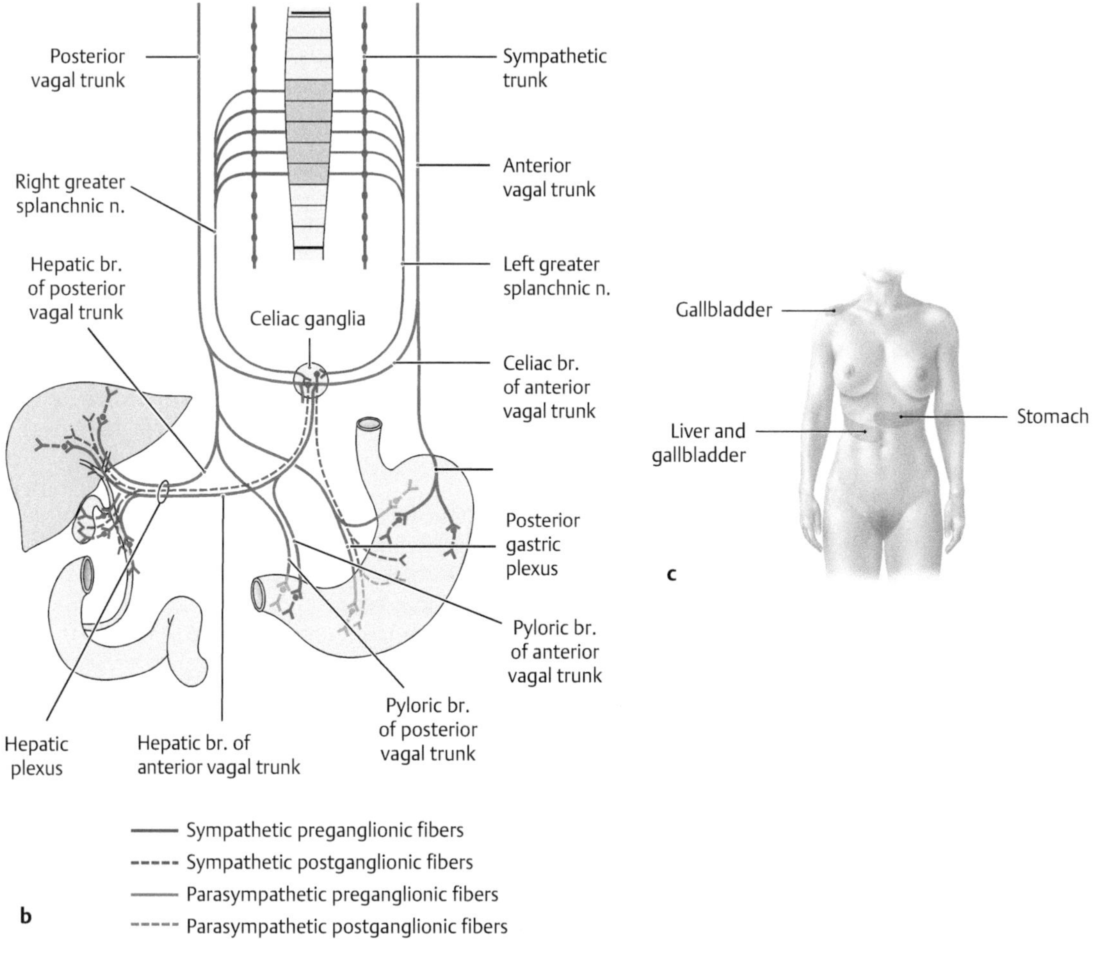

Fig. 3.99 **(a)** Innervation of the foregut and spleen. **(b)** Schematic of celiac plexus distribution to the liver, gallbladder, and stomach. **(c)** Zones of referred pain from the liver, gallbladder, and stomach. (From Schuenke M, Schulte E, Schumacher U. THIEME Atlas of Anatomy. Internal Organs. Illustrations by Voll M and Wesker K. 3rd ed. New York: Thieme Medical Publishers; 2020.)

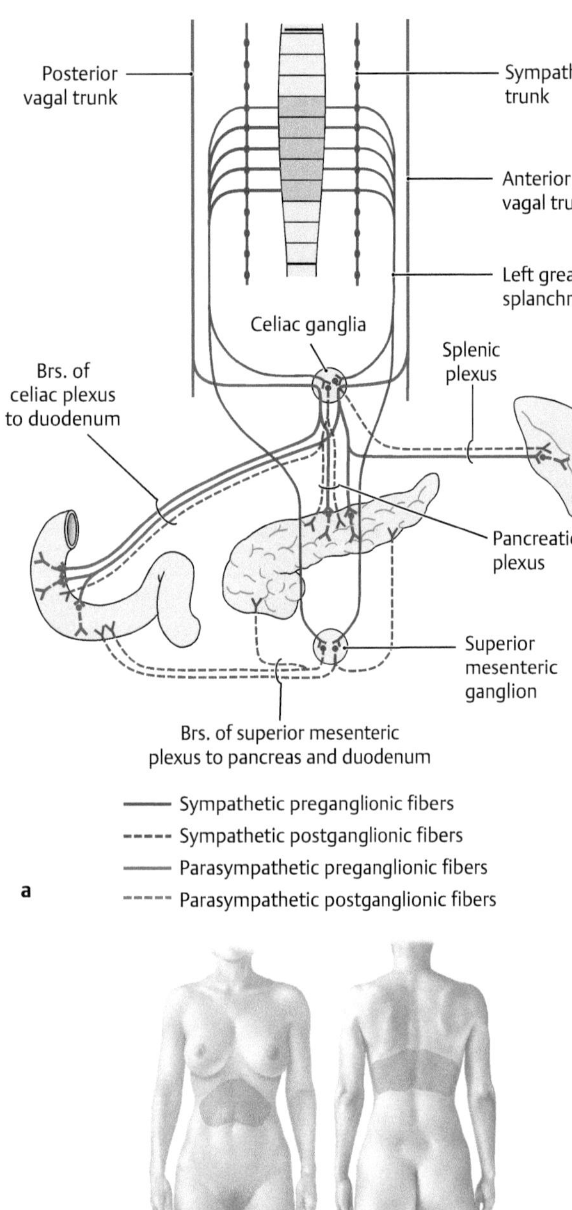

Fig. 3.100 **(a)** Schematic of celiac distribution to the pancreas, duodenum, and spleen. **(b)** Zones of referred pain from the pancreas. There are no zones associated with the duodenum and spleen. (From Schuenke M, Schulte E, Schumacher U. THIEME Atlas of Anatomy. Internal Organs. Illustrations by Voll M and Wesker K. 3rd ed. New York: Thieme Medical Publishers; 2020.)

targeting mainly midgut and posterior abdominal wall viscera (**Fig. 3.101; Fig. 3.102b**).

- **Lumbar splanchnic nerves (L1-L4)**: their sym/pre fibers synapse primarily at the inferior mesenteric ganglion. The sym/post fibers from the inferior mesenteric ganglion course along an artery targeting hindgut viscera (**Fig. 3.102**).

3.45.3 Sympathetic Pathway to the Medulla of the Suprarenal Gland

Similar to the previous pathways the sym/pre fibers (mostly from T10-L2 but contributions extend from T5-L2) enter the sympathetic trunk without synapsing before continuing through splanchnic nerves. Once these sym/pre fibers have reached mostly the upper portions of the aortic plexus, they bypass synapsing at a pre-aortic ganglion and continue their course along the peri-arterial plexuses of arteries supplying the suprarenal gland (**Fig. 3.85**). At the suprarenal medulla, the sym/pre fibers synapse on the modified postganglionic neurons called chromaffin cells. These cells secrete mostly epinephrine but also norepinephrine into the general circulation.

3.45.4 Parasympathetic Autonomic Innervation

Parasympathetic preganglionic fibers are delivered to the GI Tract by the *anterior vagal trunk* and *posterior vagal trunks* directly and the *pelvic splanchnic nerves* indirectly. The VE-para/pre fibers that pass through the vagus nerve and ultimately the vagal trunks originate from the *dorsal motor nucleus of vagus* in the brainstem. The para/pre fibers that eventually pass through the pelvic splanchnic nerves originate from the lateral horn-like region of the S2-S4 spinal segments. They then travel through the ventral roots of S2-S4 (cauda equina branches) before exiting through the ventral rami of S2-S4. The pelvic splanchnics branch off the S2-S4 ventral rami just after the ventral rami exit the sacral foramina and lead directly to the inferior hypogastric plexus.

- **Anterior vagal trunk**: the continuation of the left vagus nerve passes through the esophageal hiatus and courses along the anterior surface of the stomach near the lesser curvature before branching off the hepatic, celiac, duodenal and anterior gastric branches. Its parasympathetic fibers supply a portion of the foregut viscera.
- **Posterior vagal trunk**: the continuation of the right vagus nerve passes through the esophageal hiatus, and courses along the posterior surface of the stomach. It gives off multiple celiac and posterior gastric branches and delivers the bulk of parasympathetics associated with midgut and to a lesser degree foregut and posterior abdominal wall structures.
- **Pelvic splanchnic nerves (S2-S4)**: are branches off the ventral rami of S2-S4 and connect to the inferior hypogastric plexus located in the pelvis. They deliver the para/pre fibers to the *inferior hypogastric plexus* but these fibers do not synapse until they reach their target organ (**Fig. 3.85**). From the inferior hypogastric plexus, para/pre fibers can travel to the hindgut by passing through:

1. The left side only and directly to hindgut structures by way of the **retroperitoneal parasympathetic fibers**.
2. The left and right (minimal if any) hypogastric nerves, through the superior hypogastric plexus, and then to hindgut structures by way of the **inferior mesenteric peri-arterial plexus**.

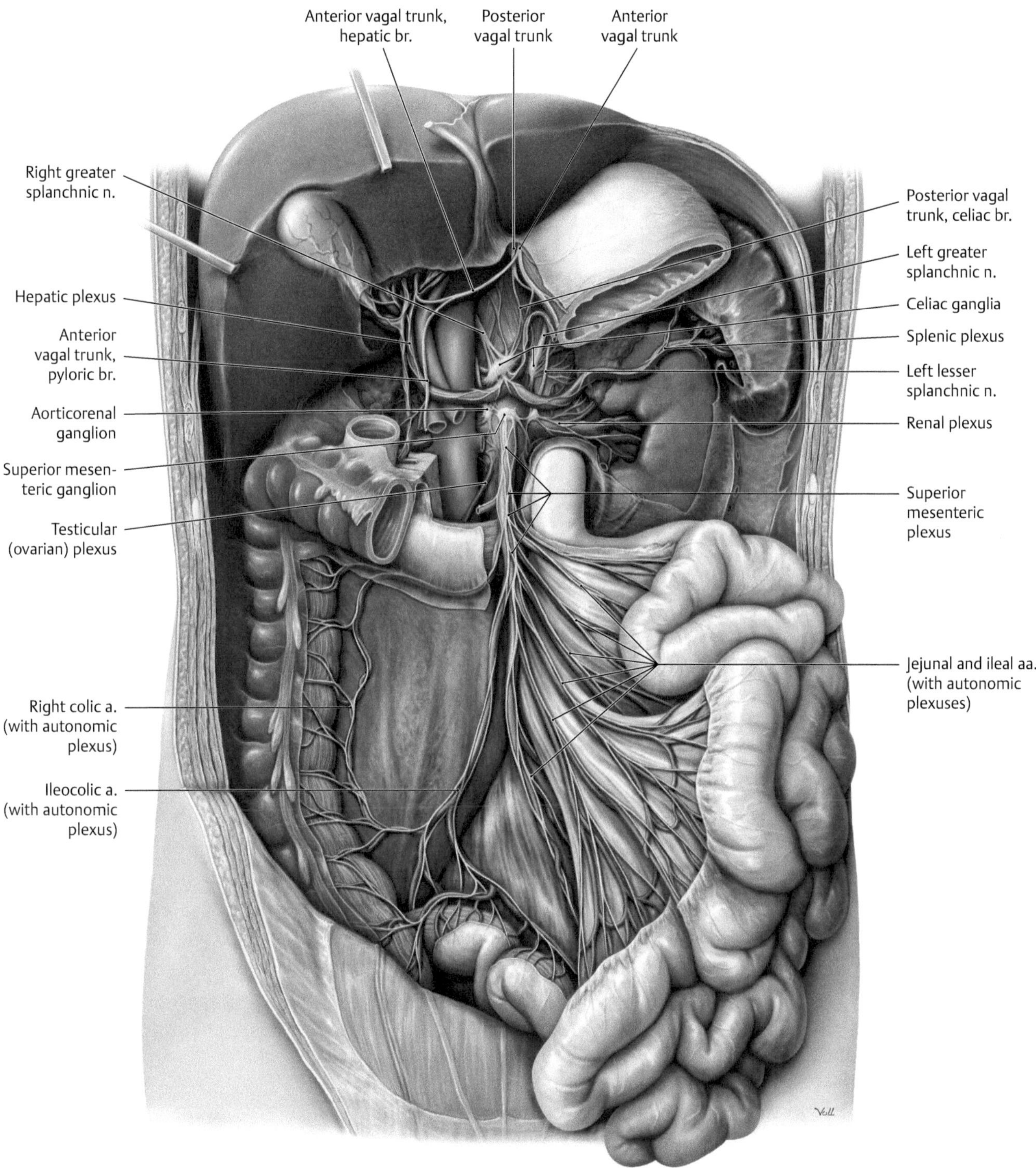

Fig. 3.101 Innervation of midgut structures such as the small intestine and proximal portion of the large intestine. (From Schuenke M, Schulte E, Schumacher U. THIEME Atlas of Anatomy. Internal Organs. Illustrations by Voll M and Wesker K. 3rd ed. New York: Thieme Medical Publishers; 2020.)

3.46 Enteric Nervous System

The overall nervous system has a great influence over digestive processes such as motility, blood flow, and ion transport that is associated with secretion and absorption of our nutrition. This control is maintained by connections between the **enteric nervous system (ENS)** of the digestive system and the central nervous system (CNS). The ENS has been shown to have its own independent reflex activity thus it is no longer considered a part of the autonomic nervous system (ANS). However, the parasympathetic and sympathetic portions of the ANS help modulate the activity of the ENS. Due to the complexity of the ENS it is sometimes referred to as the second brain in the body.

The ENS is embedded in the lining of the GI tract beginning at the esophagus and extending all the way down to the anal canal and conatins around half a billion neurons. There are two principal components or plexuses of neurons associated with the ENS and they are both embedded in the wall of the digestive tract (**Fig. 3.103**):

- **Submucous (*Meissner's*) plexus**: located deep within the submucosa layer and its principal role is to sense the environment within the lumen, in order to control epithelial cell function and regulate the blood flow of the GI tract. The submucous plexus is fairly sparse in areas such as the esophagus and stomach but becomes quite extensive from the small intestine through the anal canal.
- **Myenteric (*Auerbach's*) plexus**: is located between the inner circular and outer longitudinal layers of muscularis externa and primarily controls the motility of the GI tract. It is consistently found from the esophagus all the way through to the anal canal.

There are about 20 types of enteric neurons defined by their function. The functions of these neurons are classified as either a *motor*, *sensory* (IPANs) or an *interneuron*.

- **Motor neurons**: control GI motility and secretion and even possibly absorption of nutrients. The motor neurons act directly on a large number of effector cells that include smooth muscle, GI endocrine cells and an extensive amount of secretory cells such as mucous, chief, parietal, enterocytes and pancreatic exocrine cells. These neurons are multipolar.
- **Sensory neurons** (or *intrinsic primary afferent neurons* - **IPANs**): receive information from sensory receptors in the mucosa and smooth muscle. They can interpret information about the current gut contents and the state of the overall GI tract or the amount of stretch and tension being placed on the GI tract. Multiple sensory receptors have been identified within the mucosa and they are known to respond to mechanical, chemical, thermal and even osmotic stimulation. The lumen of the GI tract can test the food bolus passing through it to gauge its importance and this can be done by chemoreceptors that are sensitive to glucose and amino acids for example. These neurons are either pseudo-unipolar or bipolar.
- **Interneurons**: integrate information from sensory neurons and provide an effect on the motor neurons or facilitate reflexes. These neurons are multipolar.

The enteric neurons secrete as many as thirty neurotransmitters and many of them are the ones seen in the brain. One of these, acetylcholine can stimulate smooth muscle contraction, increase intestinal secretions, vasodilate blood vessels and release enteric hormones. About 90% of all serotonin and 50% of all dopamine found in the body is located in the gut. They both have an effect on the regulation of intestinal movements.

3.47 Visceral Sensory Innervation

The visceral sensory (GVA) fibers are divided into *visceral pain* or *visceral reflex fibers*. The visceral pain fibers are paired with sympathetic fibers and they are associated with the phenomenon known as *referred pain*. Visceral reflex fibers pair with the parasympathetic fibers and are related to reflex arcs that control secretion and peristaltic movements of the GI tract (**Fig. 3.104**).

3.48 Referred Pain

The visceral pain fibers passing through sympathetic fibers that originally innervated the foregut, midgut and hindgut structures travel retrograde through the corresponding splanchnic nerve before reaching the sympathetic trunk. These fibers continue through the adjacent white rami communicans, ventral rami, spinal nerve, and the dorsal root before finally terminating on the dorsal horn of the spinal cord. Their cell bodies are located in dorsal root ganglion.

With the GVA fibers ending so close to where somatic sensory (GSA) fibers terminate on the dorsal horn of the spinal cord, the GSA fibers falsely interpret the GVA fibers as originating from a somatic nerve and thus the patient perceives this pain on defined regions of the outer body wall. This is known as **referred pain** (**Fig. 3.105**). The visceral reflex fibers of the parasympathetics are not associated with referred pain. Below the ***pelvic pain line***, parasympathetics in addition to their visceral reflex fibers contain visceral pain fibers, but these details are discussed further in the next chapter.

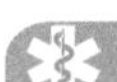
Clinical Correlate 3.54

Minimally Invasive Surgery

Surgical procedures are performed in three settings; noninvasive, open and minimally invasive. *Noninvasive procedures* do not break the skin or go past a normal body opening. An example includes LASIK eye surgery and this entails using a laser to reshape the cornea in order to correct vision problems. *Open surgery* includes any procedure that would involve cutting the skin or tissue to directly access an organ as in a liver transplant.

Minimally invasive surgery involves making much smaller incisions compared to open surgery. Examples include laparoscopic, endoscopic, endovascular and robotic surgery. In *laparoscopic surgery* a laparoscope is inserted into the abdominal wall and it has a small video camera allowing the surgeon to view the inside of a patient. This image is projected onto a monitor and with the use of additional gripping or cutting tools passing through the abdominal wall, structures are then able to be manipulated and excised as seen in a laparoscopic cholecystectomy. *Endoscopic surgery* makes use of an endoscope which is a thin tube with a small camera and light attached. This type of surgery can be used to diagnose and treat conditions such as nerve compression of the spine. *Endovascular surgery* is used to treat problems involving clogged blood vessels and stents or inflatable balloons can be inserted into nearby blood vessels in order to fix an abdominal aortic aneurysm for example. *Robotic surgery* uses the da Vinci® surgical system that employs robotic arms equipped with endoscopes. These arms respond to the precise movements of surgeon's hands and have been used in a robotic prostatectomy for example.

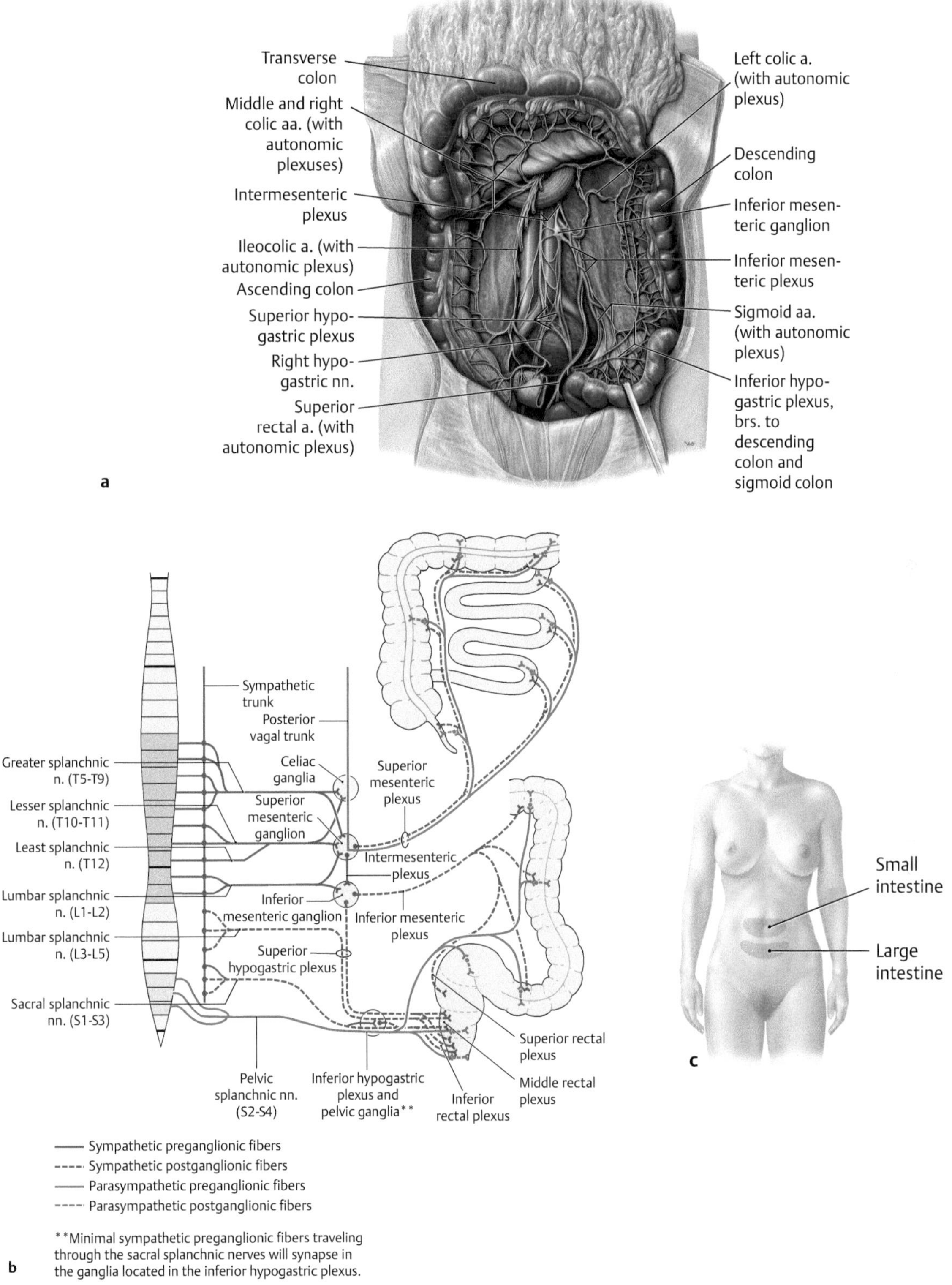

Fig. 3.102 **(a)** Innervation of the large intestine. **(b)** Schematic of superior mesenteric, inferior mesenteric, and inferior hypogastric plexuses distribution. **(c)** Zones of referred pain from the small and large intestines. (From Schuenke M, Schulte E, Schumacher U. THIEME Atlas of Anatomy. Internal Organs. Illustrations by Voll M and Wesker K. 3rd ed. New York: Thieme Medical Publishers; 2020.)

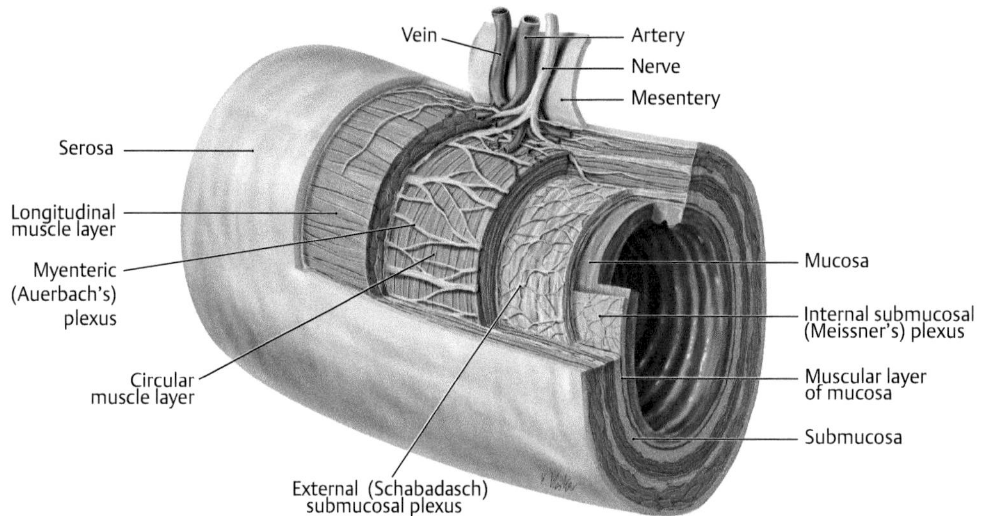

Fig. 3.103 Enteric nervous system in the small intestine. (From Schuenke M, Schulte E, Schumacher U. THIEME Atlas of Anatomy. Head, Neck, and Neuroanatomy. Illustrations by Voll M and Wesker K. 3rd ed. New York: Thieme Medical Publishers; 2020.)

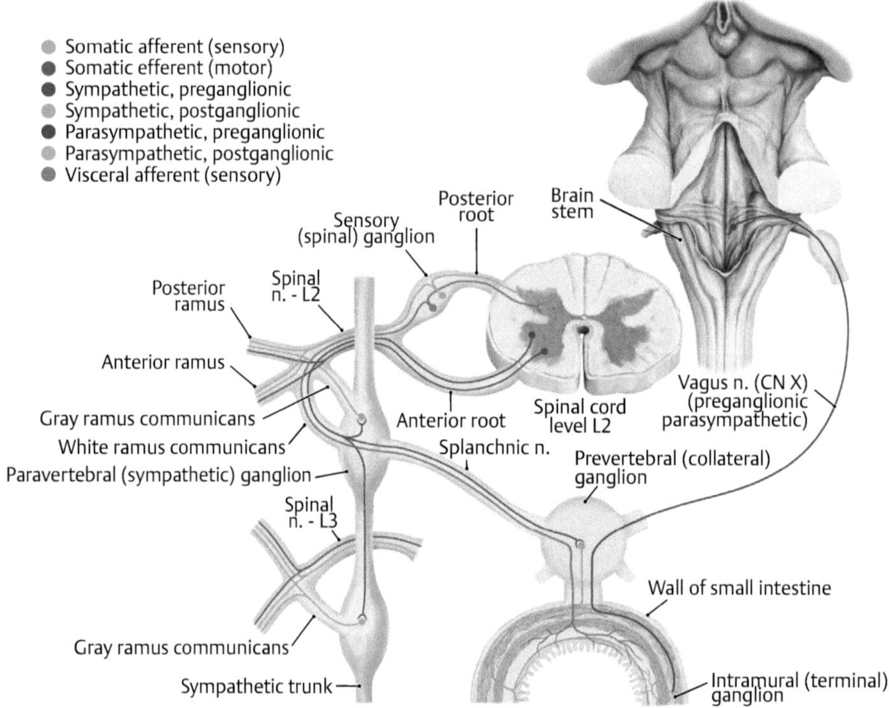

Fig. 3.104 Autonomic nervous system circuitry and visceral sensory innervation. (From Gilroy AM et al. Atlas of Anatomy. 4th ed. New York: Thieme Medical Publishers 2020. Based on Schuenke M, Schulte E, Schumacher U. THIEME Atlas of Anatomy. Head, Neck, and Neuroanatomy. Illustrations by Voll M and Wesker K. 3rd ed. New York: Thieme Medical Publishers; 2020.)

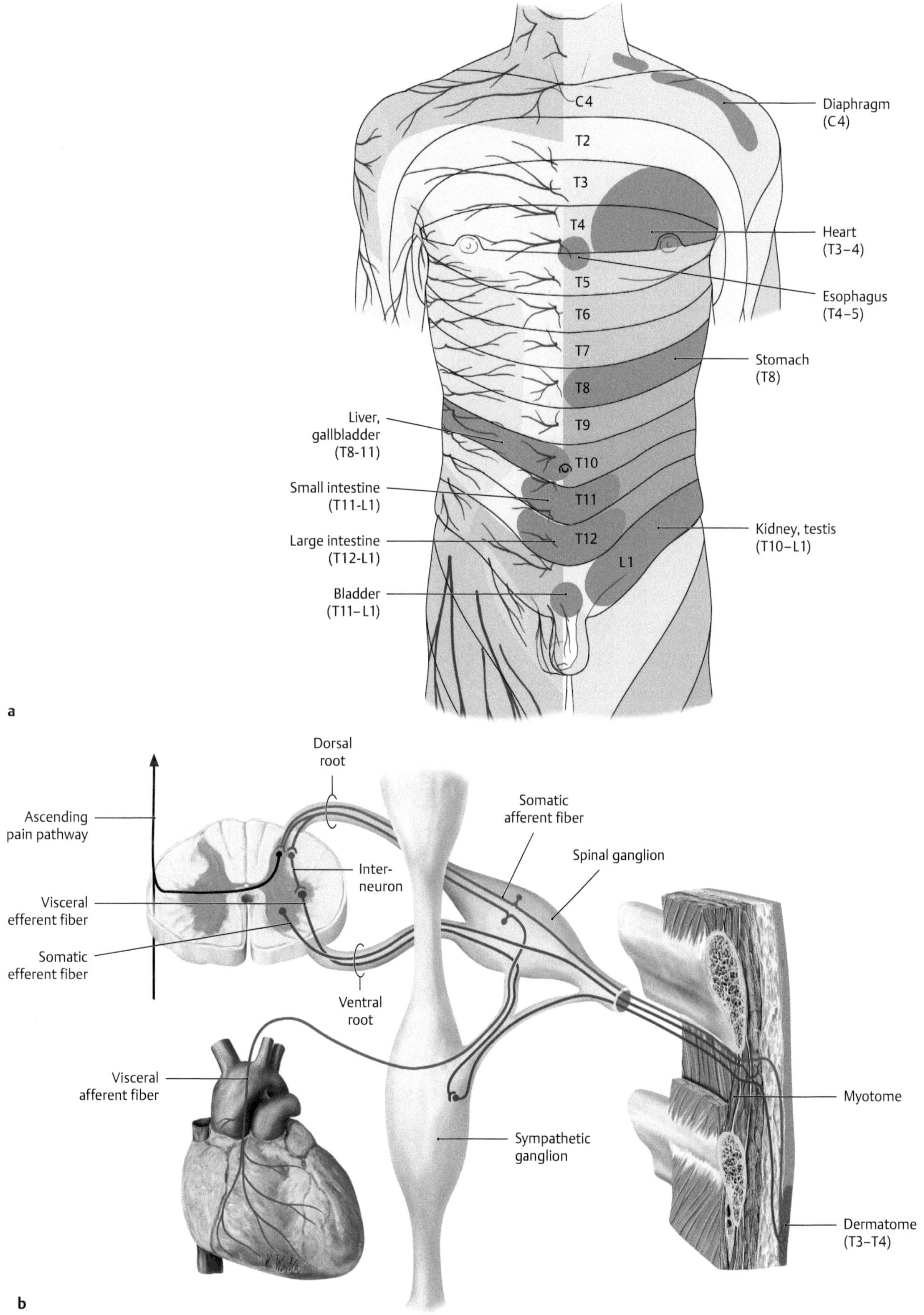

Fig. 3.105 **(a)** Referred pain of multiple visceral organs. **(b)** Convergence of somatic and visceral afferent fibers. (From Schuenke M, Schulte E, Schumacher U. THIEME Atlas of Anatomy, Head, Neck, and Neuroanatomy. Illustrations by Voll M and Wesker K. 3rd ed. New York: Thieme Medical Publishers; 2020.)

3.49 Radiology of the Abdomen

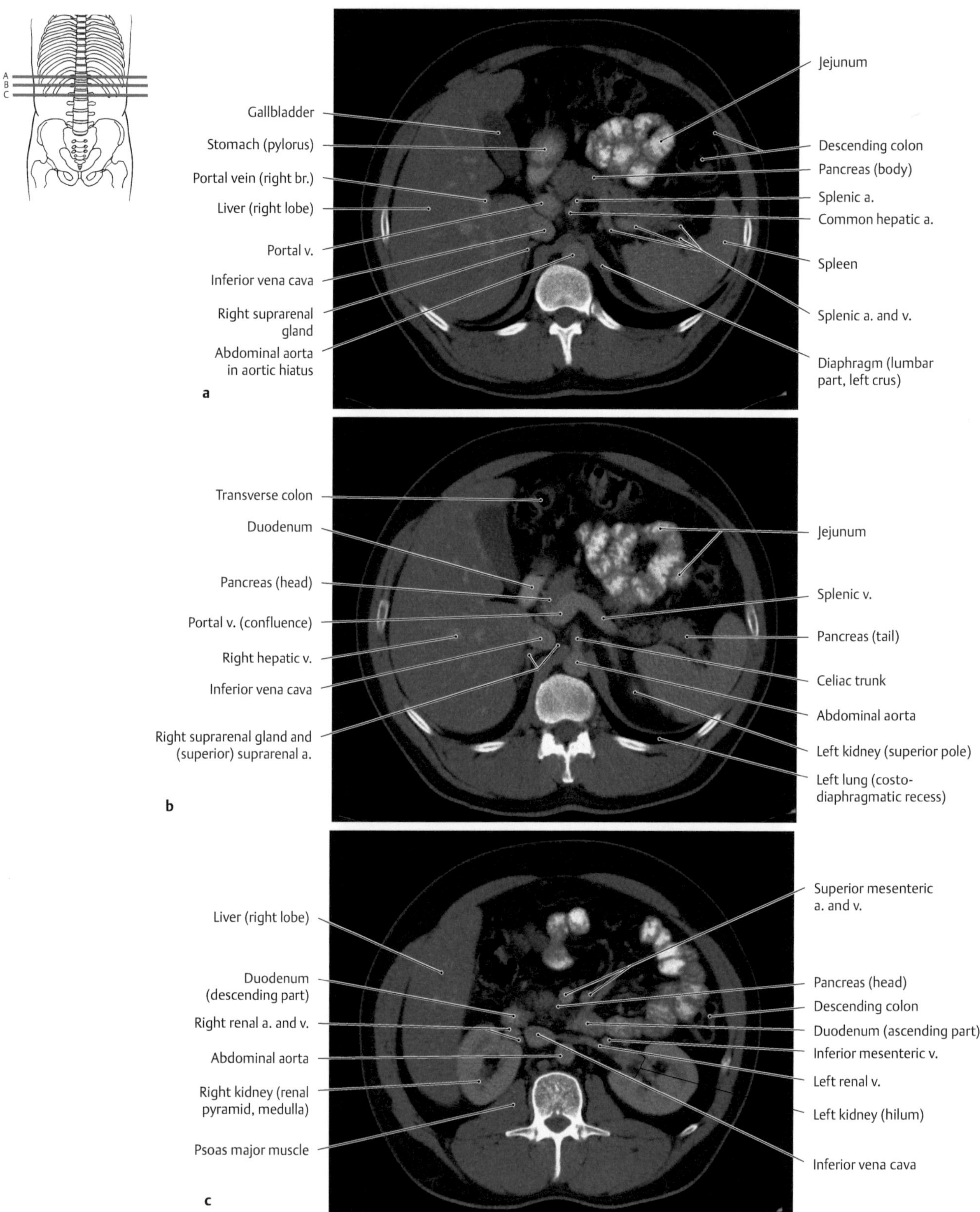

Fig. 3.106 **(a)** Transverse section through T12 vertebral level. **(b)** Transverse section through L1 vertebral level. **(c)** Transverse section though L2 vertebral level. (*continued*) (From Moeller TB, Reif E. Pocket Atlas of Sectional Anatomy, Vol 2, 4th ed. New York, NY: Thieme; 2014.)

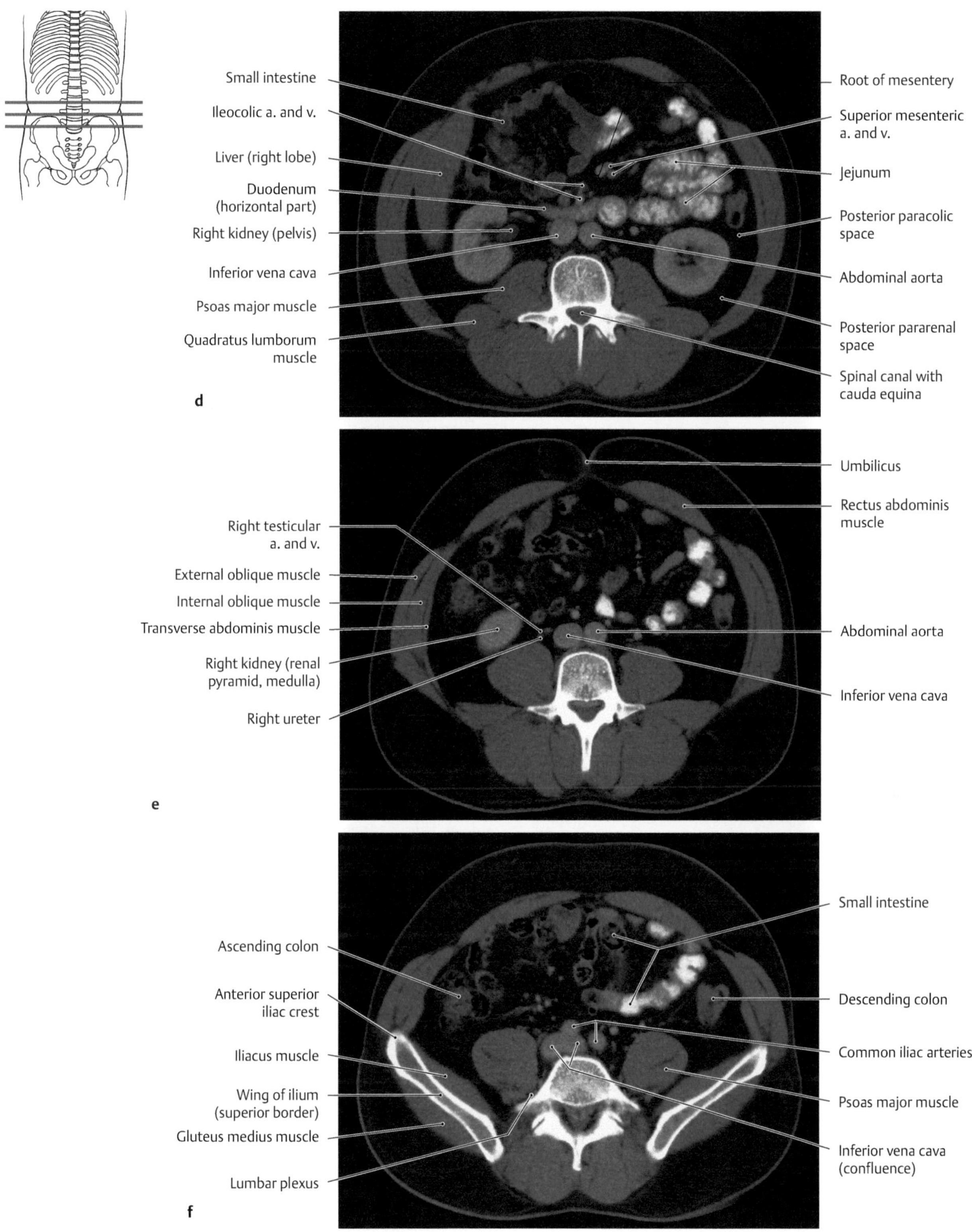

Fig. 3.106 (*continued*) **(d)** Transverse section through L3 vertebral level. **(e)** Transverse section through L4 vertebral level. **(f)** Transverse section through L5 vertebral level. (From Moeller TB, Reif E. Pocket Atlas of Sectional Anatomy, Vol 2, 4th ed. New York, NY: Thieme; 2014.)

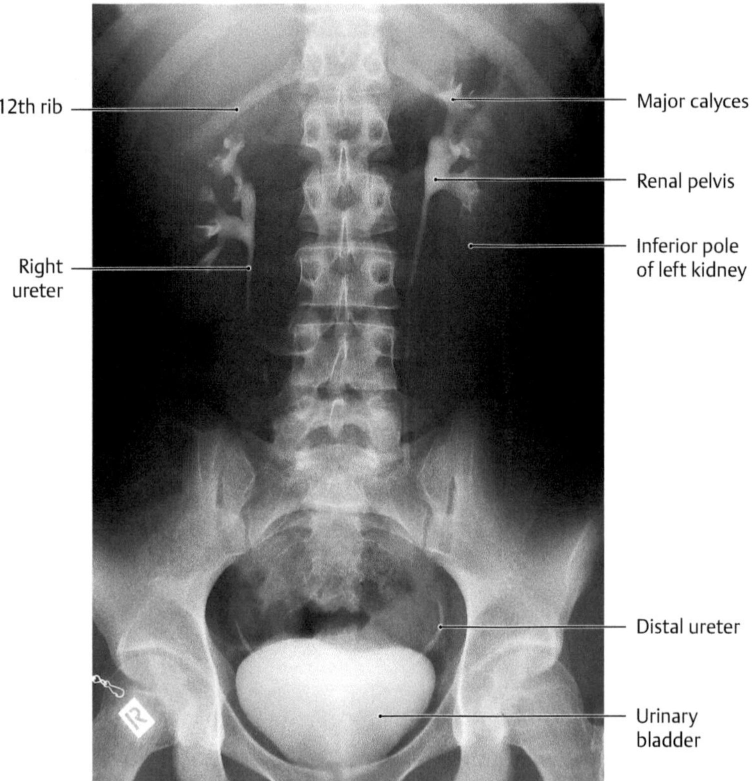

Fig. 3.107 Radiograph of intravenous pylegram. (From Gilroy AM et al. Atlas of Anatomy. 3rd ed. New York: Thieme Medical Publishers; 2016.)

PRACTICE QUESTIONS

1. A surgeon has just completed repairing an inguinal hernia on a male patient. However, two days post-op, the patient demonstrates no active elevation of the testes during a cremasteric reflex test. Which nerve is involved in the efferent limb of this particular reflex?
   A. Iliohypogastric nerve.
   B. Ilioinguinal nerve.
   C. Genital branch of genitofemoral nerve.
   D. Subcostal nerve.
   E. Femoral nerve.
2. Which statement about the rectus sheath is CORRECT?
   A. The posterior layer above the arcuate line, consists of the external oblique and the internal oblique aponeuroses.
   B. The posterior layer below the arcuate line, consists of the external oblique, internal oblique & transversus abdominis aponeuroses.
   C. The posterior layer above the arcuate line, consists of ½ the internal oblique and all the transversus abdominis aponeuroses.
   D. The anterior layer above the arcuate line, consists of ½ the internal oblique and all the transversus abdominis aponeuroses.
   E. The anterior layer below the arcuate line, consists of the external oblique and transversus abdominis aponeuroses.
3. A bar fight breaks out and one patron is stabbed by another. The knife wound is about 3 inches below the umbilicus (definitely below the arcuate line), but medial to the semilunar line separating the rectus abdominis from the external oblique muscles. In what order would the tip of the knife pass before reaching the abdominal cavity?
   A. Skin, Campers's, Scarpa's, Ext. oblique aponeurosis, 1/2 Int. oblique aponeurosis, Rectus abdominis, 1/2 Int. oblique aponeurosis, Transversus abdominis aponeurosis, Transversalis fascia, Extraperitoneal fat, Parietal peritoneum.
   B. Skin, Scarpa's, Campers's, Ext. oblique aponeurosis, Int. oblique aponeurosis, Rectus abdominis, Transversus abdominis aponeurosis, Transversalis fascia, Extraperitoneal fat, Parietal peritoneum.
   C. Skin, Scarpa's, Campers's, Ext. oblique aponeurosis, Rectus abdominis, Int. oblique aponeurosis, Transversus abdominis aponeurosis, Transversalis fascia, Extraperitoneal fat, Parietal peritoneum.
   D. Skin, Campers's, Scarpa's, Ext. oblique aponeurosis, Int. oblique aponeurosis, Transversus abdominis aponeurosis, Rectus abdominis, Transversalis fascia, Extraperitoneal fat, Parietal peritoneum.
   E. Skin, Campers's, Scarpa's, Ext. oblique aponeurosis, Int. oblique aponeurosis, Transversus abdominis aponeurosis, Rectus abdominis, Extraperitoneal fat, Transversalis fascia, Parietal peritoneum.
4. Which statement about the inguinal region is CORRECT?
   A. The roof of the inguinal canal is formed by the inguinal ligament.
   B. The medial border of Hesselbach's triangle is formed by the inferior epigastric vessels.
   C. Direct inguinal hernias pass laterally to the inferior epigastric vessels.

D. Indirect inguinal hernias account for about 25-30% of all inguinal hernias.
E. The hernial sac of a direct inguinal hernia is covered by transversalis fascia.

5. During a laparoscopic cholecystectomy, a surgeon makes an incision through the hepatoduodenal ligament to expose the cystohepatic (Calot) triangle. The borders of this triangle are formed by the cystic duct, common hepatic duct and inferior border of the liver. Before ligating the cystic artery that generally courses through this triangle, the clamp or suture would be placed at the proximal cystic artery near what other artery in order to prevent excessive bleeding?
A. Hepatic proper artery.
B. Left hepatic artery.
C. Right hepatic artery.
D. Common hepatic artery.
E. Gastroduodenal artery.

6. A radiograph of a 45-year-old woman reveals a perforation in the posterior wall of the stomach in which the gastric contents have spilled into the lesser sac. The surgeon notices the gastric juices have eroded parts of the splenorenal ligament. Which artery is at risk of being damaged?
A. Splenic artery.
B. Gastroduodenal artery.
C. Left gastric artery.
D. Right gastric artery.
E. Left gastro-omental (gastroepiploic) artery.

7. After passing through the bile canaliculi, bile next passes through what structure?
A. (Common) bile duct.
B. Left or right hepatic ducts.
C. Cystic duct.
D. (Interlobular) bile ducts.
E. Common hepatic duct.

8. An individual has a history of chronic or recurring stomach ulcers. The surgeon decides that a vagatomy involving the anterior vagal trunk will be performed. A reduced level of parasympathetics that normally course through the anterior vagal trunk could have an effect on which listed structure?
A. 2nd part of the duodenum.
B. Jejunum.
C. Distal one third of the Transverse colon.
D. 4th part of the duodenum.
E. Sigmoid colon.

9. A 21-year-old woman presents to the emergency department with pain in the right lower quadrant. It is believed that she has a ruptured appendix and is sent to surgery. While performing the appendectomy, and assuming there is no collateral circulation, a surgeon can ligate the ______ artery to cut off blood supply to the appendix.
A. Left colic artery.
B. Ileocolic artery.
C. Middle colic artery.
D. Right colic artery.
E. Inferior mesenteric artery.

10. Which statement about the small intestine is CORRECT?
A. Peyer's patches are located primarily in the jejunum.
B. The ileum contains large, tall and closely packed circular folds (plicae circulares).
C. The ileum accounts for ~40% of the total length of the small intestine.
D. The jejunum is located primarily in the right lower quadrant.
E. The jejunum has long vasa recta (straight arteries) and few arcade loops.

11. Which statement regarding the midgut or hindgut is CORRECT?
A. The sigmoid colon ends up rotating 270 degrees counterclockwise during development.
B. Parasympathetics that innervate the proximal 2/3 of the transverse colon originated from the pelvic splanchnics.
C. Sympathetics that innervate the jejunum originated from the lumbar splanchnics.
D. Diverticulosis is commonly found in the ileum.
E. The ascending colon receives blood directly from the right colic artery.

12. A 31-year-old man receives a penetrating knife wound in the abdomen and is injured in both the superior mesenteric artery and the posterior vagal trunk. Which portion of the colon would most likely be impaired by this injury?
A. Ascending and descending colons.
B. Distal 1/3 of transverse colon and sigmoid colon.
C. Proximal 2/3 of transverse colon and sigmoid colon.
D. Cecum and ascending colon.
E. Cecum and distal 1/3 of transverse colon.

13. The villi of the small intestine contain lymphatic capillaries known as lacteals and they are responsible for the absorption of dietary fat. Beginning with the lacteals, what is the order of lymph nodes in which these fats as well as lymph travel to the superior mesenteric lymph nodes?
A. Lacteals, intermediate (mesenteric), juxta-intestinal, central (superior), superior mesenteric lymph nodes.
B. Lacteals, central (superior), juxta-intestinal, intermediate (mesenteric), superior mesenteric lymph nodes.
C. Lacteals, juxta-intestinal, intermediate (mesenteric), central (superior), superior mesenteric lymph nodes.
D. Lacteals, juxta-intestinal, central (superior), intermediate (mesenteric), superior mesenteric lymph nodes.
E. Lacteals, central (superior), intermediate (mesenteric), juxta-intestinal, superior mesenteric lymph nodes.

14. Which pairing of vessels is NOT considered one of the portocaval anastomoses?
A. Colic and retroperitoneal veins.
B. Superior mesenteric and splenic veins.
C. Paraumbilical and epigastric veins.
D. Superior rectal and middle/inferior rectal veins.
E. Left gastric and esophageal veins.

15. A rare soft tissue sarcoma known as a gastrointestional stromal tumor (GIST) is identified after a CT scan is done on a 21-year-old male who has come in complaining of pain in the abdomen, infrequent bowel movements and on a more frequent basis, blood is seen in his stool. The mass is originating from the descending colon and has extended medially near the aorta and partially into the upper pelvic cavity. Surgery will be performed but it will take place near the ureter. Which statement about the ureter is INCORRECT?
A. It passes anterior to the gonadal vessels.
B. In the female it passes inferior to the uterine arteries.
C. It is considered a retroperitoneal structure.
D. They enter the pelvis near the common iliac artery bifurcation.
E. It has a constriction at the ureteropelvic junction.

16. Which statement about the posterior abdominal wall is INCORRECT?
   A. The middle suprarenal arteries branch from the renal arteries.
   B. Sym/pre fibers synapse directly with chromaffin cells in the adrenal medulla.
   C. The kidneys initial lymphatic drainage is to the lumbar lymph nodes.
   D. The right kidney lies between vertebral levels L1-L4.
   E. There is a constriction of the ureter when it traverses the bladder wall.
17. Which statement about the diaphragm is INCORRECT?
   A. Only the central portion moves when a person is inhaling air.
   B. The aorta passes through the aortic hiatus at T12.
   C. The phrenic nerve supplies motor fibers to the diaphragm.
   D. The superior phrenic artery supplies most of the blood to the diaphragm.
   E. The medial arcuate ligaments are formed by the thickening of psoas muscle fascia.
18. Which statement about the posterior abdominal wall is INCORRECT?
   A. The right middle suprarenal artery originates from the aorta.
   B. The left suprarenal vein drains into the left renal vein.
   C. The aortic hiatus allows for the passage of both the aorta & thoracic duct.
   D. The paranephric fat of the kidney lies between the renal capsule and renal fascia.
   E. The medial arcuate ligaments are made up of a thickening of psoas muscle fascia.
19. A patient has recently been diagnosed with hypertension and low potassium levels in the blood. The physician suspects a tumor may be causing the imbalance of a mineralocorticoid known as aldosterone. A CT scan is ordered and it reveals a tumor located in what part of the suprarenal gland?
   A. Zona glomerulosa of suprarenal cortex.
   B. Zona fasciculate of suprarenal cortex.
   C. Zona reticularis of suprarenal cortex.
   D. Medulla of suprarenal gland.
   E. All regions of the suprarenal gland.
20. During development, the midgut will rotate a total of ____ and in a _____ direction before the GI tract finds itself back in the abdomen.
   A. 90 degrees clockwise.
   B. 90 degrees counterclockwise.
   C. 180 degrees clockwise.
   D. 270 degrees clockwise.
   E. 270 degrees counterclockwise.
21. Which statement about a congenital diaphragmatic hernia (CDH) is CORRECT?
   A. CDH occurs in 1 in 20,000 newborns.
   B. CDH is the failure of the pleuroperitoneal membranes to form.
   C. CDH is the failure of the septum transversum to form.
   D. CDH is the failure of the dorsal mesentery of the esophagus to form.
   E. CDH is the least common cause of pulmonary hypoplasia.
22. A 27-year old woman is in the late 2nd trimester of her pregnancy when she undergoes a fetal ultrasound and an anterior abdominal wall defect is observed. She then undergoes a MRI and it is revealed that there is a defect involving a herniation of bowel loops through the abdominal wall just to the right of the umbilicus and there was no sac observed. What developmental defect is depicted on the MRI?
   A. Gastroschisis.
   B. Meckel's diverticulum.
   C. Omphalocele.
   D. Hirschsprung's disease.
   E. Imperforate anus.
23. Which statement regarding the histology of the kidney is INCORRECT?
   A. The proximal convoluted tubule (PCT) absorbs 65-80% of all the filtrate.
   B. The intercalated cells of collecting ducts modulate the acid-base balance of the body.
   C. The macula densa is specialized epithelium of the glomerulus.
   D. Countercurrent exchange is the efficient modification of ultrafiltrate into urine and involves the thick and thin limbs of the loop of Henle.
   E. Juxtaglomerular cells release the enzyme renin.
24. During the development of the collecting system of the kidney, the ureteric bud forms what structure?
   A. Ureter.
   B. Renal pelvis.
   C. Major and minor calyces.
   D. Collecting tubules.
   E. All of the above.
25. A 25 year-old male presents to the emergency department with a stab wound to the right upper quadrant (RUQ) of the abdomen. Of the listed structures, which one is NOT located in the RUQ?
   A. Right suprarenal gland.
   B. Right lobe of liver.
   C. 2nd part of the duodenum.
   D. Fundus of the stomach.
   E. Uncinate process of pancreas.
26. During development there are some structures that were originally intraperitoneal but later become fixed to the posterior abdominal wall and are reclassified as secondary retroperitoneal. Which of the following structures did not undergo this reclassification during development?
   A. Ascending colon.
   B. Pancreas.
   C. Rectum.
   D. 2-4th parts of the duodenum.
   E. Descending colon.
27. The esophagogastric junction or better known as the Z-line is an important region where an abrupt change from the esophageal stratified squamous epithelium becomes another type of epithelium. What is this new epithelium?
   A. Stratified cuboidal.
   B. Simple columnar.
   C. Stratified columnar.
   D. Pseudostratified columnar.
   E. Simple squamous.
28. A 5 year-old girl who never had a history of bed-wetting is now having that problem but her parents suspect this is the case because she is known to drink a lot of fluids during the day. The child is also losing weight, complains of fatigue, weakness, and blurred vision. Her physician suspects diabetes and orders

a glycated hemoglobin (A1C) test to be performed over two consecutive months and this will determine the percentage of blood sugar attached to the oxygen-carrying protein in red blood cells (hemoglobin). The tests are performed and she registers a larger than 6.5 percent confirming a diagnosis of type 1 diabetes. Type 1 diabetes is an autoimmune destruction of the insulin-producing cells located in the pancreas. What cells in the pancreas secrete insulin?
A. Alpha cells.
B. Beta cells.
C. Delta cells.
D. F cells.

29. Which cells are located on the luminal surfaces of the liver sinusoids, are classified as macrophages, and are responsible for digesting hemoglobin, metabolizing aged erythrocytes, destroying bacteria, and secreting proteins related to immunological processes?
A. Ito.
B. Chief.
C. Paneth.
D. Kupffer.
E. Parietal.

30. Which one of the lumbar plexus nerves listed below is correctly paired with their contributing ventral rami?
A. Lateral femoral cutaneous (L2-L3).
B. Femoral nerve (L1).
C. Obturator nerve (L1-L2).
D. Ilioinguinal nerve (L2-L3).
E. Genitofemoral nerve (L2-L4).

ANSWERS

1. **C.** The efferent limb of the cremasteric reflex involves the genital branch of the genitofemoral nerve.
2. **C.** The posterior layer above the arcuate line, consists of ½ the internal oblique and all the transversus abdominis aponeuroses.
3. **D.** The correct order would be Skin, Campers's, Scarpa's, Ext. oblique aponeurosis, Int. oblique aponeurosis, Transversus abdominis aponeurosis, Rectus abdominis, Transversalis fascia, Extraperitoneal fat, Parietal peritoneum.
4. **E.** The hernial sac of a direct inguinal hernia is covered by transversalis fascia.
A. The roof of the inguinal canal is formed by a combination of the transversalis fascia and aponeuroses of the external oblique, internal oblique and transversus abdominis.
B. The medial border of Hesselbach's triangle is formed by the rectus abdominis muscle.
C. Direct inguinal hernias pass medially to the inferior epigastric vessels.
D. Indirect inguinal hernias account for about 70-75% of all inguinal hernias.
5. **C.** In over 90% of the population the cystic artery originates from the right hepatic artery.
6. **A.** The splenic artery passes through the splenorenal ligament.
7. **D.** Bile passes through the bile canaliculi followed by the (interlobular) bile ducts.
8. **A.** The anterior vagal trunk is the continuation of the left vagus nerve and the parasympathetic fibers that run through them target foregut structures, of which the 2nd part of the duodenum is one of them.
9. **B.** The ileocolic artery has multiple branches, one of which is the appendicular artery.
10. **E.** The jejunum has long vasa recta (straight arteries) and few arcade loops.
A. Peyer's patches are located primarily in the ileum.
B. The jejunum contains large, tall and closely packed circular folds (plicae circulares).
C. The jejunum accounts for ~40% of the total length of the small intestine.
D. The ileum is located primarily in the right lower quadrant.
11. **E.** The ascending colon receives blood directly from the right colic artery.
A. The sigmoid colon is part of the hindgut and this portion of the developing gut does not necessarily rotate during development much like the foregut and midgut.
B. Parasympathetics that innervate the proximal 2/3 of the transverse colon originated from the posterior vagal trunk.
C. Sympathetics that innervate the jejunum originate primarily from the lesser and least splanchnics.
D. Diverticulosis is most commonly found in the sigmoid colon.
12. **D.** The structures that were damaged, superior mesenteric artery and posterior vagal trunk, are both associated with the midgut and that would include the cecum and ascending colon.
13. **C.** The proper order in which fat and lymph will travel from the lacteals to the superior mesenteric lymph nodes is: lacteals, juxta-intestinal, intermediate (mesenteric), central (superior), and finally the superior mesenteric lymph nodes.
14. **B.** The superior mesenteric and splenic veins unite to form the portal vein but are not considered one of the portocaval anastomoses.
15. **A.** The ureter will pass posterior to the gonadal vessels.
16. **A.** The middle suprarenal arteries originate directly off of the abdominal aorta at approximately the L1 vertebral level.
17. **D.** It is the inferior phrenic and not the superior phrenic artery that supplies most of the blood to the diaphragm.
18. **D.** The paranephric (pararenal) fat lies between the renal fascia and the fascia along the posterior abdominal wall that was a continuation of the transversalis fascia.
19. **A.** The zona glomerulosa is the region that secretes mineralocorticoids namely aldosterone.
B. The zona fasciculate is responsible for glucocorticoids namely cortisol.
C. The zona reticularis is responsible for producing precursor androgens with the primary product being dehydroepiandrosterone (DHEA).
D. The suprarenal medulla secrete the catecholamines epinephrine and norepinephrine.
E. The individual would present with more symptoms if the entire suprarenal gland were affected.
20. **E.** During development, the midgut rotates a total of 270 degrees and in a counterclockwise direction before the GI tract finds itself back in the abdomen.
21. **B.** A congenital diaphragmatic hernia (CDH) is the failure of the pleuroperitoneal membranes not forming and not that of the septum transversum or dorsal mesentery of the esophagus.

They occur in every 1/2,000 births and are the most common cause of pulmonary hypoplasia.

22. **A.** Gastroschisis is a defect involving a herniation of bowel loops through the abdominal wall usually on the right side and there is no observable sac surrounding it.
23. **C.** The macula densa is specialized epithelium of the distal convoluted tubule (DCT) near the vascular pole of the glomerulus.
24. **E.** The ureteric bud forms all of the listed structures.
25. **D.** The majority of the stomach including the fundus would be located in the left upper quadrant (LUQ). The only portion generally seen in the RUQ would be the pyloric region.
26. **C.** The upper portion of the rectum is considered a primary retroperitoneal structure while the lower portion lies subperitoneal thus neither portion of the rectum ever transitioned from being an intraperitoneal structure. Note: the tail of the pancreas is closely associated with the hilum of the spleen and can remain intraperitoneal while the rest of it undergoes the intraperitoneal to secondary retroperitoneal transition.
27. **B.** Simple columnar epithelium will be the primary epithelial layer of the GI tract until the pectinate (dentate) line of the anal canal. At this point the simple columnar epithelium will revert back to a stratified squamous epithelium.
28. **B.** The beta cells of the pancreas are responsible for secreting insulin.
    A. Alpha cells secrete glucagon.
    C. Delta cells secrete both somatostatin and gastrin.
    D. F cells secrete pancreatic polypeptide.
29. **D.** The Kupffer cells are located in the liver and serve as macrophages.
    A. Ito cells.
    B. Chief cells are located in the stomach.
    C. Paneth cells are located in the intestine.
    E. Parietal cells are located in the stomach.
30. **A.** The correct ventral rami contributions to the lateral femoral cutaneous nerve are L2-L3.
    B. Femoral nerve (L2-L4).
    C. Obturator nerve (L2-L4).
    D. Ilioinguinal nerve (L1).
    E. Genitofemoral nerve (L1-L2).

References

1. Ivanschuk G, Cesmebasi A, Sorenson EP, Blaak C, Loukas M, Tubbs SR. Amyand's hernia: a review. Med Sci Monit 2014;20:140–146 PubMed
2. Bollinger RR, Barbas AS, Bush EL, Lin SS, Parker W. Biofilms in the large bowel suggest an apparent function of the human vermiform appendix. Journal of Theoretical Biology. 2007; 249:826-831

4 Pelvis and Perineum

LEARNING OBJECTIVES

- To understand all the bones associated with the pelvis, what defines the greater versus the lesser pelvis, and obstetrically important pelvic diameters. Clinical correlates include a look at the differences between a male and female pelvis.
- To describe the joints and ligaments of the pelvic girdle. A clinical correlate takes a look at the effect of pregnancy on pelvic ligaments and joints.
- To describe the peritoneal reflections in both male and females.
- To describe the pelvic cavity wall, floor, and muscles associated with each and what is the effect of a pelvic floor injury.
- To understand the pelvic fascia with an emphasis on the endopelvic fascia.
- To describe the somatic sacral and coccygeal nerve plexuses and the individual nerves associated with each. Describe the parasympathetic and sympathetic innervation pathways to all pelvic cavity viscera.
- To describe the major arteries, veins and general lymphatic drainage of the pelvic cavity.
- To describe the neurovasculature, lymphatic drainage, and histology of the pelvic viscera.
- To describe the embryology associated with the urogenital system.
- Clinical correlates include urethral catheterization, urethral ruptures, exstrophy of the bladder, deferentectomy, prostate examination and cancer, prostate brachytherapy, birth control pills, ectopic pregnancy, hysterectomy, endometriosis, fibroids, abnormal placentas, nabothian cysts, pap smears, culdocentesis, pelvic inflammatory disease, uterus and vagina abnormalities, phimosis, paraphimosis, circumcision, impotence and erectile dysfunction, episiotomy, hypospadias, epispadias, bifid penis, pudendal nerve blocks, and lumbar epidurals.

The **pelvis** refers to the region of the trunk located inferior to the abdomen. The inferior most part of the abdominopelvic cavity is referred to as the *pelvic cavity*. From an anatomical standpoint, the pelvis refers to the part of the body surrounded by the *pelvic girdle*, which is a part of the appendicular skeleton of the lower limb.

4.1 Pelvis

There are superior and inferior boundaries that define the **pelvic cavity** and they are known respectively as the pelvic inlet and pelvic outlet. The bony edge of the pelvic inlet is called the **pelvic brim** but these two terms are used interchangeably. The **pelvic inlet** (*superior pelvic aperture*) is bounded by the **linea terminialis** and this is formed by the **(Fig. 4.1; Fig. 4.2)**:

- Pubic symphysis (superior margin).
- Pubic crest (posterior border).
- The continuation of the superior ramus of the pubis called the **pectineal line (pecten pubis)**.
- **Arcuate line** of the ilium.
- Ala of the sacrum (anterior border).
- Sacral promontory.

The **pelvic outlet** (*inferior pelvic aperture*) is bounded by:

- Pubic symphysis (inferior margin).
- Inferior rami of the pubis and ischial tuberosities.
- Sacrotuberous ligaments.
- Tip of the coccyx.

4.2 Pelvic Girdle

The **pelvic girdle** is a ring of bones connecting the vertebral column to the femurs of the thighs. The pelvic girdle is quite strong and functions to transfer the weight of the upper body from the axial to the lower appendicular skeleton during standing and walking. It also withstands compression and other forces resulting from its support of the body weight. The bony pelvis is formed by three bones:

- Left and right hip (coxal) bones that consist of an ilium, ischium and pubis (**Fig. 4.3** and in Chapter 5).
- The sacrum which is formed by the fusion of five sacral vertebrae.

4.3 Ilium

The **ilium** makes up the largest portion of the hip bone and the superior portion of the acetabulum. The **body of the ilium** represents the junction between the ischium and pubis and creates a portion of the acetabulum. The thick medial columns are responsible for weight bearing but the thin wing-like parts, or **alae**, provide large areas for attaching muscles. The **iliac crest** is the long and curved border of the ala that bridges the **anterior superior iliac spine** (ASIS) and **posterior superior iliac spines** (PSIS). The ASIS and **anterior inferior iliac spines** (AIIS) provide attachment sites for muscles. The **posterior inferior iliac spine** (PIIS) located just below the PSIS marks the superior border of the *greater sciatic notch* **(Fig. 4.4)**.

The **iliac tubercle** is located on the iliac crest approximately 5 cm posterior to the ASIS and the smooth depression found on the medial side of each ala is called the **iliac fossa**. The **anterior**, **posterior** and **inferior gluteal lines** located on the lateral side of the ala are related to attachment sites for the gluteal muscle group. On the medial side and posterior aspect of the ilium there are some rough regions, one of which is the ear-shaped articular region called the **auricular surface** and the other being the **iliac tuberosity**. This is the location of the *sacroiliac joint* and it consists of both a synovial and syndesmotic articulation **(Fig. 4.4)**.

4.4 Ischium

The **ischium** is located on the posteroinferior portion of the hip bone and contributes to the posteroinferior part of the acetabulum. Its superior portion or **body of the ischium** fuses with the ilium and pubis bones. The **ramus of the ischium** connects to the inferior ramus of the pubis and forms a combined structure known as the **ischiopubic ramus**. The larger projection seen on the inferior end of the ramus of the ischium is called the **ischial tuberosity (Fig. 4.4)**.

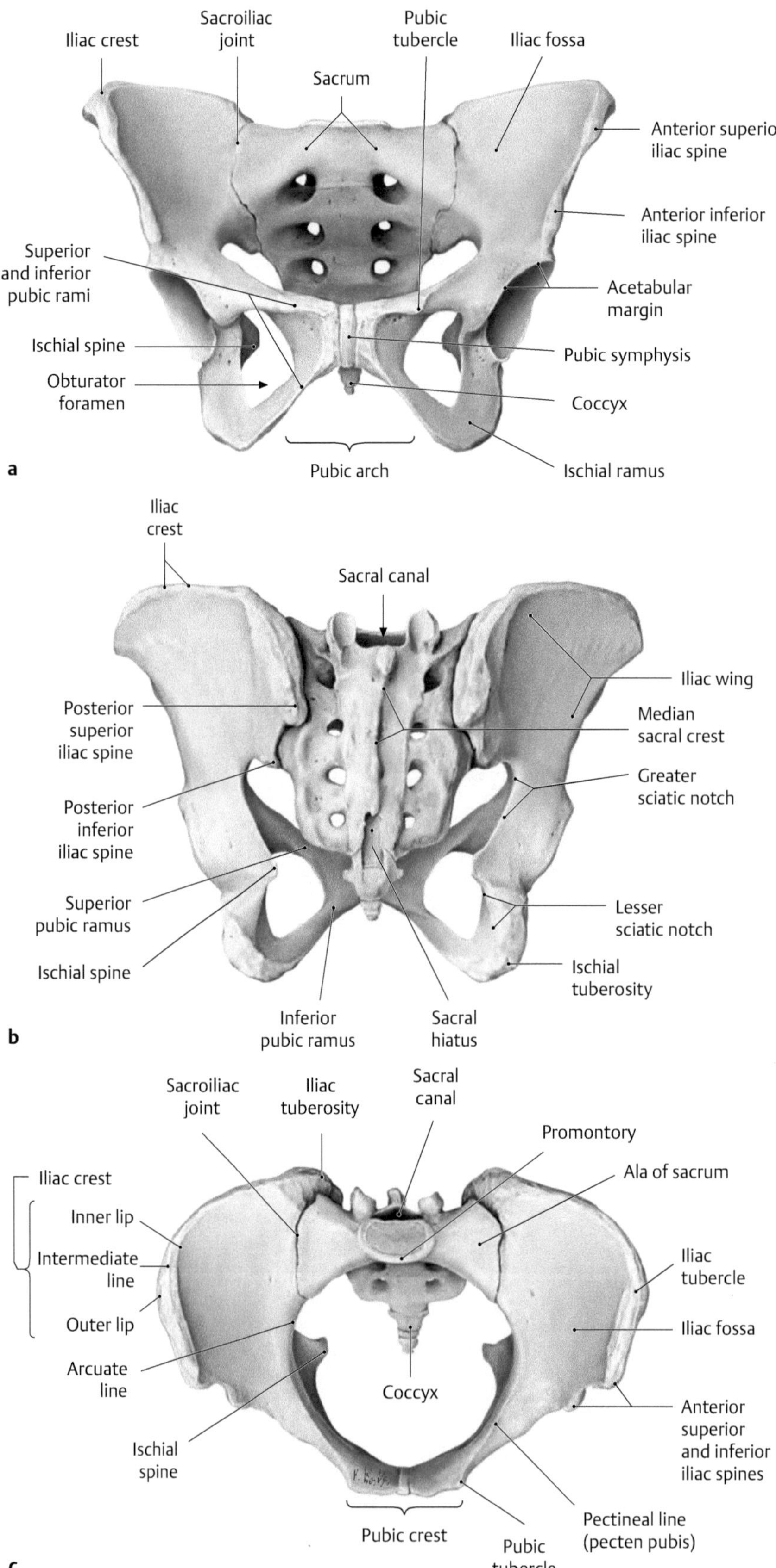

Fig. 4.1 The female pelvis. **(a)** Anterior view. **(b)** Posterior view. **(c)** Superior view. (From Schuenke M, Schulte E, Schumacher U. THIEME Atlas of Anatomy. General Anatomy and Musculoskeletal System. Illustrations by Voll M and Wesker K. 3rd ed. New York: Thieme Medical Publishers; 2020.)

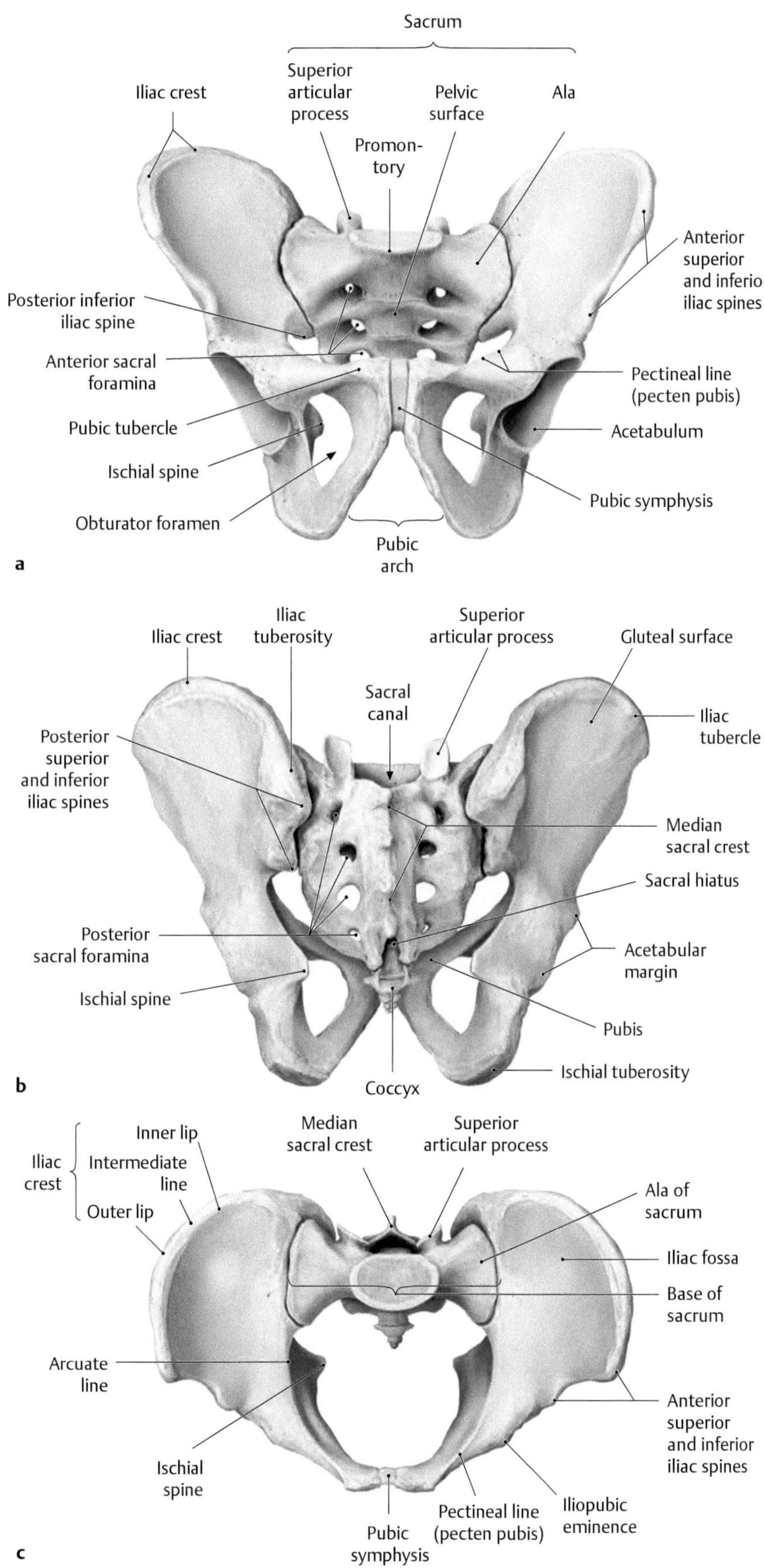

Fig. 4.2 The male pelvis. **(a)** Anterior view. **(b)** Posterior view. **(c)** Superior view. (From Schuenke M, Schulte E, Schumacher U. THIEME Atlas of Anatomy. General Anatomy and Musculoskeletal System. Illustrations by Voll M and Wesker K. 3rd ed. New York: Thieme Medical Publishers; 2020.)

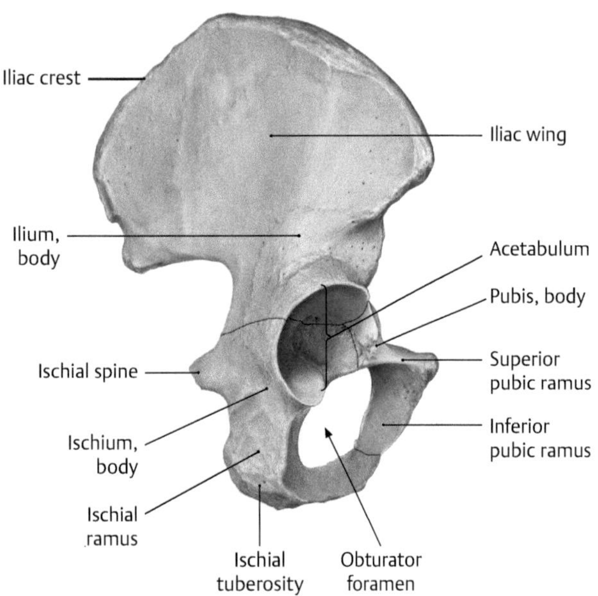

Fig. 4.3 The right hip (coxal) bone and its three parts. The black line between the three parts represents the location of the former triradiate cartilage. (From Schuenke M, Schulte E, Schumacher U. THIEME Atlas of Anatomy. General Anatomy and Musculoskeletal System. Illustrations by Voll M and Wesker K. 3rd ed. New York: Thieme Medical Publishers; 2020.)

The posterior border of the ischium forms the inferior margin of the **greater sciatic notch**. The inferior margin of this notch or the posterior projection near the junction of the ischial body and ramus is called the **ischial spine**, and it serves as a landmark for pudendal anesthesia. Inferior to both the greater sciatic notch and ischial spine is the **lesser sciatic notch (Fig. 4.4)**.

4.5 Pubis

The anteromedial portion of the hip bone is called the **pubis** and it contributes to the anterior part of the acetabulum. There is a centrally located **body of the pubis** that extends out laterally to form both the **superior** and **inferior pubic rami**. The superior pubic rami connect to both the ilium and ischium while the inferior pubic rami contribute to the ischiopubic ramus. The large oval opening bounded by parts of the pubis and ischium is known as the **obturator foramen**, most of which is closed by the **obturator membrane (Fig. 4.4)**.

The pubic bodies both have a *symphysial surface* that articulates with a fibrocartilaginous interpubic disk to help form the pubic symphysis. The **pubic crests** form the anterosuperior portion of these bones and located on the lateral aspects of the crests are the **pubic tubercles**. Extending posteriorly from near the pubic tubercles and onto the superior margin of the superior pubic rami is the **pecten pubis** (pectineal line). The combination of the ischiopubic rami meeting at the pubic symphysis forms the **pubic arch**.

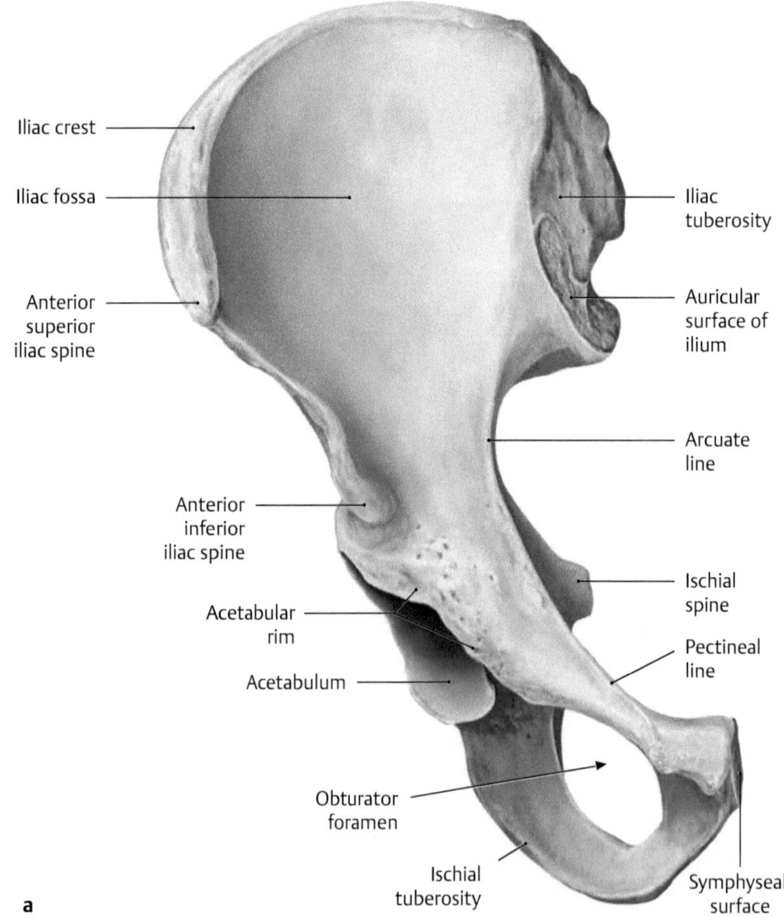

Fig. 4.4 The right hip (coxal) bone. **(a)** Anterior view. (*continued*) (From Schuenke M, Schulte E, Schumacher U. THIEME Atlas of Anatomy. General Anatomy and Musculoskeletal System. Illustrations by Voll M and Wesker K. 3rd ed. New York: Thieme Medical Publishers; 2020.)

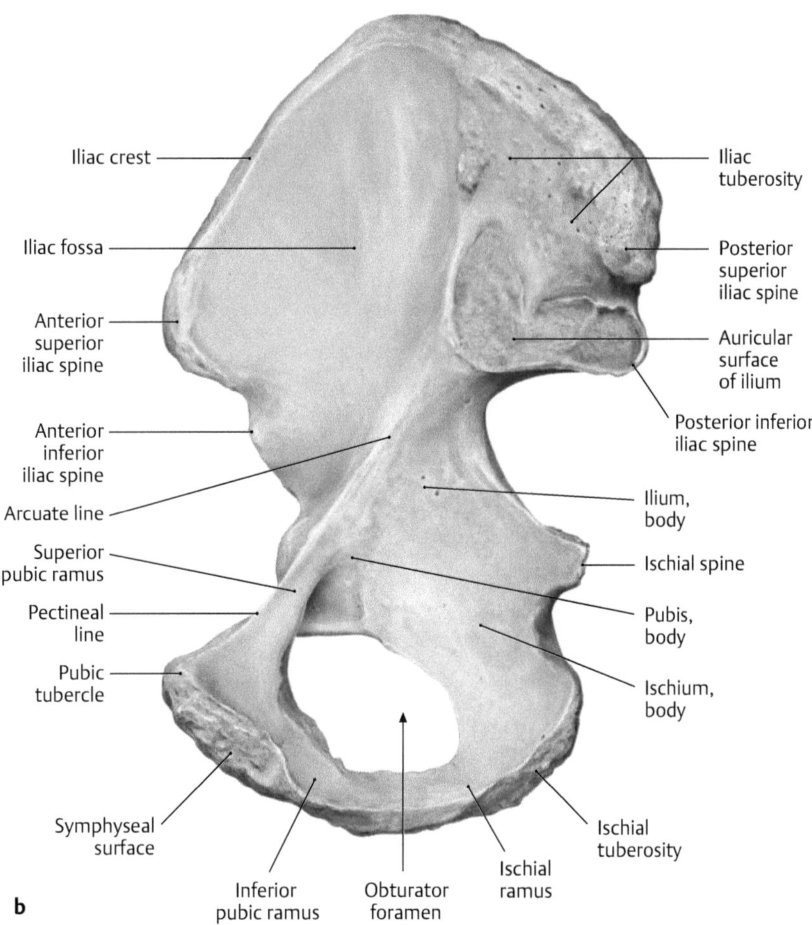

Fig. 4.4 *(continued)* The right hip (coxal) bone. **(b)** Medial view. (From Schuenke M, Schulte E, Schumacher U. THIEME Atlas of Anatomy. General Anatomy and Musculoskeletal System. Illustrations by Voll M and Wesker K. 3rd ed. New York: Thieme Medical Publishers; 2020.)

The inferior borders of the rami along with the pubic symphysis forms the **subpubic angle**, the distance between the left and right ischial tuberosities. This angle can be approximated by the angle between the abducted middle and index fingers for the male and the angle between the index finger and extended thumb for the female. In males this angle is approximately 70° and in females it is between 90-100° **(Fig. 4.5; Table 4.1)**.

4.6 Sacrum

The **sacrum** is responsible for providing strength and stability to the pelvis **(Fig. 4.1; Fig. 4.2)**. It transmits body weight through the pelvic girdle or the combination of the sacrum and hip bones and only the superior half is weight bearing. The superior surface of the S1 vertebra serves as the **base** of the sacrum and the **apex** is the portion that tapers off and articulates with the coccyx. The **sacral promontory** is the anterior projection from the superior portion of the S1 body.

The **pelvic surface** is concave and smooth while the **dorsal surface** is convex and rough. The **lateral surface** has a superior portion called the **auricular surface** and it is the site of the synovial part of the sacroiliac joint between the sacrum and ilium. Posterior to the auricular surface is a rough surface called the **sacral tuberosity** and it serves as an attachment site for the posterior sacroiliac ligaments and forms the syndesmotic portion of the sacroiliac joint. The surfaces of the sacrum are related to multiple ligaments namely the *anterior*, *interosseous* and *posterior sacroiliac*, *sacrotuberous* and *sacrospinous ligaments*.

The continuation of the vertebral canal into the sacrum is called the **sacral canal**. It allows for passage of spinal nerves associated with the cauda equina. These spinal nerves pass through the intervertebral foramen before continuing as either the anterior or posterior rami branches that pass through the **anterior** or **posterior sacral foramina**, respectively. The **sacral hiatus** is a U-shaped space and continuation of the sacral canal that the paired coccygeal (Co1) nerves along with the filum terminale pass through and is the site of a *caudal epidural block*.

The bony pelvis is divided into a **greater** and **lesser pelvis** by the *plane of the pelvic inlet*. This plane spans the superior aspect of the pubic symphysis and the sacral promontory **(Fig. 4.6)**.

- The **greater (false) pelvis** is:
  - Superior to the pelvic inlet.
  - Bounded by the abdominal wall anteriorly, the iliac alae laterally, and L5 and S1 vertebrae posteriorly.
  - The location of a portion of the ileum and sigmoid colon.
- The **lesser (true) pelvis** is:
  - Between the pelvic inlet and the pelvic outlet (plane between inferior aspect of pubic symphysis and tip of coccyx).
  - Bounded by the pelvic surfaces of the hip bones, sacrum and coccyx.

Table 4.1 Gender-specific features of the pelvis

Structure	♀	♂
False pelvis	Wide and shallow	Narrow and deep
Pelvic inlet	Transversely oval	Heart-shaped
Pelvic outlet	Roomy and round	Narrow and oblong
Ischial tuberosities	Everted	Inverted
Pelvic cavity	Roomy and shallow	Narrow and deep
Sacrum	Short, wide, and flat	Long, narrow, and convex
Subpubic angle	90–100 degrees	70 degrees

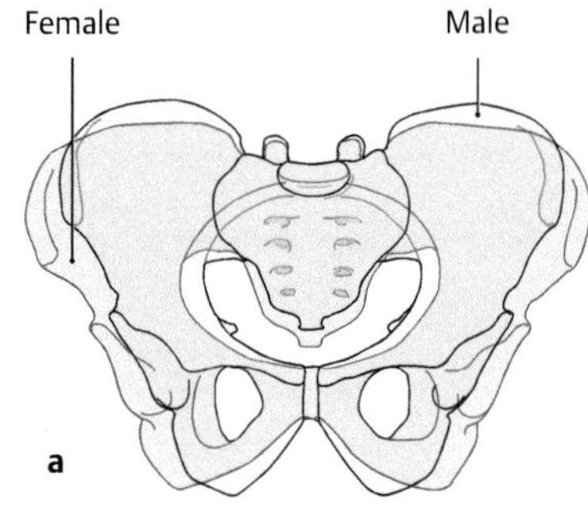

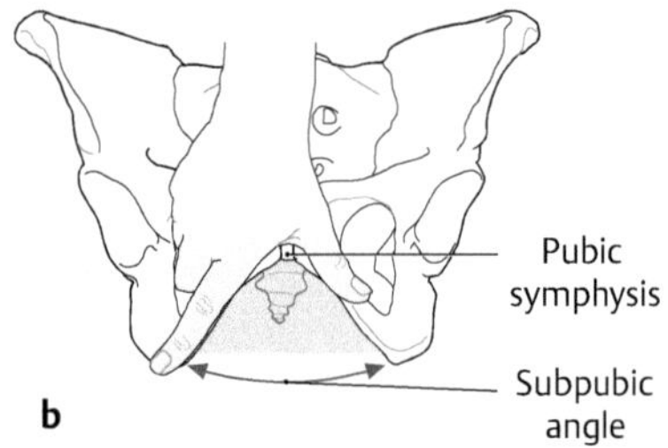

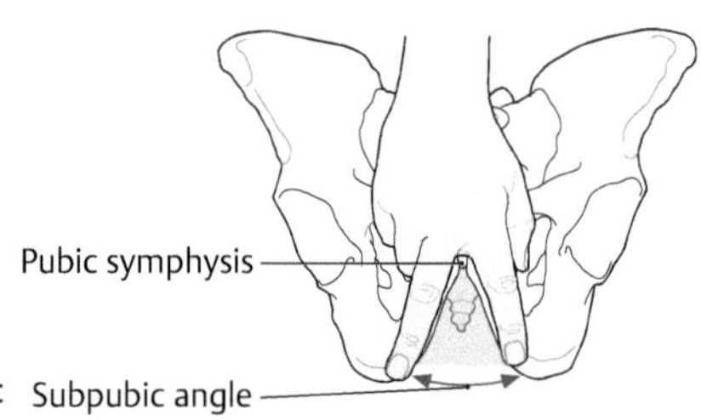

Fig. 4.5 **(a)** Gender-specific features of the pelvis, anterosuperior view. **(b)** Female pelvis. **(c)** Male pelvis. (From Schuenke M, Schulte E, Schumacher U. THIEME Atlas of Anatomy. General Anatomy and Musculoskeletal System. Illustrations by Voll M and Wesker K. 3rd ed. New York: Thieme Medical Publishers; 2020.)

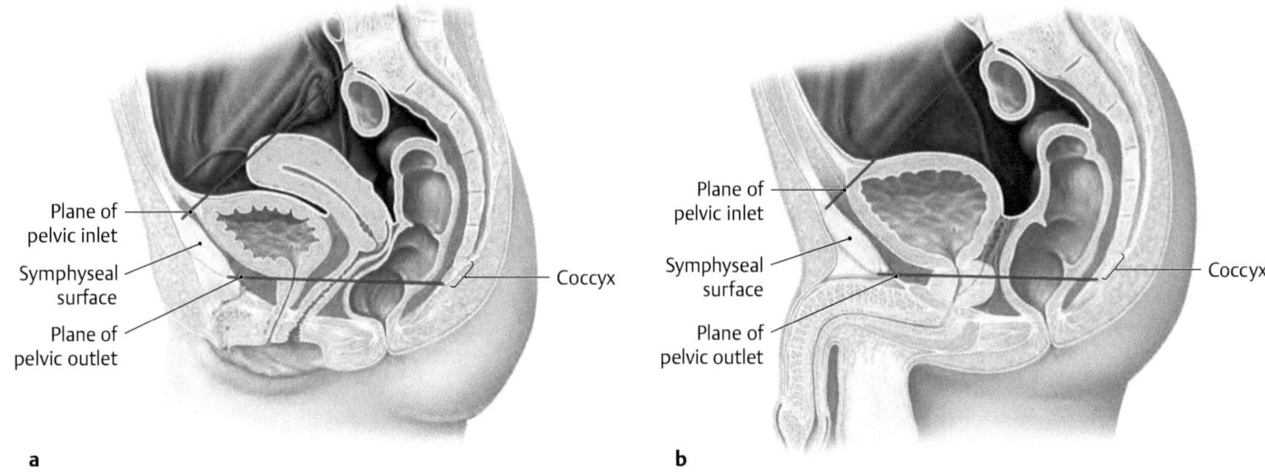

Fig. 4.6 The location of the lesser (true) pelvis. Midsagittal section viewed from left side. **(a)** Female. **(b)** Male. (From Schuenke M, Schulte E, Schumacher U. THIEME Atlas of Anatomy. Internal Organs. Illustrations by Voll M and Wesker K. 3rd ed. New York: Thieme Medical Publishers; 2020.)

- Limited inferiorly by the pelvic diaphragm.
- The location of pelvic viscera.

Certain measurements or diameters of the pelvis are obstetrically important when looking at the size of the pelvic (birth) canal. The distance between the promontory and the most posterosuperior point of the pubic symphysis is called the **true conjugate** and it is the narrowest anteroposterior diameter of the pelvic (birth) canal. A **diagonal conjugate** exists because it is hard to measure the true conjugate due to the visceral organs present and in the way. The diagonal conjugate is the distance between the promontory and inferior border of the pubic symphysis. The **transverse** and **oblique diameters** of the female pelvic inlet along with the **interspinous diameter** between the ischial spines are also obstetrically important. The interspinous diameter is the narrowest diameter of the pelvic outlet and pelvic canal. The **pelvic canal** is the passageway including the pelvic inlet, lesser pelvis and pelvic outlet of which a fetus' head will pass during delivery. Diameters applicable to both male and female include the **transtubercular distance** connecting the iliac tubercles and the **interspinous distance** connecting the anterior superior iliac spines together (**Fig. 4.7**).

Clinical Correlate 4.1

Sexual Differences between the Male and Female Pelvis
The male pelvis is thicker, heavier and displays more prominent bony processes mainly due to the presence of larger muscles. The female pelvis is wider and shallower with a larger pelvic inlet and outlet due to a fetal head passing through the lesser pelvis during child birth. The lesser pelvis diameter is a key component to establishing a safe passage for delivery of a fetus (**Fig. 4.5** and **Table 4.1**).

4.7 Joints and Ligaments of the Pelvic Girdle

The two primary joints of the pelvis are the **sacroiliac** and **pubic symphysis**, and they link the skeleton of the trunk and lower limb. There are two other joints that are directly related to the pelvic girdle, the **lumbosacral** and **sacrococcygeal joints**.

4.7.1 Sacroiliac Joints

- These are strong, weight-bearing and compound joints consisting of an anterior *synovial joint* between the auricular surfaces of the sacrum and ilium and a posterior *syndesmosis joint* located between the tuberosities of these same bones. The synovial joint auricular surfaces are irregular but are compatible and help engage the joint (**Fig. 4.8; Fig. 4.9**).

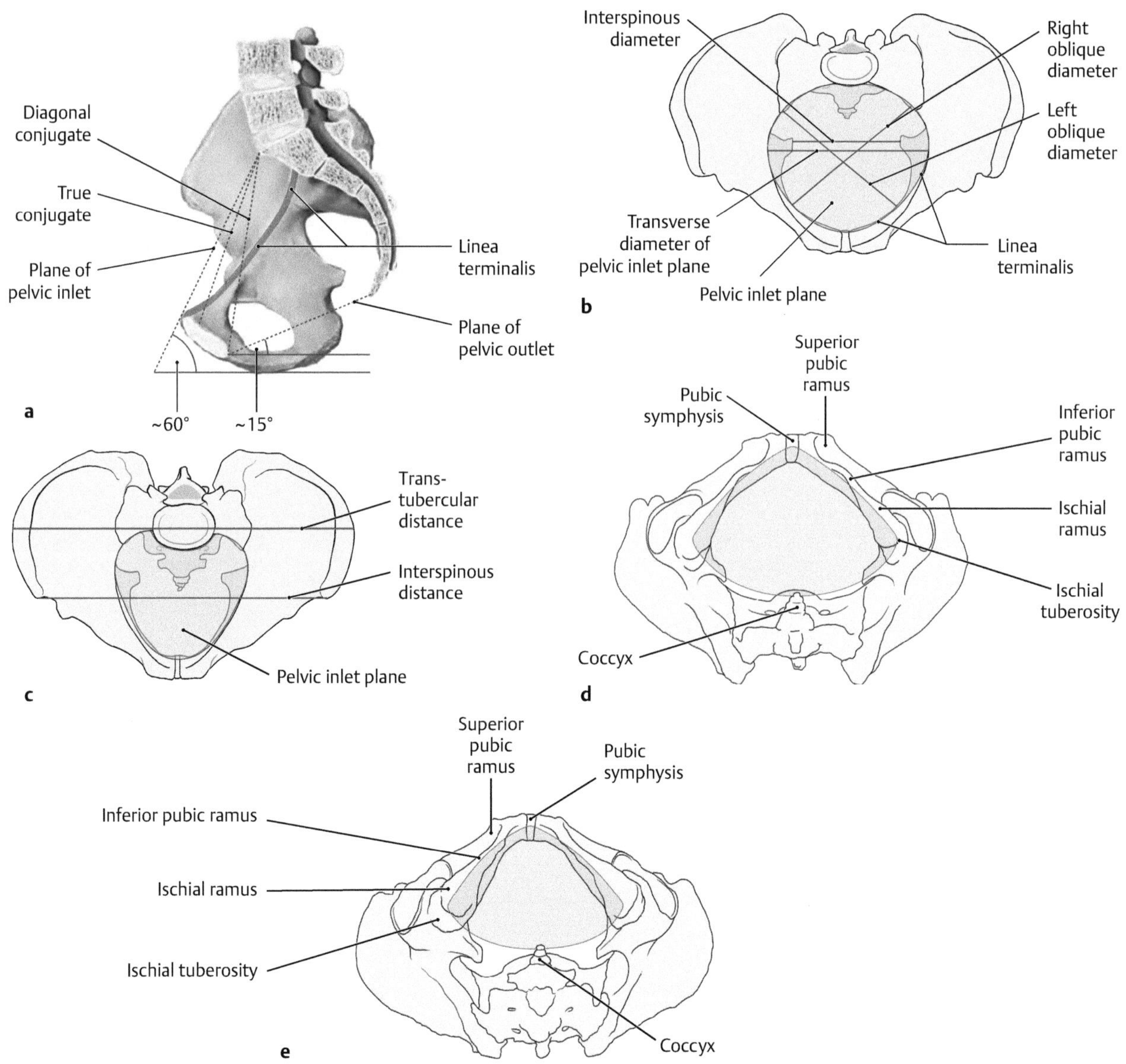

Fig. 4.7 Internal and external pelvic measurements. **(a)** Right half of a female pelvis, medial view. **(b)** Female pelvis, superior view. **(c)** Male pelvis, superior view. **(d)** Female pelvis, inferior view. **(e)** Male pelvis, inferior view. Pelvic inlet outlined in *red* (b,c). Pelvic outlet outlined in *red* (d,e). (From Schuenke M, Schulte E, Schumacher U. THIEME Atlas of Anatomy. General Anatomy and Musculoskeletal System. Illustrations by Voll M and Wesker K. 3rd ed. New York: Thieme Medical Publishers; 2020.)

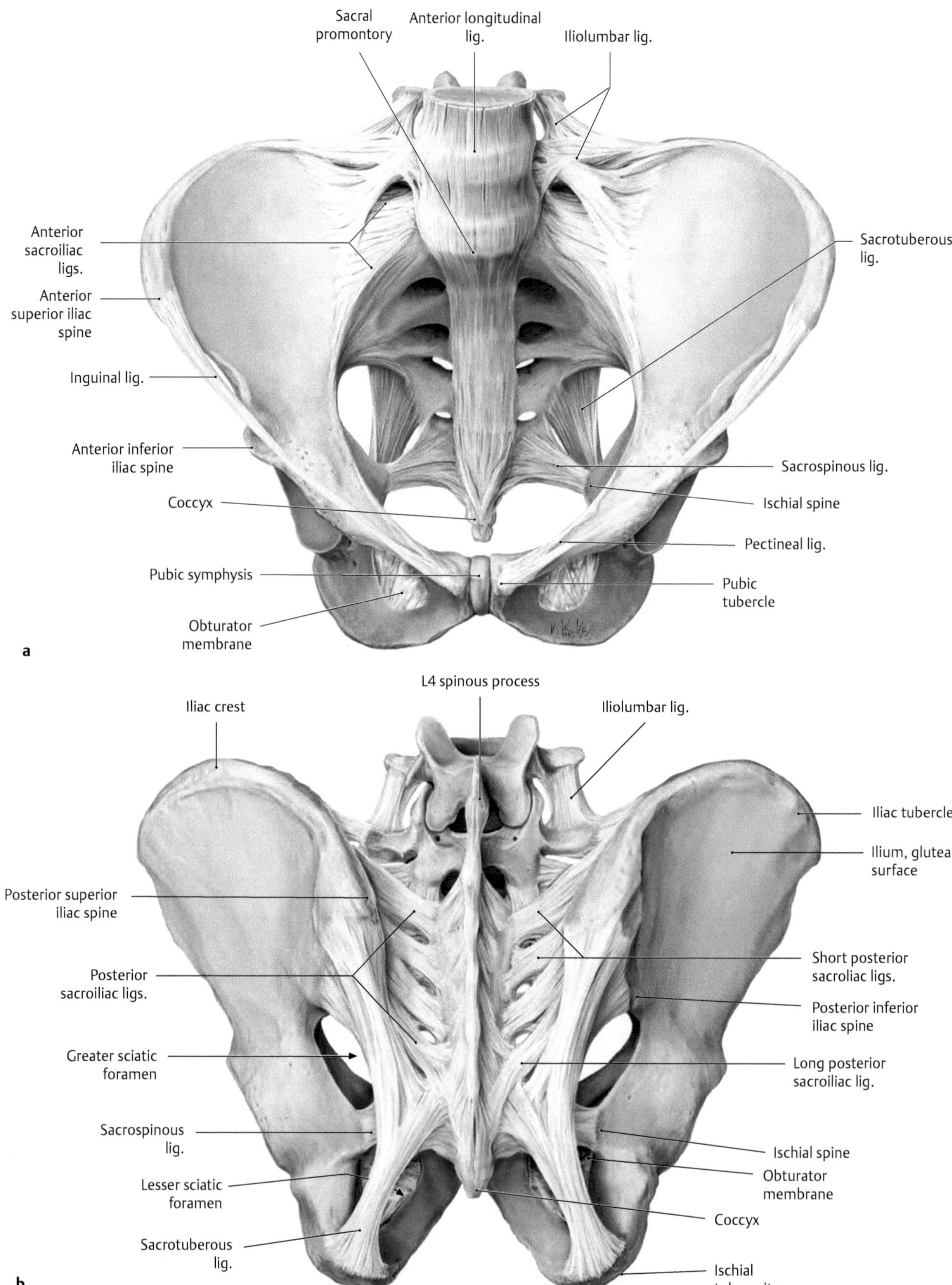

Fig. 4.8 Ligaments of the pelvis, male pelvis. **(a)** Anterosuperior view. **(b)** Posterior view. (From Schuenke M, Schulte E, Schumacher U. THIEME Atlas of Anatomy. General Anatomy and Musculoskeletal System. Illustrations by Voll M and Wesker K. 3rd ed. New York: Thieme Medical Publishers; 2020.)

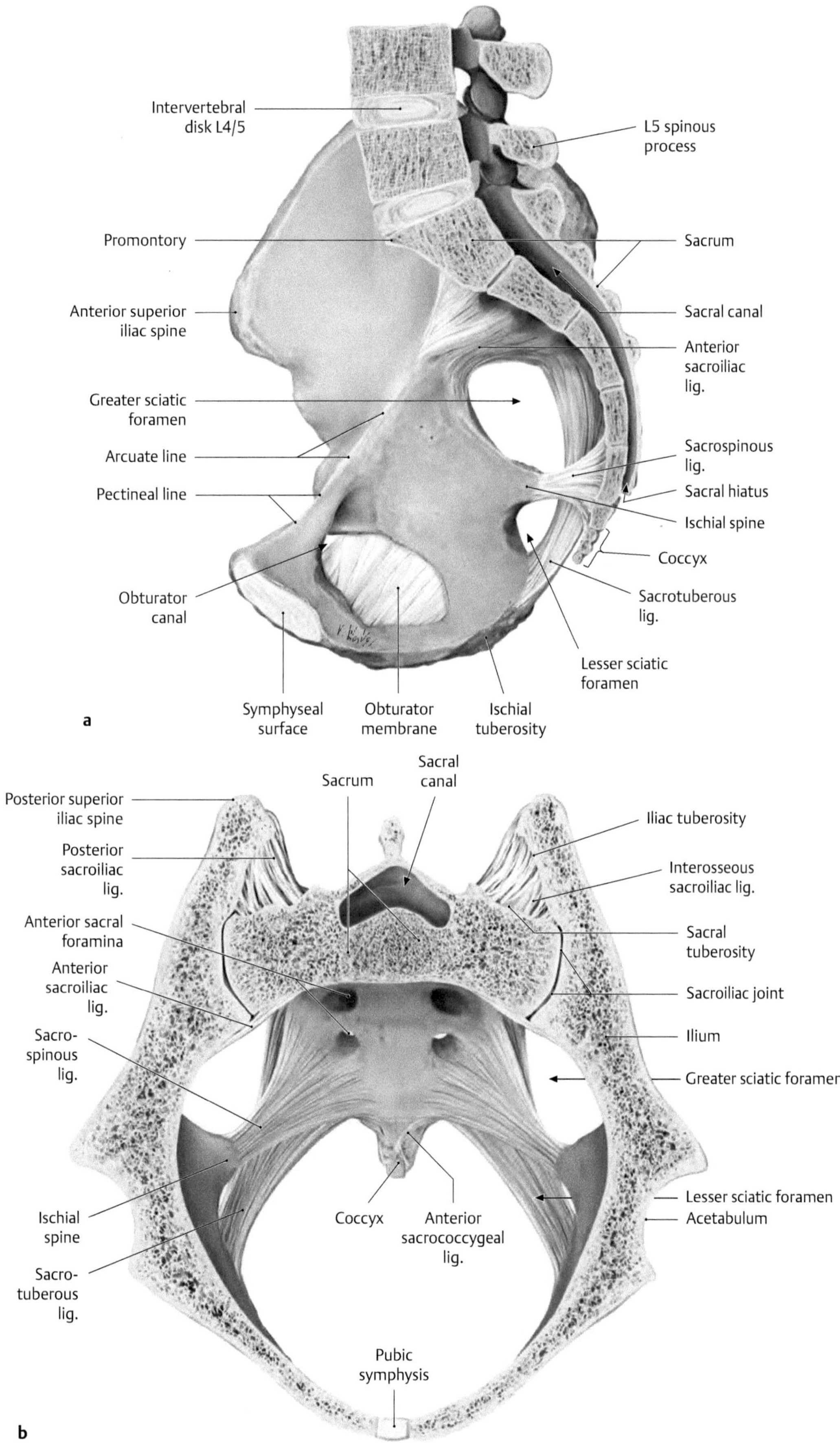

Fig. 4.9 Ligaments of the sacroiliac joint, male pelvis. **(a)** Right half of pelvis, medial half. **(b)** Oblique section, superior view. (From Schuenke M, Schulte E, Schumacher U. THIEME Atlas of Anatomy. General Anatomy and Musculoskeletal System. Illustrations by Voll M and Wesker K. 3rd ed. New York: Thieme Medical Publishers; 2020.)

- Mobility of the joint is limited, which differs from most synovial joints. This is due to their role in transmitting most of the body weight to the hip bones.
- The **anterior sacroiliac, interosseous sacroiliac** and **posterior sacroiliac ligaments** add strength to these joints.
- Movement is limited to slight gliding and rotary movements except for when considerable force is applied during late pregnancy or after a high jump. The weight of the body is transmitted through the sacrum anterior to the rotation axis. This rotates the superior part of the sacrum inferiorly while the inferior part rotates superiorly. The **sacrotuberous** and **sacrospinous ligaments** resist these rotations. These ligaments allow limited upward movement of the inferior end of the sacrum. This then provides resilience to the sacroiliac region when the vertebral column takes on sudden weight increases.

4.7.2 Pubic Symphysis

- A *secondary cartilaginous joint* formed by the union of the bodies of the pubic bones (**Fig. 4.8; Fig. 4.9**).
- Has a **fibrocartilaginous interpubic disk** that is generally wider in women.
- Decussating fibers of tendinous attachments of the rectus abdominis and external oblique muscles called the **superior/ inferior pubic ligaments** strengthen the anterior portion of the pubic symphysis.

4.7.3 Lumbosacral Joints

- A combination joint that includes the articulation between the L5 and S1 vertebrae formed by the L5/S1 intervertebral (IV) disk (*secondary cartilaginous*) and at two zygapophysial (facet) joints (*synovial*) between the articular processes of these same vertebrae (**Fig. 4.8; Fig. 4.9**).
- The **iliolumbar ligaments** join the L5 transverse processes to the ilia.

Clinical Correlate 4.2

Effect of Pregnancy on Pelvic Ligaments and Joints

Pelvic ligaments and joints relax during the late stages of pregnancy. The hormone *relaxin* along with other sex hormones is responsible for this greater mobility especially at the pubic symphysis and sacroiliac joints. The diameters increase in mostly the transverse plane which facilitates the passage of a fetus through the pelvic canal.

4.7.4 Sacrococcygeal Joint

- A *secondary cartilaginous joint* located where the sacrum meets the coccyx and it has a disk similar to an IV disk (**Fig. 4.9**).
- The **anterior/posterior sacrococcygeal ligaments** strengthen the joint

4.8 Peritoneum and Peritoneal Cavity of the Pelvis

The parietal peritoneum of the abdominal cavity extends down into the pelvic cavity but only rests over the superior aspects of most pelvic viscera. The ovaries are not covered by peritoneum although they are in the pelvic cavity. When the oocyte is expelled at ovulation it is located in the peritoneal cavity before being captured by the fimbriae of the uterine tubes. If the peritoneum rested over the ovary the oocyte would not be able to reach the uterine tube. The uterine tubes are intraperitoneal and suspended by a mesentery except for at the ostia where the oocyte would be captured. Due to the peritoneum reflecting back from most pelvic viscera, it forms folds, pouches and fossae. The peritoneum is loosely attached to the suprapubic crest and this allows the urinary bladder to expand superiorly as it fills. These reflections can include (**Fig. 4.10; Fig. 4.11**):

- **Supravesical and paravesical fossae** (male/female): fossae located on the superior and lateral aspects of the bladder respectively.
- **Rectovesical pouch** (male): pouch resting over and between the rectum, seminal vesicles and urinary bladder.
- **Vesicouterine pouch** (female): pouch between the urinary bladder and anterior uterus.
- **Rectouterine pouch** (of Douglas in females): reflection over rectum and posterior vagina.
- **Rectouterine (uterosacral) fold** (female): a fold connecting the rectum and uterine cervix.
- **Pararectal fossae** (male/female): the lateral reflections of both the rectovesical and rectouterine pouches in the male and female respectively that are now located on the lateral aspects of the rectum.
- **Broad ligament** (female): a double fold of mesentery that extends laterally from the uterus to the lateral pelvic wall.
- **Suspensory (infundibulopelvic) ligament of the ovary** (female): a fold of peritoneum resting over the ovarian neurovasculature and lymphatics.

4.9 Pelvic Cavity Walls and Floor

- Anteroinferior pelvic wall:
  - Formed by bodies and rami of the pubic bones and pubic symphysis.
  - Supports weight of the urinary bladder.
- Lateral pelvic walls:
  - Formed by hip bones and the **obturator foramen** which is mostly covered by the **obturator membrane (Fig. 4.9)**.
  - Covered by the **obturator internus muscles**. These muscles are covered medially by the **obturator fascia**, which thickens centrally as the **tendinous arch of the levator ani** and provides attachment for the levator ani muscles (**Fig. 4.12**).
  - The **obturator neurovasculature** along with numerous branches/tributaries of the internal iliac vessels are located medial to the obturator internus.
- Posterior pelvic wall:
  - Has a bony wall and roof (sacrum and coccyx) and a combo muscular and ligamentous posterolateral walls made of the sacroiliac joints, their associated ligaments and the **piriformis muscle**.
  - Site of the **sacral plexus** with piriformis forming a muscular bed for this plexus.

4.10 Muscles of the Pelvic Walls and Floor

The pelvic floor is formed by the bowl-shaped **pelvic diaphragm**, which consists of the *levator ani* muscle group and *coccygeus muscles* and fascias covering the superior and inferior aspects of these

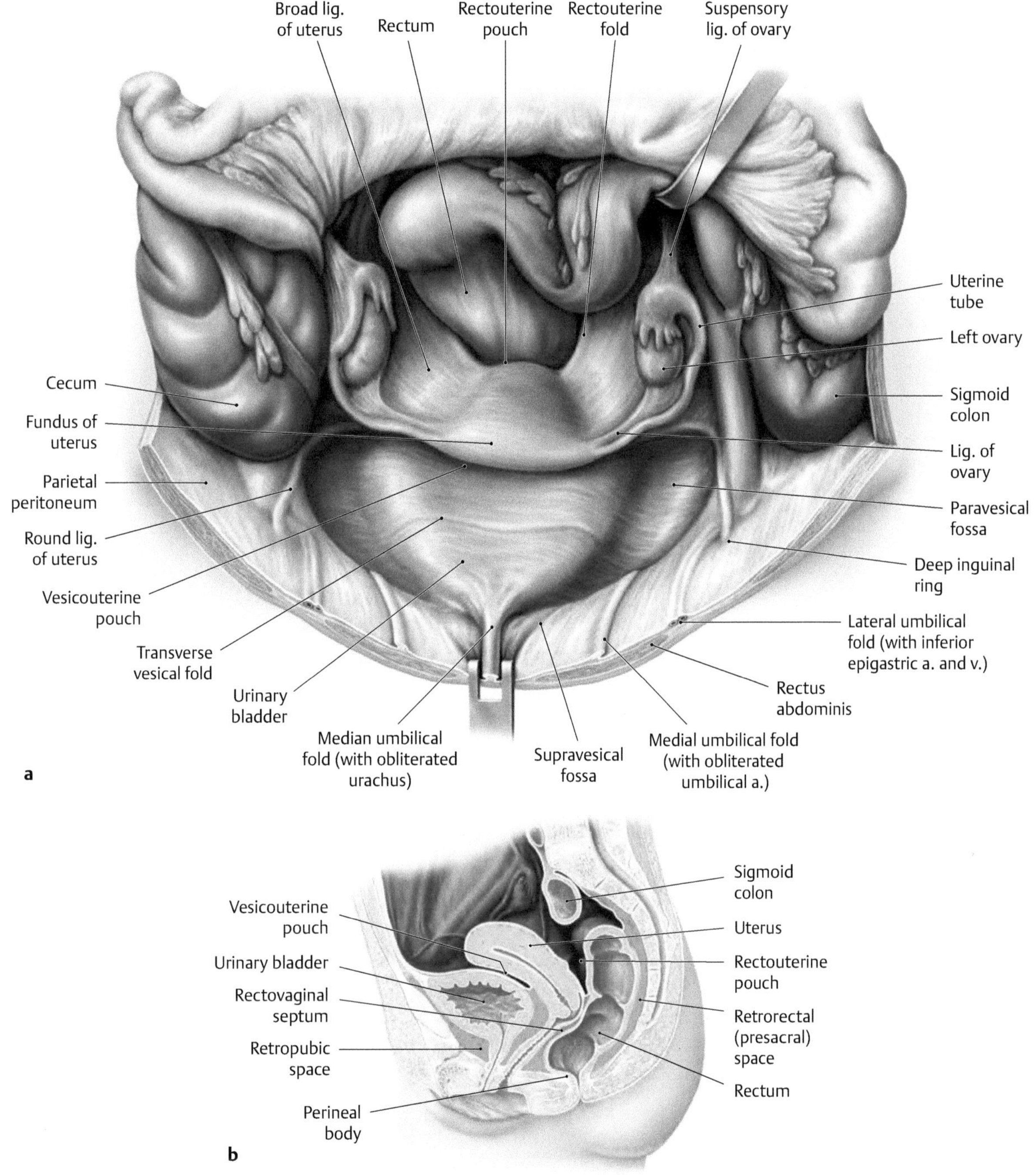

Fig. 4.10 (a) Peritoneal relationships in the female pelvis, superior view. **(b)** Peritoneal and subperitoneal spaces (green) in the female pelvis, midsagittal section viewed from the left side. (From Schuenke M, Schulte E, Schumacher U. THIEME Atlas of Anatomy. Internal Organs. Illustrations by Voll M and Wesker K. 3rd ed. New York: Thieme Medical Publishers; 2020.)

muscles. The function of these muscles is mainly to support the pelvic viscera and resist increases in intra-abdominal pressure. Descriptions of the pelvic wall and floor muscles are found in **Table 4.2**.

- **Levator ani muscles** are attached to the pubic bones anteriorly, to the ischial spines posteriorly, and to a thickening in the obturator fascia (tendinous arch of the levator ani). Innervation to these muscles is mainly from the *nerve to the levator ani (S4)*, *inferior rectal nerve* and *coccygeal plexus*. These muscles consist of 3 parts **(Fig. 4.12)**:
  - Puborectalis muscle: the medial most muscle that forms the U-shaped muscular sling (puborectal sling) that passes posterior to the anorectal junction. Maintaining fecal continence is the major function of this specific muscle. The **urogenital hiatus** is the space bordered by this muscle and allows for passage of the urethra in both sexes and the vagina in women.
  - Pubococcygeus muscle: the wider but thinner intermediate part of the levator ani that arises from the anterior part of the tendinous arch and passes posteriorly in a nearly horizontal plane. The lateral fibers attach to the coccyx posteriorly while the medial fibers merge with those of the contralateral side and form part of the **anococcygeal body/ligament**.

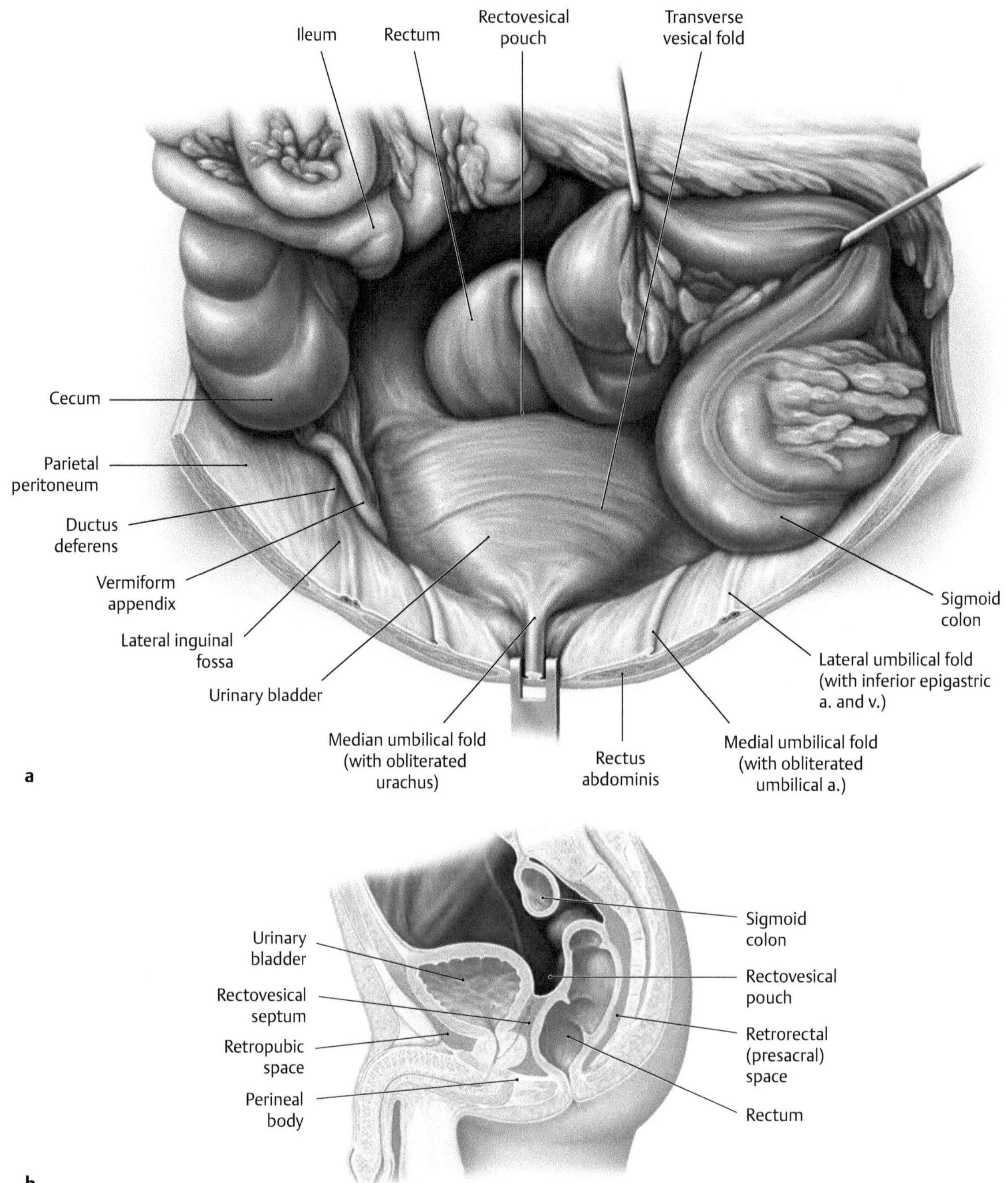

Fig. 4.11 **(a)** Peritoneal relationships in the male pelvis, superior view. **(b)** Peritoneal and subperitoneal spaces (green) in the male pelvis, midsagittal section viewed from the left side. (From Schuenke M, Schulte E, Schumacher U. THIEME Atlas of Anatomy. Internal Organs. Illustrations by Voll M and Wesker K. 3rd ed. New York: Thieme Medical Publishers; 2020.)

 - Iliococcygeus muscle: the posterolateral part of the levator ani that arises from the posterior part of the tendinous arch and ischial spine. Posteriorly it blends with the anococcygeal body/ligament.
- **Coccygeus muscle**: is not part of the levator ani but it extends from the ischial spines to the inferior sacrum and coccyx. Innervation is from *ventral rami of S4 and S5* (**Fig. 4.12**).
- The lateral and posterior pelvic walls are made up of the obturator internus and piriformis muscles respectively. In addition to forming pelvic walls these muscles have the following functions and are discussed in more detail during the *Gluteal Region* of Chapter 5.
 - **Obturator internus**: rotates the thigh laterally; assists in holding head of the femur in the acetabulum. It is innervated by the *nerve to obturator internus.*
 - **Piriformis** rotates thigh laterally; abducts thigh; assists in holding head of the femur in the acetabulum. It is innervated by *ventral rami of S1-S2* or simply the *nerve to piriformis.*

Table 4.2 **Pelvic wall and floor muscles**

Muscle	Innervation	Function(s)	Origin	Insertion
Levator ani (puborectalis, pubococcygeus and iliococcygeus)	Nerve to levator ani (S4 ventral rami br.), inferior rectal nerve (pudendal nerve br.) and coccygeal plexus (S4-Co1)	Forms the majority of the pelvic diaphragm; supports pelvic viscera; resists increases in intra-abdominal pressure	Body of pubis; tendinous arch of levator ani; ischial spine	Perineal body; coccyx; anococcygeal ligament; walls vagina, prostate, rectum and anal canal
Coccygeus	Ventral rami of S4-S5	Forms a minority of the pelvic diaphragm; supports pelvic viscera; flexes coccyx	Ischial spine	Inferior end of sacrum and coccyx
Obturator internus	Nerve to obturator internus	Abduct flexed thigh; laterally rotate extended thigh	Deep surface of obturator membrane; ischiopubic rami	Greater trochanter
Piriformis	Ventral rami of S1-S2 (or nerve to piriformis)	Abduct flexed thigh; laterally rotate extended thigh	Pelvic surface of sacrum; sacrotuberous ligament	Greater trochanter

Clinical Correlate 4.3

Pelvic Floor Injury

The pelvic floor helps support the head of the fetus while the cervix is dilating in order to allow delivery of the fetus. The pelvic fascia, levator ani and perineum are all at risk of being damaged during child birth, especially the pubococcygeus muscle of the levator ani. This muscle is especially important because it supports the urethra, vagina and anal canal. Stretching of the pelvic fascia and levator ani may alter the position of the neck of the bladder and urethra leading to urinary stress incontinence. An individual in this situation will leak urine whenever there is an increase in intra-abdominal pressure such as during coughing or strenuous exercise.

4.11 Pelvic Fascia

The connective tissue that occupies space between the membranous peritoneum and the muscular pelvic walls and floor not occupied by pelvic organs is referred to as **pelvic fascia**. This fascia layer is a continuation of the transversalis (endoabdominal) fascia that lies between the muscular walls and peritoneum of the abdominal wall superiorly. Note that endoabdominal fascia may be described as a combination of both the transversalis fascia and extraperitoneal fat layers (**Fig. 4.13**).

- The **parietal pelvic fascia** is a membranous layer of variable thickness that lines the internal aspects of the muscles forming the walls and floor of the pelvis and it is continuous with the transversalis and iliopsoas fascias. It covers the pelvic surfaces of the obturator internus, piriformis, levator ani, coccygeus, and part of the urethral sphincter muscles.
- The **visceral pelvic fascia** includes the membranous fascia that directly ensheathes the pelvic organs, forming the adventitial layer. It becomes continuous with the parietal layer where the organs penetrate the pelvic floor. The parietal fascia thicken at this point forming the **tendinous arch of the pelvic fascia**, a continuous bilateral band running from the pubis to the sacrum along the pelvic floor adjacent to the viscera (**Fig. 4.14**). The **pubovesical ligament** (female) (**Fig. 4.15**) and **puboprostatic ligament** (male) (**Fig. 4.16**) are the most anterior parts of this tendinous arch. The posterior most part of this tendinous arch is represented as the *sacrogenital ligaments*. They run from the sacrum to the side of the rectum before attaching to the vagina in females and the prostate in males.
- The **endopelvic fascia** is the filler subperitoneal connective tissue found between and continuous with the parietal and visceral pelvic fascial layers. Some of this fascia is more like loose areolar (fatty) tissue while the rest of it is more ligamentous in nature. There are potential spaces called the **retropubic** (prevesical) and **retrorectal** (presacral) **spaces** that allow for the expansion of the urinary bladder and rectum respectively (**Fig. 4.10; Fig. 4.11**).
- The **hypogastric sheath** is condensed endopelvic fascia that gives passage to essentially all the neurovasculature passing from the lateral pelvic walls to the pelvic viscera, along with the ureters and the ductus deferens in males. This sheath is divided into three laminae that pass to or between the pelvic organs conveying certain neurovasculature.
  - Anterior lamina: contains the **lateral ligament of the bladder** and conveys the *superior vesical vessels* (**Fig. 4.14; Fig. 4.17**).
  - Middle lamina: in females, it contains the **cardinal ligament** (transverse cervical or *Mackenrodt's ligament*) and it conveys the *uterine vessels*. The ureter passes inferior to the uterine vessels. (**Fig. 4.14; Fig. 4.15; Fig. 4.17**) In males, the middle lamina consists of the **rectovesical septum** located between the rectum and prostate (**Fig. 4.11**).
  - Posterior lamina: contains the **lateral rectal ligament** that conveys the *middle rectal vessels* (**Fig. 4.17**).
  - In females, the **paracolpium** suspends the vagina between the tendinous arches of the pelvic fascia. In addition, there are **rectouterine (uterosacral) fold/ligaments** consisting of thickened mounds of endopelvic fascia that extend from the sacrum to the uterine cervix. They contain the uterovaginal plexus and the ureter as it travels towards the bladder. The cardinal ligament and uterosacral ligament/folds are together referred to as the **parametrium** of the endopelvic fascia (**Fig. 4.14**).

4.12 Pelvic Somatic Nerves

The ventral rami of L4-S4 contribute to the formation of the **sacral plexus**. Most branches of this plexus leave the pelvis through the *greater sciatic foramen* and innervate muscles or skin in the gluteal region or lower extremity discussed in Chapter 5. The pudendal nerve and its branches will target the muscles and skin of the perineum. The nerves of this plexus have the functional components GSE, GSA and GVE-sym/post or GSA and GVE-sym/post if they are cutaneous nerves. Individual nerves of this plexus include (**Fig. 4.18**):

- **Lumbosacral trunk** (L4-L5)
- **Sciatic nerve** (L4-S3)
- **Superior gluteal nerve** (L4-S1)

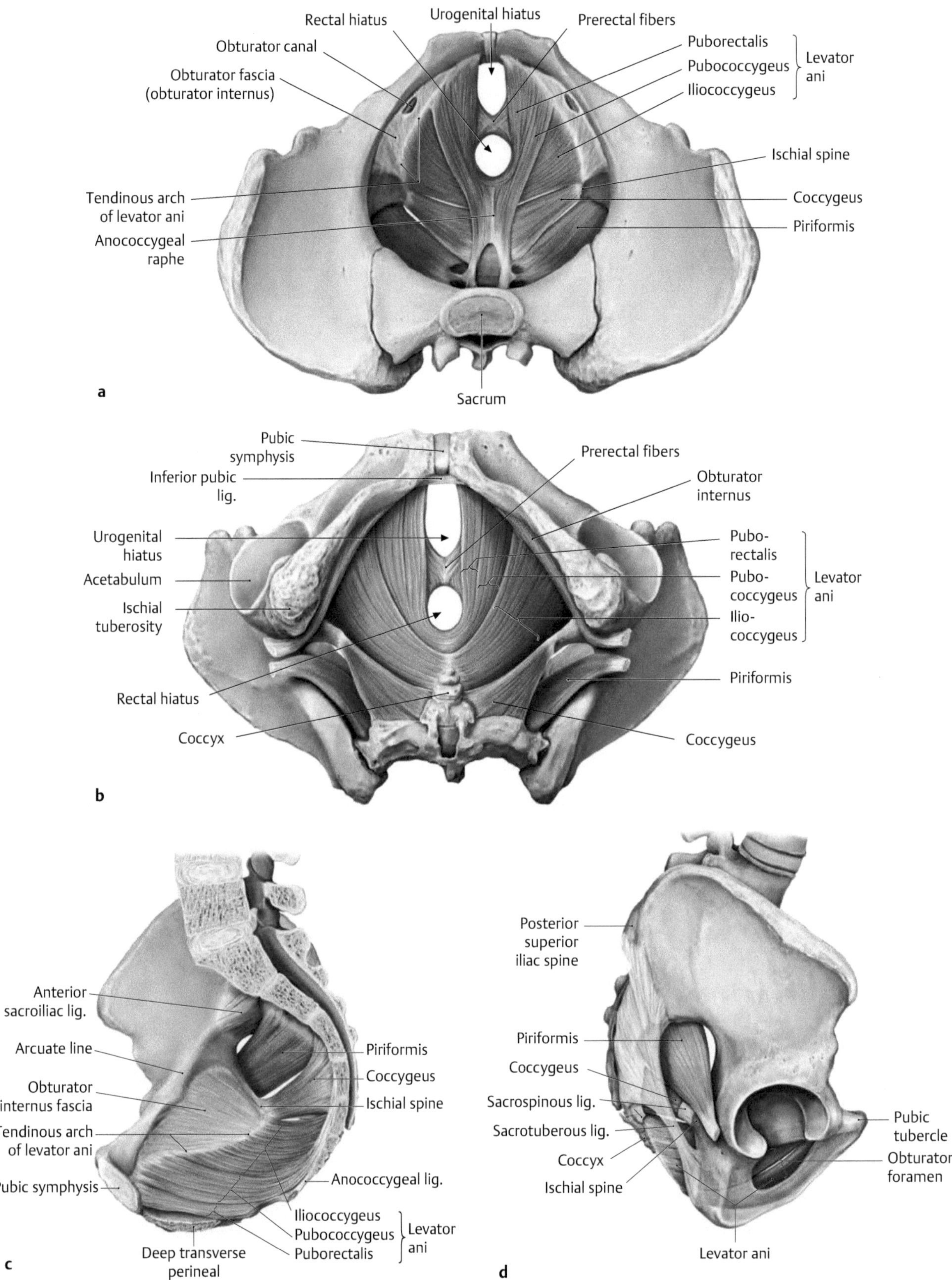

Fig. 4.12 Muscles of the pelvic walls and floor. **(a)** Superior view. **(b)** Inferior view. **(c)** Medial view of right hemipelvis; **(d)** Right lateral view. (From Schuenke M, Schulte E, Schumacher U. THIEME Atlas of Anatomy. General Anatomy and Musculoskeletal System. Illustrations by Voll M and Wesker K. 3rd ed. New York: Thieme Medical Publishers; 2020.)

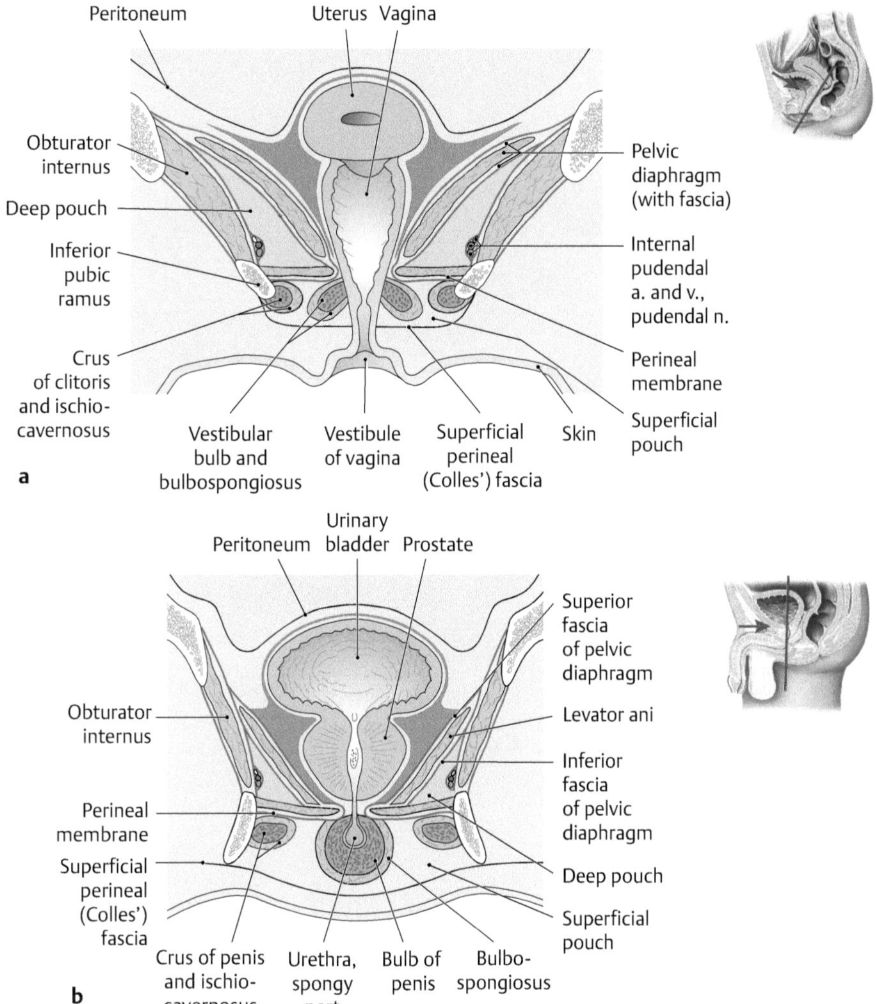

Fig. 4.13 Pelvic fascia. **(a)** Female, oblique section. **(b)** Male, coronal section. (From Schuenke M, Schulte E, Schumacher U. THIEME Atlas of Anatomy. General Anatomy and Musculoskeletal System. Illustrations by Voll M and Wesker K. 3rd ed. New York: Thieme Medical Publishers; 2020.)

- **Nerve to quadratus femoris** (L4-S1).
- **Inferior gluteal nerve** (L5-S2).
- **Nerve to obturator internus** (L5-S2).
- **Nerve to piriformis** (S1-S2).
- **Posterior femoral cutaneous nerve** (S1-S3).
- **Pudendal nerve** (S2-S4).
- Additional **perforating cutaneous nerves** (S2-S3).

The ventral rami of S4-Co1 contribute to the much smaller **coccygeal plexus**. It supplies the levator ani, coccygeus and external anal sphincter muscles, along with the sacrococcygeal joint and a small area of skin between the tip of the coccyx and the anus. The nerves of this plexus have the functional components GSE, GSA and GVE-sym/post except for the anococcygeal nerve, which is a cutaneous nerve containing the GSA and GVE-sym/post functional components. The individual nerves of this plexus include **(Fig. 4.18)**:

- **Nerve to levator ani** (S4).
- **Nerve to coccygeus** (S4-S5).
- **Anococcygeal nerve** (S4-Co1).

4.13 Pelvic Autonomic Nerves

Autonomic innervation plays a pivotal role in the innervation of pelvic viscera. The **sympathetics** are vasomotor to the vessels supplying the viscera, stimulate the contraction of the genital organs during orgasm as in male ejaculation, and they inhibit the peristaltic contraction of the rectum. The **parasympathetics** stimulate the expansion of the external genitalia erectile bodies leading to an erection by relaxing the helicine vessels in addition to stimulating the contraction of the rectum and bladder to allow for defecation and urination respectively. Multiple structures are involved in delivering autonomic fibers to these pelvic viscera **(Fig. 4.19; Fig. 4.20; Fig. 4.21; Fig. 4.22; Fig. 4.23)**.

- The **superior hypogastric plexus** is located just inferior to the bifurcation of the aorta and sym/post fibers primarily pass through it. Para/pre fibers from the inferior hypogastric plexus pass back up through the hypogastric nerves, through this plexus, and finally onto the periarterial plexus paired with sym/post fibers wrapped around the inferior mesenteric artery responsible for hindgut structures.
- The **left** and **right hypogastric nerves** are the inferior extensions of the superior hypogastric plexus into the pelvis and the connection to the inferior hypogastric plexus. They predominately consist of sym/post fibers heading down to the pelvis but they also allow para/pre fibers to travel back to the hindgut structures.
- The **inferior hypogastric plexuses** are located lateral to the rectum, bladder, prostate, vagina and uterus. They receive sympathetics originating from the hypogastric nerves and *sacral splanchnics* and parasympathetics from the *pelvic splanchnic*

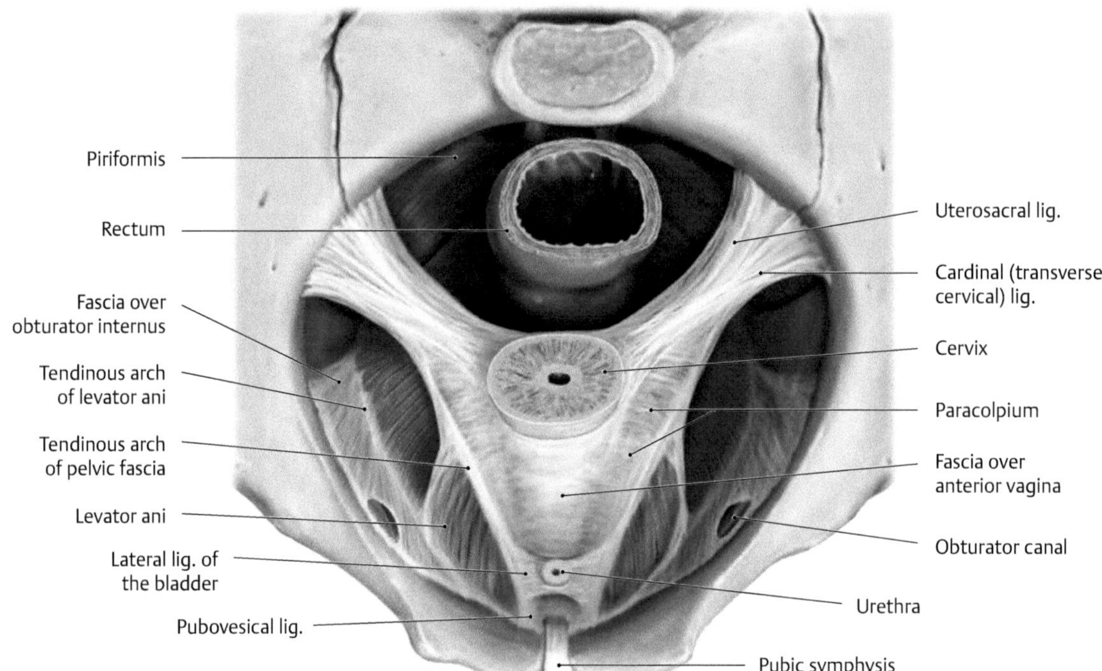

Fig. 4.14 Ligaments of the deep pelvis in the female, superior view. (From Schuenke M, Schulte E, Schumacher U. THIEME Atlas of Anatomy. General Anatomy and Musculoskeletal System. Illustrations by Voll M and Wesker K. 3rd ed. New York: Thieme Medical Publishers; 2020.)

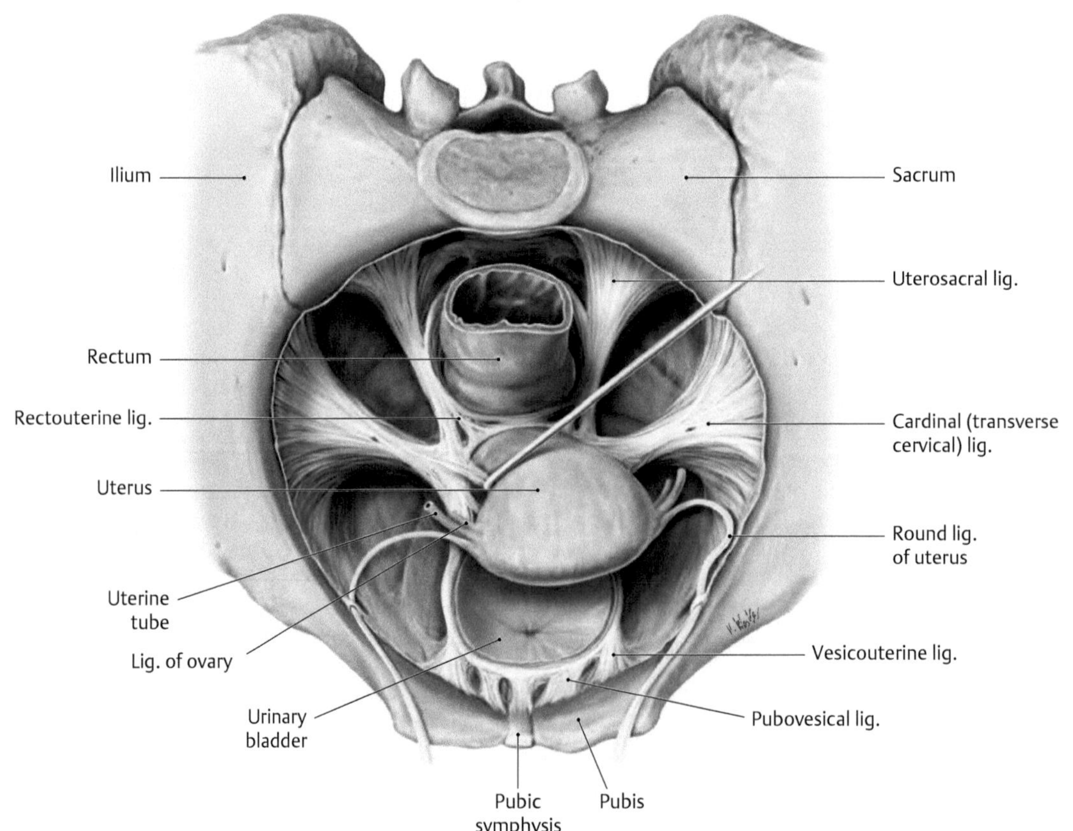

Fig. 4.15 Ligaments of the female pelvis, superior view. (From Schuenke M, Schulte E, Schumacher U. THIEME Atlas of Anatomy. Internal Organs. Illustrations by Voll M and Wesker K. 3rd ed. New York: Thieme Medical Publishers; 2020.)

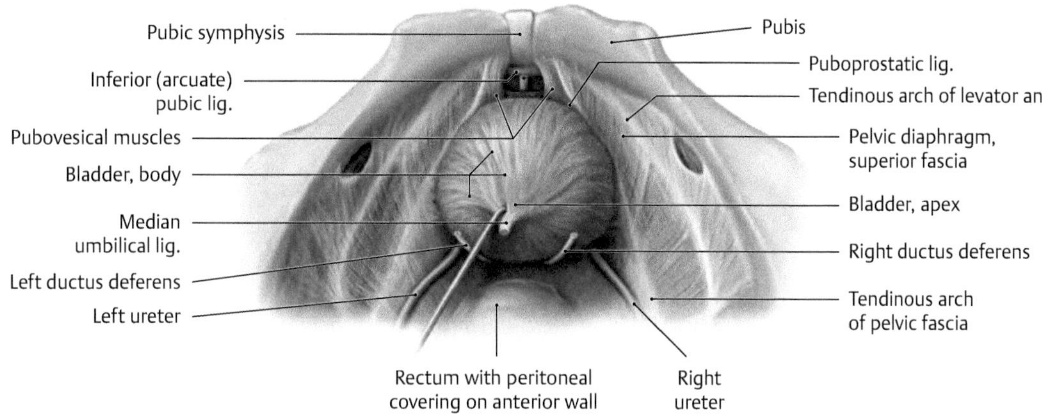

Fig. 4.16 Ligaments of the male pelvis, superior view with peritoneum removed. (From Schuenke M, Schulte E, Schumacher U. THIEME Atlas of Anatomy. Internal Organs. Illustrations by Voll M and Wesker K. 3rd ed. New York: Thieme Medical Publishers; 2020.)

Pubovesical lig.
Vesicovaginal space
Retropubic space
Medial umbilical lig.
Urinary bladder
Inferior epigastric a. and v.
Tendinous arch of pelvic fascia
Cervix
Superior vesical a. in lateral vesicular lig.
Ureter
Inferior vesical a.
Rectovaginal space
Tendinous arch of levator ani
Neurovascular bundle of the rectum (with the middle rectal a.)
Cardinal (transverse cervical) lig.
Uterosacral lig.
Ovarian a. and v.
Obturator a.
Uterine a.
Psoas major muscle
Internal iliac a. and v.
Mesorectal space
Rectum
Presacral space
Retrorectal space
Retroperitoneal space
Parietal pelvic fascia
Visceral pelvic fascia

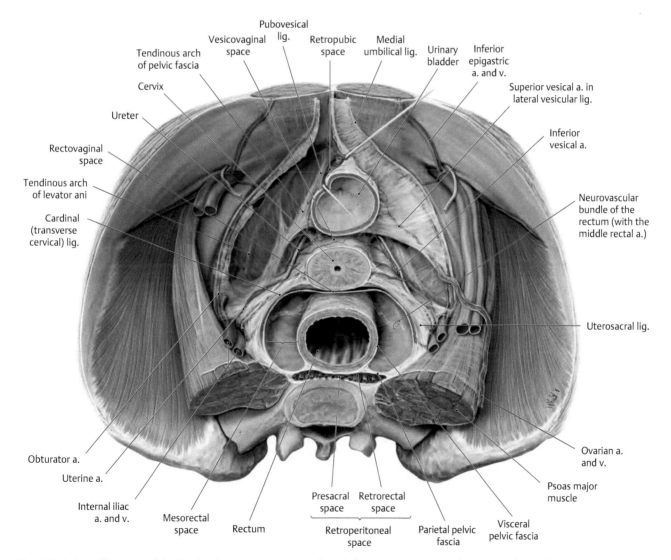

Fig. 4.17 Fasica and ligaments of the female pelvis. Transverse section through the cervix, superior view. (From Schuenke M, Schulte E, Schumacher U. THIEME Atlas of Anatomy. Internal Organs. Illustrations by Voll M and Wesker K. 3rd ed. New York: Thieme Medical Publishers; 2020.)

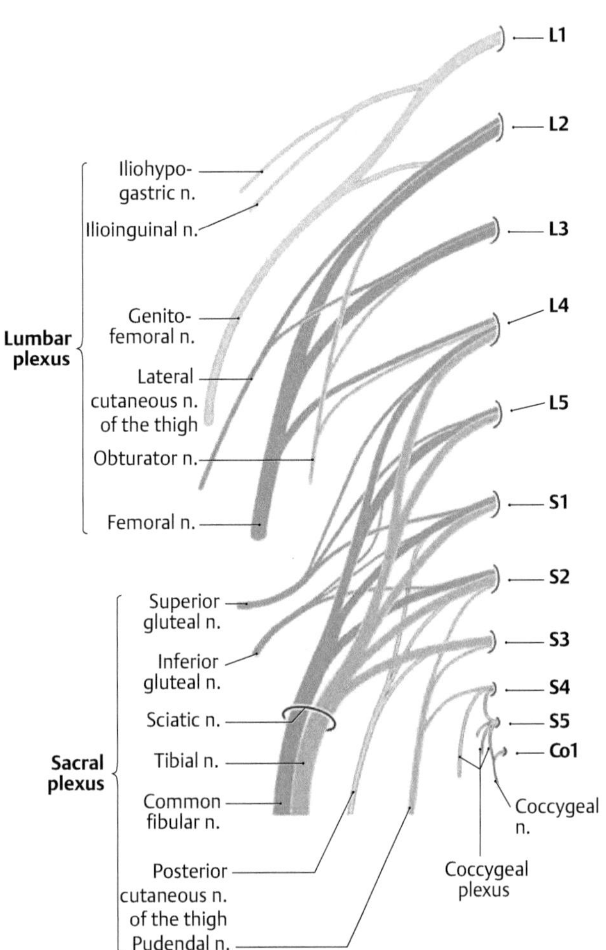

Fig. 4.18 Structure of the lumbar and sacral plexuses. (From Schuenke M, Schulte E, Schumacher U. THIEME Atlas of Anatomy. General Anatomy and Musculoskeletal System. Illustrations by Voll M and Wesker K. 3rd ed. New York: Thieme Medical Publishers; 2020.)

nerves. These plexuses have been described as having a minimal amount of ganglion-like cells where limited sym/pre fibers that made it through the sacral splanchnic nerves synapse at. A special set of **retroperitoneal parasympathetic nerves** originate from the left inferior hypogastric plexus and they extend up to the lower hindgut region.

The GVE-para/pre fibers destined for the pelvic organs and hindgut originated from the equivalent lateral horns of the S2-S4 portion of the spinal cord. These para/pre fibers pass through the **pelvic splanchnic nerves** that branch off the S2-S4 ventral rami just after the ventral rami exit the sacral foramina and they lead directly to the inferior hypogastric plexus. From this plexus, para/pre fibers can travel through:

1. Left and right hypogastric nerves, the superior hypogastric plexus, and then to hindgut structures by way of the inferior mesenteric periarterial plexus.
2. Additional visceral nerve plexuses adjoined to the inferior hypogastric plexus (i.e., rectal and vesical plexuses).
3. Redundancy to the hindgut structures by way of the retroperitoneal parasympathetic fibers (left side only).

- The **sacral sympathetic trunks** are the inferior continuations of the former lumbar sympathetic trunks with each side eventually meeting near the coccyx to form the **ganglion impar**. They allow sym/pre fibers to course to a sympathetic chain ganglion in the sacral region before synapsing. After this synapse occurs, the now sym/post fibers pass through gray ramus communicans to a spinal nerve associated with a dorsal rami branch or a sacral plexus nerve branch. These fibers continue through one of these nerve branches and innervate a muscle or skin surface. These postganglionic fibers can also continue through the **sacral splanchnic nerves** that originate from the S1-S4 level ganglions before reaching the inferior hypogastric plexus. The sacral splanchnic nerves have passing through them a limited amount of sym/pre fibers that do not synapse at a sympathetic chain ganglion but instead synapse at the ganglion-like cells of the inferior hypogastric plexus.
- The **periarterial plexuses** that follow the aorta distally to the common iliac, external iliac and internal iliac exclusively consist of sym/post fibers that continue into the lower extremity or target pelvic and structures of the perineum via the internal iliac and its branches. The gonadal and superior rectal arteries may have of a mixed autonomic periarterial plexus combination of both sym/post and para/pre fibers destined for their respective visceral structures.
- The **pelvic pain line** is an imaginary line located at the inferior limit of the peritoneum. Visceral afferent fibers conducting pain from the viscera *superior to the pelvic pain line* follow the sympathetic fibers retrogradely to inferior thoracic and superior lumbar spinal ganglia. Visceral afferents that transmit pain sensations from the viscera *inferior to the pelvic pain line* travel with parasympathetic fibers to the spinal ganglia of S2-S4. This would be in addition to the *visceral reflex fibers* already within the parasympathetic fibers.

4.14 Pelvic Blood Supply and Venous Drainage

There are four main arteries (three in the male) that enter the lesser pelvis and they include the **internal iliac**, **superior rectal**, **median sacral** and **ovarian arteries** (female only).

- **Internal iliac**: delivers most of the blood to the pelvic region. It is divided into an anterior and posterior division with the anterior division supplying most of the pelvic viscera. The *anterior division* consists of the **umbilical**, **obturator**, **inferior vesical**, **middle rectal**, **internal pudendal** and **inferior gluteal arteries**. The **uterine** and **vaginal arteries** would be additional branches seen off the anterior division in females. The inferior vesical artery generally branches off the vaginal artery but it may also be an individual branch from the internal iliac in females. Some authors still describe the inferior vesicle as a nonexistent artery in females but there is an argument for either orientation. The *posterior division* gives rise to the **iliolumbar**, **lateral sacral** and **superior gluteal arteries**.
- **Superior rectal**: branch off the inferior mesenteric artery and supplies most of the rectum.
- **Median sacral**: branches near the bifurcation of the aorta and gives off the fifth pair of lumbar arteries.
- **Ovarian**: branch off the aorta just inferior to the renal artery branches and supplies the ovaries (female only).

Multiple venous plexuses are located within the lesser pelvis. They include the **vesical**, **prostatic**, **uterine**, **vaginal** and **rectal venous plexuses** and are primarily drained by tributaries of the **internal**

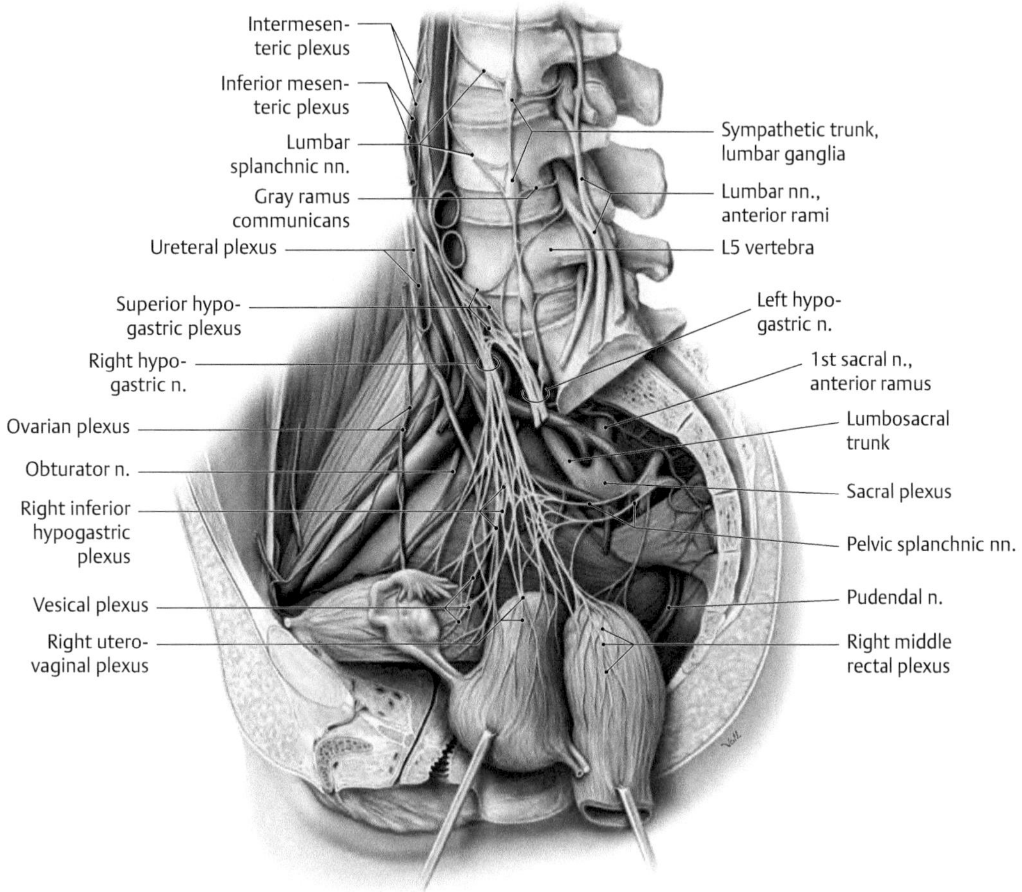

Fig. 4.19 Innervation of the female pelvis. Opened and viewed from the left side with the rectum and uterus reflected. (From Schuenke M, Schulte E, Schumacher U. THIEME Atlas of Anatomy. Internal Organs. Illustrations by Voll M and Wesker K. 3rd ed. New York: Thieme Medical Publishers; 2020.)

iliac veins. Venous blood from the internal iliac vein joins the external iliac vein and passes through the common iliac vein and IVC before finally reaching the right atrium of the heart. Additional drainage patterns include the **lateral sacral veins** draining into the *internal vertebral venous plexus*; the **left** and **right ovarian veins** draining to the *left renal* and *IVC* respectively; the **superior rectal vein** draining to the *inferior mesenteric vein* before reaching the portal venous system; and finally the **median sacral veins** draining to the *IVC* (**Fig. 4.24; Table 4.4**).

4.15 Lymph Nodes of the Pelvis

The multiple sets of lymph nodes involved in pelvic viscera lymphatic drainage are quite variable in both size and numbers and are named for the blood vessels with which they are associated. Due to the high amount of interconnections between these particular lymph nodes, cancer originating from this region has the ability to spread in multiple directions and does not have a very predictable pattern of metastasis. There are four primary groups of lymph nodes involved in lymphatic drainage of the pelvis and they include the **common iliac, external iliac, internal iliac** and **sacral lymph nodes (Table 4.5)**.

- **Common iliac**: receive lymph from the three main groups listed below before traveling to the **lumbar (caval/aortic) nodes**.
- **External iliac**: receive lymph mainly from the inguinal lymph nodes but also from the superior parts of the anterior pelvic organs.
- **Internal iliac**: receive lymph from the inferior pelvic organs, deep perineum and gluteal region.
- **Sacral**: receive lymph from the posteroinferior pelvic organs.

The other groups of lymph nodes associated with the pelvis include the **superficial inguinal**, **deep inguinal** and **preaortic** (*inferior* and *superior mesenteric*) **lymph nodes**.

The Pelvic Viscera

4.16 Ureters

The **ureters** are muscular tubes that carry urine from the kidney down to the bladder and lie retroperitoneal (**Fig. 4.16; Fig. 4.25; Fig. 4.26**). The second ureter constriction (described in Chapter 3) occurs near the bifurcation of the common iliac arteries and is the point at which the ureter enters the lesser pelvis. While in the pelvis, the ureters are near the lateral wall and travel under the uterine vessels or ductus deferens before passing obliquely through the urinary bladder. A one-way valve is formed as it passes through the bladder and with the natural filling and muscular contractions

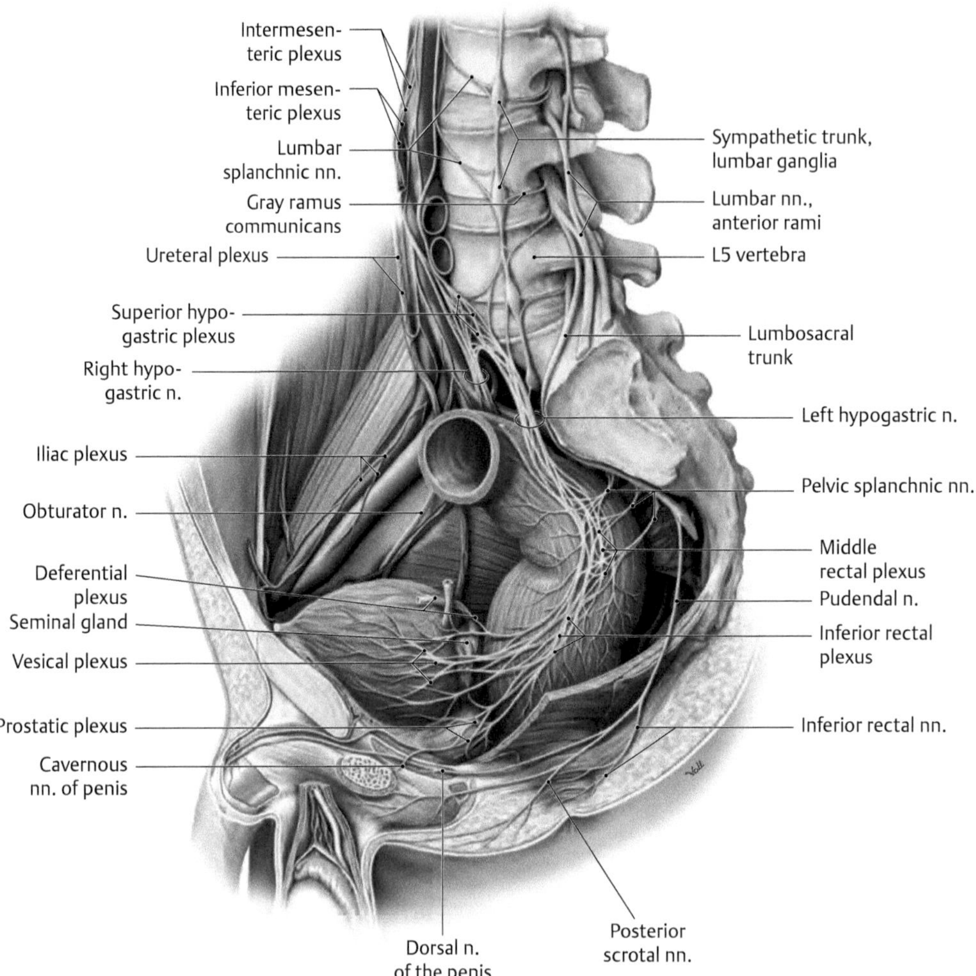

Fig. 4.20 Innervation of the male pelvis. Opened and viewed from the left side. (From Schuenke M, Schulte E, Schumacher U. THIEME Atlas of Anatomy. Internal Organs. Illustrations by Voll M and Wesker K. 3rd ed. New York: Thieme Medical Publishers; 2020.)

of the bladder during micturition, this valve closes preventing any reflux of urine. Peristaltic contractions help transport urine down towards the urinary bladder.

4.16.1 Neurovasculature and Lymphatic Drainage of the Ureters

A combination of autonomic plexuses including the aortic, renal, superior and inferior hypogastric plexuses help innervate the ureters because of their total length. The **ureteric plexus**, primarily from the renal plexus, has sympathetic fibers acting primarily as vasoconstrictors and parasympathetics involved in peristaltic movements (**Fig. 4.21**). The autonomics may have little effect on peristaltic waves in the ureter. Instead, these peristaltic contractions may originate from spontaneously depolarizing smooth muscles cells beginning at the renal pelvis. Afferent pain fibers follow the sympathetic fibers mainly because the majority of the ureters are found above the pelvic pain line. The referred ureteric pain is usually to the ipsilateral lower abdominal quadrant, especially to the groin region.

Blood supply to the ureters is segmental and from multiple smaller **ureter arteries**. The ureter artery branches can originate from the *abdominal aorta, renal, common iliac, internal iliac, superior vesical* and *gonadal arteries*. Most blood supply while in the lesser pelvis is from the uterine arteries in females and inferior vesical arteries in males. Venous drainage is by multiple smaller **ureter veins** that drain to the renal, ovarian or testicular veins. Lymphatic drainage is also segmental. The *upper portion* of the ureter drains to the **lumbar lymph nodes**. The *middle portion* of the ureter drains mostly to the **common iliac lymph nodes** while the *lower portion* drains to the **external iliac** and **internal iliac lymph nodes** (**Fig. 4.24; Table 4.3; Table 4.4; Table 4.5**).

4.16.2 Histology of the Ureter

The mucosa has a stellate-shaped lumen lined with *transitional epithelium* and a lamina propria. The muscularis layer includes an inner longitudinal followed by outer circular layer for the proximal two-thirds (**Fig. 4.27**). This is opposite of what was seen in the GI tract. The distal one-third has a third layer and they are now orientated as the inner longitudinal, middle circular and the newly added outer longitudinal muscle layer. The main function of the muscularis layer is to produce peristalsis and help propel the urine toward the urinary bladder. The mucosa creates the one-way valve near the ureter/bladder junction preventing urine reflux.

4.17 Urinary Bladder

The **urinary bladder** is a hollow reservoir for urine with strong muscular walls and is located just below the peritoneum (**Fig. 4.28; Fig. 4.29**). It is separated from the pubic symphysis by the *retropubic*

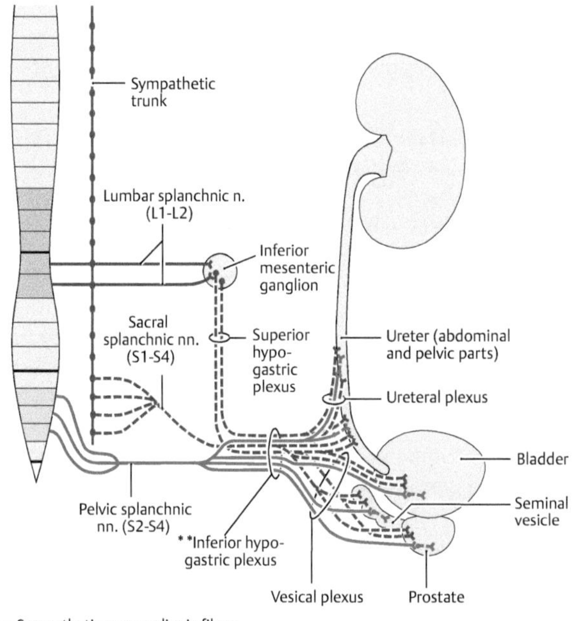

Fig. 4.21 Autonomic innervation schematic of the urinary bladder and ureter. (From Schuenke M, Schulte E, Schumacher U. THIEME Atlas of Anatomy. Internal Organs. Illustrations by Voll M and Wesker K. 3rd ed. New York: Thieme Medical Publishers; 2020.)

space. The bladder has a somewhat tetrahedral shape when empty and is made up of an apex, body, fundus and neck. The **apex** points anteriorly towards the pubic symphysis while the **fundus** faces posteriorly. In males, the fundus is closely related to the rectum while in females it is closely related to the anterior wall of the vagina. The **body** lies between the apex and fundus. When full, the bladder can be located in the greater pelvis. The **neck** is where the fundus and inferolateral surfaces of the bladder meet inferiorly. The bladder is a relatively free structure except for at the neck region. Here it is firmly attached by the *lateral ligaments of the bladder* and the *puboprostatic ligament* in males and *pubovesical ligament* in females.

The walls of the bladder are composed mainly of the **detrusor muscle.** Near the neck, its muscle fibers form the involuntary **internal urethral sphincter**. In males, these fibers are continuous with the fibromuscular tissue of the prostate and in females these fibers are continuous with muscle fibers in the wall of the urethra.

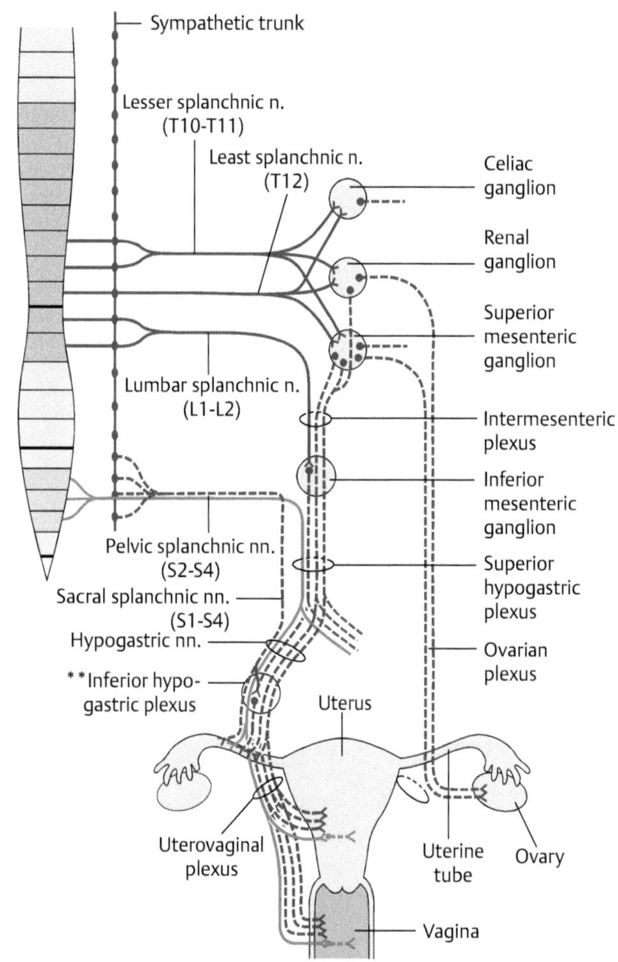

Fig. 4.22 Autonomic innervation schematic of female organs and genitalia. (From Schuenke M, Schulte E, Schumacher U. THIEME Atlas of Anatomy. Internal Organs. Illustrations by Voll M and Wesker K. 3rd ed. New York: Thieme Medical Publishers; 2020.)

4.17.1 Neurovasculature and Lymphatic Drainage of the Urinary Bladder

Innervation is from the autonomic **vesical plexus** where sympathetic fibers contract the internal urethral sphincter preventing reflux of semen while these same fibers simultaneously stimulate ejaculation. Parasympathetic fibers are motor to the detrusor muscle and inhibitory to the internal urethral sphincter **(Fig. 4.21)**.

Blood supply to the superior portion of the urinary bladder is from the **superior vesical artery** in both male and females. The **inferior vesical** supplies the inferior portion of the bladder. The **vaginal artery** may also contribute to the inferior portion of the bladder in females **(Fig. 4.24; Table 4.3)**. Venous drainage travels from the **vesical venous plexus** to the internal iliac veins **(Fig. 4.24; Table 4.3)**. Lymphatic drainage of the superior portion is to the **external iliac lymph nodes** while the inferior portion drains to the **internal iliac lymph nodes (Fig. 4.30)**.

4.17.2 Histology of the Urinary Bladder

The mucosa is arranged in numerous folds that disappear when the bladder becomes distended with urine. The large dome-shaped cells of *transitional epithelium* become stretched and flattened with distension and also act as an osmotic barrier between the urine and lamina propria **(Fig. 4.31)**. Cell shape accommodation is due to a feature of the epithelium's cell plasmalemma composed of unique thickened regions called **plaques**. It is these plaques that are impermeable to water and salts, thus creating the osmotic barrier. The **trigone** is a portion of the bladder whose apices are the **ureteric orifices** and the **internal urethral orifice**. The **uvula of the bladder** is a slight elevation of the trigone in the internal urethral orifice. The muscularis is composed of three

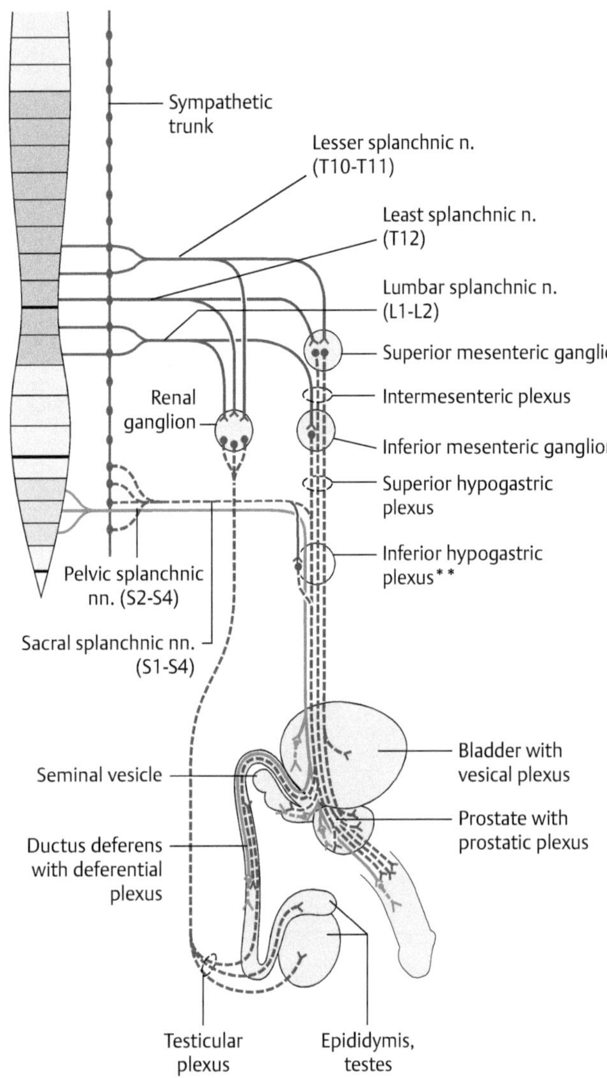

Fig. 4.23 Autonomic innervation schematic of male organs and genitalia. (From Schuenke M, Schulte E, Schumacher U. THIEME Atlas of Anatomy. Internal Organs. Illustrations by Voll M and Wesker K. 3rd ed. New York: Thieme Medical Publishers; 2020.)

interlaced smooth muscle layers commonly referred to as the **detrusor muscle**, and can only be separated near the neck of the bladder. Here they are arranged as inner longitudinal, middle circular and outer longitudinal layers with the middle layer forming the **internal urethral sphincter**. The peritoneum only covers the superior portion of the bladders adventitia **(Fig. 4.28; Fig. 4.29)**.

4.18 Female Urethra

The **female urethra** passes anteroinferiorly from the *internal urethral orifice* of the urinary bladder, posterior and then inferior to the pubic symphysis to the *external urethral orifice* in the vestibule of the vagina **(Fig. 4.28)**. It lies anterior to the vagina and averages about 3.5-4 cm in total length. The superior part of the urethra contains **paraurethral** (*Skene's*) **glands** that are homologous to the prostate and they drain into or near the opening of the urethra.

4.18.1 Neurovasculature and Lymphatic Drainage of the Female Urethra

Innervation of the female urethra is primarily from the autonomic nerves that arise from the **vesical nerve plexus**. Additional innervation near the external orifice comes from distal branches of the **pudendal nerve**.

The blood supply is primarily from the **vaginal artery** along with the **internal pudendal arteries** (both internal iliac brs.) **(Fig. 4.24; Table 4.3)**. Venous drainage runs parallel with arterial supply. Lymph drains mainly to the **sacral** and **internal iliac lymph nodes**. A minimal amount will drain to the **superficial** and **deep inguinal lymph nodes (Fig. 4.30)**.

4.18.2 Histology of the Female Urethra

The female urethra is lined by a *transitional epithelium* closest to the bladder and then a *stratified squamous non-keratinized epithelium* throughout the remainder of its length. The epithelium does display interspersed sections of *pseudostratified columnar epithelium*. The **urethral glands** extend from the lamina propria and secrete mucus. The muscularis is composed of an inner longitudinal and outer circular smooth muscle layer. At the level of the urogenital diaphragm, skeletal muscle forms the **external urethral sphincter**.

4.19 Male Urethra

The **male urethra** is the muscular tube that conveys both urine and semen (sperm and glandular secretions) and is approximately 20 cm in total length. It is divided into four parts **(Fig. 4.32)**:

- **Intramural (preprostatic)**: the most proximal part and surrounded by the *internal urethral sphincter.*
- **Prostatic**: is surrounded by the *prostate gland.*
- **Intermediate (membranous)**: is surrounded by the *external urethral sphincter.*
- **Spongy (penile)**: is the longest part and expands to form the **navicular fossa** near the *external urethral orifice.*

Urine passes through the internal urethral orifice of the urinary bladder before entering the most proximal intramural part while semen first enters the urethra at the prostatic part of the urethra. The **bulbourethral glands** open into the proximal part of the spongy urethra. There are many minute duct openings of mucus-secreting **urethral glands** (of *Littré*) into the spongy urethra.

4.19.1 Neurovasculature and Lymphatic Drainage of the Male Urethra

Innervation to the male urethra is primarily from autonomic nerves that arise from the **prostatic nerve plexus**. The **dorsal nerve of the penis** may also contribute to the innervation **(Fig. 4.20; Fig. 4.23)**. The blood supply is from the **urethral** (internal pudendal br.), **inferior vesical** (internal iliac br.), **middle rectal** (internal iliac br.) and **dorsal artery of the penis** (internal pudendal br.) **(Fig. 4.24; Table 4.3)**. Venous drainage mirrors the blood supply before reaching the **vesical** and **prostatic venous plexuses** **(Fig. 4.24; Table 4.4)**.

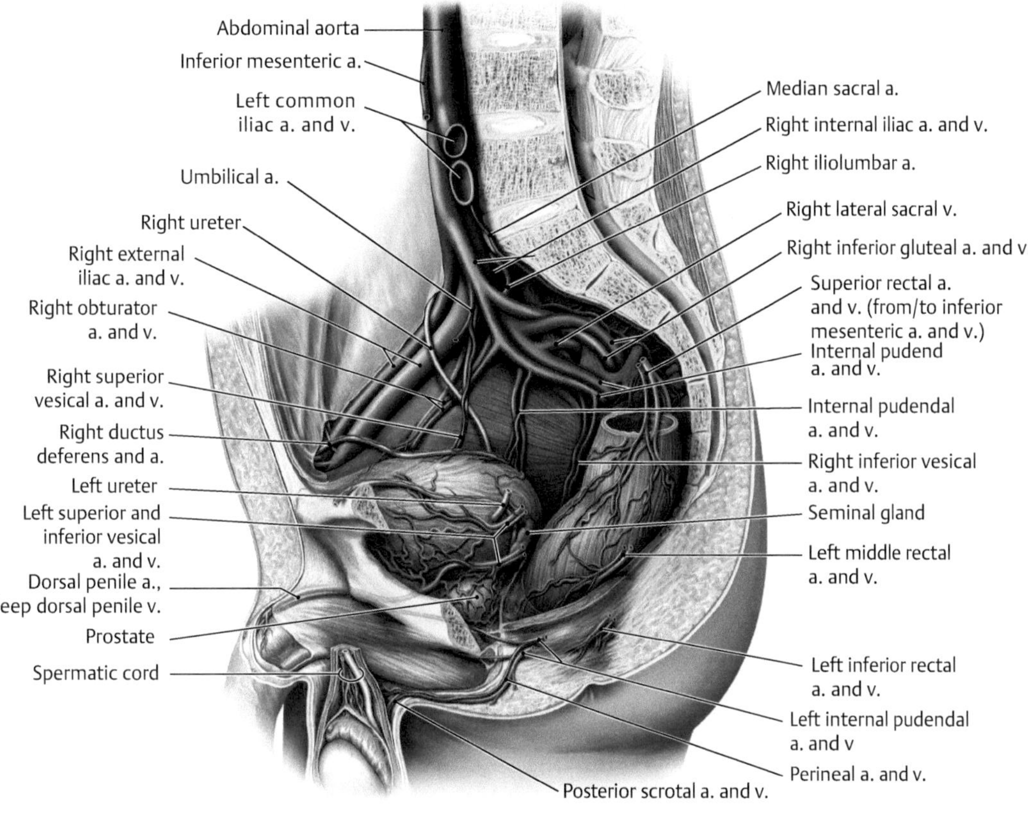

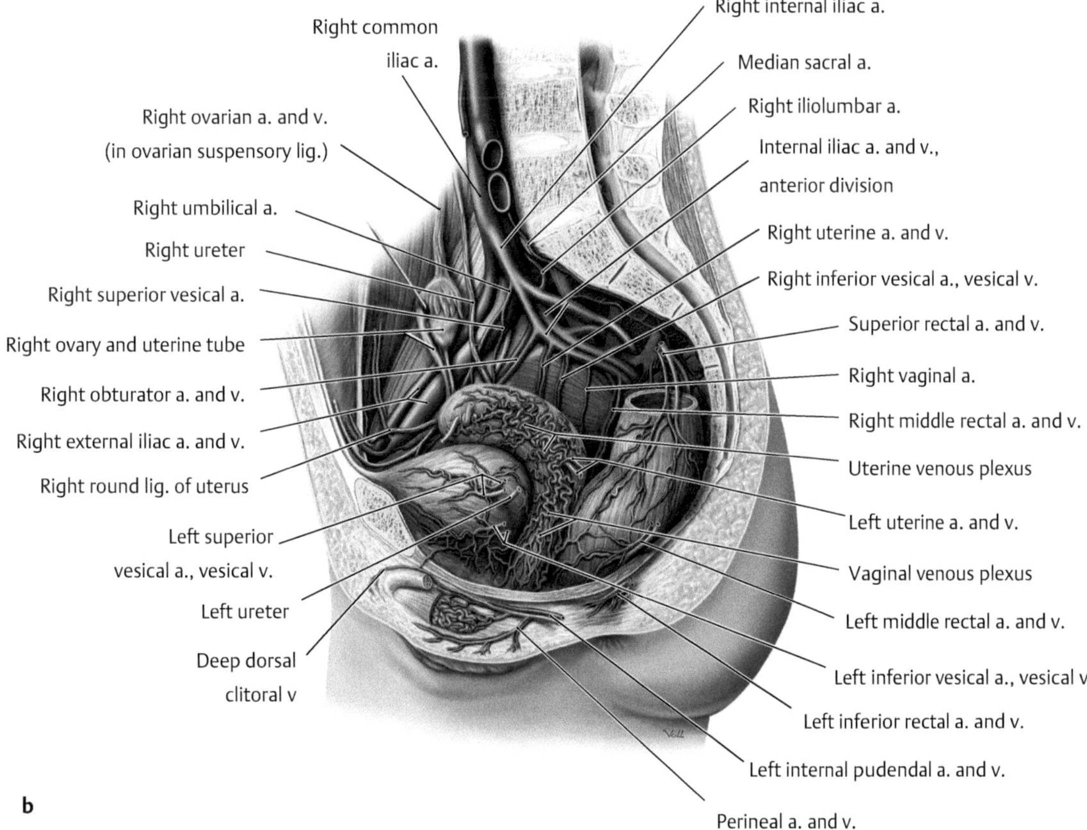

Fig. 4.24 Blood vessels of the **(a)** male pelvis and **(b)** female pelvis. (From Schuenke M, Schulte E, Schumacher U. THIEME Atlas of Anatomy. Internal Organs. Illustrations by Voll M and Wesker K. 3rd ed. New York: Thieme Medical Publishers; 2020.)

Table 4.3 Branches of the internal iliac artery

The internal iliac artery gives off five parietal (pelvic wall) and four visceral (pelvic organs) branches.* Parietal branches are shown in italics.

Branches		
①	*Iiolumbar a.*	
②	*Superior gluteal a.*	
③	*Lateral sacral a.*	
④	Umbilical a.	A. of ductus deferens
		Superior vesical a.
⑤	*Obturator a.*	
⑥	Inferior vesical a.	
⑦	Middle rectal a.	
⑧	Internal pudendal a.	Inferior rectal a.
		Dorsal penile a.
		Posterior scrotal aa.
⑨	*Inferior gluteal a.*	

* In the female pelvis, the uterine and vaginal arteries arise directly from the anterior division of the internal iliac artery.

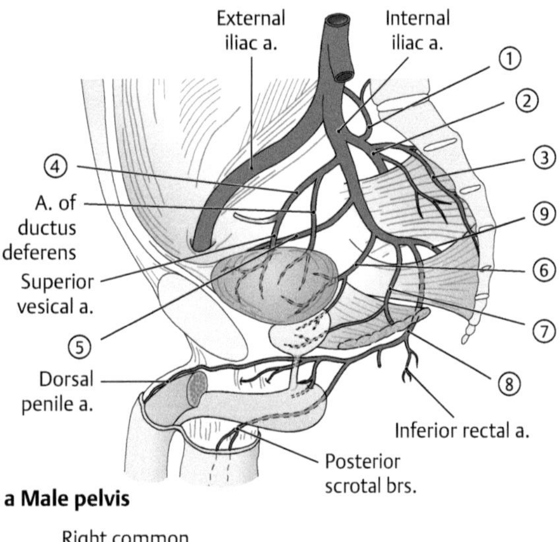

a Male pelvis

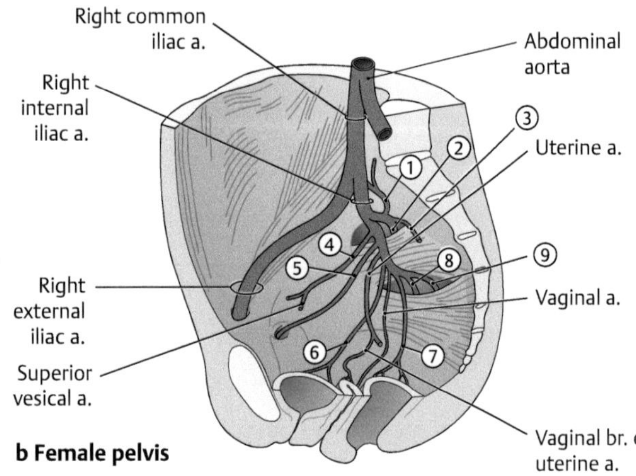

b Female pelvis

(From Schuenke M, Schulte E, Schumacher U. THIEME Atlas of Anatomy. Internal Organs. Illustrations by Voll M and Wesker K. 2nd ed. New York: Thieme Medical Publishers; 2016.)

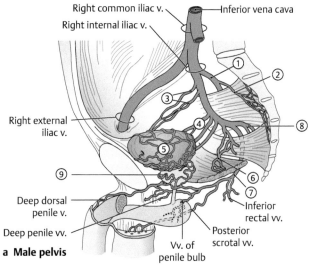

Table 4.4 Venous drainage of the pelvis

Tributaries	
①	Superior gluteal v.
②	Lateral sacral v.
③	Obturator vv.
④	Vesical vv.
⑤	Vesical venous plexus
⑥	Middle rectal vv. (rectal venous plexus) (also superior and inferior rectal vv., not shown)
⑦	Internal pudendal v.
⑧	Inferior gluteal vv.
⑨	Prostatic venous plexus
⑩	Uterine and vaginal venous plexus

The male pelvis also contains veins draining the penis and scrotum.

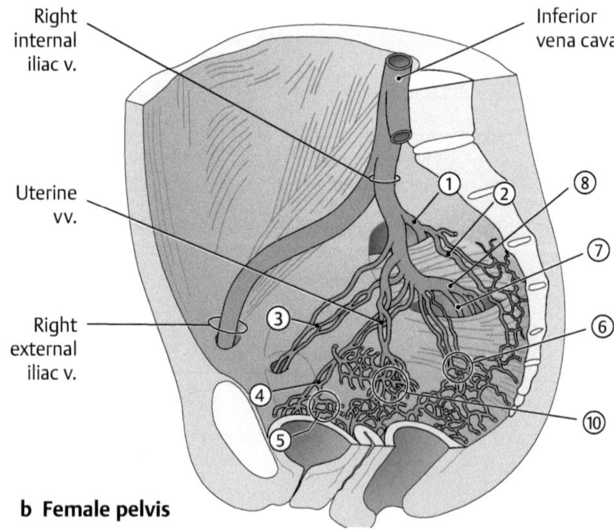

a Male pelvis

b Female pelvis

(From Schuenke M, Schulte E, Schumacher U. THIEME Atlas of Anatomy. Internal Organs. Illustrations by Voll M and Wesker K. 3rd ed. New York: Thieme Medical Publishers; 2020.)

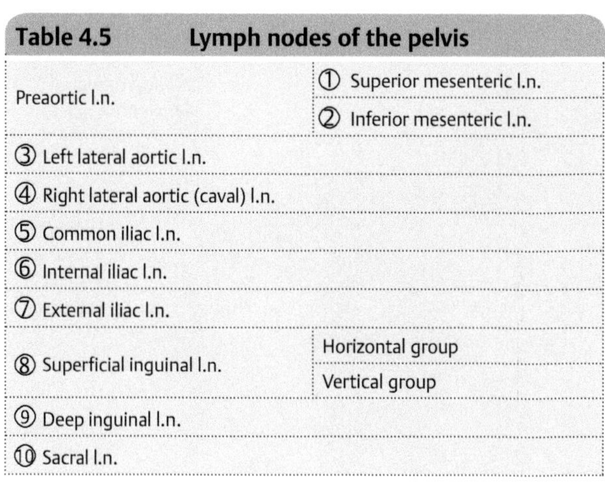

Table 4.5 Lymph nodes of the pelvis	
Preaortic l.n.	① Superior mesenteric l.n.
	② Inferior mesenteric l.n.
③ Left lateral aortic l.n.	
④ Right lateral aortic (caval) l.n.	
⑤ Common iliac l.n.	
⑥ Internal iliac l.n.	
⑦ External iliac l.n.	
⑧ Superficial inguinal l.n.	Horizontal group
	Vertical group
⑨ Deep inguinal l.n.	
⑩ Sacral l.n.	

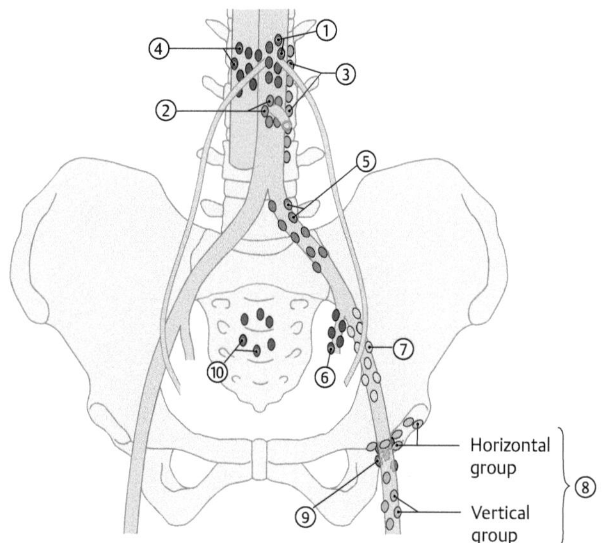

(From Schuenke M, Schulte E, Schumacher U. THIEME Atlas of Anatomy. Internal Organs. Illustrations by Voll M and Wesker K. 3rd ed. New York: Thieme Medical Publishers; 2020.)

Clinical Correlate 4.4

Urethral Catheterization

For individuals unable to micturate or urinate, urethral catheterization is done to remove urine from the bladder. Additional reasons for performing this procedure are for obtaining an uncontaminated sample of urine, monitoring the total urine output, or imaging the urinary tract. When inserting catheters into a male patient, the overall length and its curvatures must be considered. The female urethra is a little easier to work with because it is short and has a direct course from the bladder. It is also more distensible due to its larger content of elastic tissue and smooth muscle.

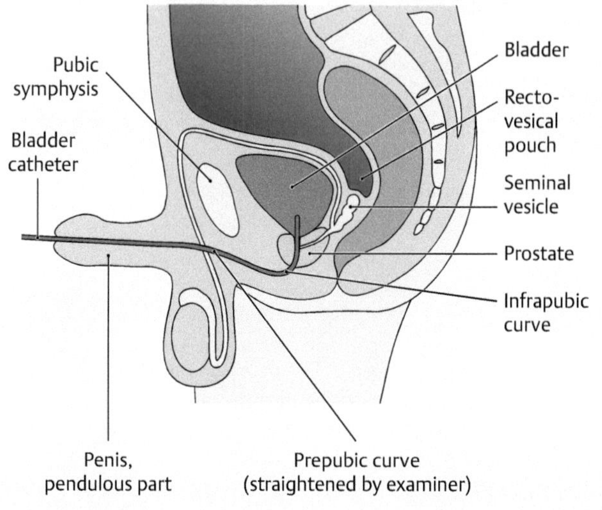

(From Schuenke M, Schulte E, Schumacher U. THIEME Atlas of Anatomy. Internal Organs. Illustrations by Voll M and Wesker K. 3rd ed. New York: Thieme Medical Publishers; 2020.)

Clinical Correlate 4.5

Urethral Ruptures

A rupture of the spongy urethra occurs generally at the bulb of the penis, and urine and blood are capable of passing (or extravasating) into the superficial perineal space. These fluids may pass into the loose connective tissue of the scrotum, around the penis, or superiorly and deep to the membranous (Scarpa's) layer of subcutaneous connective tissue of the lower anterior abdominal wall. Fluids are unable to pass into the thighs because Colles' fascia blends with the fascia lata of the thigh. A rupture of the intermediate (membranous) portion of the urethra could result in the extravasation of urine and blood into the deep perineal pouch. Any of these fluids would pass superiorly through the urogenital hiatus and distribute extraperitoneally around the prostate and bladder. Urethra ruptures could be due to pelvic fractures or improper urethra catheterizations.

Clinical Correlate 4.6

Exstrophy of the Bladder

Exstrophy of the bladder is an anterior body wall defect characterized by the exposure and protrusion of the mucosal surface of the posterior wall of the bladder. The trigone and ureteric orifices are exposed and urine dribbles intermittently from the everted bladder. It primarily occurs in males with a frequency of around 1 in 50,000 births. Complete exstrophy of the bladder may be accompanied by epispadias and a wide separation of the pubic bones. The penis may be divided into two parts with the scrotum split as well. The cause is believed to be due to the failure of the mesoderm cells migrating between the ectoderm and endoderm of the cloacal membrane during the 4th week of development.

Lymph from the *intramural, prostatic* and *intermediate* parts drains to the **internal iliac lymph nodes.** Additional drainage from the *prostatic* urethra along with the *proximal spongy* part drains to the **external iliac lymph nodes.** The **deep inguinal lymph nodes** receive lymph from the *distal spongy part* (**Fig. 4.30**).

4.19.2 Histology of the Male Urethra

The **intramural (preprostatic)** and **prostatic parts** have *transitional epithelium*; the **intermediate (membranous)** and **spongy (penile) parts** have a *stratified columnar epithelium* interspersed

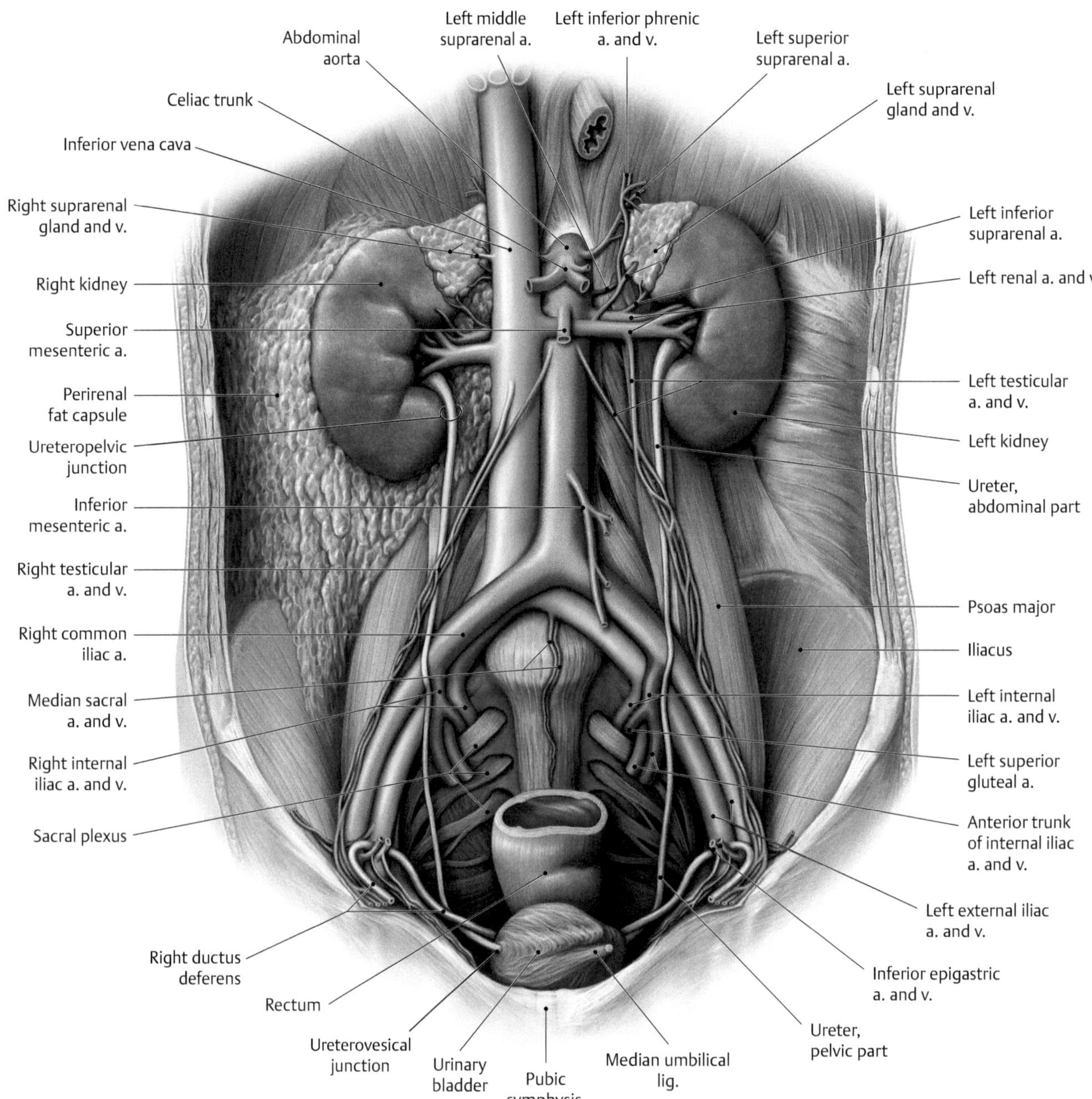

Fig. 4.25 Ureters in situ. (From Schuenke M, Schulte E, Schumacher U. THIEME Atlas of Anatomy. Internal Organs. Illustrations by Voll M and Wesker K. 3rd ed. New York: Thieme Medical Publishers; 2020.)

with sections of *pseudostratified columnar epithelium*. The **navicular fossa**, part of the spongy urethra, is lined with a *squamous non-keratinized epithelium*. The prostatic part receives the openings of the ejaculatory ducts and prostatic utricle, while the **urethral glands** extend from the lamina propria and open into the spongy urethra. At the level of the urogenital diaphragm, skeletal muscle wraps around the intermediate (membranous) part of the urethra to form the **external urethral sphincter**.

4.20 Urinary Bladder and Urethra Development

Sometime during the 4th-7th weeks of development, the **urorectal septum** divides the **cloaca** into the **urogenital sinus** anteriorly and the **rectum/anal canal** posteriorly. The urogenital sinus can be divided into three parts **(Fig. 4.33)**:

- Vesical (cranial) part: forms the majority of the urinary bladder.
- Pelvic (middle) part: forms the intramural (preprostatic), prostatic and intermediate (membranous) parts of the male urethra and the entire urethra of the female.
- Phallic (caudal) part: projects toward the genital tubercle and forms the spongy urethra in males.

The most distal portion of the male urethra coursing through the glans penis is derived from a solid cord of ectodermal cells that grows from the glans penis to meet the spongy urethra derived from the phallic portion of the urogenital sinus. The ectodermal cords canalize to open into the spongy urethra **(Fig. 4.34)**. The bladder is initially continuous with the **allantois** but the connection soon becomes a thick, fibrous cord called the **urachus** and it is present in an adult as the *median umbilical ligament*. It is the distal and inferior parts of the mesonephric ducts that become incorporated into the posterior wall of the bladder and form the **trigone of the bladder (Fig. 4.35)**.

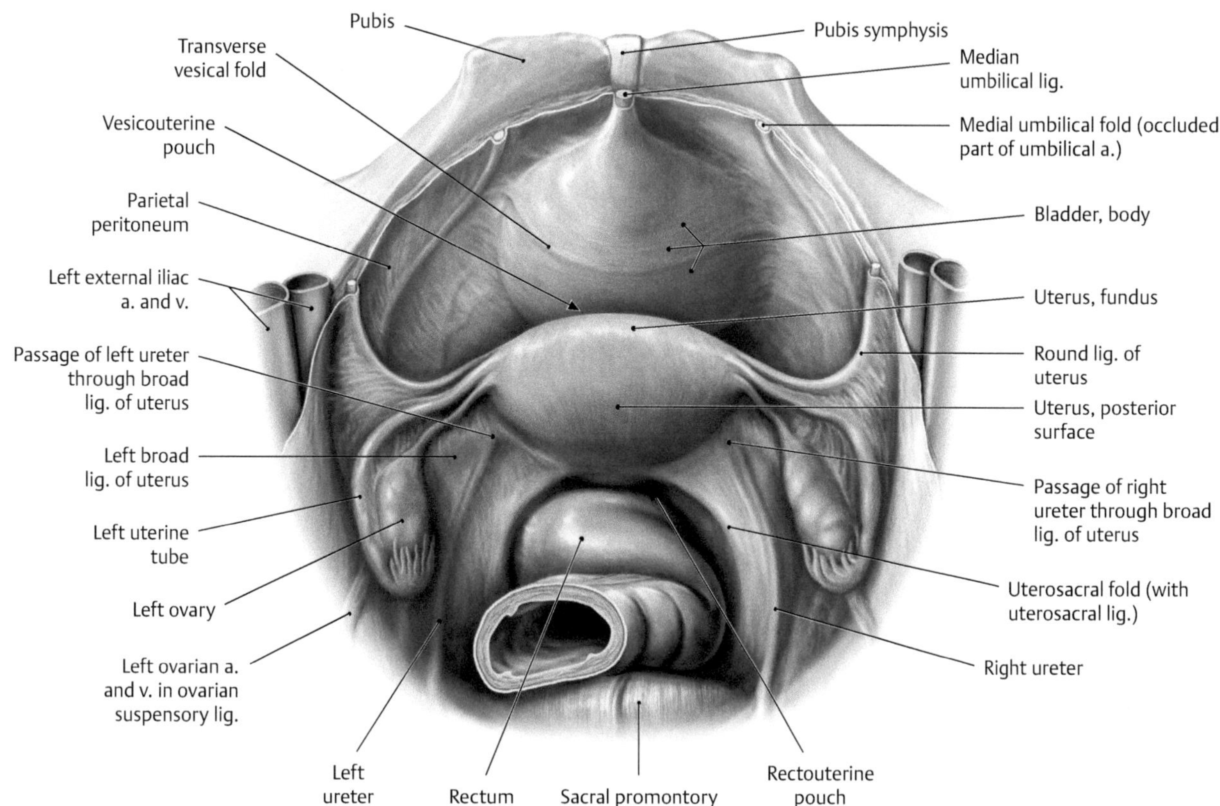

Fig. 4.26 Ureter in the female pelvis. (From Schuenke M, Schulte E, Schumacher U. THIEME Atlas of Anatomy. Internal Organs. Illustrations by Voll M and Wesker K. 3rd ed. New York: Thieme Medical Publishers; 2020.)

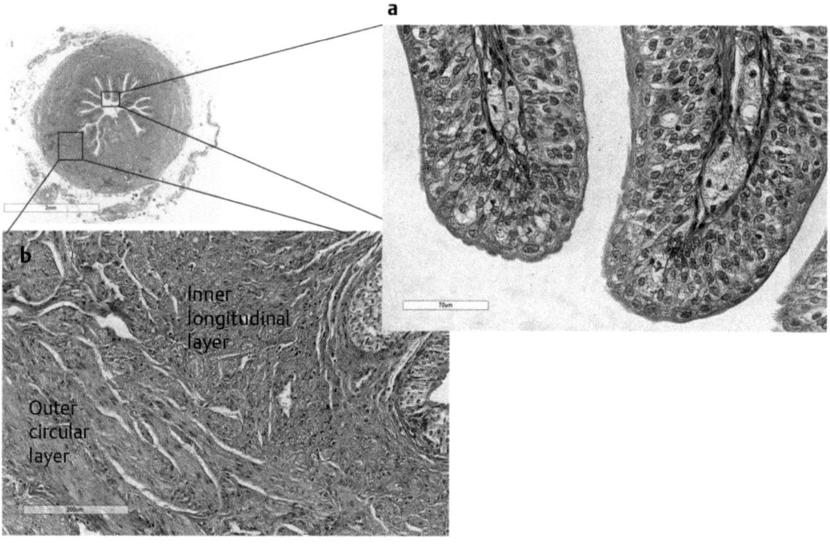

Fig. 4.27 Histology of the ureter. **(a)** Transitional epithelium lining the lumen. **(b)** Smooth muscle layers of the muscularis externa. (From Lowrie DJ. Histology: An Essential Textbook. New York: Thieme Medical Publishers; 2020.)

4.21 Ductus Deferens

The **ductus (vas) deferens** is the continuation of the duct of the epididymis (**Fig. 4.36**). It is the primary structure of the spermatic cord and has a relatively thick muscular wall but a small lumen. It ascends posterior to the testis and medial to the epididymis before entering the anterior abdominal wall through the deep inguinal ring. It crosses over the external iliac vessels and continues on the lateral wall of the pelvis before enlarging to form the **ampulla of the ductus deferens** just before it terminates. There is a quick narrowing where it joins the duct of the seminal vesicle to form the ejaculatory duct.

4.21.1 Neurovasculature and Lymphatic Drainage of the Ductus Deferens

Sympathetic fibers of the **ductus deferens plexus** are derived from the larger inferior hypogastric plexus. These sympathetic fibers originate from the lateral horns of the T12-L2 spinal cord segments and stimulate a rapid peristaltic contraction propelling the sperm from the epididymis and into the pelvis. It is still unclear whether there is any parasympathetic innervation to this structure at all (**Fig. 4.23**).

The blood supply comes from the **artery of the ductus deferens** (or **deferential artery**) which forms an anastomosis with the

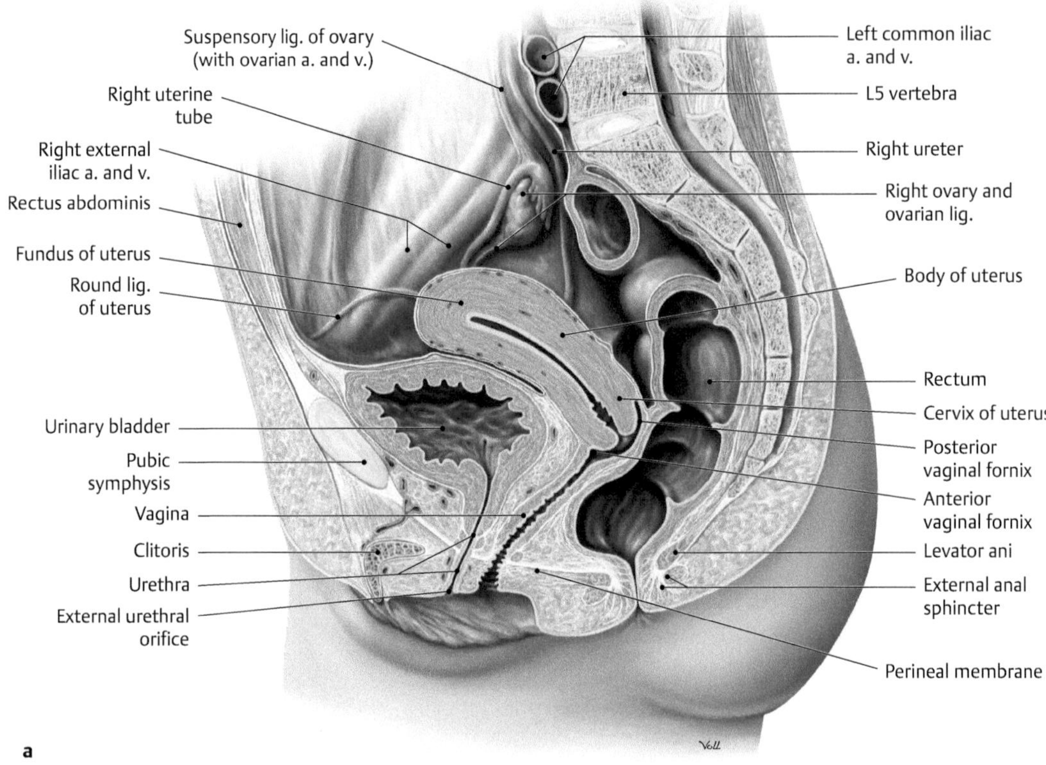

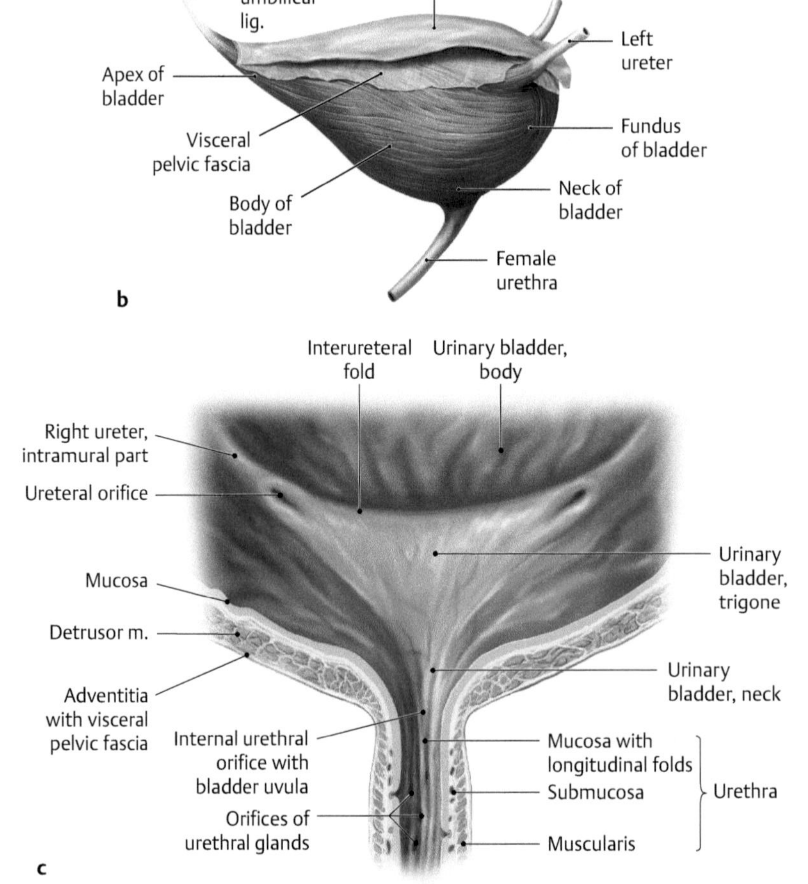

Fig. 4.28 Female urinary bladder and urethra. **(a)** Midsagittal section of pelvis. **(b)** Bladder and urethra. **(c)** Trigone and urethra. (From Schuenke M, Schulte E, Schumacher U. THIEME Atlas of Anatomy. Internal Organs. Illustrations by Voll M and Wesker K. 3rd ed. New York: Thieme Medical Publishers; 2020.)

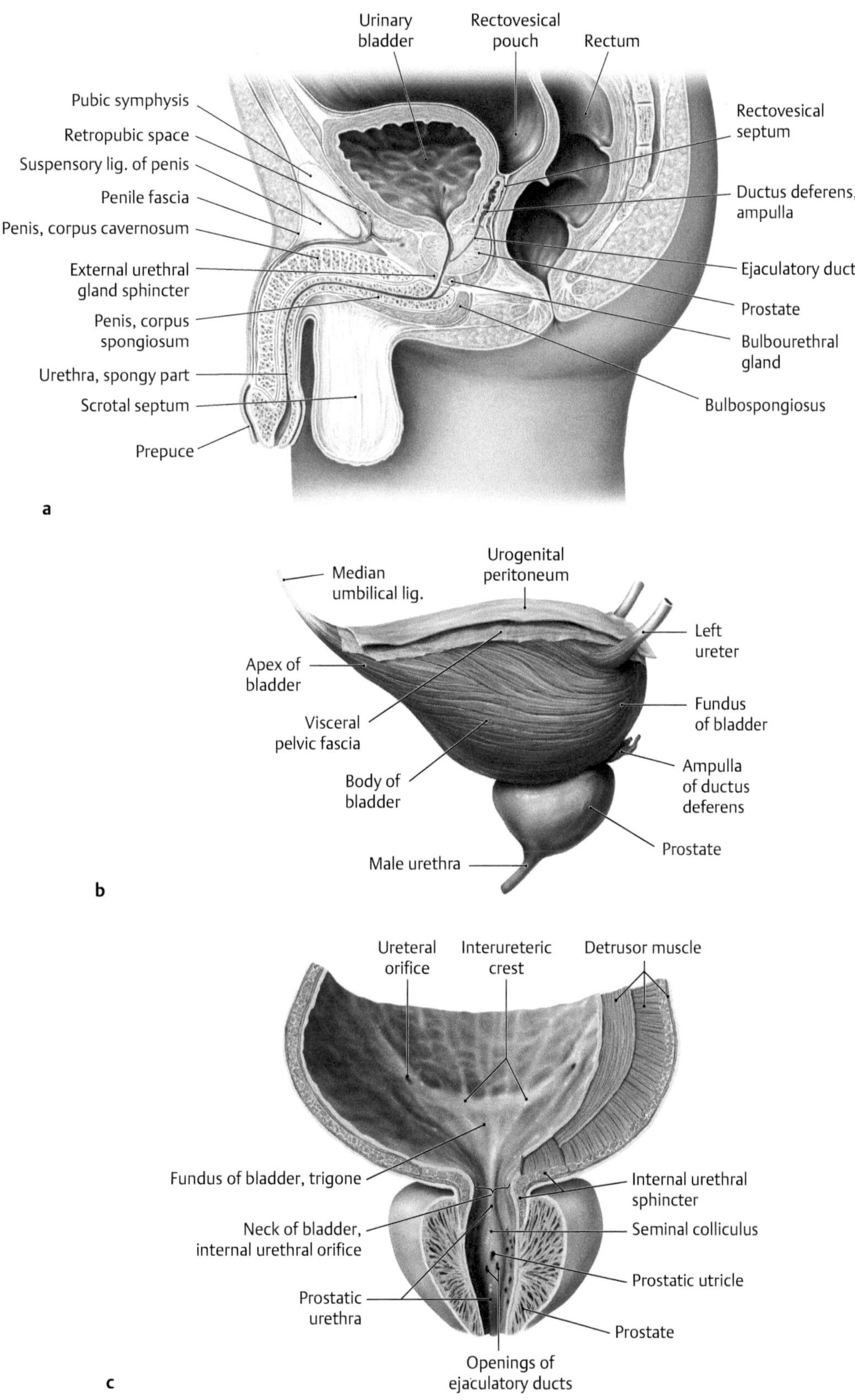

Fig. 4.29 Male urinary bladder and urethra. **(a)** Midsagittal section of pelvis. **(b)** Bladder, urethra and prostate. **(c)** Trigone, urethra, and prostate. (From Schuenke M, Schulte E, Schumacher U. THIEME Atlas of Anatomy. Internal Organs. Illustrations by Voll M and Wesker K. 3rd ed. New York: Thieme Medical Publishers; 2020.)

testicular artery. The artery of the ductus deferens is usually a branch off the *superior vesical artery* but it may also come from the *inferior vesical* or *umbilical arteries* (**Fig. 4.24; Table 4.3**). Venous drainage may run with the **testicular vein**, **internal iliac vein** or from the **vesical** and **prostatic venous plexuses** before again reaching the internal iliac vein (**Fig. 4.24; Table 4.4**). Lymphatic drainage is to the **external iliac** and **internal iliac lymph nodes** (**Fig. 4.37**).

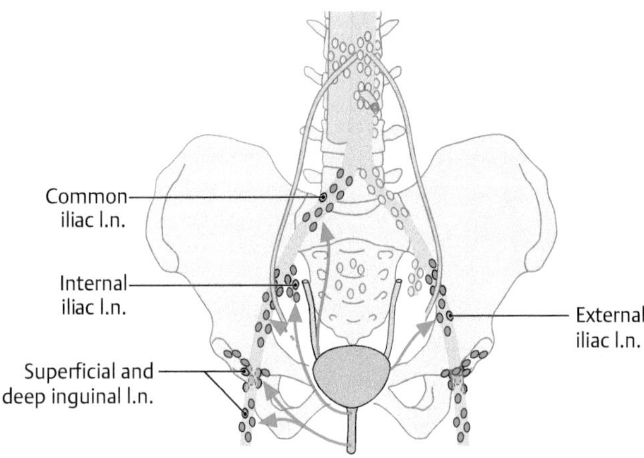

Fig. 4.30 Lymphatic drainage of the bladder and urethra. (From Schuenke M, Schulte E, Schumacher U. THIEME Atlas of Anatomy. Internal Organs. Illustrations by Voll M and Wesker K. 3rd ed. New York: Thieme Medical Publishers; 2020.)

4.21.2 Histology of the Ductus Deferens

The ductus deferens is a thick-walled muscular tube about 30 cm in total length. It has a *stereociliated pseudostratified columnar epithelium*. The muscularis has inner longitudinal, middle circular and outer longitudinal smooth muscle layers that are responsible for propulsion of the sperm during ejaculation (**Fig. 4.38**).

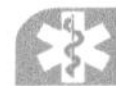

Clinical Correlate 4.7

Deferentectomy (Vasectomy)

A **deferentectomy** (more commonly referred to as a **vasectomy**) is a form of male sterilization. The procedure involves ligating and/or excising a part of the ductus (vas) deferens through an incision in the superior part of the scrotum. Ejaculated fluid is devoid of any sperm but still contains fluid from the seminal glands, prostate and bulbourethral glands. Sperm not expelled degenerate in the epididymis and proximal portion of the ductus deferens.

4.22 Seminal Glands

The **seminal glands** (vesicles) are elongated and obliquely placed superior to the prostate and lie between the fundus of the bladder and the rectum (**Fig. 4.39**). The *rectovesical septum* separates them from the rectum. They do not store sperm (like they were once thought to do) but instead produce a thick alkaline fluid that mixes with sperm as they pass into the ejaculatory ducts and urethra.

4.22.1 Neurovasculature and Lymphatic Drainage of the Seminal Glands

Sympathetic fibers from the **prostatic nerve plexus** stimulate the contraction and secretion of these glands. It is still unclear whether there is any parasympathetic innervation at all (**Fig. 4.20; Fig. 4.23**). Blood supply is from the **inferior vesical** and **middle rectal arteries** both branches of the *internal iliac artery* (**Fig. 4.24; Table 4.3**). Venous drainage is to both the **vesical** and **prostatic venous plexuses**.

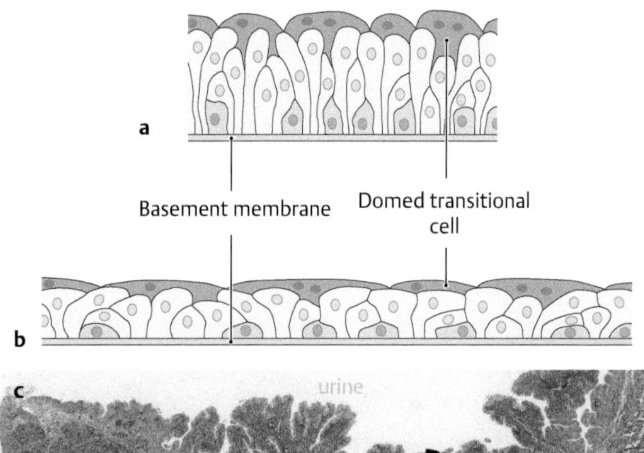

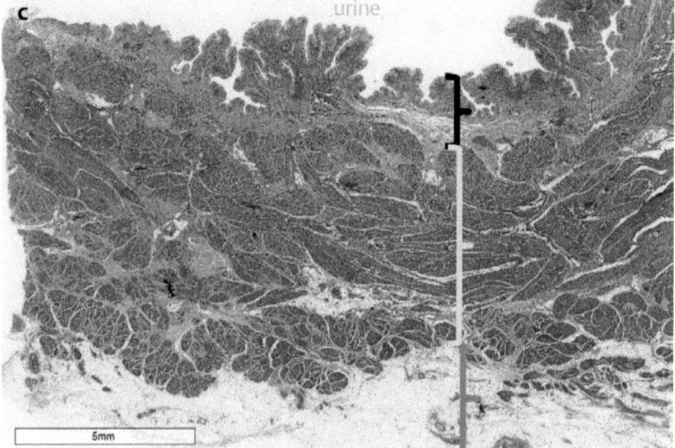

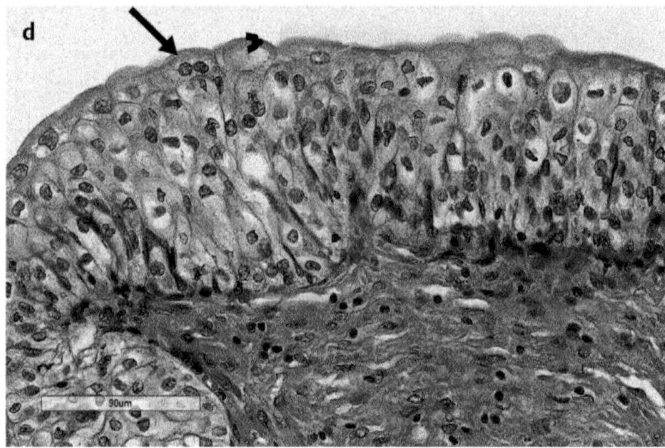

Fig. 4.31 Histology of the urinary bladder. **(a)** Bladder empty: tall epithelium. **(b)** Bladder full: flattened epithelium. **(c)** The wall of the bladder is composed of mucosa (*black bracket*), muscularis (*yellow bracket*), and adventitia (*blue bracket*). **(d)** Transitional epithelium of the bladder. The cytoplasmic band (plaque) is indicated by the bracket. Arrow shows a binucleate cell. (From Schuenke M, Schulte E, Schumacher U. THIEME Atlas of Anatomy. Internal Organs. Illustrations by Voll M and Wesker K. 3rd ed. New York: Thieme Medical Publishers; 2020.)

Lymphatic drainage is to the **external iliac** and **internal iliac lymph nodes** (**Fig. 4.37**).

4.22.2 Histology of the Seminal Glands

These highly coiled and approximately 15 cm long tubular structures have a lumen lined with a *pseudostratified columnar epithelium* that is directly dependent on blood testosterone levels. The columnar cells contain numerous short microvilli and a single flagellum. The subepithelium is fibroelastic and is surrounded by smooth muscle arranged as inner circular and outer longitudinal layers (**Fig. 4.40**). These glands produce a viscous, alkaline and fructose-rich secretion that makes up over 70% of the total ejaculate or semen. This secretion also contains ascorbic acid, prostaglandins, amino acids and proteins and is the source of energy for spermatozoa.

4.23 Ejaculatory Ducts

The **ejaculatory ducts** are slender tubes that arise by the union of the ductus deferens and seminal gland. The short and straight ejaculatory ducts pass through the prostate and terminate at the level of the seminal colliculus (**Fig. 4.36; Fig. 4.39b; Fig. 4.41**). Histologically, there are no smooth muscle fibers wrapped around them, but the lumen is lined by a *simple columnar epithelium*.

4.23.1 Neurovasculature and Lymphatic Drainage of the Ejaculatory Ducts

These ducts are very short with no surrounding smooth muscle thus they have no real innervation. The blood supply is from the **artery to the ductus deferens** (superior vesical br.) with venous drainage to both the **vesical** and **prostatic venous plexuses (Fig. 4.24; Table 4.3; Table 4.4)**. Lymphatic drainage is to the **external iliac lymph nodes (Fig. 4.37)**.

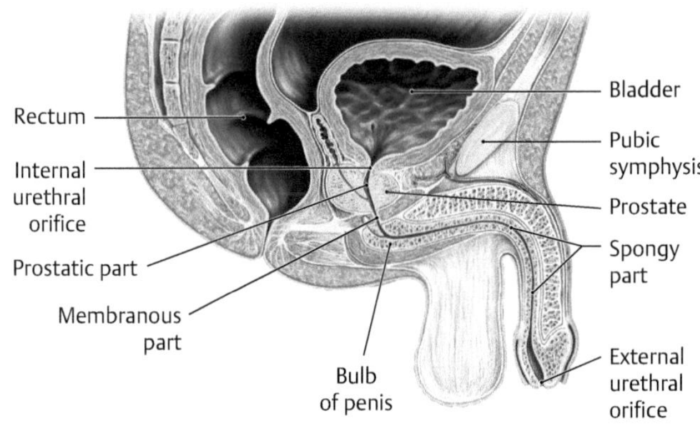

Fig. 4.32 Course of the male urethra. (From Schuenke M, Schulte E, Schumacher U. THIEME Atlas of Anatomy. General Anatomy and Musculoskeletal System. Illustrations by Voll M and Wesker K. 3rd ed. New York: Thieme Medical Publishers; 2020.)

4.24 Prostate Gland

The **prostate** is a walnut-sized gland the surrounds the prostatic urethra and is about two-thirds glandular and one-third fibromuscular. The prostate is a collection of 30-50 branched tubuloalveolar glands embedded in a fibromuscular stroma. There is no true anatomical capsule surrounding the prostate; instead, the smooth muscle of the prostatic stroma gradually extends into fibrous tissue and ends as loose connective and adipose tissue. At the apex and anteriorly, even this minimally distinct border is

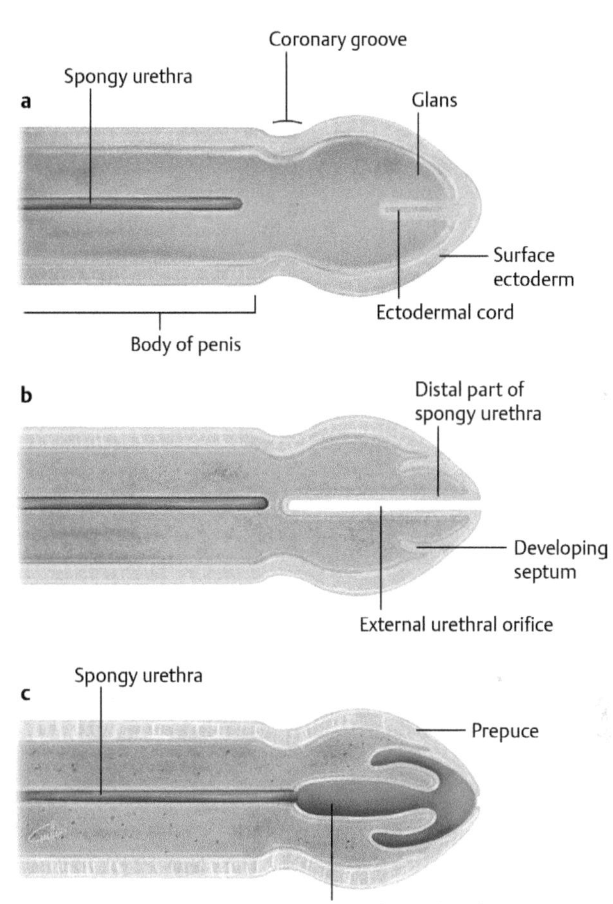

Fig. 4.34 Development of the distal spongy urethra. Illustration by Calla Heald.

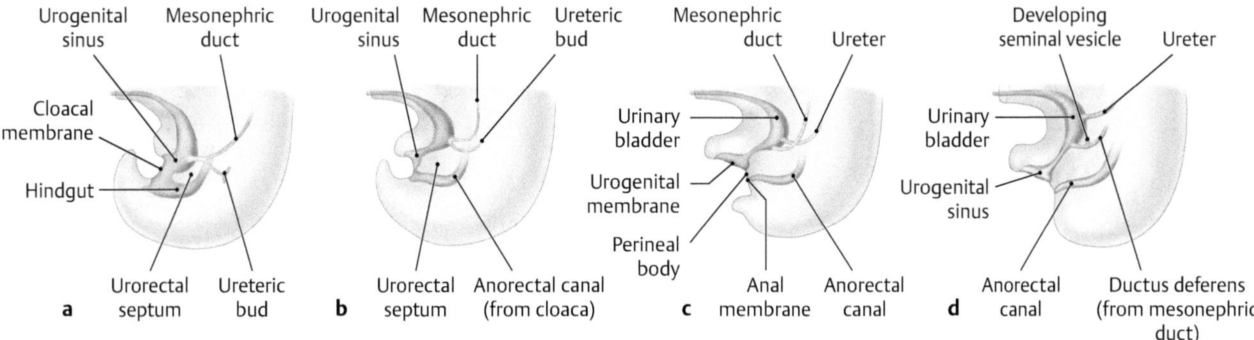

Fig. 4.33 Development of the urinary bladder and urethra. Embryo viewed from left side: **(a)** 5 weeks; **(b)** 7 weeks; **(c)** 8 weeks; **(d)** ~10 weeks. (From Schuenke M, Schulte E, Schumacher U. THIEME Atlas of Anatomy. Internal Organs. Illustrations by Voll M and Wesker K. 3rd ed. New York: Thieme Medical Publishers; 2020.)

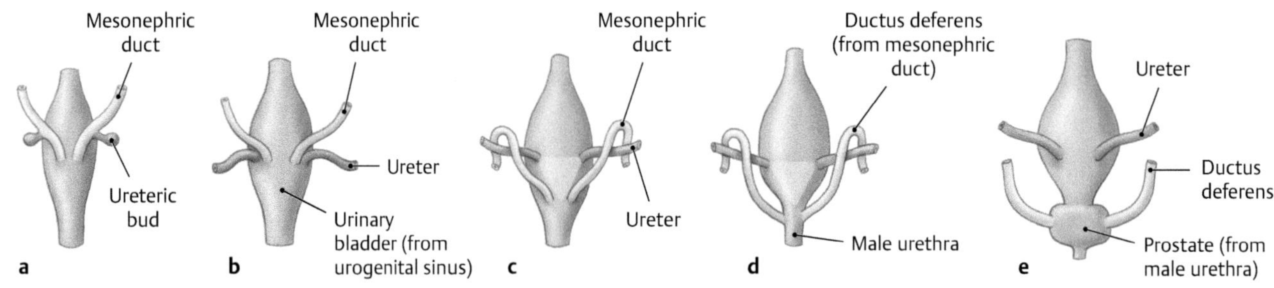

Fig. 4.35 (a-e) Development of the connection between the ureters and urinary bladder and the trigone. (From Schuenke M, Schulte E, Schumacher U. THIEME Atlas of Anatomy. Internal Organs. Illustrations by Voll M and Wesker K. 3rd ed. New York: Thieme Medical Publishers; 2020.)

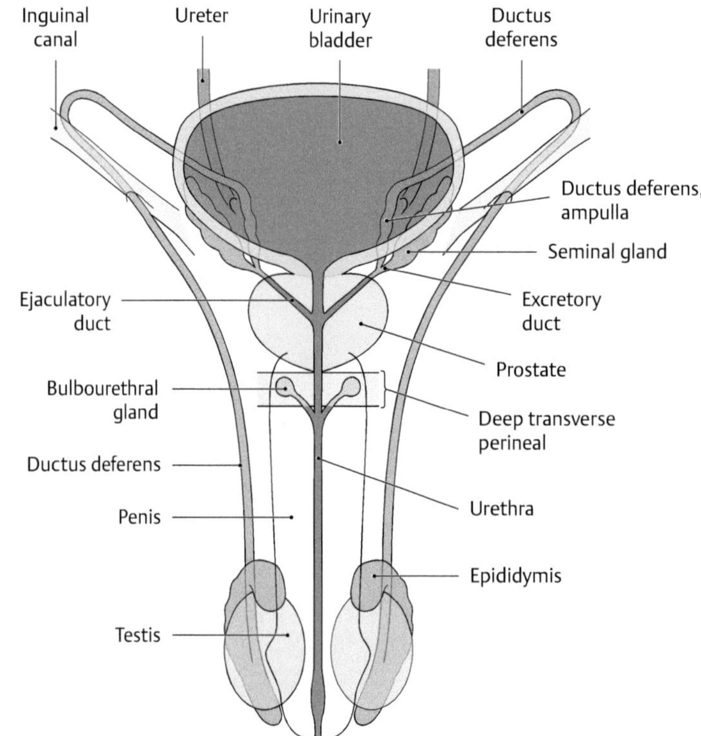

Fig. 4.36 Male genital organs. (From Schuenke M, Schulte E, Schumacher U. THIEME Atlas of Anatomy. Internal Organs. Illustrations by Voll M and Wesker K. 3rd ed. New York: Thieme Medical Publishers; 2020.)

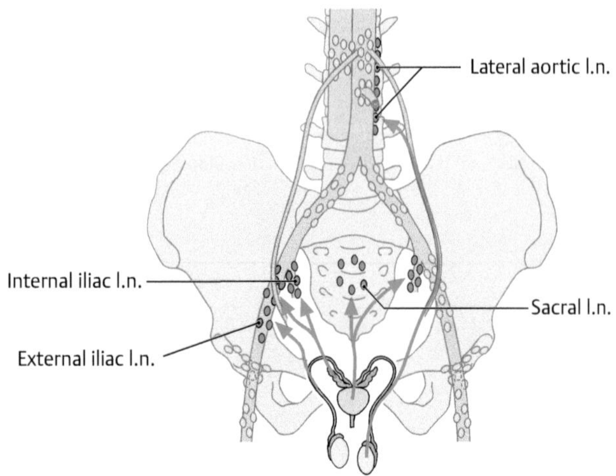

Fig. 4.37 Lymphatic drainage of the male genitalia. (From Schuenke M, Schulte E, Schumacher U. THIEME Atlas of Anatomy. Internal Organs. Illustrations by Voll M and Wesker K. 3rd ed. New York: Thieme Medical Publishers; 2020.)

lost. The visceral layer of the pelvic fascia forms a fibrous *prostatic sheath* that is thin anteriorly, is continuous anterolaterally with the *puboprostatic ligaments*, and is dense posteriorly where it is continuous with the *rectovesical septum*.

Prostatic fluid passes through the **prostatic ducts** that mainly open into the **prostatic sinuses,** which lie on either side of the **seminal colliculus**. The seminal colliculi are on the posterior wall of the prostatic urethra. The ducts of these glands empty into the prostatic urethra. The prostate is described as having lobes and lobules but they are not distinct anatomically. From a clinical prospective the prostate is better defined as having 4-5 distinct zones (**Fig. 4.41**):

- Periurethral/Transition zone (can be considered separate zones): surrounds the proximal prostatic urethra and is the zone associated with *benign prostatic hypertrophy*. It accounts for approximately 5% of the total gland.
- Central zone: surrounds the ejaculatory ducts and accounts for 20-25% of the total gland. The more aggressive prostate cancers originate from this zone but these account for less than 5% of all prostate cancers.

Clinical Correlate 4.8

Prostate Examination and Cancer

The benign enlargement or benign hypertrophy of the prostate (BHP) is common after middle age especially in men over 55 years of age. When the prostate becomes enlarged it begins to project into the bladder and impede urination by distorting the prostatic urethra associated with the periurethral/transition zones. Most prostate cancers develop in the posterolateral region of the peripheral zone and in advanced stages, cancer cells may initially metastasize to the internal iliac and sacral lymph nodes before reaching additional lymph nodes or bone. If a prostatectomy is the chosen course of treatment, the *prostatic plexus* is of major concern. It closely surrounds the prostatic sheath and gives rise to the *cavernous nerves* that convey parasympathetic fibers responsible for the penile erection. If this plexus or the set of nerves that extend from it are damaged it may lead to impotence.

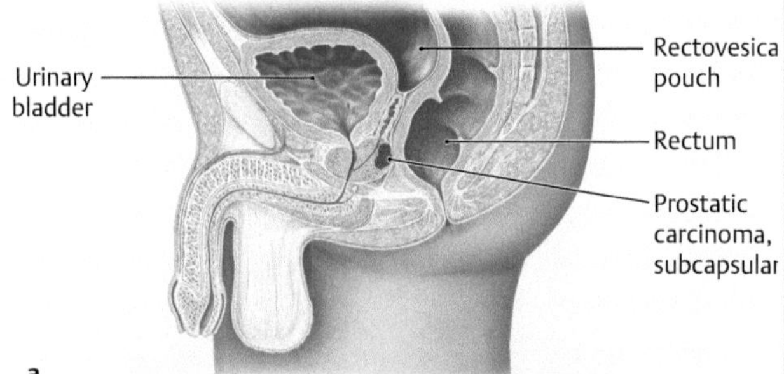

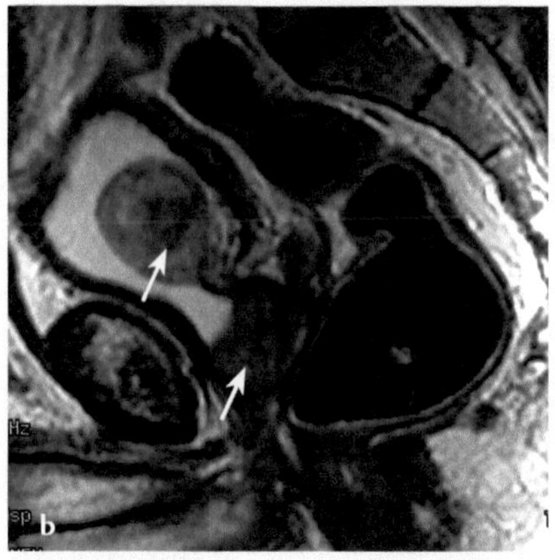

(a) Most common site of prostatic carcinoma. **(b)** Prostatic carcinoma (*arrows*) with bladder infiltration. (From Schuenke M, Schulte E, Schumacher U. THIEME Atlas of Anatomy. Internal Organs. Illustrations by Voll M and Wesker K. 3rd ed. New York: Thieme Medical Publishers; 2020.)

Clinical Correlate 4.9

Prostate Brachytherapy

Brachytherapy (or internal radiation) is a procedure that involves placing radioactive and permanent seed implants or high-dose rate temporary material inside the body to treat prostate cancer. Brachytherapy allows doctors to deliver higher doses of radiation to more-specific areas of the body such as the prostate, compared with the conventional form of radiation therapy (external beam radiation) that projects radiation from a machine outside of your body. This form of therapy may cause fewer side effects than conventional radiation, and the overall treatment time is usually shorter.

- Peripheral zone: it makes up about 70% of the total gland, surrounds the distal prostatic urethra, and is the origination site of 70-80% of all prostate cancers.
- Anterior (fibromuscular) zone: contains no glandular tissue and is composed of only fibrous and muscular tissue. It accounts for approximately 5% of the total gland.

4.24.1 Neurovasculature and Lymphatic Drainage of the Prostate

Sympathetic fibers from the **prostatic nerve plexus** stimulate the contraction and secretion of this gland. It is still unclear whether there is any parasympathetic innervation at all (**Fig. 4.20; Fig. 4.23**). Blood supply is from smaller **prostatic arteries** that originate mainly from the **inferior vesical artery**. They may also branch directly from the **middle rectal** or **internal pudendal arteries** (**Fig. 4.24; Table 4.3**). The paired veins of the arteries drain to the **prostatic venous plexus** that also drain the *deep dorsal vein of the penis* (**Fig. 4.24; Table 4.4**). Lymphatic drainage is primarily to the **internal iliac lymph nodes** but may also include the **sacral lymph nodes** (**Fig. 4.37**).

4.24.2 Histology of the Prostate

The active form of testosterone, dihydrotestosterone, is responsible for the formation, synthesis and release of prostatic secretions. The *simple cuboidal* to *pseudostratified columnar epithelium* secretes this acidic secretion that constitutes 25-30% of the total ejaculate. It is a serous fluid containing acid phosphatase, prostate-specific antigen, fibrinolysin, citric acid, lipids and proteolytic enzymes. In older men, calcified prostatic concretions, or **corpora amylacea**, are often found in the prostatic alveoli (**Fig. 4.42**).

4.25 Bulbourethral Glands

The **bulbourethral (Cowper) glands** lie posterolateral to the intermediate part of the urethra and are embedded within the external urethral sphincter. Their ducts penetrate the perineal membrane before opening into the most proximal portion of the spongy urethra (**Fig. 4.36; Fig. 4.39b; Fig. 4.41**). Histologically, these small glands have a fibroelastic capsule that has septa dividing the gland into several lobules. The epithelium varies from *simple cuboidal* to

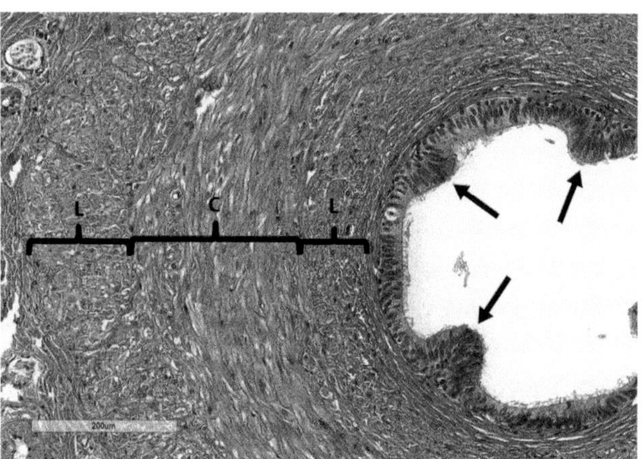

Fig. 4.38 Histology of the ductus deferens showing the inner pseudostartified epithelium with ridges (*arrows*), and three layers of muscle in the muscularis (L = longitudinal, C = circular). (From Lowrie DJ. Histology: An Essential Textbook. New York: Thieme Medical Publishers; 2020.)

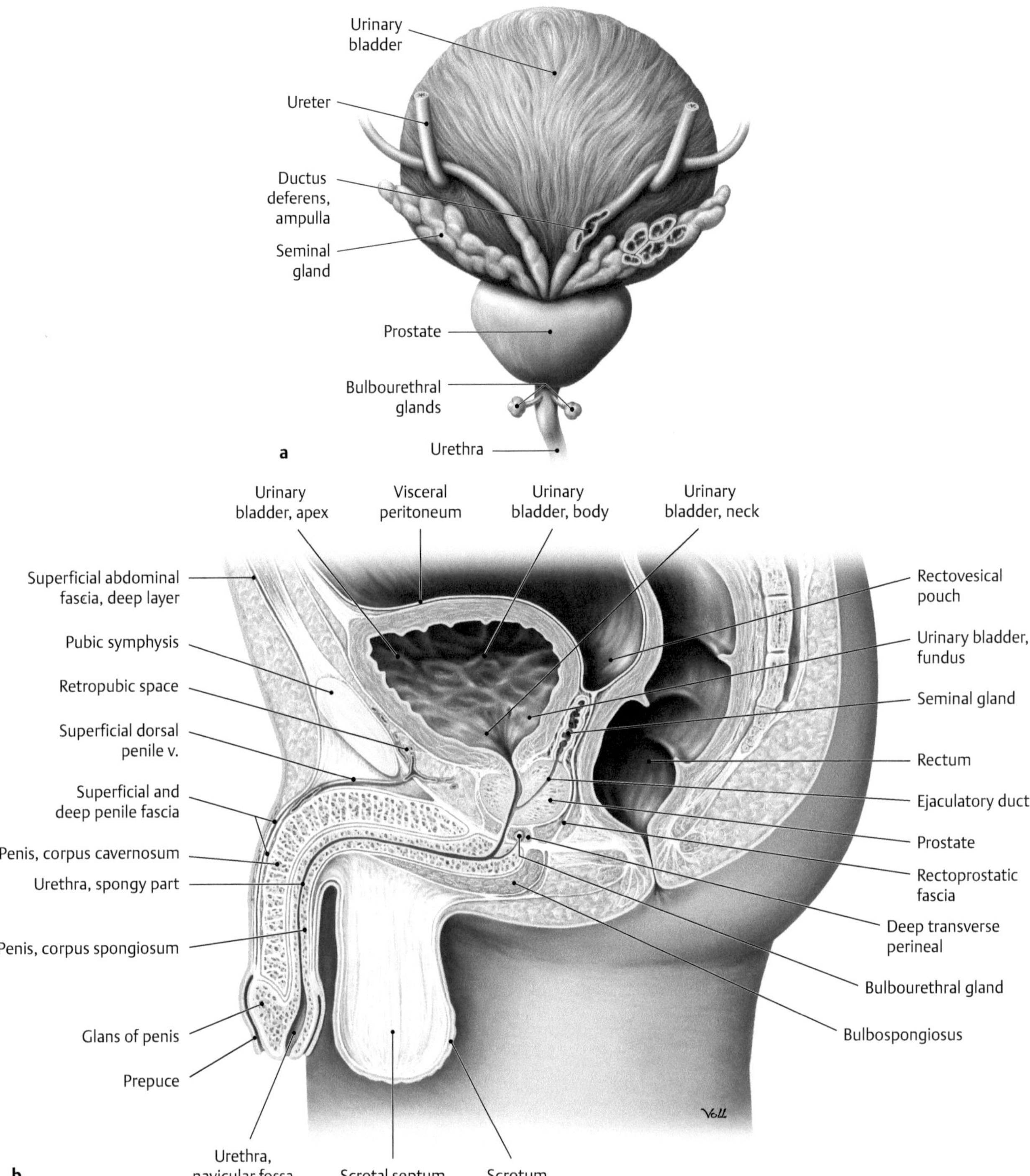

Fig. 4.39 **(a)** Male accessory sex glands, posterior view. **(b)** Sagittal section through the male pelvis, left lateral view. (From Schuenke M, Schulte E, Schumacher U. THIEME Atlas of Anatomy. Internal Organs. Illustrations by Voll M and Wesker K. 3rd ed. New York: Thieme Medical Publishers; 2020.)

simple columnar. Their mucus-like secretions lubricate the lumen of the urethra during sexual arousal and prior to ejaculation.

4.25.1 Neurovasculature and Lymphatic Drainage of the Bulbourethral Glands

Sympathetic fibers from the **prostatic nerve plexus** stimulate the contraction and secretion of this gland. It is still unclear whether there is any parasympathetic innervation at all. The blood supply is from the **artery to the bulb of the penis** (internal pudendal br.) with venous drainage following the **internal pudendal vein** or involving the **prostatic venous plexus** (**Fig. 4.24; Table 4.3; Table 4.4**). Lymphatic drainage is to the **external iliac** and **internal iliac lymph nodes**.

4.26 Genital Duct Development of the Male

Male and female embryos initially have two pairs of genital ducts called the **mesonephric (Wolffian)** and **paramesonephric (Müllerian) ducts**. The **mesonephric ducts** play an essential role

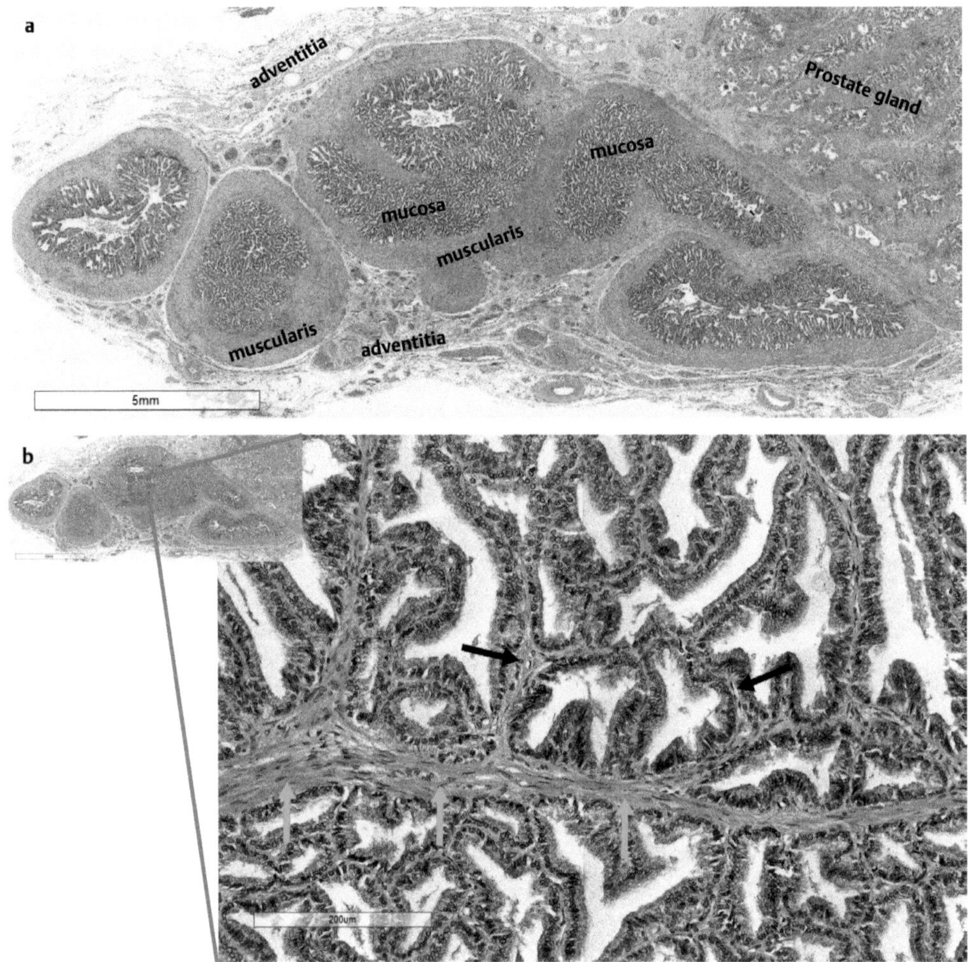

Fig. 4.40 Histology of the seminal gland. **(a)** Scanning magnification showing the mucosa, muscularis, and adventitia of the seminal gland and with a portion of the prostate shown. **(b)** Medium magnification showing thin projections of the muscularis (*green arrows*) and loose connective tissue of the mucosa (*black arrows*). (From Lowrie DJ. Histology: An Essential Textbook. New York: Thieme Medical Publishers; 2020.)

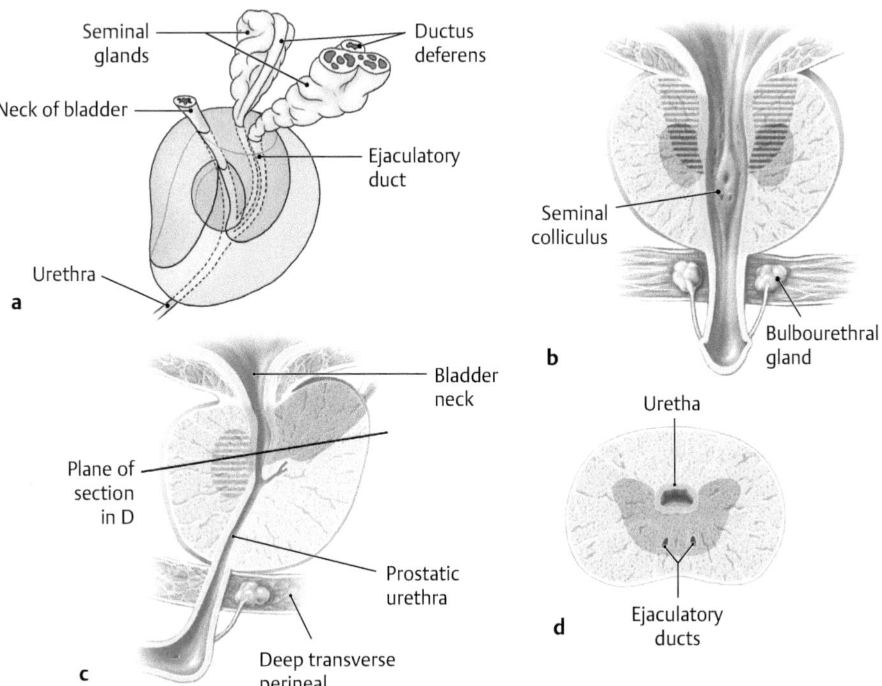

Fig. 4.41 Clinical divisions of the prostate. **(a)** Prostate and seminal glands. **(b)** Coronal section, anterior view. **(c)** Sagittal section, left lateral view. **(d)** Transverse section, superior view. (From Schuenke M, Schulte E, Schumacher U. THIEME Atlas of Anatomy. Internal Organs. Illustrations by Voll M and Wesker K. 3rd ed. New York: Thieme Medical Publishers; 2020.)

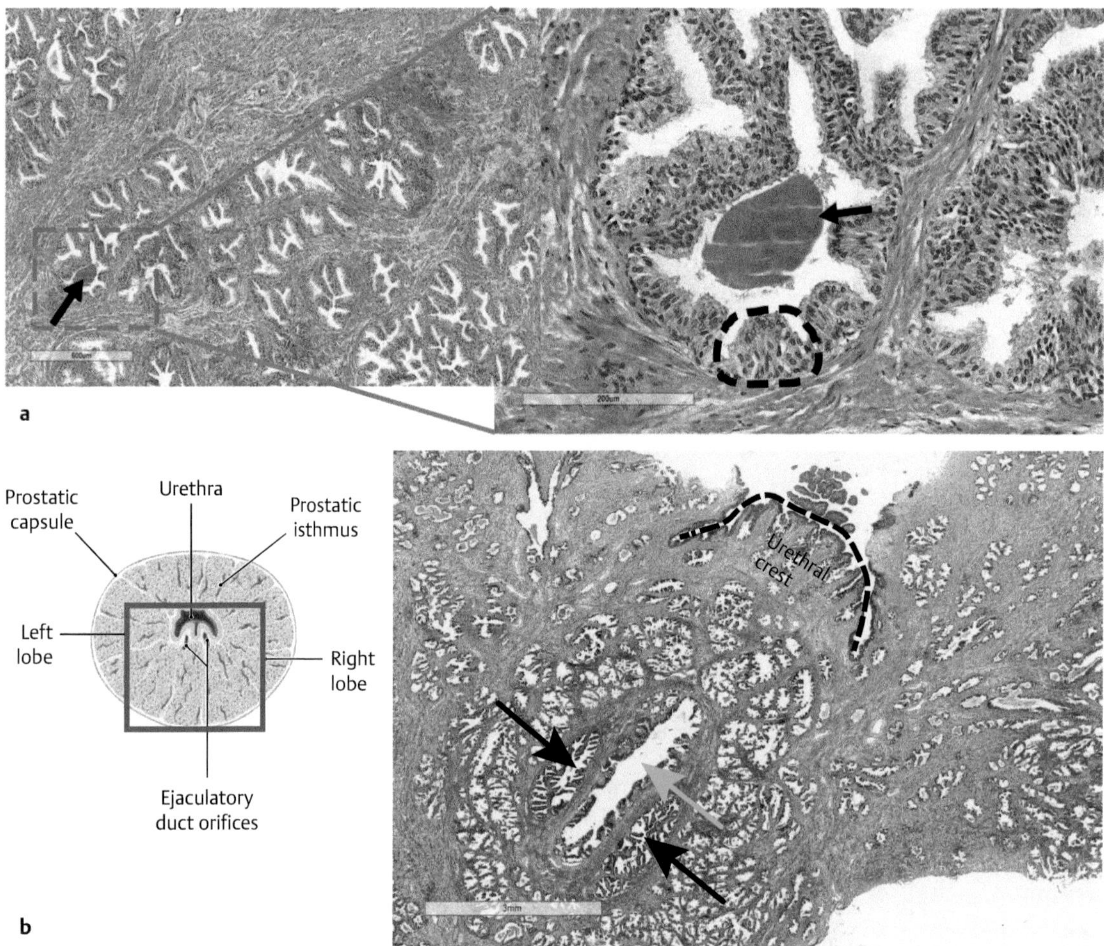

Fig. 4.42 Histology of the prostate gland. **(a)** Low-medium magnification: the epithelium is pseudostratified, with taller regions that appear stratified (*outlined*). A corpora amylacea is noted by the *black arrow*. **(b)** Prostate gland including posterior wall of prostatic urethra, showing the urethral crest. Lumen of the prostatic urethra (*dotted line*). The ejaculatory ducts (*black arrows*) and prostatic utricle (*green arrow*) are shown. (From Lowrie DJ. Histology: An Essential Textbook. New York: Thieme Medical Publishers; 2020.)

in the development of the male reproductive system **(Fig. 4.43)**. The testes produce **testosterone** while Sertoli cells produce **Müllerian-inhibiting substance (MIS)**. Testosterone stimulates the mesonephric ducts to form male genital ducts while MIS causes the paramesonephric ducts to disappear. As the mesonephros of the nephrogenic cord degenerates, some of the mesonephric tubules contained within it remain to form the efferent ductules. The efferent ductules open into the mesonephric duct, which has been transformed into the **duct of the epididymis** in this region. Distal to the epididymis the mesonephric duct becomes the **ductus deferens**. At the caudal ends of each duct, lateral outgrowths represent the **seminal vesicles**. The **ejaculatory duct** originates from the part of the mesonephric duct located between the duct of the seminal vesicle and the urethra.

The **prostate gland** originates from multiple endodermal outgrowths from the prostatic urethra while paired endodermal outgrowths from the proximal spongy urethra give rise to the **bulbourethral glands**.

4.27 Ovaries

The female gonads or **ovaries** are almond-shaped and suspended by the mesovarium. They are endocrine glands producing reproductive hormones and are the location of oocyte development **(Fig. 4.44; Fig. 4.45)**. The ovarian neurovasculature passes under the **suspensory (infundibulopelvic) ligament of the ovary**. The **ovarian ligament** attaches the ovary to the fundus of the uterus at the uterotubal junction and is a remnant of the *gubernaculum*. During a pelvic or ultrasonic examination the ovaries are generally found laterally between the uterus and lateral pelvic wall. The oocyte expelled at ovulation passes into the peritoneal cavity but is trapped by the fimbriae of the uterine tube and carried to the ampulla. There is no peritoneum covering the ovary thus this is the reason an oocyte is capable of being expelled and picked up by the fimbriae.

4.27.1 Neurovasculature and Lymphatic Drainage of the Ovaries

Autonomic fibers originating from both the **ovarian periarterial plexus** and **uterovaginal plexus** are responsible for innervating the ovaries. Sympathetic fibers vasoconstrict and parasympathetic fibers may dilate the blood vessels **(Fig. 4.19; Fig. 4.22)**. The blood supply is from the **ovarian artery** (abdominal aorta br.) **(Fig. 4.24; Table 4.3)**. Venous drainage originates from the **pampiniform plexus**, near the ovary, before draining to the **ovarian vein**. The left ovarian vein drains to the *left renal vein* and the right ovarian vein drains to the *IVC*. Lymphatic drainage is to the **lumbar (caval/aortic) lymph nodes (Fig. 4.46)**.

Mesonephric (Wolffian) duct
Paramesonephric (Müllerian) duct
Primordium of prostate
Urogenital sinus
Gonad primordium
Caudal gonadal ligament (gubernaculum)
Primordia of bulbourethral or greater vestibular glands
Seminal vesicle
Ductus deferens
Prostatic utricle
Prostate
Bulbourethral gland
Epididymis
Appendix of testis
Testis
Uterus
Uterine tube
Epoophoron
Suspensory ligament of ovary
Ovary
Ovarian lig.
Gartner's duct (remnant of the mesonephric duct)
Round ligament of the uterus
Vagina
Greater vestibular gland
Paraurethral gland

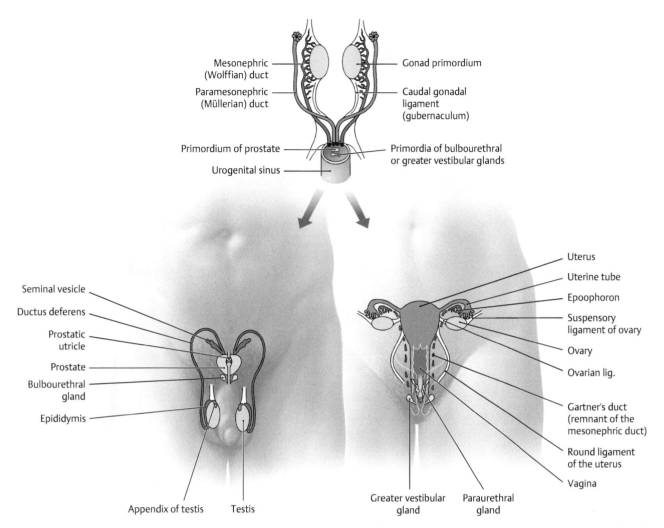

Fig. 4.43 Genital duct development. (From Schuenke M, Schulte E, Schumacher U. THIEME Atlas of Anatomy. Internal Organs. Illustrations by Voll M and Wesker K. 3rd ed. New York: Thieme Medical Publishers; 2020.)

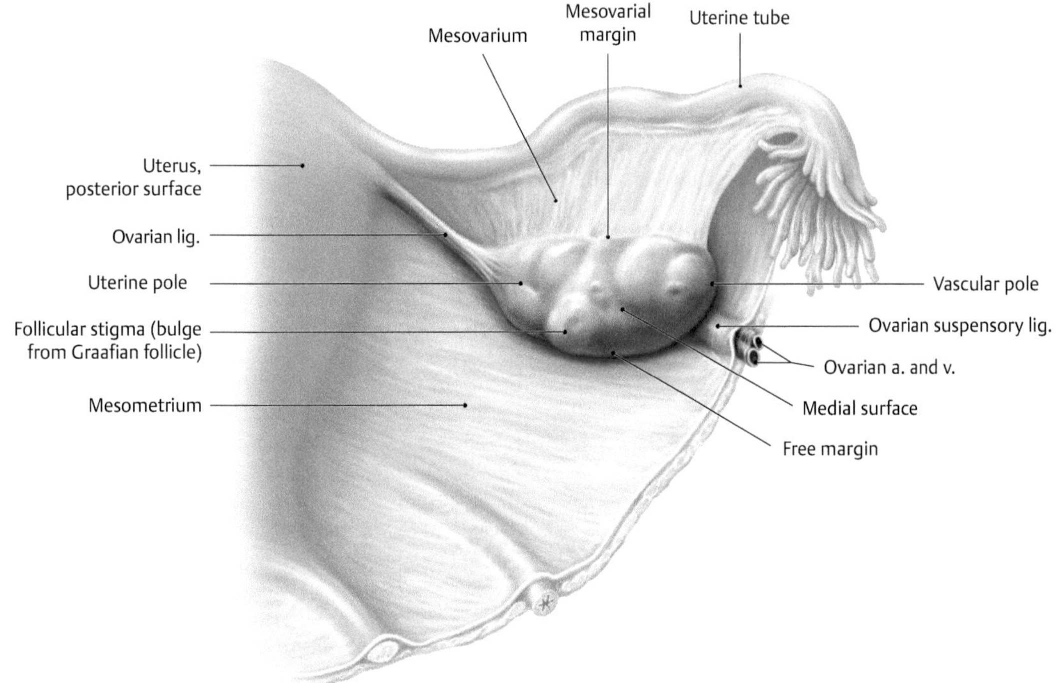

Fig. 4.44 Right ovary, posterior view. (From Schuenke M, Schulte E, Schumacher U. THIEME Atlas of Anatomy. Internal Organs. Illustrations by Voll M and Wesker K. 3rd ed. New York: Thieme Medical Publishers; 2020.)

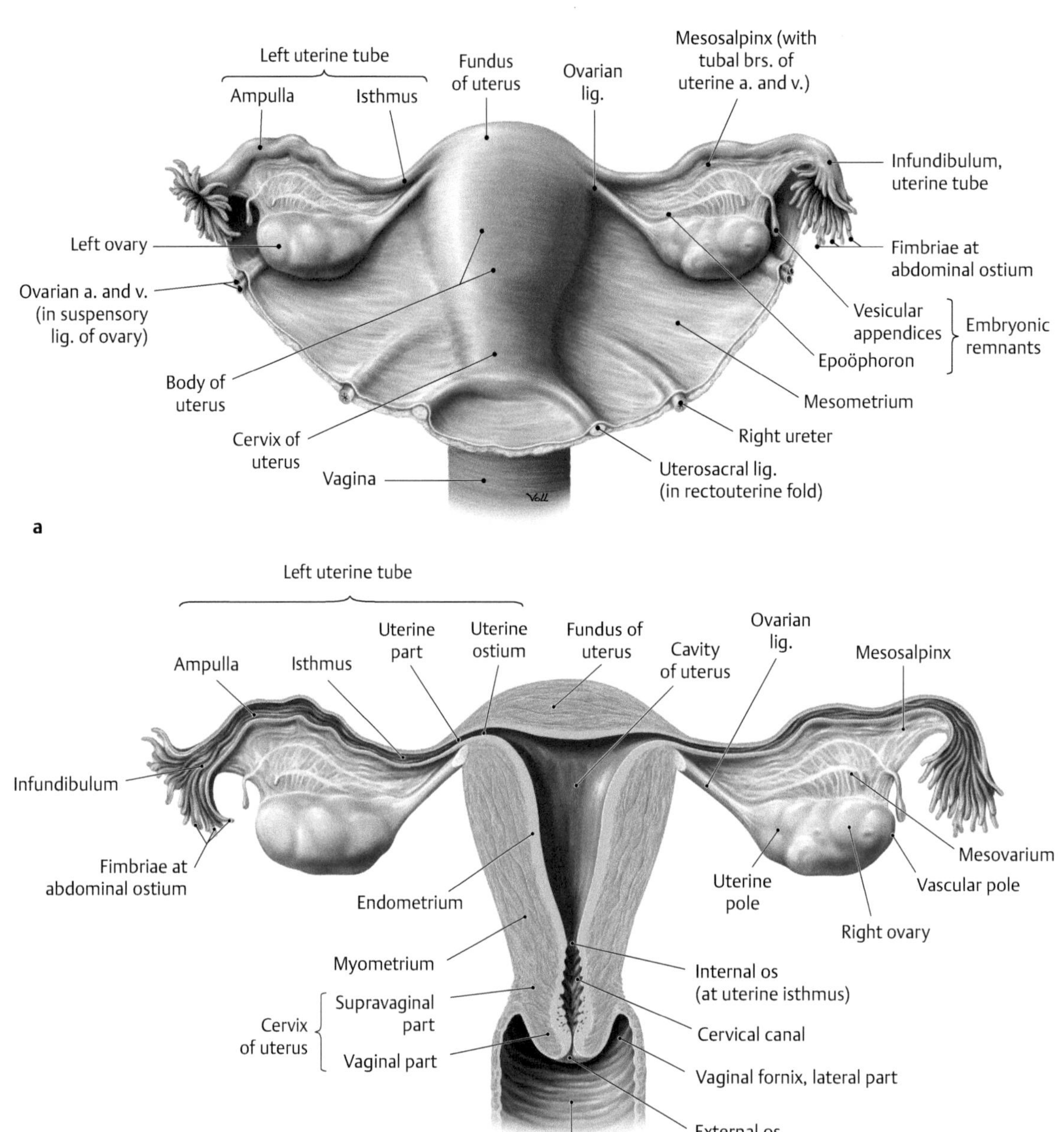

Fig. 4.45 (a) Posterosuperior view of the uterus, ovaries, uterine tubes, and broad ligaments. **(b)** Posterior view of a coronal section with the uterus straightened and the mesometrium removed. (From Schuenke M, Schulte E, Schumacher U. THIEME Atlas of Anatomy. Internal Organs. Illustrations by Voll M and Wesker K. 3rd ed. New York: Thieme Medical Publishers; 2020.)

4.27.2 Histology of the Ovaries

The ovaries are attached and vascularized along their anterior margins by the mesovarium, the ovarian ligament, and the suspensory ligament. The ovary increases in size by 30-fold from infancy to puberty and has an outer **cortex**, inner **medulla** and **hilum**. Follicular structures are typically seen in the cortex.

A *simple squamous* or *cuboidal epithelium* that is continuous with the peritoneal infolding at the hilum covers the surface or **germinal epithelium**. Lying just deep to the germinal layer is the tunica albuginea and it is responsible for the whitish color of the ovary. The ovarian follicles of all stages of their development are embedded in the stroma of the cortex. The cortex functions in providing structural support for the ova, differentiating into internal and external thecal layers that surround the developing follicles, and secreting hormones. The inner medulla has a rich supply of neurovasculature within a loose connective tissue that enters or leaves at the hilum **(Fig. 4.47)**.

There are small populations of **primordial germ cells** near the end of the first month of embryonic development that migrate from the yolk sac and to the primordial gonads. While in the gonads these cells divide and become **oogonia**. By the seventh month of embryonic development, division has been so fast that there are around seven million oogonia. However, it is during the third month of development that the oogonia become arrested in prophase of the first meiotic division. After being surrounded by follicular (granulosa) cells (*simple squamous*), these cells become the **primary oocytes**. Many of these primary oocytes undergo atresia and as a result there may only be 300,000-600,000 remaining at the first sign of puberty (menarche). Only one oocyte is normally released at ovulation and this means that during the entire reproductive life of a woman (~35 years), she may only release a total of 450 oocytes.

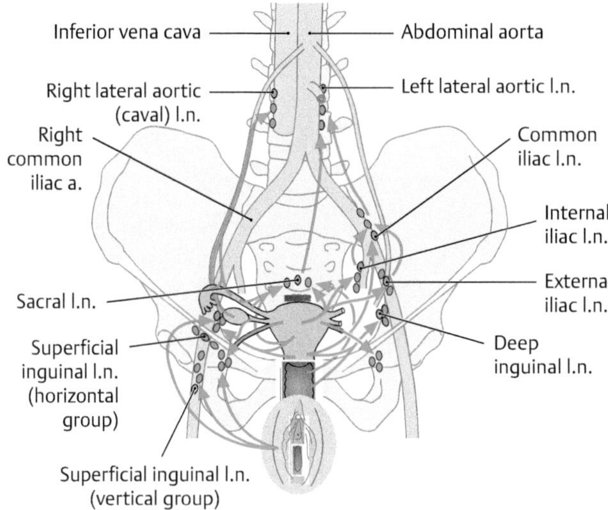

Fig. 4.46 Lymphatic drainage of the female genitalia. (From Schuenke M, Schulte E, Schumacher U. THIEME Atlas of Anatomy. Internal Organs. Illustrations by Voll M and Wesker K. 3rd ed. New York: Thieme Medical Publishers; 2020.)

4.27.3 Folliculogenesis

A small group of primordial follicles begins the process of follicular growth. This consists of modifications to the oocyte, follicular cells and the stromal fibroblasts that surround the follicles (**Fig. 4.48**). The follicular growth is stimulated by follicle-stimulating hormone (FSH) secreted by the pituitary gland. Oocyte growth is most rapid during early follicular growth. The follicular cells will divide by mitosis and form a single cuboidal cell layer at which point this is known as the **unilaminar primary follicle** and represents initiation of follicular maturation. With continued proliferation, the follicular cells become more stratified and are referred to as the **granulosa cell layer**. The follicle is now called the **multilaminar primary (preantral) follicle**. Concurrently, a noticeable and thick amorphous **zona pellucida** now surrounds the oocyte.

As the multilaminar primary follicles increase in size, the granulosa cells secrete the **liquor folliculi** and it begins to accumulate between the follicular cells. Granulosa cells rearrange themselves to form a larger cavity or **antrum** and the follicles are now called **secondary (antral) follicles**. Follicular fluid contains components of the plasma, steroid-binding proteins, progesterone, androgens, estrogens and glycosaminoglycans. The fibroblasts of the stroma surrounding the follicle form the **theca folliculi** which

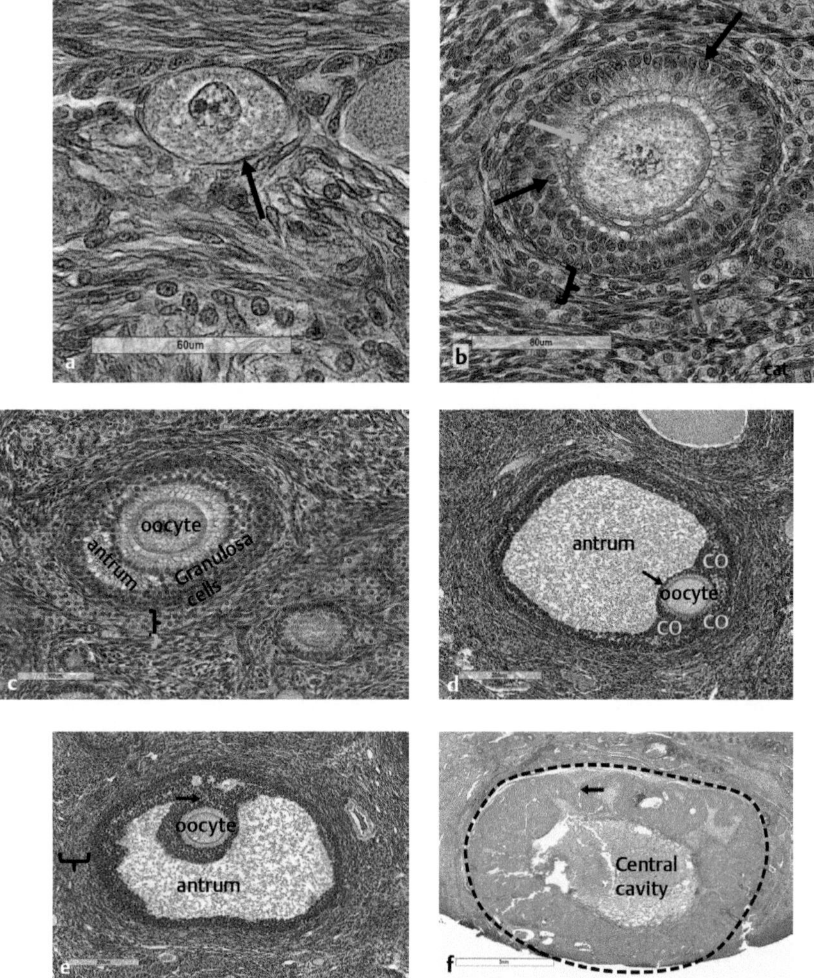

Fig. 4.47 Histology of the ovary. **(a)** Primordial follicles with squamous follicular cells (*black arrow*). **(b)** Late primary follicles: granulosa cells (*black arrows*), zona pellucida (*blue arrow*), theca (*black bracket*), and basement membrane (*red arrow*). **(c)** Secondary follicle: theca interna (*black bracket*) and theca externa (*blue bracket*). **(d)** Late secondary follicle: cumulus oophorus (CO and arrow). **(e)** Graafi an follicle: zona pellucida *(purple arrow*), corona radiata (*yellow arrows*); cumulus oophorus (*green arrows*), basement membrane (*black arrows*), theca interna (*blue arrow*), and theca externa (*orange arrow*). **(f)** Corpus luteum (*outlined*). Folds of the corpus luteum (*arrows*) contain thecal cells. (From Lowrie DJ. Histology: An Essential Textbook. New York: Thieme Medical Publishers; 2020.)

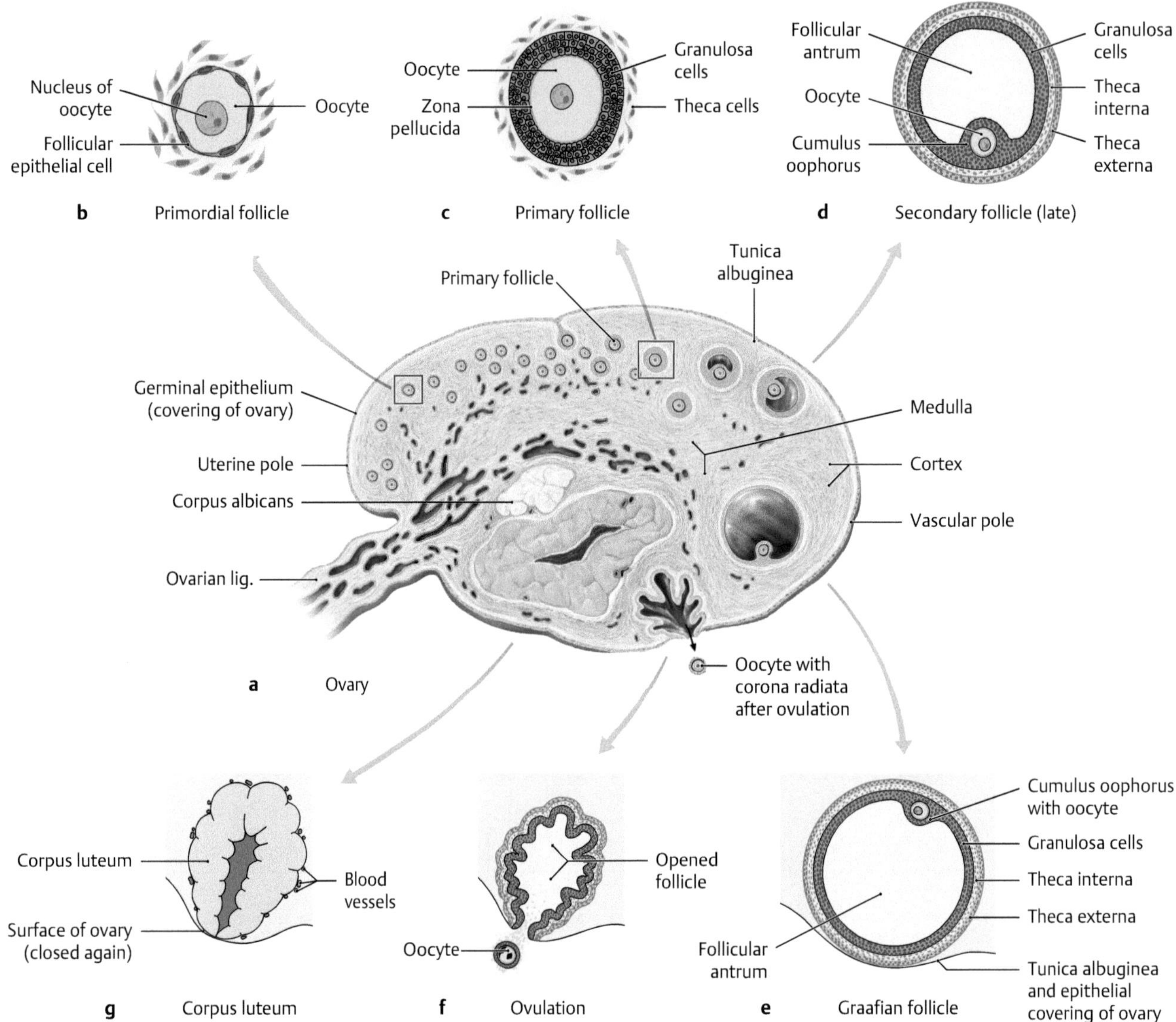

Fig. 4.48 (a-g) Follicular maturation in the ovary. (From Schuenke M, Schulte E, Schumacher U. THIEME Atlas of Anatomy. Internal Organs. Illustrations by Voll M and Wesker K. 3rd ed. New York: Thieme Medical Publishers; 2020.)

subsequently begin differentiating into the **theca interna** and **theca externa** layers.

As the granulosa cells reorganize to form the antrum, some of these cells concentrate at a specific site on the follicular wall and form the **cumulus oophorus**. This structure protrudes toward the interior of the antrum and contains the oocyte. A small concentration of granulosa cells that surround the oocyte are known as the **corona radiata**. After the development of these two structures and the further differentiation of the theca interna and externa, this follicle is now referred to as a **tertiary (mature** or **graafian) follicle**. FSH stimulates the theca interna to secrete a steroid called *androstenedione*, which is then transported to the granulosa layer. FSH also causes the granulosa cells to secrete *aromatase*, an enzyme that transforms androstenedione into *estrogen*. Estrogen then returns to the stroma before reaching the blood vessels so that it can be distributed to the body.

4.27.4 Ovulation

In the days immediately preceding ovulation and under the influence of FSH and luteinizing hormone (LH), the follicle grows rapidly to become a tertiary (mature or graafian) follicle. An abrupt increase in LH causes the primary oocyte to complete meiosis I, forming a **secondary oocyte** and a polar body. This oocyte begins the second meiotic division but stops at metaphase approximately three hours before ovulation. It does not complete the second meiotic division unless fertilization occurs.

As the follicle continues to enlarge, a localized bulge forms on the surface of the ovary. At the apex of this bulge, a small and avascular spot called the **stigma** appears. High levels of LH increase the collagenase activity resulting in digestion of the collagen fibers surrounding the follicle. Muscular contractions of the ovarian wall are due to increases in prostaglandin levels in response to LH. The secondary oocyte is then released along with the surrounding granulosa cells located near the cumulus oophorus before ultimately rearranging themselves to form the corona radiata near the zona pellucida (**Fig. 4.48**).

4.27.5 Corpus Luteum

After ovulation, the granulosa and theca interna cells of the ovulated follicle begin to reorganize and form a temporary endocrine gland called the **corpus luteum (Fig. 4.47; Fig. 4.48)**. Blood from the theca interna coagulates after entering the follicular lumen and forms the **corpus hemorrhagicum**. Granulosa cells do not divide after ovulation but increase in size and contribute up to 80% of the parenchyma of the corpus luteum. They are now known as **granulosa lutein cells** and secrete progesterone. The theca interna cells give rise to smaller **theca lutein cells** and they secrete progesterone and some estrogens. Increased progesterone inhibits *gonadotropin-releasing hormone* (GnRH) from the hypothalamus and LH and FSH release from the pituitary gland, thereby inhibiting folliculogenesis but stimulating the endometrium to thicken and prepare for implantation of the embryo.

- Corpus luteum of pregnancy: after implantation of a fertilized ovum, the syncytiotrophoblast of the developing embryos placenta begins to secrete *human chorionic gonadotropin* (hCG) and this spares the corpus luteum from degeneration of which it is now known as the corpus luteum of pregnancy (CLP). The hormone hCG also causes further growth of the corpus luteum and stimulates the secretion of progesterone, which helps maintain the uterine mucosa throughout pregnancy.
- Corpus luteum of menstruation: when fertilization does not occur, hCG from the embryonic placenta does not prevent the corpus luteum from degenerating. The collapsed follicle that participated in ovulation becomes the corpus luteum of menstruation (CLM). The breakdown of the CLM does not occur for 8-9 days following ovulation and there is a progressive fibrosis and shrinkage of the CLM over multiple months. The CLM eventually becomes more fibrotic and is then referred to as the **corpus albicans**.

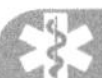 *Clinical Correlate 4.10*

Birth Control Pills

Birth control pills can prevent pregnancy through several mechanisms, but mainly they are for preventing ovulation. Simply put, if there is no oocyte present, there is nothing for the sperm to fertilize and the woman is unable to become pregnant. Most birth control pills contain synthetic forms of estrogen and progestin. These synthetic hormones stabilize the natural hormone levels in a woman and prevent estrogen from peaking mid-cycle. This mid-cycle peak normally triggers the pituitary gland to produce FSH and LH, but synthetic estrogen prevents this and it also supports the endometrium, preventing any breakthrough bleeding mid-cycle.

The synthetic progestin prevents the pituitary gland from producing LH, which is crucial for ovulation of the oocyte. It also makes the uterine wall inhospitable to a fertilized egg and thickens the cervical mucus hindering sperm movement.

There are two main types of hormonal birth control pills: a combination pill that contains estrogen and progestin or a progestin-only pill. The combo pills are more effective than progestin-only pills and tend to have less breakthrough bleeding. Progestin-only pills are especially useful for patients who cannot tolerate estrogen.

4.28 Gonad Development

The key to sexual dimorphism is the Y chromosome, which contains the testis-determining gene called the **sex-determining region on Y (SRY) gene** on its short arm (Yp11). The SRY protein is the **testis-determining factor (TDF)** and under its influence a male will develop instead of a female. The sex of an individual is determined genetically at the time of fertilization; however, the gonads do not acquire male or female characteristics until the seventh week of development.

The superior portion of the posterior abdominal wall contains the **urogenital ridges** that originate from the intermediate mesoderm. The gonads initially appear as a pair of longitudinal **gonadal (genital) ridges** that proliferated from the urogenital ridges.

During the 3rd week of development, the **primordial germ cells** that originate from the epiblast migrate through the primitive streak before residing among the endoderm of the yolk sac wall near the allantois. Around the 4th week, these cells migrate to the dorsal mesentery of the hindgut before arriving at the primitive gonads in the 5th week. Invasion of these germ cells into the gonadal ridges occurs during the 6th week. The gonads do not develop if the primordial germ cells fail to reach the gonadal ridges. This demonstrates that the primordial germ cells have an inductive influence on gonad development (**Fig. 4.49**).

Shortly before and during the arrival of these cells, the epithelium of the gonadal ridge proliferates and epithelial cells penetrate the underlying mesoderm, forming many irregularly shaped **primary sex cords**. In both sexes, these cords are connected to the surface epithelium but it is impossible to differentiate between a male or female gonad and this is known as an **indifferent gonad** (**Fig. 4.49**).

A genetically male embryo has primordial germ cells that carry the XY sex chromosome complex and under the influence of the SRY gene, which encodes TDF, the primary sex cords continue to proliferate and penetrate deep into the medulla to form the **testis** or **medullary cords**. Near the hilum of the gland, the cords break up into a network of tiny cell strands that give rise to tubules of the **rete testis**. With further development, the **tunica albuginea** develop and separate the medullary cords from the surface epithelium (**Fig. 4.50a,b**).

During the 4th month of development, the medullary cords become horseshoe shaped and continuous with the rete testis. The medullary cords are now composed of primitive germ cells and **Sertoli cells** derived from the surface epithelium. The **Leydig cells** are derived from the gonadal ridge and lie between the medullary cords. They begin their development shortly after the onset of cord differentiation but by the 8th week these cells are capable of producing **testosterone**. Medullary cords are solid throughout development, until puberty, when they obtain a lumen forming the **seminiferous tubules**. Once canalized, they join the rete testis tubules, which in turn enter the **efferent ductules**. These are the remaining parts of the excretory tubules of the mesonephric system and they link the rete testis and the mesonephric duct, which becomes the **ductus deferens** (**Fig. 4.50a,b**).

The **primary sex cords** of a genetically female embryo with the XX sex chromosome complement dissociate into irregular cell clusters. These clusters contain the primitive germ cells and occupy the medullary part of the ovary. They disappear soon after and are replaced by a vascular stroma that forms the **ovarian medulla**. The surface epithelium of the gonad continues to proliferate and during the seventh week of development it gives rise to the **secondary sex cords** (cortical cords), which penetrate the underlying mesenchyme but remain close to the surface. In the third month of development, these cords split into isolated cell clusters that proliferate and begin to surround each oogonium with a layer of epithelial cells called **follicular cells**. The follicular cells along with the oogonia constitute a **primordial follicle** (**Fig. 4.50c,d**).

Descent of the testes and ovaries from the posterior abdominal wall were discussed in Chapter 3.

4.29 Uterine Tubes

The **uterine tubes** (formally fallopian) are approximately 10-12 cm in total length and extend laterally from the uterine horns before opening into the peritoneal cavity near the ovaries. They lie in the mesosalpinx in the free edge of the broad ligament. Their course extends posterolaterally towards the lateral pelvic walls before ascending and arching over the ovaries. Positioning of the tubes is variable and often asymmetrical from one side to

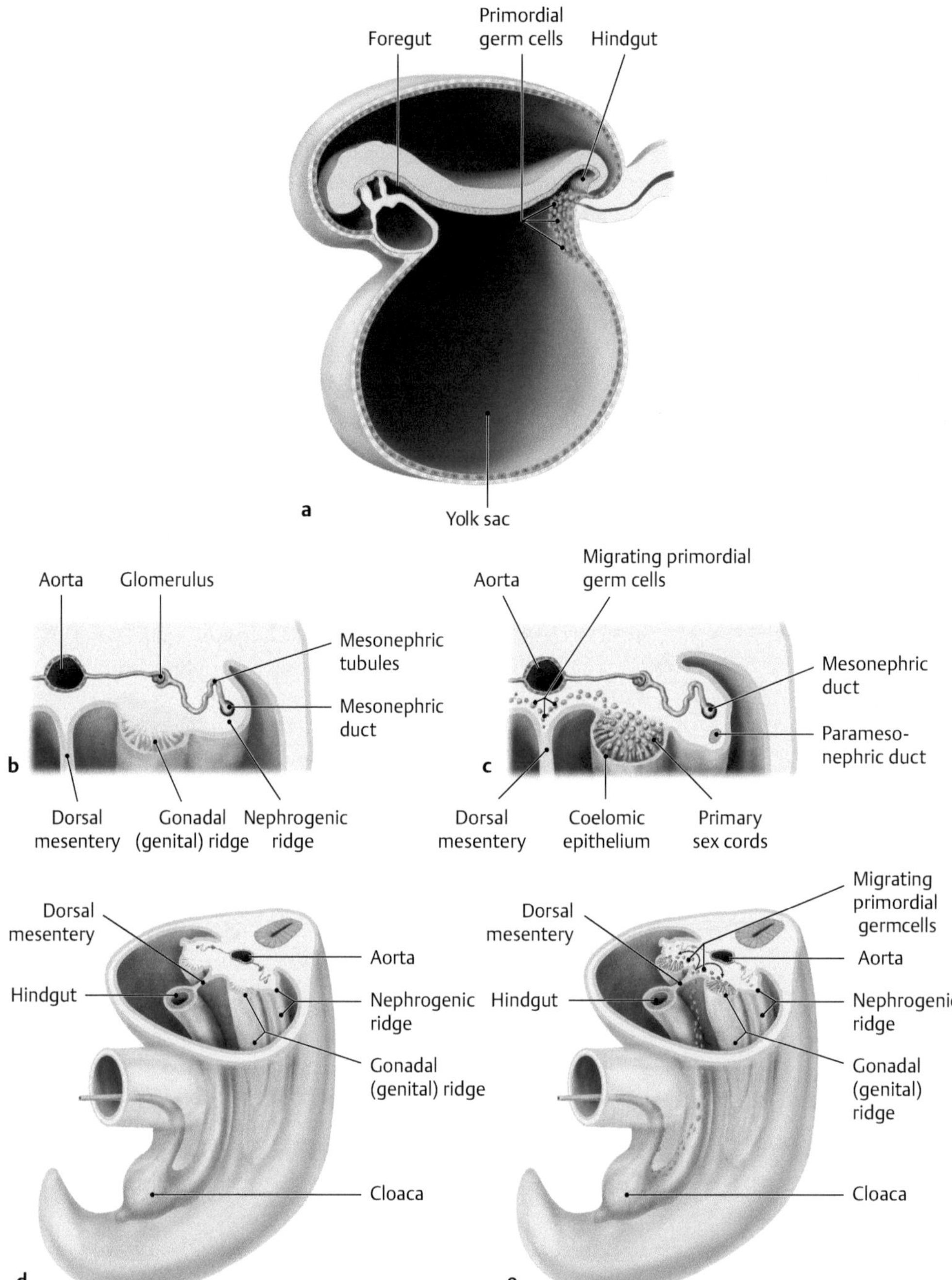

Fig. 4.49 Development of the genital ridges and gonad primordia; germ cell migration. **(a)** With yolk sac, viewed from left side. **(b-c)** Horizontal sections, superior view. **(d-e)** Spatial representations of **b** and **c**. (From Schuenke M, Schulte E, Schumacher U. THIEME Atlas of Anatomy. Internal Organs. Illustrations by Voll M and Wesker K. 3rd ed. New York: Thieme Medical Publishers; 2020.)

the next. There are four parts to the uterine tubes (from distal to proximal) **(Fig. 4.44; Fig. 4.45)**.

- **Infundibulum**: the funnel-shaped part that opens into the peritoneal cavity through the *abdominal ostium*. The **fimbriae** are finger-like processes that extend from the infundibulum, rest on the medial surface of the ovary, and draw in the ovulated oocyte **(Fig. 4.51)**.
- **Ampulla**: the longest and widest part and where most oocytes become fertilized.
- **Isthmus**: the thicker walled part that enters the uterine horn.
- **Uterine**: the short intramural portion that passes through the wall of the uterus and opens into the uterine cavity through the *uterine ostium*.

4.29.1 Neurovasculature and Lymphatic Drainage of the Uterine Tubes

Autonomic fibers originating from both the **ovarian periarterial plexus** and **uterovaginal plexus** are responsible for innervating the uterine tubes. Sympathetic fibers constrict and parasympathetic fibers may dilate the blood vessels **(Fig. 4.19; Fig. 4.22)**. The blood supply to the uterine tubes is from the **uterine artery** (internal iliac br.) and **ovarian artery** (abdominal aorta br.) **(Fig. 4.24; Table 4.3)**. Venous drainage originates from the **pampiniform plexus** near the ovary before draining to the **ovarian vein**. The left ovarian vein drains to the *left renal vein* and the right ovarian vein drains to the *IVC*. Additional venous drainage follows the **uterine vein** to the *internal iliac vein* (**Fig. 4.24; Table 4.4**). Lymphatic drainage is primarily to the **lumbar (caval/aortic) lymph nodes** (**Fig. 4.46**).

4.29.2 Histology of the Uterine Tubes

The uterine tubes have a *simple columnar epithelium* consisting of two cell types. The *Peg cells* secrete a nutritive fluid while the *ciliated cells* force the released ova toward the uterus. During the menstrual cycle, ciliated cells increase during the proliferative (follicular) phase due to estrogen and the peg cells increase during the secretory (luteal) phase due to increased progesterone. The longitudinal mucosal folds, or *plicae*, are most numerous within the ampulla and can have secondary or tertiary branching. The least amount is seen in the isthmus (**Fig. 4.52**).

The muscularis layer consists of an inner circular and outer longitudinal layer and rhythmic contractions move the ova towards the uterus. Visceral peritoneum serves as the serosa layer and it covers the uterine tubes. A benign cluster of epithelial cells most commonly found in the connective tissue of the uterine tubes is known as **Walthard cell rests**. They may also be seen in the mesosalpinx or mesovarium of the broad ligament. They appear as white or yellowish cysts with elliptical nuclei that have the appearance of a coffee bean. They may be the precursor to **Brenner tumors**, a rare type of ovarian surface epithelial tumor.

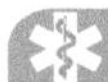 ***Clinical Correlate 4.11***

Ectopic Pregnancy

An **ectopic pregnancy** refers to any implantation that takes place outside the uterus and about 95% of these occur in the uterine tube. Approximately 80% of all uterine tube implantations occur in the ampulla part. Other locations include, and these tend to be rare, the rectouterine pouch (of Douglas), internal os, and ovarian implantations.

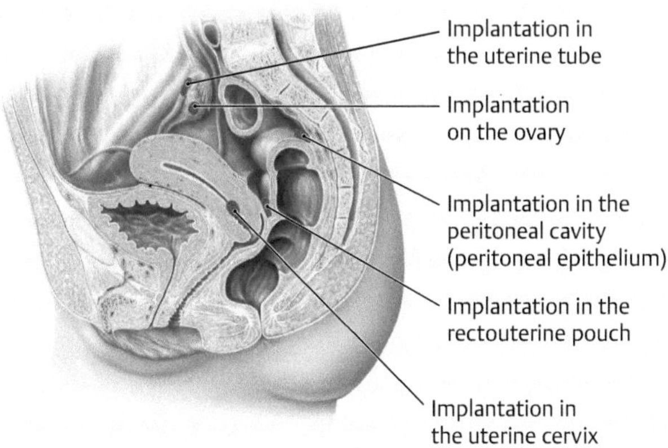

(From Schuenke M, Schulte E, Schumacher U. THIEME Atlas of Anatomy. Internal Organs. Illustrations by Voll M and Wesker K. 3rd ed. New York: Thieme Medical Publishers; 2020.)

4.30 Uterus

The **uterus** (or womb) is a thick, pear-shaped, and hollow muscular organ that generally leans anteriorly up against the urinary bladder. It consists mostly of a **body** that forms the superior two-thirds of the uterus and includes the **fundus**, **isthmus** and **uterine horns**. The body terminates as the **cervix of the uterus** (**Fig. 4.45**). The **cervix** is divided into a *supravaginal* and *vaginal part*. The supravaginal part is located between the isthmus and the vagina while the vaginal part protrudes into the vagina and surrounds the external os. The adult uterus is generally in the *anteverted* and *anteflexed* position. Anteverted refers to the longitudinal cervical axis being tipped anteriorly relative to the longitudinal axis of the vagina and anteflexed is the angle created between the longitudinal uterine body axis relative to the longitudinal cervical axis (**Fig. 4.53**). A nongravid (not pregnant) uterus is found in the lesser pelvis.

There are ligaments associated with the uterus. The **broad ligament** is a double layer of peritoneum that extends from the lateral walls of the uterus to the lateral walls of the pelvis where they become continuous with the peritoneum. The two layers are continuous with each other at a free edge via the uterine fundus and separate near the superior surfaces of the levator ani. It has three main parts (**Fig. 4.44; Fig. 4.45; Fig. 4.54**):

- **Mesometrium**: or the mesentery of the uterus. It is the largest part of the broad ligament and it extends from the pelvic floor to the ovarian ligament and uterine body. The uterine artery passes between the two layers near the cervix.
- **Mesosalpinx**: or mesentery of the uterine tube. Between the uterine tube and ovary the mesosalpinx contains vascular anastomoses involving the uterine and ovarian vessels.
- **Mesovarium**: portion of broad ligament that suspends the ovary.

The broad ligament extends superolaterally as the **suspensory (infundibulopelvic) ligament of the ovary** and it overlies the ovarian neurovasculature. The **ovarian ligament** lies between the layers of the broad ligament. The **round ligament** attaches at the uterotubal junction and connects the uterus to the labia majora. This is another remnant of the *gubernaculum* and it passes between the layers of the broad ligament as it extends toward the deep inguinal ring prior to entering the inguinal canal (**Fig. 4.26; Fig. 4.45**).

The pelvic diaphragm is able to provide *dynamic support* to the uterus because of its active contraction when there is increased intra-abdominal pressure and by its tonicity or continuous contraction during sitting and standing. The natural anteverted and anteflexed position of the uterus provides a *passive support* to this organ. The least mobile part of the uterus is at the cervix and this is because of the passive support provided by the attached endopelvic fascial ligaments. These include (**Fig. 4.15**):

- **Transverse cervical (cardinal** or ***Mackenrodt's*) ligaments**: attach the lateral parts of the cervix to the lateral pelvic walls. They arefound between the two layers of peritoneum forming the mesometrium of the broad ligament and contains the uterine vessels. The ureters pass just below these ligaments.

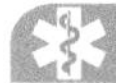 ***Clinical Correlate 4.12***

Hysterectomy

A **hysterectomy** is the surgical removal of the uterus and means a woman is unable to become pregnant. It may be used to treat uterine fibroids (most common reason for a hysterectomy), uterine cancer, uterine prolapse, chronic pelvic pain or abnormal uterine bleeding. It can be performed through the lower abdominal wall or through the vagina. There are different types of hysterectomies. A *total hysterectomy* includes the entire uterus and cervix. A *partial (supracervical) hysterectomy* involves removing the upper uterus and not the cervix. A *radical hysterectomy* involves the removal of the uterus, cervix and additional structures such as the ovaries and uterine tubes. The ureter is in danger of being damaged because it passes deep to the uterine artery, a structure that is clamped during this procedure.

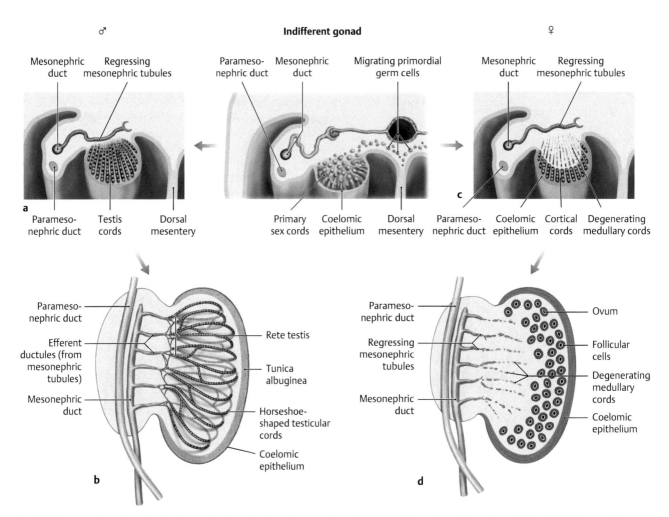

Fig. 4.50 Cross-section of the developing testis and genital ducts in the male embryo; viewed from above **(a)** and from the front **(b)**. Cross-section of the developing ovary and genital ducts in a female embryo; viewed from the above **(c)** and from the front **(d)**. (From Schuenke M, Schulte E, Schumacher U. THIEME Atlas of Anatomy. Internal Organs. Illustrations by Voll M and Wesker K. 3rd ed. New York: Thieme Medical Publishers; 2020.)

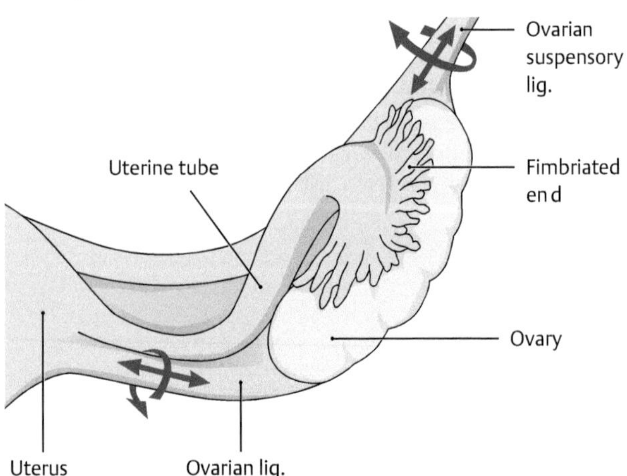

Fig. 4.51 Ovum collection mechanism: Rotational and longitudinal movements of the tube make it easier for the fimbriated end of the tube to contact the entire ovary. (From Schuenke M, Schulte E, Schumacher U. THIEME Atlas of Anatomy. Internal Organs. Illustrations by Voll M and Wesker K. 3rd ed. New York: Thieme Medical Publishers; 2020.)

- **Uterosacral ligaments**: pass posteriorly from the cervix to the middle sacrum and are palpable during a rectal examination. The ureters are located just lateral to these ligaments.

4.30.1 Neurovasculature and Lymphatic Drainage of the Uterus

Autonomic fibers passing through the **uterovaginal plexus** are responsible for innervating the uterus. Sympathetic fibers stimulate smooth muscle contraction of the uterine wall and vasoconstriction of blood vessels. Parasympathetic fibers inhibit smooth muscle contraction and vasodilate the blood vessels. Hormone levels effecting the uterine wall may dictate overall autonomic control (**Fig. 4.19; Fig. 4.22**).

The blood supply is primarily from the **uterine arteries** (internal iliac br.) with a potential collateral supply from both the *ovarian* and *vaginal arteries* (**Fig. 4.24; Table 4.3**). Most venous drainage leads back to the **uterine venous plexus** before passing through the **uterine veins** and finally the internal iliac vein. Lymphatic drainage from the *fundus* and *superior body* is to the **lumbar (caval/aortic)** via the ovarian vessels and **superficial inguinal lymph nodes** via the round ligament; the *middle portion* drains to the **internal iliac lymph nodes**; the *majority of the uterine body*

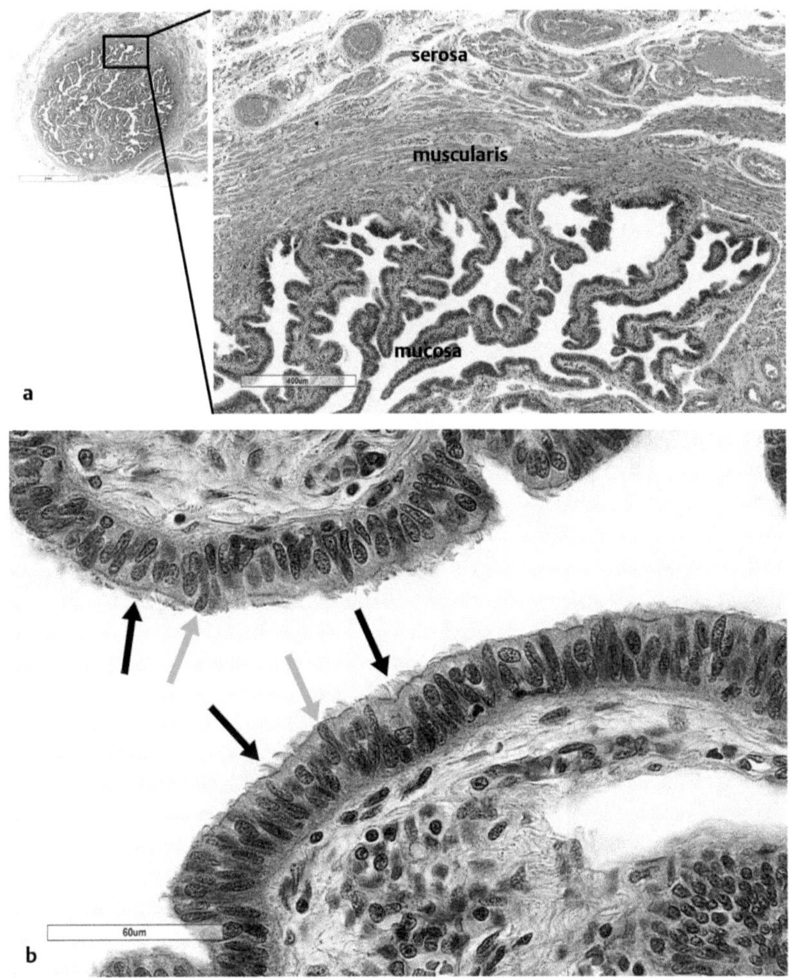

Fig. 4.52 Histology of the uterine tube: **(a)** low magnification, showing mucosa, muscularis, and serosa. **(b)** epithelium showing ciliated cells (*black arrows*) and peg cells (*green arrows*). (From Lowrie DJ. Histology: An Essential Textbook. New York: Thieme Medical Publishers; 2020.)

drains to the **external iliac lymph nodes**; and finally the *uterine cervix* drains to the **internal iliac lymph nodes** via the transverse cervical (cardinal) ligament and the **sacral lymph nodes** via the uterosacral ligaments (**Fig. 4.46**).

4.30.2 Histology of the Uterus

The uterine wall is composed of a spongy mucosa called the *endometrium*; a thick muscularis known as the *myometrium*; and either an adventitia or serosa called the *perimetrium* depending on the location (**Fig. 4.55**).

- Endometrium: it consists of a *simple columnar epithelium* and a lamina propria (stroma) containing simple tubular glands that may branch closer to the myometrium. The surface epithelial cells are a mix of secretory and rare ciliated cells. This layer undergoes cyclic morphologic changes during the menstrual cycle. The outer layer of mucosa is called the **stratum functionalis** and it is the layer that undergoes cyclic hyperplasia and degeneration. This layer may also be referred to as the compact and spongy layer that shed during menstruation or parturition. The innermost layer is called the **stratum basalis** and it is adjacent to the myometrium and remains mostly unchanged during the menstrual cycle. Stromal cells are small during the proliferative phase but are stimulated to enlarge by progesterone during the secretory phase of the menstrual cycle.

There is an abundance of blood vessels supplying the endometrium. **Arcuate arteries** located in the myometrium give rise to two sets of arteries that supply the endometrium: the **straight arteries** that supply the stratum basalis and the **spiral arteries** which supply the stratum functionalis.

Clinical Correlate 4.13

Endometriosis

Endometriosis is the growth of the endometrial tissue outside of the uterus. The endometrial tissue can be located anywhere in the peritoneal cavity and adjacent to other pelvic organs. There may be inflammation, fibrosis or even adhesions of the surrounding tissue that are due to the responses of normal circulating hormones. Difficult or painful menstruation (*dysmenorrhea*) and even infertility could occur because of this. It occurs primarily during the reproductive years in less than 10% of all women. Family history and genetics play a role but the exact cause is unknown. The use of combined oral contraceptives (birth control) may reduce the risk but treatments could include hormone therapy and surgery in extreme cases.

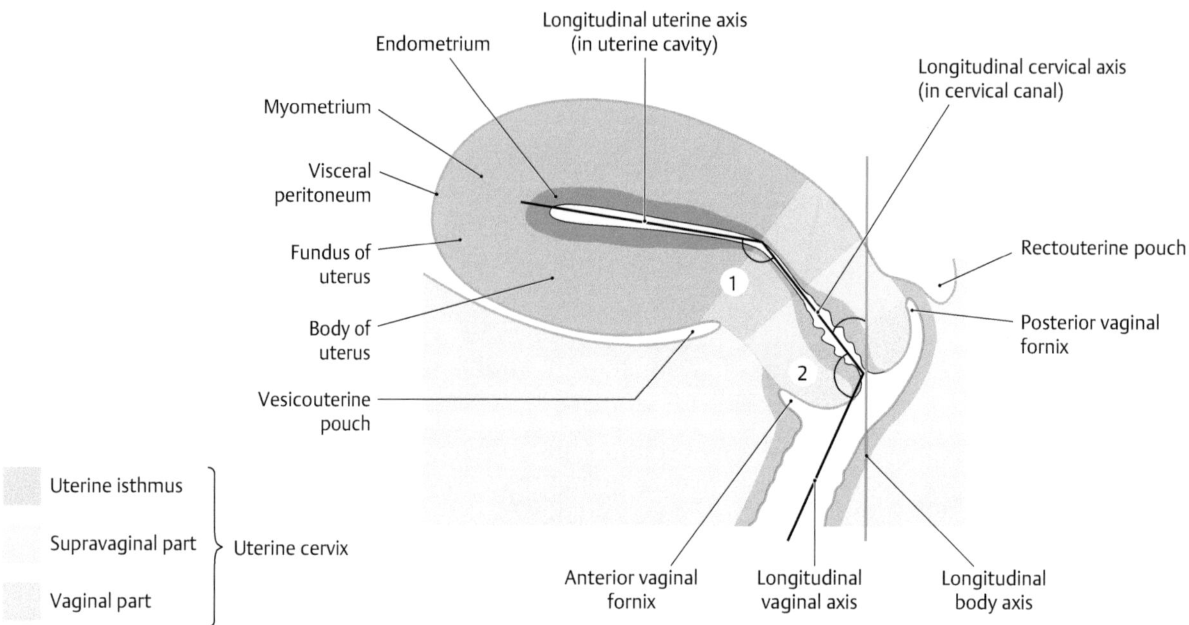

Fig. 4.53 Curvature of the uterus. (From Schuenke M, Schulte E, Schumacher U. THIEME Atlas of Anatomy. Internal Organs. Illustrations by Voll M and Wesker K. 3rd ed. New York: Thieme Medical Publishers; 2020.)

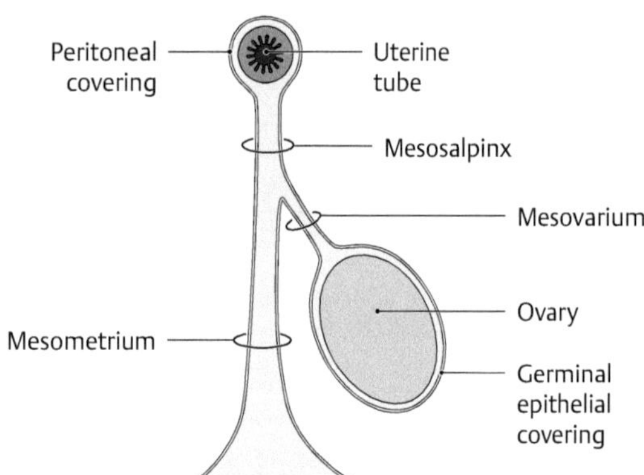

Fig. 4.54 Sagittal section through the regions of the broad ligament. (From Schuenke M, Schulte E, Schumacher U. THIEME Atlas of Anatomy. Internal Organs. Illustrations by Voll M and Wesker K. 3rd ed. New York: Thieme Medical Publishers; 2020.)

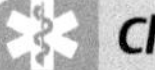

Clinical Correlate 4.14

Fibroids

Fibroids are non-cancerous growths appearing on the uterus and they are not associated with an increased risk of uterine cancer. They develop from the myometrium, where a single cell may begin dividing uncontrollably, creating a mass. They may shrink or disappear on their own and can vary greatly in overall size. As much as 75% of women may have fibroids during their lifetime but most are unaware of them because they are generally asymptomatic. The cause is unknown but may be associated with hormones or genetic changes in the tissue. They rarely interfere with pregnancy. Treatments include periodic observations, medications or surgery in extreme situations.

- Myometrium: this is the thickest layer and it contains mostly smooth muscle cells separated by connective tissue. There is an inner and outer longitudinal layer but the middle is thick, has a circular fiber pattern, and contains larger blood vessels. During pregnancy the myometrium undergoes *hyperplasia* (greater number of cells) and *hypertrophy* (larger individual cells) and results in a 20-fold increase in size.
- Perimetrium: the outer most layer of the uterus that is approximately three-quarters covered by a serosa (connective tissue and mesothelium) while the rest is covered by an adventitia (connective tissue).

4.30.3 Menstrual Cycle

The menstrual cycle follows a precise schedule of morphologic and physiologic events characterized by proliferation, secretory differentiation, degeneration and regeneration of the uterine wall (**Fig. 4.56**). These events are controlled by cyclically released estrogen and progesterone related to the discharge of FSH and LH by the anterior pituitary thereby linking the ovarian and uterine cycles. The menstrual cycle usually begins between the ages of 12-15 and continues until about age 45-50. This means the female is fertile only during the years she is having menstrual cycles. The beginning of the menstrual cycle for practical purposes begins when menstrual bleeding is first observed (day 1). Ovulation will take place on day 14 of this presumed 28 day cycle. Menstrual discharge is a mix of degenerating endometrium and blood from ruptured blood vessels. The cycle includes the *menstrual phase* (3-4 days), the *proliferative phase* (~10 days), and the *secretory phase* (~14 days).

- Menstrual phase: the onset of bleeding defines this phase. Before menstruation, estrogen and progesterone secretion from the corpus luteum decreases 8-12 days after ovulation if fertilization of the oocyte does not occur. This leads to a prolonged contraction of the spiral arteries resulting in ischemic necrosis of the stratum functionalis layer of the endometrium. Detachment of the stratum functionalis layer begins at the fundus and extends inferiorly toward the cervix.

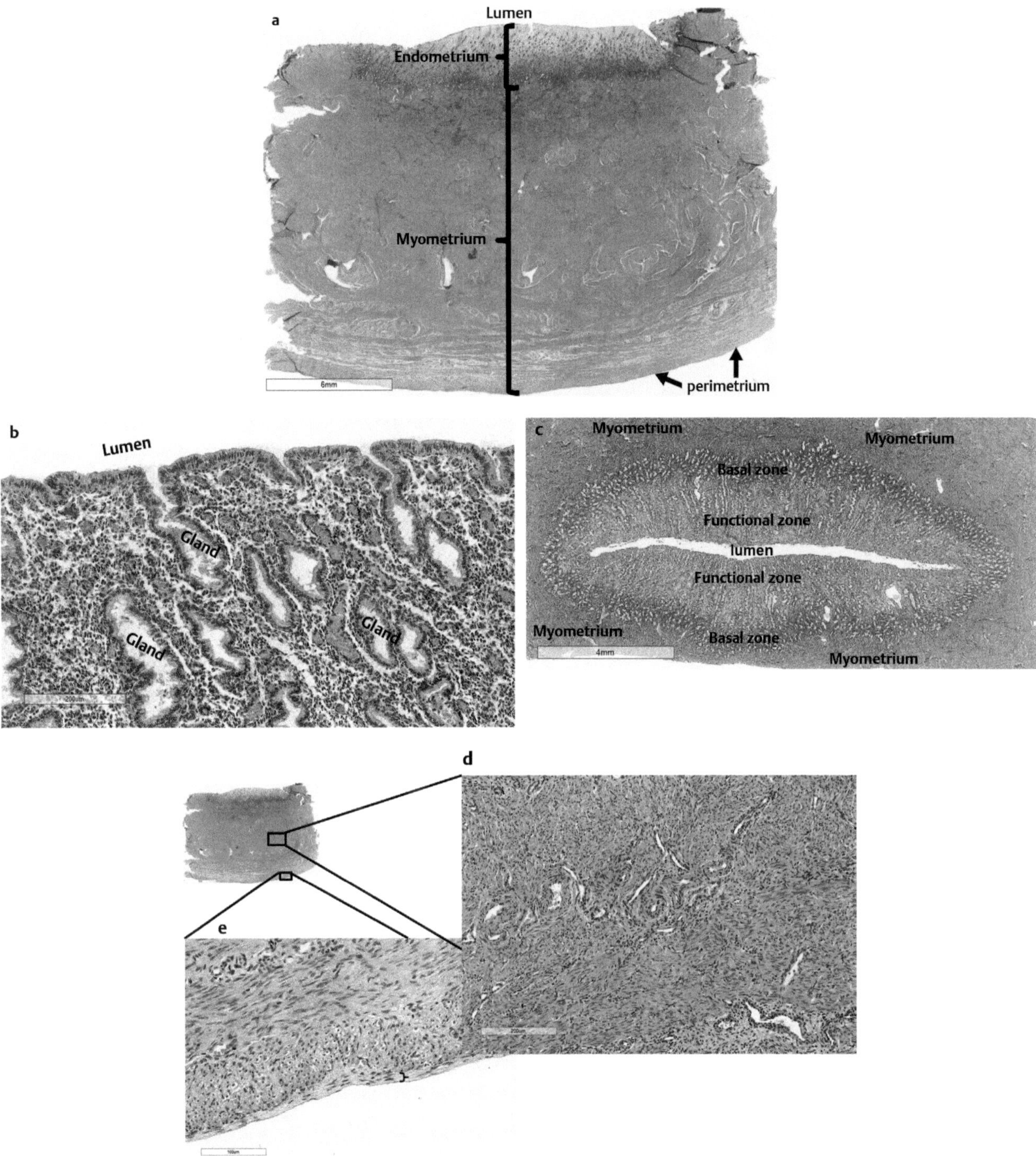

Fig. 4.55 Histology of the uterus. **(a)** Scanning magnification showing endometrium, myometrium, and perimetrium. **(b)** Surface endometrium showing the uterine glands. **(c)** Endometrium showing the stratum functionalis (functional) zone and stratum basalis (basal) zone. **(d)** Closer view of the myometrium. **(e)** Closer view of the perimetrium. (From Lowrie DJ. Histology: An Essential Textbook. New York: Thieme Medical Publishers; 2020.)

- Proliferative phase: this phase is driven by estrogen which has an effect on the proliferation of epithelial glandular, lamina propria and endothelial cells of the stratum functionalis. This phase coincides with the theca interna actively secreting estrogen from a select few ovarian follicles probably transitioning between the multilaminar primary and secondary stages.
- Secretory (luteal) phase: after ovulation, the endometrium undergoes a rapid secretory differentiation under the influence of progesterone secreted by the corpus luteum. This stimulates the gland cells to secrete glycoproteins and they become highly coiled and the epithelial cells begin to accumulate glycogen. If fertilization has taken place, the blastocyst attaches to the uterine wall during this phase approximately 7 days after ovulation. If a blastocyst does not implant, the stratum functionalis begins to degenerate due to localized ischemia around the spiral arteries because of decreased progesterone and estrogen secretion from the corpus luteum.

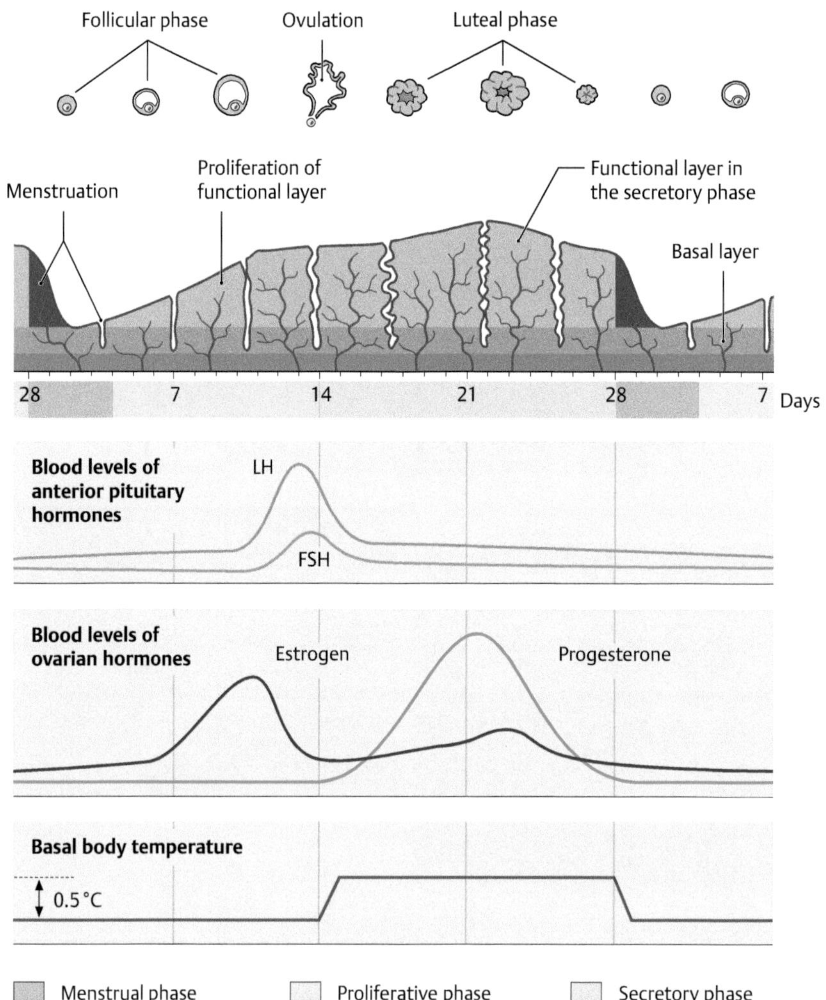

Fig. 4.56 Menstrual cycle. (From Schuenke M, Schulte E, Schumacher U. THIEME Atlas of Anatomy. Internal Organs. Illustrations by Voll M and Wesker K. 3rd ed. New York: Thieme Medical Publishers; 2020.)

4.30.4 Implantation

Multiple cell divisions occur 3-4 days after the ovum is fertilized in the uterine tube before it reaches the uterus. Once it has reached 16 cells or **blastomeres** it is called a **morula**. A **blastocystic cavity** forms as fluid begins to enter with the degeneration of the **zona pellucida** resulting in an inner cell mass called the **embryoblast** and an outer cell mass called the **trophoblast**. The embryo is now known as a **blastocyst**. The zona pellucida must be absent for implantation to occur.

Six to seven days after fertilization is when implantation, the embedding of a blastocyst in the endometrial wall of the uterus, takes place **(Fig. 4.57)**. The most common site for implantation of a blastocyst is on the posterior wall of the uterus. The trophoblast differentiates into an inner **cytotrophoblast** and an outer **syncytiotrophoblast**. The syncytiotrophoblast of the embryos developing placenta begins to secrete *human chorionic gonadotropin* (hCG) and this spares the early termination of the corpus luteum thus preventing menstruation. The embryoblast differentiates into a **bilaminar embryonic disk** composed of an **epiblast** and **hypoblast**. The bilaminar disk becomes a **trilaminar disk** that subsequently leads to the formation of the three germ layers through a process known as **gastrulation**. These germ layers give rise to specific tissues and organs and are called the *ectoderm*, *mesoderm* and *endoderm* **(Fig. 4.58)**.

- Ectoderm: gives rise to the epidermis, nervous system, retina and teeth enamel, among other things.
- Mesoderm: gives rise to connective tissue, smooth muscular coats and vessels associated with the tissues and organs, most of the cardiovascular system, blood cells, bone marrow, the skeleton, striated muscles, reproductive and excretory organs, among other things.
- Endoderm: gives rise to the epithelial linings of the digestive and respiratory tracts, glands that open into the GI tract and the glandular cells of the pancreas and liver, among other things.

At the non-embryonic pole, flattened cells of the hypoblast form a thin **exocoelomic (*Heuser's*) membrane** that lines the internal surface of the cytotrophoblast but on the opposite side lines the **primitive yolk sac**. A new population of cells derived from the yolk sac cells appears between the inner surface of the cytotrophoblast and the outer surface of the primitive yolk sac to form the **extraembryonic mesoderm**. Large spaces develop in the extraembryonic mesoderm to form a new space known as the **chorionic cavity**. The **secondary yolk sac** displaces the primitive yolk sac as it is being pinched by the expansion of the chorionic cavity. The extraembryonic mesoderm lining the cytotrophoblast and amnion is known as the **extraembryonic somatic mesoderm** (or **chorionic plate**), while the layer covering the yolk sac is known as **extraembryonic splanchnic mesoderm (Fig. 4.59)**.

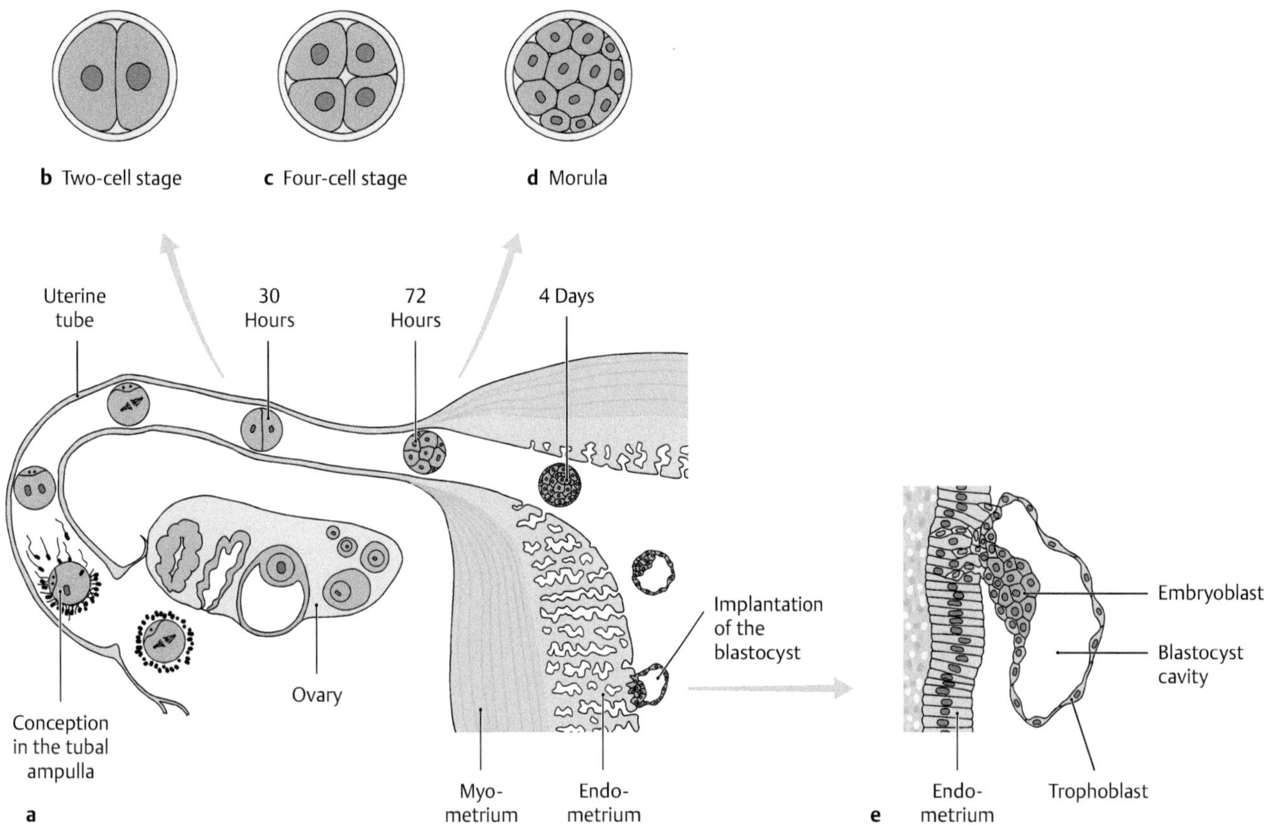

Fig. 4.57 Phases in the migration of the fertilized ovum. **(a)** Fertilization of the ovum. **(b-e)** The development of the two- and four-cell stages of development (30 hours), a morula with 16 cells (3 days), and the zygote after implantation **(e)**. (From Schuenke M, Schulte E, Schumacher U. THIEME Atlas of Anatomy. Internal Organs. Illustrations by Voll M and Wesker K. 3rd ed. New York: Thieme Medical Publishers; 2020.)

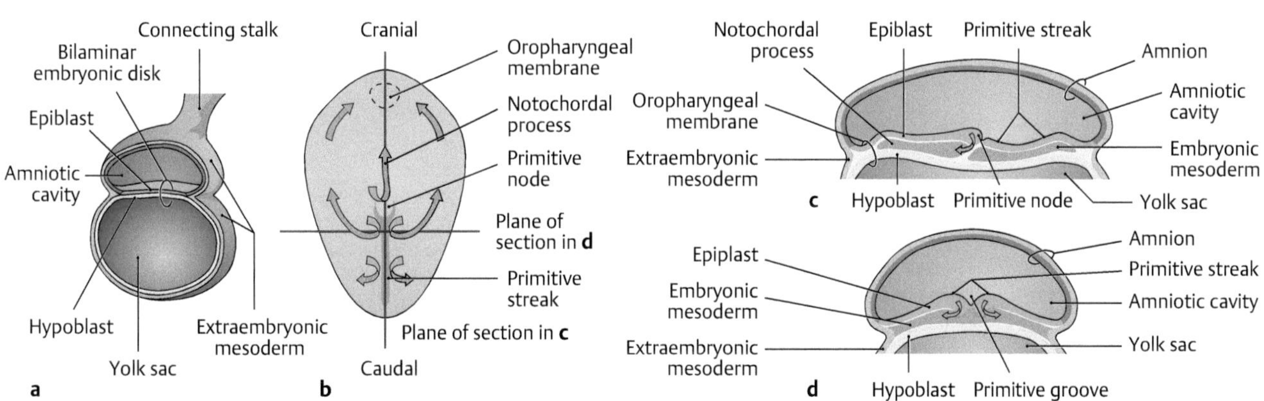

Fig. 4.58 Gastrulation: the formation of the trilaminar disk. **(a)** Sagittal section through the bilaminar disk at 2 weeks. **(b)** Dorsal view of the embryonic disk at the start of gastrulation. **(c)** Sagittal section along the notochordal process; **(d)** Cross section at the level of the primitive groove. (From Schuenke M, Schulte E, Schumacher U. THIEME Atlas of Anatomy. General Anatomy and Musculoskeletal System. Illustrations by Voll M and Wesker K. 3rd ed. New York: Thieme Medical Publishers; 2020.)

As the syncytiotrophoblast erodes and invades the endometrium, lacunae form and they are filled with maternal blood. These lacunae and their associated networks are the precursors to the **intervillous spaces** of the placenta. Cells of the cytotrophoblast proliferate and penetrate the syncytiotrophoblast forming trabecular columns called **primary chorionic villi**. Shortly after the primary chorionic villi are formed, they begin to branch and be penetrated by mesoderm and are now known as **secondary chorionic villi**. After fetal blood vessels have penetrated the mesoderm, they become **tertiary chorionic villi**. The blood vessels in the tertiary chorionic villi make contact with capillaries that are developing in the mesoderm of the chorionic plate and **connecting stalk** (future umbilical cord) and establish an intraembryonic circulatory system. The cytotrophoblastic cells of the villi at the level of the maternal endometrium form a thin cytotrophoblastic shell and this gradually surrounds the trophoblast entirely. This attaches the **chorionic sac** or just **chorion** firmly to the maternal endometrial tissue. The chorionic sac is defined as the combination of the chorionic plate (extraembryonic somatic mesoderm), cytotrophoblast and syncytiotrophoblast (**Fig. 4.60**).

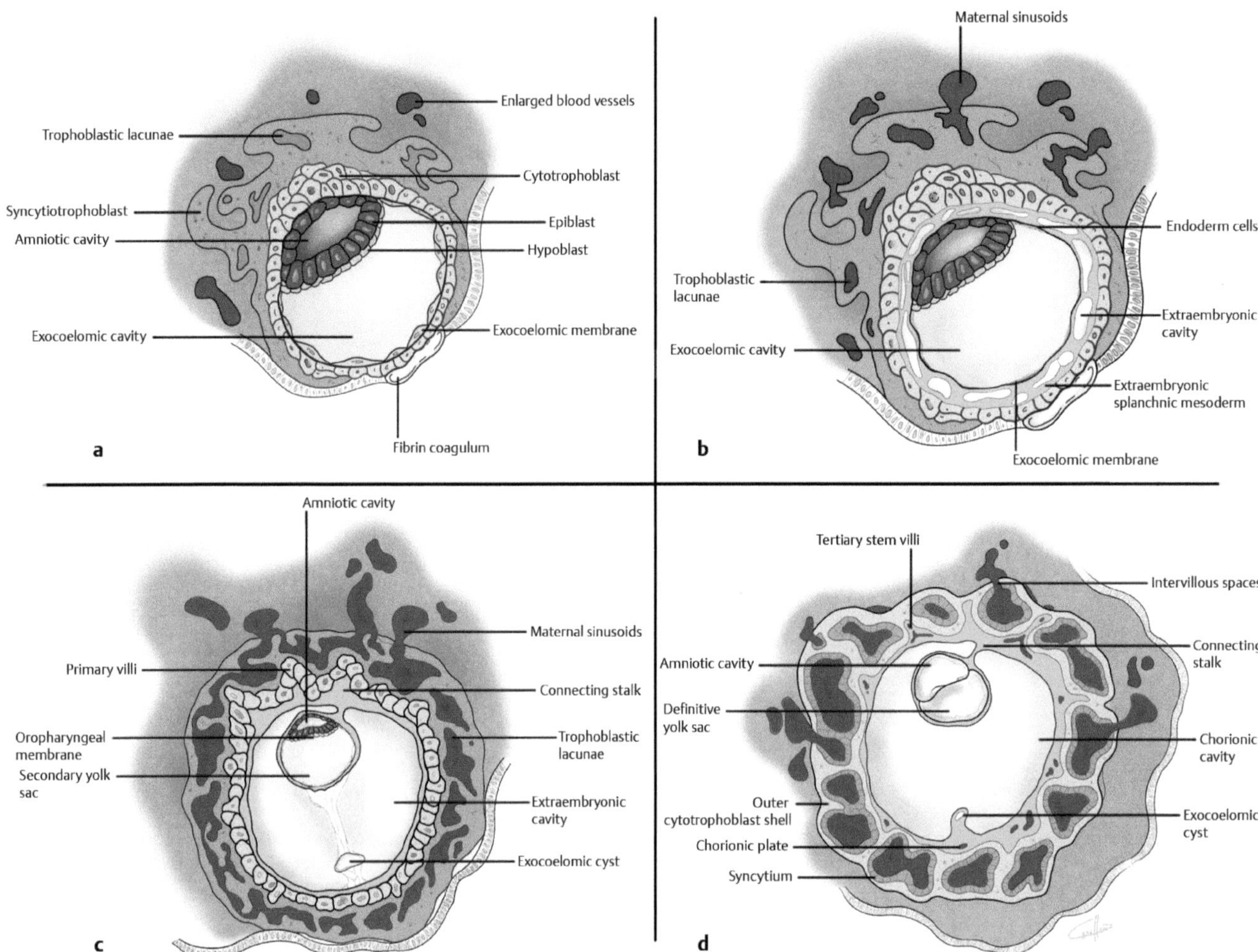

Fig. 4.59 (a-d) Implantation and early placenta development. Illustration by Calla Heald.

4.30.5 Maternal Placenta

The endometrium undergoes further morphological changes to form the **decidua** of the maternal placenta. There are a total of three decidua layers (**Fig. 4.60**):

- Decidua basalis: lies over the *chorion frondosum* of the fetal placenta and consists of decidual cells that have an abundant amount of lipids and glycogen. It is also referred to as the *decidual plate.*
- Decidua capsularis: overlies the non-embryonic pole of the embryo and becomes stretched and degenerates with growth of the embryo.
- Decidua parietalis: all of the remaining endometrium that does not involve the area of the placenta. After about 3 months, the chorionic sac containing the embryo has become so large it fuses the decidua capsularis to the decidua parietalis.

The entire surface of the chorionic sac is covered with chorionic villi; however the non-embryonic side, which is the opposite side of the embryo that first makes contact with the uterus at the initial implantation site, becomes smooth and is called the **chorion laeve**. The remainder of the chorionic sac adjacent to the decidua basalis has villi that continue to grow and this part constitutes the fetal part of the placenta called the **chorion frondosum**. The chorion frondosum and decidua basalis essentially make up the placenta.

Clinical Correlate 4.15

Abnormal Placentas

Abnormal development of the placenta could lead to medical issues during labor and delivery and these include:

- **Placenta previa**: the placenta overlies the internal os and blocks the cervical canal. It is the leading cause of prepartum hemorrhage and is the result of the placenta being unable to expand and stretch properly so parts may be torn loose which disrupts large vessels. It is considered a medical emergency because the mother can bleed to death. A cesarean delivery would be necessary in this situation.
- **Placenta accreta**: an abnormal but superficial adherence of the chorionic villi to the myometrium because the decidua basalis is absent. The placenta fails to separate from the uterine wall after delivery of the newborn and causes profuse hemorrhaging with manual removal. This is the collective term for an adherent placenta and accounts for about 75% of these types of clinical cases. Women are at a greater risk of this if they have had a previous cesarean delivery.
- **Placenta increta**: when chorionic villi penetrate only the myometrium. It accounts for less than 20% of adherent placenta cases.
- **Placenta percreta**: when chorionic villi penetrate the myometrium all the way to the perimetrium. If it passes through the perimetrium, the placenta may attach to another organ such as the bladder. It accounts for less about 5% of adherent placenta cases.

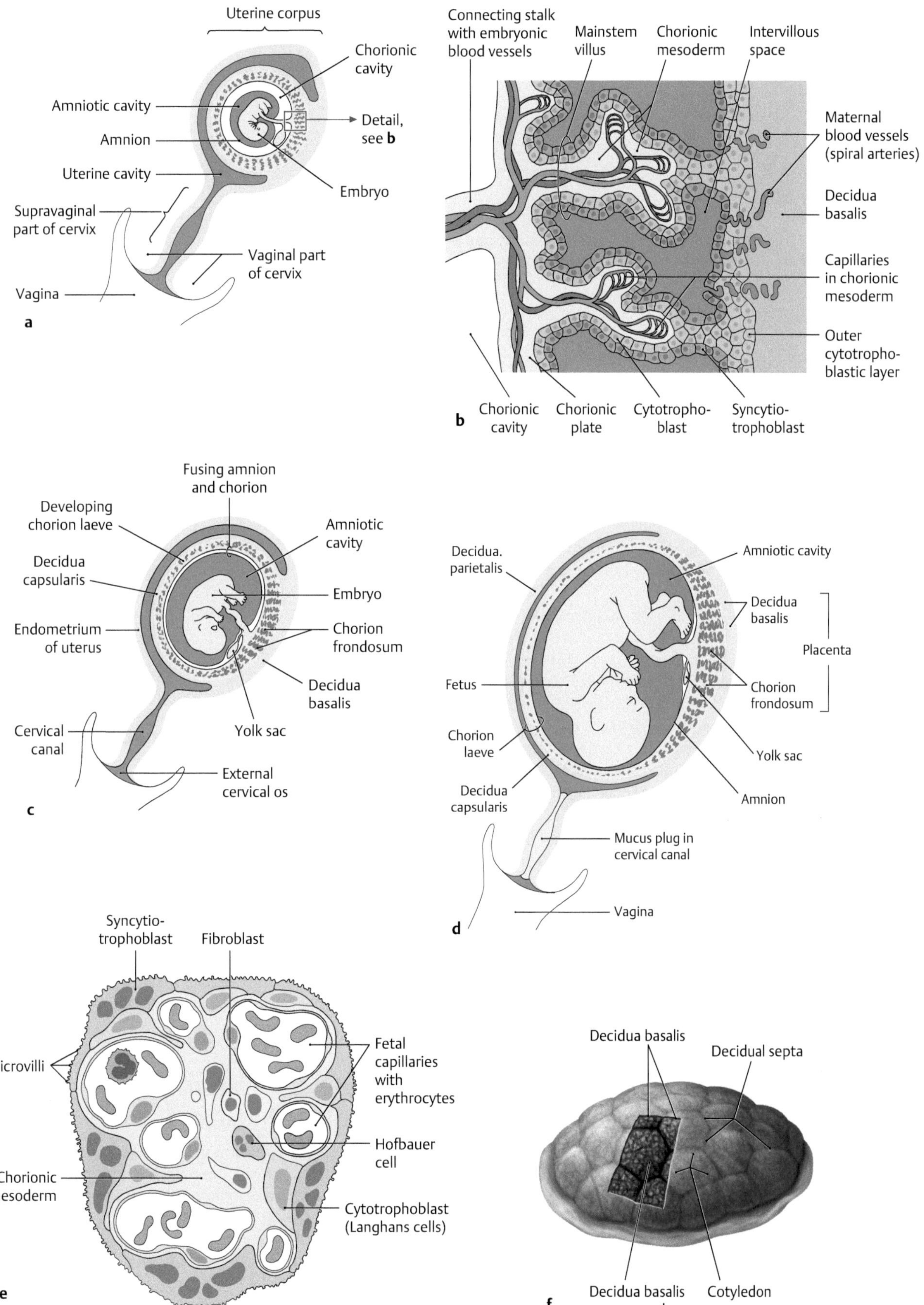

Fig. 4.60 Development of the fetal membranes and placenta. **(a)** Embryo at 5 weeks. **(b)** Detail from **a**. **(c)** Embyro at 8 weeks. **(d)** Fetus at 20 weeks. **(e)** Cross section through a terminal villus. **(f)** Postpartum placenta. (From Schuenke M, Schulte E, Schumacher U. THIEME Atlas of Anatomy. General Anatomy and Musculoskeletal System. Illustrations by Voll M and Wesker K. 3rd ed. New York: Thieme Medical Publishers; 2020.)

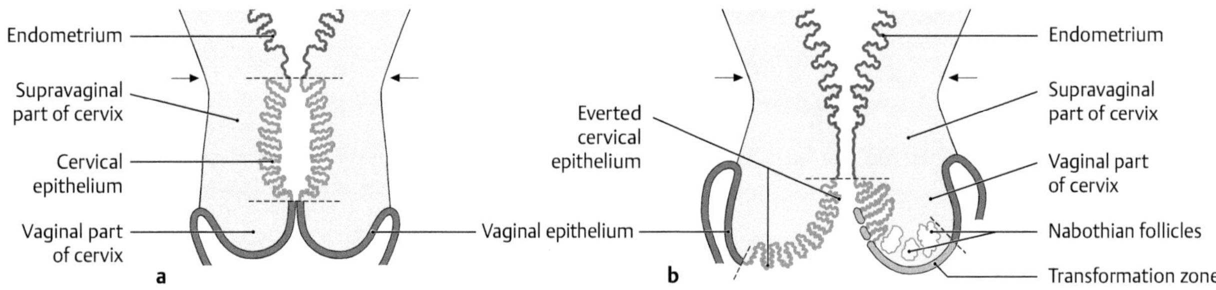

Fig. 4.61 Uterine cervix epithelium **(a)** before puberty and **(b)** during reproductive age. (From Schuenke M, Schulte E, Schumacher U. THIEME Atlas of Anatomy. Neck and Internal Organs. Illustrations by Voll M and Wesker K. 1st ed. New York: Thieme Medical Publishers; 2010.)

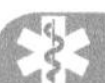

4.30.6 Uterine Cervix

The **cervix** differs histologically from the rest of the uterus. It has a **cervical canal** that opens to the uterus through the **internal os** and to the vagina through the **external os (Fig. 4.45)**. The lumen of the cervical canal (endocervix) is lined by a mucous-secreting *simple columnar epithelium* while the portion protruding into the vagina (ectocervix) is lined by a *stratified squamous non-keratinized epithelium*. There are few smooth muscle fibers and it consists of about 85% dense connective tissue. The hormone *relaxin* targets this part of the cervix and induces lysis of the collagen fibers to facilitate cervical dilation.

The mucosa of the cervix changes during the menstrual cycle however it will not slough off during menstruation. The cervical glands near ovulation and under the direction of estrogen begin to secrete a more serous and alkaline fluid to facilitates the entry of the sperm. Progesterone during the mid-secretory (luteal) phase and pregnancy cause a more viscous and acidic fluid to be secreted and this will prevent the entry of sperm and microorganisms.

The cervical squamo-columnar epithelial junction is located near the external os from birth and until menarche **(Fig. 4.61a)**. With the onset of puberty, the endocervical columnar epithelium moves out and onto the ectocervix. After menarche, the gradual replacement of columnar with squamous epithelium is called the **transformation zone (Fig. 4.61b)**. This zone is clinically important because almost all cervical squamous cell carcinomas occur here and because of this a *Pap smear* should sample the entire transformation zone. Two mechanisms are responsible for transforming this to squamous epithelium. Squamous epithelialization involves the direct ingrowth of mature squamous cells from the ectocervix. Squamous metaplasia refers to the non-cancerous change of surface sub-columnar reserve cells into fully mature squamous epithelium.

Clinical Correlate 4.16

Nabothian Cysts

A mucous-filled cyst formed where the stratified squamous epithelium of the ectocervix grows over the simple columnar epithelium of the endocervix is called a **nabothian cyst**. Rarely do they cause symptoms and are usually found during routine gynecological visits. If they look abnormal a biopsy would be performed but generally these are benign and cause no problems.

Clinical Correlate 4.17

Pap Smears

A Pap smear (Pap test) is a cervical cancer screening procedure. The primary cause of cervical cancer is the human papillomavirus (HPV), specifically HPV 16 and 18. A pap smear does not test for HPV but does identify cellular changes brought on by HPV. While lying on an examination table, a speculum is used to open the vagina and access the cervix. A tool called a spatula is then used to scrape a small sample of cells from the cervix for testing. Pap tests are very accurate and have led to reducing cervical cancer rates and mortality.

4.31 Vagina

The **vagina** is a musculomembranous tube located posterior to the urethra and anterior to the anal canal and rectum **(Fig. 4.45; Fig. 4.62; Fig. 4.63)**. It extends from the uterine cervix to the *vestibule*, a region of the perineum located between the labia minora. The vagina, urethra and greater vestibular glands all open into the vestibule. The vagina receives the penis and ejaculate during intercourse and serves as the inferior portion of the birth canal as well as the canal for passing menstrual fluid.

The vagina is normally collapsed except for the recess located around the protruding cervix called the **vaginal fornix**. It is composed of **anterior**, **posterior** and **lateral fornices** with the posterior fornix closely related to the rectouterine pouch (of *Douglas*). The *bulbospongiosus*, *pubovaginalis* and *urethrovaginal sphincter* (part of the *external urethral sphincter*) are capable of acting like sphincters and compressing the vagina.

4.31.1 Neurovasculature and Lymphatic Drainage of the Vagina

The innervation to the inferior portion of the vagina is somatic in nature and comes from the **deep perineal nerves** (pudendal br.). The rest of the vagina is innervated by autonomics originating from the **uterovaginal plexus**. Sympathetic fibers stimulate smooth muscle contraction and vasoconstriction of blood vessels while parasympathetics are involved in transudation **(Fig. 4.19; Fig. 4.22)**.

Blood supply to the *upper 1/5* is from the **uterine artery**; the *middle 3/5* is from the **vaginal artery**; and the *inferior 1/5* is supplied

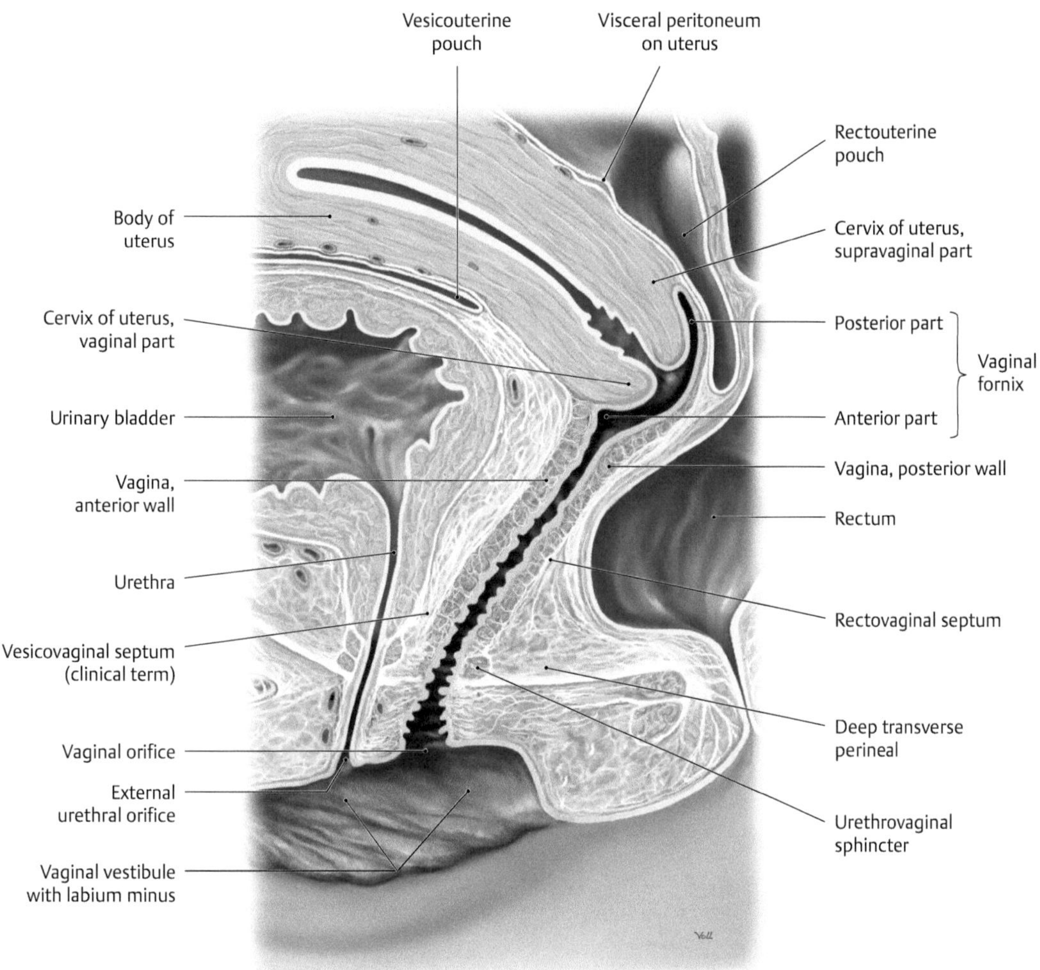

Fig. 4.62 Location of the vagina. Midsagittal section viewed from the left side. (From Schuenke M, Schulte E, Schumacher U. THIEME Atlas of Anatomy. Internal Organs. Illustrations by Voll M and Wesker K. 3rd ed. New York: Thieme Medical Publishers; 2020.)

by the **internal pudendal artery**. All of these branches originate from the *internal iliac artery* (**Fig. 4.24; Table 4.3**). Venous drainage is primarily from the **vaginal venous plexus** but the **uterine venous plexuses** may also contribute before they both continue to the **internal iliac veins**. Lymphatic drainage from the *upper portion* is to the **internal** and **external iliac lymph nodes**; the *middle portion* drains to the **internal iliac lymph nodes**; the *inferior portion* drains to the **sacral** and **common iliac lymph nodes**; and finally the *external orifice* drains to the **superficial inguinal lymph nodes** (**Fig. 4.46**).

4.31.2 Histology of the Vagina

The mucosa is thick and demonstrates rugae (folds) and has a *stratified squamous epithelium*. It is devoid of glands and is instead lubricated by mucus produced by the glands of the uterine cervix. The epithelial cells proliferate in response to estrogen (preovulatory phase) and thereby attain the maximal mucosal thickness with the superficial cells containing a large amount of cytoplasmic glycogen. Bacteria located in the vagina metabolize this glycogen and produce lactic acid, decreasing the pH. Progesterone limits epithelial proliferation during the post-ovulatory phase of the menstrual cycle and pregnancy. The muscularis smooth muscle is arranged as an inner longitudinal and outer circular layer. The longitudinal layers are continuous with those of the uterus. The outer adventitia is rich in thick elastic fibers and merges with the stroma of the adjacent tissues.

Clinical Correlate 4.18

Culdocentesis

A **culdocentesis** is a procedure where an endoscopic instrument or culdoscope is inserted through an incision made in the posterior fornix and into the peritoneal cavity to drain a pelvic abscess in the rectouterine pouch (*of Douglas*).

Vesicouterine pouch
Posterior vaginal fornix
Rectouterine pouch (cul-de-sac)

(From Schuenke M, Schulte E, Schumacher U. THIEME Atlas of Anatomy. Internal Organs. Illustrations by Voll M and Wesker K. 1st ed. New York: Thieme Medical Publishers; 2010.)

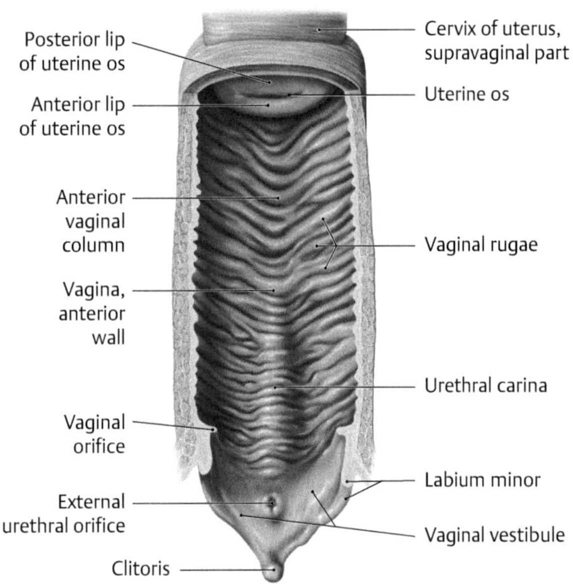

Fig. 4.63 Structure of the vagina, posterior view. (From Schuenke M, Schulte E, Schumacher U. THIEME Atlas of Anatomy. Internal Organs. Illustrations by Voll M and Wesker K. 3rd ed. New York: Thieme Medical Publishers; 2020.)

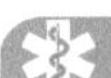

Clinical Correlate 4.19

Pelvic Inflammatory Disease

Pelvic inflammatory disease (PID) is due to an infection affecting the reproductive organs of a woman. It is most commonly caused by a sexually transmitted disease such as *gonorrhea* or *chlamydia*. Pain may present in the lower abdomen and include a burning sensation while urinating. An unusual discharge or smell from the vagina, pain and/or bleeding during sex or between periods are additional symptoms. Tenderness of the uterus, cervix or uterine tubes may be noted during a physical examination. There is no specific test for PID but it can be more successfully treated with antibiotics the earlier it is diagnosed. If left untreated, infertility may be an issue due to scarring of the uterine tubes and the individual may experience chronic pelvic pain.

4.32 Genital Duct Development of the Female

The **paramesonephric ducts** play an important role in the development of the female reproductive system. In females, the mesonephric ducts regress because of the lack of testosterone, while the paramesonephric ducts flourish due to the absence of MIS. The paramesonephric ducts arise from the anterolateral surface of the urogenital ridge as a longitudinal invagination of the epithelium (**Fig. 4.43**). The ducts open cranially as a funnel shaped structure and this region is where the **uterine tubes** originate. As they extend caudally they first run laterally to the mesonephric duct before crossing over anteriorly and terminating medially to them. The two ducts are initially separated by a **uterine septum**, but with degeneration of the septum the **uterovaginal primordium** or **uterine canal** forms and serves as the structure that gives rise to the **uterus**, **cervix** and the **superior one-third of the vagina** (**Fig. 4.64**). The caudal tip of the combined ducts projects into the posterior wall of the urogenital sinus, creating a small swelling called the **paramesonephric tubercle**. The mesonephric ducts open into the urogenital sinus on either side of this tubercle. Fusion of the paramesonephric ducts draws together two peritoneal folds that form both sides of the **broad ligament** and results in the creation of the **rectouterine** and **vesicouterine pouches**.

Contact between the uterovaginal primordium and the urogenital sinus, resulting in the formation of the **sinus tubercle**, also induces the formation of the **sinovaginal bulbs**, the paired endodermal outgrowths that extend from the urogenital sinus to the caudal end of the uterovaginal primordium. The sinovaginal bulbs fuse to form the **vaginal plate**, which eventually canalizes to form the **inferior two-thirds of the vagina**. The epithelial lining of the entire vagina is of endodermal origin although the vagina originates from two sources (**Fig. 4.64**).

Until late in fetal life, the **hymen** separates the lumen of the vagina from the cavity of the urogenital sinus. It is formed by an invagination of the posterior wall of the urogenital sinus.

The **urethral** and **paraurethral (Skene) glands** originate from buds that extend from the urethra and into the surrounding mesenchyme and outgrowths from the urogenital sinus form the **greater vestibular glands (of Bartholin)** located in the lower one-third of the labia minora.

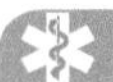

Clinical Correlate 4.20

Uterus and Vagina Abnormalities

Developmental abnormalities of the uterus and vagina are caused primarily by the persistence of the uterine septum or obliteration of the lumen of the uterine canal. When the paramesonephric ducts demonstrate a lack of fusion in a local area or throughout their normal line of fusion this results in duplications of the uterus. The presence of a double uterus is called uterus didelphys and it is the result of the lack of fusion of the paramesonephric ducts; it may present with a double vagina. A mild variant includes an indentation near the fundus of the uterus and this is called uterus arcuatus. A relatively common anomaly in which the uterus has two horns entering a common vagina and is the result of a partial fusion of the paramesonephric ducts is called uterus bicornis. The failure of the sinovaginal bulbs to fuse or to develop entirely results in a double vagina or vaginal atresia respectively.

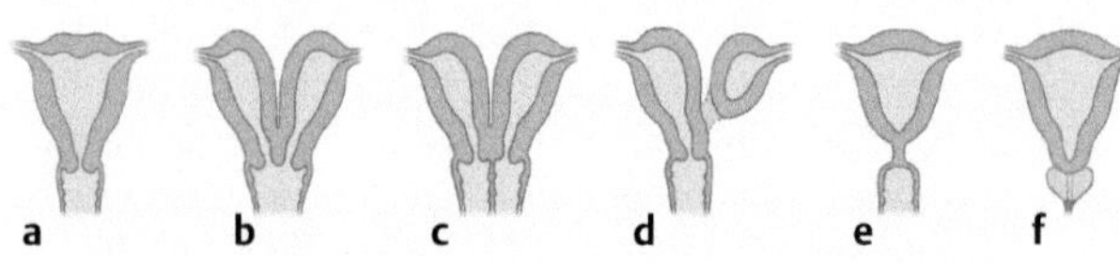

(a-c) Incomplete fusion with double uterus (and/or double vagina). **(d)** Rudimentary horn on one side of the uterus. **(e)** Atresia of the cervix. **(f)** Vaginal atresia. (From Schuenke M, Schulte E, Schumacher U. THIEME Atlas of Anatomy. Internal Organs. Illustrations by Voll M and Wesker K. 3rd ed. New York: Thieme Medical Publishers; 2020.)

4.33 Perineum

The diamond-shaped external surface and shallow compartment of the body that lies inferior to the inferior pelvic aperture and is separated from the pelvic cavity by the pelvic diaphragm is known as the **perineum** (**Fig. 4.65**). The borders of this region include the *pubic symphysis* (anteriorly), *ischiopubic rami* (anterolaterally),

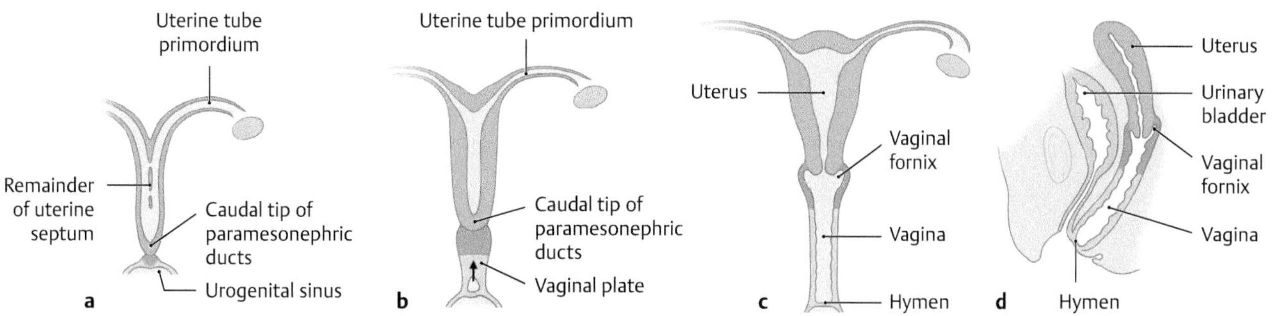

Fig. 4.64 Formation of the uterus and vagina. **(a-c)** Anterior view. **(d)** Midsagittal section viewed from the left side. (From Schuenke M, Schulte E, Schumacher U. THIEME Atlas of Anatomy. Internal Organs. Illustrations by Voll M and Wesker K. 3rd ed. New York: Thieme Medical Publishers; 2020.)

ischial tuberosities (laterally), *sacrotuberous ligaments* (posterolaterally), and finally the inferior most portions of the *sacrum* and *coccyx* (posteriorly).

The perineum is divided into two separate triangles by a transverse line that connects each ischial tuberosity and passes through the *perineal body*. The **urogenital triangle** is anterior to this line and contains the vulva in females and the root of the scrotum and penis in males. The **anal triangle** is posterior to this line and contains the anal canal and anus surrounded by ischioanal fat. The **perineal body** is a fibromuscular mass located in the median plane posterior to the vestibule of the vagina or bulb of the penis and anterior to the anus. It is the convergence site of multiple muscles and these include the *bulbospongiosus, external anal sphincter, superficial transverse perineal, deep transverse perineal*, and slips of skeletal or smooth muscle from the *external urethral sphincter, levator ani* and *muscular coats of the rectum*.

4.33.1 Muscles of the Perineum

The muscles of the perineum can help support the perineal body and pelvic floor, maintain an erection, constricts the anal canal or compresses the urethra. All of these muscles receive their innervation from branches of the pudendal nerve but can be subdivided into a superficial or deep layer of muscles. The *superficial muscles of the perineum* of both sexes are the bulbospongiosus, ischiocavernosus, superficial transverse perineal, and external anal sphincter **(Fig. 4.66; Table 4.6)**.

- The **superficial transverse perineal muscles** fix and support the perineal body and pelvic floor to resist increased intra-abdominal pressure.
- The **bulbospongiosus** and **ischiocavernosus muscles** function primarily in constricting venous outflow from the erectile bodies and thus they maintain an erection by simultaneously pushing blood from the root of the penis/crura of the clitoris into the body of the penis/clitoris. The bulbospongiosus fixes and supports the perineal body and pelvic floor in both sexes. In males, the bulbospongiosus also helps expel the last few drops of urine or semen. It acts like a sphincter for the vagina and compress the bulb of the vestibule and greater vestibular glands in females.
- The **external anal sphincter** mainly constricts the anal canal during peristalsis and resists defecation. It is only a part of the anal triangle.

The *deep muscles of the perineum* of both sexes are the deep transverse perineal and external urethral sphincter (compressor portion only) **(Fig. 4.66; Table 4.6)**.

- The **deep transverse perineal muscles** are purely skeletal in males but are replaced with smooth muscle in females. Much like their superficial counterpart, these muscles fix and support the perineal body and resist increased intra-abdominal pressure.
- The **external urethral sphincter** is a tube-like structure oriented perpendicular rather than parallel to the *perineal membrane*. It contains separate fibers called the **compressor urethrae muscles** that extend from the ischiopubic ramus to each side of the neck of the bladder. In males, only a small part of the muscle forms a true sphincter and that is at the intermediate (membranous) portion of the urethra inferior to the prostate. The majority of it extends vertically to the neck of the bladder, investing the prostatic urethra on both the anterior and anterolateral sides. For females, the external urethral sphincter not only contains the compressor urethrae muscle but it consists of another band-like portion that encircles both the vagina and urethra known as the **urethrovaginal sphincter (Fig. 4.66)**.

Urogenital Triangle Fasciae and Pouches

The **urogenital triangle** is closed by the perineal membrane. The **perineal membrane** is a thin sheet of tough deep fascia that stretches between the left and right sides of the pubic arch. It will cover the anterior portion of the pelvic outlet and the urethra of both sexes along with the vagina of a woman perforate it.

4.33.2 Perineal Fasciae

There is both a superficial and deep layer of **perineal fascia**. The subcutaneous tissue of the perineum, or **superficial perineal fascia**, consists of a fatty superficial layer and a membranous deep layer similar to that of the anterior abdominal wall. In females, the **fatty superficial layer** of superficial perineal fascia which continues into the labia majora, originates from *Camper's fascia* of the abdomen and is connected posteriorly with the ischioanal fat bodies. The **membranous deep layer (*Colles' fascia*)** of superficial perineal fascia passes superior to the fatty layer forming the labia majora and becomes continuous with *Scarpa's fascia* of the abdomen **(Fig. 4.67)**.

For males, the **fatty superficial layer** of superficial perineal fascia is greatly reduced in the urogenital triangle and replaced in the penis and scrotum with **dartos fascia**. It is continuous between the scrotum and thighs with *Camper's fascia* of the abdomen and posteriorly with the ischioanal fat bodies. The **membranous deep**

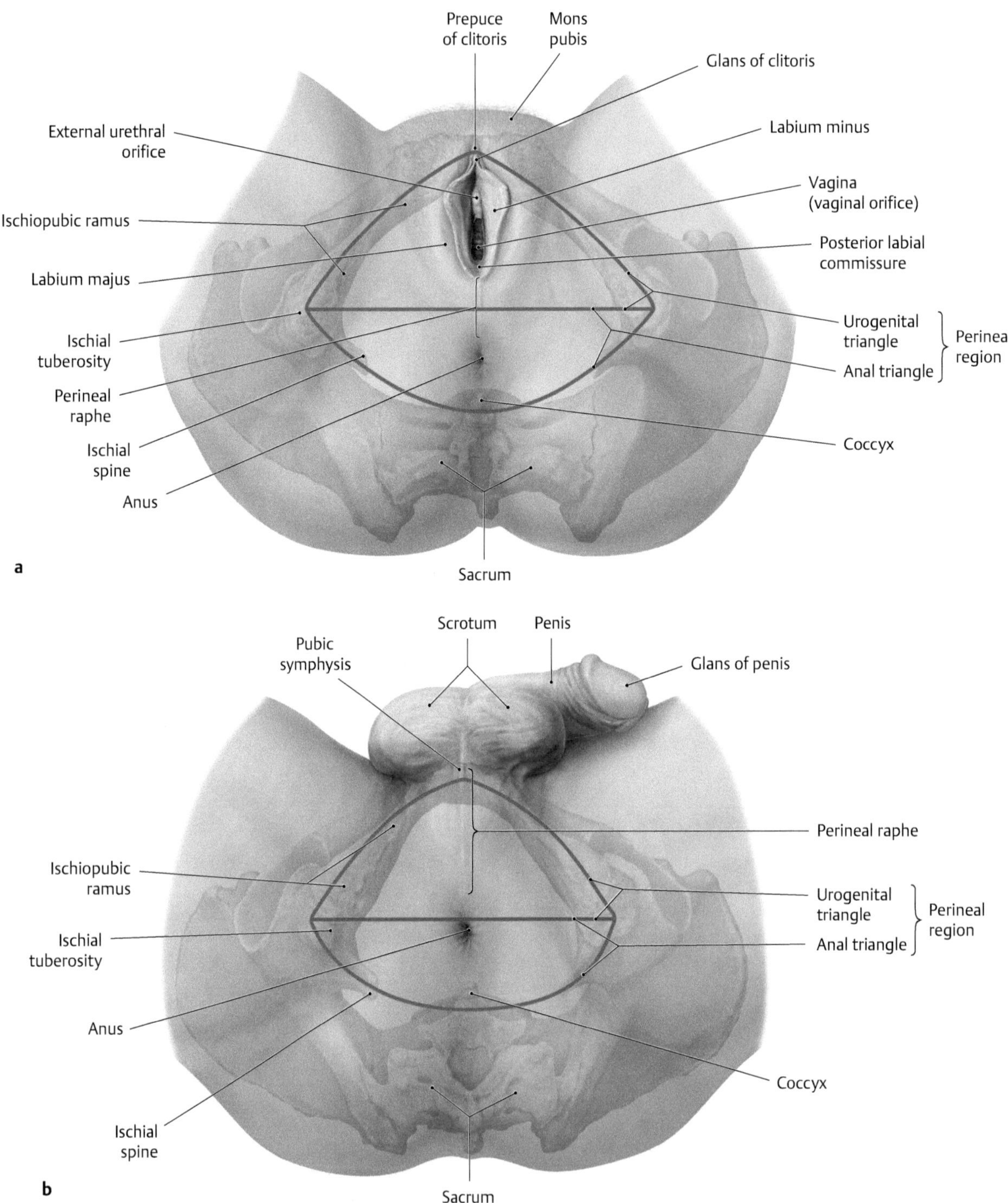

Fig. 4.65 Lithotomy position. **(a)** Female perineum. **(b)** Male perineum. (From Schuenke M, Schulte E, Schumacher U. THIEME Atlas of Anatomy. Internal Organs. Illustrations by Voll M and Wesker K. 3rd ed. New York: Thieme Medical Publishers; 2020.)

layer (*Colles' fascia*) of superficial perineal fascia is attached posteriorly to the posterior margin of the perineal membrane and the perineal body. Anteriorly the *Colles'* fascia is continuous with dartos fascia in the scrotum. On each side of and anterior to the scrotum the *Colles'* fascia becomes continuous with *Scarpa's fascia* of the abdomen. It attaches laterally to the *fascia lata of the thigh* (**Fig. 4.68**).

The **deep perineal fascia** (***Gallaudet*** or **investing fascia**) invests the bulbospongiosus, ischiocavernosus and superficial transverse perineal muscles. It attaches laterally to the ischiopubic rami and is continuous with the deep fascia covering the external oblique muscle and rectus sheath. In females it is fused with the **suspensory ligament of the clitoris** while in males it is fused to the **suspensory ligament of the penis**.

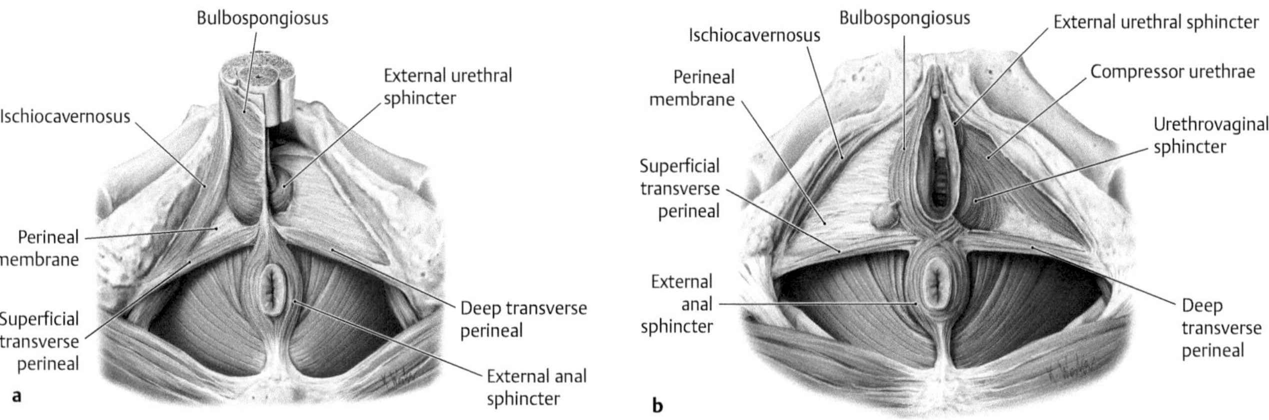

Fig. 4.66 Muscles of the perineum. **(a)** Male. **(b)** Female. (From Schuenke M, Schulte E, Schumacher U. THIEME Atlas of Anatomy. Internal Organs. Illustrations by Voll M and Wesker K. 3rd ed. New York: Thieme Medical Publishers; 2020.)

Table 4.6 **Muscles of the perineum**

Muscle	Innervation	Function(s)	Origin	Insertion
Bulbospongiosus	Deep perineal nerve (pudendal nerve br.)	Constrict venous outflow from the erectile bodies to maintain an erection; fix and support perineal body and pelvic floor	Male: perineal body; median raphe on ventral surface of bulb of penis. Female: perineal body	Male: wraps lateral aspects of bulb and proximal part of penis to insert into perineal membrane, fascia of bulb of penis, and dorsal aspects of corpora cavernosa and corpus spongiosum. Female: wraps around each side of lower vagina enclosing the bulb and greater vestibular gland before inserting into the pubic arch and fascia of the corpora cavernosa of clitoris
Ischiocavernosus	Deep perineal nerve (pudendal nerve br.)	Constrict venous outflow from the erectile bodies to maintain an erection	Internal surface of the ischiopubic ramus and ischial tuberosity	Crus of penis or clitoris
Superficial transverse perineal	Deep perineal nerve (pudendal nerve br.)	Fix and support perineal body and pelvic floor against intra-abdominal pressure	Internal surface of the ischiopubic ramus and ischial tuberosity	Perineal body
Deep transverse perineal	Deep perineal nerve (pudendal nerve br.)	Fix and support perineal body and pelvic floor against intra-abdominal pressure	Internal surface of the ischiopubic ramus and ischial tuberosity	Perineal body and external anal sphincter
External urethral sphincter	Dorsal nerve of penis/ clitoris (pudendal nerve br.)	Compresses urethra to maintain urinary continence	Encircles urethra; In males: ascends anteriorly to the neck of the bladder; In females: some fibers surround the vagina as the urethrovaginal sphincter; compressor urethrae in both sexes originates from the ischiopubic ramus	Encircles urethra; In males: ascends anteriorly to the neck of the bladder; In females: some fibers surround the vagina as the urethrovaginal sphincter; compressor urethrae in both sexes blends with fibers located around the urethra
External anal sphincter	Inferior rectal (anal) nerve (pudendal nerve br.)	Constricts the anal canal during peristalsis and resists defecation; fixes and supports perineal body and pelvic floor	Skin and fascia surrounding the anus; to the coccyx via the anococcygeal ligament	Wraps around the lateral aspects of anal canal before inserting into perineal body

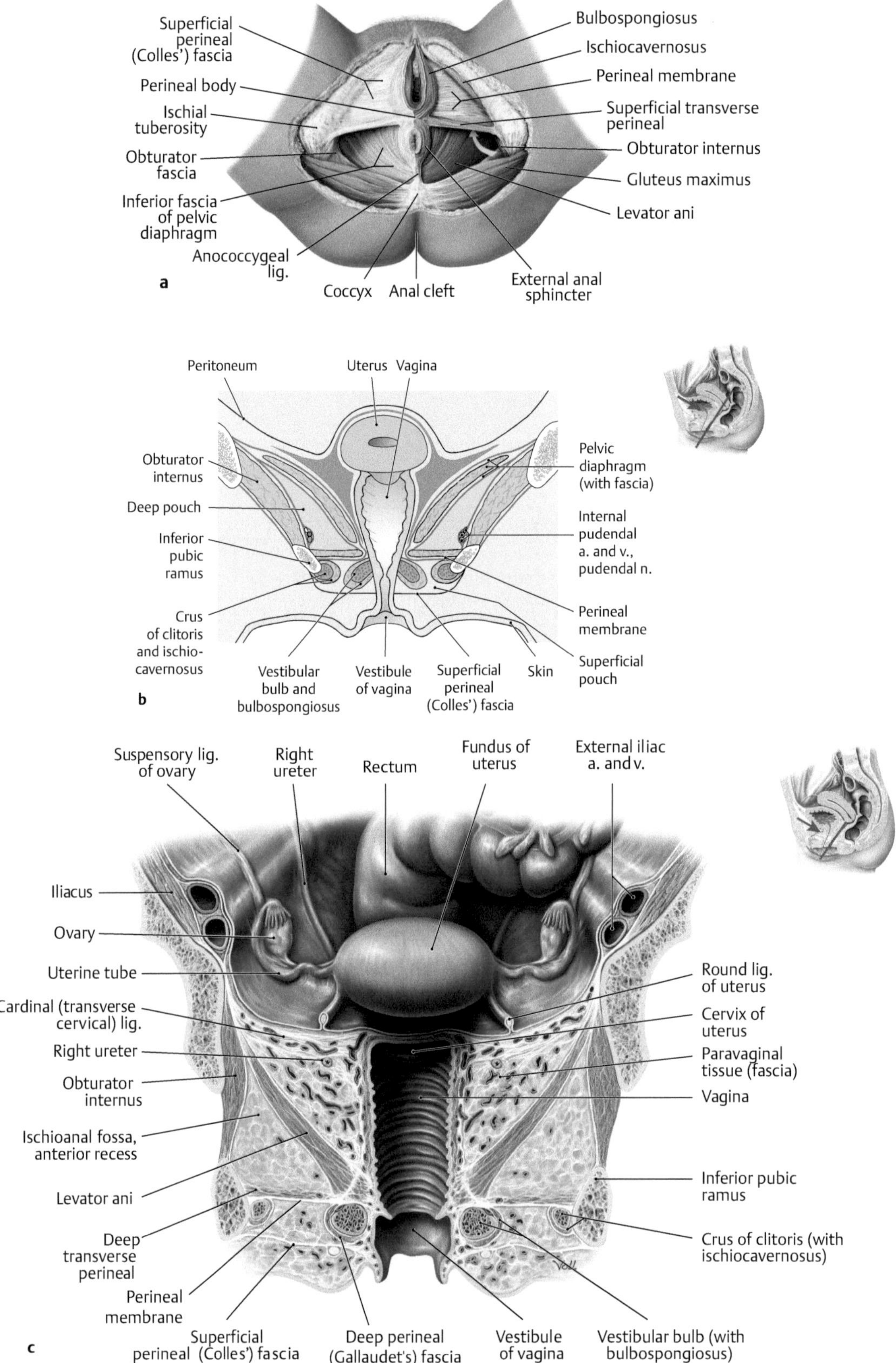

Fig. 4.67 Perineal fasica of the female. **(a)** Lithotomy position. Removed on left side: superficial perineal (Colles') fascia, inferior fascia of the pelvic diaphragm, and obturator fascia. Note: green arrow is pointing to anterior recess of the ischial anal fossa. **(b)** Oblique section. **(c)** Oblique section of pelvis, anterior view. (From Schuenke M, Schulte E, Schumacher U. THIEME Atlas of Anatomy. Internal Organs. Illustrations by Voll M and Wesker K. 3rd ed. New York: Thieme Medical Publishers; 2020.)

4.33.3 Perineal Pouches

The **superficial perineal pouch** is a potential space between *Colles' fascia* and the *perineal membrane*, bounded laterally by the *ischiopubic rami.*

- In males, this pouch contains **(Fig. 4.69)**:
  - **Root of the penis** (bulb and crura) and their associated bulbospongiosus and ischiocavernosus muscles.
  - **Superficial transverse perineal muscles.**
  - *Proximal (of bulb) portion* of **spongy urethra.**
  - **Perineal branches** of the *pudendal nerve* and *internal pudendal vessels.*
- In females, this pouch contains **(Fig. 4.70)**:
  - **Root of the clitoris** (crura) and their associated ischiocavernosus muscles.
  - **Bulbs of the vestibule** and **greater vestibular glands** and their adjacent bulbospongiosus muscle.
  - **Superficial transverse perineal muscles.**
  - **Perineal branches** of the *pudendal nerve* and *internal pudendal vessels.*

The **deep perineal pouch** has borders that include the *perineal membrane* (inferiorly), the *inferior pelvic fascia of the pelvic diaphragm* (superiorly), and the inferior portion of the *obturator fascia* (laterally). This pouch includes the anterior recesses of the ischioanal fossae. However, it is not an enclosed space and is open superiorly.

- In males, this pouch contains **(Fig. 4.69)**:
  - *Intermediate (membranous) portion* of the **urethra**
  - **External urethral sphincter muscle**
  - **Bulbourethral glands**
  - **Deep transverse perineal muscles**
  - **Deep perineal branches** and the **dorsal nerve/vessels of the penis**, branches of the *pudendal nerve* and *internal pudendal vessels*
- In females, this pouch contains **(Fig. 4.70)**:
  - *Proximal part* of the **urethra**
  - **External urethral sphincter muscle**
  - **Deep transverse perineal muscles**
  - **Deep perineal branches** and the **dorsal nerve/vessels of the clitoris**, branches of the *pudendal nerve* and *internal pudendal vessels*

4.34 Male Perineum

The male perineum includes the penis, the intermediate (membranous) and spongy urethra, scrotum, perineal muscles and the anal canal **(Fig. 4.65)**. The anal canal is detailed in the *Anal Triangle* section of this chapter.

4.34.1 Penis

The male organ of copulation and the outlet for both urine and semen is the **penis.** It consists of a root, body and glans penis. There are three cylindrical bodies of erectile cavernous tissue that make up the bulk of the penis. These are the paired **corpora cavernosa** located dorsally and the isolated **corpus spongiosum** located ventrally. The corpora cavernosa are fused until they separate to form the **crura of the penis**. The corpus spongiosum is continuous with the **bulb** and **glans penis** and contains the spongy urethra. The **root of the penis** includes the bulb and crura **(Fig. 4.71)**.

The fibrous outer covering or capsule surrounding each cavernous body is known as the **tunica albuginea**. Superficial to this outer covering is the **deep (*Buck's*) fascia of the penis**, a continuation of the *deep perineal (Galludet's) fascia* that forms a membranous covering binding the corpora together. The deep (Buck's) fascia extends from the body to cover both the bulb and crura at the root of the penis.

The **body of the penis** is free and suspended from the pubic symphysis. The **suspensory ligament of the penis**, which is a condensation of the deep fascia that arises from the anterior surface of the pubic symphysis, splits and forms a sling that is attached to the deep fascia of the penis near the junction of its root and body. The **glans penis** is the expansion of erectile tissue that extends distally from the corpus spongiosum. The **corona of the glans** is the margin of the glans that projects beyond the ends of the corpora cavernosa and it overhangs the **neck of the glans**, which separates the glans from the body of the penis. The thin skin and fascia of the penis that forms a double layer covering the glans to variable extents is called the **prepuce** (foreskin). The median fold that passes from the prepuce to the urethral surface of the glans is called the **frenulum of the prepuce**.

4.34.2 Neurovasculature of the Penis

Somatic sensation and sympathetic innervation of the skin and glans penis is primarily from the **dorsal (penile) nerve of the penis**, a terminal **pudendal nerve** (ventral rami of S2-S4) branch. The **ilioinguinal nerve** supplies skin near the root of the penis. An **erection of the penis** is a hemodynamic process that is controlled by autonomic neural input. The maintenance of a fully erect penis is attributed to somatic innervation of specific perineal muscles. When the male is erotically stimulated, parasympathetic innervation passing through the **cavernous nerves** that originate from the **prostatic plexus**, close the arteriovenous anastomoses that are normally open near the sinuses of the corpora when the penis is in a flaccid state **(Fig. 4.20)**. Simultaneously the tonic contraction of the smooth muscle in the fibrous trabeculae and coiled **helicine arteries** is inhibited. As a result, the arteries dilate and allow blood flow into the sinuses of the corpora. The ischiocavernosus and bulbospongiosus muscles are innervated by perineal branches of the pudendal nerve and when they contract while overlying the crura and bulb regions respectively, they compress and impede the return of any venous blood. This, along with the rush of blood filling the erectile cavernous tissues, results in an **erection** as the corpora cavernosa and corpus spongiosum become engorged with blood causing elevation of the penis **(Fig. 4.72)**.

The process of **emission** is sympathetically driven and it is when semen is delivered to the prostatic urethra through the ejaculatory ducts after peristalsis of the ductus deferens and seminal vesicles and the contraction of prostate smooth muscle releasing prostatic fluid. The process of **ejaculation** is when semen is expelled from the external urethral orifice. It involves the prevention of retrograde ejaculation into the bladder by contraction of the internal urethral sphincter (sympathetic innervation); contraction of the bulbospongiosus muscle (from pudendal nerve); and contraction of the urethral smooth muscle (parasympathetic innervation). The process of **remission** occurs after ejaculation when the penis gradually returns to a flaccid state. This results from sympathetic

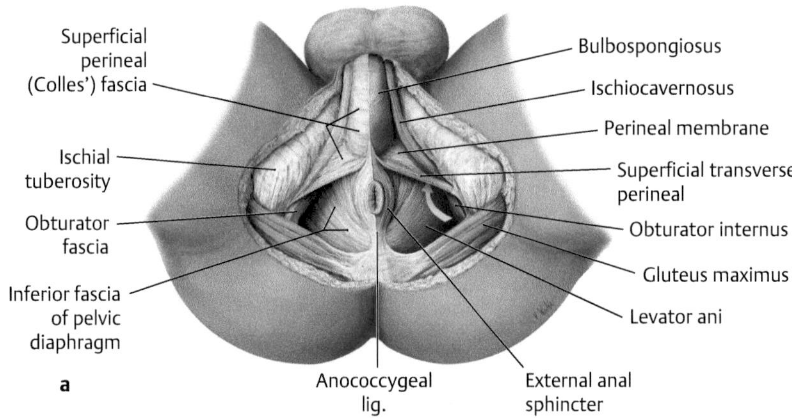

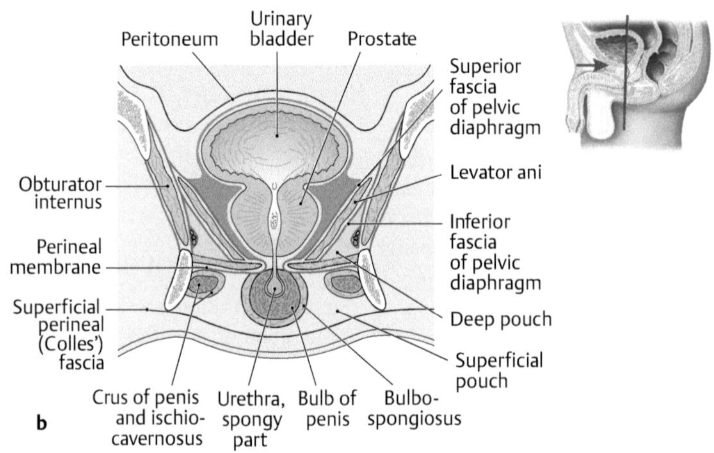

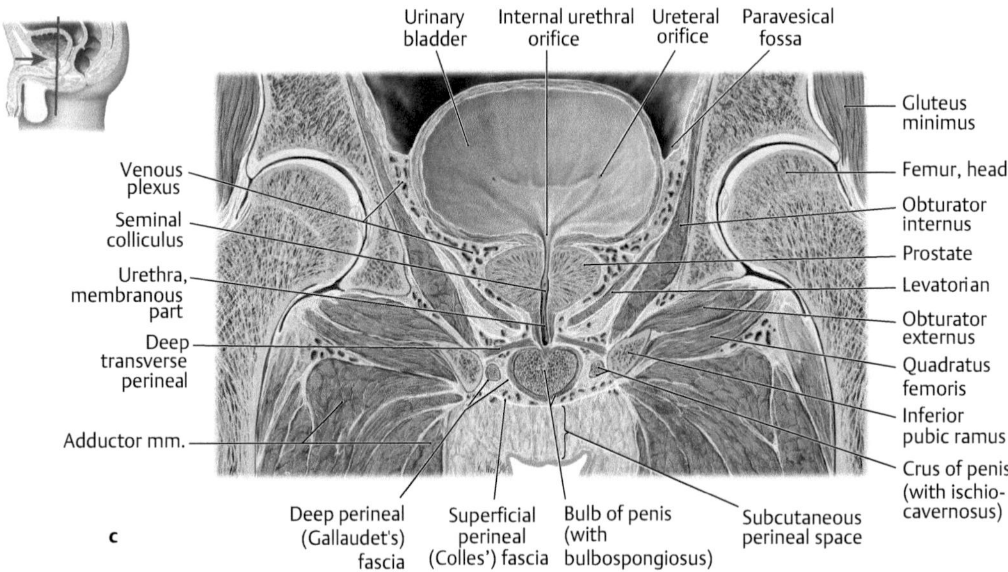

Fig. 4.68 Perineal fascia of the male. **(a)** Lithotomy position. Removed on left side: superficial perineal (Colles') fascia, inferior fascia of the pelvic diaphragm, and obturator fascia. Note: green arrow is pointing to anterior recess of the ischial anal fossa. **(b)** Coronal section. **(c)** Coronal section of pelvis, anterior view. (From Schuenke M, Schulte E, Schumacher U. THIEME Atlas of Anatomy. Internal Organs. Illustrations by Voll M and Wesker K. 3rd ed. New York: Thieme Medical Publishers; 2020.)

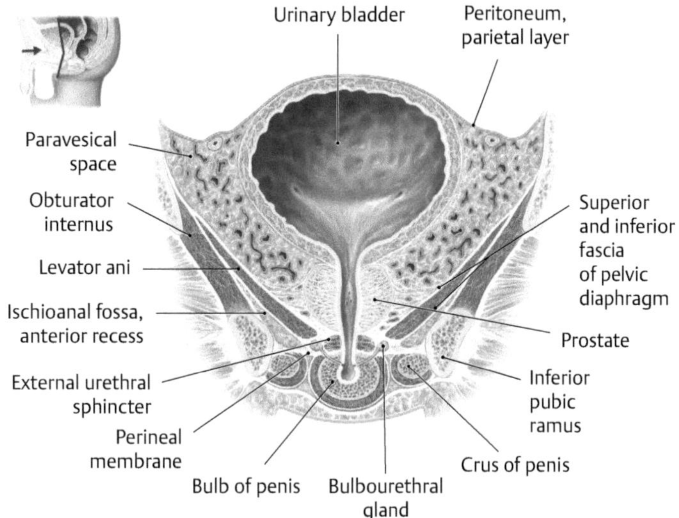

Fig. 4.69 Perineal pouches of the male. Coronal section, anterior view. (From Schuenke M, Schulte E, Schumacher U. THIEME Atlas of Anatomy. Internal Organs. Illustrations by Voll M and Wesker K. 3rd ed. New York: Thieme Medical Publishers; 2020.)

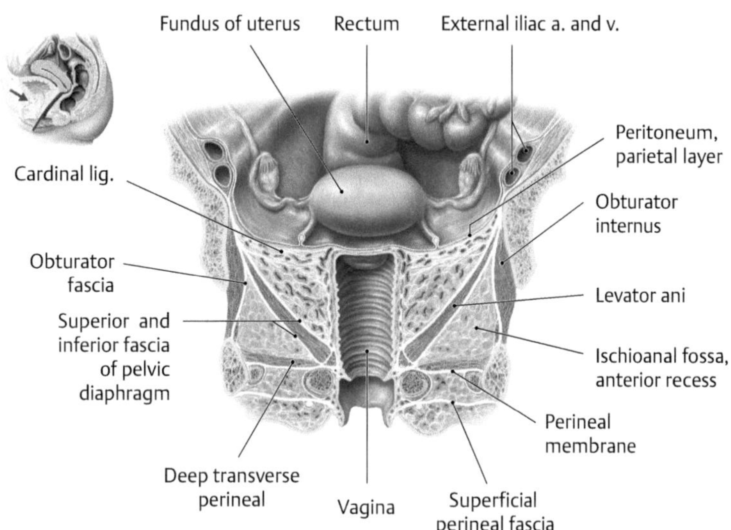

Fig. 4.70 Perineal pouches of the female. Oblique section, anterior view. (From Schuenke M, Schulte E, Schumacher U. THIEME Atlas of Anatomy. Internal Organs. Illustrations by Voll M and Wesker K. 3rd ed. New York: Thieme Medical Publishers; 2020.)

innervation that opens the arteriovenous anastomoses and causes contraction of the helicine artery smooth muscle thus recoiling them. Relaxation of the ischiocavernosus and bulbospongiosus muscles allows for uncompromised venous drainage.

The blood supply for much of the penis is from the **internal pudendal artery** and its branches (**Fig. 4.73**). The **dorsal arteries of the penis** run between the deep (*Buck's*) fascia and tunica albuginea of the corpora cavernosa lateral to the **deep dorsal vein of the penis**. The deep dorsal vein drains the bulk of the erectile tissue after an erection and the vein passes deep to the suspensory ligament before passing anterior to the perineal membrane where it ultimately drains to the **prostatic venous plexus**. The *dorsal nerves of the penis* run just laterally to these arteries. The **deep arteries of the penis** pierce the crura and run through the center of the corpora cavernosa and have **helicine artery** branches. The **arteries of the bulb of the penis** and **urethral arteries** supply the bulb, the main corpus spongiosum and glans penis along with the bulbourethral gland. They also have helicine artery branches. The **external pudendal artery** (femoral artery br.) divides into a superficial and deep branch itself and helps supply the penile and scrotal skin and anastomoses with branches of the internal pudendal arteries. Their paired veins drain back to the femoral or great saphenous veins. The **superficial dorsal veins of the penis** drain the prepuce and superficial skin regions of the penis. These veins are tributaries of the superficial external pudendal vein (**Fig. 4.71; Fig. 4.73; Fig. 4.74**).

Lymphatic drainage from the skin of the penis drains to the **superficial inguinal lymph nodes**. The glans penis and distal spongy urethra drains to the **deep inguinal** and **external iliac lymph nodes**. Lymph from the erectile cavernous tissue and proximal spongy urethra drains to the **internal iliac lymph nodes**.

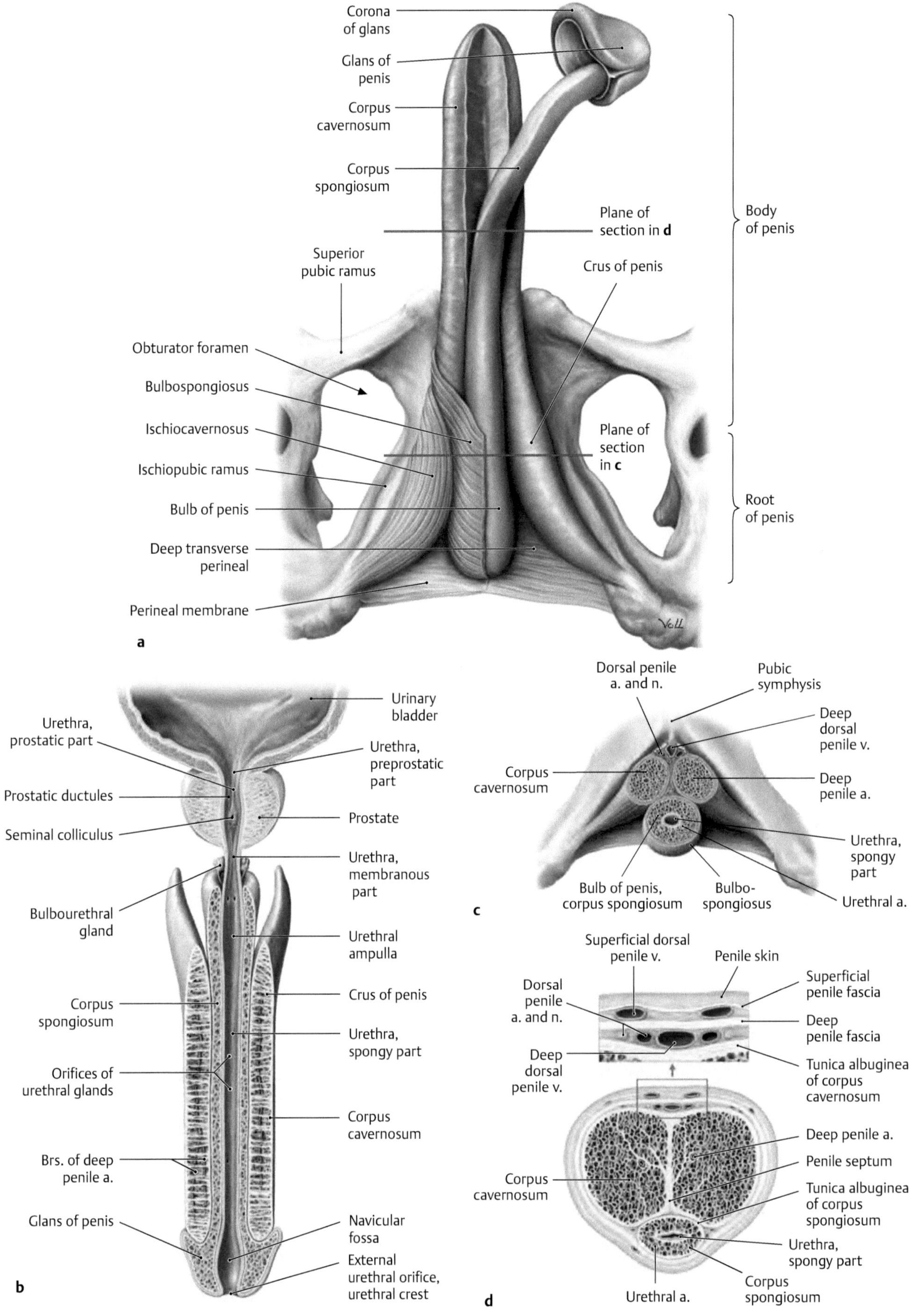

Fig. 4.71 Penis. **(a)** Inferior view. **(b)** Longitudinal section. **(c)** Cross section through the root of the penis. **(d)** Cross section through the body of the penis. (From Schuenke M, Schulte E, Schumacher U. THIEME Atlas of Anatomy. Internal Organs. Illustrations by Voll M and Wesker K. 3rd ed. New York: Thieme Medical Publishers; 2020.)

Clinical Correlate 4.21

Phimosis, Paraphimosis and Circumcision

An uncircumcised prepuce covers all or most of the glans penis. However it is usually sufficiently elastic to allow for a smooth retraction over the glans. If the prepuce is tight and unable to retract easily over the glans this is referred to as **phimosis.** If the retraction results in a constriction of the neck of the glans and interferes with the venous and lymphatic drainage thus enlarging the glans this is called **paraphimosis.** A circumcision would have to be performed in this case. A **circumcision** is the surgical excision of the prepuce and exposes most if not all of the glans. It is the most common minor surgical procedure performed on male infants.

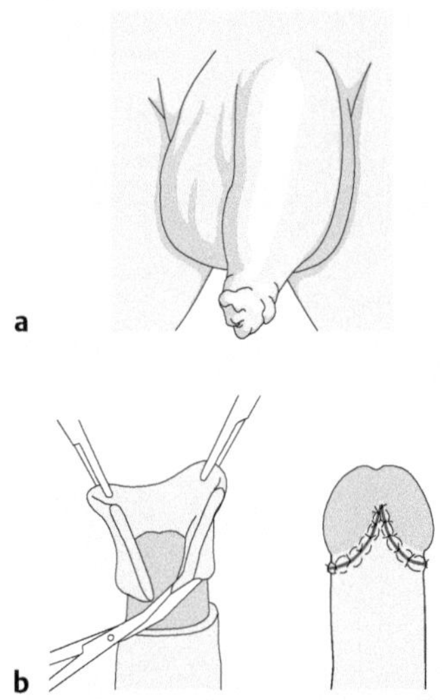

(a-b) Circumcision being performed. (From Schuenke M, Schulte E, Schumacher U. THIEME Atlas of Anatomy. General Anatomy and Musculoskeletal System. Illustrations by Voll M and Wesker K. 3rd ed. New York: Thieme Medical Publishers; 2020.)

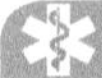
Clinical Correlate 4.22

Impotence and Erectile Dysfunction

The inability to obtain an erection or **impotence** may be due to several causes. A lesion could be present on the prostatic plexus or cavernous nerves, affecting the normal autonomic innervation that stimulates the erectile tissues and blood vessels that fill them. In this case, a surgically implanted and inflatable penile prosthesis may assume the role of the erectile tissue. **Erectile dysfunction (ED)** can be related to testosterone levels and not just damage to the nervous tissue and these reduced testosterone levels may be the result of hypothalamic, testicular or pituitary disorders. In many cases, an erection can still be achieved with the assistance of oral medications that increase blood flow into the cavernous sinusoids by causing a relaxation of the smooth muscle that surround them.

4.35 Scrotum

Details of the scrotum were addressed in Chapter 3. The **scrotum** is a double-chambered, suspended sac made up of an outer, pigmented skin layer and an internal, fat-free **dartos fascia** with **dartos muscle** layer (**Fig. 4.75**). The dartos fascia is continuous with the *membranous layer of subcutaneous tissue of the perineum (Colles' fascia)* and the *membranous layer of subcutaneous tissue of the abdomen (Scarpa's fascia)*. The **septum of the scrotum**, a central continuation of the dartos fascia, separates the testes. The external demarcation of the septum is displayed by the **scrotal raphe**, a fusion of the embryonic *labioscrotal swellings*.

4.35.1 Neurovasculature of the Scrotum

The **anterior scrotal nerve** (ilioinguinal br.) supplies the anterior surface and the **posterior scrotal nerve** (pudendal br.) supplies the posterior surface of the scrotum. The **genital branch of the genitofemoral nerve** not only innervates the cremaster muscle but it can also supply the anterolateral surface of the skin. The **perineal nerves** (posterior femoral cutaneous br.) supply the posteroinferior surface of the skin. Dartos muscle is innervated by GVE-sym/post fibers that pass through the nerves listed above (**Fig. 4.76**).

Blood supply to the scrotum includes the **anterior scrotal** (external pudendal br.), **posterior scrotal** (perineal br.), and the **cremasteric arteries** (inferior epigastric br.) (**Fig. 4.76**). These vessels all have paired venous drainage and their lymphatic drainage is to the **superficial inguinal lymph nodes**.

4.36 Female Perineum

The female perineum includes the mons pubis, labia majora, labia minora, clitoris, bulbs of the vestibule, greater (Bartholin) glands, paraurethral (lesser vestibular or Skene) glands, urethra, and the anal canal. With the female perineum, the terms **pudendum** and **vulva** are synonymous. The pudendum has multiple functions serving as sensory and erectile tissue for sexual arousal and intercourse, directing the flow of urine, and preventing the entry of foreign material into the urogenital tract.

The **mons pubis** is a fatty eminence located anterior to the pubic symphysis, pubic tubercle and superior pubic rami. The amount of fat in the mons pubis increases at puberty but decreases after menopause. The prominent folds of skin called the **labia majora** indirectly provide protection for the urethral and vaginal orifices and are largely filled with fat. They are covered with pubic hair and each side joins the opposite side at the **anterior** and **posterior commissures**. The two sides meet at the midline and form the **pudendal cleft**. The round ligament of the uterus terminates in the labia majora. The **labia minora** are folds of fat-free, hairless skin that are thinner than the labia majora and have a core of spongy connective tissue containing erectile tissue with many sensory nerve endings and small blood vessels. They establish the borders of the **vestibule**, a space that contains the opening of the urethra, vagina and the greater vestibular and paraurethral glands. The vaginal orifice may still have a **hymen** present closing off the lumen. The labia minora are connected posteriorly by a small transverse fold known as the **frenulum of the labia minora** in younger women (**Fig. 4.77**).

The labia minora form two laminae: the medial laminae that unite to form the **frenulum of the clitoris** and the lateral laminae that merge to form the **prepuce of the clitoris**. The **clitoris** is an erectile organ located where the labia minora meet anteriorly. It will consist of a **root** and a **body**, which are composed of two **crura** and the **glans of the clitoris**. The prepuce of the clitoris covers the glans. The clitoris is highly sensitive with the glans being the most highly innervated portion and enlarges on tactile stimulation (**Fig. 4.77**).

The **bulbs of the vestibule** are paired, elongated masses of erectile tissue that are located along the sides of the vaginal orifice

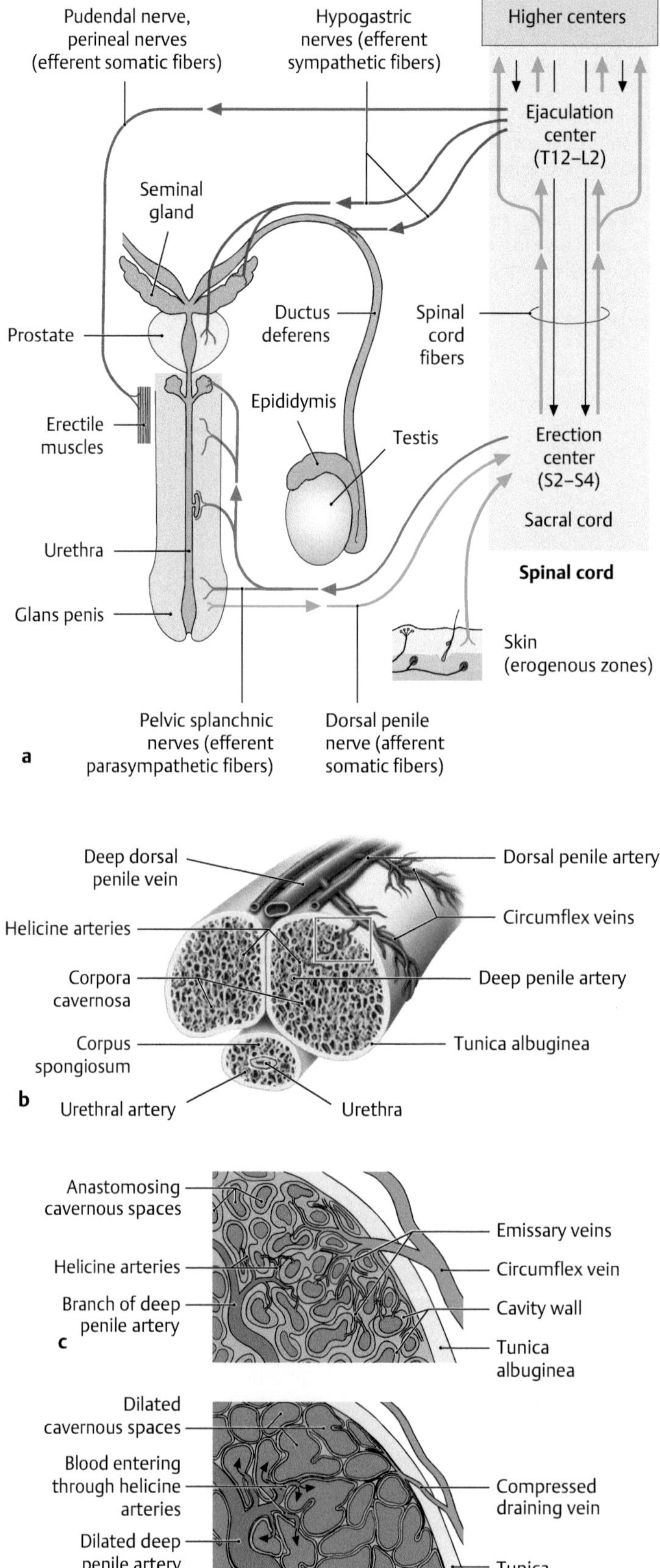

Fig. 4.72 **(a)** Overview of the male sexual reflexes. **(b)** Penis is cross section showing the blood vessels involved in erection. **(c)** Corpus cavernosum in the flaccid state. **(d)** Corpus cavernosum in the erect state. (From Schuenke M, Schulte E, Schumacher U. THIEME Atlas of Anatomy. General Anatomy and Musculoskeletal System. Illustrations by Voll M and Wesker K. 3rd ed. New York: Thieme Medical Publishers; 2020.)

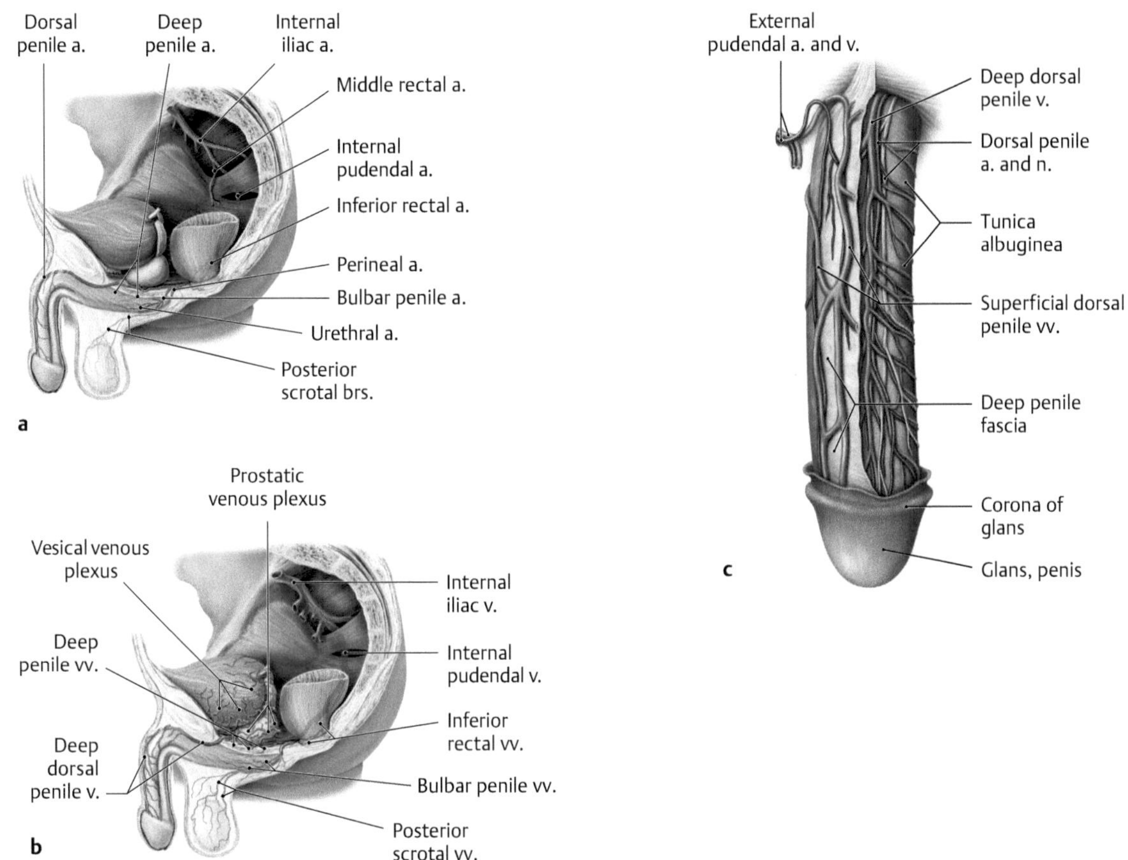

Fig. 4.73 Vasculature of the penis. **(a)** Arterial supply. **(b)** Venous drainage. **(c)** Dorsal vasculature of the penis. (From Schuenke M, Schulte E, Schumacher U. THIEME Atlas of Anatomy. Internal Organs. Illustrations by Voll M and Wesker K. 2nd ed. New York: Thieme Medical Publishers; 2016.)

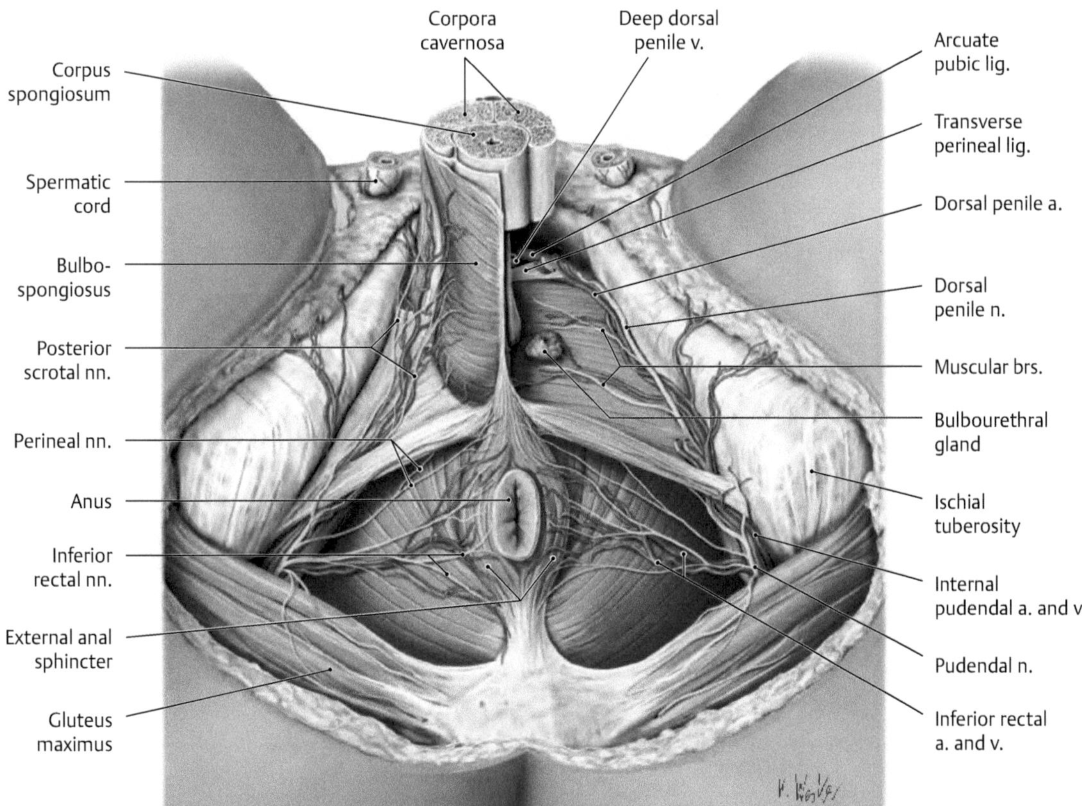

Fig. 4.74 Neurovasculature of the male perineum. (From Schuenke M, Schulte E, Schumacher U. THIEME Atlas of Anatomy. Internal Organs. Illustrations by Voll M and Wesker K. 3rd ed. New York: Thieme Medical Publishers; 2020.)

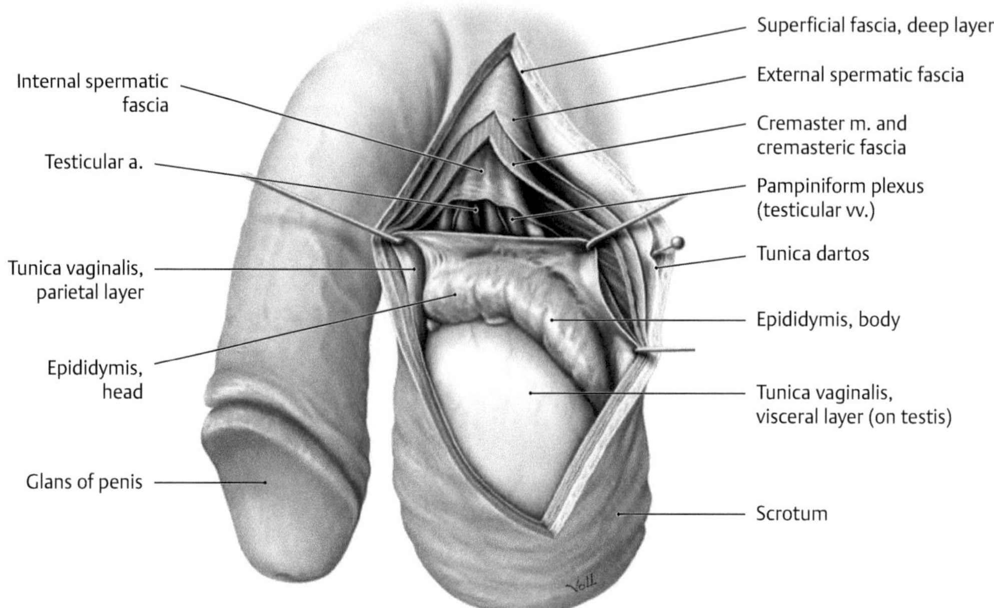

Fig. 4.75 Lateral view of the penis, testis, epididymis, and scrotum. (From Schuenke M, Schulte E, Schumacher U. THIEME Atlas of Anatomy. Internal Organs. Illustrations by Voll M and Wesker K. 3rd ed. New York: Thieme Medical Publishers; 2020.)

and are covered by the bulbospongiosus muscles. They are homologous with the glans penis and corpus spongiosum. The **greater vestibular (*Bartholin*) glands** are located posterolateral to the vaginal orifice and on each side of the vestibule. These round glands are partially overlapped by the bulbs of the vestibule as well as the bulbospongiosus muscles and secrete mucus into the vestibule during sexual arousal (**Fig. 4.77**).

4.36.1 Neurovasculature of the Female Perineum

The **anterior labial nerve** (ilioinguinal br.) and the **genital branch of the genitofemoral nerve** supply the anterior skin of the pudendum. The **posterior labial nerves** (pudendal br.) and **perineal nerves** (posterior cutaneous nerve of the thigh br.)

Clinical Correlate 4.23

Episiotomy

An **episiotomy** is a surgical incision of the perineum and inferoposterior vaginal wall that is done to enlarge the vaginal orifice during labor or vaginal surgery. The intent is to decrease the chance of any excessive and unwanted tearing of the perineum and perineal muscles to occur. This procedure is declining in frequency but may still be used when descent of the fetus is arrested or to expedite delivery when fetal distress is detected.

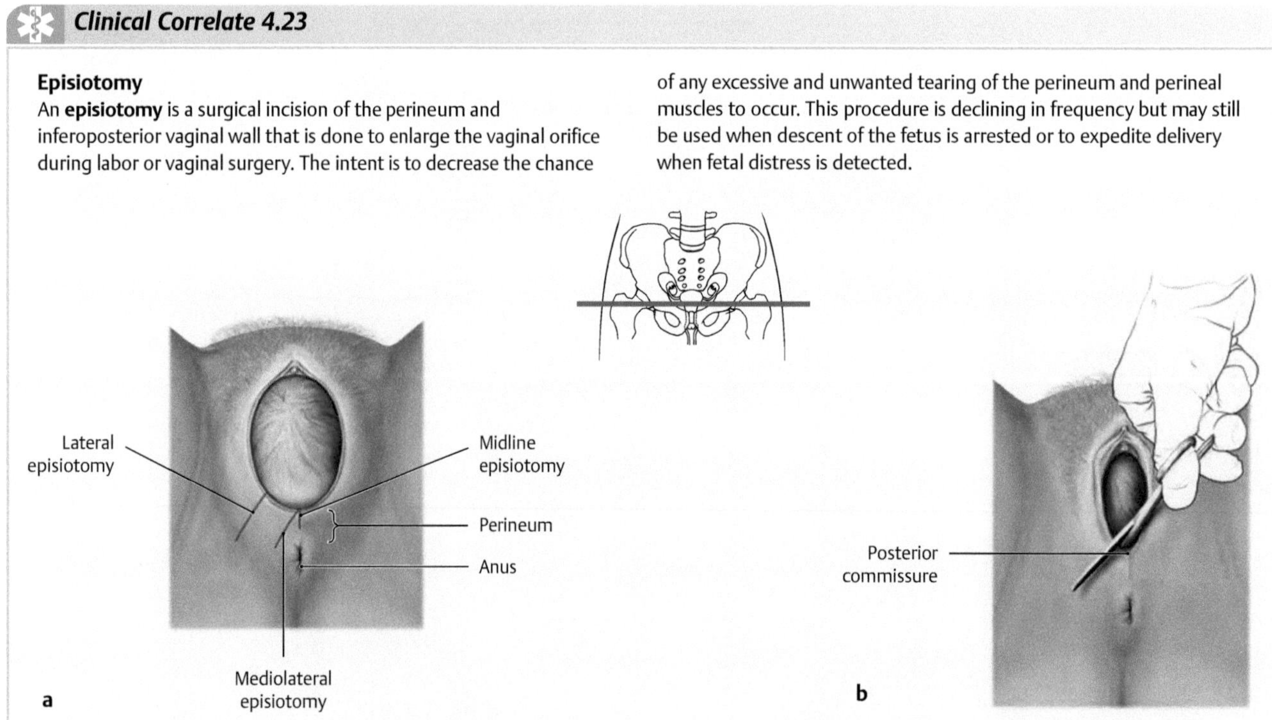

(a) Types of eipsiotomy: midline, mediolateral, and lateral. **(b)** Mediolateral episiotomy performed at the height of a contraction. (From Schuenke M, Schulte E, Schumacher U. THIEME Atlas of Anatomy. Internal Organs. Illustrations by Voll M and Wesker K. 3rd ed. New York: Thieme Medical Publishers; 2020.)

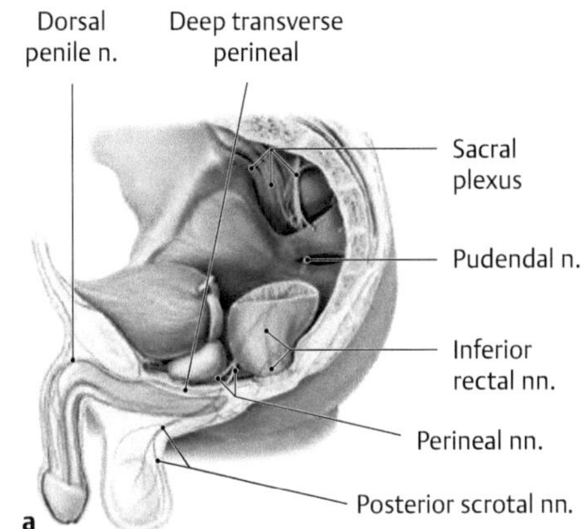

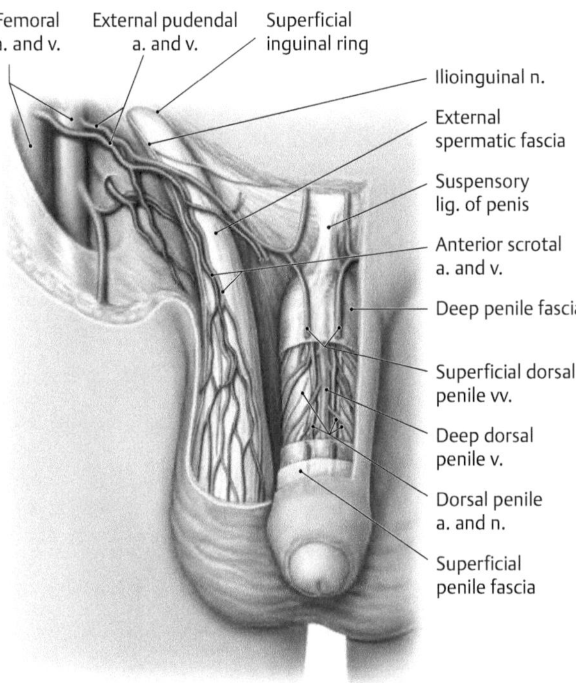

Fig. 4.76 **(a)** Nerve supply of the penis and scrotum. **(b)** Cutaneous innervation of the anterior scrotum and dorsum penis. (From Schuenke M, Schulte E, Schumacher U. THIEME Atlas of Anatomy. Internal Organs. Illustrations by Voll M and Wesker K. 2nd ed. New York: Thieme Medical Publishers; 2016.)

supply the posterior skin of the pudendum. The **deep** and **superficial perineal nerves** (pudendal brs.) supply the superficial perineal muscles and orifice of the vagina. The **dorsal (clitoral) nerve of the clitoris** (pudendal br.) supplies the sensation of the clitoris and innervation to some deep perineal muscles. The **cavernous nerves** via the **uterovaginal plexus** deliver parasympathetics to the bulb of the vestibule and the erectile tissue of the clitoris (**Fig. 4.78**).

The blood supply to the pudendum is primarily from the **internal pudendal** artery with its branches suppling most of the skin, external genitalia and perineal muscles. These branches can include the **perineal**, **dorsal (clitoral) artery of the clitoris**, **artery of the vestibular bulb** and **posterior labial arteries**. Branches of the **external pudendal artery** supply the mons pubis and anterior labial regions. Venous drainage mirrors the blood supply (**Fig. 4.79**). Lymphatic drainage of the pudendum is primarily to the **superficial inguinal lymph nodes**. The glans of the clitoris and anterior labia minora drain to the **deep inguinal** or **internal iliac lymph nodes**.

4.37 External Genitalia Development

The external genitalia are sexually undifferentiated from the 4th – 7th weeks of development. Distinguishing sexual characteristics begin to appear during the 9th week, but the external genitalia are not fully differentiated until the 12th week of development. During the 3rd week, proliferating mesenchyme from near the primitive streak migrate around the cloacal membrane and form **cloacal folds**, and these folds during the 4th week unite to form the **genital tubercle** in both sexes at the cranial end of the cloacal membrane. **Genital (urogenital) folds** and **genital swellings** soon develop on each side of the cloacal membrane (**Fig. 4.80**).

Masculinization of the indifferent external genitalia is induced by **testosterone**. The genital tubercle elongates to form a **phallus** that ultimately becomes the **glans penis, corpus spongiosum** and **corpora cavernosa**. The genital folds form the lateral walls of the **urethral groove** on the ventral surface of the penis. This groove is lined by a proliferation of endodermal cells, the **urethral plate**, which extends from the phallic portion of the urogenital sinus. The genital folds fuse with each other to form the **spongy urethra** and the **penile raphe**. The genital swellings in the male are known as the **scrotal swellings** and they fuse along the **scrotal raphe** to form the **scrotum**. An ingrowth of ectoderm near the periphery of the glans eventually breaks down and forms the **prepuce** (foreskin).

The development of a **phallus** is similar in the female; however, it gradually decreases in its overall size and becomes the clitoris. Both the glans and crura of the clitoris along with the bulb of the vestibule originate from the phallus. The **genital folds** only fuse posteriorly and form the **frenulum of the labia minora**. The unfused parts of the genital folds form the **labia minora**. The **labial swellings** form the **labia majora, mons pubis**, and the **anterior** and **posterior labial commissures**.

4.38 Anal Triangle

The **anal triangle** is located between the lines connecting the ischial tuberosities and the coccyx. It contains the anal canal and anus surrounded by ischioanal fat or fat bodies. The **fat bodies** fill the larger wedge-shaped and fascia-lined spaces known as the **ischioanal fossae** located between the skin of the anal region and pelvic diaphragm. The fat bodies support the anal canal and permit expansion of the anal canal during the passage of feces. A communication exists between them by way of the deep postanal space superior to the **anococcygeal ligament**. The borders of these fossae are (**Fig. 4.65; Fig. 4.66; Fig. 4.81**):

- Anteriorly: bodies of the pubic bones, inferior to the origin of the puborectalis. These parts of the fossae are known as the **anterior recesses of the ischioanal fossae** and they extend into the urogenital triangle superior to the perineal membrane.
- Posteriorly: the sacrotuberous ligament and gluteus maximus.
- Medially: the external anal sphincter and the sloping medial wall or roof formed by the levator ani.
- Laterally: the ischium and inferior part of obturator internus covered with obturator fascia.
- Apex: where the levator ani and obturator internus muscles meet.

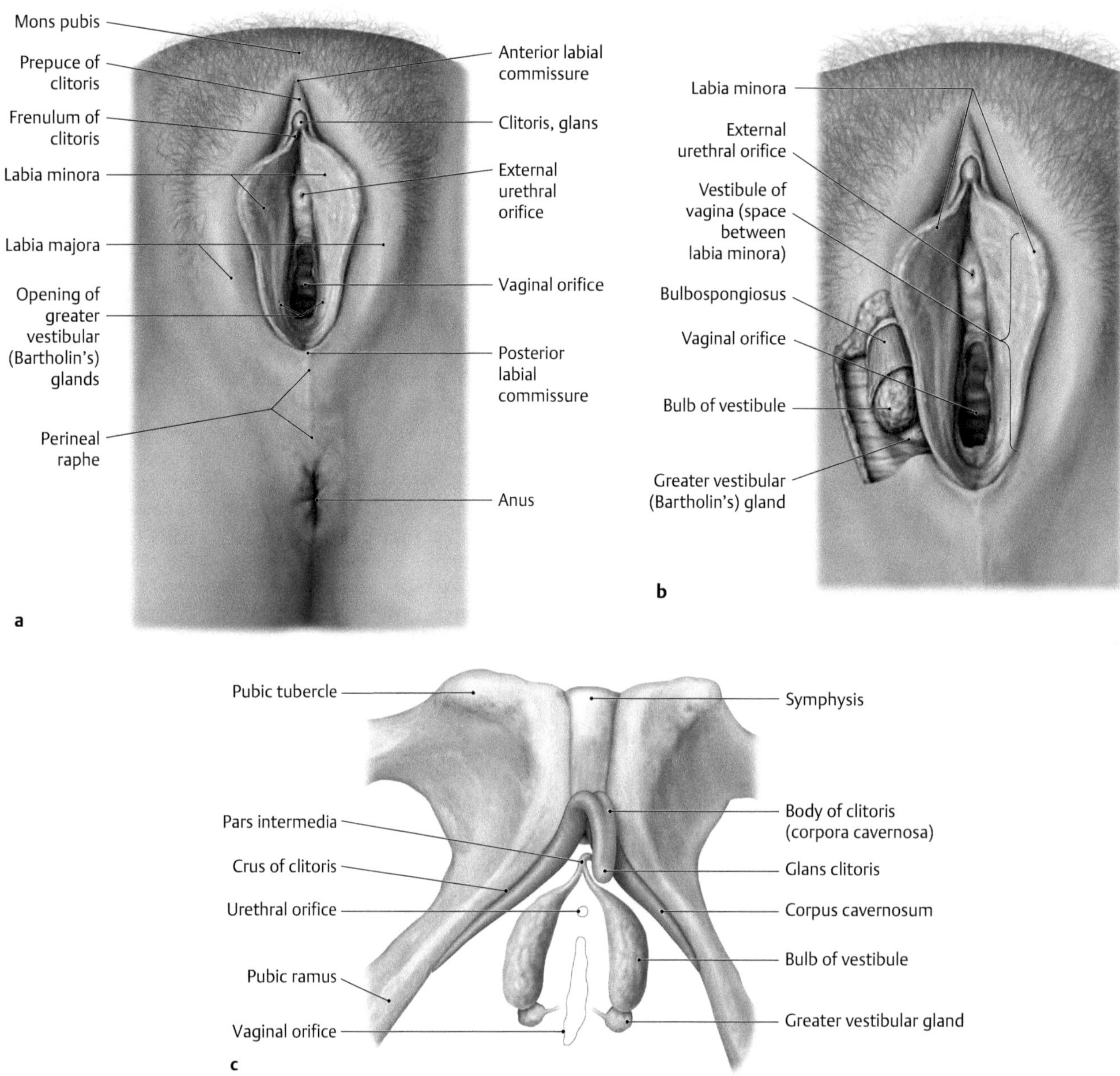

Fig. 4.77 **(a)** Female external genitalia with the labia minora separated and in the lithotomy position. **(b)** Exposure of the vestibule and vestibular glands. **(c)** Erectile tissue in the female perineum. (From Schuenke M, Schulte E, Schumacher U. THIEME Atlas of Anatomy. Internal Organs. Illustrations by Voll M and Wesker K. 3rd ed. New York: Thieme Medical Publishers; 2020.)

Clinical Correlate 4.24

Male Genitalia Defects

When the fusion of the urethral folds is incomplete and abnormal openings of the urethra occur along the inferior aspect of the penis, usually near the glans, along the shaft, or near the base of the penis this is known as hypospadias. When the urethral meatus is found on the dorsum of the penis this is called epispadias. It is rare and is most often associated with *exstrophy of the bladder* and abnormal closure of the anterior body wall. If the genital tubercle splits it may result in a bifid penis (double penis) and if there is not enough androgen stimulation due to a pituitary dysfunction or hypogonadism this may lead to the development of a micropenis.

4.38.1 Pudendal Canal

The **pudendal canal** (Alcock's canal) is the horizontal passageway found on the lateral walls of the ischioanal fossae within the obturator fascia covering the medial aspect of the obturator internus muscle (**Fig. 4.81**). It originates at the posterior border of the ischioanal fossa and runs from the lesser sciatic notch adjacent to the ischial spine to the posterior edge of the perineal membrane. The contents include the **pudendal nerve**, **internal pudendal vessels** and the **nerve to obturator internus**. The pudendal nerve and internal pudendal vessels are the primary source of neurovasculature to the perineum. Just as they enter the pudendal canal, they give rise to the **inferior rectal artery/nerve**, structures that supply the external anal sphincter and peri-anal skin.

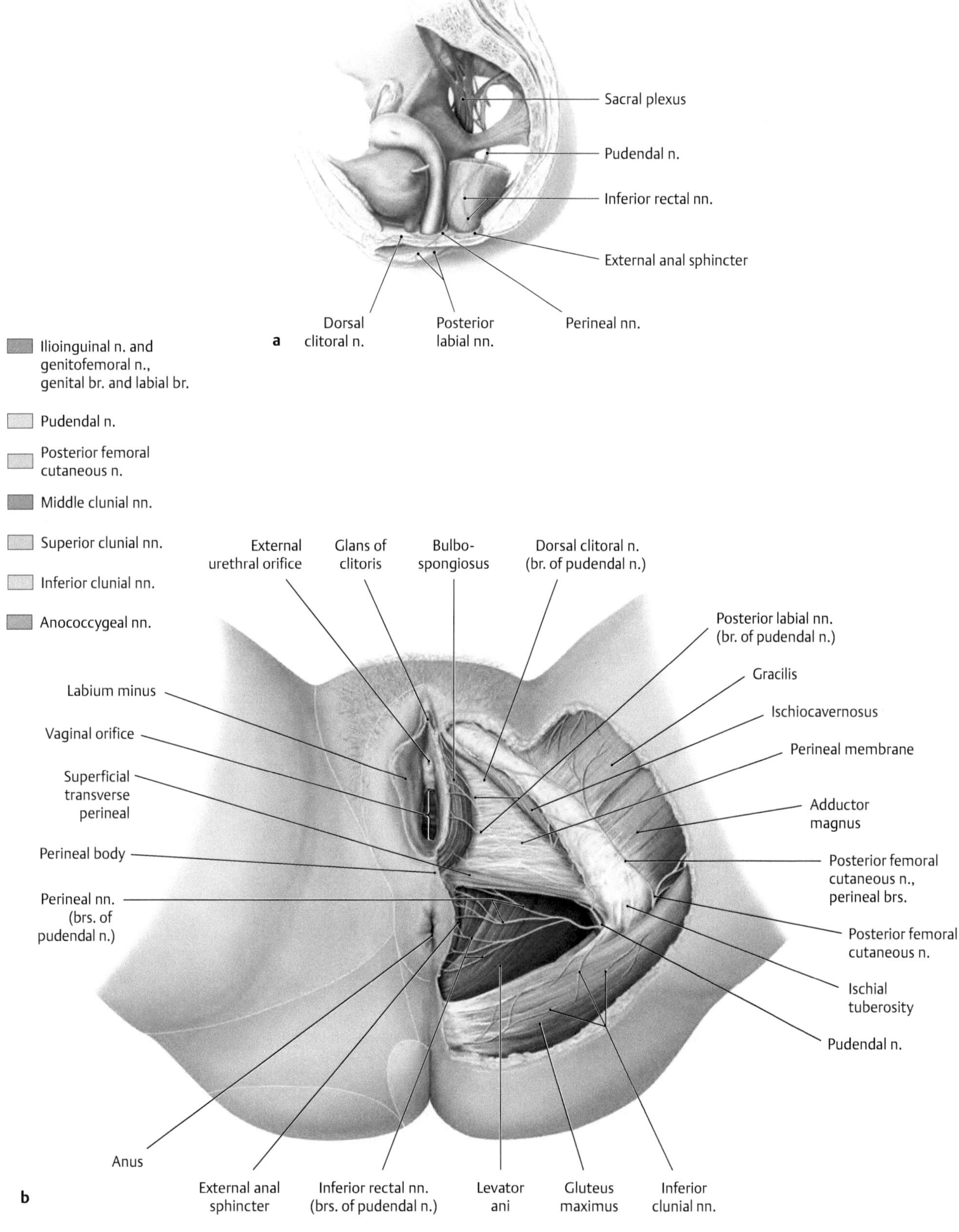

Fig. 4.78 **(a)** Nerves of the female genitalia and perineum. **(b)** Innervation of the female perineum. (From Schuenke M, Schulte E, Schumacher U. THIEME Atlas of Anatomy. Internal Organs. Illustrations by Voll M and Wesker K. 2nd ed. New York: Thieme Medical Publishers; 2016.)

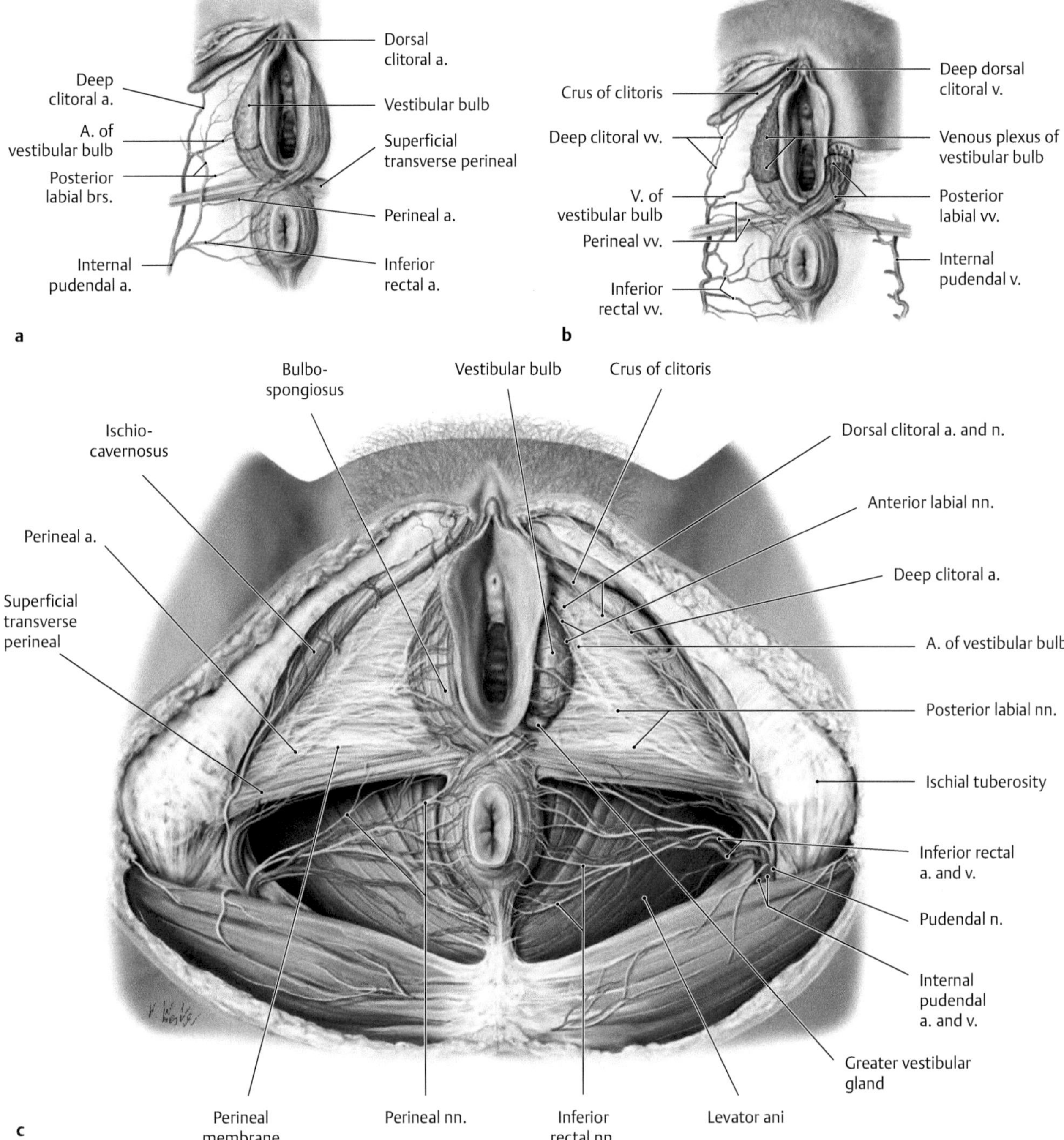

Fig. 4.79 **(a, b)** Blood vessels of the female external genitalia. **(c)** Neurovasculature of the female perineum. Bulbospongiosus and ischiocavernous muscles removed from left side. (From Schuenke M, Schulte E, Schumacher U. THIEME Atlas of Anatomy. Internal Organs. Illustrations by Voll M and Wesker K. 2nd ed. New York: Thieme Medical Publishers; 2016.)

Near the distal end of the pudendal canal, the pudendal nerve and internal pudendal artery give rise to the **perineal nerve/artery** and **dorsal nerve/artery of the penis/clitoris**. The perineal branches distribute mostly to the superficial pouch while the dorsal nerve/artery branches pass through the deep pouch **(Fig. 4.74; Fig. 4.79)**.

Near the perineal membrane, the perineal nerve bifurcates into the superficial and deep perineal nerves. The **superficial perineal nerve** gives rise to the **posterior scrotal/labial** cutaneous branches while the **deep perineal nerve** supplies muscles of the deep and superficial perineal pouches, skin of the vestibule, and mucosa of the inferiormost vagina. The **perineal artery** terminates as the **posterior scrotal/labial** and **artery of the bulb of penis/vestibule**. The **dorsal nerve/artery of the penis/clitoris** passes through deep perineal pouch before reaching the dorsum of the penis or clitoris. These are the primary sensory nerves serving the male or female organ especially the distal glans region **(Fig. 4.78; Fig. 4.79; Fig. 4.82)**.

4.39 Anal Canal

The **anal canal** is the terminal portion of the large intestine and has been discussed extensively in Chapter 3. To summarize, the anal canal begins where the ampulla of the rectum narrows at the level of the U-shaped sling called the **anorectal flexure**. This flexure is roughly 80° and it is an important mechanism for fecal continence. The flexure is maintained during the resting state by

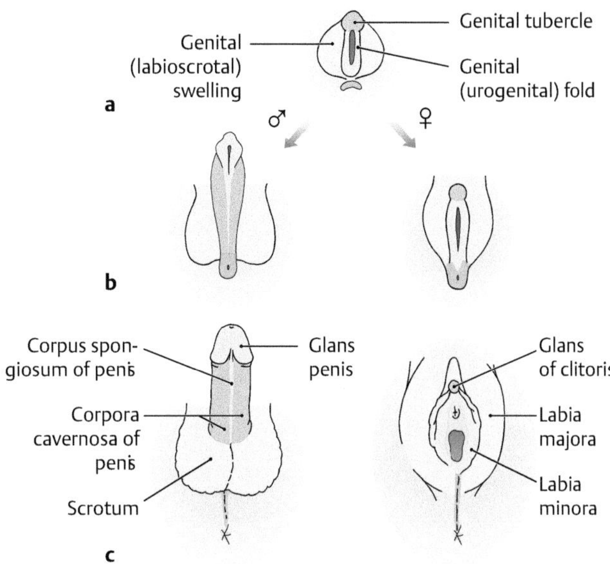

Fig. 4.80 Development of the external genitalia. **(a)** Undifferentiated external genitalia in a six-week-old embryo. **(b)** Differentiation of the external genitalia along male and female lines in a 10-week-old fetus. **(c)** Differentiated external genitalia in the newborn. (From Schuenke M, Schulte E, Schumacher U. THIEME Atlas of Anatomy. Internal Organs. Illustrations by Voll M and Wesker K. 3rd ed. New York: Thieme Medical Publishers; 2020.)

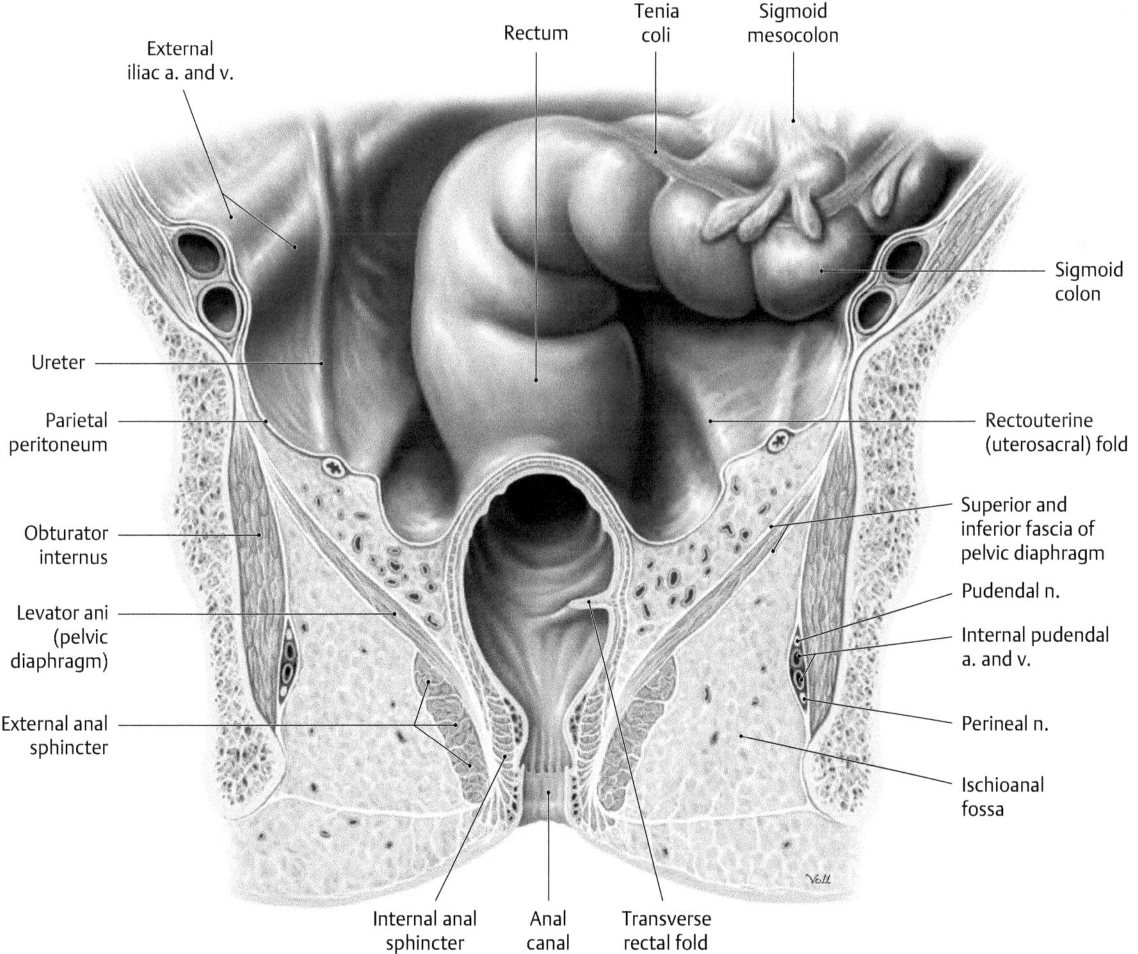

Fig. 4.81 Anal triangle and pudendal canal. (From Schuenke M, Schulte E, Schumacher U. THIEME Atlas of Anatomy. Internal Organs. Illustrations by Voll M and Wesker K. 3rd ed. New York: Thieme Medical Publishers; 2020.)

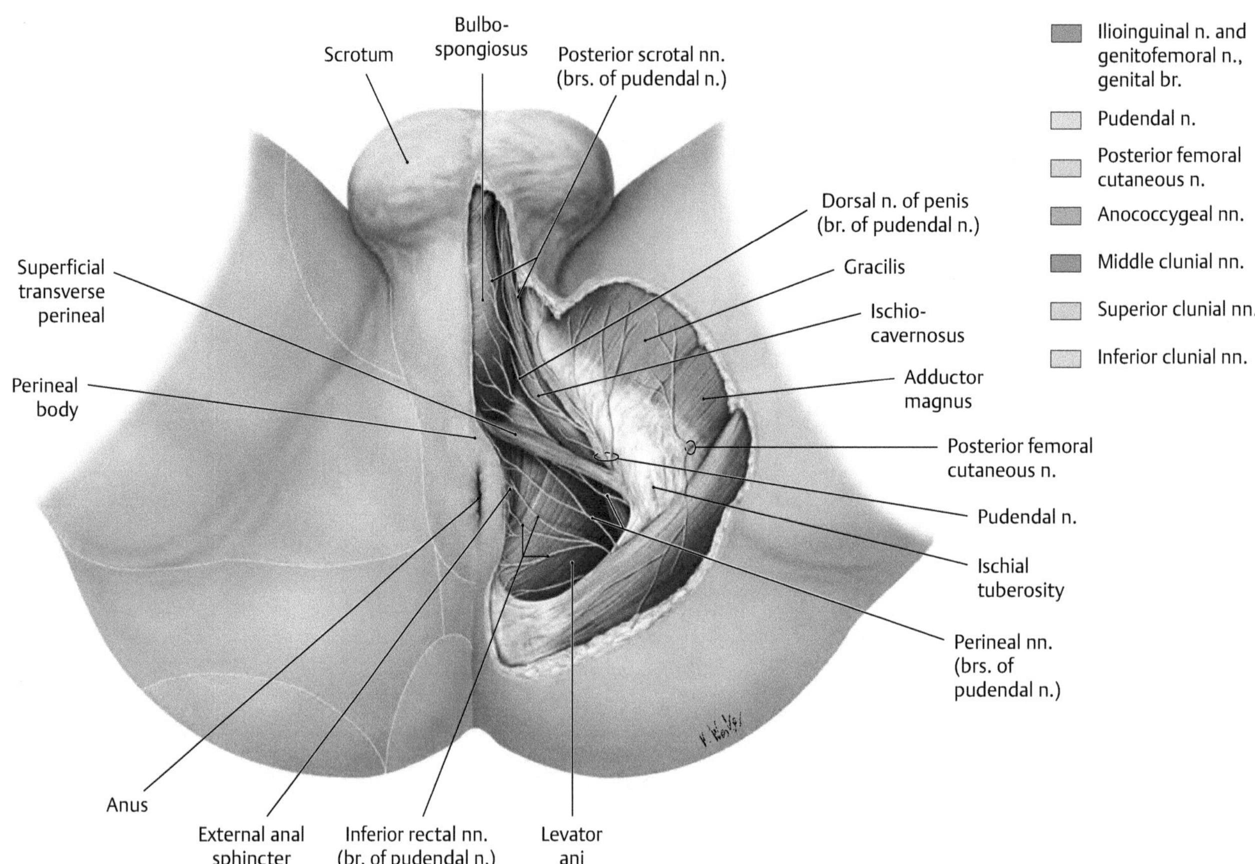

Fig. 4.82 Nerves of the male perineum and genitalia. (From Schuenke M, Schulte E, Schumacher U. THIEME Atlas of Anatomy. Internal Organs. Illustrations by Voll M and Wesker K. 3rd ed. New York: Thieme Medical Publishers; 2020.)

Clinical Correlate 4.25

Pudendal Nerve Block

A pudendal nerve block is performed by injecting a local anesthetic agent into the tissues surrounding the pudendal nerve in order to relieve pain associated with child birth. The ischial spine is first palpated transvaginally before a needle can be inserted adjacent to the fingers already present in the vagina (transvaginal approach) or guided to the ischial spine through the external perineum (perineal approach). The injection site is where the pudendal nerve crosses the lateral aspect of the sacrospinous ligament near its attachment to the ischial spine. This type of nerve block anesthetizes most of the perineum but the anterior perineum is still innervated by the ilioinguinal nerve, thus an ilioinguinal nerve block can be done to fully knock out pain to the perineum.

Clinical Correlate 4.26

Anesthesia for Childbirth

There are several types of regional anesthesia used to reduce pain during childbirth. A **lumbar epidural** or **spinal block via lumbar puncture** (into the subarachnoid space) anesthetizes somatic and visceral efferent fibers distributed below the waist level and this essentially anesthetizes the uterus, entire birth canal, perineum and in addition the lower limbs. For participatory childbirth, a **caudal epidural block** can be used but it must be administered in advance of childbirth, which is not possible with precipitous birth. The anesthesia is administered using an indwelling catheter through the sacral canal enabling additional anesthetic agent to be administered for a longer effect. It anesthetizes areas from the level of the *pelvic pain line* and inferiorly. The birth canal is anesthetized with this approach but the uterine contractions are still felt.

the tonus of the puborectalis muscle and by its active contraction during peristaltic contractions if defecation is not to occur (**Fig. 4.83**). The anal canal terminates at the external outlet of the GI tract known as the **anus.**

The superior portion is characterized by a series of longitudinal ridges called **anal columns** and they contain the terminal branches of the superior rectal vessels. The superior ends of the anal columns serve as the border between the rectum and anal canal known as the **anorectal junction. Anal valves** join the inferior ends of the anal columns and superior to these valves are the small recesses called **anal sinuses**. The **pectinate (dentate) line** is located at the inferior limit of the anal valves and indicates the junction of the *superior part* (derived from hindgut) and *inferior part* (derived from embryonic proctodeum) of the anal canal. Histologically, the *simple columnar epithelium* of the upper anal canal abruptly changes to a *stratified squamous epithelium* at the pectinate line (**Fig. 4.84**).

The anal canal is surrounded by the internal and external anal sphincters and descends posteroinferiorly between the **anococcygeal ligament** and **perineal body**. The **internal anal sphincter** is an involuntary smooth muscle that forms around the superior two-thirds of the anal canal. It is a thickening of the circular muscle layer. Sympathetics stimulate and maintain contraction while parasympathetics inhibit the muscle and allow passive expansion so defecation can occur. The anal canal is generally collapsed but both sphincters must relax before defecation can occur. The **external anal sphincter** is a voluntary skeletal muscle that forms a broad band around the inferior two-thirds of the anal canal. It is made up of three zones called the **subcutaneous**, **superficial** and **deep zones** and it blends superiorly with the puborectalis muscle **(Fig. 4.84)**.

4.39.1 Neurovasculature and Lymphatic Drainage of the Anal Canal

Superior to the pectinate line, autonomic fibers from the **rectal plexus** (sym/post and para/pre) innervate the smooth muscle of the internal anal sphincter and this region is sensitive to stretching only. *Inferior to the pectinate line*, the **inferior rectal nerves** innervate the skeletal muscle of the external anal sphincter and this region is sensitive to touch, pain and temperature **(Fig. 4.85)**.

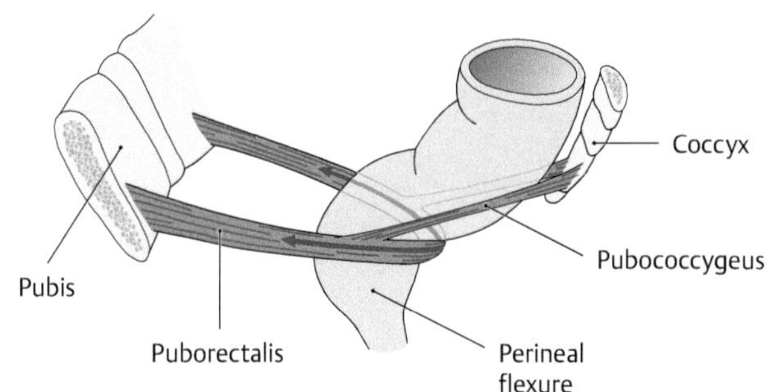

Fig. 4.83 Anorectal flexure. (From Schuenke M, Schulte E, Schumacher U. THIEME Atlas of Anatomy. Internal Organs. Illustrations by Voll M and Wesker K. 3rd ed. New York: Thieme Medical Publishers; 2020.)

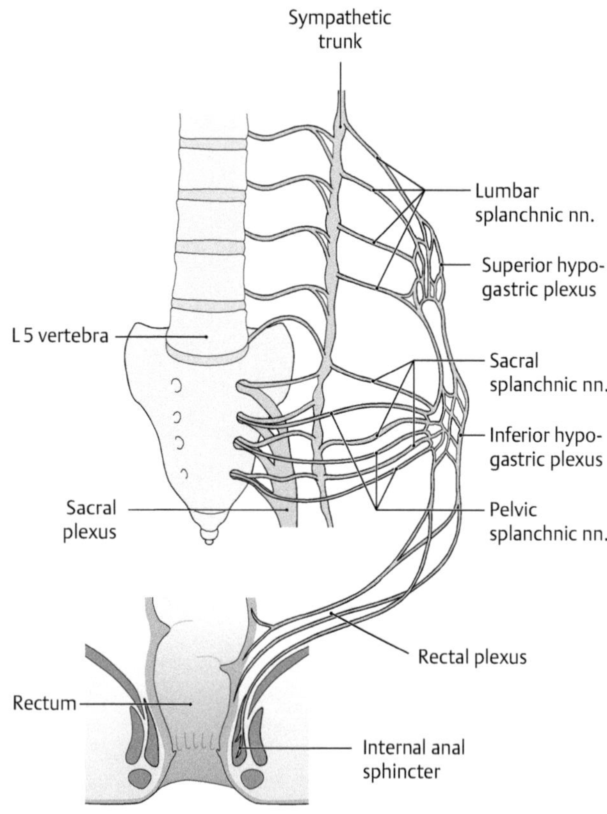

Fig. 4.85 Visceromotor and viscerosensory innervation of the rectum and anal canal. (From Schuenke M, Schulte E, Schumacher U. THIEME Atlas of Anatomy. Internal Organs. Illustrations by Voll M and Wesker K. 3rd ed. New York: Thieme Medical Publishers; 2020.)

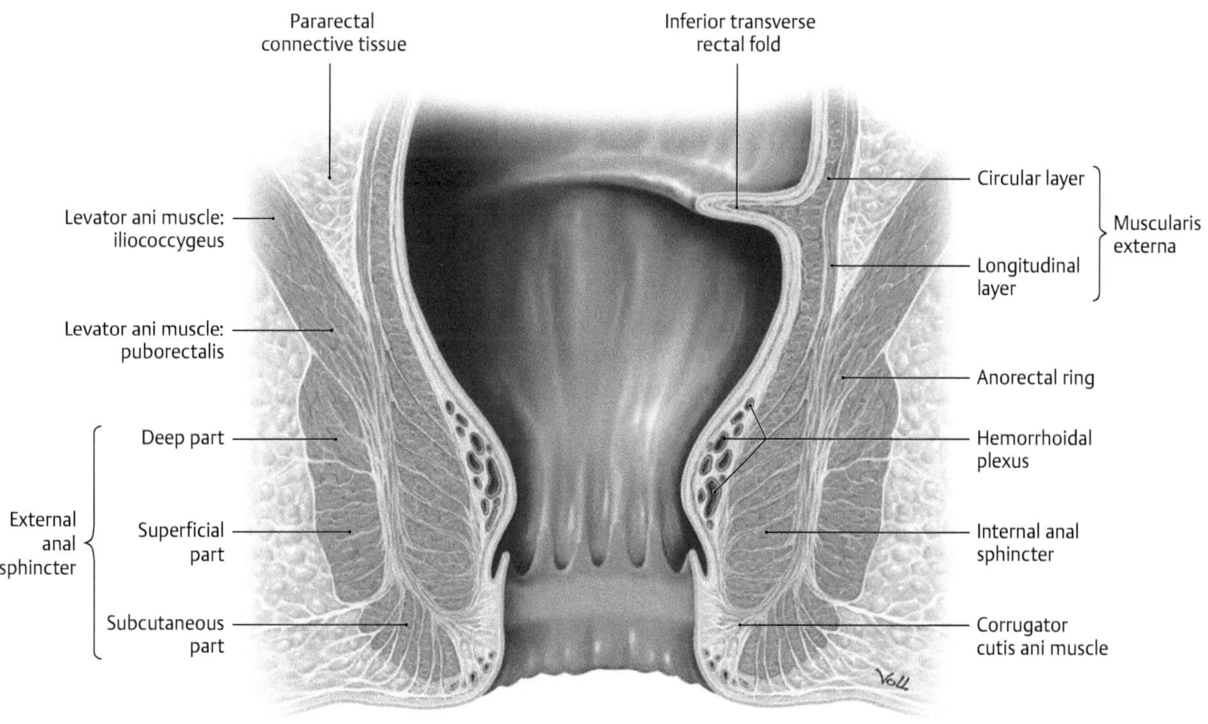

Fig. 4.84 Anal canal. (From Schuenke M, Schulte E, Schumacher U. THIEME Atlas of Anatomy. Internal Organs. Illustrations by Voll M and Wesker K. 1st ed. New York: Thieme Medical Publishers; 2010.)

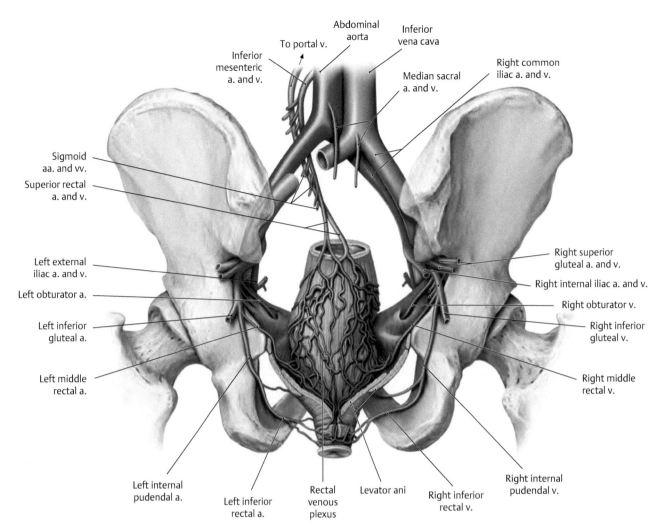

Fig. 4.86 Blood vessels of the rectum, posterior view. (From Schuenke M, Schulte E, Schumacher U. THIEME Atlas of Anatomy. Internal Organs. Illustrations by Voll M and Wesker K. 3rd ed. New York: Thieme Medical Publishers; 2020.)

Blood supply *superior to the pectinate line* is from the **superior rectal artery** while *inferior to the pectinate line* it is the **inferior rectal artery**. The **middle rectal artery** forms an anastomosis with the superior and inferior rectal arteries resulting in redundant blood supply **(Fig. 4.86)**. The venous drainage originates from the **external rectal** and **internal rectal venous plexuses** before mirroring the blood supply and it drains to the portal system above the pectinate line and the caval system below the pectinate line. Lymph drainage superior to pectinate line is to the **internal iliac lymph nodes** and while inferior to the pectinate line lymph drains to the **superficial inguinal lymph nodes (Fig. 4.87)**.

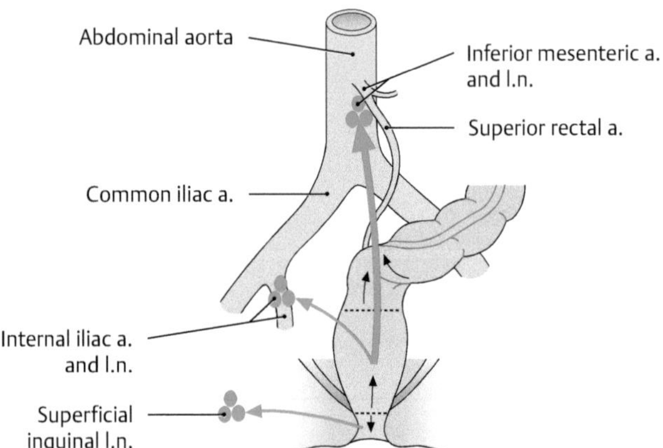

Fig. 4.87 Lymphatic drainage of the rectum and anal canal. (From Schuenke M, Schulte E, Schumacher U. THIEME Atlas of Anatomy. Internal Organs. Illustrations by Voll M and Wesker K. 3rd ed. New York: Thieme Medical Publishers; 2020.)

4.40 Radiology of the Pelvis

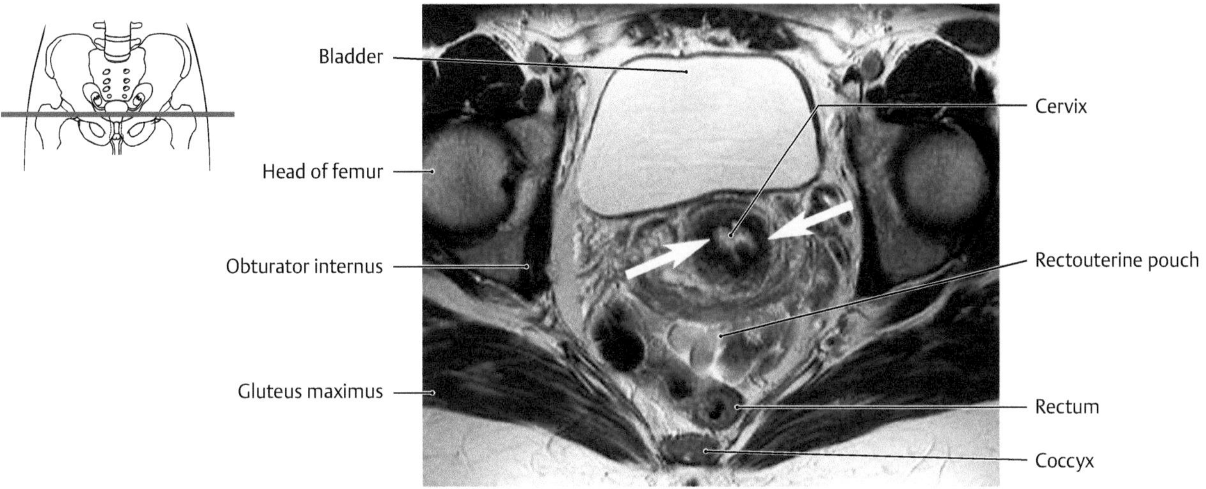

Fig. 4.88 MRI of female pelvis: Transverse section, inferior view. (From Hamm B. et al. MRT von Abdomen und Becken, 2nd ed. Stuttgart: Thieme; 2006.)

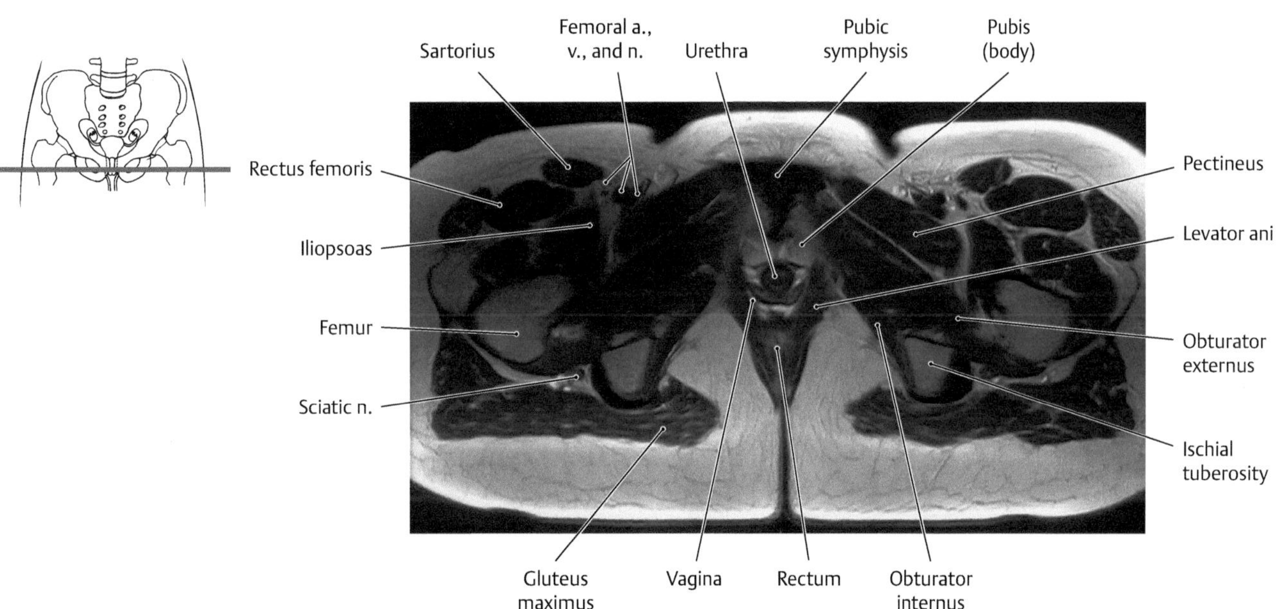

Fig. 4.89 MRI of female pelvis: Transverse section, inferior view. (From Moeller TB, Reif E. Pocket Atlas of Sectional Anatomy, Vol. 2, 4th ed. New York, NY: Thieme; 2014.)

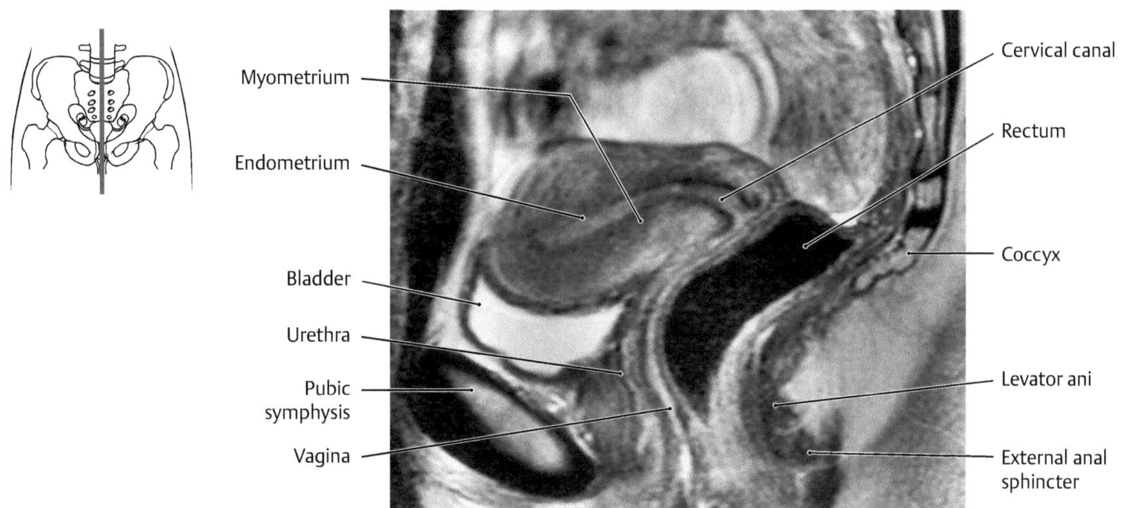

Fig. 4.90 MRI of female pelvis: Transverse section, inferior view. (From Hamm B. et al. MRT von Abdomen und Becken, 2nd ed. Stuttgart: Thieme; 2006.)

Rectus abdominis
Prostate
Seminal gland
Sacrum
Bladder
Rectovesical (Denonvillier) fascia
Ampulla of rectum
Pubic symphysis
Corpus cavernosum of penis
Anal canal
Corpus spongiosum of penis
Bulb of penis

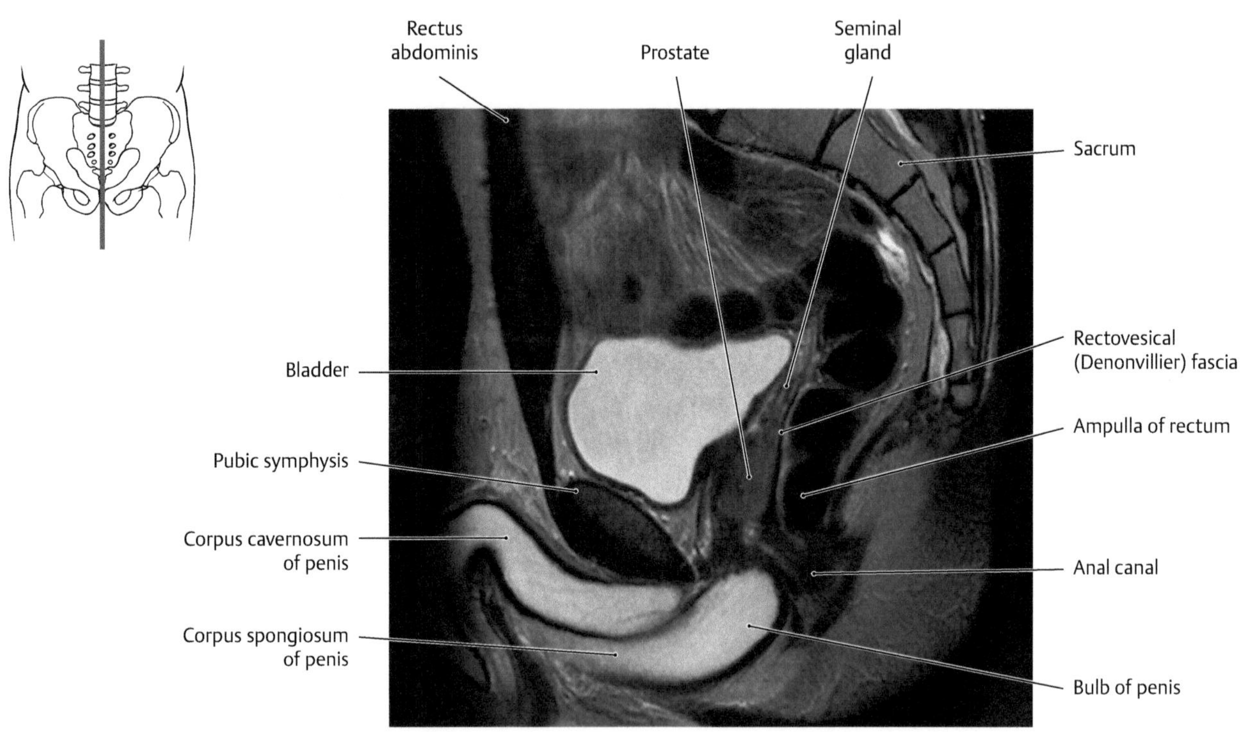

Fig. 4.91 MRI of male pelvis: Sagittal section, left lateral view. (From Hamm B. et al. MRT von Abdomen und Becken, 2nd ed. Stuttgart: Thieme; 2006.)

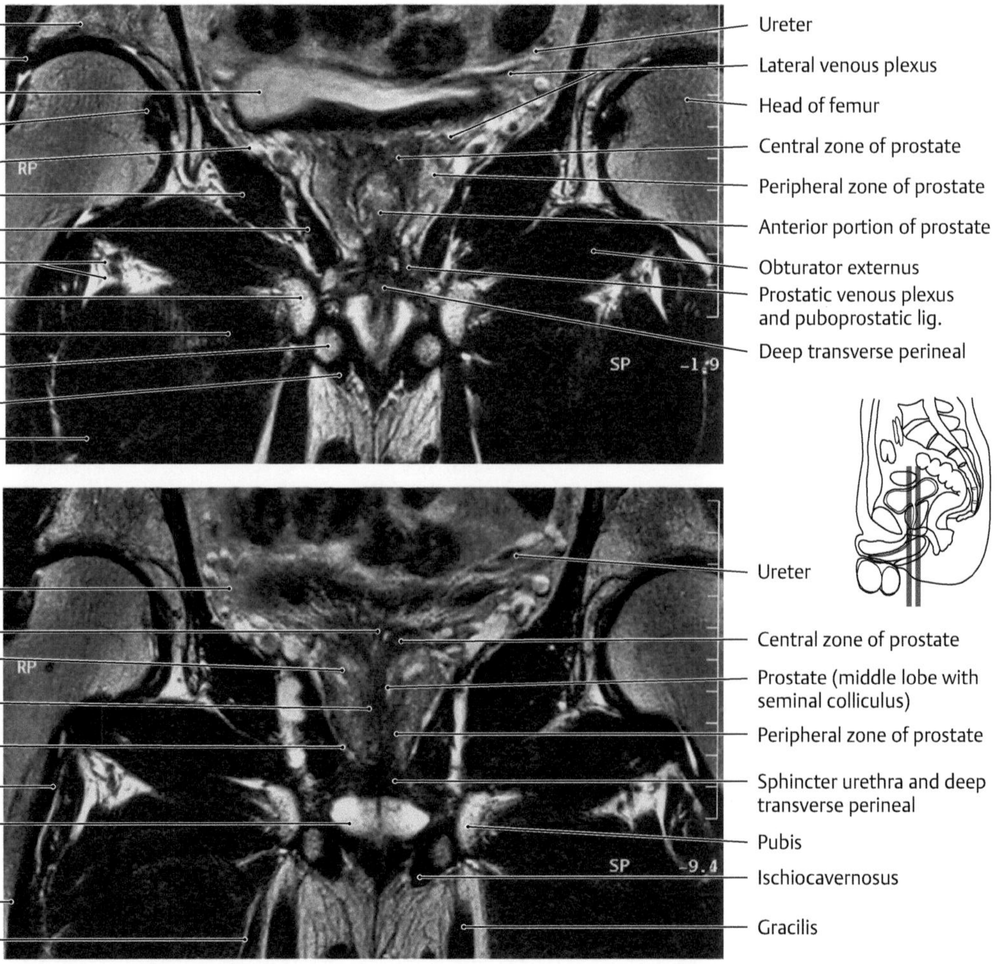

Ilium (acetabular roof)
Hip joint
Urinary bladder
Lig. of head of femur
Seminal vesicle
Obturator internus
Levator ani
Medial circumflex femoral a.
Pubis
Adductor minimus
Corpus cavernosum
Ischiocavernosus
Adductor brevis
Ureter
Lateral venous plexus
Head of femur
Central zone of prostate
Peripheral zone of prostate
Anterior portion of prostate
Obturator externus
Prostatic venous plexus and puboprostatic lig.
Deep transverse perineal
RP
SP
-1.9
Lateral venous plexus
Urethra
Ejaculatory duct
Seminal colliculus
Capsule of prostate
Pectineus
Corpus spongiosum
Iliopsoas
Adductor magnus
Ureter
Central zone of prostate
Prostate (middle lobe with seminal colliculus)
Peripheral zone of prostate
Sphincter urethra and deep transverse perineal
Pubis
Ischiocavernosus
Gracilis
RP
SP
-9.4

Fig. 4.92 Coronal sections, anterior views. (From Gilroy AM et al. Atlas of Anatomy. 3rd ed. New York: Thieme Medical Publishers; 2016.)

PRACTICE QUESTIONS

1. A 41-year-old woman complains of a deep sensation that feels to be pushing down into her vagina and this is leading her to also have frequent but burning sensations when urinating. On examination it is confirmed that she has a uterine prolapse. Which of the following structures provides the main passive support for the uterus?
   A. Round ligament of the uterus.
   B. Cardinal (transverse cervical) ligaments.
   C. Mesosalpinx of broad ligament.
   D. Suspensory (infundibulopelvic) ligaments.
   E. Uterosacral ligaments.
2. Which of the following statements regarding the innervation of the pelvic structures is INCORRECT?
   A. Parasympathetics are inhibitory to the internal urethral sphincter.
   B. Cells bodies of visceral pain fibers below the pelvic pain line are located in the S2-S4 dorsal root ganglion.
   C. Cell bodies of visceral pain fibers above the pelvic pain line are located in the thoracic and lumbar dorsal root ganglion.
   D. Sympathetics are motor to the detrusor muscle of the bladder.
   E. The functional components of the pudendal nerve are GSE, GSA, and GVE-sym/post.
3. Which zone of the prostate do the ejaculatory ducts initially pass through before reaching the prostatic urethra?
   A. Anterior zone.
   B. Peripheral zone.
   C. Central zone.
   D. Periurethral zone.
   E. Transition zone.
4. Which statement regarding the overall pelvic cavity is INCORRECT?
   A. The subpubic angle of a female is between 90-100 degrees.
   B. The urogenital hiatus is formed by the puborectalis muscle of the levator ani.
   C. The interspinous diameter is the narrowest diameter of the pelvic outlet and pelvic canal.
   D. The sacroiliac joint is a combined synovial and syndesmosis joint.
   E. Superior to pelvic pain line – parasympathetic fibers transmit visceral pain fibers.
5. A physician is inserting a catheter into the male urethra and is initially too forceful with it. The catheter pierces the spongy (penile) urethra near the bulb of the penis. Into what space would leaking urine or blood (extravasation) pass through?
   A. Deep perineal space.
   B. Superficial perineal space.
   C. Retrorectal (presacral) space.
   D. Rectouterine space.
   E. Retropubic (prevesical) space.
6. The adult uterus is usually ____ (longitudinal cervical axis being tipped anteriorly relative to the longitudinal axis of the vagina) and ____ (angle created between the longitudinal uterine body axis relative to the longitudinal cervical axis)?
   A. Retroflexed and Anteverted.
   B. Anteflexed and Anteverted.
   C. Retroflexed and Retroverted.
   D. Anteverted and Anteflexed.
   E. Retroverted and Anteflexed.
7. Walthard cell rests are benign clusters of epithelial cells that appear as white or yellowish cysts. The connective tissue of which pelvic organ would primarily display these epithelial cell clusters?
   A. Uterus.
   B. Prostate.
   C. Urinary bladder.
   D. Uterine tubes.
   E. Vagina.
8. Which statement about the prostate is INCORRECT?
   A. Two-thirds of the prostate is glandular with the other one-third fibromuscular.
   B. Prostatic fluid accounts for approximately 25% of total semen volume.
   C. The peripheral zone is the origination site of 70-80% of all prostate cancers.
   D. The prostate is a collection of 30-50 branched tubuloalveolar glands.
   E. Benign prostatic hypertrophy is associated with the anterior fibromuscular zone.
9. Which set of lymph nodes WOULD NOT be involved in the lymphatic drainage of the penis?
   A. Sacral.
   B. Deep inguinal.
   C. Internal iliac.
   D. External iliac.
   E. Superficial inguinal.
10. If a needle passed through the skin covering the superficial perineal space of the UG triangle and headed back to the erectile tissue of the bulb of the penis, in which order of structures/fascia would the needle pass? (Note: disregard any subcutaneous or dartos fascia because the scrotum is reflected superiorly).
    A. Skin, Colles', bulbospongiosus, Gallaudet's, tunica albuginea, Buck's.
    B. Skin, Gallaudet's, bulbospongiosus, Colles', Buck's, tunica albuginea.
    C. Skin, Colles', Gallaudet's, bulbospongiosus, Buck's, tunica albuginea.
    D. Skin, Colles', Gallaudet's, bulbospongiosus, tunica albuginea, Buck's.
    E. Skin, Colles', bulbospongiosus, Gallaudet's, Buck's, tunica albuginea.
11. Which statement about penis innervation during intercourse is INCORRECT?
    A. The cavernous nerves originate from the prostatic nerve plexus.
    B. Contraction of the urethral smooth muscle is due to sympathetic innervation.
    C. Prostatic fluid is released due to sympathetic innervation.
    D. Perineal nerves innervate the bulbospongiosus muscle.
    E. Parasympathetic fibers from the cavernous nerves innervate the helicine arteries.
12. A newborn baby boy presents with abnormal openings of the urethra on the ventral side of his penis and it is noted there was no exstrophy of the bladder. You recall from your anatomy course that this situation is due to the incomplete fusion of the urethral folds. What is your diagnosis?
    A. Hypospadias.
    B. Paraphimosis.
    C. Epispadias.
    D. Phimosis.
    E. Circumcision.

13. During development of the genital ducts, which structure would not originate from the paramesonephric (Müllerian) duct in the female?
    A. Uterine tubes.
    B. Superior one-third of vagina.
    C. Inferior two-thirds of vagina.
    D. Cervix of uterus.
    E. Fundus and body of uterus.

14. Which statement regarding structures of the anal canal is INCORRECT?
    A. The internal anal sphincter surrounds the inferior one-third of the anal canal.
    B. The nerve to the obturator internus passes through the pudendal (Alcock's) canal.
    C. The inferior rectal artery is a branch of the internal pudendal artery.
    D. The external anal sphincter is innervated by the inferior rectal nerve.
    E. The anterior recesses of the ischioanal fossa extend over the deep perineal pouch.

15. Superior to the pectinate line, lymphatic drainage of the anal canal drains to the ________ lymph nodes?
    A. Superficial inguinal.
    B. Internal iliac.
    C. External iliac.
    D. Common iliac.
    E. Pararectal.

16. A pregnant woman comes into the hospital to deliver her baby. The physician decides to perform a pudendal block using the transvaginal approach. What bony structure is the physician trying to locate for orientation purposes so that they may perform the pudendal block correctly?
    A. Tip of the coccyx.
    B. Posterior inferior iliac spine.
    C. Inferior pubic ramus.
    D. Ischial tuberosity.
    E. Ischial spine.

17. Which statement regarding the overall structure of the uterus is INCORRECT?
    A. Detachment of the stratum basalis layer occurs during normal menstruation.
    B. Cervical squamous cell carcinomas predominately occur in the transformation zone.
    C. The endometrium consists of a simple columnar epithelium.
    D. Cervical glands near ovulation secrete a serous and alkaline fluid that facilitates sperm entry.
    E. The proliferative phase of the menstrual cycle is driven by the presence of estrogen.

18. Which statement regarding the overall structure of the ovaries is INCORRECT?
    A. Ovulation is due to an abrupt increase in luteinizing hormone (LH).
    B. After becoming fibrotic the corpus luteum of pregnancy is called the corpus albicans.
    C. The left ovarian vein drains to the left renal vein.
    D. The secondary oocyte begins the second meiotic division but stops at prophase approximately three hours before ovulation.
    E. The ovarian ligament is a remnant of the gubernaculum.

19. A 27-year-old woman trying to conceive has begun to experience occasional sharp abdominal pains but for the past couple of weeks the pain has been more dull or cramping-like. She has also noticed some heavy vaginal bleeding that has promoted her to visit her gynecologist. A transvaginal ultrasound had determined that she has an ectopic pregnancy. What is the most common location for an ectopic pregnancy to occur?
    A. Isthmus of the uterine tube.
    B. Rectouterine pouch (of Douglas).
    C. Ampulla of the uterine tube.
    D. Internal os of cervix.
    E. Ovary.

20. Which of the following structures DOES NOT originate from the pelvic (middle) part of the urogenital sinus?
    A. Female urethra.
    B. Spongy (penile) urethra in males.
    C. Prostatic urethra in males.
    D. Intermediate (membranous) urethra in males.
    E. Intramural (preprostatic) urethra in males.

21. Which one of the sacral plexus nerves listed below is correctly paired with their contributing ventral rami?
    A. Sciatic nerve (L4-L5).
    B. Nerve to quadratus femoris (S1-S2).
    C. Superior gluteal nerve (L4-S1).
    D. Inferior gluteal nerve (S1-S3).
    E. Lumbosacral trunk (L4-S3).

22. A surgeon is working in the area of the posterior laminae of the hypogastric sheath (thick bands of condensed endopelvic fascia) in a female. What structure is at highest risk of being damaged, due to proximity, if the surgeon is not careful?
    A. Uterosacral ligament.
    B. Lateral ligament of the bladder.
    C. Suspensory ligament.
    D. Cardinal ligament.
    E. Lateral ligament of the rectum.

23. A 55 year-old female visits her physician because she has had prolonged pelvic pain, fatigue, loss of appetite, and bloating. An ultrasound has identified fluid in the peritoneal cavity and a structurally normal uterus. The treating physician suspects an epithelial ovarian cancer as a possible diagnosis but would like to obtain a sample of peritoneal fluid by way of a procedure called a culdocentesis. A culodocentesis involves inserting a needle through which space or structure to reach the rectouterine pouch (of Douglas) to obtain this sample?
    A. Posterior fornix of the vagina.
    B. External os of the cervix.
    C. Urethra.
    D. Anterior fornix of the vagina.
    E. Anterior surface of the rectum.

24. The stellate-shaped lumen of the ureter is lined with what type of epithelium?
    A. Simple columnar.
    B. Transitional.
    C. Stratified squamous.
    D. Pseuostratified columnar.
    E. Simple cuboidal.

25. A 35 year-old woman is currently pregnant with her second child and she had a cesarean delivery with her first child. She begins to have bright red vaginal bleeding without pain at 22 weeks and an ultrasound is performed. The images demonstrate that

the bleeding is due to the placenta overlying the internal os of the cervix, which in turn is blocking the cervical canal. What type of abnormal placenta does this individual currently have?
A. Placenta previa.
B. Placenta increta.
C. Placenta percreta.
D. Placenta accreta.

ANSWERS

1. **B.** The main passive support for the uterus is the cardinal (transverse cervical) ligaments.
2. **D.** Parasympathetics are the fibers that are motor to the detrusor muscle of the bladder.
3. **C.** The ejaculatory ducts initially pass through the central zone of the prostate before reaching the prostatic urethra.
4. **E.** Sympathetic fibers transmit visceral pain fibers if you are superior to the pelvic pain line.
5. **B.** Urine or blood leaking through the spongy (penile) urethra due to a urethral tear will pass into the superficial perineal space.
6. **D.** Anteverted and Anteflexed.
7. **D.** The uterine tubes are associated most with Walthard cell rests. They may also be seen in the mesosalpinx or mesovarium of the broad ligament but they may be the precursor to Brenner tumors, a rare type of ovarian surface epithelial tumor.
8. **E.** The periurethral/transitional zone is associated with benign prostatic hypertrophy.
9. **A.** Sacral lymph nodes are not associated with lymphatic drainage of the penis.
10. **C.** If a needle passed from the skin covering the superficial perineal space of the UG triangle and headed back to the erectile tissue of the bulb of the penis, the correct order the needle passes through would be skin, Colles', Gallaudet's, bulbospongiosus muscle, Buck's, and finally the tunica albuginea.
11. **B.** Parasympathetic innervation is responsible for contraction of the urethral smooth muscle during intercourse/ejaculation.
12. **A.** The proper diagnosis would be hypospadias.
13. **C.** The uterine tubes, the entire uterus, and the superior one-third of the vagina all originate from the paramesonephric duct. The inferior two-thirds of the vagina originates from the canalization of the vaginal plate that were originally formed by the fusion of the sinovaginal bulbs.
14. **A.** The internal anal sphincter will surround the superior two-thirds of the anal canal.
15. **B.** Lymphatic drainage of the anal canal superior to the pectinate line is to the internal iliac lymph nodes.
16. **E.** The ischial spine is used for orientation to correctly perform a pudendal nerve block.
17. **A.** During normal menstruation the stratum functionalis layer detaches.
18. **D.** The secondary oocyte will begin the second meiotic division but it will stop at metaphase approximately three hours before ovulation. It does not complete the second meiotic division until after fertilization occurs.
19. **C.** The most common location for an ectopic pregnancy to occur is the ampulla of the uterine tube. An ectopic pregnancy refers to any implantation that takes place outside the uterus and about 95% of all ectopic pregnancies occur in the uterine tube with approximately 80% of those occurring in the ampulla.
20. **B.** The spongy (penile) urethra in males originates from the phallic (caudal) part of the urogenital sinus.
21. **C.** The correct ventral rami contributions to the superior gluteal nerve are L4-S1.
A. Sciatic nerve (L4-S3).
B. Nerve to quadratus femoris (L4-S1).
D. Inferior gluteal nerve (L5-S2).
E. Lumbosacral trunk (L4-L5).
22. **E.** The posterior laminae contain the lateral ligament of the rectum along with the middle rectal vessels.
23. **A.** A needle would be inserted through the posterior fornix of the vagina in order to reach the rectouterine pouch and obtain a sample of peritoneal fluid.
24. **B.** The ureters are lined by a transitional epithelium.
25. **A.** When the placenta overlies the internal os of the cervix this is known as placenta previa. In this situation it will be recommended that the individual refrain from excessive physical activity and possible bed rest. The goal is to get as close to the due date as possible and there is a good chance a cesarean delivery will need to be performed in order to prevent major hemorrhaging or blood loss.

5 Lower Extremities

LEARNING OBJECTIVES

- To understand all the bones associated with the lower extremity and major fractures associated with them.
- To describe the fascial layers of the lower extremity. Clinical correlates include compartment syndromes related to the leg and a fasciotomy.
- To describe the somatic and cutaneous nerve innervation and how the dermatome and myotomes are associated with these nerves.
- To describe the major arteries, veins and general lymphatic drainage of the lower extremity. Clinical correlates include varicose veins, deep vein thrombosis and great saphenous vein grafting.
- To describe the muscles and neurovasculature of the gluteal region. Clinical correlates will include superior gluteal and sciatic nerve injuries, intragluteal injections and bursitis of this region.
- To understand the hip joint and the architecture of the joint capsule, and the ligaments and neurovasculature related to it. Clinical correlates include the difference between posterior and anterior dislocations.
- To describe the muscles and neurovasculature of the posterior thigh and popliteal fossa. Clinical correlates include hamstring injuries and Baker cysts.
- To describe the muscles, neurovasculature, femoral sheath and adductor canal of the anterior thigh region. Clinical correlates include femoral hernias and the reason for cannulation of the femoral vessels.
- To describe the muscles and neurovasculature of the medial thigh region. Clinical correlates include groin pulls, transplantation of the gracilis muscle, and a replaced versus accessory obturator artery.
- To understand the knee joint and the architecture of the joint capsule, and the ligaments and neurovasculature related to it. Clinical correlates include genu varum, genu valgum, the patellar tendon reflex, patellofemoral pain syndrome, chondromalacia patellae, the unhappy triad, knee replacement surgery, prepatellar bursitis and Osgood-Schlatter disease.
- To describe the muscles and neurovasculature of the anterior, lateral and posterior leg compartments. Clinical correlates include shin splints, different nerve entrapments, foot drop, sural nerve grafts, gastrocnemius strains, calcaneal tendon reflex and rupture.
- To understand the tibiofibular articulations and the ankle joint. Describe the ligaments and neurovasculature related to both structures. Clinical correlates include ankle sprains and Pott fractures.
- To describe the muscles, neurovasculature, joints, and arches of the foot. Clinical correlates include plantar fasciitis, plantar reflex, medial planter nerve entrapment, gout, hallux valgus, pes planus, hammer and claw toe.
- To understand the gait cycle.
- To understand lower extremity development. Clinical correlates include the difference between amelia and meromelia, cleft foot, congenital talipes and osteogenesis imperfecta.

5.1 Lower Extremity Overview

The lower extremities are extensions of the trunk region and are responsible for supporting the head and neck, trunk, and upper extremities and are also involved in locomotion and gait. They are divided into regions, which include the gluteal, thigh, knee, leg, ankle (talocrural) and 21 bones of the foot (**Fig. 5.1**).

The bones of the lower extremities are divided into two functional components and they include the pelvic girdle and free lower extremity. The pelvic girdle is the bony ring composed of the bilateral hip bones (ilium, ischium and pubis) and the sacrum which was discussed in detail last chapter. Recall that the sacrum of the pelvic girdle is part of the axial skeleton and the pelvic girdle thus serves as the bridge between the axial and lower portion of the appendicular skeleton. The free lower extremity bones consist of the femur, patella, tibia, fibula, and the numerous foot bones.

The body weight of an individual is transferred from the vertebral column through the sacro-iliac joints, through the pelvic girdle, and then through the hip joints before continuing down through the femurs and beyond. In order to support an erect position more efficiently, the femurs are directed inferomedially as they extend through the thighs so when a person is standing their knees are adjacent and placed directly inferior to the trunk. This will return the center of gravity to the vertical lines of the supporting legs and feet (**Fig. 5.2**).

5.1.1 Hip Bones

The **hip bones**, as mentioned previously, are formed by the fusion of three bones called the ilium, ischium and pubis. The lateral-most features are associated with the lower extremities and thus are described in this section. Up until puberty these three bones are still separated by the Y-shaped **triradiate cartilage** that is found in the center of the acetabulum. Fusion of these three bones does not occur until a person reaches their early to mid-twenties. The **acetabulum** is made of all three hip bones and serves as the socket with which the head of the femur articulates (**Fig. 5.3; Fig. 5.4**).

5.1.2 Ilium

The **ilium** makes up the largest portion of the hip bone and the superior portion of the acetabulum (**Fig. 5.5**). The **body of the ilium** is the junction between the ischium and pubis that help create a portion of the acetabulum. It has thick medial columns responsible for weight bearing but thin and wing-like parts, or **alae**, which provide large areas for attaching muscles. The **anterior superior iliac** (ASIS) and **anterior inferior iliac spines** (AIIS) provide attachment sites for muscles such as the sartorius and rectus femoris respectively. The **iliac crest** is the long and curved border of the ala that bridges the ASIS and **posterior superior iliac spines** (PSIS). The posterior inferior iliac spine (PIIS) located just below the PSIS marks the superior border of the *greater sciatic notch*.

The **iliac tubercle** is located on the iliac crest approximately 5 cm posterior to the ASIS and is associated with the *transtubercular plane* located at the L5 vertebral body. The smooth depression

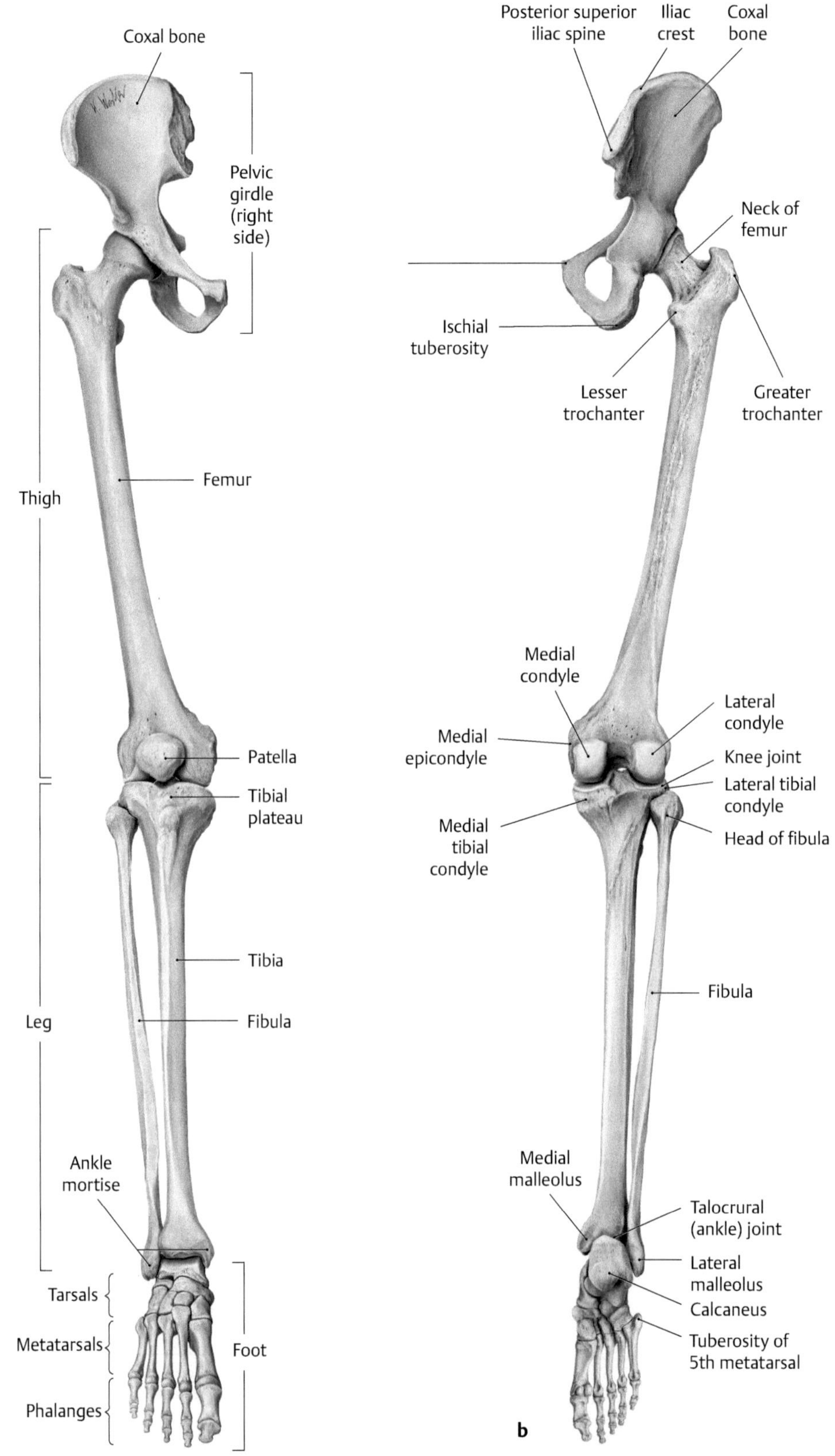

Fig. 5.1 **(a)** Anterior view. **(b)** Posterior view. (From Schuenke M, Schulte E, Schumacher U. THIEME Atlas of Anatomy. General Anatomy and Musculoskeletal System. Illustrations by Voll M and Wesker K. 3rd ed. New York: Thieme Medical Publishers; 2020.)

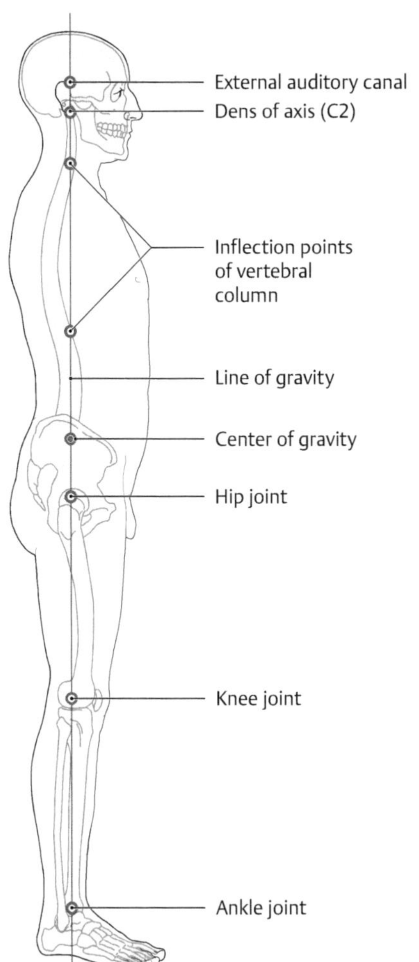

Fig. 5.2 The line of gravity runs vertically from the whole-body center of gravity to the ground. (From Schuenke M, Schulte E, Schumacher U. THIEME Atlas of Anatomy. General Anatomy and Musculoskeletal System. Illustrations by Voll M and Wesker K. 3rd ed. New York: Thieme Medical Publishers; 2020.)

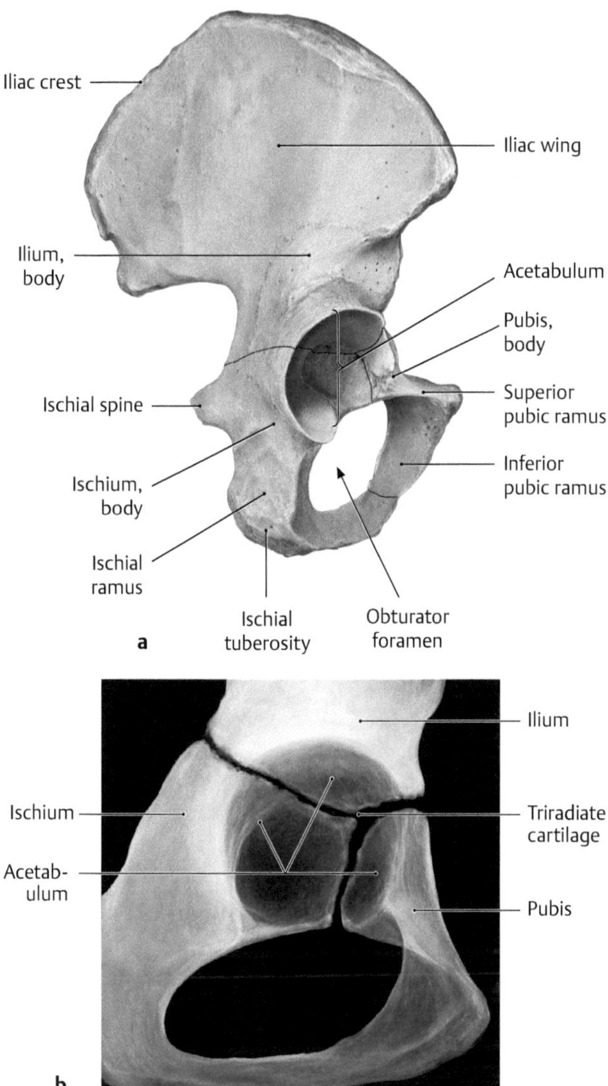

Fig. 5.3 **(a)** Hip bones and junction of triradiate cartilage. **(b)** Radiograph of a child's acetabulum. (From Schuenke M, Schulte E, Schumacher U. THIEME Atlas of Anatomy. General Anatomy and Musculoskeletal System. Illustrations by Voll M and Wesker K. 3rd ed. New York: Thieme Medical Publishers; 2020.)

area found on the medial side of each ala is called the **iliac fossa** and this serves as an attachment point for the iliacus muscle. The **anterior**, **posterior** and **inferior gluteal lines** located on the lateral side of the ala are related to attachment sites for the gluteal muscle group. On the medial side and posterior aspect of the ilium there are some rougher regions one of which is the ear-shaped articular region called the auricular surface and the other is the iliac tuberosity. This is the location of the *sacroiliac joint* and it consists of both a synovial and syndesmotic articulation.

5.1.3 Ischium

The posteroinferior portion of the hip bone is called the **ischium** (**Fig. 5.5**). Its superior portion or **body of the ischium**, fuses with the ilium and pubis bones and contributes to the posteroinferior part of the acetabulum. The **ramus of the ischium** merges with the inferior ramus of the pubis to form a combined structure known as the **ischiopubic ramus**. The larger projection seen on the inferior end of the ramus of the ischium is called the **ischial tuberosity**. It represents the common attachment point for the hamstring muscles and is the structure people technically sit on.

The posterior border of the ischium forms the inferior margin of the **greater sciatic notch**. The inferior margin of this notch elongates and is called the **ischial spine** and serves as the attachment site for the sacrospinous ligament and a few muscles and is a landmark for pudendal anesthesia. Inferior to both the greater sciatic notch and ischial spine is the **lesser sciatic notch** that serves as the trochlea for the obturator internus.

5.1.4 Pubis

The anteromedial portion of the hip bone is called the **pubis** and it contributes to the anterior part of the acetabulum (**Fig. 5.5**). There is a centrally but medial **body of the pubis** and extending out laterally from the body are the **superior** and **inferior pubic rami**.

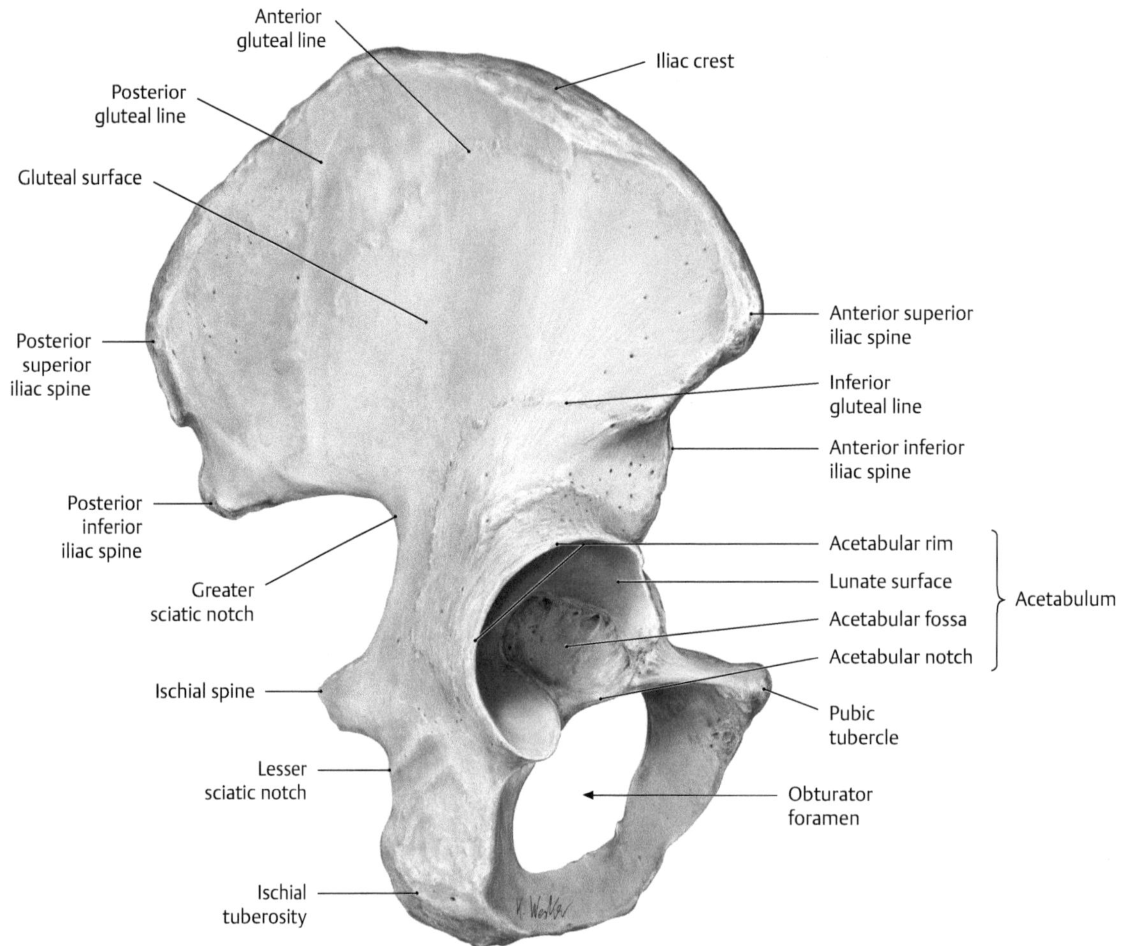

Fig. 5.4 Right hip bone, lateral view. (From Schuenke M, Schulte E, Schumacher U. THIEME Atlas of Anatomy. General Anatomy and Musculoskeletal System. Illustrations by Voll M and Wesker K. 3rd ed. New York: Thieme Medical Publishers; 2020.)

Clinical Correlate 5.1

Fractures of the Hip Bones

The mechanism of hip fractures centers on the elderly and is consequently feared by this population. Hip fractures can alter long-term living conditions or lead to death. Up to a third of these individuals has a one-year mortality rate over 30% after a hip fracture. These fractures generally involve a fall from a standing position. Individuals with a slower gait (as seen in the elderly) have less forward momentum and tend to buckle and fall to the side, increasing the likelihood of a hip fracture. The decrease in bone mass may be due to a number of factors such as lack of exercise, decreased calcium intake, hormone imbalance or having osteoporosis. Estrogen deficiency in postmenopausal women can lead to a decrease in as much as 35% of their cortical bone and 50% of their trabecular bone decades after menopause. Fracture lines of the femoral neck are best visualized with an X-ray when the thigh is medially rotated. CT and MRI scanning can also help identify particular hip fractures. The femoral neck is the most common (~50%) fracture site and is also considered an intracapsular femoral fracture. Treatments can include internal fixation (insertion of a plate or screws) or total hip arthroplasty that involves the removal and then replacement of the acetabulum and femoral head and neck with prosthetic components.

Clinical Correlate 5.2

Hip Pointers

When an individual refers to having a **hip pointer** they are generally referring to a contusion due to a direct blow of the anterior iliac crest or greater trochanter. An **avulsion fracture** is where a force on a tendon or ligament causes bone to break off from a larger piece but has occasionally been described as a hip pointer.

The superior pubic rami connect to both the ilium and ischium while the inferior pubic rami connect to the ischium to help form the ischiopubic ramus. The large oval opening bounded by parts of the pubis and ischium is known as the obturator foramen. Most of this foramen is closed by the **obturator membrane**, which is covered by either the obturator internus or obturator externus muscles. The small opening (obturator canal) that is left allows for the passage of the obturator nerve and vessels.

Each pubic body has a *symphysial surface* that articulates with a fibrocartilaginous interpubic disc to help form the pubic symphysis. The anterosuperior portion of the pubic bones is known as the **pubic crests** and the **pubic tubercles** are located on the lateral aspects of the crests. The pubic crests allow for attachments

Clinical Correlate 5.3

Angle of Inclination and Coxa Vara versus Coxa Valga Femoral Ante/Retroversion

The proximal femur is L-shaped and the long axis of the head and neck project superomedially at an angle to the obliquely orientated shaft and this is called the **angle of inclination**. In the adult the angle averages about 126°. The angle of inclination allows for greater mobility of the femur at the hip joint due to the femoral head and neck being more perpendicular to the acetabulum in the neutral position. It also allows for the oblique angle the femur displays while passing through the thigh region, which permits the knees to be adjacent and inferior to the trunk.

If the angle is larger and reaching as high as 140-150° (as it is when a person is first born), this is called **coxa valga**. In this situation the limb lengthens, which reduces the effectiveness of the hip abductors. This is due to a larger range of motion (ROM) at the hip joint. This also increases the load on the femoral head but reduces the load on the femoral neck. If the angle of inclination is less than 126° and approaching an angle as low as 90° this is called **coxa vara**. This ultimately shortens the limb but increases the effectiveness of the hip abductors. This occurs because there is a decrease in the ROM at the hip joint. There is a reduction in the load put on the femoral head but an increase of the load placed on the femoral neck, increasing the risk of fracture involving the femoral neck.

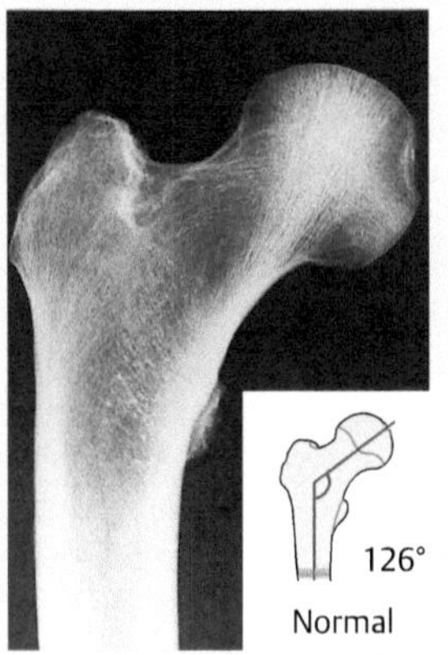

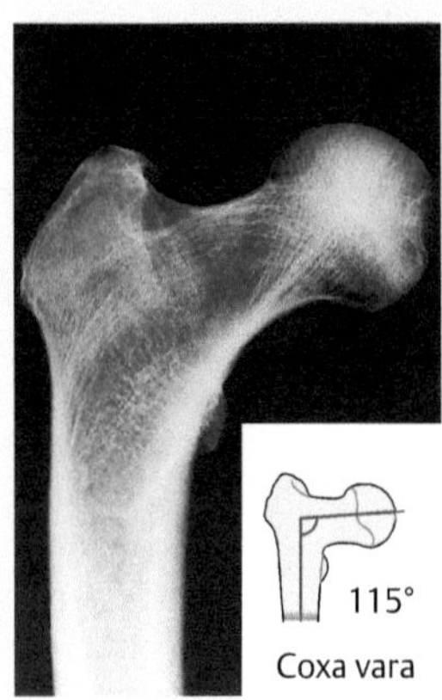

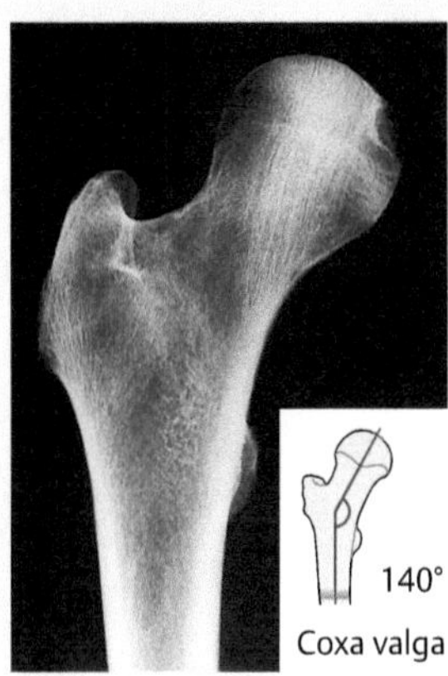

(From Schuenke M, Schulte E, Schumacher U. THIEME Atlas of Anatomy. General Anatomy and Musculoskeletal System. Illustrations by Voll M and Wesker K. 3rd ed. New York: Thieme Medical Publishers; 2020.)

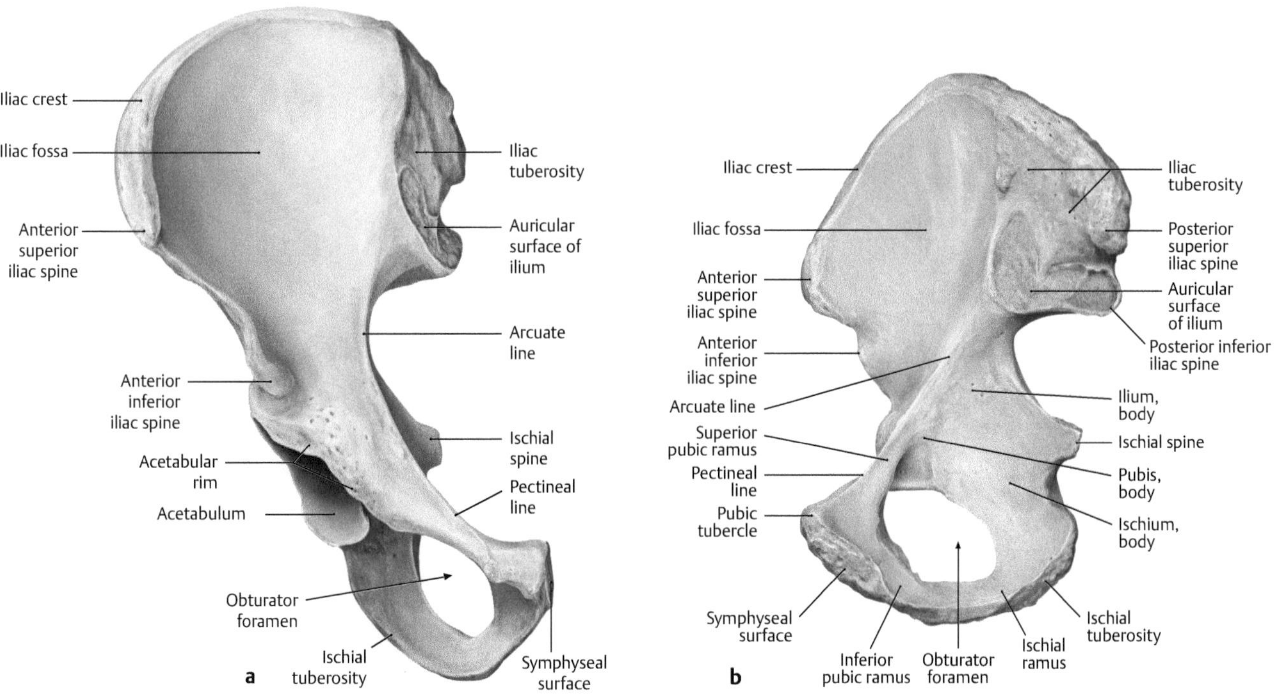

Fig. 5.5 Hip bone. **(a)** Anterior view. **(b)** Medial view. (From Schuenke M, Schulte E, Schumacher U. THIEME Atlas of Anatomy. General Anatomy and Musculoskeletal System. Illustrations by Voll M and Wesker K. 3rd ed. New York: Thieme Medical Publishers; 2020.)

> **Clinical Correlate 5.4**
>
> **Angle of Declination and Femoral Anteversion versus Retroversion**
>
> The **angle of declination (femoral torsion angle)** is assessed when looking at the femur from a superior view and it is the angle of the femoral head and neck relative to that of the shaft and femoral condyles. The angle of declination is approximately 8-15° with the larger value generally seen in females. Because of this angle, when a person is standing erect with their knees facing forward, the center of the femoral head is not located in the same frontal plane as the tip of the greater trochanter.
>
> If the angle of declination increases this is known as **femoral anteversion** and it results in a greater amount of internal (medial) rotation of the femur, demonstrating the "in-toeing" appearance. A decrease in this angle is called **femoral retroversion** and there would be a greater external (lateral) rotation of the femur with the individual displaying the "out-toeing" appearance.
>
> The combination of the angles of inclination and declination is what allows for rotatory movements of the femoral head within the obliquely placed acetabulum. This enables other movements such as flexion, extension, abduction, adduction and circumduction to occur.
>
> 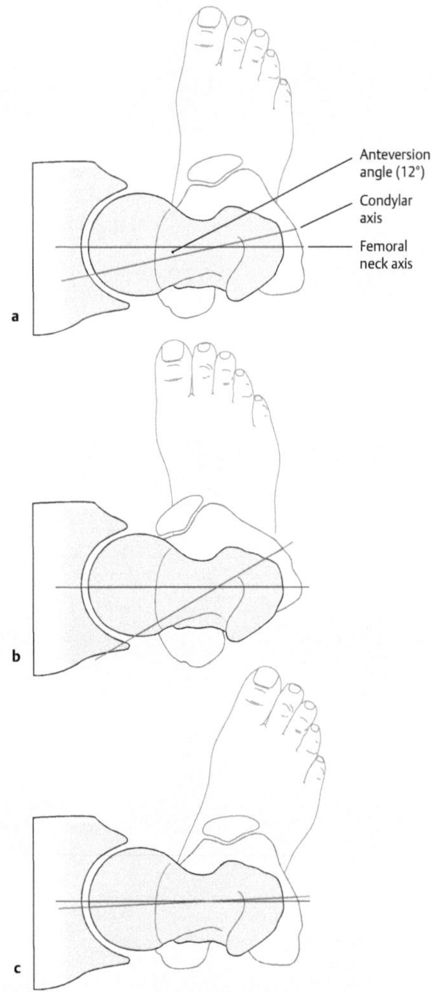
>
>
> **(a)** Normal angle of declination. **(b)** Femoral anteversion. **(c)** Femoral retroversion. (From Schuenke M, Schulte E, Schumacher U. THIEME Atlas of Anatomy. General Anatomy and Musculoskeletal System. Illustrations by Voll M and Wesker K. 3rd ed. New York: Thieme Medical Publishers; 2020.)

of abdominal muscles while the pubic tubercle is an attachment point for the *inguinal ligament*. Extending posteriorly from near the pubic tubercles onto the superior margin of the superior pubic rami is the **pecten pubis (pectineal line)**. The pecten pubis is continuous with the *arcuate line* of the ilium and together they form the *iliopectineal line*, a landmark associated with the *pelvic brim*.

In anatomical position, the acetabulum faces inferolaterally and the obturator foramen lays inferomedially to it and the acetabular notch faces directly inferior to the acetabulum. The internal portion of the pubis faces almost directly superiorly while the pelvic inlet is more vertical than horizontal.

5.2 Femur

The heaviest and longest bone in the body and the one responsible for transmitting the body weight from the hip to the knee is called the **femur** (**Fig. 5.6**). The superior (proximal) end is made up of the **head**, **neck**, and **greater** and **lesser trochanters**. The **intertrochanteric line** is located anteriorly between the two trochanters and posteriorly it is known as the **intertrochanteric crest**. The crest has a rounded elevation called the **quadrate tubercle** and serves as an attachment point for the quadratus femoris muscle. The head of the femur has a small depression known as the **fovea** and this is where the **ligament of the head of the femur** connects the femur to the acetabulum.

Extending inferomedially towards the inferior (distal) portion of the femur is the **shaft** (body) of the femur. On the posterior aspect of the shaft are two edges that make up the **linea aspera**. Superiorly the linea aspera is related to the **pectineal line** and **gluteal tuberosity** while inferiorly and closer to the knee it is related to the **lateral** and **medial supracondylar lines**. Located between the supracondylar lines is the **popliteal surface**. The inferior (distal) femur terminates as the prominent and curved **lateral** and **medial femoral condyles** that articulate with the tibia and help form the knee joint. On the lateral surface of the lateral condyle there is a **lateral epicondyle** while on the medial surface of the medial condyle there is a **medial epicondyle**. Located just superior to the medial epicondyle there is the **adductor tubercle**. From the posterior view, the **intercondylar fossa** is located between the two condyles but on the anterior surface there is a slight articular depression between the condyles called the **patellar surface**.

5.3 Patella

The large sesamoid bone located anterior to the knee joint and articulates with the patellar surface of the femur is called the **patella** (**Fig. 5.7**). The anterior surface is convex and closest to the skin while the posterior articular surface is smooth and articulates at the patellar surface of the femur. The articulating surface is divided into a lateral and medial side by a vertical ridge running down the posterior surface. The superior border is called the **base** and from here the lateral and medial borders extend inferiorly to form the **apex**.

5.4 Tibia

The **tibia** is the weight bearing bone located between the femur and talus of the foot and its anterior border is commonly referred to as the shin (**Fig. 5.8**). The **lateral** and **medial tibial condyles** have an associated **lateral** and **medial tibial plateau** that serves as the articulation point with the lateral and medial

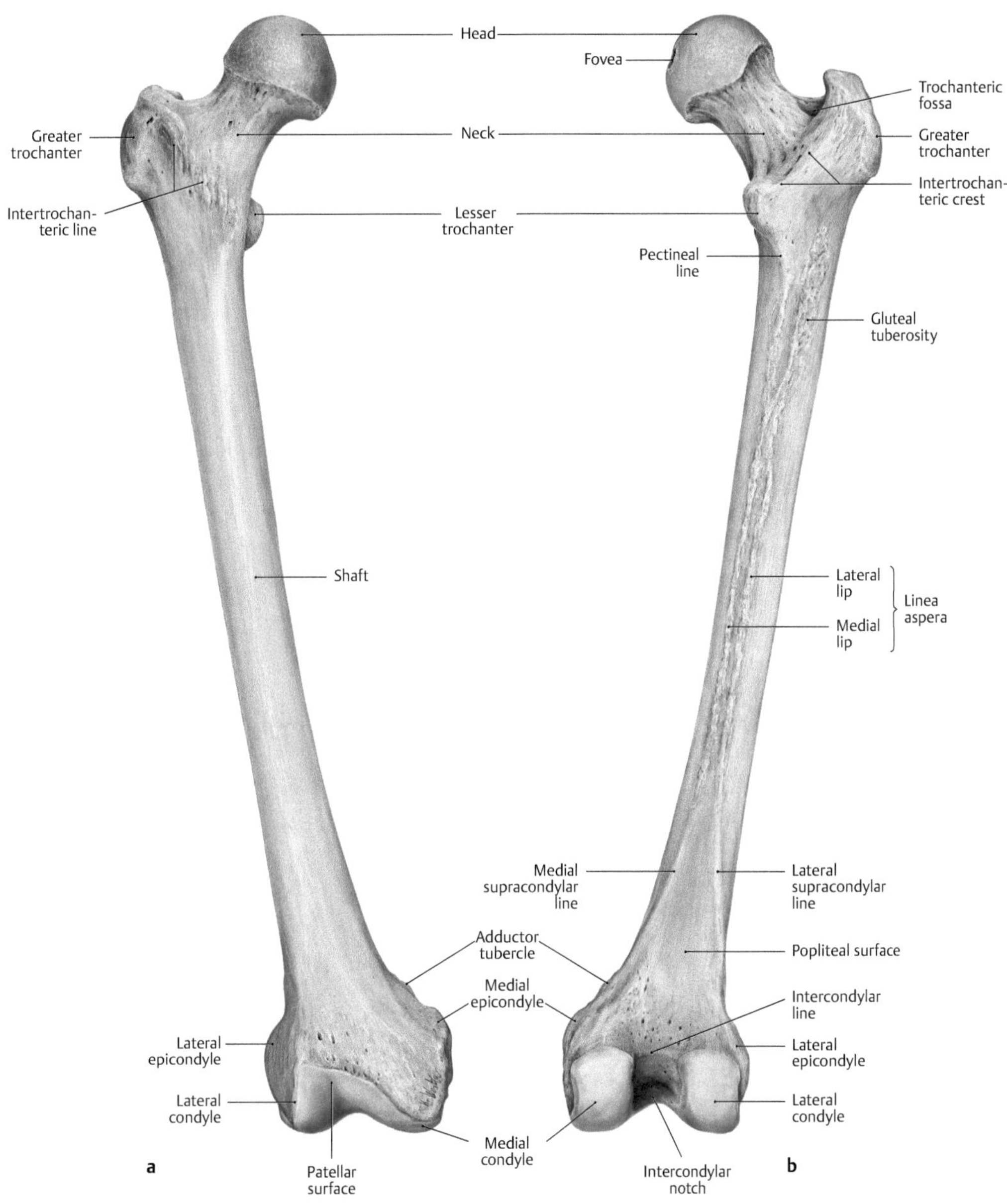

Fig. 5.6 Femur. **(a)** Anterior view. **(b)** Posterior view. (From Schuenke M, Schulte E, Schumacher U. THIEME Atlas of Anatomy. General Anatomy and Musculoskeletal System. Illustrations by Voll M and Wesker K. 3rd ed. New York: Thieme Medical Publishers; 2020.)

Clinical Correlate 5.5

Dislocation of the Femoral Head Epiphysis

The epiphysis of the femoral head in vulnerable to slipping in older children and young adolescents. Repetitive microtraumas or acute trauma especially during abduction and lateral rotation movements are responsible for placing additional shearing forces on the epiphysis. The dislocation (slipping) is generally slower in nature and results in a progressive *coxa vara*. Initial discomfort in the hip may be referred to the knee and an X-ray of the superior aspect of the femur is needed to confirm a diagnosis.

femoral condyles. Located between the tibial plateaus and articulating surfaces is the **intercondylar area** that itself has an elevated region called the **intercondylar eminence**. Protruding from the eminence are the **intercondylar tubercles** (spines). On the anterior surface of the lateral tibial condyle is the **anterolateral tibial (Gerdy's) tubercle** that serves as the attachment site for the *iliotibial tract (band)*. The broad projection located both inferior and medial to the anterolateral tibial tubercle is called the **tibial tuberosity** and it is the attachment site for the *patellar ligament*.

On the posterior surface of the tibial shaft but near the more proximal end, the **soleal line** is a diagonal ridge that runs inferomedially towards the medial border of the tibia and represents an attachment site of the soleus muscle. On the most distal portion

Clinical Correlate 5.6

Fractures of the Femur

A fracture of the femur is commonly age or sex-related. The most frequent part of the femur to fracture is the neck because it is the narrowest and weakest part of the femur that lies at a marked angle related to weight-bearing. Older females are more susceptible secondary to osteoporosis.

- Proximal femur fractures:
  - *Intracapsular fractures* occur within the capsule of the hip joint.
  - *Transcervical* (middle of neck) and *intertrochanteric fractures* are generally the result of indirect trauma such as stepping down hard on a curb. These are unstable because of the angle of inclination and the overriding of bone fragments due to the shortening of the limb called *impaction* will occur. The intertrochanteric fractures occur between the greater and lesser trochanters and are considered *extracapsular*.
  - *Greater trochanter* and *femoral shaft fractures* are the result of direct trauma. A *spiral fracture of the femoral shaft* may occur resulting in *comminuted* (several pieces) fragments that may also become *impacted*.
- Distal femur fractures: fractures in this area can affect blood supply to the leg and foot because of the popliteal artery passing through the region. If the condyles are fractured this may misalign the articular surfaces of the knee joint.

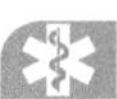

Clinical Correlate 5.7

Fracture of the Patella

A direct blow from a fall or motor vehicle accident is the most common cause of a patellar fracture. These types of fractures only account for about 1% of all fractures and often require surgery. These fractures vary from a slight crack to many small pieces. They occur at any part of the patella. Surgery is required if the fracture is displaced, comminuted or open. Long-term effects could result in arthritis (because the articular cartilage is often damaged) or quadriceps muscle weakness.

of the tibia there is a projection known as the **medial malleolus** and it is a part of the ankle. The flat and square-like **inferior articular surface (plafond)** of the distal tibia is where the tibia articulates with the talus. Near this region and on the lateral aspect of the distal tibia is the **fibular notch**. This is where the distal fibula articulates with the tibia.

5.5 Fibula

The non-weight bearing bone lying posterolateral to the tibia is called the **fibula** (**Fig. 5.8**). The proximal **head** region articulates with the lateral tibial condyle while the distal portion enlarges to form the **lateral malleolus**, which also helps form an outer wall or rectangular socket or *mortise* of the ankle joint. The **interosseous membrane** connects the medial border of the fibular shaft with that of the lateral border of the tibial shaft. The interosseous membrane forms a syndesmosis type of fibrous joint between the two bones.

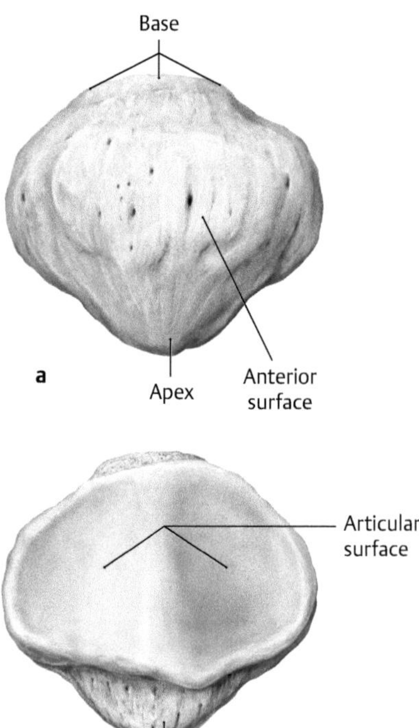

Fig. 5.7 Patella. **(a)** Anterior view. **(b)** Posterior view. (From Schuenke M, Schulte E, Schumacher U. THIEME Atlas of Anatomy. General Anatomy and Musculoskeletal System. Illustrations by Voll M and Wesker K. 3rd ed. New York: Thieme Medical Publishers; 2020.)

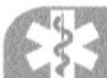

Clinical Correlate 5.8

Fractures of the Tibia

- The most common site of a tibial fracture is between the middle and inferior thirds of the bone where it is the narrowest and is also the region least vascularized. The tibial shaft is the most common site for a *compound fracture* because it lies just beneath the skin. If a fracture involves the nutrient foramen the non-union of bone fragments would occur because of damage to the nutrient artery.
- The inferior one-third is susceptible to a *transverse march (stress) fracture* in individuals who are unconditioned to long hikes for example with the fracture affecting the anterior cortex of the bone.
- A *diagonal fracture* would occur in a situation that involves severe torsion being placed on the tibia as during a high-speed and forward fall seen in skiing accidents. These fractures generally include a fracture to the fibula and both bones override their counterpart.
- A *pilon fracture* involves the distal tibia and represents as much as 10% of all lower limb fractures. They are generally due to some form of high-energy axial loading injury that causes the talus to be driven into the plafond of the tibia while also producing severe soft tissue damage. They are classified as type I-III and can present with an articular fracture with minimal to no displacement (type I) or an articular impaction displaying marked comminution or small fragments (type III).

Clinical Correlate 5.9

Fractures of the Fibula

The most common fibular fractures occur near the proximal portion of the lateral malleolus. Most occur in conjunction with an ankle or tibia injury. An isolated fibular fracture near the lateral malleolus could be due to a severely sprained ankle involving forced inversion. Stress fractures seen in long distance runners are due to repetitive stress and the pain gradually increases but may be relieved with rest. A forced eversion of the ankle can fracture either or both malleoli. Surgery to stabilize the ankle and realign the fractured bones is generally required.

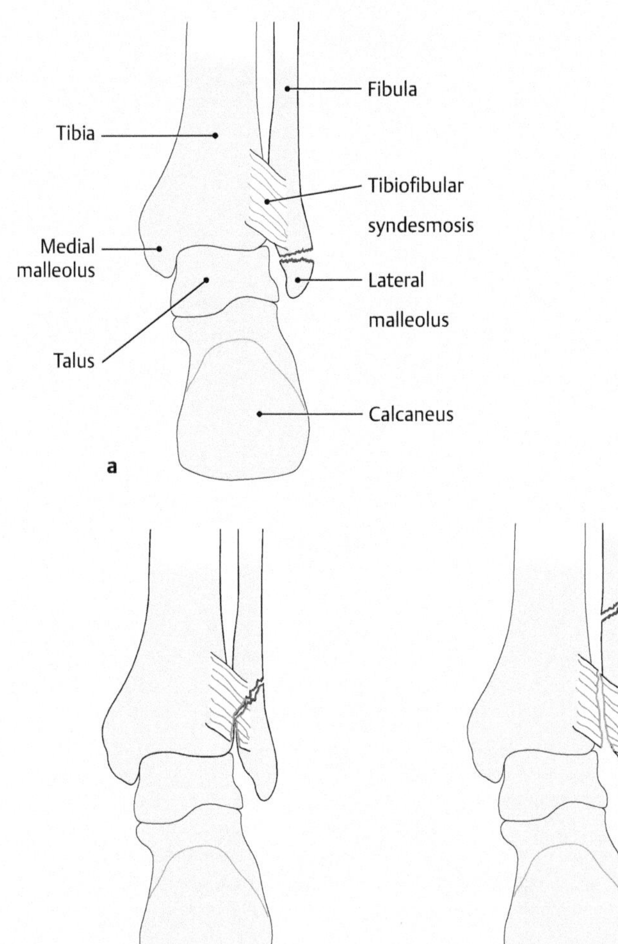

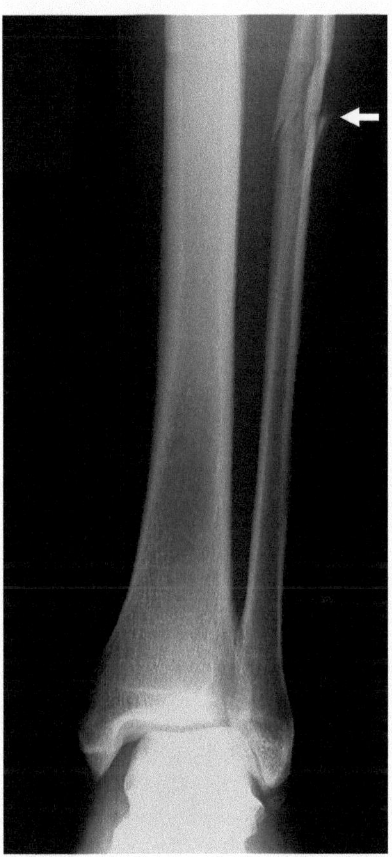

Fibular fractures may occur distal to **(a)**, level with **(b)**, or proximal to the tibiofibular syndesmosis **(c)**. Radiograph of a fibular fracture **(d)**. (From Schuenke M, Schulte E, Schumacher U. THIEME Atlas of Anatomy. General Anatomy and Musculoskeletal System. Illustrations by Voll M and Wesker K. 3rd ed. New York: Thieme Medical Publishers; 2020.)

5.6 Tarsus, Metatarsus, and Phalanges of the Foot

The foot is made up of 26 total bones that consist of 7 tarsal, 5 metatarsal and 14 phalange bones. Functionally the foot can be divided into a **hindfoot** (talus and calcaneus), **midfoot** (navicular, cuneiforms and cuboid) and the **forefoot** (metatarsals and phalanges) (**Fig. 5.9**).

5.6.1 Tarsus

There are seven tarsal bones; the calcaneus, talus, navicular, medial (1st), intermediate (2nd) and lateral (3rd) cuneiforms, and finally the cuboid (**Fig. 5.10**). The largest and strongest bone of the foot is the **calcaneus** (heel). It articulates superiorly with the talus and anteriorly with the cuboid and while standing transmits the majority of an individual's body weight from the talus to the ground. Projecting from the superior border of the medial surface is the **sustentaculum tali** (talar shelf). It supports the head of the talus and has a groove for the flexor hallucis longus tendon to pass through on its way to the distal great toe. On the lateral surface there is a **fibular trochlea**, a projection that serves as a tendon pulley for the fibularis longus and brevis muscles that are responsible for eversion of the foot. The **calcaneal tuberosity** is located on the posterior portion and it has an anterior, lateral and medial tubercle associated with it and only the medial tubercle is in contact with the ground while standing.

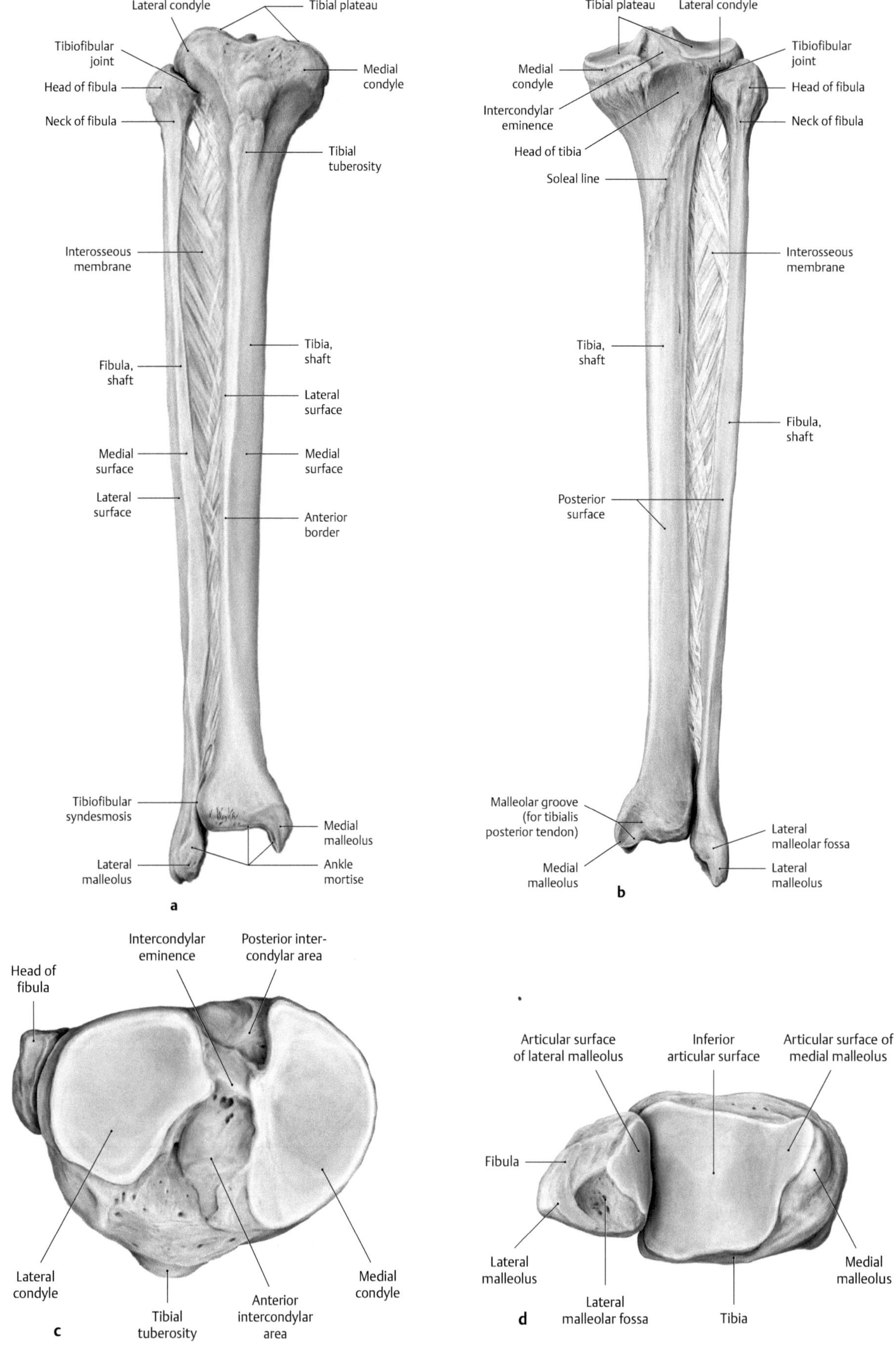

Fig. 5.8 Tibia and fibula. **(a)** Anterior view. **(b)** Posterior view. **(c)** Superior and proximal view. **(d)** Distal view. (From Schuenke M, Schulte E, Schumacher U. THIEME Atlas of Anatomy. General Anatomy and Musculoskeletal System. Illustrations by Voll M and Wesker K. 3rd ed. New York: Thieme Medical Publishers; 2020.)

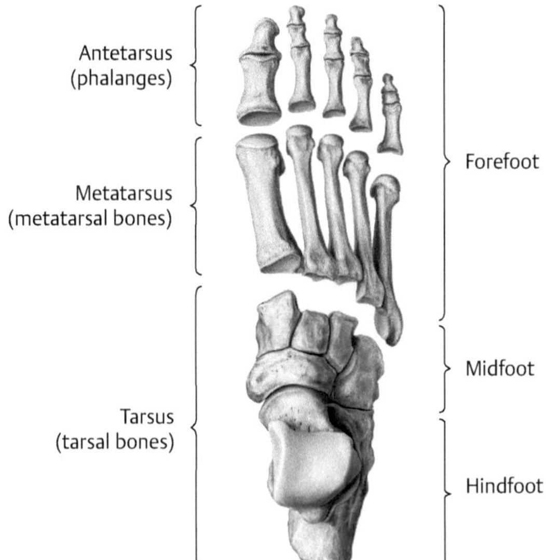

Fig. 5.9 Subdivisions of the foot. (From Schuenke M, Schulte E, Schumacher U. THIEME Atlas of Anatomy. General Anatomy and Musculoskeletal System. Illustrations by Voll M and Wesker K. 3rd ed. New York: Thieme Medical Publishers; 2020.)

The **talus** has a **head**, **neck** and **body** and is the only tarsal bone that has no muscular or tendinous attachments and is covered primarily by an articular cartilage. The superior surface called the **trochlea of the talus** receives the body weight originating from the tibia. It then distributes the weight to the calcaneus, on which the **body** of the talus lies, and then to the anterior portion of the foot that includes both the midfoot and forefoot with much of that support coming by way of the *spring ligament*. The midfoot specifically is related to the **head** of the talus and the spring ligament, which is suspended across a gap found between the sustentaculum tali and the navicular bone. A posterior process extends from the body and features a large **lateral tubercle** and smaller **medial tubercle**. Located between the two tubercles is the **groove for the flexor hallucis longus tendon**.

The **navicular** is a boat-shaped bone located between all three cuneiforms anteriorly and the head of the talus posteriorly. The **navicular tuberosity** is located on the medial surface of the bone and serves as the attachment site of the tibialis posterior muscle. This muscle and the navicular bone contribute to the *medial longitudinal arch* of the foot.

Lying anterior to the navicular bone are the **medial (1st)**, **intermediate (2nd)**, and **lateral (3rd) cuneiform bones**. The cuneiforms articulate anteriorly with the 1st, 2nd and 3rd metatarsals respectively. The medial cuneiform is the largest while the intermediate cuneiform is the smallest.

The **cuboid** is the most lateral tarsal bone and it articulates with the 4th and 5th metatarsals anteriorly and the calcaneus posteriorly. It articulates with the lateral (3rd) cuneiform and navicular bone medially. A **groove for the fibularis longus tendon** is located anterior to the **cuboid tuberosity** and this tendon travels all the way from the lateral to the medial aspect of the foot.

5.6.2 Metatarsus

There are five total metatarsals and they are a part of the forefoot (**Fig. 5.10**). They articulate with the proximal phalanges anteriorly and with the three cuneiforms and cuboid posteriorly. The posterior articulation is known as the **tarsometatarsal (*Lisfranc*) joint**. The numbering of metatarsals runs from medial to lateral with the 1st metatarsal corresponding to the 1st digit or great toe and the 5th metatarsal corresponding with the 5th digit or little toe. Each metatarsal bone has a proximal **base**, **shaft** and distal **head**. The 1st and 5th metatarsals both have a large **metatarsal tuberosity** associated with tendon attachments. On the plantar surface of the 1st metatarsal there is a **lateral** and **medial sesamoid bone** located near the head of this bone. They elevate the metatarsal head off the ground and increase the mechanical properties of the flexor hallucis brevis muscle. The flexor hallucis longus tendon runs between these sesamoid bones but there is no direct connection with them.

5.6.3 Phalanges

There are 14 total phalanges found in each foot (**Fig. 5.10**). The 2-5 digits each have a **proximal**, **middle** and **distal phalanx**. The 1st digit or great toe has only a proximal and distal phalanx. Each phalanx has a proximal **base**, **shaft** and distal **head** similar to the metatarsals.

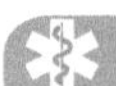

Clinical Correlate 5.10

Fractures of the Foot

- *Talus fractures*: most common area of fracture is at the neck of the talus (i.e. *aviator fracture*). Another common area of fracture is near the lateral tubercle. These fractures are seen in high-energy trauma that forces dorsiflexion of the foot at the ankle. This could include an automobile or snowboarding accident.
- *Calcaneus (lover's) fracture*: are seen in about 50-60% of all tarsal bone fractures and are associated with landing on ones heel after falling from a tall structure. The lover's terminology originates from the idea that a person will jump from great heights to escape their lover's spouse.
- *Nutcracker fracture*: a cuboid bone fracture associated with a navicular avulsion fracture. It is due to compression between the bases of 4th and 5th metatarsals and calcaneus bone. It is usually secondary to traumatic abduction of the forefoot.
- *Metatarsal fractures*:
  - *March fracture*: a fatigue or stress fracture classically involving the 2nd metatarsal. It is due to repeated or prolonged periods of marching as seen in a soldiers training.
  - *Avulsion fracture of the 5th metatarsal tuberosity* (pseudo-Jones fracture) is caused by forced inversion of the foot during plantarflexion. It is common in tennis players and is sometimes referred to as a *tennis fracture*.
  - *Jones fracture*: a transverse fracture of the 5th metatarsal distal from the tuberosity. It occurs as a result of significant force during adduction applied to the forefoot while plantarflexing. These injuries are prone to non-union.

5.7 Surface Anatomy of the Lower Extremity

During a physical examination or even in surgery, bony landmarks are important to be able to evaluate in order to detect areas of possible trauma or damaged neurovasculature. Structures located just

Clinical Correlate 5.11

Accessory Tarsal Bones

A number of accessory tarsal bones can be located in the foot. They rarely cause discomfort if present, but they must be differentiated from foot fractures. A clinically significant accessory bone would be the **external tibial bone**, which can be a source of discomfort when shoes are worn too tight. The **os trigonum** is an accessory bone that occurs in up to 25% of the population and it is seen mostly bilateral. It occurs due to the failure of the secondary ossification center of the talus to unite with the body. The structure that would have formed is the lateral tubercle.

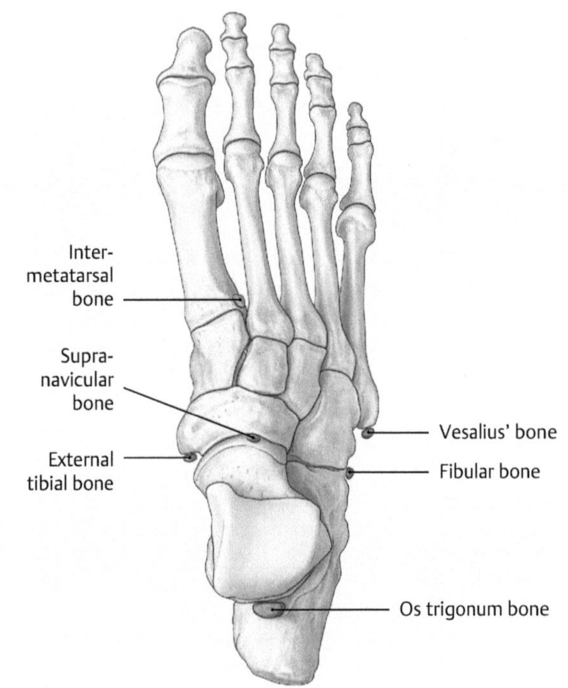

(From Schuenke M, Schulte E, Schumacher U. THIEME Atlas of Anatomy. General Anatomy and Musculoskeletal System. Illustrations by Voll M and Wesker K. 3rd ed. New York: Thieme Medical Publishers; 2020.)

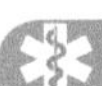

Clinical Correlate 5.12

Bone Grafting

In the case of major trauma, during a surgical procedure, or bone removal due to cancer, **bone grafts** are used to replace any missing bone. Autologous grafts can originate from the iliac crest, fibula, ribs and mandible and other sources. They will be reabsorbed and replaced as natural bone heals over multiple months. Bone tissue has the ability to regenerate completely if a space is provided to allow for its growth thus the reason bone grafting is a possibility.

below the skin with very little soft tissue or surrounding muscle are the easiest to discern (**Fig. 5.11**).

With the hip region, the **iliac crests** are where an individual rests their hands on top of the hips. The anterior portion is more subcutaneous and hence easier to palpate, especially the anterior most portion that forms the **ASIS**. To estimate the L5 vertebral level, the **iliac tubercles** can be located just a few centimeters posterior to the ASIS. The iliac crests end at the **PSIS** and may be difficult to palpate but their location is detected with the normally present dimples of the lower back region. The **ischial tuberosity** is the structure people technically sit on and it can be easily palpated near the inferior portion of the buttocks. Near the superior portion of the pubic symphysis, the **pubic bodies** and **superior pubic rami** can be palpated. Also able to be palpated are the **pubic tubercles** located about 2 cm lateral to the superior portion of the pubic symphysis and just inferior to the **pubic crests**.

In the thigh region, the parts of the femur that can be palpated quite easily would include the **greater trochanter** that is located lateral to the femoral shaft and neck junctions and near the lateral portion of the buttocks. This is the structure that causes discomfort if a person was to lie on their side for an extended period of time. The center of the **femoral head** is not as easily palpated but it can be felt deep approximately a few centimeters below the midpoint of the inguinal ligament. Down near the knees, both the **femoral condyles** and **epicondyles** can be palpated. The **adductor tubercle** can also be located just superior to the medial condyle. The **patella** is easily palpated and can be felt sliding back and forth during flexion and extension at the knee.

In the leg region, the head and lateral malleolus of the fibula are easily palpable. The head rests near the lateral condyle and **anterolateral (Gerdy's) tubercle** of the tibia. The **medial condyle** of the tibia and the very prominent **tibial tuberosity** can be felt on the medial and mid-tibial regions. The **anterior surface of the tibia** is directly below the skin and can be felt all the way inferior before becoming the **medial malleolus**. Together the medial and lateral malleoli represent the ankle region that is easily palpated.

In the foot region, the prominent **calcaneus** is easily identifiable and its **sustentaculum tali** can be felt just below the medial malleolus. The **fibular trochlea** is not very well defined thus it may or may not be able to be palpated. The **head of the talus** is most palpable anterior to the medial malleolus when the foot is everted and anteromedial to the proximal part of the lateral malleolus when the foot is inverted. On the medial foot the **navicular tuberosity** is easily palpable. However, the medial border of the medial cuneiform and the lateral border of the cuboid are really all that can be felt in that row of tarsal bones. These are best felt near the base of the adjacent 1st or 5th metatarsals respectively. The **tuberosity of the 5th metatarsal** can be palpated quite easily but overall the metatarsals and phalanges are distinguishable.

5.8 Fascia of the Lower Extremity

Just below the skin the **subcutaneous tissue**, or **superficial fascia**, consists of loose connective tissue containing a variable amount of fat, cutaneous nerves, superficial veins, their tributaries and lymph nodes with their corresponding lymphatic vessels. This layer is fairly consistent throughout the lower extremity except near the knee where there is a reduction in the fat.

A strong **deep fascia** of the lower limb can be observed extending from the gluteal and thigh regions and inferiorly to the foot. This particular fascia limits the outward expansion of contracting muscles and this in turns makes these muscular contractions more efficient as they compress the veins pumping blood back

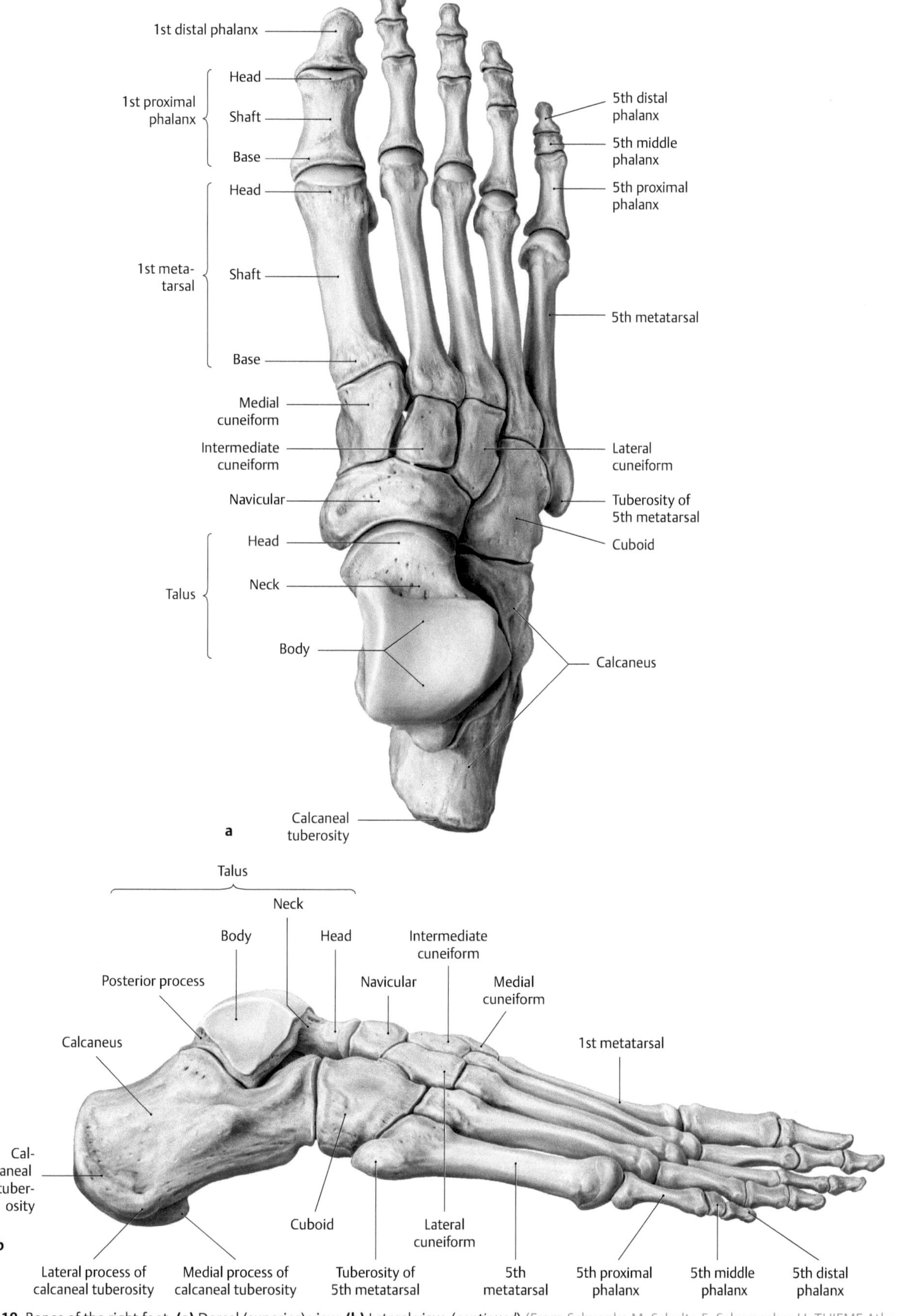

Fig. 5.10 Bones of the right foot. **(a)** Dorsal (superior) view. **(b)** Lateral view. (*continued*) (From Schuenke M, Schulte E, Schumacher U. THIEME Atlas of Anatomy. General Anatomy and Musculoskeletal System. Illustrations by Voll M and Wesker K. 3rd ed. New York: Thieme Medical Publishers; 2020.)

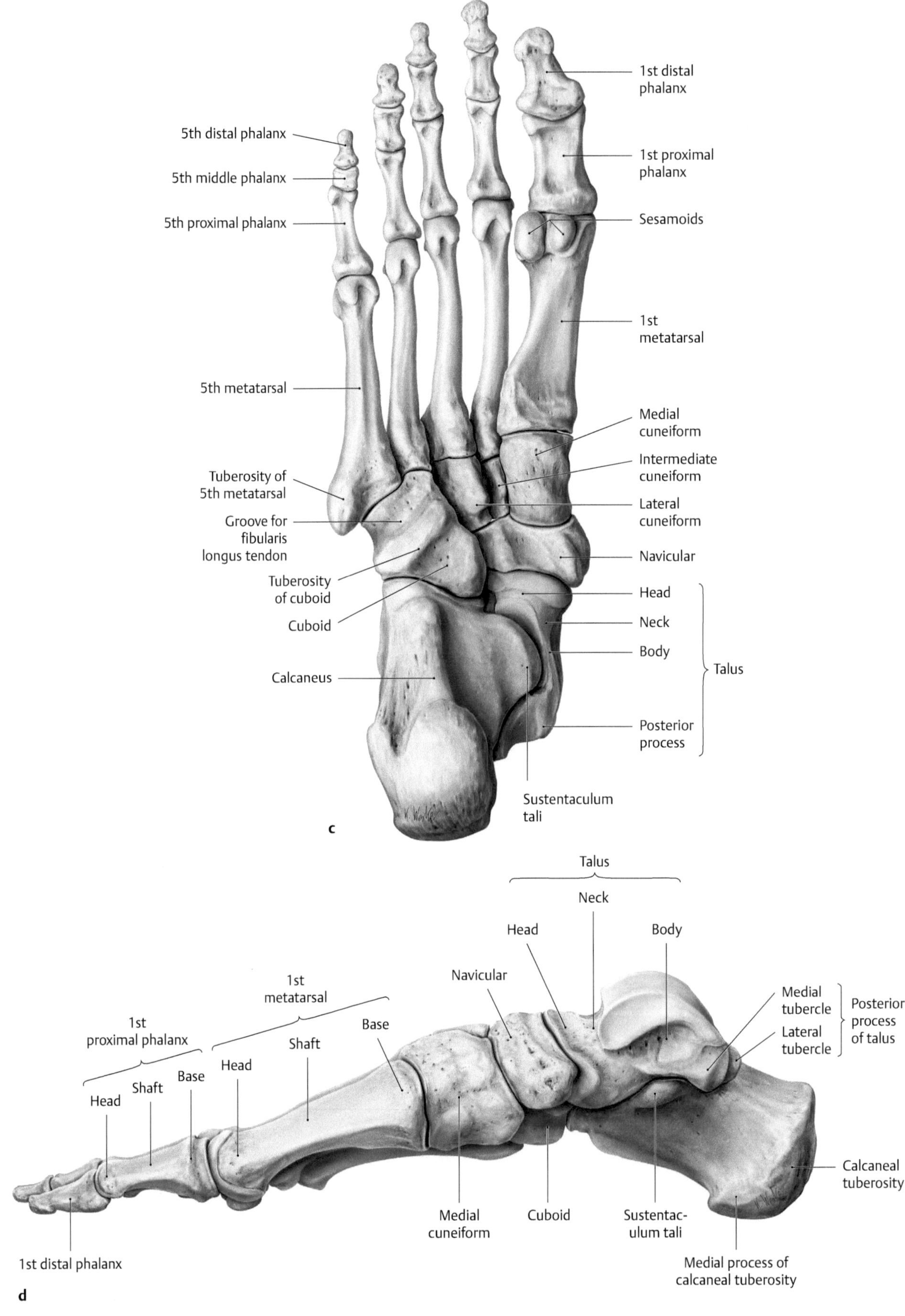

Fig. 5.10 (*continued*) Bones of the foot **(c)** Plantar (inferior) view. **(d)** Medial view. (From Schuenke M, Schulte E, Schumacher U. THIEME Atlas of Anatomy. General Anatomy and Musculoskeletal System. Illustrations by Voll M and Wesker K. 3rd ed. New York: Thieme Medical Publishers; 2020.)

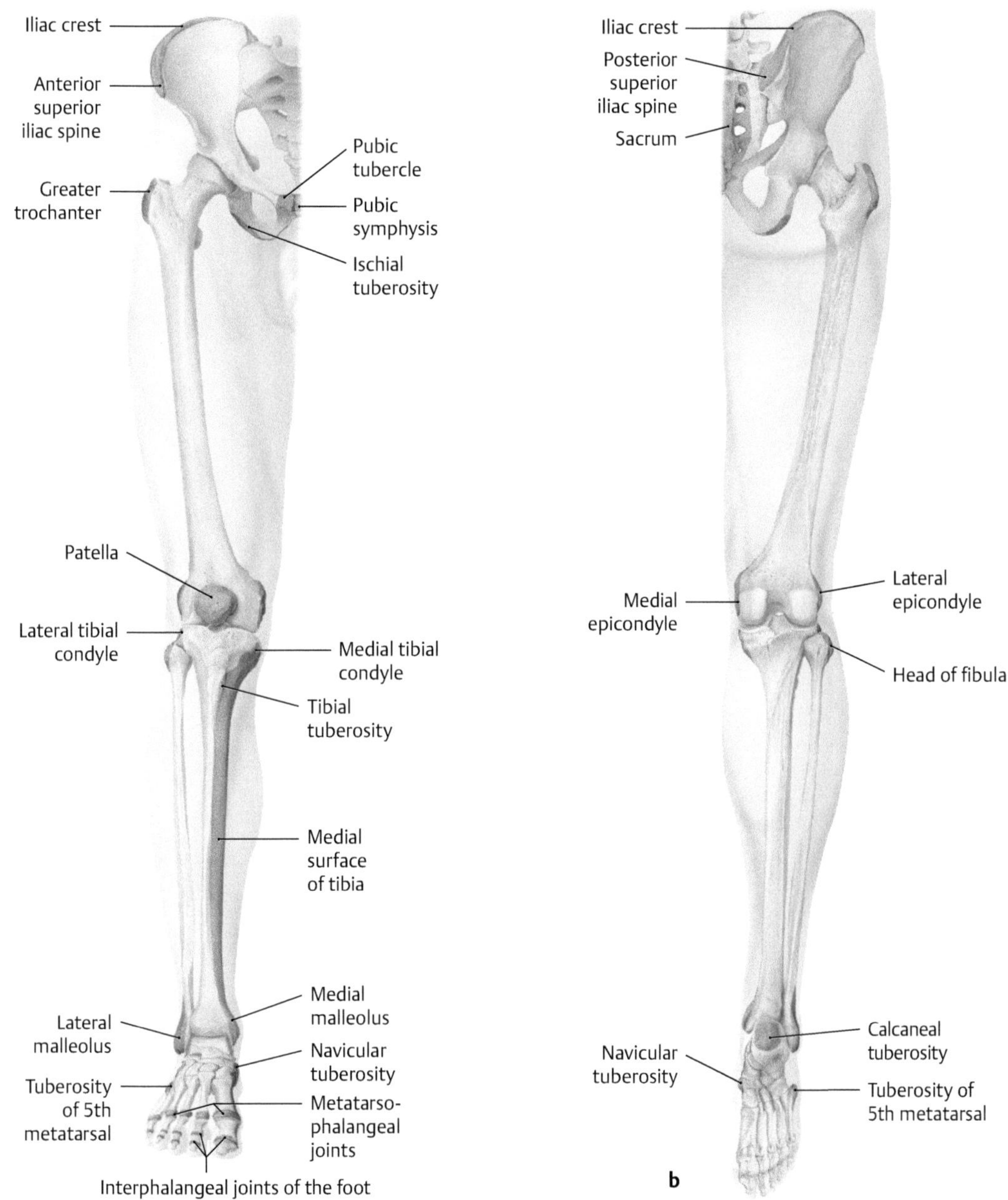

Fig. 5.11 Palpable bony prominences of the lower extremity. **(a)** Anterior view. **(b)** Posterior view. (From Schuenke M, Schulte E, Schumacher U. THIEME Atlas of Anatomy. General Anatomy and Musculoskeletal System. Illustrations by Voll M and Wesker K. 3rd ed. New York: Thieme Medical Publishers; 2020.)

to the heart. Although this fascia is continuous it is known as the *fascia lata*, *crural fascia* and general *foot fascia*.

The **deep fascia of the thigh** is also known as the **fascia lata**. It is continuous with the gluteal fascia and wraps around the entire thigh region. It extends to and connects with structures such as the pubic body, inguinal ligament, Scarpa's fascia, iliac crest, sacrum, coccyx, ischial tuberosity and ischiopubic ramus. It then extends inferiorly to the leg and become the crural fascia. Near the medial portion of the inguinal ligament and just inferior to here, there is a **saphenous opening** in the fascia lata. The more defined superior, lateral and inferior portion of this opening is referred to as the **falciform margin** but the opening is technically filled in with the **cribiform fascia** and this is a localized membranous layer of subcutaneous tissue. The great saphenous vein along with some smaller tributaries and the efferent vessels of the superficial inguinal lymph nodes pass through the cribriform fascia (**Fig. 5.12; Fig. 5.13**).

The lateral aspect of the fascia lata condense and form the **iliotibial tract (band)**, which is a shared aponeurosis of the tensor fasciae latae and gluteus maximus muscles. This is the structure that ultimately attaches to the anterolateral (Gerdy's) tubercle of the tibia. The fascia lata penetrates into the thigh at multiple areas and in doing so forms compartments (anterior, posterior and medial) and intermuscular septa. The strongest of the septa

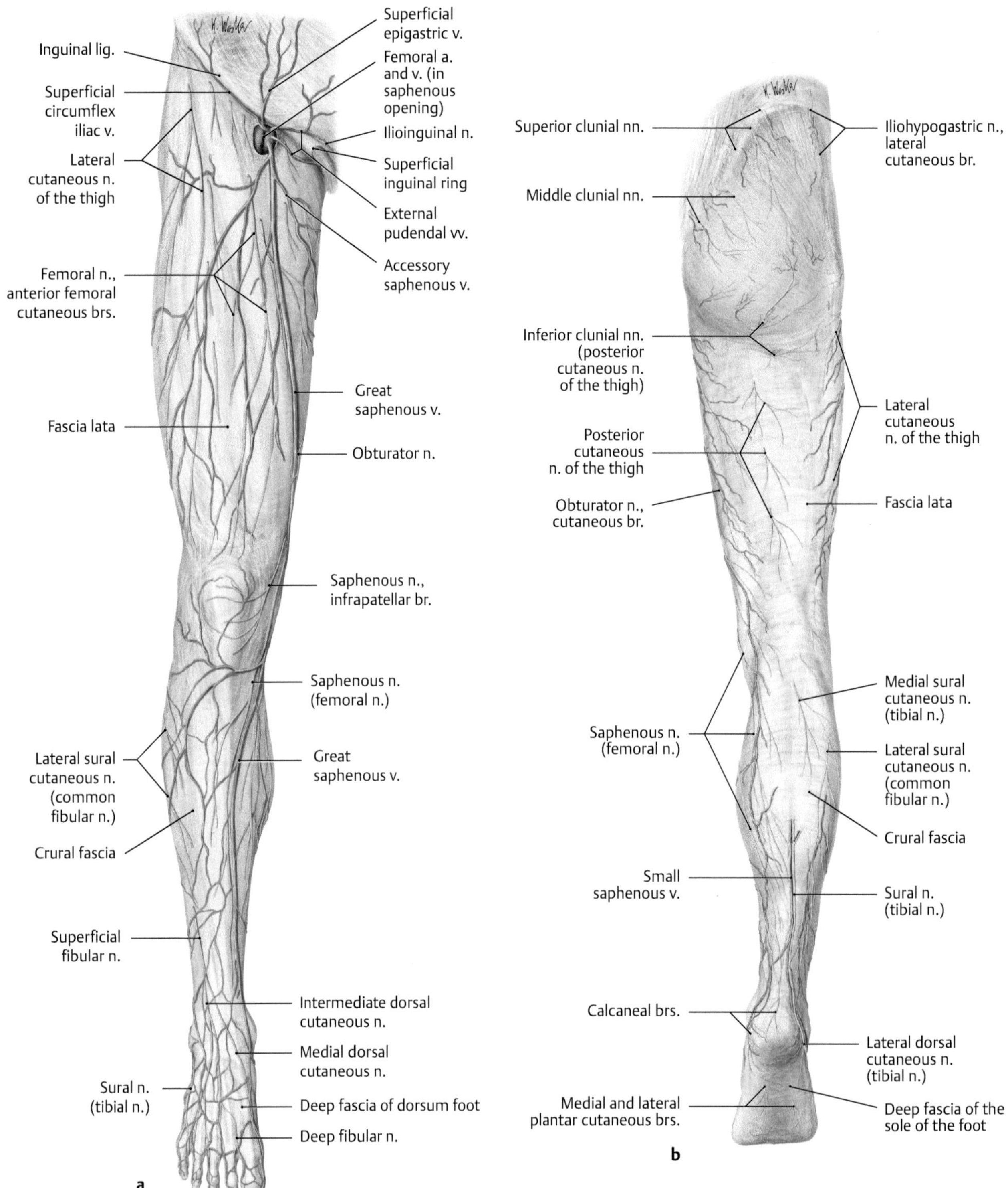

Fig. 5.12 (a, b) Fascia and superficial cutaneous veins and nerves of the right lower extremity. **(a)** Anterior view. **(b)** Posterior view. (From Schuenke M, Schulte E, Schumacher U. THIEME Atlas of Anatomy. General Anatomy and Musculoskeletal System. Illustrations by Voll M and Wesker K. 3rd ed. New York: Thieme Medical Publishers; 2020.)

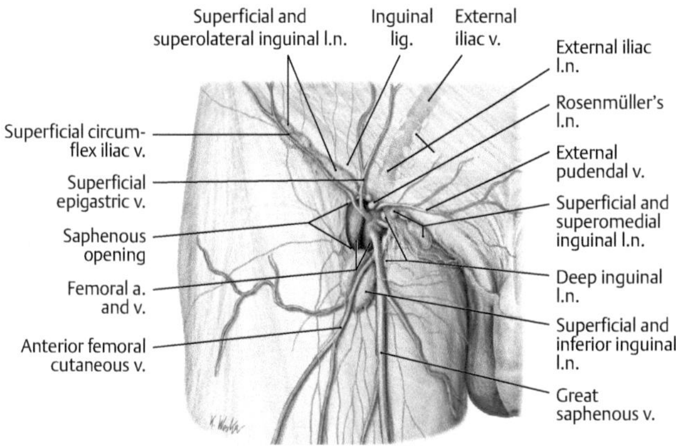

Fig. 5.13 Superficial veins and lymph nodes. (From Schuenke M, Schulte E, Schumacher U. THIEME Atlas of Anatomy. General Anatomy and Musculoskeletal System. Illustrations by Voll M and Wesker K. 3rd ed. New York: Thieme Medical Publishers; 2020.)

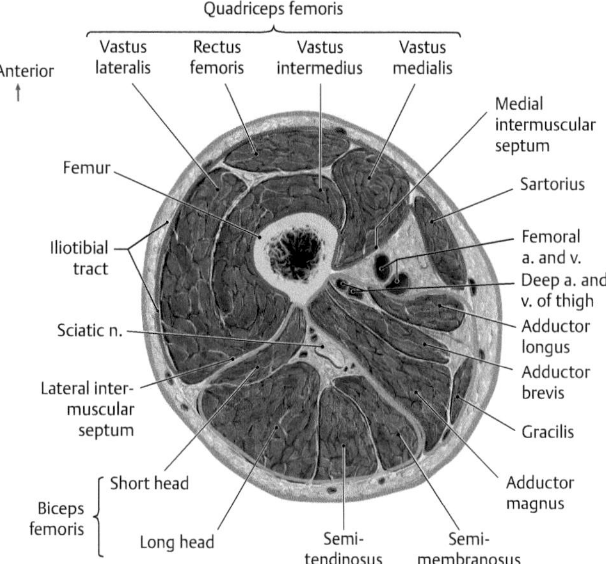

Fig. 5.14 Thigh. Anterior compartment, *red*; posterior compartment, *green*; medial compartment, *orange*. (From Schuenke M, Schulte E, Schumacher U. THIEME Atlas of Anatomy. General Anatomy and Musculoskeletal System. Illustrations by Voll M and Wesker K. 3rd ed. New York: Thieme Medical Publishers; 2020.)

is the **lateral intermuscular septum** and it extends from the iliotibial tract to the lateral lip of the linea aspera of the femur. It help separates the anterior and posterior compartments of the thigh. The **medial** and **posterior intermuscular septa** are weaker and separate the *anterior* from the *medial compartment* and the *medial* from the *posterior compartment* respectively **(Fig. 5.14)**.

The **deep fascia of the leg** is also known as the **crural fascia**. It attaches to the anterior and medial borders of the tibia and is continuous with the periosteum. The crural fascia is thicker proximally but becomes thinner as it extends down near the ankle and foot. Passing from the lateral portion of the crural fascia and attaching to corresponding margins of the fibula are the **anterior** and **posterior intermuscular septa**. The combination of these two septa forms the *lateral compartment* of the leg. The previously mentioned **interosseous membrane** spanning both the tibia and fibula, along with the anterior intermuscular septa forms the *anterior compartment* of the leg. The posterior intermuscular septum and interosseous membrane define the *posterior compartment* of the leg. Extending from the posterior intermuscular septum and back to the medial side of the crural fascia is the **transverse intermuscular septum**. This septum further divides the posterior compartment into a *superficial* versus *deep posterior compartment* **(Fig. 5.12; Fig. 5.15)**.

The **deep fascia of the foot** is continuous with the crural fascia and can be described as the **deep fascia of the dorsum of the foot** and the **deep fascia of the sole (plantar fascia) (Fig. 5.12)**. The deep fascia of the dorsum of the foot is fairly thin but the deep fascia of the sole of the foot/plantar fascia can be thin on the lateral and medial portions of the sole but has a much thicker central region that leads to the formation of the **plantar aponeurosis**.

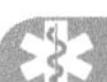 ***Clinical Correlate 5.13***

Compartment Syndrome and Fasciotomy

The fascial compartments of the lower extremities are generally closed spaces ending near joints. Increased pressure, by way of a contusion or infection, compresses small nerves and vessels, leading to ischemia of certain structures. This is referred to as a **compartment syndrome**. Infections of the anterior and posterior leg compartments spread mainly in a distal direction. Lateral compartment infections ascend proximally into the popliteal fossa by following the course of the common fibular nerve. To relieve this pressure a **fasciotomy** (opening of the fascia) can be done, which allows for debridement of any damaged of infectious tissue.

5.9 Neurovasculature of the Lower Extremity

5.9.1 Nerves of the Lower Extremity

The nerves that innervate the lower extremity originate from both the *lumbar plexus* (ventral rami of L1-L4) located in the abdomen and the *sacral plexus* (ventral rami of L4-S4) found in the pelvic region. These somatic nerve plexuses, commonly referred together as the lumbosacral plexus, allow the nerve fibers derived from different segments of the spinal cord to be arranged and distributed within different nerve trunks to various parts of the lower extremity (**Fig. 5.16; Fig. 5.17**). Like all somatic nerve plexuses the functional components of their nerves are GSE, GSA and GVE-sym/post, unless it is a cutaneous nerve, in which case it only has GSA and GVE-sym/post fibers. The nerves entering the lower extremity provide:

- Motor innervation to the muscles.
- Sensory innervation from the skin, muscles and joints.
- Sympathetic innervation to the blood vessels and sweat glands.

The **lumbar plexus** is made up of the *iliohypogastric* (L1), *ilioinguinal* (L1), *lateral femoral cutaneous* (L2-L3), *femoral* (L2-L4), *genitofemoral* (L1-L2) and the *obturator* (L2-L4) *nerves* from lateral to medial. The iliohypogastric nerve can receive contributions from the T12 spinal nerve and the femoral followed by the obturator nerve are the largest nerves of this plexus. An **accessory obturator**

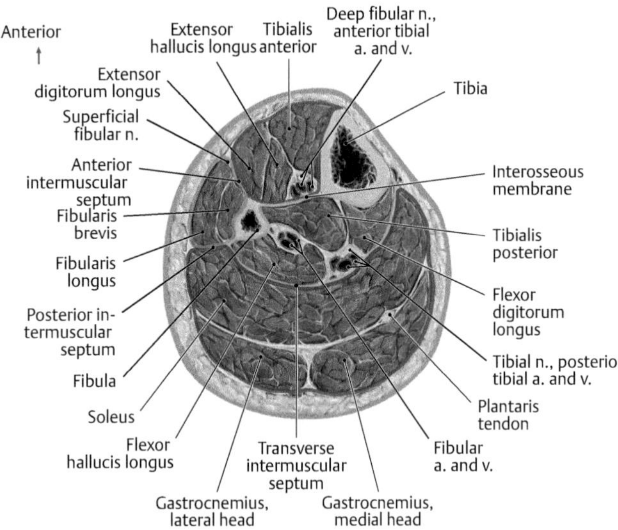

Fig. 5.15 Leg. Anterior compartment, *red*; deep posterior compartment, *green*; superficial posterior compartment, *blue*; lateral compartment, *orange*. (From Schuenke M, Schulte E, Schumacher U. THIEME Atlas of Anatomy. General Anatomy and Musculoskeletal System. Illustrations by Voll M and Wesker K. 3rd ed. New York: Thieme Medical Publishers; 2020.)

nerve may arise from the L3 and L4 spinal nerves but may only be present in about a quarter of the population **(Fig. 5.17)**.

- The **iliohypogastric** (L1) and **ilioinguinal nerves** (L1) help innervate the anterior abdominal wall muscles and supply skin near these same muscles, the inguinal and pubic regions.
- The **lateral femoral cutaneous nerve** (L2-L3) supplies skin over the anterolateral surface of the thigh.
- The **femoral nerve** (L2-L4) innervates the iliacus and anterior thigh muscles and the skin over the anterior thigh.
- The **genitofemoral nerve** (L1-L2) divides into a separate genital and femoral branch. The genital branch innervates the cremater muscle in the male spermatic cord and skin over the anterior scrotum/labia majora while the femoral branch innervates skin over the superomedial thigh in both sexes.
- The **obturator nerve** (L2-L4) innervates the medial thigh muscles and a limited portion of skin over the medial thigh.
- There are also direct muscular branches from L1-L4 and in addition from T12 that innervate the psoas major and quadratus lumborum muscles.

The **sacral plexus** is made up of the *lumbosacral trunk, superior gluteal, nerve to quadratus femoris, nerve to piriformis, inferior gluteal, nerve to obturator internus, posterior femoral cutaneous, sciatic* and both of its *tibial* and *common fibular divisions, pudendal, nerve to levator ani and coccygeus* and *pelvic splanchnic nerves*. The pudendal nerve, nerve to the levator ani and coccygeus, and the pelvic splanchnic nerves are associated with the perineum, pelvic floor or pelvic viscera and were detailed in the last chapter. All other listed branches are involved in the innervation of muscles or skin of the lower extremity and the focus of this chapter **(Fig. 5.17)**.

- The **lumbosacral trunk** (L4-L5) is a thick, cord-like combination of lumbar spinal nerves that contribute to the sacral plexus.

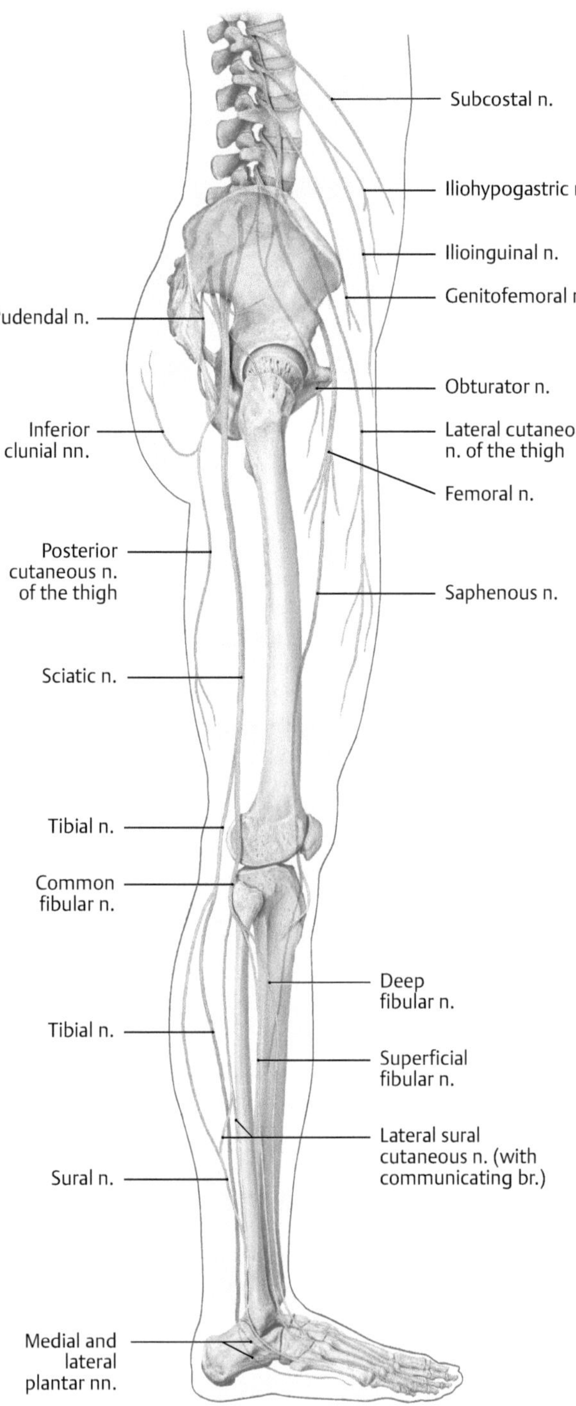

Fig. 5.16 The lumbosacral plexus, lateral view. (From Schuenke M, Schulte E, Schumacher U. THIEME Atlas of Anatomy. General Anatomy and Musculoskeletal System. Illustrations by Voll M and Wesker K. 3rd ed. New York: Thieme Medical Publishers; 2020.)

- The **superior gluteal nerve** (L4-S1) innervates the gluteus medius, gluteus minimus and tensor fasciae latae muscles.
- The **nerve to quadratus femoris** (L4-S1) innervates the quadratus femoris and inferior gemellus muscles.
- The **nerve to piriformis** (S1-S2) innervates the piriformis muscle.
- The **inferior gluteal nerve** (L5-S2) innervates the gluteus maximus muscle.

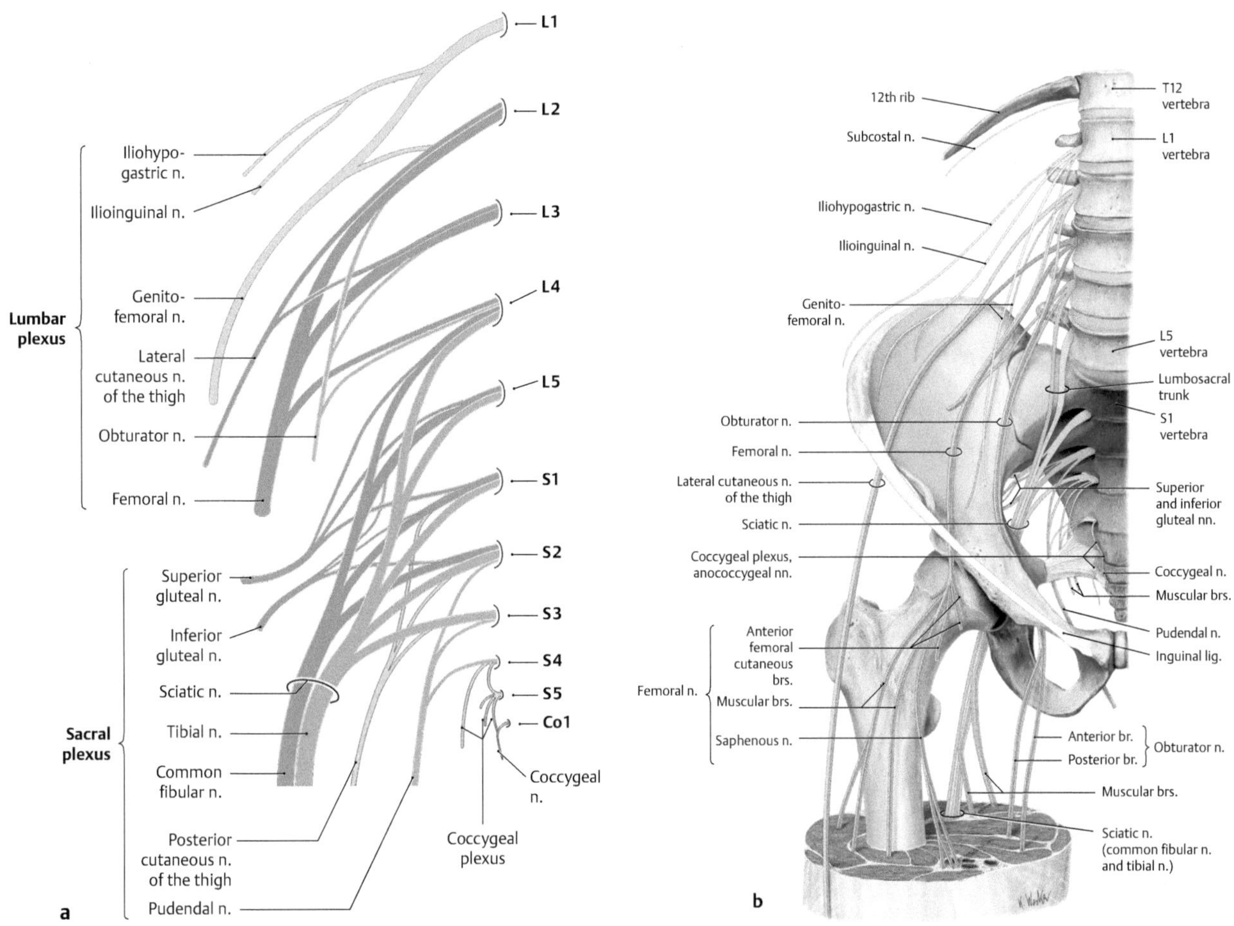

Fig. 5.17 **(a)** Structure of the lumbar and sacral plexuses. **(b)** Course of the lumbar and sacral plexuses. (From Schuenke M, Schulte E, Schumacher U. THIEME Atlas of Anatomy. General Anatomy and Musculoskeletal System. Illustrations by Voll M and Wesker K. 3rd ed. New York: Thieme Medical Publishers; 2020.)

- The **nerve to obturator internus** (L5-S2) innervates the obturator internus and superior gemellus muscles.
- The **posterior cutaneous nerve of the thigh** (S1-S3) innervates the skin of the inferior half of the buttocks (via inferior clunial nerves), posterior thigh and popliteal fossa, lateral perineum, and the upper medial thigh.
- The **sciatic nerve** (L4-S3) is the largest nerve in the body and is actually made up of two individual nerves loosely bound by the same connective tissue sheath, the *tibial* and *common fibular nerves*. The **tibial nerve** (L4-S3) is the more medial branch of the sciatic nerve and it continues through posterior thigh and leg before bifurcating into the **lateral plantar** (S1-S3) and **medial planter nerves** (L4-S3) near the ankle. The tibial nerve supplies the hamstring muscles and posterior leg compartment muscles while the paired planter nerves innervate the foot muscles and skin of the plantar surface of the foot. The **common fibular (peroneal) nerve** (L4-S2) is the more lateral branch of the sciatic nerve and it bifurcates into a **superficial fibular** (L4-S1) and **deep fibular nerve** (L5-S2) near the head and neck of the fibula. The common fibular nerve innervates the short head of the biceps femoris muscle while the superficial fibular nerve supplies the lateral leg compartment and the deep fibular nerve supplies the anterior leg compartment. These terminal plantar and fibular branches would be considered indirect branches of the sacral plexus.

5.9.2 Cutaneous Nerve Innervation of the Lower Extremity

In addition to some of the nerves listed from the lumbar and sacral plexuses, the *superior clunial, middle clunial, inferior clunial, subcostal, saphenous, lateral sural cutaneous, medial sural cutaneous, sural* and *calcaneal nerves* lie within the subcutaneous tissue and supply the skin of the lower extremity **(Fig. 5.18; Fig. 5.19)**. The **superior clunial nerves** (dorsal rami of L1-L3) innervate the skin of the superior buttocks and as far lateral as the iliac tubercle.

- The **middle clunial nerves** (dorsal rami of S1-S3) innervate the skin over the sacrum and adjacent region of the buttocks.
- The **inferior clunial nerves** (ventral rami of S1-S3) are branches of the posterior femoral cutaneous nerve and they innervate the skin of the inferior half of the buttocks and as far lateral as the greater trochanter.
- The **subcostal costal nerve** (T12) assists in the innervation of the anterior abdominal wall but its skin innervation involves the hip region inferior to the anterior part of the iliac crest and anterior to the greater trochanter.
- The **saphenous nerve** (L3-L4) is a branch of the femoral nerve that passes through the adductor (*Hunter's*) canal, bypasses the adductor hiatus, and continues down near the medial knee, leg and foot. It innervates most of the skin of the medial leg and a portion of the medial foot.

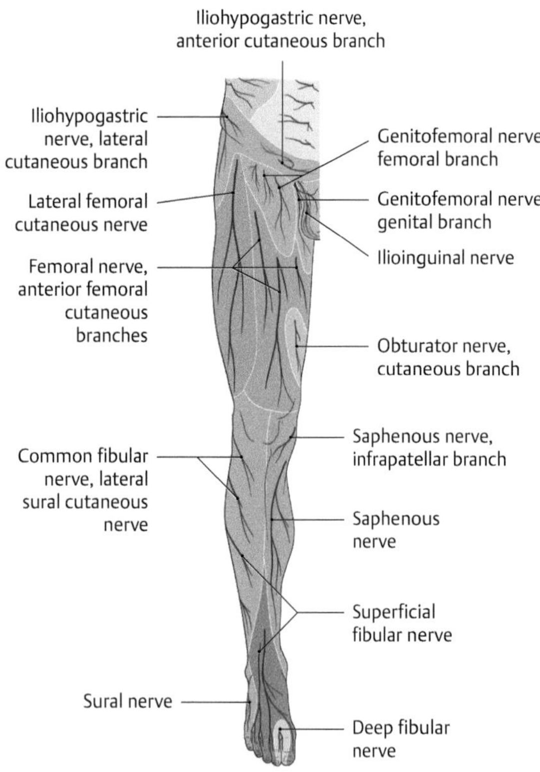

Fig. 5.18 Cutaneous innervation of the lower extremity, anterior view. (From Schuenke M, Schulte E, Schumacher U. THIEME Atlas of Anatomy. General Anatomy and Musculoskeletal System. Illustrations by Voll M and Wesker K. 3rd ed. New York: Thieme Medical Publishers; 2020.)

- The **lateral sural cutaneous nerve** (L5-S2) is a branch of the common fibular nerve and innervates most of the skin of the lateral leg.
- The **medial sural cutaneous nerve** (S1-S2) is a branch of the tibial nerve and innervates the skin of the posterior but middle portion of the leg.
- The **sural nerve** (S1-S2) is formed by the fusion of the lateral and medial sural cutaneous nerves or the fusion of the medial sural cutaneous with that of a communicating branch that originates from either the common fibular or lateral sural cutaneous nerve. It innervates the skin of the posterolateral leg, lateral malleolus and lateral aspect of the foot.
- The **calcaneal nerves** (S1-S2) originate from the tibial and sural nerves and innervate the skin of the heel.

5.9.3 Dermatomes and Myotomes of the Lower Extremity

The areas of skin supplied primarily by the T12-S3 spinal nerves contribute to the lower extremity **dermatomes**. Like any other region of the body, there is an overlap with the next adjacent dermatome except at the **axial line**, a line that demarcates a junction of dermatomes that are supplied by discontinuous spinal levels. An axial line is located on the posteromedial lower extremity between the L1-L4 and the S2 dermatomes **(Fig. 5.20)**.

Somatic motor (GSE) fibers traveling through mixed peripheral nerves are responsible for innervating the muscles of the lower extremities. The ipsilateral and embryological muscle group that receives innervation from a single spinal cord segment or spinal nerve constitutes a **myotome**. Lower extremity

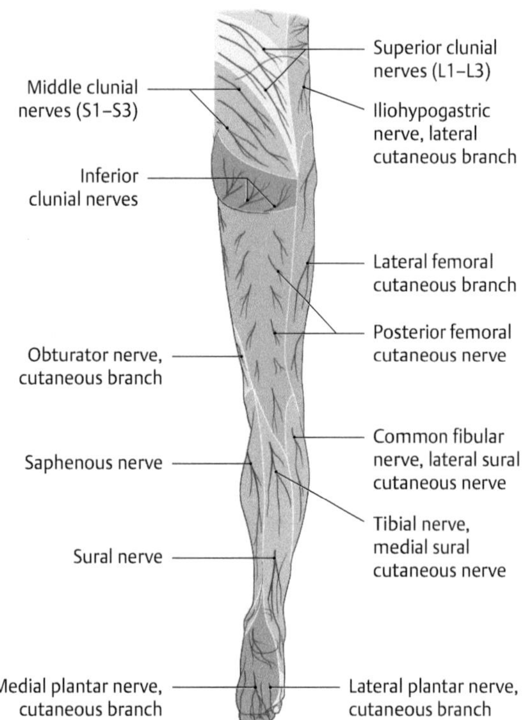

Fig. 5.19 Cutaneous innervation of the lower extremity, posterior view. (From Schuenke M, Schulte E, Schumacher U. THIEME Atlas of Anatomy. General Anatomy and Musculoskeletal System. Illustrations by Voll M and Wesker K. 3rd ed. New York: Thieme Medical Publishers; 2020.)

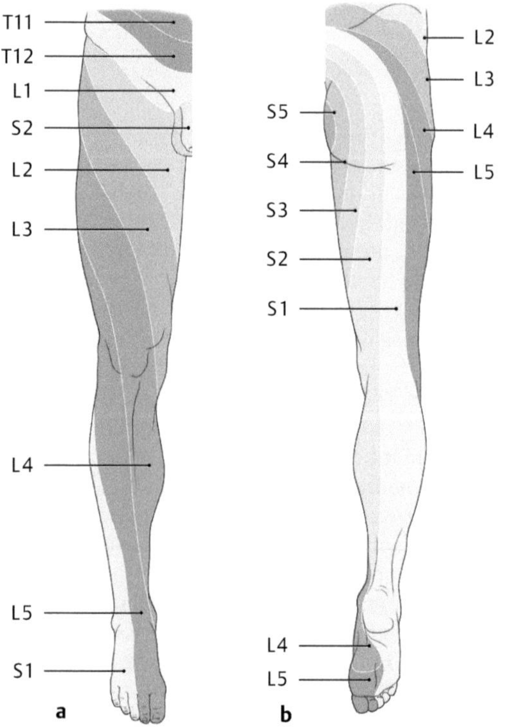

Fig. 5.20 Dermatomes of the lower extremity. **(a)** Anterior view. **(b)** Posterior view. (From Schuenke M, Schulte E, Schumacher U. THIEME Atlas of Anatomy. General Anatomy and Musculoskeletal System. Illustrations by Voll M and Wesker K. 3rd ed. New York: Thieme Medical Publishers; 2020.)

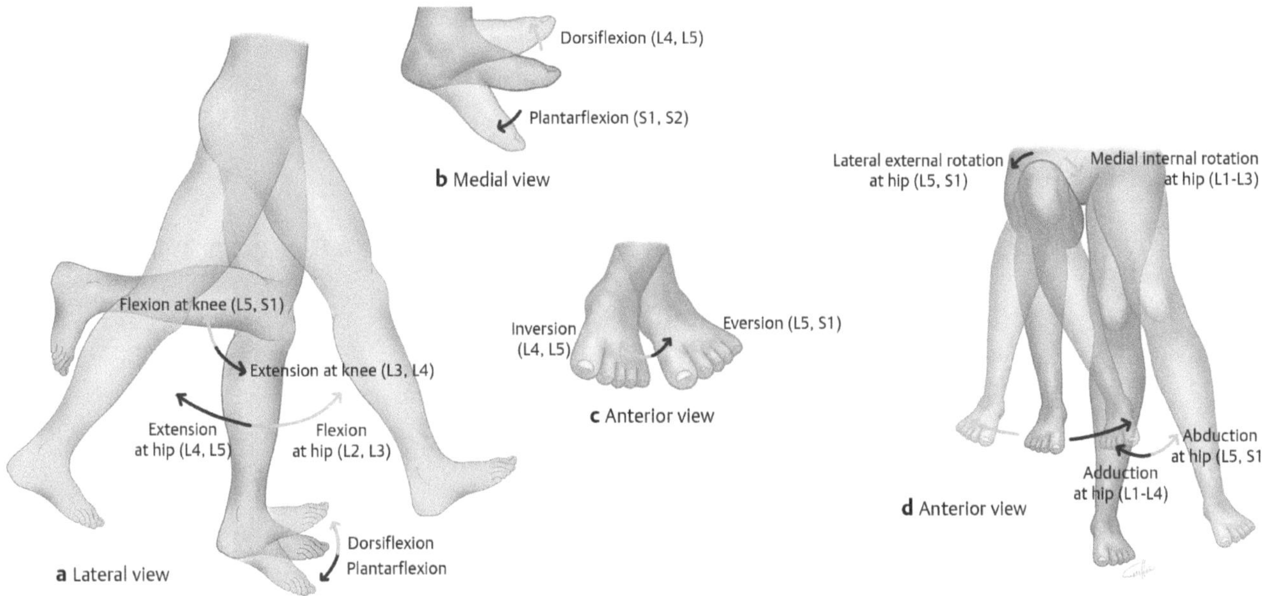

Fig. 5.21 Myotomes: segmental innervation of muscle groups. Illustration by Calla Heald.

muscles can be quite bulky and extensive thus they generally receive motor fibers from several spinal cord segments or nerves. This means that lower extremity muscles are usually composed of multiple myotomes. The segmental innervation and the movements of the lower extremity they assist with are as follows (**Fig. 5.21**):

- Adduction, flexion and medial (internal) rotation at hip joint: L1-L4.
- Abduction, extension and lateral (external) rotation at hip joint: L5-S1.
- Extension at knee joint: L3-L4.
- Flexion at knee joint: L5-S1.
- Dorsiflexion at ankle joint: L4-L5.
- Plantarflexion at ankle joint: S1-S2.
- Inversion of foot: L4-L5.
- Eversion of foot: L5-S1.
- Intrinsic muscles of foot: S2-S3.

5.9.4 Blood Supply of Lower Extremity

There are two major arteries and their branches that are responsible for distributing blood to soft tissue and muscles related to the lower extremities. They are the *internal iliac* and *femoral arteries* (**Fig. 5.22**).

The **internal iliac** is one of two branches of the *common iliac artery* and it is mostly associated with branches that supply the pelvic organs and perineum. However, the *superior gluteal, inferior gluteal* and *obturator arteries* that originate from it are responsible for supplying either the gluteal or medial thigh regions respectively. The **superior gluteal artery** passes between the lumbosacral trunk and S1 ventral rami branch and enters the buttocks through the greater sciatic foramen above the piriformis muscle. The artery itself splits into a *superficial* and *deep branch* by the gluteus medius muscle. The **inferior gluteal artery** generally passes between the S2 and S3 ventral rami branches and enters the buttocks through the greater sciatic foramen as well but below the piriformis muscle. Both gluteal arteries supply the gluteal muscles and skin of the buttocks. The inferior gluteal can form an anastomosis with the superior gluteal, internal pudendal, obturator and the medial circumflex femoral arteries that allow for additional blood supply to the posterior thigh, pelvis and hip joint regions. The **obturator artery** generally originates from the internal iliac but in a minority of individuals it arises from the external iliac or inferior epigastric arteries. It gives rise to the **artery to the head of the femur** in addition to other branches. It may form a circular anastomosis on the superficial surface of the obturator membrane before extending into the medial thigh to assist in supplying the muscles of that region.

The external iliac becomes the **femoral artery** as it passes deep to the inguinal ligament. It has a palpable pulsation just below the inguinal ligament as it enters the anterior thigh and because of its close proximity to the skin while in the femoral triangle it makes it susceptible to damage. Just after passing the inguinal ligament, there are multiple arterial branches that include the *superficial circumflex iliac, superficial epigastric, superficial external pudendal* and the *deep external pudendal arteries.* The **superficial circumflex iliac artery** supplies blood to the subcutaneous inguinal region whereas the **superficial epigastric artery** supplies blood to the subcutaneous lower anterior abdominal wall region. Both the **superficial** and **deep external pudendal arteries** have branches that supply the skin of the scrotum, labium majus and perineum regions. While in the area known as the femoral triangle, the femoral artery will give off the **profunda femoris artery** (deep artery of the thigh). This artery will have 3-4 **perforating artery** branches that help supply the posterior thigh region as well as the **lateral** and **medial circumflex femoral arteries** that supply a combination of the hip joint, anterior thigh and gluteal regions. At the apex of the femoral triangle, the femoral artery continues through the adductor canal and before reaching the adductor hiatus, give rise to the **descending genicular artery** that supplies the knee joint and medial skin of the knee region. As the femoral artery passes through the adductor hiatus it becomes the popliteal artery (**Fig. 5.22**).

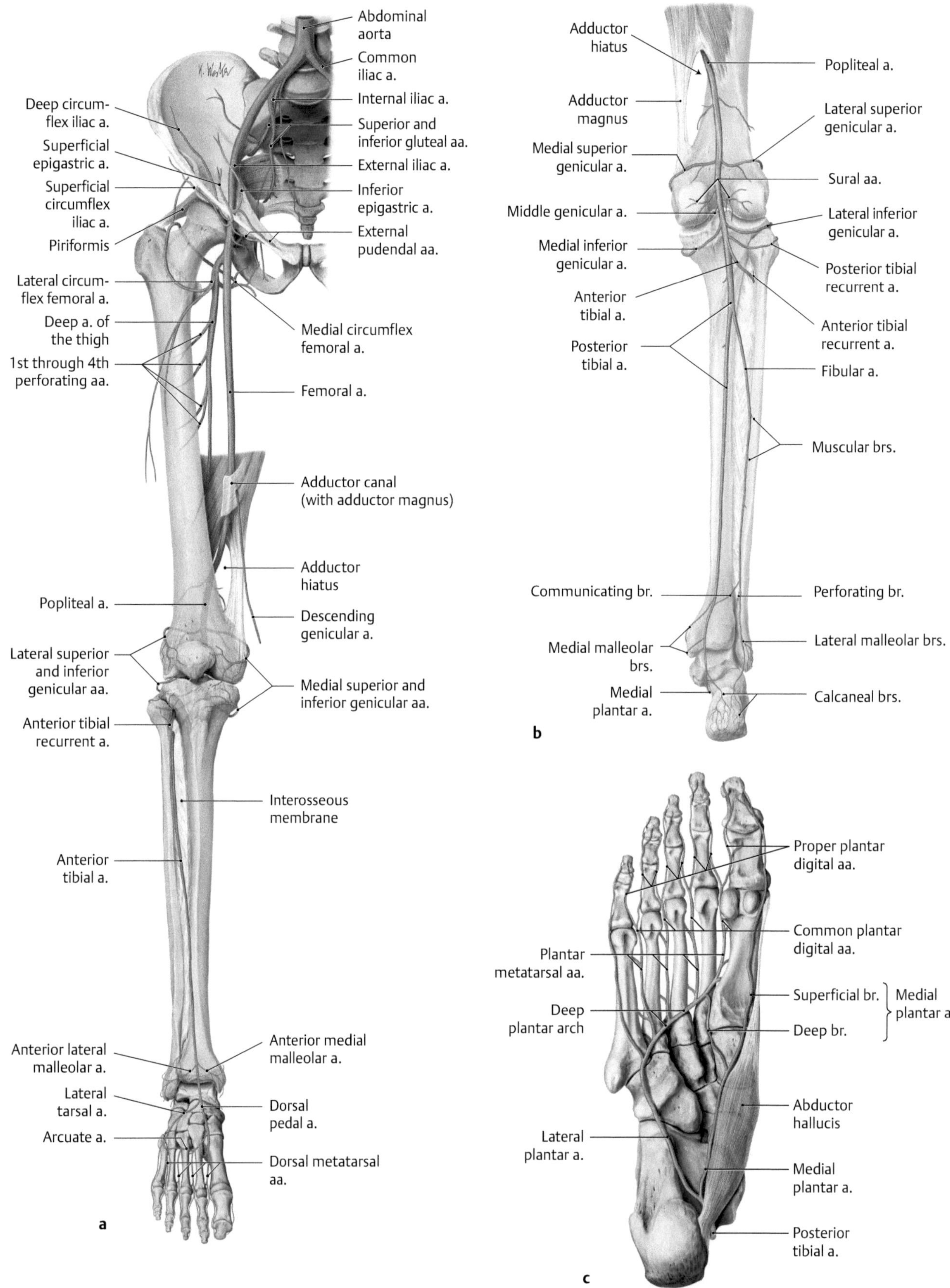

Fig. 5.22 Arteries of the lower extremity. **(a)** Right limb, anterior view. **(b)** Right leg, posterior view. **(c)** Right foot, plantar view. (From Schuenke M, Schulte E, Schumacher U. THIEME Atlas of Anatomy. General Anatomy and Musculoskeletal System. Illustrations by Voll M and Wesker K. 3rd ed. New York: Thieme Medical Publishers; 2020.)

The **popliteal artery** passes through the popliteal fossa region of the posterior knee. In this region, the popliteal artery gives rise to multiple genicular arteries that form a larger anastomosis responsible for supplying the knee joint. These include the **superior lateral genicular**, **superior medial genicular**, **middle genicular**, **inferior lateral genicular** and the **inferior medial genicular arteries.** The popliteal artery bifurcates into an anterior and posterior tibial artery near the popliteus muscle. The **anterior tibial artery** passes through a gap in the interosseous membrane and supplies the anterior leg compartment as well as both sides of the ankle. The **posterior tibial artery** continues through the tendinous arch of the soleus muscle along with the *tibial nerve*. Just after passing through the tendinous arch the **fibular (peroneal) artery** branches from the posterior tibial and helps supply the lateral compartment of the leg along with the lateral ankle region **(Fig. 5.22)**.

The posterior tibial artery bifurcates just distal to the tarsal tunnel to become the lateral and medial plantar arteries. The **lateral plantar artery** is the larger of the two branches and forms the majority of the **plantar arch** of the foot that gives rise to vessels that supply portions of all the foot digits. The **medial plantar artery** contributes to the great toe and a small portion to the plantar arch **(Fig. 5.22)**.

5.9.5 Venous Drainage of Lower Extremity

There are both superficial and deep veins responsible for draining blood from the lower extremity. Coursing through the subcutaneous tissue under the skin but above the deep fascia are the *superficial veins* and these include the numerous unnamed tributaries that drain into either the *great* or *small saphenous veins.* These veins have **venous valves** or flaps of endothelium with valvular sinuses that fill with blood from above. When full, the valve cusps occlude the lumen of the vein thereby preventing of any retrograde blood movement. These valves also break down the blood into shorter segments, reducing back pressure. Both the prevention of retrograde flow and reducing back pressure make it easier for the *musculovenous pump* to overcome gravity when returning blood towards the heart. The two major superficial veins are described below **(Fig. 5.23; Fig. 5.24)**.

- The **great saphenous vein** is the longest vein in the body, contains approximately 10-20 venous valves, and is formed by the *dorsal venous arch of the foot* and the *dorsal vein of the great toe*. It begins its ascent anterior to the medial malleolus, and passes posterior to the medial condyle about

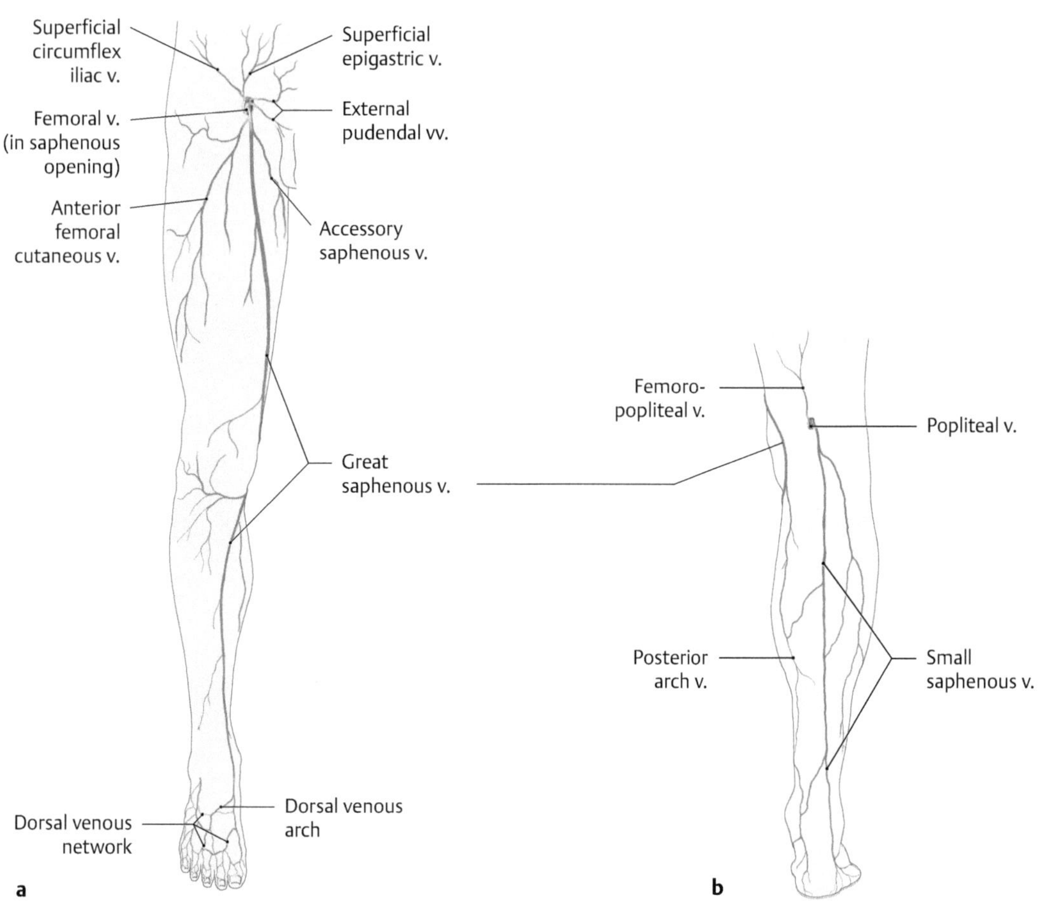

Fig. 5.23 Superficial veins of the lower extremity. **(a)** Anterior view. **(b)** Posterior view. (From Schuenke M, Schulte E, Schumacher U. THIEME Atlas of Anatomy. General Anatomy and Musculoskeletal System. Illustrations by Voll M and Wesker K. 3rd ed. New York: Thieme Medical Publishers; 2020.)

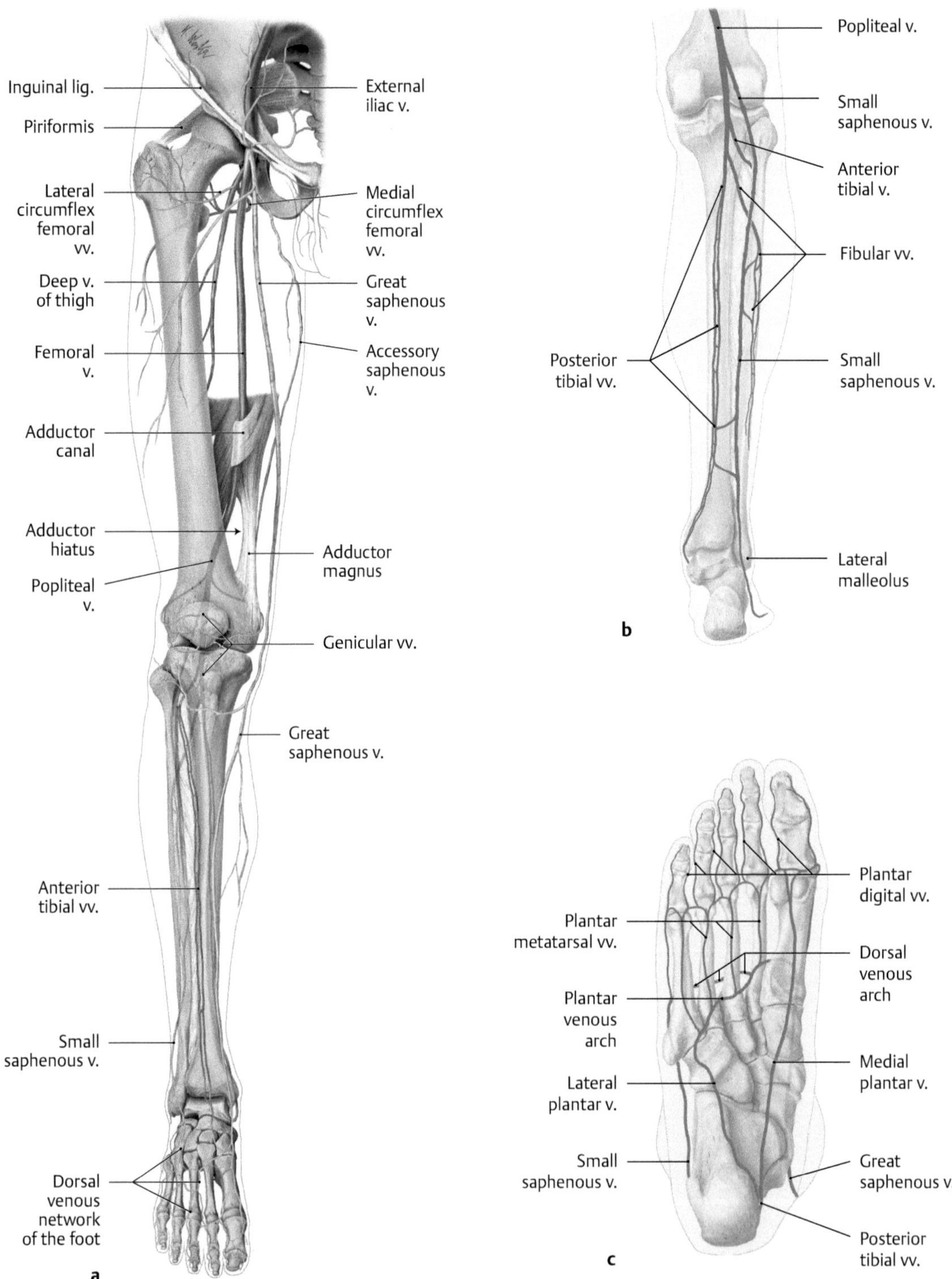

Fig. 5.24 Deep veins of the lower extremity. **(a)** Right limb, anterior view. **(b)** Right leg, posterior view. **(c)** Right foot, plantar view. (From Schuenke M, Schulte E, Schumacher U. THIEME Atlas of Anatomy. General Anatomy and Musculoskeletal System. Illustrations by Voll M and Wesker K. 3rd ed. New York: Thieme Medical Publishers; 2020.)

a hands breadth posterior to the medial border of the patella before passing through the saphenous opening and draining into the femoral vein. There are multiple tributaries that drain into the great saphenous vein and it does have an anastomosis with small saphenous vein in multiple locations. An **accessory saphenous vein** may be present and is formed primarily by tributaries of the medial and posterior thigh regions. The accessory saphenous vein may serve as the main anastomosis between the great and small saphenous veins. The great saphenous vein also receives drainage from the *anterior femoral cutaneous*, *external pudendal*, *superficial epigastric* and *superficial circumflex iliac veins* near its termination and is paired with the *saphenous nerve* in the leg region.

- The **small saphenous vein** contains approximately 10 venous valves and is formed by the *dorsal venous arch of the foot, dorsal vein of the little toe* and the *lateral marginal vein of the foot.* This vein ascends posterior to the lateral malleolus and lateral to the calcaneal tendon. After splitting the two heads of the gastrocnemius muscle, it perforates the deep fascia of the popliteal fossa and drains into the popliteal vein.

There are **perforating veins** that penetrate the deep fascia at an oblique angle starting first near their origin next to the corresponding superficial veins and they contain valves that allow for only superficial to deep blood flow. Due to their oblique angles, when muscles contract leading to pressure increases inside the deep fascia, the now compressed perforating veins prevent the blood from traveling in the direction of deep to superficial veins. The proper drainage of superficial to deep venous circulation enables the muscular contractions to pump blood back toward the heart against gravity thus contributing to the *musculovenous pump* **(Fig. 5.25)**.

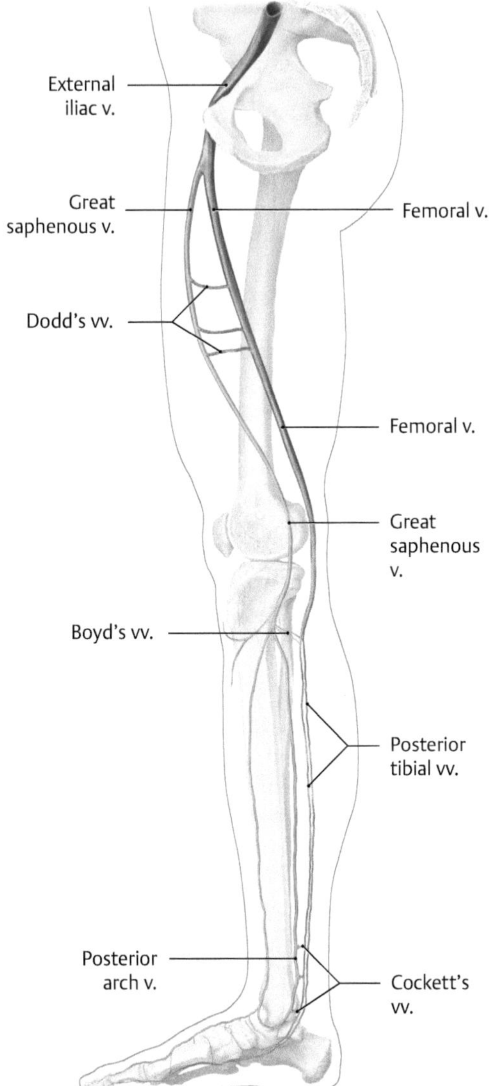

Fig. 5.25 Clinically important perforating veins include Dodd, Boyd and Cockett veins. (From Schuenke M, Schulte E, Schumacher U. THIEME Atlas of Anatomy. General Anatomy and Musculoskeletal System. Illustrations by Voll M and Wesker K. 3rd ed. New York: Thieme Medical Publishers; 2020.)

The deep veins are located below the deep fascia and are paired with the arteries. They contain valves and in many instances there are two smaller veins paired with one slightly larger artery. Beginning with the foot region, the major deep veins that would pair with the blood supply recently discussed are described **(Fig. 5.26)**.

The **lateral** and **medial plantar veins** receive blood from the **plantar digital veins** and **plantar arch of the foot** before fusing to become the posterior tibial veins. The **posterior tibial vein** receives the **fibular (peroneal) vein** just prior to the soleal line of the tibia. Just superior to the soleal line the **anterior tibial vein** joins the posterior tibial vein near the inferior border of the popliteus muscle to become the **popliteal vein**. Near the knee region there are multiple **genicular veins** that drain into the popliteal vein.

As the popliteal vein passes through the adductor hiatus it changes names to become the femoral vein. The **femoral vein** passes through the *adductor canal* of the anterior thigh and receives the great saphenous vein just deep to the *saphenous opening*. The **profunda femoris vein** receives 3-4 **perforating veins** that drain the posterior thigh region along with the **lateral** and **medial circumflex femoral veins** that are closely associated with the lateral thigh and hip joint. The profunda femoris vein drains into the femoral vein and at the level of the inguinal ligament the femoral vein becomes the **external iliac vein** and it receives the drainage of the **deep circumflex iliac** and **inferior epigastric veins**. The **obturator**, **internal pudendal**, **superior gluteal** and **inferior gluteal veins** all drain into the **internal iliac vein**. After the external iliac fuses with the internal iliac vein they become the **common iliac vein (Fig. 5.23; Fig. 5.24)**.

Clinical Correlate 5.14

Varicose Veins

When the veins of the lower extremities become enlarged and gnarled so that the cusps of the valves are unable to close properly these are known as **varicose veins**. The valves in a varicose vein are incompetent due to this dilation or venous rotation allowing blood to regurgitate causing pain, itching and possible vascular disease. Causes include normal aging that reduces the elasticity of the vein, obesity, standing for long periods of time, or during pregnancy when blood volume increases. Treatments can include wearing compression socks in mild cases or endoscopic vein surgery, vein stripping, and sclerotherapy procedures with more advanced varicose veins.

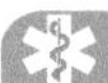

Clinical Correlate 5.15

Deep Vein Thrombosis (DVT)

A **deep vein thrombosis (DVT)** occurs when a blood clot forms in one or more of the deep veins, usually somewhere in the lower extremity. It is a serious condition because these clots can break loose and lodge themselves into the lungs resulting in a pulmonary embolism. A patient may feel pain or notice swelling in the affected leg. A sudden onset of shortness of breath, chest pain, lightheadedness and rapid pulse are warning signs of a pulmonary embolism. Risk factors include prolonged bed rest or sitting, a recent surgery, pregnancy, age, smoking or having an inflammatory bowel disease.

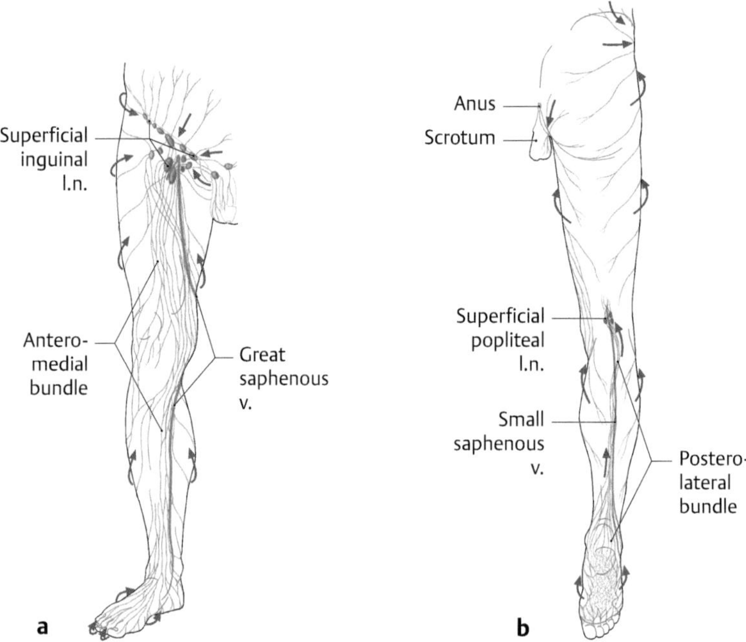

Fig. 5.26 Superficial lymph nodes of the lower extremity. Arrows indicate the main directions of lymphatic drainage. **(a)** Anterior view. **(b)** Posterior view. (From Schuenke M, Schulte E, Schumacher U. THIEME Atlas of Anatomy. General Anatomy and Musculoskeletal System. Illustrations by Voll M and Wesker K. 3rd ed. New York: Thieme Medical Publishers; 2020.)

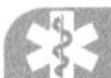 *Clinical Correlate 5.16*

Great Saphenous Vein Grafting

The great saphenous vein was originally the vessel of choice during coronary bypass surgery but the reliance of this vessel has decreased some. It was and still is for some surgeons the vessel of choice because of its accessibility; it has a larger amount of elastic and muscular fibers versus other superficial veins; and the total length of the graft is sufficient because of the distance between the tributaries and the perforating veins. The vein is inverted during a bypass so that the valves allow for free flow of the blood. The musculovenous pump may become more effective with the removal of this vein by facilitating more superficial to deep venous drainage.

5.9.6 Lymphatic Drainage of the Lower Extremity

Much like the venous drainage, the lower extremity has both superficial and deep lymphatic drainage. The superficial lymphatic vessels are seen converging towards and then coursing along the great and small saphenous veins. The lymphatic vessels that accompany the great saphenous veins drain into the **superficial inguinal lymph nodes**. These lymph nodes also receive lymph from the superficial tissues of the gluteal region. Lymph can then pass directly to the **external iliac lymph nodes** or first through the **deep inguinal lymph nodes** before reaching the external iliac lymph nodes. The lymphatic vessels that follow the small saphenous vein ultimately drain into the **popliteal lymph nodes** located near the popliteal vessels (**Fig. 5.26**).

Deep veins of the leg including the anterior tibial, posterior tibial and fibular (peroneal) veins have *deep lymphatic vessels* passing along with them. These lymphatic vessels drain into the popliteal lymph nodes. From these lymph nodes, lymph travels along the femoral vessels before reaching the deep inguinal lymph nodes. From the deep inguinal lymph nodes, lymph continues to travel superiorly to the **external iliac** and **common iliac lymph nodes** before reaching the **lumbar lymph nodes**. Lymph originating from the deeper tissues of the gluteal region travel with the superior and inferior gluteal vessels before reaching the **superior gluteal** and **inferior gluteal lymph nodes** respectively. From these lymph nodes, lymph travels to the **internal iliac lymph nodes** before reaching the common iliac and then from here the lymph continues to the lumbar lymph nodes (**Fig. 5.27**).

5.10 Lower Extremity Region Specifics

The lower extremity is separated into areas such as the gluteal region, posterior thigh and popliteal fossa, anterior thigh, medial thigh, anterior leg, lateral leg, posterior leg and the foot. These regions each have a nerve or two associated with the innervation of their muscles and certain vessels supplying the muscles and surrounding tissue and skin. A simple principle regarding muscles of the lower extremity (as well as the upper extremity) is if the muscle crosses and acts on a joint thus creating a movement, these same muscles also function to stabilize that joint.

5.11 Gluteal Region

The area located posterior to the pelvis is known as the **gluteal region** or more commonly as the buttocks. The borders of this region include the iliac crest and ASIS superiorly, the greater trochanter inferolaterally, and the gluteal fold inferiorly. The individual buttocks are separated down the midline by the **intergluteal**

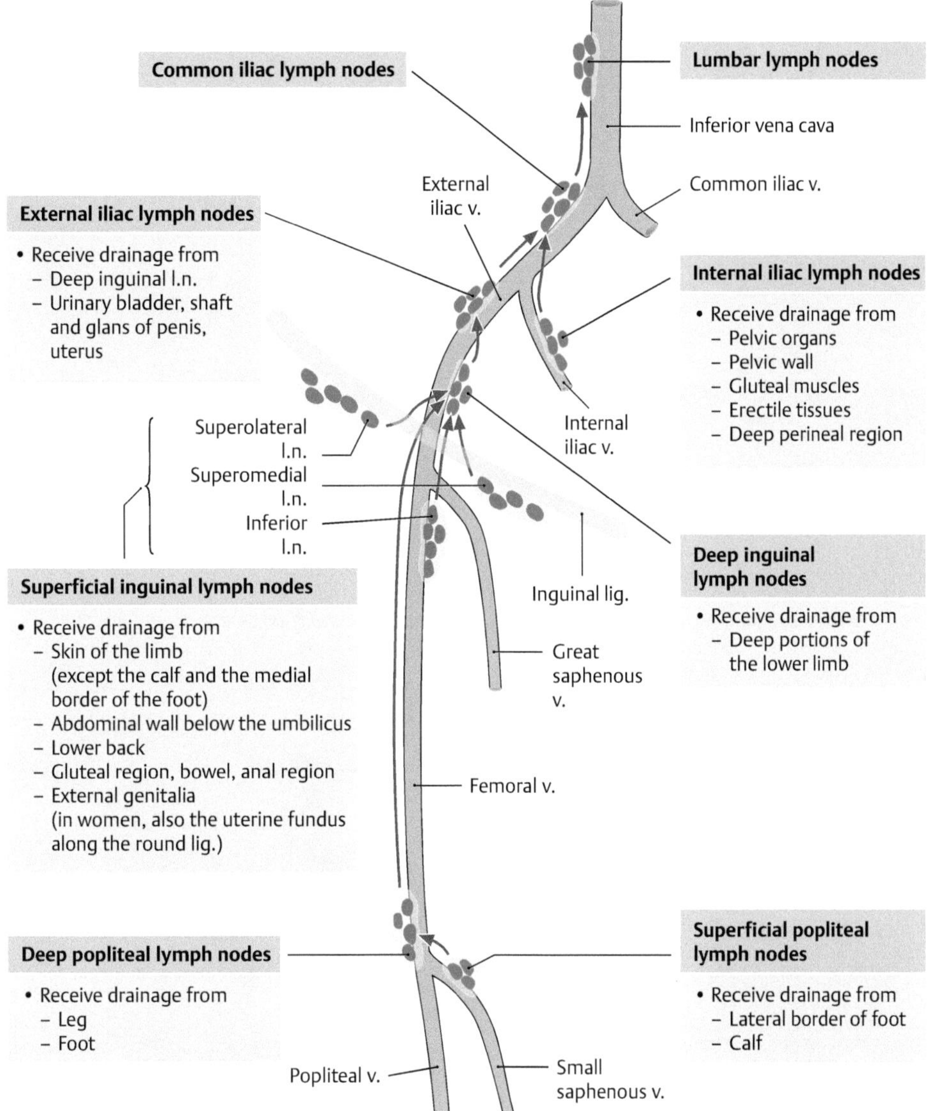

Fig. 5.27 Lower extremity lymph nodes and drainage. (From Schuenke M, Schulte E, Schumacher U. THIEME Atlas of Anatomy. General Anatomy and Musculoskeletal System. Illustrations by Voll M and Wesker K. 3rd ed. New York: Thieme Medical Publishers; 2020.)

cleft. The sacrotuberous and sacrospinous ligaments are responsible for binding together the hip bones, sacrum and coccyx, structures that make up the bony pelvis. The **sacrotuberous ligament** extends from the ischial tuberosity to the posterior iliac spines, inferior sacrum and coccyx. Along with the sacrospinous ligament, it converts the lesser sciatic notch into the **lesser sciatic foramen**, a passageway for structures passing to and from the perineum. The **sacrospinous ligament** connects the ischial spine with that of the inferior sacrum and coccyx. It converts the greater sciatic notch into the **greater sciatic foramen**, a passageway for structures that enter and exit the pelvis **(Fig. 5.28)**.

5.11.1 Gluteal Muscles

The gluteal muscles are divided into a superficial and deep muscle group. The *superficial group* consists of the much larger muscles and they include the gluteus maximus, gluteus medius, gluteus minimus and the tensor fasciae latae muscles. The gluteus maximus acts primarily in *extension* and *lateral rotation of the thigh* at the hip joint. The gluteus medius, gluteus minimus and tensor fasciae latae muscles function primarily in *abduction* and *medial rotation of the thigh*. In addition, the two gluteal muscles help *maintain a level pelvis* when the opposite leg is elevated **(Fig. 5.29)**.

The *deep group* consists of smaller muscles and they include the piriformis, obturator internus, superior and inferior gemelli that rest above or below the obturator internus, and finally the quadratus femoris. All of these muscles act as *lateral rotators of the thigh* but other functions can include *abduction of the thigh* and stabilization of the hip joint. Descriptions of gluteal region muscles are found in **Table 5.1.**

5.11.2 Gluteal Region Bursae

- There are four **gluteal bursas** and three of them are associated with the gluteus maximus muscle. The other bursa associated

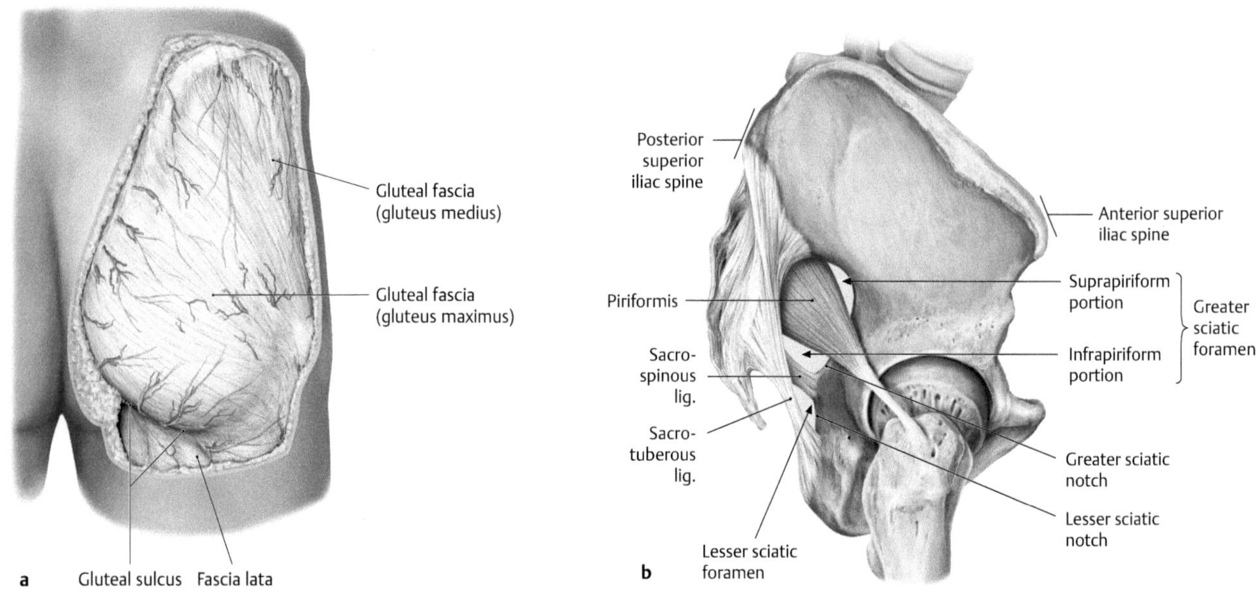

Fig. 5.28 (a) Fasciae of the gluteal region. **(b)** Sciatic foramina. (From Schuenke M, Schulte E, Schumacher U. THIEME Atlas of Anatomy. General Anatomy and Musculoskeletal System. Illustrations by Voll M and Wesker K. 3rd ed. New York: Thieme Medical Publishers; 2020.)

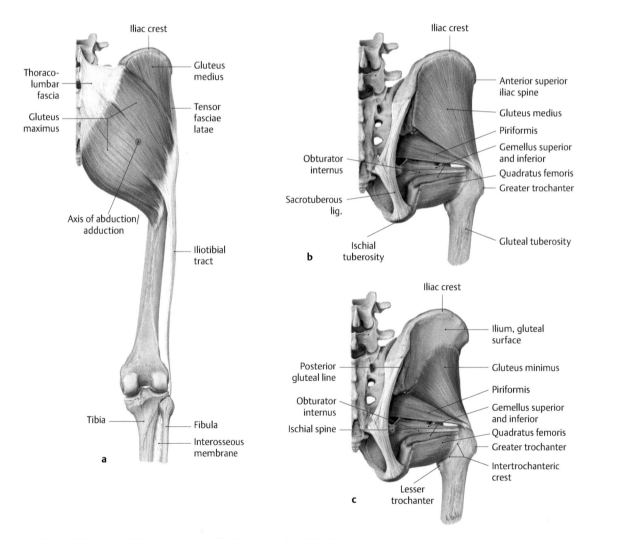

Fig. 5.29 (a) Superficial muscles of the gluteal region. **(b, c)** Deep muscles of the gluteal region. (From Schuenke M, Schulte E, Schumacher U. THIEME Atlas of Anatomy. General Anatomy and Musculoskeletal System. Illustrations by Voll M and Wesker K. 3rd ed. New York: Thieme Medical Publishers; 2020.)

Table 5.1 **Gluteal region muscles**

Muscle	Innervation	Function(s)	Origin	Insertion
Gluteus maximus	Inferior gluteal nerve	Extends thigh especially when standing; laterally rotates thigh	Posterior iliac crest; posterior surface of sacrum and coccyx; sacrotuberous ligament	Iliotibial tract and gluteal tuberosity
Gluteus medius	Superior gluteal nerve	Abducts and medially rotates thigh; keeps pelvis level when opposite lower limb is elevated during swing phase of gait	External surface of ilium between the anterior and posterior gluteal lines	Greater trochanter (lateral surface)
Gluteus minimus	Superior gluteal nerve	Abducts and medially rotates thigh; keeps pelvis level when opposite lower limb is elevated during swing phase of gait	External surface of ilium between the anterior and inferior gluteal lines	Greater trochanter (anterior surface)
Tensor fasciae latae	Superior gluteal nerve	Abducts, flexes and medially rotates thigh	Anterior iliac crest; anterior superior iliac spine	Iliotibial tract and distally at the anterolateral tubercle (Gerdy's) of tibia
Piriformis	Ventral rami of S1-S2	Abduct flexed thigh; laterally rotate extended thigh	Pelvic surface of sacrum; sacrotuberous ligament	Greater trochanter (superior border)
Superior gemellus	Nerve to obturator internus	Abduct flexed thigh; laterally rotate extended thigh	Ischial spine	Greater trochanter (trochanteric fossa)
Obturator internus	Nerve to obturator internus	Abduct flexed thigh; laterally rotate extended thigh	Deep surface of obturator membrane; ischiopubic rami	Greater trochanter (trochanteric fossa)
Inferior gemellus	Nerve to quadratus femoris	Abduct flexed thigh; laterally rotate extended thigh	Ischial tuberosity	Greater trochanter (trochanteric fossa)
Quadratus femoris	Nerve to quadratus femoris	Laterally rotate thigh	Ischial tuberosity	Quadrate tubercle on interchanteric crest

with the obturator internus muscle. They function by reducing friction and permitting unhindered movement. These include:

- **Ischial bursa**: separates the gluteus maximus from the ischial tuberosity.
- **Trochanteric bursa**: separates the gluteus maximus from the greater trochanter (**Fig. 5.31**).
- **Gluteofemoral bursa**: separates the portion of the iliotibial tract associated with the gluteus maximus from the proximal attachment of the vastus lateralis muscle.
- **Obturator internus bursa**: it underlies the tendon of the obturator internus and allows free movement over the posterior border of the ischium.

5.11.3 Neurovasculature of the Gluteal Region

The skin of this region is innervated primarily by multiple *clunial nerves* but on the lateral aspects the **iliohypogastric** and **lateral femoral cutaneous nerves** are involved. The **superior clunial nerves** originate from the dorsal rami of L1-L3 while the **middle clunial nerves** originate from the dorsal rami of S1-S3. Only the inferior clunial nerves, branches of the posterior femoral cutaneous nerve originate from ventral rami and those are of S1-S3 (**Fig. 5.30**).

The **superior gluteal nerve** is a sacral plexus branch which passes above the piriformis and between the gluteus medius and minimus muscles and is paired with the deep branch of the superior gluteal artery. This nerve innervates the gluteus medius, gluteus minimus and tensor fasciae latae muscles. The **inferior gluteal nerve** is a sacral plexus branch that passes inferior to the piriformis and is responsible for innervating the gluteus maximus muscle. Multiple branches are present in order to sufficiently innervate the gluteus maximus, which is very broad and the largest muscle of the body (**Fig. 5.31**).

The **sciatic nerve** is the largest nerve in the body and it generally passes inferior to the piriformis muscle. It is composed of both a medial *tibial* and lateral *common fibular nerve* that bifurcate near the popliteal fossa. It is the lateral most structure exiting from the greater sciatic foramen that is inferior to the piriformis muscle. The sciatic nerve innervates nothing in the gluteal region. Its tibial or common fibular nerve divisions supply the posterior thigh muscles or give off branches that ultimately innervate muscles of the leg and foot as well as the skin of most of the leg and foot (**Fig. 5.31**).

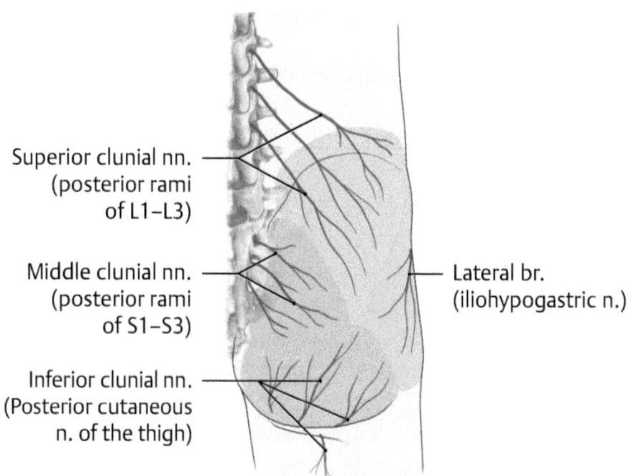

Fig. 5.30 Cutaneous innervation of the gluteal region. (From Schuenke M, Schulte E, Schumacher U. THIEME Atlas of Anatomy. General Anatomy and Musculoskeletal System. Illustrations by Voll M and Wesker K. 3rd ed. New York: Thieme Medical Publishers; 2020.)

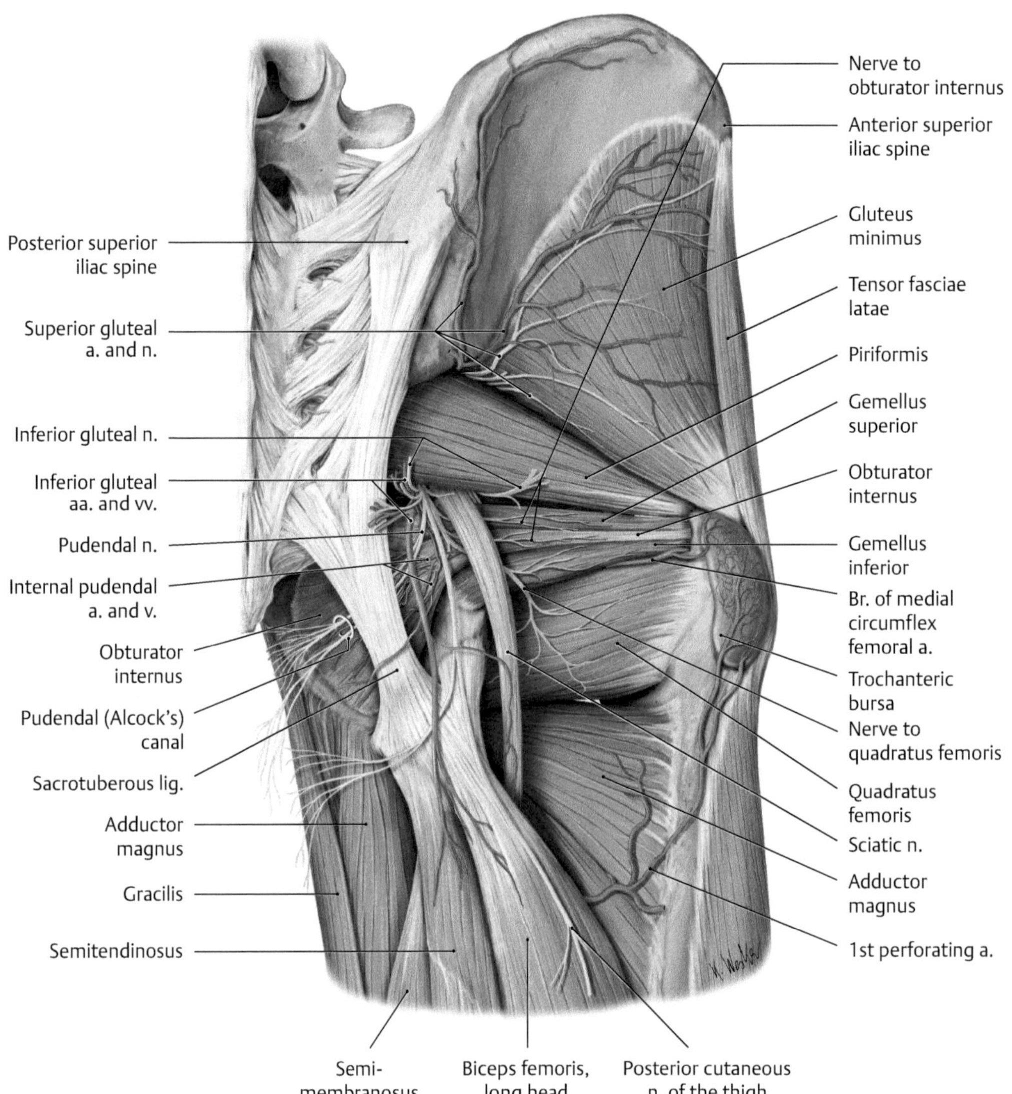

Fig. 5.31 Neurovasculature of the gluteal region. (From Schuenke M, Schulte E, Schumacher U. THIEME Atlas of Anatomy. General Anatomy and Musculoskeletal System. Illustrations by Voll M and Wesker K. 3rd ed. New York: Thieme Medical Publishers; 2020.)

Lying just medial to the sciatic nerve is the **posterior femoral cutaneous nerve.** Its inferior clunial nerve branches innervate the skin of the lower buttocks but the majority of this nerve innervates the skin of the posterior thigh and popliteal fossa.

The **nerve to obturator internus** passes between the posterior femoral cutaneous nerve and the pudendal nerve before innervating the obturator internus and superior gemellus muscles. The **pudendal nerve** is the most medial structure to exit the pelvis through the greater sciatic foramen but it does not innervate any structures related to the lower extremity. This nerve and its branches are primarily involved in the innervation of the perineum discussed in Chapter 4. The **nerve to quadratus femoris** passes anterior to the obturator internus muscle and sciatic nerve and will then continue over the posterior surface of the hip joint before innervating the quadratus femoris and inferior gemellus muscles (**Fig. 5.31**).

The blood supply to the gluteal region originates mostly from the superior and inferior gluteal arteries. Both of these arteries, along with the internal pudendal artery originate from the internal iliac artery. The **superior gluteal artery** is the largest internal iliac artery branch and it passes between the lumbosacral trunk and S1 ventral rami spinal nerve. Its deep branch courses along with the superior gluteal nerve. Branches of this artery supply the gluteus maximus, medius and minimus along with the tensor fascia latae muscles. It forms an anastomosis with both the inferior gluteal and medial circumflex femoral arteries (**Fig. 5.31**).

The **inferior gluteal artery** generally passes between the S2 and S3 ventral rami spinal nerves before pairing up with the inferior gluteal nerve. Branches of this artery supply in addition the gluteus maximus, the obturator internus, superior and inferior gemelli, quadratus femoris and superior portions of the hamstrings. The **artery of the sciatic nerve** is a branch of the inferior gluteal artery. Located just medial to the inferior gluteal artery is the **internal pudendal artery**. It is paired with the pudendal nerve and it exits the gluteal region immediately in order to enter the perineum through the lesser sciatic foramen and supplies no structures in the gluteal region (**Fig. 5.31**).

Clinical Correlate 5.17

Superior Gluteal Nerve Injury
An injury to the superior gluteal nerve results in a disabling "gluteus medius limp" which compensates for the weakened abduction of the thigh by the gluteus medius and minimus muscles. A gluteal gait may also be present and is a compensatory leaning of the body toward the weakened side. When a person stands on one leg, the gluteus medius and minimus normally contract as soon as the contralateral foot leaves the floor to prevent tipping of the pelvis to the unsupported side.

When a person stands on one leg and there is a paralysis of the superior gluteal nerve, the pelvis descends on the unsupported side, indicating that the contralateral gluteus medius and minimus are weak or nonfunctional. Clinically this referred to as a **positive Trendelenburg test**. To compensate for the unsupported side that makes the lower limb on that side too long, the individual leans away from the unsupported side raising the pelvis to allow adequate room for the foot to clear the ground as it swings forward and the patient demonstrates a *waddling gait*.

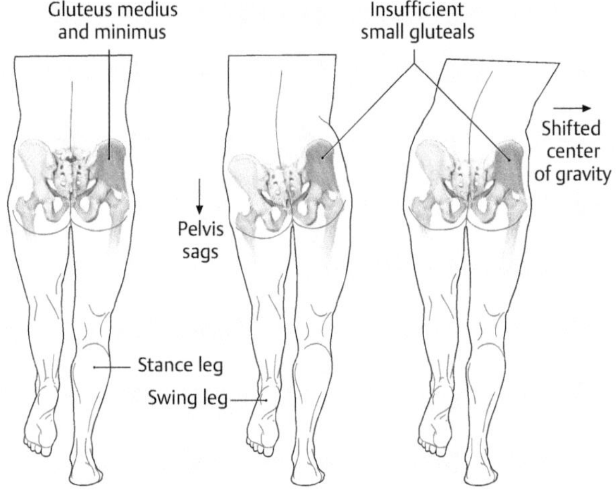

(From Schuenke M, Schulte E, Schumacher U. THIEME Atlas of Anatomy. General Anatomy and Musculoskeletal System. Illustrations by Voll M and Wesker K. 3rd ed. New York: Thieme Medical Publishers; 2020.)

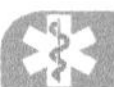

Clinical Correlate 5.18

Bursitis of the Gluteal Region
Trochanteric bursitis is described as point tenderness near the greater trochanter. It can be a diffuse deep pain located in the lateral thigh region radiating along the iliotibial (IT) tract and is due to repetitive activities such as stair climbing. **Ischial bursitis** is the result of excessive friction between the ischial bursae and ischial tuberosity while overextending oneself during cycling exercises for example. The ischial tuberosities bear the weight of the body while sitting. Over time, pressure sores can develop and become debilitating, especially in paraplegics.

Venous drainage of the gluteal region follows the arterial supply with the **superior** and **inferior gluteal veins** along with the **internal pudendal vein** draining back into the **internal iliac vein**.

Clinical Correlate 5.19

Intragluteal Injections
The gluteal region is a common place for intramuscular injections because the muscles are thick and provide a large area for venous absorption of drugs. Injections must be done in the *superolateral quadrant* of the buttock to reduce any complications that may lead to the injuring of nerves, or creating an abscess or hematoma.

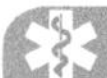

Clinical Correlate 5.20

Sciatic Nerve Injury and Nerve Blocks
If the sciatic nerve is *completely severed*, the ipsilateral lower extremity becomes mostly useless. Motor innervation to the posterior thigh, leg and foot is lost. Functions such as hip extension, knee flexion, dorsiflexion and plantarflexion of the foot are eliminated. The cutaneous innervation to the most of the leg and foot is lost, as well. The anterior and medial thigh regions are spared because the femoral and obturator nerves innervate them, respectively. *Compression of the sciatic nerve* could be the result of **piriformis syndrome**. In this case, the sciatic nerve (or a specific division of it) is compressed as it passes through the piriformis muscle. The sciatic nerve as a whole generally leaves the gluteal region just inferior to the piriformis muscle.

Anesthesia in a **sciatic nerve block** can be injected a few centimeters inferior to the midpoint of a line connecting the posterior superior iliac spine and superior border of the greater trochanter. This eliminates any paresthesia normally radiating down the posterior lower extremity down to the foot.

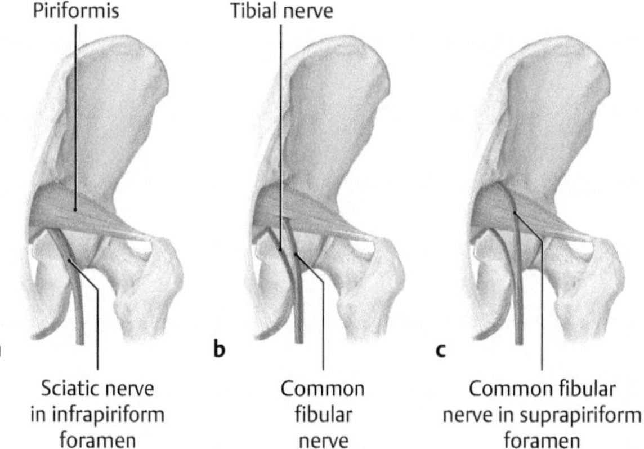

Variations of the sciatic nerve: **(a)** 85%; **(b)** ~15%; **(c)** ~0.5%.
(From Schuenke M, Schulte E, Schumacher U. THIEME Atlas of Anatomy. General Anatomy and Musculoskeletal System. Illustrations by Voll M and Wesker K. 3rd ed. New York: Thieme Medical Publishers; 2020.)

5.12 Hip Joint

The **hip joint** is located between the pelvic girdle and lower limb. It is a strong and stable *ball-and-socket type synovial joint*. The acetabulum forms the socket and the femoral head serves as the ball. Movements include flexion, extension, abduction, adduction, lateral (extortion) and medial (intortion) rotation and the combined movement known as circumduction. When an individual stands, the entire weight of the upper body is transmitted through the hip

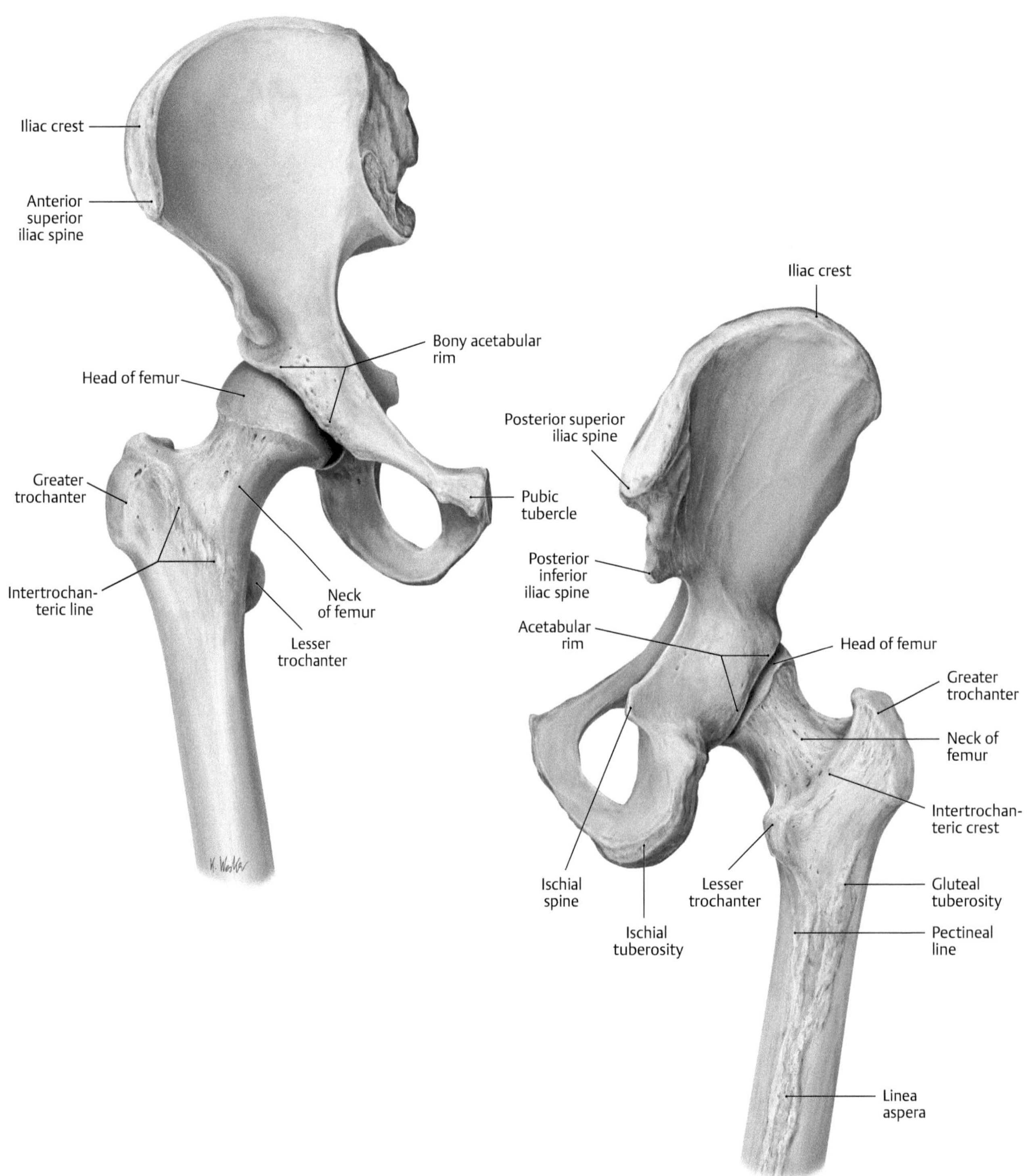

Fig. 5.32 Right hip joint. (From Schuenke M, Schulte E, Schumacher U. THIEME Atlas of Anatomy. General Anatomy and Musculoskeletal System. Illustrations by Voll M and Wesker K. 3rd ed. New York: Thieme Medical Publishers; 2020.)

bones to the heads and necks of the femurs (**Fig. 5.32; Fig. 5.33; Fig. 5.34; Fig. 5.35**).

5.12.1 Acetabulum and Articulating Surfaces

The large cup-shaped socket on the lateral aspect of the hip bones is called the acetabulum and it is where the head of the femur articulates. The acetabulum is not a complete socket and an **acetabular notch** is located on its inferior aspect. Depth of the acetabulum increases due to the fibrocartilaginous **acetabular labrum** along with the **transverse acetabular ligament** that fills in the acetabular notch. The **acetabular fossa** is the middle depression in the floor of the acetabulum that extends to the acetabular notch. A fat pad fills this fossa in the region not occupied by the ligament of the femoral head. The surface that articulates with the femur is called

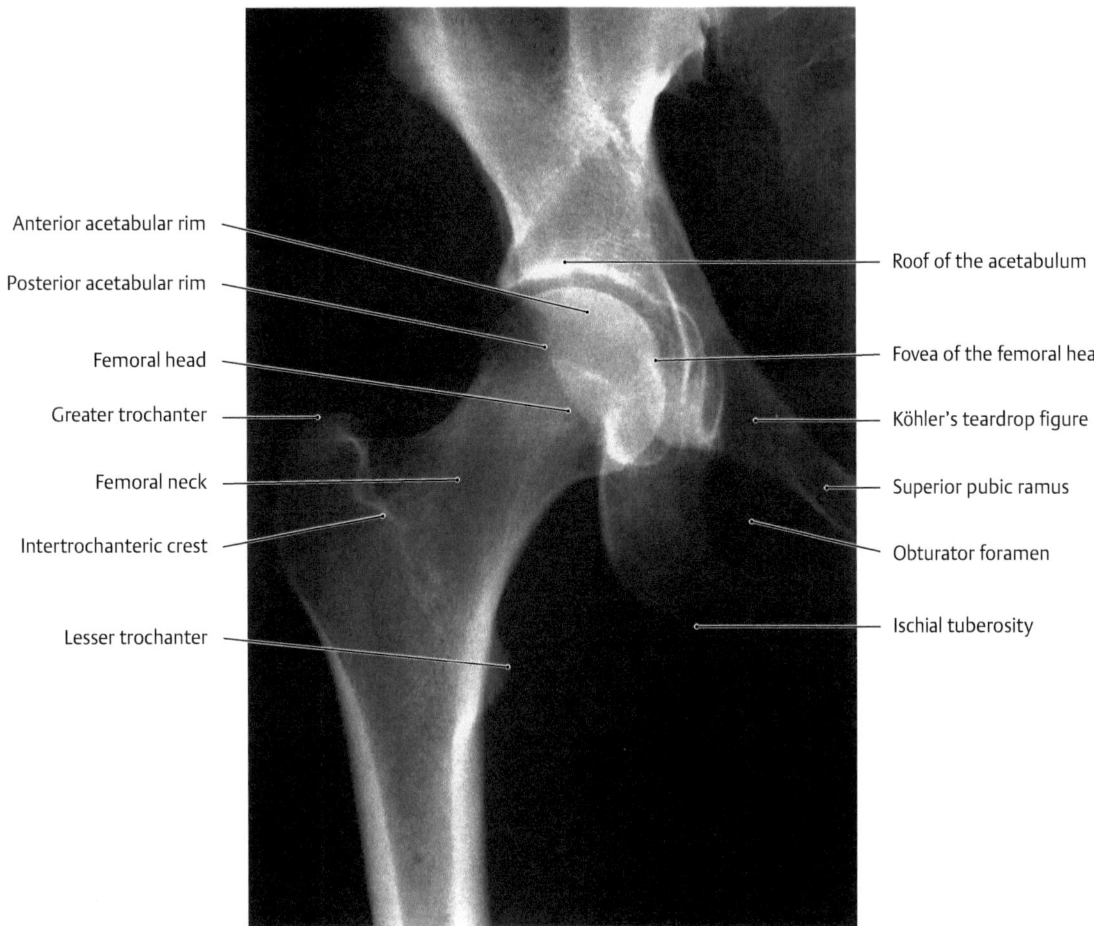

Fig. 5.33 Radiograph of the right hip joint, anteroposterior view. (From Möller TB, Reif E. Taschenatlas der Röntgenanato 2nd ed. Stuttgart: Thieme; 1998.)

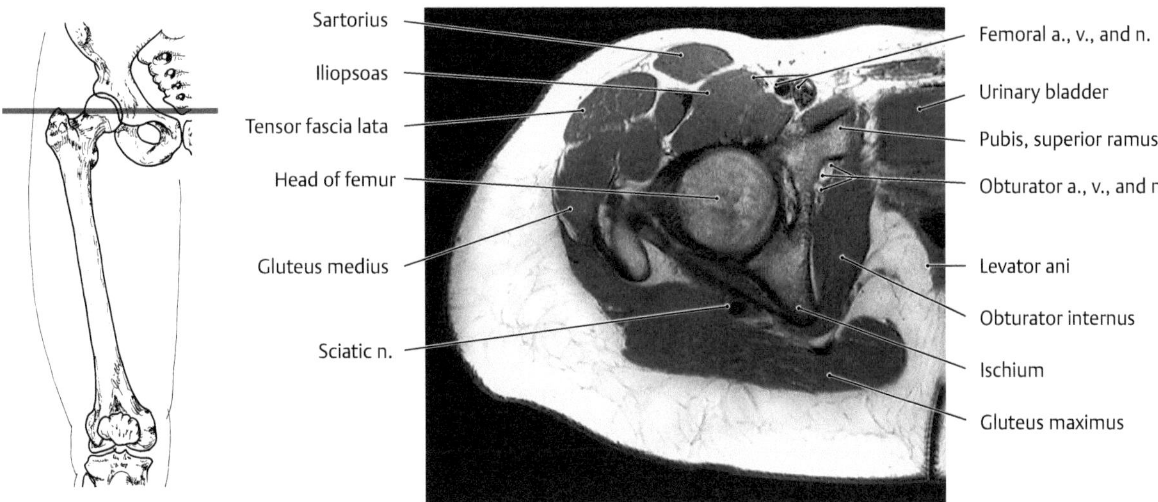

Fig. 5.34 MRI of the right hip joint. Transverse section, inferior view. (From Moeller TB, Reif E. Atlas of Sectional Anatomy: The Musculoskeletal System. New York, NY: Thieme; 2009.)

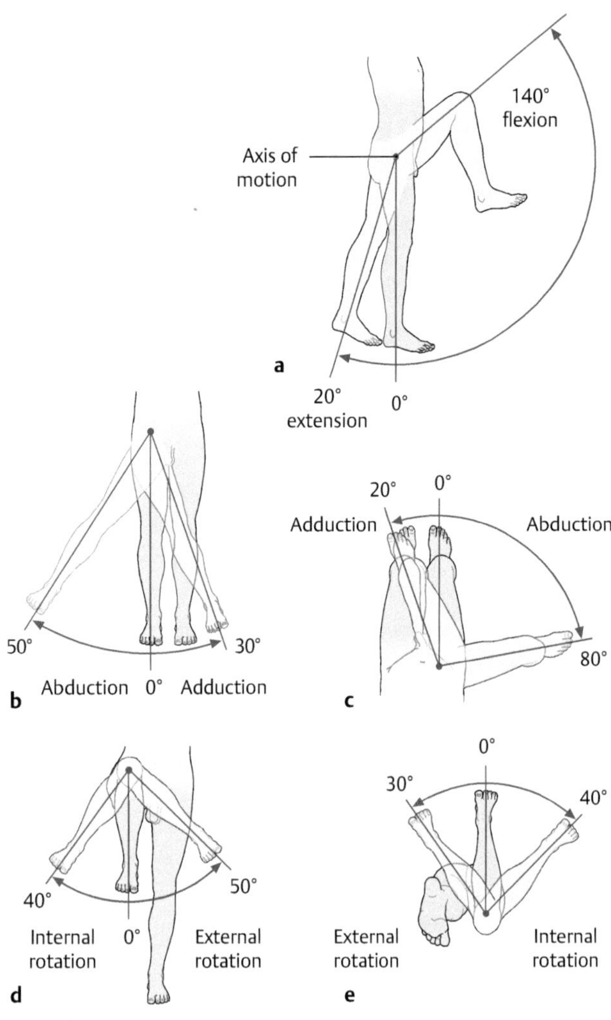

Fig. 5.35 Range of motion of the hip joint from the neutral (zero-degree) position. **(a)** Range of flexion/extension. **(b)** Range of abduction/adduction with the hip extended. **(c)** Range of abduction/adduction with hip flexed 90-degrees. **(d)** Range of internal/external rotation with the hip flexed 90-degrees. **(e)** Range of internal/external rotation in the prone position. (From Schuenke M, Schulte E, Schumacher U. THIEME Atlas of Anatomy. General Anatomy and Musculoskeletal System. Illustrations by Voll M and Wesker K. 3rd ed. New York: Thieme Medical Publishers; 2020.)

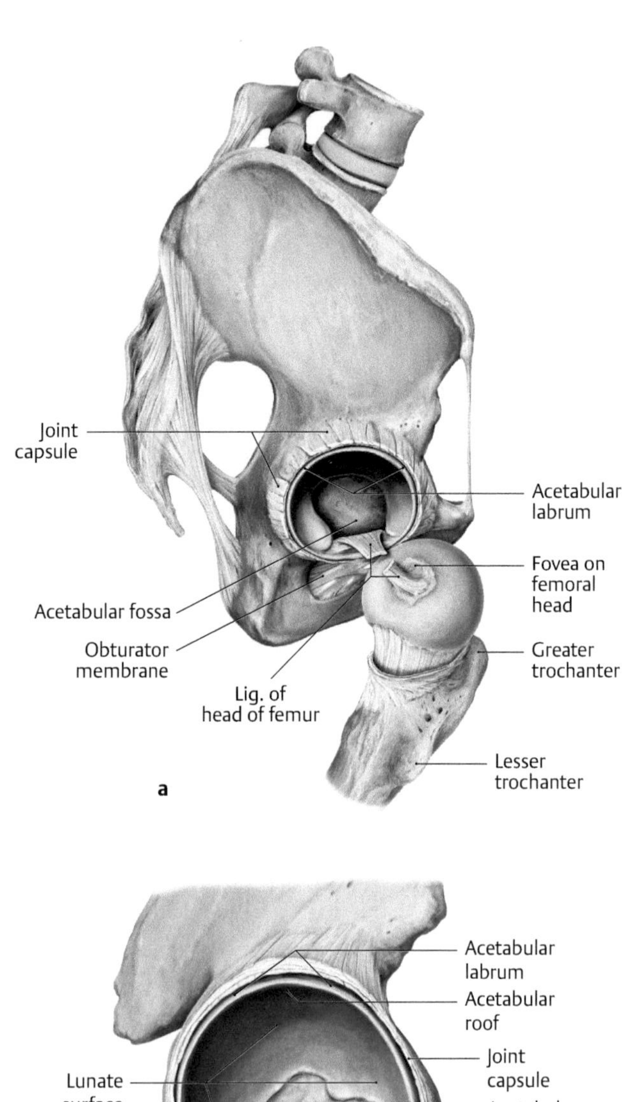

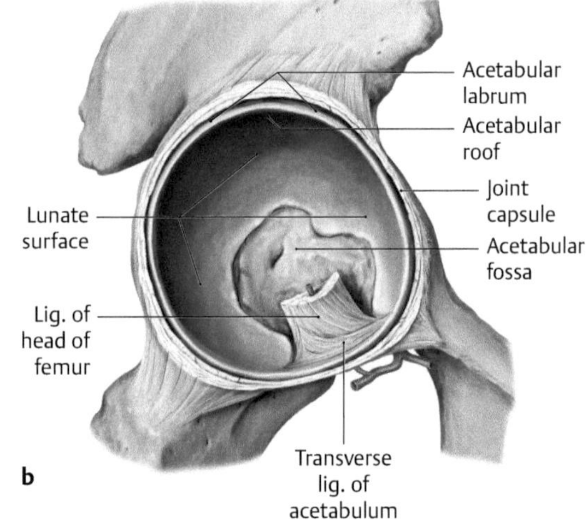

Fig. 5.36 (a, b) Lateral view of hip joint and acetabulum. (From Schuenke M, Schulte E, Schumacher U. THIEME Atlas of Anatomy. General Anatomy and Musculoskeletal System. Illustrations by Voll M and Wesker K. 3rd ed. New York: Thieme Medical Publishers; 2020.)

the **lunate surface** of the acetabulum. As mentioned previously, all three hip bones contribute to the overall structure of the acetabulum **(Fig. 5.36)**.

The **head of the femur** is round and more than half of it fits within the acetabulum. Most of the outer articulating surface is covered by hyaline cartilage except for the pit region called the **fovea for the ligament of the femoral head**. The **ligament of the femoral head** is a weak synovial fold that allows for passage of the **artery to the head of the femur** (or *acetabular branch*). It originates mostly from the obturator but also from the medial circumflex femoral artery **(Fig. 5.36)**.

5.12.2 Joint Capsule

The capsule of the hip joint is strong. It is formed by an external fibrous layer (fibrous capsule) and lined internally by the synovial membrane. The fibrous layer attaches to the peripheral acetabular rim and transverse acetabular ligament proximally. Distally it attaches to the intertrochanteric line (anteriorly) and passes over the intertrochanteric crest (posteriorly) without attaching to it. The fibrous capsule has fibers that have a spiral orientation while some of the deeper fibers are more circular and form the **orbicular zone.** The extracapsular ligaments of the hip joint make up the fibrous layer for the most part and they include **(Fig. 5.37; Fig. 5.38)**:

- **Iliofemoral ligament** (*Y ligament of Bigalow*): located anteriorly and superiorly and considered the strongest ligament of

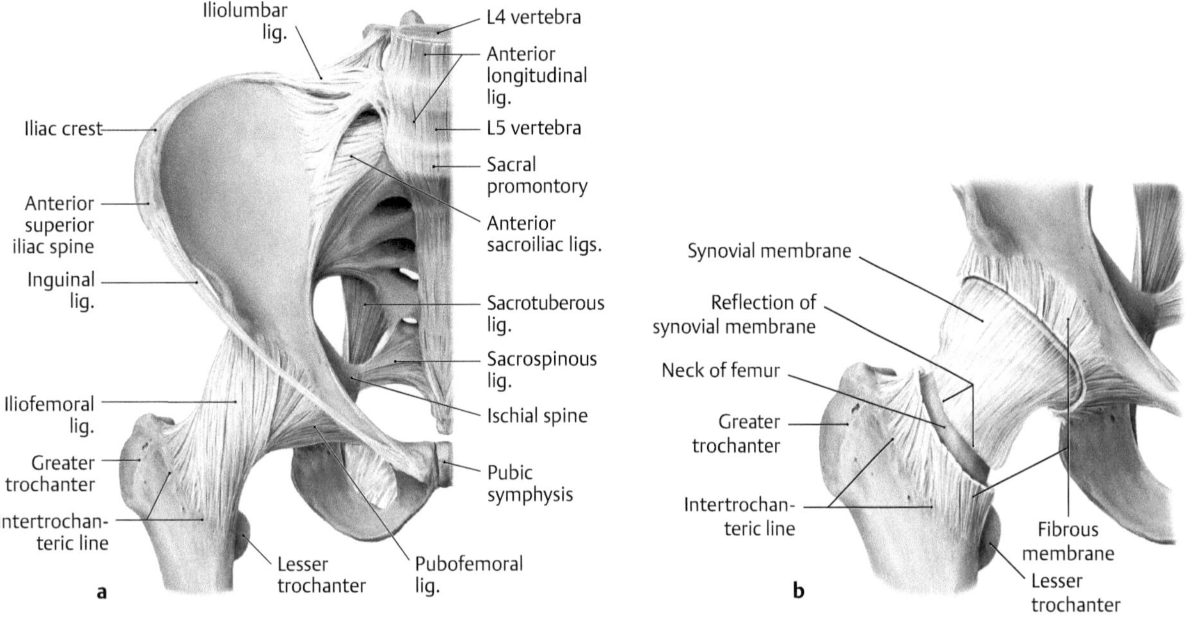

Fig. 5.37 (a, b) Anterior view of the hip joint, synovial membrane, and ligaments. (From Schuenke M, Schulte E, Schumacher U. THIEME Atlas of Anatomy. General Anatomy and Musculoskeletal System. Illustrations by Voll M and Wesker K. 3rd ed. New York: Thieme Medical Publishers; 2020.)

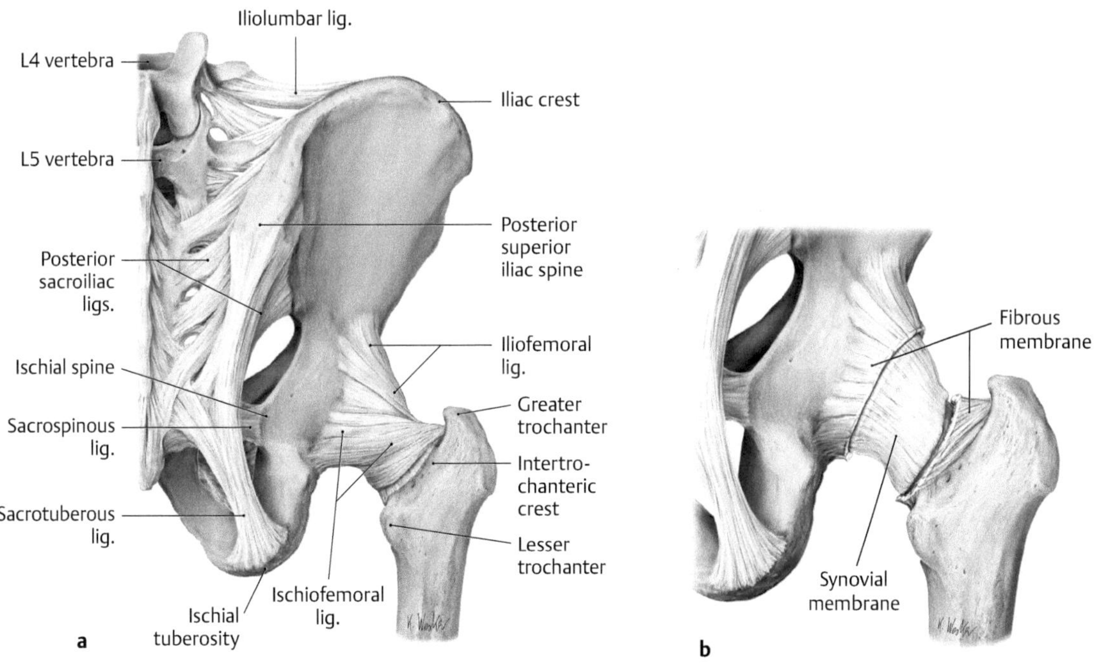

Fig. 5.38 (a, b) Posterior view of the hip joint, synovial membrane, and ligaments. (From Schuenke M, Schulte E, Schumacher U. THIEME Atlas of Anatomy. General Anatomy and Musculoskeletal System. Illustrations by Voll M and Wesker K. 3rd ed. New York: Thieme Medical Publishers; 2020.)

the body. It attaches to the AIIS and acetabular rim proximally while distally it attaches to the intertrochanteric line distally. It prevents hyperextension at the hip joint during standing by screwing the femoral head into the acetabulum and limits lateral rotation.

- **Pubofemoral ligament**: located anteriorly and inferiorly originating from the obturator crest of the pubic bone. Blends with the medial portion of the iliofemoral ligament. Prevents overabduction of the hip joint.
- **Ischiofemoral ligament** (*of Bertin*): located posteriorly and originates from the ischial part of the acetabular rim. Spirals superolaterally to the neck of the femur medial to the base of the greater trochanter. Prevents hyperextension and limits medial rotation.

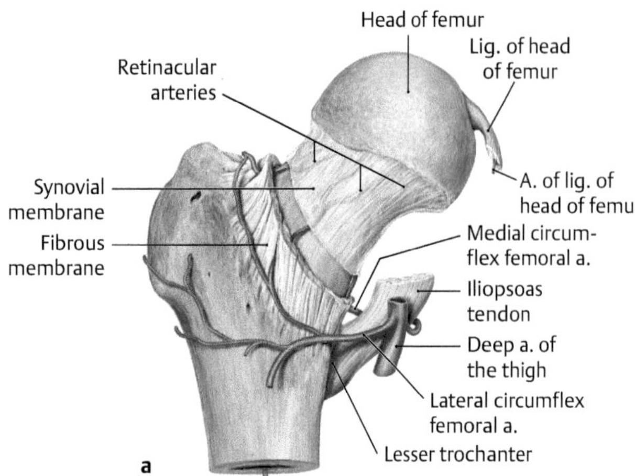

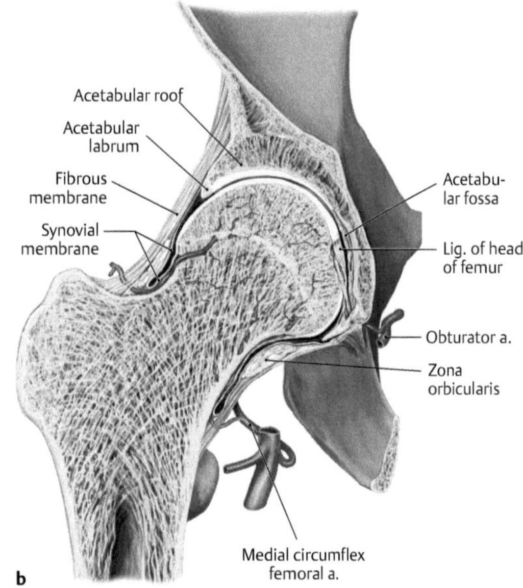

Fig. 5.39 (a) Right femur. **(b)** Right femur, coronal section. (From Schuenke M, Schulte E, Schumacher U. THIEME Atlas of Anatomy. General Anatomy and Musculoskeletal System. Illustrations by Voll M and Wesker K. 3rd ed. New York: Thieme Medical Publishers; 2020.)

The *synovial membrane*, much like all synovial joints, lines the internal surface of the fibrous layer. It extends to all parts of the intracapsular surfaces except for where there is articular cartilage. The synovial membrane of the hip joint reflects proximally along the femoral neck and to the edge of the femoral head. The membrane has synovial folds (retinacula) and they cover the femoral neck. Passing through these folds are the **retinacular arteries**, branches mainly of the medial circumflex femoral artery that supply the femoral head and neck **(Fig. 5.39)**.

5.12.3 Neurovasculature of the Hip Joint

Innervation to this joint and all others in the limbs will follow *Hilton's Law*, which states that the nerves supplying the muscles extending directly across and acting on the joint also innervate it. Thus the nerves acting on muscles that have an effect at the hip joint would include the sciatic, superior gluteal, inferior gluteal, obturator, femoral, nerve to quadratus femoris, and nerve to obturator internus. The first few have a greater effect.

The main blood supply to this joint is via the **retinacular arteries** described above. These vessels are branches of the **medial circumflex femoral** mainly but the **lateral circumflex femoral** and **artery to the head of the femur** (obturator br.) also contribute to this joint. The lateral/medial circumflex femoral arteries are branches of the profunda femoris artery. Venous drainage would pair with the arterial supply **(Fig. 5.39)**.

Clinical Correlate 5.21

Hip Joint Dislocations

Posterior hip dislocations occur through a posterior tear of the joint capsule. These account for about 90% of all hip dislocations and are commonly seen in head-on motor vehicle collisions. These dislocations occur when the femur is flexed and adducted at the hip joint. Structures damaged may include the sciatic nerve, ligament of the head of the femur, and the posterior acetabular labrum. These result in the affected lower limb being *shortened, flexed, adducted* and *medially rotated*.

Anterior dislocations of the hip joint occur through an anterior tear through the joint capsule. They occur when the femur is abducted and laterally rotated at the hip joint. Structures damaged could include the femoral neurovasculature and this type of dislocation results in the affected lower limb being *lengthened, flexed, abducted* and *laterally rotated*.

5.13 Posterior Thigh and Popliteal Fossa Regions

The area located just below the gluteal region is known as the **posterior thigh**. This region is synonymous with the hamstring muscles and *extension of thigh* and *flexion of the knee*. The sciatic nerve and posterior femoral cutaneous nerves are the major nerves of the posterior thigh. After the sciatic nerve bifurcates into the tibial and common fibular nerves near the popliteal fossa the tibial nerve travels through the popliteal fossa and the common fibular nerve makes its way toward the lateral leg. Both of these nerves then branch off cutaneous nerves that pass through the popliteal fossa and superoposterior leg region **(Fig. 5.40)**.

The **popliteal fossa**, or posterior knee region, has superficial borders formed by the biceps femoris (superolaterally), semimembranosus (superomedially), lateral head of gastrocnemius (inferolaterally) and the medial head of the gastrocnemius (inferomedially). More deeply, the lateral and medial supracondylar lines of the femur establish the superior borders while the soleal line of the tibia represents the inferior border. The anterior border is made up of the popliteal surface of the femur while the popliteal deep fascia forms the posterior border. This fossa is mainly filled with fat but its contents include the tibial, common fibular and posterior femoral cutaneous nerves, the proximal lateral and medial sural cutaneous nerves (before they penetrate the popliteal deep fascia), popliteal vessels, termination of the small saphenous vein, and the popliteal lymph nodes **(Fig. 5.41)**.

5.13.1 Posterior Thigh Muscles

All muscles found in the posterior thigh are considered the hamstring muscles except for the **short head of biceps femoris**. Therefore the

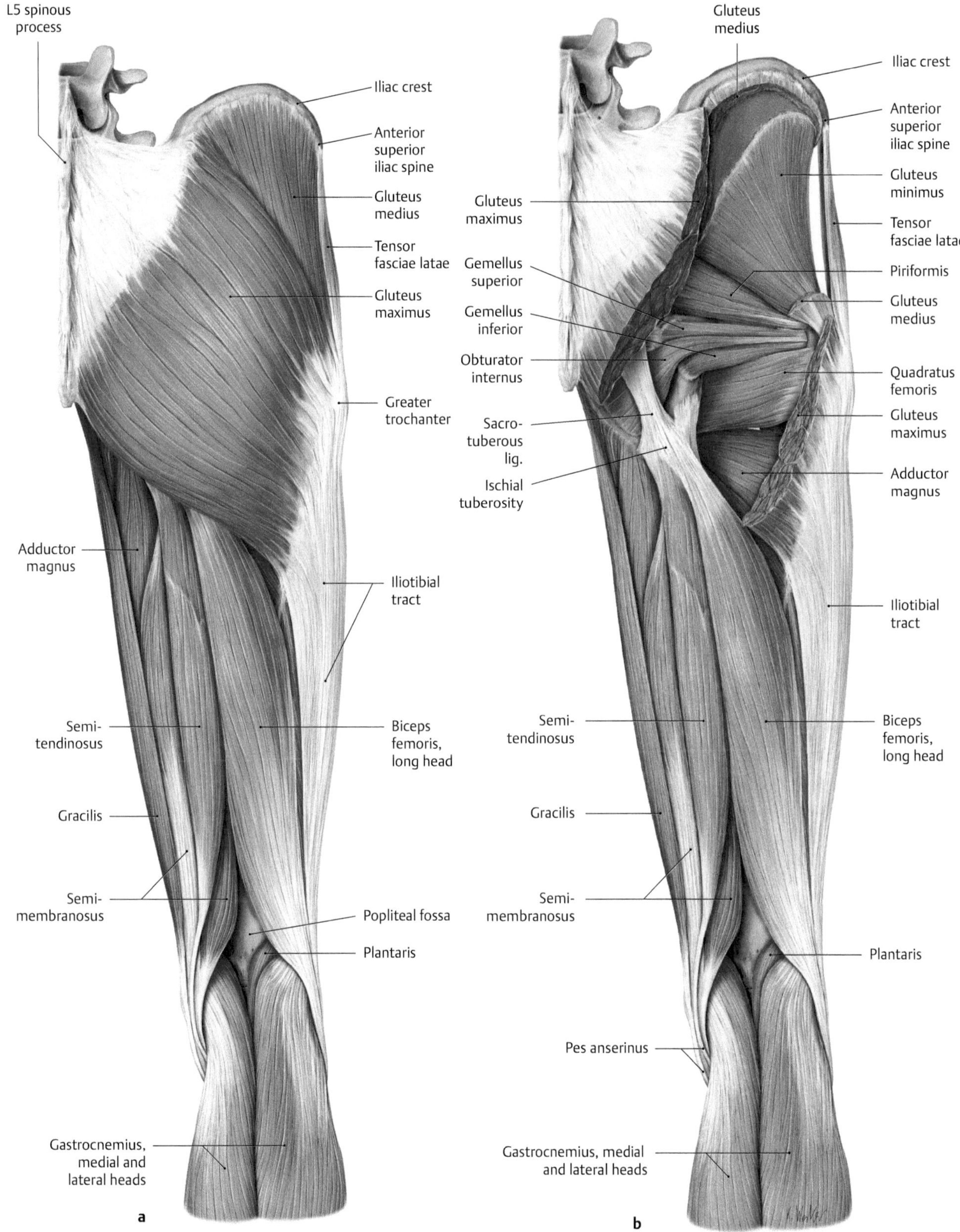

Fig. 5.40 Posterior muscles of the hip, thigh, and gluteal region. **(a)** Removed: fascia lata (to iliotibial tract). **(b)** Partially removed: gluteus maximus and medius. (From Schuenke M, Schulte E, Schumacher U. THIEME Atlas of Anatomy. General Anatomy and Musculoskeletal System. Illustrations by Voll M and Wesker K. 3rd ed. New York: Thieme Medical Publishers; 2020.)

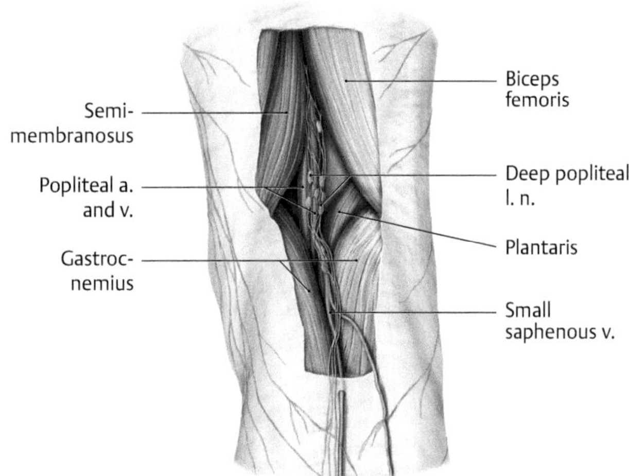

Fig. 5.41 Popliteal fossa lymph nodes. (From Schuenke M, Schulte E, Schumacher U. THIEME Atlas of Anatomy. General Anatomy and Musculoskeletal System. Illustrations by Voll M and Wesker K. 3rd ed. New York: Thieme Medical Publishers; 2020.)

"true" hamstring muscles include the **long head of biceps femoris, semitendinosus** and the **semimembranosus muscles.** These muscles are involved in both extension of the thigh at the hip joint and flexion of the leg at the knee joint. The short head of biceps femoris is only involved in flexion of the leg. Descriptions of posterior thigh muscles are found in **Table 5.2 (Fig. 5.40).**

5.13.2 Neurovasculature of the Posterior Thigh and Popliteal Fossa Regions

The **sciatic nerve** passes deep to the hamstring muscles and just above the popliteal fossa bifurcates into an isolated tibial and common fibular nerve. Branches of the **tibial division of the sciatic nerve** innervate the "true" hamstring muscles. These muscles are defined as those who act by extending the thigh and flexing the leg. The **tibial nerve** continues directly into the popliteal fossa and pairs with the popliteal vessels. Numerous muscular branches of the tibial nerve are seen in this region targeting the posterior leg muscles that act on the knee joint. The **medial sural cutaneous nerve** branches off of the tibial nerve in the popliteal fossa and contributes to the formation of the *sural nerve* (**Fig. 5.42**).

The **common fibular division of the sciatic nerve** only innervates the short head of biceps femoris in the posterior thigh. It continues as the **common fibular nerve** after separating from the sciatic nerve and then wraps around the head of the fibula before bifurcating into the **deep fibular** and **superficial fibular nerves.** The **lateral sural cutaneous nerve** branches off from it and supplies skin of the lateral leg. A **communicating branch** from either the common fibular or the lateral sural cutaneous nerve helps form the *sural nerve* of the posterior leg (**Fig. 5.42**).

The **posterior femoral cutaneous nerve** is responsible mainly for innervating the skin of the posterior thigh and popliteal fossa. This nerve runs just deep to the fascia lata, which is uncharacteristic for normal cutaneous nerves because they generally pass through the subcutaneous tissue.

The blood supply to the posterior thigh is from 3-4 **perforating arteries** that originate from the **profunda femoris artery.** The fourth branch would serve as the termination of the profunda femoris artery. These arteries are generally larger and penetrate the adductor magnus to reach the posterior thigh or can send some branches to supply the vastus lateralis muscle of the anterior thigh. The muscular branches of these vessels supply the posterior thigh muscles and can give rise to a continuous anastomotic chain that connects with the inferior gluteal, popliteal or other perforating arteries (**Fig. 5.42**).

The popliteal fossa and its contents receive blood mainly from the **popliteal artery,** which was the femoral artery before it passed through the adductor hiatus. The popliteal artery gives rise to five **genicular arteries** described with the knee joint. The *descending branch* of the **lateral circumflex femoral artery** forms an anastomosis with the superior lateral genicular artery to help supply the knee region (**Fig. 5.43**).

The venous drainage of the popliteal fossa begins with the **popliteal vein** after it receives drainage from multiple **genicular veins** supplying the knee joint. The popliteal vein becomes the femoral vein after passing through the adductor hiatus. The posterior thigh drainage follows the **perforating veins** back to the **profunda femoris vein.** From here the profunda femoris vein drains into the

Clinical Correlate 5.22

Hamstring Injuries

Sports involving a lot of running, kicking or quick starts such as soccer, baseball and football place a large amount of stress on the tendinous attachments of the hamstrings especially near the ischial tuberosity. During a forceful kick, the combined hip flexion and knee extension could result in an avulsion of the combined muscle tendon at the ischial tuberosity. Hamstring injuries occur around twice as frequently as quadriceps injuries.

Table 5.2 **Posterior thigh muscles**

Muscle	Innervation	Function(s)	Origin	Insertion
Biceps femoris	Long head: tibial division of sciatic nerve Short head: common fibular division of sciatic nerve	Extend thigh, flex and laterally rotate leg (when knee is flexed)	Long head: ischial tuberosity; Short head: linea aspera and lateral supracondylar line of femur	Head of fibula
Semitendinosus	Tibial division of sciatic nerve	Extend thigh, flex and medially rotate leg (when knee is flexed)	Ischial tuberosity	Medial surface of superior tibia (via pes anserinus)
Semimembranosus	Tibial division of sciatic nerve	Extend thigh, flex and medially rotate leg (when knee is flexed)	Ischial tuberosity	Posterior part of medial condyle of tibia; lateral femoral condyle via oblique popliteal ligament

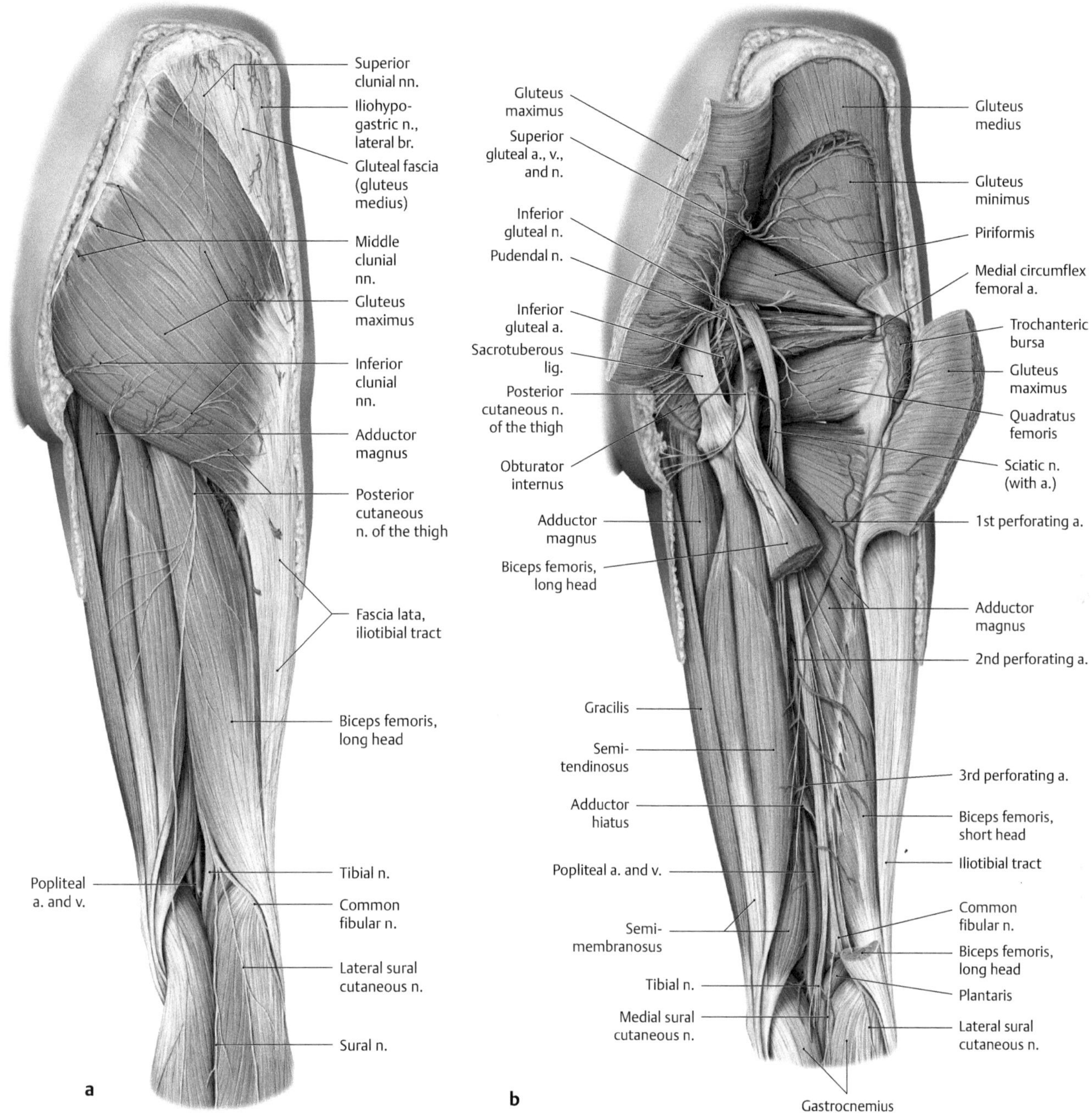

Fig. 5.42 Neurovasculature of the gluteal region and posterior thigh. **(a)** Removed: fascia lata. **(b)** Partially removed: gluteus maximus, gluteus medius, and biceps femoris. Retracted: semimembranosus. (From Schuenke M, Schulte E, Schumacher U. THIEME Atlas of Anatomy. General Anatomy and Musculoskeletal System. Illustrations by Voll M and Wesker K. 3rd ed. New York: Thieme Medical Publishers; 2020.)

femoral vein. Venous drainage from the genicular veins of the lateral knee could bypass the popliteal vein altogether and travel back with a tributary of the **lateral circumflex femoral vein** that ultimately reaches the profunda femoris vein.

5.14 Anterior Thigh Region

Deep to the inguinal ligament, the **retro-inguinal (Bogros's) space** serves as an important pathway for structures that link the trunk and abdominopelvic cavity to the lower extremity. It is created as the inguinal ligament spans the gap between the pubic tubercle and ASIS. The space itself is divided into a lateral and medial compartment by a thickening of the *iliopsoas fascia* called the **iliopectineal arch (Fig. 5.44)**.

The **lateral compartment** (lacuna musculorum) is primarily filled with the *iliopsoas muscle* but it also contains the *femoral nerve* and *lateral femoral cutaneous nerve*. The **medial compartment** (lacuna vasorum) is mostly filled with neurovasculature and these structures include the *femoral branch of the genitofemoral nerve*, *femoral artery* and *femoral vein*. This is also near the site

Clinical Correlate 5.23

Baker's Cyst

A **Baker's cyst**, also known as a *popliteal cyst*, is usually seen with almost any form of knee arthritis or cartilage tear. It is a benign swelling of the popliteal bursa between the medial head of the gastrocnemius and semimembranosus muscles and lies posterior to the medial femoral condyle. Surgical intervention is rarely needed and these cysts can be treated with rest, ice, heat or anti-inflammatory medication **(Fig. 5.51)**.

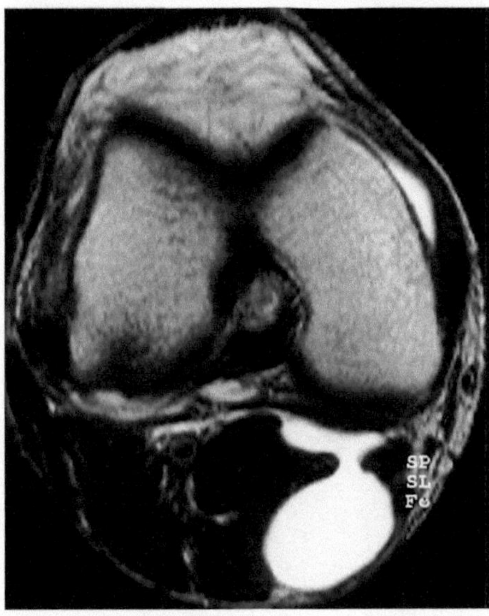

(From Schuenke M, Schulte E, Schumacher U. THIEME Atlas of Anatomy. General Anatomy and Musculoskeletal System. Illustrations by Voll M and Wesker K. 3rd ed. New York: Thieme Medical Publishers; 2020.)

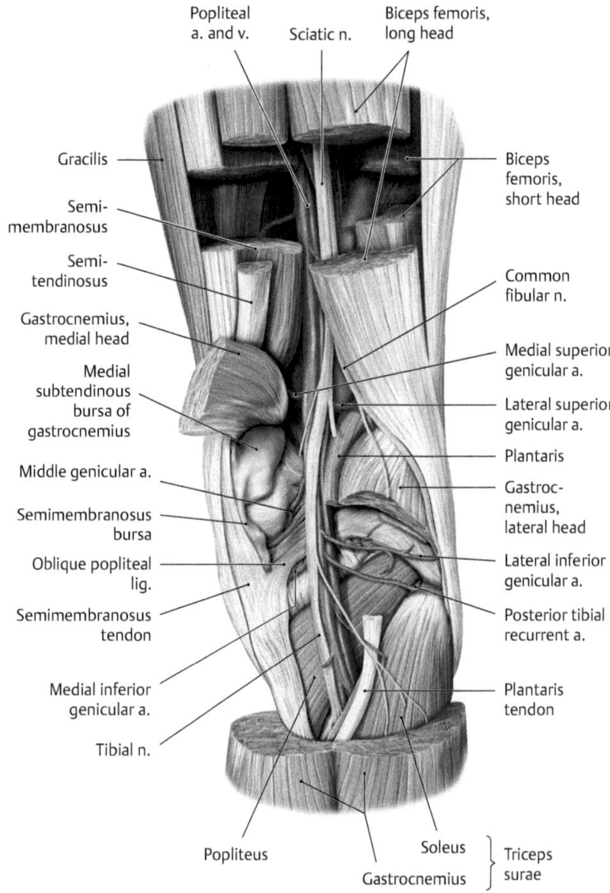

Fig. 5.43 Neurovasculature of the popliteal fossa. (From Schuenke M, Schulte E, Schumacher U. THIEME Atlas of Anatomy. General Anatomy and Musculoskeletal System. Illustrations by Voll M and Wesker K. 3rd ed. New York: Thieme Medical Publishers; 2020.)

of the femoral ring of the femoral canal, where the *Rosenmüller/Cloquet lymph node* can be found and this area generally serves as the passageway for lymphatics traveling from the anteromedial thigh region to the greater pelvis. The retro-inguinal space is closely associated with the *femoral triangle* and *femoral sheath* **(Fig. 5.44)**.

The **femoral triangle** is a sub-fascial formation appearing as a triangular depression with the inguinal ligament (superiorly), sartorius muscle (laterally) and adductor longus muscle (medially) serving as its borders. Both the iliopsoas and pectineus muscles form the floor of this triangle. The roof is formed by a combination of structures that include the fascia lata, cribriform fascia and subcutaneous tissue and skin. Contents of the femoral triangle include **(Fig. 5.45)**:

- Femoral nerve.
- Femoral artery.
- Femoral vein.
- Proximal portions of the profunda femoris vessels and great saphenous vein.
- Deep inguinal lymph nodes and their associated lymphatic vessels.

The funnel-shaped fascial tube called the **femoral sheath** is formed superiorly by transversalis and iliopsoas fascia and terminates inferiorly by incorporating itself into the tunica adventitia surrounding the femoral vessels. The femoral sheath is split into three compartments whose contents include **(Fig 5.46)**:

- *Lateral compartment*: femoral artery.
- *Intermediate (middle) compartment*: femoral vein.
- *Medial (femoral canal) compartment*: deep inguinal lymph nodes and lymphatics.

The medial compartment or **femoral canal** is the smallest of the three compartments. It allows for expansion when venous return heading back from the lower extremity has increased or if the intra-abdominal pressure has increased as when performing a *Valsalva maneuver*. The base or superior most portion of the femoral canal is called the **femoral ring** and it is closed by extraperitoneal fatty tissue that forms the **femoral septum (Fig. 5.46)**.

The location where the sartorius crosses over the adductor longus muscle is called the apex of the femoral triangle. Extending from this point and inferiorly to the adductor hiatus is the **adductor (Hunter's) canal (Fig. 5.47)**. The **adductor hiatus** is an opening between the distal aponeurotic attachment of the adductor part of the adductor magnus and its hamstring part is attached at the adductor tubercle. The borders of this canal are established by the vastus medialis muscle (anteriorly and laterally), sartorius

Clinical Correlate 5.24

Femoral Hernia

A **femoral hernia** passes through the *femoral ring* located at the superior aspect of the medial compartment of the femoral sheath. The small intestine is normally involved in this sort of hernia and enters the femoral ring before continuing through the femoral canal. It is most common in females and may enlarge after passing through the saphenous opening of the anterior thigh. If strangulation of a femoral hernia is to occur it may interfere with the blood supply to the herniated portion of intestine causing tissue death.

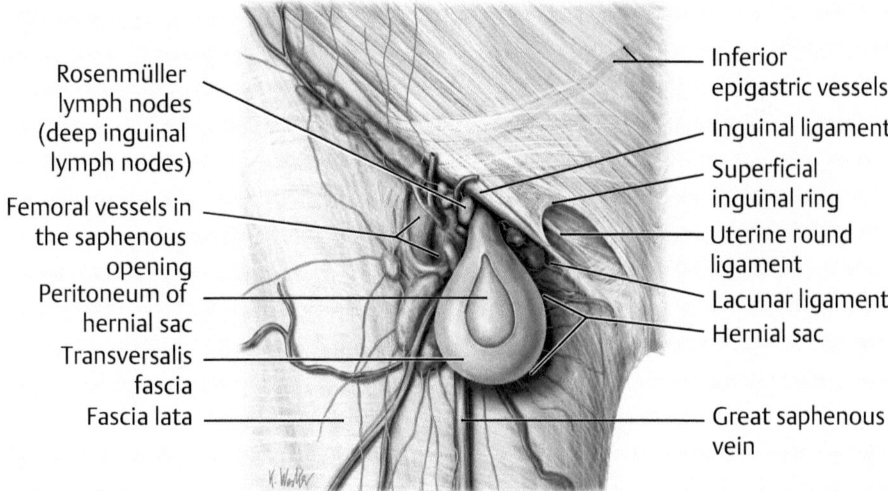

(From Schuenke M, Schulte E, Schumacher U. THIEME Atlas of Anatomy. General Anatomy and Musculoskeletal System. Illustrations by Voll M and Wesker K. 3rd ed. New York: Thieme Medical Publishers; 2020.)

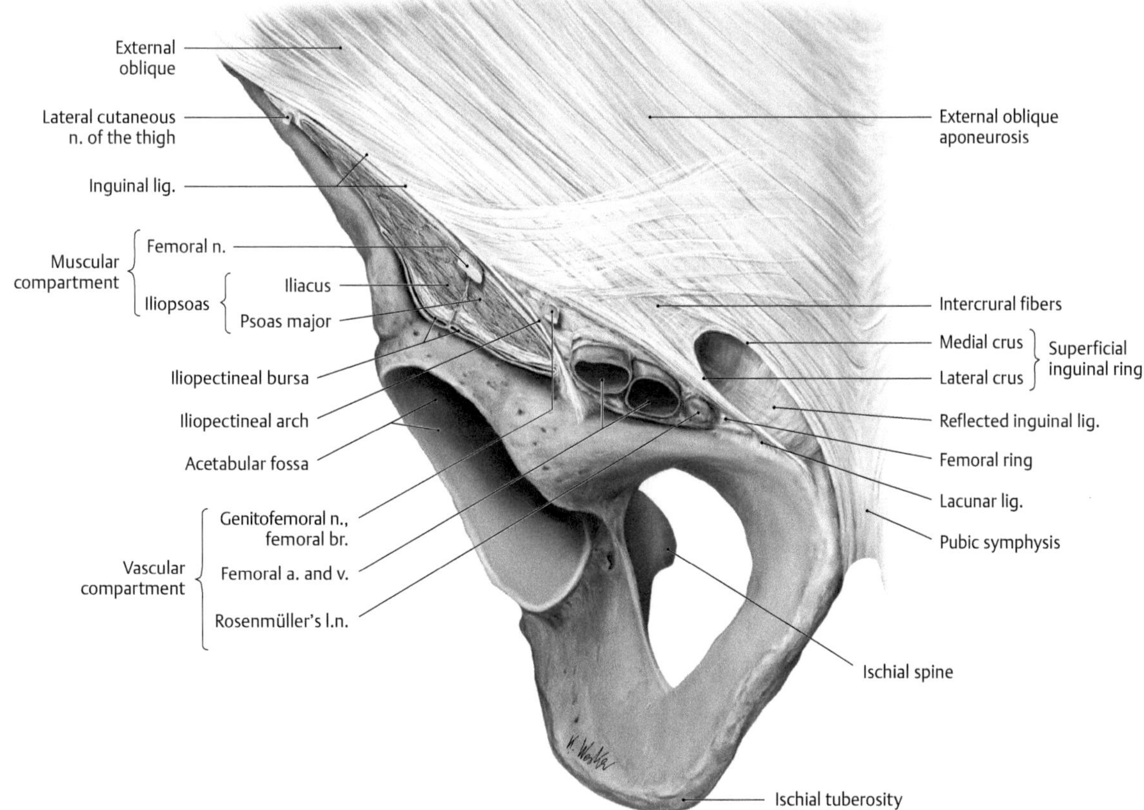

Fig. 5.44 Retro-inguinal space: muscular and vascular compartments. (From Schuenke M, Schulte E, Schumacher U. THIEME Atlas of Anatomy. General Anatomy and Musculoskeletal System. Illustrations by Voll M and Wesker K. 3rd ed. New York: Thieme Medical Publishers; 2020.)

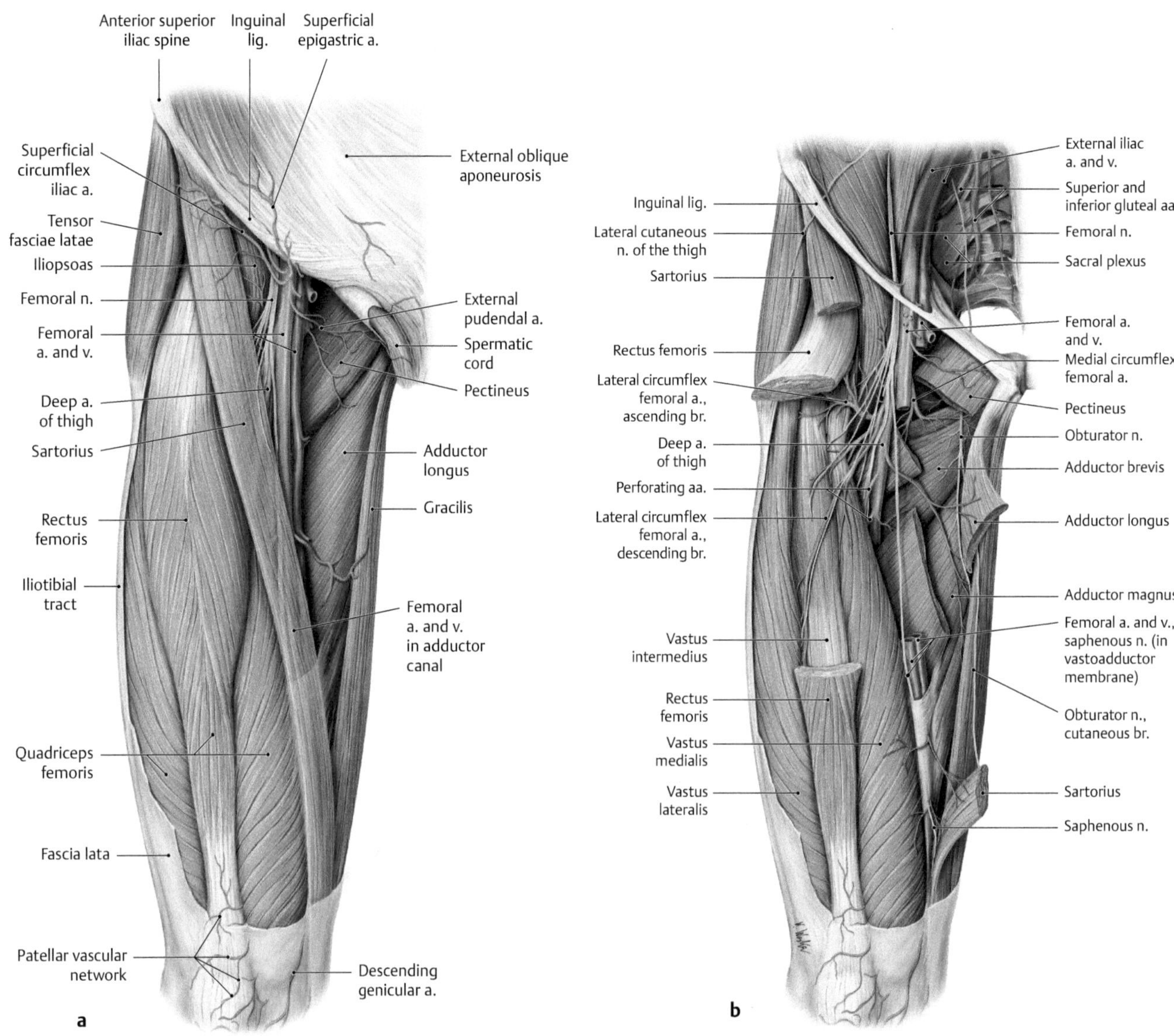

Fig. 5.45 Neurovasculature of the anterior and medial thigh. **(a)** Femoral triangle. **(b)** Deeper dissection with sections of the sartorius, rectus femoris, adductor longus, and pectineus removed. (From Schuenke M, Schulte E, Schumacher U. THIEME Atlas of Anatomy. General Anatomy and Musculoskeletal System. Illustrations by Voll M and Wesker K. 3rd ed. New York: Thieme Medical Publishers; 2020.)

muscle (medially) and the adductor longus and magnus muscles (posteriorly). Contents of the adductor canal include:

- Femoral artery.
- Femoral vein.
- Saphenous nerve (femoral nerve br.).
- Femoral nerve branch that supplies the vastus medialis muscle.

5.14.1 Anterior Thigh Muscles

The anterior thigh muscles include the sartorius, iliopsoas, pectineus, and the quadriceps muscle group **(Fig. 5.48)**. These muscles are primarily involved in *flexion at the hip joint* and *extension of the knee*. The **sartorius muscle** is known as the "tailor's muscle" and it is the longest muscle in the body. It stretches from the hip laterally to the knee medially. It can act in both flexion of the thigh and knee and abduction and lateral rotation of the thigh. The **iliopsoas** is a combination of both the iliacus and psoas major muscles. It is the most powerful muscles and thus chief flexors of the thigh. The bilateral contraction of this muscle initiates flexion of the trunk and decreases the lumbar curvature of the vertebral column. It plays a large role during the earlier swing phases of the gait cycle. The **pectineus muscle** is generally innervated by the femoral nerve but may receive dual innervation by the obturator nerve. This muscle is responsible for adduction, flexion and medial rotation of the thigh **(Fig. 5.49)**.

The **quadriceps femoris** muscle group makes up the majority of the anterior thigh. It consists of the **rectus femoris**, **vastus lateralis**, **vastus intermedius** and the **vastus medialis muscles**. All of these muscles are involved in extension of the leg at the knee joint. The rectus femoris, unlike the other three muscles, crosses the hip joint and can act as a flexor of the thigh. Due to the importance of this muscle group (for example during rising from a sitting position, walking up multiple stairs or accelerating during running),

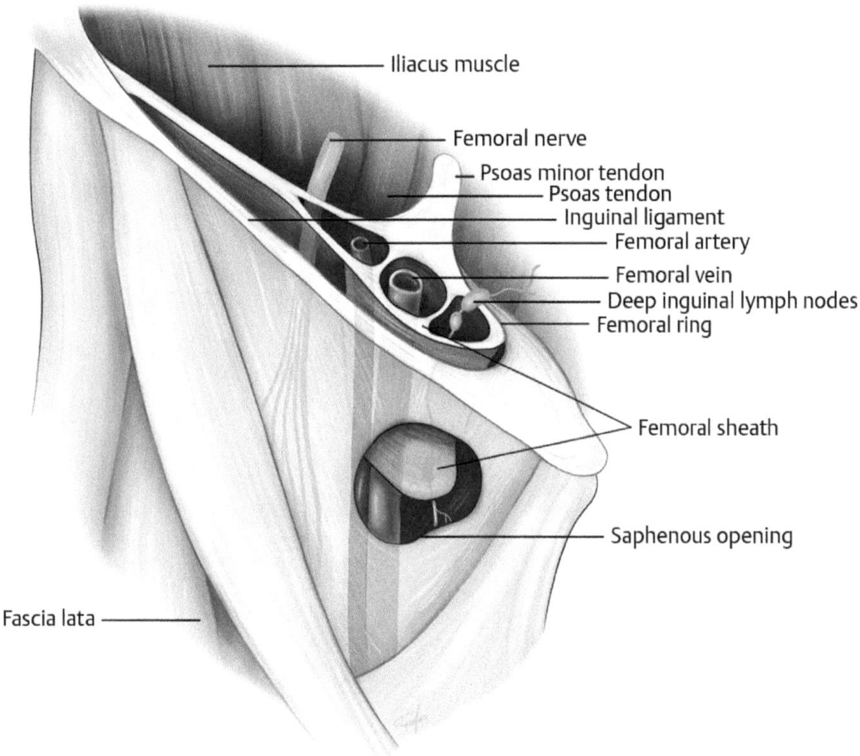

Fig. 5.46 Structure and contents of the femoral sheath. Illustration by Calla Heald.

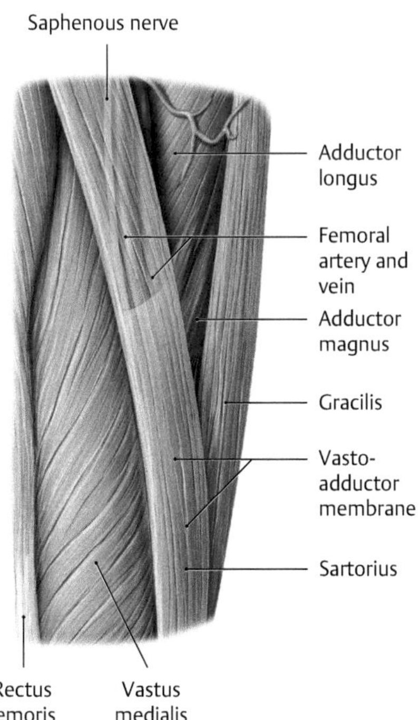

Fig. 5.47 Location of the adductor canal. (From Schuenke M, Schulte E, Schumacher U. THIEME Atlas of Anatomy. General Anatomy and Musculoskeletal System. Illustrations by Voll M and Wesker K. 3rd ed. New York: Thieme Medical Publishers; 2020.)

the quadriceps may be as much as three times stronger than its antagonist, the hamstrings. During the gait cycle, the quadriceps group becomes active during the termination of the swing phase and prepares the knee to accept weight. It is primarily responsible for absorbing shock from the heel strike and absorbs more weight during the early loading phase (**Fig. 5.48**).

The quadriceps unites distally to form the **quadriceps tendon** and it embeds the patella, the largest sesamoid bone in the body. The **patella** provides additional leverage for the quadriceps by placing the tendon more anteriorly and farther from the knee joint axis. This causes it to approach the tibia from a position of greater mechanical advantage. The patella provides a bony surface that withstands the friction of the knee being flexed and extended rapidly during running and the compression placed on it during kneeling. The continuation of the quadriceps tendon is known as the **patellar ligament** and it attaches to the tibial tuberosity. The vastus lateralis and medialis muscles attach independently to the patella and form the **lateral** and **medial patellar retinacula** respectively, and these function by reinforcing the joint capsule of the knee joint as they extend inferiorly towards the anterior border of the tibial plateau (**Fig. 5.56**).

A small and flat muscle that derives from the vastus intermedius is called the **articularis genu**. It originates from the more inferior portion of the anterior femur and during knee extension; this muscle pulls the synovial membrane and suprapatellar bursa superiorly, thereby preventing folds of the membrane from being compressed between the femur and patella. Descriptions of anterior thigh muscles are found in **Table 5.3.**

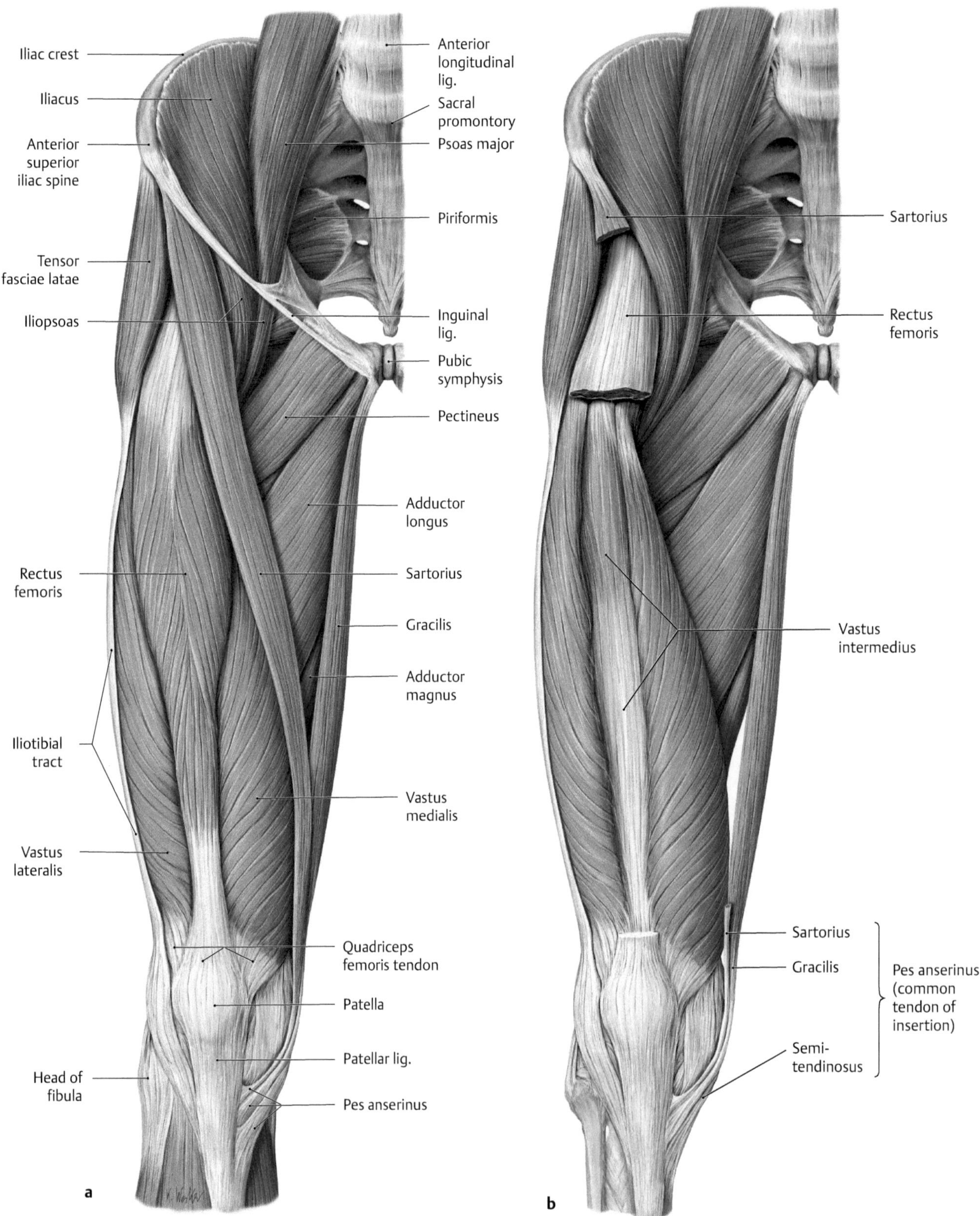

Fig. 5.48 Muscles of the anterior hip and anterior thigh compartments. **(a)** Fasica lata of the thigh was removed. **(b)** Deeper dissection with the inguinal ligament, sartorius, and rectus femoris. (From Schuenke M, Schulte E, Schumacher U. THIEME Atlas of Anatomy. General Anatomy and Musculoskeletal System. Illustrations by Voll M and Wesker K. 3rd ed. New York: Thieme Medical Publishers; 2020.)

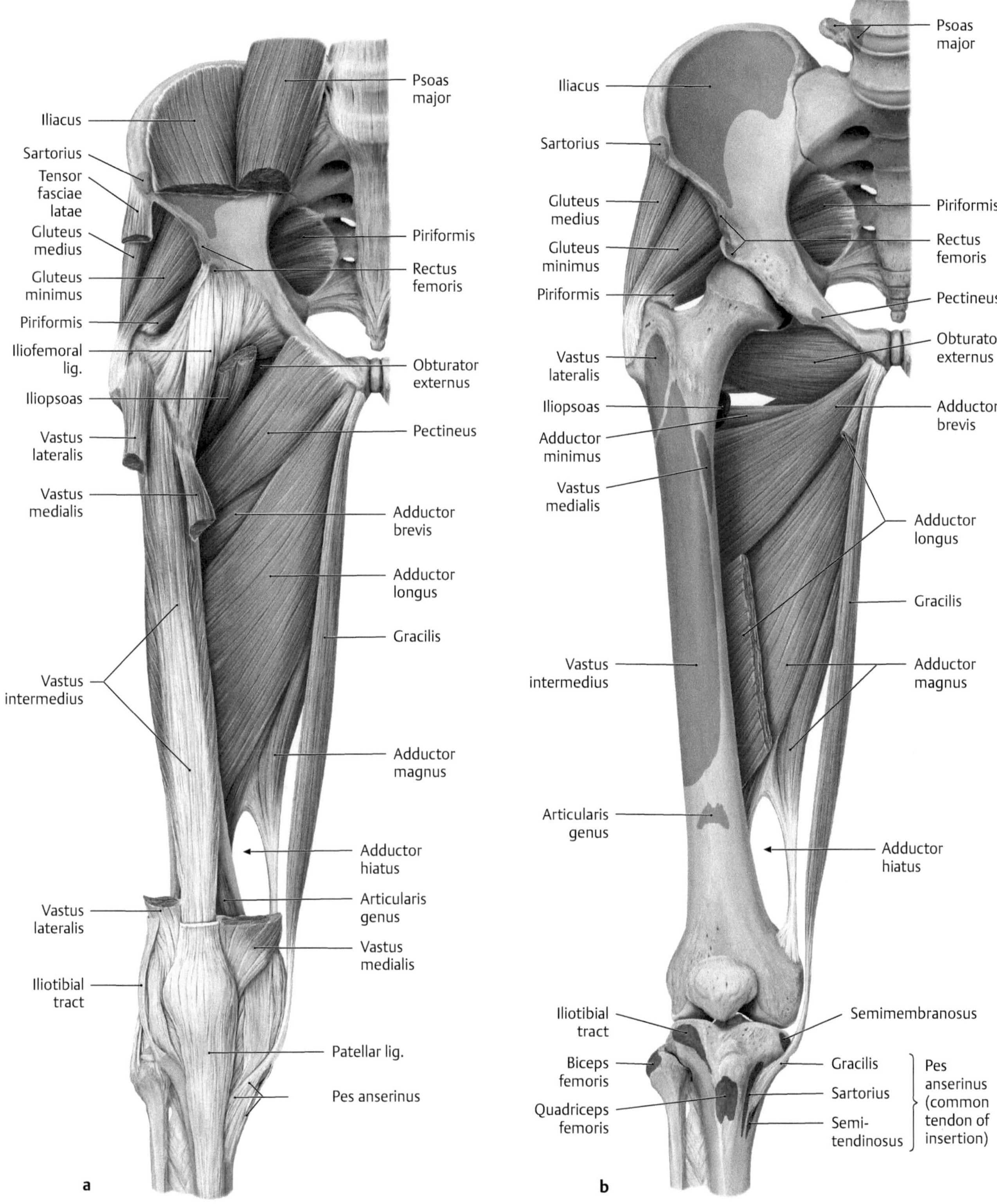

Fig. 5.49 Muscles of the medial thigh compartment. **(a)** Removed: rectus femoris, vastus lateralis, vastus medialis, iliopsoas, and tensor fasciae latae. **(b)** Removed: quadriceps femoris, iliopsoas, tensor fasciae latae, pectineus, and midportion of adductor longus. (From Schuenke M, Schulte E, Schumacher U. THIEME Atlas of Anatomy. General Anatomy and Musculoskeletal System. Illustrations by Voll M and Wesker K. 3rd ed. New York: Thieme Medical Publishers; 2020.)

Table 5.3 **Anterior thigh muscles**

Muscle	Innervation	Function(s)	Origin	Insertion
Iliopsoas: Psoas major Iliacus	Ventral rami of L1-L4, femoral nerve	Flexes thigh and trunk as combined iliopsoas muscle	Transverse process and body of T12-L4 vertebrae; IV discs between T12-L5 Superior 2/3 of iliac fossa, ala of sacrum and anterior sacro-iliac ligaments	Lesser trochanter (as iliopsoas)
Pectineus	Femoral nerve (occasionally the obturator nerve)	Adducts, flexes and assists in medial rotation of thigh	Superior ramus of pubic bone	Pectineal line of femur
Sartorius	Femoral nerve	Abducts, flexes and lateral rotation of thigh; flexes leg	Anterior superior iliac spine	Medial surface of superior tibia (via pes anserinus)
Rectus femoris	Femoral nerve	Flexes thigh; extends leg	Anterior inferior iliac spine; the ilium superior to the acetabulum	To patella (via quadriceps tendon) and tibial tuberosity (via patellar ligament)
Vastus lateralis	Femoral nerve	Extends leg	Greater trochanter; lateral lip of linea aspera	To patella (via quadriceps tendon) and tibial tuberosity (via patellar ligament)
Vastus medialis	Femoral nerve	Extends leg	Intertrochanteric line; medial lip of linea aspera	To patella (via quadriceps tendon) and tibial tuberosity (via patellar ligament)
Vastus intermedius	Femoral nerve	Extends leg	Anterior and lateral surfaces of femur	To patella (via quadriceps tendon) and tibial tuberosity (via patellar ligament)

5.14.2 Neurovasculature of the Anterior Thigh Region

The **femoral nerve** is the largest branch of the lumbar plexus and after passing (for the most part) between the individual iliacus and psoas major muscles, it continues just below the midpoint of the inguinal ligament and into the anterior thigh. Just distal to the inguinal ligament, the femoral nerve immediately splits into many smaller but visible branches. It lies laterally to all structures considered contents of the femoral triangle but it does not pass through any compartments of the femoral sheath (**Fig. 5.45**).

It provides cutaneous branches to the anteromedial thigh and sends articular branches to both the hip and knee joints. It has a terminal branch called the **saphenous nerve** that courses through the adductor canal but does not pass through the adductor hiatus like the femoral artery and vein. It then passes between the sartorius and gracilis muscles on the medial side of the knee before continuing down the medial side of the leg. It is ultimately responsible for innervating the skin of the anteromedial knee, leg and foot regions (**Fig. 5.45**).

The blood supply of the anterior and anteromedial aspects of the thigh originates from the **femoral artery**. The femoral artery is the continuation of the external iliac artery at the level of the inguinal ligament. It is located just medial to the femoral nerve but lateral to the femoral vein and passes through the lateral compartment of the femoral sheath. Just inferior to the inguinal ligament, branches that come off the femoral artery include the *superficial circumflex iliac, superficial epigastric, superficial external pudendal* and the *deep external pudendal arteries* (**Fig. 5.45a**).

The largest branch of the femoral artery is the **profunda femoris artery** and it serves as the chief artery of the thigh. It is responsible for supplying blood to the posterior, medial and lateral part of the anterior thighs. It arises mostly from the posterolateral side of the femoral artery while it is still in the femoral triangle. It gives off 3-4 **perforating arteries** that pass through the adductor magnus to reach the posterior thigh. Prior to the first perforating artery branch, the **lateral** and **medial circumflex femoral arteries** are seen making their way toward the upper most femoral shaft and anastomose with each other and other arteries (**Fig. 5.45b**).

The **lateral circumflex femoral artery** has an ascending, transverse and descending branch. The *ascending branch* supplies the anterior gluteal region. The *transverse branch* forms an anastomosis with the medial circumflex femoral artery and supplies a minimal amount of blood to the hip joint. The *descending branch* supplies mainly the lateral thigh region and forms an anastomosis with the genicular arteries of the lateral knee joint. The **medial circumflex femoral artery** is the primary blood supply to the head and neck of the femur directly through its **retinacular artery** branches. It has two other primary branches. The *ascending branch* joins the inferior gluteal artery and helps supply the gluteal region while the *descending branch* can assist in supplying blood in the medial compartment namely adductor muscles. Other branches of the medial circumflex femoral have been described but are less consistent (**Fig. 5.45b**).

The venous drainage closely follows the arterial supply. The union of all 3-4 **perforating veins** creates the **profunda femoris vein** (deep vein of the thigh) that is receiving blood from the posterior thigh region. The profunda femoris vein then receives the **lateral** and **medial circumflex femoral veins** responsible for draining areas such as the lateral anterior thigh and hip region after the first perforating vein has already established part of the profunda femoris. All of this occurs before the profunda femoris drains into the femoral vein located in the femoral triangle.

The **femoral vein** is formed after the **popliteal vein** passes through the *adductor hiatus* and continues through the *adductor* *canal* before passing through the *intermediate (middle) compartment* of the femoral sheath. Near the medial knee, an isolated **genicular vein** may extend superiorly and into the femoral vein at the level of the mid-thigh. The **great saphenous vein** passes through the saphenous opening formed in the fascia lata and drains into the femoral vein just superior to where the profunda femoris normally meets the femoral vein. The femoral vein continues through the intermediate compartment of the femoral sheath and at the level of the inguinal ligament becomes the **external iliac vein**. Just prior to this, the femoral vein receives the venous drainage passing through the *superficial epigastric, superficial circumflex iliac* and *external pudendal veins.*

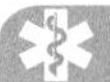 *Clinical Correlate 5.25*

Cannulation of the Femoral Artery and Vein

The **femoral artery** is located midway between the ASIS and pubic tubercle and can be cannulated just inferior to the midpoint of the inguinal ligament. This would be done for procedures such as cardioangiography-radiography of the heart and great vessels after introduction of contrast material. A long, slender catheter is inserted percutaneously into the femoral artery and passed superiorly in the aorta to the openings of the coronary arteries during a left cardiac angiography.

The **femoral vein** can be cannulated in order to secure blood samples and take pressure recordings from the chambers of the right side of the heart and/or from the pulmonary artery.

A catheter is inserted into the femoral vein for right cardiac angiography. Fluoroscopy may be used to control passage of these catheters as it extends superiorly to the openings of the coronary arteries or right atrium of the heart.

5.15 Medial Thigh Region

The medial thigh compartment is associated primarily with the *adductor muscles of the thigh.* Muscles of this region attach for the most part on the anteroinferior external surface of the bony pelvis and obturator membrane before extending distally to attach to the linea aspera, adductor tubercle or medial surface of the superior tibia. The adductor longus muscle of this region contributes a border to both the femoral triangle and adductor canal.

5.15.1 Medial Thigh Muscles

The medial thigh includes the obturator externus, adductor brevis, adductor longus, adductor magnus and the gracilis muscles. These muscles are primarily involved in adduction of the thigh at the hip joint. The **obturator externus** is an outlier in that it does not participate in adduction but only lateral rotation of the thigh. And although it inserts near it, the obturator externus is not capable of abduction like the obturator internus of the gluteal region (**Fig. 5.49**).

The **adductor brevis** lies anterior to the obturator externus but just posterior to the pectineus and adductor longus muscles. The **adductor longus** is a larger fan-shaped muscle that is the most anterior of all medial thigh muscles. The **adductor magnus** is the largest and most powerful of the medial thigh muscle group. It is made up of a lateral *adductor part* and a medial *hamstring part.* The adductor brevis, longus and adductor part of the adductor magnus all participate in adduction of the thigh. The adductor part can also flex the thigh with the hamstring part only capable of extending the thigh (**Fig. 5.49**).

The **gracilis** is a long and thin muscle that acts on both the hip and knee joints. It is the weakest of the medial thigh muscles and forms a common tendon attaching to the superior and medial aspect of the tibia called the **pes anserinus** along with the *sartorius* and *semitendinosus muscles.* It functions by adducting the thigh but also flexing and medially rotating the leg. Descriptions of medial thigh muscles are found in **Table 5.4** (**Fig. 5.49**).

5.15.2 Neurovasculature of the Medial Thigh Region

The **obturator nerve** passes along with the obturator vessels and splits into an anterior and posterior division due to the adductor brevis muscle. It supplies all muscles of the medial thigh except for the hamstring portion of the adductor magnus. Occasionally, it provides innervation to a portion or the entire pectineus muscle (**Fig. 5.45b**).

The blood supply to the medial thigh is from a combination of the profunda femoris, femoral and obturator arteries. The **obturator artery** originates from the **internal iliac artery** and passes through the obturator canal before splitting into an anterior and posterior branch much like the obturator nerve. It is not

Table 5.4 **Medial thigh muscles**

Muscle	Innervation	Function(s)	Origin	Insertion
Obturator externus	Obturator nerve	Laterally rotates thigh	Margins of obturator foramen and obturator membrane	Greater trochanter (trochanteric fossa)
Adductor brevis	Obturator nerve	Adducts and flexes thigh	Body and inferior ramus of pubic bone	Pectineal line; superior part of linea aspera
Adductor longus	Obturator nerve	Adducts thigh	Body of pubic bone below the pubic crest	Middle 1/3 of linea aspera
Adductor magnus	Adductor part: Obturator nerve Hamstring part: tibial division of sciatic nerve	Adducts thigh; flexes thigh (adductor part) and extends thigh (hamstring part)	Adductor part: ischiopubic ramus; Hamstring part: ischial tuberosity	Adductor part: gluteal tuberosity, linea aspera and medial supracondylar line; Hamstring part: adductor tubercle
Gracilis	Obturator nerve	Adducts thigh; flexes and medially rotates leg	Body and inferior ramus of pubic bone	Medial surface of superior tibia (via pes anserinus)

a substantially large set of vessels but it does assist in supplying blood to the medial compartment. Its posterior branch gives rise to the **artery to the head of the femur**.

The **obturator veins** are understated when compared to the surrounding veins, like their artery counterparts. The obturator veins are made up of an anterior and posterior tributary that eventually unite, enter through the obturator canal, and then drain into the **internal iliac vein**.

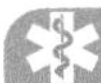 *Clinical Correlate 5.26*

Groin Pull

A "pulled groin" usually refers to a strain or tear at the proximal attachment of an adductor or flexor muscle of the anteromedial thigh. These proximal attachments are in the inguinal region (also known as the groin). Sports that require quick starts, such as track and field, or that involve extreme stretching, such as gymnastics, tend to have higher rates of groin pulls.

 *Clinical Correlate 5.27*

Gracilis Transplantation

The gracilis is a relatively weak adductor muscle and because of this it can be removed without noticeable loss of function. Transplantion of the gracilis (or portion of it) and its neurovasculature is done in order to replace a damaged muscle in the forearm, face or a nonfunctional external anal sphincter, for example.

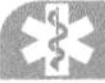 *Clinical Correlate 5.28*

Replaced and Accessory Obturator Arteries

The inferior epigastric artery may have an enlarged pubic branch that takes the place of the obturator artery. If so, the individual has a replaced obturator artery. If this branch joins the obturator artery, it is called the accessory obturator artery and this is present in approximately 20% of the population. This artery is in close relationship with the femoral ring as it courses to obturator foramen and is thus closely associated with the neck of a femoral hernia. This artery could become involved in a strangulated femoral hernia. When staples are placed during endoscopic repair of both inguinal and femoral hernias, these arterial variations must be addressed.

5.16 Knee Joint

The **knee joint** is located between the femur of the thigh and tibia of the leg. It is a *hinge-type synovial joint* and movements include primarily flexion and extension but gliding, rolling and rotational movements are also observed. The knee passively locks into place when the knee is fully extended and the foot on the ground. This is due to medial rotation of the femoral condyles on the tibial plateau. Unlocking of the knee is due to contraction of the popliteus muscle when it laterally rotates the femur 5° on the tibial plateau. It is relatively weak, with the strength of the joint to a greater degree stemming from the inferior muscle fibers of the vastus lateralis and vastus medialis (**Fig. 5.50; Fig. 5.51**).

5.16.1 Articulating Surfaces

There are three articulations involving the knee. The **femorotibial articulations** are located between both the lateral and medial condyles of the femur and tibia. The **patellofemoral articulation** is located between the patella and femur. Note that the fibula is not part of the knee joint (**Fig. 5.52; Fig. 5.53**).

5.16.2 Joint Capsule

The capsule of the knee joint is reinforced by extracapsular ligaments and has the typical external fibrous layer and an internal synovial membrane that lines all internal surfaces of the articular cavity not covered by the articular cartilage. The fibrous capsule attaches at multiple locations (**Fig. 5.54**):

- *Anteriorly*: the quadriceps tendon, patella and patellar ligament contribute to the capsule as an anchoring point because the fibrous capsule is located technically on the lateral and medial aspects of these structures.
- *Superiorly*: to the femur just proximal to the articular margins of the condyles.
- *Posteriorly*: the capsule encloses the condyles and intercondylar fossa with the popliteus tendon passing through the joint capsule to reach the tibia.
- *Inferiorly*: to the margin of the articular surface of the tibial plateau.

5.16.3 Extracapsular Ligaments of the Joint Capsule

- **Fibular/lateral collateral ligament** (FCL/LCL): a strong and cord-like structure that connects the lateral epicondyle of the femur to the lateral surface of the fibular head. The tendon of the biceps femoris is split into two parts by this ligament. The popliteus tendon passes deep to it to separate it from the lateral meniscus (**Fig. 5.55; Fig. 5.56**).
- **Patellar ligament**: a strong and thick fibrous structure that serves as the continuation of the quadriceps tendon by extending from the apex and outer margins of the patella to the tibial tuberosity. The **lateral** and **medial patellar retinacula** attach to the ligament and are aponeurotic expansions of the vastus lateralis and medialis muscles respectively. They help make up the joint capsule and are important in maintaining the alignment of the patella relative to the patellar articular surface found on the femur. Lateral displacement of the patella is much more favored. This is due to the *Q-angle*, an oblique placement of the femur versus the line of pull by the quadriceps femoris muscle group relative to the axis of the quadriceps tendon/patellar ligament and tibia (**Fig. 5.55**).
- **Tibial/medial collateral ligament** (TCL/MCL): a strong and flat structure that connects the medial epicondyle of the femur to the medial condyle and superior portion of the medial tibia. The TCL attaches to the medial meniscus and are commonly damaged together. The TCL is weaker than the FCL (**Fig. 5.55; Fig. 5.56**).
- **Oblique popliteal ligament**: the recurrent expansion of the semimembranosus tendon spanning the intracondylar fossa arising from the posterior aspect of the medial tibial condyle and passing superolaterally back to the lateral femoral condyle.

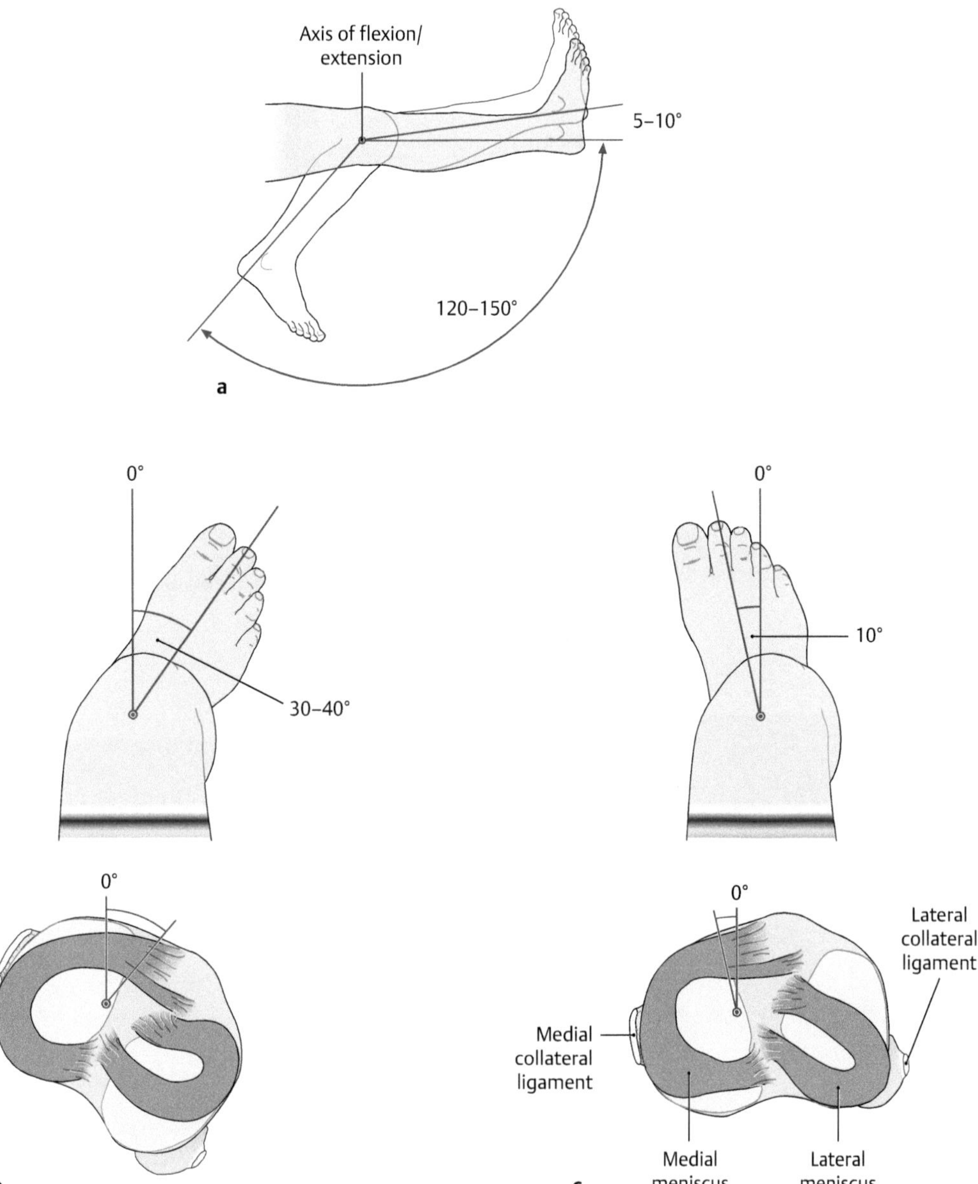

Fig. 5.50 **(a)** Flexion and extension of the knee joint. **(b)** External rotation of the flexed knee. **(c)** Internal rotation of the flexed knee. (From Schuenke M, Schulte E, Schumacher U. THIEME Atlas of Anatomy. General Anatomy and Musculoskeletal System. Illustrations by Voll M and Wesker K. 3rd ed. New York: Thieme Medical Publishers; 2020.)

It acts as reinforcement to the posterior portion of the joint capsule (**Fig. 5.55**).

- **Arcuate popliteal ligament**: arises from the posterior aspect of the fibular head and fans out to two different locations. It blends with the oblique popliteal ligament after passing over the tendon of the popliteus muscle and it attaches near the lateral epicondyle of the femur (**Fig. 5.55**).

The *synovial membrane* attaches to the periphery of the patella and the edges of the menisci. It continues to line the fibrous layer laterally and medially but becomes separated from it more centrally. It reflects superiorly to become associated with the **suprapatellar bursa** and into the intercondylar region from the posterior aspect to cover both the anterior and posterior cruciate ligaments. The anterior portion of synovial membrane reflects posteriorly toward the intercondylar region to become the **infrapatellar synovial fold**. An **infrapatellar fat pad** exists between the anterior parts of the fibrous capsule and anterior portion of the synovial membrane. Located on each side of the of the patellar ligament and internal to the fibrous layer are the fat-filled **lateral** and **medial alar fat pads** that cover the inner surface of the fat pads (**Fig. 5.54; Fig. 5.57**).

5.16.4 Intra-articular Ligaments and Menisci

- **Anterior cruciate ligament** (ACL): arises from the anterior intercondylar area of the tibia and extends superiorly, posteriorly and laterally before attaching to the posterior portion of

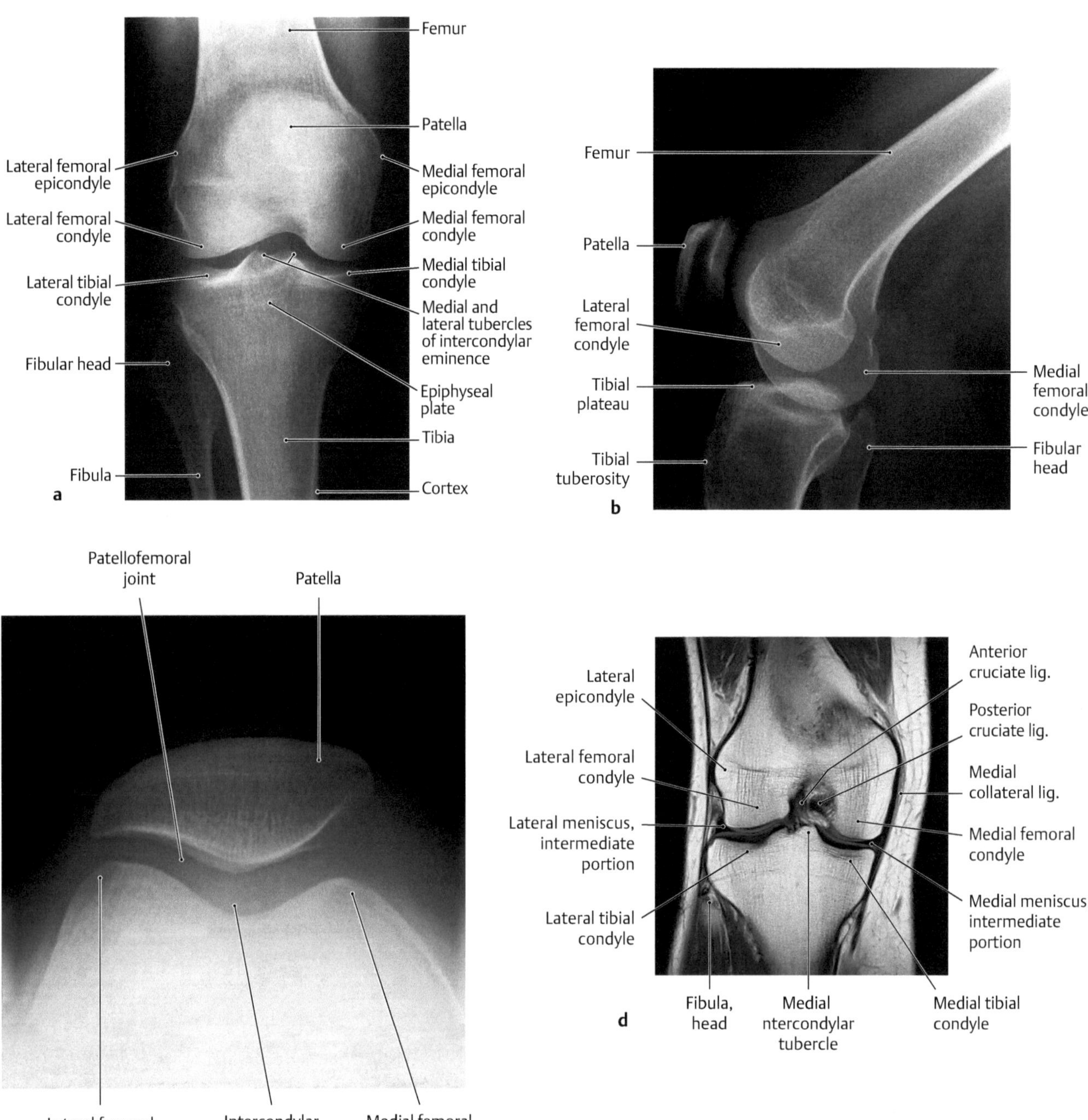

Fig. 5.51 (a) Radiograph of the right knee joint, anteroposterior view. **(b)** Radiograph of the knee in flexion, lateral view. **(c)** Right knee, sunrise view. **(d)** MRI of right knee, coronal section. (Reproduced courtesy of Klinik für Diagnostische Radiologie, Universitätsklinikum Schleswig Holstein, Campus Kiel: Prof. Dr. Med. S. Müller-Huelsbeck.)

the medial side of the lateral condyle of the femur. It prevents posterior displacement of the femur on the tibia (or anterior displacement of the tibia on the femur) and hyperextension of the knee joint. It also limits posterior rolling of the femoral condyles on the tibial plateau during flexion and converts this to spin (**Fig. 5.58; Fig. 5.59**).

- **Posterior cruciate ligament** (PCL): arises from the posterior intercondylar area of the tibia and extends superiorly and anteriorly on the medial side of the ACL before attaching to the lateral side of the medial condyle of the femur. It prevents anterior displacement of the femur on the tibia (or posterior displacement of the tibia on the femur) and hyperflexion of the knee joint. The PCL is the strongest of the two knee cruciate ligaments and is the main stabilizer of the femur when the knee is flexed and weight bearing (i.e., walking down hill) (**Fig. 5.58; Fig. 5.59**).
- **Menisci**: the crescent-shaped plates of fibrocartilage found on the articular surface of the tibia and function in shock absorption are called **menisci**. They are thicker and attached on the external margins but thin out and remain unattached at the

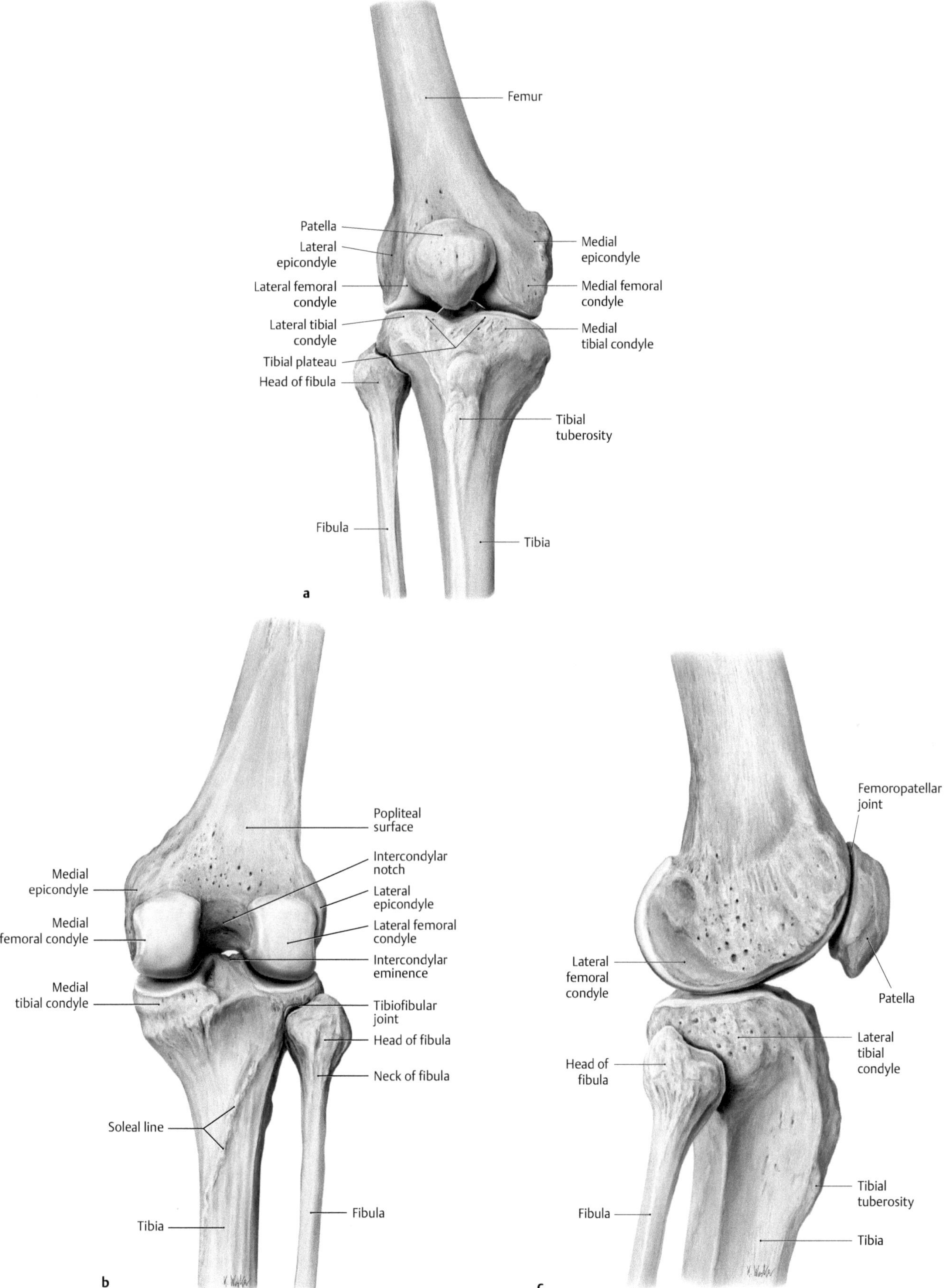

Fig. 5.52 Right knee joint. **(a)** Anterior view. **(b)** Posterior view. **(c)** Lateral view. (From Schuenke M, Schulte E, Schumacher U. THIEME Atlas of Anatomy. General Anatomy and Musculoskeletal System. Illustrations by Voll M and Wesker K. 3rd ed. New York: Thieme Medical Publishers; 2020.)

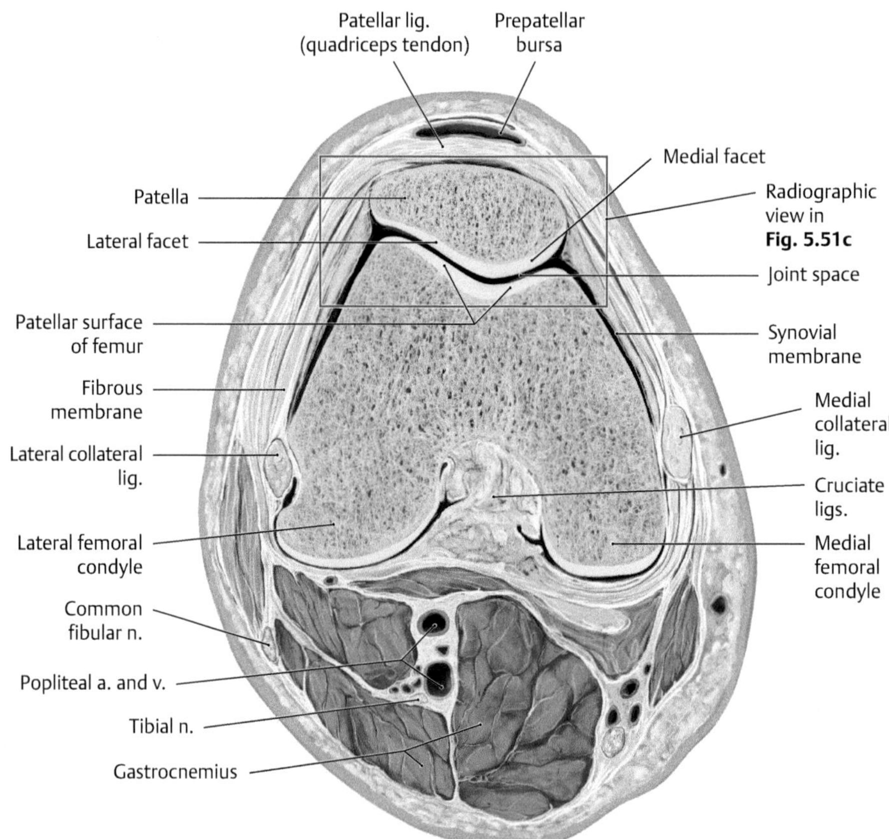

Fig. 5.53 Patellofemoral joint: transverse section. (From Schuenke M, Schulte E, Schumacher U. THIEME Atlas of Anatomy. General Anatomy and Musculoskeletal System. Illustrations by Voll M and Wesker K. 3rd ed. New York: Thieme Medical Publishers; 2020.)

internal ends. The external margins are thicker and attached to the joint capsule. The **coronary ligaments** are the parts of the joint capsule that connect the inferior edges of the menisci to the periphery of the tibial condyles. The internal margins of the menisci are thinner and attach to the intercondylar area of the tibia. A **transverse ligament** attaches the anterior edges of the menisci together as it crosses over the anterior intercondylar area. There is both a lateral and medial meniscus (**Fig. 5.59**).

- **Lateral meniscus**: smaller, more movable and nearly a complete circle. The **posterior meniscofemoral ligament** joins the lateral meniscus to the PCL and medial femoral condyle.
- **Medial meniscus**: the larger of the two menisci and C-shaped. The anterior part is attached to the anterior intercondylar area of the tibia and anterior to the ACL. The posterior part is attached to the posterior intercondylar area of the tibia but it is located anterior to the PCL. The TCL/MCL firmly attaches to the medial meniscus.

5.16.5 Bursa of the Knee Joint

There are many bursae associated with the knee joint and this is primarily because during knee movements most of the tendons run parallel to the bones and pull lengthwise across the joint (**Fig. 5.53; Fig. 5.55**). The **suprapatellar**, **popliteus**, **semimembranosus** and **gastrocnemius bursae** can communicate with the synovial cavity of the knee joint. The **subcutaneous** and **subtendinous prepatellar bursae** lie adjacent to the patella. The **subcutaneous** and **deep infrapatellar bursae** are located near the tibial tuberosity where the patellar ligament inserts. The **anserine bursa** lies just deep to the common insertion point of the sartorius, semitendinosus and gracilis muscles known as the *pes anserinus* (goose's foot).

5.16.6 Neurovasculature of the Knee Joint

Articular branches from the femoral (anteriorly), tibial (posteriorly), common fibular (laterally), obturator (medially) and saphenous nerves (medially) innervate the knee joint.

Blood supply of the knee originates from ten separate arteries and they contribute to the **genicular anastomosis (Fig. 5.22; Fig. 5.43)**. They include: **descending branch of the lateral circumflex femoral**, **descending genicular** (femoral br.), **superior lateral/medial genicular** (popliteal br.), **inferior lateral/medial genicular** (popliteal br.), **middle genicular** (popliteal br.), **anterior tibial recurrent** (anterior tibial br.), **posterior tibial recurrent** (an inconstant anterior tibial br.) and finally the **circumflex fibular** (posterior tibial br.).

Clinical Correlate 5.29

Genu Varum and Genu Valgum

The femur passes through the thigh diagonally and the tibia is nearly vertical within the leg. The angle created between a line connecting the ASIS to the middle of the patella and a line connecting the tibial tuberosity to the middle of the patella is known as the **Q-angle**. The Q-angle is approximately 14° in males and 17° in females.

If the Q-angle is decreased, it is known as **genu varum** or "bowleg." In most children under two years of age, bowing of the legs is quite normal and is referred to as physiologic genu varum. *Blount's disease* and *rickets* are known to cause bowing of the legs. If the Q-angle is increased, it is known as **genu valgum** or "knock-knee." It may naturally be present during the first few years in children but rickets or a genetic disorder such as Down's syndrome may cause it. Adolescents may demonstrate an idiopathic version that warrants no real treatment because the condition is generally benign.

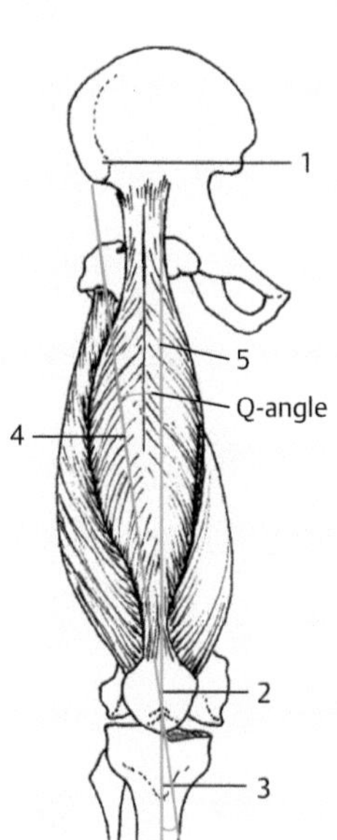

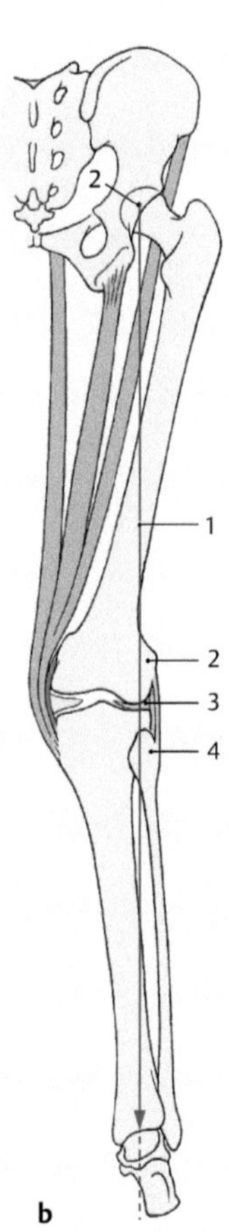

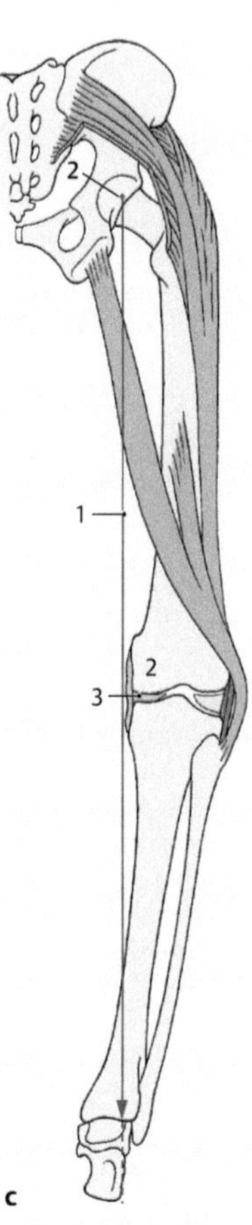

(a) Normal Q-angle and reference points: (1) anterior superior iliac spine (ASIS), (2) Midpoint of patella, (3) Tibial tuberosity, (4) Line connecting ASIS to the superior and middle part of patella, (5) Line of gravity (mechanical axis). **(b)** Genu valgum, posterior view. (1) Line of gravity, (2) Lateral condyle of femur, (3) Lateral meniscus, (4) Head of fibula. (c) Genu varum, posterior view. (1) Line of gravity, (2) Medial condyle of femur, (3) Medial meniscus. (Part **a** is from Buckup, K. Clinical Tests for the Musculoskeletal System: Examinations-Signs-Phenomena, 3rd ed. Stuttgart: Thieme Medical Publishers. Parts **b** and **c** are from Platzer, Color Atlas of Human Anatomy, Vol. 1: Locomotor System, 7th ed., Stuttgart: Thieme Medical Publishers, 2014.)

Clinical Correlate 5.30

Patellar Tendon Reflex

To elicit the **patellar reflex** or "knee jerk," you must tap the patellar ligament with a reflex hammer to cause the leg to extend. This is a myotatic (deep tendon) reflex that is routinely tested during a physical examination. This tests the integrity of the femoral nerve and the L2-L4 spinal cord segments. The absence or diminution of this reflex could be the result of a spinal cord lesion somewhere between the L2-L4 spinal segments.

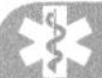

Clinical Correlate 5.31

Patellofemoral Pain Syndrome and Chondromalacia Patellae

Both **patellofemoral pain syndrome** and **chondromalacia patellae** are both generally referred to as "runner's knee" along with a few other diagnoses but they are commonly seen in marathon runners, cyclists or individuals who may have to sit for a long time with flexed knees. The soreness and aching around or deep to the patella is the result of a quadriceps muscle imbalance. There is a key distinction between the two conditions is that patellofemoral pain syndrome involves no damage to the articular surface whereas in chondromalacia patellae there is articular damage or softening.

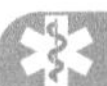

Clinical Correlate 5.32

Unhappy Triad and Cruciate Ligament Testing

The **unhappy triad** is a result of a blow to the lateral side of the extended knee or excessive lateral twisting of the flexed knee. It results in the tearing of the anterior cruciate ligament (ACL), tibial collateral ligament and the medial meniscus. The **anterior drawer sign** tests to see if the ACL is torn. If so, the tibia slides anteriorly. The **posterior drawer sign** tests to see if the posterior cruciate ligament (PCL) is torn and if this ligament is damaged, the tibia slides posteriorly.

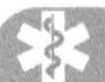

Clinical Correlate 5.33

Knee Replacement

Total knee replacement is performed on a patient's knee when it is diseased, mostly due to osteoarthritis, rheumatoid arthritis or post-traumatic arthritis. An artificial knee joint consists of a combination of removing damaged cartilage, positioning metal implants, resurfacing the patella, and, finally, inserting a plastic spacer that is situated in a position similar to the old menisci. The procedure takes approximately 1-2 hours and the components can last over fifteen years.

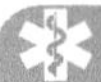

Clinical Correlate 5.34

Prepatellar Bursitis

Prepatellar bursitis or "housemaid's knee" is usually a bursitis caused by friction between the skin and the patella. A direct blow could lead to this form of bursitis but it is also commonly seen in carpet layers, gardeners, roofers or plumbers because they may spend a larger amount of time on their knees. If the inflammation is chronic, the bursa becomes distended with fluid and swelling appears anterior to the knee.

Clinical Correlate 5.35

Osgood-Schlatter Disease

Osgood-Schlatter disease is a common cause of knee pain in growing adolescents and involves the inflammation of the patellar ligament at the tibial tuberosity. Activities involving a lot of running and jumping such as soccer or basketball cause the quadriceps muscle group to pull repeatedly on the tibial tuberosity and the closely associated growth plate via the patellar ligament. Surgery is rarely needed but rest, anti-inflammatory medicine or physical therapy can be used to treat the pain.

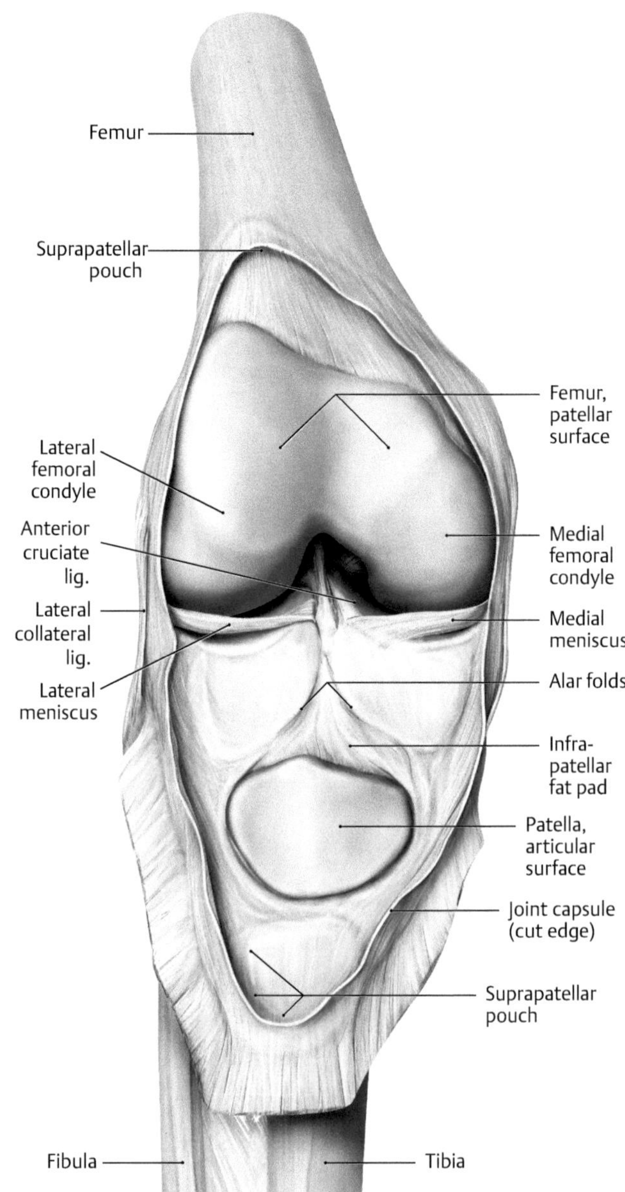

Fig. 5.54 Opened knee joint capsule. (From Schuenke M, Schulte E, Schumacher U. THIEME Atlas of Anatomy. General Anatomy and Musculoskeletal System. Illustrations by Voll M and Wesker K. 3rd ed. New York: Thieme Medical Publishers; 2020.)

5.17 Anterior Leg Compartment

The anterior leg compartment is located anterior to the interosseous membrane and between the lateral surfaces of the tibial shaft, anteromedial surface of the fibular shaft and the anterior intermuscular septum. With the addition of the crural fascia along with the surrounding bones, a tight compartment is formed. The anterior leg is the most susceptible to *compartment syndromes*. Near the ankle, two band-like thickenings of deep fascia called the superior and inferior retinacula are formed. The **superior retinaculum** attaches just above the malleoli of the ankle from the fibula to the tibia. The Y-shaped **inferior retinaculum** attaches laterally at the anterosuperior surface of the

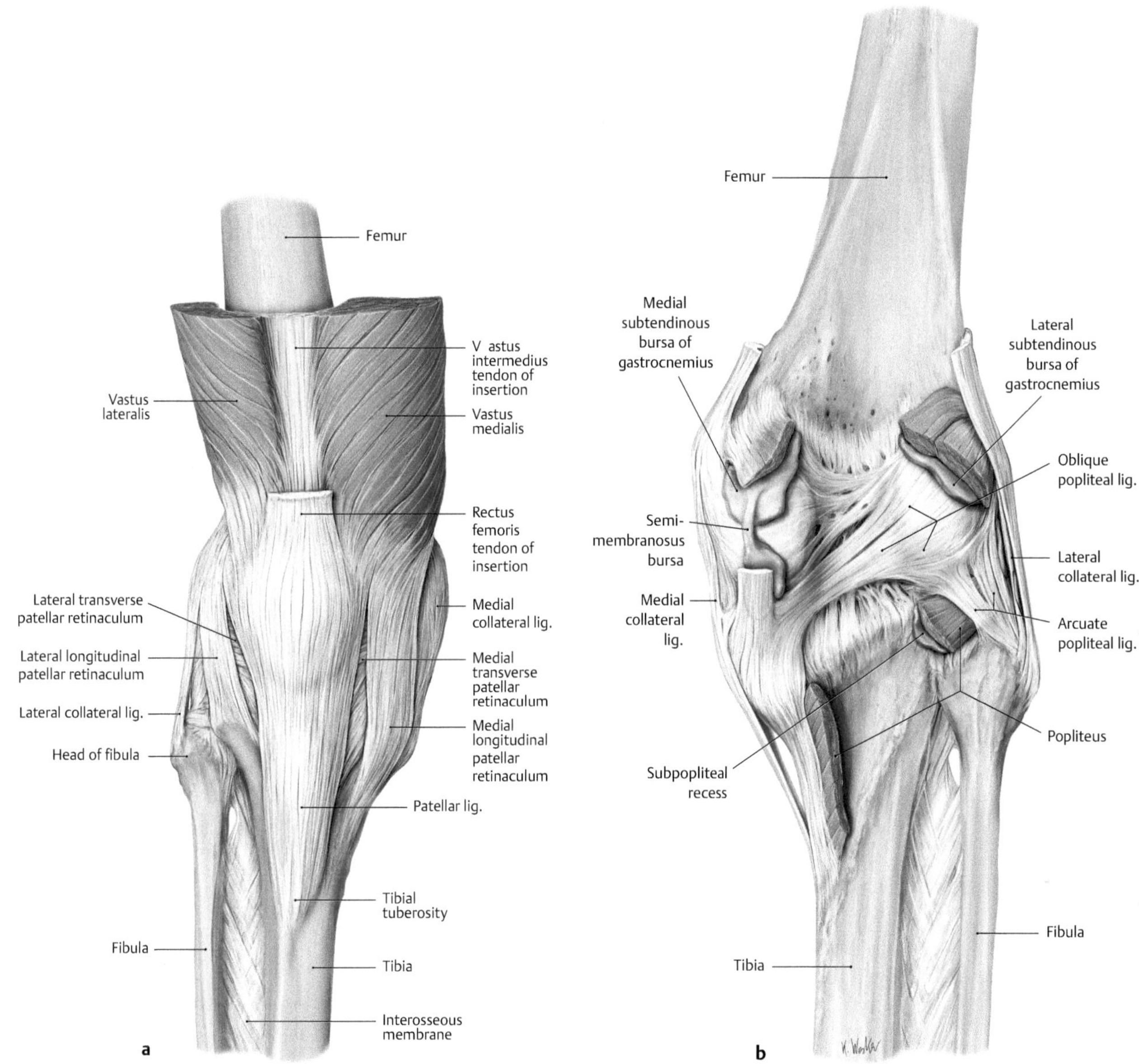

Fig. 5.55 Ligaments of the knee joint. **(a)** Anterior view of right knee. **(b)** Ligaments, capsule, and limited periarticular bursae of the knee joint, posterior view. (From Schuenke M, Schulte E, Schumacher U. THIEME Atlas of Anatomy. General Anatomy and Musculoskeletal System. Illustrations by Voll M and Wesker K. 3rd ed. New York: Thieme Medical Publishers; 2020.)

calcaneus and passes medially to attach at both the medial malleolus (superiorly) and plantar aponeurosis (inferiorly). These are responsible for binding the tendons of the anterior leg muscles and preventing bowstringing during dorsiflexion of the foot (**Fig. 5.61**).

5.17.1 Anterior Leg Muscles

The anterior leg muscles include the tibialis anterior, extensor hallucis longus, extensor digitorum longus and the fibularis tertius and pass just deep to the *extensor retinacula* (**Fig. 5.61**). These muscles are primarily involved in *dorsiflexion of the foot* at the ankle joint, in addition to *inversion* and *eversion of the foot.* The action of dorsiflexion is important because it is involved in the elevation of the forefoot during the swing phases of the gait cycle. When standing, dorsiflexion reflexively pulls the leg anteriorly on the fixed foot when the body begins to lean posteriorly and this results in a person's heel to compress against the surface and help them regain their center of balance.

The **tibialis anterior** is the most medial muscle in this compartment of the leg and it lies adjacent to the tibia. Its long tendon gives it a mechanical advantage, making it the strongest dorsiflexor muscle. Following the heel strike of the gait cycle, the tibialis anterior is important in creating a smoother lowering of the forefoot to the walking surface. This action also allows for deceleration if a person is running or walking downhill. The **extensor hallucis longus** is located between the tibialis anterior and extensor digitorum longus muscles. It primarily extends the great toe

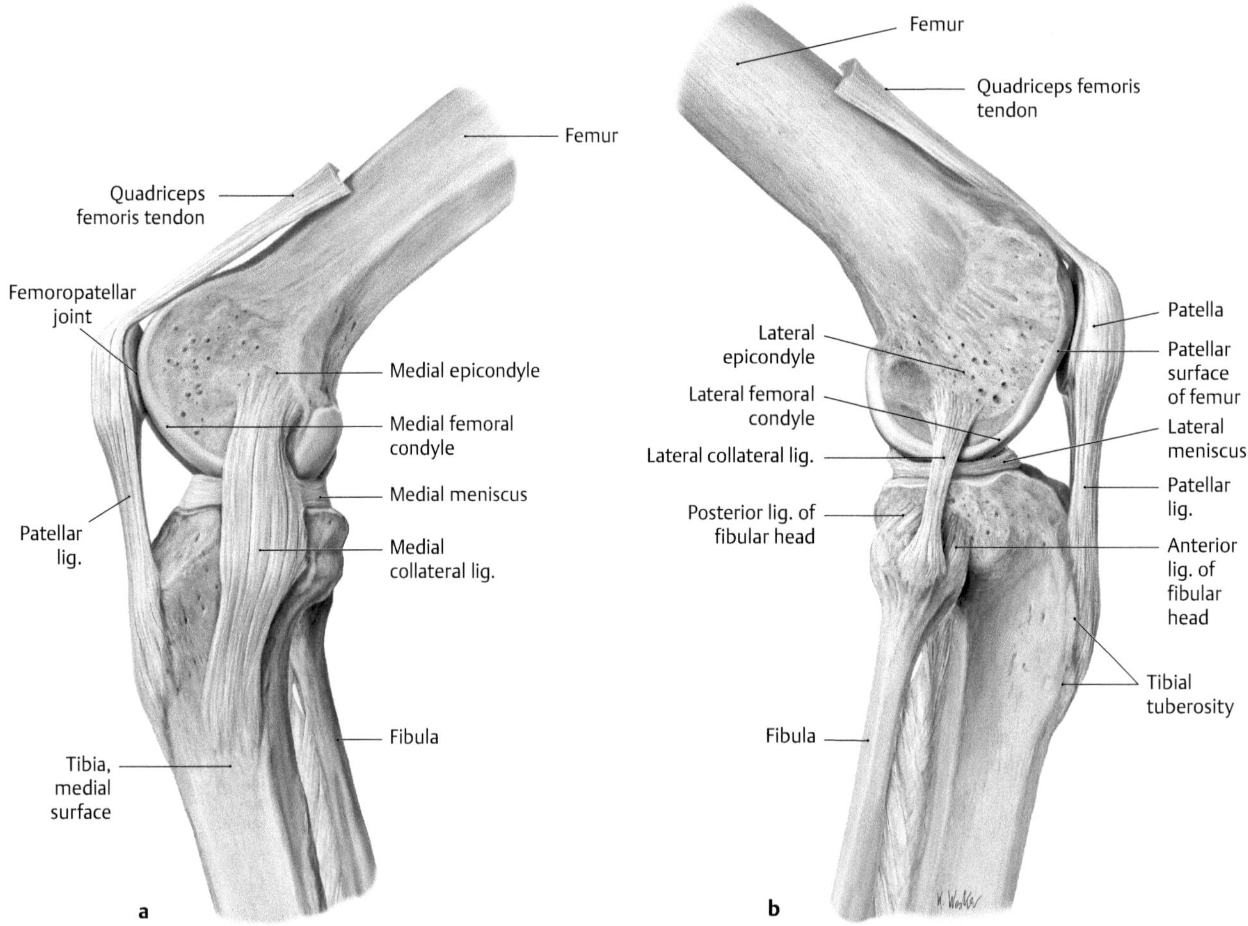

Fig. 5.56 Collateral and patellar ligaments of the knee joint. **(a)** Medial view. **(b)** Lateral view. (From Schuenke M, Schulte E, Schumacher U. THIEME Atlas of Anatomy. General Anatomy and Musculoskeletal System. Illustrations by Voll M and Wesker K. 3rd ed. New York: Thieme Medical Publishers; 2020.)

and assists in dorsiflexion and helps create the extensor expansion of the great toe. The **extensor digitorum longus** is the lateral most muscle of the anterior leg. The distal portions of its four tendons become the extensor expansions of digits 2-5. It functions by extending digits 2-5 and in dorsiflexion of the foot. The **fibularis tertius** may not always be present however it is technically a separate part of the extensor digitorum longus. It functions in eversion of the foot and has no real direct effect on the 5th digit. Descriptions of anterior leg muscles are found in **Table 5.5.**

5.17.2 Neurovasculature of the Anterior Leg Compartment

The **common fibular nerve** first wraps around the neck of the fibula before passing deep to the origin of the fibularis longus muscle. While deep to this muscle attachment, the common fibular nerve bifurcates into a **superficial** and **deep fibular nerve** just prior to reaching the *anterior intermuscular septum.* The deep fibular nerve passes through this intermuscular septum and enters the anterior leg compartment; it extends inferiorly initially between the tibialis anterior and extensor digitorum longus muscles before continuing toward the ankle between the tibialis anterior and extensor hallucis longus muscles; and then terminates on the dorsum of the foot. It is responsible for innervating muscles found in the anterior leg and dorsum of the foot regions, as well as a small area of skin between the webbing of the first and second digits (**Fig. 5.60**).

The smaller of the two terminating branches of the popliteal artery called the **anterior tibial artery** supplies blood to the anterior leg compartment (**Fig. 5.60**). It pairs along with veins of the same name and the deep fibular nerve after passing through a small gap on the superior portion of the interosseous membrane. At the ankle, it continues as the **dorsalis pedis artery** and this artery combines with a few others to supply the dorsum of the foot. Venous drainage follows these arteries back to the **popliteal vein**.

Clinical Correlate 5.36

Shin Splints

Tibialis anterior strains, more commonly known as shin splints, are a common exercise-related issue seen at the onset of a new fitness program or any vigorous athletic activity such as long distance running. Edema or pain generally in the area of the distal two-thirds of the tibia is the result of repetitive microtrauma of the tibialis anterior muscle and causes small tears in the tibial periosteum.

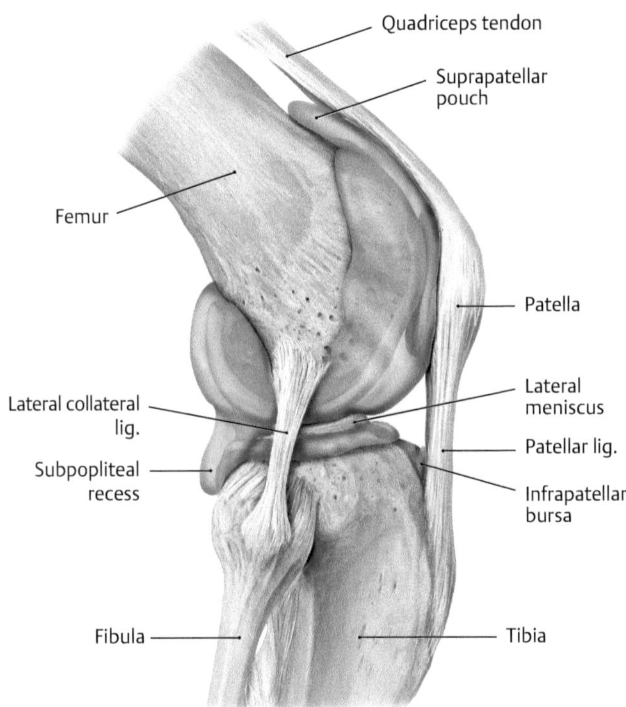

Fig. 5.57 Demonstration of the right knee joint after it had been injected with liquid plastic. (From Schuenke M, Schulte E, Schumacher U. THIEME Atlas of Anatomy. General Anatomy and Musculoskeletal System. Illustrations by Voll M and Wesker K. 3rd ed. New York: Thieme Medical Publishers; 2020.)

5.18 Lateral Leg Compartment

The lateral leg compartment is involved in *eversion of the foot*. It is the smallest leg compartment and the crural fascia, anterior and posterior intermuscular septa, and the lateral surface of the fibula establish its borders. The two muscles located in this compartment, the fibularis longus and brevis, pass deep to the **superior fibular retinaculum** and enter a common synovial sheath. This retinaculum serves as the inferior border of the lateral leg.

5.18.1 Lateral Leg Muscles

The **fibularis (peroneus) longus** continues deep to the **inferior fibular reticulum** and onto a groove on the cuboid bone. It then crosses the sole of the foot and attaches at the base of the first metatarsal and medial cuneiform, just on the opposite side of the insertion sites for the tibialis anterior muscle. Due to its length and orientation, the fibularis longus has plenty of leverage to evert the foot and help support all foot arches. When standing on one foot, the fibularis longus helps to steady the leg on the foot (**Fig. 5.62**). The **fibularis brevis** has a much wider muscle belly but only extends inferiorly to the base of the fifth metatarsal bone and only everts the foot. Both muscles can weakly plantarflex the foot at the ankle. Descriptions of lateral leg muscles are found in **Table 5.6.**

5.18.2 Neurovasculature of the Lateral Leg Compartment

After wrapping around the head of the fibula and passing just deep to the fibularis longus, the common fibular nerve bifurcates into the superficial and deep fibular nerves. The **superficial fibular nerve** travels inferiorly and tucks between the fibularis longus, fibularis brevis and extensor digitorum longus muscles before emerging as a cutaneous nerve (**Fig. 5.63**). It innervates both of the fibularis muscles and the skin on the distal part of the anterior surface of the leg along with the majority of the dorsum of the foot. There is no paired set of vessels with the superficial fibular nerve but blood supply to this compartment is from ***perforating branches*** of both the **anterior tibial** and **fibular arteries**. Venous drainage follows these arteries eventually back to the **popliteal vein** before continuing up through the **femoral vein**.

5.19 Posterior Leg Compartment

The posterior leg compartment is primarily involved in *plantarflexion of the foot* at the ankle joint, but also *inversion* at a couple of foot joints, and *flexion of the toes*. It is the largest of the leg compartments and is composed of both a *superficial* and *deep posterior leg compartment* primarily due to the *transverse intermuscular septum*. The transverse intermuscular septum terminates to help form the **flexor retinaculum** located between the calcaneus and medial malleolus.

5.19.1 Superficial Muscle Group of Posterior Leg

The **superficial muscle group** of the posterior leg is located between the deep fascia of the leg, posterior and transverse intermuscular septa. It contains the **gastrocnemius**, **soleus** and **plantaris muscles** and all three of these muscles extend inferiorly to become the **calcaneal (Achilles) tendon** (**Fig. 5.64**). The calcaneal tendon spirals approximately 90° during its descent toward the calcaneus bone. The fibers of the gastrocnemius attach laterally while the soleus attaches medially to it and it is this fiber arrangement that gives the tendon its elastic ability to absorb energy and recoil thus releasing the energy as part of the propulsive force it exerts. There are two bursas located near the attachment point to the calcaneus. The **subcutaneous calcaneal bursa** is between the skin and tendon while the **deep calcaneal bursa** is located between the tendon and calcaneus. The two heads of the gastrocnemius along with the soleus muscle are collectively known as the **triceps surae** and they are responsible for just over 90% of all plantarflexion.

The **gastrocnemius** has two muscle bellies and is the most superficial muscle of this muscle group. It acts on both the knee and ankle joints and helps define the inferior borders of the popliteal fossa. It is unable to exert its full power on both joints at the same time. It is most effective when the leg is fully extended at the knee and the foot is dorsiflexed of, for example at the start of a sprint. The **soleus** is located just deep to the gastrocnemius and is the most active muscle in plantarflexion. It has a continuous arched attachment spanning the tibia and fibula and there is a **tendinous arch of the soleus** located in the middle. Passing through this arch are the tibial nerve and popliteal vessels. Just pass the tendinous arch is generally where the popliteal artery bifurcates into the anterior and posterior tibial arteries. The soleus is considered an antigravity muscle and helps maintain balance

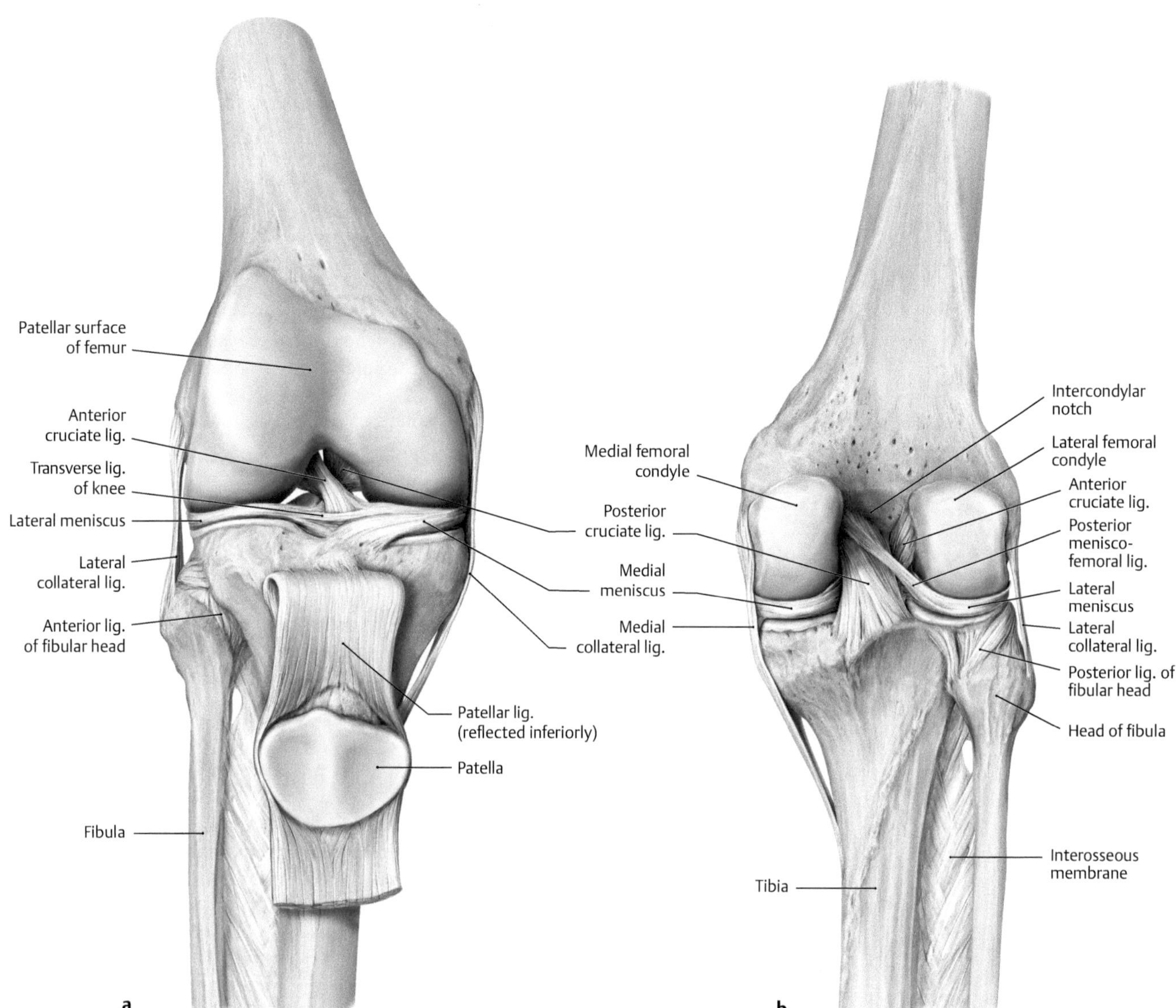

Fig. 5.58 Cruciate and collateral ligaments. **(a)** Anterior view. **(b)** Posterior view. (From Schuenke M, Schulte E, Schumacher U. THIEME Atlas of Anatomy. General Anatomy and Musculoskeletal System. Illustrations by Voll M and Wesker K. 3rd ed. New York: Thieme Medical Publishers; 2020.)

when it contracts antagonistically, but in a cooperative manner, with the dorsiflexor muscles of the leg. The **plantaris** has a short muscle belly and a long tendon. It may be absent in 10% of the population and most likely plays a larger role in proprioception versus its plantarflexion and knee flexion functions because these are quite insignificant. The tendon is commonly used for surgical grafting procedures. Descriptions of superficial posterior leg muscles are found in **Table 5.7.**

5.19.2 Deep Muscle Group of Posterior Leg

The **deep muscle group** of the posterior leg is located between the interosseous membrane, posterior and transverse intermuscular septa, and a small portion of the deep fascia of the leg. This compartment is composed of the popliteus, tibialis posterior, flexor digitorum longus and flexor hallucis longus muscles (**Fig. 5.65**).

The **popliteus** is a flat, triangular shaped muscle that helps contribute to the floor of the popliteal fossa. The **popliteus tendon** passes between the joint capsule of the knee and the *fibular (lateral) collateral ligament* from its lateral femoral condyle attachment with a **popliteal bursa** lying beneath this tendon. This muscle is insignificant in general knee flexion but is most known for unlocking the knee by laterally rotating the femur approximately 5° when a person transitions from full knee extension. When standing with the knee partially flexed, the popliteus assists the *posterior cruciate ligament (PCL)* in preventing anterior displacement of the femur. The **tibialis posterior** muscle belly lies between the fibularis digitorum longus and flexor hallucis longus muscle bellies. It extends down to the navicular bone primarily but also attaches to multiple tarsal and metatarsal bones. It acts

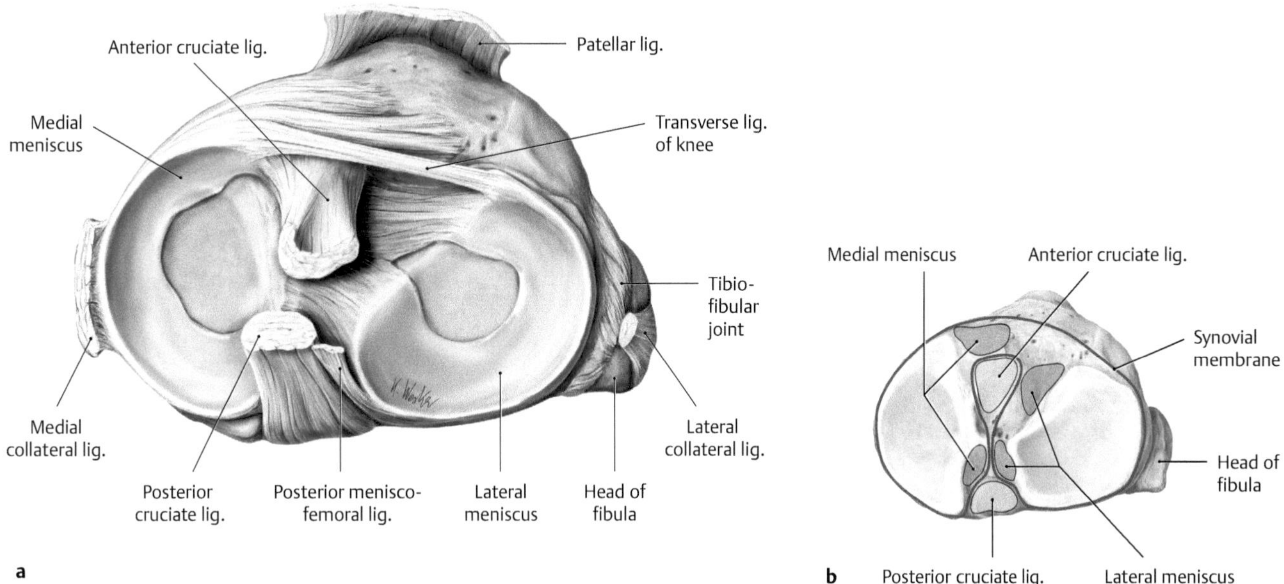

Fig. 5.59 Menisci in the knee joint. **(a)** Right tibial plateau, proximal view. **(b)** Attachment sites of menisci and cruciate ligaments. (From Schuenke M, Schulte E, Schumacher U. THIEME Atlas of Anatomy. General Anatomy and Musculoskeletal System. Illustrations by Voll M and Wesker K. 3rd ed. New York: Thieme Medical Publishers; 2020.)

mostly in support of the medial longitudinal arch of the foot while bearing weight but it also functions in plantarflexion at the ankle and inversion of the foot.

The **flexor digitorum longus** muscle belly is medial to the tibialis posterior. Its tendon crosses over the tibialis posterior, however, on its way to the foot. The *quadratus plantae*, located in the sole of the foot, attaches to the central part of the flexor digitorum longus tendon before it splits into four individual tendons. The functions of this muscle are to plantarflex the foot and flex digits 2-5. The **flexor hallucis longus** has a muscle belly lateral to the tibialis posterior and closest to the fibula. Its tendon passes posterior to the distal end of the tibia and occupies a groove on the posterior surface of the talus, which is continuous with a groove on the sustentaculum tali. It continues deep to the flexor digitorum longus tendon before splitting the sesamoid bones and attaching to the big distal phalanx of the great toe. It is involved in plantarflexion of the foot and flexion of the great toe. The flexion of the great toe is evident during the final thrust of the pre-swing phase of the gait cycle. Descriptions of deep posterior leg muscles are found in **Table 5.8.**

5.19.3 Neurovasculature of the Posterior Leg Compartment

The **tibial nerve** is a terminal branch of the **sciatic nerve** and it passes vertically from the posterior thigh and popliteal fossa into the posterior leg. It passes deep to the tendinous arch of the soleus muscle and pairs with the posterior tibial vessels before bifurcating into the lateral and medial plantar nerves that supply the foot. The tibial nerve innervates every muscle of the posterior leg compartment (**Fig. 5.66**).

The **popliteal artery** passes along with the tibial nerve just deep to the tendinous arch of the soleus muscle. Just after passing the tendinous arch, the popliteal artery bifurcates into an **anterior** and **posterior tibial artery**. The anterior tibial artery continues just above the superior part of interosseous membrane and into the anterior leg compartment. The posterior tibial artery remains paired with the tibial nerve and, a few centimeters after the popliteal artery bifurcation, the **fibular artery** branches off the posterior tibial and lies closer to the fibula with no nerve pairing. The posterior tibial continues inferiorly before passing posterior to the medial malleolus. It then passes deep to the flexor retinaculum and, near the origin of the abductor hallucis muscle, bifurcates into the **lateral** and **medial plantar arteries**, the vessels responsible for supplying the sole of the foot (**Fig. 5.66**).

The **nutrient artery of the tibia**, the largest of its kind in the body, originates from the posterior tibial artery and enters the tibia posteriorly somewhere near the proximal one-third of the bone. The **nutrient artery of the fibula** arises from the fibular artery. Near the bifurcation of the popliteal into anterior and posterior tibial arteries, the **circumflex fibular artery** arises and anastomoses with the blood supply of the knee.

5.20 Tarsal Tunnel

The **tarsal tunnel** is located between the medial malleolus and calcaneus and is covered by the flexor retinaculum (**Fig. 5.67**). Passing through this tunnel is a combination of tendons related to the tibialis posterior, flexor digitorum longus and flexor hallucis longus and the tibial nerve and posterior tibial vessels. There is a characteristic order extending from the medial malleolus back to the calcaneus. It begins with the tibialis posterior, flexor digitorum longus, posterior tibial artery and veins, tibial nerve, and finally finishes with the flexor hallucis longus tendon. Inflammation of this area is called *tarsal tunnel syndrome* and involves compression of the tibial nerve.

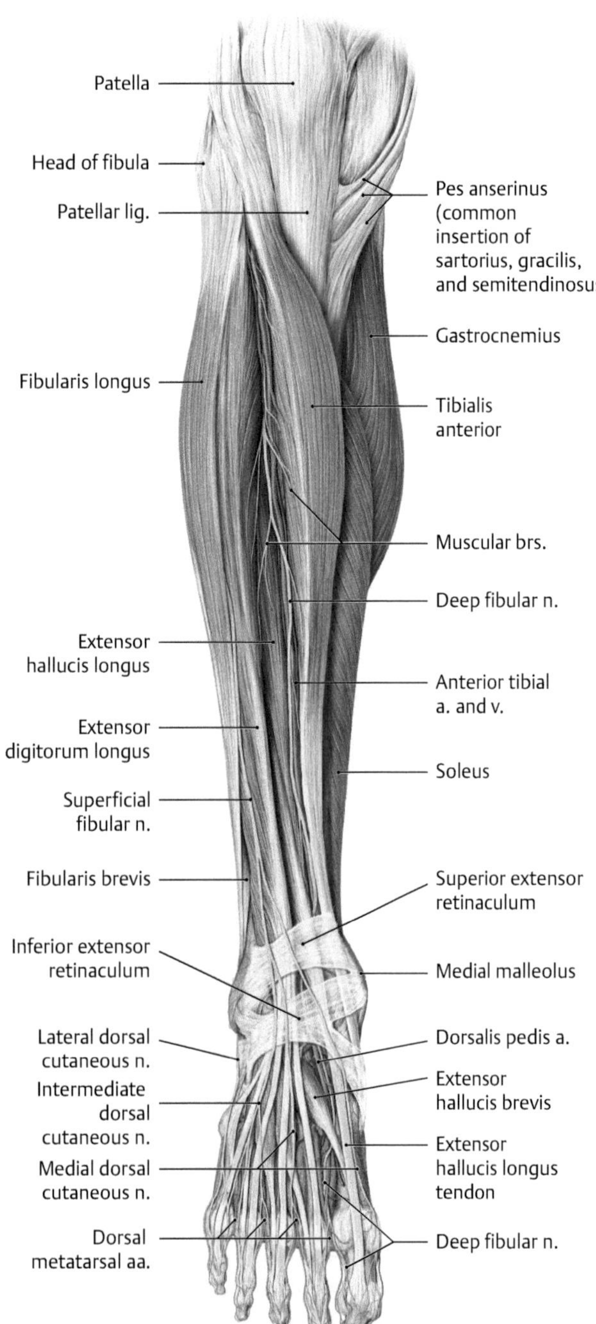

Fig. 5.60 Neurovasculature of the anterior leg compartment and dorsum foot. (From Schuenke M, Schulte E, Schumacher U. THIEME Atlas of Anatomy. General Anatomy and Musculoskeletal System. Illustrations by Voll M and Wesker K. 3rd ed. New York: Thieme Medical Publishers; 2020.)

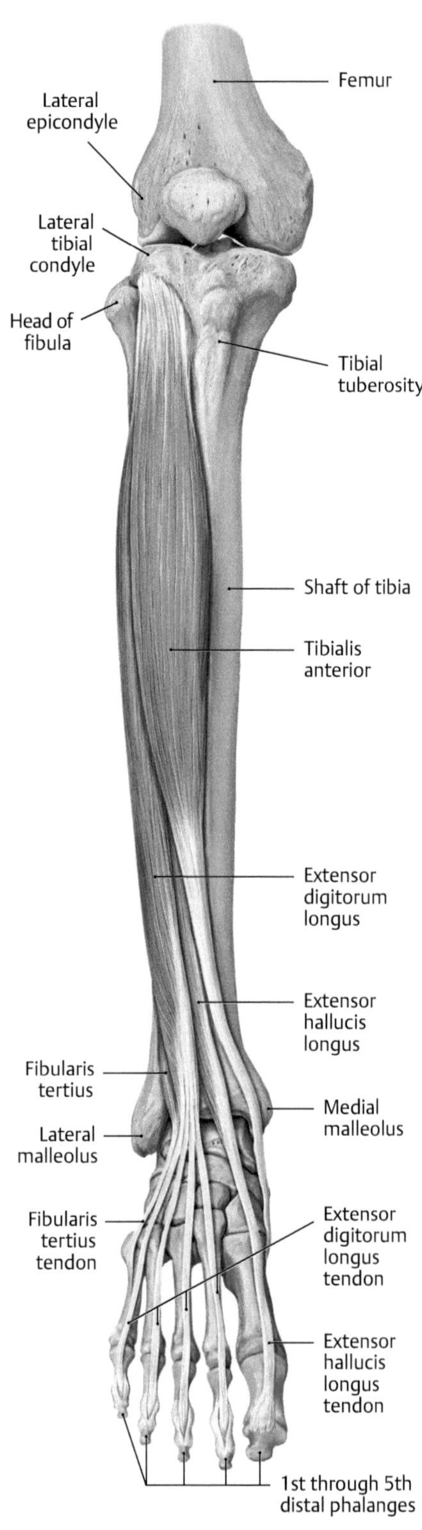

Fig. 5.61 Muscles of the anterior leg compartment. (From Schuenke M, Schulte E, Schumacher U. THIEME Atlas of Anatomy. General Anatomy and Musculoskeletal System. Illustrations by Voll M and Wesker K. 3rd ed. New York: Thieme Medical Publishers; 2020.)

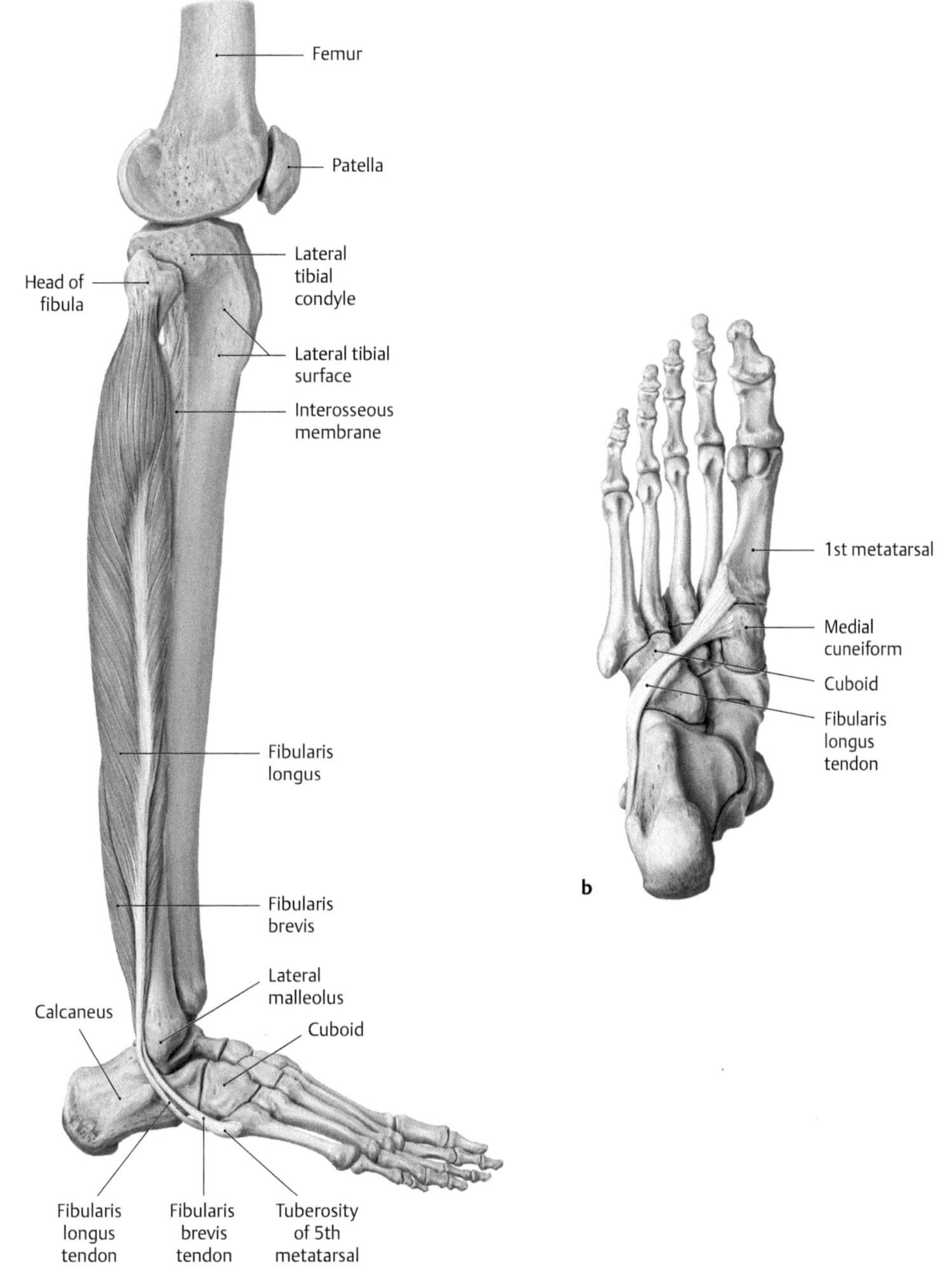

Fig. 5.62 Muscles of the lateral leg compartment. **(a)** Right lateral view. **(b)** Course of the fibularis longus tendon, plantar view. (From Schuenke M, Schulte E, Schumacher U. THIEME Atlas of Anatomy. General Anatomy and Musculoskeletal System. Illustrations by Voll M and Wesker K. 3rd ed. New York: Thieme Medical Publishers; 2020.)

5.21 Tibiofibular Articulations

There are two articulations between the tibia and fibula with one proximally at the knee and the other distally at the ankle. They are the proximal and distal **tibiofibular joints**. Movement is minimal and there are no muscles that directly act on these joints. Ligaments associated with these joints are orientated inferiorly from the tibia to the fibula and are able to resist downward movements by the muscles that attach to the fibula.

- **Proximal tibiofibular joint**: is a *plane-type synovial joint* located between the fibular head and lateral condyle of the tibia. The **anterior** and **posterior ligaments of the fibular head** strengthen the joint (**Fig. 5.56; Fig. 5.58**).
- **Distal tibiofibular joint**: is a *fibrous joint* that helps create a mortise formed by the lateral and medial malleoli. The malleoli cup the talus and stabilize the ankle joint. The primary support of the joint comes from the **interosseous tibiofibular ligament**, which is a continuation of the interosseous membrane. The **anterior**

Table 5.5 **Anterior leg muscles**

Muscle	Innervation	Function(s)	Origin	Insertion
Tibialis anterior	Deep fibular nerve	Dorsiflexes foot; inverts foot; supports medial longitudinal arch of foot	Lateral condyle and superior part of lateral surface of tibia; interosseous membrane	Medial and inferior surfaces of medial cuneiform; base of 1st metatarsal
Extensor hallucis longus	Deep fibular nerve	Extends great toe; dorsiflexes foot	Middle part of anterior surface of fibula; interosseous membrane	Base of distal phalanx of great toe
Extensor digitorum longus	Deep fibular nerve	Extends digits 2-5; dorsiflexes foot	Lateral condyle of tibia; superior 3/4 of medial surface of fibula; interosseous membrane	Middle and distal phalanges of digits 2-5
Fibularis tertius	Deep fibular nerve	Dorsiflexes and everts foot	Inferior 1/3 of anterior surface of fibula; interosseous membrane	Base of 5th metatarsal

Table 5.6 **Lateral leg muscles**

Muscle	Innervation	Function(s)	Origin	Insertion
Fibularis longus	Superficial fibular nerve	Everts foot; weak plantarflexion of foot; supports longitudinal arches of foot	Head and superior 2/3 of lateral surface of fibula	Base of 1st metatarsal; medial cuneiform
Fibularis brevis	Superficial fibular nerve	Everts foot; weak plantarflexion of foot	Inferior 2/3 of lateral surface of fibula	Base of 5th metatarsal

and **posterior tibiofibular ligaments** that are found external to the interosseous tibiofibular ligament also strengthen this joint. The inferior portion of the posterior tibiofibular ligament may be defined as the **inferior transverse (tibiofibular) ligament**, and along with the lateral and medial malleoli forms the **malleolar mortise** (**Fig. 5.8; Fig. 5.68; Fig. 5.69**).

- The **interosseous membrane** is in itself a *syndesmosis-type fibrous joint* connecting the shafts of the tibia and fibula together.

5.21.1 Neurovasculature of the Tibiofibular Joints

The *proximal tibiofibular joint* is innervated by the common fibular nerve and nerve to popliteus while the *distal tibiofibular joint* along with the interosseous membrane are innervated by the tibial, deep fibular and saphenous nerves (**Fig. 5.16**).

The blood supply to the *proximal tibiofibular joint* originates from the **anterior tibial recurrent** and **inferior lateral genicular arteries** (**Fig. 5.22**). The *distal tibiofibular joint* receives blood from **perforating branches of the fibular artery** and **lateral malleolar** branches (anterior tibial and fibular brs.). The interosseous membrane of the leg receives blood from branches of the anterior tibial and fibular arteries. Venous drainage mirrors blood supply and travels in the opposite direction.

5.22 Ankle Joint

The **ankle (talocrural) joint** is located between the distal ends of the tibia and fibula and the superior part of the talus. It is a *hinge-type synovial joint* and movements include primarily dorsiflexion and plantarflexion of the foot (**Fig. 5.70; Fig. 5.71**). The ROM when the foot is planted is 30° with dorsiflexion and 50° with plantarflexion. When non-weight bearing, the ROM of dorsiflexion is between 20-30° and plantarflexion is 40-50°. Muscles of the anterior leg compartment produce dorsiflexion while plantarflexion, a more powerful movement, is produced by the posterior leg compartment with a minor contribution from the lateral leg compartment (**Fig. 5.72**).

5.22.1 Articulating Surfaces

The *malleolar mortise* is formed by the combination of the distal tibia and fibula along with the inferior transverse (tibiofibular) ligament. The pulley-shaped *trochlea* is the round and superior articulating surface of the talus that fits within the mortise. The flat, inferior surface of the tibia forms the roof of the mortise and it articulates with the trochlea of the talus. The medial malleolus (lateral surface) of the tibia articulates with the medial surface of the trochlea. The lateral malleolus (medial surface) of the fibula articulates with the lateral surface of the trochlea (**Fig. 5.73**).

The grip on the trochlea by the malleoli is strongest during dorsiflexion of the foot at the ankle. Dorsiflexion forces the wider and anterior portion of the trochlea posteriorly thus spreading the tibia and fibula slightly apart from each other. During plantarflexion the ankle is relatively unstable and allows for the foot to wobble. The trochlea in this position is narrower posteriorly allowing it to be loose in the mortise.

5.22.2 Joint Capsule

The capsule of the ankle joint is thin both anteriorly and posteriorly but is supported laterally and medially by strong collateral ligaments. The fibrous layer of the capsule attaches to the borders of the articular surfaces of the malleoli, tibia and talus. The synovial membrane lines the fibrous layer internally and can extend superiorly as far as the interosseous tibiofibular ligament.

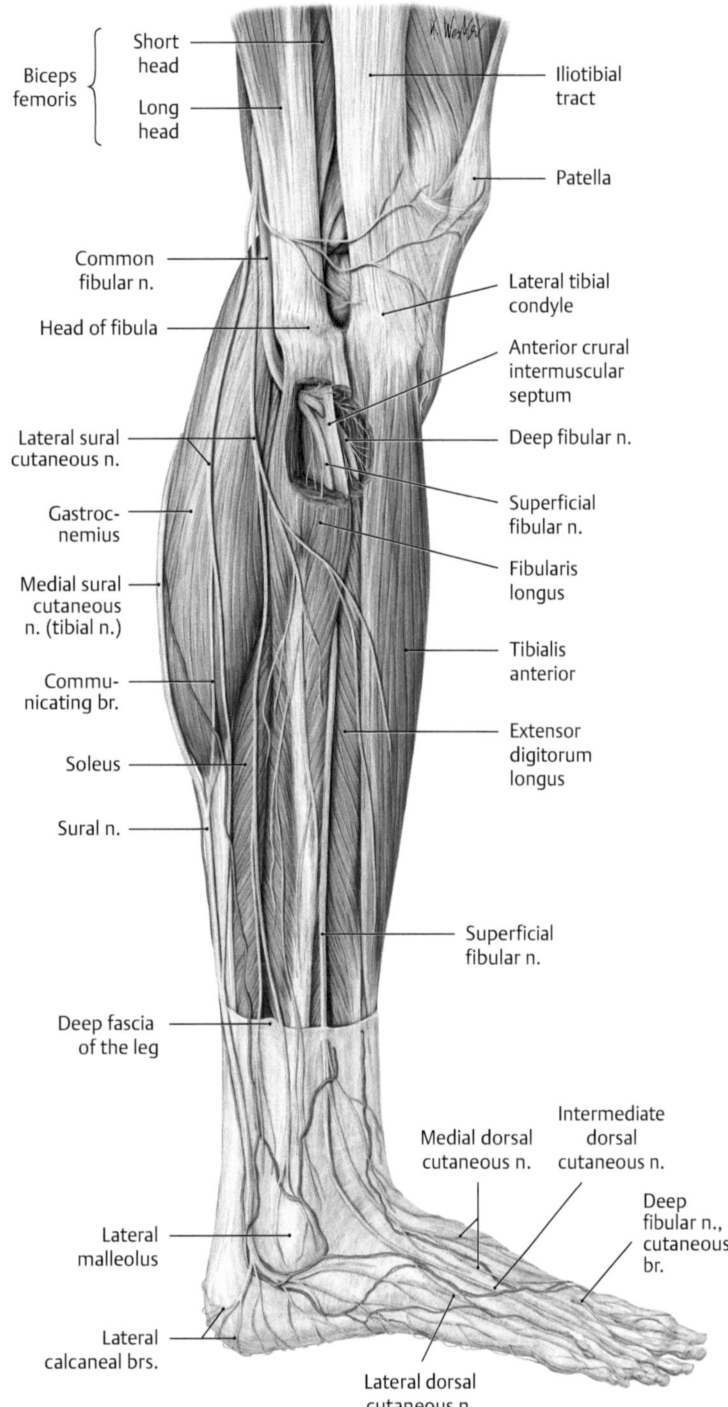

Fig. 5.63 Neurovasculature of the lateral leg compartment. (From Schuenke M, Schulte E, Schumacher U. THIEME Atlas of Anatomy. General Anatomy and Musculoskeletal System. Illustrations by Voll M and Wesker K. 3rd ed. New York: Thieme Medical Publishers; 2020.)

5.22.3 Lateral Ligaments of the Ankle Joint

- **Anterior talofibular ligament**: weaker ligament that extends anteromedially from the lateral malleolus to the neck of the talus (**Fig. 5.69**).
- **Calcaneofibular ligament**: round ligament that connects the tip of the lateral malleolus to the lateral surface of the calcaneus.
- **Posterior talofibular ligament**: stronger ligament that courses horizontally and medially from the malleolar fossa of the fibula to the lateral tubercle of the talus.

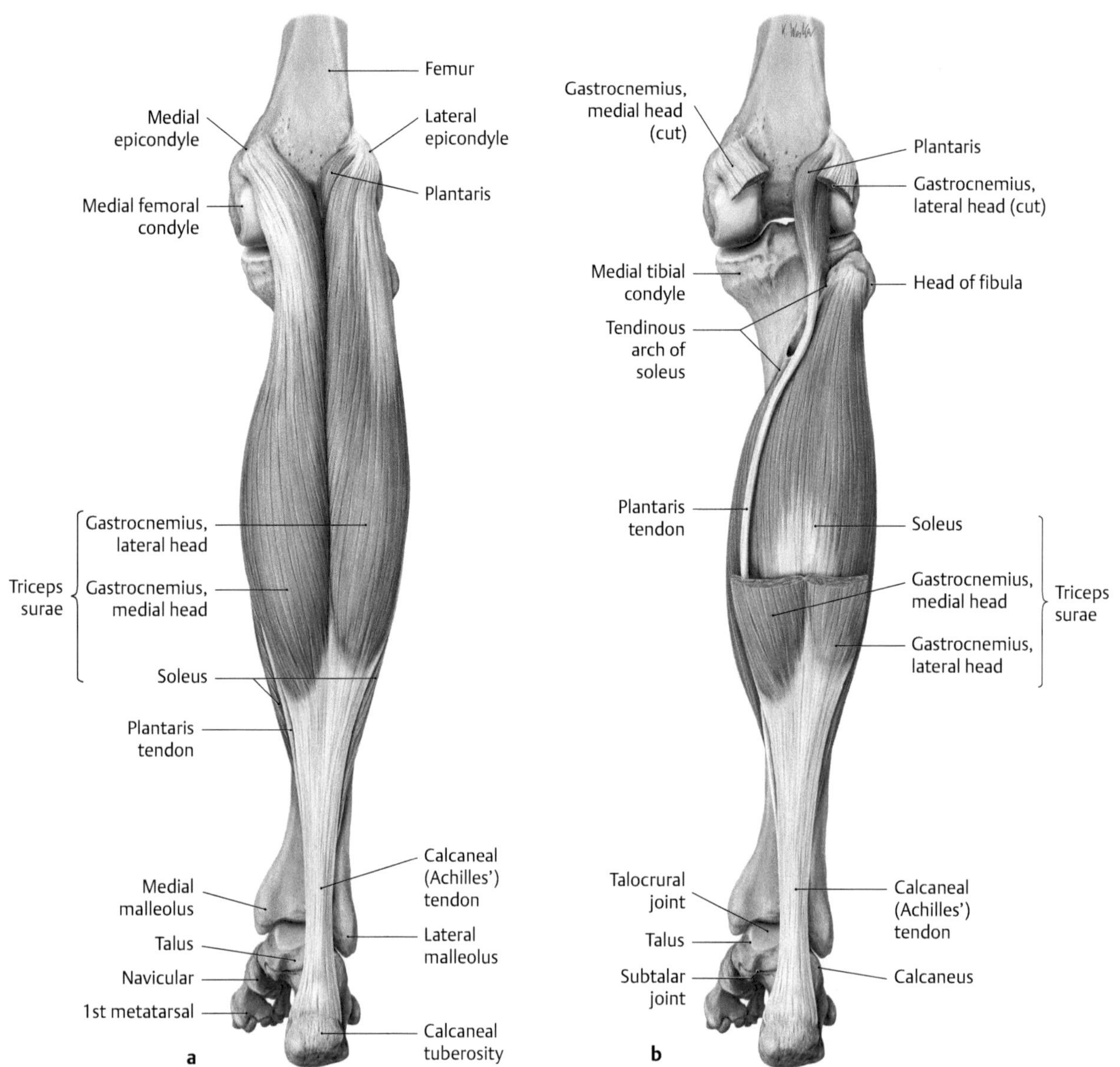

Fig. 5.64 Muscles of the posterior leg compartment. **(a)** Superficial muscle layer. **(b)** Superficial muscles with portions of the gastrocnemius removed. (From Schuenke M, Schulte E, Schumacher U. THIEME Atlas of Anatomy. General Anatomy and Musculoskeletal System. Illustrations by Voll M and Wesker K. 3rd ed. New York: Thieme Medical Publishers; 2020.)

Table 5.7 **Superficial posterior leg muscles**

Muscle	Innervation	Function(s)	Origin	Insertion
Gastrocnemius	Tibial nerve	Plantarflexion of foot; flexes leg	The non-articulating surface of the lateral (lateral head) and medial condyles (medial head)	Calcaneal tuberosity via calcaneal tendon
Soleus	Tibial nerve	Plantarflexion of foot	Posterior surface of head, neck and superior 1/4 of fibula; soleal line	Calcaneal tuberosity via calcaneal tendon
Plantaris	Tibial nerve	Negligible plantarflexion of foot and flexion of leg	Lateral supracondylar line; oblique popliteal ligament	Calcaneal tuberosity via calcaneal tendon

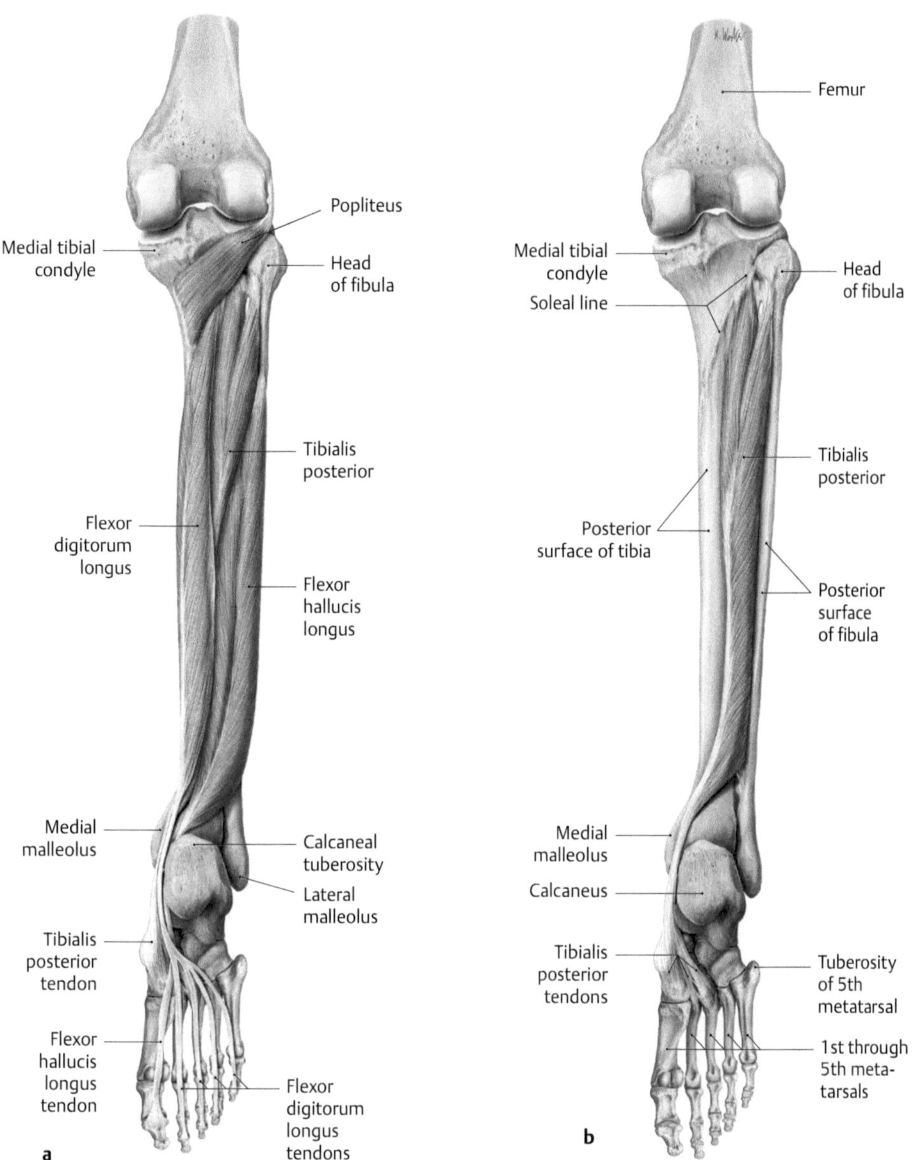

Fig. 5.65 Muscles of the posterior leg compartment. **(a)** Deep muscle layer. **(b)** Isolated tibialis posterior. (From Schuenke M, Schulte E, Schumacher U. THIEME Atlas of Anatomy. General Anatomy and Musculoskeletal System. Illustrations by Voll M and Wesker K. 3rd ed. New York: Thieme Medical Publishers; 2020.)

Table 5.8 **Deep posterior leg muscles**

Muscle	Innervation	Function(s)	Origin	Insertion
Popliteus	Tibial nerve	Weakly flexes leg and unlocks knee by laterally rotating femur 5°; medially rotates tibia when foot is off ground	Lateral femoral condyle; posterior horn of lateral meniscus	Posterior tibial surface above soleal line
Tibialis posterior	Tibial nerve	Supports the medial longitudinal and transverse arches of foot; inverts and plantarflexes foot	Interosseous membrane; adjacent superior parts of tibia and fibula	Navicular tuberosity; sustentaculum tali; all three cuneiforms; cuboid; bases of 2-4 metatarsals
Flexor digitorum longus	Tibial nerve	Flexes digits 2-5; plantarflexes foot; supports longitudinal arches of foot	Middle 1/3 of posterior tibial surface	Bases of distal phalanges of digits 2-5
Flexor hallucis longus	Tibial nerve	Flexes great toe; weak plantarflexor of foot; supports medial longitudinal arch of foot	Inferior 2/3 of posterior fibular surface; adjacent interosseous membrane	Base of distal phalanx of great toe

Clinical Correlate 5.37

Nerve Entrapments of the Leg

- *Tibial nerve entrapment* (tarsal tunnel syndrome): caused by edema or compression by the synovial sheaths of tendons passing through the tarsal tunnel of the ankle region and the flexor retinaculum on the tibial nerve. This is near the bifurcation of the lateral and medial plantar nerves and has an effect on both the sensory and motor innervation of the sole of the foot.
- *Deep fibular nerve entrapment* (ski boot syndrome): compression of this nerve reduces skin sensation of the webbing between the 1st and 2nd digits of the foot. Motor deficits include the loss of dorsiflexion of the foot at the ankle joint which could lead to *foot drop*.
- *Superficial fibular nerve entrapment*: can be caused by chronic ankle sprains that continuously stretch this nerve. Paresthesia is felt on the lateral leg and most of the dorsal foot skin. Motor deficits include loss of foot eversion.

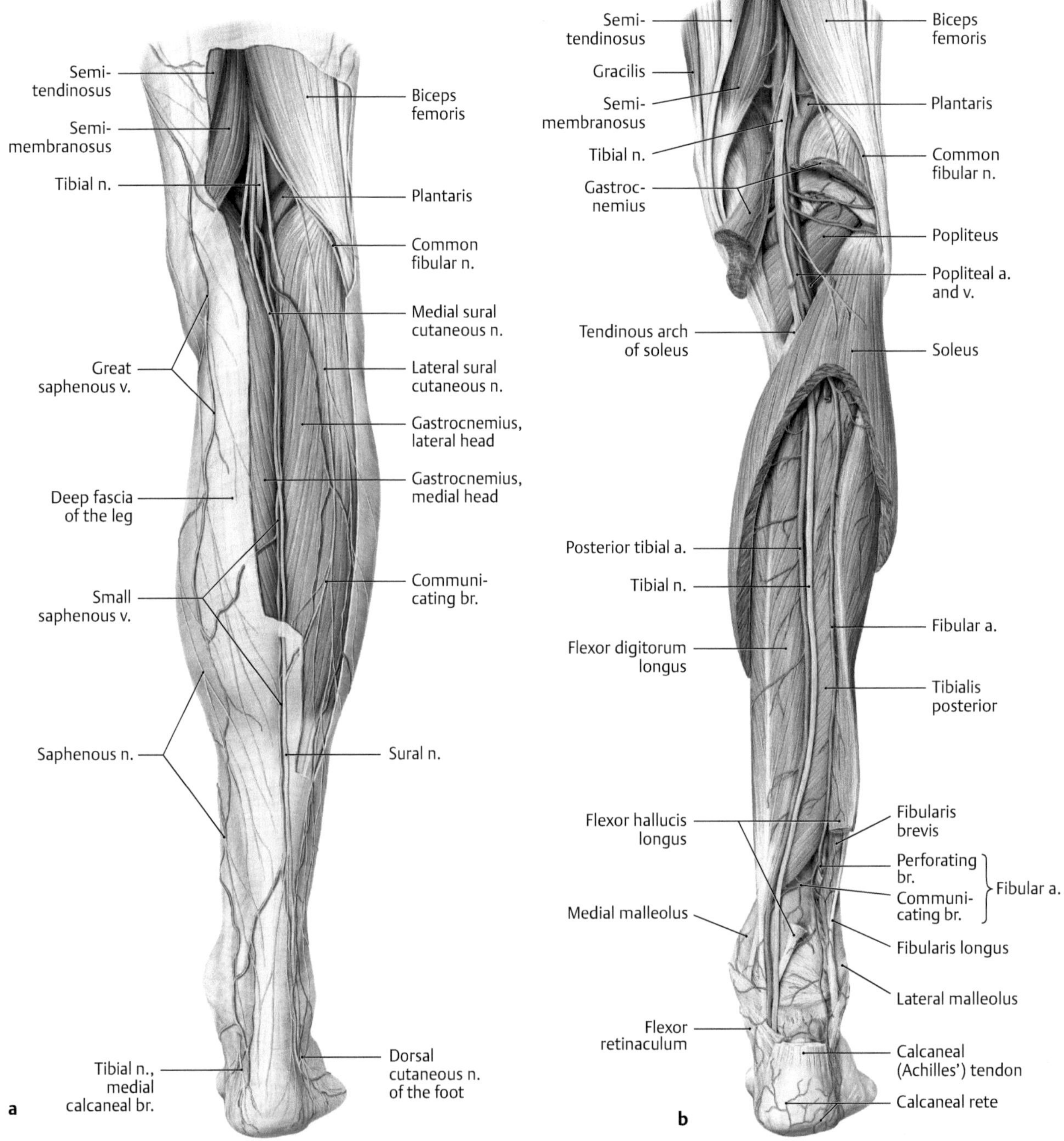

Fig. 5.66 Neurovasculature of the posterior leg compartment. **(a)** Superficial structures. **(b)** Deeper structures with the gastrocnemius removed and soleus windowed. (From Schuenke M, Schulte E, Schumacher U. THIEME Atlas of Anatomy. General Anatomy and Musculoskeletal System. Illustrations by Voll M and Wesker K. 3rd ed. New York: Thieme Medical Publishers; 2020.)

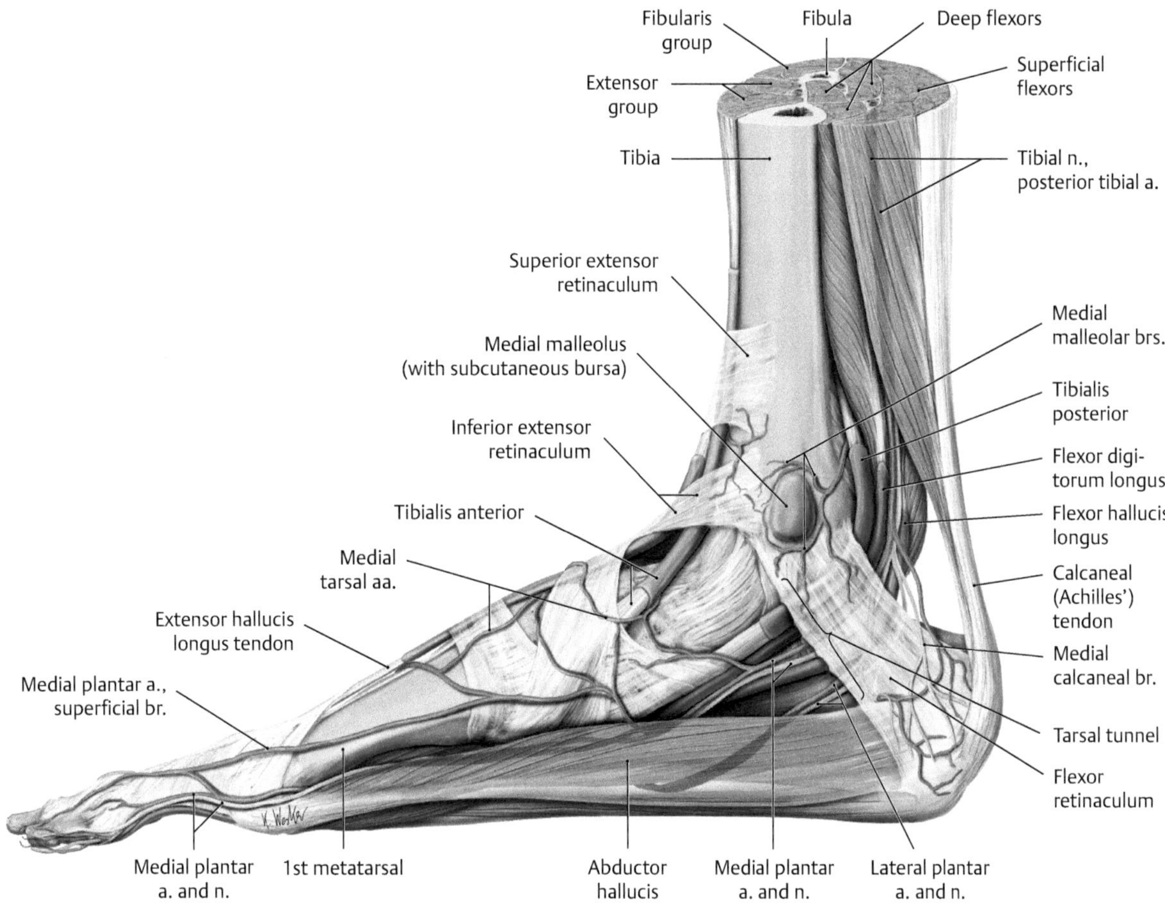

Fig. 5.67 Tarsal tunnel. Right ankle, medial view. (From Schuenke M, Schulte E, Schumacher U. THIEME Atlas of Anatomy. General Anatomy and Musculoskeletal System. Illustrations by Voll M and Wesker K. 3rd ed. New York: Thieme Medical Publishers; 2020.)

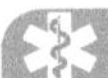 ***Clinical Correlate 5.38***

Foot Drop

An injury to the common fibular nerve can result in **foot drop** and there is primarily a loss of dorsiflexion of the foot at the ankle. The common fibular nerve is the most often injured nerve of the lower extremity and this is because it is exposed as it wraps around the lateral aspect of the fibular neck. Foot drop is exasperated by unopposed inversion of the foot which has the effect of lengthening the leg and not allowing the toes to clear the ground during the swing phase of walking. There are three different gaits that can compensate for a lengthened lower extremity:

- *Waddling gait*: an individual leans to the side opposite of the long limb to lift it up.
- *Swing-out gait*: the longer limb is swung out laterally to allow the toes to clear the ground.
- *High-steppage gait*: extra hip and knee flexion is employed to raise the foot as high as necessary to clear the ground.

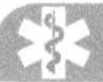 ***Clinical Correlate 5.39***

Sural Nerve Grafts

Sural nerve grafts are commonly used in procedures that require repairing nerve defects resulting from wounds. They are often used in "cable grafting" or when a nerve and the graft have different diameters, the grafts are joined in bundles with stitches. The surgeon would be able to locate this nerve adjacent to the small saphenous vein.

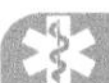 ***Clinical Correlate 5.40***

Gastrocnemius Strain

A **gastrocnemius strain** (tennis leg) is a calf injury resulting from the partial tearing of the medial belly of the gastrocnemius at or near its musculotendinous junction. Overstretching the muscle with accompanying full extension of the knee and dorsiflexion of the foot causes it. These types of strains are often seen in the occasional active athlete and are at times referred to as "weekend warrior" injuries.

Clinical Correlate 5.41

Calcaneal Tendon Reflex

To elicit the **calcaneal tendon reflex** or "ankle jerk" the calcaneal tendon is struck with a reflex hammer while a person's legs are dangling over the side of an exam table. This reflex tests the integrity of the S1 and S2 spinal cord segments. However, if the S1 nerve root is cut or damaged, this reflex is virtually absent.

Clinical Correlate 5.42

Calcaneal Tendon Rupture

Most calcaneal tendon ruptures occur about 2 inches above its insertion onto the calcaneus. Individuals are unable to plantarflex against resistance, balance on the affected side and demonstrate excessive dorsiflexion. If it is a complete tear a gap may be palpable under the skin. Surgical intervention is generally required to fix the ruptured tendon.

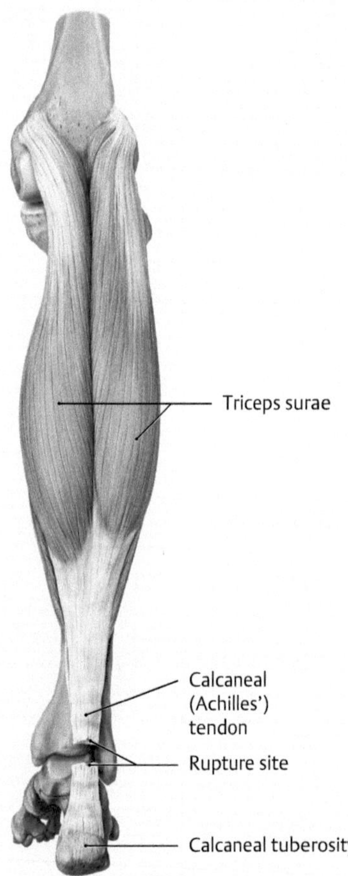

(From Schuenke M, Schulte E, Schumacher U. THIEME Atlas of Anatomy. General Anatomy and Musculoskeletal System. Illustrations by Voll M and Wesker K. 3rd ed. New York: Thieme Medical Publishers; 2020.)

5.22.4 Medial (Deltoid) Ligaments of the Ankle Joint

- **Anterior tibiotalar ligament**: extends from the medial malleolus to the talus anteriorly (**Fig. 5.69**).
- **Tibionavicular ligament**: extends inferiorly from the medial malleolus to the navicular.
- **Tibiocalcaneal ligament**: extends inferiorly from the medial malleolus to the sustentaculum tali of the calcaneus.
- **Posterior tibiotalar ligament**: extends from the medial malleolus to the talus posteriorly near the groove for the flexor hallucis longus tendon.

5.22.5 Neurovasculature of the Ankle Joint

Branches of the tibial and deep fibular nerve innervate the ankle joint. Blood supply along with venous drainage is associated with multiple malleolar vessels derived from the fibular, anterior tibial and posterior tibial vessels (**Fig. 5.67**).

Clinical Correlate 5.43

Ankle Sprains

The most common joint injuries occur at the ankle. An **ankle sprain** is mostly an inversion injury on the weight-bearing foot. The *anterior talofibular ligament* is generally injured and can be partially or completely torn, creating an unstable joint. A **high ankle (syndesmosis) sprain** occurs above the ankle and is less common than the typical ankle sprains just described. This type of sprain involves the ligaments that connect the tibia and fibula just above the ankle joint and that help form the ankle mortise. This injury occurs when the foot is planted and laterally rotated, which results in a shearing force between the tibia and fibula. This can lead to damage of the *anterior*, *interosseous* or *posterior tibiofibular ligaments*.

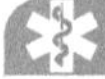

Clinical Correlate 5.44

Pott Fracture

A **Pott fracture** is an injury caused by the foot being forcibly everted at the ankle joint. This pulls on the strong medial (deltoid) ligament, frequently causing a fracture of the medial malleolus but no tearing of the medial ligament. The talus moves laterally, shearing off the lateral malleolus or breaking the fibula superior to the tibiofibular syndesmosis. When the tibia moves anteriorly, the talus bone shears off the posterior margin of its distal end.

5.23 Foot

The foot is divided into several regions. The **dorsum of the foot** is the portion that faces superiorly or the region that gets stepped on (**Fig. 5.74**). The **sole of the foot** is the region that has contact with the ground (**Fig. 5.75**). The portion of the sole related to the heads of the two most medial metatarsals is called the **ball of the foot** while the portion that rests against the calcaneus is known as the **heel**. The **big toe** is also known as the **1**st **toe** whereas the **little toe** would correspond to the **5**th **toe**.

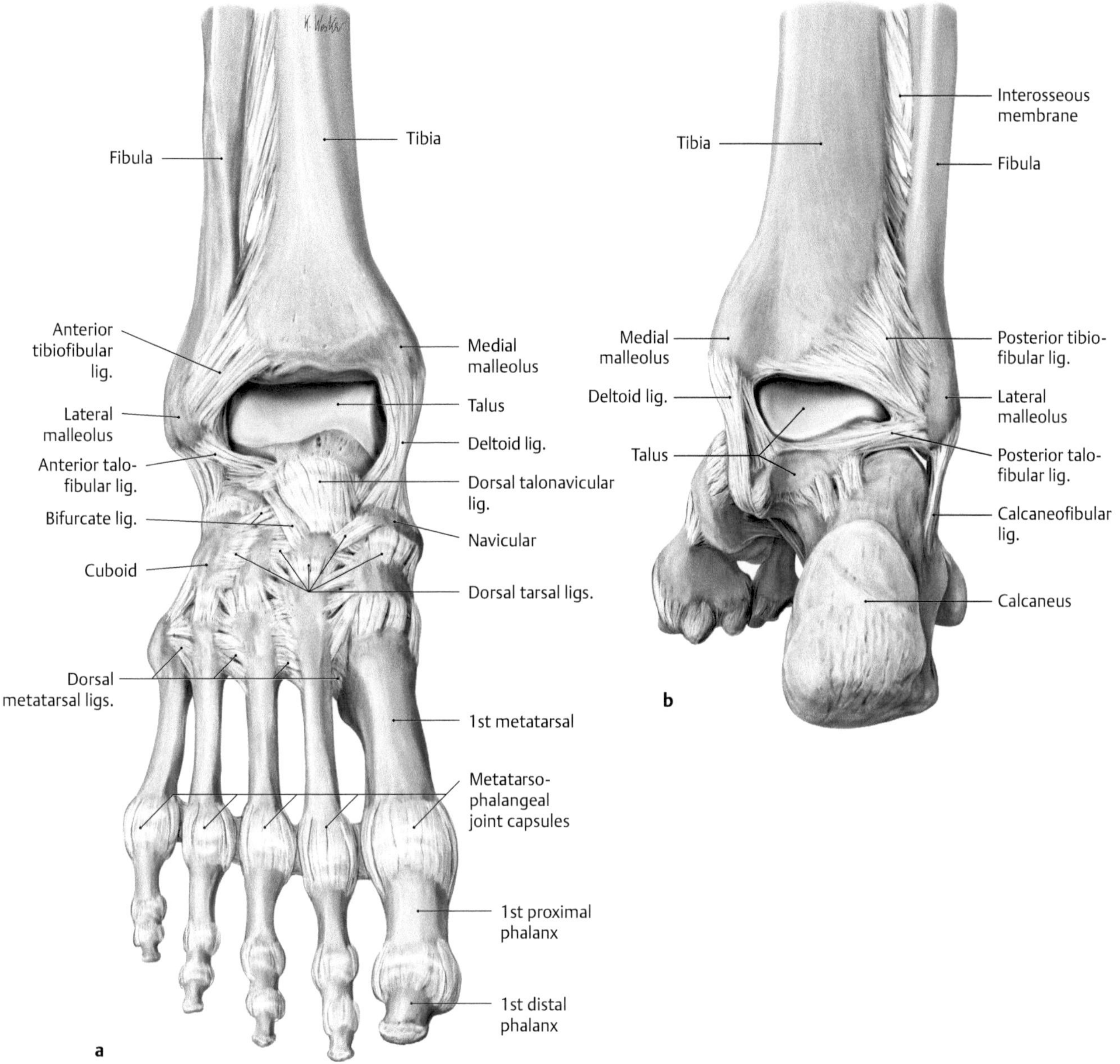

Fig. 5.68 Ligaments of the ankle and foot. **(a)** Anterior view. **(b)** Posterior view. (From Schuenke M, Schulte E, Schumacher U. THIEME Atlas of Anatomy. General Anatomy and Musculoskeletal System. Illustrations by Voll M and Wesker K. 3rd ed. New York: Thieme Medical Publishers; 2020.)

The skin and subcutaneous fascia over the dorsum of the foot is very thin compared to the sole and not very sensitive. The sole has thicker skin where natural weight bearing occurs in regions such as the ball, heel and lateral margin of the foot. The sole is hairless, very sensitive, and has many sweat glands. There are **fibrous septa** that divide the subcutaneous tissue of the sole into isolated fat-filled parts that act as shock absorbers. The fibrous septa assist in anchoring the skin to the underlying deep fascia, specifically the *plantar aponeurosis*.

The crural fascia continues into the foot as the **deep fascia of the dorsum of the foot** and the **deep fascia of the sole (plantar fascia)**. The deep fascia of the sole of the foot/plantar fascia can be thin on the lateral and medial portions of the sole but has a much thicker central region that leads to the formation of the **plantar aponeurosis**. This structure originates from the calcaneus and extends distally toward the toes. The longitudinal bundles of collagen split into five separate bands and become continuous with the **fibrous digital sheaths**. These sheaths enclose the flexor tendons that act on the toes. At the level of the metatarsal heads, the **superficial transverse metatarsal ligament** reinforces the plantar aponeurosis (**Fig. 5.76**).

The sole of the foot that is associated with the midfoot and forefoot is divided into three compartments by the vertically aligned *intermuscular septa* that pass superiorly from the plantar aponeurosis and towards the 1st and 5th metatarsals (**Fig. 5.77**).

- **Medial compartment of sole**: covered by the medial plantar fascia. Contents include the abductor hallucis and flexor

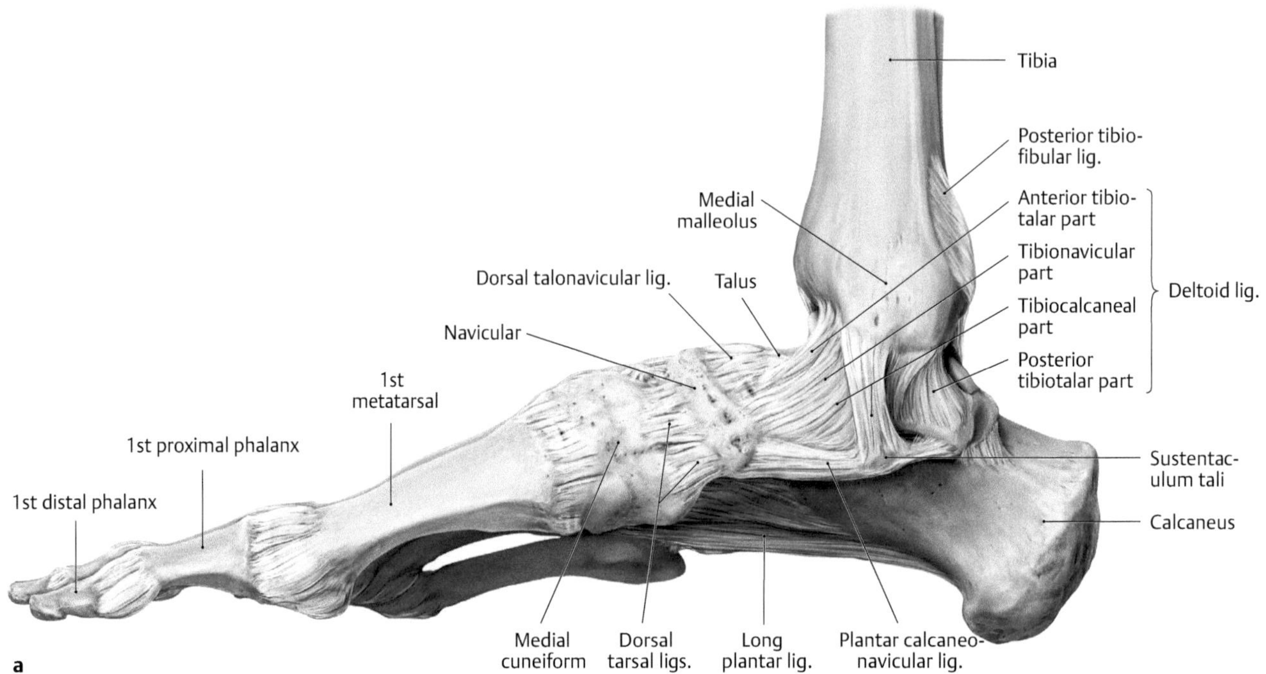

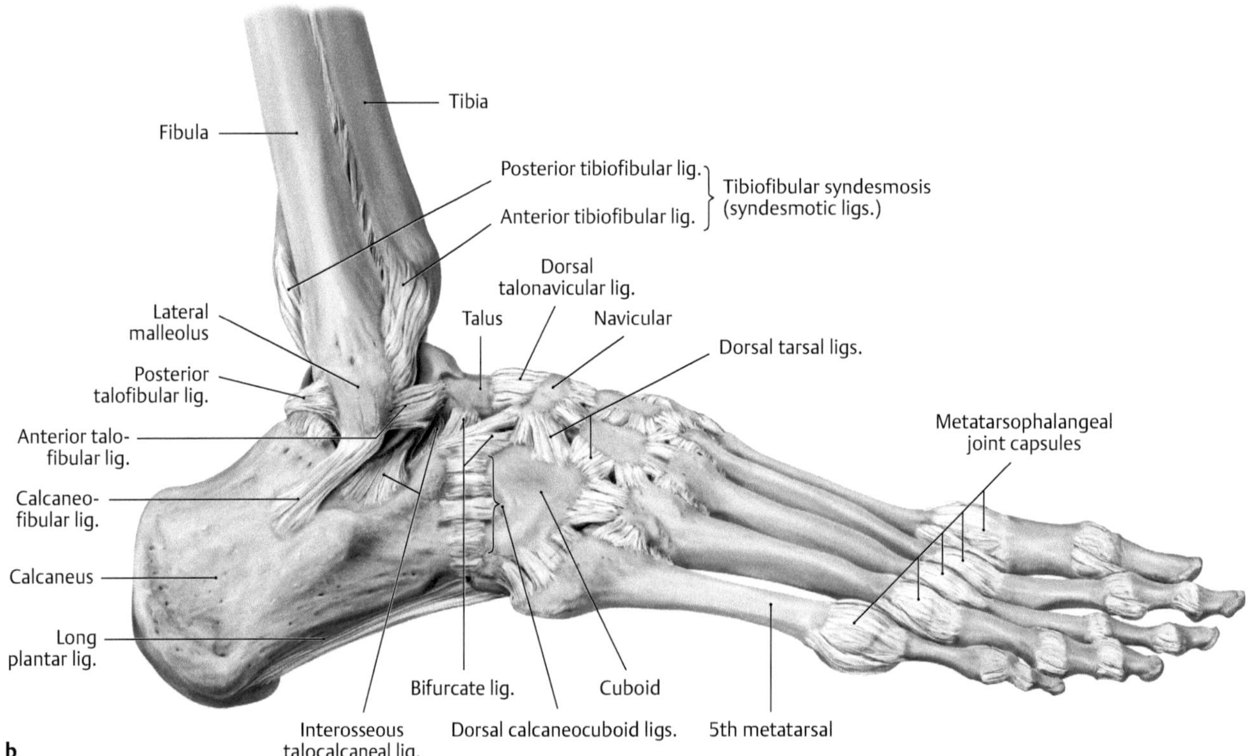

Fig. 5.69 Ligaments of the ankle and foot. **(a)** Medial view. **(b)** Lateral view. (From Schuenke M, Schulte E, Schumacher U. THIEME Atlas of Anatomy. General Anatomy and Musculoskeletal System. Illustrations by Voll M and Wesker K. 3rd ed. New York: Thieme Medical Publishers; 2020.)

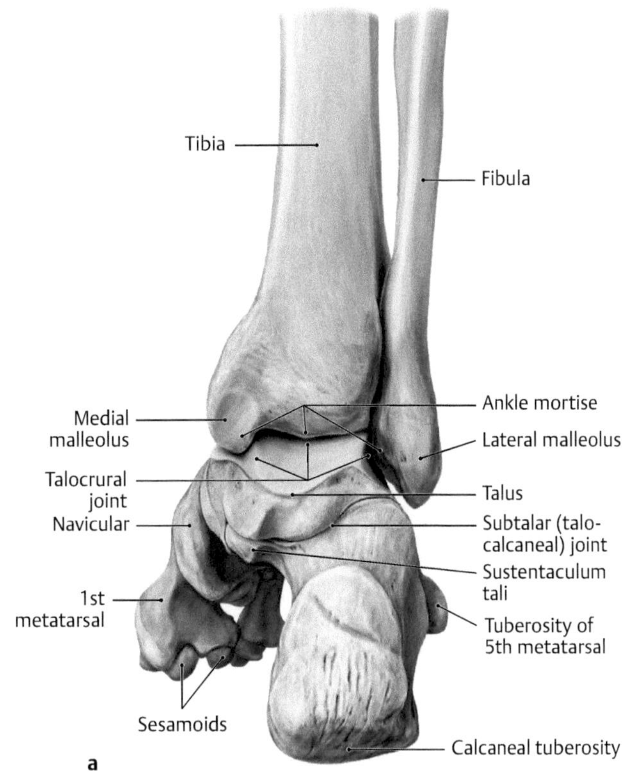

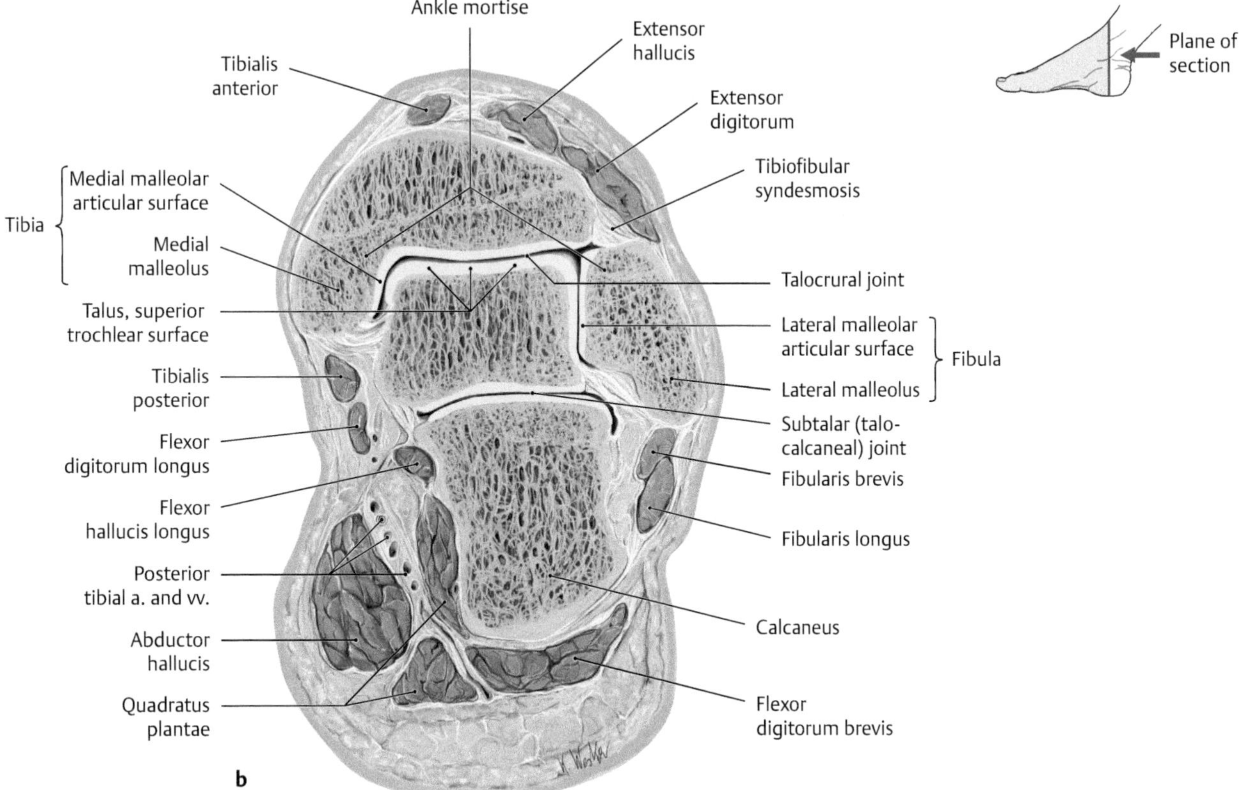

Fig. 5.70 Talocrural and subtalar joints. **(a)** Posterior view with foot in neutral (0-degree) position. **(b)** Coronal section, proximal view. (From Schuenke M, Schulte E, Schumacher U. THIEME Atlas of Anatomy. General Anatomy and Musculoskeletal System. Illustrations by Voll M and Wesker K. 3rd ed. New York: Thieme Medical Publishers; 2020.)

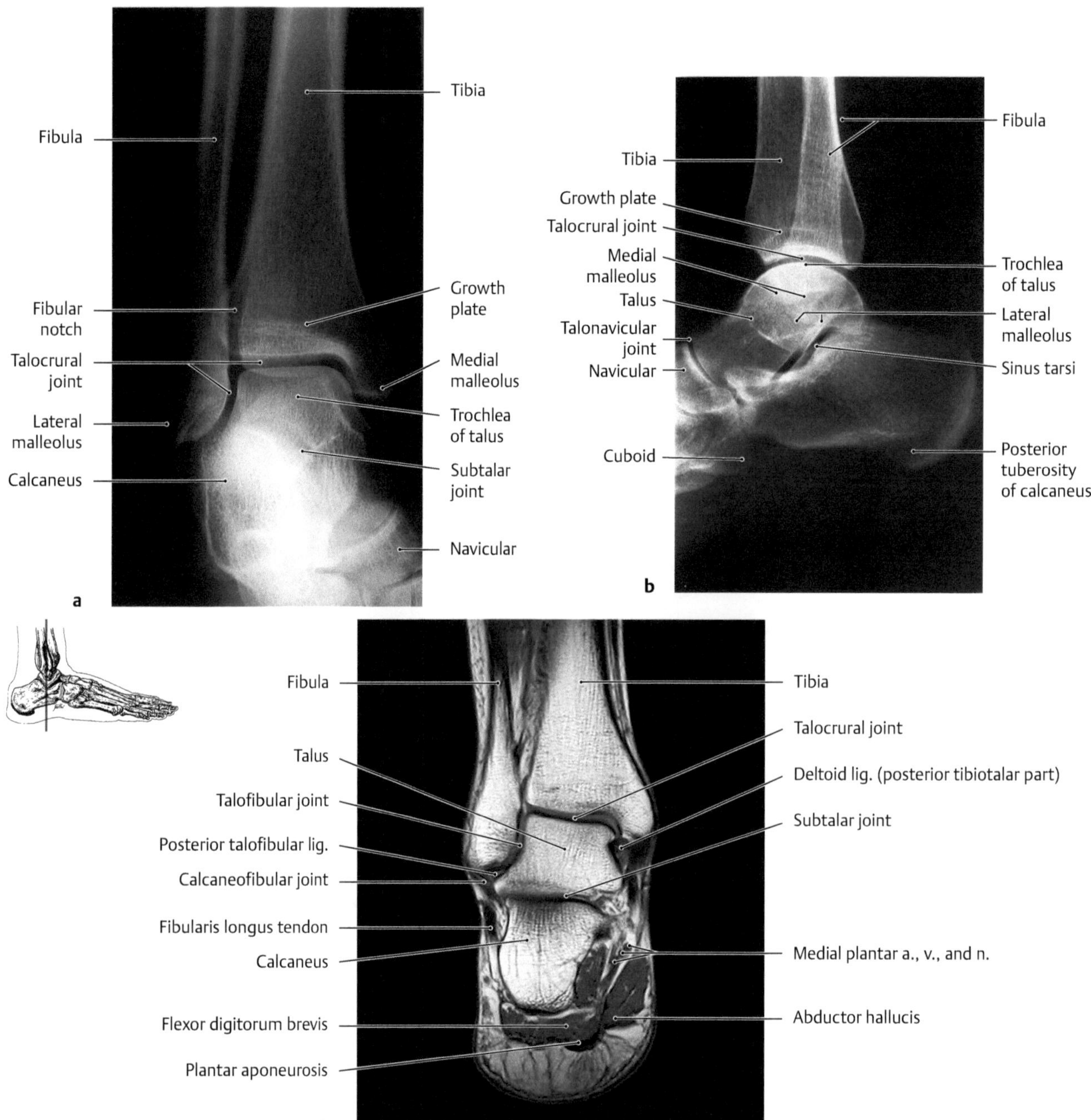

Fig. 5.71 Radiographs of the ankle. **(a)** Anteroposterior view. **(b)** Left lateral view. **(c)** MRI of the right ankle. (From Moeller TB, Reif E. Taschenatlas der Roentgenanatomie, 2nd ed. Stuttgart: Thieme; 1998.)

hallucis brevis muscles, the flexor hallucis longus tendon and the medial plantar neurovasculature.

- **Central compartment of sole**: covered by the plantar aponeurosis. Contents include the flexor digitorum brevis, flexor digitorum longus, lumbricals, quadratus plantae, and adductor hallucis muscles, tendons of the flexor hallucis longus and flexor digitorum longus, and the lateral plantar neurovasculature.
- **Lateral compartment of sole**: covered by the *lateral plantar fascia*. Contents include the abductor digiti minimi and flexor digiti minimi brevis muscles. Some authors have described an opponens digiti minimi muscle to be located in this compartment, as well.

Isolated to the forefoot of the sole, a fourth compartment called the **interosseous compartment of the foot** is located between the dorsal and plantar interosseous fascias. Contents include the dorsal and planter interosseous muscles, metatarsal bones, and the deep plantar and metatarsal vessels **(Fig. 5.77)**.

The dorsum of the foot can be considered a fifth compartment and it is located between the tarsal bones and dorsal interosseous fascia of the forefoot and midfoot and the deep fascia of the dorsum of the foot. The **extensor hallucis brevis** and **extensor digitorum brevis muscles** are located in this region and are described in **Table 5.9 (Fig. 5.78)**.

The remaining muscles of the foot are located in the sole of the foot and are organized into four separate layers **(Fig. 5.79; Fig. 5.80; Fig. 5.81; Fig. 5.82)**. These muscles do have individual functions but fine motor control of them is not necessarily important. As

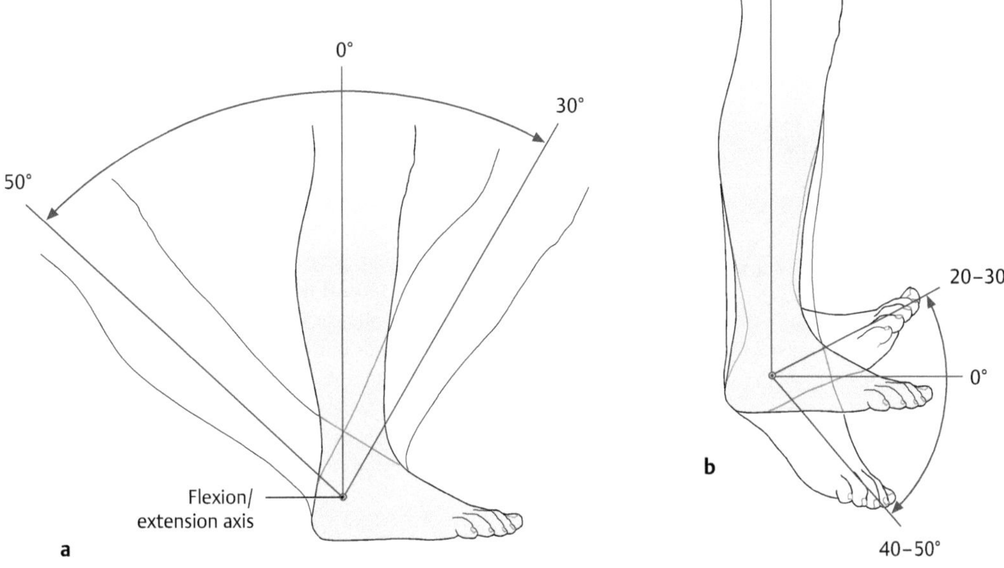

Fig. 5.72 Range of motion of the talocrural joint. **(a)** Right foot on ground (stance leg). **(b)** Right foot on ground (swing leg). (From Schuenke M, Schulte E, Schumacher U. THIEME Atlas of Anatomy. General Anatomy and Musculoskeletal System. Illustrations by Voll M and Wesker K. 3rd ed. New York: Thieme Medical Publishers; 2020.)

a group, they act during the support phase of stance and maintain the longitudinal arches of the foot. They resist weight-bearing forces that reduce primarily the medial longitudinal arch when weight is transferred from the heel back towards the ball of the foot and big toe. They are most active in fixing the foot or increasing the pressure applied against the floor to maintain balance; and near the end of the stance phase when an individual is moving into the pre-swing (push off) phase, a moment when forces flatten the transverse arch of the foot. Descriptions of the muscles belonging to certain layers are found in **Table 5.10, Table 5.11, Table 5.12,** and **Table 5.13.**

5.23.1 Neurovasculature of the Foot

Two neurovascular planes are seen in the sole of the foot and they are seen between the 1st and 2nd muscle layers and between the 3rd and 4th muscle layers. The **tibial nerve** at the level of the tarsal tunnel bifurcates into the **lateral** and **medial plantar nerves** (**Fig. 5.83**). The medial planter nerve passes through the 1st and 2nd muscle layers and into the medial compartment of the sole. The lateral planter nerve originally passes along the lateral border of the space between the 1st and 2nd muscle layers but its deeper branches extend into the space between the 3rd and 4th muscle layers. The lateral plantar nerve innervates all of the muscles of the sole of the foot except for the abductor hallucis, flexor digitorum brevis, lumbrical 1 (medial most) and the flexor hallucis brevis, which are innervated by the medial plantar nerve. The two extensor muscles of the dorsum of the foot are supplied by the **deep fibular nerve**, a branch of the common fibular nerve (**Fig. 5.84**).

5.23.2 Cutaneous Innervation of the Foot Originates from Multiple Nerves

- The **superficial fibular nerve** primarily supplies the skin of the dorsum of the foot with the exception of the webbing between the 1st and 2nd digits where the deep fibular nerve innervates this skin.
- The skin of the sole is primarily supplied by the **medial plantar** and its **common** and **proper plantar digital nerve** branches from the great toe to the medial half of the 4th toe. The remaining skin adjacent to the medial plantar innervation and including the other half of the 4th toe and the entire 5th toe are supplied by the **lateral plantar** and its **common** and **proper plantar digital nerves** branches.
- The heel is supplied by **lateral calcaneal cutaneous branch** of the *sural nerve* and the **medial calcaneal cutaneous branch** of the *tibial nerve.*
- The **sural nerve** innervates the lateral aspect of the foot and lateral malleolus.
- The **saphenous nerve** innervates the proximal medial aspect of the foot and medial malleolus.

Blood supply to the dorsum of the foot is from the **dorsalis pedis artery**, a direct continuation of the anterior tibial artery. Just proximal to where the dorsalis pedis artery begins, there is an **anterior lateral malleolar** and **anterior medial malleolar artery** branch that helps supply the ankle. Arising from the dorsalis pedis is the **lateral tarsal artery** proximally but distally it terminates as the 1st **dorsal metatarsal** and **deep plantar arteries.** The 1st dorsal metatarsal gives rise to the **dorsal digital arteries** that contribute blood to both the big and 2nd toes. The deep plantar artery passes deep and into the sole of the foot to form the *deep plantar arch* along with the lateral plantar artery.

The **arcuate artery** is located near the bases of the lateral four metatarsals and is an anastomosis between the lateral tarsal and dorsalis pedis arteries. The **2nd-4th dorsal metatarsal arteries** (and occasionally a 5th) originate from the arcuate artery before they give rise to the **dorsal digital arteries** responsible for supplying the 2nd through 5th toes. There are a few *perforating branches* connecting the arcuate artery and deep plantar arch (**Fig. 5.84**).

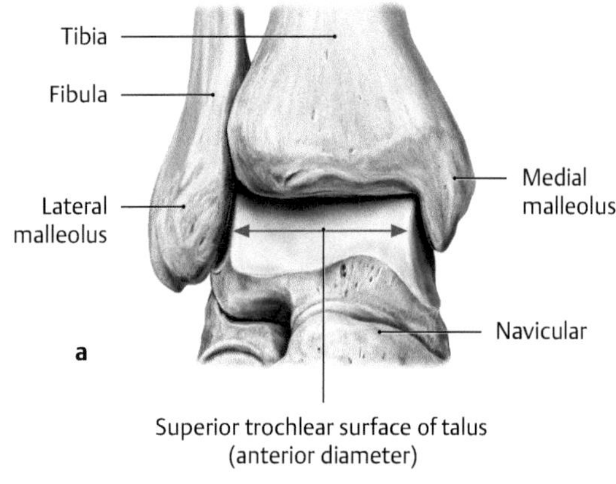

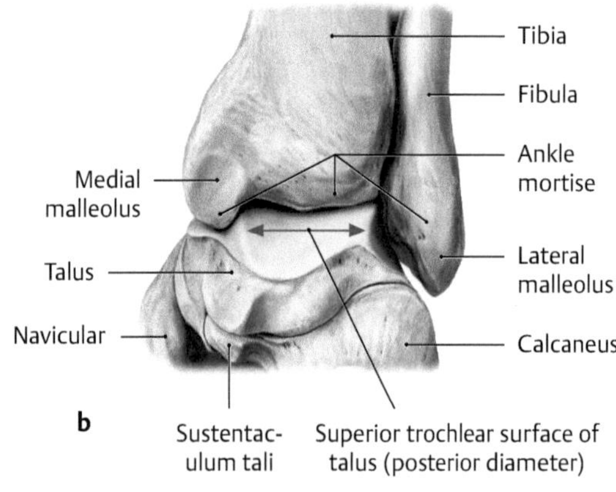

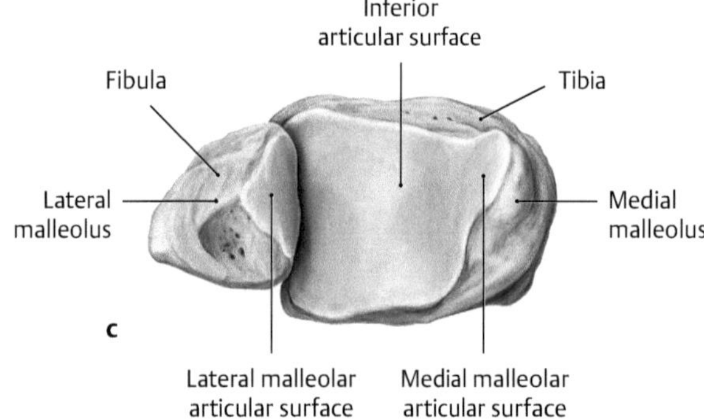

Fig. 5.73 Articulating surfaces of talocrural joint. **(a)** Anterior view. **(b)** Posterior view. **(c)** Proximal (superior) view of talus. (From Schuenke M, Schulte E, Schumacher U. THIEME Atlas of Anatomy. General Anatomy and Musculoskeletal System. Illustrations by Voll M and Wesker K. 3rd ed. New York: Thieme Medical Publishers; 2020.)

At the level of the tarsal tunnel, the **posterior tibial artery** bifurcates into the **lateral** and **medial plantar arteries** and these vessels pair with the nerve and vein of the same name. The lateral plantar artery crosses over medially back towards the great toe and proximal to the metatarsophalangeal joints to form the **deep plantar arch**. Originating from the deep plantar arch are four **plantar metatarsal** and three **perforating arteries**. The plantar metatarsals give rise to multiple **plantar digital arteries**. The **medial plantar artery** is smaller than the lateral plantar branch and is made up of a superficial and deep branch. The superficial branch may give rise to a **superficial plantar arch** that connects to the deep plantar arch (**Fig. 5.85**).

Venous drainage parallels the arterial supply and generally consists of two smaller veins. The **dorsal digital veins** continue as **dorsal metatarsal veins**, which also receive drainage from the **plantar digital veins**. These veins contribute to the formation of the **dorsal venous arch of the foot** located just distal to the **dorsal venous network**. Plantar digital veins form the **plantar metatarsal veins** before becoming the **plantar venous arch**. The arch contributes the tributaries that become the **lateral** and **medial plantar veins**. Superficially, a **plantar venous network** forms near the toes and if it passes laterally around the foot, it combines with the *dorsal venous arch* and **lateral marginal vein** to form the **small saphenous vein**. If the plantar venous network passes medially around the foot, it combines with the *dorsal venous arch* and **medial marginal vein** to form the **great saphenous vein**. The **perforating veins** form a one-way shunting of blood from the superficial to deep veins proximal to the ankle joint. Most venous drainage from the foot passes through the superficial veins (**Fig. 5.24c**).

5.23.3 Joints of the Foot

There are multiple joints of the foot and they involve the tarsals, metatarsals and phalanges. Of these, the more important ones include the subtalar and transverse tarsal joints that allow for eversion and inversion movements (**Fig. 5.70; Fig. 5.86**). The total ROM with combined joint movements in the foot is about 30° of eversion and 60° of inversion. The terms supination and pronation are often used with foot movements. *Supination* is a combination of plantarflexion, adduction and inversion while *pronation* is a combination of dorsiflexion, abduction and eversion movements (**Fig. 5.87**).

- **Subtalar joint**: the articulation between the inferior surface of the talus and superior surface of the calcaneus and the site where most eversion and inversion of the foot occurs. It is a *plane-type synovial joint* that has an anterior compartment containing the *talocalcaneal portion of the talocalcaneonavicular articulation* and a posterior compartment that contains the *posterior talocalcaneal articulation*. The especially strong **interosseous talocalcaneal ligament** is located in the *tarsal sinus* and separates the anterior and posterior parts of this joint. The subtalar joint is broken into an anatomical versus surgical joint. The anatomical version is really only between the posterior talocalcaneal articulating surfaces whereas the surgical version includes both the anterior and posterior compartments listed above. The ROM is about 10° of eversion and 20° of inversion (**Fig. 5.88; Fig. 5.91**).
- **Transverse tarsal joint**: compound joint that involves two separate articulations aligned transversely and the talus, calcaneus and navicular bones. One articulation is between the **talonavicular part of the talocalcaneonavicular joint** and the other at the **calcaneocuboid joint**. The talonavicular articulation is a *ball-and-socket-type synovial joint* that allows for gliding and rotary movements. The calcaneocuboid joint is a *plane-type synovial joint* and allows eversion, inversion and circumduction movements. The ROM of the transverse tarsal joint is about 20° of pronation and 40° of supination (**Fig. 5.86; Fig. 5.89**).

5.23.4 Additional Joints of the Foot

- **Cuneonavicular joint**: articulation between the anterior navicular and bases of the cuneiform bones. It is a *plane-type synovial joint* that has minimal movement (**Fig. 5.86**).

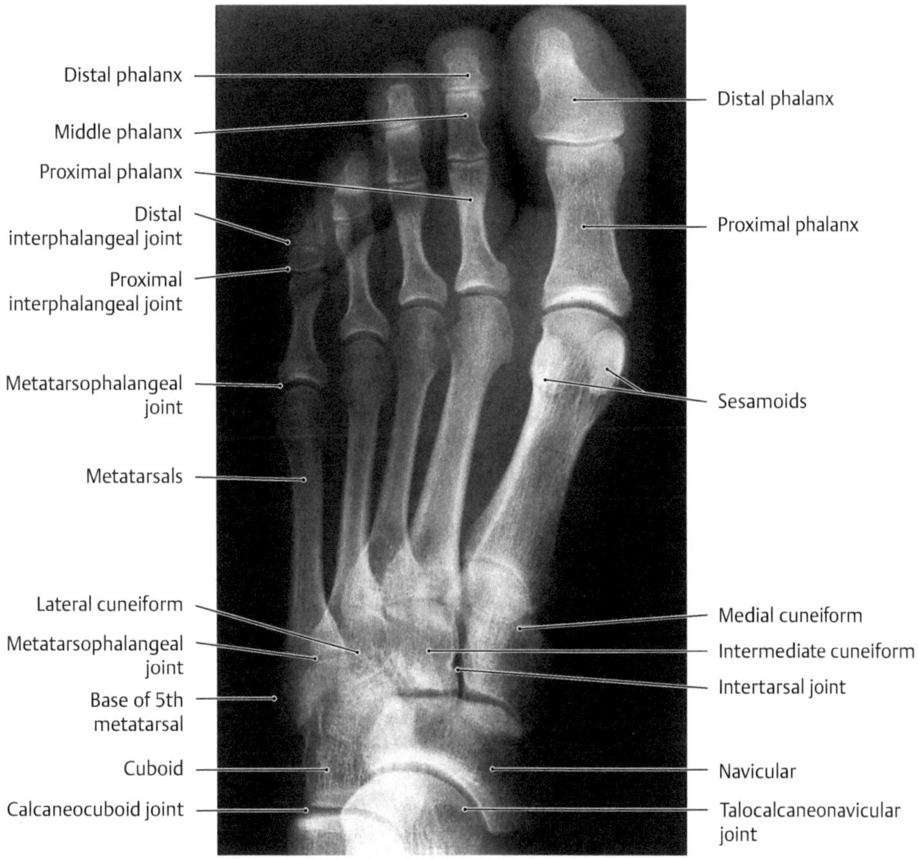

Fig. 5.74 Anterior-posterior view of the forefoot. (From Moeller TB, Reif E. Taschenatlas der Roentgenanatomie, 2nd ed. Stuttgart: Thieme; 1998.)

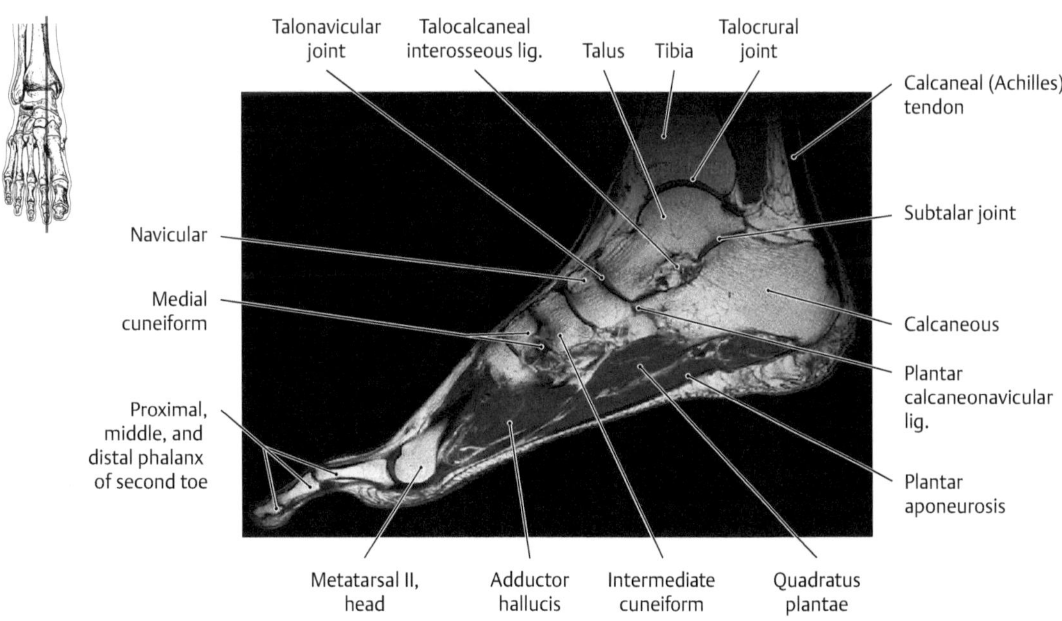

Fig. 5.75 MRI of the right foot and ankle. (From Moeller TB, Reif E. Atlas of Sectional Anatomy: The Musculoskeletal System. New York, NY: Thieme; 2009.)

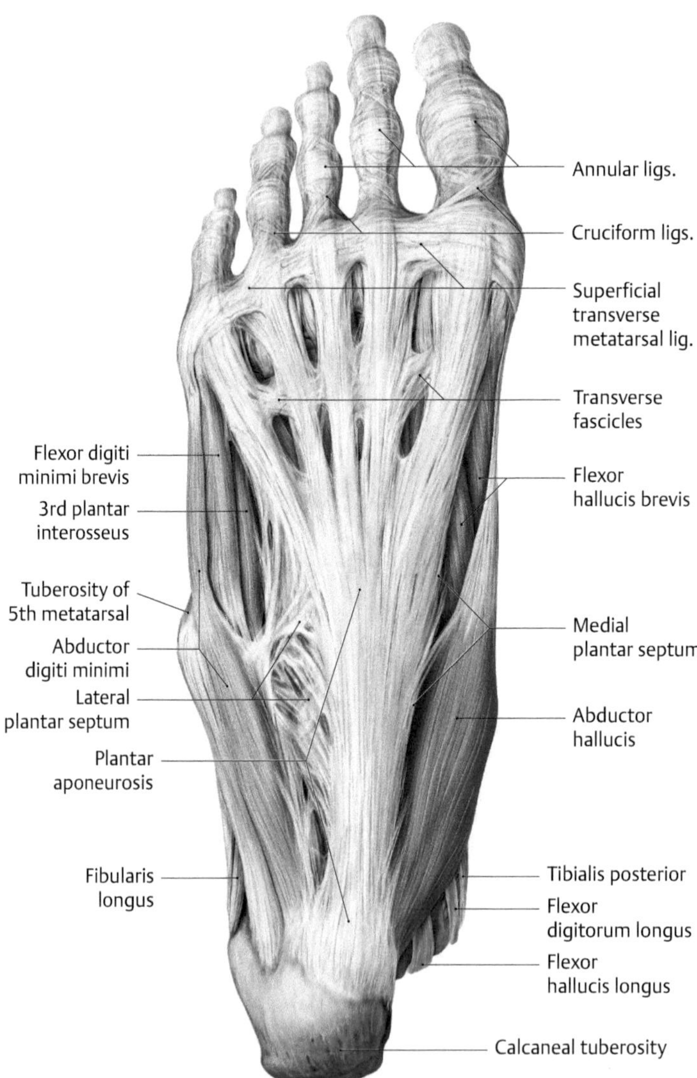

Fig. 5.76 Plantar aponeurosis. Right foot, plantar view. (From Schuenke M, Schulte E, Schumacher U. THIEME Atlas of Anatomy. General Anatomy and Musculoskeletal System. Illustrations by Voll M and Wesker K. 3rd ed. New York: Thieme Medical Publishers; 2020.)

- **Tarsometatarsal joints**: articulations between the five metatarsals, cuboid and the three cuneiform bones. They are *plane-type synovial joints* that allow for gliding and sliding movements (**Fig. 5.86**).
- **Intermetatarsal joints**: articulations between adjacent metatarsal bases. They are *plane-type synovial joints* and have minimal movement (**Fig. 5.86**).
- **Metatarsophalangeal joints**: articulations between the heads of the metatarsals and the bases of the proximal phalanges. They are *condyloid-type synovial joints* and allow for flexion and extension along with minimal abduction, adduction and circumduction movements. The 1st metatarsophalangeal joint has a ROM of up to 70° of extension and about 45° of flexion. The ROM is generally less with the 2nd-5th joints **(Fig. 5.86; Fig. 5.90)**.
- **Interphalangeal joints**: articulations between the head of one phalanx and the base of the next distal phalanx. They are *hinge-type synovial joints* and allow for flexion and extension movements. The 1st interphalangeal joint has a ROM of up to 80° of flexion but 0° of extension **(Fig. 5.86; Fig. 5.90)**.

5.23.5 Neurovasculature of Foot Joints

The subtalar, talocalcaneonavicular, calcaneocuboid, cuneonavicular and tarsometatarsal joints are innervated by the deep fibular, lateral plantar and medial plantar nerves. The sural nerve also innervates the tarsometatarsal joint. The intermetatarsal, metatarsophalangeal and interphalangeal joints receive innervation through the digital nerves that may originate from the lateral or medial plantar nerves.

Blood supply to the subtalar joint is from branches originating from the posterior tibial and fibular arteries. The talocalcaneonavicular, calcaneocuboid, cuneonavicular and tarsometatarsal joints receive blood from branches of the lateral tarsal and dorsalis pedis

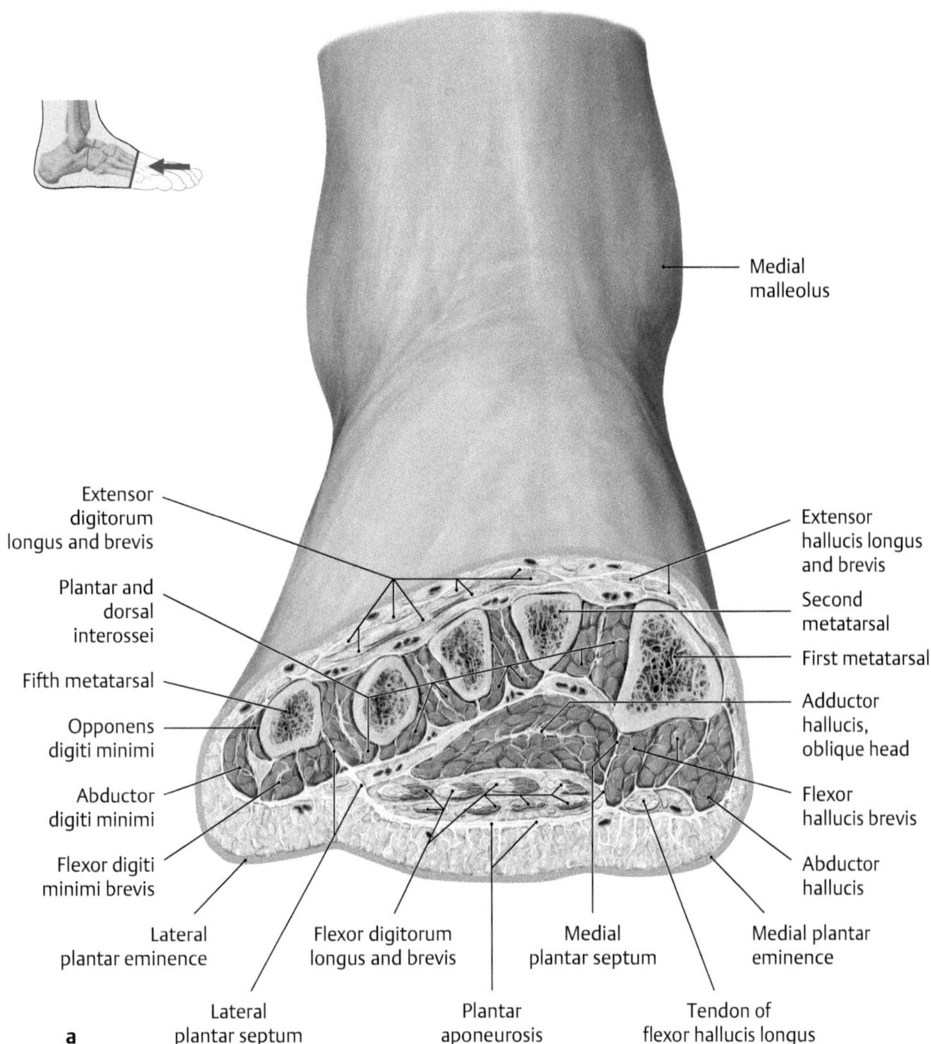

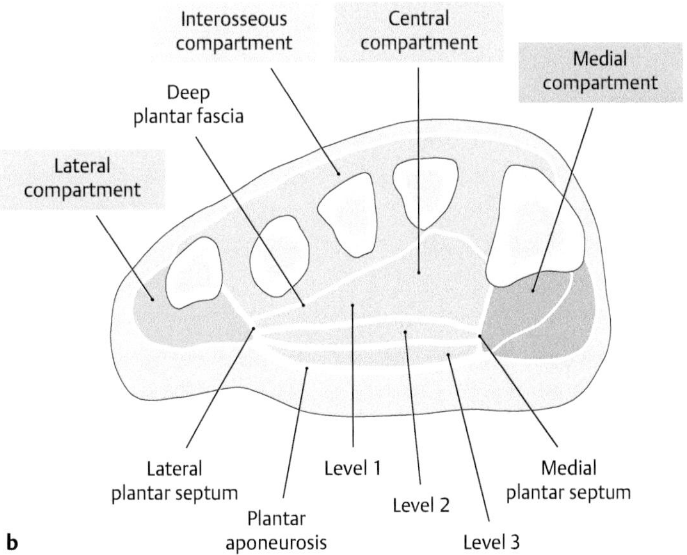

Fig. 5.77 **(a)** Cross-section through the right foot at the level of the metatarsals. View of the distal cut surface. **(b)** Location of the compartments of the foot. (From Schuenke M, Schulte E, Schumacher U. THIEME Atlas of Anatomy. General Anatomy and Musculoskeletal System. Illustrations by Voll M and Wesker K. 3rd ed. New York: Thieme Medical Publishers; 2020.)

Table 5.9 **Foot muscles: dorsum of foot (Fig. 5.78)**

Muscle	Innervation	Function(s)	Origin	Insertion
Extensor hallucis brevis	Deep fibular nerve	Extends great toe	Dorsal surface of calcaneus	Base of proximal phalanx of great toe
Extensor digitorum brevis	Deep fibular nerve	Extends digits 2-4	Dorsal surface of calcaneus	Bases of middle phalanges of digits 2-4; tendons of extensor digitorum longus

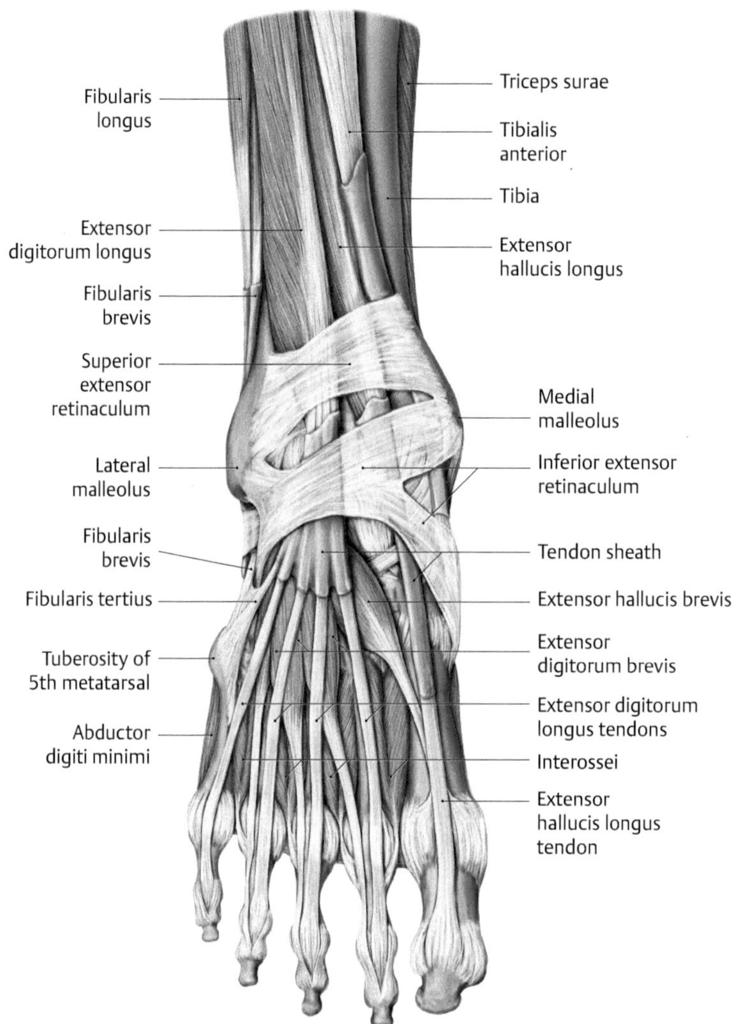

Fig. 5.78 Dorsum of the foot muscles. (From Schuenke M, Schulte E, Schumacher U. THIEME Atlas of Anatomy. General Anatomy and Musculoskeletal System. Illustrations by Voll M and Wesker K. 3rd ed. New York: Thieme Medical Publishers; 2020.)

arteries. The intermetatarsal joint receives blood from branches of the lateral tarsal, arcuate and dorsalis pedis arteries. The metatarsophalangeal joints receive blood from the dorsal metatarsal and common plantar digital arteries. Finally, the proper plantar digital arteries supply the interphalangeal joints.

5.23.6 Major Ligaments of the Plantar Foot

- **Long plantar ligament**: connects the plantar surface of the calcaneus to the groove on the cuboid and the bases of a couple of the middle metatarsals. It forms the tunnel for the fibularis longus tendon as it passes from lateral to medial and towards the base of the 1st metatarsal. It helps maintain the longitudinal arches of the foot (**Fig. 5.91; Fig. 5.92**).
- **Plantar calcaneocuboid ligament** (short plantar): located deep to the long plantar ligament and adjacent to the plantar calcaneonavicular ligament. It connects the anterior aspect of the inferior surface of the calcaneus to the inferior surface of the cuboid. It helps maintain the longitudinal arches of the foot (**Fig. 5.92**).
- **Plantar calcaneonavicular ligament** (spring ligament): extends over and fills in the gap between the sustentaculum tali and the inferior margin of the posterior articular surface of the navicular bone. It supports the head of the talus and helps

Table 5.10 **Foot muscles: sole of foot: first layer (Fig. 5.79)**

Muscle	Innervation	Function(s)	Origin	Insertion
Abductor hallucis	Medial plantar nerve	Abducts and flexes great toe; supports medial longitudinal arch of foot	Calcaneal tuberosity (medial tubercle); plantar aponeurosis	Medial side of the proximal phalanx base of great toe
Flexor digitorum brevis	Medial plantar nerve	Flexes digits 2-5; supports the transverse arch of foot	Calcaneal tuberosity (medial tubercle); plantar aponeurosis	Both sides of the middle phalanges base of digits 2-5
Abductor digiti minimi	Lateral plantar nerve	Abducts and flexes 5th digit; supports lateral longitudinal arch of foot	Calcaneal tuberosity (medial and lateral tubercles); plantar aponeurosis	Lateral side of the proximal phalanx base of 5th digit

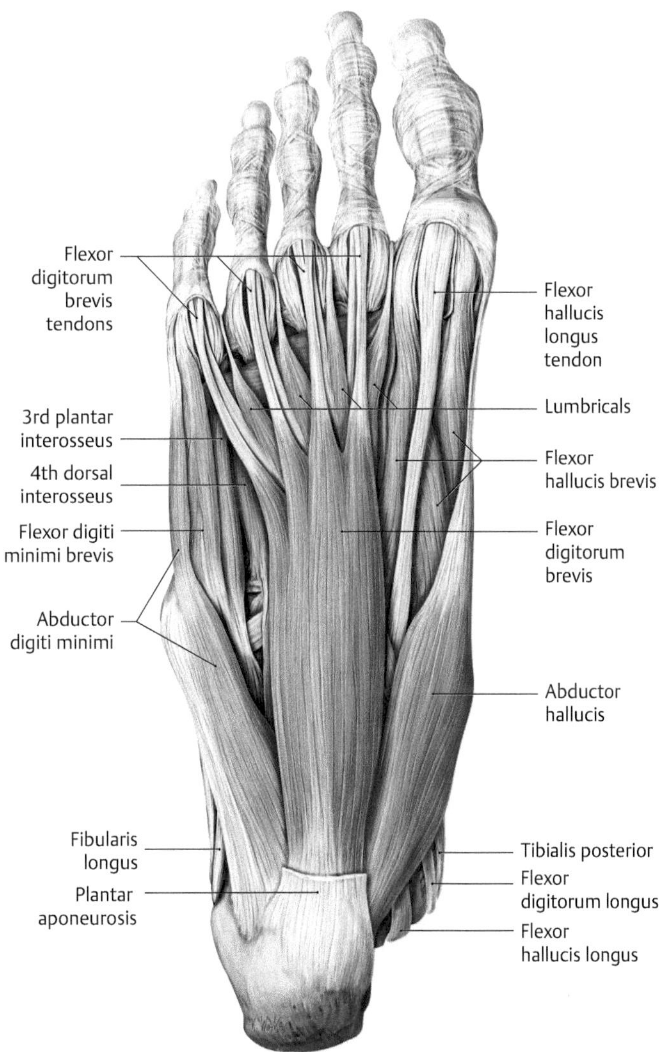

Fig. 5.79 Sole of the foot muscles: first layer. (From Schuenke M, Schulte E, Schumacher U. THIEME Atlas of Anatomy. General Anatomy and Musculoskeletal System. Illustrations by Voll M and Wesker K. 3rd ed. New York: Thieme Medical Publishers; 2020.)

Table 5.11 **Foot muscles: sole of foot: second layer (Fig. 5.80)**

Muscle	Innervation	Function(s)	Origin	Insertion
Quadratus plantae	Lateral plantar nerve	Assists flexor digitorum longus with flexing digits 2-5	Calcaneal tuberosity (medial and lateral sides of plantar surface)	Posterolateral side of flexor digitorum longus tendon
Lumbricals	Medial one (1): medial planter nerve Lateral three (2-4): lateral plantar nerve	Flex proximal phalanges; extend middle and distal phalanges of digits 2-5	Flexor digitorum longus tendons	Medial side of the expansion of digits 2-5

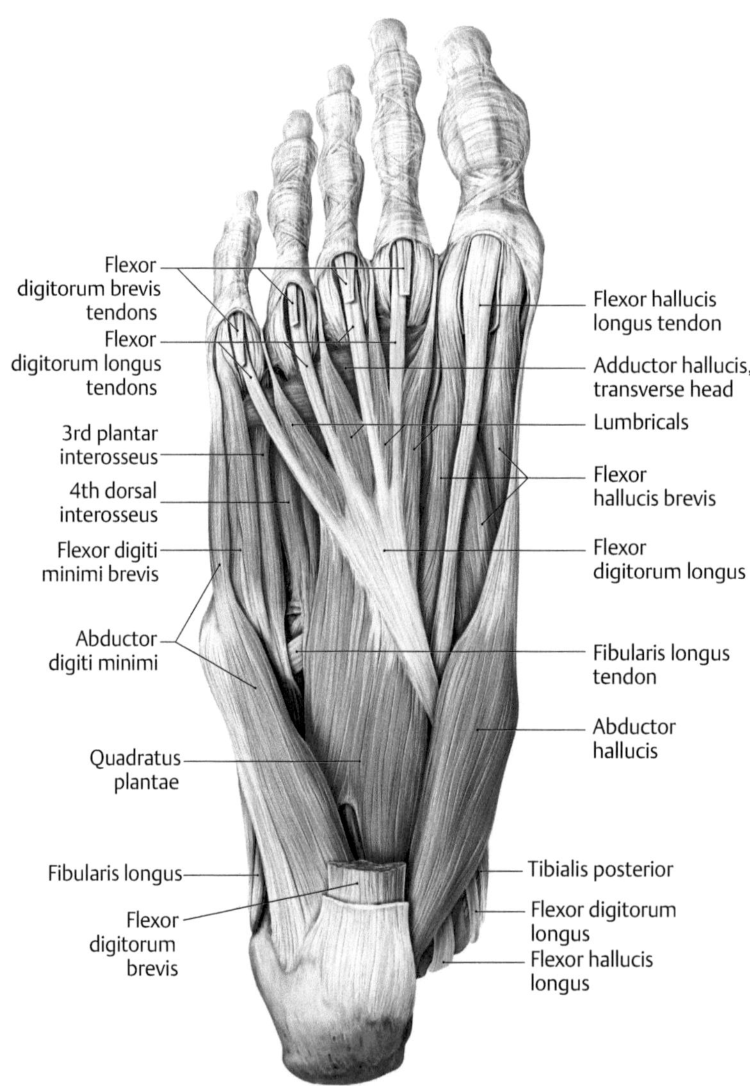

Fig. 5.80 Sole of the foot muscles: second layer. (From Schuenke M, Schulte E, Schumacher U. THIEME Atlas of Anatomy. General Anatomy and Musculoskeletal System. Illustrations by Voll M and Wesker K. 3rd ed. New York: Thieme Medical Publishers; 2020.)

Table 5.12 **Foot muscles: sole of foot: third layer (Fig. 5.81)**

Muscle	Innervation	Function(s)	Origin	Insertion
Flexor hallucis brevis	Medial plantar nerve	Flexes proximal phalanx of great toe	Cuboid; lateral (3rd) cuneiform	Both sides of the proximal phalanx base of great toe
Adductor hallucis	Medial plantar nerve	Adducts great toe; supports transverse arch of foot	Transverse head: capsule of metatarsophalangeal joints 2-5 Oblique head: Bases of metatarsals 2-4	Both heads attach to the lateral side of the proximal phalanx base of great toe
Flexor digiti minimi brevis	Lateral plantar nerve	Flexes proximal phalanx of 5th digit	Base of 5th metatarsal	Base of proximal phalanx of 5th digit

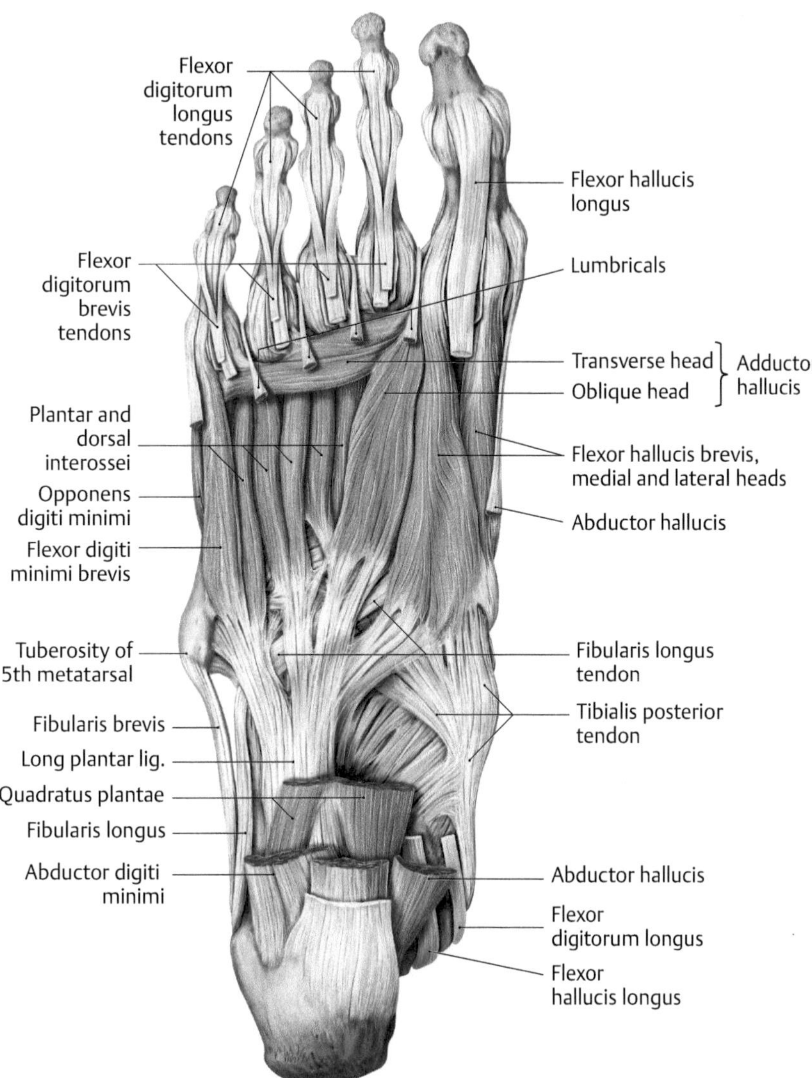

Fig. 5.81 Sole of the foot muscles: third layer. (From Schuenke M, Schulte E, Schumacher U. THIEME Atlas of Anatomy. General Anatomy and Musculoskeletal System. Illustrations by Voll M and Wesker K. 3rd ed. New York: Thieme Medical Publishers; 2020.)

Table 5.13 **Foot muscles: sole of foot: fourth layer (Fig. 5.82)**

Muscle	Innervation	Function(s)	Origin	Insertion
Plantar interossei (3) - unipennate	Lateral plantar nerve	Adduct digits 3-5; flex metatarsophalangeal joints	Plantar side of medial shafts of metatarsals 3-5	Medial side of the proximal phalanx base of digits 3-5
Dorsal interossei (4) - bipennate	Lateral plantar nerve	Abduct digits 2-4; flex metatarsophalangeal joints	Adjacent shafts of metatarsals 1-5	1st: medial side of proximal phalanx of 2nd digit 2nd-4th: lateral side of proximal phalanx of digits 2-4

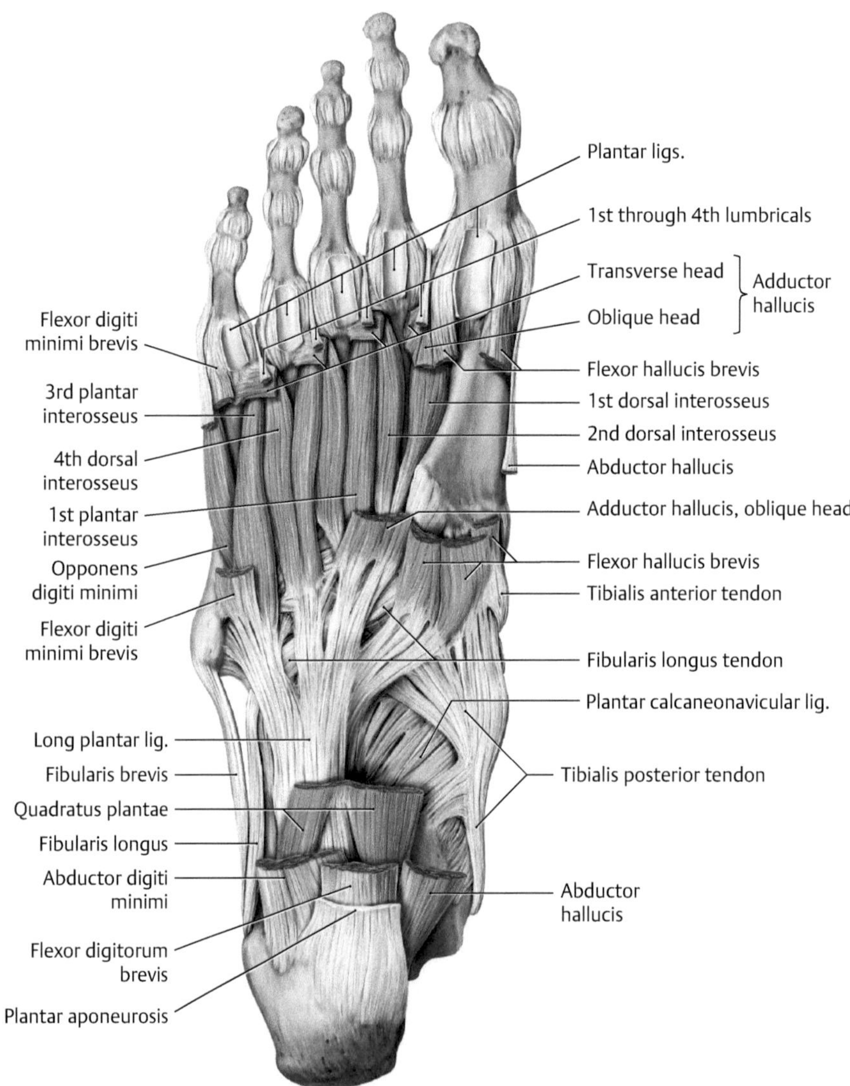

Fig. 5.82 Sole of the foot muscles: fourth layer. (From Schuenke M, Schulte E, Schumacher U. THIEME Atlas of Anatomy. General Anatomy and Musculoskeletal System. Illustrations by Voll M and Wesker K. 3rd ed. New York: Thieme Medical Publishers; 2020.)

transfer weight from the talus and maintain the longitudinal arch of the foot (**Fig. 5.91; Fig. 5.92**).

5.23.7 Arches of the Foot

The numerous bones of the foot are connected by ligaments and this gives it considerable flexibility for when it comes in contact with the ground. The tarsal and metatarsal bones are arranged in longitudinal and transverse arches. These arches are passively supported and actively restrained by tendons that add even more weight-bearing capabilities and resiliency to the foot.

The arches distribute weight over the foot when absorbing shock after striking the ground. They also serve as a springboard for walking, jumping and running movements and allow the foot to adapt to uneven surfaces. The body weight is transmitted from the tibia to the talus. After this, the weight passes posteriorly to the calcaneus and anterior to the ball of the foot, with it then being spread out to the heads of the 3rd-5th metatarsals. After the

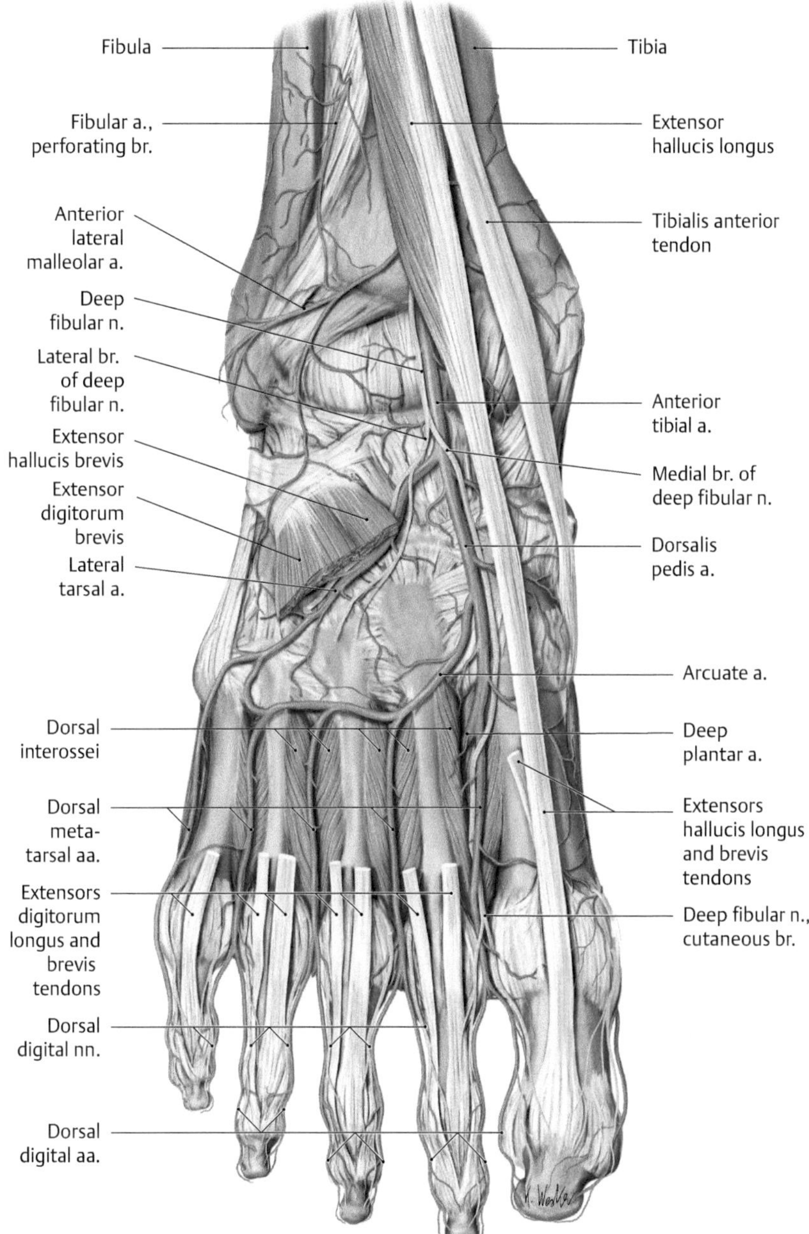

Fig. 5.83 Neurovasculature of the dorsum of the foot. (From Schuenke M, Schulte E, Schumacher U. THIEME Atlas of Anatomy. General Anatomy and Musculoskeletal System. Illustrations by Voll M and Wesker K. 3rd ed. New York: Thieme Medical Publishers; 2020.)

applied pressure is retracted the arches recoil back to their original curvatures. The arches of the foot are maintained by both passive and dynamic support systems.

The *passive support* that contributes to the arches is related to the orientation of the foot bones, and fibrous tissue associated with the plantar aponeurosis and major ligaments of the sole. From superficial to deep, the fibrous tissue includes the plantar aponeurosis, long plantar ligament, plantar calcaneocuboid ligament and plantar calcaneonavicular ligament **(Fig. 5.92)**.

The *dynamic support* of the arches is maintained by active and tonic contractions of muscles and tendons. The more reflexive but active contraction of the intrinsic foot muscles help support the longitudinal arches. Active and tonic contraction of the flexor hallucis longus and flexor digitorum longus muscle tendons can support the longitudinal arch whereas the fibularis longus and tibialis posterior are more active in supporting the transverse arch **(Fig. 5.92; Fig. 5.94)**.

The **longitudinal arch** has lateral and medial parts that function as one unit.

- **Medial longitudinal arch**: higher and considered more important than the lateral arch. It is composed of the calcaneus, talus, navicular, all three cuneiforms and metatarsals 1-3. The head of the talus is the keystone of this arch. The tibialis anterior, tibialis posterior, fibularis longus, flexor hallucis longus and flexor digitorum longus tendons strengthen this arch **(Fig. 5.93)**.
- **Lateral longitudinal arch**: is much lower than the medial side and lies on the ground when an individual is standing. It is

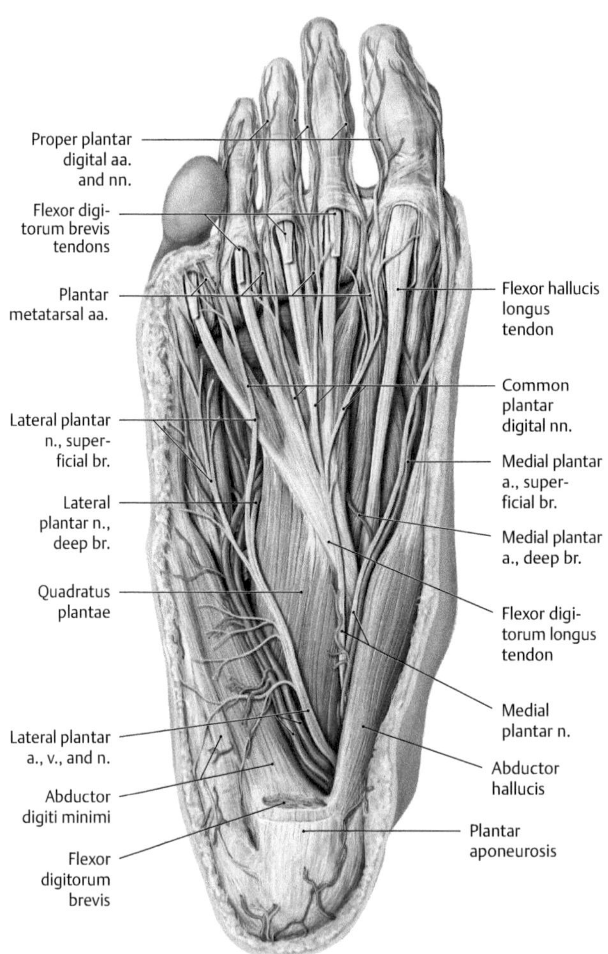

Fig. 5.84 Neurovasculature of the sole of the foot: second layer. (From Schuenke M, Schulte E, Schumacher U. THIEME Atlas of Anatomy. General Anatomy and Musculoskeletal System. Illustrations by Voll M and Wesker K. 3rd ed. New York: Thieme Medical Publishers; 2020.)

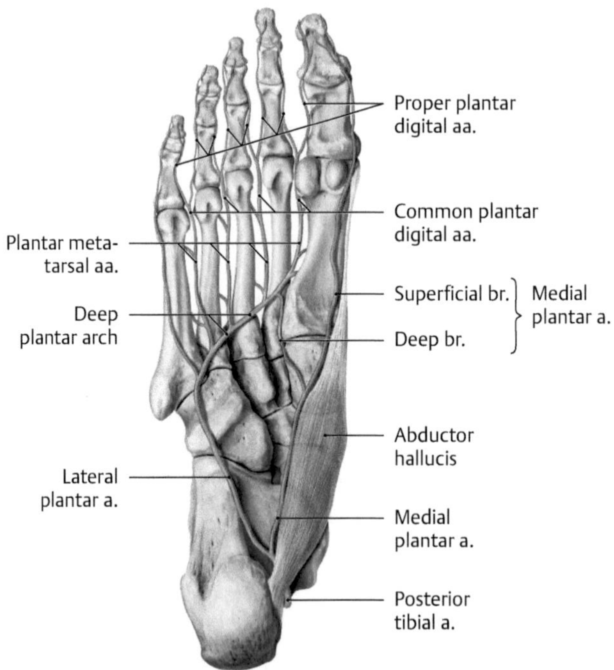

Fig. 5.85 Arteries of the sole of the foot. (From Schuenke M, Schulte E, Schumacher U. THIEME Atlas of Anatomy. General Anatomy and Musculoskeletal System. Illustrations by Voll M and Wesker K. 3rd ed. New York: Thieme Medical Publishers; 2020.)

Clinical Correlate 5.45

Plantar Fasciitis

When there is inflammation of the plantar aponeurosis it is known as **plantar fasciitis**. The pain is felt on the plantar surface of the heel and on the medial aspect of the foot. Point tenderness is located at the proximal attachment of the plantar aponeurosis to the medial tubercle of the calcaneus and on the medial surface of this bone. The pain increases with passive extension of the big toe, dorsiflexion of the ankle, and even during general weight-bearing. Running or high-impact aerobics while wearing inappropriate footwear is normally the cause. Pain is felt on the medial side of the foot when walking if a *calcaneal spur* protrudes from the medial tubercle.

formed by the calcaneus, cuboid and metatarsals 4 and 5. The cuboid can serve as the keystone of this arch. It receives some support from the fibularis longus, brevis and tertius muscle tendons **(Fig. 5.93)**.

The **transverse arch** runs from side to side and is formed by the cuboid, all three cuneiforms, and the bases of all of the metatarsals. Both longitudinal arches serve as pillars for this arch. The fibularis longus and tibialis posterior muscle tendons help maintain this curvature **(Fig. 5.94)**.

5.24 Gait Cycle

The gait cycle (**Fig. 5.95; Table 5.14**) is a complex sequence of lower extremity movements that define normal walking. It is made up of a *stance* and *swing phase*. It begins as one foot makes contact with the ground and ends when that same foot contacts the ground again. The **stance phase** begins with initial contact referred to as the heel strike and ends with the push off of the forefoot. It makes up 60% of the normal walking gait cycle. The stance phase makes up less of the gait cycle when an individual is running. The **swing phase** begins when the toes leave the ground and end at the following heel strike. It makes up 40% of the normal walking gait cycle (**Fig. 5.95**).

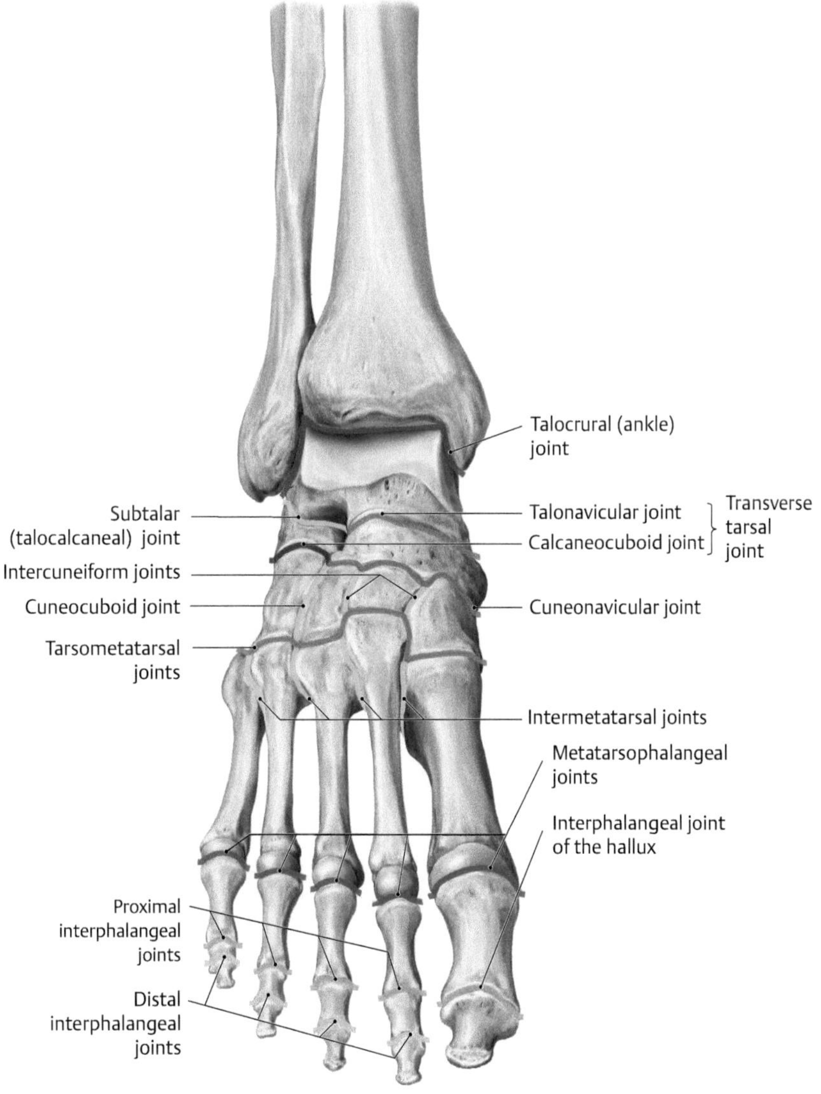

Fig. 5.86 Joints of the foot. (*continued*) (From Schuenke M, Schulte E, Schumacher U. THIEME Atlas of Anatomy. General Anatomy and Musculoskeletal System. Illustrations by Voll M and Wesker K. 3rd ed. New York: Thieme Medical Publishers; 2020.)

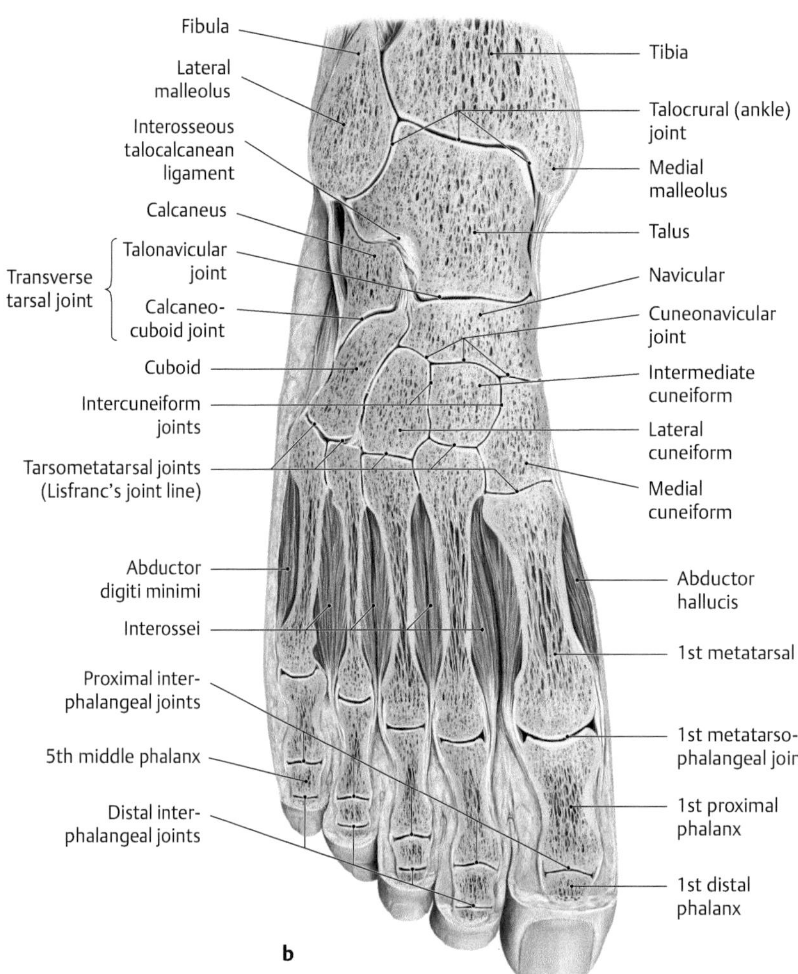

Fig. 5.86 (*continued*) Joints of the foot. **(b)** Superior view of coronal section. (From Schuenke M, Schulte E, Schumacher U. THIEME Atlas of Anatomy. General Anatomy and Musculoskeletal System. Illustrations by Voll M and Wesker K. 3rd ed. New York: Thieme Medical Publishers; 2020.)

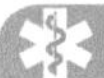 **Clinical Correlate 5.46**

Plantar Reflex
The **plantar reflex** is a myotatic (deep tendon) reflex and is associated with the L4-S2 nerve roots. To test it, a blunt object is passed over the lateral aspect of the sole beginning at the heel and crossing to the base of the big toe. Flexion of the toes is a normal response but may not be present until the child is about four years of age due to the corticospinal tracts still developing. An abnormal (*Babinski*) sign demonstrates dorsiflexion of the great toe and a slight fanning of the lateral four toes indicating a cerebral disease or brain injury except for anyone less than four years of age.

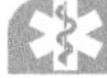 **Clinical Correlate 5.47**

Medial Plantar Nerve Entrapment
The medial plantar nerve may become compressed or entrapped deep to the flexor retinaculum or after it passes deep to the abductor halluces, causing numbness or tingling on the medial side of the foot along with weakness in muscles innervated by this nerve. This is seen frequently in long distance runners and can be referred to as *jogger's foot*. Surgical intervention is rarely needed and rest may be enough to alleviate the pain.

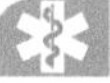 **Clinical Correlate 5.48**

Gout
Gout is characterized by the sudden and recurring painful attacks of the joints that most commonly involve the big toe. It is a form of arthritis caused by a combination of diet and genetics but the underlying mechanisms involve elevated levels of uric acid in the blood. Uric acid is produced by breaking down purines that are found naturally in the body and in foods that include meat, seafood, drinks containing fructose, and alcoholic beverages, especially beer. Treatment may involve dietary changes or taking drugs such as NSAIDs, corticosteroids or others that block uric acid production for example.

5.25 Development of the Lower Extremity

Arising from the lateral body wall during the early part of the 5th week of development, the lower limb buds develop opposite the L2-S2 segments. Each limb bud initially consists of a mesenchymal core derived from the *somatic (parietal) layer of lateral plate mesoderm* that forms the bones and connective tissues of the limb and

Clinical Correlate 5.49

Hallux Valgus

The foot deformity known as **hallux valgus** is caused by degenerative joint disease and results in the lateral deviation of the big toe (hallux). This deviation may involve the big toe overlapping the 2nd digit. These individuals are usually unable to move their big toe away from the 2nd digit. This is the result of the sesamoid bones deep to the head of the 1st metatarsal being displaced and lying in the space between the heads of the 1st and 2nd metatarsals. A subcutaneous bursa can form and when it becomes inflamed it is called a **bunion**. These are due to the pressure and friction against the shoe.

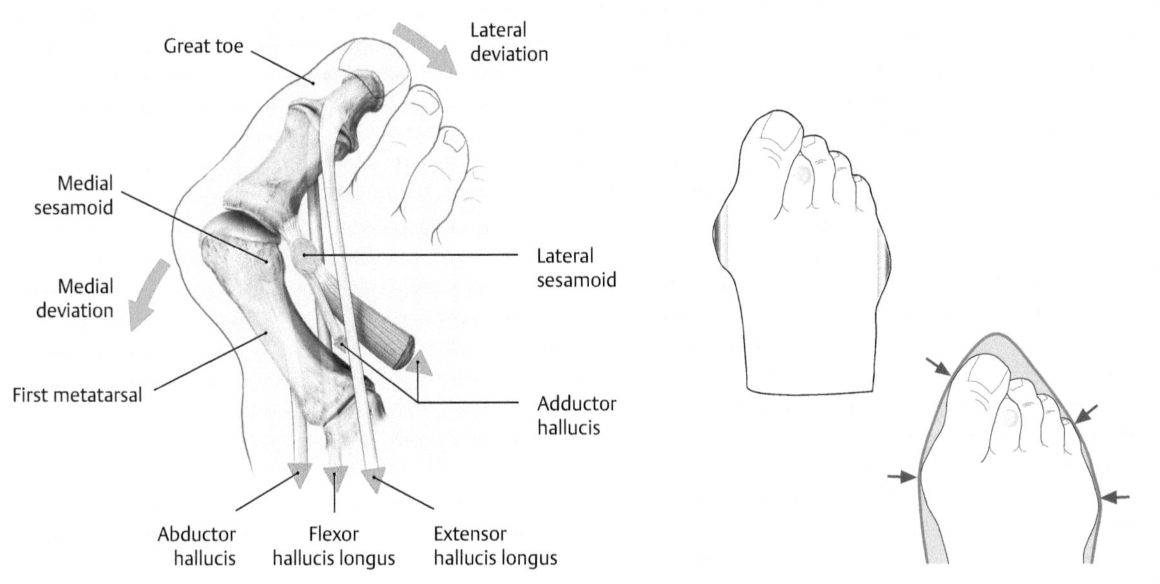

Pathogenic mechanism and etiology of hallux valgus. (From Schuenke M, Schulte E, Schumacher U. THIEME Atlas of Anatomy. General Anatomy and Musculoskeletal System. Illustrations by Voll M and Wesker K. 3rd ed. New York: Thieme Medical Publishers; 2020.)

Clinical Correlate 5.50

Pes Planus (Flatfeet)

Pes planus or flatfeet are common in older individuals who may have begun undertaking a lot of unaccustomed standing or have quickly gained weight. Pregnancy can also lead to developing pes planus. This increases stress to both the muscles and ligaments supporting the arches. Acquired flatfeet or "fallen arches" are more than likely secondary to dysfunction of the tibialis posterior because of trauma, degeneration with age or denervation. When the passive or dynamic support normally present is absent, the plantar calcaneonavicular ligament fails to support the head of the talus. This causes the talar head to displace inferomedially and become prominent. This displacement causes some flattening of the medial part of the medial longitudinal arch and lateral deviation of the forefoot.

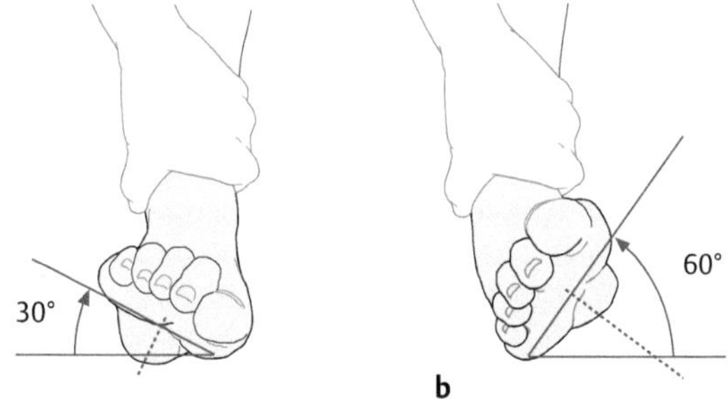

Fig. 5.87 Total range of motion of the forefoot and hindfoot. **(a)** Eversion. **(b)** Inversion. (From Schuenke M, Schulte E, Schumacher U. THIEME Atlas of Anatomy. General Anatomy and Musculoskeletal System. Illustrations by Voll M and Wesker K. 3rd ed. New York: Thieme Medical Publishers; 2020.)

this is covered by a *cuboidal ectoderm*. Later, cells from the ventrolateral portion of the dermomyotome migrate into this region.

At the apex of each limb bud the ectoderm thickens to form an **apical ectodermal ridge (AER)**. The AER promotes outgrowth of the bud in the *proximodistal axis* and exerts an inductive influence on adjacent mesenchyme, causing it to remain as a population of undifferentiated and rapidly proliferating cells called the **progress zone**. Cells differentiate into cartilage and muscle until they are far enough from the influence of the AER. A cluster of cells at the posterior border of the limb near the body wall is known as the **zone of polarizing activity (ZPA)**. The ZPA regulates growth on the *anteroposterior axis*. A *dorsoventral patterning* also takes place to differentiate the dorsal from the ventral sides of a limb (**Fig. 5.96**).

In six-week old embryos, the terminal portion of these limb buds flatten and form **footplates** and the mesenchymal tissue in these footplates condense to form **digital rays** that outline the pattern of the digits. At the tip of each ray, a part of the AER induces the development of the mesenchyme into the primordial digit bones. Intervening regions of mesenchyme undergo *apoptosis* (programmed cell death) to create individual digits. Two constrictions occur near the future knee and ankle joints and divide the limb bud into a recognizable thigh, leg and foot segment (**Fig. 5.97**).

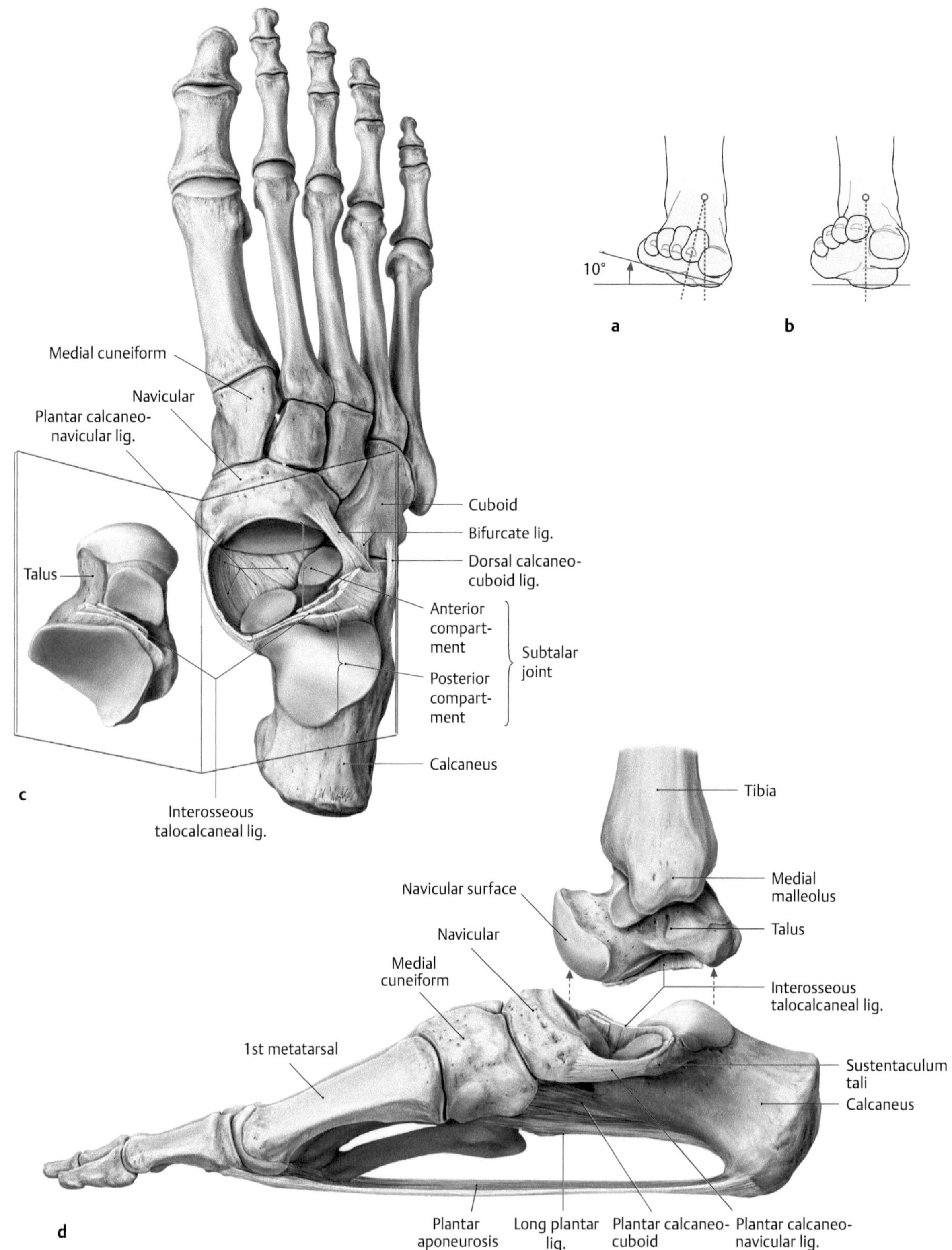

Fig. 5.88 Range of motion at the subtalar joint. **(a)** Eversion. **(b)** Inversion. Subtalar joint and ligaments. **(c)** Dorsal view. **(d)** Medial view. (From Schuenke M, Schulte E, Schumacher U. THIEME Atlas of Anatomy. General Anatomy and Musculoskeletal System. Illustrations by Voll M and Wesker K. 3rd ed. New York: Thieme Medical Publishers; 2020.)

Clinical Correlate 5.51

Hammer and Claw Toe

Hammer toe is a deformity caused by shoes not fitting correctly or by an imbalance of toe muscles and it generally affects the 2nd-4th toes. The proximal phalanx is hyperextended at the metatarsophalangeal joint and the middle phalanx is in hyperflexion at the proximal interphalangeal joint (PIP). The distal phalanx is generally hyperextended at the distal interphalangeal joint (DIP) giving the digit a hammer-like appearance. **Claw toe** is characterized by hyperextension at the metatarsophalangeal joints but hyperflexion at both the proximal (PIP) and distal interphalangeal joints (DIP). Digits 2-5 are generally the most effected.

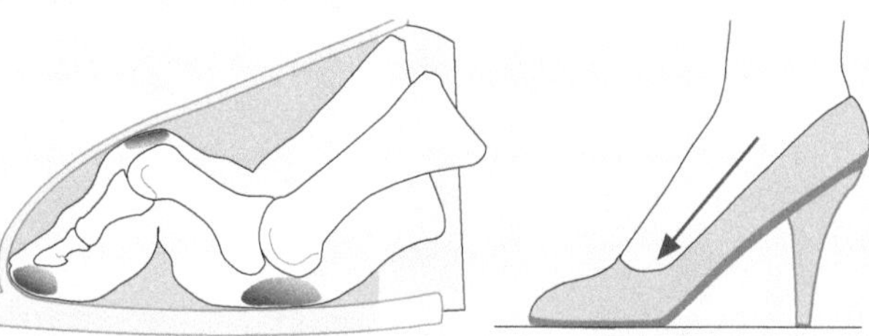

Pathogenic mechanism and etiology of hallux valgus. (From Schuenke M, Schulte E, Schumacher U. THIEME Atlas of Anatomy. General Anatomy and Musculoskeletal System. Illustrations by Voll M and Wesker K. 3rd ed. New York: Thieme Medical Publishers; 2020.)

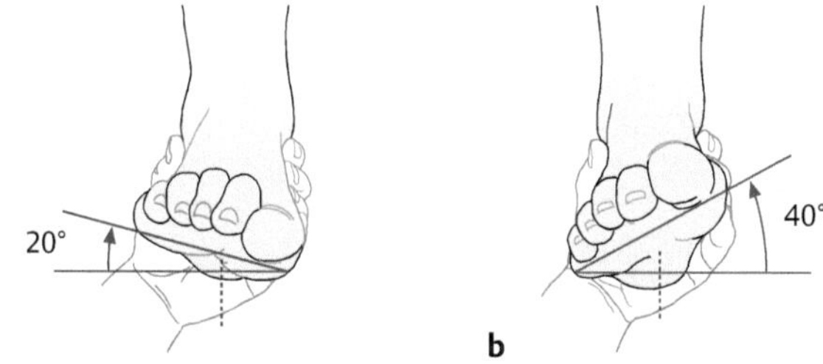

Fig. 5.89 Range of motion of the transverse tarsal joint. **(a)** Pronation. **(b)** Supination. (From Schuenke M, Schulte E, Schumacher U. THIEME Atlas of Anatomy. General Anatomy and Musculoskeletal System. Illustrations by Voll M and Wesker K. 3rd ed. New York: Thieme Medical Publishers; 2020.)

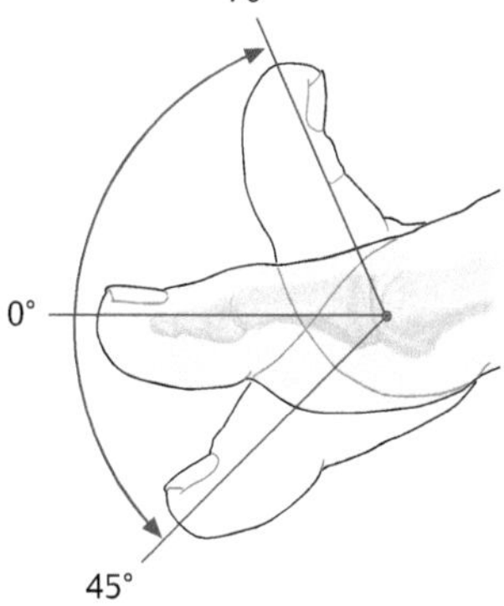

Fig. 5.90 Range of motion at the metatarsophalangeal joint of the big toe. (From Schuenke M, Schulte E, Schumacher U. THIEME Atlas of Anatomy. General Anatomy and Musculoskeletal System. Illustrations by Voll M and Wesker K. 3rd ed. New York: Thieme Medical Publishers; 2020.)

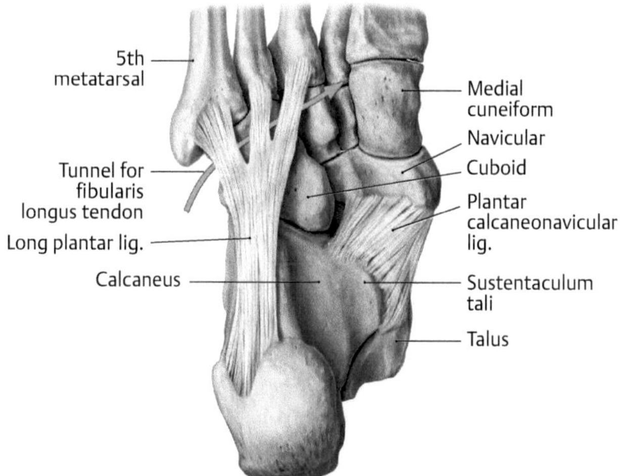

Fig. 5.91 Stabilizers of the longitudinal arches, plantar view. (From Schuenke M, Schulte E, Schumacher U. THIEME Atlas of Anatomy. General Anatomy and Musculoskeletal System. Illustrations by Voll M and Wesker K. 3rd ed. New York: Thieme Medical Publishers; 2020.).

From the *dermomyotome regions of the somites*, myogenic precursor cells migrate into the limb bud and differentiate into **myoblasts**, the precursors of muscle cells that are segmented according to the somites from which they are derived. Each myotome of a somite divides into a dorsal **epaxial division** and a ventral **hypaxial division**. The epaxial division develops into true back muscles while the hypaxial division develops into muscles of the body wall and limbs. With elongation of the limbs, myoblasts aggregate and form large muscle masses that split into extensor and ventral components. The lower limbs rotate 90° medially between weeks 6-8, thus the future knees point ventrally **(Fig. 5.98)**.

- The big toe is located on the medial side of foot.
- The extensor muscles lie ventrally and flexor muscles lie dorsally.

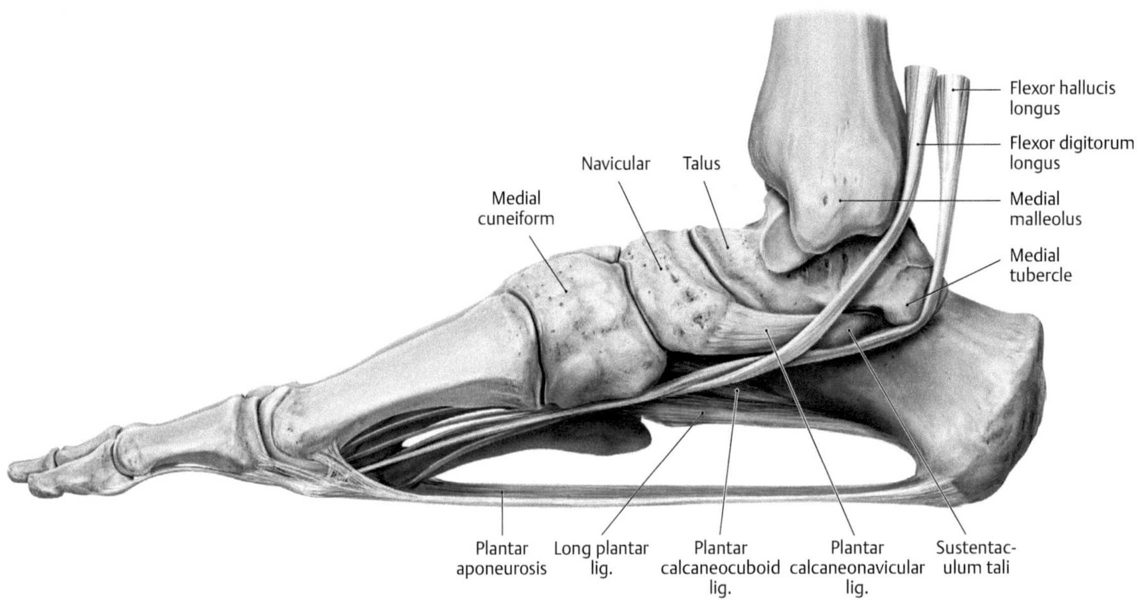

Fig. 5.92 Stabilizers of the longitudinal arches, medial view. (From Schuenke M, Schulte E, Schumacher U. THIEME Atlas of Anatomy. General Anatomy and Musculoskeletal System. Illustrations by Voll M and Wesker K. 3rd ed. New York: Thieme Medical Publishers; 2020.)

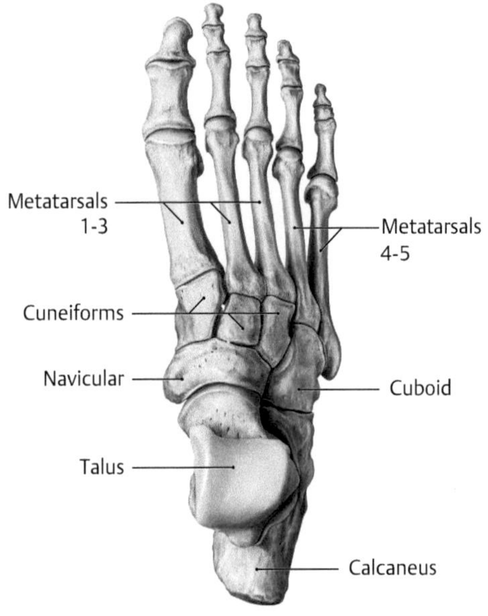

Fig. 5.93 Bone contributions to the medial and lateral longitudinal arches of the foot. (From Schuenke M, Schulte E, Schumacher U. THIEME Atlas of Anatomy. General Anatomy and Musculoskeletal System. Illustrations by Voll M and Wesker K. 3rd ed. New York: Thieme Medical Publishers; 2020.)

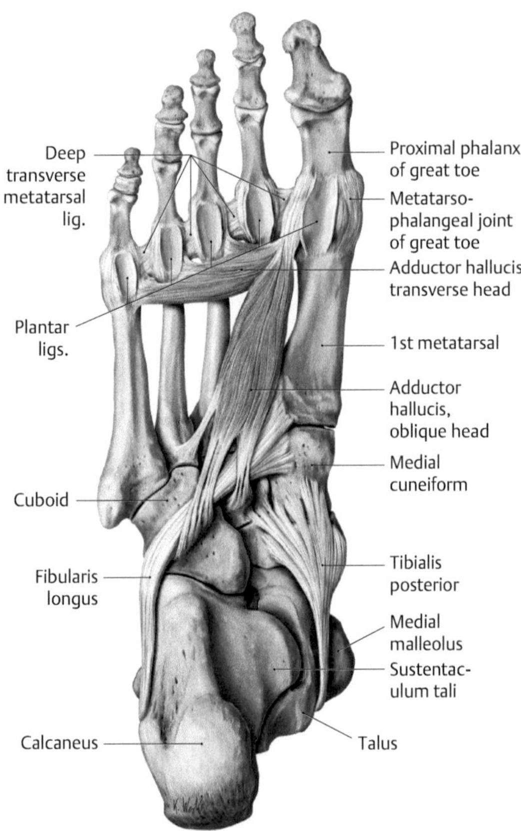

Fig. 5.94 Stabilizers of the transverse arch of the foot. (From Schuenke M, Schulte E, Schumacher U. THIEME Atlas of Anatomy. General Anatomy and Musculoskeletal System. Illustrations by Voll M and Wesker K. 3rd ed. New York: Thieme Medical Publishers; 2020.)

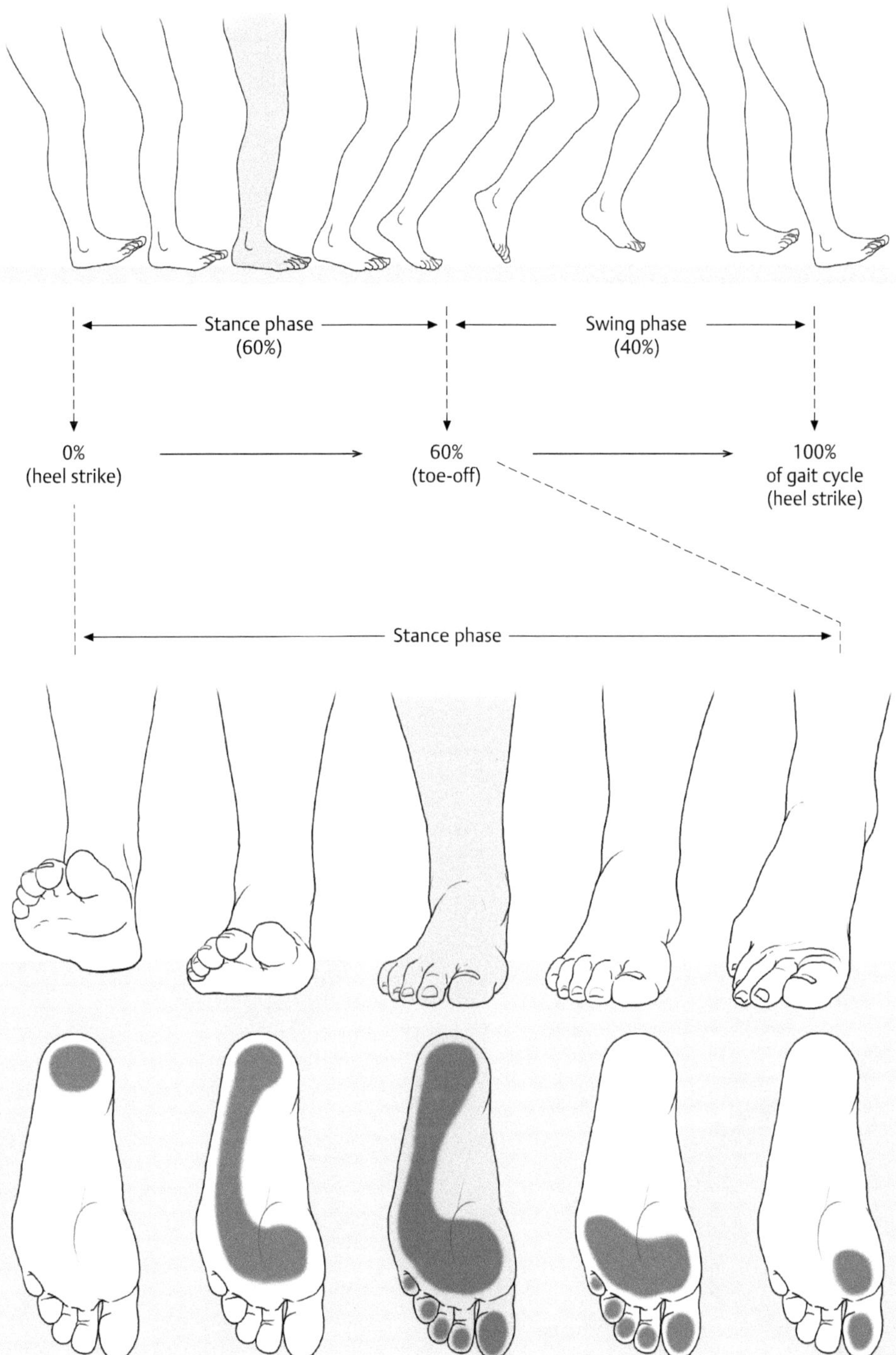

Fig. 5.95 Movements of the lower extremity during one gait cycle. (From Schuenke M, Schulte E, Schumacher U. THIEME Atlas of Anatomy. General Anatomy and Musculoskeletal System. Illustrations by Voll M and Wesker K. 3rd ed. New York: Thieme Medical Publishers; 2020.)

The **motor axons** that originate from the spinal cord enter the limb buds during the 5th week of development and grow into the ventral and dorsal muscle masses. During this same period, the peripheral nerves grow from the developing **limb plexus** (lumbosacral) and into the mesenchyme of the lower limb buds. The spinal nerves are distributed in segmental bands and supply both the ventral and dorsal surfaces of the limb buds. The **sensory axons** enter the limb buds shortly after the motor axons. The myelin sheaths and neurilemma of motor and sensory nerve fibers originate form **neural crest cells.**

The lower extremity blood supply originates from the **umbilical artery** that gives rise to the **axis artery**. The axis artery ends as a **terminal plexus** near the tip of the limb bud and becomes the **deep plantar arch** located in the sole of the foot. The axis artery initially gives off the **anterior tibial** and **posterior tibial arteries.** However, most of the axis artery undergoes regression and persists in the adult as the **inferior gluteal**, **sciatic (ischiadic)**, proximal **popliteal** and distal **fibular arteries**. The **external iliac** gives rise to the **femoral artery**, which later gives off the **profunda**

Table 5.14 **Muscle action sequence during the gait cycle**

Activity	Active Muscle Group
Stance Phase	
The initial heel strike begins the phase.	Hip extensors Dorsiflexors
The foot begins to accept the weight of the body (loading response) and the pelvis is stabilized.	Hip adductors Knee Extensors Plantarflexors
At midstance, the pelvis, knee and ankle are stabilized.	Hip abductors Knee extensors Plantarflexors
This phase ends (terminal stance) with the push off that includes the "heel lift" and "toe off." The pelvis is stabilized.	Hip abductors Plantarflexors
The arches of the foot are preserved throughout the stance phase.	Long tendons of the foot Intrinsic muscles of the foot
Swing Phase	
This phase begins with forward acceleration of the thigh. Contralateral hip abductors contract to maintain level pelvis.	Hip flexors Hip abductors
The foot must clear the ground as it swings forward. Contralateral hip abductors continue to contract to maintain level pelvis.	Dorsiflexors Hip abductors
The thigh decelerates in preparation for landing.	Hip extensors
As the foot prepares for heel strike, the knee extends and positions the foot.	Knee extensors Dorsiflexors

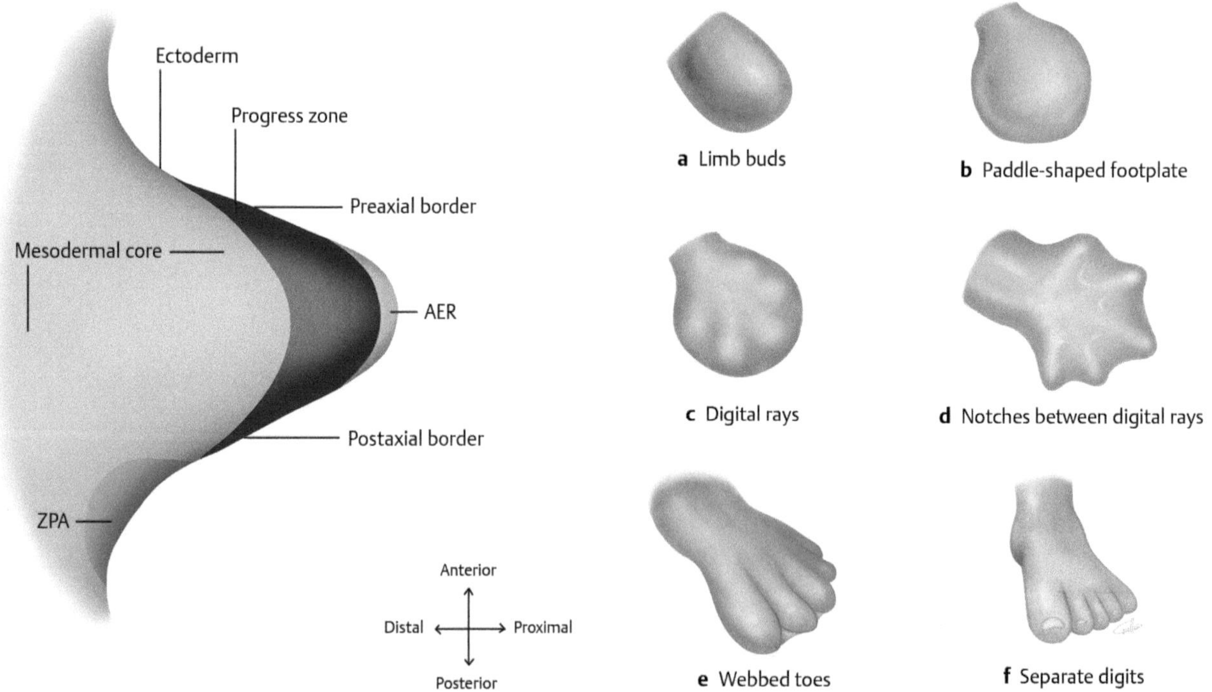

Fig. 5.96 Apical ectodermal ridge (AER) and zone of polarizing activity (ZPA). Illustration by Calla Heald.

Fig. 5.97 (a-f) Progression from limb buds to separate digits. Illustration by Calla Heald.

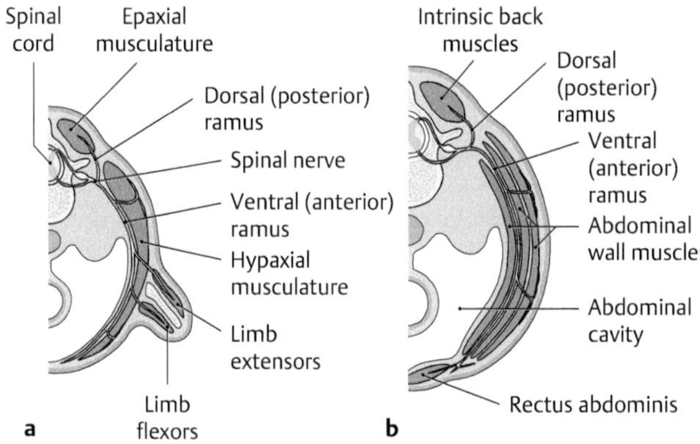

Fig. 5.98 (a, b) Epaxial and hypaxial muscle divisions. (From Schuenke M, Schulte E, Schumacher U. THIEME Atlas of Anatomy. General Anatomy and Musculoskeletal System. Illustrations by Voll M and Wesker K. 3rd ed. New York: Thieme Medical Publishers; 2020.)

femoris artery. The vascular pattern is largely due to remodeling and angiogenesis and has been described in a few different developmental patterns **(Fig. 5.99)**.

There are two main types of limb anomalies: (1) **amelia** – complete absence of a limb or (2) **meromelia** – a partial absence of a limb. These anomalies originate at different stages of development. The suppression of limb bud development during the early part of the 4th week results in amelia. An arrest or disturbance of the differentiation or growth of the limbs during the 5th week results in meromelia. Teratogen-induced limb defects are rare. Many children during the time period of 1957-1962 had mothers who were taking **thalidomide**, a drug used as a sleeping pill and anti-nauseant. This drug however was linked to an absence or gross deformities of the long bones along with intestinal atresia and cardiac anomalies.

Limb defects involving the digits are classified as:

- *Brachydactyly*: shortened digits.
- *Syndactyly*: two or more digits are fused. *Cutaneous syndactyly* is the most common limb anomaly and it presents as webbing between the fingers. This is due to the lack of normal apoptosis that occurs between early footplates separating individual digits from each other.
- *Polydactyly*: extra digits that present bilaterally and lack the proper muscle connections.
- *Ectrodactyly*: absence of a digit (usually unilateral).

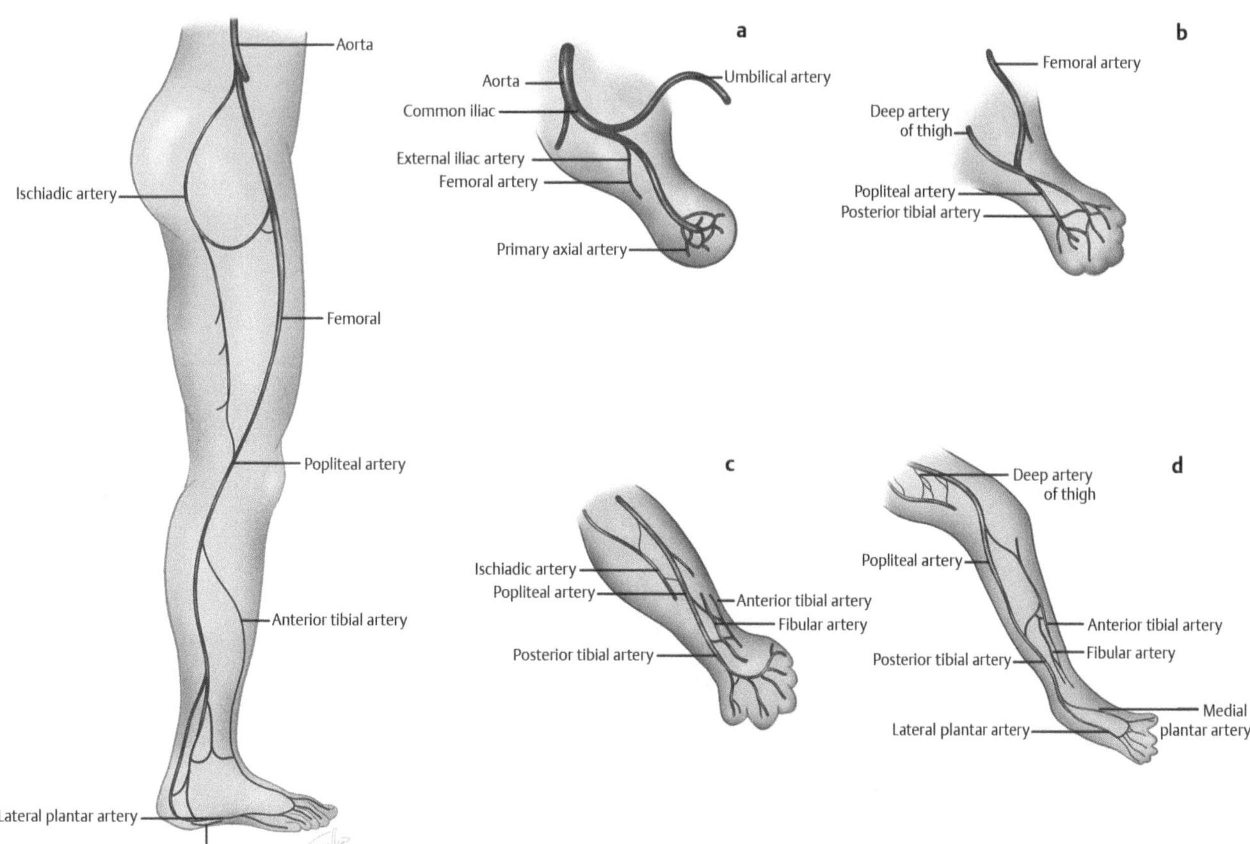

Fig. 5.99 (a-d) Development of the arteries of the lower extremity. Illustration by Calla Heald.

Clinical Correlate 5.52

Cleft Foot

Cleft foot is an abnormal conical defect that extends from the periphery towards the tarsus and is classified into six types that vary based on the amount of missing metatarsals or spacing between the present digits. It is very rare affecting only 1:1,000,000 newborns. Surgery can help correct the deformity.

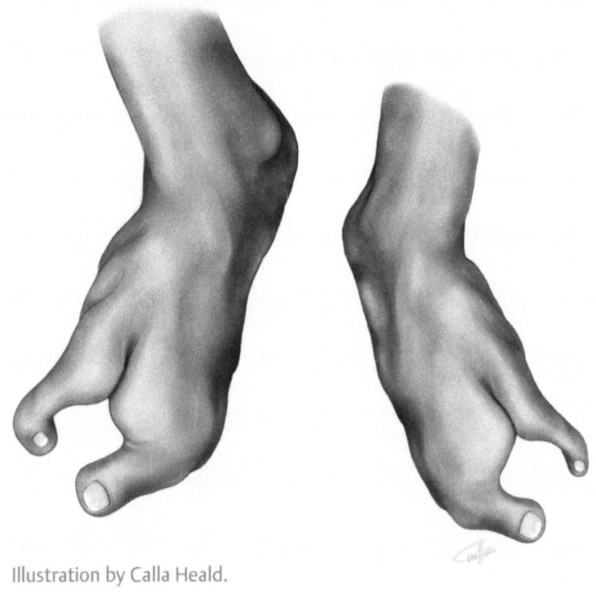

Illustration by Calla Heald.

Clinical Correlate 5.53

Congenital Talipes

Congenital talipes (clubfoot) consists of several types and all are congenital with *talipes equinovarus* being the most common type (1:1000 live births). In half of those affected, both feet are malformed. The main abnormality displays a shortness of muscles, tendons and ligaments. The articular capsule is located on the medial side and posterior aspect of the foot/ankle. The sole of the foot is turned medially and the foot is inverted. The cause is uncertain but hereditary and environmental factors are involved. Intrauterine positioning may create an abnormal positioning for the feet while in utero.

Clinical Correlate 5.54

Osteogenesis Imperfecta

Osteogenesis imperfecta is characterized by the shortening, bowing, and low mineralization of the long bones of limbs that can result in fractures and these patients can present with blue sclera of the eyes. Various versions exist and there is a link between genes responsible for the production of type 1 collagen and its existence.

PRACTICE QUESTIONS

1. The lower extremity muscles can be bulky and extensive thus they generally receive motor fibers from several spinal cord segments or nerves and this means that these muscles are usually composed of multiple myotomes. What combination of segmental innervation has control over the movements of abduction, extension and lateral (external) rotation at the hip joint?
   A. L1-L4.
   B. L5-S1.
   C. L3-L4.
   D. S1-S2.
   E. S2-S3.
2. A 46 year old patient presents with chronic hip pain that he remembers having for much of his life. The orthopedist orders a set of x-rays and notices the angle of inclination between the head and neck of the femur versus the femoral shaft is approximately 110°. What is your diagnosis?
   A. Coxa Vara.
   B. Coxa Valga.
   C. Genu Varum.
   D. Genu Valgum.
   E. A positive Trendelenburg test.
3. Which muscle listed below does not participate in both lateral rotation and abduction at the hip joint?
   A. Inferior gemellus.
   B. Obturator internus.
   C. Superior gemellus.
   D. Piriformis.
   E. Quadratus femoris.
4. After undergoing a major surgical procedure, the patient is given a course of antibiotics by gluteal intramuscular injection. In order to avoid damaging the sciatic nerve during the injection, a needle should be inserted into what location?
   A. The midpoint of the gluteal fold.
   B. Over the location of the obturator internus tendon.
   C. Inferomedial quadrant of the buttocks.
   D. Superolateral quadrant of the buttocks.
   E. Over the location of the sacrospinous ligament.
5. A patient with a deep knife wound in the buttock walks with a waddling gait that is characterized by the pelvis falling toward the "good" side at each step. Which of the following nerves is damaged?
   A. Nerve to obturator externus.
   B. Inferior gluteal nerve.
   C. Femoral nerve.
   D. Obturator nerve.
   E. Superior gluteal nerve.
6. An individual has been in a head-on collision in their car and posteriorly dislocates their hip? What feature WOULD NOT be present if a person has posteriorly dislocated their hip?
   A. Appearance of a flexed thigh at the hip.
   B. Medially rotated lower extremity.
   C. Abducted lower extremity.
   D. Injury to the sciatic nerve.
   E. Appearance of a shortened lower extremity.
7. Which statement regarding the posterior thigh and popliteal fossa is INCORRECT?
   A. Perforating arteries that supply the posterior thigh originate from the femoral artery.

B. The short head of biceps femoris is innervated by the common fibular nerve.
C. The sciatic nerve originates from the dorsal rami of L4-S3.
D. The ischial tuberosity is the structure we technically sit on.
E. The small saphenous vein drains into the popliteal vein.

8. A patient complains of paresthesia or tingling of the skin above the patella and this paresthesia extends down her medial leg to the medial malleolus. Which spinal root is most likely compressed?
A. L2.
B. L4.
C. L5.
D. S1.
E. S2.

9. Which statement regarding the anterior thigh, medial thigh or knee regions is CORRECT?
A. Muscles innervated by the obturator nerve are involved in knee extension.
B. The oblique popliteal ligament is a reflection of the semitendinosus muscle.
C. The saphenous nerve pairs up with the great saphenous vein after passing through the adductor hiatus.
D. The patellar reflex ("knee jerk") tests the L2-L4 spinal cord segments.
E. Genu valgum (or "knock-knee") involves a decrease in the Q-angle.

10. After a car accident, a lesion of the femoral nerve develops near the level of the inguinal ligament. Which function COULD NOT have been affected or lost due to this femoral nerve injury?
A. Knee flexion (flexion of leg at knee).
B. Knee extension (extension of leg at knee).
C. Hip extension (extension of thigh at hip).
D. Hip flexion (flexion of thigh at hip).
E. Lateral rotation of hip.

11. A patient is brought into the ED with a penetrating wound that has passed through the medial compartment of the retroinguinal (Bogro's) space? Which structure WOULD NOT be at risk of being damaged?
A. Femoral nerve.
B. Femoral vein.
C. Femoral artery.
D. Femoral branch of genitofemoral nerve.
E. Deep inguinal lymph nodes.

12. During a local football game, a player receives a blow to the lateral side of their extended knee resulting in an "unhappy triad". What three structures are damaged after one of these injuries?
A. Posterior cruciate ligament, Tibial/medial collateral ligament, Popliteal artery.
B. Posterior cruciate ligament, Fibular/lateral collateral ligament, Lateral meniscus.
C. Anterior cruciate ligament, Tibial/medial collateral ligament, Medial meniscus.
D. Anterior cruciate ligament, Fibular/lateral collateral ligament, Medial meniscus.
E. Anterior cruciate ligament, Tibial/medial collateral ligament, Lateral meniscus.

13. A 16-year-old volleyball player visits her physician with the chief complaint of weakness, numbness and tingling radiating down into her left foot. She is diagnosed with tarsal tunnel syndrome. Which nerve would be compressed and is leading to her discomfort?
A. Deep fibular nerve.
B. Common fibular nerve.
C. Tibial nerve.
D. Saphenous nerve.
E. Superficial fibular nerve.

14. A construction worker is struck near the ankle by a concrete block creating a deep gash and severe damage to a tendon. Damage to this tendon has reduced plantarflexion and inversion of the foot. Which muscle listed below was most likely damaged?
A. Fibularis longus.
B. Fibularis brevis.
C. Tibialis anterior.
D. Tibilais posterior.
E. Extensor hallucis longus.

15. Which statement about a lesion occurring at the proximal superficial fibular nerve near where it branched off from the common fibular is INCORRECT?
A. There would be reduced support for the transverse arch of the foot.
B. Eversion of the foot is drastically reduced.
C. Skin innervation of most of the dorsum of the foot would be lost.
D. Innervation to the fibularis longus and fibularis brevis would be lost.
E. Dorsiflexion of the foot at the ankle would be lost.

16. A 30-year old man running on the beach severely lacerates his foot and ankle region after he accidently steps in a pit that contains broken glass. The first of a few anesthetic injections before suturing occurs near the distal saphenous nerve. Where would be the best location for the ER physician to anesthetize the distal saphenous nerve?
A. Anterior to the lateral malleolus.
B. Posterior to the lateral malleolus.
C. Anterior to the medial malleolus.
D. Posterior to the medial malleous.
E. Webbing between the big toe and 2nd toe.

17. A group of students are playing a game of basketball when one of them sustains a Pott fracture or forced eversion of the foot. This particular person was spared the avulsion of the medial malleolus but the injury did result in a tear of the medial (deltoid) ligament. Which ligament is not considered part of the medial (deltoid) ligament?
A. Calcaneofibular ligament.
B. Anterior tibiotalar ligament.
C. Posterior tibiotalar ligament.
D. Tibionavicular ligament.
E. Tibiocalcaneal ligament.

18. An individual is walking barefoot on the beach and steps on a piece of broken glass penetrating the central compartment of the foot. Which muscle listed below is NOT found in the central compartment of the foot?
A. Flexor digitorum brevis.
B. Plantar interossei.
C. 1st lumbrical.
D. Adductor hallucis.
E. Quadratus plantae.

19. An active 36-year-old participates in a form of high-intensity interval training that some refer to as CrossFit. However, this individual has recently relocated for a new job and over the past three weeks has not been as active. After things have settled down they immediately start their workout regimen as if there was no break. Unfortunately, the morning after their first workout they have swelling, cramping, and are nearly unable to walk. After seeing a physician they are diagnosed with tennis leg. Which muscle is strained if a person has tennis leg?
   A. Flexor hallucis longus.
   B. Soleus.
   C. Flexor digitorum longus.
   D. Gastrocnemius.
   E. Tibialis posterior.
20. When an individual is walking, a set of muscles are responsible for the contralateral hip abduction that helps maintain a level pelvis when the opposite lower limb is elevated during the swing phase of gait. What set of muscles function in this way?
   A. Obturator internus and obturator externus.
   B. Gluteus medius and gluteus minimus.
   C. Piriformis and gluteus maximus.
   D. Superior gemellus and inferior gemellus.
   E. Gluteus maximus and tensor fasciae latae.
21. A basketball player jumps up for a rebound but sprains their ankle after the weight-bearing foot is forced into inversion. What ligament could be partially or completely torn with an ankle sprain?
   A. Plantar calcaneocuboid.
   B. Calcaneofibular.
   C. Anterior talofibular.
   D. Tibiocalcaneal.
   E. Posterior talofibular.
22. The calcaneal tendon reflex or "ankle jerk" tests the integrity of which spinal cord segments?
   A. L1/L2.
   B. L2/L3.
   C. L4/L5.
   D. S1/S2.
   E. S3/S4.
23. A 63-year-old male has over the past three days noticed that he has been tripping over his foot while on his morning walks. He visits a physician and mentions that a bicyclist had accidently ran into his leg at the level of the knee, but at the time he did not think much about it. There was some noticeable bruising and swelling and the physician diagnosed him with foot drop. Which nerve if damaged would result in foot drop?
   A. Common fibular.
   B. Superficial fibular.
   C. Tibial.
   D. Sural.
   E. Medial plantar.
24. An individual presents to the emergency department with pain in their foot after jumping down from a ladder. An X-ray is performed and the individual is told they have what is commonly referred to as a *Jones* fracture. Which bone of the foot would the fracture be seen on the X-ray?
   A. Cuboid.
   B. 2nd metatarsal.
   C. 5th metatarsal.
   D. Calcaneus.
   E. Talus.
25. After consulting their family medicine physician, a 42-year-old female decides to begin a running program to improve her cardiovascular health. After four days of light running pain, pain begins to develop near the tibia bone or shin region. After receiving an evaluation for the pain, the individual is diagnosed with shin splints. Shin splints are the result of microtrauma involving what particular muscle?
   A. Extensor digitorum longus.
   B. Fibularis tertius.
   C. Tibialis posterior.
   D. Extensor hallucis longus.
   E. Tibialis anterior.

ANSWERS

1. **B.** L5-S1.
   A. L1-L4 best describes adduction, flexion and medial (internal) rotation at the hip joint.
   C. L3-L4 best describe extension at the knee joint.
   D. S1-S2 best describes plantarflexion at the ankle joint.
   E. S2-S3 best describes intrinsic muscles of the foot.
2. **A.** When the angle of inclination is below the normal level of 125°, the individual is presenting with coxa vara.
3. **E.** The quadratus femoris is involved in only lateral rotation and has no abduction function.
4. **D.** The safest site for any gluteal injection is in the superolateral quadrant. If one were targeting the sciatic nerve for a nerve block, the location for that would be near the midpoint of a line connecting the posterior superior iliac spine and superior border of the greater trochanter.
5. **E.** The individual has a superior gluteal nerve injury and the contralateral hip would be seen leaning toward the floor when that side's leg was elevated during gait. This is because the gluteus medius and minimus on the affected side are unable to maintain a level pelvis. The individual is also said to have a positive Trendelenburg test.
6. **C.** If the lower extremity was abducted the individual would most likely have an anterior dislocation of the hip joint and are less prevalent.
7. **C.** The sciatic nerve originates from the ventral rami of L4-S3.
8. **B.** If the L4 spinal nerve was compressed, the corresponding dermatome passes over both the patella and medial malleolus.
9. **D.** Correct; the patellar reflex tests the L2-L4 spinal cord segments.
   A. The femoral nerve will innervate muscles involved in knee extension.
   B. The oblique popliteal ligament is a reflection of the semimembranosus muscle.
   C. The saphenous nerve does not pass through the adductor hiatus but will pair with the great saphenous vein near the medial part of the knee joint.
   E. Genu valgum (or "knock-knee") involves an increase in the Q-angle.
10. **C.** The femoral nerve can innervate a muscle that has the capability to function as any of the described movements except for hip extension (extension of the thigh at hip).
11. **A.** The femoral nerve passes through the lateral compartment of the retroinguinal space. All other listed structures are associated with the medial compartment.
12. **C.** The unhappy triad involves the anterior cruciate ligament, tibial/medial collateral ligament and the medial meniscus.

13. **C.** The tibial nerve is compresseD. Tarsal tunnel syndrome is also known as posterior tibial neuralgia although anatomically there are only posterior tibial vessels and not a nerve of that name.
14. **D.** The tibialis posterior is involved in both plantarflexion and inversion.
    A. Fibularis longus – eversion and weak plantarflexion.
    B. Fibularis brevis – eversion and weak plantarflexion.
    C. Tibialis anterior – dorsiflexion of foot and inversion.
    E. Extensor hallucis longus – extension of great toe and dorsiflexion of foot.
15. **E.** Dorsiflexion of the foot at the ankle is controlled by the deep fibular nerve and the muscles of the anterior leg compartment are responsible for that function. Damage of the superficial fibular nerve would have an effect on every situation described in A-D.
16. **C.** The saphenous nerve is paired with the great saphenous vein and these two structures will lie adjacent to the anterior aspect of the medial malleolus.
17. **A.** All the ligaments listed are part of the medial (deltoid) ligament except for the calcaneofibular ligament. This ligament is associated with the lateral ligament of the ankle joint.
18. **B.** The plantar interosseous muscles are located in the interosseous compartment located just superior the central compartment of the foot.
19. **D.** Tennis leg involves the gastrocnemius and is generally isolated to the medial muscle head.
20. **B.** The gluteus medius and minimus are the muscles that abduct and medially rotate the thigh but also maintain a level pelvis when the opposite lower limb is raised during the swing phase of gait.
21. **C.** The anterior talofibular ligament is at risk of damage with an ankle sprain. With a "high" ankle sprain, this type of injury involves the ligaments connecting the tibia and fibula technically above the ankle joint and could lead to the damage of the anterior tibiofibular, interosseous tibiofibular, and posterior tibiofibular ligaments.
22. **D.** The S1 and S2 spinal cord segments are involved in the calcaneal tendon reflex. S1 plays a much larger role and if cut, this reflex is nearly absent.
23. **A.** Foot drop is due to the inability to dorsiflex the foot when walking, and the nerve damaged would be the common fibular nerve. The most often injured nerve of the lower extremity is the common fibular nerve because it is exposed as it wraps around the lateral aspect of the fibular neck. Deep fibular nerve entrapment or "ski boot syndrome" could lead to foot drop as well.
24. **C.** A fracture of the 5th metatarsal is known as a *Jones* fracture.
    A. A *nutcracker* fracture involves the cuboid.
    B. A *march* fracture involves the 2nd metatarsal.
    D. A *lover's* fracture involves the calcaneus.
    E. An *aviator* fracture involves the talus.
25. **E.** Shin splints are related to microtrauma involving the tibialis anterior muscle.

6 Upper Extremities

LEARNING OBJECTIVES

- To understand all the bones associated with the upper extremity and major fractures associated with them.
- To describe the fascial layers of the upper extremity.
- To describe the somatic and cutaneous nerve innervation and how the dermatome and myotomes are associated with these nerves.
- To describe the major arteries, veins and general lymphatic drainage of the upper extremity.
- To describe the muscles and neurovasculature of the pectoral region. Clinical correlates would include winging of the scapula.
- To describe the muscles, neurovasculature and bursae of the shoulder region. Clinical correlates would include rotator cuff tears, adhesive capsulitis and scapular arterial anastomoses.
- To understand the shoulder region joints, ligaments, and neurovasculature. Clinical correlates include the difference between shoulder separations and dislocations.
- To describe the borders and major neurovasculature of the axilla. Clinical correlates include brachial plexus blocks, upper and lower brachial plexus injuries.
- To describe the muscles and neurovasculature of the arm. Clinical correlates include the bicep brachii and triceps brachii reflexes.
- To describe the borders and neurovasculature of the cubital fossa. Clinical correlates include how to measure arterial blood pressure and venipunctures.
- To understand the elbow joint, ligaments, and neurovasculature. Clinical correlates include the carrying angle of the elbow joint, olecranon fractures, dislocation and bursitis of the elbow joint, subluxation of the radial head, and ulnar collateral ligament reconstruction.
- To understand the proximal radioulnar joint, ligaments, and neurovasculature.
- To describe the muscles and neurovasculature of the anterior forearm. Clinical correlates include medial epicondylitis, median nerve palsy, pronator syndrome and ulnar nerve palsy.
- To escribe the muscles and neurovasculature of the posterior forearm. Clinical correlates include lateral epicondylitis, synovial cyst, anatomical snuff box, De Quervain tenosynovitis and mallet finger.
- To understand the distal radioulnar joint, ligaments, and neurovasculature.
- To describe the muscles, neurovasculature and flexor tendon sheaths of the hand. Clinical correlates include carpal tunnel syndrome, Dupuytren contracture and tenosynovitis.
- To understand the wrist joint, ligaments, and neurovasculature.
- To understand the multiple hand joints, ligaments, and neurovasculature.
- To understand upper extremity development.

6.1 Upper Extremity Overview and Bones

The upper extremities extend from the trunk and are used primarily to position the hands in such a way that they are capable of touching, grasping or conducting other fine motor movements. The upper extremities are not involved in normal weight bearing, thus the muscles are not as bulky, but they may still have considerable strength (**Fig. 6.1**).

They are divided into regions, which include the shoulder, axilla, arm, elbow, forearm, wrist and hand. The shoulder is a broad term and overlaps the lower neck, back and thorax. It includes the lower parts of the posterior triangle of the neck that serves as a conduit for neurovasculature that passes back and forth to the upper extremity. The shoulder may be described as a larger region including pectoral, deltoid and scapular regions. The pectoral region is treated as a separate region in this chapter.

The bones of the upper extremities are divided, much like the lower extremity, into two functional components and these include the pectoral girdle and free upper extremity. The **pectoral girdle** (or **shoulder girdle**) is a bony ring formed by the clavicles and scapulae. It is incomplete posteriorly but anteriorly it is associated with the manubrium of the sternum. The free upper extremity bones consist of the humerus, ulna, radius and the numerous hand bones. In general, the upper extremity is more mobile than the lower extremity.

6.1.1 Clavicle

The **clavicle**, more commonly known as the *collarbone*, serves as the connection between the upper extremity and trunk (**Fig. 6.2**). It is designated a long bone but it has no marrow cavity. Instead, it has a compact bone shell overlying spongy bone. The **shaft** consists of a double curve in the horizontal plane. The medial portion is convex anteriorly while the lateral end is concave anteriorly and flattened. The medially positioned **sternal end** is triangular and slightly enlarged and this is the end that articulates as the *sternoclavicular joint* with the *manubrium of the sternum*. The laterally positioned **acromial end** articulates with the acromion of the scapula at the *acromioclavicular joint*.

The **superior surface** is smooth and acts as an attachment site for skin and the platysma muscle. The **inferior surface** is rough, allowing for the attachment of certain structures. The most medial end of this inferior surface has an impression for the *costoclavicular ligament*. The **subclavian groove** is the site of attachment for the subclavius muscle. There is a **conoid tubercle** located near the acromial end that allows for the attachment of the *conoid ligament*. The **trapezoid line** located on this end also serves as an attachment site for the *trapezoid ligament*. The conoid and trapezoid ligaments are part of the *coracoclavicular ligament*.

The curvatures of the clavicle increase its resilience. The clavicle functions as a movable strut from which the scapula and upper extremity are suspended, separating them from the trunk. This strut also allows the scapula to move across the thoracic wall, increasing the range of motion of the upper extremity. This movement occurs at the so-called *scapulothoracic joint* discussed later in the *Shoulder Region Joints* section of this chapter. Elevation of the ribs during deep inspiration is enhanced when the clavicle is fixed in position especially when it is already elevated.

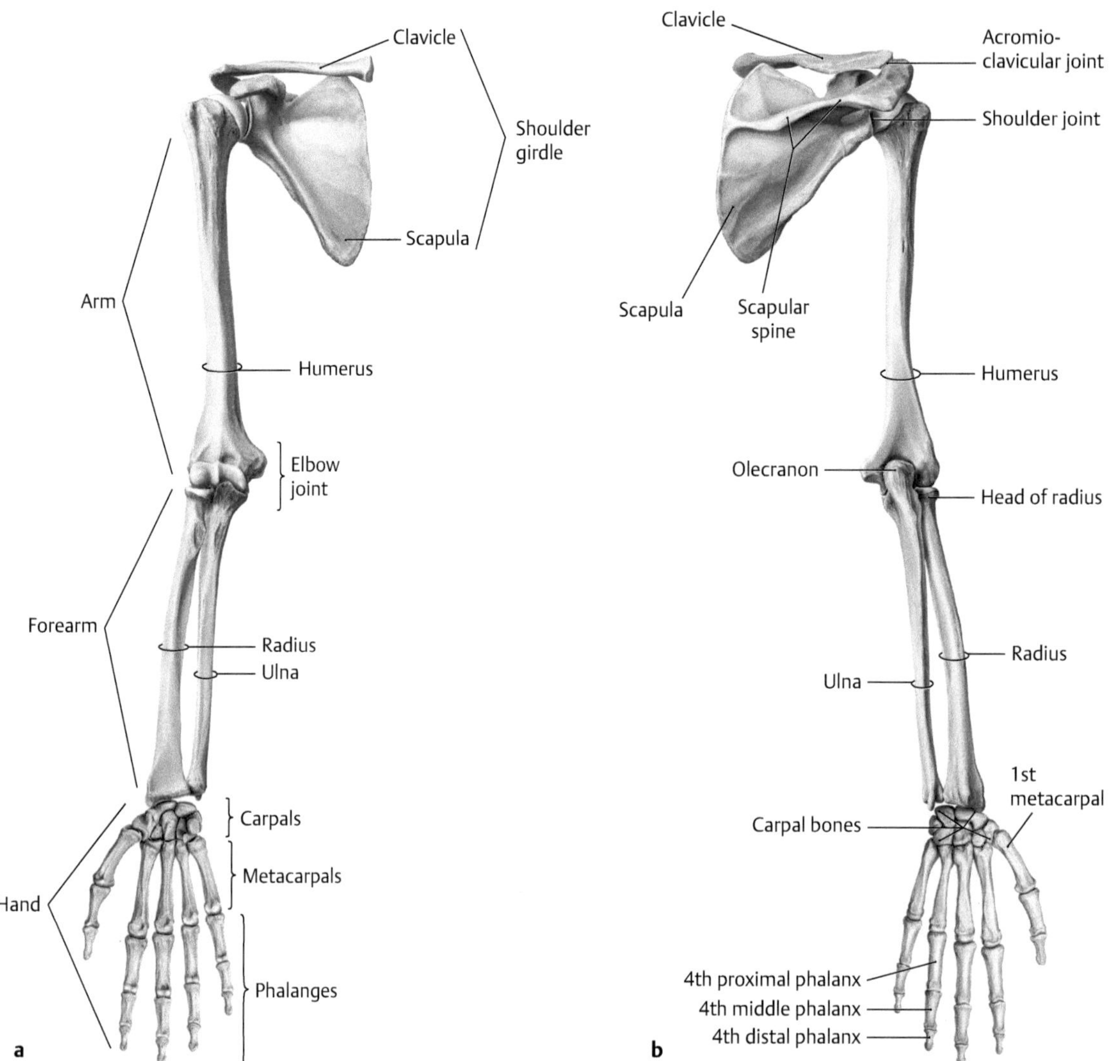

Fig. 6.1 Upper extremity overview and bones. **(a)** Anterior view. **(b)** Posterior view. (From Schuenke M, Schulte E, Schumacher U. THIEME Atlas of Anatomy. General Anatomy and Musculoskeletal System. Illustrations by Voll M and Wesker K. 3rd ed. New York: Thieme Medical Publishers; 2020.)

Clinical Correlate 6.1

Clavicle Fractures

One of the most common bones fractured is the clavicle and this often occurs due to an indirect force transmitted from an outstretched hand through the bones of the forearm and arm to the shoulder during a fall. The weakest part of the clavicle is at the junction of its middle and lateral 1/3 parts. With this type of fracture, the sternocleidomastoid muscle elevates the medial fragment of broken bone. The trapezius muscle is unable to hold up the lateral fragment of broken bone due to the weight of the upper extremity causing the shoulder to drop. The lateral fragment can be pulled medially by any muscle that functions in adduction of the arm.

The clavicle is capable of transmitting shock from the upper extremity back to the axial skeleton during a fall, for example. It also serves as protection for the axillary vessels and brachial plexus nerves, among other structures, which pass between the neck and arm regions linked to the *cervicoaxillary canal.*

6.1.2 Scapula

The **scapula,** more commonly known as the *shoulder blade*, is a triangularly shaped flat bone overlying the 2nd-7th ribs on the posterolateral aspect of the thorax (**Fig. 6.3**). The anterior *costal surface* forms the large **subscapular fossa** and is the site of the subscapularis muscle. The *posterior surface* is divided into the **supraspinous** and **infraspinous fossae** by the **spine of the scapula**. These fossae are associated with the supraspinatus and infraspinatus muscles, respectively. The spine continues laterally to become the **acromion** and together they serve as attachment sites for the trapezius and deltoid muscles. There is a **superior** and **inferior angle** closely associated with the supraspinous and infraspinous fossae respectively.

The **medial (vertebral) border** runs parallel to the spinous processes of the thoracic vertebrae and is an attachment site for the rhomboid muscles. The **lateral (axillary) border** runs superolaterally toward the apex of the axilla from the inferior angle. The thicker lateral border terminates as the lateral angle, the thickest part of the scapula and features the **head** of the scapula. The short extension leading to the head is called the **neck** of

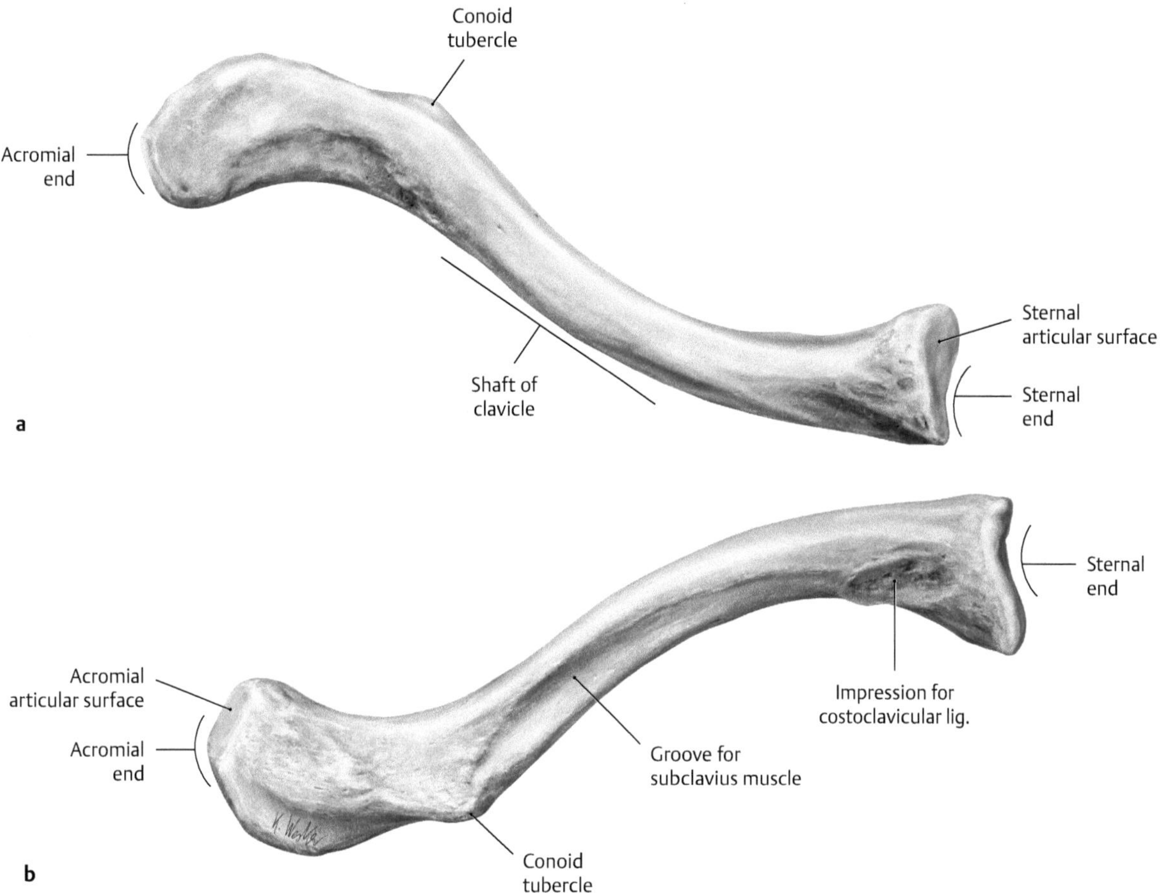

Fig. 6.2 Clavicle. **(a)** Superior view. **(b)** Inferior view. (From Schuenke M, Schulte E, Schumacher U. THIEME Atlas of Anatomy. General Anatomy and Musculoskeletal System. Illustrations by Voll M and Wesker K. 3rd ed. New York: Thieme Medical Publishers; 2020.)

the scapula. The lateral surface of the scapula has the **glenoid cavity**, a concave but shallow fossa that is the articulation site between the head of the humerus and scapula forming the *glenohumeral joint*. Just superior and inferior to the glenoid cavity are the **supraglenoid** and **infraglenoid tubercles** that serve as attachment points for both the long heads of biceps brachii and triceps respectively. Superior to the glenoid cavity and projecting anterolaterally is the **coracoid process**, a site for the attachment of the coracobrachialis, short head of biceps brachii and pectoralis minor muscles. Just medial to this process is the **scapular notch**, an indentation associated with the **superior transverse ligament of the scapula** and the suprascapular nerve and vessels. The **superior border** of the scapula is located between the superior angle and this notch.

The *acromioclavicular joint* is located lateral to the mass of the scapula and its attached muscles because of how lateral the acromion is situated in relation to the rest of the scapular parts. The *glenohumeral joint* is located inferior to this joint, which results in the scapular mass being balanced with that of the free upper extremity. The *coracoclavicular ligament* lies between these two masses and serves as the suspending structure. The scapula is involved in multiple movements involving the upper extremity such as protraction, retraction, superior and inferior rotations, and these are carried out at the "*scapulothoracic joint*".

Clinical Correlate 6.2

Scapula Fractures

Severe trauma is usually the cause of a scapula fracture as in an accident involving a pedestrian being hit by a moving vehicle. There are usually rib fractures associated with a fractured scapula. Little treatment is needed in these types of fractures because the scapula is covered by muscles on both sides. The acromion is the most fractured part of the scapula.

6.1.3 Humerus

The **humerus** or arm bone is the largest bone in the upper extremity (**Fig. 6.4**). It articulates with the scapula at the *glenohumeral joint* and the ulna and radius at the *elbow joint*. There is a head, anatomical neck, surgical neck, and greater and lesser tubercles located at it proximal end. The **head** of the humerus has an articulating surface that articulates with the glenoid cavity of the scapula and the **anatomical neck** is the groove separating the head from the greater and lesser tubercles. The **greater tubercle** is on the lateral margin of the humerus while the **lesser tubercle** is on the anterior side of the humerus medial to the greater tubercle. Both of these tubercles are located near the head and anatomical neck and serve

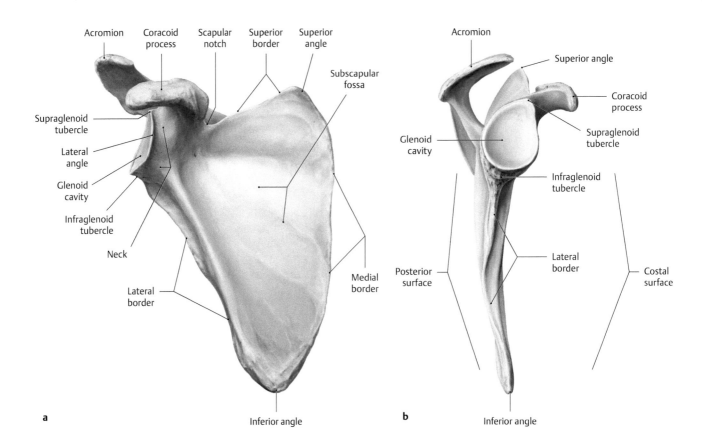

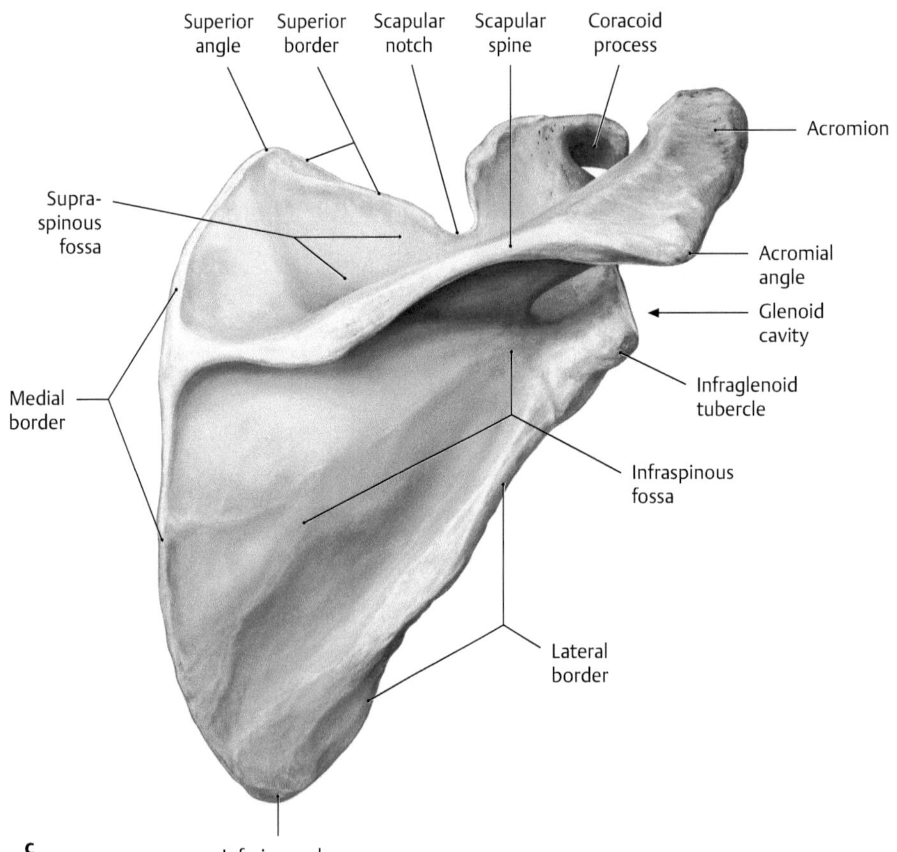

Fig. 6.3 Scapula. **(a)** Anterior view. **(b)** Right lateral view. **(c)** Posterior view. (From Schuenke M, Schulte E, Schumacher U. THIEME Atlas of Anatomy. General Anatomy and Musculoskeletal System. Illustrations by Voll M and Wesker K. 3rd ed. New York: Thieme Medical Publishers; 2020.)

as the attachment sites for the rotator cuff muscles. Splitting the two tubercles is the **intertubercular sulcus** (or **bicipital groove**) that allows for the passage of the long head of the biceps brachii. The **surgical neck** of the humerus is the slight constriction of bone just distal to the tubercles and is the most common fracture site of the proximal humerus. Fractures at this location could affect the axillary nerve and the circumflex humeral vessels.

The **deltoid tuberosity** (laterally) and **radial groove** (posteriorly) are located midway down the **shaft** of the humerus. The deltoid tuberosity is the attachment site for the deltoid muscle and the passing radial nerve and profunda brachii vessels form the radial groove. The distal portion of the humeral shaft widens to become the **lateral** and **medial supracondylar ridges** and eventually the **lateral** and **medial epicondyles**.

The most distal portion of the humerus is known as the **condyle**. It includes the coronoid, radial, and olecranon fossae, along with the trochlea and capitulum. The **coronoid** and **radial fossae** receive the coronoid process of the ulna and head of the radius respectively and are located on the anterior surface. The articulating surfaces of the condyle include the **trochlea** that articulates with the trochlear notch of the ulna and the **capitulum** that articulates with the head of the radius. The posterior surface of the condyle has the **olecranon fossa** and it receives the olecranon of the ulna.

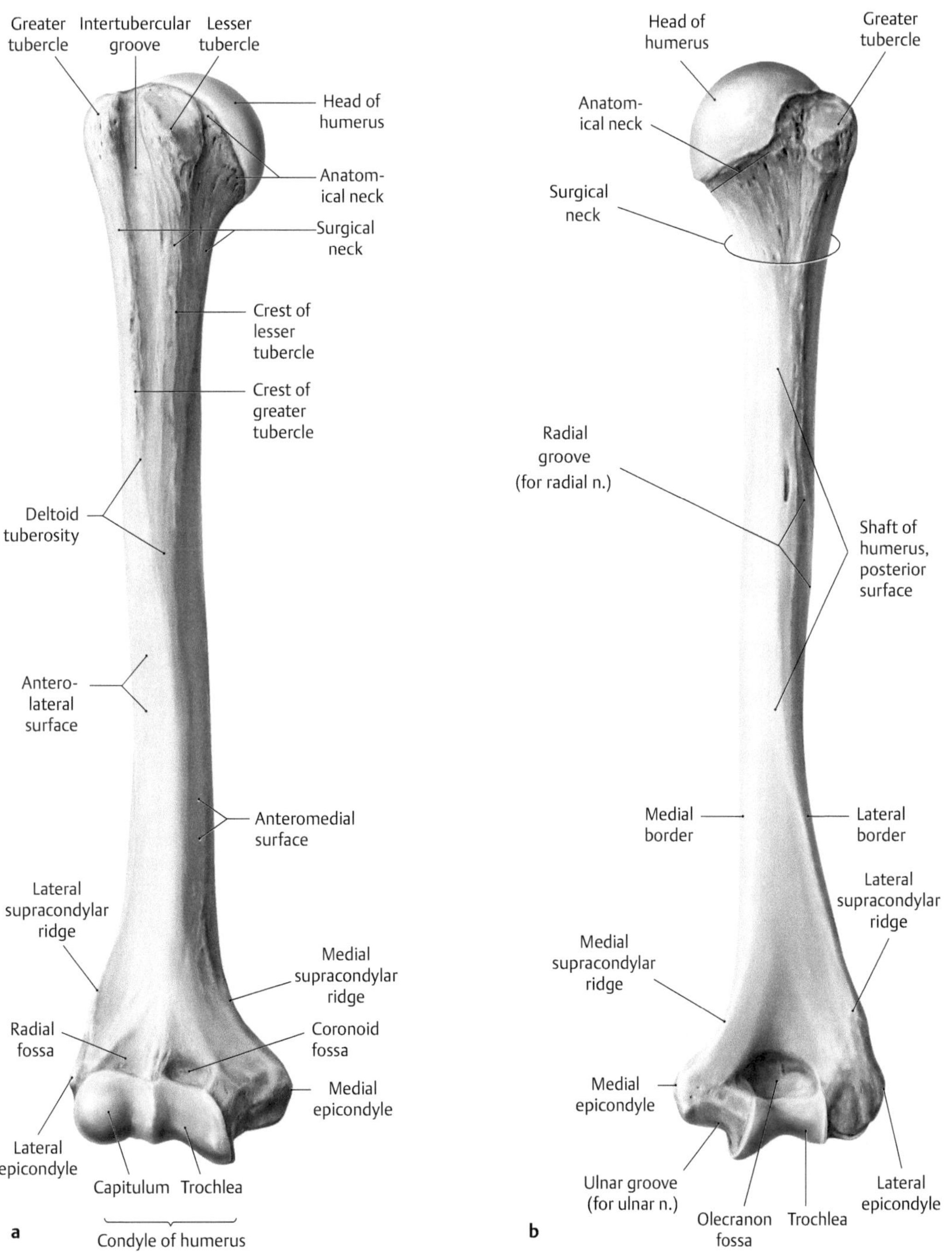

Fig. 6.4 Humerus. **(a)** Anterior view. **(b)** Posterior view. (From Schuenke M, Schulte E, Schumacher U. THIEME Atlas of Anatomy. General Anatomy and Musculoskeletal System. Illustrations by Voll M and Wesker K. 3rd ed. New York: Thieme Medical Publishers; 2020.)

Clinical Correlate 6.3

Humeral Fractures

Most injuries of the humerus are located at the surgical neck. These types of fractures commonly result in one fragment of bone being driven into the spongy bone of the other fragment and are known as *impacted fractures*. Most humeral fractures are seen in older individuals and involve that person falling onto the outstretched arms or directly onto the shoulder. Three main types of fractures are distinguishable; an *extra-articular* **(a)**, *intra-articular* **(b)**, *and a comminuted fracture* **(c)**. *Spiral fractures* of the humeral shaft may involve falling on an outstretched hand. Fractures near the surgical neck can affect the axillary nerve while mid-shaft fractures may damage the radial nerve. A *lateral epicondyle fracture* may also damage the radial nerve while a medial epicondyle fracture could result in damage to the *ulnar nerve*.

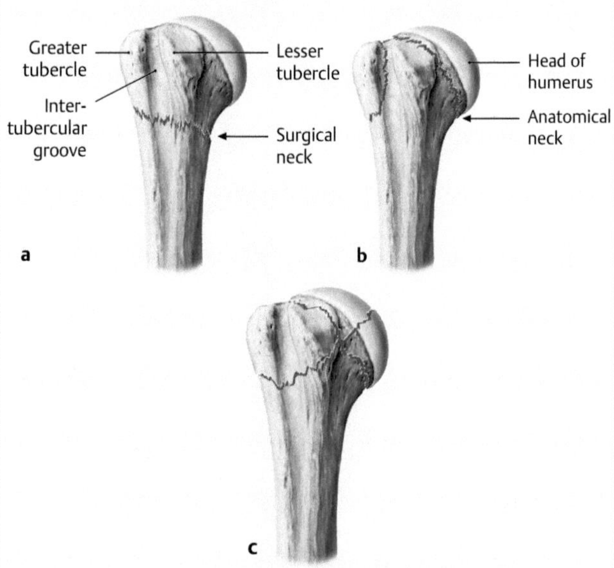

(From Schuenke M, Schulte E, Schumacher U. THIEME Atlas of Anatomy. General Anatomy and Musculoskeletal System. Illustrations by Voll M and Wesker K. 3rd ed. New York: Thieme Medical Publishers; 2020.)

6.1.4 Ulna

Of the forearm bones, the **ulna** is the most medial and longer of the two (**Fig. 6.5**). It is larger at its proximal end versus its distal end and is considered the stabilizing bone of the forearm. There are two prominent projections from the ulna. The **coronoid process** is located on the anterior side while the **olecranon** is located on the posterior surface and is commonly called the "elbow" and serves as the short lever in elbow extension. Both of these processes contribute to the walls of the **trochlear notch**, which acts to grasp the trochlea of the humerus tightly.

The radial head fits into the **radial notch** located on the lateral side of the coronoid process. The **supinator crest** and **supinator fossa** are located just below the radial notch on the lateral ulnar shaft and they act as attachment sites for the deep part of the supinator muscle. Just distal to the coronoid process is the **ulnar tuberosity** and it serves as an attachment site for the brachialis muscle. The **shaft** of the ulna becomes thinner as it moves closer to the wrist. At the distal end, there is a small enlargement known as the **head** of the ulna with a **styloid process** that extends out from it. The distal ulna does not articulate with any carpal bones thus it is not technically part of the wrist joint.

6.1.5 Radius

The shorter and lateral most of the two forearm bones is called the **radius** (**Fig. 6.5**). The proximal end is the thinner section that includes the head, neck and radial tuberosity. The **head** of the radius articulates with the capitulum of the humerus while the **radial tuberosity** is an attachment point for the biceps brachii muscle. The **shaft** of the radius gradually becomes larger before reaching its max size near the wrist joint. The lateral side of the distal ulna has a **styloid process** and the medial side has the **ulnar notch**, the articulation site with the distal ulna. On the posterior side, there is the **dorsal (*Lister's*) tubercle of the radius**. This structure acts as a pulley for the extensor pollicis longus muscle of the thumb.

The **interosseous membrane** spans the medial border of the radius and lateral border of the ulna (interosseous borders). The fibers of this membrane run in an oblique fashion and in an inferior direction from the radius down to the ulna. The articulation between the two bones by way of the interosseous membrane is a *syndesmosis type* of fibrous joint. This membrane transmits forces from the radius via the hand and back to the ulna before heading up through the humerus.

Clinical Correlate 6.4

Radius Fractures

A fracture involving the distal end of the radius is the most common fracture seen in people over 50. A complete fracture of the distal 2 cm of the radius is called a **Colles fracture** and is the most common fracture in the forearm. The distal fragment is displaced dorsally and often *comminuted* or broken into pieces. These types of fractures are the result of forced dorsiflexion of the hand while trying to ease a fall by outstretching the upper limb. The styloid process of the ulna is often *avulsed* or broken off. The styloid process of the radius normally projects further distally than the styloid process of the ulna but after a Colles fracture, this relationship is reversed and this fracture is also commonly referred to as a **dinner fork deformity**. This is due to the posterior angulation that occurs in the forearm just proximal to the wrist.

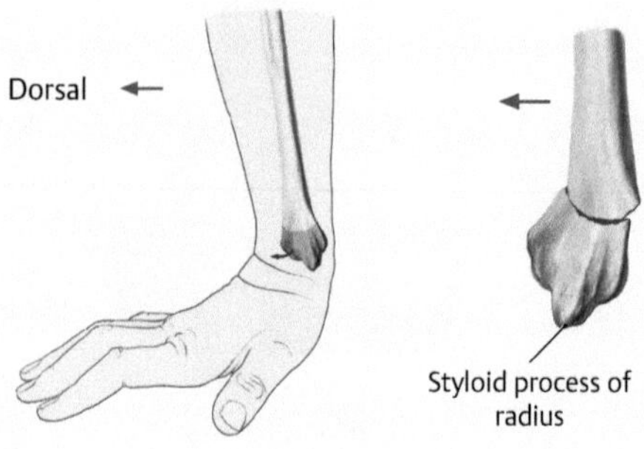

(From Schuenke M, Schulte E, Schumacher U. THIEME Atlas of Anatomy. General Anatomy and Musculoskeletal System. Illustrations by Voll M and Wesker K. 3rd ed. New York: Thieme Medical Publishers; 2020.)

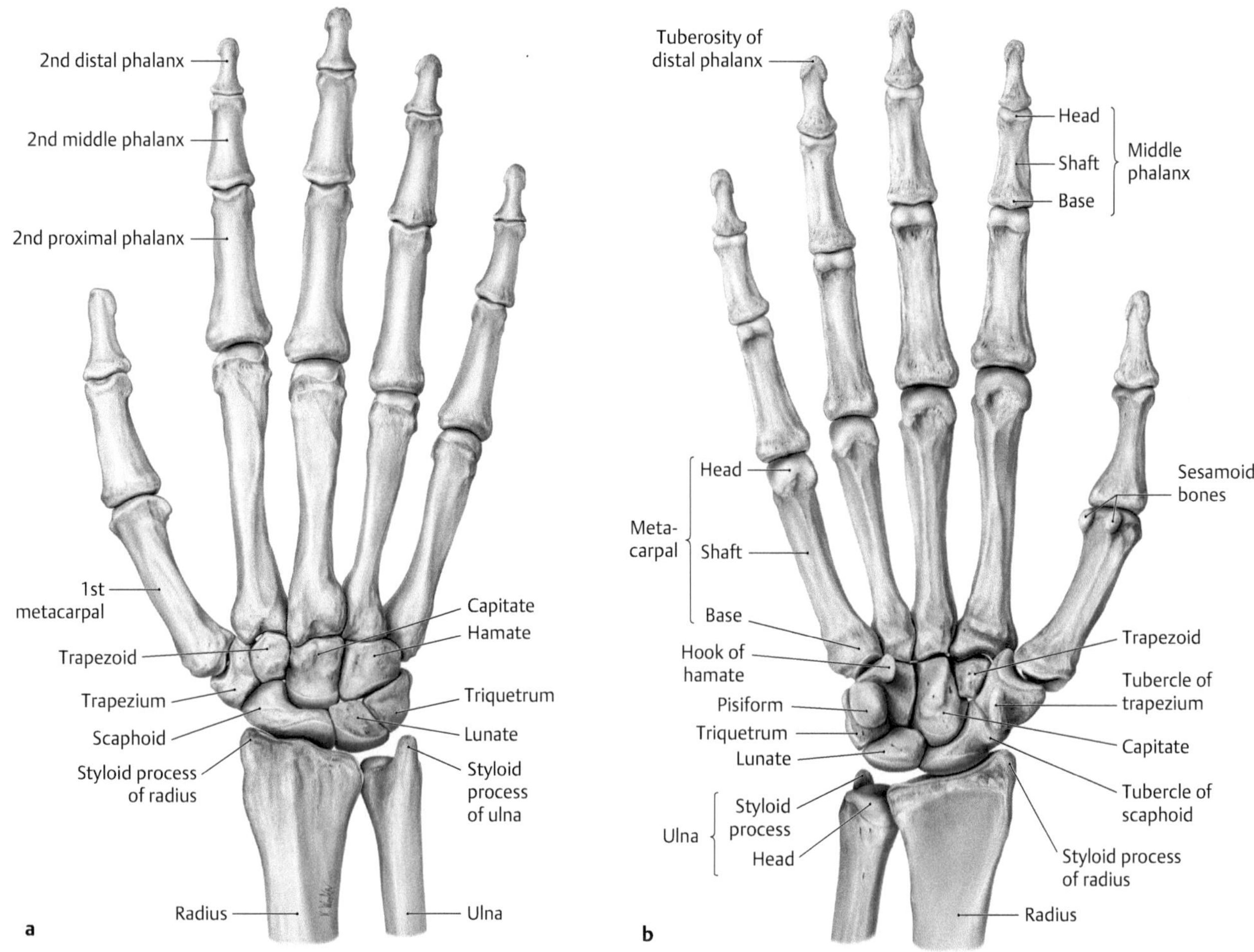

Fig. 6.5 **(a)** Dorsal view of right hand. **(b)** Palmar view of right hand. (From Schuenke M, Schulte E, Schumacher U. THIEME Atlas of Anatomy. General Anatomy and Musculoskeletal System. Illustrations by Voll M and Wesker K. 3rd ed. New York: Thieme Medical Publishers; 2020.)

6.1.6 Carpals, Metacarpals, and Phalanges of the Hand

The hand is made up of 27 total bones that consist of 8 carpal, 5 metacarpal, and 14 phalange bones (**Fig. 6.6; Fig. 6.7**). When we speak of the **wrist** or **carpus**, we are talking about the combination of all carpal bones. The *wrist (radiocarpal) joint* is the articulation between the distal radius and the proximal row of carpal bones minus the pisiform bone.

Carpus

The eight carpal bones include the scaphoid, lunate, triquetrum, pisiform, trapezium, trapezoid, capitate and hamate. There is a larger degree of flexibility to the overall wrist due to the small size of these carpal bones. The bones themselves are split into a proximal and distal row (**Fig. 6.6; Fig. 6.7**).

- Proximal row are nearest the forearm (from lateral to medial):
  - **Scaphoid**: the largest of the proximal row carpal bones and has a prominent **scaphoid tubercle** near the trapezium bone. It is boat-shaped and articulates with the radius, lunate, trapezium, trapezoid and capitate.
  - **Lunate**: articulates with the radius, scaphoid, capitate, hamate and the triquetrum.
  - **Triquetrum**: articulates with the pisiform, lunate, hamate, the radius especially during ulnar deviation (adduction), and the articular disc of the *distal radioulnar joint.*
  - **Pisiform**: very small and pea-shaped bone located on the palmar surface of the triquetrum.
- Distal row are nearest the metacarpals (from lateral to medial):
  - **Trapezium**: articulates with the scaphoid, trapezoid, and 1st and 2nd metacarpals.
  - **Trapezoid**: articulates with the scaphoid, capitate, trapezium and 2nd metacarpal.
  - **Capitate**: largest carpal bone and articulates with the scaphoid, lunate, trapezoid, hamate and 3rd metacarpal.
  - **Hamate**: has a distinctive hook of the hamate and articulates with the capitate, triquetrum, and the 4th and 5th metacarpals.

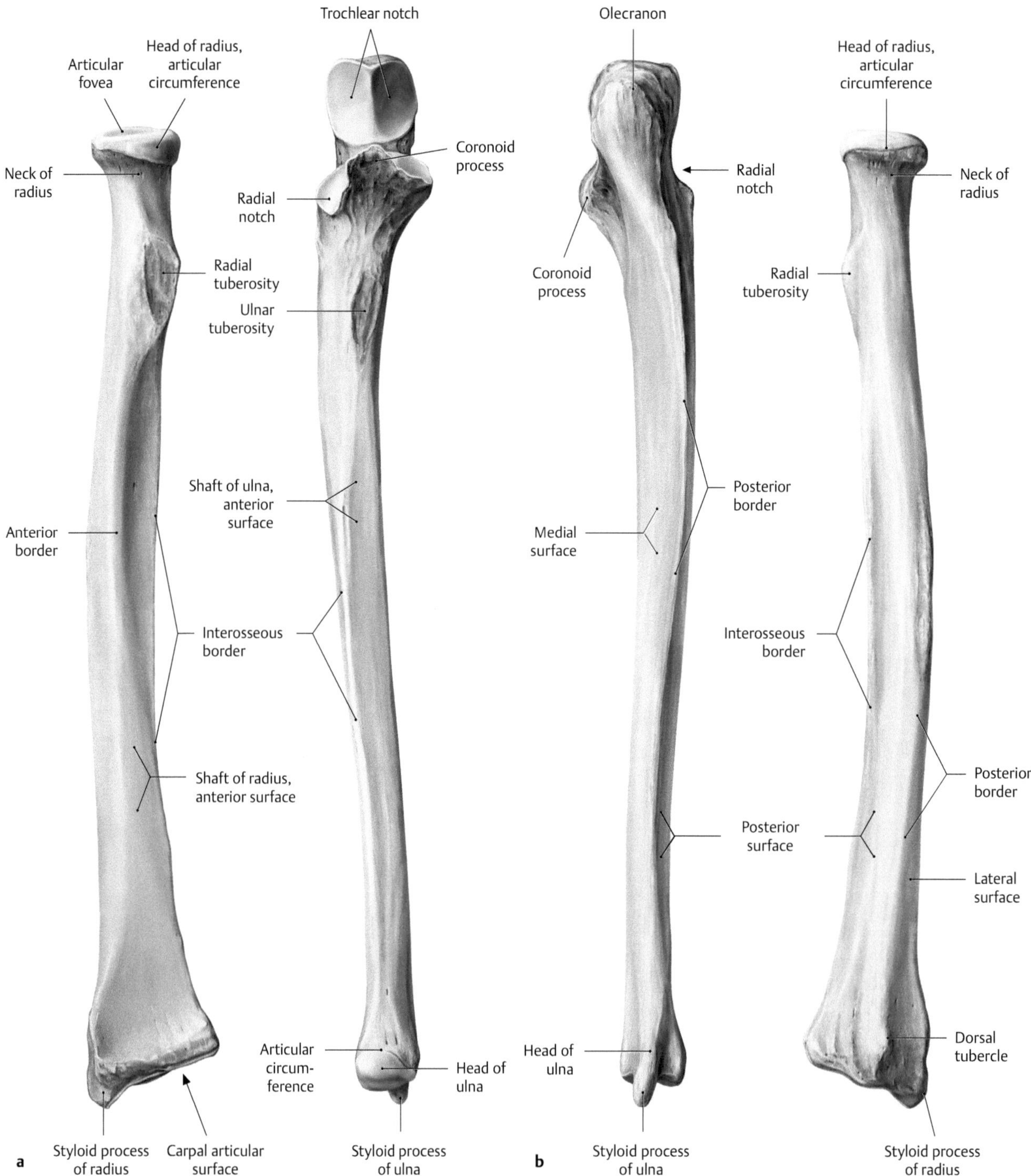

Fig. 6.6 Radius and ulna. **(a)** Anterior view. **(b)** Posterior view. (From Schuenke M, Schulte E, Schumacher U. THIEME Atlas of Anatomy. General Anatomy and Musculoskeletal System. Illustrations by Voll M and Wesker K. 3rd ed. New York: Thieme Medical Publishers; 2020.)

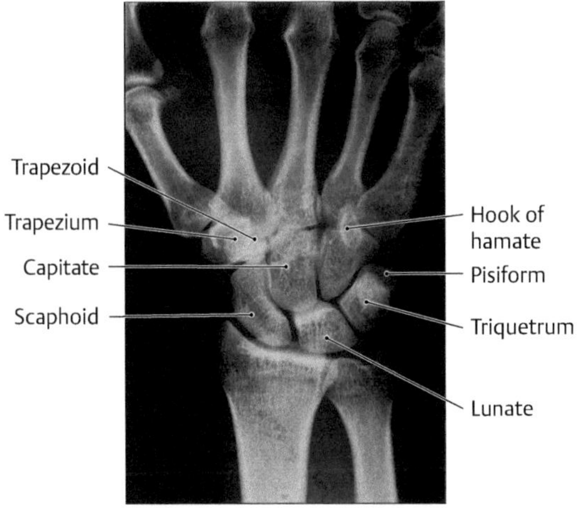

Fig. 6.7 Radiograph of the left wrist (anteroposterior view). (From Schuenke M, Schulte E, Schumacher U. THIEME Atlas of Anatomy. General Anatomy and Musculoskeletal System. Illustrations by Voll M and Wesker K. 3rd ed. New York: Thieme Medical Publishers; 2020.)

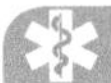

Clinical Correlate 6.5

Carpal Fractures

A **fracture of the scaphoid** generally results from a fall on the palm with the hand abducted. It is the most common carpal bone fractured and it occurs across a narrow portion of the scaphoid. Initial X-rays may not show the fracture but if a radiograph is taken a week or so after, there will be a fracture present because of bone resorption. Fractured parts may take several months to heal and lead to *avascular necrosis* of the proximal portion (blood supply is poor to this region) of the scaphoid leading to *degenerative joint disease* of the wrist.

A **fracture of the hamate** may not fully heal because of the constant traction being put on the bone by certain muscles. Due to the ulnar nerve and vessels coursing through this area known as the **ulnar tunnel** (or **Guyon's canal**), injury to the nerve would affect most of the intrinsic hand muscles.

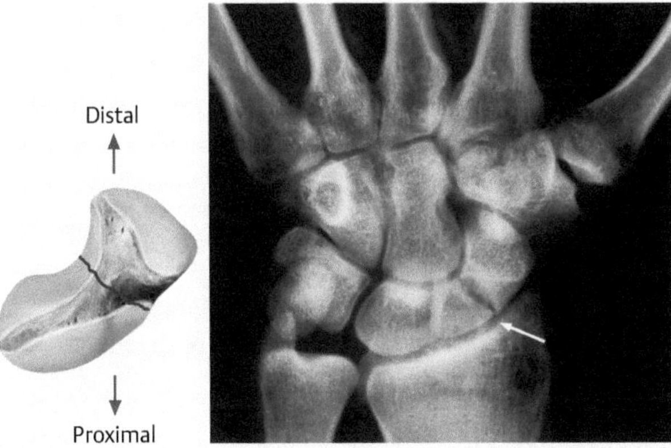

(From Schuenke M, Schulte E, Schumacher U. THIEME Atlas of Anatomy. General Anatomy and Musculoskeletal System. Illustrations by Voll M and Wesker K. 3rd ed. New York: Thieme Medical Publishers; 2020.)

Metacarpals

There are a total of five metacarpals and together they form the skeleton of the palm of the hand (**Fig. 6.6**). Much like the metatarsals of the foot, the metacarpal bones have a proximal **base**, **shaft** and distal **head**. A **styloid process** is located on the 3rd metacarpal. The bases of the metacarpals articulate with the carpal bones and the heads articulate with the proximal phalanges. These last articulations are known as the metacarpophalangeal joints or knuckles.

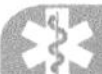

Clinical Correlate 6.6

Metacarpal Fractures

A 5th metacarpal fracture or **boxer's fracture** is common in unskilled individuals who punch something or in individuals who punch with a closed and abducted fist. Metacarpal fractures in general heal quickly because they have good blood supply.

Phalanges

Similar to the foot, there are a total of 14 phalanges found in each hand. The 2-5 digits each have a **proximal**, **middle** and **distal phalanx** (**Fig. 6.6**). The 1st digit or thumb has only a proximal and distal phalanx. Each phalanx has a proximal **base**, **shaft** and distal **head** similar to the metacarpals.

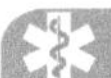

Clinical Correlate 6.7

Phalanx Fractures

Fractures involving the proximal and middle phalanges are generally the result of a hyperextension or crushing injury. In the event multiple fragments of bone are present, alignment of the bone fragments is crucial because of the close relationship they have to multiple tendons, especially of the flexor muscles. A distal phalanx fracture is generally due to a crushing injury and it is usually comminuted and painful. A local hematoma is common with these types of fractures.

6.2 Surface Anatomy of the Upper Extremity

Good portions of the upper extremity bones are palpable allowing for a thorough physical examination in order to detect possible trauma or damaged neurovasculature much like the lower extremity. These structures are generally located just deep to the skin and are easily discernable because of thin fascia and very little surrounding muscle (**Fig. 6.8; Fig. 6.9**).

Just medial to the sternoclavicular joint of the clavicle, there is the **jugular notch** of the manubrium. The articulation between the lateral portion of the clavicle and acromion of the scapula forming the acromioclavicular joint feels like a flat elevation on the lateral shoulder region. The **clavicle** is easily palpable throughout its course.

In the shoulder region and leading back from the acromion, the **spine of the scapula** can be palpated all the way back to the medial border of the scapula. The **acromion** is best felt after contraction of the deltoid muscle. The **acromion angle** is the point where both

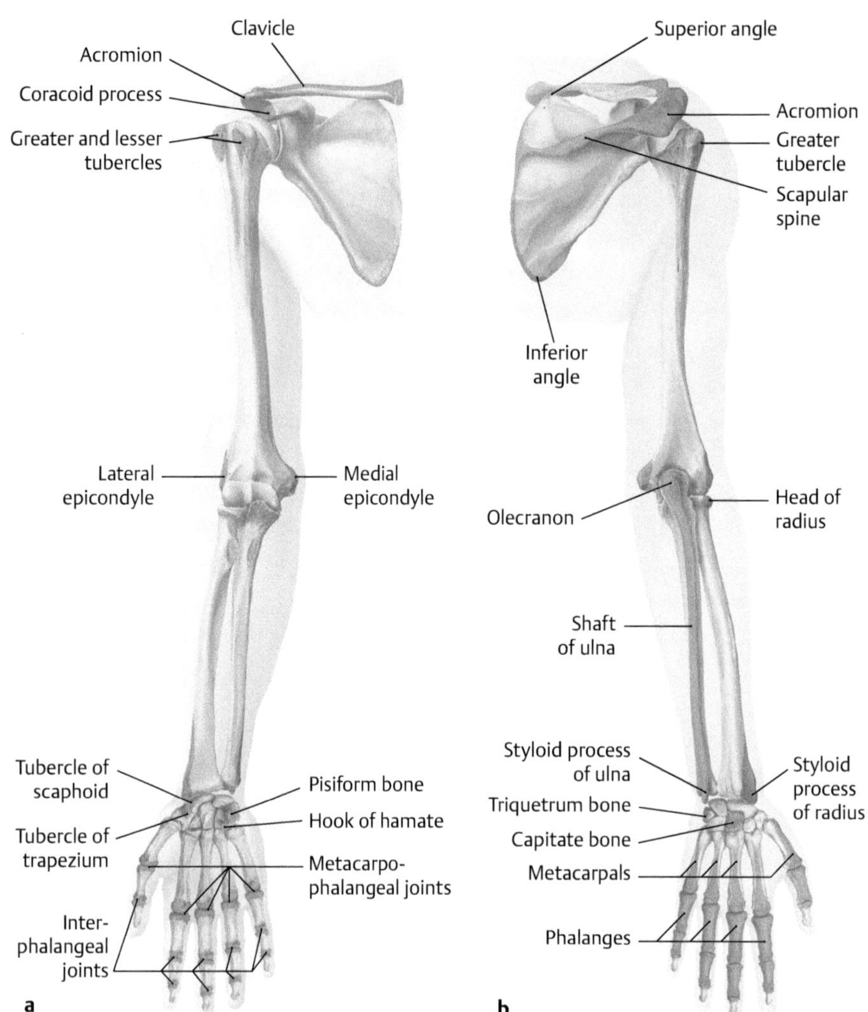

Fig. 6.8 Palpable bony prominences of the upper extremity. **(a)** Anterior view. **(b)** Posterior view. (From Schuenke M, Schulte E, Schumacher U. THIEME Atlas of Anatomy. General Anatomy and Musculoskeletal System. Illustrations by Voll M and Wesker K. 3rd ed. New York: Thieme Medical Publishers; 2020.)

the lateral and posterior borders of the acromion meet. Palpation of the **coracoid process** is done best at the lateral side of the *delto-pectoral triangle*. The rounded portion of the shoulder is formed by the deltoid muscle and articulation of the humerus in the glenoid fossa. The most superior portion of the shoulder aligns with the **superior angle** of the scapula and this lies at approximately the T2 vertebral level. The medial most portion of the spine of the scapula is located at the T3 vertebral level and the **inferior angle** can be palpated at the level of the T7 vertebra. The inferior angle may be grasped when attempting to immobilize the scapula during movements at the glenohumeral joint.

With the arm partially abducted the **head of the humerus** may be palpated with the fingers thrust well into the examinee's *axillary fossa* or armpit. The **greater tubercle** of the humerus is the most lateral bony projection and can be palpated through the deltoid if the examinee's arm is at their side. In full abduction the greater tubercle is hidden beneath the acromion. The **lesser tubercle** is generally a difficult structure to identify but rotation of the arm may facilitate better access to it. The **shaft of the humerus** is identifiable at certain locations but the epicondyles are more clearly distinct during full extension and up to half extension/half flexion. The **medial epicondyle** is much more prominent than the **lateral epicondyle** and is palpable at any level of elbow flexion/extension.

The **olecranon** of the ulna is one of the most recognized bony features of the upper extremity and is commonly referred to as ones elbow. All levels of elbow joint movements still allow for identification of the olecranon. The **posterior border** and **styloid process of the ulna** are easily felt during a wide range of movements.

On the posterolateral portion of the extended elbow joint and just distal to the lateral epicondyle, the **head of the radius** can be palpated during supination and pronation movements. Within the area known as the *anatomical snuff box* on the lateral wrist region, the **styloid process of the radius** along with the *radial artery pulse* can be felt. The **dorsal tubercle of the radius** can be palpated and is the site of a common fracture known as a *Colles' fracture*.

In the hand, the **pisiform** is easily identified on the medial border of the wrist and on the anterior side. Deep pressure applied just distal and slightly lateral to the pisiform would help a person

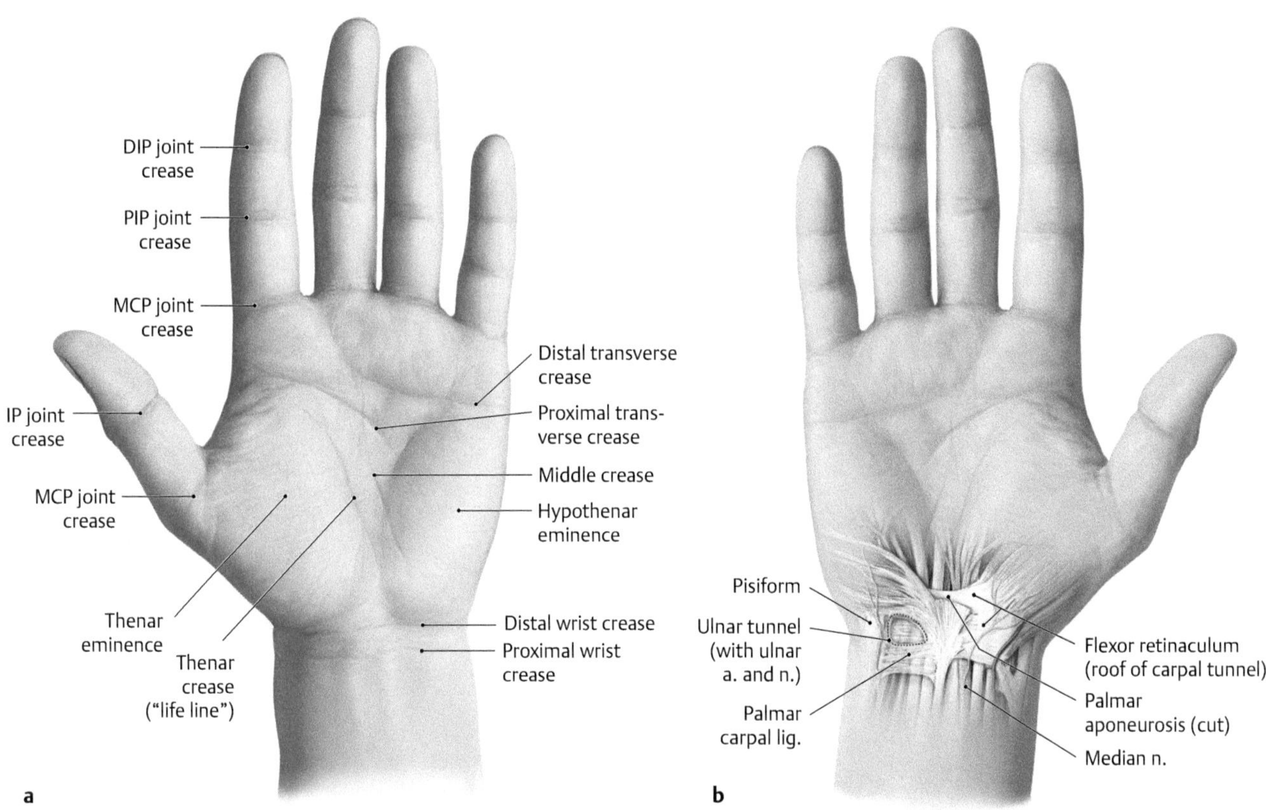

Fig. 6.9 (a, b) Surface anatomy of the wrist and hand. The locations of the carpal and ulnar tunnels are superimposed onto the image. (From Schuenke M, Schulte E, Schumacher U. THIEME Atlas of Anatomy. General Anatomy and Musculoskeletal System. Illustrations by Voll M and Wesker K. 3rd ed. New York: Thieme Medical Publishers; 2020.)

identify the **hook of the hamate**. On the lateral wrist region, the **scaphoid** and **trapezium tubercles** can be palpated on the anterior side just distal and medial to the styloid process of the radius. The **metacarpals** are easily palpable with their heads serving as the *knuckles*. On the posterior side near the wrist, the **styloid process of the 3rd metacarpal** is the most prominent projection in that area.

6.3 Fascia of the Upper Extremity

Located just below the skin is the **subcutaneous tissue** or **superficial fascia** that consists of loose connective tissue containing variable amounts of fat, cutaneous nerves, superficial veins, their tributaries and lymph nodes with corresponding lymphatic vessels similar to the lower extremities. This layer is pretty consistent in total depth except near the axillary fossa where there is generally an increase in the amount of fat.

A thicker **deep fascia** closely associated with the skeletal musculature can be observed extending from the clavicle and inferiorly down to the hands. Deep fascia limits the expansion of contracting muscles, making them more efficient while contracting, and this helps compress veins leading back to the heart. This fascia is continuous and named based on its location. It may be known as the *deltoid, pectoral, clavipectoral, axillary, brachial,* and *antebrachial fasciae*, along with the *dorsal* and *palmar fascia of the hand.*

The **deltoid fascia** passes from the clavicle and over the deltoid muscle to become continuous with the pectoral fascia anteriorly, brachial fascia distally, and the infraspinous fascia posteriorly (**Fig. 6.10**). The muscles adjacent to the scapula are covered by deep fascia and create the supraspinous, infraspinous and subscapular compartments. The **supraspinous** and **infraspinous fasciae** are fairly thick.

The **pectoral fascia** is connected to the clavicle and sternum and is continuous with the deltoid, axillary and anterior abdominal wall fasciae. It invests the pectoralis major muscle and it is at the lateral border of the pectoralis major that it becomes the axillary fascia. The **axillary fascia** forms the floor of the axilla. The **clavipectoral fascia** extends down from the subclavius muscle before investing the pectoralis minor muscle. This fascia continues inferiorly form the pectoralis minor muscle to the axillary fascia. The connection between the subclavius and pectoralis minor muscle is referred to as the **costocoracoid membrane** and the *lateral pectoral nerve* and *thoracoacromial arterial trunk* pierces it. The connection between the pectoralis minor muscle and the axillary fascia is called the **suspensory ligament of the axilla (Fig. 6.11)**.

The **brachial fascia** invests both the anterior and posterior parts of the brachium or arm. It is continuous with the pectoral, deltoid, axillary and infraspinous fascias. It attaches to both epicondyles of the humerus as well as the olecranon of the ulna before continuing as the antebrachial fascia of the forearm. The brachial fascia forms a **lateral** and **medial intermuscular septum** that extends to the central shaft and the lateral and medial supracondylar ridges to create the **anterior (flexor)** and **posterior (extensor) arm compartments (Fig. 6.10; Fig. 6.12)**.

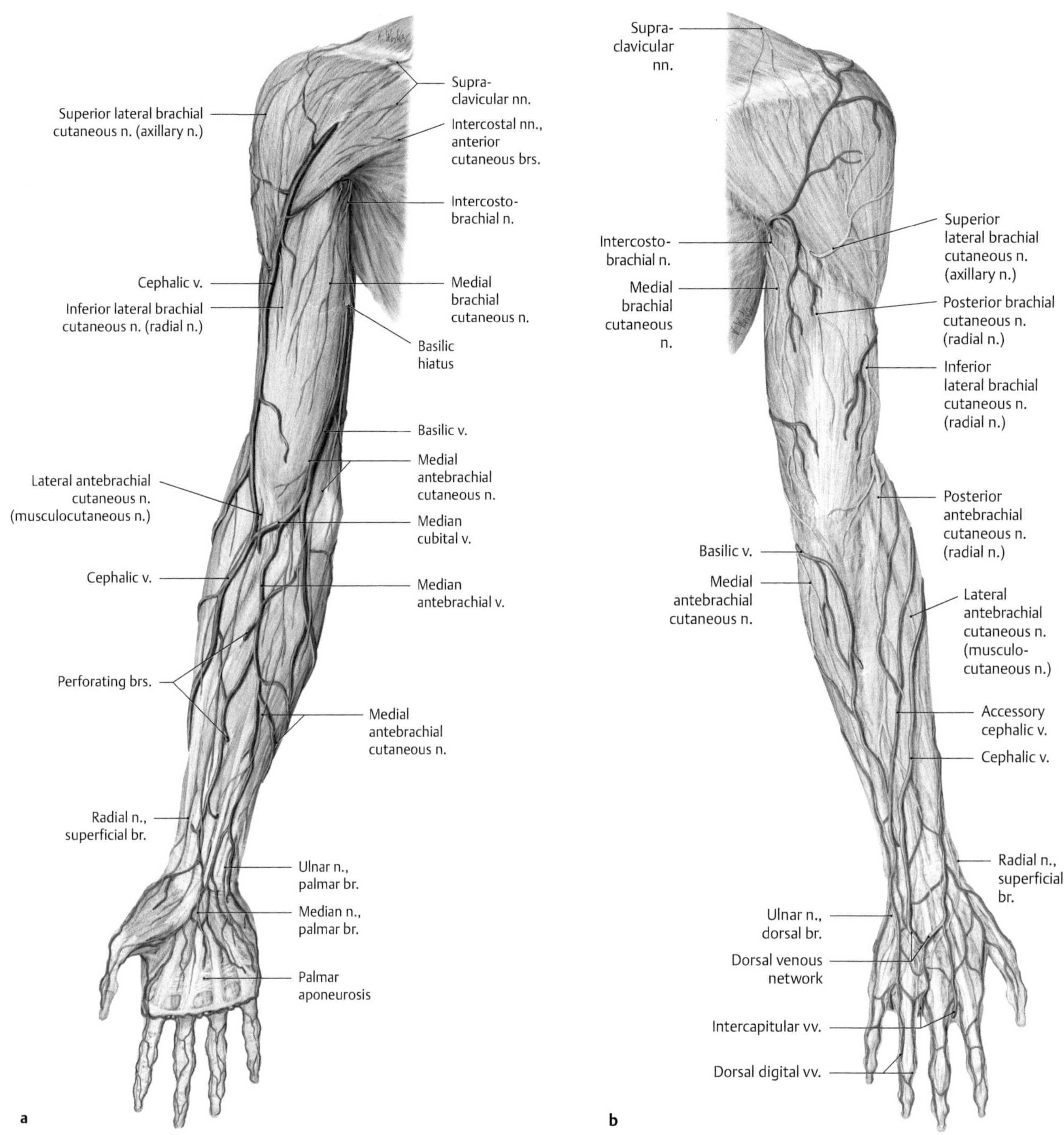

Fig. 6.10 Fascia and superficial cutaneous veins and nerves of the right upper extremity. **(a)** Anterior view. **(b)** Posterior view. (From Schuenke M, Schulte E, Schumacher U. THIEME Atlas of Anatomy. General Anatomy and Musculoskeletal System. Illustrations by Voll M and Wesker K. 3rd ed. New York: Thieme Medical Publishers; 2020.)

The **antebrachial (forearm) fascia** extends deep to the radius and ulna, and, along with the **interosseous membrane** that connects both these bones, creates the main anterior and posterior forearm compartments. The antebrachial fascia continues and thickens at the wrist as the **flexor** and **extensor retinaculum**, and also as the palmar carpal ligament anteriorly. The **palmar carpal ligament** is sometimes confused with the flexor retinaculum, but the **flexor retinaculum** (or **transverse carpal ligament**) in fact lies just deep to the palmar aponeurosis of the hand. It is not easily seen but it helps enclose the clinically significant *carpal tunnel* **(Fig. 6.10; Fig. 6.13)**.

From the extensor retinaculum, the deep fascia continues as the **dorsal fascia of the hand**. From the palmar carpal ligament and flexor retinaculum, the deep fascia continues as the **palmar fascia of the hand**. The **palmar aponeurosis** is part of this palmar fascia and is continuous with the palmaris longus muscle tendon. There are four distinct condensations of this aponeurosis that mirror digits 2-5 and extend to the bases of the

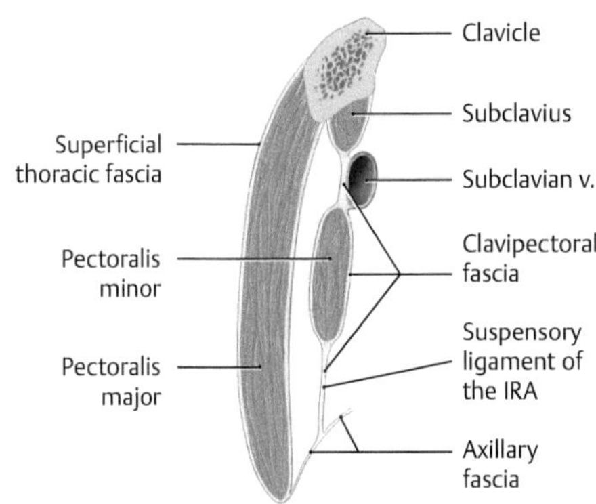

Fig. 6.11 Anterior right shoulder: sagittal section through anterior wall. (From Schuenke M, Schulte E, Schumacher U. THIEME Atlas of Anatomy. General Anatomy and Musculoskeletal System. Illustrations by Voll M and Wesker K. 3rd ed. New York: Thieme Medical Publishers; 2020.)

fingers before becoming continuous with the fibrous tendon sheaths of the digits. The **superficial transverse metacarpal ligament** traverses the four condensations at the level of the metacarpophalangeal joints or knuckles. Located between the skin and aponeurosis are very small *skin ligaments* that keep the skin close to the aponeurosis thus allowing only minimal sliding movements between these two structures (**Fig. 6.10; Fig. 6.14**).

6.4 Neurovasculature of the Upper Extremity

6.4.1 Nerves of the Upper Extremity

The nerves that innervate the upper extremity originate from the *brachial plexus* (ventral rami of C5-T1) located mainly in the posterior triangle of the neck and axilla regions (**Fig. 6.15**). One of the muscles receives innervation by way of the spinal accessory (XI) cranial nerve. Like all somatic nerve plexuses the functional components of their nerves are GSE, GSA and GVE-sym/post unless it is a cutaneous nerve, in which case it only has GSA and GVE-sym/post fibers. The brachial plexus is a somatic nerve plexus and the nerves entering the shoulder region and down into the rest of the upper extremity provide:

- Motor innervation to the muscles.
- Sensory innervation from the skin, muscles and joints.
- Sympathetic innervation to the blood vessels and sweat glands.

The brachial plexus is made up of *roots, trunks, divisions, cords* and *terminal branches* that are detailed in their entirety later in the *Axilla* portion of this chapter. Individual branches that participate in the innervation of both muscles and skin include:

- The **dorsal scapular nerve** (C5, possibly some C4) innervates both the levator scapulae and rhomboid muscles.
- The **long thoracic nerve** (C5-C7) innervates the serratus anterior muscle.
- The **suprascapular nerve** (C5-C6, possibly some C4) innervates the supraspinatus and infraspinatus muscles along with the glenohumeral joint of the shoulder.
- The **nerve to subclavius** (C5-C6) or the *subclavian nerve* by some authors innervates the subclavius muscle.
- The **lateral pectoral nerve** (C5-C7) innervates a portion of the pectoralis major muscle.
- The **medial pectoral nerve** (C8-T1) innervates all of the pectoralis minor muscle before contributing to a portion of the pectoralis major muscle.
- The **medial brachial cutaneous nerve** (T1) or the *medical cutaneous nerve of the arm* supplies the skin over the medial side of the arm.
- The **medical antebrachial cutaneous nerve** (C8-T1) or the *medial cutaneous nerve of the forearm* supplies the skin over the medial side of the forearm.
- The **upper subscapular nerve** (C5-C6) innervates a portion of the subscapularis muscle.
- The **thoracodorsal nerve** (C6-C8) innervates the latissimus dorsi muscle.
- The **lower subscapular nerve** (C5-C6) innervates a portion of the subscapularis muscle and all of the teres major muscle.
- The **musculocutaneous nerve** (C5-C7) innervates the biceps brachii, coracobrachialis and brachialis muscles. It has a cutaneous branch listed below.
- The **median nerve** (C5-T1) innervates all muscles of the anterior forearm except for the flexor carpi ulnaris and the medial part of the flexor digitorum profundus; and the flexor pollicis brevis, abductor pollicis brevis, opponens pollicis and the two-most lateral lumbricals in the hand. It has multiple cutaneous branches listed below.
- The **axillary nerve** (C5-C6) innervates the deltoid and teres minor muscles along with the glenohumeral joint of the shoulder. It has a cutaneous branch listed below.
- The **radial nerve** (C5-T1) innervates all muscles of the posterior arm and forearm. It has multiple cutaneous branches listed below.
- The **ulnar nerve** (C8-T1) innervates the flexor carpi ulnaris and medial part of flexor digitorum profundus in the anterior forearm; most intrinsic and two-most medial lumbricals of the hand. The multiple cutaneous branches are listed below.

6.4.2 Cutaneous Nerve Innervation of the Upper Extremity

In addition to some of the nerves listed as direct branches of the larger brachial plexus, the *supraclavicular, intercostobrachial, superior lateral brachial, posterior brachial, posterior antebrachial, superficial radial, lateral antebrachial,* the *palmar, common palmar digital* and *proper palmar digital* of median, the *palmar, dorsal* and *superficial branch* of ulnar all lie within the subcutaneous tissue and supply specific parts of the upper extremity skin (**Fig. 6.16**).

- The **supraclavicular nerves** (C3-C4) originate from the cervical plexus to supply skin over the neck but it overlaps onto the upper pectoral and shoulder regions.
- The **intercostobrachial nerve** (T2-T3) originates from the 2nd and 3rd intercostal nerves and supplies a small section of the skin over the upper medial arm.
- The **superior lateral brachial cutaneous nerve** (C5-C6) is a branch of the axillary nerve and supplies skin overlying the majority of the deltoid muscle.
- The **posterior brachial cutaneous nerve** (C5-C8) is a branch of the radial nerve and supplies a portion of the posterior arm.

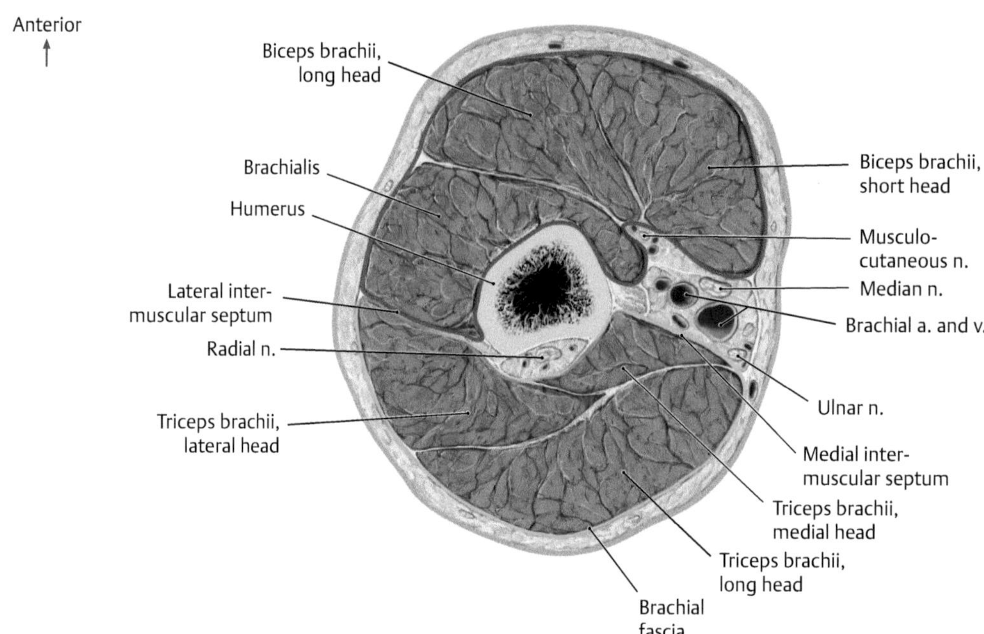

Fig. 6.12 Compartments of the arm. (From Schuenke M, Schulte E, Schumacher U. THIEME Atlas of Anatomy. General Anatomy and Musculoskeletal System. Illustrations by Voll M and Wesker K. 3rd ed. New York: Thieme Medical Publishers; 2020.)

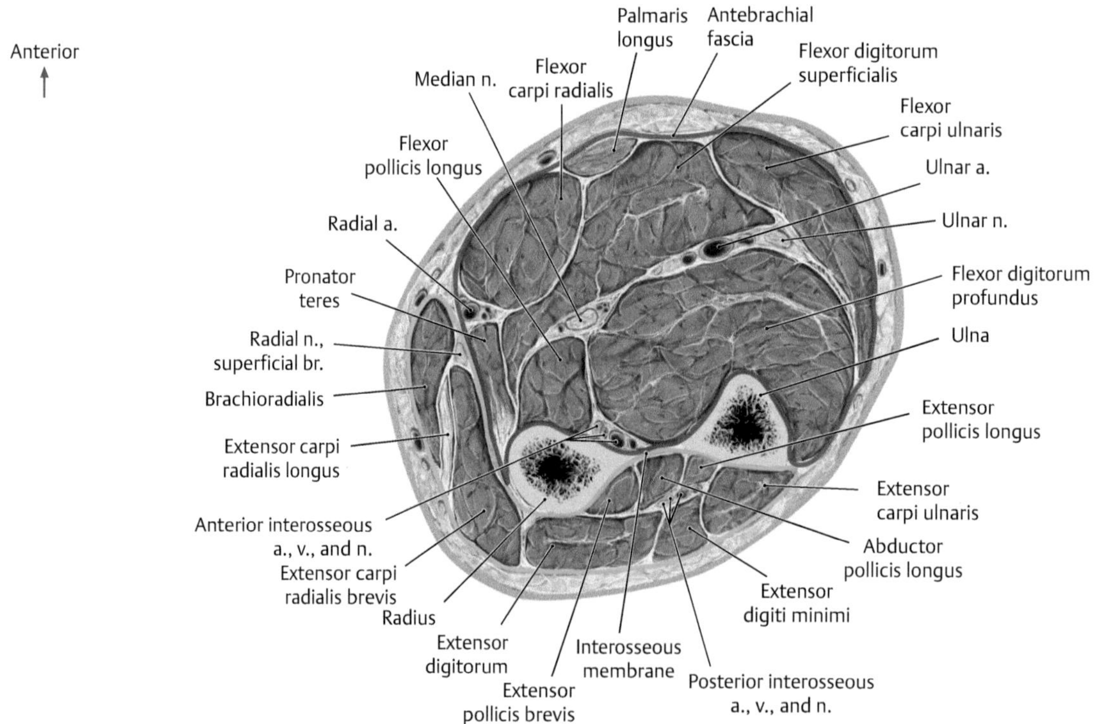

Fig. 6.13 Compartments of the forearm. (From Schuenke M, Schulte E, Schumacher U. THIEME Atlas of Anatomy. General Anatomy and Musculoskeletal System. Illustrations by Voll M and Wesker K. 3rd ed. New York: Thieme Medical Publishers; 2020.)

The **inferior lateral brachial cutaneous nerve** (also a radial nerve branch) may accompany it or originate from it.

- The **posterior antebrachial cutaneous nerve** (C5-C8) is a branch of the radial nerve and supplies the posterolateral forearm.
- The **superficial branch of radial nerve** (C6-C8) is one of the bifurcating branches of the larger radial nerve. It passes deep to the brachioradialis muscle in the forearm but only innervates skin over the dorsum hand, wrist, and thumb.

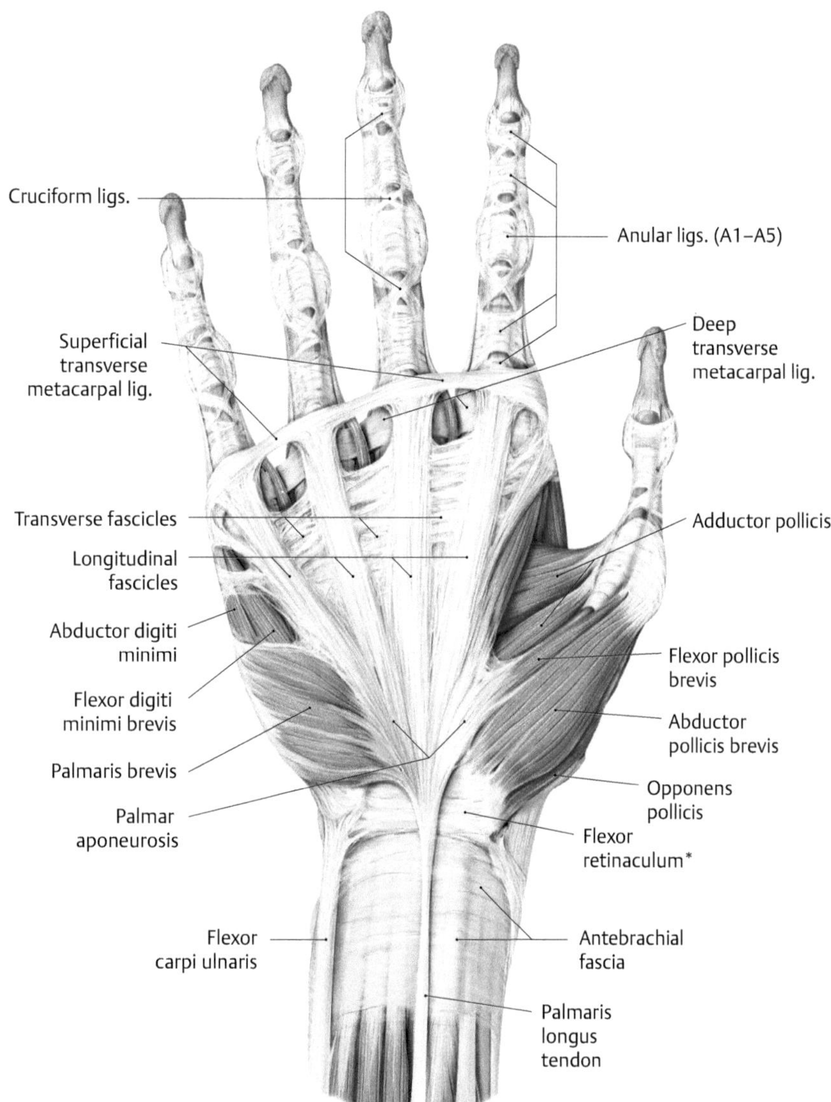

Fig. 6.14 Fascia of the hand. Right hand, palmar surface. *Also known as transverse carpal ligament. (From Schuenke M, Schulte E, Schumacher U. THIEME Atlas of Anatomy. General Anatomy and Musculoskeletal System. Illustrations by Voll M and Wesker K. 3rd ed. New York: Thieme Medical Publishers; 2020.)

- The **lateral antebrachial cutaneous nerve** (C6-C7) is the continuation of the musculocutaneous nerve at the elbow and supplies the lateral forearm.
- The **palmar branch of median** (C6-C8) supplies a small section of skin on the distal lateral forearm adjacent to the wrist as well as the central palm.
- The **common palmar digital** and **proper palmar digital nerves** (C6-C8) of the median nerve supply the central palm, majority of the 1st – 3rd digits and the lateral half of the 4th digit. The **dorsal digital nerves** of the median nerve supply the dorsum of the 1st – 3rd and lateral half of the 4th digit.
- The **palmar branch of ulnar** (C8-T1) supplies a small section of skin on the distal medial forearm adjacent to the wrist as well as the base of the medial palm.
- The **dorsal branch of ulnar nerve** (C8-T1) continues as the **dorsal digital nerves.** They supply the skin over the distal and medial wrist, dorsum of hand adjacent to digits 4-5, and the majority of dorsal skin over the 4th and 5th digits.
- The **superficial branch of ulnar nerve** (C8-T1) gives off **common palmar digital** and **proper palmar digital** branches that supply skin on the palmar side associated with the medial 4th and all of the 5th digits.

6.4.3 Dermatomes and Myotomes of the Upper Extremity

The areas of skin supplied by the C4-T1 spinal nerves contribute to the upper extremity **dermatomes (Fig. 6.17)**. Much like the lower extremity, there is an overlap with the next adjacent dermatome except at the **axial line**, a line that demarcates a junction of dermatomes that are supplied by discontinuous spinal levels. An axial line is located anteriorly separating the C5 and C6 from the T1 dermatome. On the posterior side, the axial line is separating the C4-C6 from the T1 and T2 dermatomes. Note: the axial line may vary depending on the specific dermatome map.

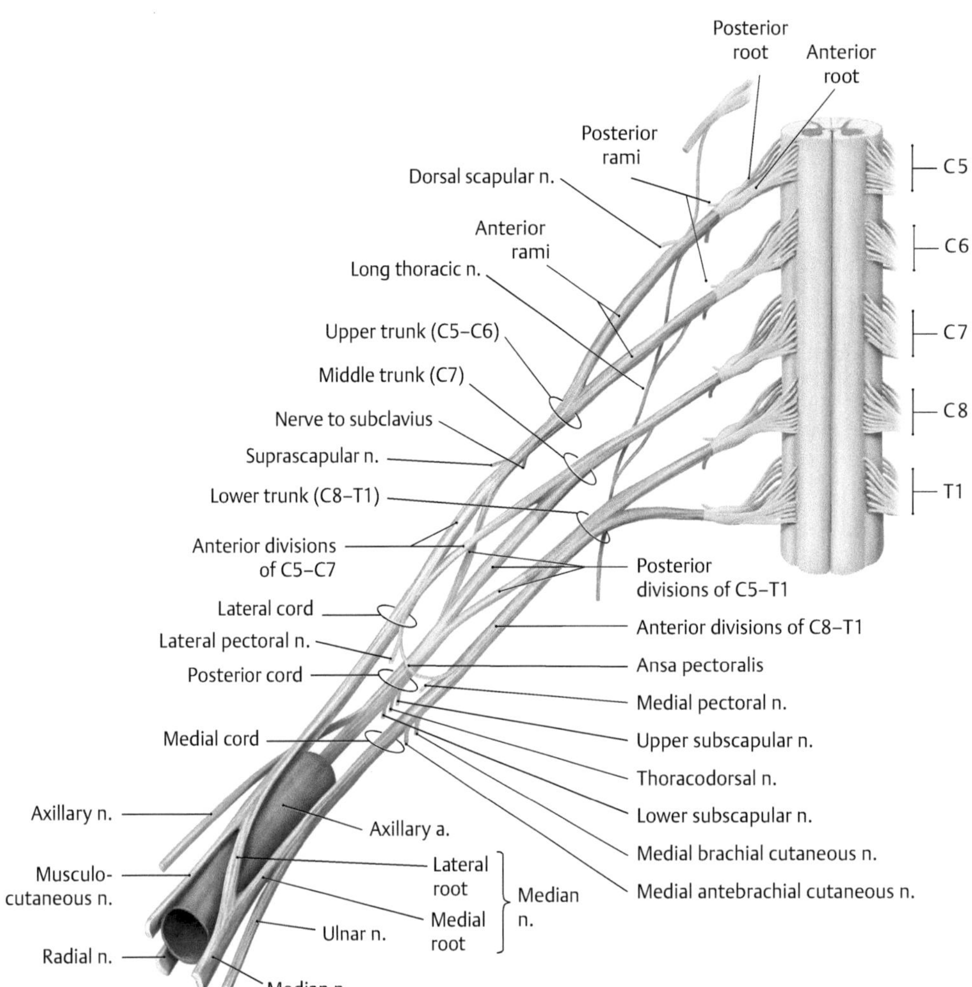

Fig. 6.15 Nerves of the upper extremity and brachial plexus. (From Schuenke M, Schulte E, Schumacher U. THIEME Atlas of Anatomy. General Anatomy and Musculoskeletal System. Illustrations by Voll M and Wesker K. 3rd ed. New York: Thieme Medical Publishers; 2020.)

Somatic motor (GSE) fibers traveling through mixed peripheral nerves are responsible for innervating the muscles of the upper extremities. The ipsilateral and embryological muscle group that receives innervation from a single spinal cord segment or spinal nerve constitutes a **myotome**. Upper extremity muscles may not be as bulky and extensive as the lower extremity but they still generally receive motor fibers from several spinal cord segments or nerves. Much like the lower extremity, the upper extremity muscles are usually composed of multiple myotomes. The segmental innervation and the movements of the upper extremity they assist with are as follows (**Fig. 6.18**):

- Abduction, flexion and lateral (external) rotation at glenohumeral joint: C5.
- Adduction, extension and medial (internal) rotation at glenohumeral joint: C6-C8.
- Flexion at elbow joint: C5-C6.
- Extension at elbow joint: C6, C7.
- Supination of forearm at radioulnar joints: C6.
- Pronation of forearm at radioulnar joints: C7-C8.
- Flexion at wrist joint: C6-C7.
- Extension at wrist joint: C6-C7.
- Flexion and extension of digits by forearm muscles: C7-C8.
- Intrinsic muscles of hand: C8-T1.

6.4.4 Blood Supply of the Upper Extremity

There are two major arteries and their branches that are responsible for distributing blood to the soft tissue and muscles related to the upper extremities. They are the *subclavian* and *axillary arteries* (**Fig. 6.19; Fig. 6.20; Fig. 6.21**).

The **subclavian artery** originates from the *aortic arch* on the left side but from the bifurcation of the *brachiocephalic trunk* on the right side. The subclavian artery on both sides is divided into three parts with the first two having branches. Details of the subclavian artery are described in Chapter 7. However, the second part has multiple branches and its thyrocervical trunk has 3-4 branches of itself. One of these branches is called the **suprascapular artery** and it passes posterolaterally toward the scapula and over the *superior transverse ligament of the scapula*. Another branch from this trunk is called the **transverse cervical artery** (or cervicodorsal) and it has two branches called the **superficial cervical** and **dorsal scapular arteries**. The dorsal scapular in a minority of individuals may originate from the 3rd part of the subclavian artery (**Fig. 6.20**).

At the lateral border of the first rib, the subclavian artery becomes the **axillary artery**. The axillary artery has three parts that are defined by the pectoralis minor muscle. The *first part*

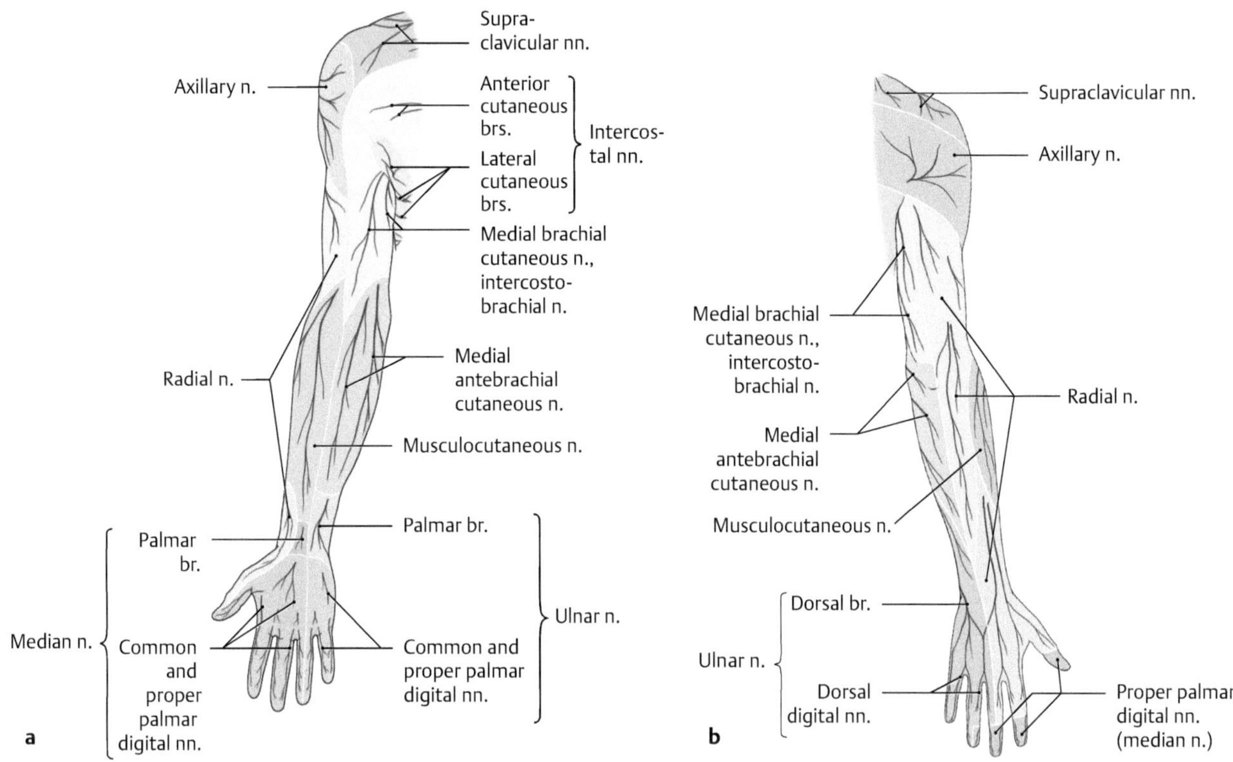

Fig. 6.16 Cutaneous innervation of the upper extremity. **(a)** Anterior view. **(b)** Posterior view. (From Schuenke M, Schulte E, Schumacher U. THIEME Atlas of Anatomy. General Anatomy and Musculoskeletal System. Illustrations by Voll M and Wesker K. 3rd ed. New York: Thieme Medical Publishers; 2020.)

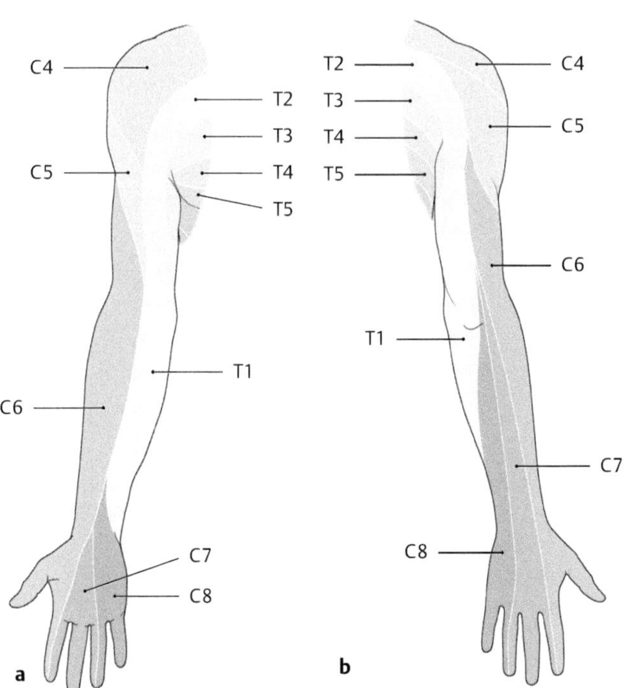

Fig. 6.17 Dermatomes of the upper extremity. **(a)** Anterior view. **(b)** Posterior view. (From Schuenke M, Schulte E, Schumacher U. THIEME Atlas of Anatomy. General Anatomy and Musculoskeletal System. Illustrations by Voll M and Wesker K. 3rd ed. New York: Thieme Medical Publishers; 2020.)

lies between the lateral border of the 1st rib and lateral border of pectoralis minor and has one branch (*superior thoracic*); the *second part* is located posterior to the pectoralis minor and has two branches (*thoracoacromial trunk* and *lateral thoracic*); and the *third part* is located between the lateral border of pectoralis minor and the inferior border of the teres major muscles and has three branches (*subscapular*, *anterior*, and *posterior circumflex humeral*) **(Fig. 6.19; Fig. 6.20)**

At the inferior border of the teres major muscle, the axillary artery becomes the **brachial artery**. The **profunda brachii** (deep artery of the arm) branches of the brachial artery are just distal to the teres major muscle. The brachial artery continues posteroinferiorly toward the elbow and terminates as the **middle** and **radial collateral arteries.** At the mid-humeral area and medially, a **superior ulnar collateral artery** is given off and just distal to that an **inferior ulnar collateral artery** branches off the brachial artery. These two arteries form an anastomosis with the *posterior* and *anterior ulnar recurrent arteries* respectively, while in the *cubital fossa* the brachial artery bifurcates into the radial and ulnar arteries (**Fig. 6.19; Fig. 6.21**).

The **radial artery** is located laterally on the forearm and almost immediately branches off the **recurrent radial artery** that forms an anastomosis with the radial collateral artery. The radial artery continues toward the wrist and hand before giving off the **dorsal carpal** and **princeps pollicis arteries** and a small contribution to the *superficial palmar arch* before becoming the *deep palmar arch*. The **ulnar artery** is on the medial side of the forearm and very quickly the **anterior** and **posterior ulnar recurrent arteries** along with the **common interosseous artery** branch from it. The common interosseous artery is short but when it lies just adjacent

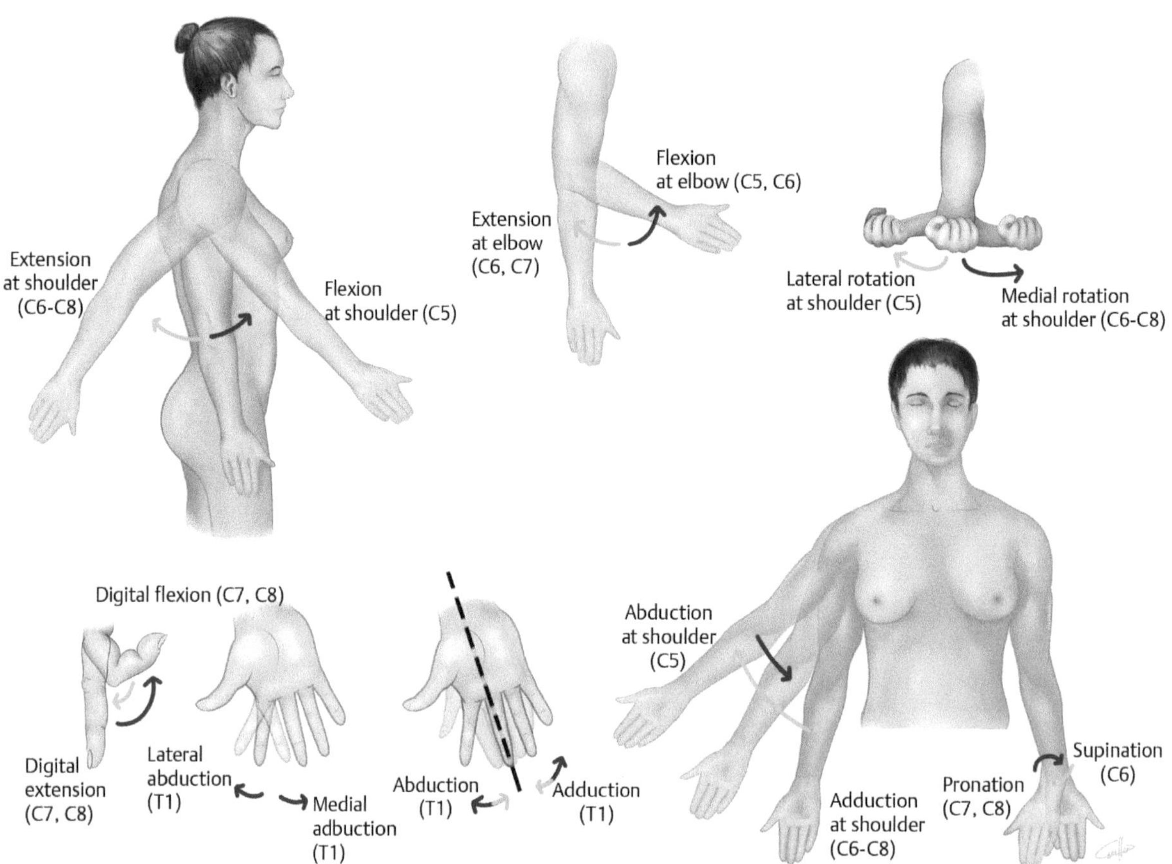

Fig. 6.18 Myotomes: segmental innervation of muscle groups. Illustration by Calla Heald.

to the interosseous membrane it bifurcates into an **anterior** and **posterior interosseous artery**. The ulnar artery continues toward the hand before it branches off a small contribution to the *deep palmar arch* and then it terminates as the *superficial palmar arch*. The radial, anterior interosseous, ulnar and posterior interosseous arteries all contribute to the **palmar** and **dorsal carpal network (arches)** of arteries that supply blood adjacent to the carpal bones **(Fig. 6.19; Fig. 6.22)**.

The **superficial palmar arch** branches off multiple **common palmar digital arteries** that then become the **proper palmar digital arteries**. The deep palmar arch has **palmar metacarpal artery** branches that form an anastomosis with the common palmar digital arteries. The **dorsal carpal arch** has **dorsal metacarpal arteries** extending out from it and they eventually become the **dorsal digital arteries**. The 1st digit (thumb) and 2nd digit (index finger) have individual arteries specified to them. The **princeps pollicis** and **dorsalis pollicis arteries** specifically target the thumb while the **radialis indicis** and **dorsalis indicis arteries** help supply the index finger **(Fig. 6.22)**.

6.4.5 Venous Drainage of the Upper Extremity

Similar to the lower extremity there are both superficial and deep veins that are responsible for draining blood back to the heart from the limb. The **perforating veins** form communications between the superficial and deep veins similar to the lower extremity. The *superficial veins* course through the subcutaneous tissue located between the skin and deep fascia. Many of the superficial veins are unnamed but the major ones originate from the **dorsal venous network** of the hand to become the *basilic* and *cephalic veins* and are described below **(Fig. 6.23a; Fig. 6.24; Fig. 6.25)**.

- The **basilic vein** is located on the medial side of the forearm and arm before uniting with the *brachial veins* to become the *axillary vein* at the inferior border of the teres major muscle. In the arm, it pierces the brachial fascia at the **basilic hiatus** and lies near the brachial veins prior to forming the axillary vein. It is paired with the *medial antebrachial cutaneous nerve (medial cutaneous of the forearm)* for much of its course.
- The **cephalic vein** is located on the lateral side of the forearm and arm. Near the elbow it is connected to the highly variable vein **median cubital vein** that passes obliquely across the *cubital fossa* before draining into the basilic vein. While still in the forearm, the cephalic vein is paired with the *lateral antebrachial nerve (lateral cutaneous nerve of the forearm)*. At the level of the arm, this vein passes between the deltoid and pectoralis major muscles in the **deltopectoral groove** before entering the **clavipectoral triangle**.
- The **median antebrachial vein** is another highly variable superficial vein but if it is present it begins at the base of the dorsum side of the thumb before curving around the lateral side of the wrist and ascending across the middle of the anterior forearm between the basilic and cephalic veins. It may form the intermediate **median basilic** and/or **median**

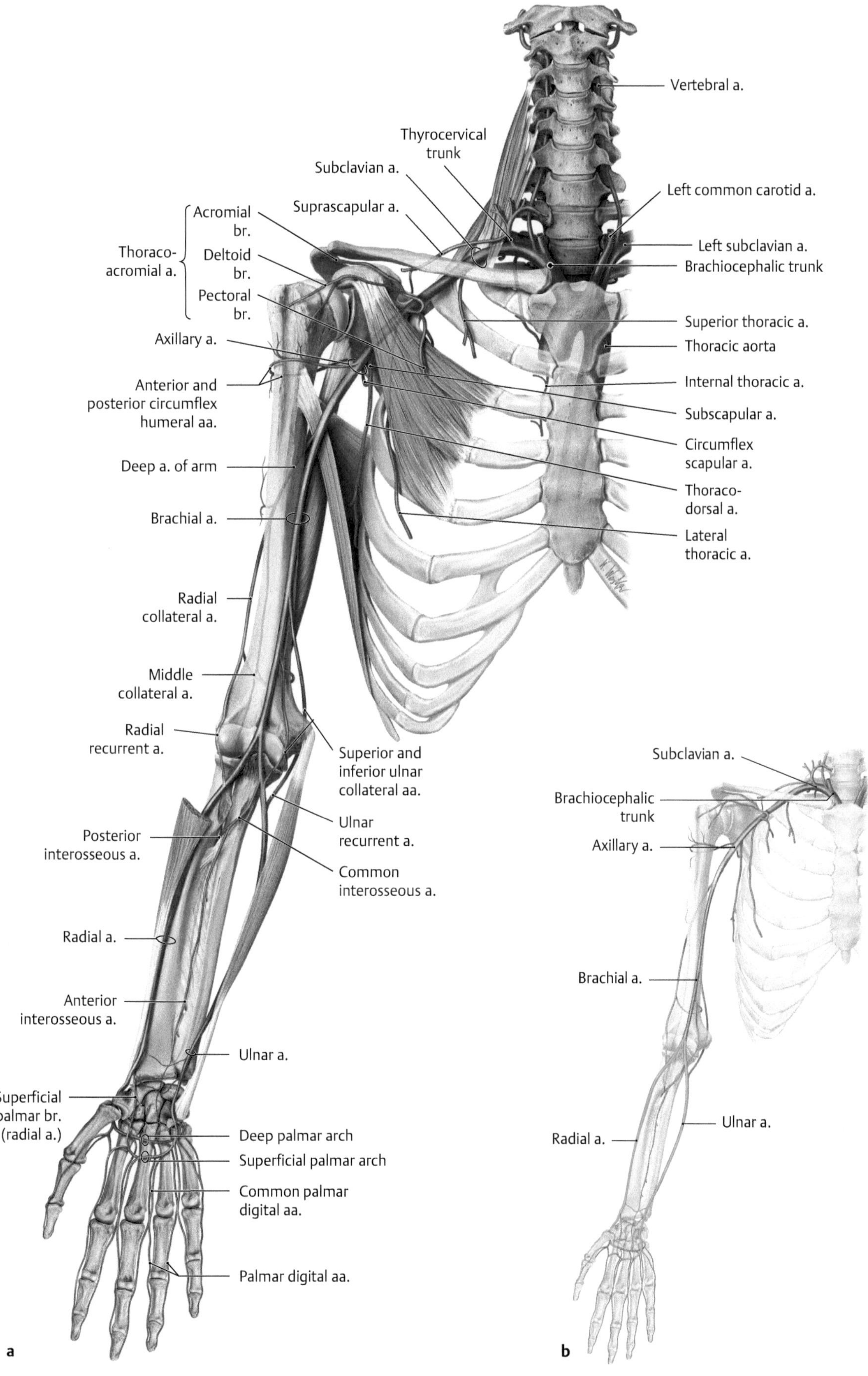

Fig. 6.19 (a, b) Arteries of the upper extremity. (From Schuenke M, Schulte E, Schumacher U. THIEME Atlas of Anatomy. General Anatomy and Musculoskeletal System. Illustrations by Voll M and Wesker K. 3rd ed. New York: Thieme Medical Publishers; 2020.)

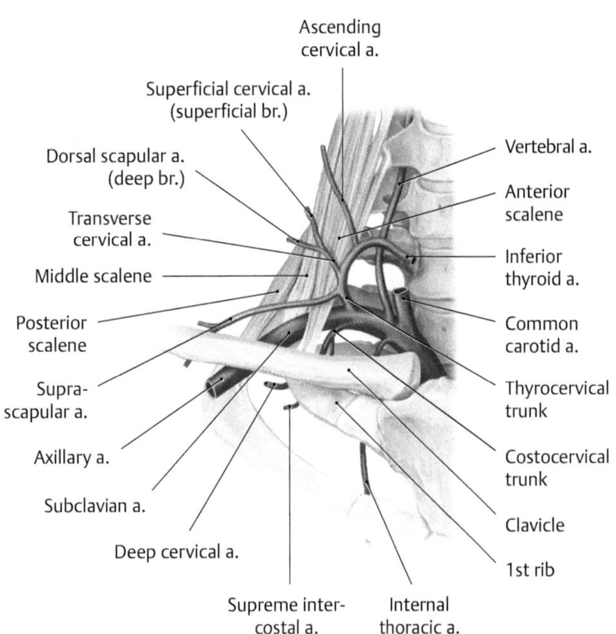

Fig. 6.20 Branches of the subclavian artery, right side, anterior view. (From Schuenke M, Schulte E, Schumacher U. THIEME Atlas of Anatomy. General Anatomy and Musculoskeletal System. Illustrations by Voll M and Wesker K. 3rd ed. New York: Thieme Medical Publishers; 2020.)

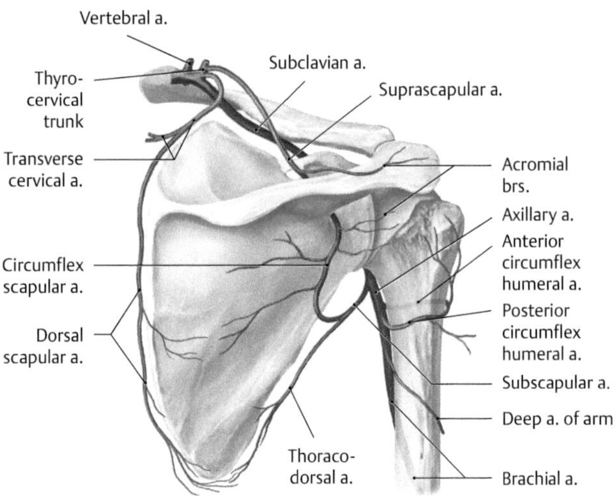

Fig. 6.21 Scapular arcade, right side, posterior view. (From Schuenke M, Schulte E, Schumacher U. THIEME Atlas of Anatomy. General Anatomy and Musculoskeletal System. Illustrations by Voll M and Wesker K. 3rd ed. New York: Thieme Medical Publishers; 2020.)

cephalic vein before draining into the basilic and/or cephalic vein respectively.

The *deep veins* are located below the deep fascia and are paired with the arteries. There are two smaller veins paired with only one larger artery. Beginning with the hand region, the **dorsal digital veins** unite with the **dorsal metacarpal veins** before these veins become the **dorsal venous network**. The **proper palmar digital veins** drain into the **common palmar digital (palmar metacarpal) veins**. Blood from these veins may enter either the **superficial venous palmar arch** or **deep venous palmar arch**. Venous drainage from these arches continues through deep veins of the forearm such as the radial, ulnar and anterior interosseous (**Fig. 6.23b**).

From the dorsal venous network or dorsal carpal veins, the **posterior interosseous veins** ascend before reaching another network of veins associated with the elbow region. The radial and ulnar veins may have smaller tributaries that originate from this venous network as well. However, the majority of the **radial** and **ulnar veins** originate from the deep and superficial venous palmar arches. The venous drainage is similar to the blood supply where

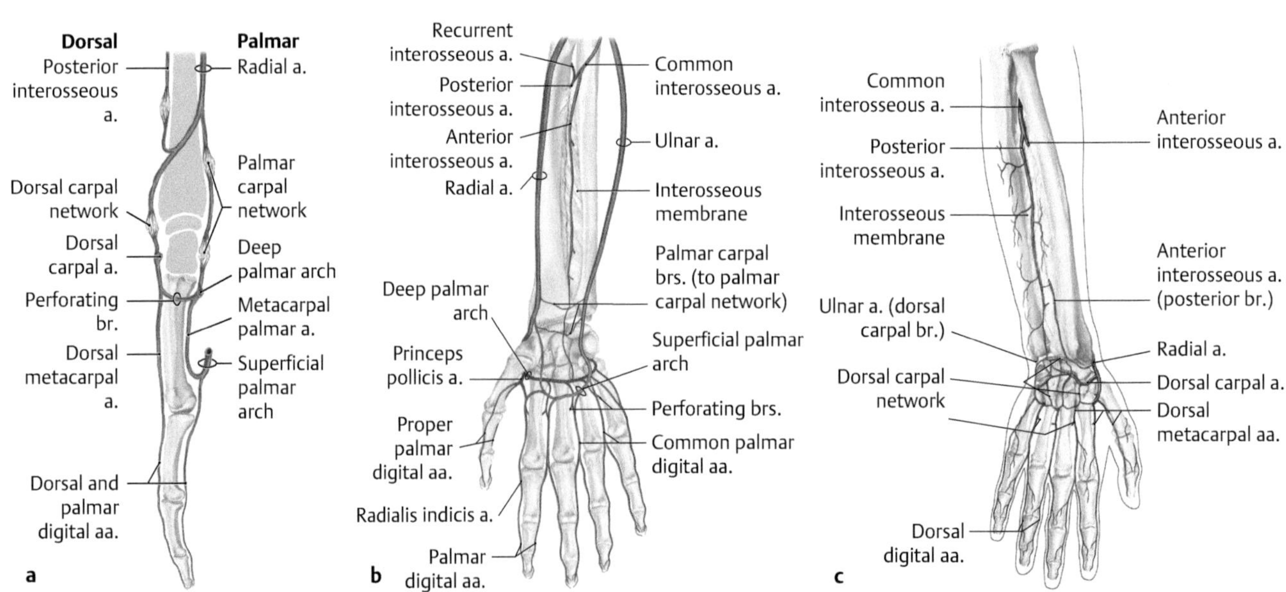

Fig. 6.22 Arteries of the forearm and hand: **(a)** Right middle finger, lateral view. **(b)** Anterior (palmar) view. **(c)** Posterior (dorsal) view. (From Schuenke M, Schulte E, Schumacher U. THIEME Atlas of Anatomy. General Anatomy and Musculoskeletal System. Illustrations by Voll M and Wesker K. 3rd ed. New York: Thieme Medical Publishers; 2020.)

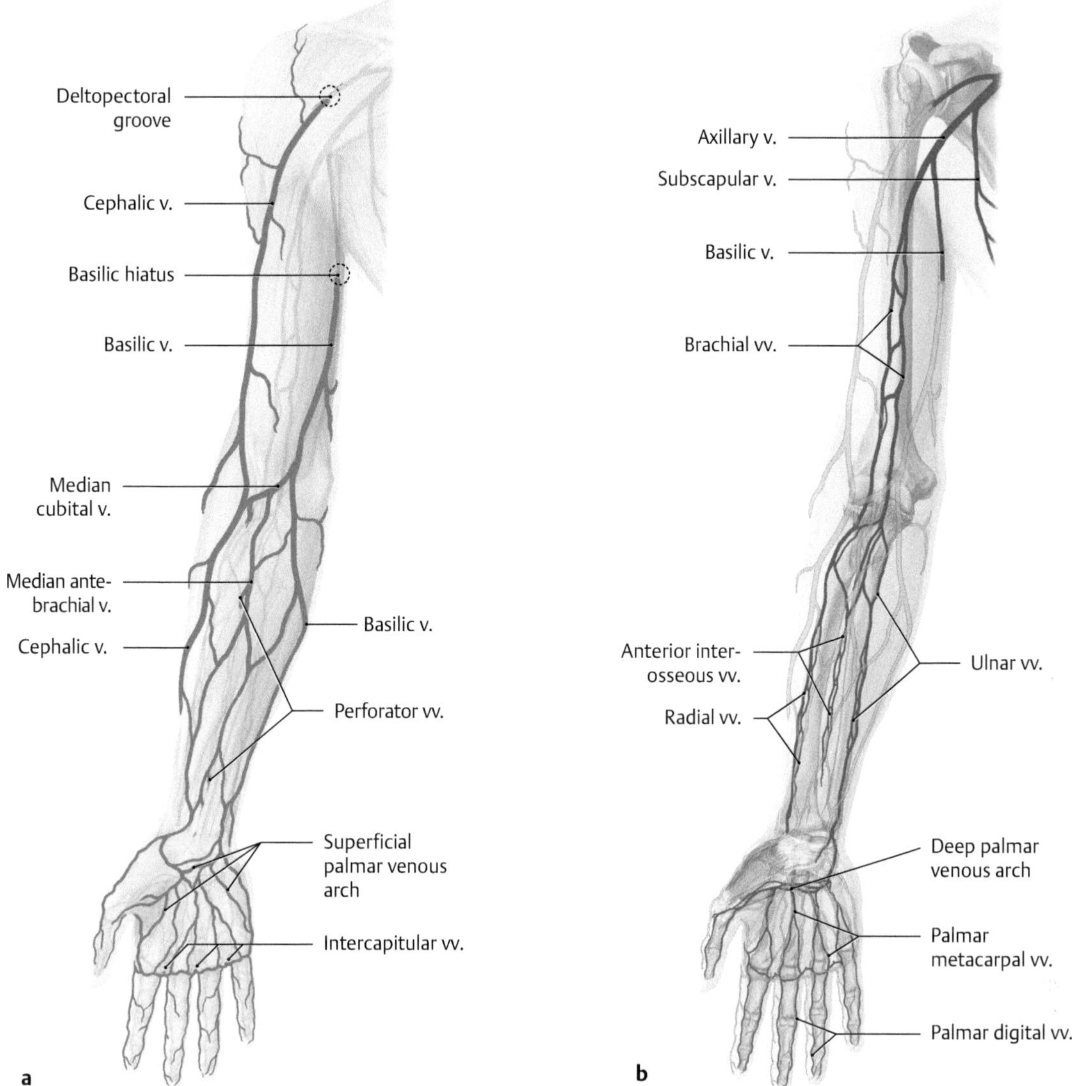

Fig. 6.23 Veins of the upper limb. Right extremity, anterior view. **(a)** Superficial veins. **(b)** Deep veins. (From Schuenke M, Schulte E, Schumacher U. THIEME Atlas of Anatomy. General Anatomy and Musculoskeletal System. Illustrations by Voll M and Wesker K. 3rd ed. New York: Thieme Medical Publishers; 2020.)

the radial vein is associated most with the deep venous palmar arch and the ulnar vein primarily drains the superficial venous palmar arch. The **anterior interosseous veins** may also receive blood from the deep and superficial palmar arches before coursing through the anterior forearm to reach the elbow venous drainage (**Fig. 6.23b**).

The radial, ulnar, anterior and posterior interosseous veins eventually reach the elbow region where they drain into a multitude of veins including the **radial recurrent**, **anterior** and **posterior ulnar recurrent**, **superior** and **inferior ulnar collateral**, **brachial** and **profunda brachii veins**.

The deeper structures of the arm are drained by the **brachial** and **profunda brachii veins** (deep vein of the arm). The profunda brachii eventually drains into the brachial vein before the brachial along with the basilic vein merge to form the axillary vein (**Fig. 6.23b**).

6.4.6 Lymphatic Drainage of the Upper Extremity

The lymphatic drainage of the upper extremity has both a superficial and deep drainage pattern (**Fig. 6.26; Fig. 6.27**). The superficial lymph drainage mirrors the superficial venous drainage, especially the major veins located in this region such as the basilic and cephalic veins. They are more numerous than their deep lymphatic drainage counterparts.

Lymph drainage from the medial hand and forearm that lie adjacent to the basilic vein may drain into the **cubital lymph nodes** before continuing to the **humeral (lateral) axillary lymph nodes**. Lymph drainage associated with more the lateral hand, forearm and arm travel closest to the cephalic vein and pass over the anterior shoulder region before primarily reaching the **apical axillary lymph nodes**.

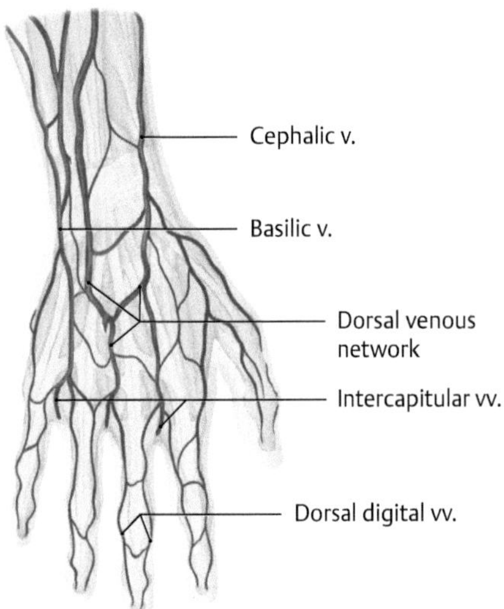

Fig. 6.24 Veins of the dorsum hand, right hand, posterior view. (From Schuenke M, Schulte E, Schumacher U. THIEME Atlas of Anatomy. General Anatomy and Musculoskeletal System. Illustrations by Voll M and Wesker K. 3rd ed. New York: Thieme Medical Publishers; 2020.)

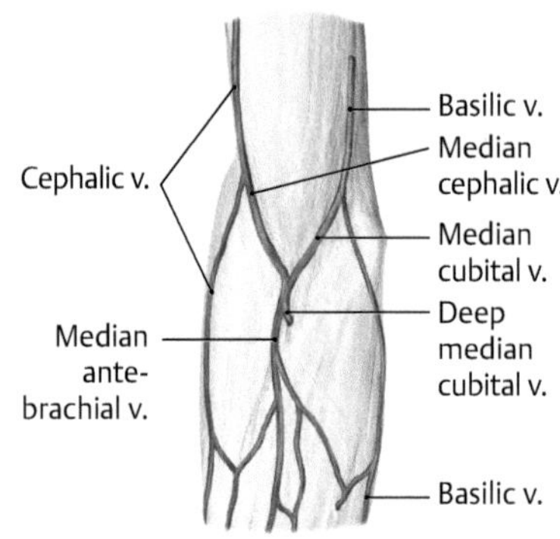

Fig. 6.25 Veins of the cubital fossa, right limb, anterior view. (From Schuenke M, Schulte E, Schumacher U. THIEME Atlas of Anatomy. General Anatomy and Musculoskeletal System. Illustrations by Voll M and Wesker K. 3rd ed. New York: Thieme Medical Publishers; 2020.)

The deep lymphatic drainage follows the deeper veins such as the radial, ulnar and brachial before primarily draining into the humeral (lateral) axillary lymph nodes. It is important to note that there are numerous anastomoses that exist between the superficial and deep lymphatic systems. Lymph progresses through the axillary lymph node system before following the *clavicular* and *subclavian* lymph nodes and trunks. Eventually lymph reaches the *thoracic duct* on the left side and the *right lymphatic duct* on the right side. These ducts are mostly found draining near the venous angles created by the junction of the internal jugular and subclavian veins. Details of axillary lymph nodes and beyond are discussed in the *Axilla* section of this chapter.

6.5 Upper Extremity Region Specifics

The upper extremity is separated into areas such as the pectoral and shoulder regions, axilla, arm, anterior forearm, posterior forearm and the hand. These regions each have a nerve or two associated with the innervation of their muscles and certain vessels supplying the muscles and surrounding tissue and skin. A simple principle regarding muscles of the upper extremity (much like the lower extremity) is this: If some muscles crosses and acts on a joint thus creating a movement, those same muscles also function to stabilize that joint.

6.6 Pectoral Region

6.6.1 Pectoral Region Muscles

There are four pectoral or anterior axio-appendicular region muscles responsible for moving the pectoral girdle. The **pectoralis major** is a fan-shaped muscle that covers the superior portion of the thorax. It consists of a clavicular, sternocostal and abdominal muscle head. It acts primarily in *adduction* and *medial rotation of the humerus* at the glenohumeral joint of the shoulder but it is capable of both *flexion* and *extension* at the shoulder. For surface anatomy, it forms the *anterior axillary fold*. The **pectoralis minor** is located deep to the pectoralis major and functions primarily as a *stabilizer of the scapula* (**Fig. 6.28; Fig. 6.29**).

The **serratus anterior** is a broad and thick sheet of muscle that overlies most of the lateral thorax. The muscle near the thorax appears more as individual slips or serrations of muscle versus the portion attached to the scapula. It functions mainly in *protraction* and *superior rotation of the scapula* but can also inferiorly rotate the scapula. The **subclavius** is a small muscle that lies almost horizontally with the clavicle on its inferior surface. It helps to some degree to protect the brachial plexus and subclavian vessels from damage if the clavicle was broken. It functions to *anchor* and *depress the clavicle* (**Fig. 6.28; Fig. 6.29bc**). Descriptions of the pectoral region muscles are found in **Table 6.1**.

6.6.2 Neurovasculature of the Pectoral Region

The skin of this region is innervated for the most part by the **intercostal nerves** but the **supraclavicular nerves** of the cervical plexus extend just past the clavicle. The **lateral** and **medial pectoral nerves** originate from the lateral and medial cords of the brachial plexus respectively (**Fig. 6.49; Fig. 6.51**). The lateral pectoral nerve penetrates the *costocoracoid membrane* of the *clavipectoral fascia* before reaching the pectoralis major. The medial pectoral nerve pierces the pectoralis minor muscle before reaching the pectoralis major. The **nerve to subclavius** originates from the superior trunk of the brachial plexus and has a short path before reaching the subclavius muscle. The **long thoracic nerve** passes deep in the axilla and rests on the superficial surface of the serratus anterior. It is at risk of being damaged or compressed due to its superficial course (**Fig. 6.29c**).

The blood supply to this region is from multiple artery branches. The **superior thoracic artery** comes from the 1st part of the axillary artery while the **lateral thoracic artery** originates directly from the 2nd part of the axillary and gives rise to the **lateral**

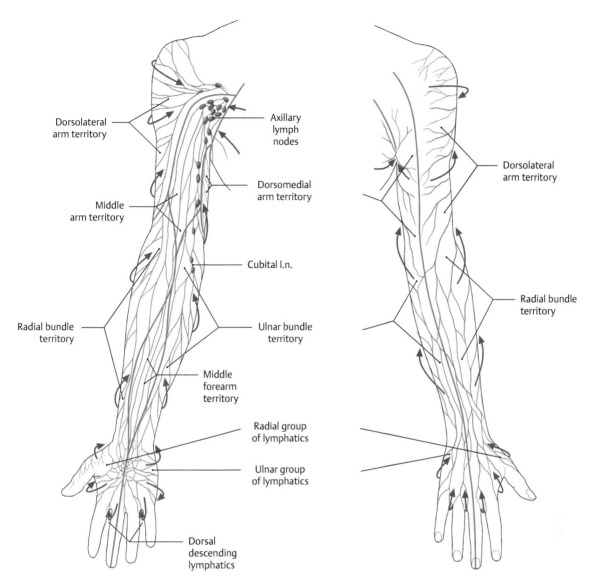

Fig. 6.26 Lymphatic drainage of the upper extremity. (From Schuenke M, Schulte E, Schumacher U. THIEME Atlas of Anatomy. General Anatomy and Musculoskeletal System. Illustrations by Voll M and Wesker K. 3rd ed. New York: Thieme Medical Publishers; 2020.)

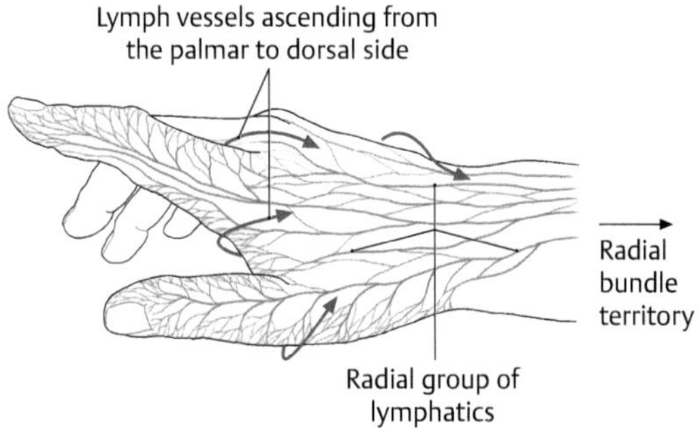

Fig. 6.27 Lymphatic drainage of the hand. (From Schuenke M, Schulte E, Schumacher U. THIEME Atlas of Anatomy. General Anatomy and Musculoskeletal System. Illustrations by Voll M and Wesker K. 3rd ed. New York: Thieme Medical Publishers; 2020.)

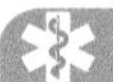 ***Clinical Correlate 6.8***

Winging of the Scapula

Damage to the long thoracic nerve causes the medial border of the scapula to move laterally and posteriorly away from the thoracic wall because the serratus anterior muscle is unable to function properly. When the arm is raised, the medial border and inferior angle pull markedly away from the posterior thoracic wall, a deformation known as a **winged scapula** because the scapula now has the appearance of a wing. Abduction of the arm above the horizontal position cannot be done because the serratus anterior is unable to rotate the glenoid cavity superiorly to complete abduction of the upper limb.

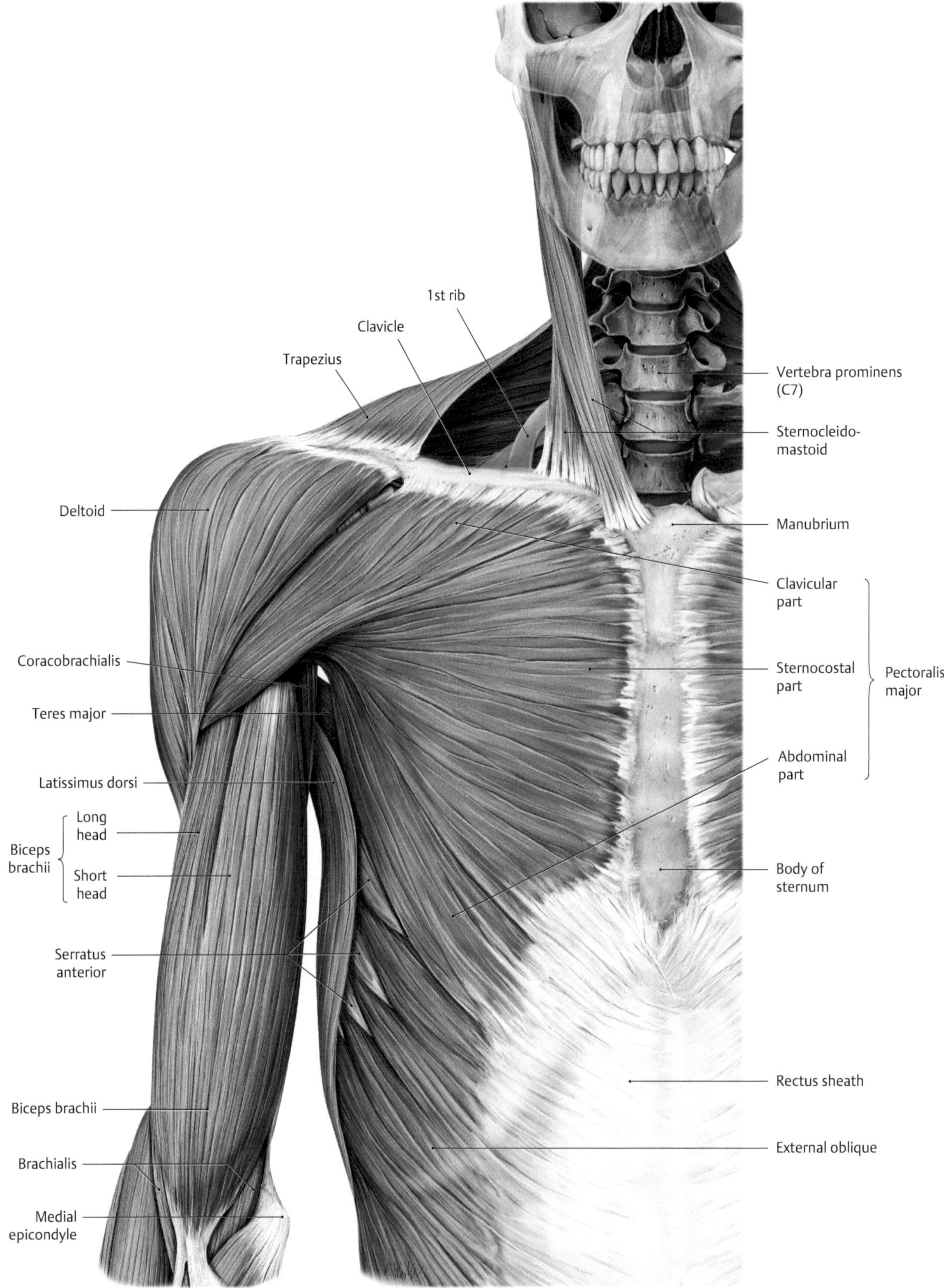

Fig. 6.28 Anterior muscles of the shoulder and arm. (From Schuenke M, Schulte E, Schumacher U. THIEME Atlas of Anatomy. General Anatomy and Musculoskeletal System. Illustrations by Voll M and Wesker K. 3rd ed. New York: Thieme Medical Publishers; 2020.)

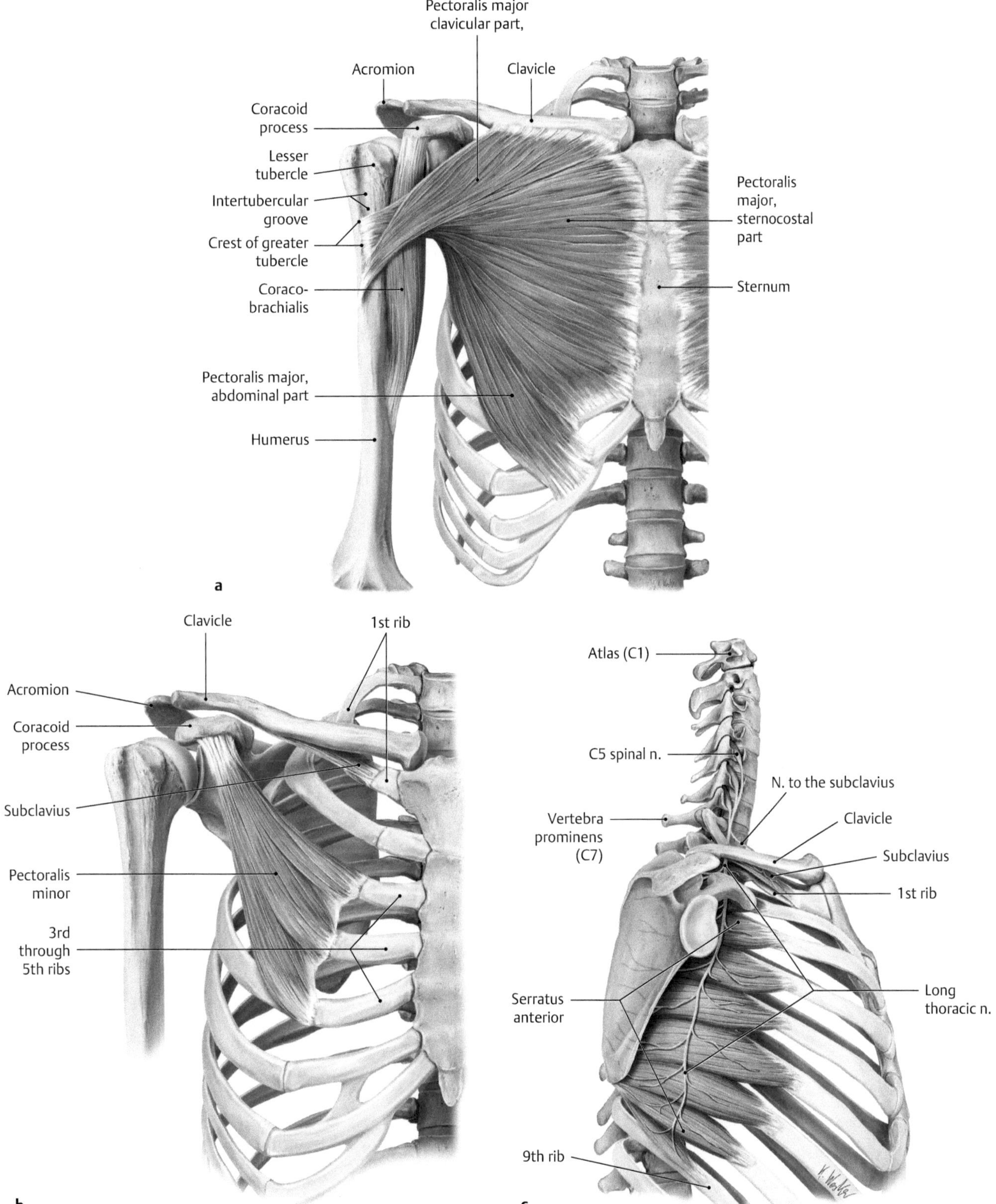

Fig. 6.29 **(a)** Pectoralis major and coracobrachialis, anterior view. **(b)** Pectoralis minor and subclavius, anterior view. **(c)** Serratus anterior and subclavius muscles along with the long thoracic nerve and nerve to subclavius. Right lateral view. (From Schuenke M, Schulte E, Schumacher U. THIEME Atlas of Anatomy. General Anatomy and Musculoskeletal System. Illustrations by Voll M and Wesker K. 3rd ed. New York: Thieme Medical Publishers; 2020.)

Table 6.1 **Pectoral region muscles (anterior axio-appendicular)**

Muscle	Innervation	Function(s)	Origin	Insertion
Pectoralis major	Lateral and medial pectoral nerves	Adducts, flexes (clavicular head) and medially rotates arm. Extension from the flexed position (sternocostal head)	Clavicle (medial half); sternum and costal cartilage 1-6; and anterior layer of rectus sheath	Lateral lip of intertubercular sulcus of humerus (or crest of greater tubercle)
Pectoralis minor	Medial pectoral nerve	Stabilizes scapula. Does this by a downward and anterior movement toward the thoracic wall	External surface of 3rd-5th ribs	Coracoid process
Serratus anterior	Long thoracic nerve	Protracts scapula; rotates scapula superiorly (to elevate arm past 90°) and inferiorly (as in lowering arm)	External surfaces of 1st-8th/9th ribs	Anterior surface of medial border of scapula
Subclavius	Nerve to subclavius (subclavian nerve)	Depresses and steadies clavicle	1st rib	Inferior surface of clavicle

mammary arteries. The **thoracoacromial trunk** has up to four branches and originates from the 2nd part of the axillary artery. These include the *clavicular*, *acromial*, *pectoral* and *deltoid* artery branches but the clavicular and pectoral branches supply the most blood to this region. *Perforating branches* from the **internal thoracic artery** along with the **medial mammary** branches supply the medial portion of the thorax. Distal branching from both the **anterior** and **posterior intercostal arteries** contributes to the blood supply as well. Venous drainage mirrors the blood supply back mainly to the **axillary vein** more laterally and **subclavian vein** on the medial side (**Fig. 6.30**).

6.7 Shoulder Region

6.7.1 Shoulder Region Muscles

The shoulder muscles are divided into either a posterior axio-appendicular/extrinsic or scapulohumeral/intrinsic muscle group. The extrinsic muscles have been discussed previously as a superficial group of "back" muscles in Chapter 1. The extrinsic shoulder muscles include the trapezius, latissimus dorsi, levator scapulae and rhomboids.

The **trapezius** creates a direct attachment between the pelvic girdle with that of the vertebral column and cranium. It has a

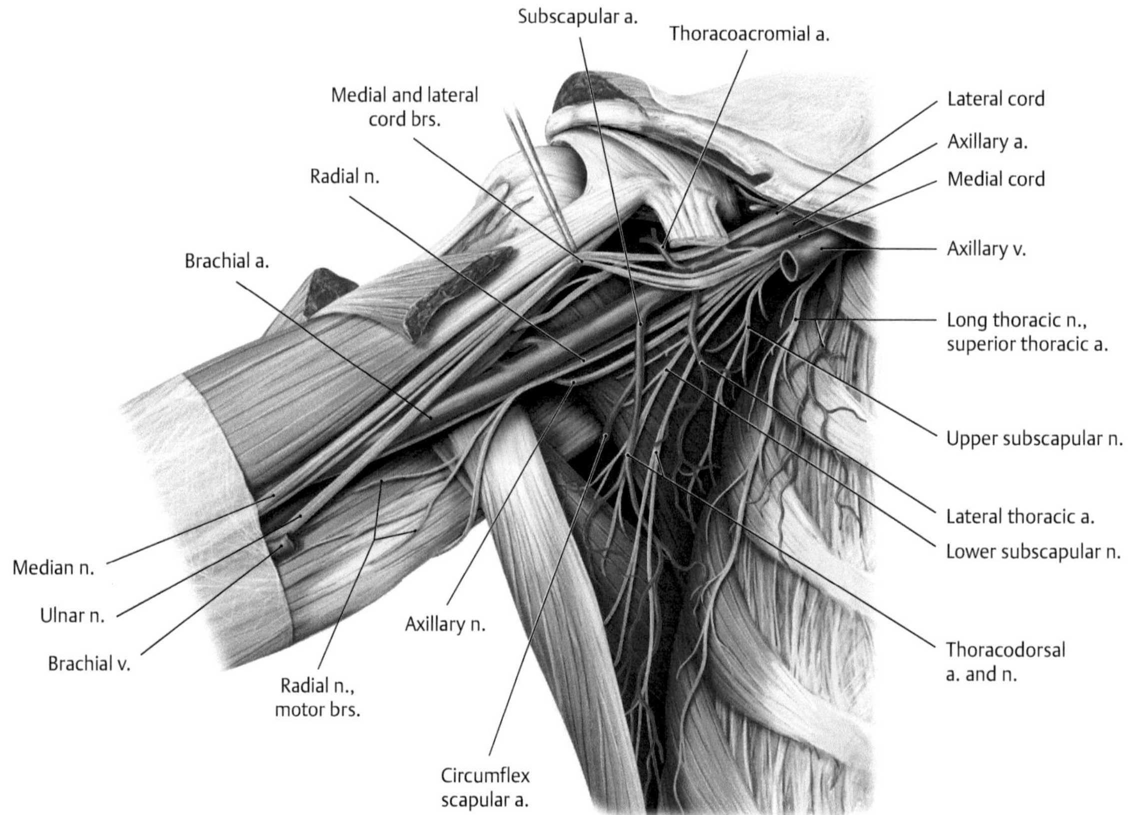

Fig. 6.30 Deep axilla dissection. Right shoulder, anterior view. Pectoralis major and minor have been removed. (From Schuenke M, Schulte E, Schumacher U. THIEME Atlas of Anatomy. General Anatomy and Musculoskeletal System. Illustrations by Voll M and Wesker K. 3rd ed. New York: Thieme Medical Publishers; 2020.)

combination of superior, middle and inferior muscle fibers that lead to functions such as *elevation, retraction, depression,* and *superior rotation of the scapula.* Tonic contraction of the trapezius fixes the shoulders against the thoracic wall. Drooping of the shoulders indicates that the trapezius has become weak. The **latissimus dorsi** extends from the trunk to the humerus where it acts directly on the glenohumeral joint and indirectly on the scapulothoracic joint of the pelvic girdle. It functions in *adduction, extension* and *medial rotation of the humerus.* It helps play a role in restoring the upper extremity to anatomical position from an abducted position. Major activities that are associated with latissimus dorsi actions include doing chin-ups and climbing. For surface anatomy, it forms the *posterior axillary fold* (**Fig. 6.31**).

The **levator scapulae** rests at some point during its course deep to both the sternocleidomastoid and trapezius muscles. It functions in *elevation of the scapula* and along with the rhomboids, *inferior rotation of the scapula.* A bilateral action can result in extension of the neck. The **rhomboids** lie deep to the trapezius in the same plane as the levator scapulae and are divided into a major and minor component. The minor belly is superior and thicker to the major belly. The major belly is much wider and thinner than the minor. The muscle as a whole *retracts the scapula* and with the assistance of the levator scapulae, *inferiorly rotates the scapula.* The rhomboids assist the serratus anterior in holding and fixing the scapula against the thorax during upper extremity movements (**Fig. 6.31; Fig. 6.32**). Descriptions of the extrinsic shoulder region muscles are found in **Table 6.2**.

The scapulohumeral or intrinsic shoulder muscles include the deltoid, subscapularis, supraspinatus, infraspinatus, teres minor and teres major and they all act on the glenohumeral joint. The **deltoid** is a thicker muscle that consists of an anterior (clavicular), middle (acromial) and posterior (spinal) belly. These bellies can function individually or as a larger group. Individually, the anterior belly *flexes* and *medially rotates the arm* while the posterior belly *extends* and *laterally rotates the arm.* All three muscles together *abduct the arm,* with the bulk of the action originating from the middle belly. The **teres major** muscle is round and thick and functions primarily in *adduction* and *medial rotation of the arm.* It helps stabilize the head of the humerus in the glenoid cavity (**Fig. 6.31b; Fig. 6.33**).

The next set of muscles is referred to as the **rotator cuff muscles** and they include the subscapularis, supraspinatus, infraspinatus and teres minor. These muscles as a group form a musculotendinous rotator cuff around the glenohumeral joint. All of the tendons of these muscles reinforce the fibrous layer of the glenohumeral joint capsule and help stabilize the joint. In addition, as a group they help rotate the arm (except for the supraspinatus). The **subscapularis** is triangular and the only rotator cuff muscle located anteriorly. It is the primary *medial rotator of the arm* in addition to being an *adductor of the arm* (**Fig. 6.31b; Fig. 6.34**).

The **supraspinatus** is located in the supraspinous fossa before passing over the glenohumeral joint. It initiates *abduction of the arm* for the first 15°. At that point the deltoid becomes the primary abductor of the arm and continues from the 15-90° range. For any angle greater than 90°, abduction is done by a combination of the serratus anterior, trapezius and deltoid muscles. The **infraspinatus** is triangular, much like the subscapularis, but it is found posteriorly on the scapula. A good portion of it is hidden and deep to the trapezius and deltoid muscles. In addition to stabilizing the glenohumeral joint it functions in *lateral rotation of the arm.* The **teres minor** is short and located just inferior to the infraspinatus. It acts similarly to the infraspinatus by stabilizing the glenohumeral joint and *laterally rotating the arm* (**Fig. 6.31; Fig. 6.34**). Descriptions of the intrinsic shoulder region muscles are found in **Table 6.3**.

Clinical Correlate 6.9

Rotator Cuff Tears

Repetitive use of the upper extremity above the horizontal plane commonly results in an injury to the rotator cuff. Individuals at a greater risk include baseball and tennis players, swimmers and even weight lifters. Recurrent inflammation, especially at the relatively avascular region of the *supraspinatus tendon*, is the most common cause of torn rotator cuffs and this occurs near its greater tubercle insertion site. Repetitive use may also cause the humeral head and rotator cuff to impinge on the coracoacromial arch, thus producing irritation at both the arch and rotator cuff. The initial 15° of upper limb abduction would be lost due to a rotator cuff tear.

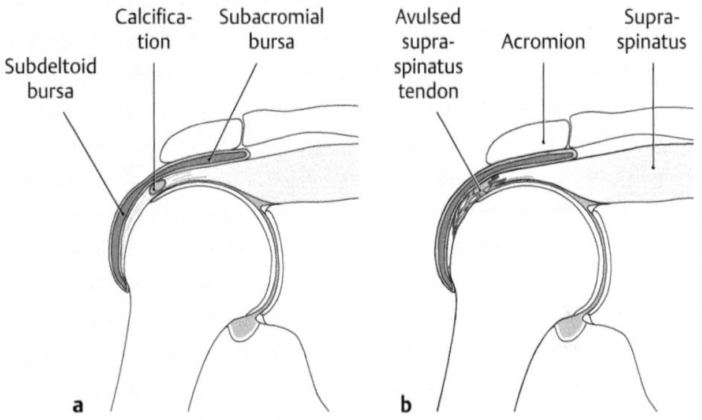

(a) Calcification (calcifying tendinitis) and related degenerative changes. **(b)** Rotator cuff tear (supraspinatus tendon avulsion). (From Schuenke M, Schulte E, Schumacher U. THIEME Atlas of Anatomy. General Anatomy and Musculoskeletal System. Illustrations by Voll M and Wesker K. 3rd ed. New York: Thieme Medical Publishers; 2020.)

6.7.2 Shoulder Region Bursae

The **subacromial/subdeltoid bursa** is a synovial-lined sac that has two parts. The portion of this bursa deep to the acromion is called the **subacromial bursa**. The part deep to the deltoid is called the **subdeltoid bursa** (**Fig. 6.35; Fig. 6.36**). These parts may fuse or remain separate. With either orientation, the bursa lies between the supraspinatus tendon and deltoid muscle in the subacromial space. It facilitates movement of the supraspinatus tendon under the coracoacromial arch reducing friction during movements of the arm.

Clinical Correlate 6.10

Adhesive Capsulitis

When there is adhesive fibrosis and scarring between the inflamed capsule of the glenohumeral joint, subacromial bursa, deltoid and rotator cuff, this can lead to **adhesive capsulitis** ("frozen shoulder"). With this condition, a patient typically has difficulty abducting the arm but can obtain as much as 45° of abduction by elevating and rotating the scapula. Injuries that may initiate such a condition include glenohumeral dislocations, calcific supraspinatus tendinitis, a partial rotator cuff tear, or bicipital tendinitis.

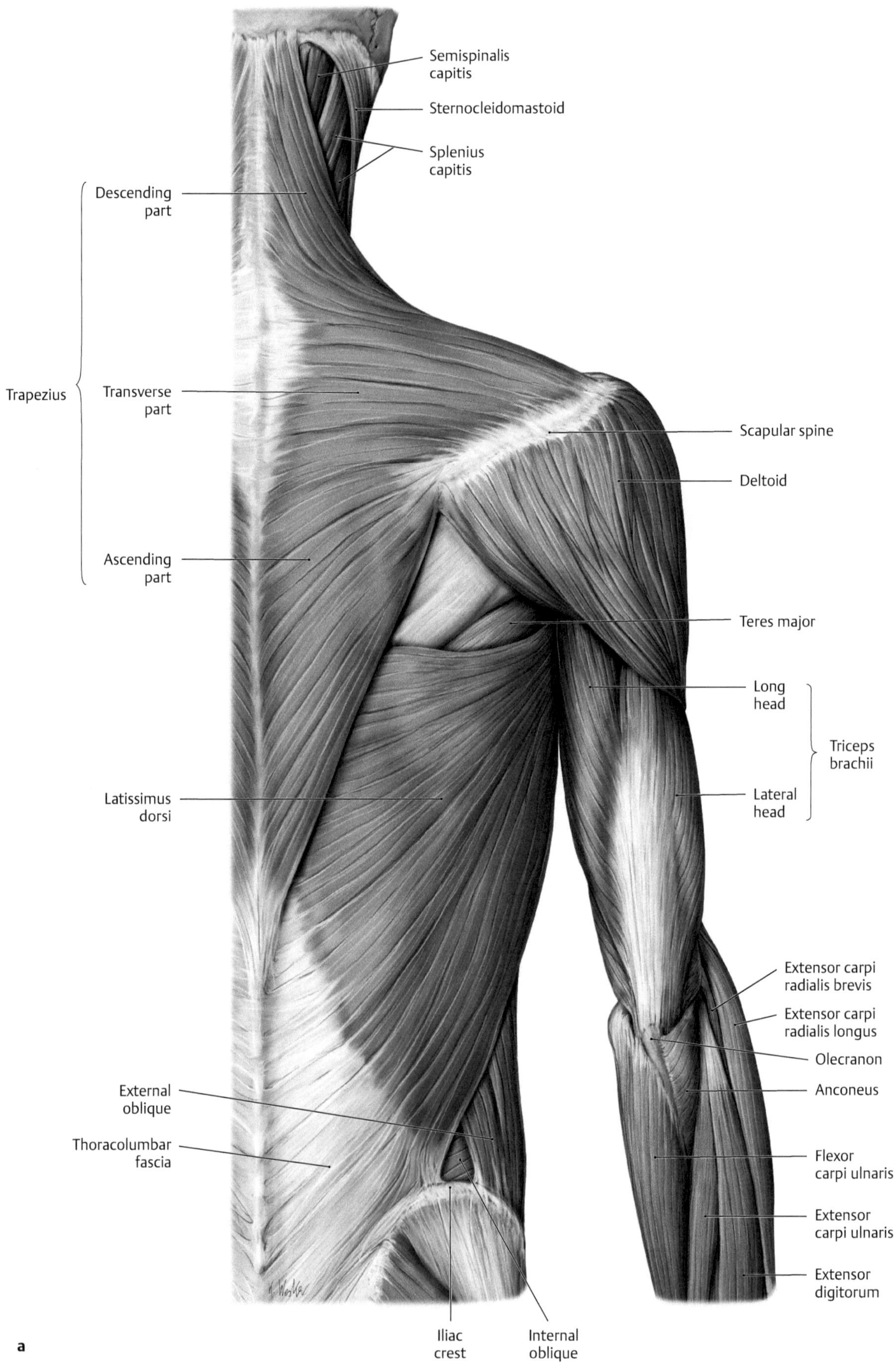

Fig. 6.31 Posterior muscles of the shoulder and arm. Right side, posterior view. **(a)** Superficial view. (*continued*) (From Schuenke M, Schulte E, Schumacher U. THIEME Atlas of Anatomy. General Anatomy and Musculoskeletal System. Illustrations by Voll M and Wesker K. 3rd ed. New York: Thieme Medical Publishers; 2020.)

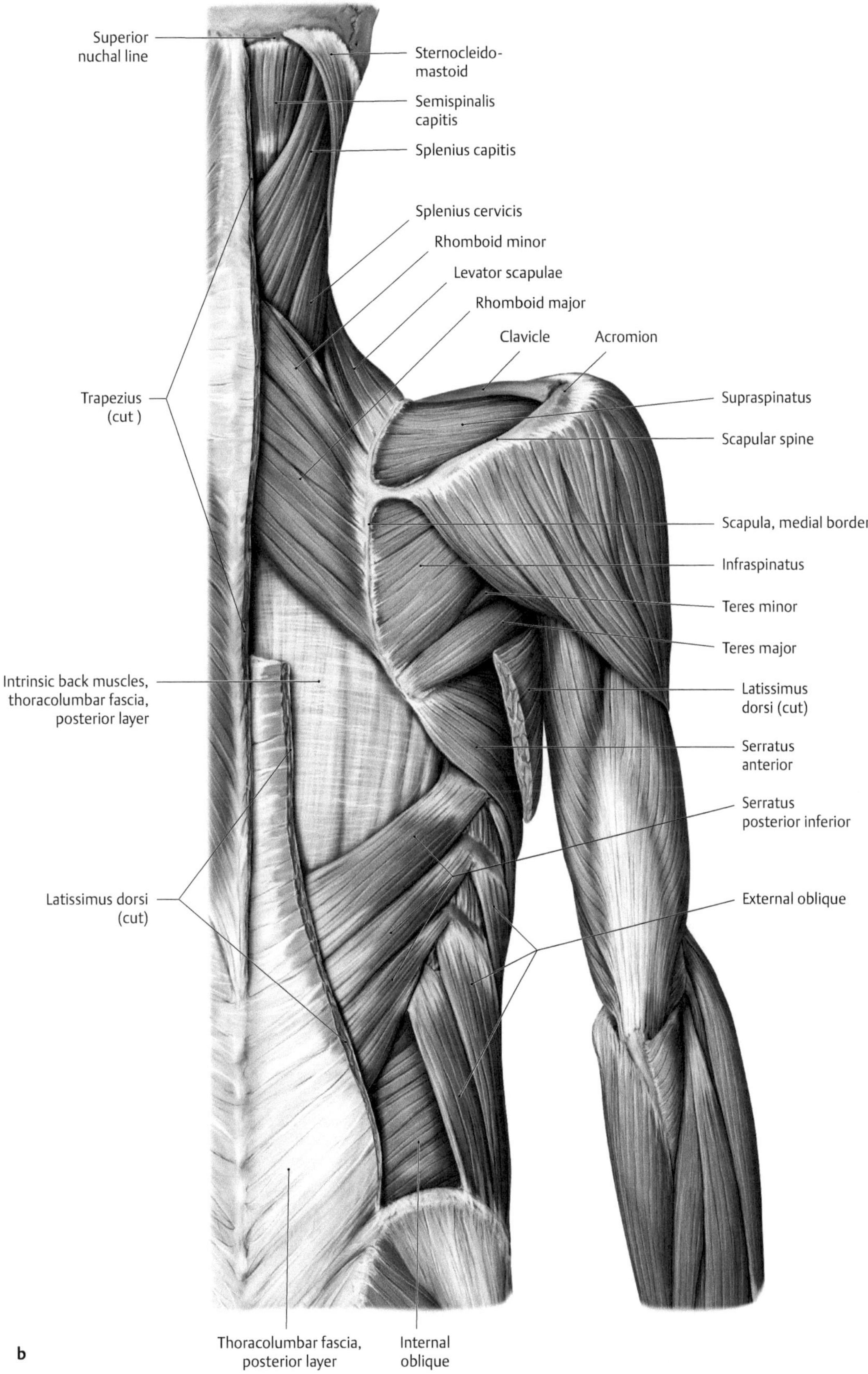

Fig. 6.31 (*continued*) Posterior muscles of the shoulder and arm. Right side, posterior view. **(b)** Deep view. (From Schuenke M, Schulte E, Schumacher U. THIEME Atlas of Anatomy. General Anatomy and Musculoskeletal System. Illustrations by Voll M and Wesker K. 3rd ed. New York: Thieme Medical Publishers; 2020.)

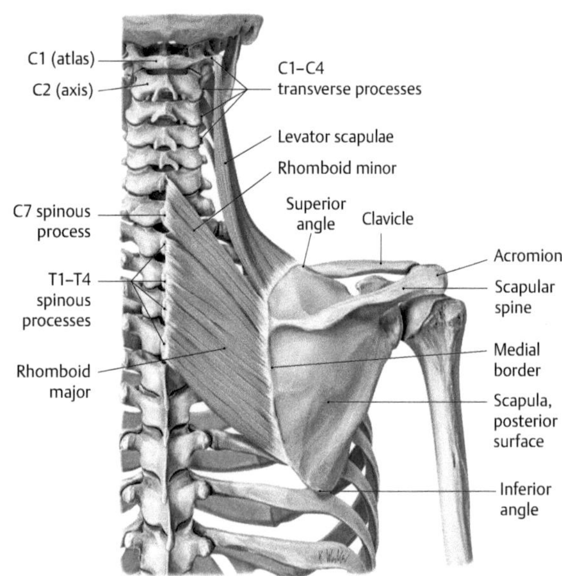

Fig. 6.32 Levator scapulae with rhomboids major and minor. (From Schuenke M, Schulte E, Schumacher U. THIEME Atlas of Anatomy. General Anatomy and Musculoskeletal System. Illustrations by Voll M and Wesker K. 3rd ed. New York: Thieme Medical Publishers; 2020.)

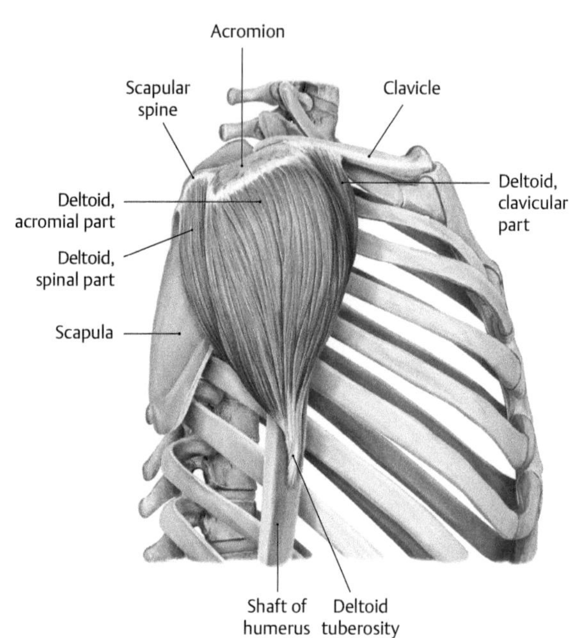

Fig. 6.33 Deltoid and its anterior (clavicular), middle (acromial), and posterior (spinal) parts. (From Schuenke M, Schulte E, Schumacher U. THIEME Atlas of Anatomy. General Anatomy and Musculoskeletal System. Illustrations by Voll M and Wesker K. 3rd ed. New York: Thieme Medical Publishers; 2020.)

Table 6.2 **Shoulder region muscles (posterior axio-appendicular/extrinsic shoulder)**

Muscle	Innervation	Function(s)	Origin	Insertion
Trapezius	Spinal accessory nerve (CN XI) and ventral rami of C3, and C4 for pain and proprioception	*Superior fibers*: elevate scapula; *Middle fibers*: retract scapula; *Inferior fibers*: depress scapula; *superior and inferior fibers* together superiorly rotate the scapula	Medial 1/3 of superior nuchal line; external occipital protuberance; nuchal ligament; C7-T12 spinous processes	Lateral 1/3 of clavicle; acromion and spine of scapula
Latissimus dorsi	Thoracodorsal nerve	Adducts, extends and medially rotates humerus	T7-T12 spinous processes; thoracolumbar fascia; iliac crest; inferior 3-4 ribs	Floor of intertubercular sulcus (bicipital groove) of humerus
Levator scapulae	Dorsal scapular nerve	Elevates and inferiorly rotates scapula	C1-C4 transverse processes	Superior angle and superomedial border of scapula
Rhomboids (major and minor)	Dorsal scapular nerve	Retracts and inferiorly rotates scapula	*Minor*: nuchal ligament, C7-T1 spinous processes; *Major*: T2-T5 spinous processes	*Minor*: medial border of scapula (above scapular spine); *Major*: medial border of scapula (below scapular spine)

Table 6.3 **Shoulder region muscles (scapulohumeral/intrinsic shoulder)**

Muscle	Innervation	Function(s)	Origin	Insertion
Deltoid	Axillary nerve	*Anterior fibers*: abduct, flex and medially rotate arm; *Middle fibers*: abduct arm; *Posterior fibers*: abduct, extend and laterally rotate arm	Lateral 1/3 of clavicle; acromion and spine of scapula	Deltoid tuberosity
Subscapularis	Upper and lower subscapular nerves	Stabilize glenohumeral joint; adduct and medially rotate arm	Scapular fossa	Lesser tubercle
Supraspinatus	Suprascapular nerve	Stabilize glenohumeral joint; initiates the first 15° of arm abduction	Supraspinous fossa	Greater tubercle
Infraspinatus	Suprascapular nerve	Stabilize glenohumeral joint; laterally rotates arm	Infraspinous fossa	Greater tubercle
Teres minor	Axillary nerve	Stabilize glenohumeral joint; laterally rotates arm	Middle portion of lateral border of scapula	Greater tubercle
Teres major	Lower subscapular nerve	Adducts and medially rotates arm	Posterior surface of inferior angle of scapula	Medial lip of intertubercular sulcus of humerus

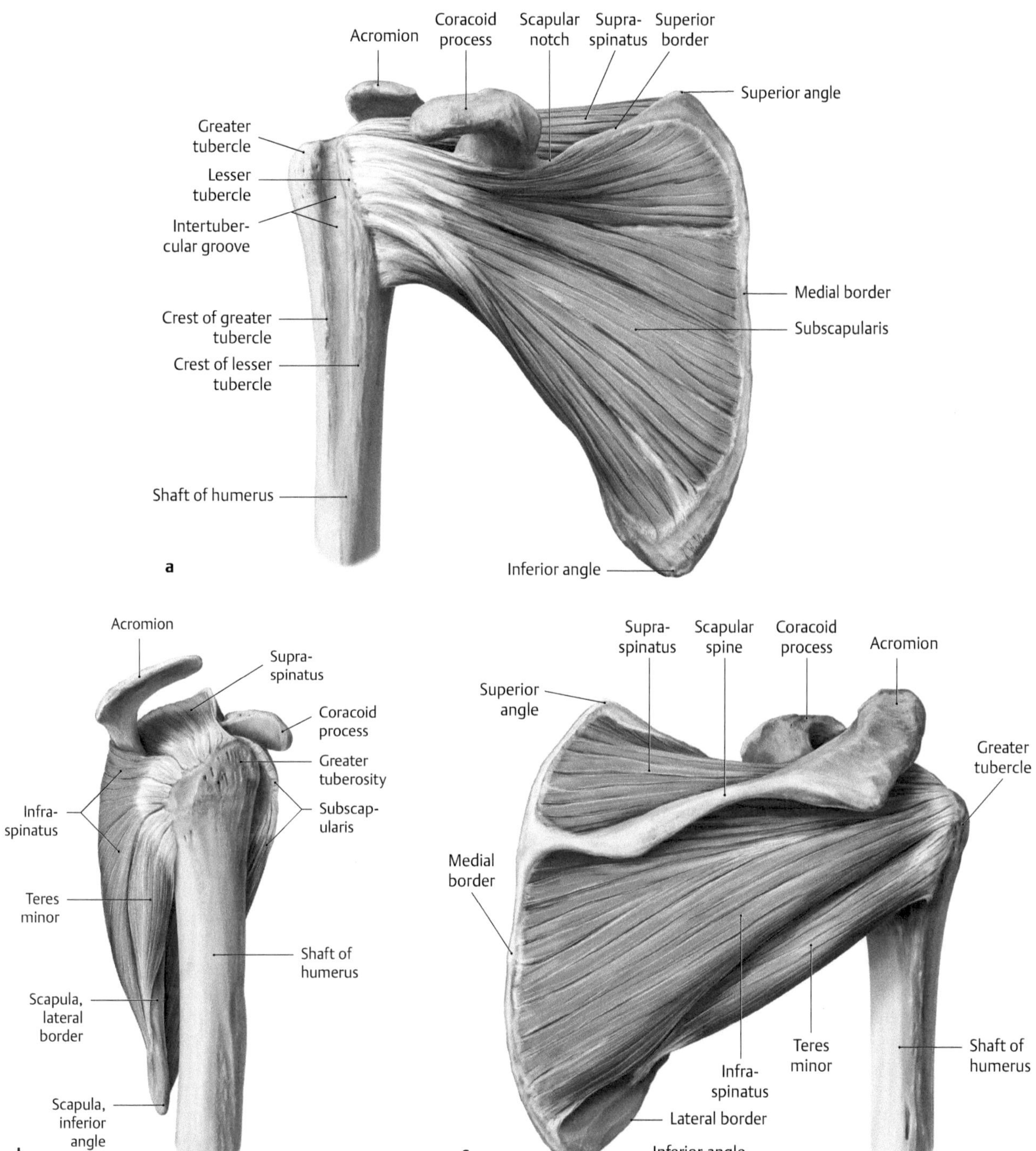

Fig. 6.34 Rotator cuff muscles. **(a)** Anterior view. **(b)** Lateral view. **(c)** Posterior view. (From Schuenke M, Schulte E, Schumacher U. THIEME Atlas of Anatomy. General Anatomy and Musculoskeletal System. Illustrations by Voll M and Wesker K. 3rd ed. New York: Thieme Medical Publishers; 2020.)

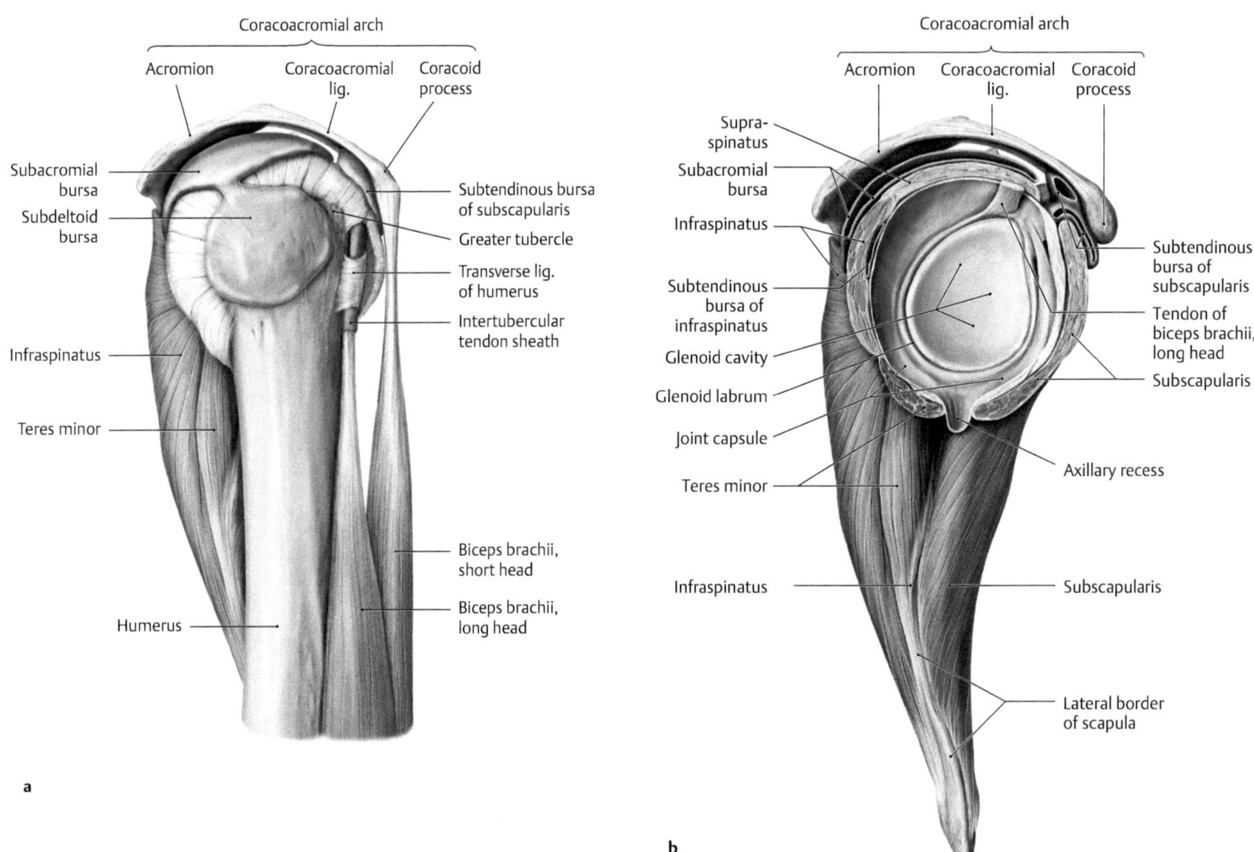

Fig. 6.35 **(a)** Subacromial space, lateral view. **(b)** Subacromial bursa and glenoid cavity, lateral view. (From Schuenke M, Schulte E, Schumacher U. THIEME Atlas of Anatomy. General Anatomy and Musculoskeletal System. Illustrations by Voll M and Wesker K. 3rd ed. New York: Thieme Medical Publishers; 2020.)

The **subtendinous bursa of subscapularis** is located between the subscapularis tendon and neck of the scapula. This bursa protects the tendon where it passes inferior to the root of the coracoid process and over the neck of the scapula. It may communicate with the glenohumeral joint through an opening in the fibrous layer of the joint capsule.

6.7.3 Neurovasculature of the Shoulder Region

The **spinal accessory nerve** (CN XI) passes through the jugular foramen of the skull before splitting into two parts, one responsible for innervating the sternocleidomastoid muscle, the other responsible for innervating the trapezius muscles (course of nerve shown in chapter 1). The **dorsal scapular nerve** arises mostly from the C5 ventral rami branch of the brachial plexus and innervates the levator scapulae and rhomboid muscles. The **suprascapular nerve** originates from the superior/upper trunk of the brachial plexus and extends posterolaterally with the paired vessels of the same name before passing ***underneath*** the superior transverse ligament of the scapula. It innervates the supraspinatus and infraspinatus muscles (**Fig. 6.37; Fig. 6.51**).

The **axillary nerve** originates from the posterior cord of the brachial plexus before passing through the *quadrangular space* along with the posterior circumflex vessels. It innervates the deltoid and teres minor muscles. The **upper** and **lower subscapular nerves** arise from the posterior cord of the brachial plexus and, located between them and originating from the same cord, is the **thoracodorsal nerve**. The lower subscapular nerve contributes to both the subscapularis and teres major innervation but the upper subscapular only adds to the innervation of the subscapularis muscle. The thoracodorsal nerve innervates the latissimus dorsi.

The **subclavian artery** has a **thyrocervical trunk** that has multiple branches including the suprascapular and transverse cervical arteries. The **suprascapular artery** extends posterolaterally before passing *over* the superior transverse ligament of the scapula and then continues deep to both the supraspinatus and infraspinatus muscles before meeting the circumflex scapular artery. The **transverse cervical artery** passes posteriorly before bifurcating into a superficial cervical and dorsal scapular artery. The **superficial cervical artery** continues with the spinal accessory nerve (CN XI) deep to the trapezius muscle while the **dorsal scapular artery** pairs up with the dorsal scapular nerve and travels deep to the levator scapulae and rhomboid muscles near the medial border of the scapula. The dorsal scapular artery in a third of the population may originate from the third part of the subclavian artery. It also forms an anastomosis with the posterior intercostal arteries (**Fig. 6.20**).

The **third part of the axillary artery** has a **subscapular artery** branch that bifurcates into a thoracodorsal and circumflex

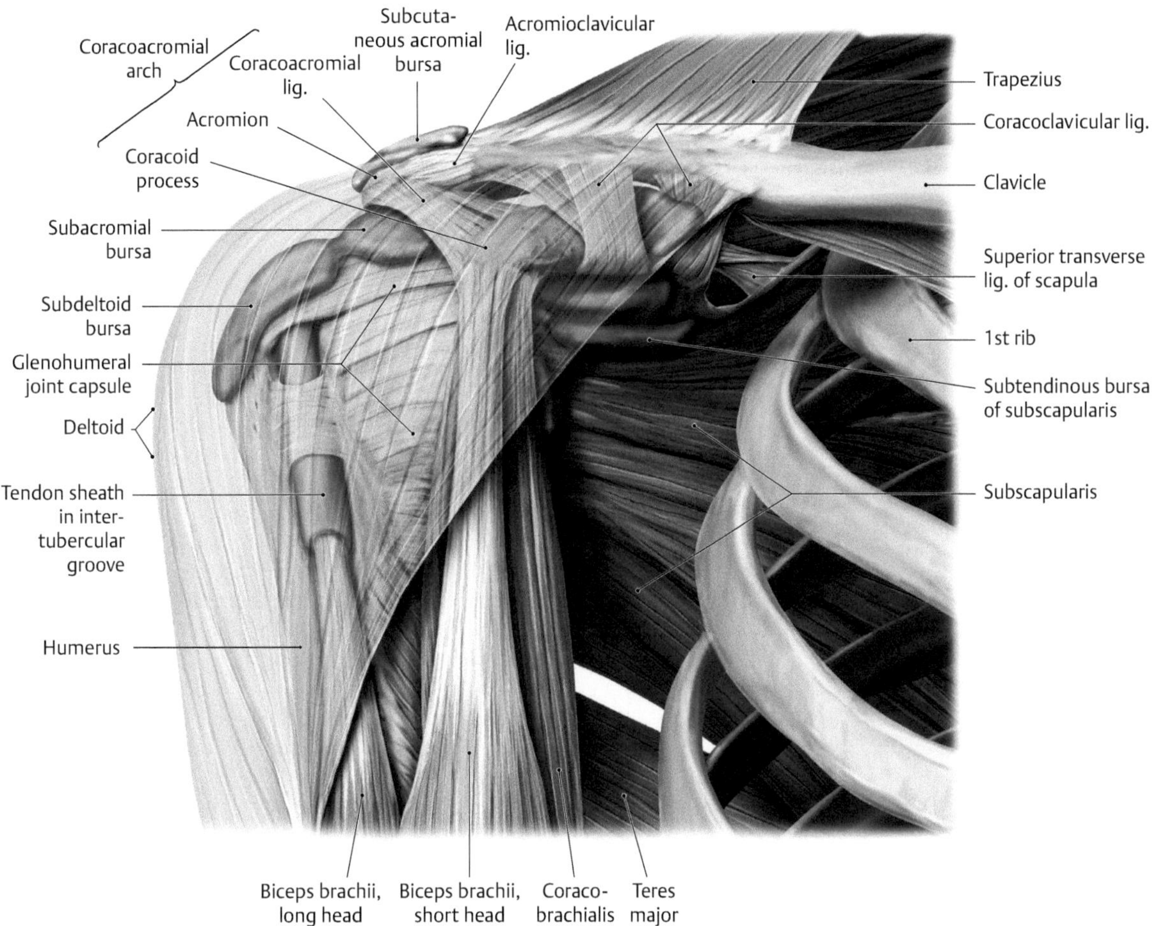

Fig. 6.36 Shoulder region bursae. (From Schuenke M, Schulte E, Schumacher U. THIEME Atlas of Anatomy. General Anatomy and Musculoskeletal System. Illustrations by Voll M and Wesker K. 3rd ed. New York: Thieme Medical Publishers; 2020.)

scapular artery. The **thoracodorsal artery** pairs with the thoracodorsal nerve and helps supply the latissimus dorsi muscle. The **circumflex scapular artery** forms an anastomosis with the suprascapular and dorsal scapular arteries and passes through the *triangular space* (**Fig. 6.21**).

Clinical Correlate 6.11

Scapular Arterial Anastomosis

There are multiple arteries that supply the shoulder region and they ultimately form a larger scapular arterial anastomosis. This anastomosis create a collateral circulation that is vitally important in the case of a lacerated subclavian or axillary artery so that blood is able to bypass the occluded artery and still supply the upper extremity. The suprascapular, dorsal scapular, circumflex scapular and posterior intercostal arteries all take part in this scapular anastomosis. A trauma situation does not allow the collateral circulation enough time to produce sufficient blood flow to structures dependent on this blood. Hence any damage must be fixed in a timely manner. Slower occlusions that build up over time allow for the collateral circulation to establish itself and ultimately supply blood to this region without any disturbances. A surgical ligation distal to the 3rd part of the axillary artery would cut off any blood traveling to the rest of the upper extremity.

6.7.4 Spaces of the Shoulder Region

- The **quadrangular space** allows for passage of the **axillary nerve** and **posterior circumflex humeral vessels.** It has 4 borders (**Fig. 6.38**):
  - Lateral: surgical neck of humerus.
  - Medial: long head of triceps brachii.
  - Superior: teres minor.
  - Inferior: teres major.
- The **triangular space** allows for the passage of only the **circumflex scapular artery** and **vein** and involves no major nerve passing through it. It has three borders:
  - Lateral: long head of triceps brachii.
  - Superior: teres minor.
  - Inferior: teres major.
- The **triangular hiatus** is considered more a part of the posterior arm but is closely associated with the last two spaces. The **profunda brachii vessels** and **radial nerve** pass through it. It has three borders:
  - Lateral: proximal humerus.
  - Medial: long head of triceps brachii.
  - Superior: teres major.

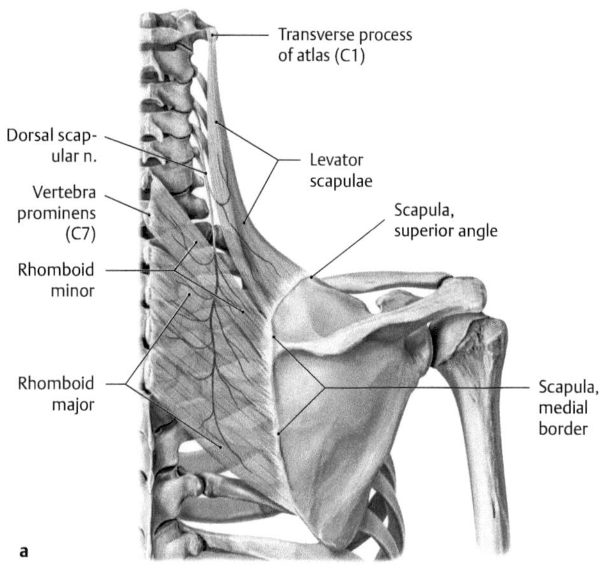

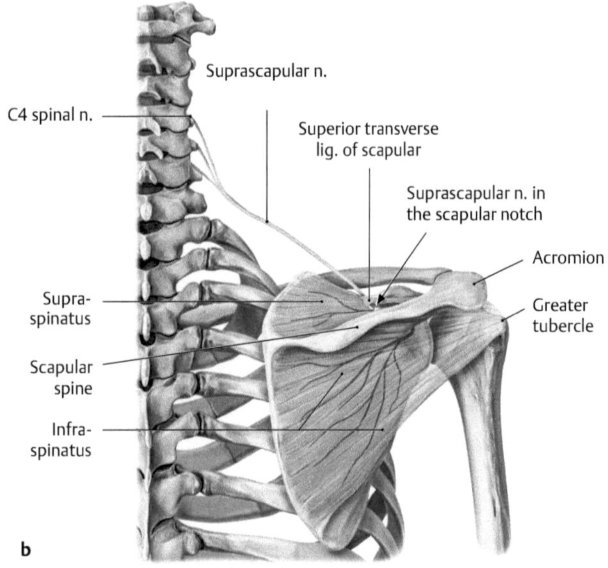

Fig. 6.37 **(a)** Course of the dorsal scapular nerve, posterior view. (b) Course of the suprascapular nerve, posterior view. (From Schuenke M, Schulte E, Schumacher U. THIEME Atlas of Anatomy. General Anatomy and Musculoskeletal System. Illustrations by Voll M and Wesker K. 3rd ed. New York: Thieme Medical Publishers; 2020.)

6.7.5 Shoulder Region Joints

The range of motion of the upper extremity is quite dependent on the mobility of the scapula. The shoulder includes three true articulating joints called the **sternoclavicular, acromioclavicular** and **glenohumeral joints.** Generally it is the simultaneous movement of all three of these joints that is responsible for moving the pectoral girdle. In addition, there are two "articulations" that are not true joints but are referred to as "joints." These are the **subacromial** and **scapulothoracic joints (Fig. 6.39).**

The **scapulohumeral rhythm** refers to the integrated movement of the scapula and humerus together. This movement is involved in any movement of the upper extremity that results in placement of the hand in a functional position. When abducting or elevating the arm for example, there is a simultaneous movement of the humerus at the glenohumeral joint accompanied by rotation of the scapula at the scapulothoracic joint. The initial 30° degrees of movement may occur without motion of the scapula but it is recognized that scapular movement occurs in a 2:1 ratio. For every 2° of abduction or elevation at the glenohumeral joint, there will be 1° of scapular rotation. Thus when the arm is abducted 90°, 60° occurred at the glenohumeral joint and the other 30° occurs from scapular rotation **(Fig. 6.40).**

Sternoclavicular Joint

The **sternoclavicular (SC) joint** is a *saddle-type synovial joint* that functions more like a ball and socket synovial joint. It is the articulation between the sternal end of the clavicle and the manubrium of the sternum and first costal cartilage. It is the only joint located between the pectoral girdle and axial skeleton. There is a **joint capsule** that is reinforced by the **anterior** and **posterior sternoclavicular ligaments.** The joint is divided into two separate cavities because of an **articular disc** located deep to the capsule and this disc attaches to both sternoclavicular ligaments. The **interclavicular ligament** spans both SC joints to add more support to the capsules superiorly and the articular disc attaches to it as well **(Fig. 6.41).**

The SC joint is very strong and dislocations are rare here. It is quite mobile to allow movements of the pectoral girdle. Elevation at this joint is limited by the **costoclavicular ligament** that attaches the inferior surface at the sternal end of the clavicle to the first ribs and its costal cartilage. The clavicle can be elevated about 40-45°, depressed about 10°, and can move in an anterior or posterior direction of up to 25-30° **(Fig 6.41).**

Neurovasculature of the sternoclavicular joint

The SC joint is innervated by the **nerve to subclavius** and **supraclavicular nerves** and receives blood from the **internal thoracic** (subclavian br.) and **suprascapular arteries** (thyrocervical trunk br.).

Acromioclavicular Joint

The **acromioclavicular (AC) joint** is a *plane-type synovial joint* and it is the articulation between the acromion of the scapula and the acromial end of the clavicle. It is a relatively weak joint that allows gliding movements. The **joint capsule** is fairly loose and has an *incomplete articular disk* internally. It is strengthened by the **superior** and **inferior acromioclavicular ligaments** with the superior portion being much thicker.

The **coracoclavicular ligament** has two parts, the *conoid* and *trapezoid*, and it supplies most of the strength to the AC joint along with providing the means by which the free extremity and scapula are passively suspended from the clavicle. The **conoid ligament** attaches to the *conoid tubercle* of the clavicle and *coracoid process* of the scapula. The **trapezoid ligament** attaches to the *coracoid process* and the *trapezoid line* located on the inferior surface of the clavicle **(Fig. 6.42; Fig. 6.43).**

Neurovasculature of the acromioclavicular joint

The AC joint is innervated by the **supraclavicular, lateral pectoral** and **axillary nerves.** It receives blood from branches of the **thoracoacromial trunk** (2nd part of axillary br.) and **suprascapular arteries** (thyrocervical trunk br.).

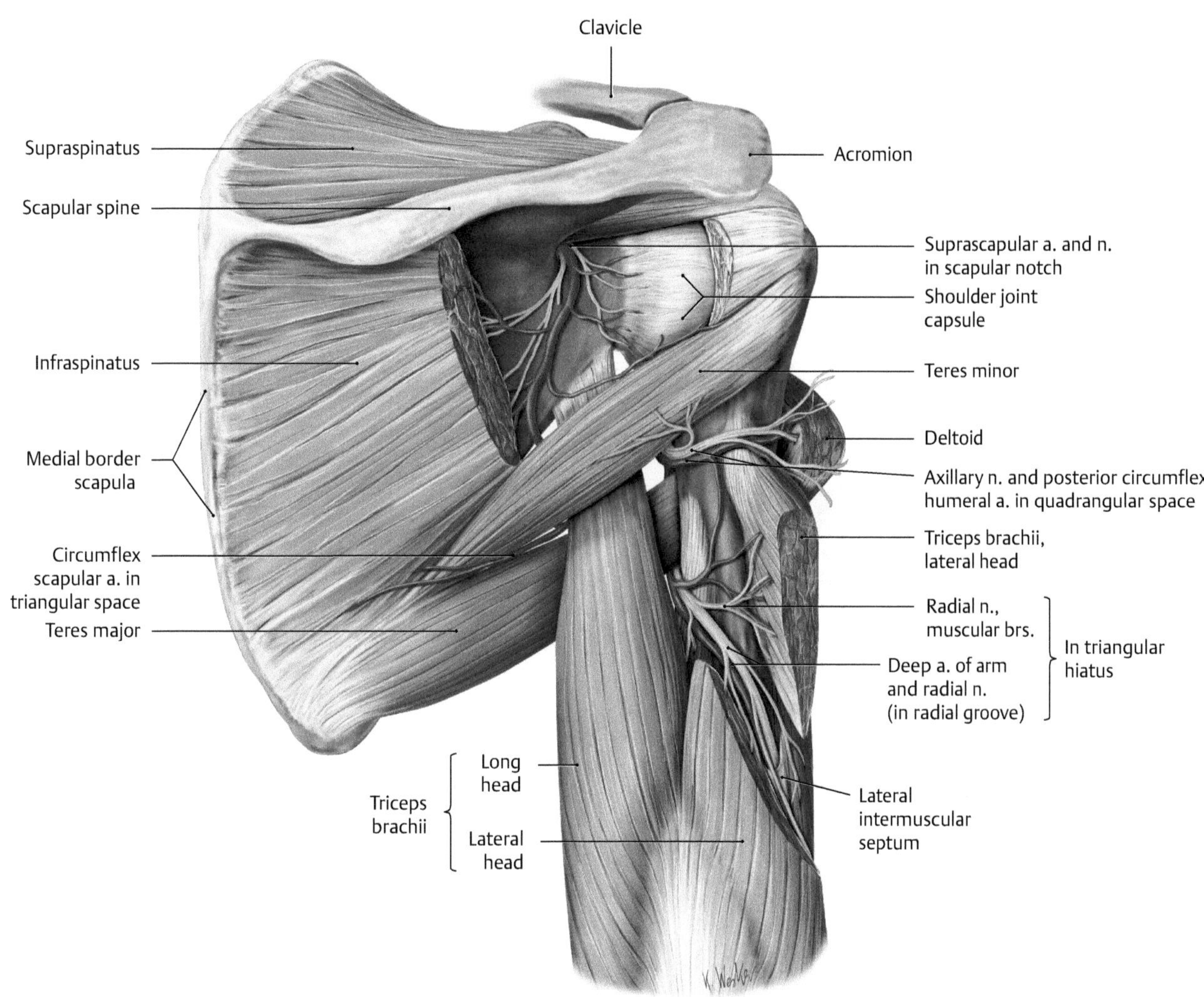

Neurovascular tracts of the scapula

	Passageway	Boundaries	Transmitted structures
①	Scapular notch	Superior transverse lig. of scapula, scapula	Suprascapular a. and n.
②	Medial border	Scapula	Dorsal scapular a. and n.
③	Triangular space	Teres major and minor Long head of triceps brachii	Circumflex scapular a.
④	Triangular hiatus	Triceps brachii, humerus, teres major	Deep a. of arm and radial n.
⑤	Quadrangular space	Teres major and minor, triceps brachii, humerus	Posterior circumflex humeral a. and axillary n.

①
②
Superior transverse lig. of scapula
Inferior transverse lig. of scapula
⑤
④
③

Fig. 6.38 Spaces of the shoulder region. (From Schuenke M, Schulte E, Schumacher U. THIEME Atlas of Anatomy. General Anatomy and Musculoskeletal System. Illustrations by Voll M and Wesker K. 3rd ed. New York: Thieme Medical Publishers; 2020.)

Glenohumeral Joint

The **glenohumeral (shoulder) joint** is a *ball and socket synovial joint* that serves as the articulation between the hyaline cartilage of the head of the humerus and the glenoid cavity of the scapula.

This joint allows for a large range of functional movements but is a fairly unstable joint. The **joint capsule** surrounds the glenohumeral joint and attaches medially to the margin of the glenoid cavity and laterally to the humerus at the level of the anatomical neck. It is loose but reinforced anteriorly by the **glenohumeral**

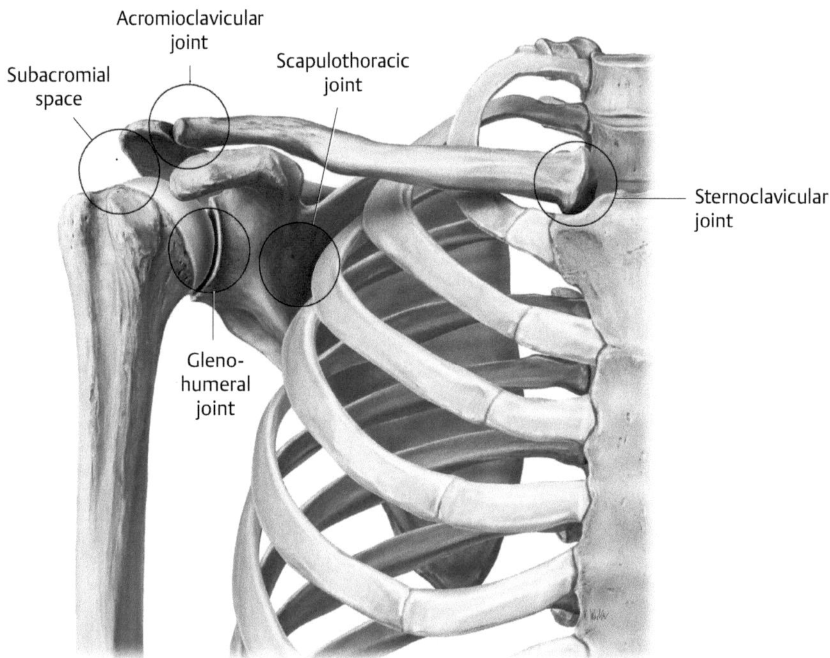

Fig. 6.39 Joints of the shoulder region. (From Schuenke M, Schulte E, Schumacher U. THIEME Atlas of Anatomy. General Anatomy and Musculoskeletal System. Illustrations by Voll M and Wesker K. 3rd ed. New York: Thieme Medical Publishers; 2020.)

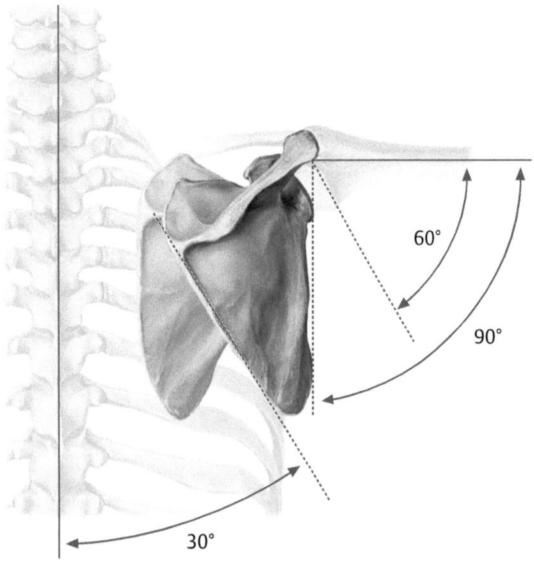

Fig. 6.40 Scapulohumeral rhythm. (From Schuenke M, Schulte E, Schumacher U. THIEME Atlas of Anatomy. General Anatomy and Musculoskeletal System. Illustrations by Voll M and Wesker K. 3rd ed. New York: Thieme Medical Publishers; 2020.)

ligaments and superiorly and posteriorly by the rotator cuff tendons. The inferior portion is the weakest area and is where the joint capsule is lax when the arm is adducted but taut when the arm is abducted. The **glenohumeral ligaments** are made up of individual *superior, middle* and *inferior ligaments* but there is a weakness between the superior and middle ligaments known as the *foramen of Weitbrecht* (**Fig. 6.43; Fig. 6.44; Fig. 6.45; Fig. 6.46**).

The **glenoid labrum** is a fibrocartilagenous ring that surrounds the glenoid fossa and helps deepen the socket of the shoulder joint. The fibrous joint capsule attaches to the labrum, so any injury of the joint capsule can potentially involve the labrum. There are two apertures located on the joint capsule. One located between the greater and lesser tubercles of the humerus that allow for the *tendon of the long head of the biceps brachii* to invaginate the joint capsule (*intracapsular*) but remain outside the synovial cavity (*extrasynovial*). The other is an opening located anterior and inferior to the coracoid process that permits communication between the synovial cavity of the joint and the *subtendinous bursa of subscapularis* (**Fig. 6.35**).

The large range of motion is the greatest of any other joint in the body but it has a lower degree of stability and this can lead to an increased risk of dislocation. This joint allows movement on three different axes and it permits abduction-adduction, flexion-extension, lateral (external) and medial (internal) rotation, along with circumduction. Circumduction is an orderly sequence of flexion followed by abduction, extension and adduction or it can be in the opposite direction. The range of motions related to the glenohumeral joint is summarized in **Fig. 6.47**.

Neurovasculature of the glenohumeral joint

The **glenohumeral joint** is innervated by the axillary, suprascapular and lateral pectoral nerves. It receives blood from the **anterior** and **posterior circumflex humeral** (3rd part of axillary brs.) and **suprascapular arteries** (thyrocervical trunk br.).

Subacromial and Scapulothoracic Joints

The **subacromial joint** is not a true joint but refers to the space between the head of the humerus, acromion and coracoacromial ligament. It is also known as the *suprahumeral joint*. This

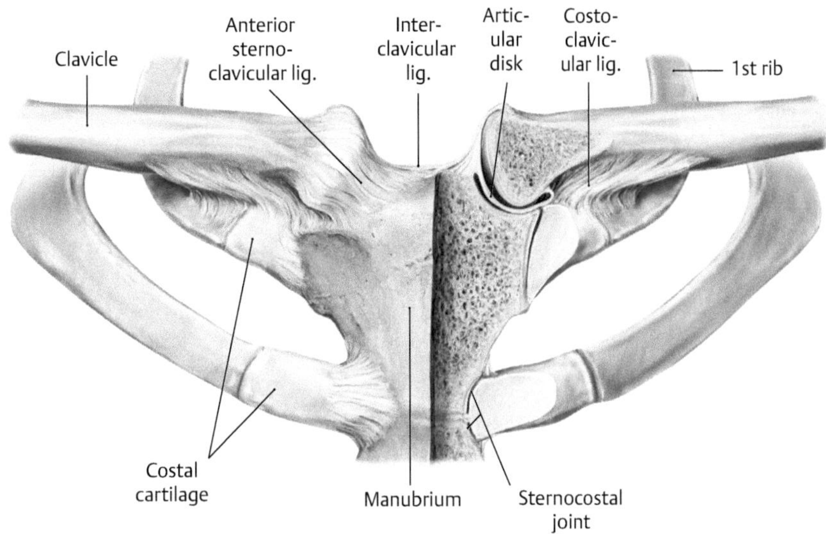

Fig. 6.41 The sternoclavicular joint and its ligaments. (From Schuenke M, Schulte E, Schumacher U. THIEME Atlas of Anatomy. General Anatomy and Musculoskeletal System. Illustrations by Voll M and Wesker K. 3rd ed. New York: Thieme Medical Publishers; 2020.)

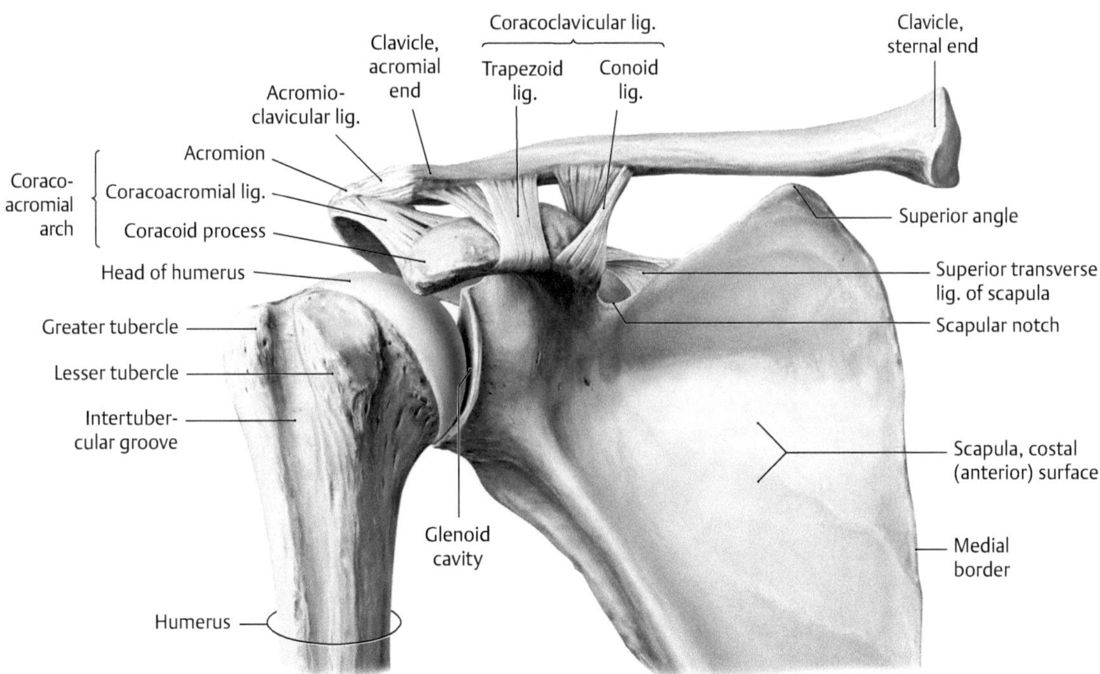

Fig. 6.42 The acromioclavicular joint and its ligaments. (From Schuenke M, Schulte E, Schumacher U. THIEME Atlas of Anatomy. General Anatomy and Musculoskeletal System. Illustrations by Voll M and Wesker K. 3rd ed. New York: Thieme Medical Publishers; 2020.)

joint/space contains the *tendon of the long head of bicep brachii, rotator cuff tendons, subacromial/subdeltoid bursa* and the *glenohumeral joint capsule* (**Fig. 6.35; Fig. 6.39**). The **scapulothoracic joint** is also not a true articulating joint but is primarily the loose connective tissue between the subscapularis and serratus anterior muscles that allows gliding of the scapula over the chest wall (**Fig. 6.39; Fig. 6.48**).

6.7.6 Additional Ligaments of the Shoulder Region

- The **coracoacromial ligament** connects the coracoid and acromial processes of the scapula and together these structures form the **coracoacromial arch**. The arch prevents superior displacement of the humerus (**Fig. 6.44a**).

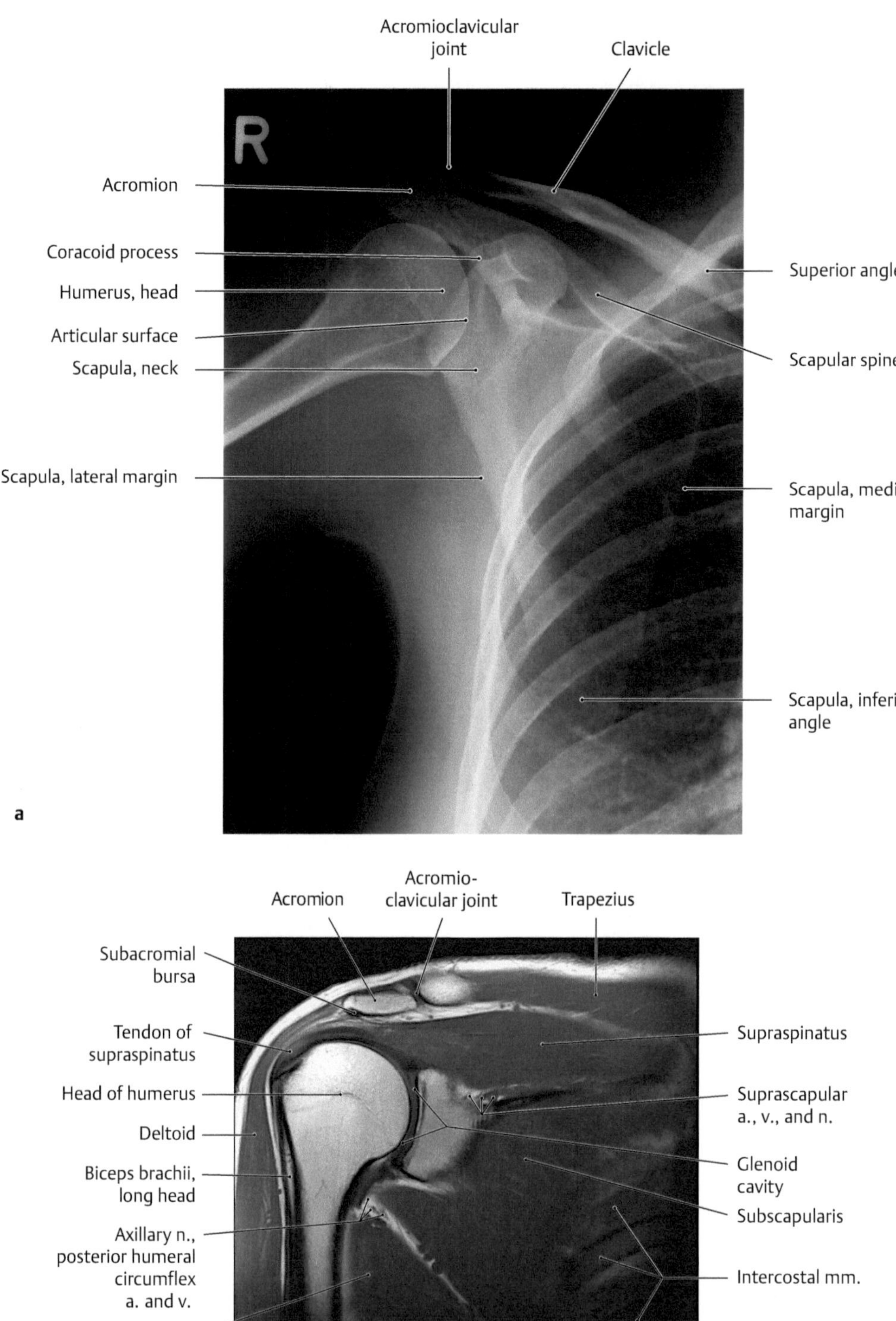

Fig. 6.43 **(a)** Radiograph of the scapula, anteroposterior view. (From Moeller TB, Reif E. Pocket Atlas of Radiographic Anatomy, 3rd ed. New York, NY: Thieme; 2010.) **(b)** MRI of the right shoulder joint, coronal section, anterior view. (From Schuenke M, Schulte E, Schumacher U. THIEME Atlas of Anatomy. General Anatomy and Musculoskeletal System. Illustrations by Voll M and Wesker K. 3rd ed. New York: Thieme Medical Publishers; 2020.)

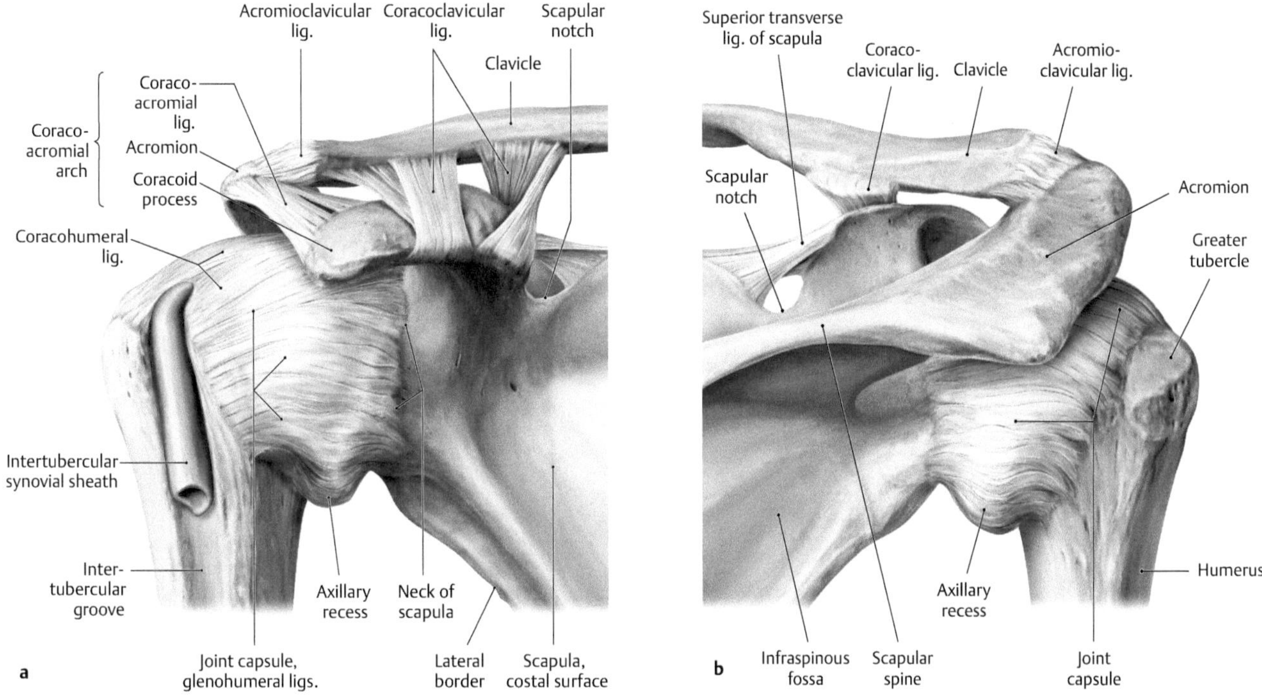

Fig. 6.44 Glenohumeral joint: capsule and ligaments. **(a)** Anterior view. **(b)** Posterior view. (From Schuenke M, Schulte E, Schumacher U. THIEME Atlas of Anatomy. General Anatomy and Musculoskeletal System. Illustrations by Voll M and Wesker K. 3rd ed. New York: Thieme Medical Publishers; 2020.)

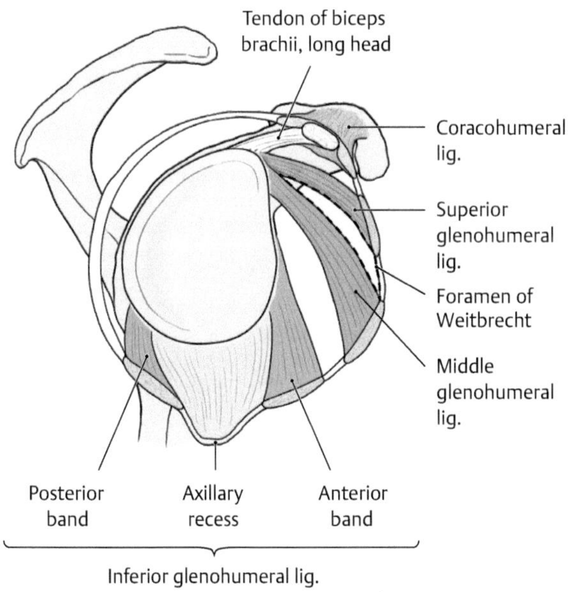

Fig. 6.45 Ligaments reinforcing capsule, lateral view. (From Schuenke M, Schulte E, Schumacher U. THIEME Atlas of Anatomy. General Anatomy and Musculoskeletal System. Illustrations by Voll M and Wesker K. 3rd ed. New York: Thieme Medical Publishers; 2020.)

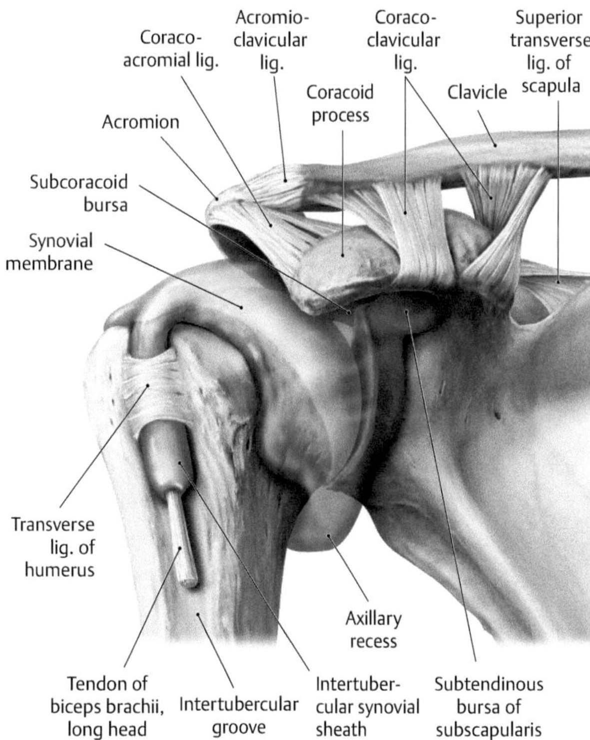

Fig. 6.46 Glenohumeral joint cavity with capsule removed, anterior view. (From Schuenke M, Schulte E, Schumacher U. THIEME Atlas of Anatomy. General Anatomy and Musculoskeletal System. Illustrations by Voll M and Wesker K. 3rd ed. New York: Thieme Medical Publishers; 2020.)

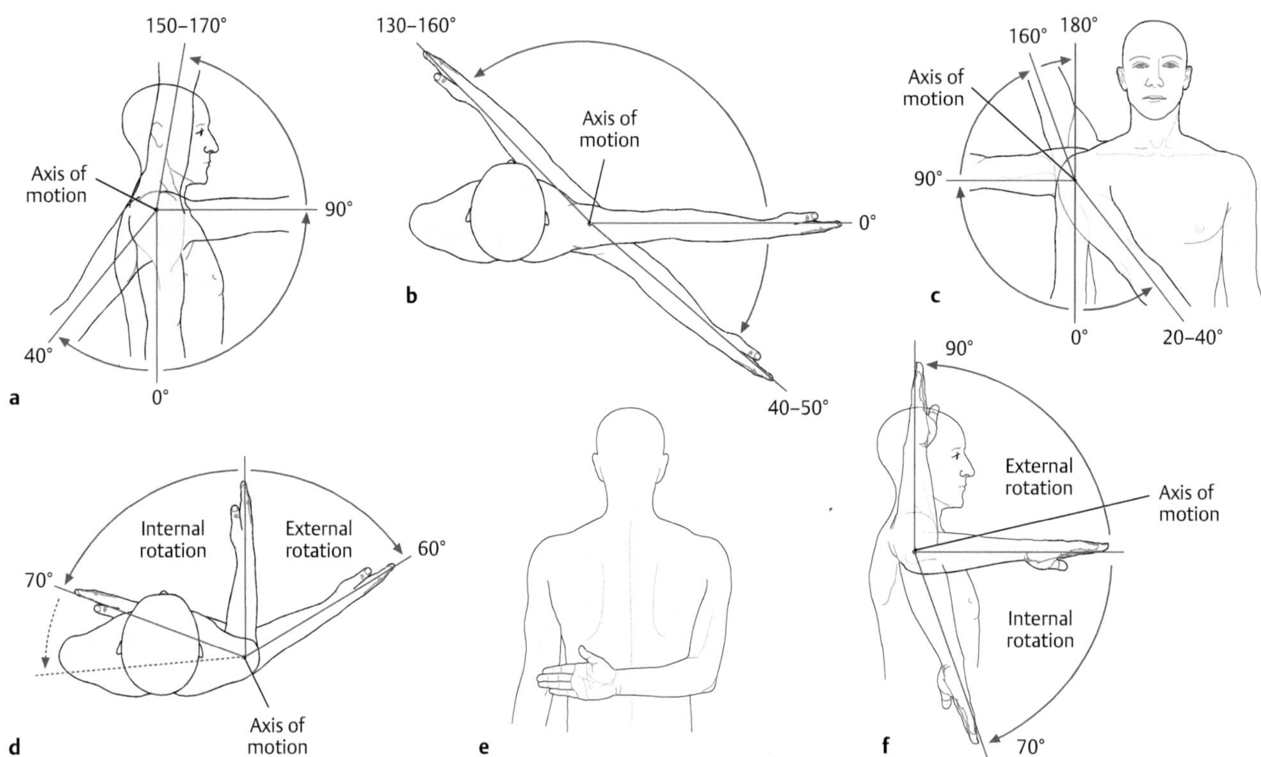

Fig. 6.47 **(a)** Flexion and extension on a horizontal axis. **(b)** Flexion and extension while the arm is raised to 90 degrees abduction. **(c)** Abduction and adduction. **(d-f)** Lateral (external) and medial (internal) rotation. (From Schuenke M, Schulte E, Schumacher U. THIEME Atlas of Anatomy. General Anatomy and Musculoskeletal System. Illustrations by Voll M and Wesker K. 3rd ed. New York: Thieme Medical Publishers; 2020.)

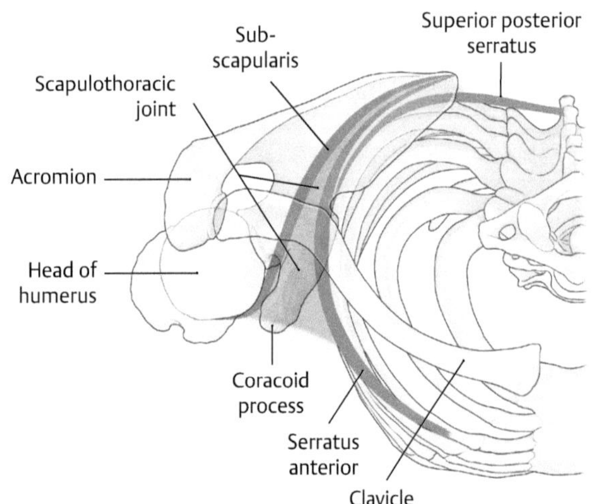

Fig. 6.48 Scapulothoracic joint. (From Schuenke M, Schulte E, Schumacher U. THIEME Atlas of Anatomy. General Anatomy and Musculoskeletal System. Illustrations by Voll M and Wesker K. 3rd ed. New York: Thieme Medical Publishers; 2020.)

Clinical Correlate 6.12

Shoulder Separation vs. Shoulder Dislocation

Shoulder separations occur at the acromioclavicular (AC) joint and involve tearing of the AC ligament, coracoclavicular ligament or both. The severity of separation is measured by grades (depending on source 1-3, 1-4, or 1-6) with grade 1 being the least affected.

Shoulder dislocations occur at the glenohumeral joint. Dislocations occur in an anterior (95%), posterior (< 5%) or inferior (~1%) fashion. Anterior displacement of the humerus represents a weakness in the joint capsule between the superior and middle glenohumeral ligaments known as the *foramen of Weitbrecht* **(Fig. 6.45)**.

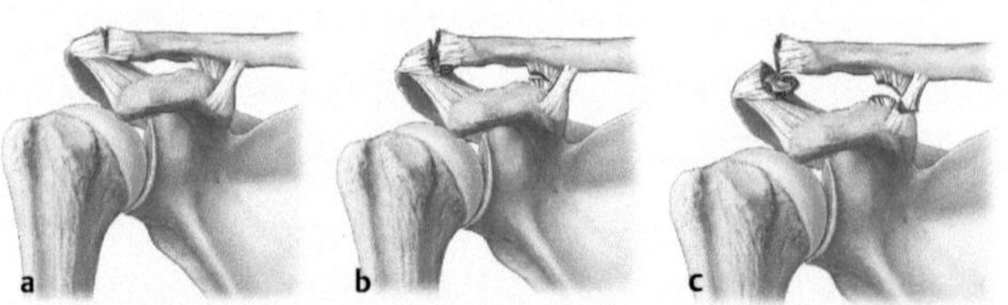

(a) Acromioclavicular and coracoclavicular ligaments are stretched but still intact. **(b)** Rupture of the acromioclavicular ligament allowing for subluxation of the joint. **(c)** All ligaments are disrupted allowing for complete separation of the acromioclavicular joint. (From Schuenke M, Schulte E, Schumacher U. THIEME Atlas of Anatomy. General Anatomy and Musculoskeletal System. Illustrations by Voll M and Wesker K. 3rd ed. New York: Thieme Medical Publishers; 2020.)

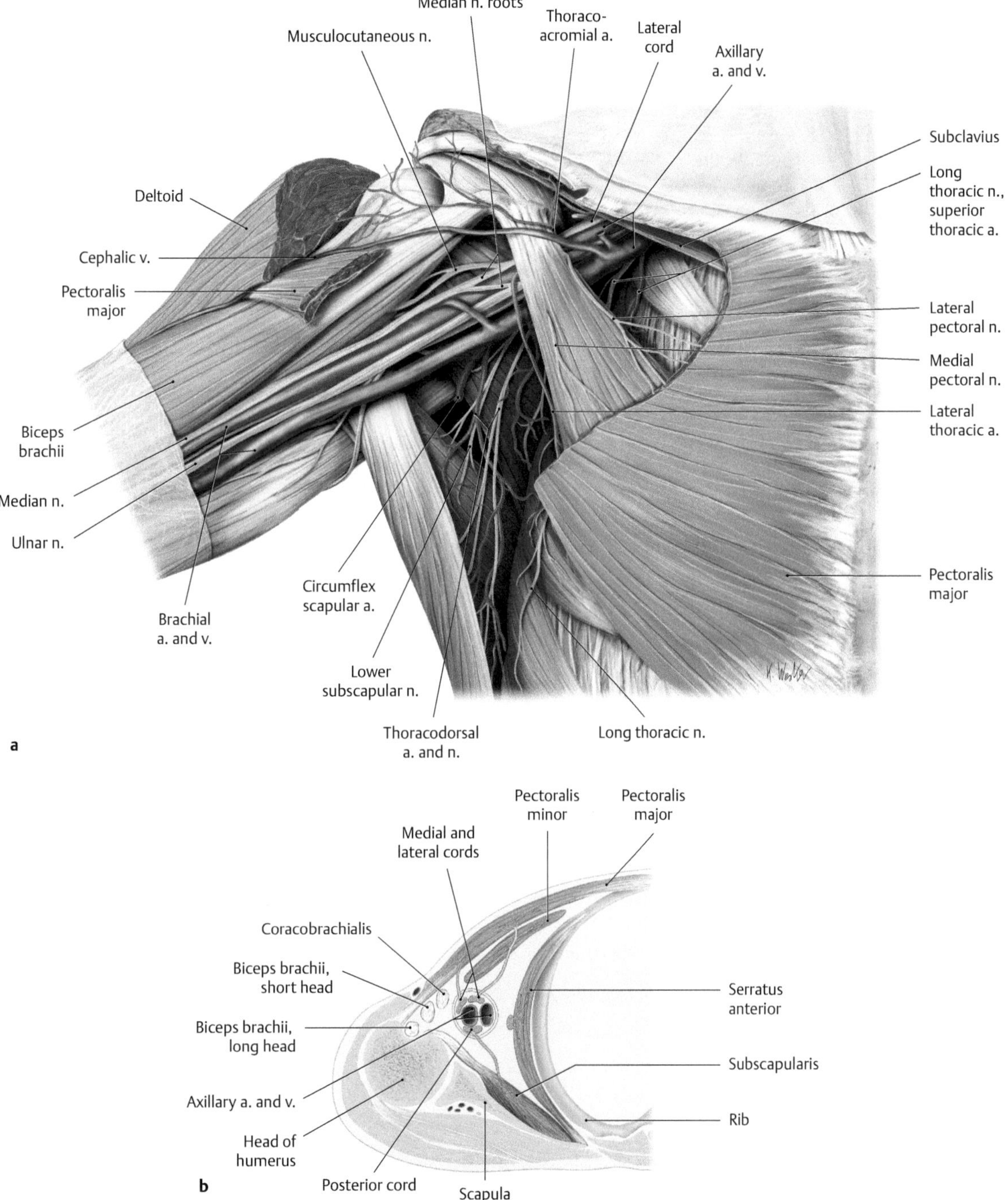

Fig. 6.49 **(a)** Right shoulder, anterior view. Lateral portion of pectoralis major has been removed. **(b)** Walls of the axilla. (From Schuenke M, Schulte E, Schumacher U. THIEME Atlas of Anatomy. General Anatomy and Musculoskeletal System. Illustrations by Voll M and Wesker K. 3rd ed. New York: Thieme Medical Publishers; 2020.)

- The **coracohumeral ligament** is a strong band that passes from the base of the coracoid process to the anterior aspect of the greater tubercle. It strengthens the glenohumeral joint capsule superiorly (**Fig. 6.44a**).
- The **transverse humeral ligament** runs from the greater to the lesser tubercle forming a bridge over the intertubercular sulcus and holds the tendon of the long head of bicep brachii in place. Fibers of this ligament may fuse with the glenohumeral ligaments (**Fig. 6.46**).

6.8 Axilla

Inferior to the glenohumeral joint and superior to the axillary fascia is the **axilla**. It is the passageway for which neurovascular structures pass to and from the upper extremity, neck, thoracic wall, and scapular and pectoral regions. The axilla is defined as having an apex, a base, and four walls. The more proximal neurovasculature is enclosed in a sleeve-like extension of the cervical fascia called the **axillary sheath** (**Fig. 6.49**).

- Apex: formed by the passageway between the axilla and neck called the **cervicoaxillary canal**. This passage is bounded by the clavicle, 1st rib and superior edge of the scapula.
- Base: formed by a combination of skin, subcutaneous fascia and the deep axillary fascia found between the thoracic wall and arm forming the **axillary fossa**. Referred to as the armpit.
- Anterior wall: formed by the pectoralis major and minor muscles and the clavipectoral fascia. The *anterior axillary fold* formed by the pectoralis major serves as the inferior most part of this wall.
- Posterior wall: formed primarily by the subscapularis muscle and scapula. The *posterior axillary fold* formed by the latissimus dorsi and teres major serves as the inferior most part of this wall.
- Lateral wall: the bony wall formed by the intertubercular sulcus of the humerus.
- Medial wall: formed by the serratus anterior muscle and thoracic wall.

6.8.1 Brachial Plexus

The major network of somatic nerves that supply the upper extremity is called the **brachial plexus**. It begins in the posterior triangle of the neck and extends into the axilla. It is formed by the union of the ventral rami of C5-T1 nerves, which constitute the roots of the brachial plexus. Sympathetic fibers that are carried by each root of the plexus are received from gray rami communicantes of the middle and inferior cervical ganglia. The brachial plexus is divided into **five roots**, **three trunks**, **six divisions**, **three cords** and **five terminal branches (Fig. 6.50)**.

The **roots** are formed by the last four cervical (C5-C8) and first thoracic (T1) ventral rami. They originate from between the anterior and middle scalene muscles and it is the roots that form the trunks. The *dorsal scapular nerve* originates from C5 root but may receive a contribution from C4. The *long thoracic nerve* originates from the C5-C7 roots.

The union of the C5 and C6 roots forms the **upper trunk**. The **middle trunk** is just a continuation of the C7 root. Lastly, the union of the C8 and T1 roots forms the **lower trunk**. The middle and lower trunks do not have any direct branches that originate from them but the upper trunk gives rise to the *suprascapular nerve* and *nerve to subclavius*.

Each trunk has an **anterior** and **posterior division** as the plexus continues through the cervicoaxillary canal, so there are three anterior and three posterior divisions. The anterior divisions supply the anterior or flexor compartments while the posterior divisions

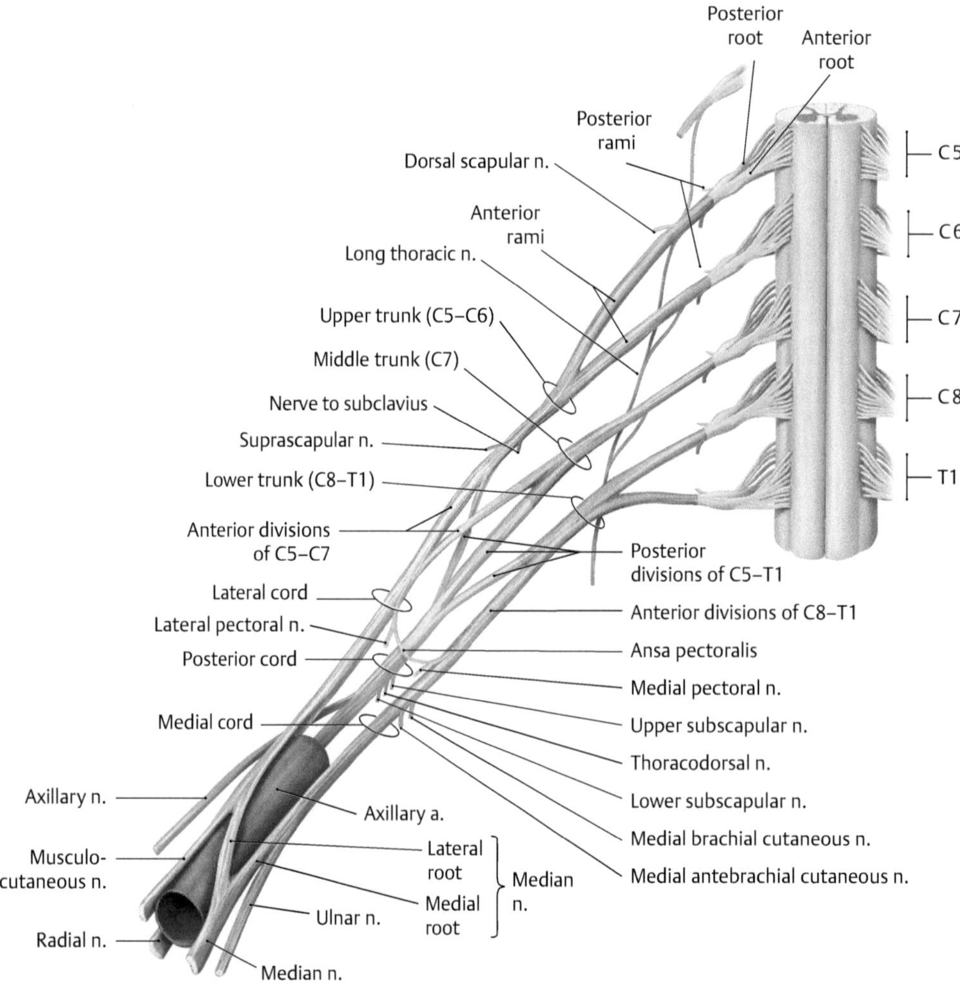

Fig. 6.50 Nerves of the upper extremity and brachial plexus. (From Schuenke M, Schulte E, Schumacher U. THIEME Atlas of Anatomy. General Anatomy and Musculoskeletal System. Illustrations by Voll M and Wesker K. 3rd ed. New York: Thieme Medical Publishers; 2020.)

supply the posterior or extensor compartments of the upper extremity. The anterior divisions from both the upper and middle trunks merge to form the *lateral cord*. The anterior division of the lower trunk continues as the *medial cord*. The **posterior divisions** of all three trunks unite and form the *posterior cord*. There are no direct nerve branches that originate from the divisions (**Fig. 6.50**).

The **lateral cord** bifurcates into the **musculocutaneous nerve** and the **lateral root of the median nerve**. The **lateral pectoral nerve** originates just proximal to the lateral cord's bifurcation. The **medial cord** bifurcates into the **medial root of the median nerve** and **ulnar nerve**. Prior to this bifurcation, the medial cord branches off the **medial pectoral**, **medial brachial cutaneous** and **medial antebrachial cutaneous nerves** from proximal to distal respectively. The **posterior cord** bifurcates into the **axillary** and **radial nerves**. The **upper subscapular**, **thoracodorsal** and **lower subscapular nerves** originate from the posterior cord just prior to the bifurcation from proximal to distal respectively (**Fig. 6.30**). The cords are named based on their location to the axillary artery. The **terminal branches** of the brachial plexus are considered to be the musculocutaneous, median, ulnar, axillary and radial nerves (**Fig. 6.51**).

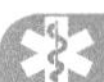

Clinical Correlate 6.13

Brachial Plexus Blocks

Injecting an anesthetic solution into or immediately surrounding the axillary sheath interrupts nerve impulses to structures supplied by the branches or cords of the brachial plexus. These types of nerve blocks allow surgeons to operate on the upper extremity without using a general anesthetic. These blocks could include an interscalene, supraclavicular, infraclavicular or an axillary approach.

The location of the clavicle helps divide the brachial plexus into a **supraclavicular** and **infraclavicular part**. Branches of the supraclavicular part include the *dorsal scapular, long thoracic, nerve to subclavius, suprascapular nerves* in addition to the *phrenic nerve* and numerous unnamed *muscular branches* that supply the diaphragm and related prevertebral muscles of the posterior triangle of the neck respectively. The infraclavicular branches include the *lateral pectoral, medial pectoral, medial brachial, medial antebrachial, upper subscapular, thoracodorsal* and *lower subscapular nerves* (**Fig. 6.50; Fig. 6.51**).

6.8.2 Axillary Artery and Vein

The **axillary artery** extends from the lateral edge of the 1st rib to the inferior border of the teres major muscle. The axillary artery begins at the termination of the subclavian artery and ends as the brachial artery. It has 3 parts:

- **1st part**: located between the lateral edge of the 1st rib and the medial border of pectoralis minor. It is enclosed in the axillary sheath and has one branch called the **superior thoracic artery**. This artery is small, highly variable, and arises just inferior to the subclavius muscle. It supplies the subclavius, intercostal muscles between the 1st and 2nd intercostal spaces, and portions of the pectoral and serratus anterior muscles. The internal thoracic and upper intercostal arteries anastomose with it (**Fig. 6.52**).

Clinical Correlate 6.14

Upper Brachial Plexus Injury

The **upper brachial plexus injury** (***Erb-Duchenne palsy***) involves damage to the *superior trunk* of the brachial plexus that is made up of the C5 and C6 roots. The superior trunk can be damaged by a stab wound, stretching of the neck during the delivery of a neonate, or when the head and trunk is separated from the shoulder during a head-first fall. The major nerves damaged by this injury are the suprascapular, axillary and musculocutaneous nerves. The major muscles affected by disruption of these nerves are the supraspinatus, infraspinatus, deltoid, teres minor, biceps brachii and brachialis. This injury results in the limb hanging limply by the side, medially rotated and with the forearm pronated due to loss of the supinating action of the biceps brachii. Hence the reason this type of injury is also referred to as a "waiter's tip" injury.

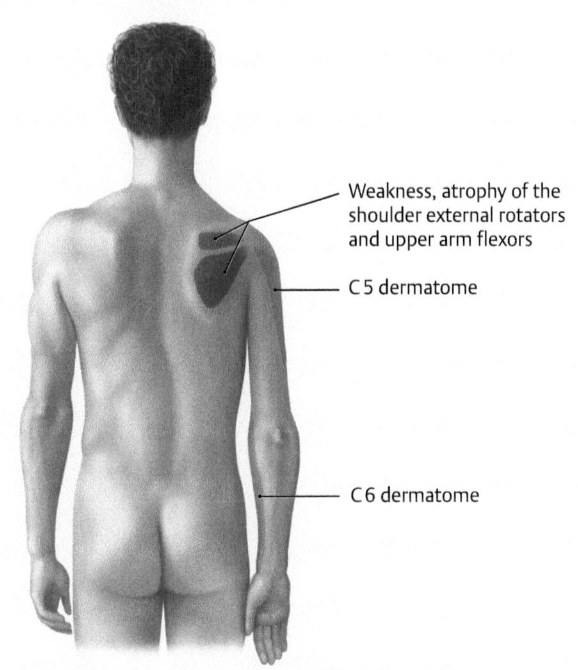

(From Schuenke M, Schulte E, Schumacher U. THIEME Atlas of Anatomy. General Anatomy and Musculoskeletal System. Illustrations by Voll M and Wesker K. 3rd ed. New York: Thieme Medical Publishers; 2020.)

- **2nd part**: located posterior to the pectoralis minor and has two branches called the thoracoacromial trunk and lateral thoracic artery. The **thoracoacromial trunk** is located near the medial border of the pectoralis minor and pierces the costocoracoid membrane before dividing into four branches (*acromial, clavicular, deltoid* and *pectoral*). Structures supplied can include the deltoid, pectoral and subclavius muscles along with the breast and sternoclavicular joint. The **lateral thoracic artery** is generally said to originate distal to the thoracoacromial trunk near the lateral border of the pectoralis minor and descend near the serratus anterior and long thoracic nerve. However, its origin is quite variable and may arise from the subscapular, thoracoacromial or suprascapular arteries. It supplies the serratus anterior, pectoral and intercostal muscles along with the lateral breast and axillary lymph nodes (**Fig. 6.52**).
- **3rd part**: located between the lateral border of pectoralis minor and inferior border of the teres major muscle. It has

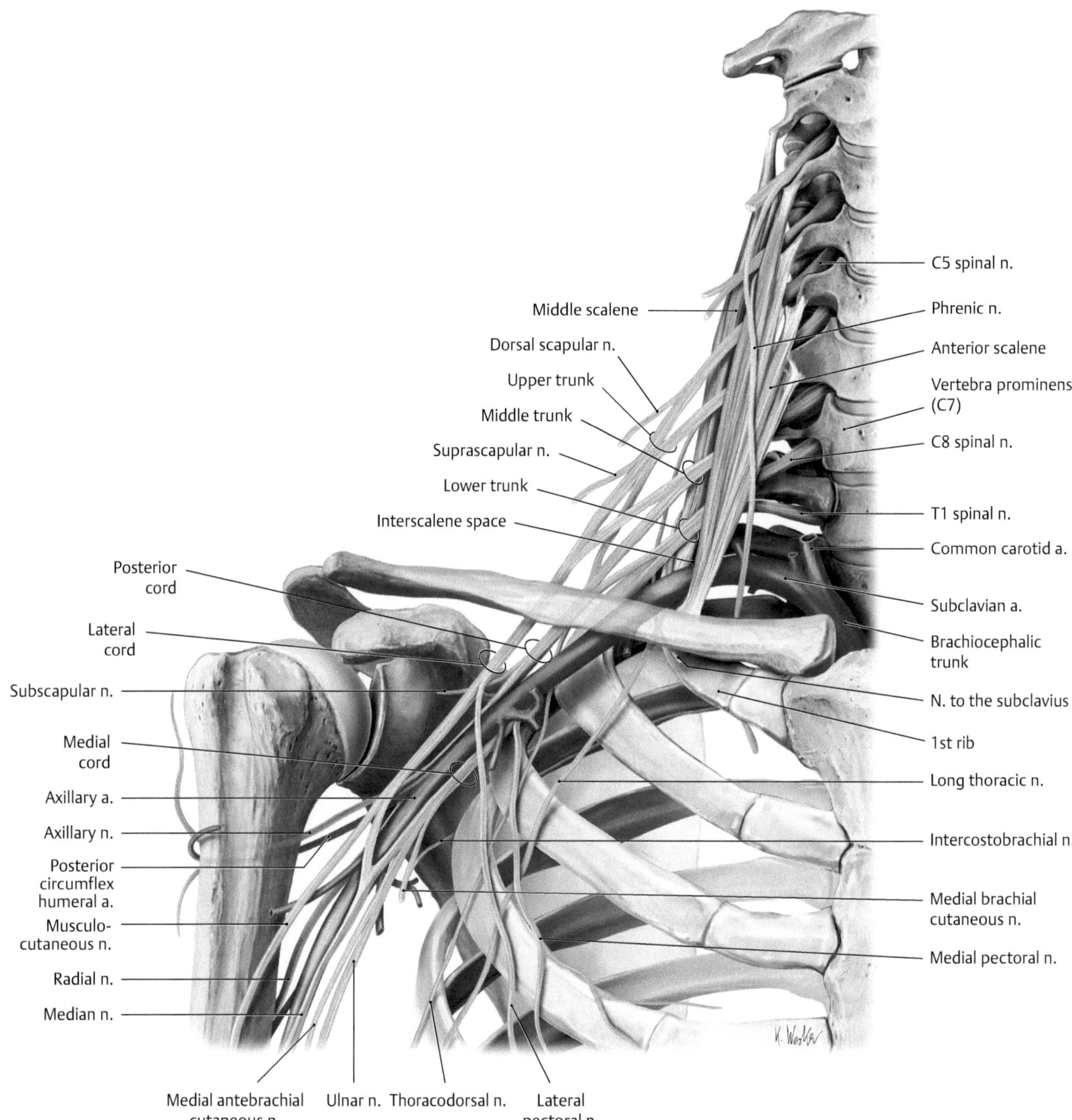

Fig. 6.51 Course of the brachial plexus and its relation to the thorax after passing through the interscalene space. Right side, anterior view. (From Schuenke M, Schulte E, Schumacher U. THIEME Atlas of Anatomy. General Anatomy and Musculoskeletal System. Illustrations by Voll M and Wesker K. 3rd ed. New York: Thieme Medical Publishers; 2020.)

three branches called the subscapular, anterior and posterior circumflex humeral arteries. The **subscapular artery** descends along the lateral border of the subscapularis muscle on the posterior axillary wall before bifurcating as the circumflex scapular and thoracodorsal arteries. The **circumflex scapular artery** curves posteriorly around the lateral border of the scapula and in between the subscapularis and teres major muscles initially. It forms an anastomosis with the suprascapular and dorsal scapular arteries before continuing through the *triangular space*. It helps supply muscles on the dorsum of the scapula. The **thoracodorsal artery** pairs with the nerve of the same name and is the principal blood supply to the latissimus dorsi muscle (**Fig. 6.52**).

The **anterior circumflex humeral artery** is about half the size of the posterior branch and passes laterally and deep to the biceps brachii and coracobrachialis muscles to help supply the shoulder region. The **posterior circumflex humeral artery** passes through the quadrangular space along with the axillary nerve and supplies blood to the surrounding muscles and glenohumeral joint.

The **axillary vein** lies mostly anterior to the axillary artery. The union of the *basilic* and *brachial veins* forms it and it has three parts that correspond to the arterial parts. The axillary vein

Clinical Correlate 6.15

Lower Brachial Plexus Injury

The **lower brachial plexus injury** (***Klumpke's paralysis***) involves damage to the inferior trunk of the brachial plexus that is made up of the C8 and T1 roots. A version of "claw hand" can actually occur if damage is located at the inferior trunk, medial epicondyle of the humerus (*cubital tunnel syndrome*), or the ulnar tunnel near the wrist (*ulnar tunnel syndrome*). The severity in a sense decreases as you move closer to the wrist. The inferior trunk can be damaged by excessive abduction of the arm such as when a person grasps onto something to prevent a fall. The major nerve fibers from this trunk run in the median & ulnar nerves which supply all the small muscles of the hand and anterior forearm muscles. The ulnar nerve fibers are generally affected the most. Paralysis of the intrinsic muscles of the hand causes the fingers to assume this "claw hand" position. This position is exaggerated by the unopposed action of the extensor digitorum muscle (innervated by the radial nerve).

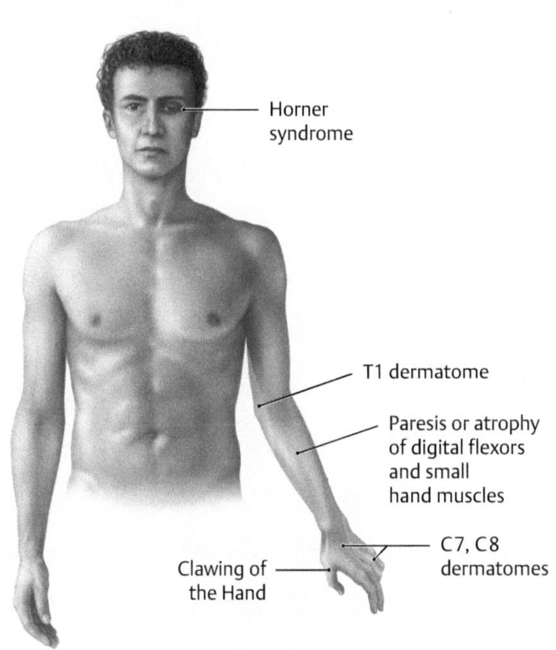

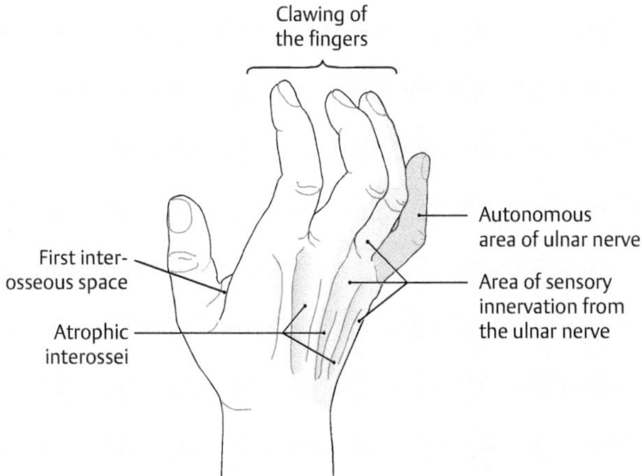

(From Schuenke M, Schulte E, Schumacher U. THIEME Atlas of Anatomy. General Anatomy and Musculoskeletal System. Illustrations by Voll M and Wesker K. 3rd ed. New York: Thieme Medical Publishers; 2020.)

terminates as the **subclavian vein** at the lateral border of the 1st rib. The venous tributaries that correspond to the branches of the axillary arteries drain into the axillary vein except for the veins related to the thoracoacromial trunk, which drain either directly into the axillary vein or into the cephalic vein. In addition, the **thoracoepigastric vein(s)** that originate from some superficial periumbilical veins near the umbilicus and inguinal region drain into the axillary vein (**Fig. 6.23a; Fig. 6.53**).

6.8.3 Axillary Lymph Nodes

There are six principal groups of axillary lymph nodes and they lie within the pyramidal borders of the axilla. The principle groups of axillary lymph nodes are the pectoral (anterior), humeral (lateral), subscapular (posterior), central, interpectoral and apical lymph nodes (**Fig. 6.54**).

- **Pectoral (anterior)** (~4 nodes): receive lymph mainly from the anterior thoracic wall and this includes most of the breast.
- **Humeral (lateral)** (~5 nodes): receive nearly all the lymph from the upper limb. However, lymphatic vessels accompanying the cephalic vein drain primarily to the apical and infraclavicular nodes.
- **Subscapular (posterior)** (~6 nodes): receive lymph from the scapular region and posterior aspect of the thoracic wall.
- **Central** (~3 large nodes): receive efferent lymphatic vessels from the *pectoral, humeral* and *subscapular lymph nodes*. They drain to the apical lymph nodes.
- **Interpectoral (*Rotter's*)** (range from 1-4): are located between the pectoralis major and minor muscles and may drain to either the central or apical nodes. Some authors do not consider them to be part of the larger axillary node group.
- **Apical**: receive lymph from all the axillary lymph node groups as well as that near the proximal cephalic vein. The efferent vessels from these nodes pass through the cervicoaxillary canal and unite to form the **subclavian lymphatic trunk**, with some drainage heading towards the **supra/infraclavicular nodes**. The jugular and bronchomediastinal trunks on the right side may join the subclavian trunk to help form the **right lymphatic duct**. On the left side the subclavian trunk generally drains directly into the **thoracic duct**.

Previously described in Chapter 2, these groups of lymph nodes can be divided into three different levels surgically and can be used to determine the 5-year survival rate for patients with breast cancer. The **level I** or **lower axillary group** is located lateral to the pectoralis minor and consists of the *pectoral (anterior), humeral (lateral)* and *subscapular (posterior)* lymph nodes. The **level II** or **middle axillary group** is located at the level of the pectoralis minor and consists of the *central* and *interpectoral* lymph nodes. The **level III** or **upper infraclavicular group** is located medial to the pectoralis minor and consists of the *apical* lymph nodes (**Fig. 6.55**).

6.9 Arm

6.9.1 Arm Region Muscles

The *anterior arm* consists of three muscles associated primarily with flexion. The **biceps brachii**, as indicated in its name, has two heads that arise from the scapula and insert primarily on the radius. Although it courses over the humerus, it has no direct attachment to this bone (**Fig. 6.28; Fig. 6.56**). A minority of individuals may have a smaller third head that extends from

Thyrocervical trunk
Scalene muscles
Acromial, clavicular, and deltoid branches
Suprascapular artery
Vertebral artery
Common carotid artery
Subclavian artery
Brachiocephalic trunk
Internal thoracic artery
Axillary artery
Superior thoracic artery
Thoracoacromial artery
Pectoral branch
Pectoralis minor
Posterior circumflex humeral artery
Circumflex scapular artery
Subscapular artery
Anterior circumflex humeral artery
Latissimus dorsi
Thoracodorsal artery
Lateral thoracic artery
Brachial artery
Deep artery of arm
Triceps brachii, long head

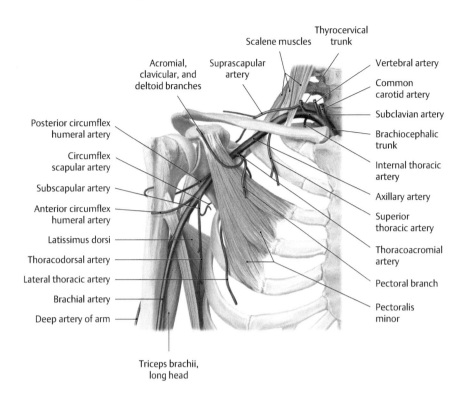

Fig. 6.52 Origin and branches of the axillary artery. (From Schuenke M, Schulte E, Schumacher U. THIEME Atlas of Anatomy. General Anatomy and Musculoskeletal System. Illustrations by Voll M and Wesker K. 3rd ed. New York: Thieme Medical Publishers; 2020.)

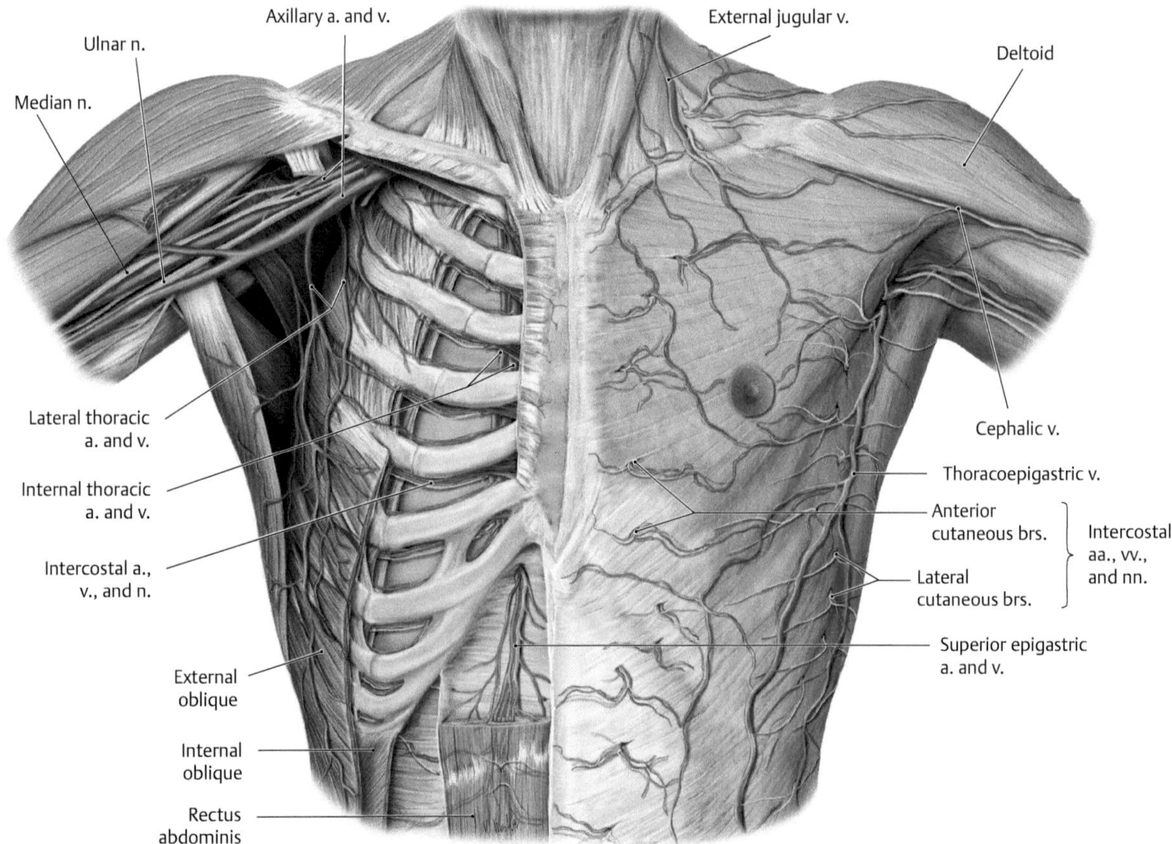

Fig. 6.53 Neurovasculature of the thoracic wall. (From Schuenke M, Schulte E, Schumacher U. THIEME Atlas of Anatomy. General Anatomy and Musculoskeletal System. Illustrations by Voll M and Wesker K. 3rd ed. New York: Thieme Medical Publishers; 2020.)

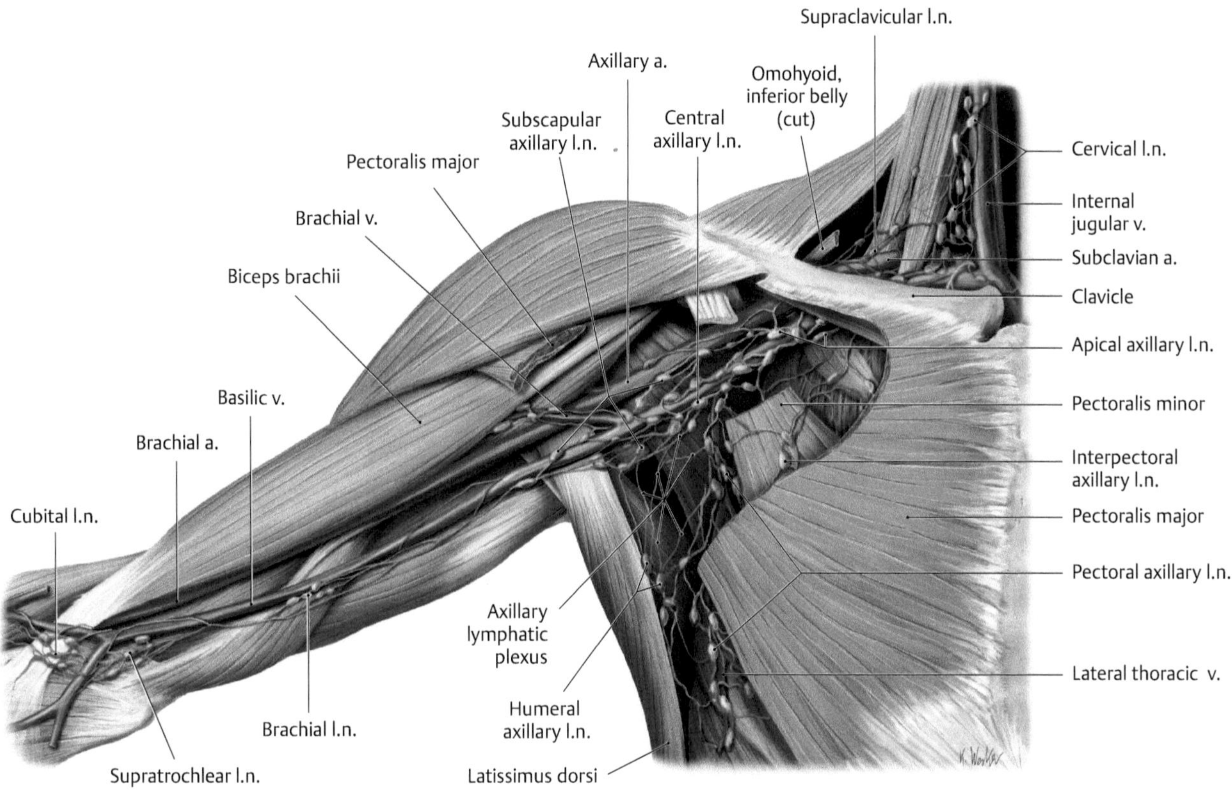

Levels of axillary lymph nodes

Level		Position	Lymph nodes (l.n.)
I	Lower axillary group	Lateral to pectoralis minor	Pectoral axillary l.n.
			Subscapular axillary l.n.
			Humeral axillary l.n.
II	Middle axillary group	Along pectoralis minor	Central axillary l.n.
			Interpectoral axillary l.n.
III	Upper infraclavicular group	Medial to pectoralis minor	Apical axillary l.n.

Fig. 6.54 Axillary lymph nodes. (From Schuenke M, Schulte E, Schumacher U. THIEME Atlas of Anatomy. General Anatomy and Musculoskeletal System. Illustrations by Voll M and Wesker K. 3rd ed. New York: Thieme Medical Publishers; 2020.)

the superomedial portion of the brachialis. This muscle functions in *flexion of the arm (weak) and forearm* and as the most powerful *supinator of the forearm*. When the elbow is fully extended the biceps brachii is primarily a flexor of the forearm. Arm flexion at the shoulder is weak in any position. When the elbow is near 90° flexion and the forearm is supinated, the biceps is a forearm flexor. If the forearm is pronated, the biceps mostly supinates. The **bicipitoradial bursa** reduces friction between the biceps tendon and radial tuberosity.

The **coracobrachialis** only crosses the shoulder joint and thus has no action at the elbow joint. The musculocutaneous nerve pierces it and the nutrient artery of the humerus enters the bone near its distal attachment. It functions in *adduction* and *flexion of the arm*. The **brachialis** is flat and functions in *flexion of the forearm*. It is the strongest flexor of the forearm and the orientation of the forearm in either supination or pronation does not affect it (**Fig. 6.28; Fig. 6.56; Fig. 6.57**).

The *posterior arm* consists of two muscles, the triceps brachii and anconeus, although the anconeus muscle belly is found mostly in the posterior forearm. The **triceps brachii** has three heads, as indicated by its name, which arise from either the scapula or humerus but insert as a common tendon on the olecranon of the ulna. It is the main muscle for *extension of the forearm* and the medial head of the muscle participates the most during this action. The long head also participates in *adduction* and *extension of the arm* but it is the least active head of the three. Supination and pronation of the forearm does not affect its functions. The **anconeus** is a small muscle that really only assists the triceps brachii in *extension of the forearm* but it also tenses the joint capsule during elbow extension. This prevents any pinching of the joint capsule, a function similar to what the articularis genu does at the knee. It may abduct the ulna during forearm pronation (**Fig. 6.31b; Fig. 6.58**). Descriptions of the arm region muscles are found in **Table 6.4**.

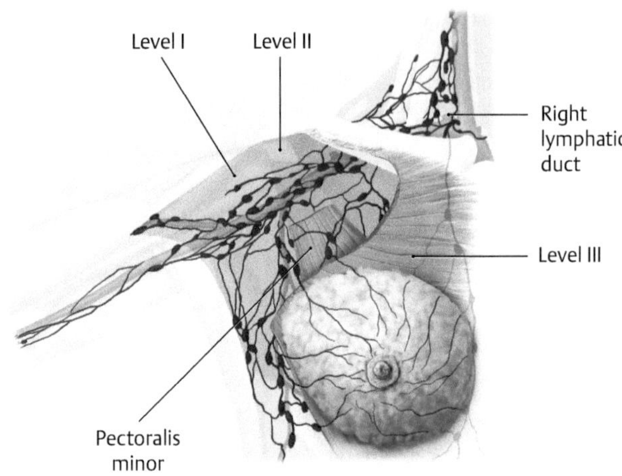

Fig. 6.55 Axillary lymph node levels. Refer to **Fig. 6.54** for list of individual nodes located at each level. (From Schuenke M, Schulte E, Schumacher U. THIEME Atlas of Anatomy. General Anatomy and Musculoskeletal System. Illustrations by Voll M and Wesker K. 3rd ed. New York: Thieme Medical Publishers; 2020.)

6.9.2 Neurovasculature of the Arm Region

The **musculocutaneous nerve** innervates all muscles of the anterior arm and it pierces the coracobrachialis before passing between the biceps brachii and brachialis muscles. Near the level of the cubital fossa there are no longer any motor fibers coursing through this nerve and it continues as the *lateral antebrachial cutaneous nerve*. The **radial nerve** enters the arm posterior to the brachial artery and medial to the humerus. It continues anterior to the long head of the triceps brachii and pairs with the profunda brachii vessels (viewed through the *triangular hiatus*) before advancing inferolaterally against the *radial groove* to the lateral humeral shaft. It then pierces the *lateral intermuscular septum* and progresses between the brachialis and brachioradialis muscles before reaching the cubital fossa. The radial nerve innervates the triceps brachii and anconeus of the posterior arm compartment **(Fig. 6.59; Fig. 6.60)**

The **median** and **ulnar nerves** pass down the medial portion of the arm but do not innervate any structures located in either compartment of the arm. The median nerve follows the brachial artery into the cubital fossa while the ulnar nerve pierces the *medial intermuscular septum* and descends between the septum and medial head of the triceps brachii. It then passes medial to the olecranon and posterior to the medial epicondyle through the *cubital tunnel* before entering the forearm **(Fig. 6.59)**.

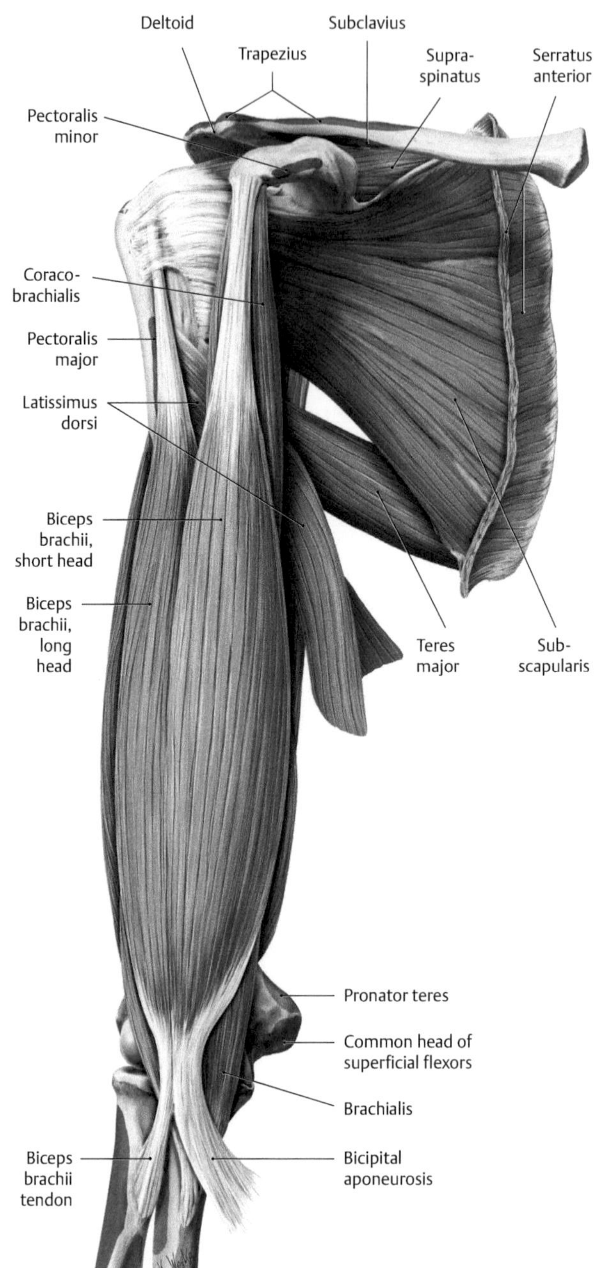

Fig. 6.56 Anterior muscles of the shoulder and arm. (Red = origin; blue = insertion). (From Schuenke M, Schulte E, Schumacher U. THIEME Atlas of Anatomy. General Anatomy and Musculoskeletal System. Illustrations by Voll M and Wesker K. 3rd ed. New York: Thieme Medical Publishers; 2020.)

Clinical Correlate 6.16

Biceps Brachii and Triceps Brachii Reflexes

There are monosynaptic and ipsilateral (same side) muscle stretch reflexes routinely tested during a physical examination of the upper extremity. They consist of an afferent and efferent limb that travel to and from the spinal cord but are incorrectly referred to as deep tendon reflexes. A normal (positive) response is the involuntary and brief jerk-like contraction of a particular muscle at a particular joint. A positive response of the **biceps brachii reflex** confirms the integrity of the musculocutaneous nerve and the C5 and C6 spinal cord segments. A positive response of the **triceps brachii reflex** confirms the integrity of the radial nerve and the C7 and C8 spinal cord segments.

Blood supply to the anterior arm is from the **brachial artery**, a continuation of the axillary artery. It is paired with multiple **brachial veins**, which, along with the basilic vein, form the axillary vein. Just distal to the inferior border of the teres major muscle, the **profunda brachii artery** (deep artery of the arm) branches from the brachial artery and continues posteroinferiorly toward the elbow before terminating as the middle and radial collateral arteries. The **humeral nutrient artery** originates from the brachial artery near the mid-arm and supplies the humerus. At the mid-humeral area and medially, the **superior ulnar collateral**

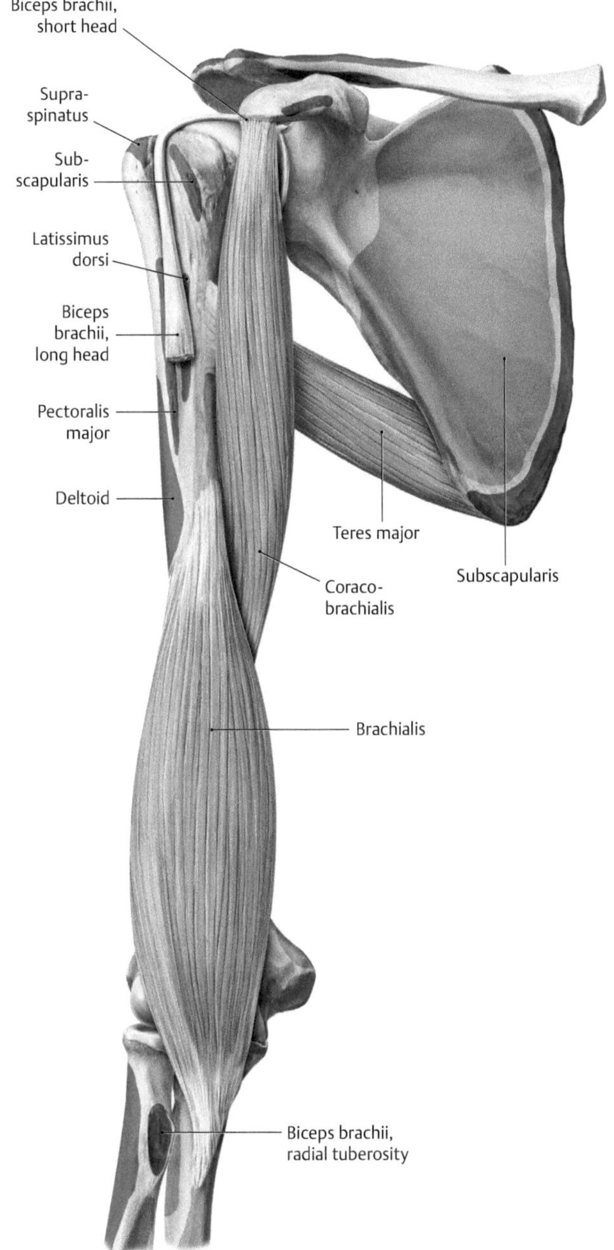

Fig. 6.57 Brachialis and coracobrachialis. (Red = origin; blue = insertion) (From Schuenke M, Schulte E, Schumacher U. THIEME Atlas of Anatomy. General Anatomy and Musculoskeletal System. Illustrations by Voll M and Wesker K. 3rd ed. New York: Thieme Medical Publishers; 2020.)

artery arises from the brachial artery and distally from that location the **inferior ulnar collateral artery** is given off (**Fig. 6.61**).

6.10 Cubital Fossa

The triangular-shaped superficial depression located on the anterior side of the elbow is known as the **cubital fossa**. This fossa has three borders, a roof and a floor (**Fig. 6.62**):

- Superior border: the imaginary line connecting the lateral and medial epicondyles.
- Lateral border: brachioradialis muscle.

> ***Clinical Correlate 6.17***
>
> **Wrist Drop**
>
> Damage to the radial nerve at a point generally before the deep and superficial branches causes patients to in lose the ability to actively extend their hands at the wrist. This is referred to as **wrist drop**. Most patients with damage to the proximal or mid-level radial nerve display wrist drop and sensory loss over a large portion of the dorsum hand (where the superficial branch of the radial nerve is responsible for innervating the skin).
>
> 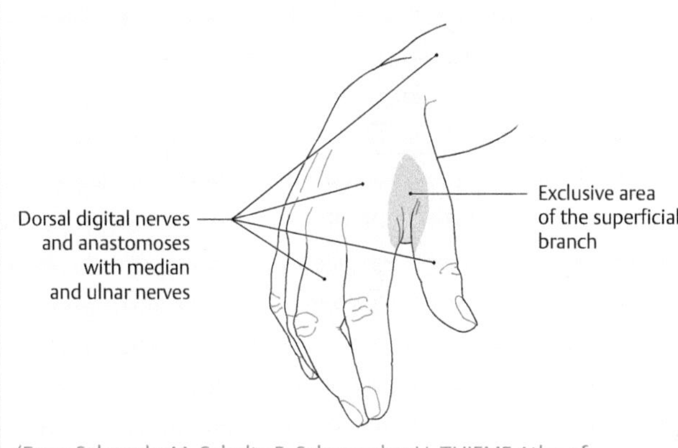
>
>
> (From Schuenke M, Schulte E, Schumacher U. THIEME Atlas of Anatomy. General Anatomy and Musculoskeletal System. Illustrations by Voll M and Wesker K. 3rd ed. New York: Thieme Medical Publishers; 2020.)

- Medial border: pronator teres muscle.
- Roof: junction between the brachial and antebrachial fascia.
- Floor: brachialis and supinator muscles.

Contents of the cubital fossa include the **median nerve**, which is adjacent to the brachial vessels in the arm and visible through the fossa before it passes between the two heads of the pronator teres muscle. As the radial nerve emerges from between the brachialis and brachioradialis muscles and anterior to the lateral epicondyle, it bifurcates into a **deep branch** and **superficial branch of the radial nerve**. The deep branch pierces the supinator muscle and on the opposite side of this muscle it becomes the **posterior interosseous nerve**. The superficial branch continues towards the wrist tucked between the brachioradialis and extensor carpi radialis longus muscles (**Fig. 6.62b**).

The **brachial artery** reaches the fossa and bifurcates into the radial and ulnar arteries. All three arterial branches are paired with two slightly smaller veins of the same name. The **radial artery** branches off the **radial recurrent artery** deep to the brachioradialis muscle and just lateral to the lateral border of this fossa before continuing down the lateral aspect of the anterior forearm. The **ulnar artery** branches off the **anterior ulnar recurrent**, **posterior ulnar recurrent** and **common interosseous arteries** before continuing down the medial aspect of the anterior forearm. These branches occur just outside the borders of the cubital fossa (**Fig. 6.61**).

The **median cubital vein** is located in the subcutaneous tissue overlying the cubital fossa. Due to the high level of variability of the veins in this area there may be some additional tributaries of the basilic and cephalic veins over the fossa. The **lateral antebrachial cutaneous** and **medial antebrachial cutaneous nerves** can pass over the cubital fossa before they rest adjacent to the cephalic and basilic veins in the forearm respectively (**Fig. 6.63**).

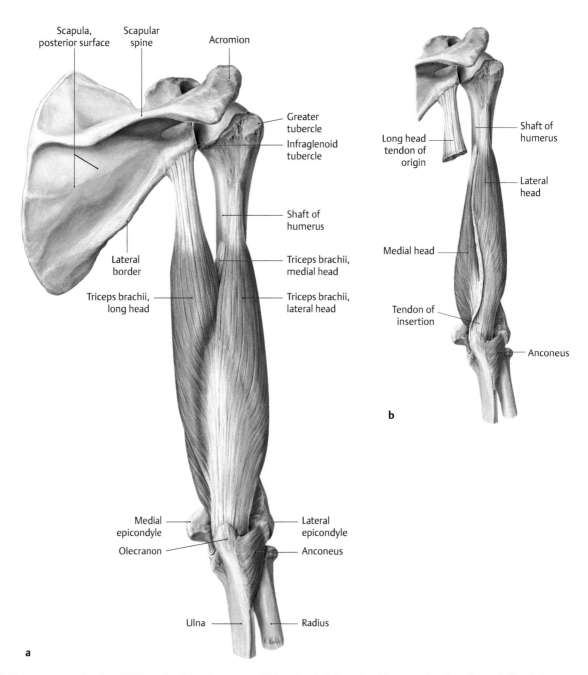

Fig. 6.58 Right arm, posterior view. **(a)** Triceps brachii and anconeus. **(b)** Long head of triceps brachii removed to show the medial head. (From Schuenke M, Schulte E, Schumacher U. THIEME Atlas of Anatomy. General Anatomy and Musculoskeletal System. Illustrations by Voll M and Wesker K. 3rd ed. New York: Thieme Medical Publishers; 2020.)

Clinical Correlate 6.18

Measuring Arterial Blood Pressure

To measure arterial blood pressure a **sphygmomanometer** is used. This is done by placing a cuff around the arm and inflating it with air until it compresses and occludes the brachial artery. A stethoscope is placed over the brachial artery in the cubital fossa prior to its bifurcation. The pressure from the cuff is gradually released and the first audible spurt of blood indicates **systolic blood pressure**. With continued pressure release, the point at which the pulse can no longer be heard indicates **diastolic blood pressure**.

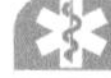

Clinical Correlate 6.19

Venipuncture

The cubital fossa is a common site for both blood sampling and transfusion along with the introduction of intravenous fluids. The median cubital vein is the most commonly targeted for venipuncture. This vein lies directly on the deep fascia before crossing over the bicipital aponeurosis which provides some protection from accidently puncturing the brachial artery or median nerve. A tourniquet is applied to the arm so that venous return is occluded resulting in distension and more visible veins. The tourniquet is removed after the vein is punctured so that bleeding will be minimal after the removal of the needle.

Table 6.4 **Arm region muscles**

Muscle	Innervation	Function(s)	Origin	Insertion
Biceps brachii	Musculocutaneous nerve	Flex arm; flex and supinate forearm	*Long head*: supraglenoid tubercle *Short head*: coracoid process	Radial tuberosity and antebrachial fascia via bicipital aponeurosis.
Coracobrachialis	Musculocutaneous nerve	Adduct and flex arm	Coracoid process	Medial surface of middle 1/3 of humerus
Brachialis	Musculocutaneous nerve	Flex forearm	Anterior surface of distal 1/2 of humerus	Ulnar tuberosity and coronoid process
Triceps brachii	Radial nerve	Adducts and extends arm; extends forearm	*Long head*: infraglenoid tubercle *Lateral head*: posterior surface of humerus proximal to radial groove *Medial head*: posterior surface of humerus distal to radial groove	Olecranon
Anconeus	Radial nerve	Extends forearm (assists triceps brachii); may abduct ulna during forearm pronation	Lateral epicondyle	Lateral (radial) surface of olecranon

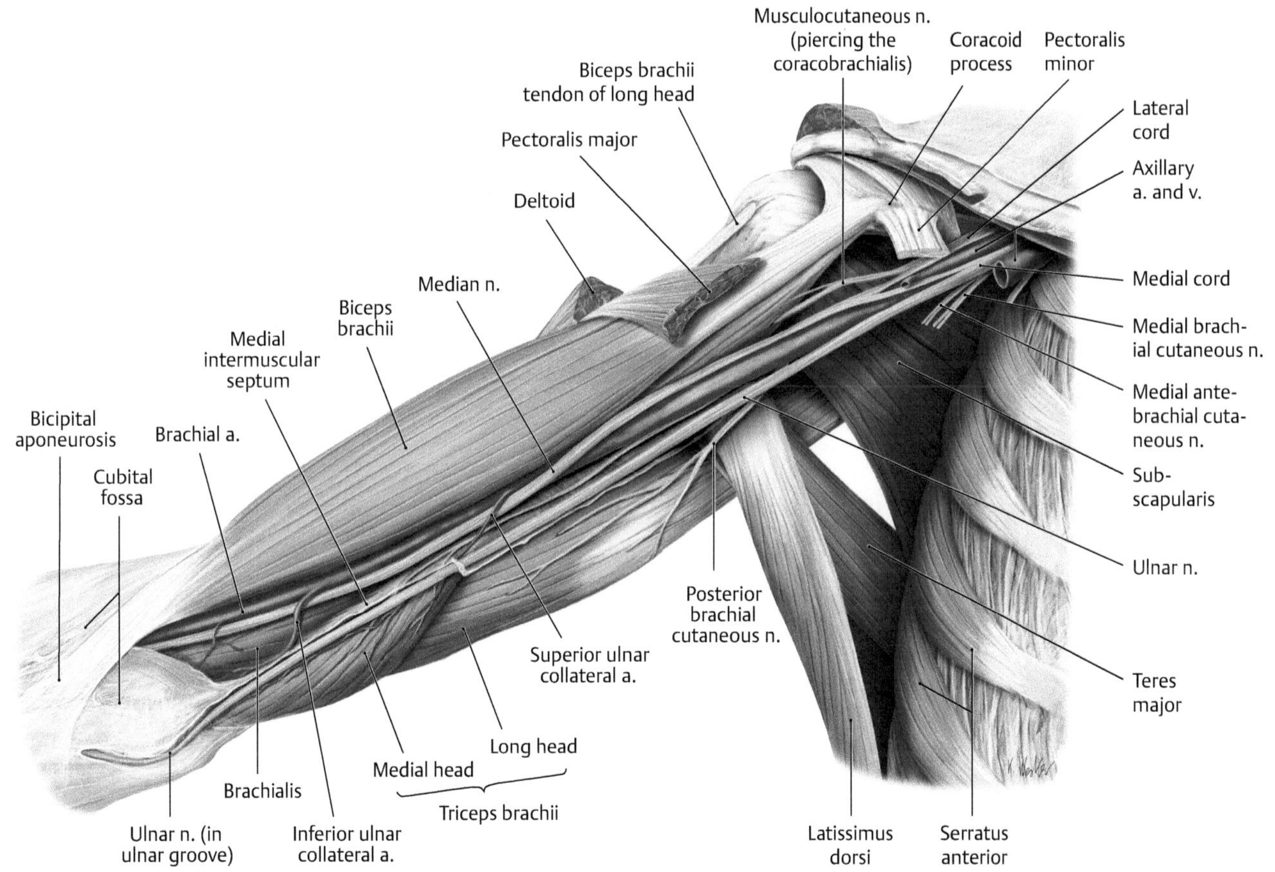

Fig. 6.59 Brachial region. Right arm, anterior view. Removed: deltoid, pectoralis major and minor. (From Schuenke M, Schulte E, Schumacher U. THIEME Atlas of Anatomy. General Anatomy and Musculoskeletal System. Illustrations by Voll M and Wesker K. 3rd ed. New York: Thieme Medical Publishers; 2020.)

6.11 Elbow Joint

The **elbow joint** is a *hinge-type synovial joint* and it consists of two articulations. The humeroradial articulation involves the capitulum of the humerus and the radial head while the humeroulnar articulation between the trochlea of the humerus and trochlear notch of the ulna is the other. This joint allows for extension and flexion movements. Range of motion is approximately 130-150° of flexion and 0-10° of extension (**Fig. 6.64**). The triceps brachii is the primary extensor and the brachialis and biceps brachii serve as the major flexors (**Fig. 6.65; Fig. 6.66; Fig. 6.67**).

6.11.1 Joint Capsule

The **joint capsule** is attached anteriorly to the humerus near the margins of the lateral and medial ends of the articular

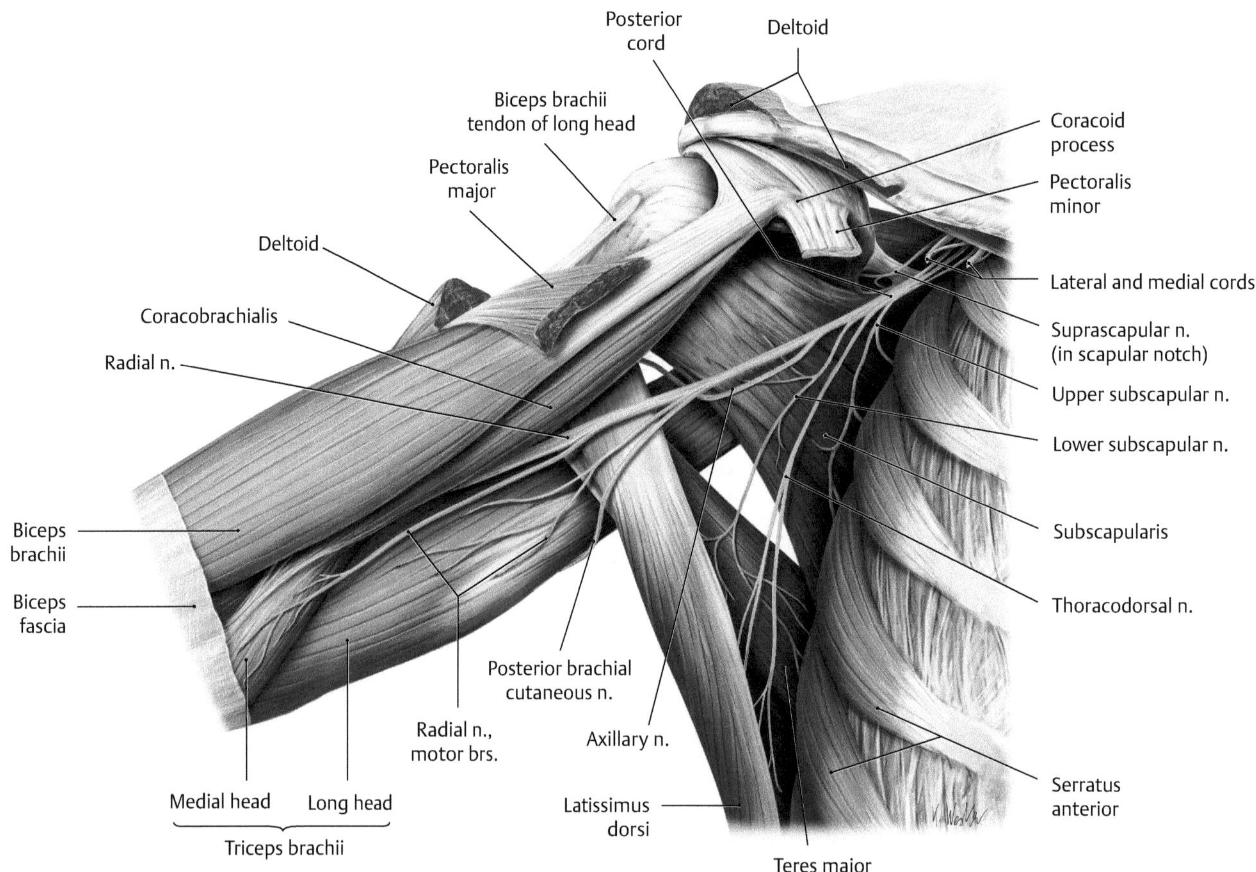

Fig. 6.60 Axilla with posterior cord exposed. Right side, anterior view. Removed: lateral and medial cords, and axillary vessels. (From Schuenke M, Schulte E, Schumacher U. THIEME Atlas of Anatomy. General Anatomy and Musculoskeletal System. Illustrations by Voll M and Wesker K. 3rd ed. New York: Thieme Medical Publishers; 2020.)

surfaces of the capitulum and trochlea, the medial epicondyle, and just superior to the coronoid and radial fossae. Posteriorly, it attaches to the superior portion of the olecranon fossa and near the coronoid process of the ulna and radial neck. Ligaments located on the lateral and medial sides strengthen the capsule (**Fig. 6.68**).

Laterally, the **radial collateral ligament** extends from the lateral epicondyle before blending with the anular ligament. The **anular ligament** holds the radial head against the radial notch, a location that represents the proximal radioulnar joint. Medially and extending from the medial epicondyle to both the coronoid process and olecranon is the **ulnar collateral ligament**. It consists of three parts: an *anterior*, *posterior* and *transverse (oblique) part*. The anterior part is the strongest and the posterior part is the weakest (**Fig. 6.69**).

6.11.2 Neurovasculature of the Elbow Joint

The **musculocutaneous**, **radial** and **ulnar nerves** innervate the elbow joint. The larger anastomosis of arteries including the **middle** and **radial collateral** (profunda brachii brs.), **superior** and **inferior ulnar collateral** (brachial brs.), **anterior** and **posterior ulnar recurrent** (ulnar brs.), **radial recurrent** (radial br.) and

Clinical Correlate 6.20

Carrying Angle

The long axis of the fully extended ulna makes an angle of approximately 170° with the long axis of the humerus bone. This is known as the **carrying angle** of the elbow. The male carrying angle is 10-15°. The female carrying angle is >15°.

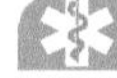

Clinical Correlate 6.21

Olecranon Fracture

Commonly referred to as a "fractured elbow" generally occur when an individual falls on their elbow and this is combined with a sudden and powerful contraction of the triceps brachii muscle. The fractured olecranon is avulsed and pulled away by the active contraction of the triceps brachii. Surgical pinning is required in most instances and healing occurs slowly.

Clinical Correlate 6.22

Dislocation of the Elbow Joint

If a person falls on their hands with their elbows in a flexed position this could result in a *posterior dislocation* of the elbow joint. Hyperextension or a blow to the elbow that forces the ulna posteriorly or posterolaterally can result in a dislocation. The distal end of the humerus is forced through the weaker anterior part of the joint capsule as the radius and ulna dislocate posteriorly.

Clinical Correlate 6.23

Bursitis of the Elbow Joint

Subcutaneous olecranon bursitis can be the result of excessive friction and pressure or an infection due to a deep abrasion or cut. The excessive friction between the triceps brachii tendon and the olecranon can result in a **subtendinous olecranon bursitis**.

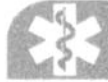

Clinical Correlate 6.24

Subluxation of the Radial Head

A **subluxation** (temporary and incomplete dislocation) of the radial head is commonly seen when a child is suddenly lifted or jerked by the upper extremity while their forearm is pronated. This sudden pulling tears the distal attachment of the anular ligament near the neck of the radius. The radial head then moves distally and partially out of the anular ligament. The proximal portion of the torn ligament can become trapped between the radial head and the capitulum of the humerus with the source of pain coming from the pinched anular ligament. It is commonly referred to as nursemaid's elbow and treatment involves a patient's forearm being left in supination while the elbow is flexed and in a sling for a couple of weeks.

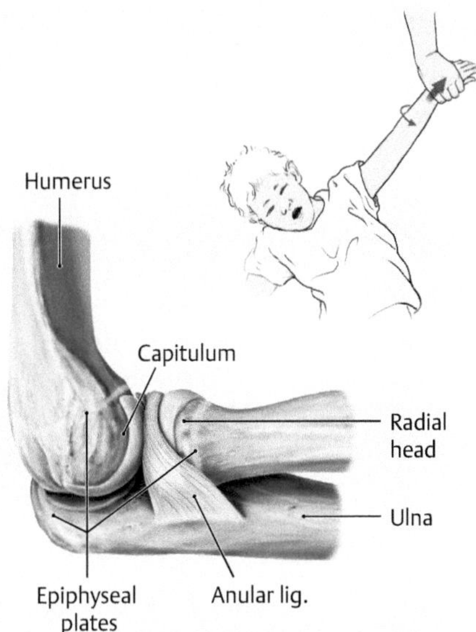

(From Schuenke M, Schulte E, Schumacher U. THIEME Atlas of Anatomy. General Anatomy and Musculoskeletal System. Illustrations by Voll M and Wesker K. 3rd ed. New York: Thieme Medical Publishers; 2020.)

Clinical Correlate 6.25

Ulnar Collateral Ligament Reconstruction

Ulnar collateral ligament (UCL) reconstruction, more commonly known as "*Tommy John surgery*," is the reconstruction of the UCL after a rupture or tearing of this ligament seen in athletes like baseball pitchers. Throwing sports have the highest rate of these injuries. The procedure involves an autologous transplant of a long tendon from the contralateral forearm or leg (palmaris longus or plantaris tendon). The tendon graft is passed through holes drilled through the medial epicondyle of the humerus and the lateral aspect of the coronoid process of the ulna.

recurrent interosseous (posterior interosseous br.) all supply blood to the elbow joint (**Fig. 6.61**).

6.11.3 Elbow Joint Bursae

There are multiple bursae associated with attachment sites of muscles located near the elbow joint. Of these, only three are considered clinically significant:

- **Subcutaneous olecranon bursa**: located in the subcutaneous tissue overlying the olecranon (**Fig. 6.70**).
- **Intratendinous olecranon bursa**: located within the triceps tendon near the attachment site of the olecranon.
- **Subtendinous olecranon bursa**: located between the triceps tendon and olecranon near the tendons attachment to the olecranon.

6.12 Proximal Radioulnar Joint

The **proximal radioulnar joint** is a *pivot-type synovial joint* and is the articulation between the radial head and the radial notch of the ulna. This joint allows for pronation and supination movements (**Fig. 6.71**). The pronator quadratus and pronator teres are the muscles that produce pronation and the supinator and biceps brachii muscles produce supination.

The joint capsule of the elbow is continuous over this joint and is specifically strengthened by the **anular ligament** that attaches anterior and posterior to the radial notch of the ulna. The synovial membrane of the elbow joint extends into the proximal radioulnar joint and past the radial head and anular ligament to form the **sacciform recess**. This recess prevents any tearing of the synovial membrane when the radius is rotating during pronation and supination movements (**Fig. 6.68; Fig. 6.72**).

6.12.1 Neurovasculature of the Proximal Radioulnar Joint

The **musculocutaneous**, **median** and **ulnar nerves** innervate the proximal radioulnar joint. The arterial supply is from the **middle** and **radial collateral** (profunda brachii brs.), and **radial recurrent** (radial br.) and **recurrent interosseous arteries** (posterior interosseous br.).

6.13 Distal Radioulnar Joint

The **distal radioulnar joint** is a *pivot-type synovial joint* and is the articulation between the ulnar head and the ulnar notch of

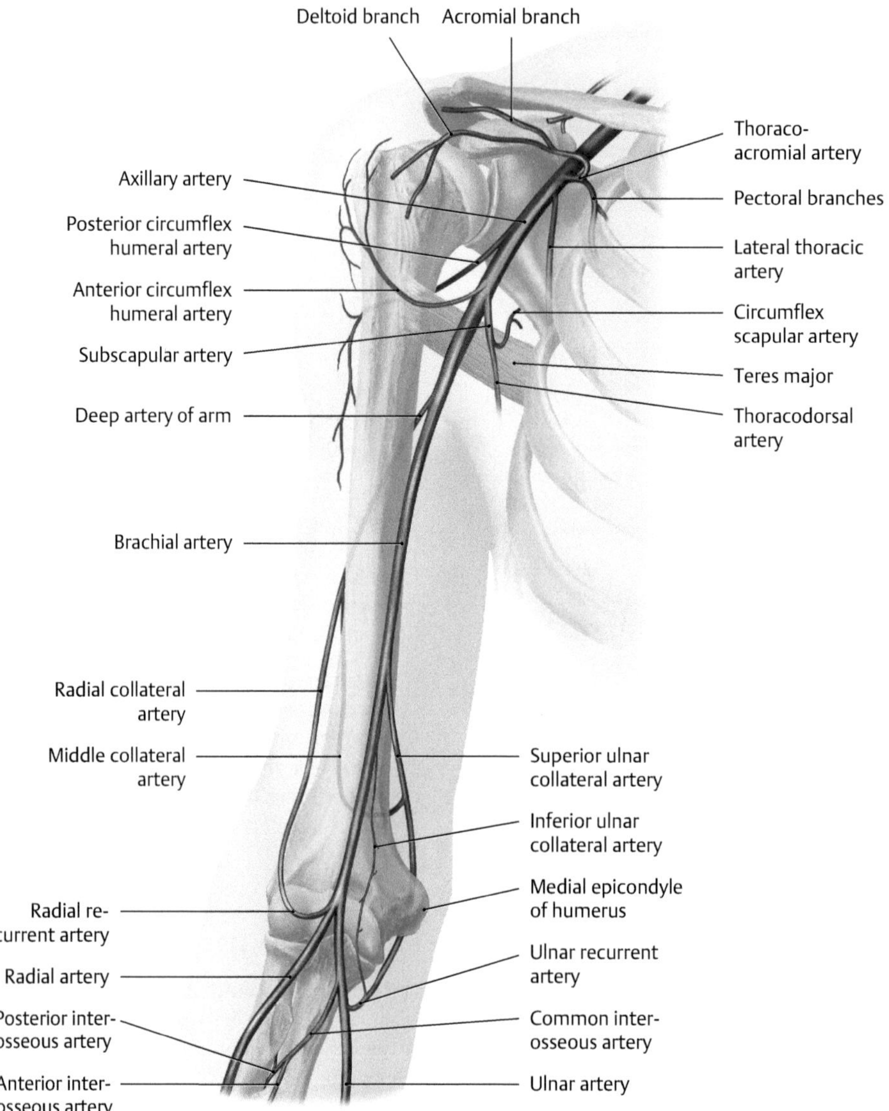

Fig. 6.61 Course of the brachial artery in the arm. (From Schuenke M, Schulte E, Schumacher U. THIEME Atlas of Anatomy. General Anatomy and Musculoskeletal System. Illustrations by Voll M and Wesker K. 3rd ed. New York: Thieme Medical Publishers; 2020.)

the radius. A fibrocartilaginous **ulnocarpal disc** (or "*triangular ligament*") binds the ends of the radius and ulna together and separates this joint from the wrist joint (**Fig. 6.100; Fig. 6.102**). In a coronal section, the joint is L-shaped because the apex of the articular disc attaches to the lateral side of the base of the styloid process of the ulna and the base of the disc is attached to the medial edge of the ulnar notch of the radius. This joint allows for pronation and supination movements (**Fig. 6.71**). Much like the proximal radioulnar joint, the pronator quadratus and pronator teres are the muscles that produce pronation and the supinator and biceps brachii muscles produce supination at this joint.

The **joint capsule** encloses the joint except on its superior aspect. The **dorsal** and **palmar radioulnar ligaments** add strength to the capsule (**Fig. 6.71**).

6.13.1 Neurovasculature of the Distal Radioulnar Joint

The **anterior** and **posterior interosseous nerves** innervate the distal radioulnar joint. The arterial supply is from the **anterior** and **posterior interosseous arteries** (common interosseous brs.).

6.14 Anterior Forearm

The anterior forearm contains flexor and pronator muscles that act on the hand or the forearm. The muscles of this compartment are divided into a superficial, intermediate and deep layer. Tendons of the muscles that extend past the wrist are mostly

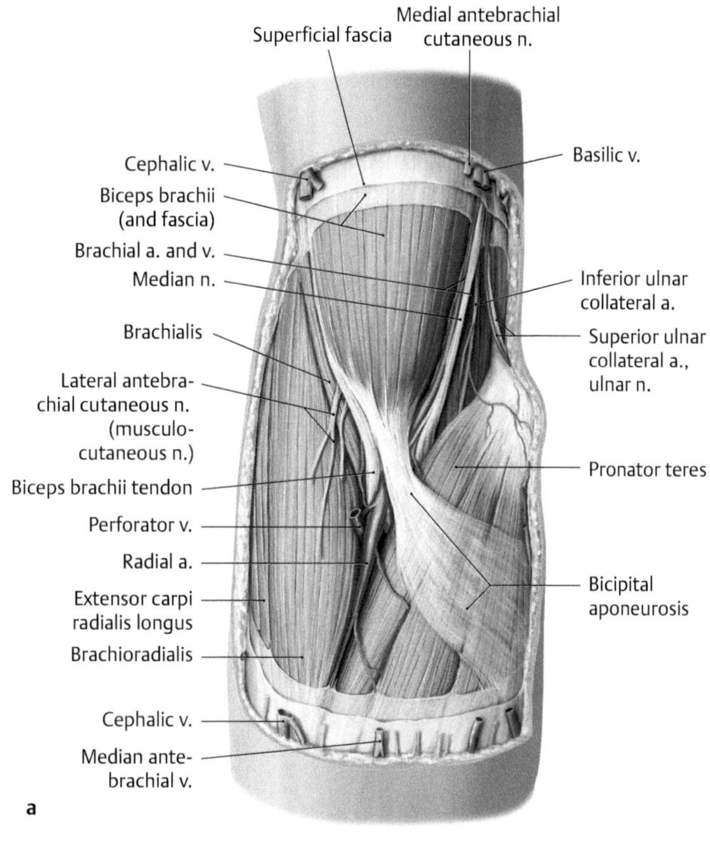

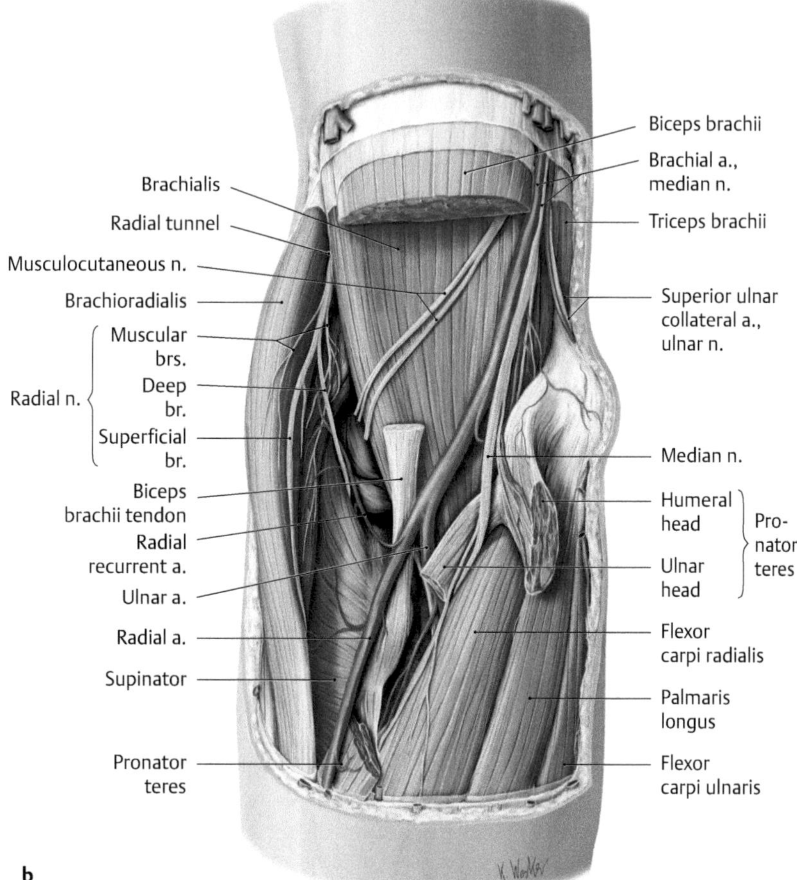

Fig. 6.62 **(a)** Superficial cubital fossa. **(b)** Deep cubital fossa. (From Schuenke M, Schulte E, Schumacher U. THIEME Atlas of Anatomy. General Anatomy and Musculoskeletal System. Illustrations by Voll M and Wesker K. 3rd ed. New York: Thieme Medical Publishers; 2020.)

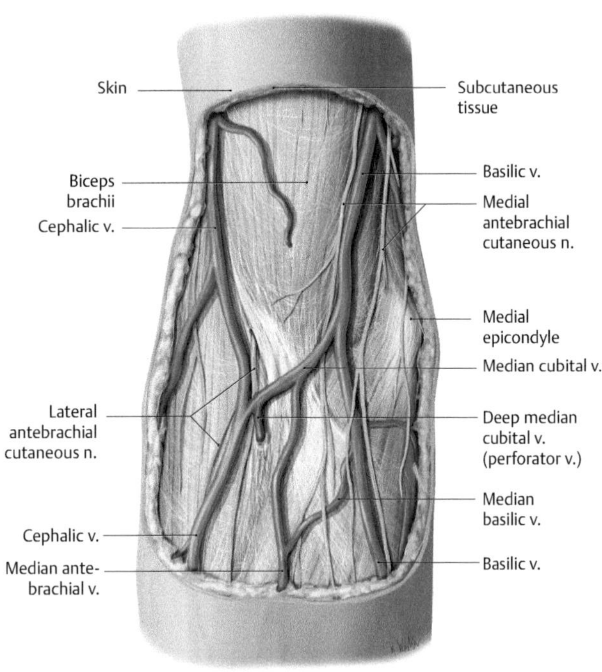

Fig. 6.63 Cutaneous neurovasculature of the cubital fossa. (From Schuenke M, Schulte E, Schumacher U. THIEME Atlas of Anatomy. General Anatomy and Musculoskeletal System. Illustrations by Voll M and Wesker K. 3rd ed. New York: Thieme Medical Publishers; 2020.)

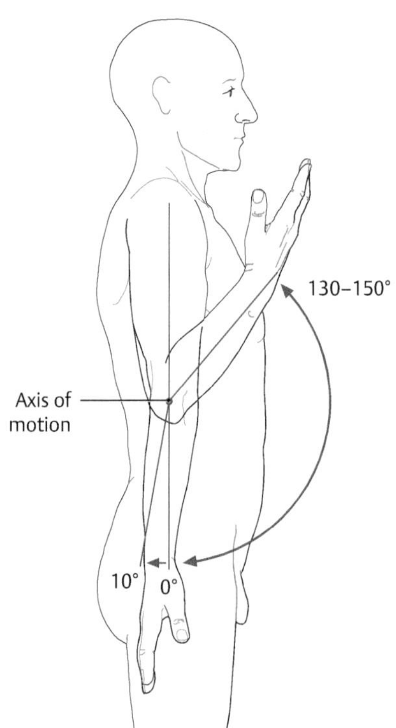

Fig. 6.64 Range of motion at in the humeroradial and humeroulnar joints of the elbow. (From Schuenke M, Schulte E, Schumacher U. THIEME Atlas of Anatomy. General Anatomy and Musculoskeletal System. Illustrations by Voll M and Wesker K. 3rd ed. New York: Thieme Medical Publishers; 2020.)

held in place by thickenings of the *antebrachial fascia* called the **flexor retinaculum** and **palmar carpal ligament**. Muscles that originate from the medial epicondyle help form a **common flexor tendon (Fig. 6.73)**.

The superficial layer consists of the pronator teres, flexor carpi radialis, palmaris longus and flexor carpi ulnaris from lateral to medial. The **pronator teres** muscle has a humeral and ulnar head that extends distally and laterally toward the radius. It functions mainly in *pronation* but also *flexion of the forearm*. The **flexor carpi radialis** is just medial to pronator teres and functions in both *flexion* and *abduction (radial deviation) of the hand*. The **palmaris longus** is a thin muscle that attaches to the palmar aponeurosis. A small percentage of individuals may not have this muscle either on one side or bilaterally, but its function in *flexion of the hand* at the wrist is minimal at best; thus, if not present, the effect is minimal. If the palmaris longus tendon is present, the median nerve is located just lateral to it. The **flexor carpi ulnaris** has a humeral and ulnar head that fuse and continue as a tendon that attaches to the pisiform, hook of the hamate and 5th metacarpal in the hand. It functions in both *flexion* and *adduction (ulnar deviation) of the hand*. The ulnar nerve and vessels lie just lateral to its tendon (**Fig. 6.73**).

The intermediate layer has only one muscle and that is the **flexor digitorum superficialis**. It originates from the humeroulnar and radial heads, and, near the wrist, this muscle gives rise to four individual tendons that become enclosed in the *common flexor synovial sheath* before continuing distally and eventually inserting onto the middle phalanges of the 2-5 digits. This muscle *flexes the middle phalanx of the 2-5 digits* at the proximal interphalangeal joint and it can assist in flexing joints proximally towards the wrist joint when increased muscle fibers are stimulated. All four of its tendons pass through the carpal tunnel (**Fig. 6.73**).

The deep layer consists of the flexor pollicis longus, flexor digitorum profundus and pronator quadratus muscles. The **flexor pollicis longus** is the most lateral muscle of the deep layer and it functions in *flexion of the first digit (thumb)*. The tendon, before inserting onto the distal phalanx of the first digit, passes through the carpal tunnel. The **flexor digitorum profundus** is the most medial muscle of this deep layer and it consists of four tendons near the wrist. It is divided into lateral and medial parts that receive innervation from the median and ulnar nerves, respectively. The tendons of the lateral part act on the 2nd and 3rd digits while the medial part acts on the 4th and 5th digits. The tendons are enclosed in the *common flexor synovial sheath* before continuing distally and eventually inserting onto the distal phalanges of the 2nd-5th digits. This muscle *flexes the distal phalanx of digits 2-5* at the distal interphalangeal joint and it can assist flexing joints back proximally towards the wrist joint when increased muscle fibers are stimulated, much like its superficialis counterpart. All four of its tendons pass through the carpal tunnel. The **pronator quadratus** is almost square-shaped and is located near the wrist, deeper than the previous two muscles (**Fig. 6.74**). It is the main *pronator of the forearm*. Descriptions of the anterior forearm muscles are found in **Table 6.5**.

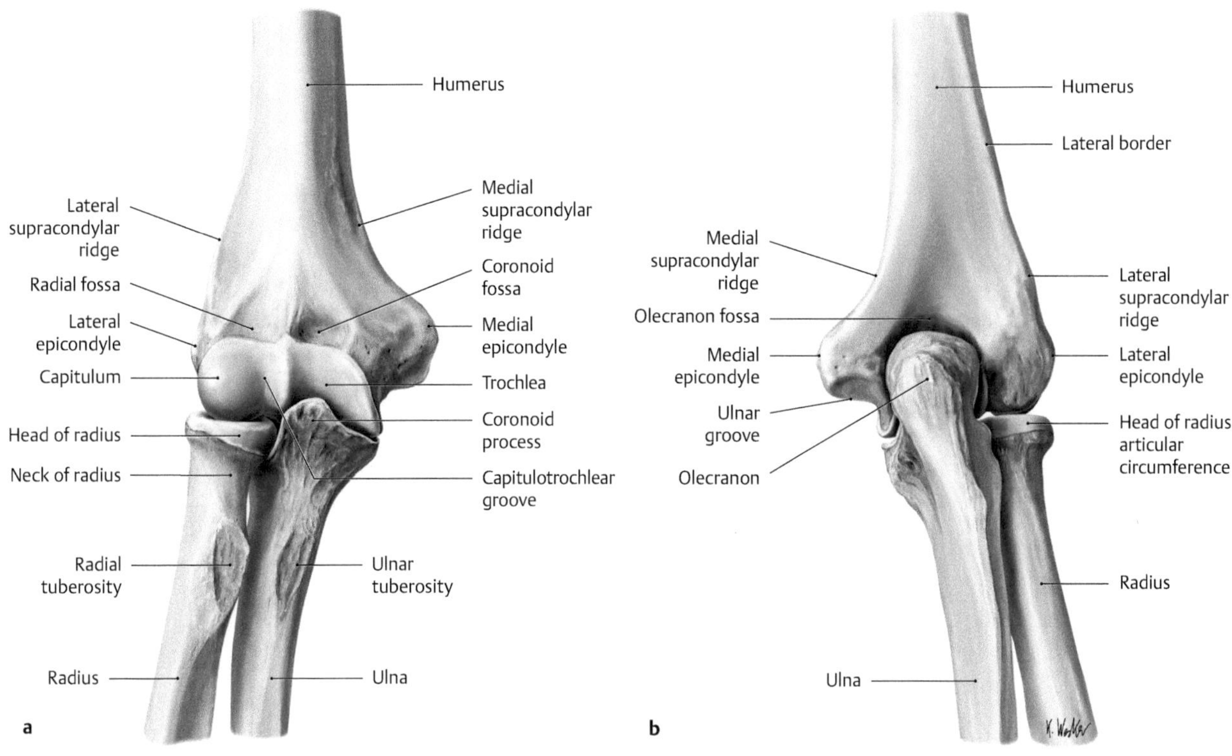

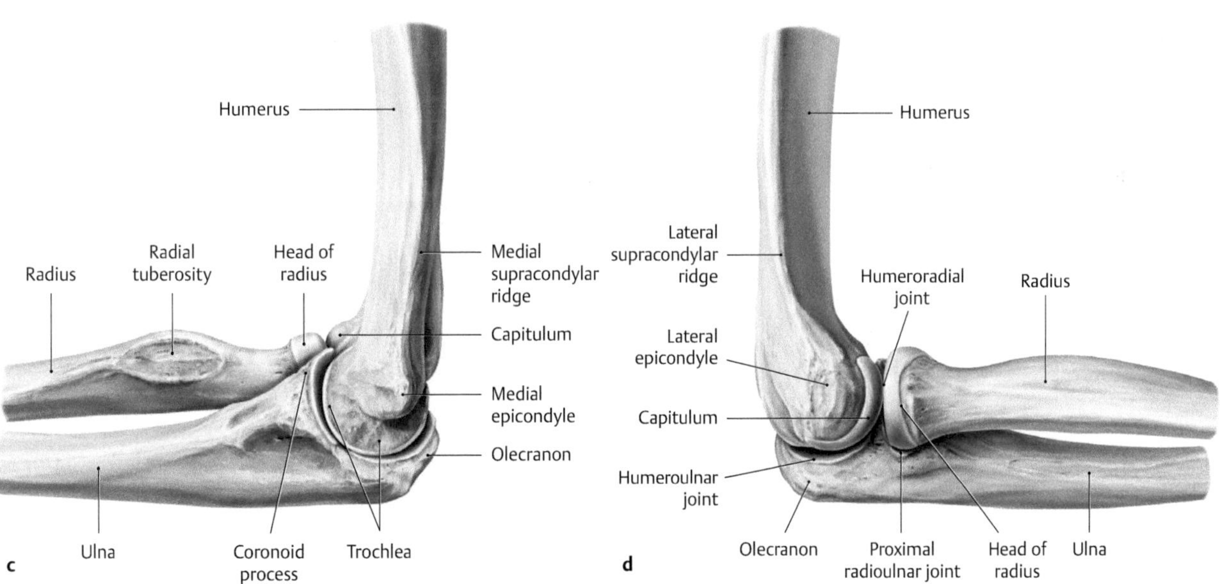

Fig. 6.65 Elbow joint. **(a)** Anterior view. **(b)** Posterior view. **(c)** Medial view. **(d)** Lateral view. (From Schuenke M, Schulte E, Schumacher U. THIEME Atlas of Anatomy. General Anatomy and Musculoskeletal System. Illustrations by Voll M and Wesker K. 3rd ed. New York: Thieme Medical Publishers; 2020.)

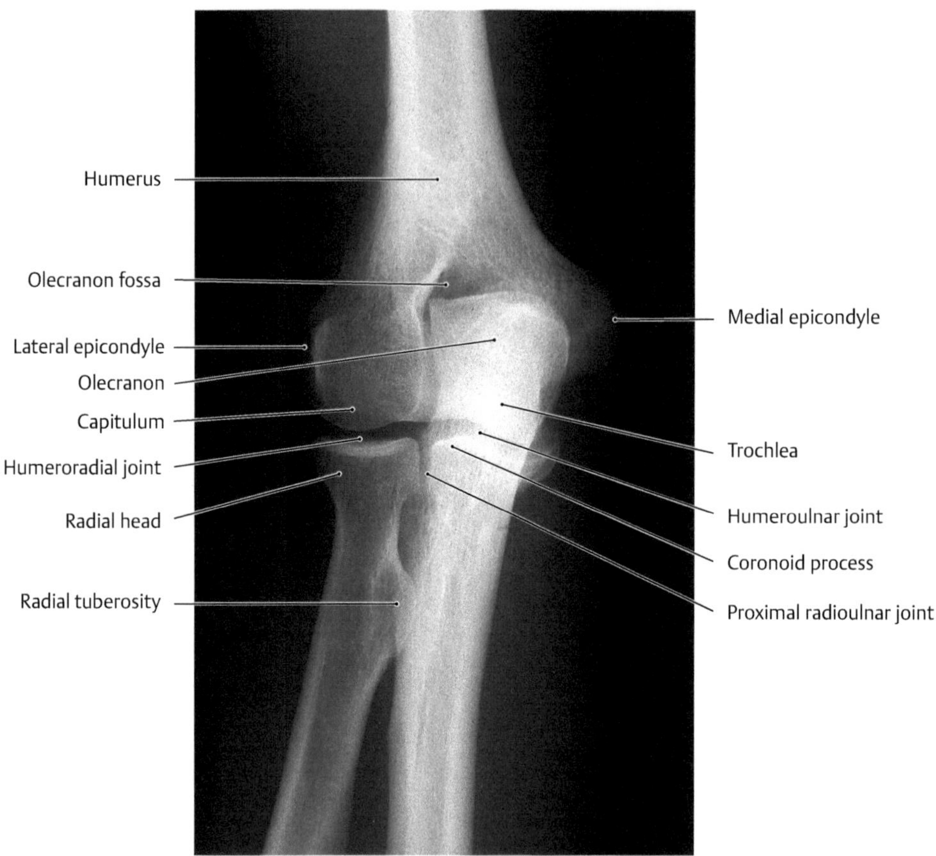

Fig. 6.66 Radiograph of the elbow, anteroposterior view. (From Moeller TB, Reif E. Pocket Atlas of Radiographic Anatomy, 3rd ed. New York, NY: Thieme; 2010.)

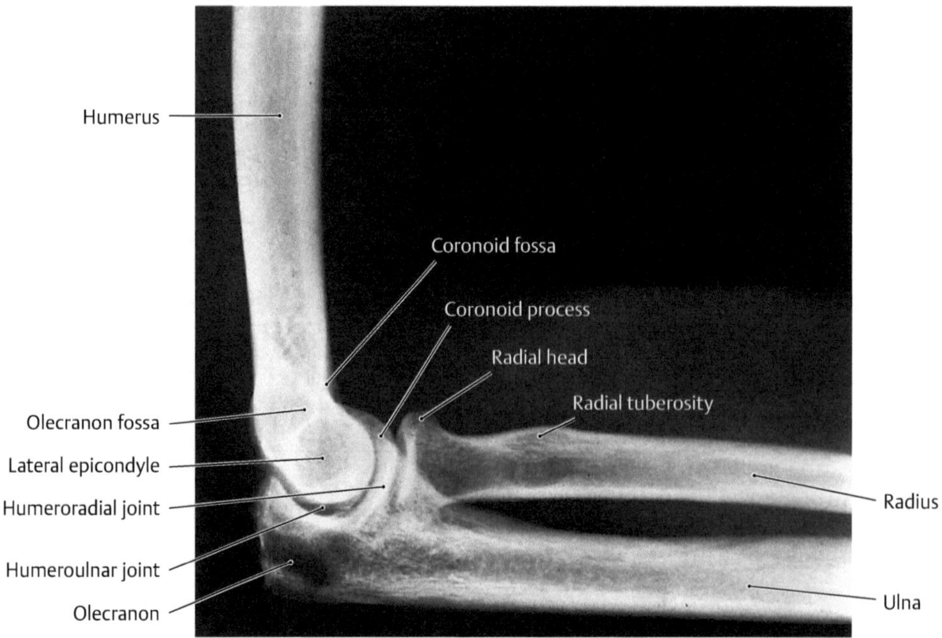

Fig. 6.67 Radiograph of the elbow, lateral view. (From Moeller TB, Reif E. Pocket Atlas of Radiographic Anatomy, 3rd ed. New York, NY: Thieme; 2010.)

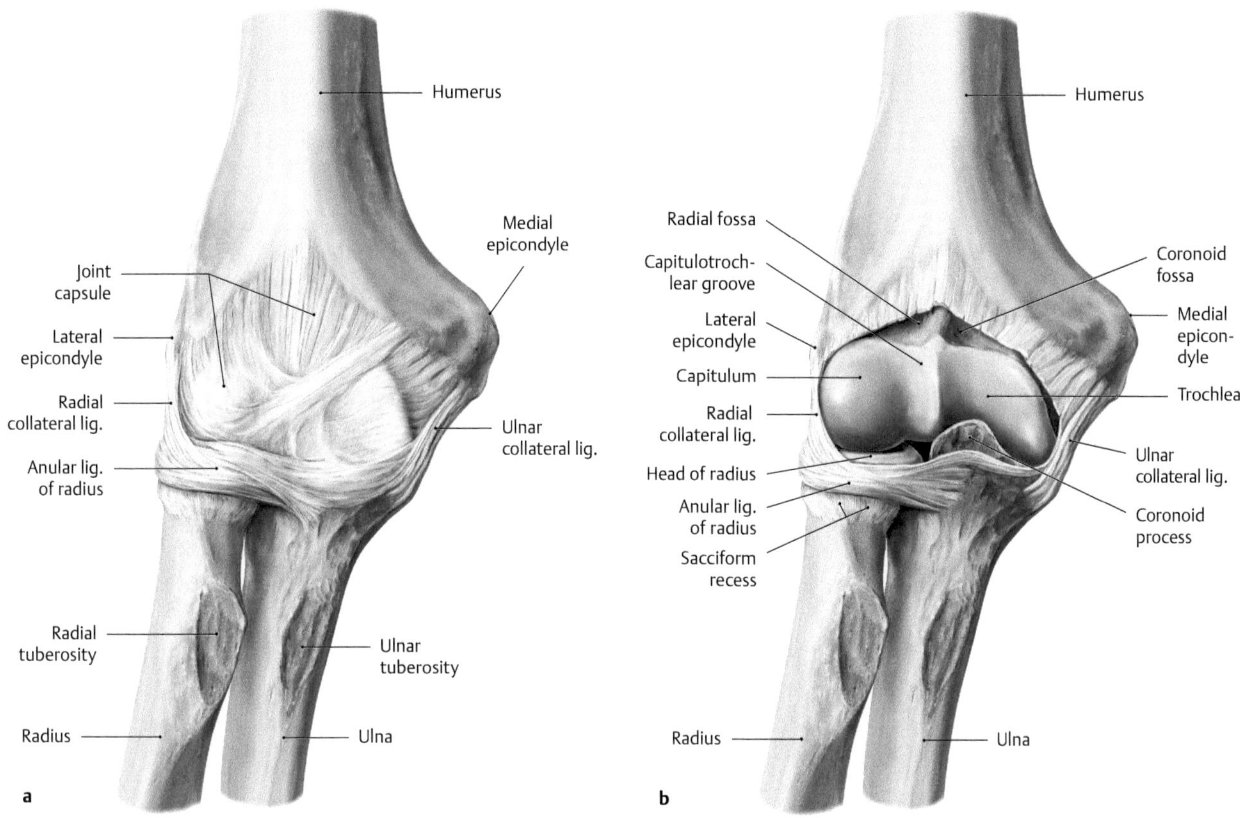

Fig. 6.68 Joint capsule of the elbow joint. Right elbow in extension, anterior view. **(a)** Intact joint capsule. **(b)** Windowed joint capsule. (From Schuenke M, Schulte E, Schumacher U. THIEME Atlas of Anatomy. General Anatomy and Musculoskeletal System. Illustrations by Voll M and Wesker K. 3rd ed. New York: Thieme Medical Publishers; 2020.)

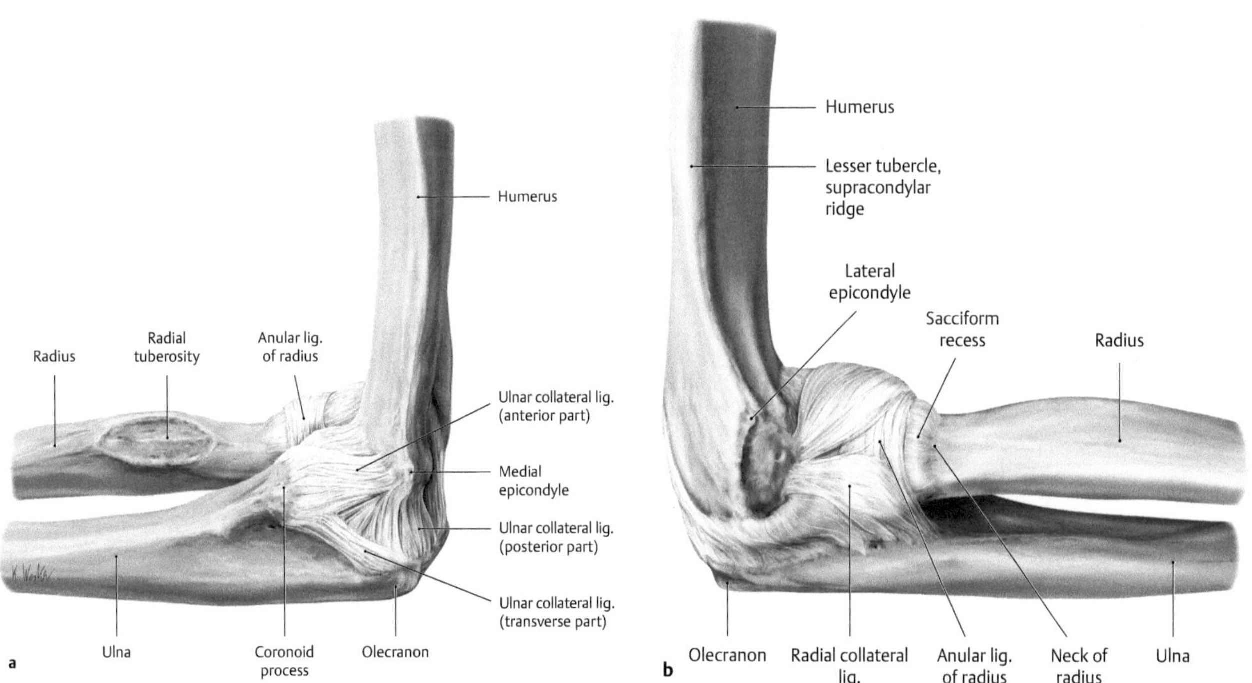

Fig. 6.69 Ligaments of the elbow joint. **(a)** Medial view. **(b)** Lateral view. (From Schuenke M, Schulte E, Schumacher U. THIEME Atlas of Anatomy. General Anatomy and Musculoskeletal System. Illustrations by Voll M and Wesker K. 3rd ed. New York: Thieme Medical Publishers; 2020.)

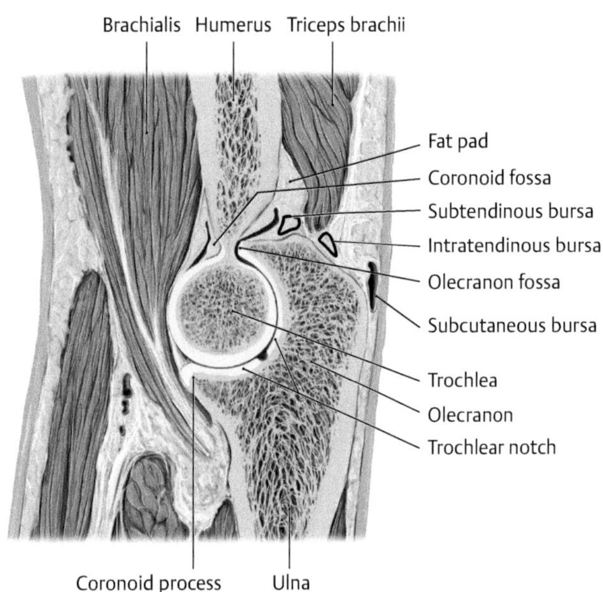

Fig. 6.70 Elbow joint bursae. Sagittal section through the humeroulnar joint, medial view. (From Schuenke M, Schulte E, Schumacher U. THIEME Atlas of Anatomy. General Anatomy and Musculoskeletal System. Illustrations by Voll M and Wesker K. 3rd ed. New York: Thieme Medical Publishers; 2020.)

6.14.1 Neurovasculature of the Anterior Forearm

The primary neurovascular plane of the anterior forearm is located between the intermediate and deep layers. The **median nerve** leaves the cubital fossa and passes between the two heads of the pronator teres muscle. It then continues distally toward the wrist between the flexor digitorum superficialis and profundus muscles before entering the carpal tunnel and into the hand. The median nerve supplies all muscles of the anterior forearm except for the flexor carpi ulnaris and the medial part of the flexor digitorum profundus. The **anterior interosseous nerve** branch of this nerve technically supplies all the muscles of the deep layer except the medial part of the flexor digitorum profundus. Prior to reaching the wrist, the median nerve gives rise to a **palmar cutaneous branch** that helps supply skin of the lateral proximal palm (**Fig. 6.74**).

The **ulnar nerve** travels posterior to the medial epicondyle through the *cubital tunnel* before passing between the two heads of the flexor carpi ulnaris to enter the medial part of the forearm. Near the wrist it journeys over the flexor retinaculum and through the *ulnar tunnel* (*Guyon's canal*) before entering the hand as either a deep or superficial branch (**Fig. 6.73; Fig. 6.98**). Similar to the median nerve and prior to reaching the wrist, the ulnar nerve gives rise to a **palmar cutaneous branch** that helps supply skin of the medial proximal palm.

Table 6.5 **Anterior forearm muscles**

Muscle	Innervation	Function(s)	Origin	Insertion
Superficial layer				
Pronator teres	Median nerve	Pronates and flexes forearm	Medial epicondyle (common flexor tendon); coronoid process	Middle of and lateral part of radius
Flexor carpi radialis	Median nerve	Flexes and abducts hand	Medial epicondyle (common flexor tendon)	Base of 2nd metacarpal
Palmaris longus	Median nerve	Flexes hand and tenses palmar aponeurosis	Medial epicondyle (common flexor tendon)	Distal half of flexor retinaculum; palmar aponeurosis
Flexor carpi ulnaris	Ulnar nerve	Flexes and adducts hand	Olecranon and posterior border of ulna	Base of 5th metacarpal; hook of hamate; pisiform
Intermediate layer				
Flexor digitorum superficialis	Median nerve	Flexes at the PIP joints of 2nd-5th digits; acting more strongly it flexes MCP joints of same digits along with wrist joint	Medial epicondyle (common flexor tendon); coronoid process; superior half of anterior border of radius	Shaft of middle phalanges of 2nd-5th digits
Deep layer				
Flexor pollicis longus	Anterior interosseous nerve (of median nerve)	Flexes 1st digit at IP, MCP and CMC joints and wrist joint	Anterior surface of radius; interosseous membrane	Base of distal phalanx of 1st digit
Flexor digitorum profundus	*Lateral part*: anterior interosseous nerve (of median nerve) *Medial part*: ulnar nerve	*Lateral part*: flex 2nd and 3rd digits at DIP joints and wrist *Medial part*: flex 4th and 5th digits at DIP joints and wrist	Proximal 3/4 of anterior and medial surfaces of ulna; interosseous membrane	*Lateral part*: base of distal phalanges of 2nd and 3rd digits *Medial part*: base of distal phalanges of 4th and 5th digits
Pronator quadratus	Anterior interosseous nerve (of median nerve)	Pronates forearm	Distal 1/4 of anterior surface of ulna	Distal 1/4 of anterior surface of radius

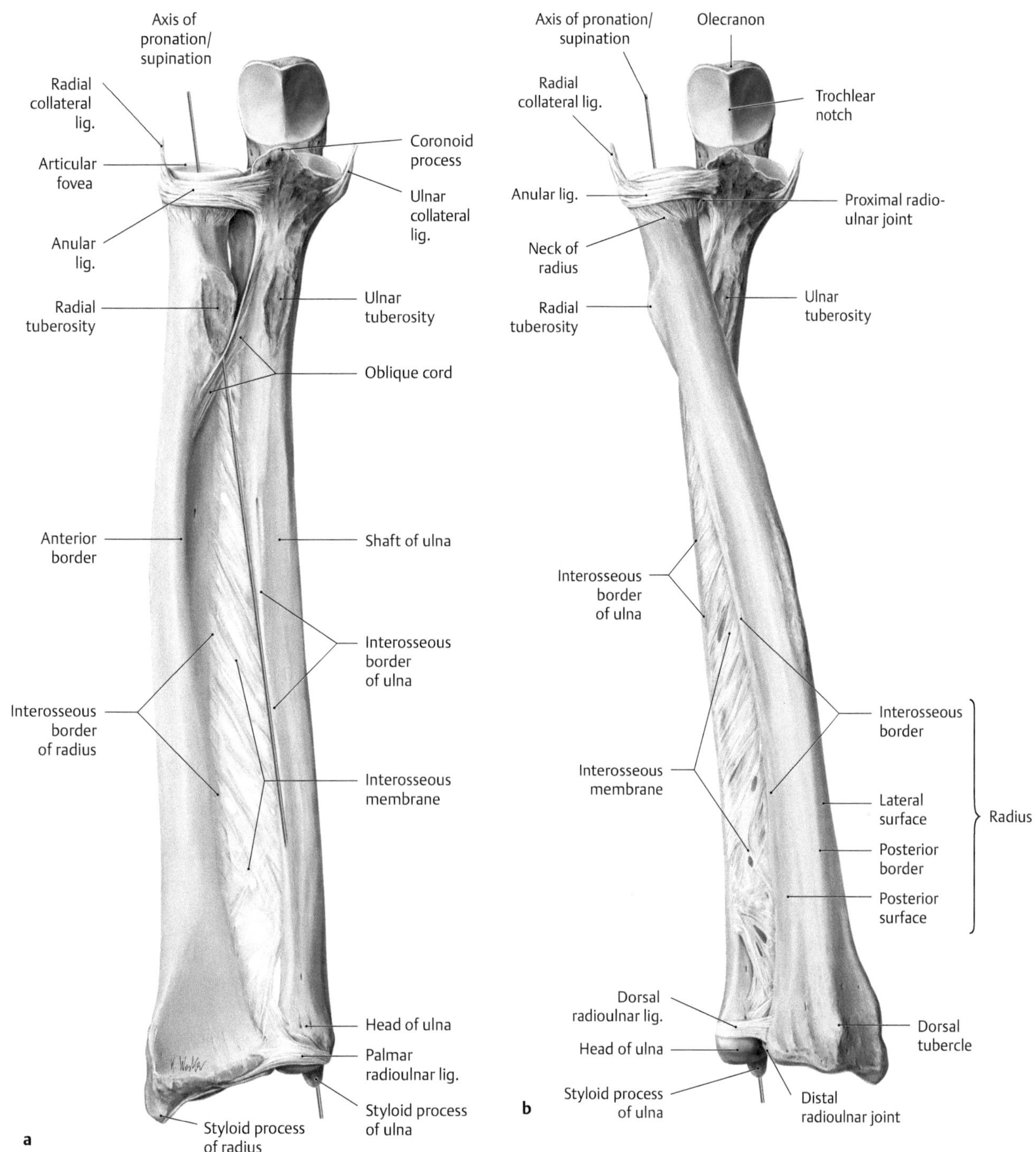

Fig. 6.71 Right forearm, anterior view. **(a)** Supination at the radioulnar joints. **(b)** Pronation at the radioulnar joints. (From Schuenke M, Schulte E, Schumacher U. THIEME Atlas of Anatomy. General Anatomy and Musculoskeletal System. Illustrations by Voll M and Wesker K. 3rd ed. New York: Thieme Medical Publishers; 2020.)

The radial and ulnar arteries bifurcate from the brachial artery just outside the cubital tunnel. The **radial artery** gives rise to the *radial recurrent artery* before continuing down the lateral aspect of the anterior forearm. It leaves the forearm by wrapping around the lateral portion of the wrist and continuing against the floor of the *anatomical snuff box*. The **ulnar artery** gives rise to the *anterior ulnar recurrent, posterior ulnar recurrent* and *common interosseous arteries* before continuing down the medial aspect of the anterior forearm. The artery follows the ulnar nerve to the ulnar tunnel and has deep and superficial branches that mirror the corresponding nerves. The **common interosseous artery** has both an anterior and posterior interosseous artery branch **(Fig. 6.73b; Fig. 6.74)**.

The **anterior interosseous artery** runs distally toward the wrist on the anterior side of the interosseous membrane and helps supply blood to this portion of the forearm. It is paired with the anterior interosseous nerve. The radial, ulnar and anterior interosseous arteries all contribute varying degrees of blood to the **deep**

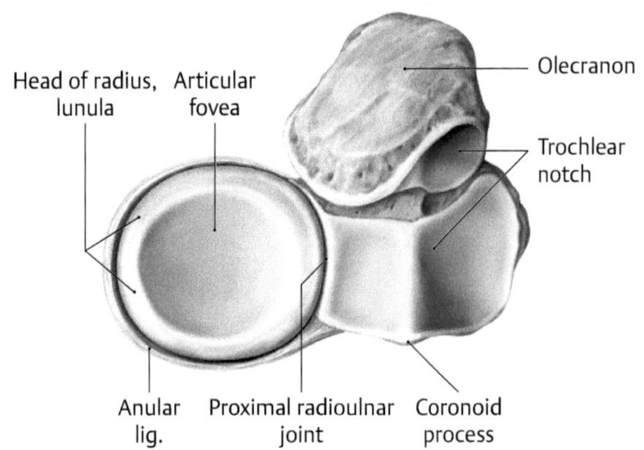

Fig. 6.72 Proximal radioulnar joint. Right elbow, proximal (superior) view. (From Schuenke M, Schulte E, Schumacher U. THIEME Atlas of Anatomy. General Anatomy and Musculoskeletal System. Illustrations by Voll M and Wesker K. 3rd ed. New York: Thieme Medical Publishers; 2020.)

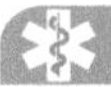 *Clinical Correlate 6.26*

Medial Epicondylitis

Medial epicondylitis (or **"golfer's elbow")** is inflammation, soreness or pain on the medial side of the humerus near the elbow. There may be a partial tear of the common flexor tendon fibers near the medial epicondyle of the humerus.

Clinical Correlate 6.27

Median Nerve Palsy

When the median nerve is injured within the cubital fossa it is referred to as a **median nerve palsy**. Damage to the median nerve at this location results in: a loss of pronation of the forearm, reduced flexion of the wrist, digits and thumb, and a loss of opposition of the thumb. Only the flexor carpi ulnaris and the medial half of the flexor digitorum profundus muscles still function in the anterior forearm. When the patient tries to make a fist, the 2nd and 3rd digits remain straight, while the 4th and 5th digits flex. This is the so-called "hand of benediction."

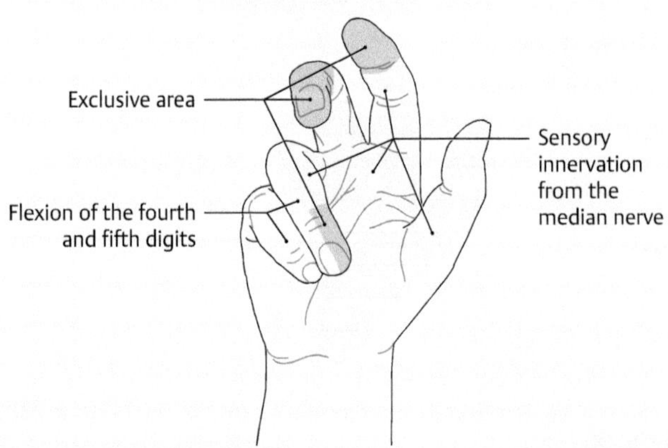

(From Schuenke M, Schulte E, Schumacher U. THIEME Atlas of Anatomy. General Anatomy and Musculoskeletal System. Illustrations by Voll M and Wesker K. 3rd ed. New York: Thieme Medical Publishers; 2020.)

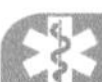 *Clinical Correlate 6.28*

Pronator Syndrome

A median nerve entrapment between the two heads of the pronator teres due, for example, to muscle hypertrophy or trauma, is called **pronator syndrome**. Hypoesthesia and activity-based paresthesia of the first three and a half digits on the palmar side along with tenderness and pain at the proximal anterior forearm are symptoms identified by a patient.

Clinical Correlate 6.29

Ulnar Nerve Palsy

When the ulnar nerve is injured, mostly at the medial epicondyle of the humerus (hitting your "funny bone"), this is referred to as **ulnar nerve palsy**. Ulnar nerve damage at this location leads to paralysis of the flexor carpi ulnaris, medial half of the flexor digitorum profundus, and all of the small muscles of the hand except for the thenar muscles and the first two lumbricals. A person is unable to flex the ring or little finger, abduct or adduct the digits, or adduct the thumb. There is hyperextension of the metacarpophalangeal joints due to the paralysis of the lumbricals and interossei muscles. With atrophy of the hypothenar and interossei muscles there is wasting of the hypothenar eminence and hollowing between the metacarpal bones.

palmar, **superficial palmar** and **palmar carpal arches** located in the hand and wrist regions. All arteries are generally paired with two smaller corresponding veins (**Fig. 6.22**).

6.15 Posterior Forearm

The posterior forearm contains the extensors, a flexor, a supinator and an abductor muscle that can act on the hand, first digit, or forearm. The muscles of this forearm compartment are divided into a superficial and deep layer. Tendons of the extensor muscles and the first digit abductor are held in place by a thickening of the *antebrachial fascia* called the **extensor retinaculum**. Muscles that originate from the lateral epicondyle help form a **common extensor tendon**.

The superficial layer from lateral to medial consists of the brachioradialis, extensor carpi radialis longus, extensor carpi radialis brevis, extensor digitorum, extensor digiti minimi, and the extensor carpi ulnaris. The **brachioradialis** is located on the anterolateral forearm surface and is special in the sense that it helps *flex the forearm* at the elbow and does not participate in extension like most of the muscles that make up the posterior forearm. This muscle does not extend pass the wrist, hence it can only act at the elbow joint and it is quite prominent when the forearm is in mid-pronation/supination. The **extensor carpi radialis longus** is partly overlapped by the brachioradialis and extends past the wrist enclosed by a synovial sheath just deep to the extensor retinaculum before reaching the 2nd metacarpal. It functions in both *extension* and *abduction (radial deviation) of the hand* and is very active during fist clenching. The **extensor carpi radialis brevis** is overlapped by the extensor carpi radialis longus and similarly extends past the wrist enclosed in a synovial sheath just deep to the extensor retinaculum before reaching the 3rd metacarpal. Much like its longus counterpart, it functions in both *extension* and *abduction (radial*

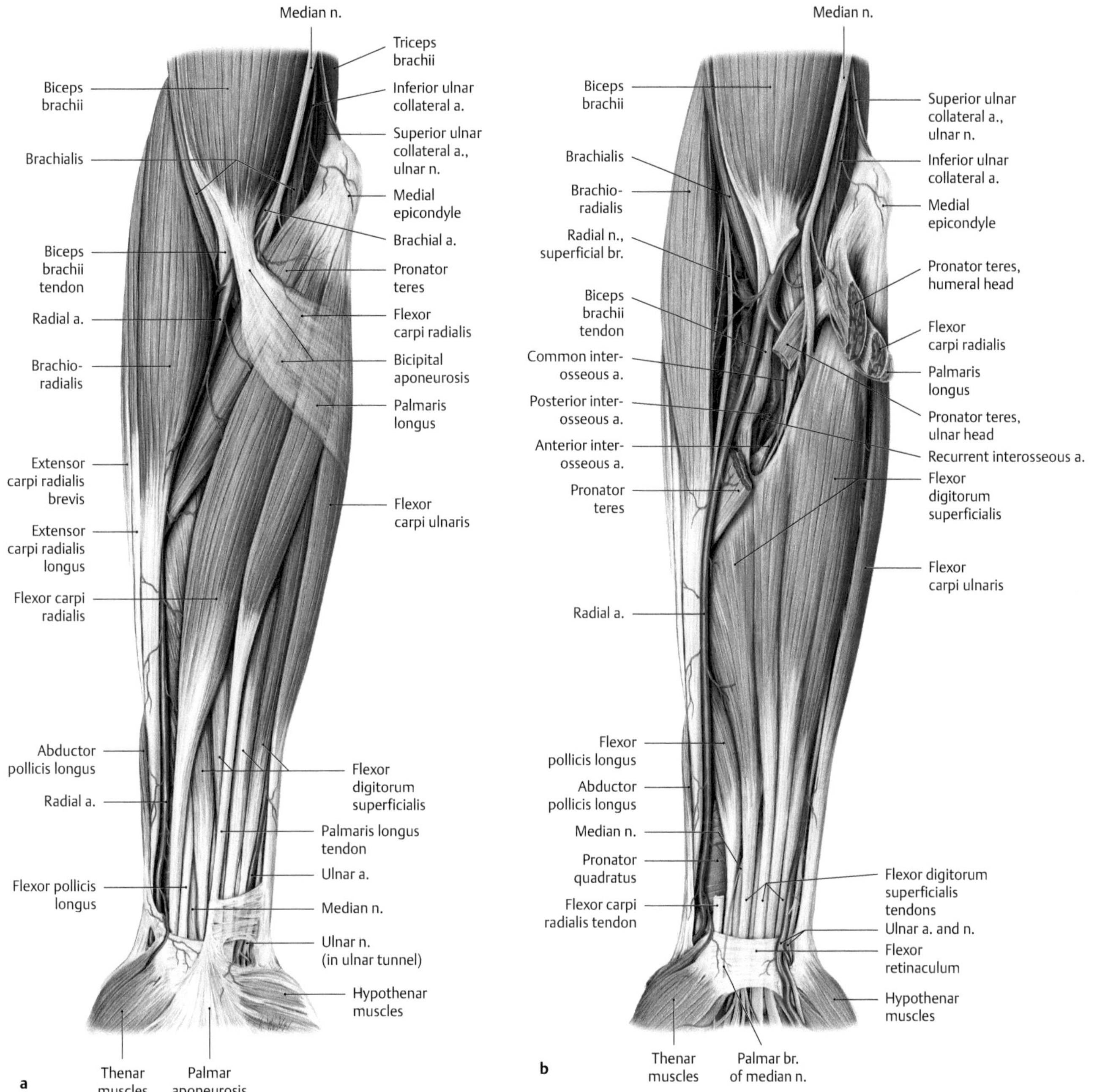

Fig. 6.73 Anterior forearm compartment muscles and neurovasculature. **(a)** Superficial layer. **(b)** Intermediate/middle layer. (From Schuenke M, Schulte E, Schumacher U. THIEME Atlas of Anatomy. General Anatomy and Musculoskeletal System. Illustrations by Voll M and Wesker K. 3rd ed. New York: Thieme Medical Publishers; 2020.)

deviation) of the hand and is active during fist clenching **(Fig. 6.75; Fig. 6.80)**.

The **extensor digitorum** is not broken up into a superficial or profundus portion like the flexors in the anterior forearm. This is the main *extensor muscle of the 2-5 digits* but it also participates in *extension of the hand.* The four tendons pass through a *common extensor synovial sheath* just deep to the extensor retinaculum before flattening out and contributing to the formation of the **extensor expansions (Fig. 6.75a)**. Each one is a triangular, tendinous aponeurosis that wraps around the posterior part and sides of the head of the metacarpal and proximal phalanx. This hood-like structure over the head of the metacarpal is anchored on each side by the **palmar ligament (Fig. 6.76b)**. The median and lateral bands that originate from the extensor digitorum tendons also contribute to the extensor expansion. The **central (median) band** travels to the base of the middle phalanx while the **lateral bands** pass to the base of the distal phalanx. The interossei and lumbrical muscle tendons join the lateral bands **(Fig. 6.76)**.

The **extensor digiti minimi** is a partially detached part of the extensor digitorum that courses through a separate synovial sheath, medial to that of the common extensor synovial sheath, before reaching the extensor expansion of the 5th digit. It functions

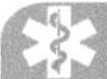

Clinical Correlate 6.30

Lateral Epicondylitis

Lateral epicondylitis (or **"tennis elbow")** is the inflammation or pain felt on the lateral side of the upper arm near the elbow. There may be a partial tear of the common extensor tendon fibers near the lateral epicondyle of the humerus.

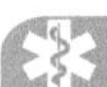

Clinical Correlate 6.31

Synovial Cyst

A cystic swelling appears most commonly on the dorsum of the wrist. The thin-walled cyst is clinically known as a *ganglion*. Synovial cysts (*Gideon's disease* or *bible cysts*) are close to and often communicate with the synovial sheaths. The distal attachment of the extensor carpi radialis brevis tendon is a common site for these types of cysts.

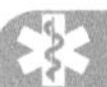

Clinical Correlate 6.32

Anatomical Snuff Box

The **anatomical snuff box** is a clinically significant region (**Fig. 6.80**). The lateral border is formed by the abductor pollicis longus and extensor pollicis brevis while the medial border is formed by the extensor pollicis longus. The floor is formed by the scaphoid and trapezium bones and the radial artery lies on the floor and courses through the snuff box. The styloid process of the radius can be palpated proximally while the base of the first metacarpal can be palpated distally. The scaphoid is the most frequently fractured carpal bone—it is often fractured when an individual trips and braces their fall by extending their hands. Scaphoid fractures can lead to a puncture wound of the radial artery.

Clinical Correlate 6.33

De Quervain Tenosynovitis

Excessive friction leading to inflammation of the tendinous sheath shared by the abductor pollicis longus and extensor pollicis brevis is called **De Quervain tenosynovitis**. The *Finkelstein test* is used to test for this. An individual makes a fist with their thumb tucked under the other fingers and bends their hand toward the 5th digit. If there is pain, the individual has a positive *Finkelstein test* and De Quervain tenosynovitis.

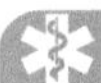

Clinical Correlate 6.34

Mallet Finger

Mallet finger or "baseball finger" is a condition in which the DIP joint of a finger bends but does not straighten by itself. Support is needed to keep the finger in a straight position. The extensor digitorum tendon may be torn or it may be pulled away from its attachment site on the bone due to a forceful flexion or a crushing injury (when sliding into a base head first, for example). A long-term deformity may result if left untreated.

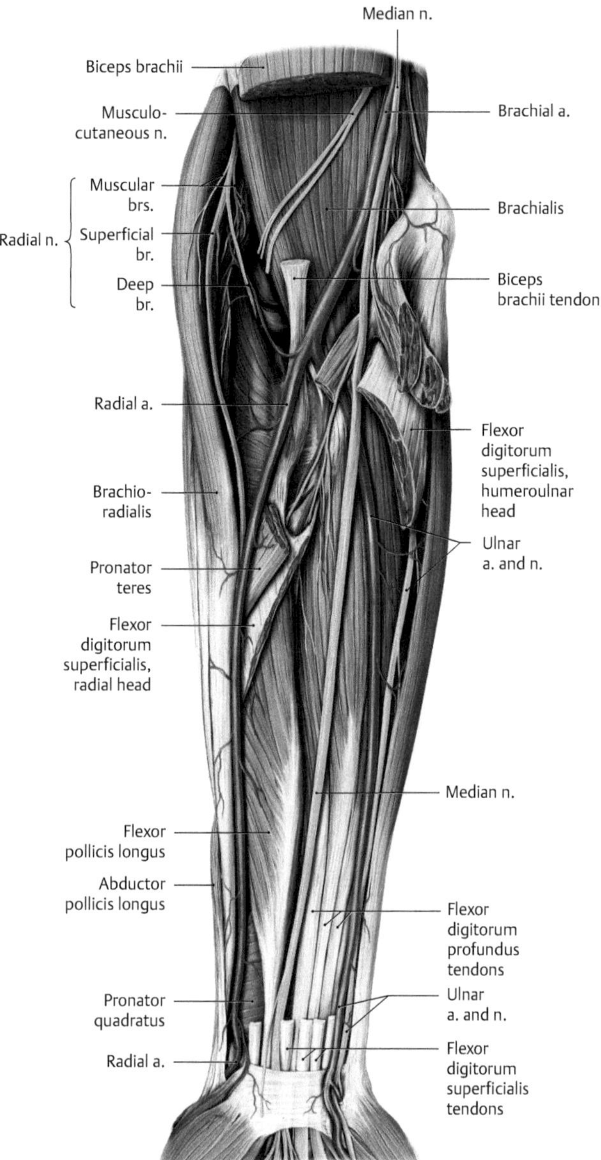

Fig. 6.74 Anterior forearm deep compartment muscles and neurovasculature. (From Schuenke M, Schulte E, Schumacher U. THIEME Atlas of Anatomy. General Anatomy and Musculoskeletal System. Illustrations by Voll M and Wesker K. 3rd ed. New York: Thieme Medical Publishers; 2020.)

in *extension of the 5th digit* and *hand*. The **extensor carpi ulnaris** has a humeral and ulnar head and the tendon that is enclosed in a synovial sheath deep to the extensor retinaculum and running in a groove between the head and styloid process of the ulna. It functions in *extension* and *adduction (ulnar deviation) of the hand* but also contributes to clenching of the fist (**Fig. 6.75a**).

The deep layer consists of the supinator, abductor pollicis longus, extensor pollicis brevis, extensor pollicis longus and the extensor indicis muscles. The **supinator** is a sheet-like muscle that is located deep in the cubital fossa. It spirals medially and distally from the lateral epicondyle and proximal ulna to the proximal shaft and neck of the radius. It functions in *supination of the forearm*. If supination is slow and subtle, the supinator is the main muscle involved here, but when supination is quick and forceful, the biceps brachii is the main supinating muscle (**Fig. 6.77**).

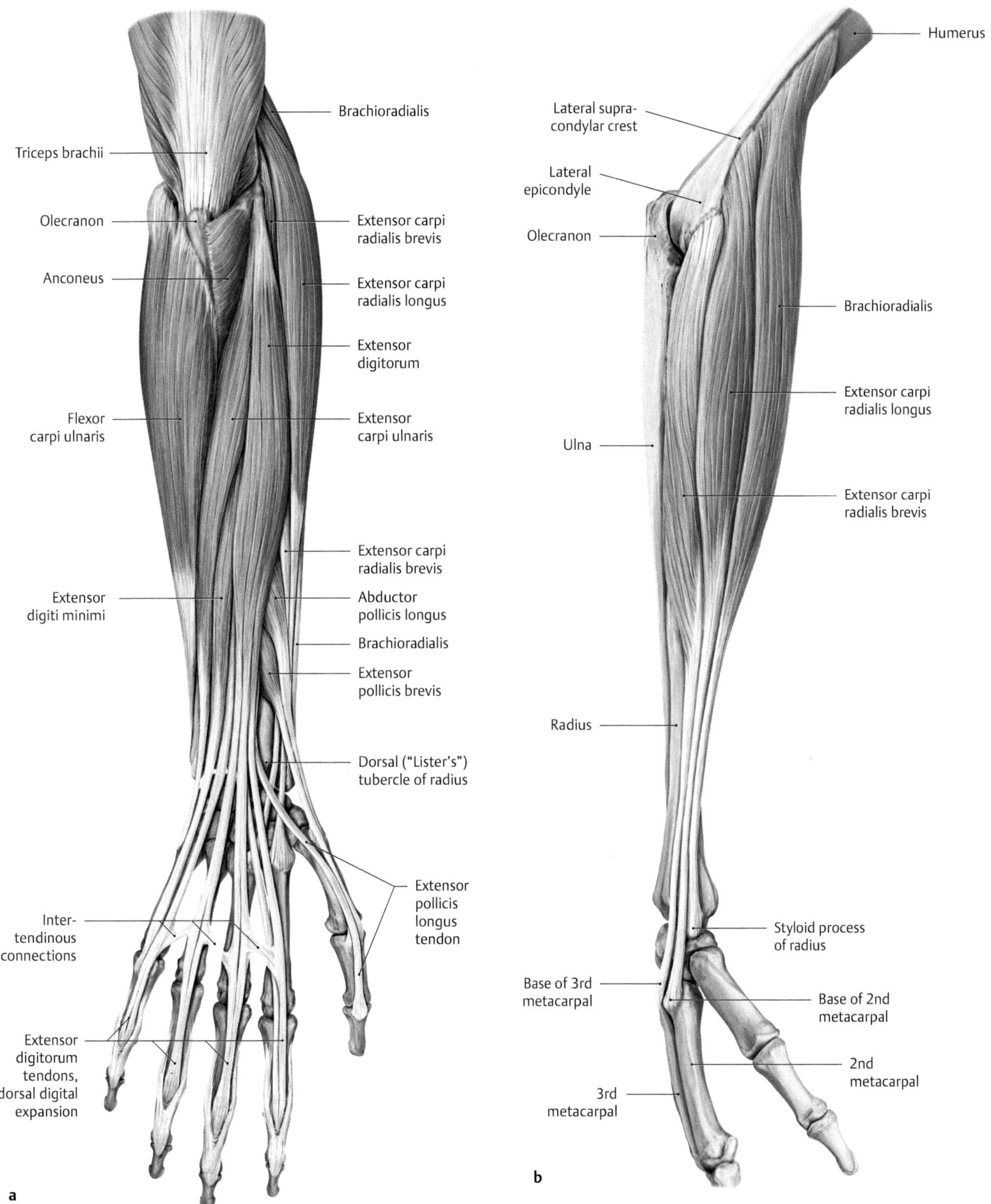

Fig. 6.75 Posterior forearm muscles, superficial layer. **(a)** Posterior view. **(b)** Lateral view. (From Schuenke M, Schulte E, Schumacher U. THIEME Atlas of Anatomy. General Anatomy and Musculoskeletal System. Illustrations by Voll M and Wesker K. 3rd ed. New York: Thieme Medical Publishers; 2020.)

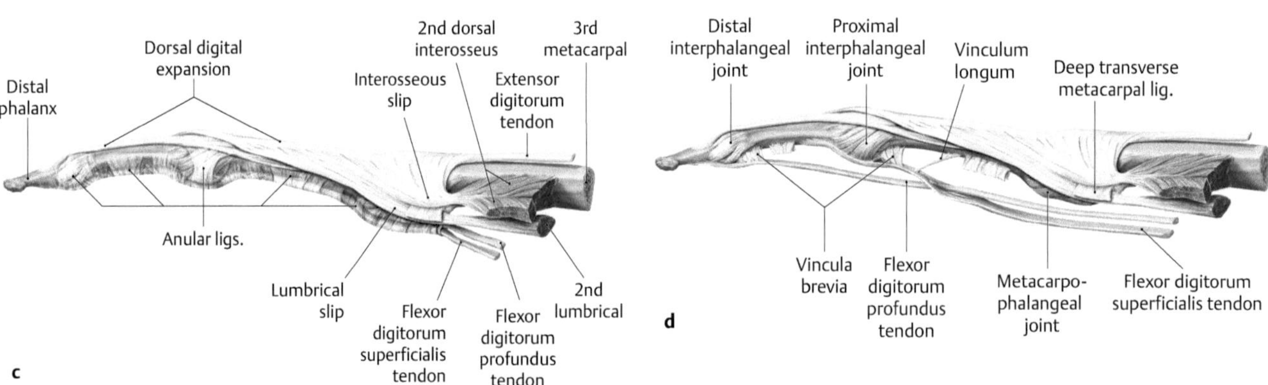

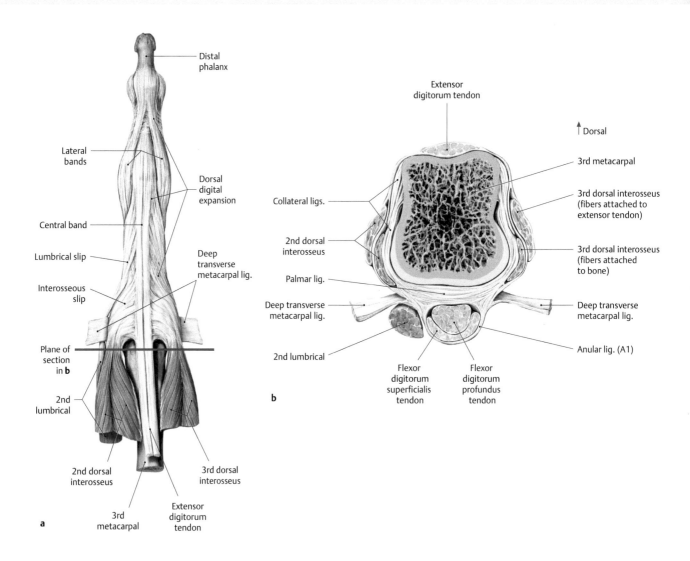

Fig. 6.76 Extensor expansions and supporting ligaments. **(a)** Posterior view. **(b)** Cross section at the level of the metacarpal head. **(c)** Radial view. **(d)** Radial view with common tendon sheath of flexor digitorum superficialis and profundus opened. (From Schuenke M, Schulte E, Schumacher U. THIEME Atlas of Anatomy. General Anatomy and Musculoskeletal System. Illustrations by Voll M and Wesker K. 3rd ed. New York: Thieme Medical Publishers; 2020.)

The **abductor pollicis longus** originates just distal to the supinator and inserts at the base of the first metacarpal. It functions in both *abduction* and *extension of the first digit.* Adjacent to this muscle is the **extensor pollicis brevis** that attaches to the base of the proximal phalanx of the thumb. It functions in *extension of the thumb.* The tendons of these muscles pass through a common synovial sheath deep to the extensor retinaculum before reaching their final attachment site. The **extensor pollicis longus** emerges fairly straight out from the deep layer before making an abrupt change in direction and traveling to the thumb. This directional change is due to the **dorsal tubercle of the radius** and this is approximately where the tendon passes through the related synovial sheath deep to the extensor retinaculum. This muscle functions in *extension of the thumb*. The abductor pollicis longus and both extensor pollicis muscles pass over the tendons of the extensor carpi radialis longus and brevis before reaching the thumb. This gives the appearance that these muscles are emerging from the forearm and have been referred to as *outcropping muscles of the thumb* (**Fig. 6.77; Fig. 6.80**).

The **extensor indicis** extends distally from the ulna and interosseous membrane before passing through the common extensor synovial sheath along with the tendons of the extensor digitorum. It continues and attaches to the extensor expansion of the 2nd digit and function in both *extension of the 2nd digit* and *hand* (**Fig. 6.77**). Descriptions of the posterior forearm muscles are found in **Table 6.6**.

6.15.1 Extensor Tendon Sheaths

Most tendons of the muscles originating from the posterior forearm act on the hand or specific digits. As these tendons travel deep to the extensor retinaculum, they are wrapped by an **extensor synovial sheath**. Tendons are normally wrapped individually by a synovial sheath, except for those of the extensor digitorum and extensor indicis tendons, which share the **common extensor synovial sheath**. Synovial sheaths allow frictionless passage of the tendons during movements of the fingers (**Fig. 6.78**).

6.15.2 Neurovasculature of the Posterior Forearm

As the **radial nerve** emerges from between the brachialis and brachioradialis muscles and anterior to the lateral epicondyle, it bifurcates into a **deep branch** and **superficial branch of the radial nerve** near the cubital fossa. The deep branch pierces the supinator, but on the opposite side of this muscle, it is known as the **posterior interosseous nerve** and it innervates the majority of the posterior forearm compartments. The superficial branch lies tucked between the brachioradialis and extensor carpi radialis longus muscles before surfacing near the wrist. This nerve specifically supplies cutaneous innervation to the majority of the dorsum hand (**Fig. 6.62b; Fig. 6.79**).

The **posterior interosseous artery** (common interosseous br.) passes posterior to the interosseous membrane and eventually pairs with the posterior interosseous nerve. It supplies blood to the posterior forearm and is continuous with the **dorsal carpal arch** near the wrist. The anterior interosseous may also pierce the interosseous membrane distally and contribute to the dorsal carpal arch (**Fig. 6.22**).

6.16 Hand

The manual part of the upper extremity distal to the forearm is the **hand** and it is separated from the forearm by the **wrist**. The skeleton of the hand consists of 8 carpals, 5 metacarpals and 14 phalanges (**Fig. 6.81**).

When the digits forcibly act against or towards the palm this is called the **power grip**. When an object is compressed between the thumb and 2nd digit (index finger) this is referred to as **pinching**. A posture or positioning of the hand due to the natural contraction of the long flexor tendons that ultimately uses little energy is

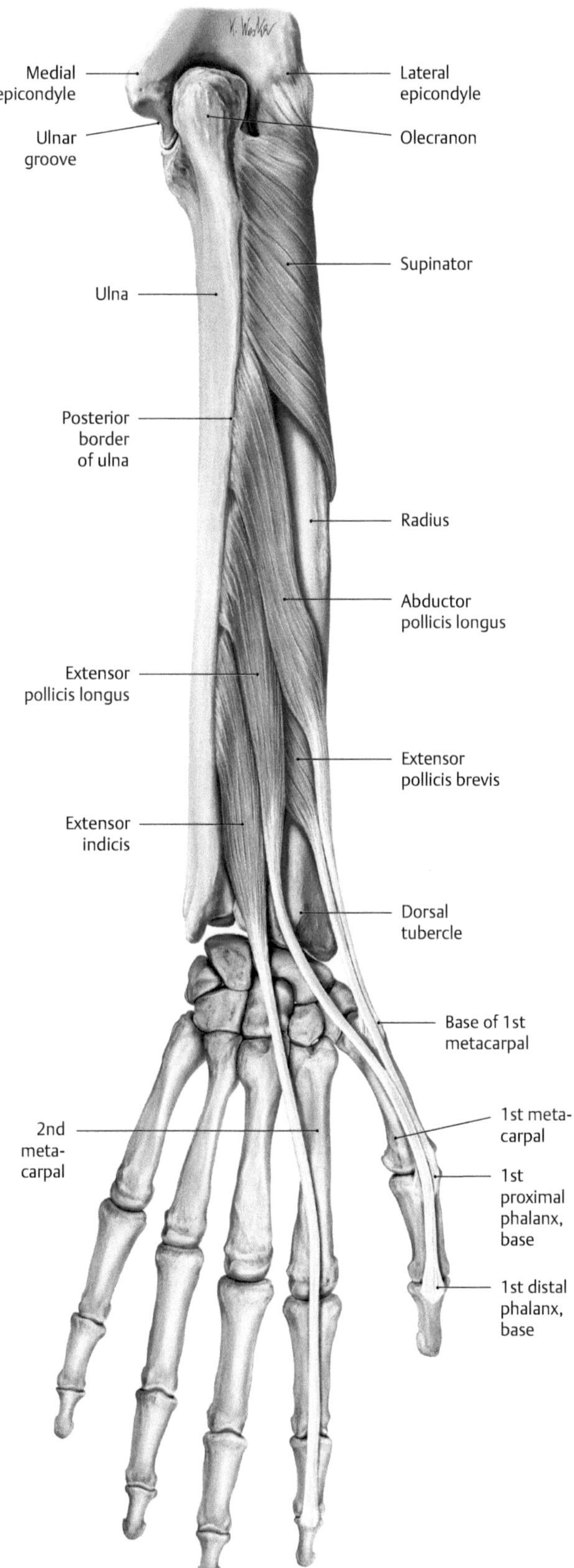

Fig. 6.77 Posterior forearm muscles, deep layer. (From Schuenke M, Schulte E, Schumacher U. THIEME Atlas of Anatomy. General Anatomy and Musculoskeletal System. Illustrations by Voll M and Wesker K. 3rd ed. New York: Thieme Medical Publishers; 2020.)

Table 6.6 **Posterior forearm muscles**

Muscle	Innervation	Function(s)	Origin	Insertion
Superficial layer				
Brachioradialis	Radial nerve	Weak flexion of forearm	Proximal 2/3 of supracondylar ridge; lateral intermuscular septum	Lateral surface of distal radius proximal to the styloid process
Extensor carpi radialis longus	Radial nerve	Extends and abducts hand	Lateral supracondylar ridge; lateral intermuscular septum	Base of 2nd metacarpal
Extensor carpi radialis brevis	Deep branch of radial nerve	Extends and abducts hand	Lateral epicondyle (common extensor tendon)	Base of 3rd metacarpal
Extensor digitorum	Posterior interosseous nerve (of deep branch of radial nerve)	Extends the 2nd-5th digits at the DIP, PIP and MCP joints; extends hand	Lateral epicondyle (common extensor tendon)	Extensor expansion of 2nd-5th digits
Extensor digiti minimi	Posterior interosseous nerve (of deep branch of radial nerve)	Extends the 5th digit at the DIP, PIP and MCP joints; extends hand	Lateral epicondyle (common extensor tendon)	Extensor expansion of 5th digit
Extensor carpi ulnaris	Posterior interosseous nerve (of deep branch of radial nerve)	Extends and adducts hand	Lateral epicondyle (common extensor tendon); posterior border of ulna	Base of 5th metacarpal
Deep layer				
Supinator	Deep branch of radial nerve	Supinates forearm	Lateral epicondyle; supinator crest and fossa of ulna; radial collateral and anular ligaments	Lateral, posterior and anterior surfaces of proximal 1/3 of radius
Abductor pollicis longus	Posterior interosseous nerve (of deep branch of radial nerve)	Abducts 1st digit and extends it at the CMC joint; assist in hand abduction	Posterior surface of proximal half of both radius and ulna; interosseous membrane	Base of 1st metacarpal
Extensor pollicis brevis	Posterior interosseous nerve (of deep branch of radial nerve)	Extends 1st digit at MCP and CMC joints; assists in hand extension and abduction	Posterior surface of distal 1/3 of radius; interosseous membrane	Base of proximal phalanx of 1st digit
Extensor pollicis longus	Posterior interosseous nerve (of deep branch of radial nerve)	Extends 1st digit at IP, MCP and CMC joints; assists in hand extension and abduction	Posterior surface of middle 1/3 of ulna; interosseous membrane	Base of distal phalanx of 1st digit
Extensor indicis	Posterior interosseous nerve (of deep branch of radial nerve)	Extends the 2nd digit at the DIP, PIP and MCP joints; extends hand	Posterior surface of distal 1/3 of ulna; interosseous membrane	Extensor expansion of 2nd digit

called the **hook grip**. A **precision handling grip** is one where the digits and wrist are held firmly together by the long extensor and flexor muscles and the intrinsic hand muscles carry out all fine movements of the digits.

When the hand is inactive it is in a *position of rest* and it can resemble a hook grip. The normal relaxed position of the hand differs from that of an anatomical positioned hand. At rest, the forearm is in a mid-supination/pronation position while the wrist is slightly extended, the thumb is in a neutral position, and the fingers form a flexion arcade (**Fig. 6.82**).

The extensor retinaculum continues as the **dorsal fascia of the hand** and from the palmar carpal ligament and flexor retinaculum, the deep fascia continues as the **palmar fascia of the hand**. The **palmar aponeurosis** is part of this palmar fascia and it is continuous with the palmaris longus muscle tendon (if present). The four distinct condensations of the aponeurosis mirror digits 2-5 and extend to the bases of the fingers before becoming continuous with the fibrous tendon sheaths of the digits. The **superficial transverse metacarpal ligament** traverses the four condensations at the level of the metacarpophalangeal joints or knuckles. Located just below and connecting the metacarpophalangeal joints are the **deep transverse metacarpal ligaments** (**Fig. 6.14**).

The hand is divided into five compartments, the *thenar*, *hypothenar*, *adductor*, *central* and *interosseous* (**Fig. 6.83**). The **thenar compartment** is associated with the thumb (first digit) and contains the flexor pollicis brevis, abductor pollicis brevis and opponens pollicis muscles. The *tendon of the flexor pollicis longus* may also be considered part of this compartment. The **flexor pollicis brevis** has two bellies that are located on each side of the flexor pollicis longus tendon and this muscle *flexes the thumb*. The **abductor pollicis brevis** *abducts the thumb* and *helps oppose it*. The **opponens pollicis** *opposes the thumb* by flexing and rotating the first metacarpal medially at the carpometacarpal joint (**Fig. 6.84**).

The **hypothenar compartment** is related to the little finger or 5th digit and contains the abductor digiti minimi, flexor digiti minimi brevis and opponens digiti minimi muscles. The palmaris

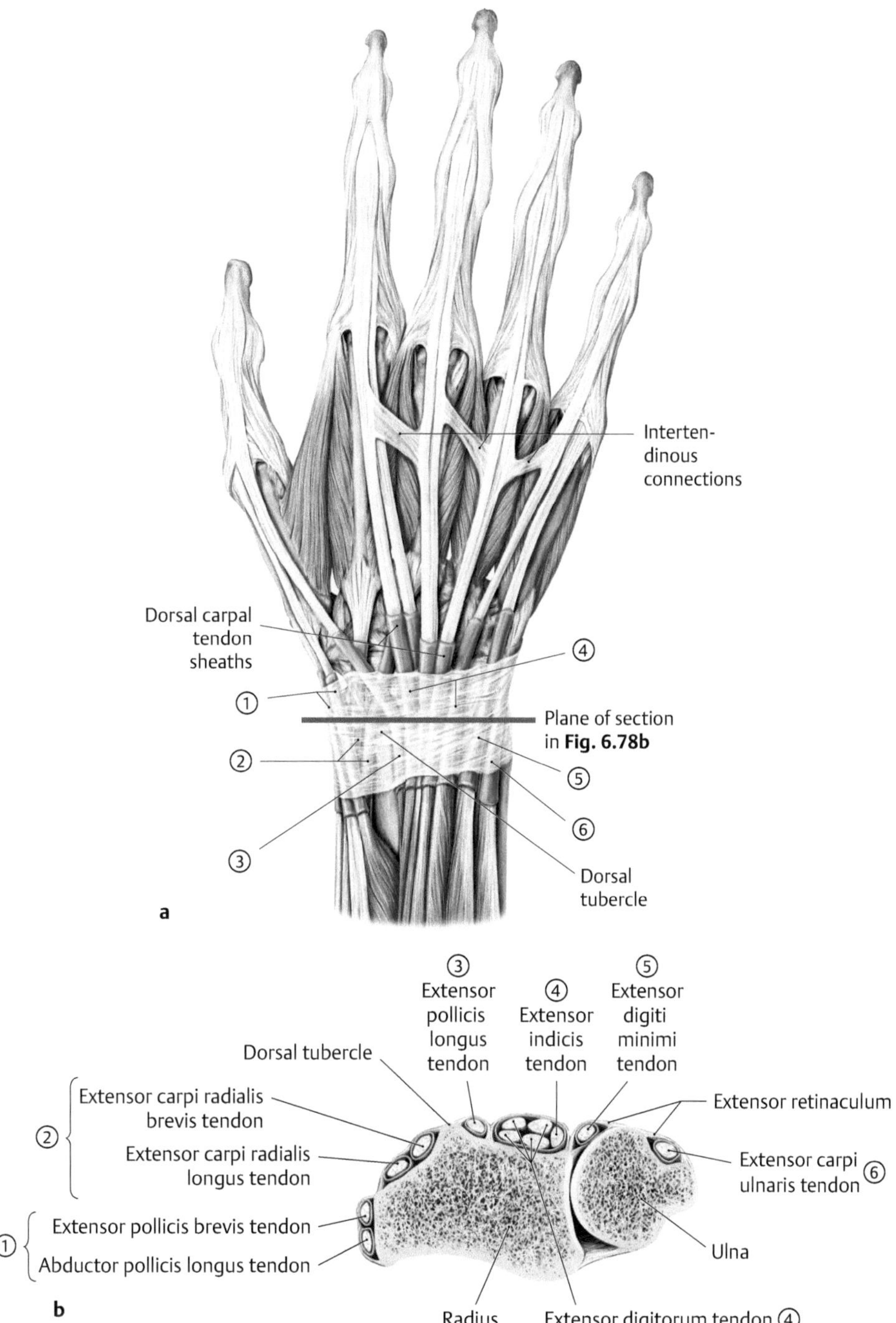

Fig. 6.78 Extensor retinaculum and synovial sheaths. **(a)** Right hand, posterior (dorsal) view. **(b)** Posterior (dorsal) compartments, proximal view of section in a. (From Schuenke M, Schulte E, Schumacher U. THIEME Atlas of Anatomy. General Anatomy and Musculoskeletal System. Illustrations by Voll M and Wesker K. 3rd ed. New York: Thieme Medical Publishers; 2020.)

brevis muscle is located in the subcutaneous tissue over the hypothenar eminence and is not considered part of this compartment. The **abductor digiti minimi** *abducts the 5th digit* and assists in flexion of its proximal phalanx. The **flexor digiti minimi brevis** (there is no longus belly) *flexes the 5th digit* at the proximal phalanx. The **opponens digiti minimi** draws the 5th metacarpal anteriorly and rotates it laterally in order to *oppose the 5th digit* with the first digit. The **palmaris brevis** covers the ulnar neurovasculature, wrinkles the skin of the hypothenar eminence, and aids in the palmar grip (**Fig. 6.84; Fig. 6.85**).

The **adductor compartment** contains only the adductor pollicis muscle. The **adductor pollicis** has an oblique and transverse head separated by the radial artery as it enters the palm to form the deep palmar arch. It functions by *adducting the first digit* and this action can increase the power of a handgrip (**Fig. 6.84; Fig. 6.85**).

The **central compartment** contains the lumbricals and the tendons of both the flexor digitorum superficialis and profundus muscles. The four **lumbricals** *flex at the metacarpophalangeal joints* and simultaneously *extend the interphalangeal joints of the 2nd-5th digits*. The **flexor digitorum superficialis** will first *flex*

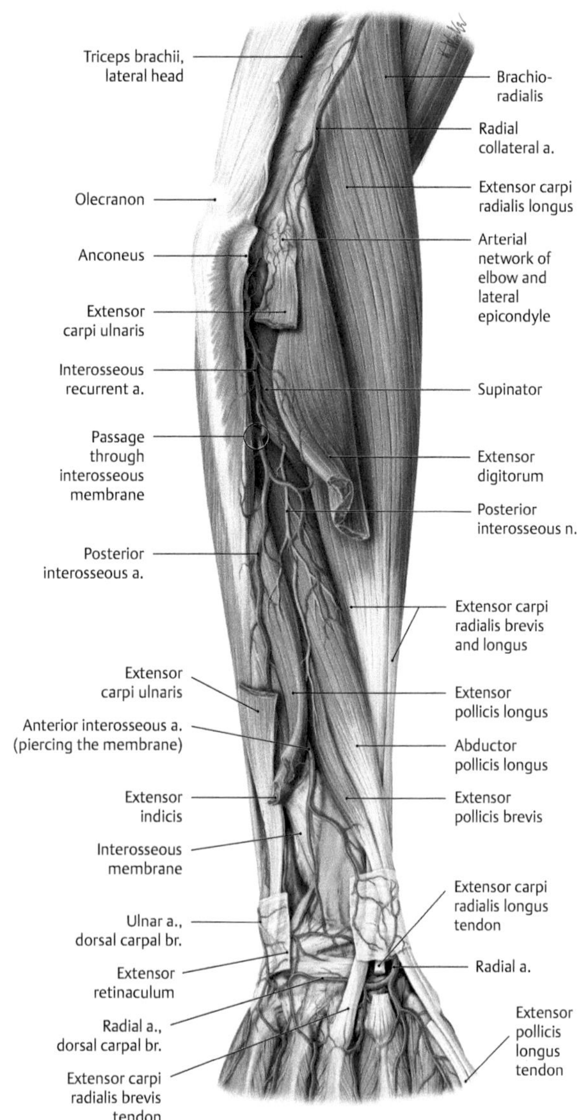

Fig. 6.79 Neurovasculature of the posterior forearm compartment. (From Schuenke M, Schulte E, Schumacher U. THIEME Atlas of Anatomy. General Anatomy and Musculoskeletal System. Illustrations by Voll M and Wesker K. 3rd ed. New York: Thieme Medical Publishers; 2020.)

the middle phalanx of the 2nd-5th digits at the proximal interphalangeal joint but can also flex more proximal joints when more muscle fibers are recruited. The **flexor digitorum profundus** *flexes the distal phalanx of digits 2-5* at the distal interphalangeal joint and it can assist flexing joints back proximally towards the wrist joint with increased muscle fiber recruitment (**Fig. 84**).

The **interosseous compartment** contains the palmar and dorsal interossei muscles. The three **palmar interossei** *adduct the 2nd, 4th and 5th digits* toward the axial line of the hand. The four **dorsal interossei** *abduct the 2nd-4th digits* away from the axial line. Both the palmar and dorsal interossei assist the lumbricals in flexing at the metacarpophalangeal and extending at the interphalangeal joints (**Fig. 6.86**). Descriptions of the hand muscles are found in **Table 6.7**.

Located between the flexor tendons and fascia covering the deep palmar muscles are two potential spaces. These are the thenar and midpalmar spaces. The **thenar space** is located between the thenar and adductor compartments while the **midpalmar space** is tucked between the central, hypothenar, adductor and interosseous compartments and is continuous with the anterior compartment of the forearm via the carpal tunnel. Fibrous septa that pass from the edges of the palmar aponeurosis to the metacarpals help constrain these spaces (**Fig. 6.83**).

6.16.1 Flexor Tendon Sheaths

As the tendons of the flexor digitorum superficialis and profundus muscles proceed through the wrist and into the central compartment of the hand they pass through the **common flexor synovial sheath** located deep to the flexor retinaculum and within the carpal tunnel. From this common sheath, the tendons fan out and enter their respective **digital synovial sheaths** (**Fig. 6.87**). These synovial sheaths allow tendons to move freely past each other during movements of the fingers. The flexor digitorum superficialis tendons split near the base of the proximal phalanx to allow the profundus tendons to pass through and the crossing of the tendons is called the **tendinous chiasm**. The flexor pollicis longus tendon courses deep to the flexor retinaculum and through the carpal tunnel as well but it generally does this in its own synovial sheath.

The digital synovial sheaths and their corresponding tendons are enclosed by ligamentous tubes called **fibrous digital sheaths** (**Fig. 6.88**). The fibrous sheaths are made of 5 **anular** and 3-4 **cruciform ligaments** (**Fig. 6.89; Fig. 6.90**). These ligaments are

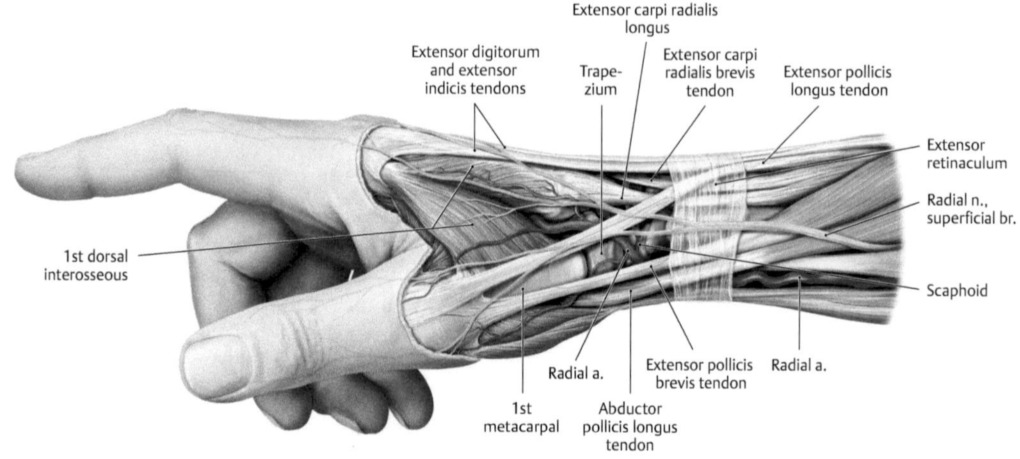

Fig. 6.80 Anatomical snuff box. (From Schuenke M, Schulte E, Schumacher U. THIEME Atlas of Anatomy. General Anatomy and Musculoskeletal System. Illustrations by Voll M and Wesker K. 3rd ed. New York: Thieme Medical Publishers; 2020.)

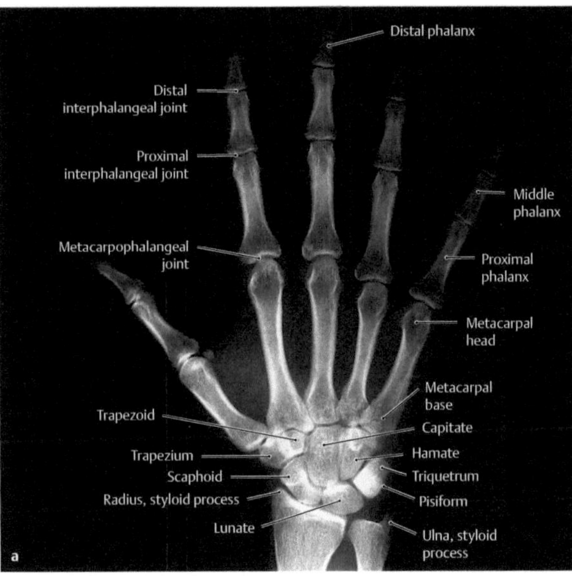

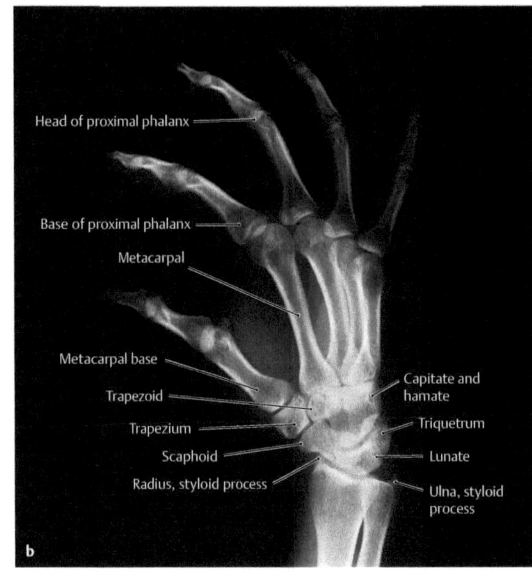

Fig. 6.81 Radiograph of the hand. **(a)** Anteroposterior view. **(b)** Oblique view. (From Moeller TB, Reif E. Pocket Atlas of Radiographic Anatomy, 3rd ed. New York, NY: Thieme; 2010.)

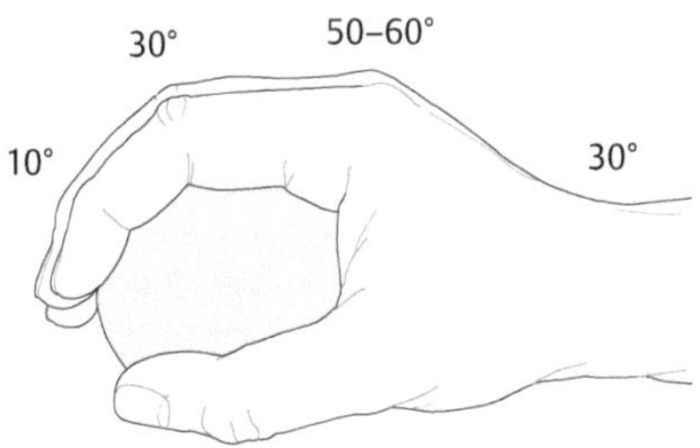

Fig. 6.82 Functional position of the hand. (From Schuenke M, Schulte E, Schumacher U. THIEME Atlas of Anatomy. General Anatomy and Musculoskeletal System. Illustrations by Voll M and Wesker K. 3rd ed. New York: Thieme Medical Publishers; 2020.)

thickened reinforcements of the sheath that attach to the bones and form an incomplete **osseofibrous tunnel** through which the tendons pass. The fibrous sheaths prevent bow-stringing of the tendons from the digits. Small blood vessels that originate from the periosteum of the phalanges course through the **vincula brevia** and **longa** (synovial folds) to supply the long flexor tendons (**Fig. 6.91**).

6.16.2 Neurovasculature of the Hand

The **median**, **ulnar** and **radial nerves** are responsible for innervation of the hand. The **median nerve** passes through the carpal tunnel and supplies the thenar muscles (via the *recurrent branch*) and the most lateral lumbricals 1 and 2. It also supplies the skin of the lateral and proximal palmar surface (via the *palmar cutaneous branch*), the sides of the first three digits, the lateral half of the 4th digit and the dorsum of the distal halves of these same digits (**Fig. 6.92; Fig. 6.93a; Fig. 6.98**).

The **ulnar nerve** passes through the *ulnar tunnel (Guyon's canal)* (**Fig. 6.92; Fig. 6.93b**) and has multiple branches that supply the skin of the hand. Innervation of the skin includes the medial side of the palm (via the *palmar cutaneous branch*); medial half of the posterior hand, the 5th digit, and medial half of the 4th digit (via the *dorsal cutaneous* and *dorsal digital branches*); and the anterior surface of the entire 5th digit and medial half of the 4th digit (via the *superficial branches*). The *deep branch* is responsible for innervating the hypothenar, adductor pollicis, medial most lumbricals 3 and 4, and all of the interossei muscles. The deep head of the flexor pollicis brevis muscle may occasionally be innervated by the ulnar nerve.

The **radial nerve** does not innervate any hand muscles but its *superficial branch* (via the *dorsal digital branches*) supplies the skin and fascia over the lateral 2/3 of the posterior hand, and the proximal parts of the 1st, 2nd, and 3rd digits with some possible overlap with the 4th digit (**Fig. 6.92; Fig. 6.94**).

The ulnar and radial arteries contribute all of the blood that supplies the hand. The **ulnar artery** is located anterior to the flexor retinaculum, just like the ulnar nerve, and passes through the ulnar tunnel. It has two terminal branches and they are the superficial and deep palmar arches. Most of the terminating ulnar artery contributes to the **superficial palmar arch**, which branches off multiple **common palmar digital arteries** before terminating as the **proper palmar digital arteries (Fig. 6.96)**.

The **radial artery** curves posteriorly around the scaphoid and trapezium in the floor of the anatomical snuff box and then enters the palm by passing the first dorsal interosseous and adductor pollicis muscles. The radial artery is the main contributor to the **deep palmar arch** with only a small portion leading to the superficial palmar arch. The deep palmar arch lies near the bases of the metacarpals and gives rise to three **palmar metacarpal arteries** that form an anastomosis with the common palmar digital arteries (**Fig. 6.96b; Fig. 6.97**).

The **dorsal carpal arch** has **dorsal metacarpal arteries** extending out from it and they eventually become the **dorsal digital arteries (Fig. 6.22)**. The first and second digits have individual arteries specified to them. The **princeps pollicis** and **dorsalis pollicis arteries** specifically target the first digit while the **radialis indicis** and **dorsalis indicis arteries** help supply the second digit. The **radialis indicis artery** may branch off the radial or princeps pollicis artery **(Fig. 6.96)**.

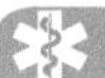

Clinical Correlate 6.35

Carpal Tunnel Syndrome

Any lesion that significantly reduces the size of the carpal tunnel, leading to compression of the median nerve, or, more commonly, increasing the size of some of the structures that pass through the tunnel, is known as **carpal tunnel syndrome**. The median nerve is the most sensitive structure in the carpal tunnel. It is accompanied by the four tendons from each of the flexor digitorum superficialis/ profundus muscles and one tendon of the flexor pollicis longus muscle. The median nerve has two terminal cutaneous branches that supply the skin of the hand, so *paresthesia, hypoesthesia* or *anesthesia* could occur in the lateral three and a half digits on the palmar side. Central palm sensation remains unaffected with carpal tunnel syndrome because the *palmar cutaneous branch (of median)* does not travel through the carpal tunnel. Wasting of the thenar muscles can occur because they are innervated by the median (recurrent branch). A partial or complete cut of the flexor retinaculum **(carpal tunnel release)** can help alleviate pain and muscle weakness associated with this syndrome.

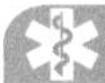

Clinical Correlate 6.36

Ulnar Tunnel Syndrome

Compression of the ulnar nerve at the ulnar tunnel is called **ulnar tunnel syndrome**. Most common causes are a benign lesion or cyst originating from the wrist or chronic pressure, from riding a bike or using a jackhammer, for example. Weakness of the hand muscles and sensory loss or paresthesia involving the medial aspect of the hand and digits are common. Treatment may involve the surgical removal of the cyst or adding protective padding if it is due to a normal leisure or work activity. The ulnar tunnel is located above the flexor retinaculum, thus a carpal tunnel syndrome cannot contribute to ulnar tunnel syndrome.

Clinical Correlate 6.37

Dupuytren Contracture

A disease of the palmar fascia resulting in the progressive shortening, thickening or even fibrosis of the palmar fascia and palmar aponeurosis is called **Dupuytren contracture**. Due to the fibrous degeneration of the longitudinal digital bands of the aponeurosis on the medial side of the hand, this pulls the 4th and 5th fingers into partial flexion at the MCP and PIP joints. Treatment may involve the complete removal of the palmar aponeurosis.

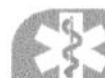

Clinical Correlate 6.38

Tenosynovitis

Tenosynovitis is the inflammation of a tendon or synovial sheath. When this occurs the digit swells and movement becomes painful. An infection of the 2nd-4th digits is usually confined because they have separate synovial sheaths. An infection of the common flexor sheath could spread to the 5th digit and possibly to the first digit because their synovial sheaths can connect to the common flexor sheath.

If enlargement of the flexor digitorum superficialis/profundus tendinous sheaths occur proximal to the osseofibrous tunnel, the patient is unable to extend their finger. When the finger is extended passively, a snap can be heard. Flexion produces another snap as the thickened tendon moves. This is known as **digital tenosynovitis stenosans ("trigger finger")** and can affect any of the digits individually or as multiples.

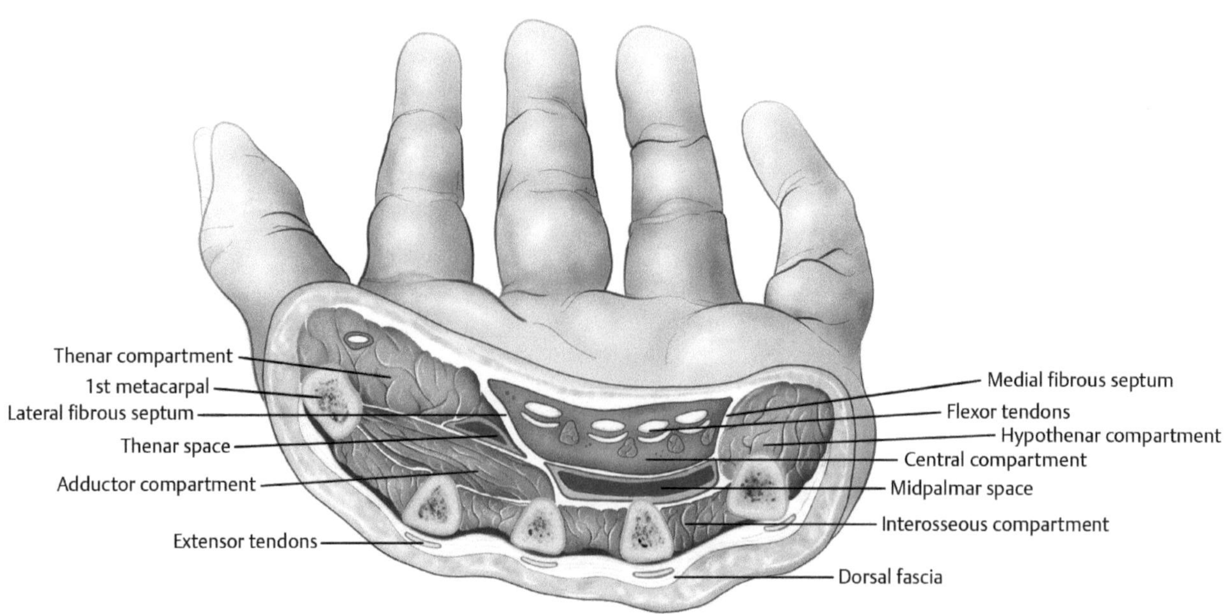

Fig. 6.83 Compartments of the hand. Illustration by Calla Heald.

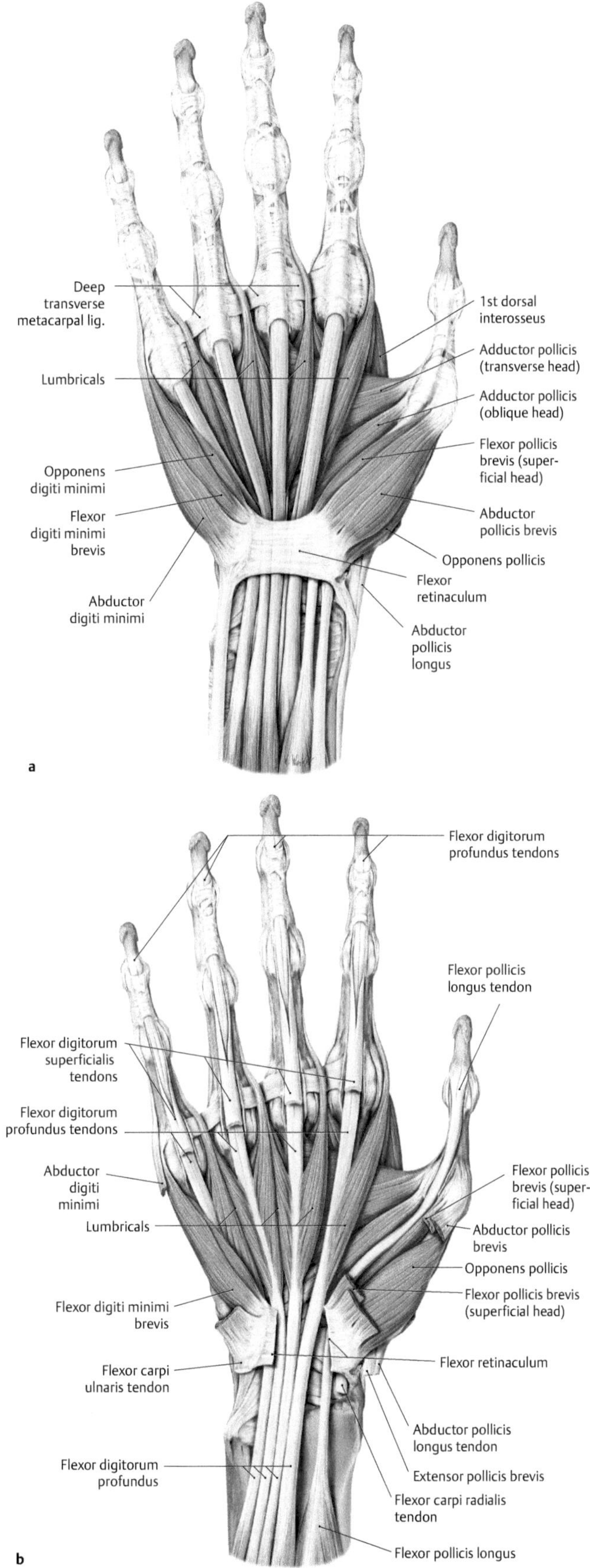

Fig. 6.84 Superficial and intermediate muscles of the right hand. **(a)** Superfical layer with tendon sheaths removed. **(b)** Intermediate layer with the flexor digitorum superficialis, flexor carpi radialis and ulnaris, and pronator quadratus removed. (From Schuenke M, Schulte E, Schumacher U. THIEME Atlas of Anatomy. General Anatomy and Musculoskeletal System. Illustrations by Voll M and Wesker K. 3rd ed. New York: Thieme Medical Publishers; 2020.)

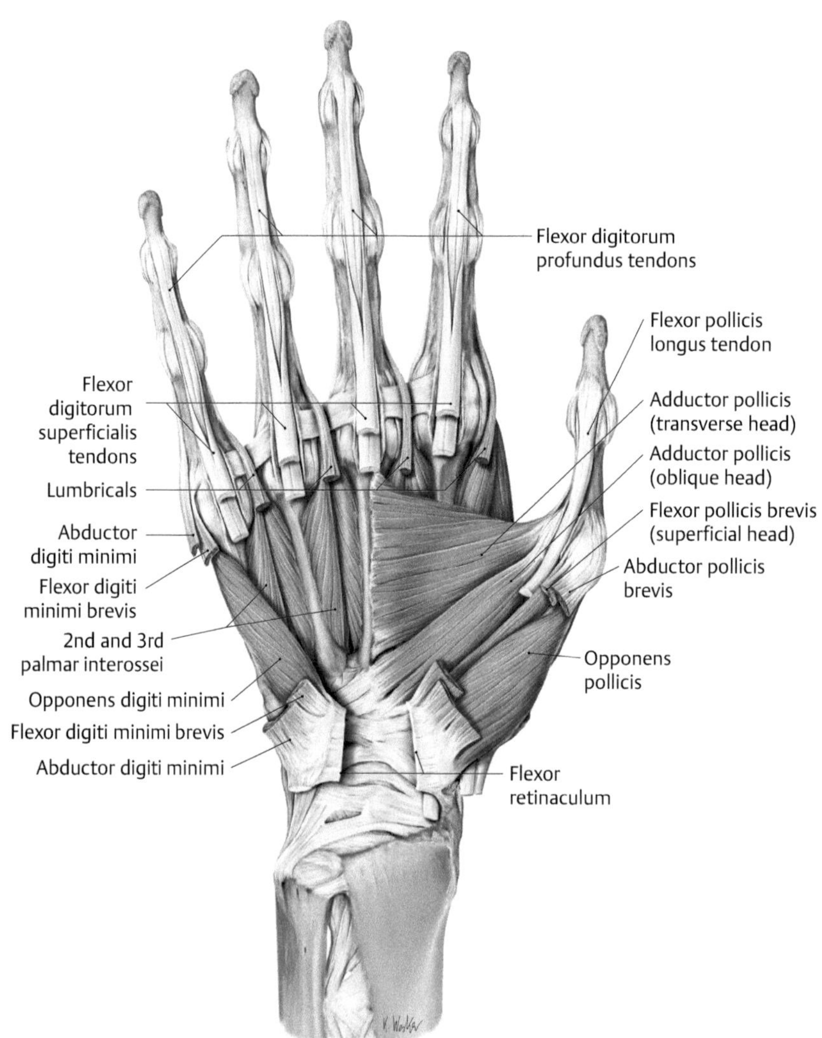

Fig. 6.85 Intrinsic muscles of the right hand. Cut: flexor digitorum profundus, lumbricals, flexor pollicis longus, and flexor digiti minimi brevis. (From Schuenke M, Schulte E, Schumacher U. THIEME Atlas of Anatomy. General Anatomy and Musculoskeletal System. Illustrations by Voll M and Wesker K. 3rd ed. New York: Thieme Medical Publishers; 2020.)

Beginning with the hand region, the **dorsal digital veins** unite with the **dorsal metacarpal veins** before these veins become the **dorsal venous network**. The **proper palmar digital veins** drain into the **common palmar digital (palmar metacarpal) veins**. Blood from these veins may enter either the **superficial venous palmar arch** or **deep venous palmar arch**. Venous drainage from these arches continues through deep veins of the forearm such as the radial, ulnar and interosseous veins **(Fig. 6.23; Fig. 6.24)**.

6.17 Wrist Joint

The **wrist (carpus)** is the proximal portion of the hand and it is made up of eight carpal bones. Certain bones of the wrist articulate with the metacarpals of the hand or the radius of the forearm. However, the **wrist (radiocarpal) joint** is a *condyloid-type synovial joint* that involves the articulation between the distal radius and three of the proximal carpal bones (*scaphoid, lunate* and *triquetrum*) **(Fig. 6.99)**.

The **joint capsule** surrounds the wrist and attaches to the proximal row of carpal bones (except the pisiform) along with the distal ends of the radius and ulna. The normally present synovial membrane is known for having numerous synovial folds. The strong palmar radiocarpal and dorsal radiocarpal ligaments strengthen the joint capsule. The **palmar radiocarpal ligaments** pass from the radius to both rows of carpal bones. They allow the hand to follow the radius during supination of the forearm. The **dorsal radiocarpal ligaments** pass obliquely from the distal tubercle of the radius to the dorsal aspect of the lunate and triquetrum. They allow the hand to follow the radius during pronation of the forearm **(Fig. 6.100)**. The carpal tunnel is located just superficial and distal to the wrist **(Fig. 6.98)**.

The **radial collateral ligament** that spans from the styloid process of the radius to the scaphoid and trapezium bones strengthens the lateral part of the joint capsule. The medial part of the capsule is strengthened by the **ulnar collateral ligament** that spans the styloid process of the ulna and the triquetrum and pisiform bones **(Fig. 6.100; Fig. 6.101)**.

This joint allows flexion-extension, abduction (radial deviation)-adduction (ulnar deviation), and circumduction movements. Movements at the intercarpal and midcarpal joints of the hand may augment these movements. Circumduction is an

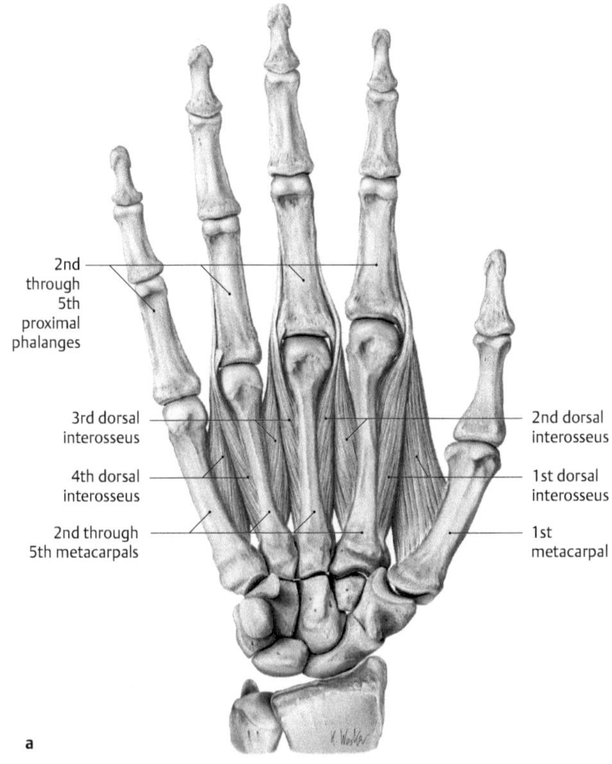

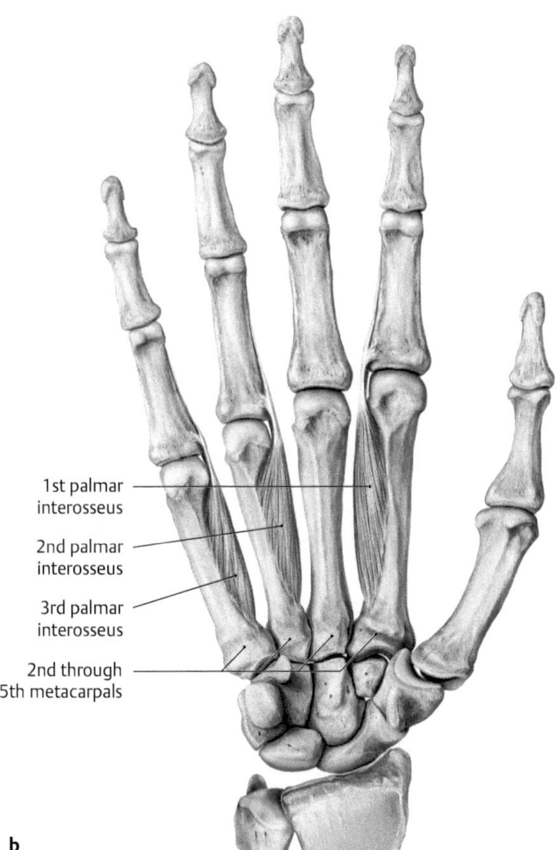

Fig. 6.86 (a) Dorsal interossei. **(b)** Palmar interossei. (From Schuenke M, Schulte E, Schumacher U. THIEME Atlas of Anatomy. General Anatomy and Musculoskeletal System. Illustrations by Voll M and Wesker K. 3rd ed. New York: Thieme Medical Publishers; 2020.)

orderly sequence of flexion, followed by adduction, extension and abduction. Most abduction occurs at the midcarpal joint while adduction primarily occurs at the wrist joint. Abduction is limited to about 15-20° because of the styloid process of the radius. Range of motion is described in **Fig. 6.102**.

6.17.1 Neurovasculature of the Wrist Joint

Innervation of the wrist joint is from the **anterior** and **posterior interosseous nerves** along with the **dorsal** and **deep branches of the ulnar nerve**. The arterial supply is from the **palmar** and **dorsal carpal arches**.

6.18 Hand Joints

6.18.1 Intercarpal Joints

The **intercarpal (IC) joints** are *plane-type synovial joints* and serve as multiple articulations interconnecting the carpal bones. These joints are located between the individual carpal bones of both the distal and proximal rows; these joints include the **midcarpal joint**, located between the complete distal and proximal row of carpal bones, and the articulation between the pisiform and palmar surface of the triquetrum called the **pisotriquetral joint (Fig. 6.99; Fig. 6.101)**.

The **joint capsule** surrounds the IC joints and has a corresponding synovial membrane. There are multiple subsets of individual, named ligaments that connect adjacent carpal bones that will not be discussed here, but know that they are grouped into the **palmar**, **dorsal**, and **interosseous intercarpal ligaments (Fig. 6.100)**.

The gliding movements observed at these joints occur concomitantly with wrist joint movements. The midcarpal joint is where flexion and extension of the hand are initiated and where most abduction occurs. The bulk of overall adduction and flexion of the hand occurs at the wrist joint.

Neurovasculature of the Intercarpal Joints

Innervation to these IC joints is from the **anterior interosseous nerve** and a combination of both the **dorsal** and **deep branches of the ulnar nerve**. Blood supply is from both the **palmar** and **dorsal carpal arches**.

6.18.2 Carpometacarpal and Intermetacarpal Joints

The **carpometacarpal (CMC)** and **intermetacarpal (IM) joints** are *plane-type synovial joints*. The CMC joint of the first digit (thumb) is a *saddle-type synovial joint*. The CMC joints are the articulations between the distal row of carpal bones and the bases of the metacarpals (**Fig. 6.99; Fig. 6.100**). The CMC joint of the first digit has a separate joint cavity. The IM joints are located at the bases of the 2nd-5th metacarpals.

There is a **common joint capsule** lined with a common synovial membrane that includes the four CMC (thumb not included) and the three IM joints. The **palmar** and **dorsal carpometacarpal ligaments** and the **palmar** and **dorsal metacarpal ligaments** strengthen the CMC and IM joint capsules respectively **(Fig. 6.101)**.

Table 6.7 **Hand muscles**

Muscle	Innervation	Function(s)	Origin	Insertion
Thenar compartment				
Flexor pollicis brevis	Recurrent branch of median nerve	Flexes 1st digit	*Superficial head*: flexor retinaculum *Deep head*: capitate and trapezium	Base of proximal phalanx of 1st digit via lateral sesamoid bone
Abductor pollicis brevis	Recurrent branch of median nerve	Abducts 1st digit and helps oppose it	Scaphoid, trapezium, and flexor retinaculum	Base of proximal phalanx of 1st digit via lateral sesamoid bone
Opponens pollicis	Recurrent branch of median nerve	Opposes the 1st digit	Trapezium	Lateral part of 1st metacarpal
Hypothenar compartment				
Abductor digiti minimi	Deep branch of ulnar nerve	Abducts 5th digit and flexes at MCP joint	Pisiform	Medial part of base of proximal phalanx of 5th digit
Flexor digiti minimi brevis	Deep branch of ulnar nerve	Flexes 5th digit at MCP joint	Hook of hamate and flexor retinaculum	Medial part of base of proximal phalanx of 5th digit
Opponens digiti minimi	Deep branch of ulnar nerve	Draws 5th metacarpal in palmar direction into opposition with 1st digit	Hook of hamate and flexor retinaculum	Medial side of 5th metacarpal
Adductor compartment				
Adductor pollicis	Deep branch of ulnar nerve	Adducts 1st digit	*Oblique head*: Bases of 2nd and 3rd metacarpals, capitate *Transverse head*: palmar surface of 3rd metacarpal	Base of proximal phalanx of 1st digit via medial sesamoid bone
Central compartment				
Lumbricals	1st and 2nd: median nerve 3rd and 4th: deep branch of ulnar nerve	Flexes 2nd-5th MCP joints; extends 2nd-5th DIP and PIP joints	1st and 2nd: unipennate bellies from tendon of flexor digitorum profundus; 3rd and 4th: bipennate bellies from tendon of flexor digitorum profundus	Lateral sides of 2nd-5th digit extensor expansions
Interosseous compartment				
Palmar interossei (3)	Deep branch of ulnar nerve	Adduct 2nd, 4th and 5th digits; act with lumbricals to flex MCP and extend DIP and PIP joints	Unipennate bellies from palmar surfaces of 2nd, 4th, and 5th metacarpals	Bases of proximal phalanges; 2nd, 4th, and 5th digit extensor expansions
Dorsal interossei (4)	Deep branch of ulnar nerve	Abduct 2nd-4th digits; act with lumbricals to flex MCP and extend DIP and PIP joints	Bipennate bellies from adjacent metacarpals	Bases of proximal phalanges; 2nd-4th digit extensor expansions

The CMC joint of the first digit permits flexion-extension, abduction-adduction and circumduction movements along with the movement of opposition (**Fig. 6.103**). The CMC joint of the 2nd and 3rd digits are immovable with only slight gliding movements are allowed at the 4th and 5th CMC joints. The IM joints are similar to the 4th and 5th CMC joints in that they are limited to slight gliding movements sufficient enough to permit limited flexion and extension.

Neurovasculature of the Carpometacarpal and Intermetacarpal Joints

Innervation to the CMC and IM joints is from the **anterior interosseous**, **posterior interosseous** and a combination of both the **dorsal** and **deep branches of the ulnar nerve**. Blood supply originates from a combination of the **palmar carpal**, **dorsal carpal** and **deep palmar arches** along with the **metacarpal arteries**.

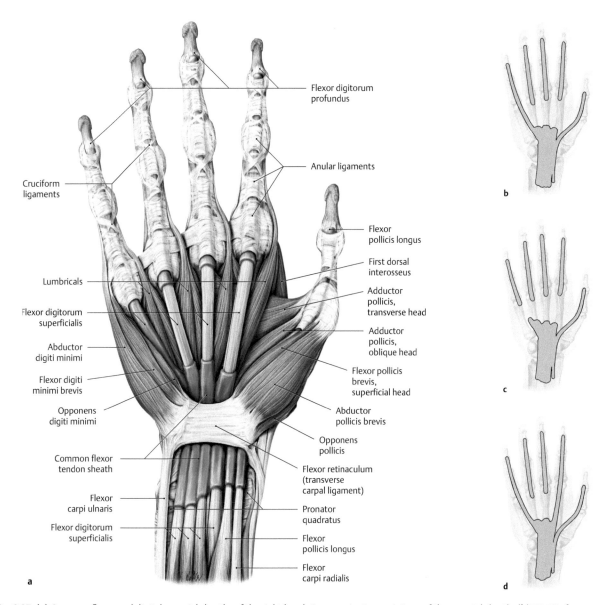

Fig. 6.87 **(a)** Common flexor and digital synovial sheaths of the right hand. Communication variations of the synovial sheath: **(b)** 71.4% of cases; **(c)** 17.4% of cases; **(d)** ~3-3.5% of cases. (From Schuenke M, Schulte E, Schumacher U. THIEME Atlas of Anatomy. General Anatomy and Musculoskeletal System. Illustrations by Voll M and Wesker K. 3rd ed. New York: Thieme Medical Publishers; 2020.)

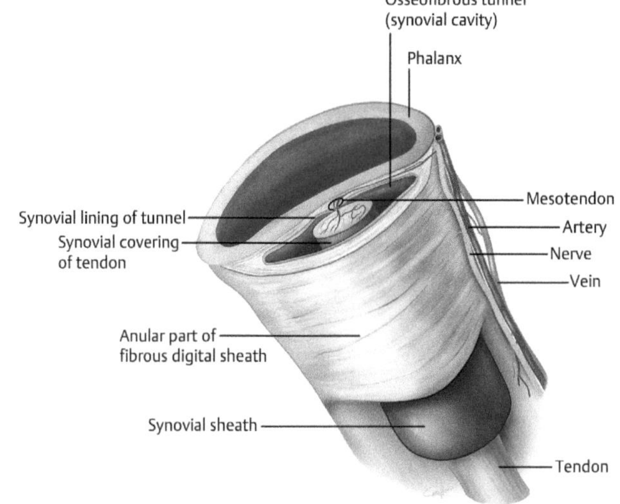

Fig. 6.88 Fibrous digital sheaths. Illustration by Calla Heald.

6.18.3 Metacarpophalangeal and Interphalangeal Joints

The **metacarpophalangeal (MCP) joints** are *condyloid-type synovial joints* and are the articulations between the heads of the metacarpals and the bases of the proximal phalanges. The **interphalangeal (IP) joints** are *hinge-type synovial joints* and are articulations found between the proximal and middle phalanges (*proximal IP*) or the middle and distal phalanges (*distal IP*). The first digit has only one IP joint located between its proximal and distal phalanges (**Fig. 6.100**).

The **joint capsule** enclosing both types of joints attaches to the margins of each joint and has a corresponding synovial membrane. **Lateral** and **medial collateral ligaments** strengthen both of the MCP and IP joint capsules. These ligaments are divided into two parts. There is a dense *cord-like* part that passes distally from the head of a metacarpal or phalange to the adjacent base of a phalange. The thinner *fan-like* part passes distally and anteriorly from the head of a metacarpal or phalange and onto a fibrocartilaginous

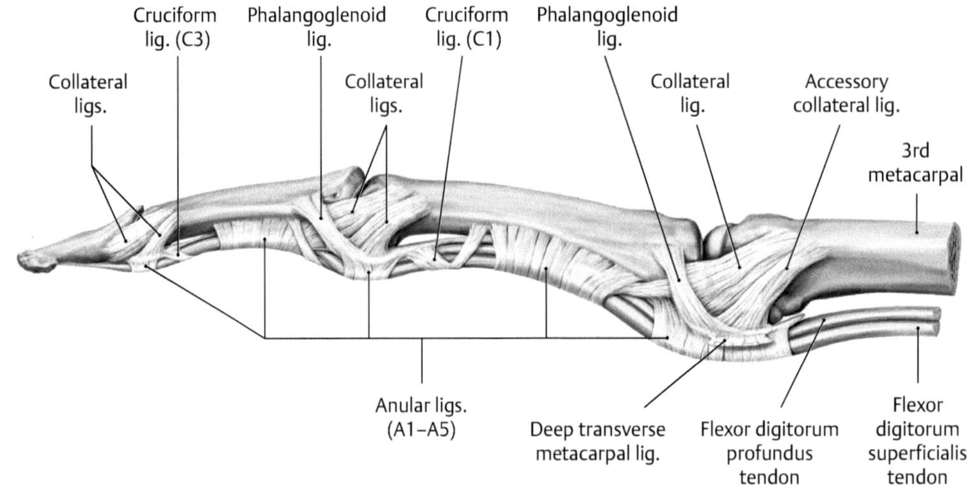

Fig. 6.89 The joint capsules, ligaments, and fibrous sheaths of the right middle finger. Lateral view. (From Schuenke M, Schulte E, Schumacher U. THIEME Atlas of Anatomy. General Anatomy and Musculoskeletal System. Illustrations by Voll M and Wesker K. 3rd ed. New York: Thieme Medical Publishers; 2020.)

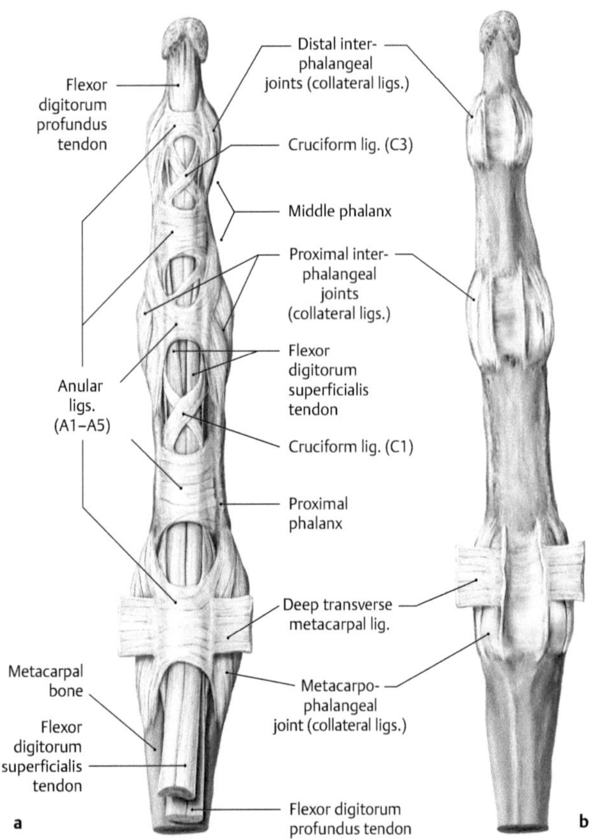

Fig. 6.90 Ligaments of the right middle finger: anterior (palmar) view. **(a)** Superficial ligaments. **(b)** Deep ligaments with flexor digitorum tendons removed. (From Schuenke M, Schulte E, Schumacher U. THIEME Atlas of Anatomy. General Anatomy and Musculoskeletal System. Illustrations by Voll M and Wesker K. 3rd ed. New York: Thieme Medical Publishers; 2020.)

palmar ligament (or **plate**). The palmar ligaments blend with the *fibrous digital sheaths* and are united by **deep transverse metacarpal ligaments** between the 2nd-5th MCP joints. The *cord-like* parts at the MCP joints are slack during extension and taut during flexion and limit any attempted abduction of the fingers when the MCP joints are fully flexed (**Fig. 6.100**).

Movement at the first MCP joint is limited to flexion-extension while movements at the 2nd-5th MCP joints include flexion-extension, abduction-adduction and circumduction. The IP joints allow only for flexion-extension movements. Range of motion of these joints is described in **Fig. 6.104**.

Neurovasculature of the Metacarpal and Interphalangeal Joints

Innervation to the MC and IP joints is from **digital nerve** branches of both the median and ulnar nerves. Blood supply is from the **deep digital arteries** of the superficial palmar arch.

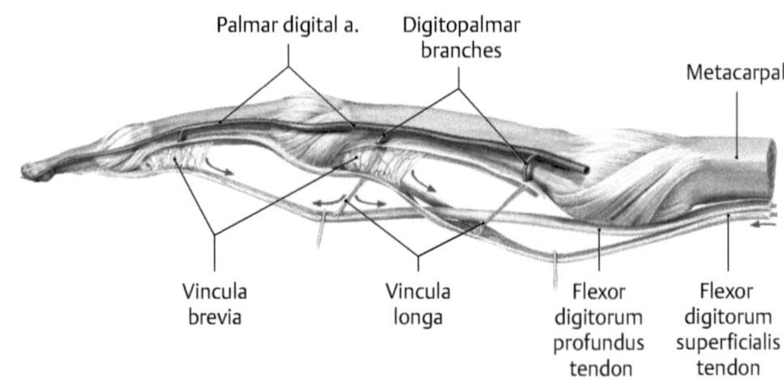

Fig. 6.91 Blood supply to the flexor tendons of the finger. (From Schuenke M, Schulte E, Schumacher U. THIEME Atlas of Anatomy. General Anatomy and Musculoskeletal System. Illustrations by Voll M and Wesker K. 3rd ed. New York: Thieme Medical Publishers; 2020.)

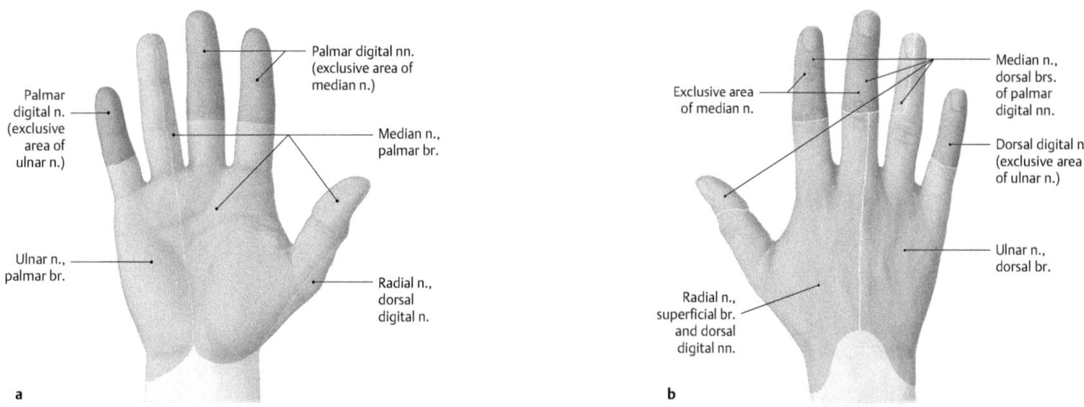

Fig. 6.92 Cutaneous nerve supply to the right hand. **(a)** Palmar surface. **(b)** Dorsum of the hand. (From Schuenke M, Schulte E, Schumacher U. THIEME Atlas of Anatomy. General Anatomy and Musculoskeletal System. Illustrations by Voll M and Wesker K. 3rd ed. New York: Thieme Medical Publishers; 2020.)

Median nerve
Medial epicondyle
Articular br.
Pronator teres, humeral head
Flexor carpi radialis
Pronator teres, ulnar head
Palmaris longus
Flexor digitorum superficialis
Anterior interosseous n.
Flexor pollicis longus
Flexor digitorum profundus
Pronator quadratus
Recurrent br.
Median n., palmar br.
Flexor retinaculum
Common palmar digital nn.
1st and 2nd lumbricals
Proper palmar digital nn.
a

Median nerve
Medial epicondyle
Ulnar groove
Flexor digitorum profundus
Flexor carpi ulnaris
Flexor retinaculum
Dorsal br.
Palmar br.
Superficial br.
Deep br.
4th common palmar digital n.
Interossei
Proper palmar digital nn.
b

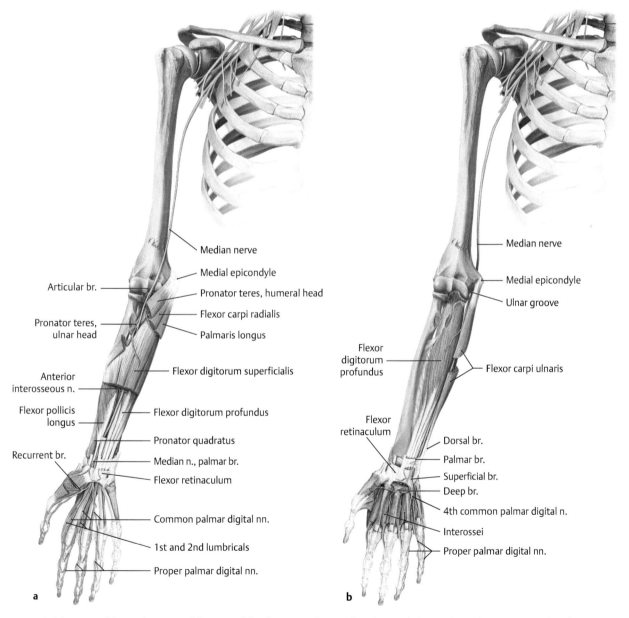

Fig. 6.93 **(a)** Course of the median nerve. **(b)** Course of the ulnar nerve. (From Schuenke M, Schulte E, Schumacher U. THIEME Atlas of Anatomy. General Anatomy and Musculoskeletal System. Illustrations by Voll M and Wesker K. 3rd ed. New York: Thieme Medical Publishers; 2020.)

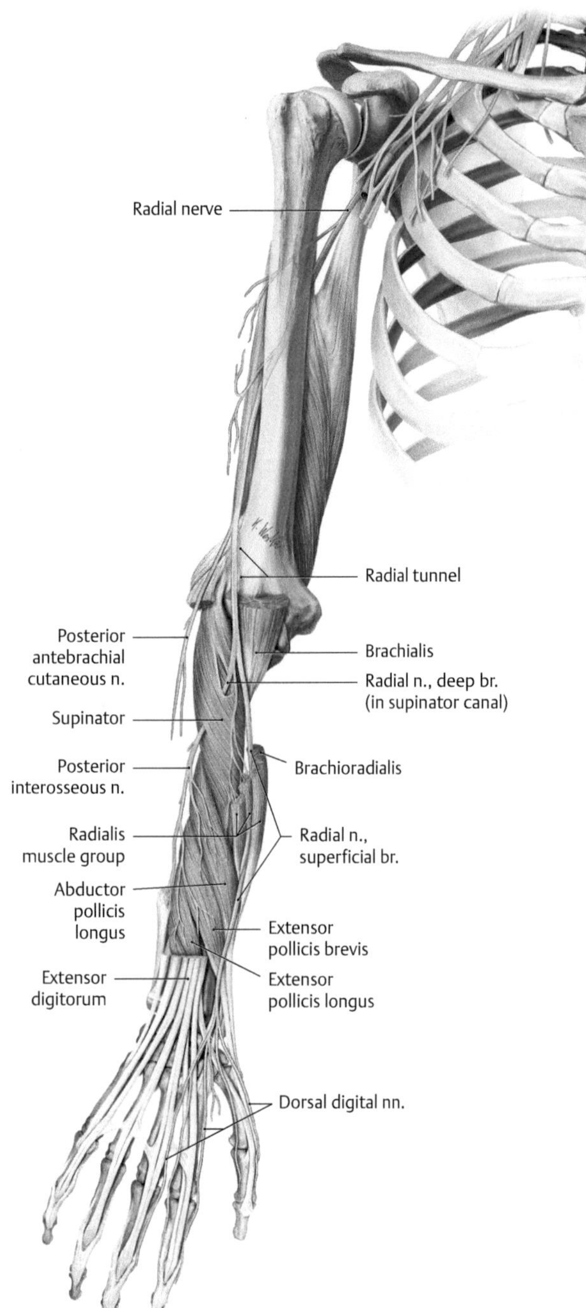

Fig. 6.94 Course of the radial nerve. (From Schuenke M, Schulte E, Schumacher U. THIEME Atlas of Anatomy. General Anatomy and Musculoskeletal System. Illustrations by Voll M and Wesker K. 3rd ed. New York: Thieme Medical Publishers; 2020.)

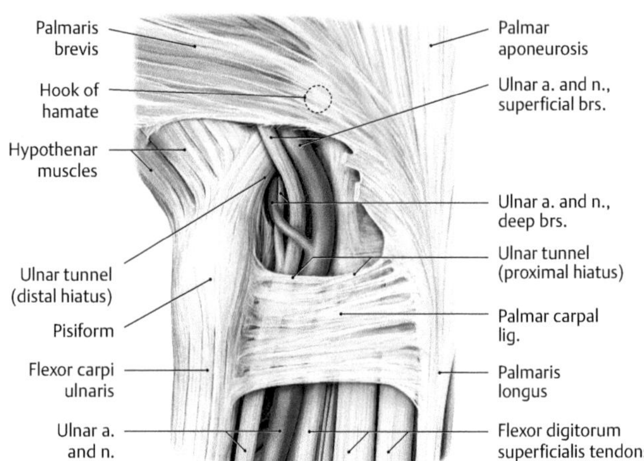

Fig. 6.95 Ulnar tunnel. (From Schuenke M, Schulte E, Schumacher U. THIEME Atlas of Anatomy. General Anatomy and Musculoskeletal System. Illustrations by Voll M and Wesker K. 3rd ed. New York: Thieme Medical Publishers; 2020.)

6.19 Development of the Upper Extremity

Arising from the lateral body wall during the last part of the 4th week of development, the upper limb buds develop opposite the C4-T2 segments. Similar to lower extremity development, each of the limb buds initially consists of a mesenchymal core derived from the *somatic (parietal) layer of lateral plate mesoderm* that is responsible for forming the bones and connective tissues of the limb and is covered by a *cuboidal ectoderm*. At a later time, cells from the ventrolateral portion of the dermomyotome migrate into this region.

Development of the upper extremity closely mirrors that of the lower extremity thus the formation of the apical ectodermal ridge (AER), progress zone, zone of polarizing activity (ZPA) and the patterning of the digits can be referenced in Chapter 5.

From the *dermomyotome regions of the somites*, myogenic precursor cells migrate into the limb bud and differentiate into **myoblasts**, the precursors of muscle cells that are segmented according to the somites from which they are derived. Each myotome of a somite divides into a dorsal **epaxial division** and a ventral **hypaxial division**. The hypaxial division develops into muscles of the body wall and limbs. With elongation of the limbs, myoblasts aggregate and form large muscle masses that split into extensor and flexor components. The upper limbs rotate laterally 90° during weeks 6-8, thus (**Fig. 6.105**):

- The future elbows point dorsally.
- The thumb is located on the lateral side of the hand.
- The extensor muscles lie dorsally and flexor muscles lie ventrally.

The **motor axons** originate from the spinal cord and enter the limb buds during the 5th week of development, extending into both the ventral and dorsal muscle masses. During this same period, the peripheral nerves grow from the developing **limb plexus** (brachial) and into the mesenchyme of the upper limb buds. Spinal nerves are distributed in segmental bands and supply both the ventral and dorsal surfaces of the limb buds. The motor axons enter the limb buds shortly before the **sensory axons**. The myelin sheaths and neurilemma of motor and sensory nerve fibers originate form **neural crest cells**.

The upper extremity blood supply originates from the **subclavian artery** and it continues into the limb bud as the **axis artery**. The axis artery ends as a **terminal plexus** near the tip of the limb bud and it contributes to both the **superficial** and **deep palmar arches** located in the hand. The axis artery initially gives off the **posterior interosseous** and **median arteries** but later it gives rise to the **radial** and **ulnar arteries**. Most of the axis artery undergoes remodeling and regression and persists in the adult as the **axillary**, **brachial** and the **anterior interosseous arteries** along with the **deep palmar arch**. The median artery regresses and loses

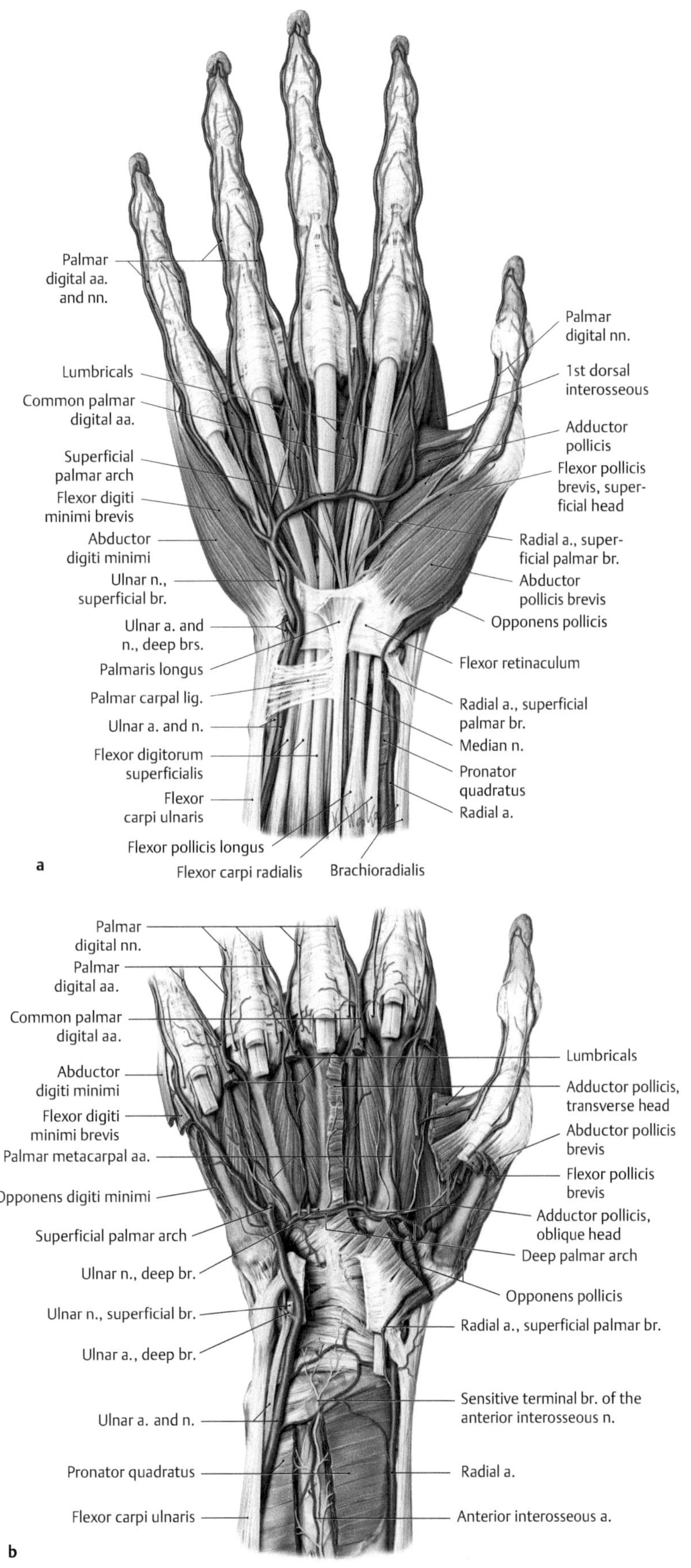

Fig. 6.96 (a) Superficial palmar arch. **(b)** Deep palmar arch. (From Schuenke M, Schulte E, Schumacher U. THIEME Atlas of Anatomy. General Anatomy and Musculoskeletal System. Illustrations by Voll M and Wesker K. 3rd ed. New York: Thieme Medical Publishers; 2020.)

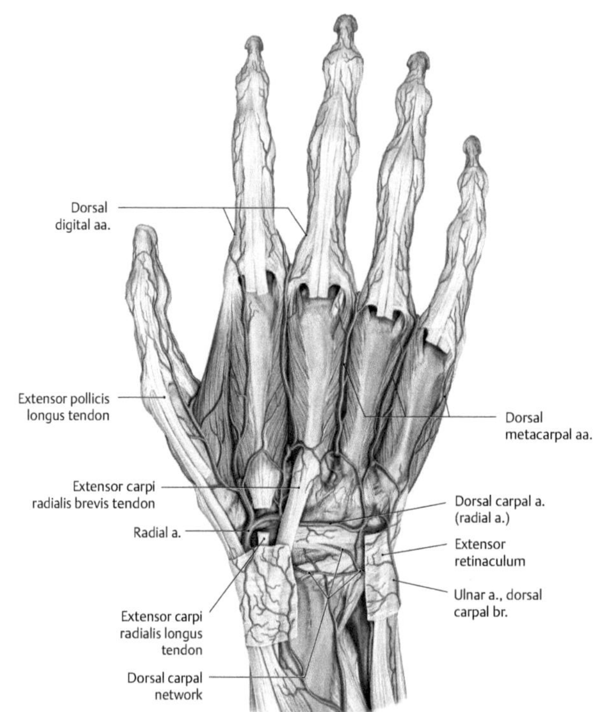

Fig. 6.97 Blood supply to the dorsum of the hand and wrist. (From Schuenke M, Schulte E, Schumacher U. THIEME Atlas of Anatomy. General Anatomy and Musculoskeletal System. Illustrations by Voll M and Wesker K. 3rd ed. New York: Thieme Medical Publishers; 2020.)

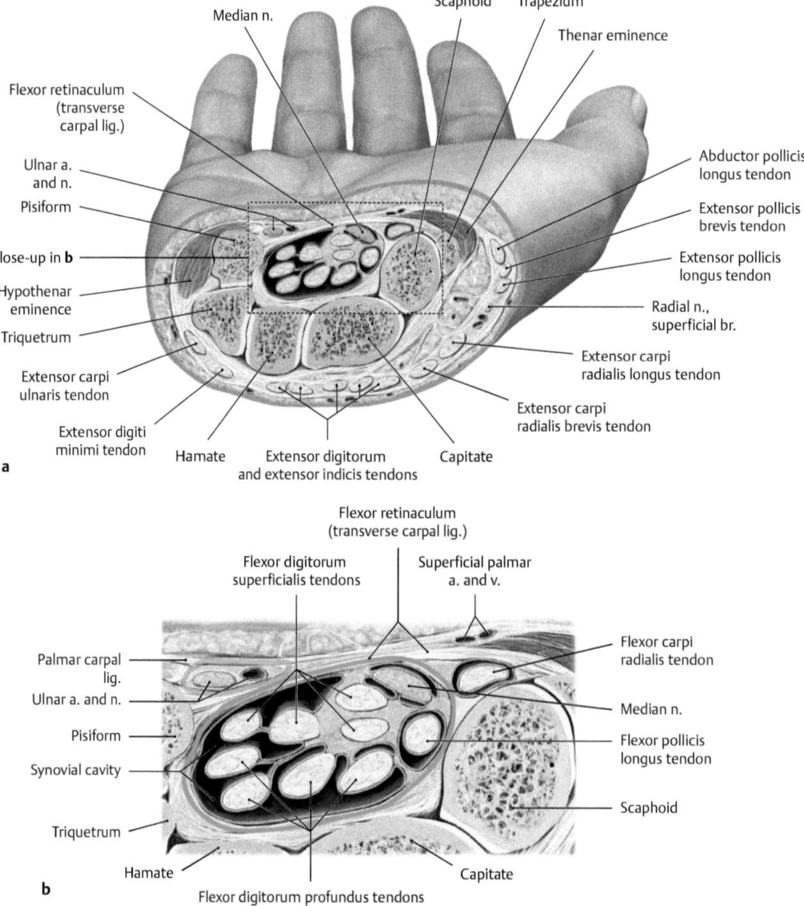

Fig. 6.98 **(a)** Cross section through the right wrist demonstrating the carpal tunnel. The four tendons and synovial sheaths of each the flexor digitorum superficialis and profundus; the tendon and synovial sheath of the flexor carpi radialis; and the median nerve traverse this tunnel. **(b)** Closer examination of the carpal tunnel (*blue circle*) and the ulnar tunnel (*green circle*). (From Schuenke M, Schulte E, Schumacher U. THIEME Atlas of Anatomy. General Anatomy and Musculoskeletal System. Illustrations by Voll M and Wesker K. 3rd ed. New York: Thieme Medical Publishers; 2020.)

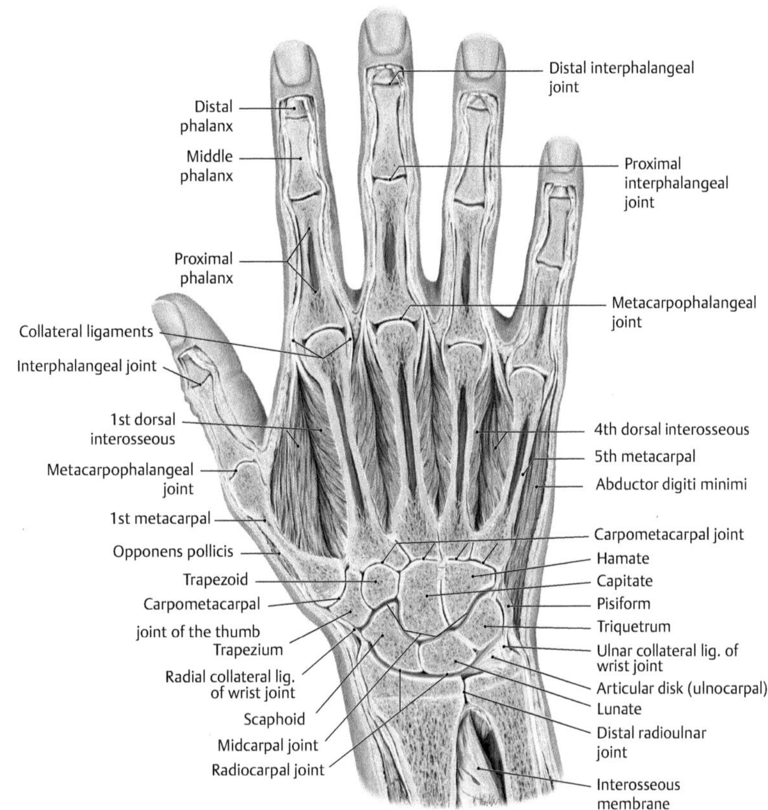

Fig. 6.99 Joints of the wrist and hand: coronal section, posterior (dorsal) view. (From Schuenke M, Schulte E, Schumacher U. THIEME Atlas of Anatomy. General Anatomy and Musculoskeletal System. Illustrations by Voll M and Wesker K. 3rd ed. New York: Thieme Medical Publishers; 2020.)

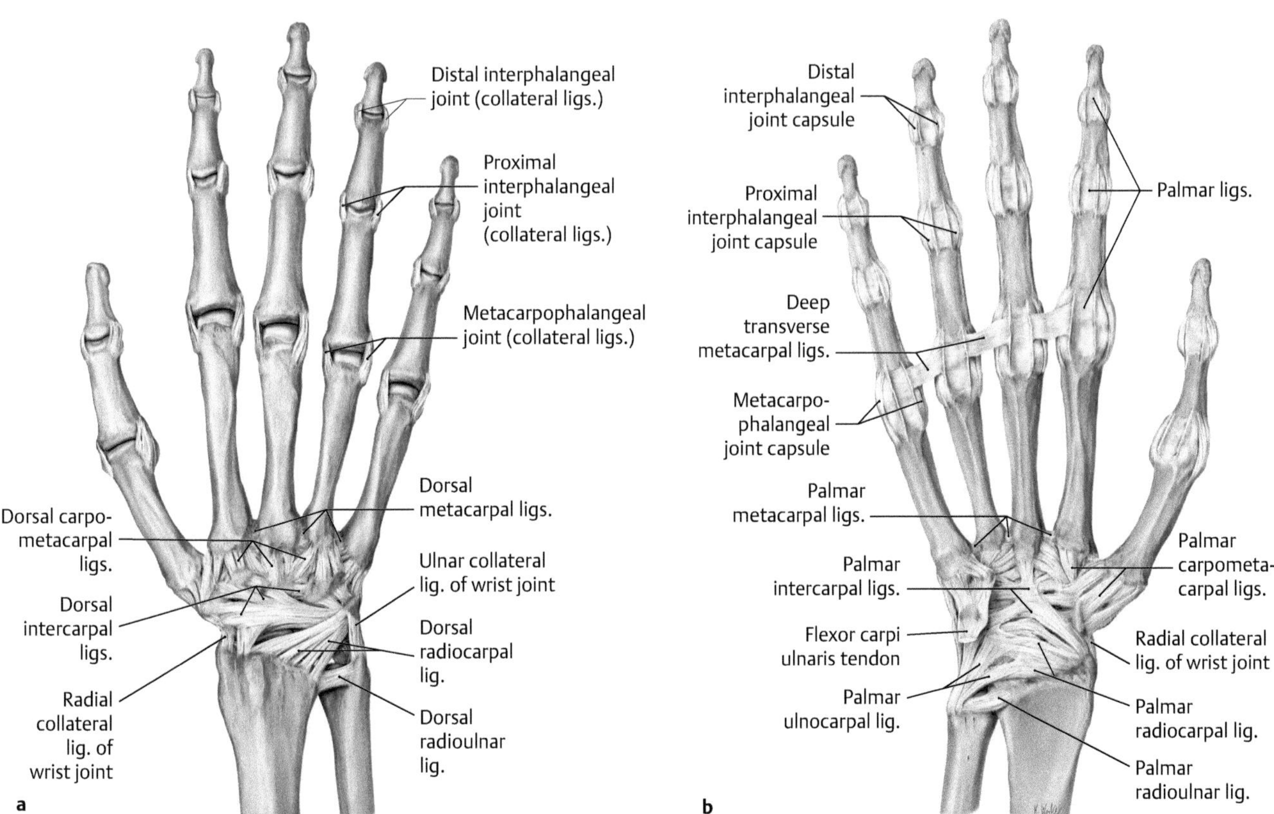

Fig. 6.100 Ligaments of the hand and wrist. **(a)** Posterior (dorsal) view. **(b)** Anterior (palmar) view. Cut: flexor retinaculum. (From Schuenke M, Schulte E, Schumacher U. THIEME Atlas of Anatomy. General Anatomy and Musculoskeletal System. Illustrations by Voll M and Wesker K. 3rd ed. New York: Thieme Medical Publishers; 2020.)

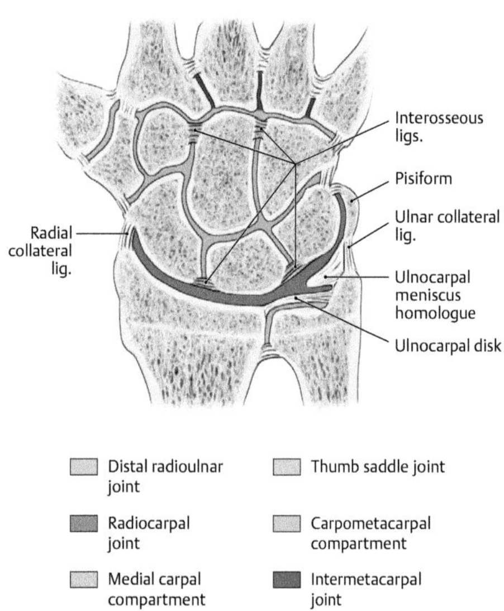

Fig. 6.101 Compartments of the wrist. Right wrist, posterior view, schematic. (From Schuenke M, Schulte E, Schumacher U. THIEME Atlas of Anatomy. General Anatomy and Musculoskeletal System. Illustrations by Voll M and Wesker K. 3rd ed. New York: Thieme Medical Publishers; 2020.)

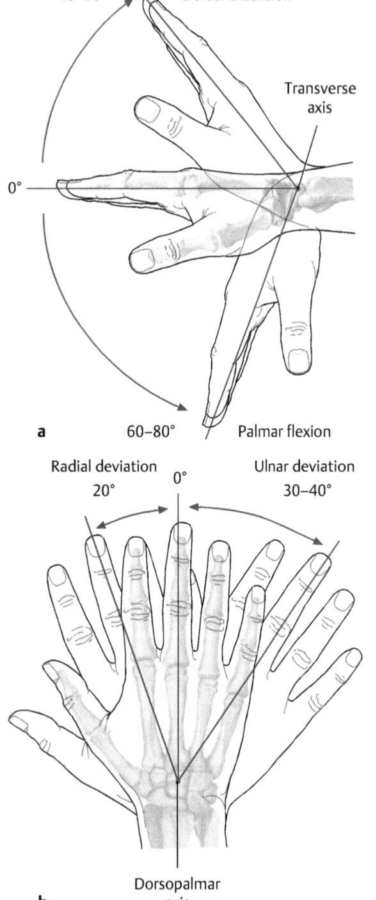

Fig. 6.102 Range of motion of the radiocarpal **(a)** and midcarpal **(b)** joints. The transverse axis runs through the lunate bone for the radiocarpal joint and the capitate bone for the midcarpal joint. (From Schuenke M, Schulte E, Schumacher U. THIEME Atlas of Anatomy. General Anatomy and Musculoskeletal System. Illustrations by Voll M and Wesker K. 3rd ed. New York: Thieme Medical Publishers; 2020.)

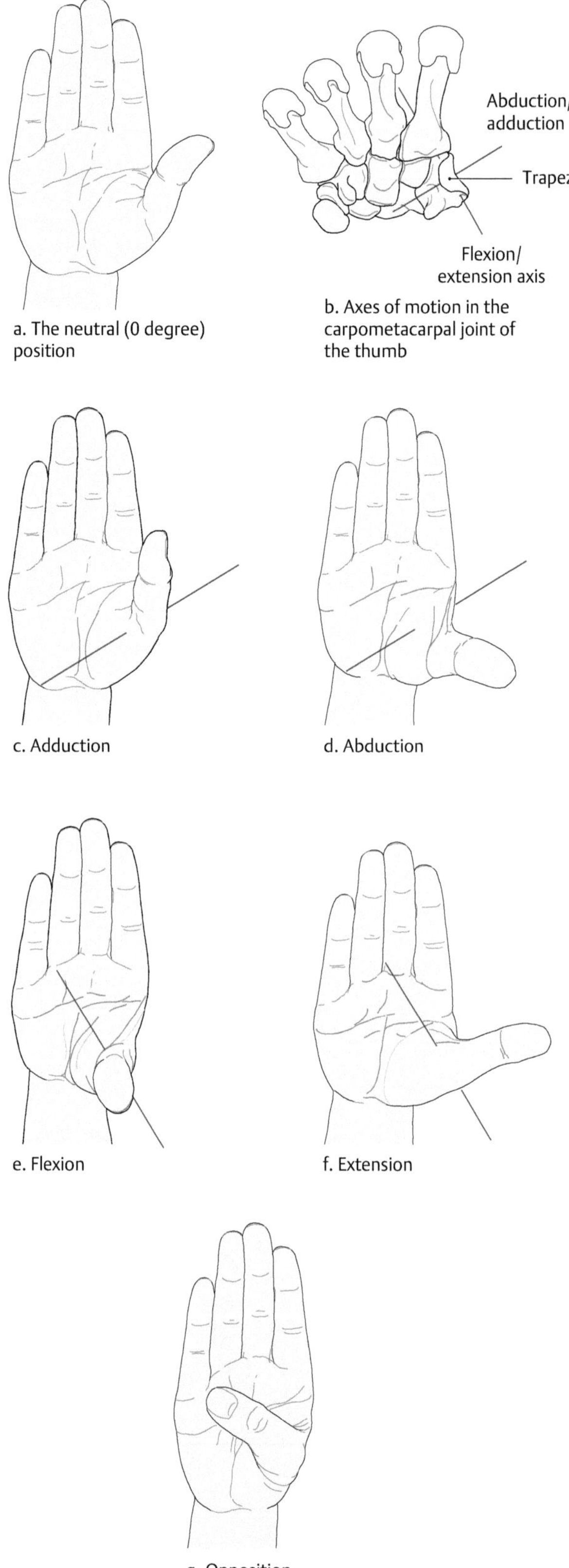

Fig. 6.103 (a-g) Movements of the carpometacarpal joint of the thumb. Right hand, palmar view. (From Schuenke M, Schulte E, Schumacher U. THIEME Atlas of Anatomy. General Anatomy and Musculoskeletal System. Illustrations by Voll M and Wesker K. 3rd ed. New York: Thieme Medical Publishers; 2020.)

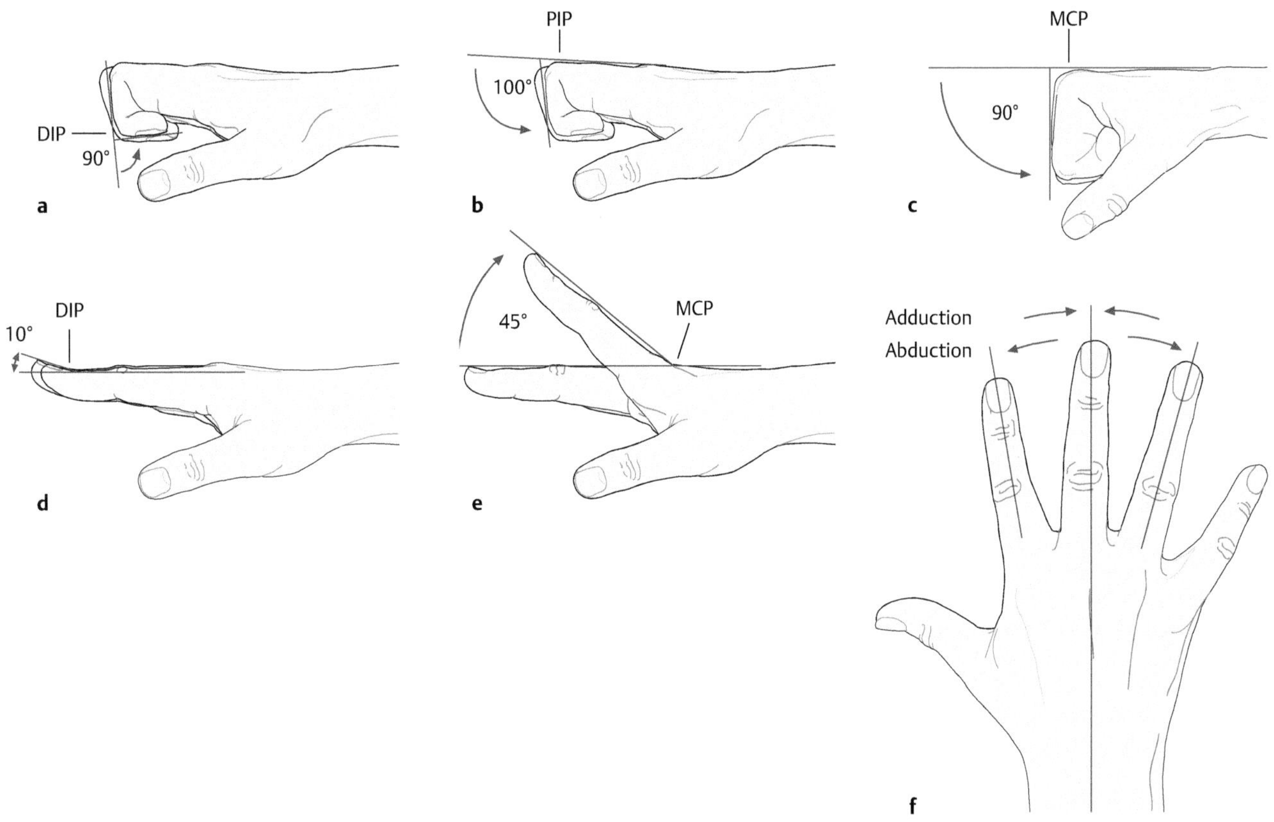

Fig. 6.104 Range of motion of the finger joints. **(a)** Flexion at the DIP joint. **(b)** Flexion at the PIP joint. **(c)** Flexion at the MCP joint. **(d)** Extension at the DIP joint. **(e)** Extension at the MCP joint. **(f)** Abduction and adduction at the MCP joint. (From Schuenke M, Schulte E, Schumacher U. THIEME Atlas of Anatomy. General Anatomy and Musculoskeletal System. Illustrations by Voll M and Wesker K. 3rd ed. New York: Thieme Medical Publishers; 2020.)

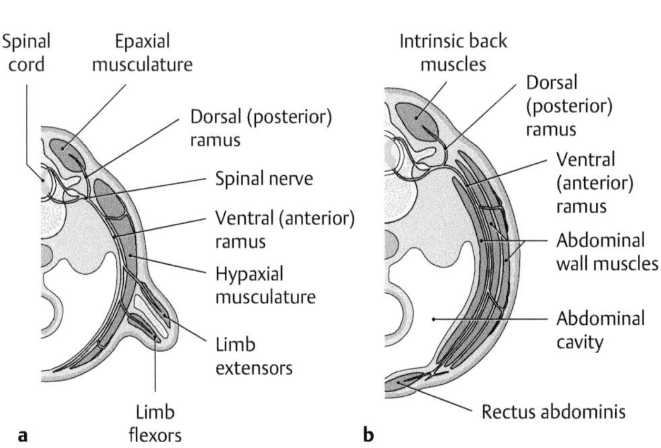

Fig. 6.105 Epaxial and hypaxial muscle divisions. (From Schuenke M, Schulte E, Schumacher U. THIEME Atlas of Anatomy. General Anatomy and Musculoskeletal System. Illustrations by Voll M and Wesker K. 3rd ed. New York: Thieme Medical Publishers; 2020.)

its connection with the terminal plexus but it may be found in a small percentage of adults. The vascular pattern of both extremities is largely due to remodeling and angiogenesis and has been described from multiple developmental patterns **(Fig. 6.106)**.

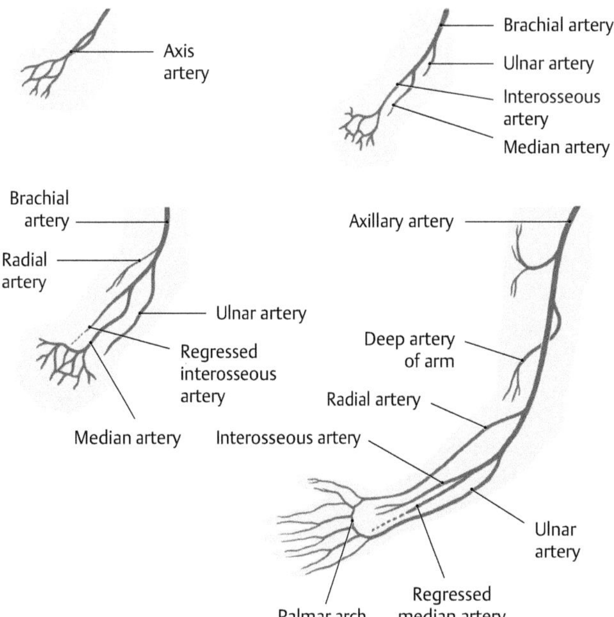

Fig. 6.106 Development of the arteries of the upper extremity. (From Schuenke M, Schulte E, Schumacher U. THIEME Atlas of Anatomy. General Anatomy and Musculoskeletal System. Illustrations by Voll M and Wesker K. 3rd ed. New York: Thieme Medical Publishers; 2020.)

PRACTICE QUESTIONS

1. Initially the _____ of the brachial plexus are located between the _____ and _____ muscles.
   A. Cords, anterior scalene, middle scalene.
   B. Roots, anterior scalene, middle scalene.
   C. Trunks, middle scalene, posterior scalene.
   D. Roots, middle scalene, posterior scalene.
   E. Divisions, anterior scalene, middle scalene.
2. While cleaning out the gutters around his home, Bill slips and awkwardly twists his neck after hitting the ground. He is diagnosed with a severely damaged C7 root. What major function would be greatly reduced due to this injury?
   A. Elbow flexion.
   B. Supination of forearm.
   C. Shoulder abduction.
   D. Elbow extension.
   E. Intrinsic muscles of the hand.
3. Which statement regarding the shoulder region is INCORRECT?
   A. The circumflex scapular vessels pass through the triangular hiatus.
   B. The clavipectoral fascia invests the pectoralis minor muscle.
   C. The serratus anterior muscle is innervated by the long thoracic nerve.
   D. The levator scapulae & rhomboid muscles act together to inferiorly rotate the scapula.
   E. The suprascapular nerve passes deep to the superior transverse scapular ligament.
4. Which statement regarding the shoulder region is INCORRECT?
   A. Clinically, 95% of all shoulder dislocations are anterior dislocations through the glenohumeral ligament.
   B. The supraspinatus tendon is the most common rotator cuff tendon torn.
   C. The latissimus dorsi adducts, medially rotates & extends the humerus/arm.
   D. Clinically, shoulder separations occur at the acromioclavicular (AC) joint.
   E. Paralysis of the pectoralis major results in a "winged scapula"
5. A patient presents in the ED with a stab wound that has resulted in the suprascapular nerve being severed. Which combination of functions would be affected?
   A. Shoulder flexion, Medial rotation of arm.
   B. Adduction of arm, Shoulder extension.
   C. Adduction of arm, Medial rotation of arm.
   D. Initiation of Abduction, Lateral rotation of arm.
   E. Shoulder extension, Medial rotation of arm.
6. A 17 year-old high school football player presents to you with a scapula that protrudes from the back when he protracts the shoulder girdle. He explains this occurred after his opponent's helmet hit him while being tackled in his last game. Where did the helmet strike?
   A. The mid-scapular line.
   B. On the superior thoracic cage at the mid-axillary line.
   C. Mid-sternum.
   D. On the lateral aspect of the shoulder.
   E. On the medial side of the upper arm.
7. A lesion of the upper trunk of the brachial plexus will result in all of the following deficits EXCEPT?
   A. Weakened rotator cuff.
   B. Reduced skin sensation over shoulder.
   C. Inability to oppose the 5th digit.
   D. Weakened strength in elbow flexion.
   E. Weakened triceps brachii.
8. A professional rodeo cowboy falls off his bull and fractures his humerus? While waiting for the x-ray to come back, a physical exam is done and the patient displays wrist drop and an inability to extend his forearm at the elbow. Which nerve has been damaged?
   A. Radial.
   B. Ulnar.
   C. Axillary.
   D. Musculocutaneous.
   E. Median.
9. Which artery is NOT a direct branch from the axillary artery?
   A. Lateral thoracic.
   B. Thoracodorsal.
   C. Anterior circumflex humeral.
   D. Thoracoacromial.
   E. Subscapular.
10. Which statement about the brachial plexus is INCORRECT?
    A. The long thoracic nerve originates from the C5-C7 roots.
    B. All 3 posterior divisions form the posterior cord.
    C. C6-C8 spinal segments make up the thoracodorsal nerve.
    D. The functional components of the ulnar nerve are GSE, GSA and GVE-sym/post.
    E. The median nerve is formed by the medial and posterior cords.
11. A lesion of the median nerve near the cubital fossa results in what clinical correlate?
    A. Golfer's elbow.
    B. Wrist drop.
    C. Tennis elbow.
    D. Hand of Benediction.
    E. Claw hand.
12. A construction worker was involved in an accident while at work and now has difficulty adducting (ulnar deviation) the hand at the wrist. Which combination of nerves is likely damaged?
    A. Median and Radial.
    B. Musculocutaneous and Median.
    C. Radial and Ulnar.
    D. Ulnar and Median.
    E. Musculocutaneous and Axillary.
13. Which function would likely be reduced if the ulnar nerve were impinged at the cubital tunnel near the medial epicondyle of the humerus?
    A. Adduction of wrist.
    B. Extension of wrist.
    C. Abduction of wrist.
    D. Flexion of the DIP joints of digits 2 & 3.
    E. Supination.
14. The median nerve passes between the two heads of the _________ muscle and lies just deep to the _________ muscle on its way to the carpal tunnel.
    A. Biceps brachii and pronator teres.
    B. Biceps brachii and brachialis.
    C. Pronator teres and flexor digitorum superficialis.
    D. Flexor carpi ulnaris and flexor digitorum profundus.
    E. Flexor carpi ulnaris and pronator quadratus.

15. Which muscle listed below is NOT innervated by the recurrent branch of the median nerve?
    A. Abductor pollicis brevis.
    B. Flexor pollicis brevis.
    C. Opponens pollicis
    D. Adductor pollicis.
    E. All of the above are innervated by the recurrent branch of the median nerve.
16. A patient has carpal tunnel syndrome and the flexor retinaculum is opened up to relieve pressure. Which structure WOULD NOT have been affected by increased pressure in the carpal tunnel?
    A. Flexor digitorum superficialis tendons.
    B. Flexor digitorum profundus tendons.
    C. Median nerve.
    D. Flexor pollicis longus tendon.
    E. Flexor carpi radialis tendon.
17. Dupuytren contracture of the palmar fascia is characterized by____ and resembles the hand of benediction?
    A. Partial flexion at the MCP joint of the 2nd and 3rd fingers.
    B. Partial flexion at the IP joint of the thumb.
    C. Partial flexion at the MCP and PIP joints of the 2nd and 3rd fingers.
    D. Partial flexion at the MCP and PIP joints of the 4th and 5th fingers.
    E. Partial flexion at the DIP and PIP of the 2nd and 4th fingers.
18. A young girl falls and hits her hand in such a way that there is now trauma resulting in compression of the ulnar nerve (deep branch) in Guyon's canal. This compression of the ulnar nerve would have no effect on which muscle of the hand?
    A. Opponens digiti minimi.
    B. Lumbrical #3.
    C. Palmar interossei.
    D. Adductor pollicis.
    E. Lumbrical #2.
19. What is the most frequent carpal bone fractured and could lead to the radial artery being lacerated?
    A. Scaphoid.
    B. Pisiform.
    C. Lunate.
    D. Hamate.
    E. Capitate.
20. Which statement regarding the posterior forearm and hand is INCORRECT?
    A. The extensor pollicis longus is in the deep layer of the dorsal forearms posterior compartment
    B. The anatomical snuff box floor is formed by the scaphoid and trapezoid bones.
    C. Dorsal interossei are innervated by the ulnar nerve.
    D. The extensor carpi ulnaris is innervated by the radial nerve.
    E. The abductor pollicis longus abducts & extends the thumb.
21. An individual comes into the clinic and describes pain near the wrist that radiates proximally to the forearm and distally to the thumb. You suspect that excessive friction of the abductor pollicis longus and extensor pollicis brevis tendons, which share the same tendinous sheath, are causing stenosis of this osseofibrous tunnel. What is your diagnosis?
    A. Carpal tunnel.
    B. Digital tenovaginitis stenosans.
    C. De Quervain tenovaginitis stenosans.
    D. Lateral epicondylitis.
    E. Mallet finger.
22. A laceration occurs and it involves the abductor pollicis longus of the anatomical snuffbox. What function(s) would be affected by this injury?
    A. Abduction of thumb only.
    B. Abduction and extension of thumb.
    C. Abduction and flexion of thumb.
    D. Abduction and extension of thumb; supination of wrist.
    E. Abduction and flexion of thumb; flexion of wrist.
23. Which disorder is classified as one involving the "fusion of digits"?
    A. Brachydactyly.
    B. Ectrodactyly.
    C. Syndactly.
    D. Polydactyly.
    E. Talipes.
24. The upper limb buds rotate how many degrees and in what direction during development?
    A. 90 degrees medially.
    B. 90 degrees laterally.
    C. 180 degrees laterally.
    D. 45 degrees medially.
    E. 45 degrees laterally.
25. A 49-year-old office worker has noticed a radiating pain running down his right arm and to his thumb, and what seems to be a general weakness when extending his wrist. An MRI revealed a herniated disc between the C5 and C6 vertebrae. What spinal nerve is affected when there is a herniation between C5/C6?
    A. C4.
    B. C5.
    C. C6.
    D. C7.
    E. C8.

ANSWERS

1. **B. Initially the** roots of the brachial plexus are located between the anterior scalene and middle scalene muscles.
2. **D.** Elbow extension involves the C7 root.
   A. Elbow flexion involves the C5-C6 roots.
   B. Supination of forearm involves the C6 root.
   C. Shoulder abduction involves the C5 root.
   E. Intrinsic muscles of the hand the C8-T1 roots.
3. **A.** The circumflex scapular vessels pass through the triangular space.
4. **E.** Paralysis of the serratus anterior muscle results in a "winged scapula"
5. **D.** If the suprascapular nerve was severed functions involving the initiation of abduction and lateral rotation of the arm would be affected.
6. **B.** This patient is presenting with a "winged scapula" and the long thoracic nerve is damaged affecting the serratus anterior. This nerve is located on the superior thoracic cage at the mid-axillary line.
7. **C.** The inability to oppose the 5th digit or little finger would be affected if the lower trunk was damaged. The lower trunk has contributions from C8 and T1 while all the other functions listed are innervated by nerves that have a fair amount

to C5 and C6 fibers that originally course through the upper trunk.

8. **A.** Wrist drop is associated with damage to the radial nerve.
9. **B.** All arteries listed are direct branches of the axillary artery except for the thoracodorsal artery, which is a branch of the subscapular artery.
10. **E.** The median nerve is formed by the medial and lateral cords.
11. **D.** A lesion of the median nerve near the cubital fossa could result in the formation of the Hand of Benediction.
12. **C.** If an individual had difficulty adducting (ulnar deviation) the hand at the wrist the combination of damaged nerves would include the radial and ulnar nerves.
13. **A.** Of the listed functions, adduction of wrist would be reduced if the ulnar nerve were impinged at the cubital tunnel.
14. **C.** The median nerve passes between the two heads of the pronator teres muscle and lies just deep to the flexor digitorum superficialis muscle on its way to the carpal tunnel.
15. **D.** The adductor pollicis is innervated by the deep branch of the ulnar nerve.
16. **E.** The flexor carpi radialis tendon is not affected by inflammation caused by increased pressure in the carpal tunnel.
17. **D.** Dupuytren contracture of the palmar fascia is characterized by partial flexion at the MCP and PIP joints of the 4th and 5th fingers.
18. **E.** Compression of the ulnar nerve would not affect the second lumbrical.
19. **A.** The most frequent carpal bone fractured is the scaphoid and this could lead to a laceration of the radial artery.
20. **B.** The floor of the anatomical snuff box is formed by the scaphoid and trapezium bones.
21. **C.** Excessive friction of the abductor pollicis longus and extensor pollicis brevis tendons is called De Quervain tenovaginitis stenosans.
22. **B.** A laceration involving the abductor pollicis longus would affect both abduction and extension of the thumb or 1st digit.
23. **C.** The disorder classified as one involving the "fusion of digits" is called syndactly.
24. **B.** The upper limb buds rotate 90 degrees laterally during development.
25. **C.** The cervical spinal nerves exit superior to the vertebra of the same number, thus a herniated disc protruding between C5 and C6 would affect the C6 spinal nerve. This information was described initially in Chapter 1.

7 Head and Neck

LEARNING OBJECTIVES

- To understand the difference between the neurocranium and viscerocranium, development of the cranium, and primarily the suture joints of the cranium. Fontanelles seen between suture joints in newborns and infants will be emphasized. The clinical correlate called craniosynostosis will be explored.
- To understand the features or spaces and the structures that pass through them from the anterior, superior, posterior, lateral, external, and internal surfaces of the cranium. Clinical correlates will include different skull fractures, LeFort fractures, craniotomies, pterion fracture, and eagle syndrome.
- Explore the different cranial meninges. Clinical correlates will include dural arteriovenous fistulas, danger triangle of the face, cavernous sinus syndrome, headaches, epidural hematomas, subdural hematomas, and subarachnoid hematomas.
- To describe the muscles and neurovasculature of the scalp and superficial face. Clinical correlates will include trigeminal neuralgia, infraorbital nerve block, Bell's palsy, and scalp lacerations.
- To describe the structure and neurovasculature of the parotid gland. Clinical correlates will include viral and bacterial infections and tumors of the parotid gland and gustatory sweating.
- To describe the muscles and neurovasculature of the temporal and infratemporal fossae along with the temporomandibular joint (TMJ).
- To describe the structures, histology, muscles, neurovasculature, and development of the oral cavity. Structures include the lips, cheeks, gingivae, teeth, tongue, and salivary glands. Clinical correlates will include viral and bacterial infections and tumors of the parotid gland and gustatory sweating.
- To describe the muscles and neurovasculature of the palate.
- To understand the borders, structures, and communications related to the pterygopalatine fossa. Identify the nerves that originate from the pterygopalatine ganglion.
- To describe the structures, histology, and neurovasculature of the nose, nasal cavity, and paranasal sinuses.
- To understandhow the face, palate, and nasal cavity develop. Clinical correlates include cleft palate and lips.
- To describe the structures, histology, muscles, neurovasculature, and development of the orbit and eye. Structures will also include the eyelids and lacrimal apparatus. Clinical correlates will include preseptal and orbital cellulitis, palpebral gland inflammation, detached retina, presbyopia, cataracts, glaucoma, oculomotor, trochlear and abducent nerve palsies, and corneal and pupillary light reflexes.
- To describe the structures, histology, muscles, neurovasculature, and development of the ear. Clinical correlates will include otitis media, Meniere syndrome, and conductive and sensorineural hearing loss.
- To describe the different fascias of the neck.
- To describe the superficial muscles of the neck and congenital muscular torticollis.
- To understandthe structures located in the submental, submandibular, muscular, and carotid triangles of the larger anterior triangle of the neck.
- To describe the structure, histology, development, and neurovasculature of the thyroid and parathyroid glands. Clinical correlates will include hyperthyroidism, hypothyroidism, hyperparathyroidism, hypoparathyroidism, and thyroglossal duct cysts.
- To understandthe internal and external carotid arteries and the major branches of them. Describe the importancethe importance between the carotid body and carotid sinus and the carotid endarterectomy procedure.
- To describe the location and function of the superior laryngeal, internal laryngeal, external laryngeal, spinal accessory, hypoglossal, and ansa cervicalis nerves.
- To understandthe structures and neurovasculature located in the posterior (lateral cervical) triangle of the neck. Be able to describe a cervical nerve plexus block.
- To understandthe muscles and neurovasculature of the prevertebral region and root of the neck. Clinical correlates include a cervicothoracic ganglion block and Horner syndrome.
- To describe the cartilages, membranes, spaces, muscles, histology, and neurovasculature of the larynx. Clinical correlates will include laryngitis, vocal fold/cord nodules, laryngoscopy, tracheostomy, cricothyrotomy, and laryngeal nerve blocks and injury.
- To describe the structure, muscles, wall gaps, neurovasculature, and histology of the pharynx and cervical region of the esophagus. Clinical correlates will include the pharyngeal (gag) reflex, Waldeyer tonsillar ring, adenoiditis, and tonsillitis.
- To understandthe three stages involved in deglutition (swallowing).
- To describethe venous and lymphatic drainage of the neck. Clinical correlates will include central venous catheters, external jugular vein prominence, Virchow node, and zones of penetrating and blunt neck traumas.
- To describe the larger development of the head and neck, which centers on structures called the pharyngeal arches, pouches, groove, and membrane. Clinical correlates include first arch syndromes, pharyngeal fistula and cysts, and DiGeorge syndrome.

The superior most part of the human body is known as the **head** and it is attached to the trunk by the neck. The major function of the head is to support and protect the brain. The head is also the location for special sensory receivers such as the eyes, ears, nose, and mouth. The intake of food and fluids; the transport of oxygen and carbon dioxide; and production of sound all occur at the head. The anterior aspect of the head is the location of the face and the source of our unique identity.

Our **neck** is the structure that bridges the base of our head to the clavicles of the trunk region. It serves as the passageway of structures heading to and from the head. The neck demonstrates great flexibility but does not have much in the way of bony protection; thus, structures coursing through the neck are vulnerable to damage. The multiple regions of the head and neck are

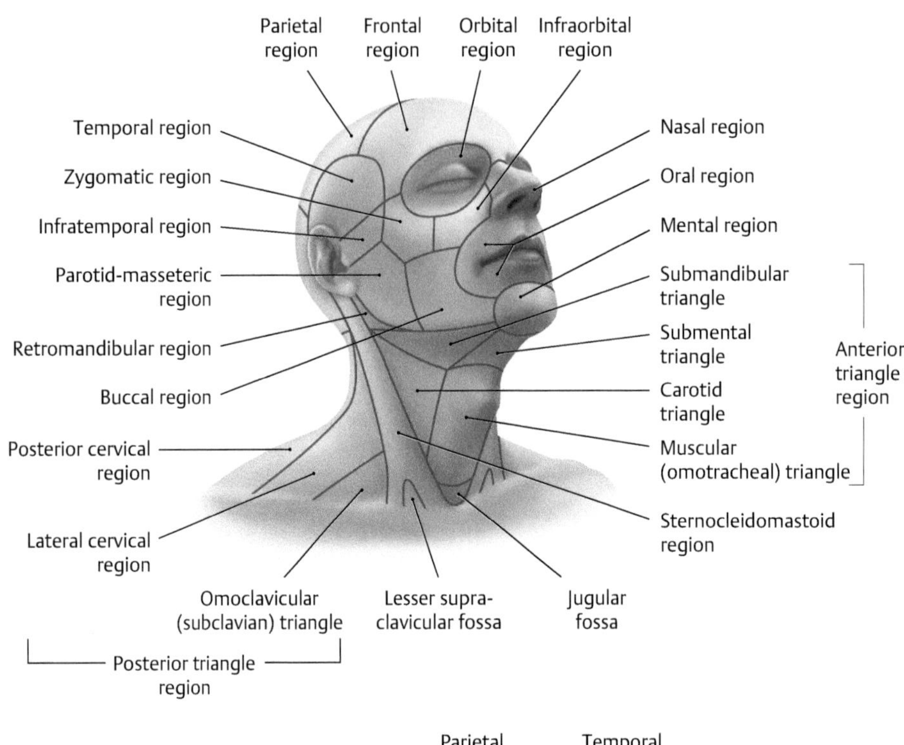

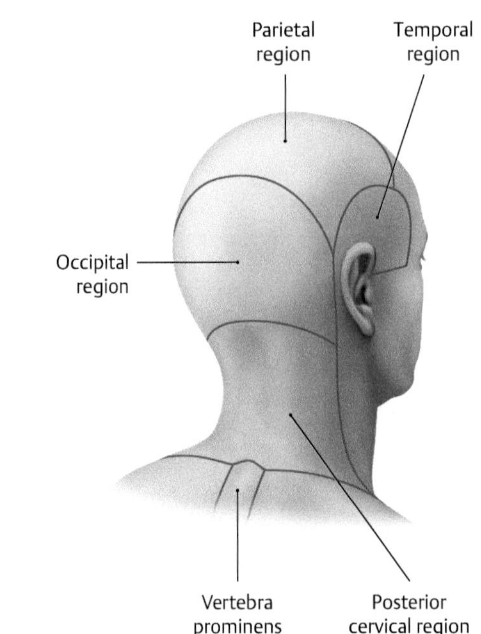

Fig. 7.1 Regions of the head and neck. (From Schuenke M, Schulte E, Schumacher U. THIEME Atlas of Anatomy. Head, Neck, and Neuroanatomy. Illustrations by Voll M and Wesker K. 3rd ed. New York: Thieme Medical Publishers; 2020.)

demonstrated (**Fig. 7.1**) but our study of head and neck will begin with the cranium.

7.1 Cranium

The cranium is defined as the skeleton of the head. It is generally considered the most complex osseous structure of the human body (**Fig. 7.2; Fig. 7.3**). In anatomical position, the cranium is orientated in such a way that the inferior margin of the orbit and the superior margin of the external acoustic meatus lie on the same horizontal plane and this is known as the **orbitomeatal plane** (*Frankfort horizontal plane*).

The cranium is divided into a neurocranium and viscerocranium. The **neurocranium** encloses the brain and cranial meninges, along with the vasculature of the brain and proximal portions of the cranial nerves. Eight bones form the neurocranium: four singular bones (*frontal, ethmoid, sphenoid*, and *occipital*) and two sets of bilaterally paired bones (*parietal* and *temporal*). The neurocranium can be subdivided into a **calvaria** (or *skullcap*) and **cranial base** (or *basicranium*). The calvaria is formed by the *frontal, parietal*, and *occipital* bones while the cranial base is formed primarily by the *sphenoid* and *occipital* bones. The *ethmoid* bone is mostly associated with the viscerocranium and only a small portion of the neurocranium (**Fig. 7.4**).

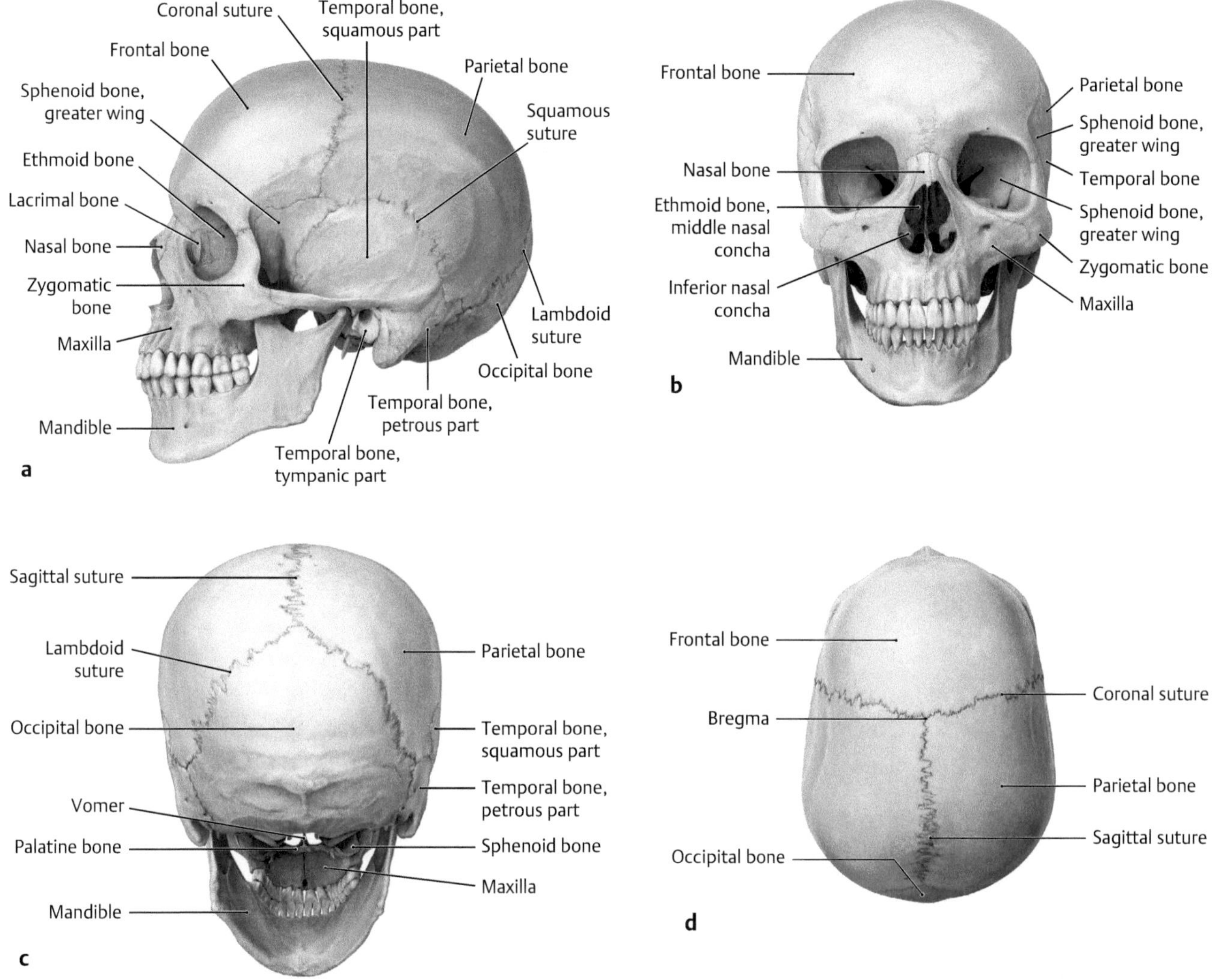

Fig. 7.2 (a) Lateral view of cranial bones. **(b)** Anterior view. **(c)** Posterior view. **(d)** Superior view. (From Schuenke M, Schulte E, Schumacher U. THIEME Atlas of Anatomy. Head, Neck, and Neuroanatomy. Illustrations by Voll M and Wesker K. 3rd ed. New York: Thieme Medical Publishers; 2020.)

The **viscerocranium** (facial skeleton) forms the anterior aspect of the cranium and is comprised of bones that make up most of the orbits, nose, and nasal cavity as well as the upper and lower jaws. Fifteen bones form the viscerocranium: the individual *vomer, ethmoid* and *mandible* bones, and the paired *nasal, lacrimal, zygomatic, maxillae, palatine,* and *inferior nasal conchae* bones **(Fig. 7.4)**.

Females, children, and the elderly tend to have thinner cranial cavity walls than adult males. And these thinner regions are deep to and near attaching muscles. This is quite evident in the temporal regions where these thinner regions are more prone to fracture. The flat bones of the cranium are made up of an **external layer** and **internal layer (or "table") of compact bone**. Between these layers is the **diploë**, which is spongy bone containing red bone marrow. The major cranial flat bones include the frontal, parietal, and occipital bones **(Fig. 7.5)**.

The cranium must also deal with high traction forces that transmit masticatory pressure exerted on the maxillae back to the calvaria. The thicker bones form **buttresses** or "pillars" and function by transmitting forces that will bypass the orbit and pneumatized paranasal sinuses. These buttresses develop along principal lines of force in response to local mechanical stresses. The major buttresses are grouped into either a **vertical** or **horizontal buttresses** **(Fig. 7.6)**.[1,2]

- ***Vertical buttresses:***
  - Nasomaxillary (anteromedial)
  - Zygomaticomaxillary (lateral)
  - Pterygomaxillary (posterior)
  - Vertical mandible
- ***Horizontal buttresses:***
  - Supraorbital-frontal (superior)
  - Infraorbital (middle)
  - Maxillary-alveolar (inferior)

Suture joints are fibrous joints that interlock bones and allow for growth during cranial development. The majority of cranial bones are held together by suture joints and some of these include the **coronal**, **sagittal**, **squamous,** and **lambdoid sutures (Fig. 7.2).** Fusion of these joints (synostosis) generally begins during the early parts of the third decade of life; progresses from the internal to external surfaces of the cranium; and the sagittal suture will be the first

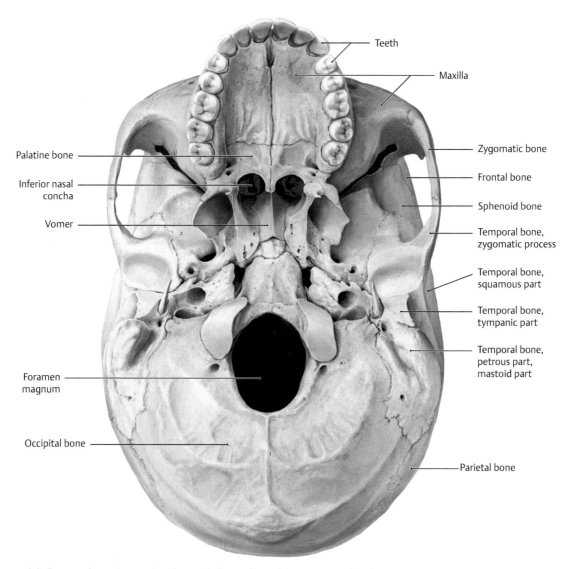

Teeth
Maxilla
Palatine bone
Inferior nasal concha
Vomer
Zygomatic bone
Frontal bone
Sphenoid bone
Temporal bone, zygomatic process
Temporal bone, squamous part
Temporal bone, tympanic part
Temporal bone, petrous part, mastoid part
Foramen magnum
Occipital bone
Parietal bone

Fig. 7.3 Base of skull, external view. (From Schuenke M, Schulte E, Schumacher U. THIEME Atlas of Anatomy. Head, Neck, and Neuroanatomy. Illustrations by Voll M and Wesker K. 3rd ed. New York: Thieme Medical Publishers; 2020.)

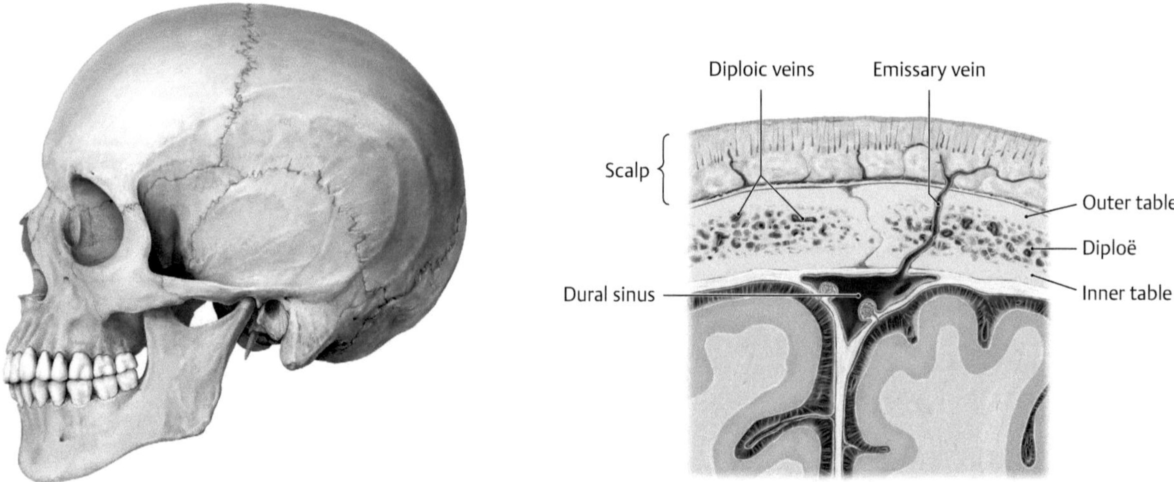

Fig. 7.4 Bones of the neurocranium (*gray*) and viscerocranium (*orange*). (From Schuenke M, Schulte E, Schumacher U. THIEME Atlas of Anatomy. Head, Neck, and Neuroanatomy. Illustrations by Voll M and Wesker K. 3rd ed. New York: Thieme Medical Publishers; 2020.)

Fig. 7.5 The three-layered structure of the calvaria. Coronal section near the superior sagittal sinus. (From Schuenke M, Schulte E, Schumacher U. THIEME Atlas of Anatomy. Head, Neck, and Neuroanatomy. Illustrations by Voll M and Wesker K. 3rd ed. New York: Thieme Medical Publishers; 2020.)

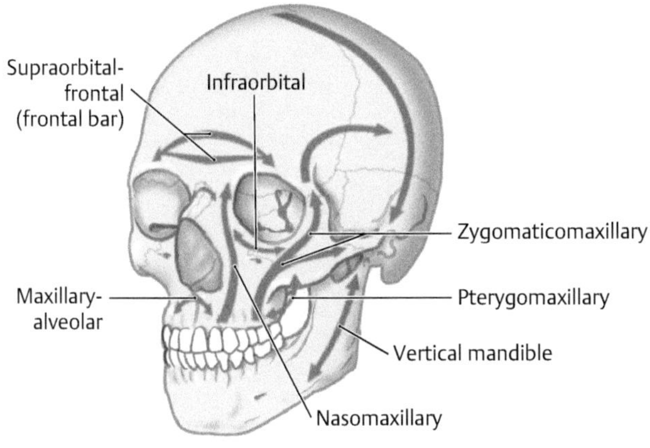

Fig. 7.6 Vertical and horizontal buttresses. (From Ernst, A, Herzog, M, and Seidl RO. Head and Neck Trauma: An Interdisciplinary Approach. Stuttgart: Thieme Medical Publishers; 2006.)

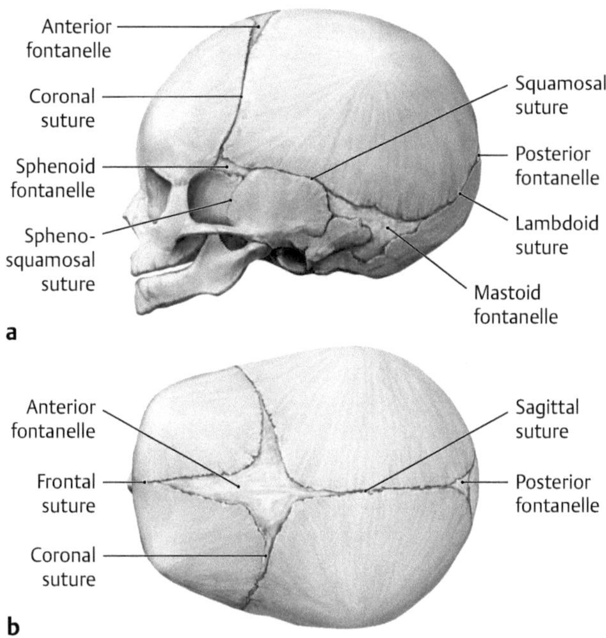

Fig. 7.7 Lateral **(a)** and superior **(b)** view of the neonatal skull. (From Schuenke M, Schulte E, Schumacher U. THIEME Atlas of Anatomy. Head, Neck, and Neuroanatomy. Illustrations by Voll M and Wesker K. 3rd ed. New York: Thieme Medical Publishers; 2020.)

joint affected. Cranial base bones are primary cartilaginous (synchondroses) joints and are united by hyaline cartilage but allow for slight movements during development. The spheno-occipital synchondrosis fuses earlier than most cranial joints at 13 to 18 years of age. There are only two synovial joint articulations involving the external cranium and they are the **atlanto-occipital** and **temporomandibular (TMJ) joints**. The atlanto-occipital joint is located between the C1 vertebra (atlas) and occipital condyles of the occipital bone while the TMJ is the articulation between the mandibular fossa of the temporal bone and head of the mandible. **Sutural bones** may be present along the lambdoid, squamous, sagittal, or coronal (frontal) sutures and can be more prevalent in some diagnoses such as Down syndrome and rickets.

A **fontanelle** is the anatomical "soft spot" associated with the neurocranium of an infant's head and are present because of the normal but incomplete formation of cranial bones. During childbirth, fontanelles allow for the movement of cranial bones resulting in an easier passage through the birth canal. The brain during the first few years of a child's life enlarges faster than the surrounding bone thus they allow for the early expansion of the cranium to allow for this brain growth **(Fig. 7.7)**.

- **Anterior fontanelle**: is located between the split frontal and parietal bones and at the junction of the future osteometric point *bregma*. This is generally the last fontanelle to close and this occurs by 18 months of age but can be as late as 36 months of age. It can serve as a site to access cerebrospinal fluid (CSF) in infants if meningitis was suspected.
- **Posterior fontanelle**: is located between the parietal and occipital bones and generally closes first between 1 and 3 months of age.
- **Sphenoid fontanelles**: are paired and located between the sphenoid, frontal, parietal, and temporal bones on each side of the neurocranium. They close at around 6 months of age.
- **Mastoid fontanelles**: are paired and located between the temporal, parietal, and occipital bones on each side of the neurocranium. They close between 6 and 18 months of age.

Clinical Correlate 7.1

Fontanelle Presentations

If fontanelles bulge outward and indicate increased intracranial pressure, it could be a sign of meningitis (infection of the meninges), encephalitis (swelling of the brain), or hydrocephalus (abnormal accumulation of CSF). If fontanelles appear to have sunk or become depressed, this may be a sign of dehydration in the child. A premature birth or children with Down syndrome have been shown to have larger fontanelles.

7.1.1 Anterior (Facial) Surface Features of the Cranium

Features of this surface include the forehead, orbits, nasal region, zygomatic, maxilla, and mandible bones. The squamous portion of the frontal bone forms the forehead. The **supraorbital margin** represents the boundary between the squamous and orbital portions of the frontal bone and it contains a **supraorbital foramen/notch**. The **superciliary arches** are located just above the supraorbital margin and they extend laterally from each side of the glabella. The **glabella** is an osteometric point located between the superciliary arches and **frontal (metopic) suture** and represents the smooth, most anterior projection of the forehead (**Fig. 7.8**).

The **nasion** is an osteometric point where the **frontonasal suture** and **internasal suture** intersect and it is related to the *bridge of the nose*. The opening inferior to the nasal bones and bordered on both sides laterally by the maxilla is known as the **piriform (nasal) aperture**. The **middle nasal conchae, inferior nasal**

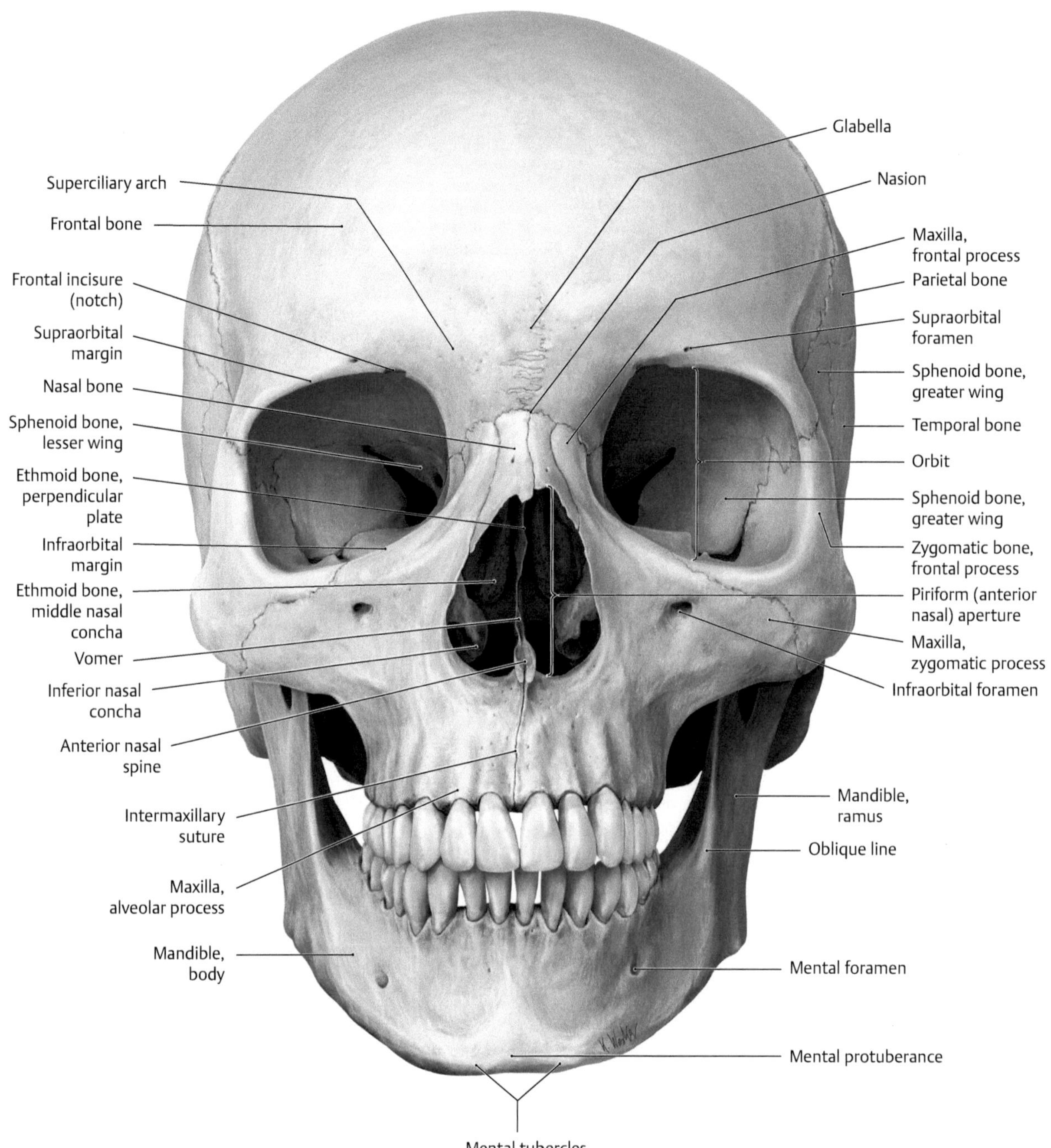

Fig. 7.8 Anterior view of the skull. (From Schuenke M, Schulte E, Schumacher U. THIEME Atlas of Anatomy. Head, Neck, and Neuroanatomy. Illustrations by Voll M and Wesker K. 3rd ed. New York: Thieme Medical Publishers; 2020.)

conchae, and **nasal septum** can be identified within the piriform aperture (**Fig. 7.8**).

The **zygomatic bones** are located on the lateral aspect of the face and represent the cheeks. They have a small opening on the lateral surface of the bone known as the **zygomaticofacial foramen**. A **zygomaticotemporal foramen** pierces the zygomatic bone from its temporal surface. The zygomatic bones form a portion of the orbit and articulate with the maxilla, temporal, frontal, and sphenoid bones. The two halves of the maxilla that form the upper jaw fuse at the **intermaxillary suture** and are known together as the **maxillae**. The **alveolar processes** of the maxillae include the tooth sockets or alveoli and support the **maxillary teeth**. The **infraorbital foramen** pierces both sides of the maxillae just below the orbit.

The individual **mandible** forms the lower jaw and consists of a mental tubercle, body, coronoid process, ramus, neck, and head. Alveolar processes of the mandible contain the **mandibular teeth**, similar to how the maxillae have their maxillary teeth (**Figs. 7.8, 7.9**).

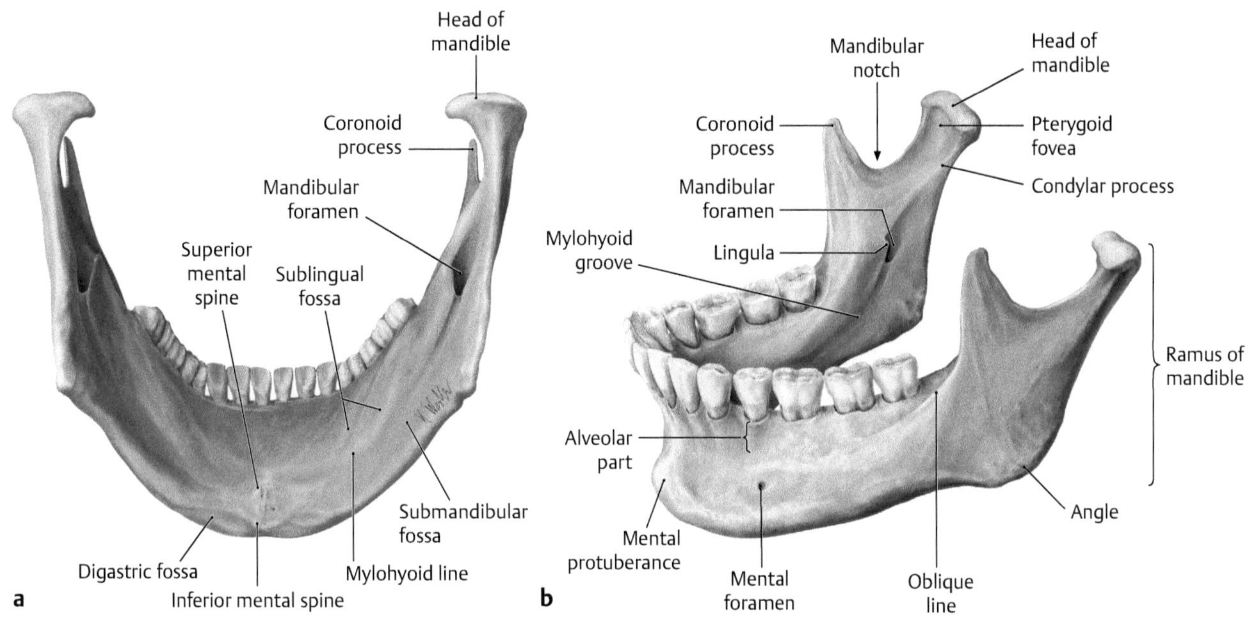

Fig. 7.9 Mandible. **(a)** Posterior view. **(b)** Oblique left lateral view. (From Schuenke M, Schulte E, Schumacher U. THIEME Atlas of Anatomy. Head, Neck, and Neuroanatomy. Illustrations by Voll M and Wesker K. 3rd ed. New York: Thieme Medical Publishers; 2020.)

7.1.2 Superior (Calvaria) Surface Features of the Cranium

The calvaria forms the superior aspect of the cranium. It is oval and broadens posterolaterally at the **parietal eminences**. Multiple sutures are located on this surface. The **coronal suture** divides the frontal and parietal bones from one another while the **sagittal suture** creates a separation between the left and right parietal bones. The **bregma** is an osteometric point located at the junction of the coronal and sagittal sutures. Another osteometric point known as the **vertex** is located at the midpoint of the sagittal suture and represents the superior most point of the human body. The **lambdoid suture** separates the paired parietal and temporal bones from the individual occipital bone (**Fig. 7.2d**). The inconstant **parietal foramina** are located on the parietal bones near the sagittal suture and can allow for an emissary vein to pass through.

7.1.3 Posterior (Occiput) Surface Features of the Cranium

The squamous portion of the occipital bone, posterior parietal bones, and the mastoid portion of the temporal bones represent the posterior aspect or **occiput** of the head. As mentioned earlier, the **lambdoid suture** separates the paired parietal and temporal bones from the individual occipital bone. The junction between the sagittal and lambdoid sutures represents the osteometric point **lambda**.

The bony process in the median plane on the back of one's head is known as the **external occipital protuberance**. Extending inferiorly from the protuberance down to the foramen magnum is the **external occipital crest**. Extending laterally from the protuberance are the **superior nuchal lines** and they represent the superior limit of the neck. The less distinct **inferior nuchal lines** represent the attachment points for the majority of the *suboccipital triangle* muscles. The **condylar canal** and **mastoid foramen** may also be present and allow for the passage of emissary veins (**Fig. 7.10; Fig. 7.12**).

7.1.4 Lateral Surface Features of the Cranium

Portions of the neurocranium and viscerocranium contribute to the lateral surface of the cranium. The **temporal fossa**, which is filled by the majority of the temporalis muscle and is bounded superiorly and posteriorly by the **superior temporal** and **inferior temporal lines**, also is the site of the clinically important osteometric point known as the **pterion**. This is the H-shaped formation of sutures binding the thinner portions of the frontal, greater wing of the sphenoid, temporal, and parietal bones. The pterion is the general location for an extradural (epidural) hematoma to occur and is the result of a torn anterior branch of the middle meningeal artery.

The **zygomatic arch** that is formed by the **temporal process of the zygomatic bone** and the **zygomatic process of the temporal bone** extends posteriorly from the cheek region. The **external acoustic (auditory) meatus** leads to the tympanic membrane (eardrum) and lies within the **tympanic portion of the temporal bone** (**Fig. 7.11**).

7.1.5 External Surface Features of the Cranial Base

The cranial base represents the inferior portion of the neurocranium and viscerocranium minus the mandible. Just posterior to the medial most incisor teeth is the **incisive foramen/fossa**. The free border of the alveolar processes supporting the maxillary teeth is known as the **alveolar arch of the maxillae**. The **palatine processes of the maxillae** along with the **horizontal plates**

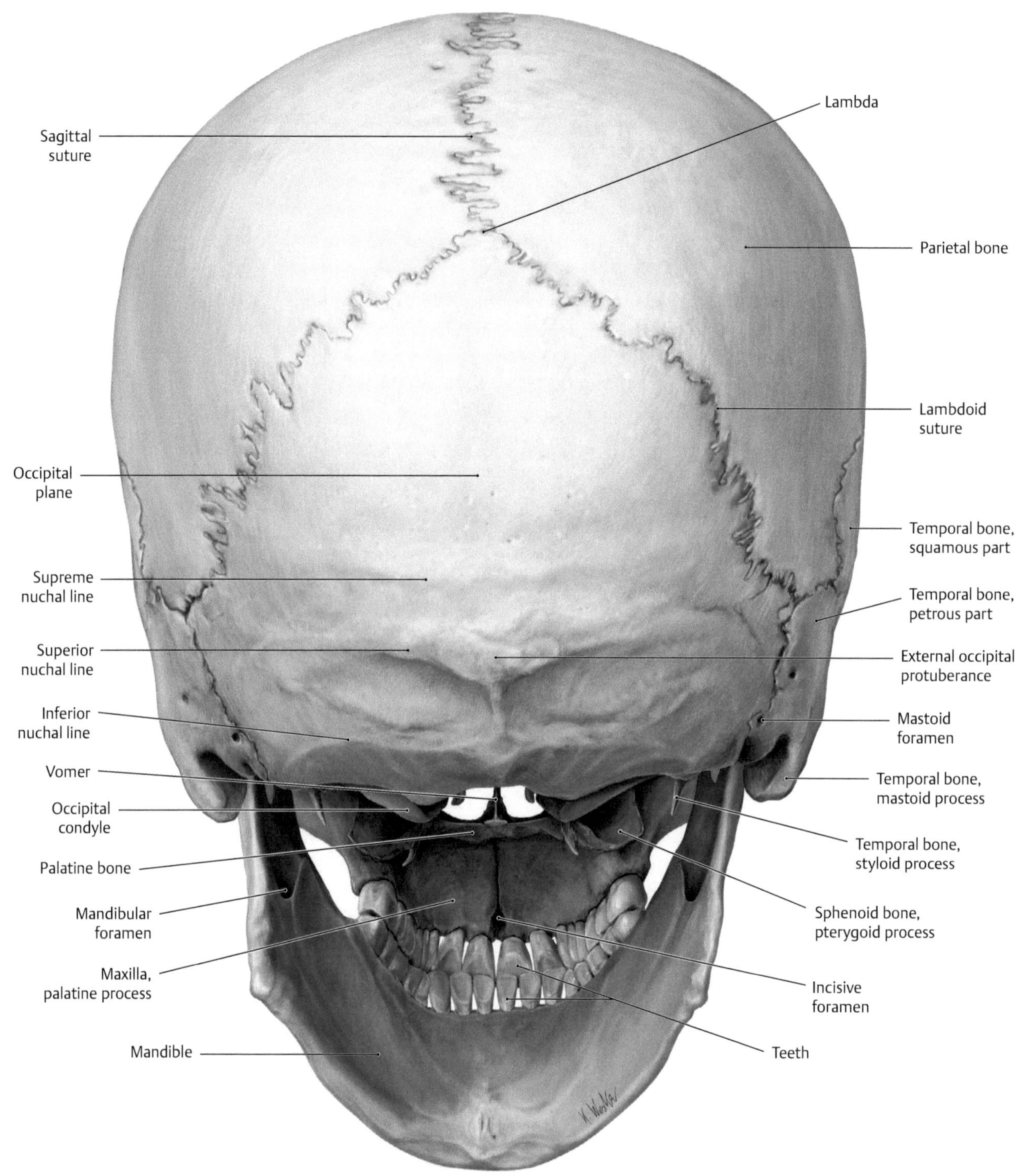

Fig. 7.10 Posterior view of the skull. (From Schuenke M, Schulte E, Schumacher U. THIEME Atlas of Anatomy. Head, Neck, and Neuroanatomy. Illustrations by Voll M and Wesker K. 3rd ed. New York: Thieme Medical Publishers; 2020.)

of the palatine bones constitute the *hard palate*. The **posterior nasal spine** projects from the posterior border of the hard palate. Located near the lateral edges of the maxillae and palatine bone articulations are the **greater/lesser palatine foramen**. Located at the posterior edge of the hard palate and extending superiorly to the sphenoid bone are the **posterior nasal apertures** (or choanae). These open spaces represent the border between the nasal cavity and nasopharynx. The **vomer** is an unpaired bone that contributes to the nasal septum and the division of the nasal cavity into a left and right half **(Fig. 7.12)**.

The **sphenoid bone** is located between the frontal, occipital, and temporal bones and consists of a **lesser wing**, **greater wing,** and

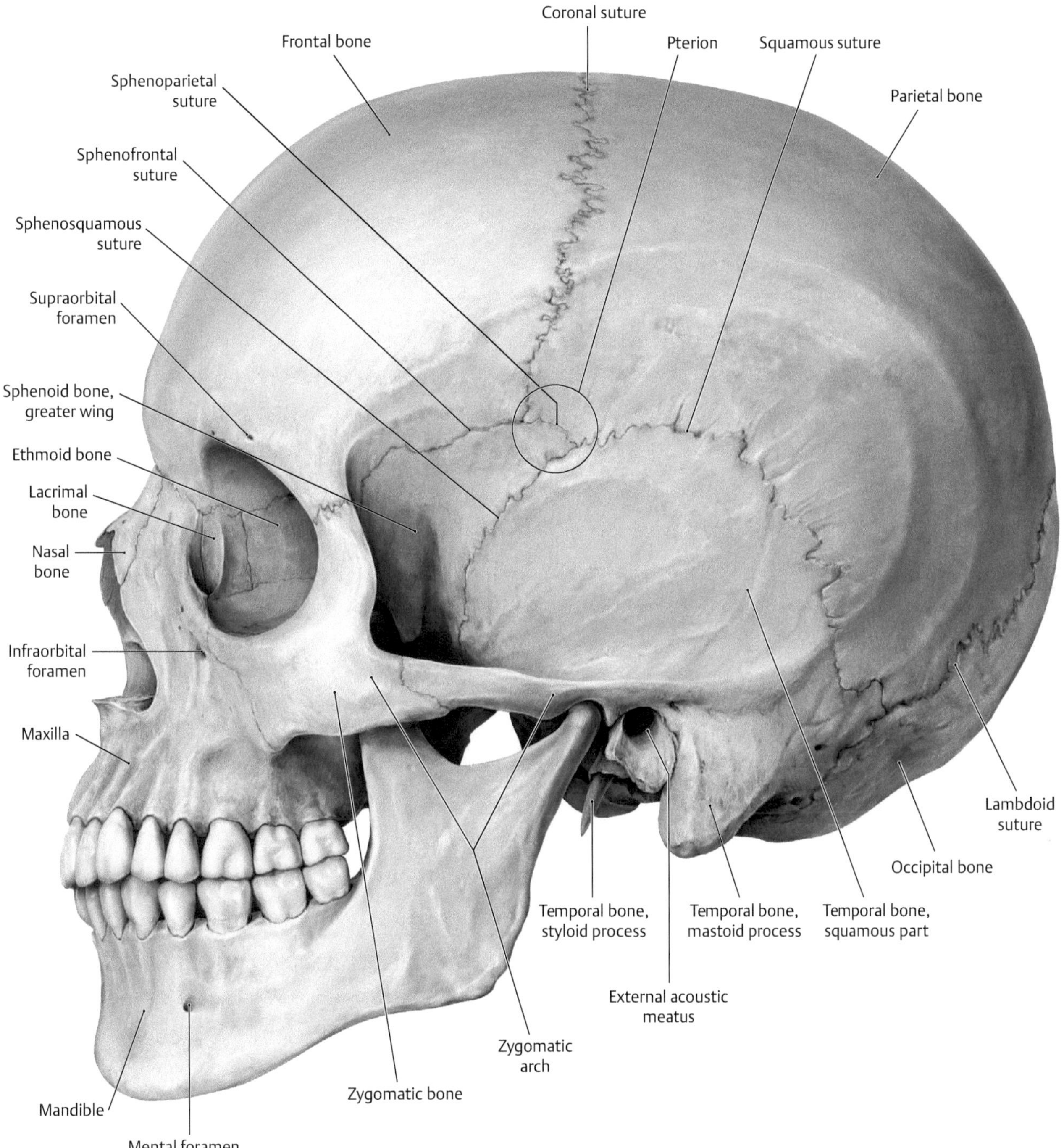

Fig. 7.11 Lateral view of the skull. (From Schuenke M, Schulte E, Schumacher U. THIEME Atlas of Anatomy. Head, Neck, and Neuroanatomy. Illustrations by Voll M and Wesker K. 3rd ed. New York: Thieme Medical Publishers; 2020.)

pterygoid processes. The pterygoid processes are each divided into a **lateral/medial pterygoid plate**. The **spine of the sphenoid** is located anterior to the carotid canal but posterolateral to the opening of the bony portion of the pharyngotympanic (auditory) tube and the sulcus for the cartilaginous part of the auditory tube.

The heads of the mandible articulate with the **mandibular fossae** located on the **squamous portion of the temporal bones**. The **petrotympanic fissure** is located near the posterior border of the mandibular fossae and allows for the passage of the chorda tympani nerve. The **styloid process** and **mastoid process** originate from the **petrous portion of the temporal bone** and act as attachment sites for a ligament or muscles. The **stylomastoid foramen** is located between these processes and allows for the passage of the motor root of the facial nerve (CN VII). The **carotid canal** also courses through the petrous portion of the temporal bone and allows for the initial passage of the internal carotid artery (ICA) (**Fig. 7.11**).

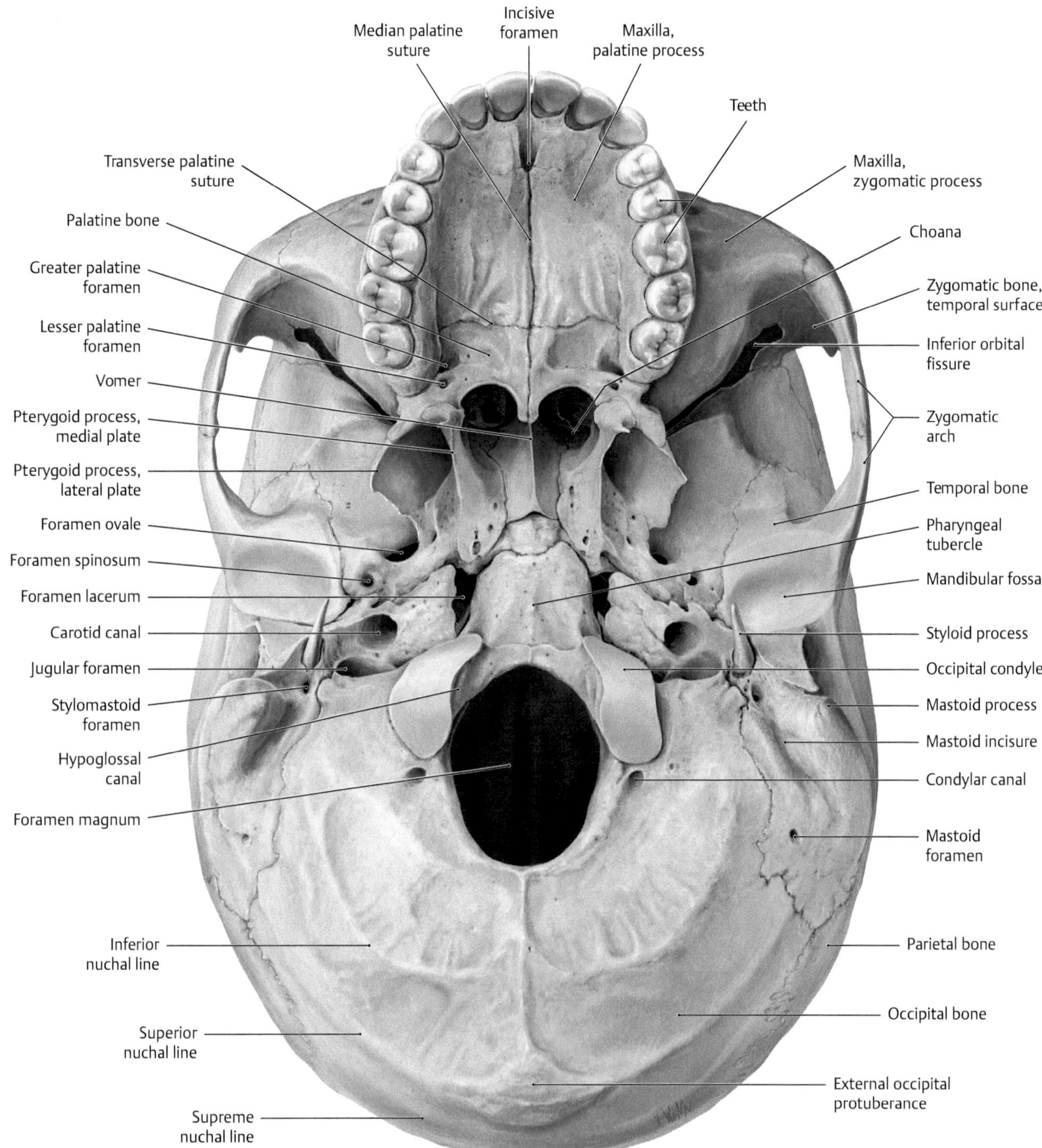

Fig. 7.12 The external surface of the cranial base. (From Schuenke M, Schulte E, Schumacher U. THIEME Atlas of Anatomy. Head, Neck, and Neuroanatomy. Illustrations by Voll M and Wesker K. 3rd ed. New York: Thieme Medical Publishers; 2020.)

7.1.6 Internal Surface Features of the Cranium

When looking at the internal surface of the cranium, three depressions known as the anterior, middle, and posterior cranial fossae are seen. These fossae constitute the cranial cavity that has its high point with the anterior cranial fossa and a low point with the posterior cranial fossa (**Fig. 7.13**).

7.1.7 Anterior Cranial Fossa

Portions of the frontal, ethmoid, and the sphenoid bones form this fossa. The **orbital plates of the frontal bone** support the frontal lobes of the brain and near the midline there is a **frontal crest**. The **cribriform plate of the ethmoid bone** contains **olfactory foramina** but on the lateral borders of this plate there are **anterior/posterior ethmoidal foramina**. The cribriform

Clinical Correlate 7.2

Skull Fractures

Skull fractures may involve one or more skull bones and can result in damage to the brain or meninges leading to a concussion, hematoma, or leaking of CSF. Blunt force trauma to the head can be minimized to some extent due to the convexity of the calvaria and how it is able to distribute forces acting on the skull. A *coup fracture* is located under the site of trauma but a *contrecoup fracture* occurs on the opposite side of the cranium and not at the site of impact. A coup fracture is usually the result of an object hitting the skull but a contrecoup fracture would be the result of the head striking an object. The four types of skull fractures:

1. **Linear:** these are the most common skull fractures that involve a break in the bone but it does not move the bone. Observation at a hospital may only take place for a short period of time and normal activities can be resumed in a few days.
2. **Depressed:** the skull is sunken or displaced inward (comminuted) from the trauma and may present with or without a cut in the scalp. Surgical intervention may be needed to correct the deformity because of intracranial pressure put on the brain.
3. **Basilar:** rare but the most serious of skull fractures because it involves the base of the skull resulting in blood in the sinuses, CSF leakage, retroauricular, and periorbital ecchymosis (hemorrhagic spot).
4. **Diastatic:** fractures that occur along the suture lines and generally result in widening of the sutures. They are most often seen in newborns or older infants.

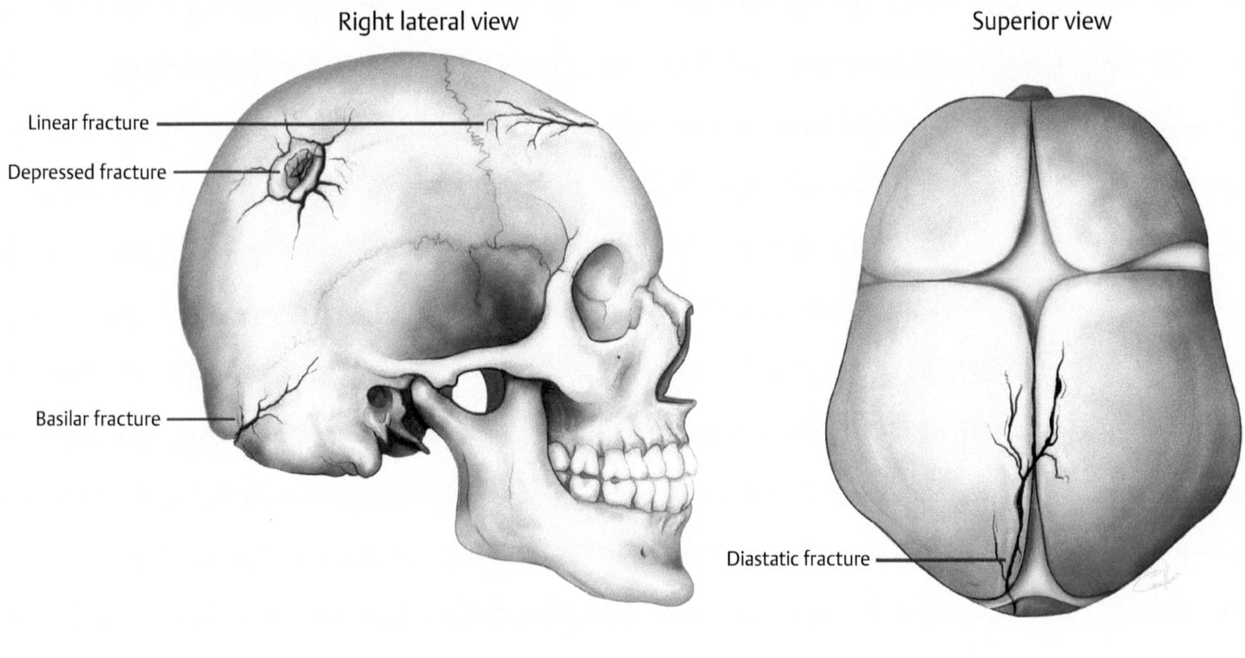

Illustration by Calla Heald.

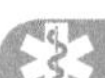

Clinical Correlate 7.3

Le Fort Fractures

There are three particular fractures involving the face that were first described by French surgeon Dr. René Le Fort. These fractures center on the midface and maxillary bone. Le Fort 1 (horizontal or floating palate) is described as being a horizontal maxillary fracture that separates the palate from the upper face. The fracture passes above the alveolar processes of the maxilla, inferior wall of the maxillary sinus, nasal septum, and possibly the pterygoid plates of the sphenoid bone. Le Fort 2 (pyramidal or floating maxilla) has a fracture line that passes through the posterolateral walls of the maxillary sinuses, inferior orbital rim, and nasal bones. Le Fort 3 (transverse or floating face) has a fracture line that passes through the superior orbital fissures, orbital walls, greater wings of the sphenoid bone, and zygomatic arches.

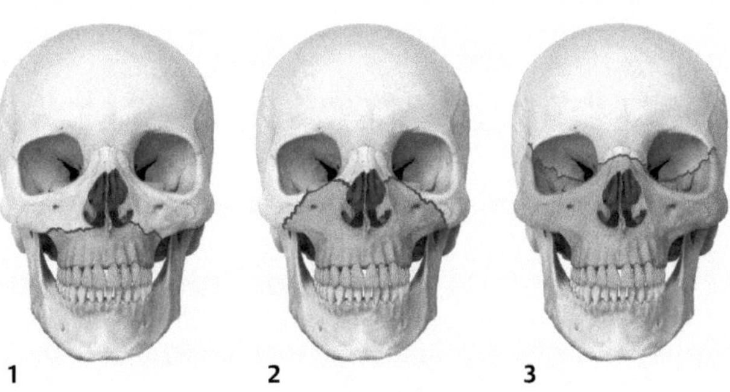

(From Schuenke M, Schulte E, Schumacher U. THIEME Atlas of Anatomy. Head, Neck, and Neuroanatomy. Illustrations by Voll M and Wesker K. 3rd ed. New York: Thieme Medical Publishers; 2020.)

Clinical Correlate 7.4

Craniotomy

A craniotomy is the surgical removal of a portion of the skull in order to expose the brain. A bone flap is elevated or temporarily removed but replaced after the brain surgery has been performed. The adult pericranium has poor bone forming (osteogenic) properties; thus, little regeneration of the bone occurs after the surgery, and it is fastened into place by wire or metal plates. A craniotomy may be done for brain tumor removal or an aneurysm clipping. A craniectomy refers to the permanent removal of a portion of the skull but the missing section will be replaced with a metal or plastic plate.

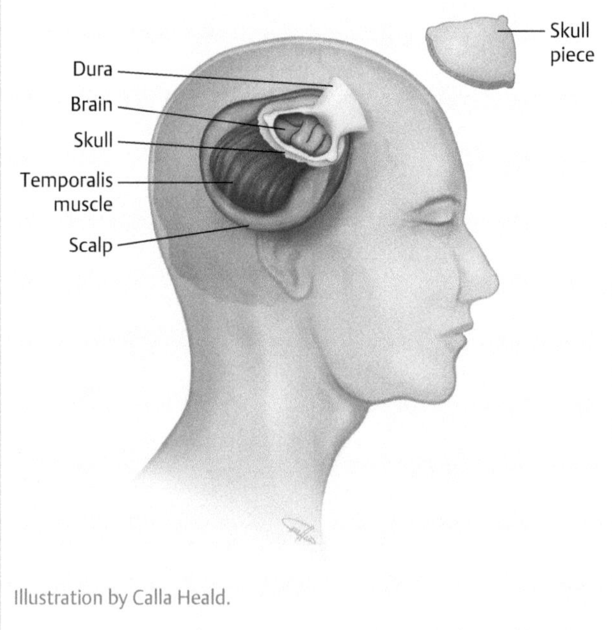

Illustration by Calla Heald.

Clinical Correlate 7.5

Pterion Fracture

The pterion **(Fig. 7.11)** is an osteometric point on the skull that represents the juncture of the frontal, sphenoid, parietal, and temporal bones. It is generally described as being two finger's breadth superior to the zygomatic arch and a thumbs breadth posterior to the frontal process of the zygomatic bone. Blunt force trauma to this region resulting in a fracture can damage the anterior branch of the middle meningeal artery and lead to an epidural hematoma. Lack of treatment could result in death in as little as a few hours.

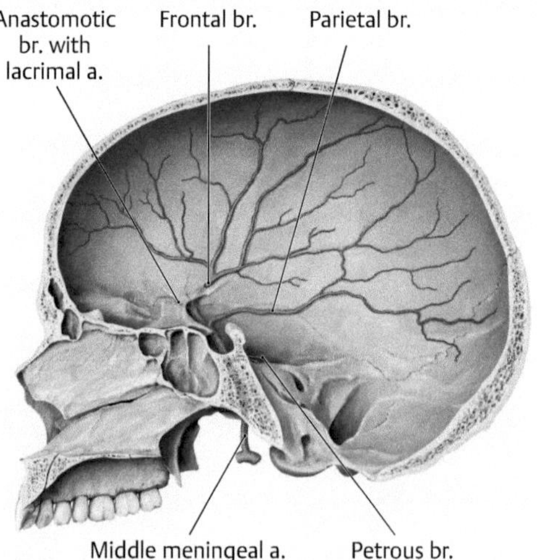

(From Gilroy AM et al. Atlas of Anatomy. 4th ed. 2020. Based on: Schuenke M, Schulte E, Schumacher U. THIEME Atlas of Anatomy. Head, Neck, and Neuroanatomy. Illustrations by Voll M and Wesker K. 3rd ed. New York: Thieme Medical Publishers; 2020.)

plate is where the *olfactory bulbs* rest. The superior projection from the ethmoid bone is known as the **crista galli**. The *falx cerebri* is a dural reflection that attaches to both the frontal crest and crista galli. Foramen of this fossa includes the olfactory foramina, anterior/posterior ethmoidal foramina, and foramen cecum. Major structures that pass through are listed (**Fig. 7.14; Fig. 7.15**).

- **Olfactory foramina**: branches of the olfactory nerve (CN I).
- **Anterior/posterior ethmoidal foramina**: anterior/posterior ethmoidal vessels and nerves.
- **Foramen cecum**: nasal emissary vein.

7.1.8 Middle Cranial Fossa

Portions of the sphenoid and the temporal bones form this fossa. The central portion is composed of the **sella turcica** (*Turkish saddle*) and it lies on the body of the sphenoid bone. The sella turcica is composed of three parts: tuberculum sellae, hypophysial fossa, and dorsum sellae.

- **Tuberculum sellae**: a slight elevation anterior to the hypophysial fossa.
- **Hypophysial (pituitary) fossa**: a saddle-like depression where the pituitary gland rests.
- **Dorsum sellae**: a square-plate of sphenoid bone posterior to the hypophysial fossa.

Clinical Correlate 7.6

Eagle Syndrome

Excessive length of a styloid process is known as eagle syndrome. A patient may present with neck pain while turning their head, difficulty swallowing (*dysphagia*), an earache (*otalgia*), or ringing of the ear (*tinnitus*). A CT scan is used to confirm the diagnosis and treatment may simply involve the partial or complete removal of the styloid process.

The sella turcica is surrounded by structures that look similar to bedposts called the anterior/posterior clinoid processes. The **anterior clinoid processes** are bony projections originating from the **sphenoidal crests** of the lesser wing of the sphenoid bone. The **posterior clinoid processes** are the superolateral angles of the dorsum sellae. The **prechiasmatic sulcus** is located just anterior to the tuberculum sellae and extends between the left and right optic canals.

Foramen of this fossa include the optic canals, superior orbital fissure, foramen rotundum, foramen ovale, foramen spinosum, foramen lacerum, and the hiatus of both the greater petrosal and lesser petrosal nerves. Major structures that pass through are listed (**Fig. 7.14; Fig. 7.15**):

- **Optic canal**: optic nerve (CN II) and ophthalmic artery.
- **Superior orbital fissure**: oculomotor nerve (CN III), trochlear nerve (CN IV), ophthalmic nerve (CN V_1), abducent nerve (CN VI), and superior ophthalmic vein.

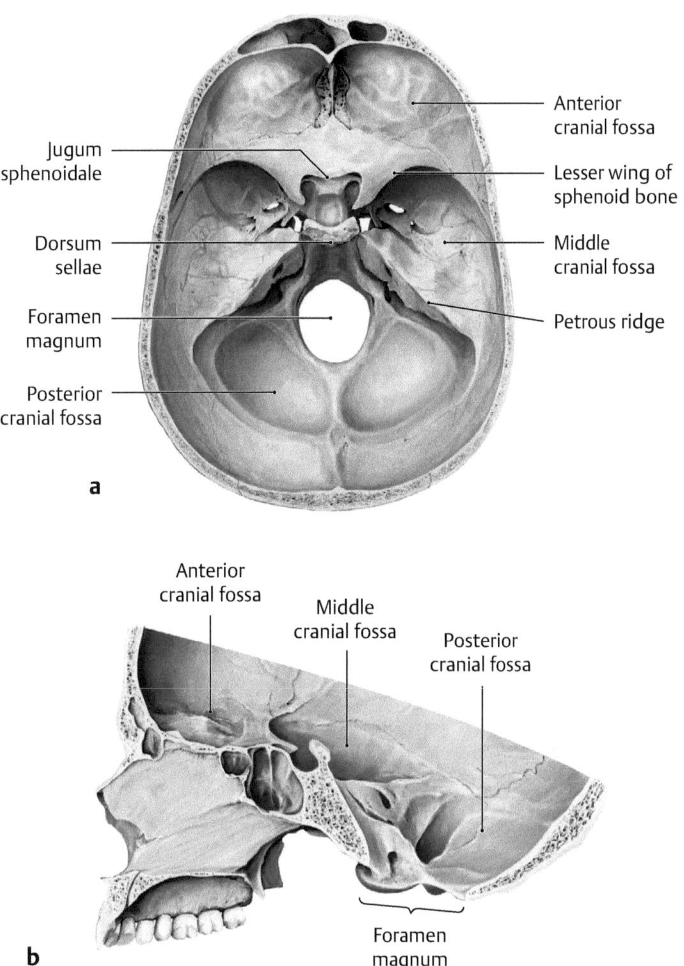

Fig. 7.13 (a) The inferior and midsagittal view of the cranial fossae. **(b)** Interior view of the base of the skull. (From Schuenke M, Schulte E, Schumacher U. THIEME Atlas of Anatomy. Head, Neck, and Neuroanatomy. Illustrations by Voll M and Wesker K. 3rd ed. New York: Thieme Medical Publishers; 2020.)

- **Foramen rotundum**: maxillary nerve (V_2).
- **Foramen ovale**: mandibular nerve (V_3), lesser petrosal nerve, and accessory meningeal vessels.
- **Foramen spinosum**: middle meningeal vessels and meningeal branch of V_3.
- **Foramen lacerum**: this is not a true foramen and is sealed with fibrocartilage during life. It is only seen as an artifact in a dry skull.
- **Hiatus of greater/lesser petrosal nerves**: passageway for the greater/lesser petrosal nerves.

7.1.9 Posterior Cranial Fossa

This fossa is formed primarily by the occipital bone but also from portions of the sphenoid and temporal bones. It is the largest and deepest cranial fossa and contains the cerebellum, pons, and medulla oblongata. Extending inferiorly from the dorsum sellae of the sphenoid and to the foramen magnum is the **clivus** of the occipital bone. There are two larger **cerebellar fossae** that correspond to the left and right portions of the cerebellum. Extending superiorly from the posterior portion of the foramen magnum and meeting the **internal occipital protuberance** is the **internal occipital crest**. This crest is also responsible for dividing the cerebellar fossae into two separate regions. Grooves for the transverse and sigmoid sinuses can be seen in this fossa. Foramen of this fossa includes the internal acoustic meatus, foramen magnum, jugular foramen, and hypoglossal canal. Major structures that pass through are listed (**Fig. 7.14; Fig. 7.15**):

- **Internal acoustic meatus**: facial nerve (CN VII), vestibulocochlear nerve (CN VIII), and the labyrinthine vessels.
- **Foramen magnum**: meninges, medulla oblongata, spinal cord, spinal accessory nerve (CN XI), anterior/posterior spinal arteries, spinal vein, and the vertebral artery.
- **Jugular foramen**: superior bulb of internal jugular vein (IJV), glossopharyngeal nerve (CN IX), vagus nerve (CN X), and spinal accessory nerve (CN XI).
- **Hypoglossal canal**: hypoglossal nerve (CN XII).

7.2 Cranial Meninges

Lying immediately internal to the cranium are the membranous connective tissue layers known as the **cranial meninges**. Similar to the spinal cord, there is a dura, arachnoid, and pia mater. They function as (**Fig. 7.16**):

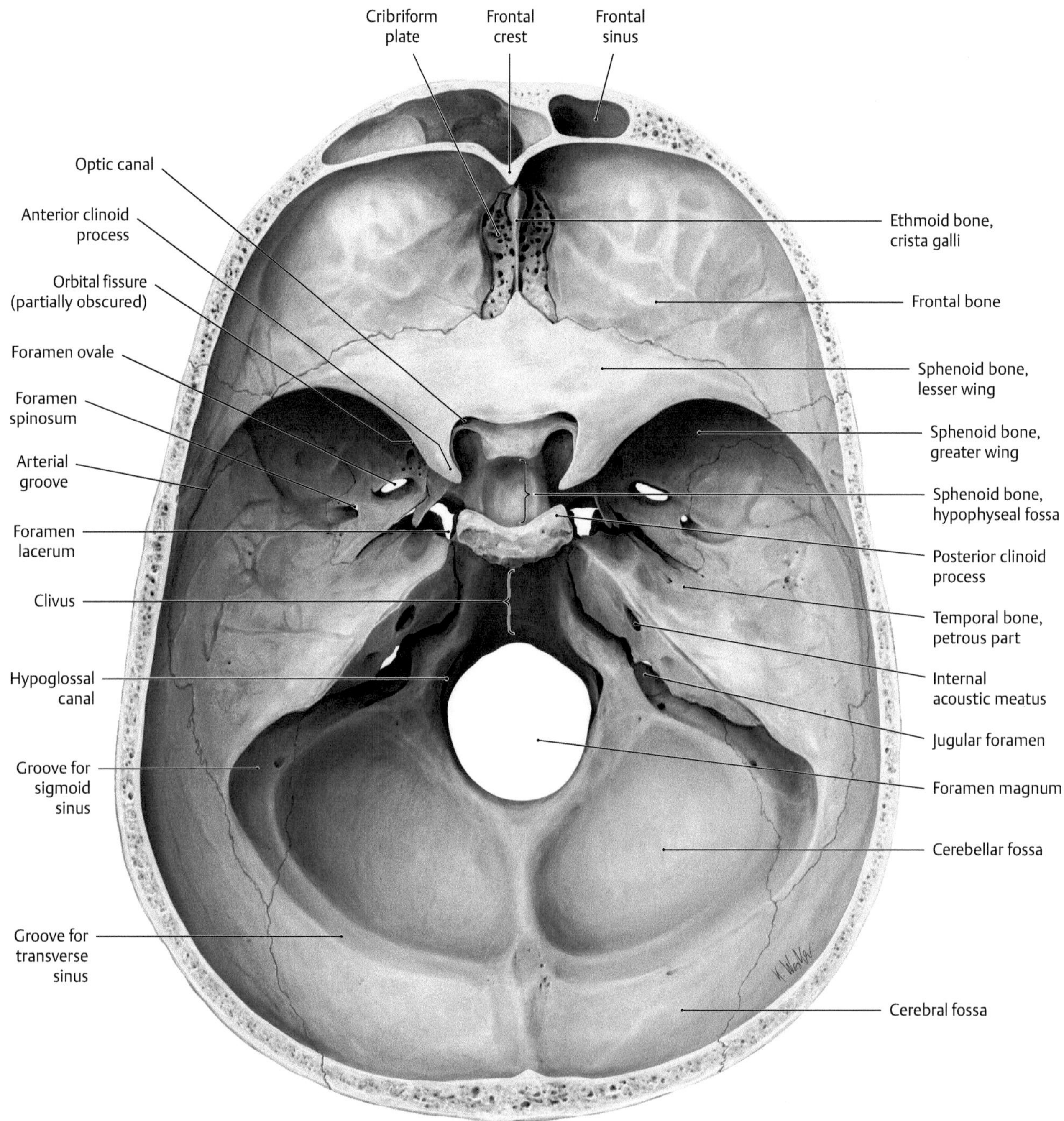

Fig. 7.14 Interior of the base of the skull. (From Schuenke M, Schulte E, Schumacher U. THIEME Atlas of Anatomy. Head, Neck, and Neuroanatomy. Illustrations by Voll M and Wesker K. 3rd ed. New York: Thieme Medical Publishers; 2020.)

- Protect the brain from mechanical injury.
- The formation of the subarachnoid space allowing for the flow of CSF.
- The formation of the supporting infrastructure for blood vessels and dural venous sinuses.

The **dura mater** of the cranium consists of two layers: the external periosteal layer and the inner meningeal layer. The **periosteal layer** adheres to the internal surface of the cranium and has a firm attachment especially at the cranial base and suture joints. It is continuous at the cranial foramina with the periosteum on the external surface of the calvaria. The **meningeal layer** is a supporting layer of dura that is fused with the periosteal layer except for when it reflects away from the periosteal layer to form dural reflections; it allows for venous drainage to flow through the dural venous sinuses; and is the only dural layer continuous with the dura associated with the spinal cord. Dural reflections divide the cranial cavity into compartments and provide support for other structures. These reflections are called **(Fig. 7.17)**:

- **Falx cerebri**: is a vertical reflection located in the longitudinal cerebral fissure and separates the left and right cerebral

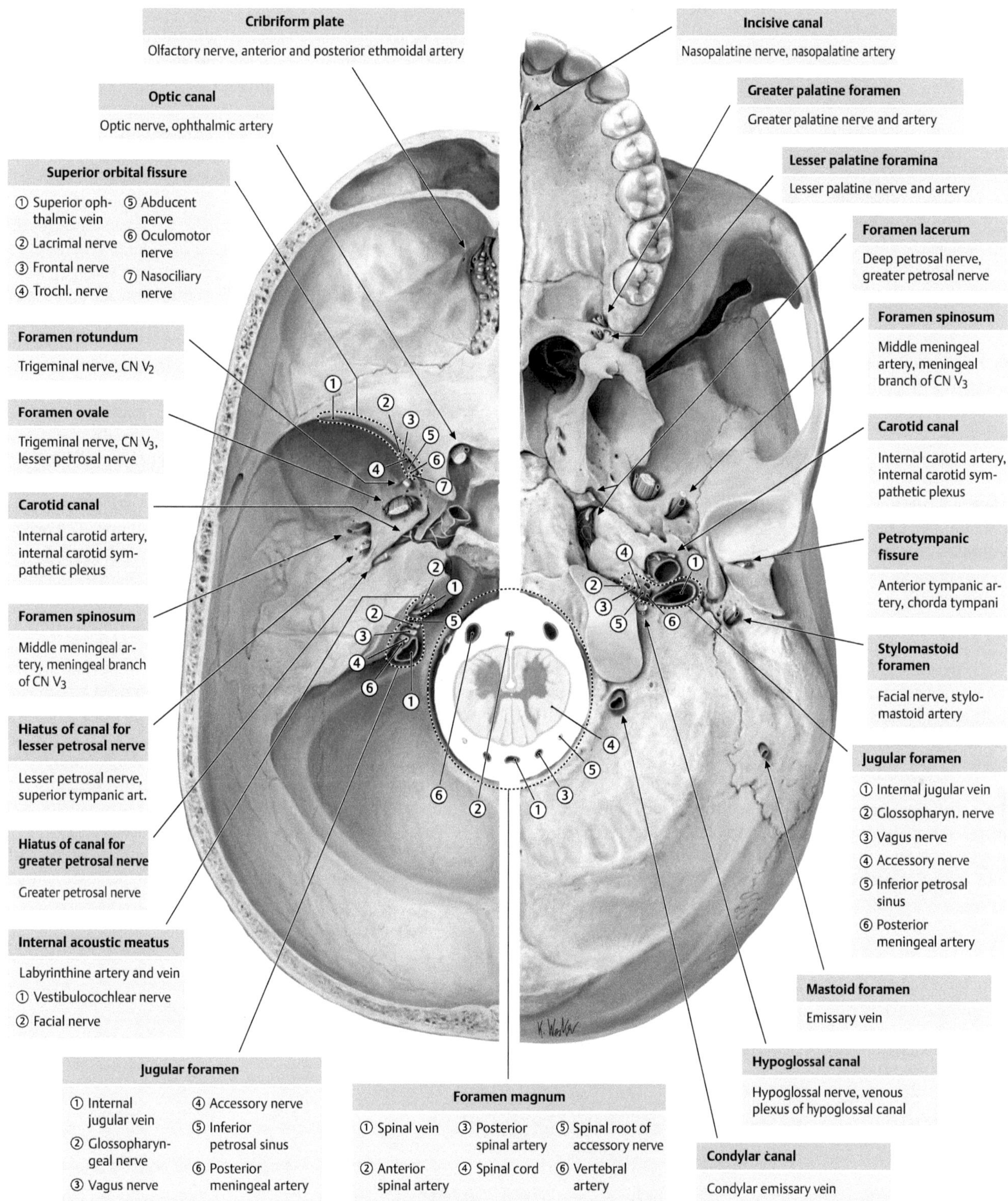

Fig. 7.15 Sites where nerves and vessels pass through the skull base. (From Schuenke M, Schulte E, Schumacher U. THIEME Atlas of Anatomy. Head, Neck, and Neuroanatomy. Illustrations by Voll M and Wesker K. 3rd ed. New York: Thieme Medical Publishers; 2020.)

hemispheres. It attaches to the frontal crest of the frontal bone, crista galli of the ethmoid bone, and the internal occipital protuberance. It will become continuous with the tentorium cerebelli and is the largest dural reflection.

- **Tentorium cerebelli**: is a horizontal, tentlike reflection that separates the cerebellum from the occipital lobes of the cerebral hemisphere. It attaches to the anterior/posterior clinoid processes, petrous portion of the temporal bone, and the

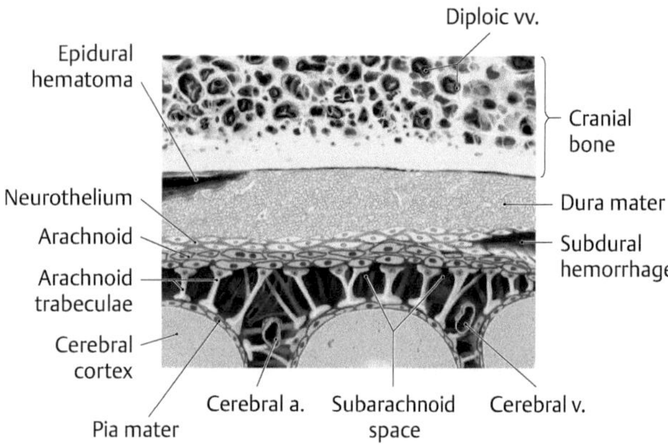

Fig. 7.16 Coronal section through the meninges, anterior view. (From Schuenke M, Schulte E, Schumacher U. THIEME Atlas of Anatomy. Head, Neck, and Neuroanatomy. Illustrations by Voll M and Wesker K. 3rd ed. New York: Thieme Medical Publishers; 2020.)

internal surfaces of both the parietal and occipital bones. The anteromedial border is free and produces a gap known as the **tentorial notch**. It is the second largest dural reflection.

- **Falx cerebelli**: a vertical reflection that adds minimal separation between the cerebellar hemispheres; attaches to the internal occipital crest and tentorium cerebelli; and contains the occipital sinus.
- **Diaphragma sellae**: is a circular sheet with a center aperture suspended between the clinoid processes forming a roof over the hypophysial fossa. The center opening allows for the passage of the infundibulum of the pituitary gland and hypophysial veins.

The separation between the periosteal and meningeal layers creates **dural venous sinuses**. These sinuses are veinlike with an endothelium but lack both a tunica media and valves. Larger veins from the surface of the brain drain into these sinuses and ultimately drain to the *internal jugular vein*. However, venous channels exist from these larger venous sinuses to venous plexuses such as the *internal vertebral, basilar,* and *pterygoid venous plexuses*. The **arachnoid granulations** are small protrusions of arachnoid through the meningeal layer of dura mater and are primarily found in the *lateral venous lacunae* of the *superior sagittal venous sinus*. Larger arachnoid granulations can erode bone and form pits called **granular foveolae** in the calvaria. Arachnoid granulations act as one-way valves for the transfer of CSF. CSF pressure is higher than venous pressure so CSF passes through the granulations to enter the venous blood of a dural venous sinus. The numerous dural venous sinuses are discussed next **(Fig. 7.18)**.

The **superior sagittal** and **inferior sagittal sinuses** are located on the superior and inferior borders of the falx cerebri, respectively. The **lateral venous lacunae** are lateral expansions of the superior sagittal sinus and are the site of most arachnoid granulations. The inferior sagittal sinus and **great cerebral vein** (*of Galen*) join to form the **straight sinus**. The straight sinus drains inferoposteriorly along the attachment site of the falx cerebri and tentorium cerebelli to join the **confluence of sinuses (Fig. 7.17; Fig. 7.19)**.

The confluence of sinuses is the anastomosis site for the superior sagittal, occipital, straight, and transverse sinuses. The **occipital sinus** runs along the attached border of the falx cerebelli and has a communication with the internal vertebral venous plexus discussed in Chapter 1. The **transverse sinuses** extend laterally from the internal occipital protuberance and confluence of sinuses and along the posterolateral attachments of the tentorium cerebelli. Venous drainage of the confluences of sinuses by the transverse sinus is not equal because the left transverse sinus is generally larger and is considered the dominant side. When the *superior petrosal sinus* meets the transverse sinus it is known as the sigmoid sinus. The **sigmoid sinus** has an S-shaped course and after joining the *inferior petrosal sinus* at the jugular foramen it is known as the internal jugular vein (IJV). The transverse and sigmoid sinuses form deep grooves within the adjacent bone.

The **superior petrosal** and **inferior petrosal sinuses** both originate at the cavernous sinus. The superior petrosal sinuses

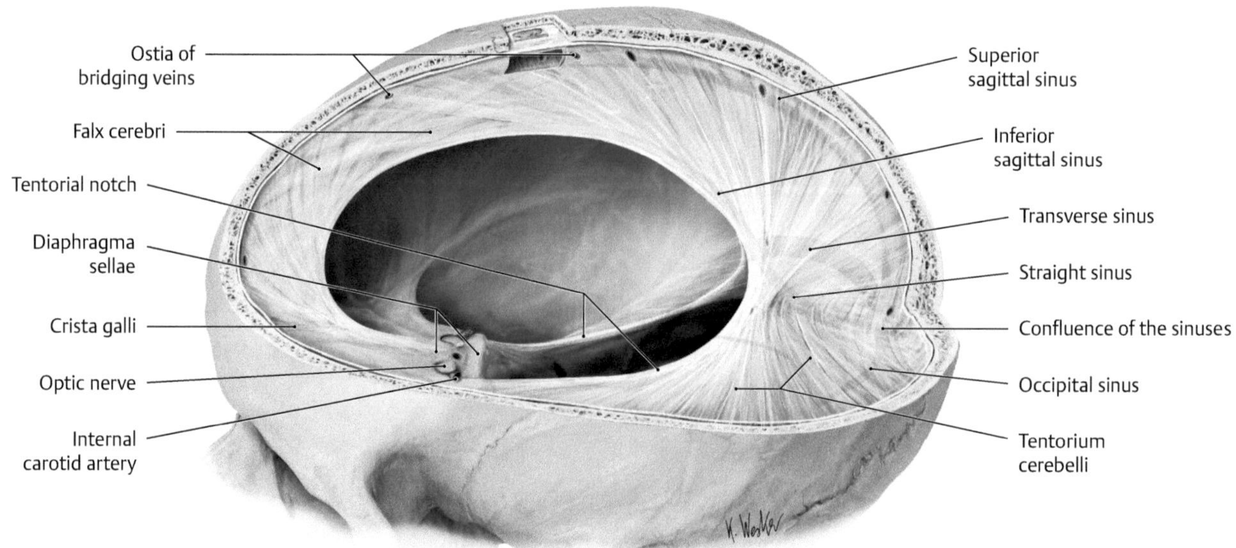

Fig. 7.17 Dural reflections. (From Schuenke M, Schulte E, Schumacher U. THIEME Atlas of Anatomy. Head, Neck, and Neuroanatomy. Illustrations by Voll M and Wesker K. 3rd ed. New York: Thieme Medical Publishers; 2020.)

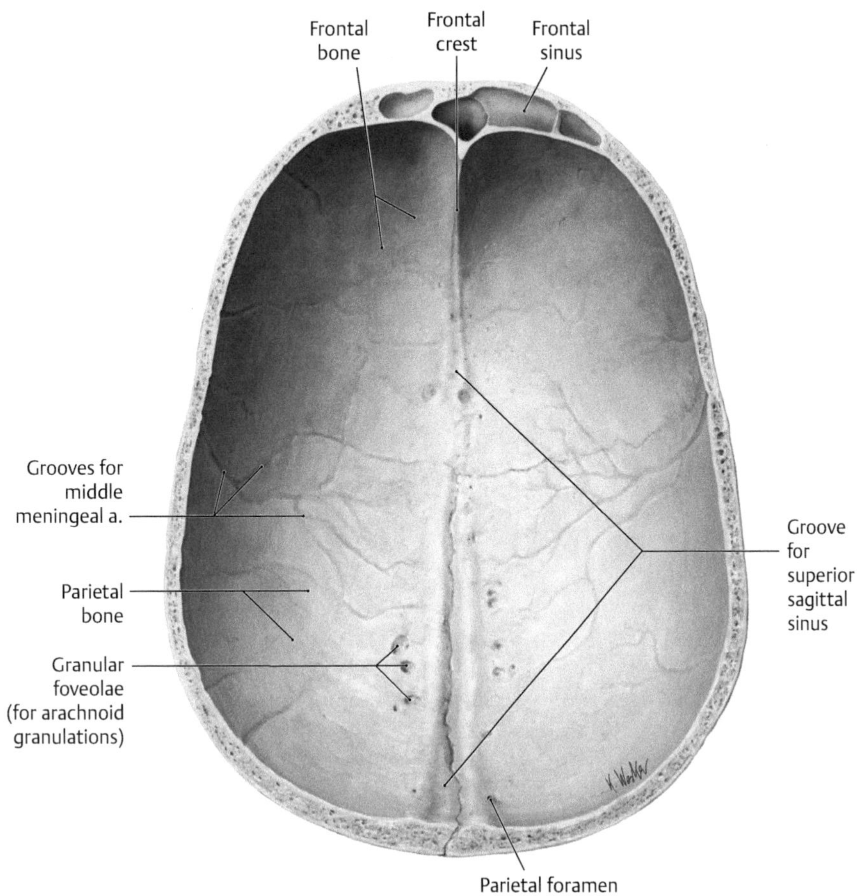

Fig. 7.18 Internal calvaria, inferior view. (From Schuenke M, Schulte E, Schumacher U. THIEME Atlas of Anatomy. Head, Neck, and Neuroanatomy. Illustrations by Voll M and Wesker K. 3rd ed. New York: Thieme Medical Publishers; 2020.)

will course along the anterolateral border of the tentorium cerebelli located on the superior border of the petrous portion of the temporal bone before joining the transverse sinus. The inferior petrosal sinuses will course within a groove between the petrous portion of the temporal bone and the basilar portion of the occipital bone before reaching the sigmoid sinus. The **basilar plexus** is located between the inferior petrosal sinuses along the clivus of the occipital bone. This plexus communicates with the internal vertebral plexus, inferior petrosal sinuses, and the **marginal sinus** located near the foramen magnum **(Fig. 7.19)**.

The **cavernous sinus** is located on each side of the sella turcica and is connected by the **anterior/posterior intercavernous sinuses**. The cavernous sinus receives venous blood from the superior ophthalmic veins, occasionally the inferior ophthalmic veins, *sphenoparietal sinus,* and the *superficial middle cerebral vein.* These sinuses then drain posteroinferiorly through the superior/inferior petrosal sinuses and through *emissary veins* to the basilar and pterygoid venous plexuses. Embedded in the dura mater of the lateral wall of the cavernous sinus is the oculomotor nerve (CN III), trochlear nerve (CN IV), ophthalmic nerve (CN V_1), and the maxillary nerve (CN V_2). The cavernous portion of the internal carotid artery (ICA), along with the carotid plexus of sym/post fibers, passes through the middle of the cavernous sinus and follows an S-shaped pattern known as the *carotid siphon.* The abducent nerve (CN VI) rests near the lateral border of the ICA within the cavernous sinus and not on the lateral wall. Along with gravity, pulsations from the ICA are thought to promote the propulsion of venous blood from the cavernous sinus **(Fig. 7.20)**.

Clinical Correlate 7.7

Cranial Dural Arteriovenous Fistula

A **dural arteriovenous fistula (DAVF)** is an abnormal connection of vessels in the tissues around the brain or spinal cord that may affect one or more arteries directly connected to one or more veins or venous sinuses. With DAVF, there is a direct connection between one or more arteries and veins or sinuses that result in numerous problems. They are most frequently seen at the cavernous and transverse sinuses although they can involve any of the cranial dural venous sinus. The most serious problem associated with DAVFs is that they transfer high-pressure arterial blood into the veins or venous sinuses, resulting in an increase in pressure of the venous system around the brain or spinal cord. They are generally classified as a type I, II, or III DAVF and can be treated with either minimally invasive endovascular embolization or microsurgical resection or both procedures simultaneously. DAVFs differ from an arteriovenous malformation (AVM), in that AVMs are found within the tissue of the brain or spinal cord, whereas DAVFs are found in the dura or arachnoid maters.

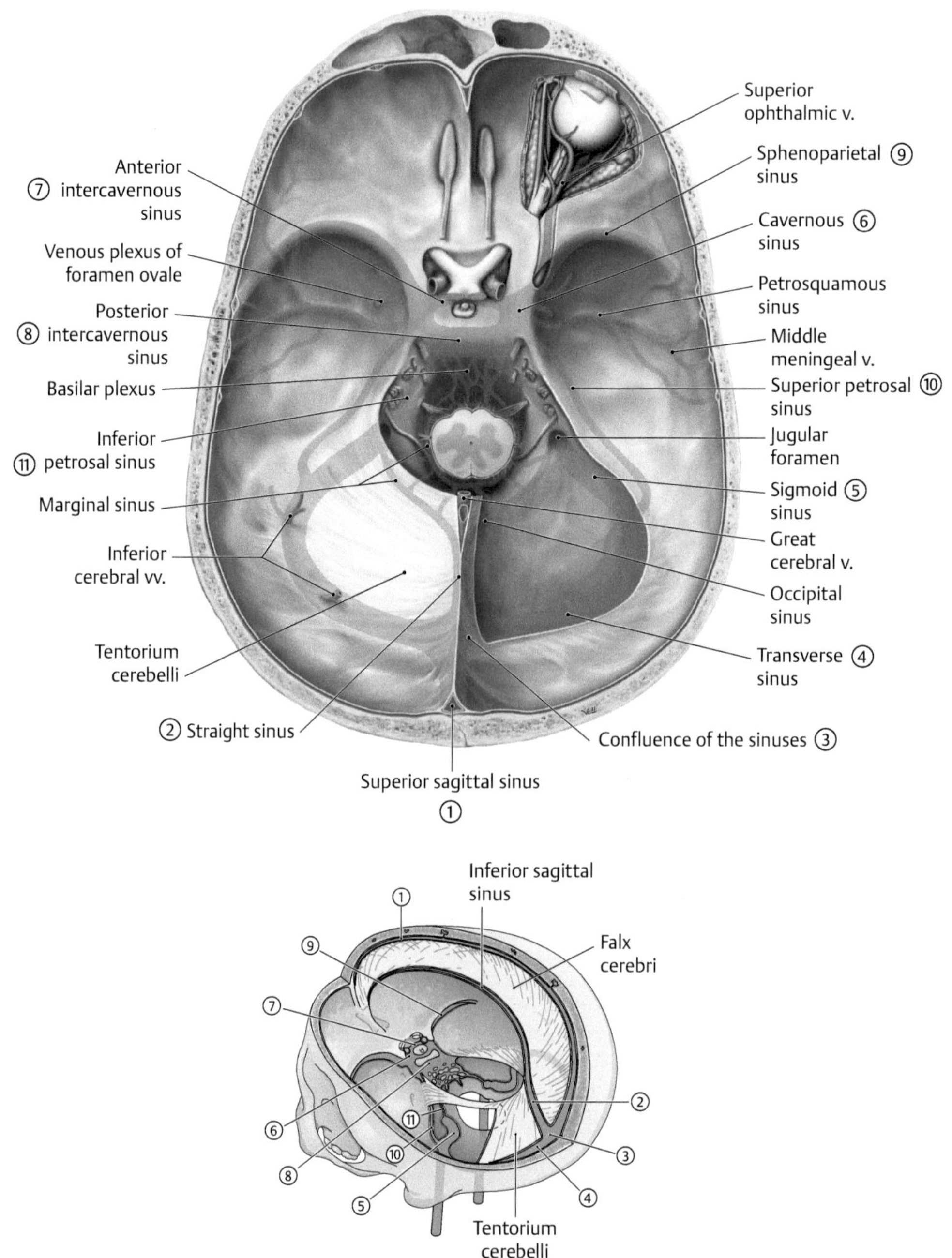

Fig. 7.19 Dural venous sinuses in the cranial cavity. (From Schuenke M, Schulte E, Schumacher U. THIEME Atlas of Anatomy. Head, Neck, and Neuroanatomy. Illustrations by Voll M and Wesker K. 3rd ed. New York: Thieme Medical Publishers; 2020.)

The **arachnoid mater** of the cranium is adjacent to the dura mater. Pressure of the CSF is what holds the arachnoid layer up against the dura. The **arachnoid trabeculae** are weblike extensions that extend to the pia mater. As seen in Chapter 1, the space between the arachnoid and pia maters is known as the **subarachnoid space** and the location of CSF. The arachnoid mater is avascular and has no direct innervation **(Fig. 7.16; Fig. 7.21)**.

The **pia mater** of the cranium is a thin, transparent membrane that adheres to the surface of the brain and all its contours. Pia mater follows the cerebral arteries as they penetrate the cerebral cortex for a short distance creating a **pial coat** and a **periarterial space**. The pia mater is highly vascularized but not innervated **(Fig. 7.16; Fig. 7.21)**.

7.2.1 Meningeal Spaces

There are generally three meningeal "spaces" described in the cranium; however, only one of them is a true space. The other two only occur when pathology is present.

- **Epidural/extradural space**: is a potential space located between the periosteal layer of dura and the cranium and is also known as the *dura-cranial interface*. Clinically, an *epidural hematoma* would create an epidural/extradural "space." This type of hematoma generally involves trauma that ruptures the anterior branch of the middle meningeal artery near the *pterion*. A cranial epidural hematoma cannot extend into the naturally occurring epidural space of the vertebral column

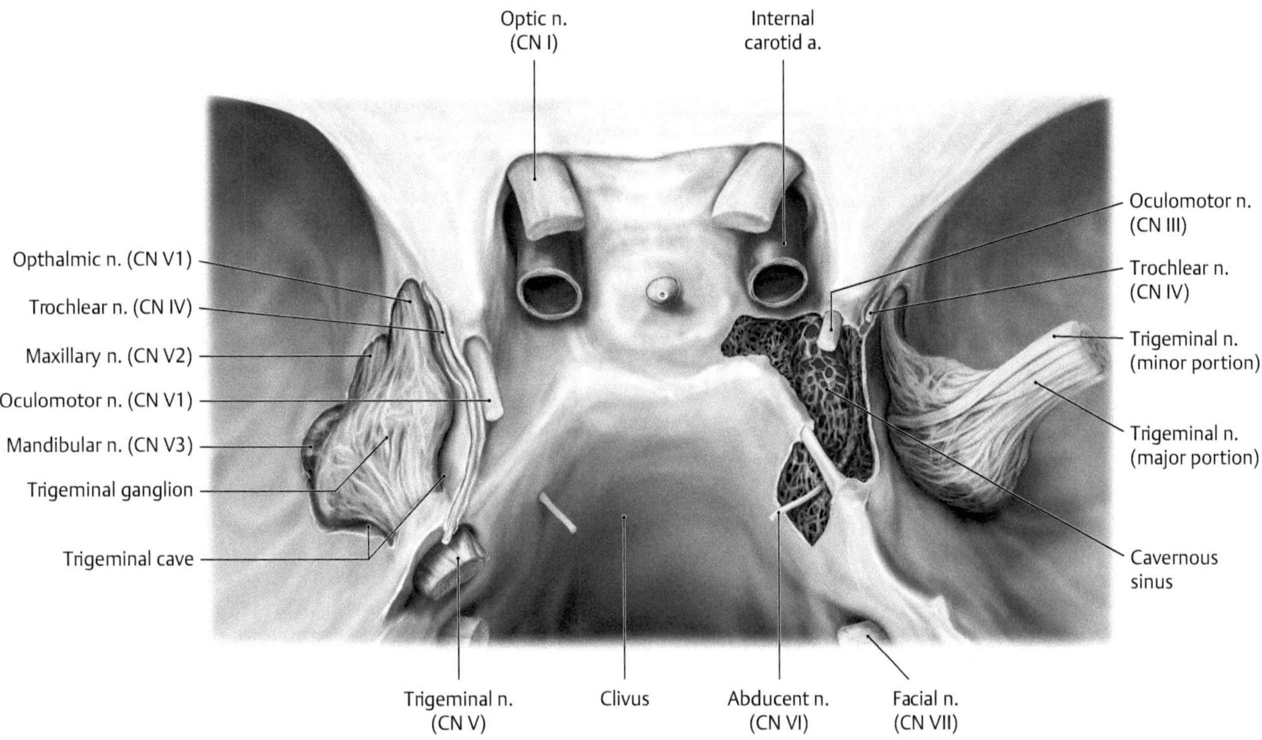

Fig. 7.20 Cavernous sinus and associated cranial nerves. Superior view of the right anterior and middle cranial fossae. (From Schuenke M, Schulte E, Schumacher U. THIEME Atlas of Anatomy. Head, Neck, and Neuroanatomy. Illustrations by Voll M and Wesker K. 3rd ed. New York: Thieme Medical Publishers; 2020.)

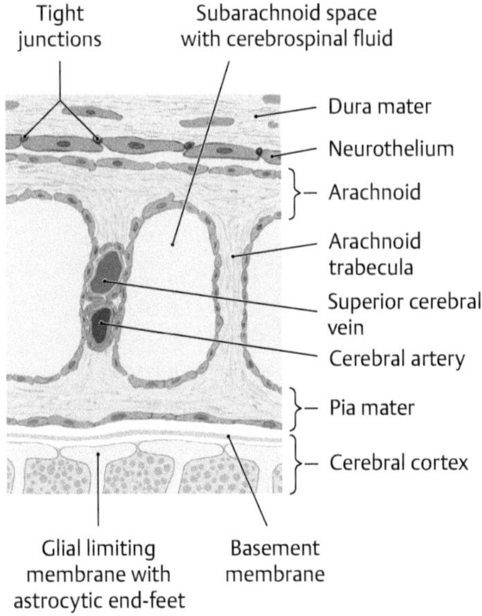

Fig. 7.21 A schematic close-up of the meninges, coronal view. (From Schuenke M, Schulte E, Schumacher U. THIEME Atlas of Anatomy. Head, Neck, and Neuroanatomy. Illustrations by Voll M and Wesker K. 3rd ed. New York: Thieme Medical Publishers; 2020.)

because the meningeal layer of dura continues into the vertebral column and not the periosteal layer **(Fig. 7.22)**.

- **Subdural space**: is a potential space located between the meningeal layer of dura and the arachnoid mater and is also known as the *dura-arachnoid interface*. Clinically, a *subdural hematoma* is generally venous in nature and commonly involves trauma

Clinical Correlate 7.8

Danger Triangle of the Face and Cavernous Sinus Syndrome

The facial vein is connected to the cavernous sinus by the superior ophthalmic vein and the pterygoid venous plexus by way of the deep facial and inferior ophthalmic veins. A bacterial infection due to a laceration or infected pimple in a particular area of the face known as the **danger triangle** could lead to this bacterial infection reaching the cavernous sinus because these venous pathways lead from the face to a dural venous sinus. An infected thrombus (clot) could drain back to the cavernous sinus and would be known as *thrombophlebitis of the cavernous sinus* of **cavernous sinus syndrome (CIS)**. A CIS diagnosis is confirmed by the loss of eyeball movements of which abduction is the first movement to be affected. This is due to compression of the abducent nerve (CN VI). Movements controlled by the oculomotor (CN III) and trochlear nerves (CN IV) will soon follow. If left untreated, individuals could die from CIS.

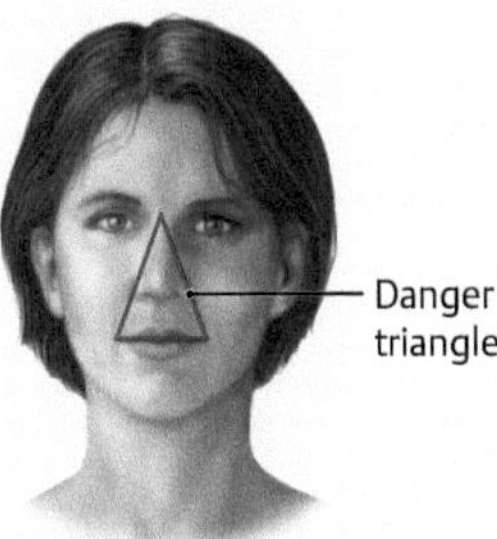

(From Schuenke M, Schulte E, Schumacher U. THIEME Atlas of Anatomy. Head, Neck, and Neuroanatomy. Illustrations by Voll M and Wesker K. 3rd ed. New York: Thieme Medical Publishers; 2020.)

Clinical Correlate 7.9

Headaches

A headache is sharp or throbbing sensation or pain in the head region and may occur on one or both sides of the head, certain location, or radiate across from one spot to another. Most headaches are not the symptoms of underlying disease but are mostly caused by overactivity of pain sensitive sensory neurons in structures such as the dura mater of the cranium. Meningeal branches of the trigeminal nerve primarily innervate the dura and most headaches appear to be dural in origin. They can be classified as cluster, tension, or migraine for most headaches. Secondary headaches are symptoms of disease and can be related to acute sinusitis, brain aneurysms, concussions, meningitis, glaucoma, and dehydration among many others.

to the superior cerebral vein as it enters the superior sagittal sinus (**Fig. 7.22**).

- **Subarachnoid space**: is a naturally occurring space located between the arachnoid and pia maters. The main contents are CSF but arteries, veins, and arachnoid trabeculae are also present. Clinically, a *subarachnoid hemorrhage* generally involves the rupture of a *saccular (or berry) aneurysm* of a cerebral artery. These are the most common cerebral artery aneurysms (**Fig. 7.22**).

7.3 Development of the Skull

The skull is associated with the axial skeleton and it is divided into two parts, the *neurocranium* and the *viscerocranium*. The **neurocranium** forms the protective surrounding around the brain and its cranial meninges but it is divided into two parts: a **membranous portion** consisting of flat bones that represent the **calvaria** (**skullcap**) and **cartilaginous portion** that represents the **cranial base (basicranium)**.

The *membranous portion* is derived from neural crest cells and the paraxial mesoderm. The mesenchyme from both of these sources invests the brain and it undergoes **intramembranous ossification**. The flat bones are characterized by *bone spicules* that radiate from the primary ossification centers and toward the periphery. From fetal and into postnatal life, these membranous bones will enlarge by apposition or the deposition of successive layers externally while being reabsorbed internally (**Fig. 7.23**).

The *cartilaginous portion (chondrocranium)* is formed by a combination of neural crest cells and mesodermal sclerotome and initially consists of numerous separate cartilages. These multiple cartilages located in front of the rostral limit of the notochord or at the level of the pituitary gland and sella turcica are derived of neural crest and form the **prechordal chondrocranium**. The individual cartilages located posterior to this location are derived from paraxial mesoderm that contributes to the occipital sclerotomes and they form what is called the **chordal chondrocranium**. Endochondral ossification is what fuses these cartilages in order to form the base of the skull (**Fig. 7.24**).

The **viscerocranium** consists of bones that help form the face, derived from neural crest cells, and is formed mainly from the first two pharyngeal arches but is divided into a *membranous* and *chondral viscerocranium*. The **membranous viscerocranium** of the first pharyngeal arch has a **dorsal part (maxillary process)** that undergoes intramembranous ossification and extends anteriorly beneath the eye and gives rise to the maxilla, zygomatic, and squamous temporal bones but the squamous temporal bones will later become part of the neurocranium. The **ventral part (mandibular process)** contains *Meckel cartilage* and this region will become surrounded by mesenchyme that condenses and ossifies by intramembranous ossification to form the mandible.

The **chondral viscerocranium** consisting of all of supporting cartilages undergoes endochondral ossification. *Meckel cartilage*

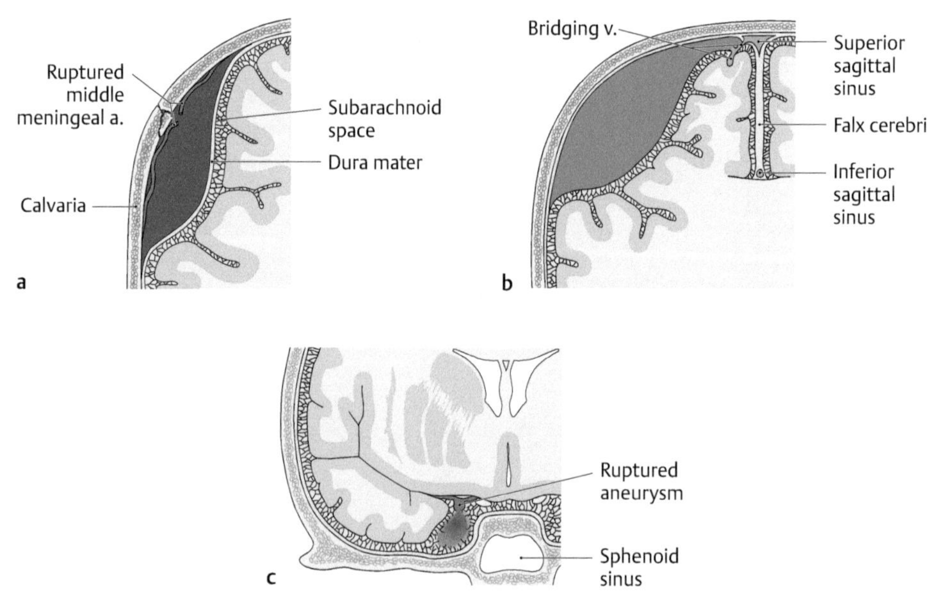

Fig. 7.22 Cerebral hemorrhages. **(a)** Epidural hematoma. **(b)** Subdural hematoma. **(c)** Subarachnoid hemorrhage. (From Schuenke M, Schulte E, Schumacher U. THIEME Atlas of Anatomy. Head, Neck, and Neuroanatomy. Illustrations by Voll M and Wesker K. 3rd ed. New York: Thieme Medical Publishers; 2020.)

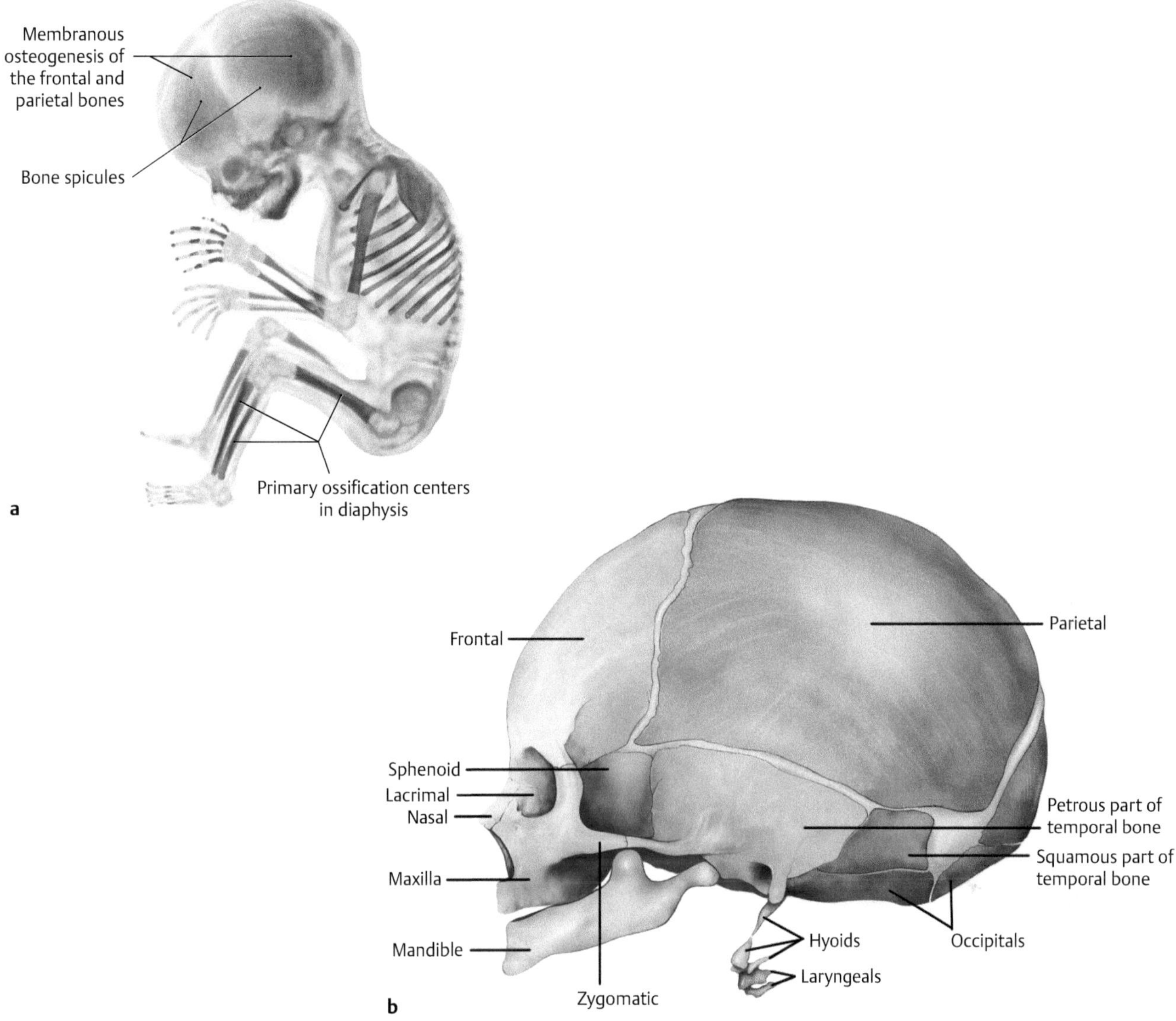

Fig. 7.23 Development of the skull. **(a)** Bone spicules radiate from the primary ossification centers toward the periphery. **(b)** Mesenchyme for these structures is derived from either neural crest cells (blue), paraxial mesoderm (purple), or lateral plate mesoderm (orange). (Part a from Schuenke M, Schulte E, Schumacher U. THIEME Atlas of Anatomy. General Anatomy and Musculoskeletal System. Illustrations by Voll M and Wesker K. 3rd ed. New York: Thieme Medical Publishers; 2020. Part b illustration by Calla Heald.)

will disappear except for its dorsal end, which ossifies to become the malleus and incus bones. The middle section's perichondrium regresses to form the sphenomandibular ligament and anterior ligament of the malleus. The dorsal end of *Reichert cartilage* in the second pharyngeal arch ossifies to become the stapes and styloid process of the temporal bone. Its perichondrium forms the stylohyoid ligament while the ventral end ossifies to become the upper body and lesser horns of the hyoid bone. The third pharyngeal arch completes the remainder of the hyoid bone while the fourth and sixth pharyngeal arches produce laryngeal cartilages (Detailed in **Table 7.13**).

7.4 Scalp and Superficial Face

The **scalp** is made up of skin and subcutaneous tissue that covers the neurocranium from to the supraorbital margins of the frontal bone anteriorly, over the temporal fascia to the zygomatic arches laterally, and the superior nuchal lines of the occipital bone posteriorly.

The scalp consists of five layers. The first three layers are connected to one another and are known as the **scalp proper**. The five layers are arranged in order to spell the word SCALP (**Fig. 7.25**).

- *Skin (S)*: generally thin except for the occipital region. The scalp contains numerous hair follicles, and sweat and sebaceous (oil) glands.
- *Connective tissue (C)*: a dense subcutaneous layer that is highly vascularized and contains numerous cutaneous nerves.
- *Aponeurosis (or epicranial aponeurosis) (A)*: the strong and broad tendinous sheet that covers the calvaria and serves as the attachment site for both the frontal and occipital muscle bellies of the **occipitofrontalis muscle**, as well as the **temporoparietalis** and **superior auricular muscles**.
- *Loose areolar tissue (L)*: the sponge-like connective tissue that allows for the scalp proper to move freely. It may also distend with fluid in the event of an infection or injury.
- *Pericranium (P)*: a dense layer of connective tissue adjacent to the external layer of compact bone of the neurocranium.

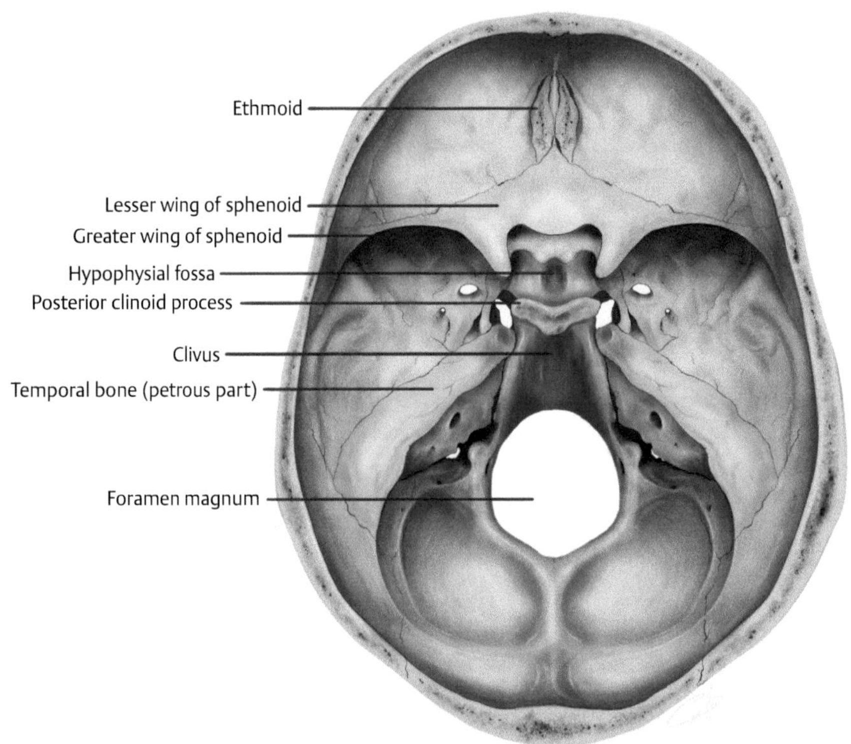

Fig. 7.24 Skull development, dorsal view: This view of the chondrocranium of the and adult demonstrates bones formed by endochondral ossification. The bones that arise from neural crest and form the prechordal chondrocranium are labeled purple. Bones derived from paraxial mesoderm and form the chordal chondrocranium are labeld blue. Illustration by Calla Heald.

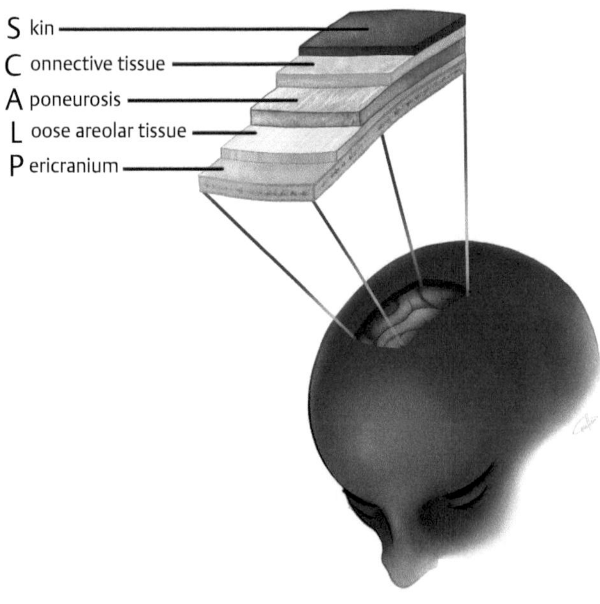

Fig. 7.25 Layers of the scalp. Illustration by Calla Heald.

7.4.1 Muscles of the Scalp, Face, Ear, and Neck

Facial muscles are also known as the facial expression (mimetic) muscles. These muscles are located in the subcutaneous tissue layer of the scalp, orbit, nose, mouth, ear, and neck regions. Movement of the skin in these regions helps convey an individual's mood while others serve as a dilator or sphincter. All muscles of facial expression are innervated by the facial nerve (CN VII). These muscles all originate from mesoderm of the *second pharyngeal arches* during development **(Fig. 7.26)**. Descriptions of these muscles are found in **Table 7.1**.

7.4.2 Neurovasculature of the Scalp and Superficial Face

As previously discussed, all the muscles of facial expression are innervated by the facial nerve (CN VII) branches and these branches contain functional components SVE (or branchiomotor/BM) and GSA. However, cutaneous innervation of the skin (somatic sensory/GSA) over the scalp and face is done primarily by the trigeminal nerve (CN V). Combinations of both ventral and dorsal rami branches supply the posterior half of the head and neck. The trigeminal nerve (CN V) consists of three divisions known as the ophthalmic (V_1), maxillary (V_2), and mandibular (V_3) nerves. All three divisions have GSA fibers but the mandibular nerve also contains SVE/BM fibers responsible for innervating the muscles of mastication along with a few other muscles.

The GSA cell bodies of these pseudounipolar neurons are located in a large **trigeminal ganglion** near the cavernous sinus. The trigeminal nerve divisions display a dermatome-like pattern on the face. CN V_1: forehead, upper eyelids, bridge, and tip of nose; CN V_2: lower eyelids, nostrils, upper lip, cheeks, and anterior temporal fossa; CN V_3: lower lip, chin, mandible, anterior ear, and most of the posterior temporal fossa. The skin innervated by ophthalmic nerve branches originates from the *frontonasal prominence*, which differs from the maxillary and mandibular innervated skin that originates from the *first pharyngeal arches* **(Fig. 7.27)**.

Clinical Correlate 7.10

Craniosynostosis

A birth defect involving the premature closure of one or more cranial sutures is known as **craniosynostosis**. This diagnosis is also a feature in over hundred genetic syndromes but for the most part the underlying cause is unknown. Surgery is usually the course of action and involves separating the fused bones to reduce increased intracranial pressure from within the skull that affects the normal brain development and growth. Multiple examples are shown but the most common form involves the sagittal suture (*scaphocephaly*) and it will force the head to grow long and narrow.

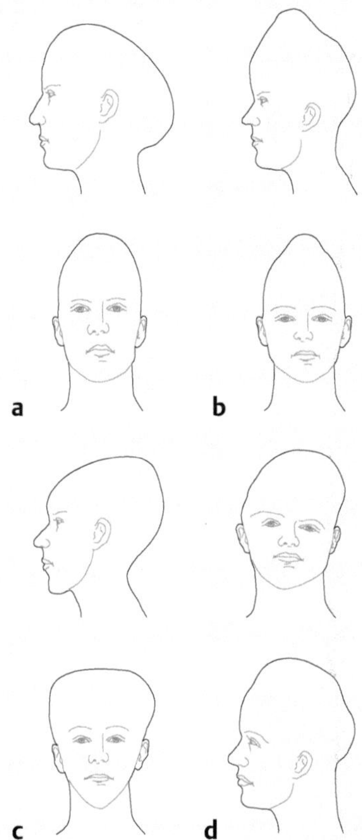

The following sutures may close prematurely, resulting in various shapes. **(a)** Sagittal suture: scaphocephaly. **(b)** Coronal suture: oxycephaly. **(c)** Frontal suture: trigonocephaly. **(d)** Asymetrical closure usually involing the coronal suture: plagiocephaly. (From Schuenke M, Schulte E, Schumacher U. THIEME Atlas of Anatomy. Head, Neck, and Neuroanatomy. Illustrations by Voll M and Wesker K. 3rd ed. New York: Thieme Medical Publishers; 2020.)

The **ophthalmic nerve (CN V_1)** is the smallest of the trigeminal nerve divisions and after passing through the superior orbital fissure has three of its own initial branches. These are the nasociliary, frontal, and lacrimal nerves **(Fig. 7.28; Fig. 7.29)**.

- The **nasociliary nerve** branches into the **sensory root of the ciliary ganglion**, **long ciliary**, **posterior/anterior ethmoidal,** and terminates as the **infratrochlear nerve**. The infratrochlear and the **external nasal nerve** (termination of anterior ethmoidal) serve as the cutaneous nerves of the nasociliary nerve and supply areas such as the *lacrimal sac, lacrimal caruncle, skin and conjunctiva of the medial upper eyelid,* and *root and tip of the nose.* All these nerves contain GSA fibers. The long ciliary nerve also contains sympathetic postganglionic (sym/post) fibers that originated from the periarterial plexus of the ICA and are responsible for innervating the *dilator pupillae muscle.* The anterior and posterior ethmoidal nerves help innervate the nasal cavities while the long ciliary is associated with a portion of the eyeball sensory innervation.
- The **frontal nerve** runs along the roof of the orbit and bifurcates into a **supratrochlear** and **supraorbital nerve** (itself having a medial and lateral branch). These nerves contain GSA fibers and are responsible for cutaneous innervation of the *scalp, forehead,* and *upper eyelid.* These nerves also innervate the conjunctiva of the upper eyelid and mucosa of the frontal sinus (supraorbital).
- The **lacrimal nerve** runs alongside the lateral wall of the orbit before reaching the lacrimal gland. Near the halfway point of its distal course, it receives the communicating branch of the zygomatic nerve (or zygomaticotemporal) and the parasympathetic preganglionic (para/pre) and sym/post fibers targeting the lacrimal gland. The entire nerve contains GSA fibers responsible for cutaneous innervation for a small area of skin and conjunctiva of the *lateral superior eyelid.*

The **maxillary nerve (CN V_2)** leaves the cranium through the *foramen rotundum* to reach the *pterygopalatine fossa.* It will then enter the orbit through the *inferior orbital fissure.* The maxillary nerve has numerous branches but the infraorbital, zygomaticofacial, and zygomaticotemporal nerves serve as the cutaneous branches of CN V_2 and contain GSA fibers. The maxillary nerve and infraorbital nerves for a short distance contain para/post and sym/post fibers that course through their posterior superior alveolar, middle superior alveolar, and anterior superior alveolar nerve branches. These details will be presented with the hard palate and upper teeth section **(Fig. 7.28; Fig. 7.30)**.

- The **infraorbital nerve** is the continuation of the maxillary nerve after it passes through the inferior orbital fissure and it is responsible for cutaneous innervation of the *lower eyelid, lateral nose, upper cheek,* and *upper lip.* Additional areas of innervation by this nerve or branches of it include the conjunctiva of the lower eyelid; mucosa of the maxillary sinus and upper lip; incisor, canine, and premolar maxillary teeth.
- The **zygomaticofacial nerve** is a branch of the **zygomatic nerve** and it innervates the skin of the *upper cheek* near zygomatic arch.
- The **zygomaticotemporal nerve** is a branch of the **zygomatic nerve** and innervates the skin of the *anterior temporal fossa region.*

The **mandibular nerve (CN V_3)** leaves the cranium through the *foramen ovale* and is the only trigeminal nerve division to contain motor fibers; SVE or branchiomotor (BM) fibers that target muscles of mastication among others. The auriculotemporal, buccal, and mental nerves serve as the cutaneous branches of CN V_3 and contain GSA fibers. Note: the auriculotemporal nerve also contains para/post and sym/post fibers important in parotid gland innervation **(Fig. 7.28; Fig. 7.31)**.

- The **auriculotemporal nerve** innervates the skin of the *anterior ear region, posterior temporal fossa region, roof of the external acoustic meatus,* and *superior tympanic membrane.*
- The **buccal nerve** innervates skin of the *lower cheek*; it also innervates the *buccal gingivae* and *oral mucosa of the cheek.*
- The **mental nerve** (continuation of inferior alveolar nerve) innervates the skin of the *chin* and the *oral mucosa of the lower lip.*

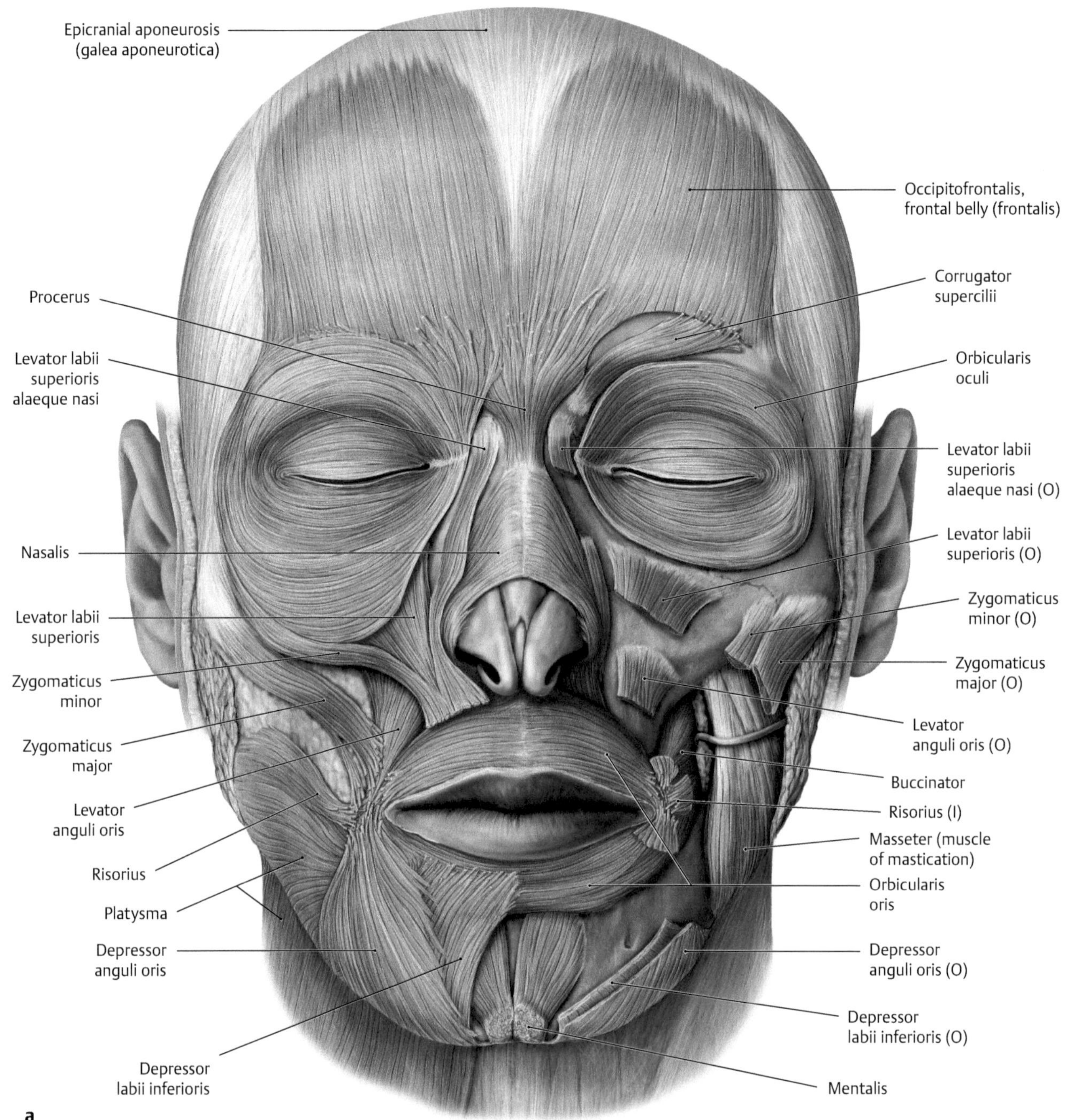

Fig. 7.26 Muscles of facial expression. **(a)** Anterior view. (*continued*) (From Schuenke M, Schulte E, Schumacher U. THIEME Atlas of Anatomy. Head, Neck, and Neuroanatomy. Illustrations by Voll M and Wesker K. 3rd ed. New York: Thieme Medical Publishers; 2020.)

Clinical Correlate 7.11

Trigeminal Neuralgia

Trigeminal neuralgia (or tic douloureux) is a neuropathic disorder associated with the sensory root of CN V and characterized by episodes of sudden sharp pains (*paroxysm*) involving the face. Individual attacks of pain can last for a few seconds to several minutes or more. Multiple attacks can occur in one day or occur in cycles with many months between attacks. The most affected part is V_2, followed by V_3. Theories exist to how it is caused and these include compression of the sensory root by an aberrant artery or demyelination of sensory axons. Symptoms generally do not begin until middle age and can be triggered by simply the wind blowing on ones face, brushing their teeth, or chewing food. Treatment may begin first with anticonvulsant medications but with continued episodes surgical intervention would be inevitable. Psychological issues may arise due to the constant pain felt by the individual and this has led to a high rate of suicide associated with this diagnosis.

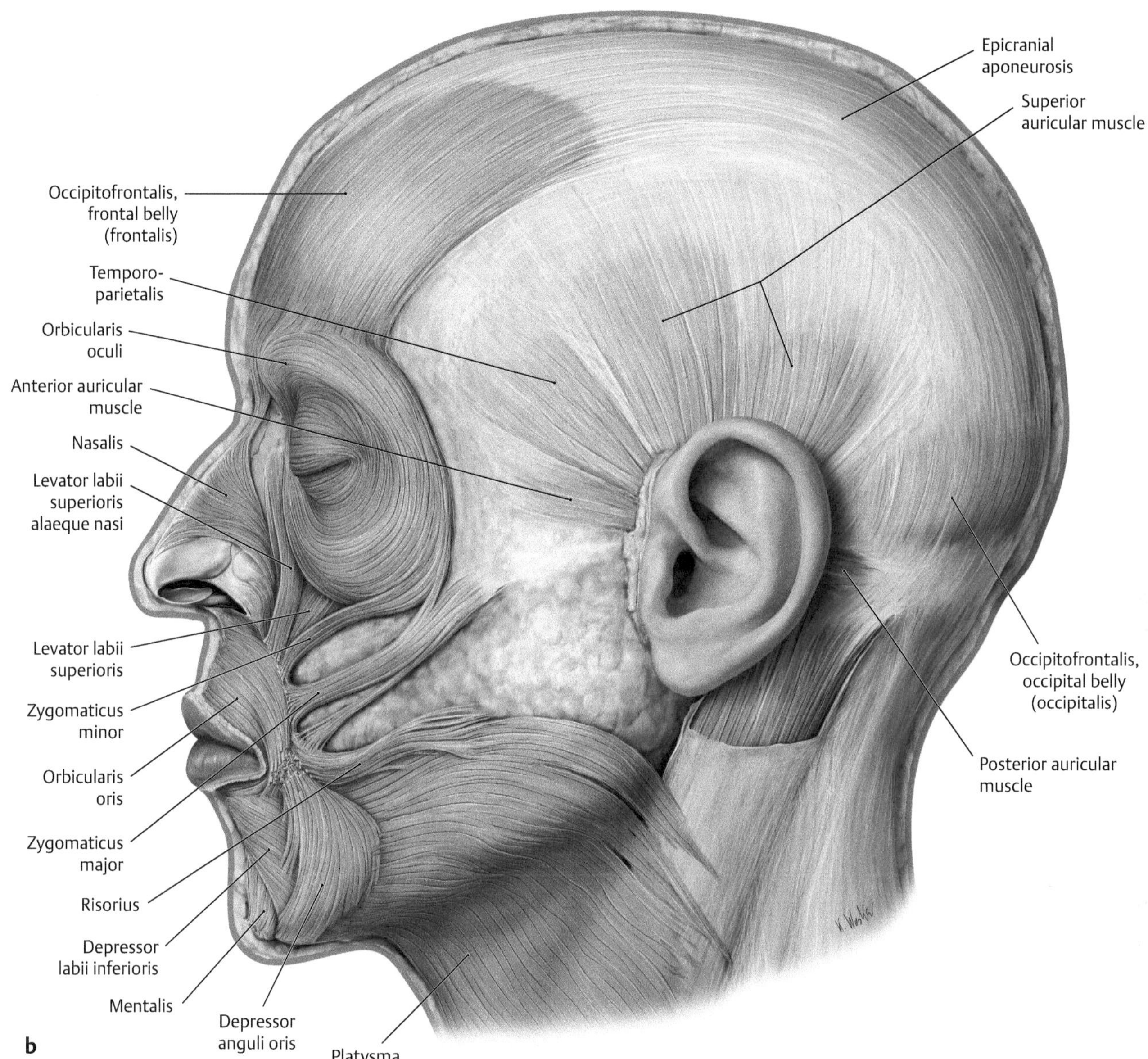

Fig. 7.26 (*continued*) Muscles of facial expression. **(b)** Left lateral view. (From Schuenke M, Schulte E, Schumacher U. THIEME Atlas of Anatomy. Head, Neck, and Neuroanatomy. Illustrations by Voll M and Wesker K. 3rd ed. New York: Thieme Medical Publishers; 2020.)

The **facial nerve (CN VII)** is made up of a larger motor root and an intermediate nerve. The motor root contains the branchiomotor (BM) fibers responsible for innervating the facial expression, posterior belly of digastric, stylohyoid, auricular (ear), stapedius, and scalp muscles. The motor root and its distal branches also contain SA fibers associated with proprioception of these muscles. After giving off all the other facial nerve branches, the motor root exits through the *stylomastoid foramen* and immediately gives off the **posterior auricular nerve**. The remainder of the motor root passing anteriorly becomes the **parotid plexus** located just deep or within the parotid gland. The parotid plexus terminates as five branches and their names refer to the region they supply. These branches are the **temporal**, **zygomatic**, **buccal**, **marginal mandibular,** and **cervical (Fig. 7.32)**.

Blood supply to the face and scalp originates primarily from the **external carotid artery (ECA)** and its branches. A smaller percentage of blood originates indirectly from branches of the ICA. The external carotid artery has six direct branches (superior thyroid, ascending pharyngeal, occipital, posterior auricular, lingual, and facial) and two terminal branches (superficial temporal and maxillary).

The **facial artery** provides the majority of the blood to the face. It consists of a **superior labial** and **inferior labial artery** that is responsible for supplying blood to the superior and inferior lips, respectively. Near the level of the nostrils the facial artery bifurcates into a smaller **lateral nasal** and a larger terminating **angular artery**. The angular artery will continue to ascend up the lateral side of the nose and form the **dorsal nasal artery.** The dorsal nasal artery forms an anastomosis with the supraorbital and supratrochlear arteries (branches of the ophthalmic artery which itself originated from the ICA). This represents an indirect connection between branches of the ECA and ICA **(Fig. 7.33; Fig. 7.34)**.

Table 7.1 **Muscles of the scalp, face, ear, and neck**

Region	Muscle	Function(s)
Scalp	• Occipitofrontalis (occipital and frontal bellies) • Temporoparietalis	• Elevates eyebrows; wrinkles the skin of the forehead; protracts scalp (indicates curiosity or surprise) • Assists the frontal belly, anterior and superior auricular muscles; tense fascia over temporal region
Orbit	• Orbicularis oculi (orbital, palpebral, and lacrimal parts) • Corrugator supercilii	• Closes eyelid and palpebral fissure tightly (orbital); closes eyelid gently and involves in palpebral reflex (palpebral); acts on lacrimal sac to aid in tear drainage (lacrimal) • Draws the eyebrows medially and inferiorly (show worry or concern)
Nose	• Procerus • Nasalis • Levator labii superioris alaeque nasii	• Depresses medial edge of eyebrow; wrinkles the root of the nose (show disdain or dislike) • Compresses the naris and dilates anterior nasal apertures (flaring nostrils) • Elevates the upper lip and ala of the nose; dilates anterior nasal apertures (flaring nostrils)
Mouth	• Orbicularis oris • Buccinator • Zygomaticus major • Zygomaticus minor • Risorius • Levator labii superioris • Levator anguli oris • Depressor anguli oris • Depressor labii inferioris • Mentalis	• Closes oral fissure and purses/protrudes lips (kissing) • Presses cheek against molar teeth and works with tongue to keep food between teeth during chewing; resists distension when blowing • Draws angle of mouth superiorly and laterally (smiling) • Elevates upper lip • Widens oral fissure (smiling or grimacing) • Elevates upper lip • Elevates angle of mouth • Depresses angle of mouth • Depresses lower lip • Elevates and protrudes lower lip/chin (showing doubt or indecision)
Ear	• Articularis (anterior, superior, and posterior parts)	• Protract, elevate, and retract the ear
Neck	• Platysma	• Tense skin over the anterior neck and inferior face; depress mandible

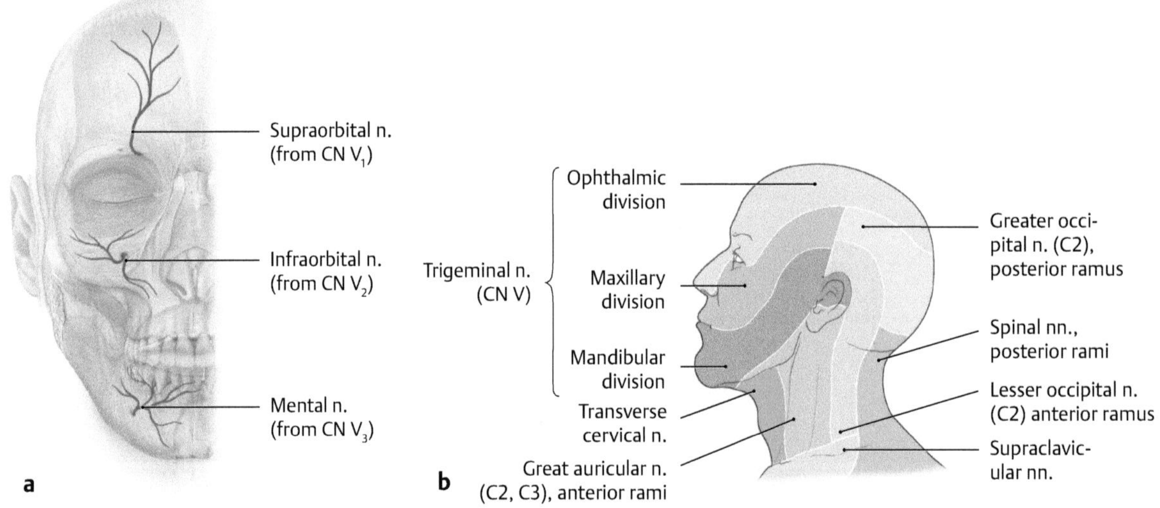

Fig. 7.27 Sensory innervation of the face. **(a)** Select sensory branches of the trigeminal nerve, anterior view. **(b)** Innervation of the head and neck, left lateral view. (From Schuenke M, Schulte E, Schumacher U. THIEME Atlas of Anatomy. Head, Neck, and Neuroanatomy. Illustrations by Voll M and Wesker K. 3rd ed. New York: Thieme Medical Publishers; 2020.)

Clinical Correlate 7.12

Sensory Nerve Blocks of the Trigeminal Nerve

An **infraorbital nerve block** would be done to anesthetize the tissue associated with the upper lip and maxillary teeth, namely the incisors. Infraorbital foramen access is obtained by elevating the upper lip and passing a needle between the border of the gingiva and oral mucosa before injecting anesthetic near the superior part of the oral vestibule. To anesthetize one side of the skin and mucous membrane of either the cheek or lower lip and chin, anesthetic is injected near the buccal and mental nerves, respectively.

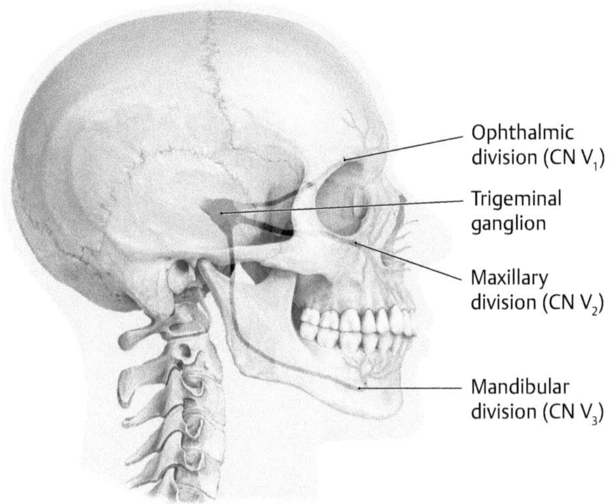

Fig. 7.28 Divisions of the trigeminal nerve (CN V). (From Schuenke M, Schulte E, Schumacher U. THIEME Atlas of Anatomy. Head, Neck, and Neuroanatomy. Illustrations by Voll M and Wesker K. 3rd ed. New York: Thieme Medical Publishers; 2020.)

Clinical Correlate 7.13

Bell Palsy

The most common cause of unilateral facial paralysis is Bell Palsy, also known as *idiopathic facial paralysis* or *facial palsy*. Its cause is unknown but gradually resolves itself over time. It is believed to be caused by a viral infection such as viral meningitis or even *herpes simplex*, which is closely associated with a common cold sore. Symptoms include facial muscle weakness and drooping of the affected side. A decrease in taste sensation along with reduced saliva and tear production on the affected side would occur.

The **superficial temporal artery** divides into a *frontal* and *parietal branch* and they supply blood to the temporal fossa and scalp. Near the level of the zygomatic arch closest to the auricle, the superficial temporal branches off the **transverse facial artery** and this artery will supply blood to the cheek and parotid gland **(Fig. 7.33; Fig. 7.34)**.

The blood supply to the scalp is found primarily in the second or "connective tissue" layer of the scalp. The *frontal* and *parietal branches of the superficial temporal, posterior auricular, occipital, supraorbital,* and *supratrochlear arteries* supply blood to the scalp.

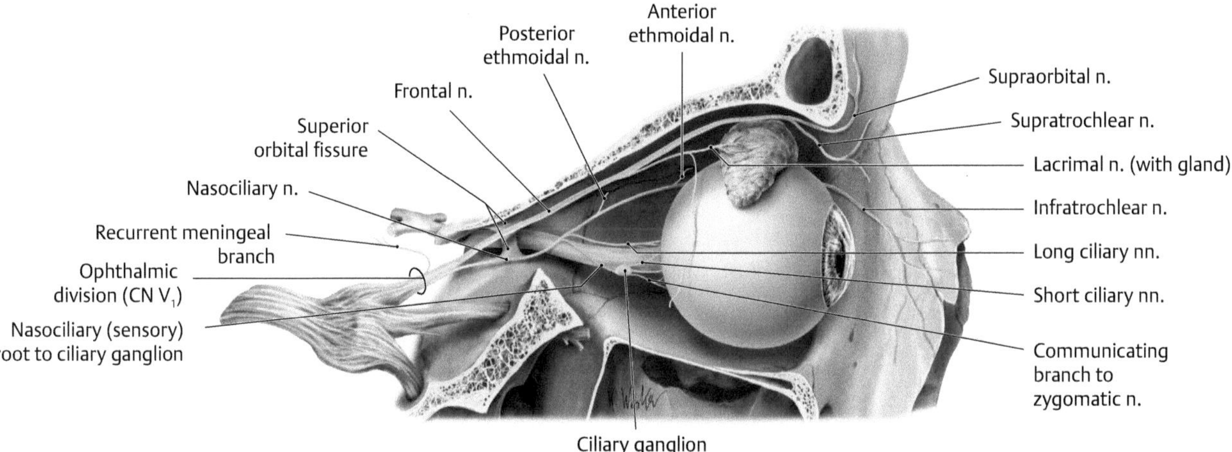

Fig. 7.29 Ophthalmic division (CN V_1). Partially opened right orbit. (From Schuenke M, Schulte E, Schumacher U. THIEME Atlas of Anatomy. Head, Neck, and Neuroanatomy. Illustrations by Voll M and Wesker K. 3rd ed. New York: Thieme Medical Publishers; 2020.)

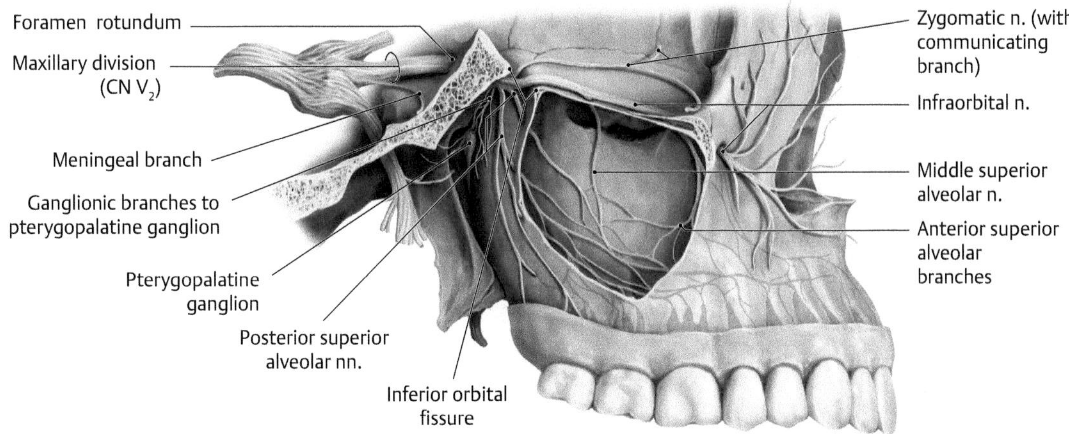

Fig. 7.30 Maxillary division (CN V_2). Partially opened right maxillary sinus with the zygomatic arch removed. (From Schuenke M, Schulte E, Schumacher U. THIEME Atlas of Anatomy. Head, Neck, and Neuroanatomy. Illustrations by Voll M and Wesker K. 3rd ed. New York: Thieme Medical Publishers; 2020.)

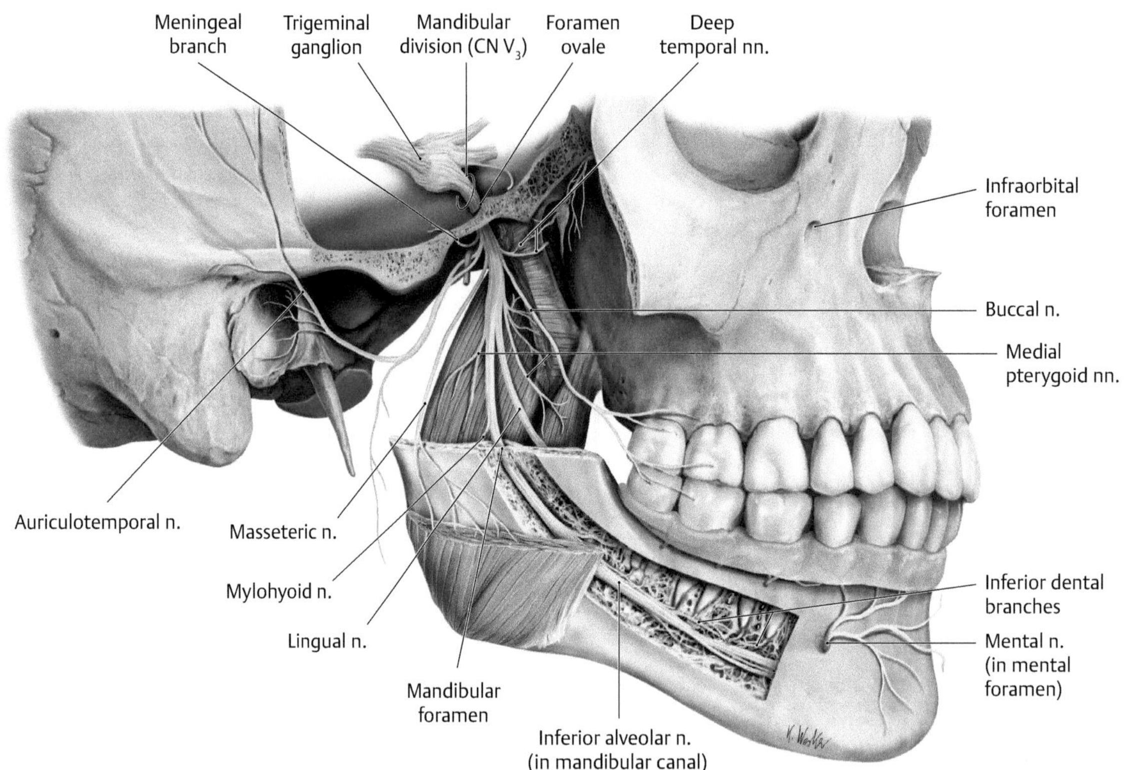

Fig. 7.31 Mandibular division (CN V_3). Partially opened mandible with the zygomatic arch removed. (From Schuenke M, Schulte E, Schumacher U. THIEME Atlas of Anatomy. Head, Neck, and Neuroanatomy. Illustrations by Voll M and Wesker K. 3rd ed. New York: Thieme Medical Publishers; 2020.)

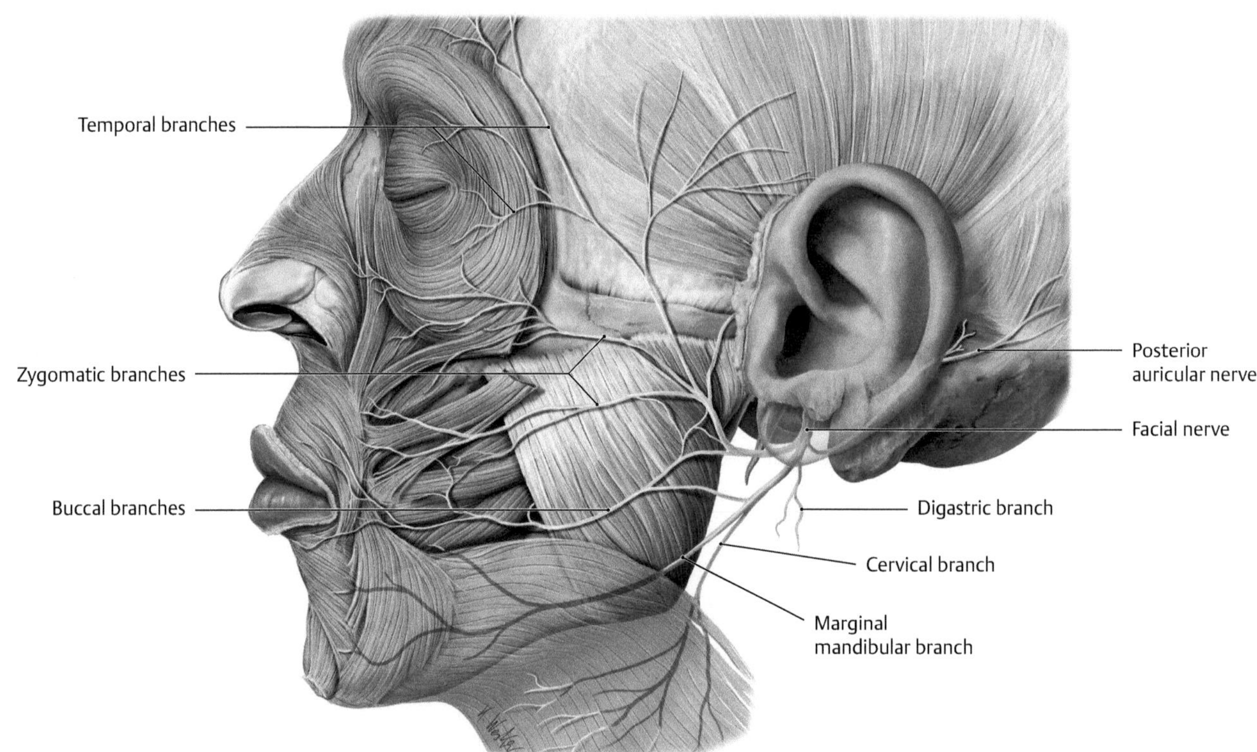

Fig. 7.32 Facial nerve branches of the parotid plexus. (From Schuenke M, Schulte E, Schumacher U. THIEME Atlas of Anatomy. Head, Neck, and Neuroanatomy. Illustrations by Voll M and Wesker K. 3rd ed. New York: Thieme Medical Publishers; 2020.)

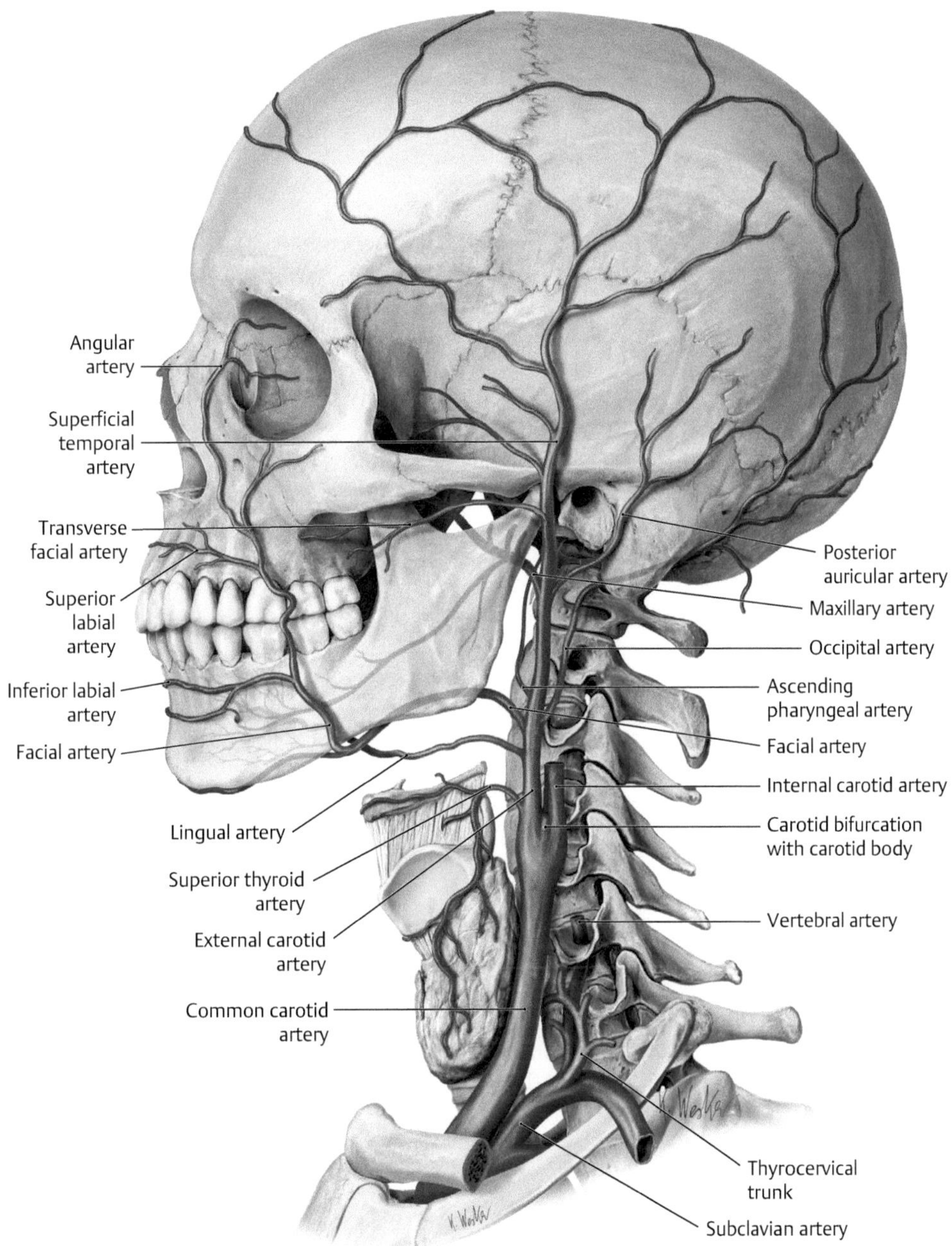

Fig. 7.33 Overview of the arteries of the head. (From Schuenke M, Schulte E, Schumacher U. THIEME Atlas of Anatomy. Head, Neck, and Neuroanatomy. Illustrations by Voll M and Wesker K. 3rd ed. New York: Thieme Medical Publishers; 2020.)

Venous drainage of the face is generally from superficial tributaries that can anastomose with a deep vein, venous plexus, or dural venous sinus. The primary superficial venous drainage of the face is by way of the valveless **facial vein**. The **angular** and facial veins communicate with the *superior/inferior ophthalmic veins* that lead to the *cavernous sinus*. The **deep facial vein**, which is a tributary of the facial vein, drains to the *pterygoid venous plexus* located in the infratemporal fossa. The *superficial temporal* and *maxillary veins* come together and form the **retromandibular vein**. This vein is generally found posterior to the mandibular ramus, deep to the facial nerve but superficial to the external carotid artery, and coursing through the substance of the parotid gland. The *posterior auricular vein* and the **posterior tributary of the retromandibular vein** form the **external jugular vein (EJV)**. The *facial vein* and **anterior tributary of the retromandibular vein** form the **common facial vein** which then drains into the **internal jugular vein (IJV)**. This venous drainage is highly variable and at times the posterior auricular vein merely drains into the retromandibular vein while the *occipital vein* and *posterior tributary of the retromandibular vein* form the EJV (**Fig. 7.35**).

The venous drainage of the superficial scalp involves multiple veins that were paired with a corresponding artery. These include the **occipital**, **superficial temporal**, **posterior auricular**, **supraorbital,** and **supratrochlear veins**. The posterior auricular and occipital veins may receive a *mastoid emissary vein* from the *sigmoid (dural venous) sinus*. Deeper aspects of the scalp's temporal

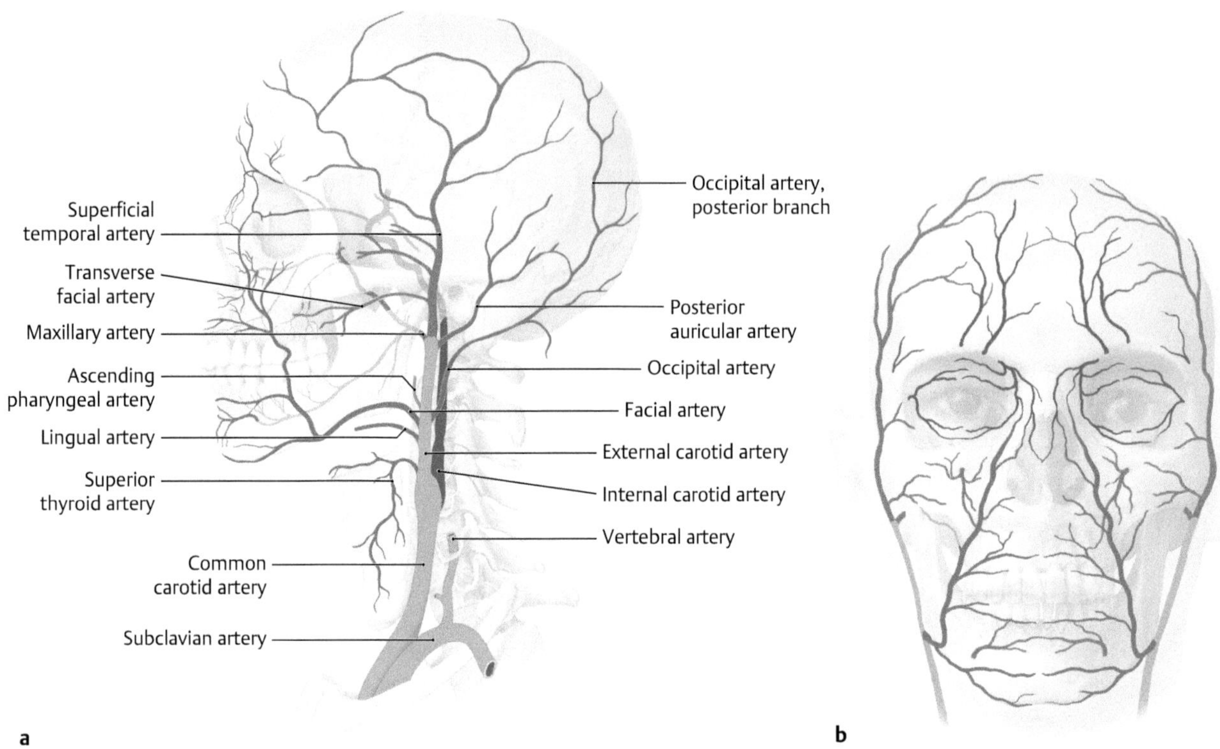

Fig. 7.34 **(a)** Branches of the external carotid artery, left lateral view. **(b)** Extracerebral branches of the internal carotid supplying the orbit are shown in blue. (From Schuenke M, Schulte E, Schumacher U. THIEME Atlas of Anatomy. Head, Neck, and Neuroanatomy. Illustrations by Voll M and Wesker K. 3rd ed. New York: Thieme Medical Publishers; 2020.)

region will drain to the **deep temporal veins** which are tributaries of the *pterygoid venous plexus*.

Emissary veins connect or establish a communication with superficial scalp veins through the skull to the dural venous sinuses. They generally flow away from the brain although flow in either direction is possible. These valveless veins vary in total number, many of which are unnamed and some of which serve as venous plexuses. These veins are clinically important because they may allow for bacteria from the scalp to enter the skull and infect the meningeal layers resulting in *meningitis*. These emissary veins include **(Fig. 7.5; Fig. 7.36)**:

- **Frontal emissary**: passes through the *foramen cecum* connecting the superior sagittal sinus with the veins of the frontal sinus and nasal cavities.
- **Parietal emissary**: passes through the *parietal foramen* and connects with the superior sagittal sinus.
- **Condyloid emissary**: passes through the *condyloid canal* and connects the sigmoid sinus with the suboccipital venous sinus.
- **Mastoid emissary**: passes through the *mastoid foramen* and connects the sigmoid sinus with the occipital vein or posterior auricular vein.
- **Venous plexuses**: a venous plexus found in the *hypoglossal canal* connecting the occipital sinus with the IJV. A venous plexus found in the *foramen ovale* connects the cavernous sinus with the pterygoid venous plexus.

Diploic veins communicate with the scalp and dural venous sinuses by way of the emissary veins. This serves as an additional route for the spread of an infection. The diploic veins are valveless and located between the external and internal layers of cranial compact bone. There are four major diploic veins located bilaterally **(Fig. 7.5; Fig. 7.37)**:

1. **Frontal diploic**: drains the anterior portion of the frontal bone into the superior sagittal sinus and supraorbital vein.
2. **Anterior temporal diploic**: drains the posterior portion of the frontal and anterior portions of the temporal and parietal bones into the temporal veins and the sphenoparietal sinus.
3. **Posterior temporal diploic**: drains the posterior portions of the temporal and parietal bones into the sigmoid sinus, transverse sinus, and mastoid emissary vein.
4. **Occipital diploic**: drain the occiput into the confluence of sinuses, transverse sinus, mastoid emissary, and occipital veins.

7.4.3 Lymphatic Drainage of the Scalp, Superficial Face, and Neck

A general principle with lymphatics of the scalp, face, and neck is that they will drain from a superior to inferior and superficial to deep direction, eventually reaching the *deep cervical lymph nodes* located near the IJV. There are no lymph nodes in the scalp and only a few located in the buccal and parotid regions of the face but there are numerous lymphatic vessels in these two regions. The lymph nodes serving the scalp and face regions form a *superficial ring/pericervical collar of lymph nodes*. These lymph nodes are named according to the region they serve and include the **submental**, **submandibular**, **buccal**, **superficial/deep parotid**, **mastoid (retroauricular)**, and **occipital lymph nodes**. The **superficial cervical lymph nodes** include the lymph

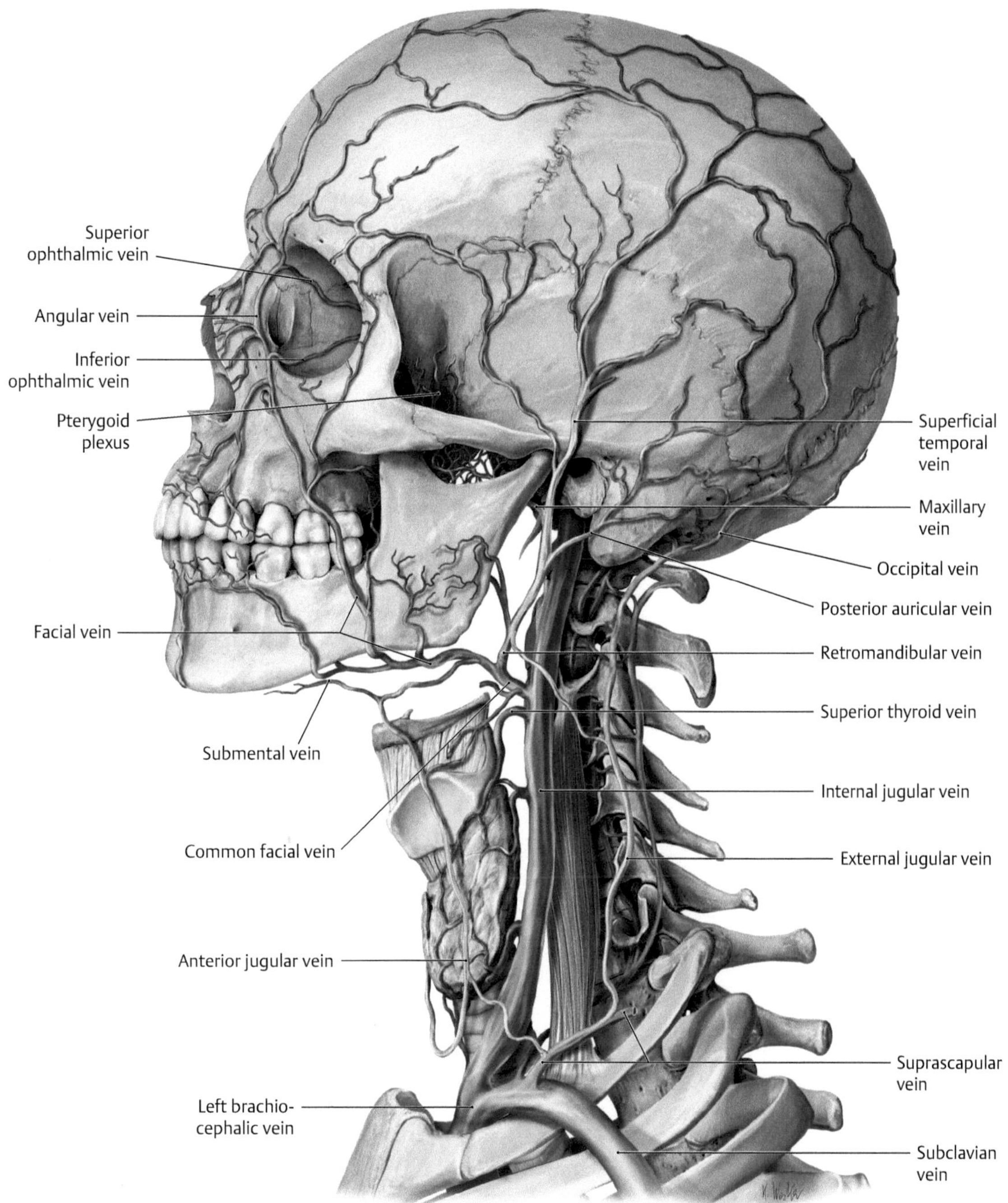

Fig. 7.35 Superficial head and neck veins and their drainage to the brachiocephalic vein. Left lateral view. (From Schuenke M, Schulte E, Schumacher U. THIEME Atlas of Anatomy. Head, Neck, and Neuroanatomy. Illustrations by Voll M and Wesker K. 3rd ed. New York: Thieme Medical Publishers; 2020.)

Clinical Correlate 7.14

Scalp Injuries

The first three layers of the scalp are clinically regarded as a single layer and are referred to as the **scalp proper**. These three layers can slide as a unit due to the loose connective tissue layer adjacent to the periosteum. Vessels supplying the scalp have little to do with the cranium; thus, removal of it would not result in any necrosis of these bones. *Scalp lacerations* result in wounds bleeding profusely because the arteries supplying the scalp bleed from both ends due to an abundant anastomotic network. The arteries will not retract because they are held open by the connective tissue of the second scalp layer. If a *superficial scalp wound* is present, the margins of the wound are held together and will not expand because of the strength of the epicranial aponeurosis. *Deep scalp wounds* will involve a laceration of the epicranial aponeurosis and will form a wide gap between the edges of laceration. The action of the occipitofrontalis muscle will prevent the wound from closing, thus necessitating suturing of the wound.

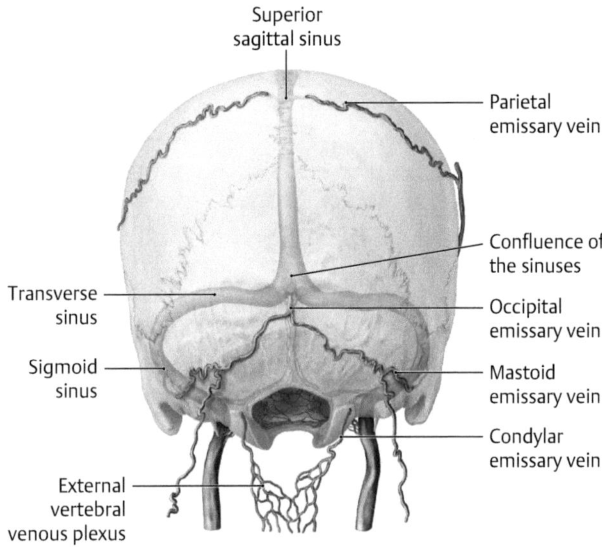

Fig. 7.36 Emissary veins of the skull. (From Schuenke M, Schulte E, Schumacher U. THIEME Atlas of Anatomy. Head, Neck, and Neuroanatomy. Illustrations by Voll M and Wesker K. 3rd ed. New York: Thieme Medical Publishers; 2020.)

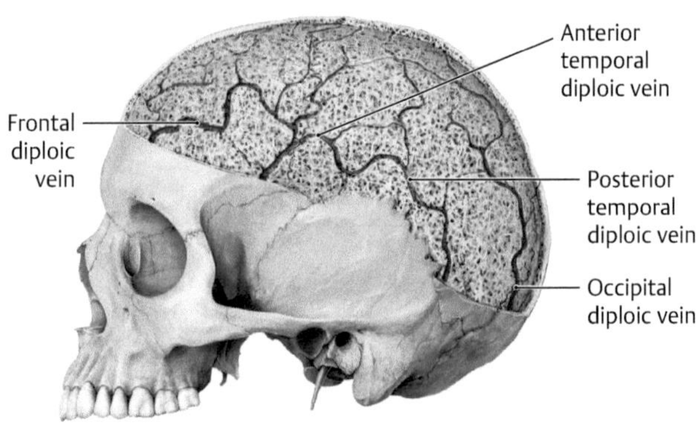

Fig. 7.37 Diploic veins in the calvaria. (From Schuenke M, Schulte E, Schumacher U. THIEME Atlas of Anatomy. Head, Neck, and Neuroanatomy. Illustrations by Voll M and Wesker K. 3rd ed. New York: Thieme Medical Publishers; 2020.)

nodes adjacent to the external jugular and anterior jugular veins (**Fig. 7.38**).

Deep cervical lymph nodes include the **superior deep cervical** and **inferior deep cervical lymph nodes** resting near the superior or inferior level of the IJV. They also include the **retropharyngeal**, **jugulodigastric**, **jugulo-omohyoid**, **infrahyoid**, **prelaryngeal**, **pretracheal**, **paratracheal**, and **supraclavicular lymph nodes**.

7.4.4 Parotid Gland

The **parotid gland** rests within the parotid region of the superficial face. The boundaries of the parotid region include (**Fig. 7.39**):

- Mandibular ramus (medially).
- Anterior border of the masseter muscle (anteriorly).
- External ear and anterior border of sternocleidomastoid muscle (posteriorly).
- Zygomatic arch (superiorly).
- Angle and inferior border of mandible (inferiorly).

Contents of the parotid region include:

- Parotid gland.
- Parotid duct.
- Parotid plexus (of CN VII).
- Masseter muscle.
- External carotid artery.
- Retromandibular vein.

The parotid gland is the largest of the three paired salivary glands and is enclosed by a tough fascial capsule known as the **parotid sheath**. This sheath originates from the *investing layer of deep cervical fascia*. The *apex* of the gland is located posterior to the angle of the mandible while the *base* is associated with the zygomatic arch. The parotid gland's unusual shape is due to how it rests on the **parotid bed**. This bed region is located between the anteroinferior aspect of the external acoustic meatus, mastoid process, and mandibular ramus. Fatty tissue between the "lobes" of the gland allows for flexibility when there is movement of the mandible. Adipocytes increase within the parotid tissue as we become older. An **accessory parotid gland** may be present lying on the masseter muscle between the zygomatic arch and parotid duct. Smaller connections to the parotid duct allow this accessory gland to release.

The **parotid (Stensen) duct** courses horizontally from the anterior border of the gland, and after passing the anterior border of the masseter muscle turns in medially and pierces the buccinator muscle to enter the oral cavity at the level of the upper second molar tooth. A *sialolith* or *salivary calculi*, a calcified mass that prevents the secretion of saliva rarely blocks the parotid duct.

7.4.5 Neurovasculature of the Parotid Gland

Secretomotor innervation of the parotid gland involves parasympathetic fibers coursing through branches of two different cranial nerves. Para/pre fibers destined for the parotid gland originate from the **inferior salivatory nucleus of the brainstem** and follow the **tympanic nerve of CN IX** to the **tympanic plexus** located on the promontory of the middle ear cavity. No synapse occurs at this plexus but the para/pre fibers will continue through the **lesser petrosal nerve**, pass through the *foramen ovale*, and finally synapse at the **otic ganglion** resting against the mandibular nerve (V_3). Para/post fibers then pass through the **auriculotemporal nerve**, a branch of V_3, to finally reach the parotid gland (**Fig. 7.40**).

The GSA fibers of the auriculotemporal nerve along with the great auricular nerve (cervical plexus branch) innervate the surrounding skin and parotid sheath. Sym/post fibers that were part of the periarterial plexus wrapped around the external carotid artery, along with the sym/post fibers that can course through the auriculotemporal nerve, vasoconstrict nearby vessels, and may reduce secretion of the gland but they tend to have a larger effect on mucous secreting glands.

Blood supply to the parotid gland includes the **transverse facial** and **posterior auricular arteries** while venous drainage will pass back to the **retromandibular vein** before reaching the *external jugular vein*. Lymphatic drainage of the parotid gland is to the **parotid lymph nodes** prior to reaching the **superior deep cervical lymph nodes**.

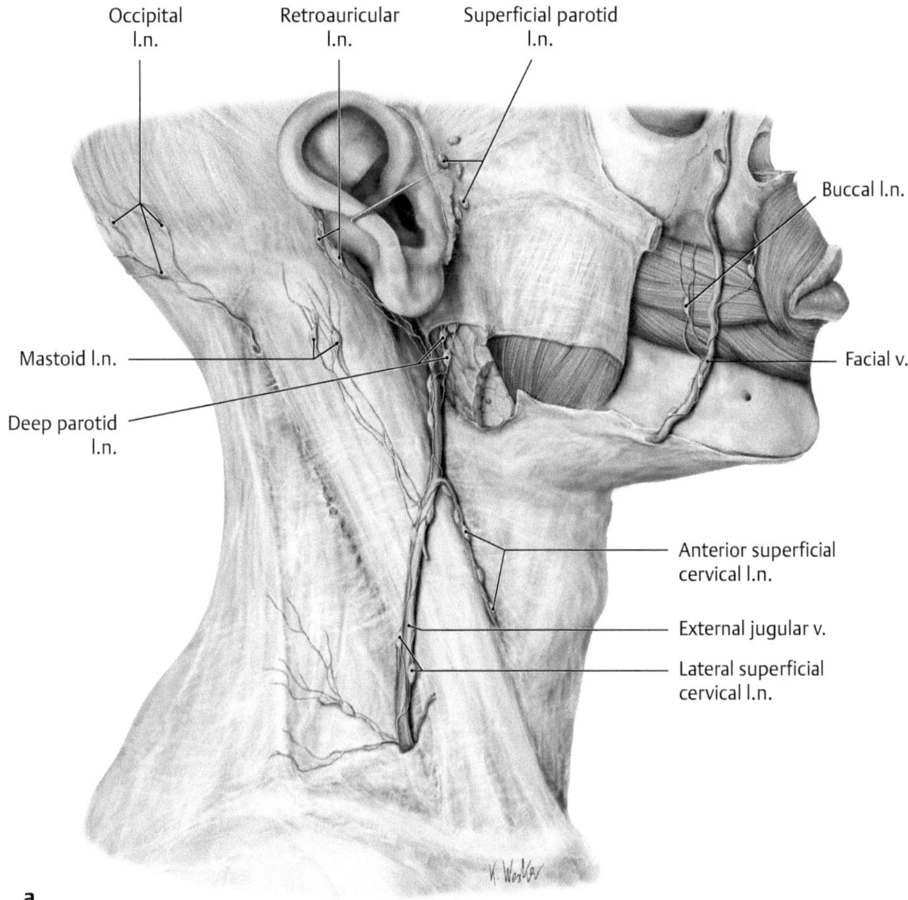

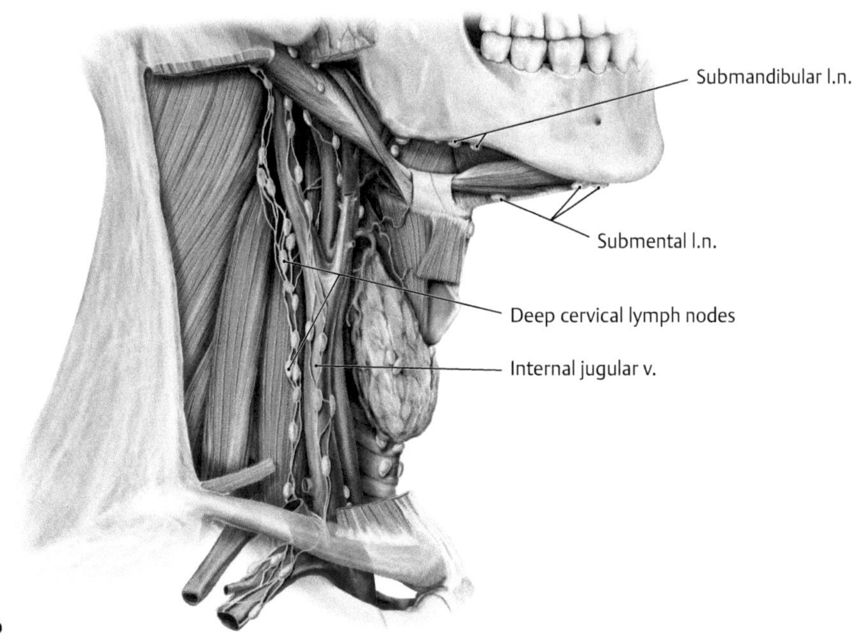

Fig. 7.38 Lymphatics of the neck. **(a)** Superficial cervical lymph nodes. **(b)** Deep cervical lymph nodes. (From Schuenke M, Schulte E, Schumacher U. THIEME Atlas of Anatomy. Head, Neck, and Neuroanatomy. Illustrations by Voll M and Wesker K. 3rd ed. New York: Thieme Medical Publishers; 2020.)

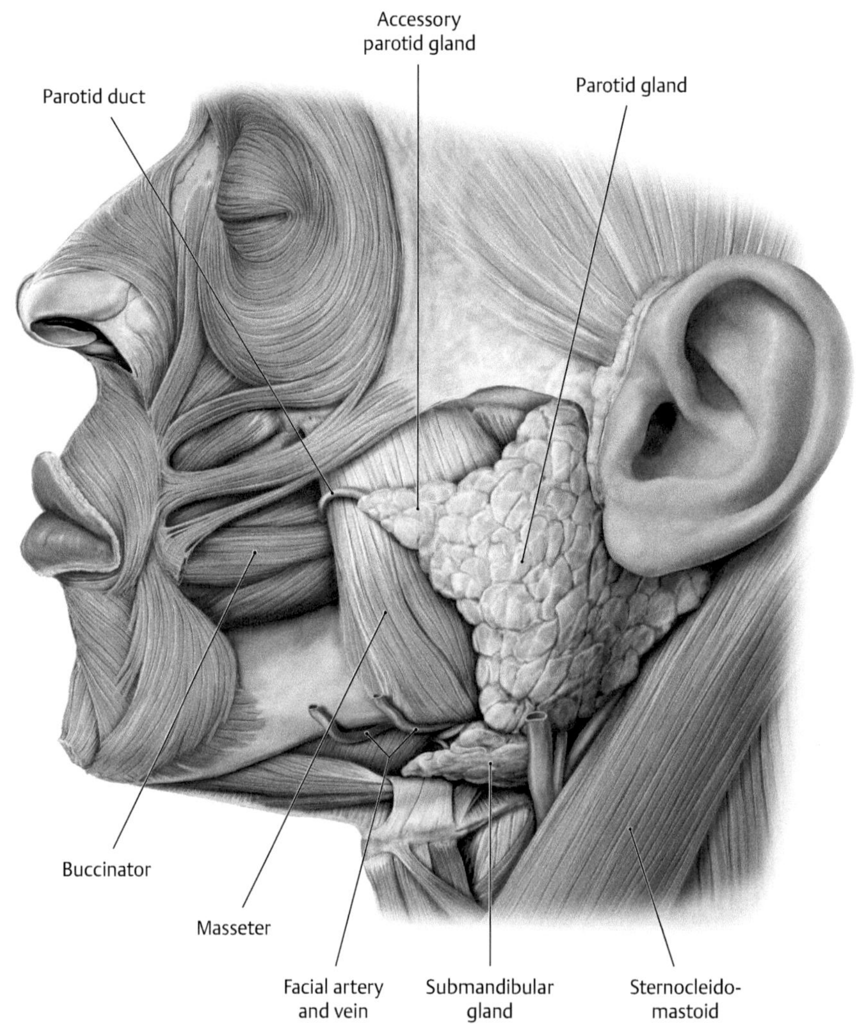

Fig. 7.39 Parotid and submandibular glands, left lateral view. (From Schuenke M, Schulte E, Schumacher U. THIEME Atlas of Anatomy. Head, Neck, and Neuroanatomy. Illustrations by Voll M and Wesker K. 3rd ed. New York: Thieme Medical Publishers; 2020.)

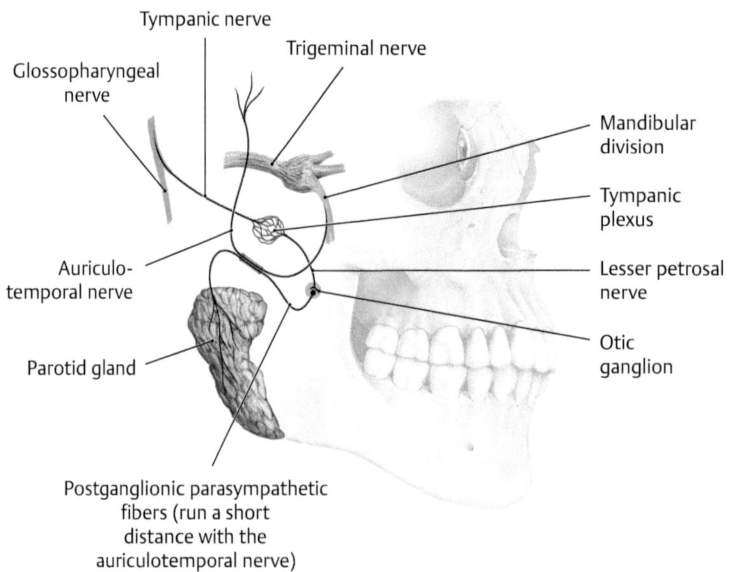

Fig. 7.40 Parotid gland innervation pathway. (From Schuenke M, Schulte E, Schumacher U. THIEME Atlas of Anatomy. Head, Neck, and Neuroanatomy. Illustrations by Voll M and Wesker K. 3rd ed. New York: Thieme Medical Publishers; 2020.)

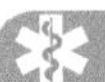 Clinical Correlate 7.15

Viral and Bacterial Infections of the Parotid Gland

Infection of the parotid gland is possible by way of the *mumps* virus. It is a contagious disease spread through coughing, sneezing, or contact with respiratory secretions such as saliva. It causes swelling of the salivary glands especially the parotid gland. Fever, headache, rash, or malaise is common in these patients. In males, a painful testicular swelling (*orchitis*) may be present, but this generally does not lead to infertility. Mumps outbreaks are generally rare because of the mumps vaccine. This vaccine is a combined measles-mumps-rubella (MMR) inoculation and has been used in its combined form since 1971. The first dose of the MMR vaccine is administered to children around their first birthday, with the second dose being administered prior to them starting school.

Poor dental hygiene could lead to a *bacterial infection* of the parotid gland producing an abscess and pus formation. The infection spreads through the parotid duct to reach the glandular tissue. If a diseased parotid gland is suspected, a cannula can be inserted through the opening of the parotid duct within the oral cavity and a radiopaque fluid (contrast medium) will be injected. This is known as *sialography* and a conventional X-ray for observation will follow it.

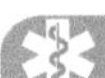 Clinical Correlate 7.16

Parotid Gland Tumors

Parotid gland cancer accounts for 70% of all salivary gland cancers. In general, most salivary gland tumors are benign and treated with surgery. The most common benign tumor is a *pleomorphic adenoma* (~70%) while the most common malignant tumor is known as a *mucoepidermoid carcinoma*. A procedure known as a *parotidectomy* is the surgical excision of the parotid gland. This procedure involves the identification, dissection of surrounding tissue, and isolation of the parotid plexus of the facial nerve while removing diseased tissue. If care is not taken in preserving the parotid plexus, an individual could have extensive paralysis of the ipsilateral facial expression muscles.

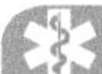 Clinical Correlate 7.17

Gustatory Sweating

Gustatory sweating (*Frey* or auriculotemporal syndrome) can be a side effect following the opening of the parotid sheath (capsule) during a surgical procedure or even trauma. It is believed that abnormal innervation of sweat glands on the face has occurred due to the regrowth of parasympathetic fibers that previously innervated the parotid gland. Hence, at the area of trauma or surgical intervention, an individual could have sweating, redness, and warmth of the face as a result of salivary stimulation due to smell or taste of food. There is no effective treatment, but symptoms can be managed with an auriculotemporal nerve avulsion or injection of botulinum toxin A (Botox®).

7.5 Temporal and Infratemporal Fossae

7.5.1 Temporal Fossa

The **temporal fossa** is the region occupied primarily by the superior portion of the *temporalis muscle*. The boundaries of the temporal fossa include (**Fig. 7.41**):

- Temporal fascia of the temporalis muscle (roof).
- The four bones forming the pterion: frontal, greater wing of sphenoid, temporal, and parietal (floor).
- Frontal and zygomatic bones (anteriorly).
- Temporal lines (superiorly/posteriorly).
- Infratemporal crest (inferiorly).
- Zygomatic arch (laterally).

The strong temporal fascia of the temporalis muscle attaches superiorly to the superior temporal line, and as it extends down inferiorly, this fascia will split into two layers. These two layers will attach to the lateral and medial surfaces of the zygomatic arch. When the masseter muscle contracts, the temporal fascia provides resistance to the downward pressure applied to the zygomatic arch by this muscle.

7.5.2 Infratemporal Fossa

The infratemporal fossa (or deep face) is a region that communicates with the temporal fossa and is located posterior to the maxilla, deep and inferior to the zygomatic arch, and deep to the mandibular ramus. The boundaries of the infratemporal fossa include (**Fig. 7.41**):

- Mandibular ramus (laterally).
- Posterior aspect of maxilla (anteriorly).
- Inferior surface of the greater wing of the sphenoid bone (superiorly).
- Tympanic plate, mastoid process, and styloid process of temporal bone (posteriorly).
- Medial pterygoid muscle attachment at the angle of the mandible (inferiorly).
- Lateral pterygoid plate (medially).

Contents of the infratemporal fossa include (**Fig. 7.42**):

- Temporalis muscle (inferior portion).
- Lateral and medial pterygoid muscles.
- Mandibular nerve and its inferior alveolar, lingual, and buccal branches.
- Otic ganglion.
- Chorda tympani (CN VII branch).
- Maxillary artery and the majority of its branches.
- Pterygoid venous plexus.

7.5.3 Muscles of Mastication

There are four muscles of mastication and they are all innervated by branches associated with the **motor root of the mandibular nerve (CN V_3)**. The **temporalis** (majority of) and **masseter** are outside the infratemporal fossa, while the *inferior portion of the temporalis*, **lateral pterygoid** and **medial pterygoid muscles** are

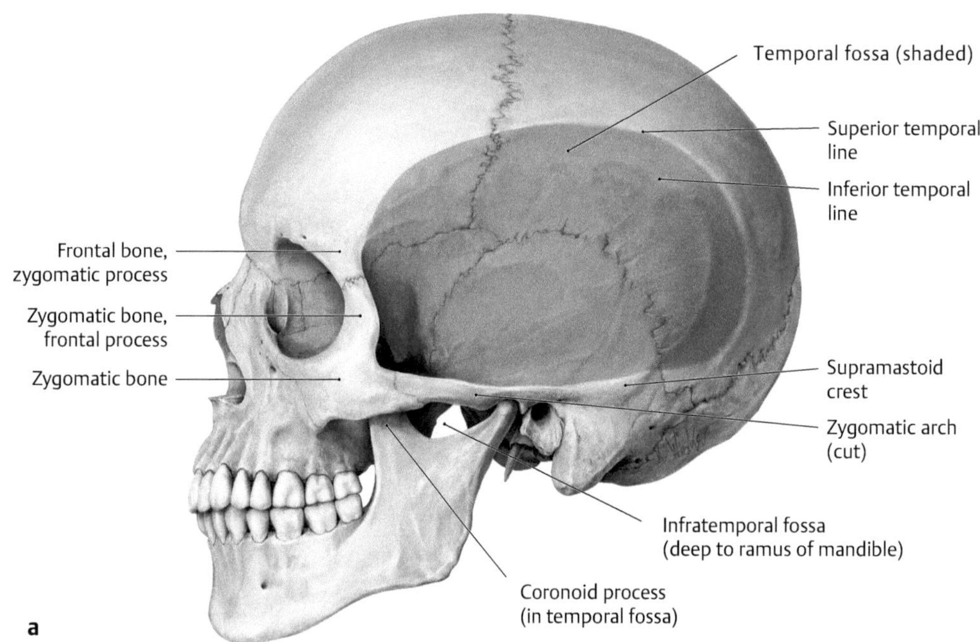

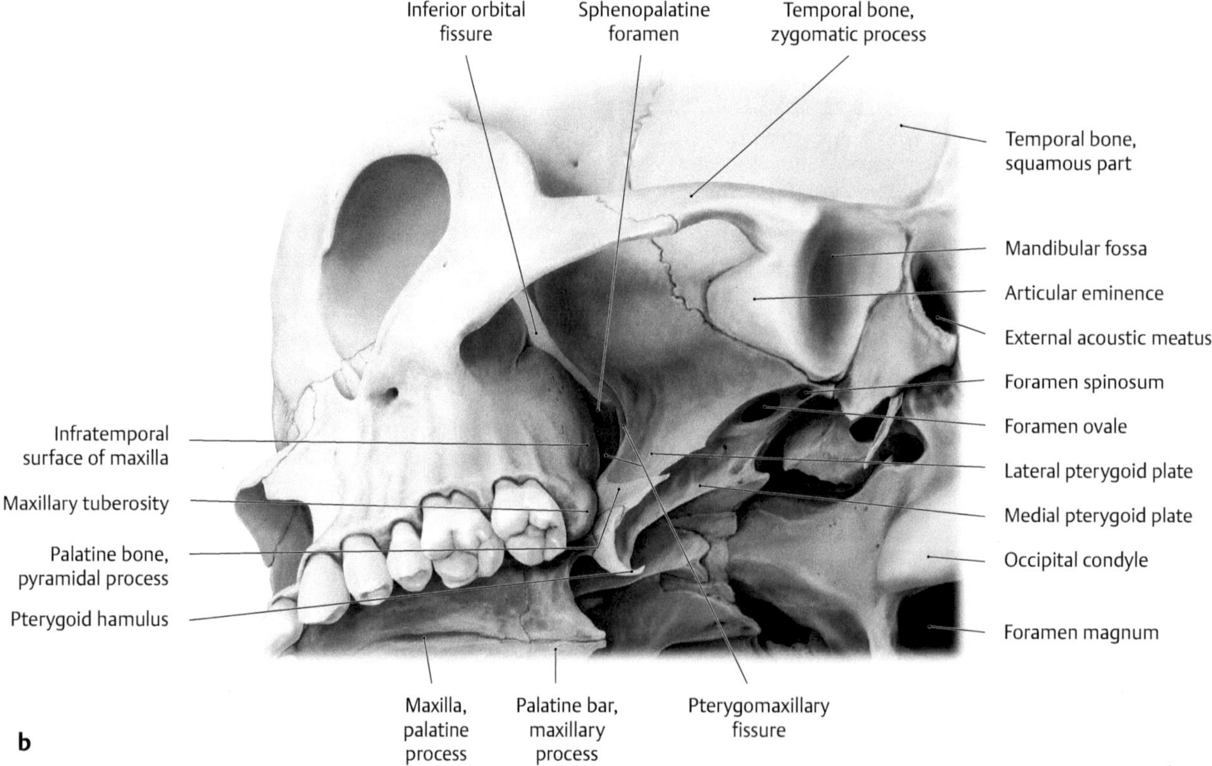

Fig. 7.41 Boundaries of the temporal fossa **(a)** and infratemporal fossa **(b).** (From Schuenke M, Schulte E, Schumacher U. THIEME Atlas of Anatomy. Head, Neck, and Neuroanatomy. Illustrations by Voll M and Wesker K. 3rd ed. New York: Thieme Medical Publishers; 2020.)

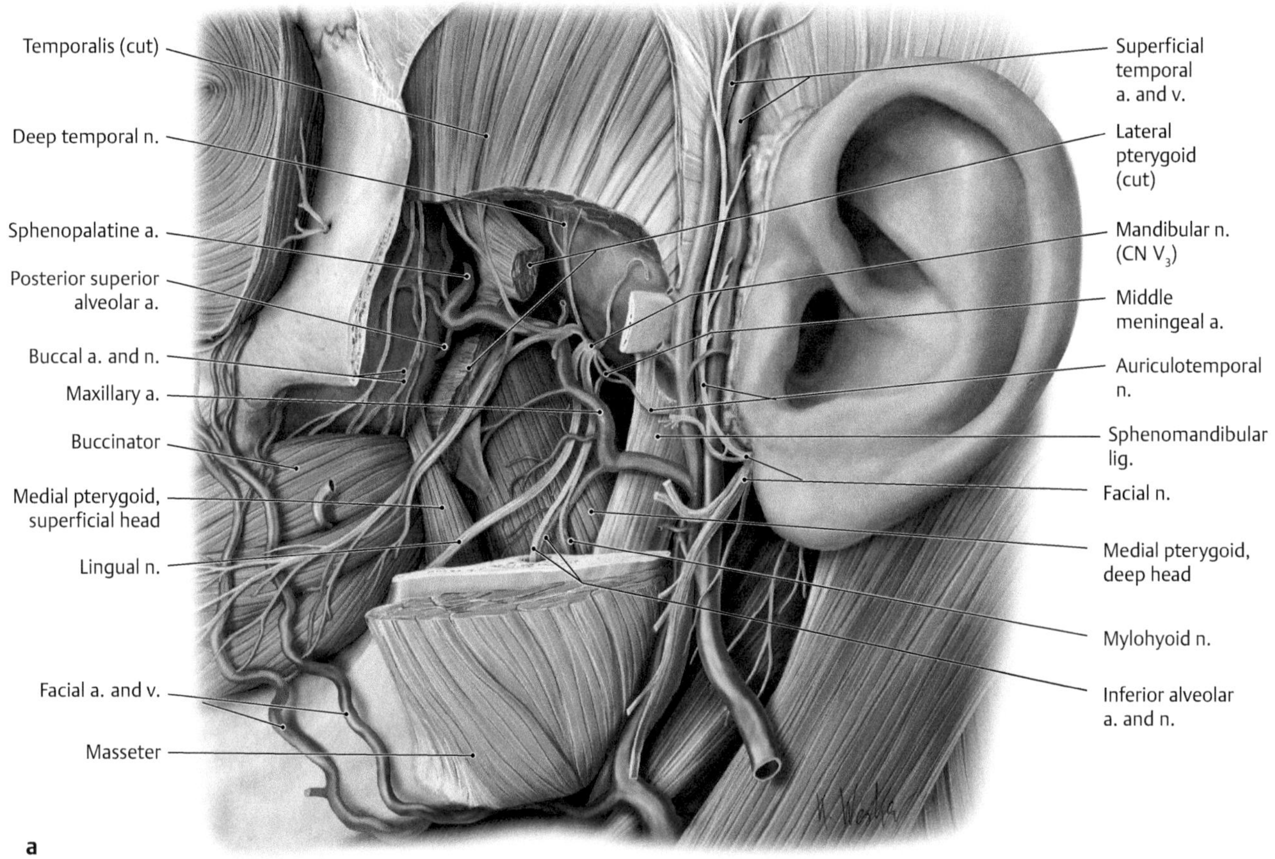

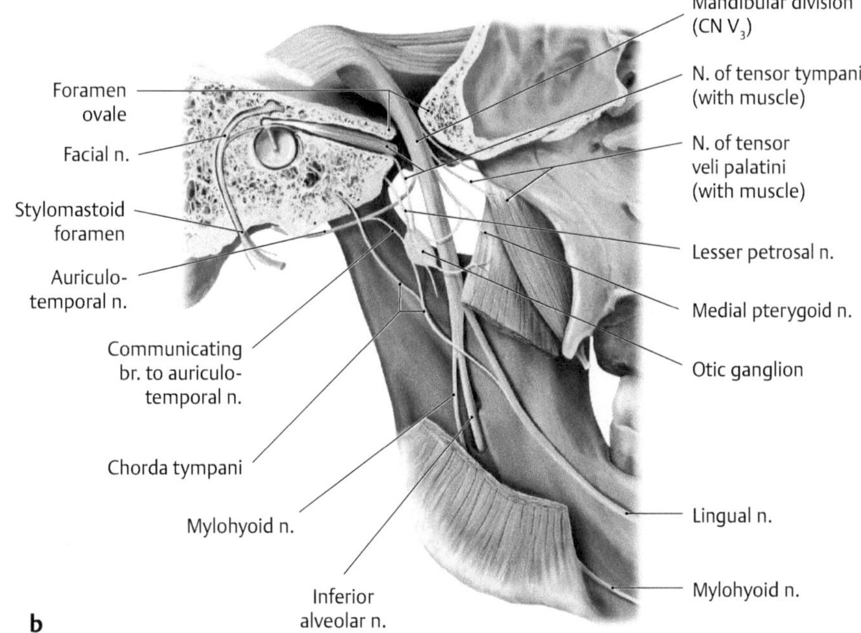

Fig. 7.42 **(a)** Contents of the infratemporal fossa. **(b)** Mandibular nerve (CN V_3) branches located in the infratemporal fossa, left medial view. (From Schuenke M, Schulte E, Schumacher U. THIEME Atlas of Anatomy. Head, Neck, and Neuroanatomy. Illustrations by Voll M and Wesker K. 3rd ed. New York: Thieme Medical Publishers; 2020.)

within the infratemporal fossa. The primary function of these muscles is to close the mouth and create a grinding action during mastication by moving the lower and upper teeth closer to one another to breakdown a food bolus. Although the lateral pterygoid muscle depresses or opens the mandible, gravity plays a larger role in opening one's mouth (**Fig. 7.43**). The description of the muscles of mastication is found in **Table 7.2**.

7.5.4 Temporomandibular Joint

The **temporomandibular joint (or TMJ)** is a modified *hinge-type synovial joint* that allows for *gliding* (translation), *hinge* and *pivoting movements*. The articulating surfaces include the *mandibular fossa* and the *articular tubercle* of the temporal bone along with the *head of the mandible*. The **fibrous layer of the joint capsule** is loose, allows for movement in three different planes, and attaches around the head of the mandible and near the articular and postglenoid tubercles. The **lateral ligament (TMJ ligament)** is a thickened portion of the joint capsule that strengthens the joint laterally and along with the postglenoid tubercle prevents posterior dislocation of the mandible (**Fig. 7.44**).

Deep to the joint capsule, an **articular disk** made of fibrocartilage, separates the articulating surfaces of the temporal bone and mandible into a **superior** and **inferior joint compartments.**

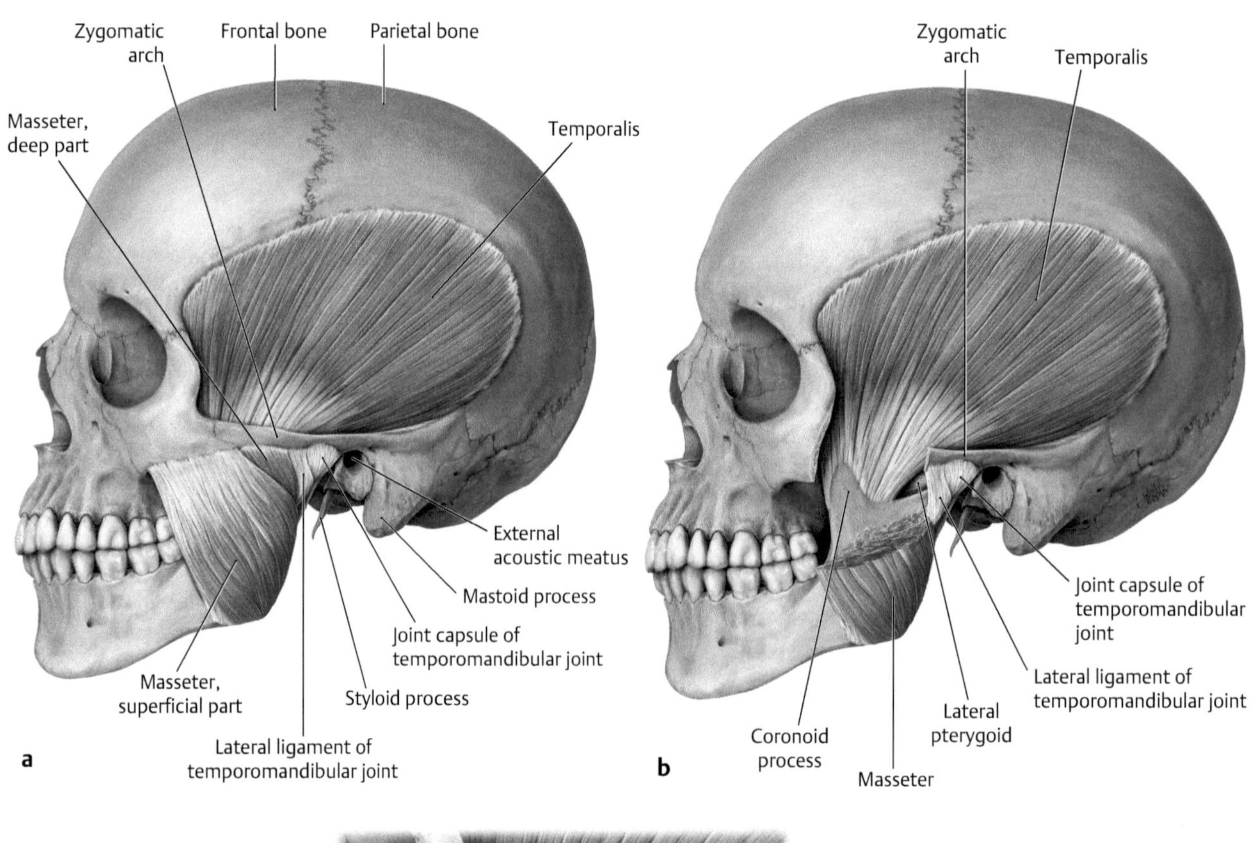

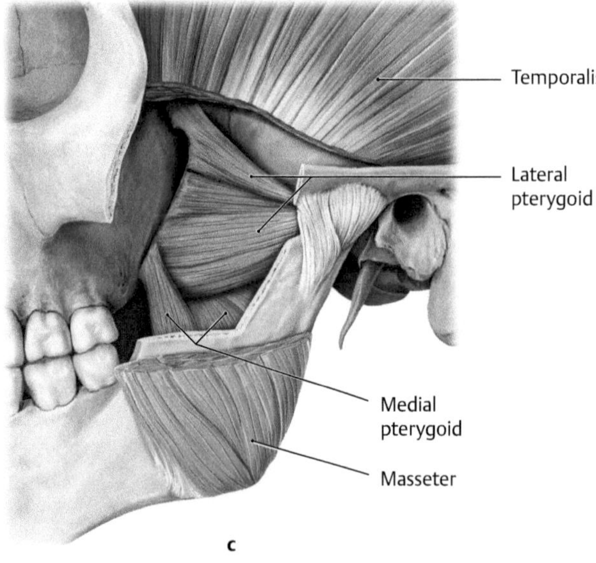

Fig. 7.43 Muscles of mastication. **(a)** Left lateral view. **(b)** Left lateral view with full temporalis muscle exposure. **(c)** Coronoid process of mandible removed to expose the lateral and medial pterygoid muscles. (From Schuenke M, Schulte E, Schumacher U. THIEME Atlas of Anatomy. Head, Neck, and Neuroanatomy. Illustrations by Voll M and Wesker K. 3rd ed. New York: Thieme Medical Publishers; 2020.)

Table 7.2 **Muscles of mastication**

Muscle	Function(s)	Origin	Insertion
Temporalis	Elevates (closes) and retracts mandible (posterior fibers)	Temporal fossa and deep surface of temporal fascia	Coronoid process and anterior border of mandibular ramus
Masseter	Elevates (closes) and protracts mandible (superficial head)	Inferior border and medial surface of zygomatic arch	Lateral surface of mandibular ramus and mandibular angle, lateral surface of coronoid process
Lateral pterygoid	Protracts and depresses (opens) mandible; swings jaw to contralateral side contributing to chewing motion (lateral deviation)	*Superior head*: infratemporal surface of sphenoid; *inferior head*: lateral surface of lateral pterygoid plate of sphenoid	*Superior head*: articular disk and joint capsule of TMJ; *inferior head*: pterygoid fovea and condylar process of mandible
Medial pterygoid	Elevates (closes) and protracts; swings jaw to contralateral side contributing to chewing motion (lateral deviation)	*Superficial head*: tuberosity of maxilla; *deep head*: medial surface of lateral pterygoid plate and pyramidal process of palatine bone	Medial surface of mandibular ramus and mandibular angle

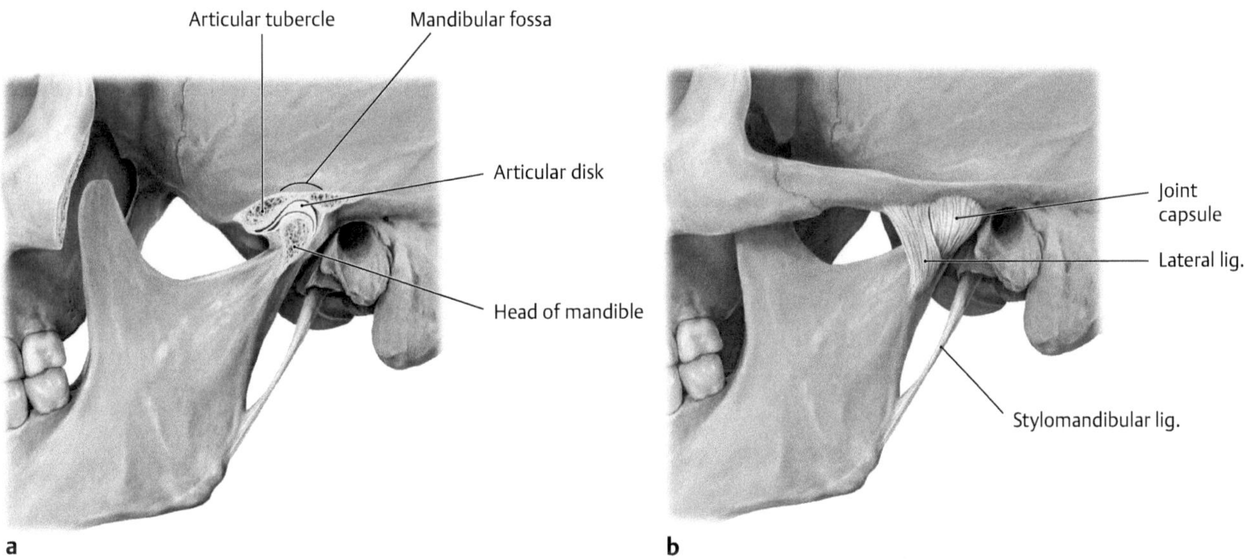

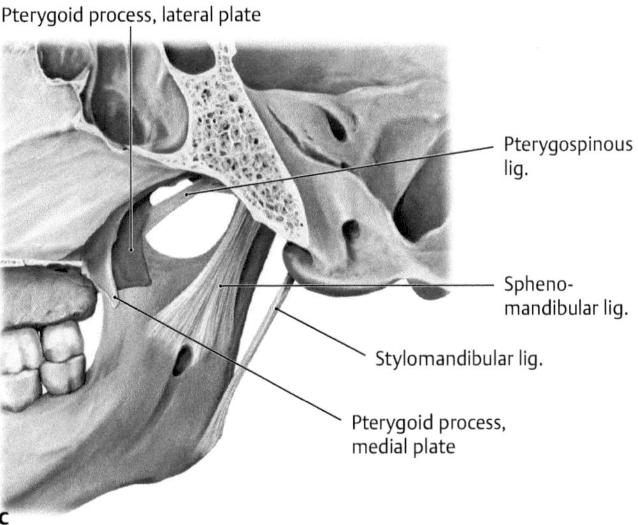

Fig. 7.44 **(a)** Opened, left temporomandibular joint (TMJ). **(b)** TMJ with associated capsule and ligaments. **(c)** Right TMJ, medial view. (From Schuenke M, Schulte E, Schumacher U. THIEME Atlas of Anatomy. Head, Neck, and Neuroanatomy. Illustrations by Voll M and Wesker K. 3rd ed. New York: Thieme Medical Publishers; 2020.)

These compartments are lined with a **superior** and **inferior synovial membrane**. The articular disk itself has attachment points with the joint capsule and the superior head of the lateral pterygoid muscle. The superior joint compartment grants gliding movements (protraction/retraction) while the inferior joint compartment allows for hinge (elevation/depression) and pivoting (side-to-side) movements. An individual may naturally open their mouth with just simple depression occurring at the inferior joint compartment. However, to open the mouth wider and at the level of the superior joint compartment, protraction of the head of the mandible and articular disk across the articular surface until the head lies up against the articular tubercle is needed **(Fig. 7.45)**. If protraction of the head and disk occurs unilaterally, the contralateral head pivots (rotates) on the inferior surface of the articular disk in the retracted position allowing for side-to-side chewing movements.

There are two minor extrinsic ligaments known as the sphenomandibular and stylomandibular ligaments. The **sphenomandibular ligament** connects the spine of the sphenoid to the lingual of the mandible. It provides passive support for the mandible and serves as a fulcrum and check ligament for movements of the mandible at the TMJ. It is derived from *Meckel cartilage*. The **stylomandibular ligament** extends from the styloid process to the angle of the mandible and is a thickening of the parotid sheath. It does not contribute much to the overall strength of the TMJ. Both of these ligaments become taut during protraction of the mandible **(Fig. 7.44)**.

7.5.5 Neurovasculature of the Infratemporal Fossa

The **mandibular nerve (CN V$_3$)** originates from the ***trigeminal ganglion*** located in the middle cranial fossa and descends through the *foramen ovale* to reach the infratemporal fossa. This nerve contains mostly GSA fibers along with SVE or BM fibers that innervate muscles of mastication among others. The major branches of the mandibular nerve include the auriculotemporal, inferior alveolar,

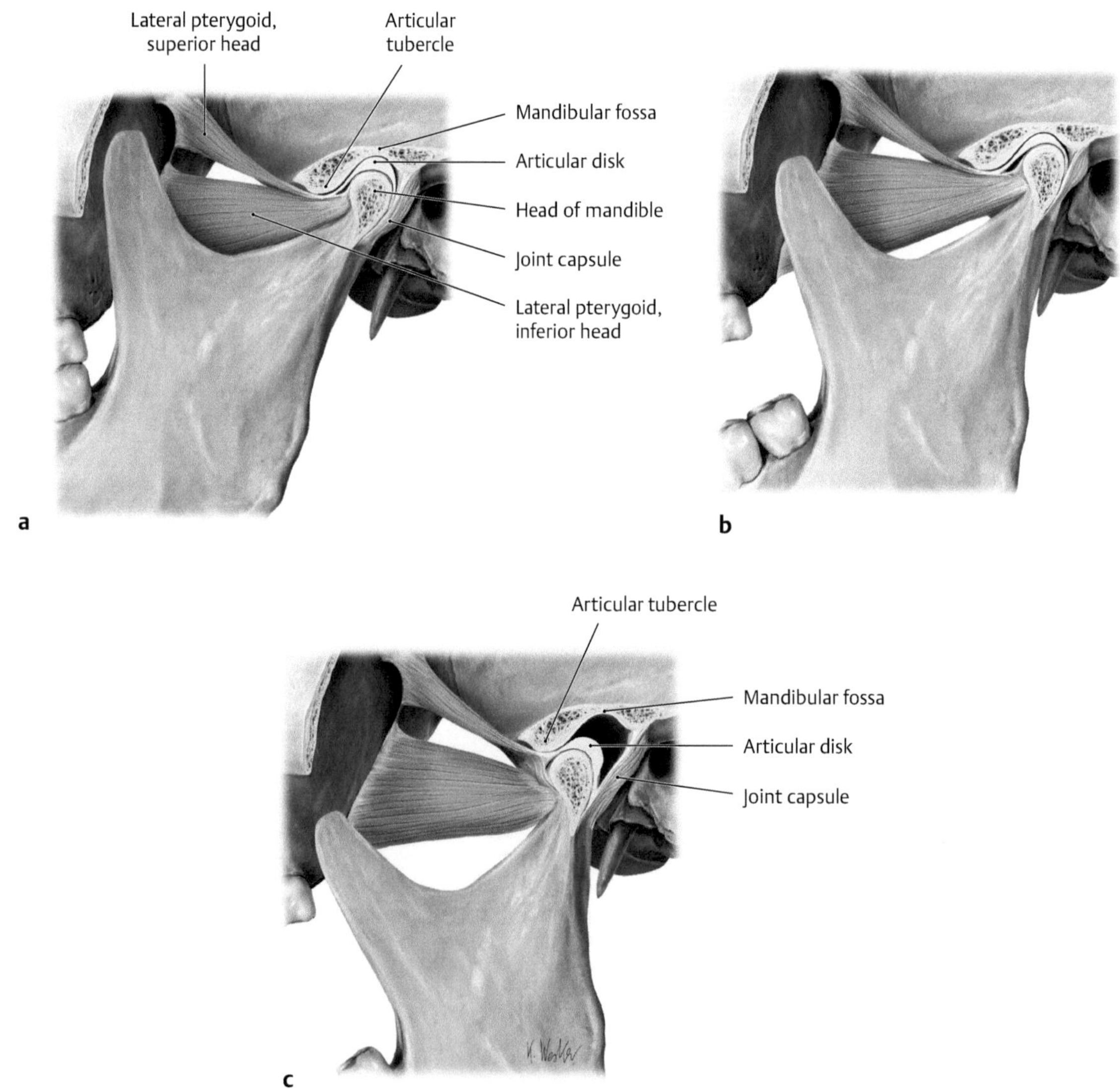

Fig. 7.45 Movement of the temporomandibular joint. **(a)** Mouth closed. **(b)** Mouth opened to 15 degrees. **(c)** Mouth opened more than 15 degrees. (From Schuenke M, Schulte E, Schumacher U. THIEME Atlas of Anatomy. Head, Neck, and Neuroanatomy. Illustrations by Voll M and Wesker K. 3rd ed. New York: Thieme Medical Publishers; 2020.)

lingual, buccal, and muscular branches. The smaller muscular branches (SVE and GSA) will innervate muscles of mastication, tensor tympani, tensor palatini, and anterior belly of digastric and mylohyoid muscles (**Fig. 7.42**).

- **Auriculotemporal nerve**: is located deep to the lateral pterygoid muscle and neck of the mandible before passing posterior to the mandible and superior to reach the external ear and temporal regions. This nerve has an initial circular portion that wraps around the *middle meningeal artery* before extending posteriorly toward the external ear. It carries GSA, GVE-para/post, and sym/post fibers responsible for innervating the skin of specific ear regions and the posterior temporal fossa, sensory of the TMJ joint, and secretomotor activity of the parotid gland.
- **Inferior alveolar**: is located anterior to the auriculotemporal nerve and passes through the mandibular foramen. Prior to entering this foramen, the **mylohyoid nerve** is given off and innervates the *mylohyoid* and *anterior belly of digastric muscles*. The inferior alveolar continues through the mandibular canal and forms the *inferior dental plexus* and terminates as the **mental nerve** as it passes through the mental foramen. The inferior alveolar nerve initially contains GSA and SVE/BM fibers but loses the BM fibers after branching off the mylohyoid nerve.
- **Lingual**: is located anterior to the inferior alveolar nerve. It passes between the medial pterygoid muscle and medial and inferior to the lower third molar tooth before reaching the tongue. Near its final extension into the mouth, the **submandibular ganglion** can be located attached to this nerve. This nerve is primarily a sensory nerve carrying GSA fibers responsible for innervating the floor of the mouth, anterior two-thirds of the tongue, and lingual gingivae. The **chorda tympani nerve** joins the lingual nerve posteriorly and contains GVE-para/pre and SVA-taste fibers (anterior two-third of the tongue).
  - The lingual nerve can be broken down into three parts with the initial portion located nearest the tongue and submandibular ganglion. It contains GSA, GVE-para/post, sym/post, and SVA-taste fibers (anterior two-third of the tongue).
  - The second portion located between the submandibular ganglion and the chorda tympani nerve attachment contains GSA, GVE-para/pre, and SVA-taste fibers (anterior two-third of the tongue).
  - The third portion located between the chorda tympani nerve attachment and foramen ovale contains only GSA fibers.
- **Buccal**: is located anterior to the lingual nerve and innervates the skin of the lower cheek, buccal gingivae, and oral mucosa of the cheek. The buccal nerve is generally thought of as carrying only GSA fibers but there may be some para/post fibers coursing through it to innervate the buccal glands.
- **Otic ganglion**: is located on the medial side of the initial mandibular nerve segment just after it passes through the foramen ovale. It is the site of GVE-para/pre fibers from the lesser petrosal nerve synapsing on the para/post cell bodies of this ganglion. The para/post fibers primarily course with the auriculotemporal nerve and target the parotid gland (**Fig. 7.42**).

The major artery of this region is the **maxillary artery** and is one of two terminal branches of the external carotid artery (superficial temporal is the other). It lies posterior to the neck of the mandible, and based on its anatomical relationship to the lateral pterygoid muscle, it is divided into three parts. These three parts of the maxillary artery will give rise to 15 individual artery branches (**Fig. 7.46**).

The **first (mandibular) part of the maxillary artery** is located proximal to the lateral pterygoid muscle, runs horizontally and deep to the neck of the mandible, but lateral to the stylomandibular ligament. It supplies blood to areas such as the ear, dura mater, periosteum, trigeminal ganglion, and mandibular teeth. It gives off five branches: the **deep auricular**, **anterior tympanic**, **middle meningeal**, **accessory meningeal**, and **inferior alveolar**.

The **second (pterygoid) part of the maxillary artery** is located either deep or superficial to the lateral pterygoid muscle and will ascend anterosuperiorly prior to becoming the third part. It supplies blood primarily to the surrounding muscles and cheek region. It gives off four branches: the **masseteric**, **pterygoid**, **deep temporal**, and **buccal**.

The **third (pterygopalatine) part of the maxillary artery** is located distal to the lateral pterygoid muscle and possibly splitting the heads of this muscle before passing through the pterygomaxillary fissure and into the pterygopalatine fossa. It supplies blood to areas such as palate, maxillary teeth, skin of the infraorbital face, nasopharynx, nasal cavity, and paranasal sinuses. The sphenopalatine branch serves as the termination of the maxillary artery. It gives off six branches: the **descending palatine**, **posterior superior alveolar**, **infraorbital**, **pharyngeal**, **artery of pterygoid canal**, and **sphenopalatine** (**Fig. 7.46; Fig. 7.70**).

The **pterygoid venous plexus** is situated between the temporalis and pterygoid muscles. This plexus is the equivalent of maxillary vein tributaries but does drain into the retromandibular vein by way of a very short maxillary vein. This plexus also forms an anastomosis with the cavernous sinus and inferior ophthalmic vein via emissary veins and also with the facial vein via the deep facial vein (**Fig. 7.47**).

7.6 Oral Cavity

The **oral cavity** is the region where food is ingested and prepared for early digestion. When food is chewed, the teeth and saliva from the salivary glands creates a manageable food bolus. The food bolus is then compressed against the palate along with movement of the bolus toward the oropharynx by tongue muscles constitutes the **first stage of deglutition (swallowing)** which is a voluntary movement.

The oral vestibule and oral cavity proper make up the two parts of the oral cavity. The **oral vestibule** is the space located between the upper/lower lips/cheeks and the upper/lower *dental arches* (or lateral edge of teeth). The **oral cavity proper** is the space medial and posterior to the upper and lower *dental arches*. The oral cavity proper has a roof (palate), floor (muscles, glands, and neurovasculature), is filled by the tongue, and extends back to the oropharynx (**Fig. 7.48**).

7.6.1 Lips and Cheeks

The **lips** are mobile, musculofibrous folds surrounding the mouth. They are covered externally by skin and internally by a mucous membrane (**Fig. 7.49**). The *orbicularis oris* is the principle muscle of the lips and they contain the *superior* and *inferior labial vessels*. They function as **oral fissure** valves and control what enters and exits the mouth, grasping of food, suckling, and contributes

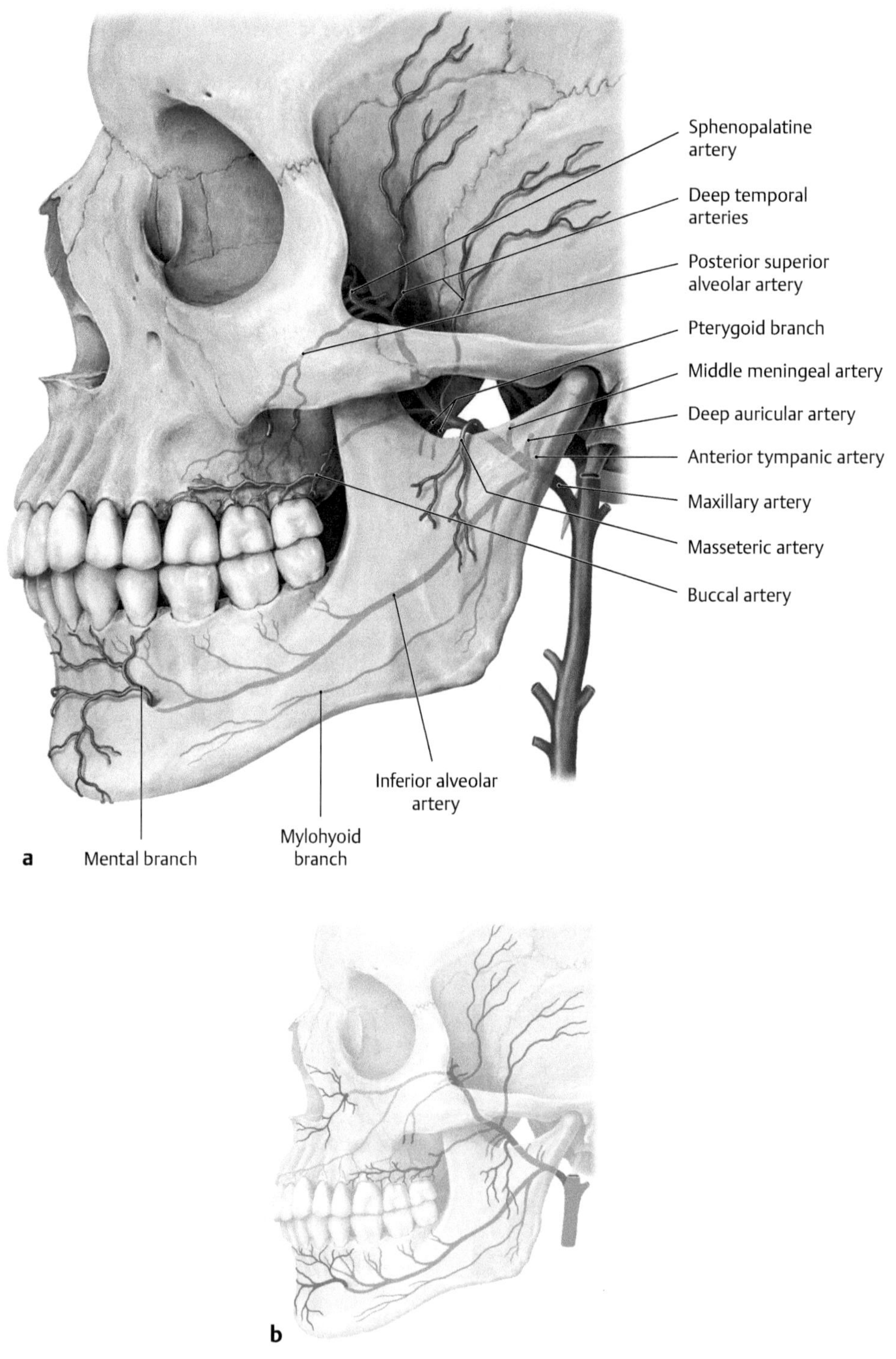

Fig. 7.46 **(a)** Maxillary artery and its branches. **(b)** Three parts of the maxillary artery: mandibular (*blue*), pterygoid (*green*), and pterygopalatine (*yellow*). (From Schuenke M, Schulte E, Schumacher U. THIEME Atlas of Anatomy. Head, Neck, and Neuroanatomy. Illustrations by Voll M and Wesker K. 3rd ed. New York: Thieme Medical Publishers; 2020.)

to speech formation. The **transitional zone of the lip** (*vermilion border*) and its reddish appearance is continuous with the labial mucosa of the inner lip. The transitional zone is clearly distinguishable from an individual's normal skin tone. The **labial frenula** are folds of mucous membrane in the midline of both lips extending from the vestibular gingiva to the mucosa of the upper and lowers (**Fig. 7.48**).

The **cheeks** are made up of skin, buccinator muscle, and oral mucosa from superficial to deep. They are the movable walls of the oral cavity and correspond with the *buccal region*. The junction of the zygomatic and buccal regions is known as the *prominence of the cheek* while the prominence of the zygomatic arch is commonly known as the *cheek bone*. The **buccinator muscle** located within the cheek is responsible for pressing the cheek against

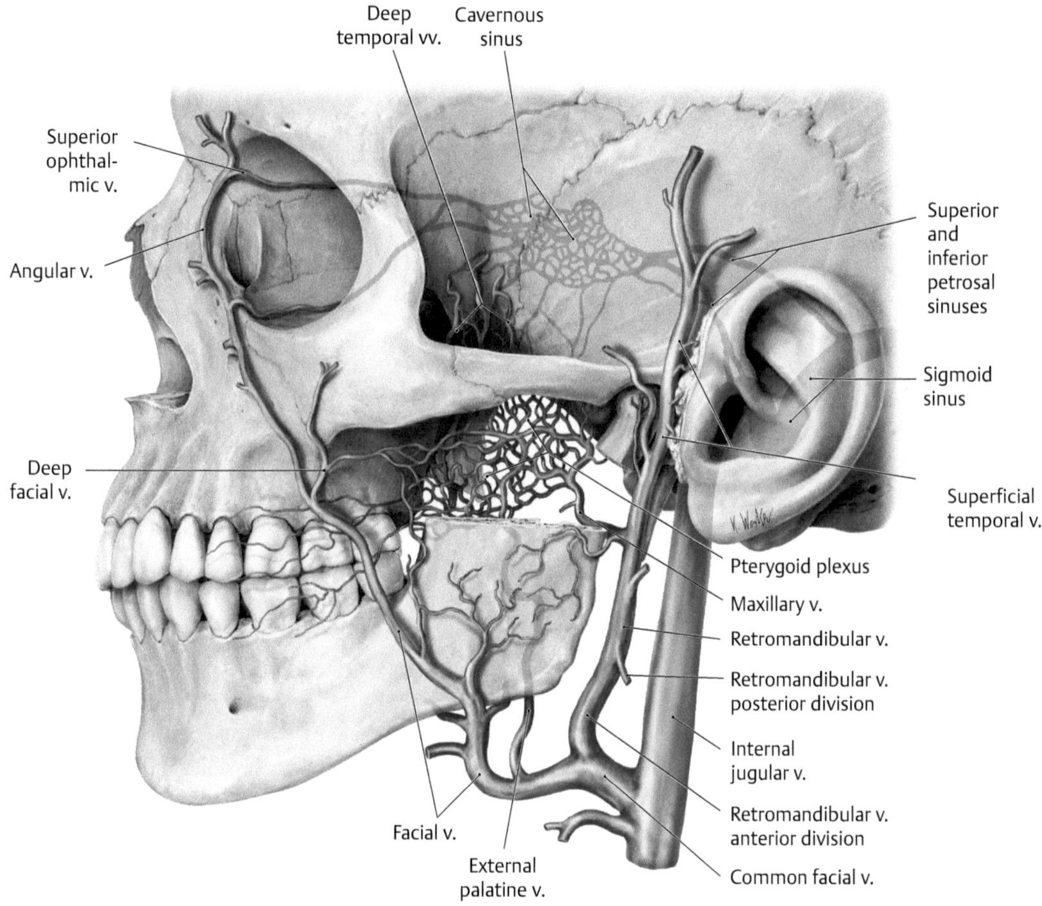

Fig. 7.47 Deep veins and pterygoid plexus of the head. (From Schuenke M, Schulte E, Schumacher U. THIEME Atlas of Anatomy. Head, Neck, and Neuroanatomy. Illustrations by Voll M and Wesker K. 3rd ed. New York: Thieme Medical Publishers; 2020.)

molar teeth and along with the tongue, keeps food between the teeth during mastication. This muscle is innervated by the facial nerve (CN VII). The **buccal fat pads**, which are larger in infants and presumably reinforce the walls of the cheek, are found superficial to the buccinator muscles. Located between the buccinator muscle and mucous membranes are the **buccal glands**.

Neurovasculature of the Lips and Cheeks

The **superior labial nerve** branches that originate from the infraorbital nerve (V_2 branch) innervate the upper lip. The **inferior labial nerve** branches originate from the mental nerve and innervate the lower lip. The superior and inferior labial vessels supply the upper and lower lips, respectively. The **superior labial artery** originates mainly from the facial artery but branches of the same name come from the infraorbital artery. The **inferior labial artery** originates primarily from the facial artery as well but branches of the same name originate from the mental artery near the chin (**Fig. 7.33**). Lymphatic drainage of the *upper lip and lateral aspect of the lower lip* drains to the **submandibular lymph nodes** while the *chin and central portion of the lower lip* drains to the **submental lymph nodes**.

The **buccal nerve** (V_3 branch) is responsible for innervating the mucous membrane and skin of the cheek region. The **buccal artery** branches originating from the maxillary artery (second part) supply blood to this region. Lymphatic drainage of the cheeks will drain to the **buccal lymph nodes** followed by the **submandibular lymph nodes** before draining to **deep cervical lymph nodes (Fig. 7.50)**.

7.6.2 Gingivae, Types of Teeth, and Dental Arches

The **gingivae**, commonly known as the *gums*, are *stratified squamous epithelium* composed of fibrous tissue covered with mucous membrane but lacking glands and a submucosa. The **gingiva proper** presents pink and keratinized and is bound tightly to the periosteum of the alveolar processes of the maxilla and mandible as well as the necks of the teeth. The gingivae proper adjacent to the cheeks is known as the superior/inferior **buccal gingiva**. Adjacent to the lips it is known as either the **maxillary (superior) labial** or **mandibular (inferior) labial gingiva**. If it is adjacent to the tongue it is known as the **maxillary (superior) lingual** and **mandibular (inferior) lingual gingiva**. The **alveolar mucosa** presents red and is the nonkeratinized, unattached gingivae.

The adult human generally has 32 teeth. **Teeth** are the small and calcified structures that function in breaking down a food bolus and assist in the pronunciation or articulation of speech. The teeth are described as being **deciduous (primary)** or **permanent (secondary)**, by the type or characteristics of the tooth, and by its proximity to the midline of the mouth. In children, there are 20 deciduous teeth that reside in the alveolar arches as

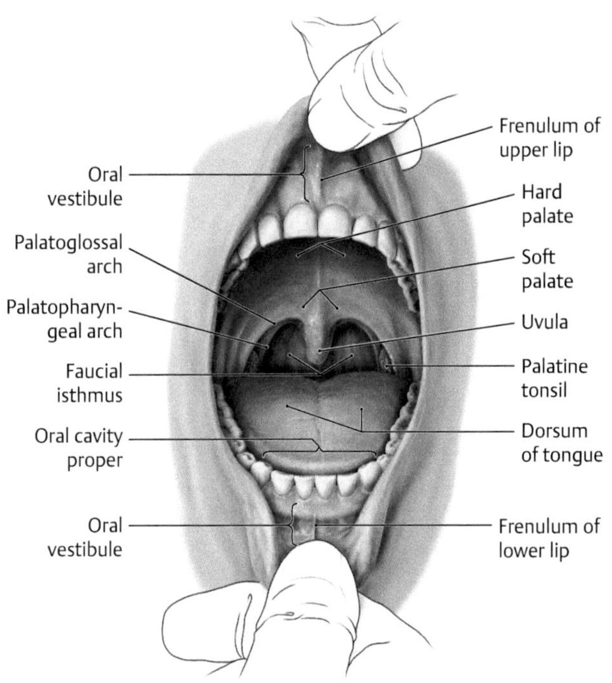

Fig. 7.48 Divisions of the oral cavity. (From Schuenke M, Schulte E, Schumacher U. THIEME Atlas of Anatomy. Head, Neck, and Neuroanatomy. Illustrations by Voll M and Wesker K. 3rd ed. New York: Thieme Medical Publishers; 2020.)

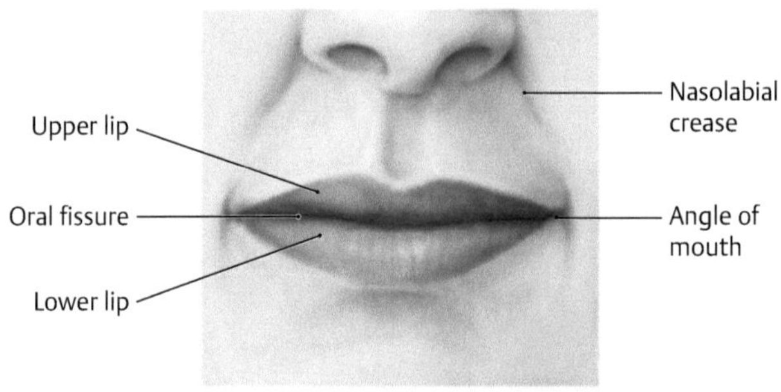

Fig. 7.49 Lips and labial creases. (From Schuenke M, Schulte E, Schumacher U. THIEME Atlas of Anatomy. Head, Neck, and Neuroanatomy. Illustrations by Voll M and Wesker K. 3rd ed. New York: Thieme Medical Publishers; 2020.)

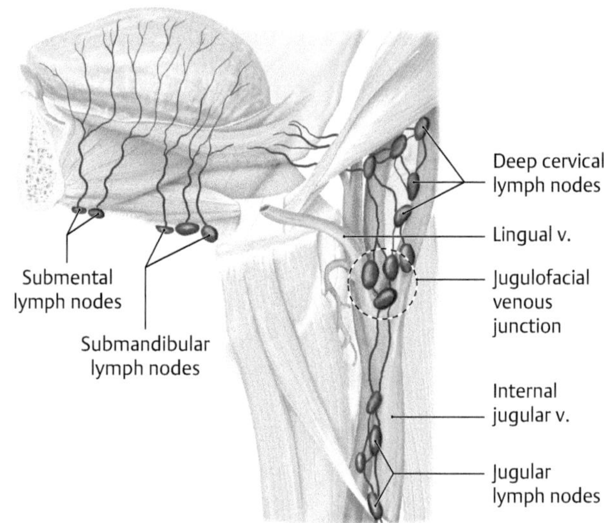

Fig. 7.50 Lymphatic drainage of the tongue and oral floor. (From Schuenke M, Schulte E, Schumacher U. THIEME Atlas of Anatomy. Head, Neck, and Neuroanatomy. Illustrations by Voll M and Wesker K. 3rd ed. New York: Thieme Medical Publishers; 2020.)

tooth buds prior to erupting into the mouth. They will be followed by the permanent teeth with all being present by the middle of the second decade of life. The permanent teeth are numbered from 1-32 with number 1 being the right third upper molar. The sequential numbering continues until the left third upper molar represents tooth number 16. Tooth number 17 is the left third lower molar with number 32 represented by the right third lower molar (**Fig. 7.51**).

The types of teeth include the **incisors** (thin cutting edges), **canines** (sharp and cone like), **premolars** (two cusps), and **molars** (three or more cusps). There are 8 incisors, 4 canines, 8 premolars, and 12 molars in total. The space between the teeth and the location of where an individual flosses is the **interalveolar septum**. The **labial surface** (of incisors and canines) and **buccal surface** (of premolars and molars) face outward toward the lips and cheeks, respectively. The labial and buccal surfaces are collectively known as *vestibular* surfaces. The **palatal surface** (of maxillary teeth) and **lingual surface** (of mandibular teeth) are directed inward toward the palate and tongue, respectively. The **mesial surface** is directed toward the anterior midline of the dental arch while the **distal surface** is directed away from the anterior midline and toward the location of the third molars. The **occlusal (top) surface** is the surface that aids in the breakdown of food (**Fig. 7.52**).

The maxillary and mandibular teeth are arranged into **dental (alveolar) arches**. The **upper (maxillary) dental arch** forms a semiellipse while the **lower (mandibular) dental arch** looks more like a parabola. When the mouth is closed the maxillary teeth are apposed to their mandibular teeth counterparts. The cusps of one tooth fit into the fissures of the two opposing teeth. Due to this arrangement, every tooth comes into contact with two opposing teeth. This is the result of the slightly greater width of the maxillary incisors. The dental arches contain the **dental alveoli (tooth sockets)** and are covered by gingivae (gums). Teeth insert into dental alveoli which themselves are located specifically in the **alveolar processes** of either the maxilla or mandible. The dental alveoli are a *fibrous syndesmosis joint* known as a **gomphosis**.

Structure and Histology of a Tooth

The principal parts of a tooth include the *crown*, *neck*, and *root*. The **crown** projects from the gingiva and is covered with enamel. The **neck** lies between the crown and root. The **root** (total number varies) begins near the *cementoenamel junction* and is fixed in the dental alveoli by the periodontium (**Fig. 7.53**). Individual roots within the dental alveoli are separated by **interradicular septa**. The **periodontium** are the tissues that invest and support a tooth and they include the gingiva, alveolar wall, cementum, and periodontal ligament.

Adult teeth consist of four structural components: *enamel*, *dentin*, and *cementum*, and a loose connective tissue filled *pulp cavity*.

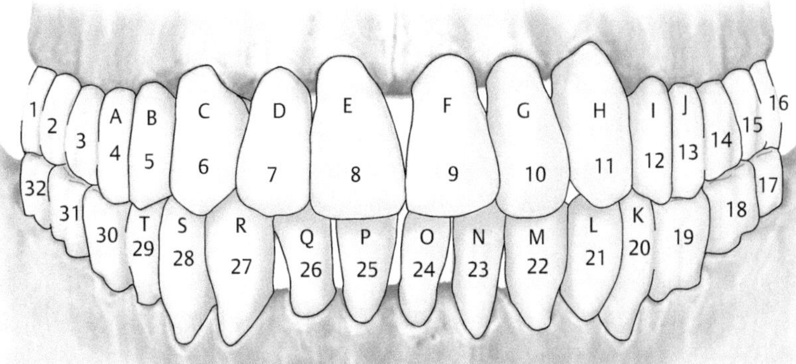

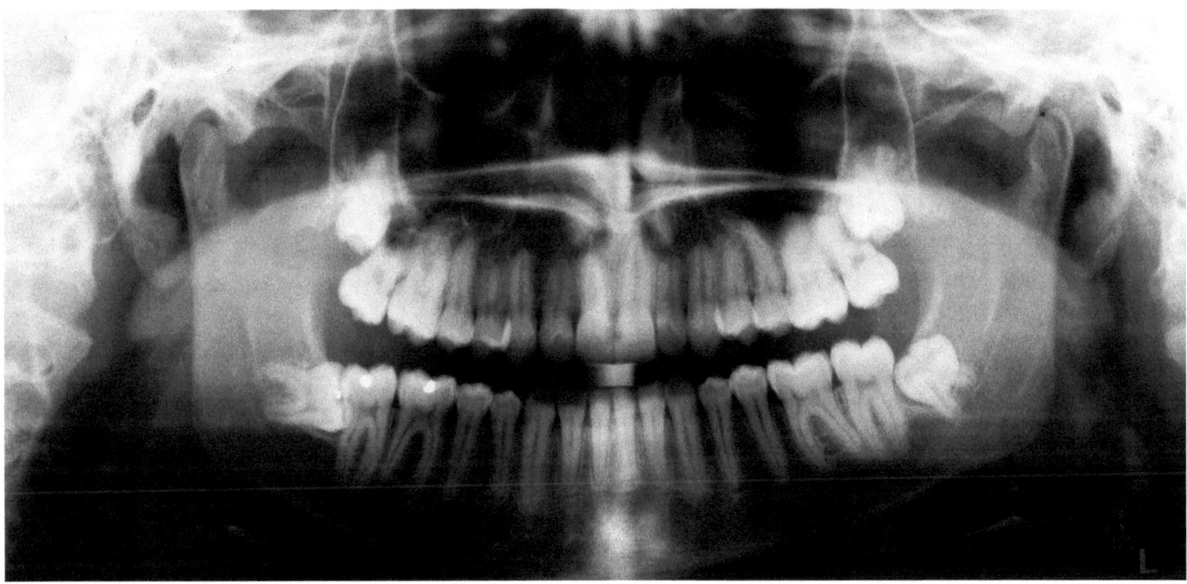

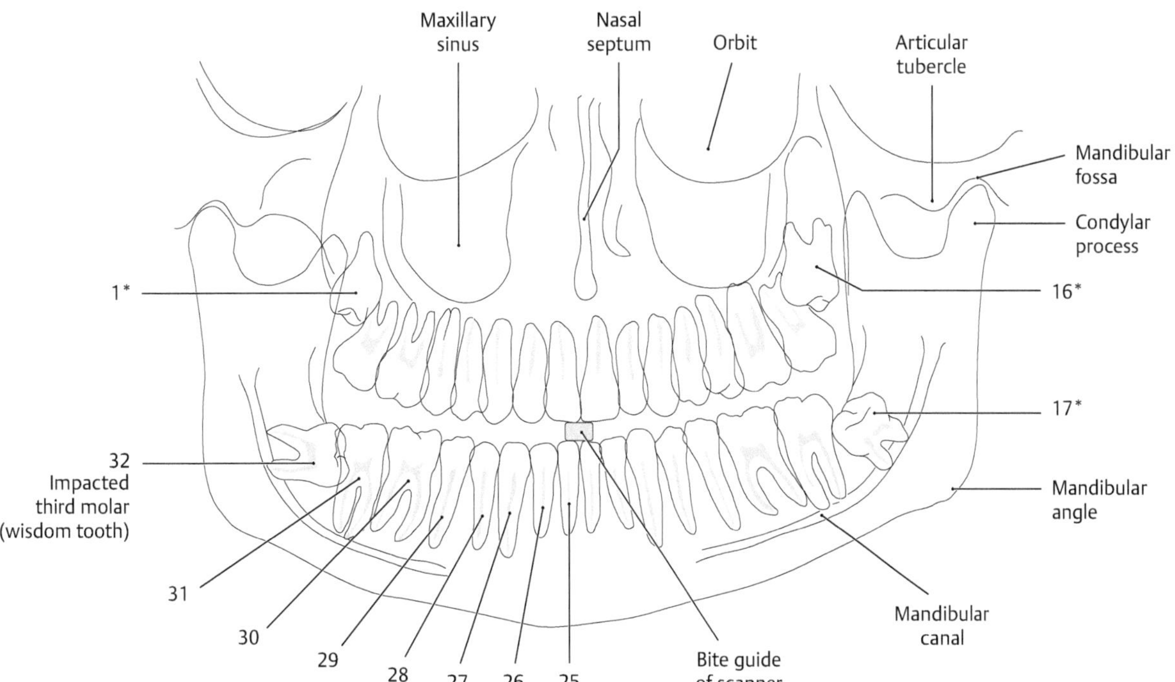

Fig. 7.51 Coding of the teeth and a dental panoramic tomogram. (From Schuenke M, Schulte E, Schumacher U. THIEME Atlas of Anatomy. Head, Neck, and Neuroanatomy. Illustrations by Voll M and Wesker K. 3rd ed. New York: Thieme Medical Publishers; 2020.)

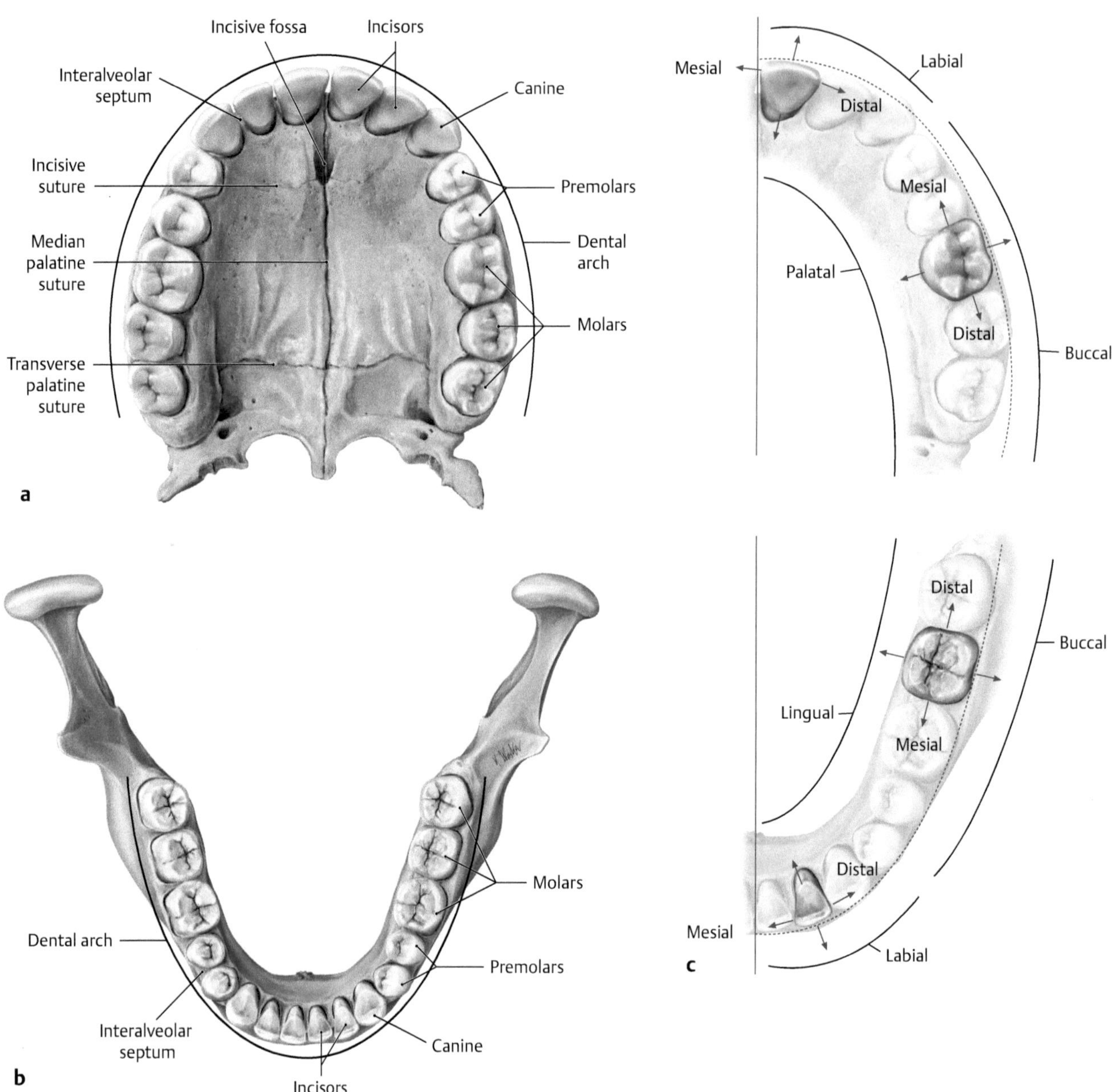

Fig. 7.52 (a) Maxillary teeth. Inferior view of the maxilla. **(b)** Mandibular teeth. Superior view of the mandible. **(c)** Tooth surfaces. (From Schuenke M, Schulte E, Schumacher U. THIEME Atlas of Anatomy. Head, Neck, and Neuroanatomy. Illustrations by Voll M and Wesker K. 3rd ed. New York: Thieme Medical Publishers; 2020.)

The first three parts are calcified. The **enamel** covers the crown and is a cell-free, extracellular, mineralized tissue consisting of almost all calcium salts (95% hydroxyapatite) and is the hardest substance in the human body. **Ameloblasts** are tall columnar, enamel-producing cells that are ectodermal in origin. The enamel is organized as crystalline rods spanning the full thickness of the enamel layer produced by a *Tomes' process* of a single secretory ameloblast. The rhythmic growth of a tooth is represented by *striae (striations) of Retzius*. Ameloblasts degenerate after a tooth has erupted; thus, enamel cannot be repaired naturally later in life if damaged.

The **dentin** forms the bulk of the tooth, is the first mineralized component of the tooth to be deposited, and is made up of approximately 70% calcium salts. **Odontoblasts** are the cells that synthesize and secrete the organic components for dentin. Odontoblasts are columnar cells located on the inner surface of the dentin within the pulp cavity and originate from neural crest cells. Production of dentin can continue into adult life to compensate for tooth damage and will slowly infiltrate the pulp cavity. The dentin contains a central chamber known as the **pulp chamber** and it is filled with soft tissue called **pulp**. The pulp chamber opens at the **apical foramen** and into the bony dental alveoli by the **root canal**. Neurovasculature along with lymphatics of a tooth pass to and from the pulp chamber through the apical foramen.

The **cementum** is bonelike mineralized tissue that covers the outer surface (dentin) of the root. It contains osteocyte-like cells

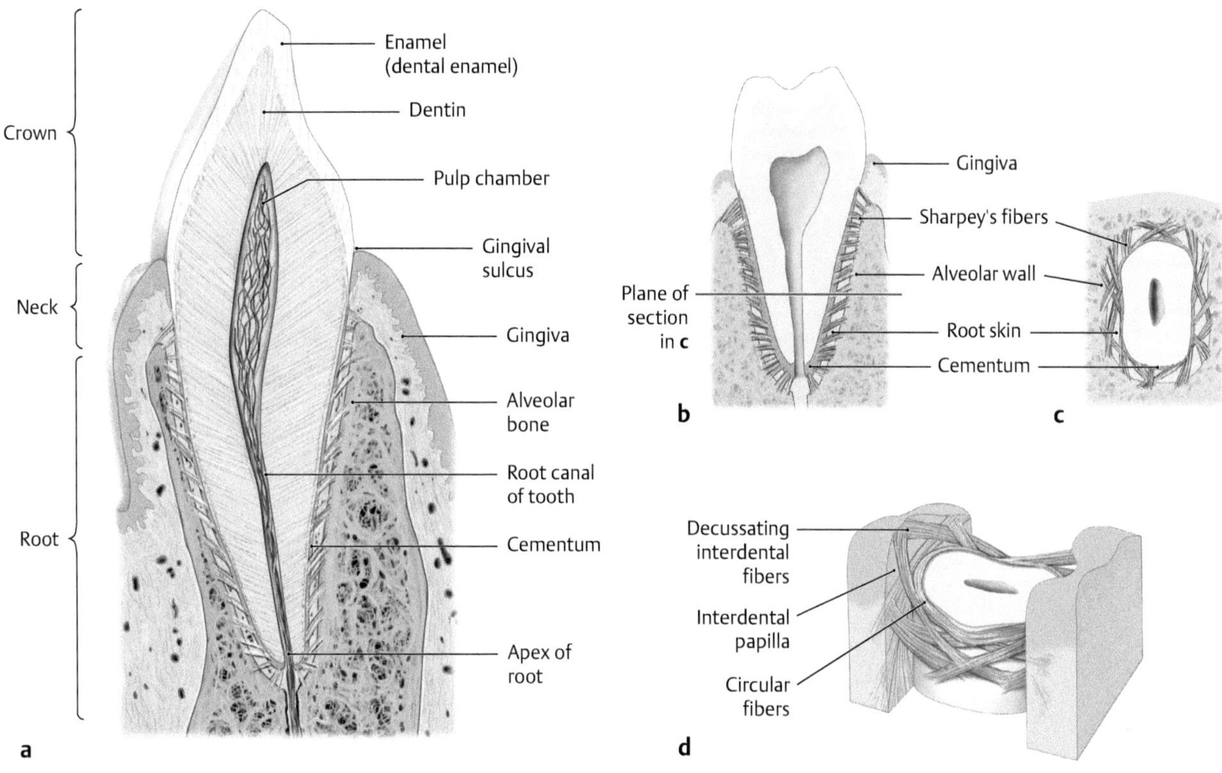

Fig. 7.53 **(a)** Histology of a tooth. **(b,c)** Longitudinal and cross section of the tooth. **(d)** Schematic course of gingival fibers. (From Schuenke M, Schulte E, Schumacher U. THIEME Atlas of Anatomy. Head, Neck, and Neuroanatomy. Illustrations by Voll M and Wesker K. 3rd ed. New York: Thieme Medical Publishers; 2020.)

known as **cementocytes** that are derived from mesenchyme and is similar to bone where it can be produced and reabsorbed. The outermost layer is uncalcified and is produced by cementoblasts. It contacts the **periodontal ligament**, a suspensory ligament that holds the tooth in the dental alveoli. *Sharpey fibers* of this ligament penetrate the cementum of the tooth and connect it to the bony wall of the tooth sockets. The periodontal ligament serves as periosteum to alveolar bone and prevents the direct transfer of forces on the tooth to the bone, thus preventing localized reabsorption of the alveolar bone.

Neurovasculature of the Gingivae and Teeth

Multiple nerve branches originating from either the maxillary or infraorbital nerves innervate the gingiva adjacent to the *labial* and *buccal* (collectively *vestibular*) *surfaces* of the maxillary teeth. The **anterior superior alveolar nerves** (infraorbital br.) innervate gingiva near the eighth and ninth teeth. The **middle superior alveolar nerves** (infraorbital br.) innervate the gingiva near the 4th and 13th teeth. Direct branches off the **infraorbital nerve** overlap the innervation of both the anterior and middle superior alveolar branches and help supply the gingiva of the 5th to 7th and 10th to 12th teeth. The **posterior superior alveolar nerves** (maxillary br.) innervate the gingiva of the 1st to 3rd and 14th to 16th teeth. The gingiva on the *palatal surface* of these maxillary teeth are innervated by the **nasopalatine** (6–11th teeth) and **greater palatine nerves** (1st–5th and 12–16th) (**Fig. 7.54**).

The **mental branch of the inferior alveolar nerve** innervates gingiva on the *labial surface* of the 20 to 29th teeth while the **buccal nerve** (CN V_3 br.) innervates the gingiva on the *buccal surface* of the 17 to 19th and 30th to 32nd teeth. The gingiva of the *lingual surface* of the mandibular teeth is innervated solely by the **lingual nerve** (17th–32nd teeth).

The teeth, along with the tooth pulp, periodontal ligament and alveolar processes, are innervated as follows. For maxillary teeth, the **anterior superior alveolar nerves** innervate the 6th to 11th teeth. The **middle superior alveolar nerves** innervate the 3rd to 5th and 12th to 14th teeth. The **posterior superior alveolar nerves** innervate the 1st to 3rd and 14th to 16th teeth (**Fig. 7.54**). Note the middle and posterior superior alveolar nerves overlap innervation. This is due to the formation of the **superior dental plexus**. Note: on occasion, the middle superior alveolar nerves may not be present. For the mandibular teeth, the **incisive branches of the inferior alveolar nerve** innervate the 22nd to 27th teeth while the **dental branches of the inferior alveolar nerve** innervate the 17th to 21st and 28th to 32nd teeth.

For maxillary teeth, the **posterior superior alveolar artery** (3rd part of maxillary br.) supplies the molars and premolars while the **anterior superior alveolar artery** (infraorbital br.) supplies the canines and incisors. If the **middle superior alveolar artery** is present (infraorbital br.) it will form an anastomosis between the posterior and anterior superior alveolar branches. For mandibular teeth, the **dental branches of the inferior alveolar artery** (1st part of maxillary br.) supply the molars and premolars. The **incisive branches of the inferior alveolar artery** supply the

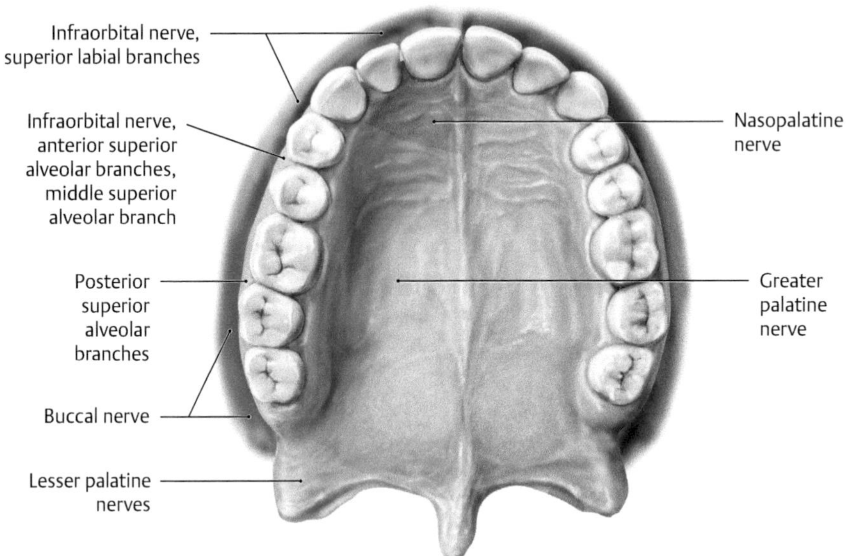

Fig. 7.54 Sensory innervation of the palatal mucosa, upper teeth and lip, cheeks, and gingiva. (From Schuenke M, Schulte E, Schumacher U. THIEME Atlas of Anatomy. Head, Neck, and Neuroanatomy. Illustrations by Voll M and Wesker K. 3rd ed. New York: Thieme Medical Publishers; 2020.)

canines and incisors. Smaller blood vessel branches that originally supplied alveolar bone and periodontal ligaments will supply the gingiva. The lymphatic drainage for the majority of teeth and gingiva is to the **submandibular lymph nodes**. Lymph from the mandibular incisors and nearby gingiva will drain to the **submental lymph nodes**.

7.6.3 Tongue

The **tongue** is a muscular but highly mobile structure covered by a mucous membrane. It is located mainly in the oral cavity proper and partly within the oropharynx. The tongue functions in mastication; squeezing food into the oropharynx during the first step in deglutition (swallowing); special sense of taste; formation of words during speaking; and oral cleansing.

The tongue is made up of an *apex*, *body*, and *root*. It is also divided into an **anterior two-third portion** that includes both the apex and body and is located in the oral cavity proper. The **posterior one-third portion** consists of the root and is located in the oropharynx. The superior and posterior surfaces of the tongue are known as the **dorsum of the tongue**. The **sulcus terminalis** is a V-shaped groove just posterior to the *vallate lingual papillae* and divides the dorsum of the tongue into an anterior two-third and posterior one-third portion. The posterior angle formed by the sulcus terminalis marks the location of the **foramen cecum**, a small pit that is the remnant of the proximal portion of the *thyroglossal duct* associated with thyroid gland development. The **median furrow** divides the anterior portion of the dorsum of the tongue into a left and right half (**Fig. 7.55**).

The **inferior/ventral surface of the tongue** is lined by a thin and transparent mucous membrane. The **lingual frenulum** connects the inferior/ventral surface to the floor of the mouth but also allows this surface of the tongue to move freely. On each side and near the base of the lingual frenulum, a **sublingual caruncle** is present and marks the opening of the *submandibular duct*. The deep lingual veins are visible through the thin mucous membrane and are important in quick absorption of drugs such as *nitroglycerin* in the case of an individual having chest pain (*angina pectoris*).

Histology of the Tongue

The dorsal surface of the tongue is covered by a nonkeratinized stratified squamous epithelium. Mucous and serous glands extend across the lamina propria with their ducts emptying into the vallate papillae and lingual tonsils, respectively. The mucosa of the anterior two-third of the tongue is relatively thin and closely attached to underlying muscle. However, the texture is fairly rough due to the numerous **lingual papillae (Fig. 7.55; Fig. 7.57)**.

The **fungiform papillae** are mushroom-shaped protrusions with a central core of connective tissue and have taste buds located on their dorsal surface. They have the appearance of a pink or red spot on the tongue and are widely distributed but most numerous near the apex and margins of the tongue. The **foliate papillae** are the small, lateral folds of lingual mucosa near the palatoglossal arches. They do contain taste buds but are poorly developed in humans. The **vallate papillae** are the large, flat-topped papillae located just anterior to the sulcus terminalis and arranged in a V-shaped row. They have a large connective tissue core with deep circular trenches that contain taste buds. The ducts of **von Ebner glands** (serous glands) open into these trenches and act to remove food from near the taste buds in order to prepare them for new stimuli. The **filiform papillae** are the long, conical, and cornified projections of the stratified squamous epithelium located on the majority of the dorsal surface of the tongue. These papillae contain afferent nerve endings but no taste buds (**Fig. 7.55; Fig. 7.57**).

The majority of the lingual papillae have **taste buds** which are barrel-shaped epithelial structures containing chemosensory cells called **gustatory (taste) receptor cells** and have a life span on average of 12 days. The human tongue has approximately 4600 taste buds. The narrow end of the taste bud is located at the free surface of the epithelium. The taste bud projects into an opening called the **taste pore** that itself is formed by the nonkeratinized

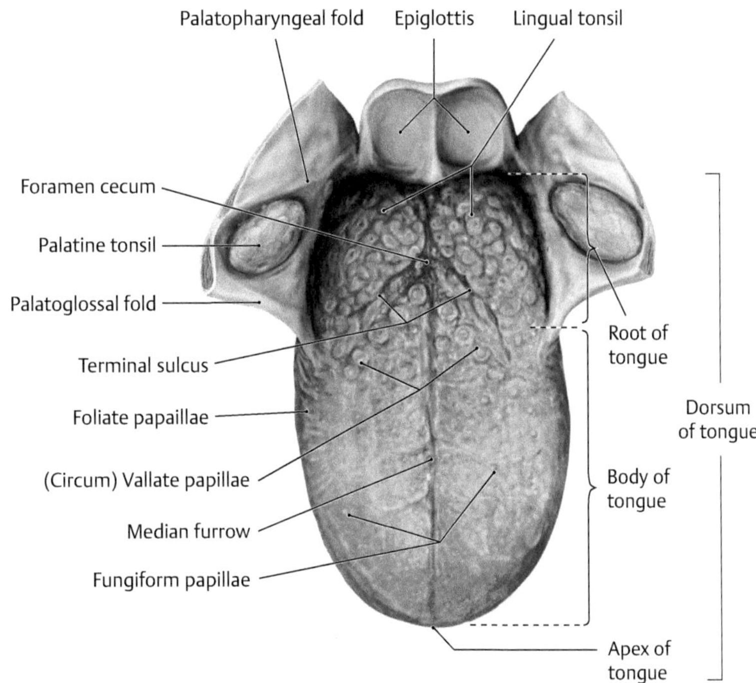

Fig. 7.55 Structure of the tongue. (From Schuenke M, Schulte E, Schumacher U. THIEME Atlas of Anatomy. Head, Neck, and Neuroanatomy. Illustrations by Voll M and Wesker K. 3rd ed. New York: Thieme Medical Publishers; 2020.)

squamous epithelium that overlies the taste bud. There are four types of cells that constitute a taste bud: **dark cells** (type I), **light cells** (type II), **intermediate cells** (type III), and **basal cells** (type IV). Dark, light, and intermediate cells project microvilli (*taste hairs*) into the taste pore and are all connected to nerve fibers. It is generally thought that basal cells give rise to dark cells, which then mature into light cells. The light cells then become intermediate cells and die (**Fig. 7.56**).

There are four basic taste sensations and they include *sweet*, *salty*, *bitter*, and *sour*. The apex is where sweetness is detected. Saltiness is detected near the lateral edges of the tongue. Both bitterness and sourness are detected at the posterior portion of the tongue. A debated fifth taste known as *umami* is picked up by receptors specific to glutamate and is commonly associated with the food additive monosodium glutamate (MSG). Many authors state the above information but there is evidence that indicates all areas of the tongue are responsive to these taste stimuli.

The mucosa of the posterior one-third of the tongue is fairly thick and freely movable. There are no lingual papillae present but there are lymphoid nodules known as the **lingual tonsils** that give this region a cobblestone-like appearance (**Fig. 7.55**).

Muscles of the Tongue

The tongue is primarily made up of a combination of extrinsic and intrinsic muscles. Muscles of the tongue are dynamic movers and often have multiple functions and do not act in isolation. The **extrinsic muscles** will *alter the position* of the tongue and include the **genioglossus**, **styloglossus**, **hyoglossus,** and **palatoglossus muscles**. The **intrinsic muscles** *alter the shape* of the tongue and include the **superior longitudinal**, **inferior longitudinal**, **vertical**, and **transverse muscles** (**Fig. 7.58**). A midline fibrous **lingual septum** separates the extrinsic and intrinsic muscles into a left versus right side. All muscles of the tongue, either extrinsic or intrinsic, are innervated by the **hypoglossal nerve (CN XII)**, except for the palatoglossus muscle that is innervated by **pharyngeal branches of the vagus nerve (CN X)**. Tongue muscles are detailed in **Table 7.3**.

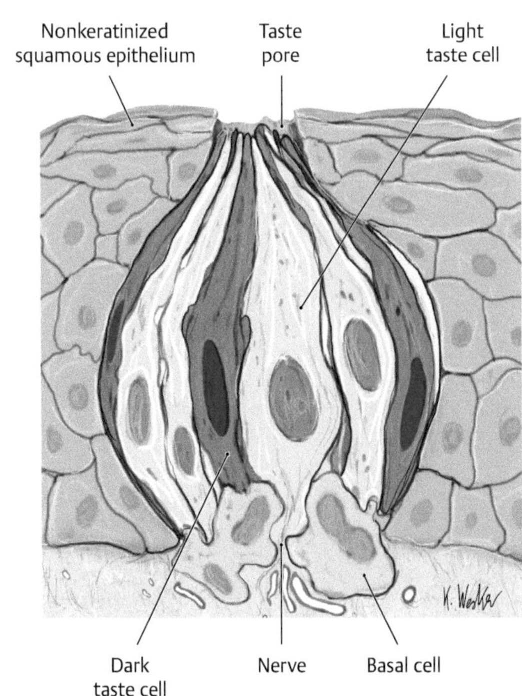

Fig. 7.56 Histology of a taste bud. (From Schuenke M, Schulte E, Schumacher U. THIEME Atlas of Anatomy. Head, Neck, and Neuroanatomy. Illustrations by Voll M and Wesker K. 3rd ed. New York: Thieme Medical Publishers; 2020.)

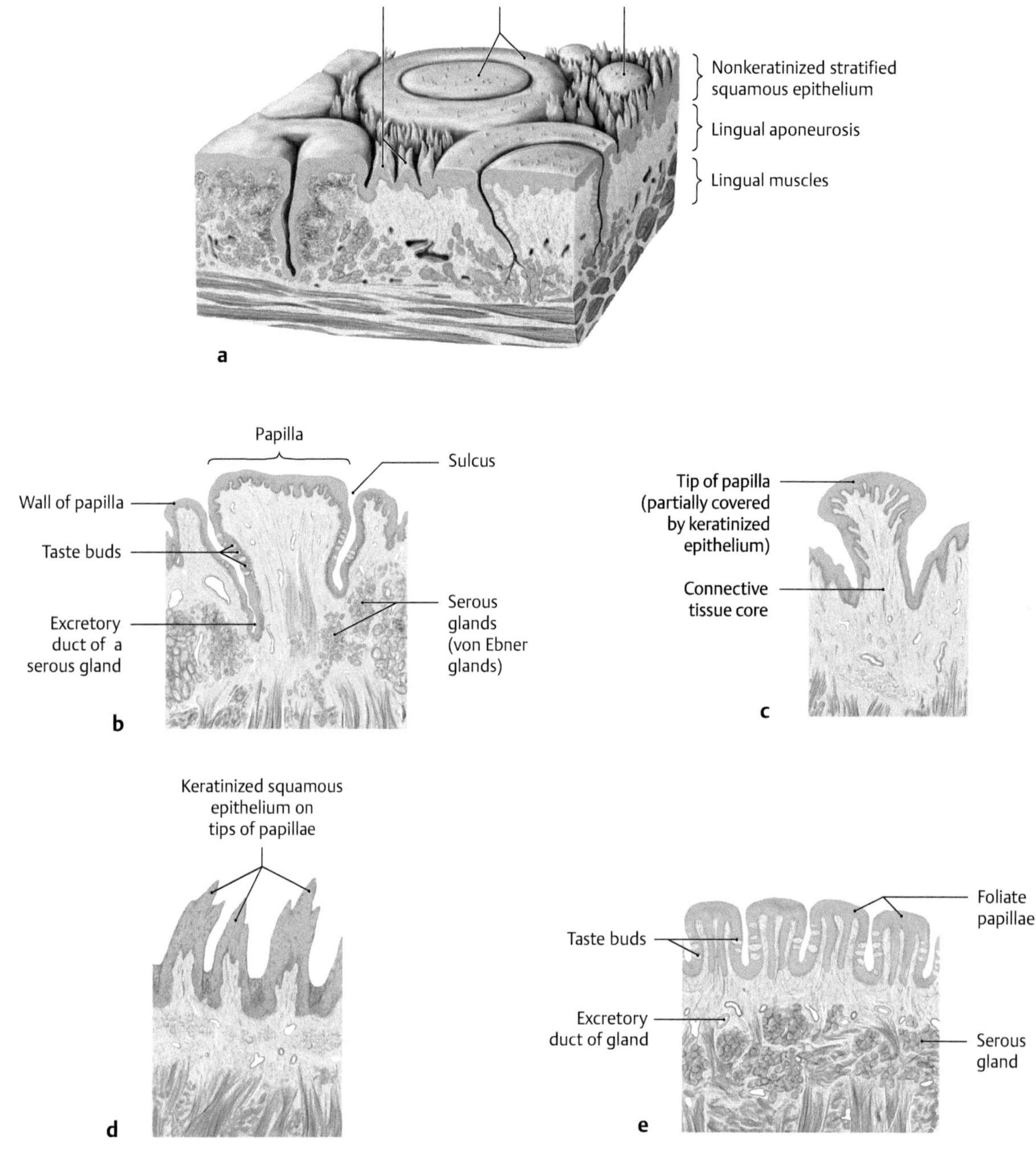

Fig. 7.57 The papillae of the tongue. **(a)** Sectional block diagram of the lingual papillae. **(b)** (Circum) Vallate papillae. **(c)** Fungiform papillae. **(d)** Filiform papillae. **(e)** Foliate papillae. (From Schuenke M, Schulte E, Schumacher U. THIEME Atlas of Anatomy. Head, Neck, and Neuroanatomy. Illustrations by Voll M and Wesker K. 3rd ed. New York: Thieme Medical Publishers; 2020.)

Neurovasculature of the Tongue

Innervation of the tongue muscles has been discussed. However, this section will focus on the general somatic sensation (GSA-touch and temperature) of the mucosa and the special sense of taste (SVA) involving multiple areas of the tongue. These regions include the anterior two-third, posterior one-third, and the anterior epiglottic regions **(Fig. 7.59)**.

- *GSA innervation of anterior two-third of tongue*: the mucosa is supplied by the **lingual nerve** (CN V_3 branch).
- *SVA innervation of anterior two-third of tongue*: taste from this general region and involving the fungiform and foliate papillae are supplied by the **chorda tympani nerve**. The chorda tympani fuses with the lingual nerve in the infratemporal fossa.
- *GSA innervation of posterior one-third of tongue*: the mucosa is supplied by the *lingual branch* of the **glossopharyngeal nerve (CN IX)**.
- *SVA innervation of posterior one-third of tongue*: taste fibers from this general region and the vallate papillae are supplied by the *lingual branch* of **glossopharyngeal nerve**.

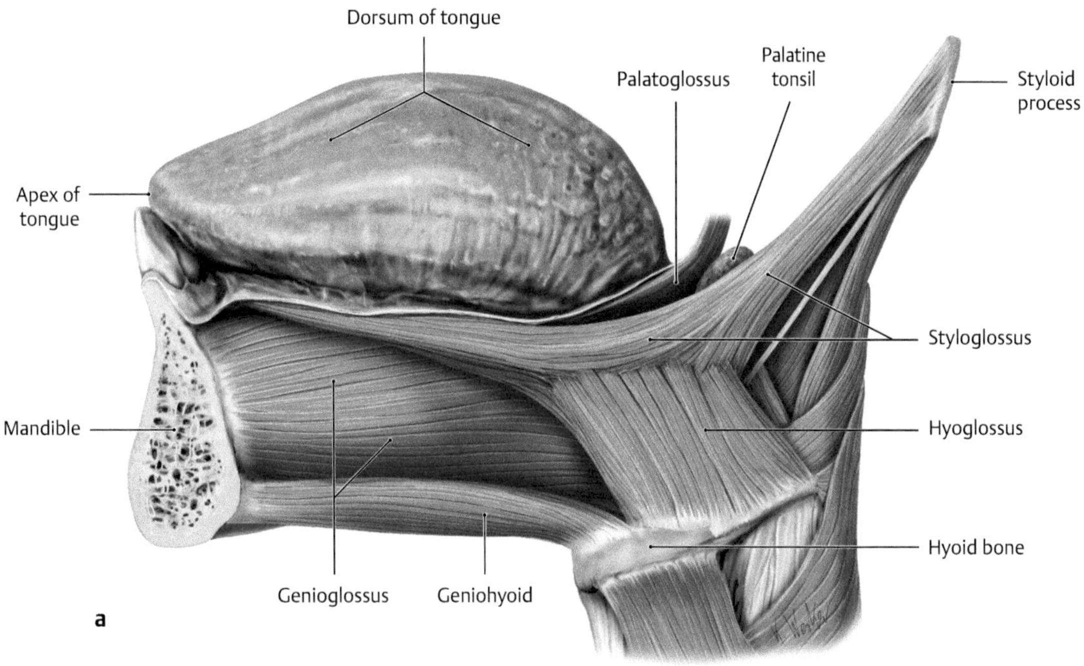

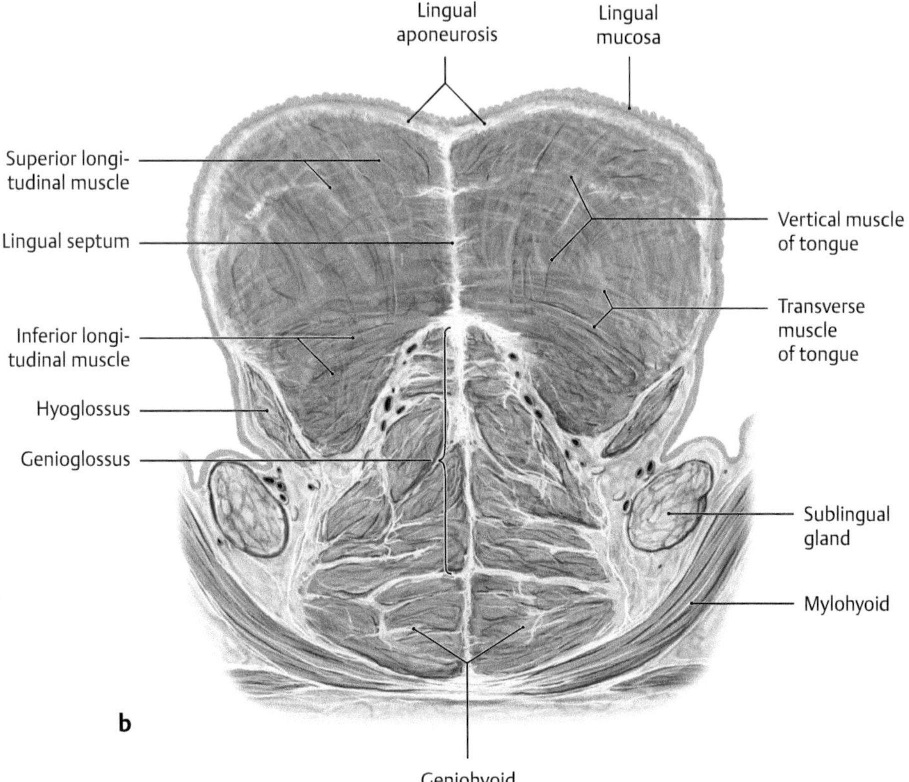

Fig. 7.58 Muscles of the tongue. **(a)** Left lateral view. **(b)** Anterior view of a coronal section. (From Schuenke M, Schulte E, Schumacher U. THIEME Atlas of Anatomy. Head, Neck, and Neuroanatomy. Illustrations by Voll M and Wesker K. 3rd ed. New York: Thieme Medical Publishers; 2020.)

Table 7.3 **Muscles of the tongue**

Muscle	Function(s)	Origin	Insertion
Genioglossus	Depresses (bilaterally); retracts apex of protracted tongue (anterior part); protracts (posterior part); deviates tongue to contralateral side (unilateral contraction)	Upper mental spines of mandible (mental spines collectively are known as genial tubercles)	Entire dorsum of the tongue; body of hyoid
Styloglossus	Retracts and elevates tongue	Anterior border of distal styloid process and the stylohyoid ligament	Superior aspect of the lateral sides of posterior tongue; fibers interdigitate with hyoglossus
Hyoglossus	Retracts and depresses tongue	Body and greater horn of hyoid bone	Inferior aspect of the lateral sides of posterior tongue; fibers interdigitate with styloglossus
Palatoglossus	Elevates posterior part of tongue (while depressing soft palate)	Palatine aponeurosis of soft palate	Intrinsic transverse muscle fibers
Superior longitudinal	Curls tongue longitudinally upward, elevating the apex and sides of the tongue	Submucosal layer and lingual septum	Margins of the tongue and mucous membrane
Inferior longitudinal	Curls tongue longitudinally downward, depressing apex; retracts tongue	Body of hyoid bone and root of tongue	Apex of tongue
Vertical	Flattens tongue	Submucosal layer of dorsum of the tongue	Inferior surfaces of borders of the tongue
Transverse	Narrows and protracts (elongates) tongue	Lingual septum	Fibrous tissue at the lateral margins

- *GVA innervation of anterior epiglottic region*: GVA fibers innervate the mucosa lining the anterior aspect of the epiglottis. These fibers are supplied by the **internal laryngeal nerve**, a branch off the *superior laryngeal nerve* and associated with the *vagus nerve (CN X)*. Some authors will describe this as GSA innervation.
- *SVA innervation of anterior epiglottic region*: the minimal amount of taste fibers in this region course back with the **internal laryngeal nerve**.

Blood supply to the tongue and floor of the mouth originates from the **lingual artery**, a branch of the external carotid artery. Near the posterior border of the hyoglossus muscle, the lingual artery gives off the **dorsal lingual artery**. The lingual artery continues toward the tongue and passes between the hyoglossus and middle constrictor muscles before bifurcating into a **sublingual** and **deep lingual artery** near the anterior border of the hyoglossus muscle. The deep lingual artery serves as the terminal portion of the original lingual artery and forms an anastomosis with its counterpart on the opposite side. These arteries have paired veins with the **lingual vein** draining directly into the IJV or forming a common trunk with the facial and retromandibular (anterior division) veins **(Fig. 7.60)**.

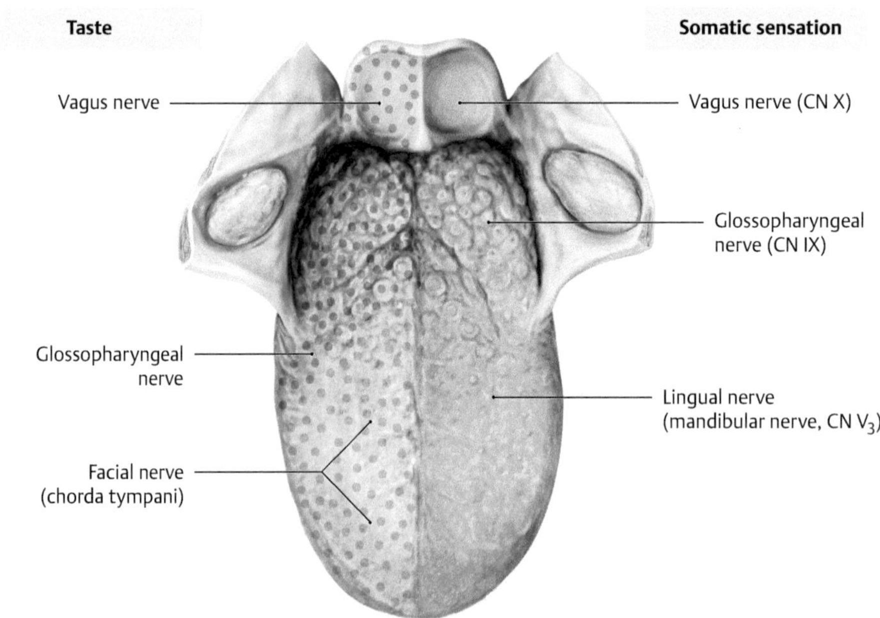

Fig. 7.59 Somatosensory innervation (left side) and special sense taste innervation (right side) of the tongue. (From Schuenke M, Schulte E, Schumacher U. THIEME Atlas of Anatomy. Head, Neck, and Neuroanatomy. Illustrations by Voll M and Wesker K. 3rd ed. New York: Thieme Medical Publishers; 2020.)

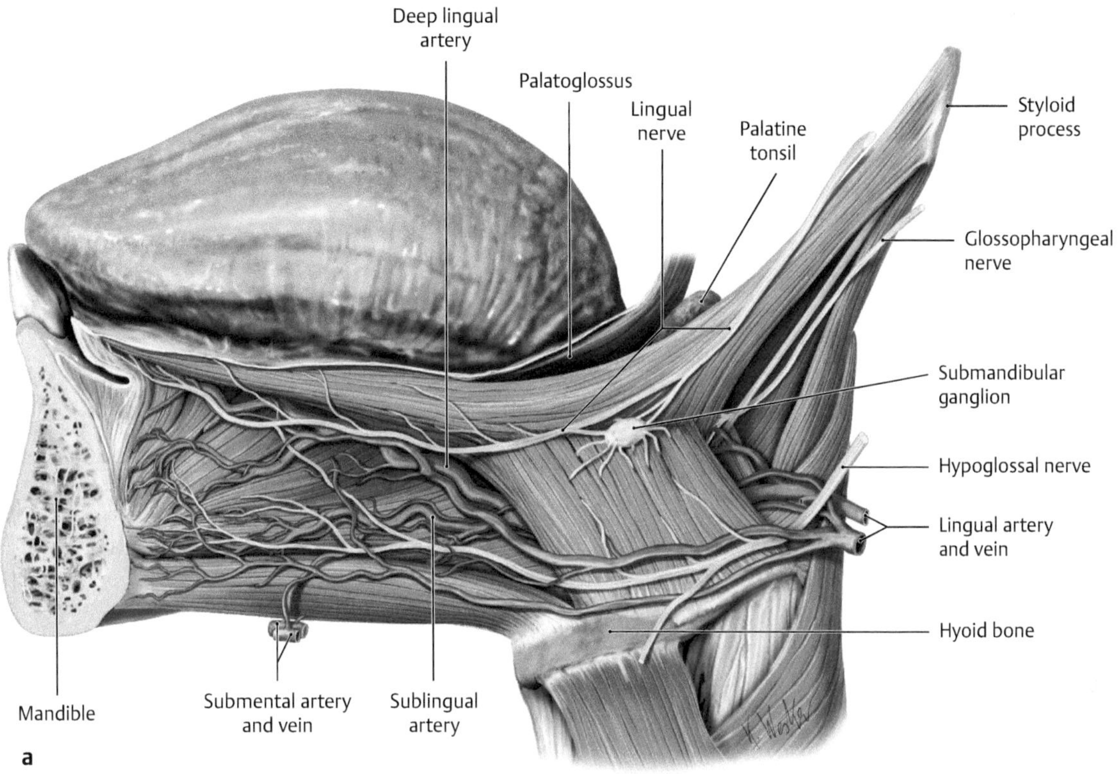

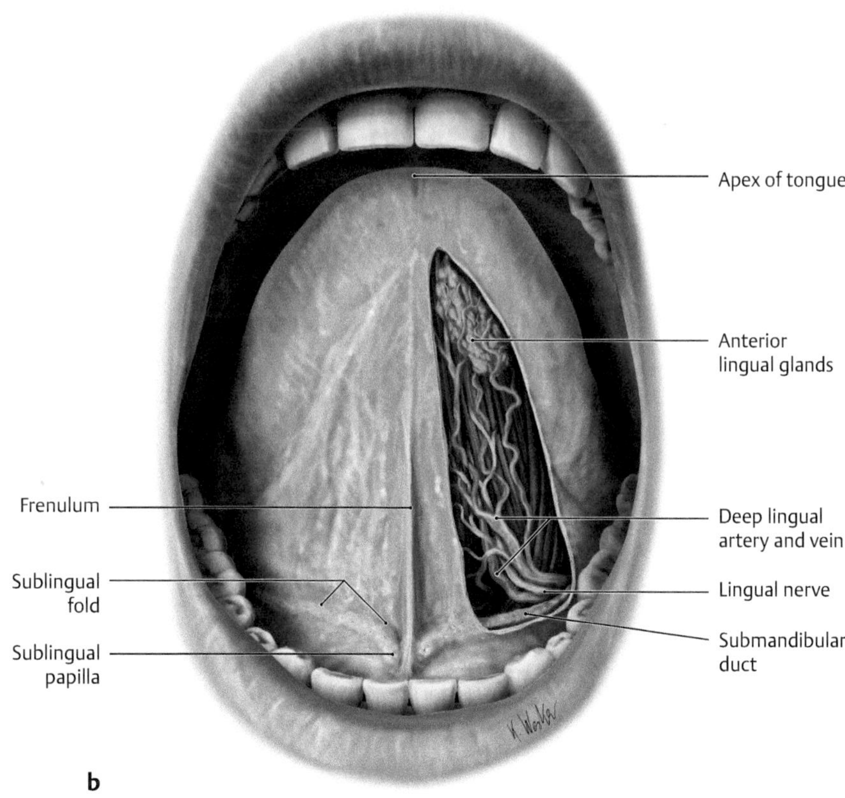

Fig. 7.60 Neurovasculature of the tongue. **(a)** Left lateral view. **(b)** View of the inferior surface of the tongue. (From Schuenke M, Schulte E, Schumacher U. THIEME Atlas of Anatomy. Head, Neck, and Neuroanatomy. Illustrations by Voll M and Wesker K. 3rd ed. New York: Thieme Medical Publishers; 2020.)

The lymphatic drainage of the tongue is region specific and has many routes. The *apex* and *frenulum* will drain to the **submental lymph nodes** with the tissue closest to the midline draining bilaterally. The *medial portion of the body* drains to the **inferior deep cervical lymph nodes** bilaterally. The *lateral portions of the body* drain to the ipsilateral **submandibular lymph nodes**. Finally the *root of the tongue* drains to the **superior deep cervical lymph nodes** bilaterally **(Fig. 7.50)**.

Development of the Tongue

At the end of the fourth week, the **median lingual swelling (tuberculum impar)** appears in the floor of the early pharynx just rostral to the foramen cecum. It is the first sign of tongue development but it will not form any recognizable part of the adult tongue. Two **lateral lingual swellings** develop on both sides of the median lingual swelling. These lateral swellings overgrow the median lingual swelling and form the anterior two-third of the tongue (oral part). The **midline groove** is formed by the fusion of the two lateral lingual swellings. The median and lateral lingual swellings originate from mesoderm associated with the first pharyngeal arch. GSA innervation is from the **lingual nerve** (V_3 br.) while SVA-taste innervation is associated with the **chorda tympani nerve** (CN VII br.) **(Fig. 7.61)**.

The **copula** (second pharyngeal arch) and **hypopharyngeal eminence** (third and portion of fourth pharyngeal arches) are two additional midline swellings but they are associated with development of the posterior one-third of the tongue (pharyngeal part). Similar to development of the oral part of the tongue, a tissue (hypopharyngeal eminence) will overgrow another (copula) to form the posterior one-third of the tongue. The anterior and posterior tongues meet at the **terminal sulcus**. Both GSA and SVA/SS-taste innervation is from the **glossopharyngeal nerve**.

A fourth midline swelling called the **epiglottic swelling** (rest of fourth pharyngeal arch) leads to the development of the epiglottis. Both GVA and SVA/SS-taste (minimal) innervation of this region is from the **internal laryngeal nerve**.

Tongue muscles originate from myoblasts that migrate from **somites 2-5** (or the occipital group). The **hypoglossal nerve** accompanies these myoblasts during their migration and will innervate all tongue muscles (except palatoglossus—CN X). By the end of the eighth week **lingual papillae** begin to appear. The **vallate** and **foliate papillae** appear first and these will be close to the terminal branches of the glossopharyngeal nerve. The **fungiform papillae** appear a little later and near the terminal branches of the chorda tympani nerve. Finally, the **filiform papillae** develop during the 10th to 11th weeks and contain afferent nerve endings sensitive to touch.

The floor of the oral cavity proper consists of a couple of muscles, the neurovasculature supplying mainly the tongue and the submandibular and sublingual glands. The **mylohyoid** and **geniohyoid muscles** establish a muscular base for the oral cavity and assist in elevating and shortening the floor of the mouth. These muscles are considered *suprahyoid muscles* and the details surrounding these muscles will be discussed during the "Anterior Triangle of the Neck" section of this chapter **(Fig. 7.62)**.

7.6.4 Salivary Glands

The major **salivary glands** include the **parotid**, **submandibular**, and **sublingual glands**. These glands are classified according to their location, function, and predominance for either **serous** or **mucous acini**, the functional secretory structures. There are also minor salivary glands that include the buccal, palatine, lingual, and labial glands. The focus will be on the major glands. Salivary glands are responsible for producing about one liter of **saliva** per day, a clear, odorless, hypotonic solution consisting of 99.5% water and containing mucus, enzymes (amylase, lysozyme, and others), electrolytes, glycoproteins, and IgA **(Fig. 7.64)**.

Saliva acts by lubricating food during mastication, begins the digestion of starches, keeps the mucous membrane of the oral cavity moist reducing friction, and helps intensify the sense of taste among other functions. Saliva can be divided into a digestive and protective function. The *digestive function* is based on

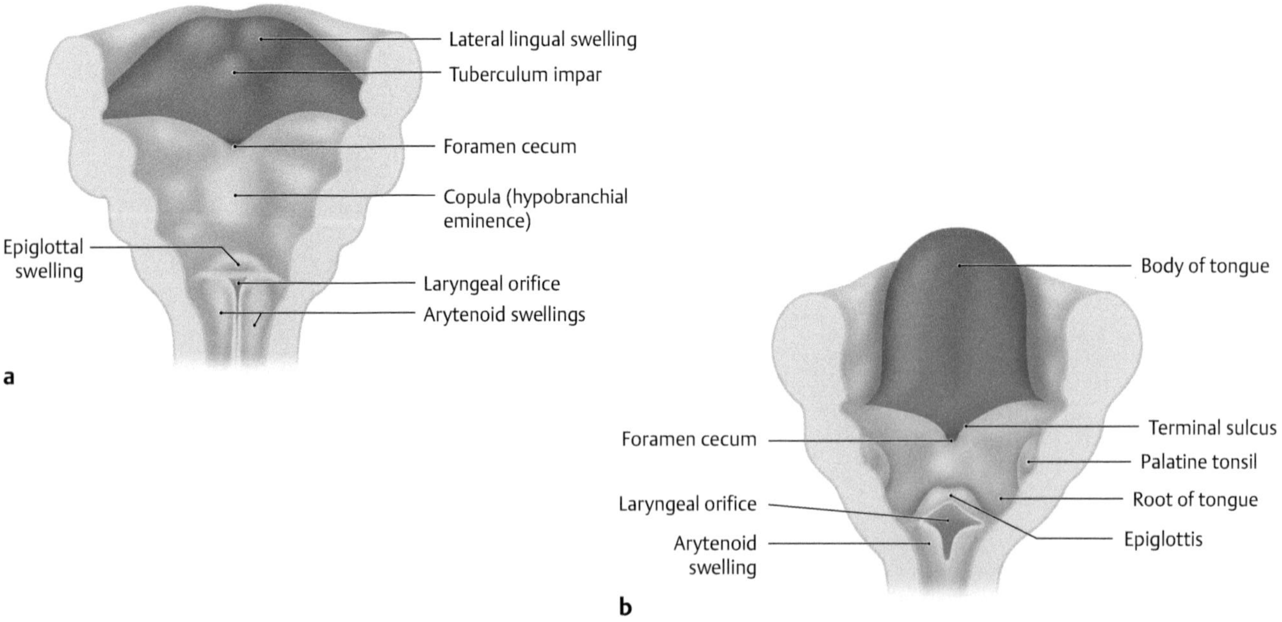

Fig. 7.61 Development of the tongue. **(a)** Near week 4. **(b)** Near week 8. (From Baker EW. Anatomy for Dental Medicine. 2nd ed. 2015. Based on the work of: Schuenke M, Schulte E, Schumacher U. THIEME Atlas of Anatomy. Illustrations by Voll M and Wesker K.)

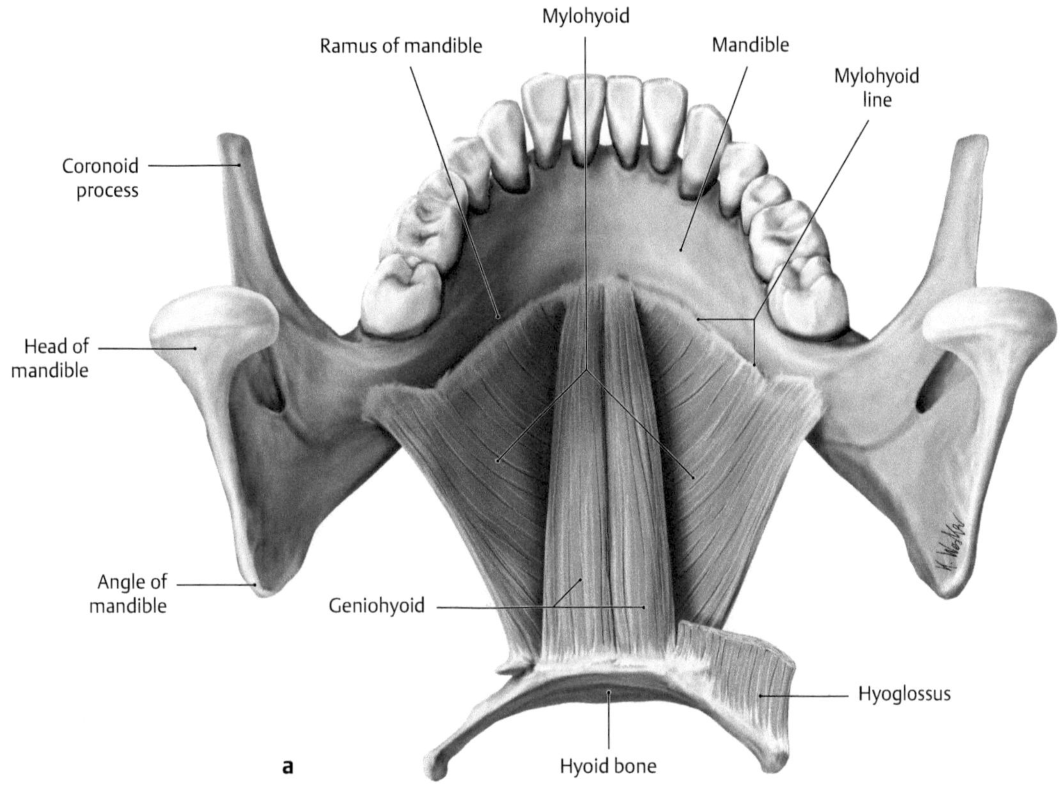

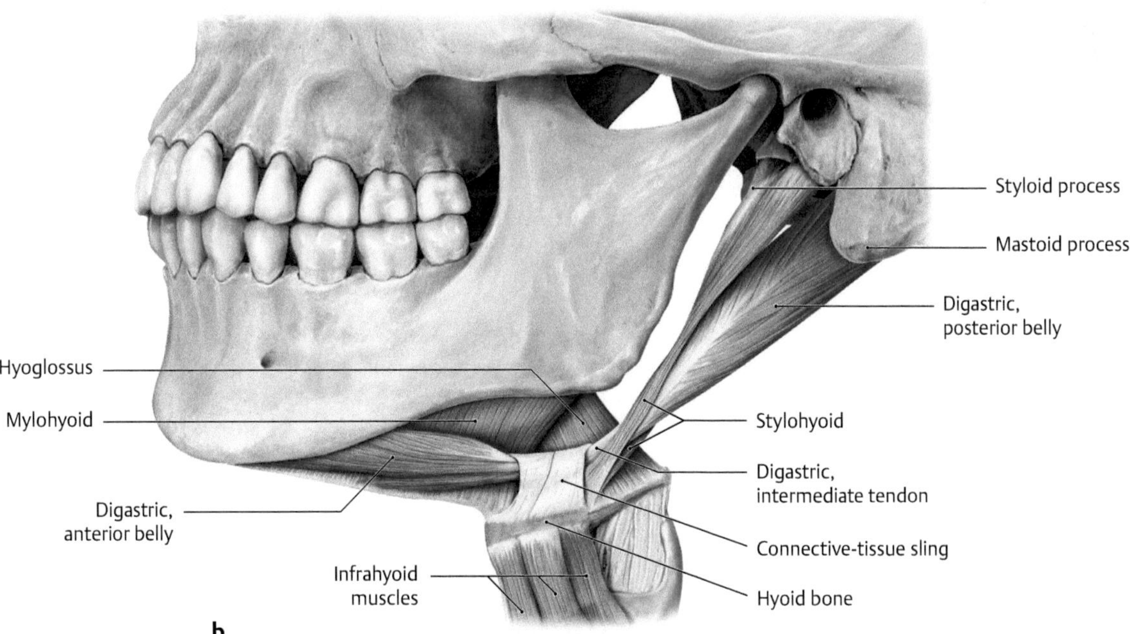

Fig. 7.62 Muscles of the oral floor. **(a)** Superior view. **(b)** Left lateral view. (From Schuenke M, Schulte E, Schumacher U. THIEME Atlas of Anatomy. Head, Neck, and Neuroanatomy. Illustrations by Voll M and Wesker K. 3rd ed. New York: Thieme Medical Publishers; 2020.)

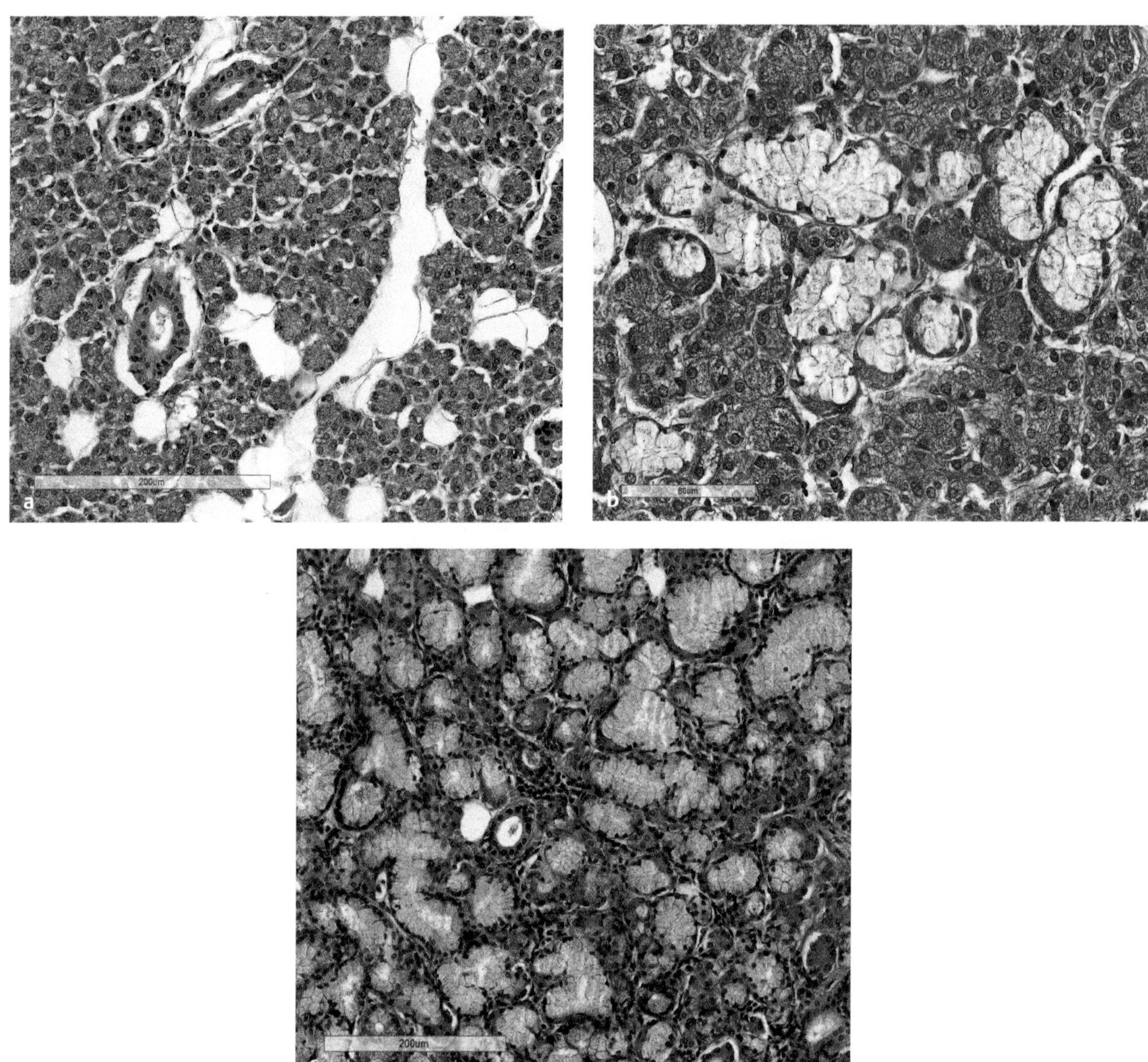

Fig. 7.63 Histology of the salivary glands. **(a)** Parotid. **(b)** Submandibular. **(c)** Sublingual. (From Lowrie DJ. Histology: An Essential Textbook. New York: Thieme Medical Publishers; 2020.)

the activity of enzymes such as **amylase**—initiates the digestion of carbohydrates (starch); **lingual lipase**—participates in hydrolysis of dietary lipids. The *protective function* centers on an antibacterial function involving **IgA**—neutralizes bacteria and viruses; **lysozyme**—breaks down bacterial walls; and **lactoferrin**—chelates the iron necessary for bacterial growth. Salivary glands also secrete the enzyme **kallikrein** into the connective tissue and bloodstream where it cleaves *kininogen* to produce *bradykinin*, which is important in vasodilation of vessels.

The autonomic nervous system controls the production of saliva. The parasympathetics stimulate the secretion of a water-rich (serous) saliva while the sympathetics stimulate the release of a protein-rich (mucous) saliva.

Histology of the Salivary Glands

The **parotid glands (Fig. 7.63)** were discussed during the "Scalp and Superficial Face" section of this chapter but are the largest of the salivary glands and only produce a serous or watery secretion. A connective tissue capsule or septa surround it and this represents a component of the stroma or supporting tissue of the gland. The septa help divide the gland into "lobes" and provide support for the neurovasculature supplying the acini or parenchyma of the gland. The parotid gland is made up exclusively of serous acini but only contributes to 20 to 25% of the total saliva volume. Its serous secretion includes products such as amylase, IgA, peroxidase, lysozyme, and the antimicrobial enzyme histatin.

The **submandibular glands (Fig. 7.63)** are located along the body of the mandible and can be subdivided into a superficial versus deep part due to its position against the posterior aspect of the mylohyoid muscle. It produces a mixed serous (mostly) and mucous secretion. Like the parotid gland it has a connective tissue capsule and septa that help divide the gland into "lobes." This gland is made of mostly serous acini (80–90%), is much smaller than the parotid gland but contributes 60 to 70% of the total saliva volume. The **submandibular (Wharton's) duct** arises from the portion of

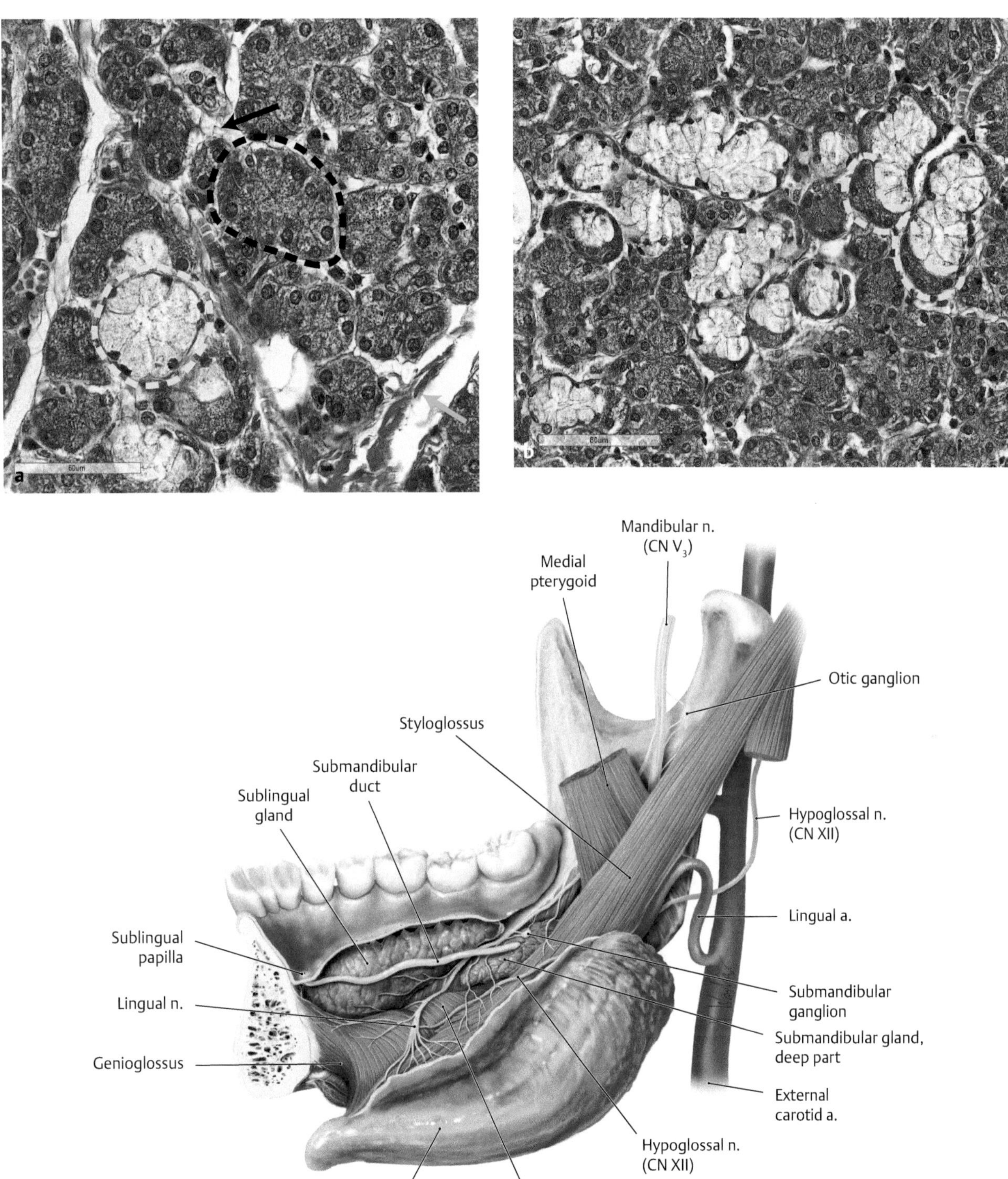

Fig. 7.64 (a) The serous or mucous acini surround a lumen. Mucous (*yellow outline*) and serous (*black outline*) acini are surrounded by loose (*black arrow*) and dense irregular connective tissue (*green arrow*). **(b)** Select serous cells are associated with a mucous acinus and are called serous demilunes (*yellow outline*). **(c)** Floor of the mouth with tongue pulled from midline: right mandible, medial view. (Parts a and b from Lowrie DJ. Histology: An Essential Textbook. New York: Thieme Medical Publishers; 2020. Part c from Schuenke M, Schulte E, Schumacher U. THIEME Atlas of Anatomy. Head, Neck, and Neuroanatomy. Illustrations by Voll M and Wesker K. 3rd ed. New York: Thieme Medical Publishers; 2020.)

the gland located between the mylohyoid and hyoglossus muscles and has a total length of approximately 5 cm. It extends anteriorly and lateral to the tongue but medial to the sublingual gland before terminating at the **sublingual caruncle** near the lingual frenulum. The *lingual nerve* passes underneath the submandibular duct from lateral to medial before reaching the tongue. Its serous secretion includes amylase while its mucous secretion can include sialomucin and sulfomucin.

The **sublingual glands (Fig. 7.63)** are the smallest of the three major salivary glands and are flat, anterior to the submandibular glands and located between the mandible and genioglossus muscle of the tongue. It also produces a mixed serous and mucous (mostly) secretion. The sublingual gland does not have a defined capsule but still has septa that divide the gland into "lobes." This gland consists mostly of mucous acini (60–65%) capped by serous demilunes (which are limited in the submandibular gland). It only contributes 3 to 5% of the total saliva volume. There are 8 to 20 smaller **sublingual ducts (of Rivinus)** that drain this gland and they open above and onto the mucous membrane. An isolated but larger sublingual duct (*of Bartholin*) may be present and joins the submandibular duct before it drains through the sublingual caruncle. Its secretions can include mucin, sialomucin, sulfomucin, and lingual lipase.

Ductule System of a Salivary Gland

Salivary glands are exocrine glands because they secrete their products through a duct system but these secretions originate from either a *serous*, *mucous*, or mixed seromucous acini known as a *serous demilunes* (**Fig. 7.64**). The branching ductule system of a salivary gland is composed of different sequential segments broken down into intralobular (intercalated, striated, and excretory ducts) and interlobular ducts. Together the acinus, intercalated, striated, and excretory ducts are known as the **salivon**, the functional unit of a salivary gland. Intralobular ducts are located in the parenchymal tissue while interlobular ducts are found in the septa. From the acinus to the oral cavity, the duct system progresses in this particular segmental order (**Fig. 7.65**):

- The **intercalated duct** receives the secretion from the acinus and is lined with a low squamous-to-cuboidal epithelium. The epithelial cells of these ducts can absorb chloride and secrete bicarbonate. The parotid gland has the longest intercalated ducts.
- The **striated duct** continues after the intercalated duct and has a simple cuboidal-to-columnar epithelium. These ducts transport secretions, modify the electrolyte balance by absorbing sodium and secreting potassium, as well as secrete kallikrein. These are well developed in the parotid and submandibular glands but not the sublingual gland.
- The **excretory duct** follows the striated duct and is initially lined by simple columnar epithelium then turning to pseudostratified columnar epithelium before joining the interlobular duct.
- The **interlobular ducts** follow the excretory ducts and initially are pseudostratified columnar, then become stratified columnar (rare epithelium) as the diameter increases, before joining the main duct which is a nonkeratinized stratified squamous epithelium prior to opening into the oral cavity.

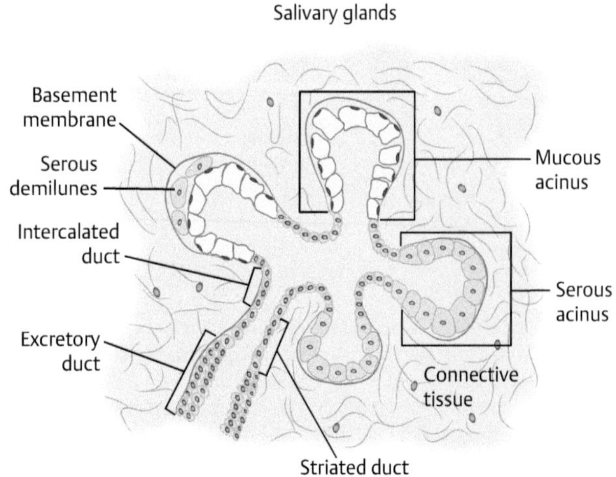

Fig. 7.65 Histology of the ductule system. (From Lowrie DJ. Histology: An Essential Textbook. New York: Thieme Medical Publishers; 2020.)

Neurovasculature of the Submandibular and Sublingual Glands

Secretomotor innervation of the submandibular and sublingual glands involves parasympathetic fibers being conveyed from the **chorda tympani nerve** (CN VII br.) to the **lingual nerve** (CN V_3 br.) before synapsing at the **submandibular ganglion** attached to the lingual nerve. Para/pre fibers destined for these glands originated from the **superior salivatory nucleus** of the brainstem. Para/post fibers then pass directly to the submandibular gland from the ganglion or hop back on the lingual nerve and course anteriorly to reach the sublingual gland. Sym/post fibers generally from the facial artery periarterial plexus pass through the submandibular ganglion before reaching the glands. These sym/post fibers initially reach the submandibular gland directly from the ganglion. However, fibers destined for the sublingual gland may continue on the lingual nerve (similar to parasympathetics) or on blood vessels that directly supply the gland. These sym/post fibers increase mucous secretion and vasoconstrict arteries supplying the glands **(Fig. 7.66)**.

Blood supply to the submandibular gland is from the **submental arteries** (facial artery br.) and these arteries have accompanying veins that drain back to the facial or anterior jugular veins. The sublingual gland is supplied by both the **submental** and **sublingual arteries** (lingual artery br.) with the accompanying veins draining back to either the facial or lingual veins **(Fig. 7.60)**.

Lymphatic drainage of the submandibular gland drains first to the **submandibular lymph nodes** followed by the **superior deep cervical lymph nodes** but has a propensity to drain to the **jugulo-omohyoid lymph nodes**. Lymph from the sublingual gland passes primarily to the **submandibular lymph nodes** prior to the **deep cervical lymph nodes**.

Development of the Salivary Glands

Salivary gland development begins as solid epithelial buds that originate from the early oral cavity. The ends of these epithelial buds will then grow into the underlying mesenchyme. The parenchymal tissue (portion that secretes) is derived from proliferations of the oral cavity epithelium. The supporting connective tissue of these glands originates from *neural crest cells*.

- The **parotid glands** develop first at the beginning of the sixth week and they originate from the oral *ectoderm* near the angles

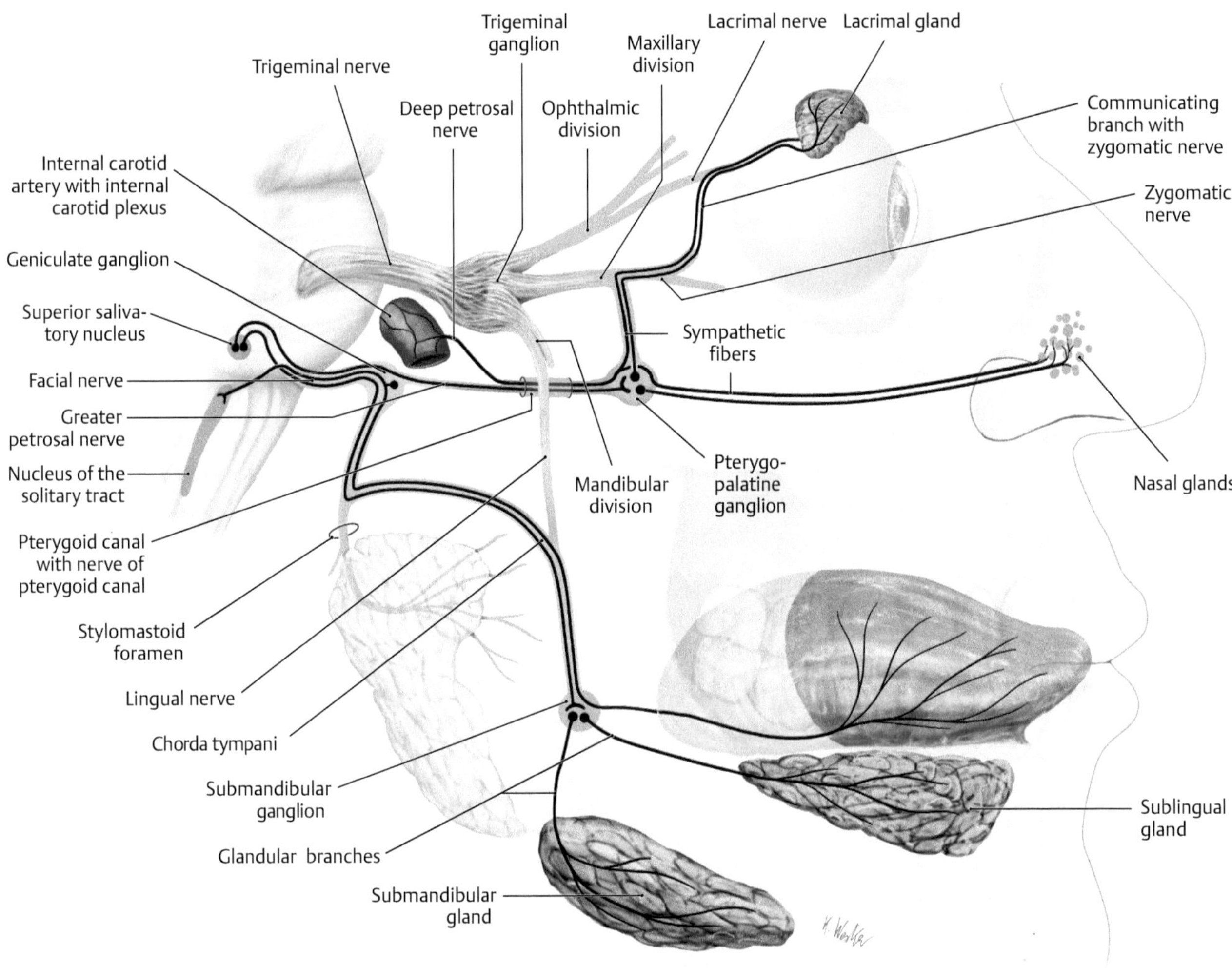

Fig. 7.66 Parasympathetic visceral efferents and special visceral afferents (taste fibers) of the facial nerve. (From Schuenke M, Schulte E, Schumacher U. THIEME Atlas of Anatomy. Head, Neck, and Neuroanatomy. Illustrations by Voll M and Wesker K. 3rd ed. New York: Thieme Medical Publishers; 2020.)

of the **stomodeum**. The buds develop in the posterior direction toward the ears and branch to form solid cords with rounded ends. The *solid cords* will canalize and become ducts by the 10th week. The *rounded ends* become acini and begin secreting during the 18th week of development. The capsule develops from the surrounding mesenchyme.

- The **submandibular glands** begin developing at the end of the sixth week and they originate from *endodermal* buds located in the floor of the stomodeum. The *cords* grow posteriorly and lateral to the tongue and will canalize shortly after. Secretory acini begin to develop during the 12th week but will not become active until the 16th week. Mucous acini do not form until after birth and will contribute to the continued growth of the gland. The *submandibular duct* forms when a linear groove just lateral to the tongue closes.
- The **sublingual glands** do not appear until the eighth week and originate from multiple *endodermal* buds located in the *paralingual sulcus*. The *cords* will canalize and form 8 to 20 sublingual ducts that open independently into the floor of the oral cavity. The *rounded ends* of these cords will become predominately mucous acini.

7.6.5 Palate

The palate is divided into a hard and soft palate. The palate separates the oral cavity from the nasal cavity and nasopharynx. Just deep to the mucosa are the **palatine glands** and they secrete mucus. The mucosa of the palate may display multiple holes due to how the palatine ducts open onto the surface. Some surface features exist and can be felt with a person's tongue. The **incisive papilla** is an elevation of mucosa located just posterior to the maxillary incisor and represents the position of the underlying incisive canal/fossa. Just lateral to the incisive papilla are the **transverse palatine folds** that can assist in food manipulation during chewing. A **palatine raphe** exists and marks the fusion of the *palatine shelves*, the structures responsible for the formation of the *secondary palate*. The secondary palate forms the majority of the hard palate and all of the soft palate.

7.6.6 Hard Palate

The **hard palate** is formed by the **horizontal plates of the palatine bones** and the **palatine processes of the maxillae**. It is the larger, anterior most portion of the overall palate and it is covered with mucosa. The tongue lies against the hard palate when it is at rest. The upper dental arch contains 16 permanent teeth and they will be numbered 1 to 16 beginning at the right third upper molar (**Fig. 7.67**).

Neurovasculature of the Hard Palate

Neurovasculature of the teeth and surrounding gingiva of the upper dental arch have been discussed previously. The **nasopalatine nerve** and distal **sphenopalatine artery** supply the mucosa near the palatal surface of the incisor and canine teeth and pass through the **incisive canal/fossa** to reach this mucosa. The **greater palatine neurovasculature** supplies the majority of the mucosa and palatine glands overlying the maxillae and palatine bones of the hard palate. There is an overlap of innervation and blood supply near the posterior aspect of the hard palate with the **lesser palatine neurovasculature**. The greater palatine neurovasculature passes through the **greater palatine foramen** to reach the hard palate. The nasopalatine and greater palatine nerves are direct branches from the pterygopalatine ganglion, and thus contain the functional components GSA, GVE-para/post, and sym/post (**Fig. 7.54; Fig. 7.68**).

The sphenopalatine artery is the terminal branch of the maxillary artery and originally passes through the sphenopalatine foramen before finding the incisive canal/fossa. The greater palatine artery is a branch of the *descending palatine artery*, which is one of the six arteries that branches from the third part of the maxillary artery. Distal branches of the aforementioned neurovasculature of the hard palate, minus the lesser palatine neurovasculature, form an anastomosis at the incisive canal/fossa. Lymphatic drainage of the hard palate is to the **submandibular**, **superior deep cervical**, or **retropharyngeal lymph nodes**.

7.6.7 Soft Palate

The **soft palate** is the movable, posterior portion of the palate. It is suspended from the posterior border of the hard palate and extends posteroinferiorly as a curved free margin from which hangs a conical process, the uvula. The soft palate is strengthened by the **palatine aponeurosis** that is formed by the tensor veli palatini muscle.

The **fauces** is the aperture leading from the oral cavity into the oropharynx. Its borders include the soft palate (superiorly), palatoglossal arches (laterally), and the dorsum of the tongue (inferiorly). Laterally, the soft palate is continuous with the wall of the pharynx and is joined to the tongue and pharynx by the **palatoglossal** and **palatopharyngeal arches**. The mucosa of these arches lies over the **palatoglossus** and **palatopharyngeus muscles**. Between the arches, the **palatine tonsils** (clinically known as just "the tonsils") rest within the **tonsillar sinus/fossa**.

Muscles of the Soft Palate

The soft palate is comprised of five pairs of muscles, **tensor veli palatini**, **levator veli palatini**, **palatoglossus**, **palatopharyngeus**, and the **musculus uvulae** (**Fig. 7.69**). The palatoglossus muscle serves as both a muscle of the tongue and of the soft palate. When a person swallows, the soft palate is initially tensed to allow the tongue to press up against it, squeezing the bolus of food toward the back of the oral cavity. It is then elevated posteriorly and superiorly against the wall of the pharynx, thereby preventing passage of food into the nasal cavity by sealing off the nasopharynx from the oropharynx. These muscles (along with the suprahyoid and longitudinal pharyngeal muscles) help elevate the larynx and shorten the pharynx. This is the **second stage of deglutition (swallowing)** and this is *involuntary and rapid*. All muscles of the

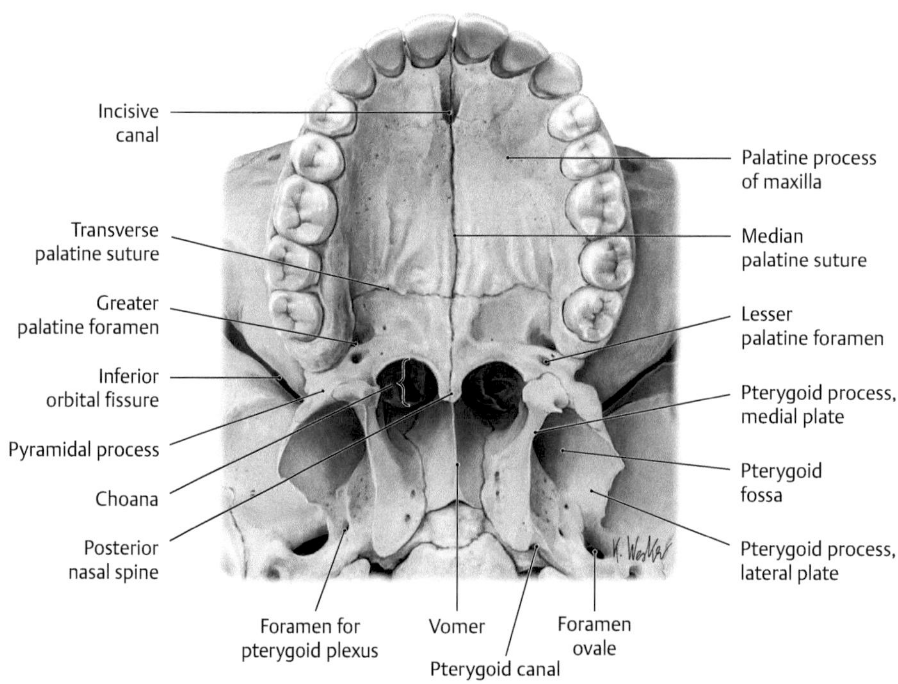

Fig. 7.67 Inferior view of the hard palate. (From Schuenke M, Schulte E, Schumacher U. THIEME Atlas of Anatomy. Head, Neck, and Neuroanatomy. Illustrations by Voll M and Wesker K. 3rd ed. New York: Thieme Medical Publishers; 2020.)

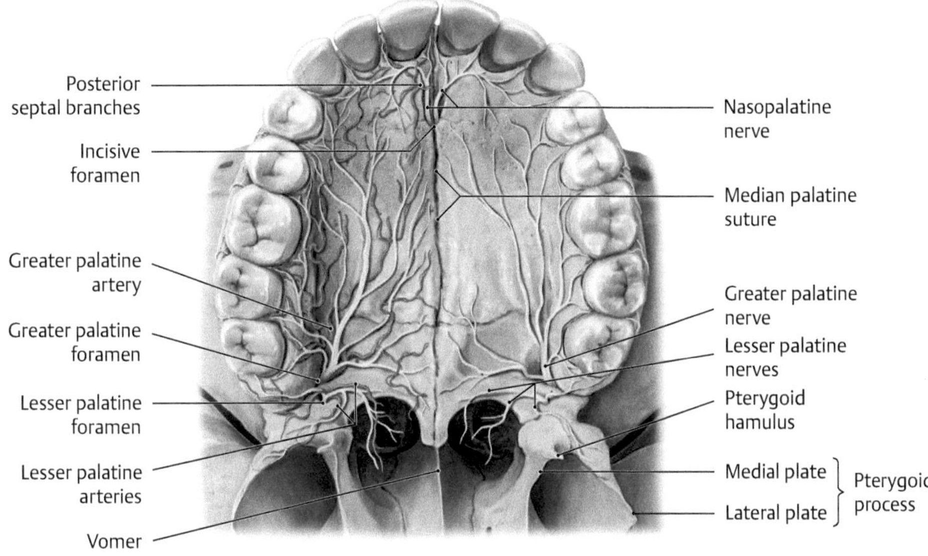

Fig. 7.68 Neurovasculature of the hard palate. (From Schuenke M, Schulte E, Schumacher U. THIEME Atlas of Anatomy. Head, Neck, and Neuroanatomy. Illustrations by Voll M and Wesker K. 3rd ed. New York: Thieme Medical Publishers; 2020.)

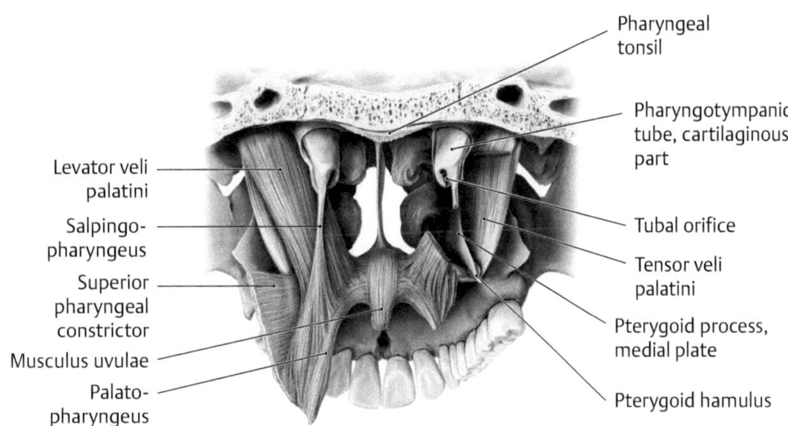

Fig. 7.69 Muscles of the soft palate: posterior view. (From Schuenke M, Schulte E, Schumacher U. THIEME Atlas of Anatomy. Head, Neck, and Neuroanatomy. Illustrations by Voll M and Wesker K. 3rd ed. New York: Thieme Medical Publishers; 2020.)

soft palate are innervated by the **pharyngeal branches of the vagus nerve (CN X)** except for the tensor veli palatini that receives its innervation from **CN V_3**. Muscles of the soft palate are detailed in **Table 7.4**.

Neurovasculature of the Soft Palate

The **lesser palatine nerve** supplies the mucosa of the soft palate and has no direct innervation to soft palate muscles. The special sense of taste (SVA) fibers from taste buds located on the soft palate also course through this nerve. The lesser palatine nerve is a direct branch from the pterygopalatine ganglion, and thus normally contains the functional components GSA, GVE-para/post, and sym/post in addition to the SVA-taste that will later become associated with the facial nerve (CN VII) **(Fig. 7.54; Fig. 7.68)**.

Blood supply to the soft palate is from the **lesser palatine** and **ascending palatine arteries**. The lesser palatine originates from the *descending palatine artery* while the ascending palatine originates from the *facial artery* **(Fig. 7.68)**. Lymphatic drainage of the soft palate is similar to the hard palate with drainage to the **submandibular**, **superior deep cervical**, or **retropharyngeal lymph nodes**.

7.7 Pterygopalatine Fossa and Ganglion

The **pterygopalatine fossa** is a small pyramidal space located inferior to the apex of the orbit, medial to the infratemporal fossa and lateral to the nasal cavity. Contents include the maxillary nerve (V_2), the pterygopalatine ganglion (PPG), and the third part of the maxillary artery and its branches. The boundaries of the pterygopalatine fossa include **(Fig. 7.70)**:

- Greater wing of the sphenoid bone (roof).
- Posterior surface of the maxilla (anterior wall).

Table 7.4 **Muscles of the soft palate**

Muscle	Function(s)	Origin	Insertion
Tensor veli palatini	Tenses the soft palate; opens the pharyngotympanic tube during swallowing and yawning to equalize air pressure	Scaphoid fossa of medial pterygoid plate; spine of sphenoid; cartilaginous part of pharyngotympanic tube	Palatine aponeurosis (after coursing around the pterygoid hamulus)
Levator veli palatini	Elevates the soft palate	Petrous part of temporal bone; cartilaginous part of pharyngotympanic tube	Palatine aponeurosis
Palatoglossus	Elevates root of tongue; closes off oral cavity from oropharynx	Palatine aponeurosis	Lateral side of posterior tongue
Palatopharyngeus	Elevates the pharynx during swallowing	Posterior border of hard palate; palatine aponeurosis	Lateral wall of pharynx; posterior border of thyroid cartilage
Musculus uvulae	Elevates and shortens uvula	Posterior nasal spine; palatine aponeurosis	Mucous membrane of uvula

- Pterygoid process of the sphenoid bone (posterior wall).
- Pyramidal process of the palatine bone (floor).
- Pterygomaxillary fissure (lateral wall).
- Perpendicular plate of the palatine bone (medial wall).

The pterygopalatine fossa can communicate with multiple regions of the head and these include **(Fig. 7.71)**:

- Anteriorly through the *inferior orbital fissure* to reach the *orbit.*
- Posterosuperiorly through the *foramen rotundum* and *pterygoid canal* to reach the *middle cranial fossa* and base of the skull, respectively.
- Posteroinferiorly through the *palatovaginal (pharyngeal) canal* to reach the *nasopharynx.*
- Laterally through the *pterygomaxillary fissure* to reach the *infratemporal fossa.*
- Medially through the *sphenopalatine foramen* to reach the *nasal cavity.*
- Inferiorly through the *greater palatine canal* (pterygopalatine) to reach the *palate.*

The **pterygopalatine (Meckel) ganglion (PPG)** is one of four major parasympathetic ganglion found in the head. Cell bodies of parasympathetic postganglionic fibers are located here. The nerve fibers that course through this ganglion control the blood flow to the nasal mucosa associated with humidifying and warming the air that passes through the nasal cavity. Nerve branches and the fibers that course through them also innervate mucosa of the paranasal sinuses, both palates and superior nasopharynx along with the lacrimal and palatine glands.

The **maxillary nerve (CN V_2)** enters the pterygopalatine fossa through the foramen rotundum. Within the fossa, the maxillary nerve will give off the **zygomatic nerve** which itself branches into the **zygomaticofacial** and **zygomaticotemporal nerves** (inconstant). The maxillary nerve continues through this fossa until passing through the inferior orbital fissure to become the infraorbital nerve. A **communicating branch** connects the zygomaticotemporal nerve to the **lacrimal nerve** (CN V_1 branch). Note: If the zygomaticotemporal nerve is not present, the communicating branch will branch off of the zygomatic nerve. The communicating branch conveys para/post (along with sym/post) fibers to the lacrimal gland. The maxillary nerve will also give off two smaller **pterygopalatine (sphenopalatine) nerves** that suspend the **PPG (Fig. 7.70)**.

The autonomic fibers that are associated with this ganglion originate from the **nerve of the pterygoid canal (Vidian nerve)**. The greater petrosal and deep petrosal nerves form the nerve of the pterygoid canal. The **greater petrosal nerve** is a branch off the facial nerve (CN VII) and conveys GVE-para/pre and SVA-taste fibers from the soft palate that originated in the lesser palatine nerve. It is these para/pre fibers that synapse at the PPG. The **deep petrosal nerve** originates from the internal carotid sympathetic periarterial plexus and conveys sym/post fibers. Thus, the functional components of the nerve of the pterygoid canal are GVE-para/pre, sym/post and SVA-taste from the soft palate.

Somatic (GSA) sensation from the nasal cavity, paranasal sinuses, palate, gingivae, and the superior nasopharynx passes back through all of the direct branches of the PPG. Once they reach the PPG, the GSA fibers will continue up through the pterygopalatine nerves to the maxillary nerve. The GSA fibers have their cell bodies located in the trigeminal ganglion. Note: GSA fibers do not pass back through the nerve of the pterygoid canal **(Fig. 7.66)**. The PPG has many branches, all of which contain the functional components GSA, GVE-para/post, and sym/post. Direct branches off the PPG include **(Fig. 7.72):**

- Orbital (multiple).
- Nasopalatine.
- Posterior superior medial/lateral nasal.
- Greater palatine.
- Lesser palatine.
- Pharyngeal.
- Pterygopalatine (also considered branches of the maxillary nerve).

The PPG does have a parasympathetic (motor) root, sympathetic root, and two sensory roots. The nerve of the pterygoid canal represents the parasympathetic and sympathetic roots. The greater petrosal nerve delivered the parasympathetic (para/pre) fibers while the deep petrosal nerve delivered the sympathetic (sym/post) fibers prior to both nerves fusing to become the nerve of the pterygoid canal. The pterygopalatine nerves serve as the sensory roots.

7.8 Nose and Nasal Cavities

The **nose** is a combination of structures and includes an external nose and a left and right nasal cavity. It is a part of the upper respiratory tract located superior to the hard palate and is lined primarily by *pseudostratified ciliated columnar epithelium.* The functions include respiration, filtration of dust and larger particles,

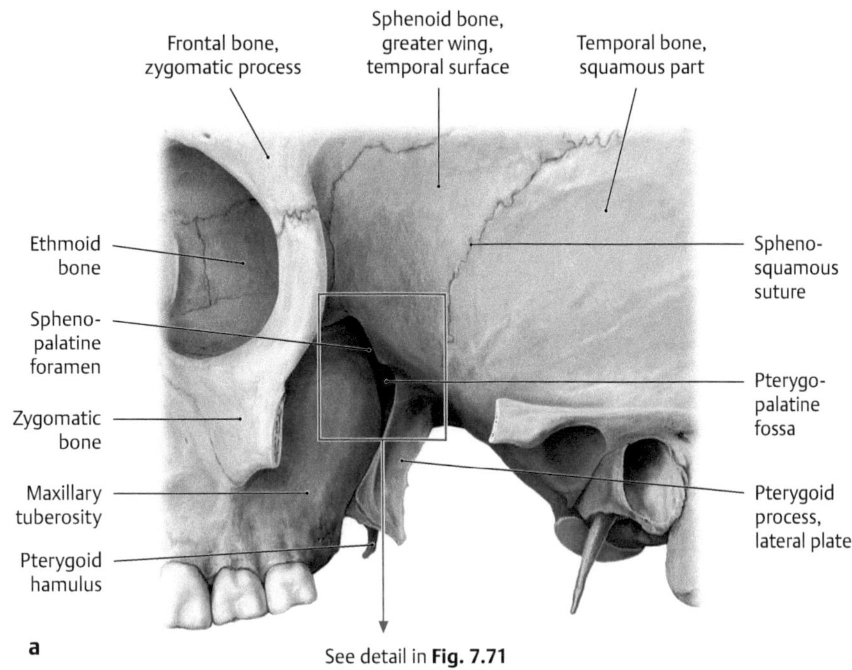

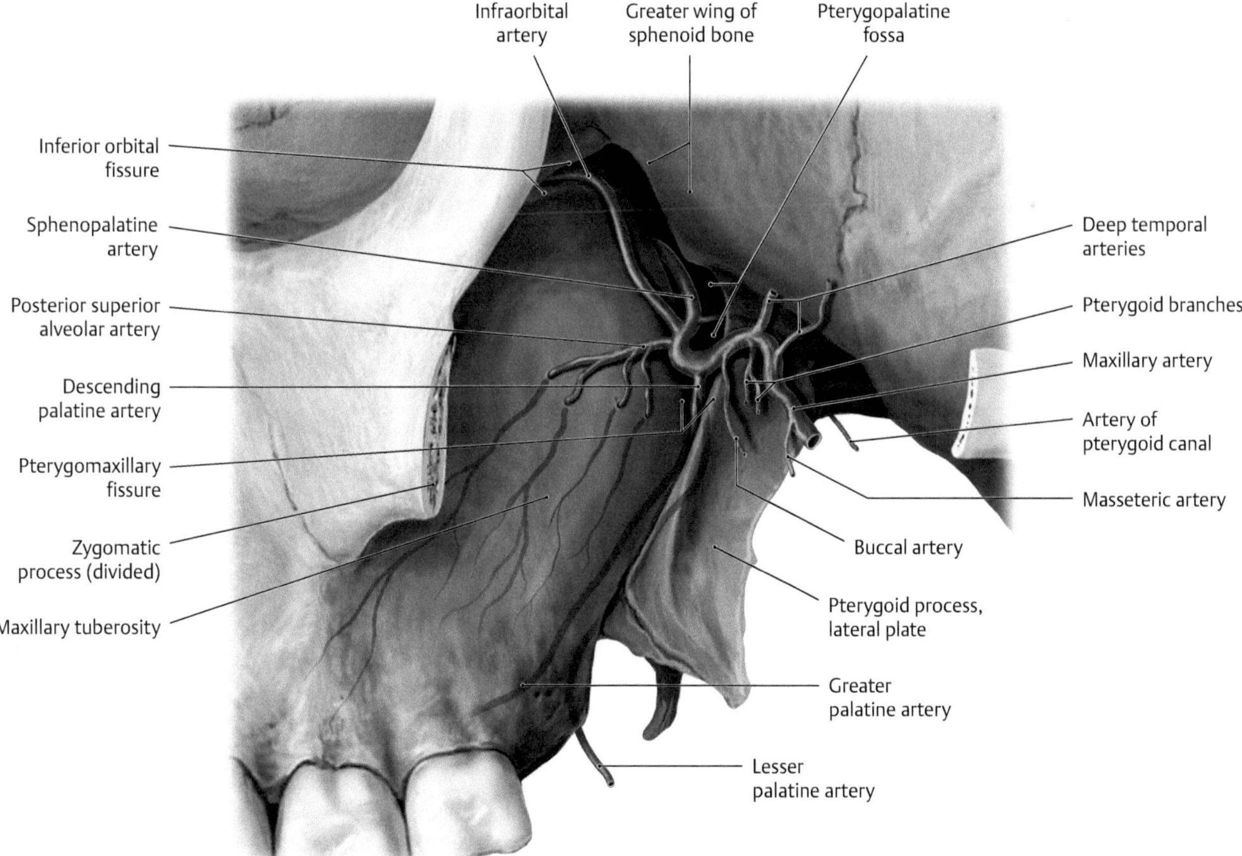

Fig. 7.70 **(a)** Pterygopalatine fossa. **(b)** Arteries of the pterygopalatine fossa. (*continued*) (From Schuenke M, Schulte E, Schumacher U. THIEME Atlas of Anatomy. Head, Neck, and Neuroanatomy. Illustrations by Voll M and Wesker K. 3rd ed. New York: Thieme Medical Publishers; 2020.)

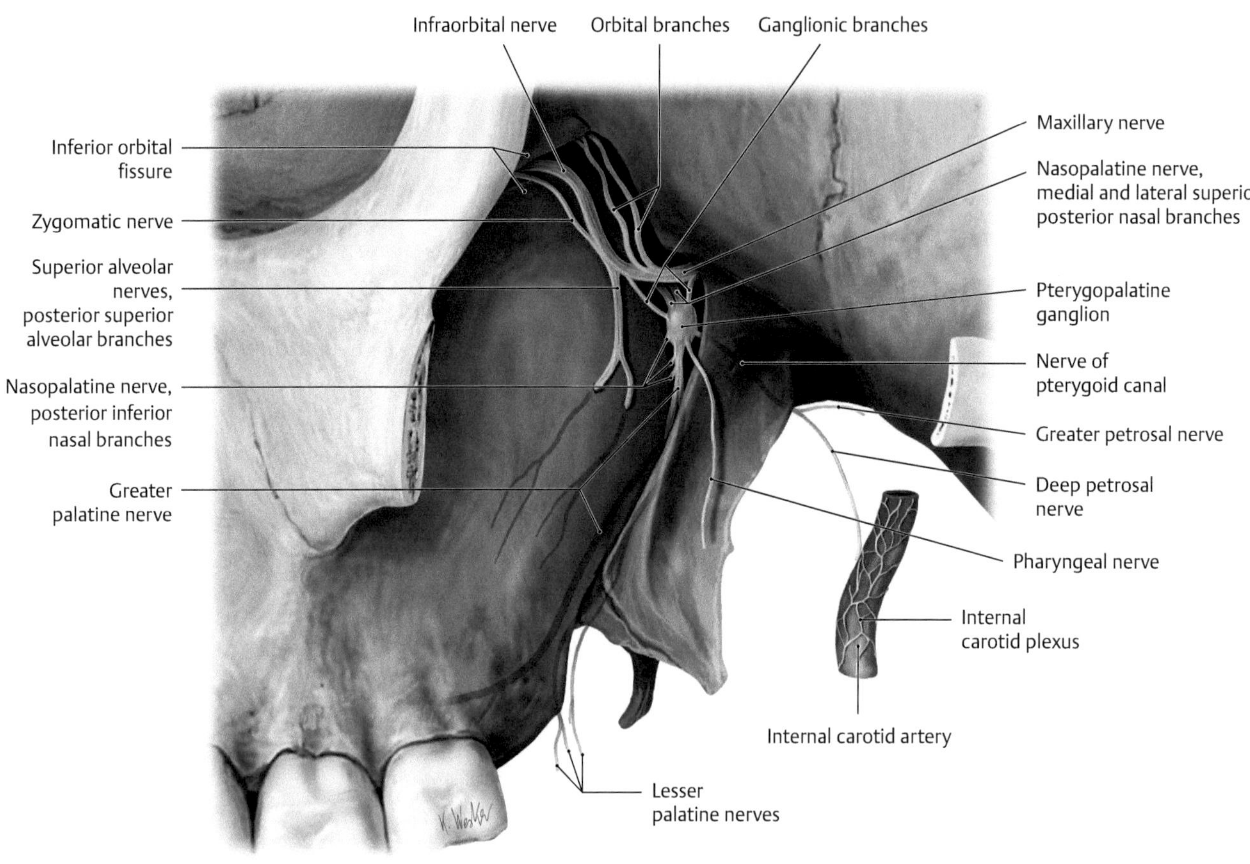

Fig. 7.70 *(continued)* **(c)** Nerves of the pterygopalatine fossa. (From Schuenke M, Schulte E, Schumacher U. THIEME Atlas of Anatomy. Head, Neck, and Neuroanatomy. Illustrations by Voll M and Wesker K. 3rd ed. New York: Thieme Medical Publishers; 2020.)

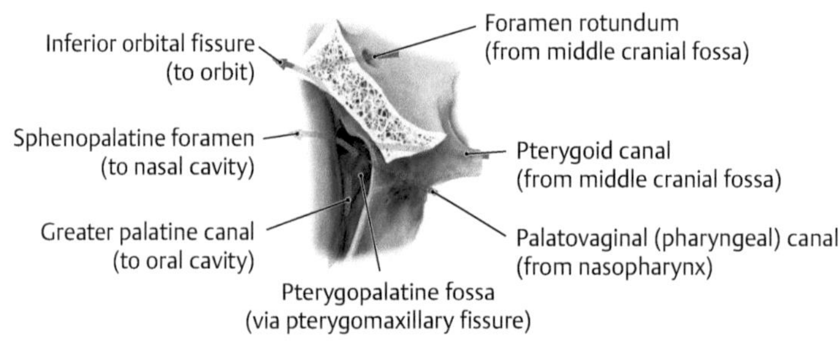

Fig. 7.71 Connections of the left pterygopalatine fossa with adjacent structures. (From Schuenke M, Schulte E, Schumacher U. THIEME Atlas of Anatomy. Head, Neck, and Neuroanatomy. Illustrations by Voll M and Wesker K. 3rd ed. New York: Thieme Medical Publishers; 2020.)

humidification of the air, drainage sites for paranasal sinuses and the nasolacrimal duct, and olfaction (sense of smell).

7.8.1 External Nose

The external nose projects anteriorly from the face and consists primarily of cartilage. The **dorsum of the nose** will extend from the **root** down to the **apex** (tip). The two nasal apertures on the inferior surface of the external nose are called **nares** (nostrils) and are bound laterally by the **alae**. Skin of the nose continues into the **vestibule** where thicker hairs called *vibrissae* are located. These are the hairs responsible for trapping larger dust particles before they can enter the nasal cavities. Cartilaginous structures that make up the external nose include: a midline **septal cartilage**, **lateral processes of the septal cartilage**, **major (greater) alar**, and three to four **minor (lesser) alar cartilages**. The alar cartilages are free and mobile and move when muscles acting on the nose contract **(Fig. 7.73)**.

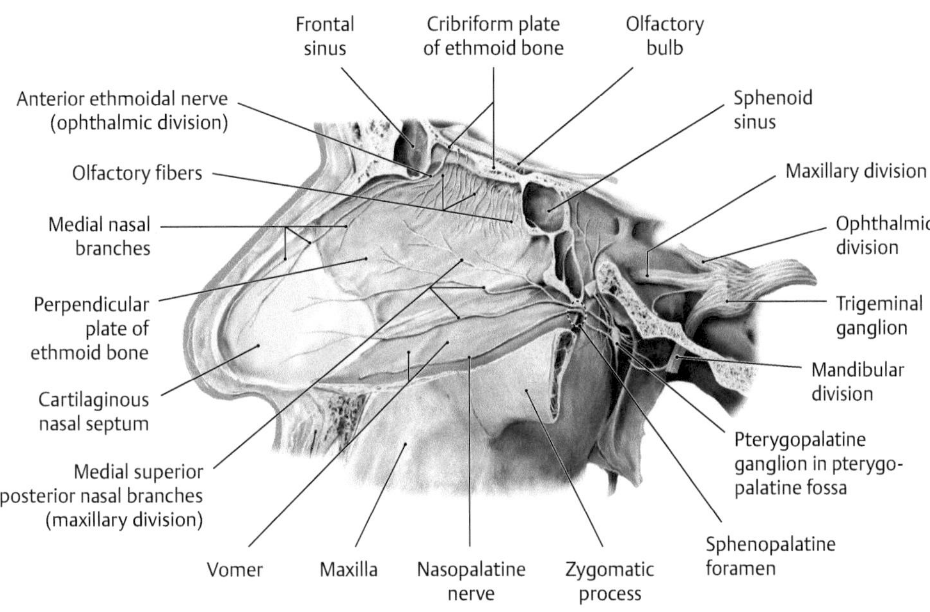

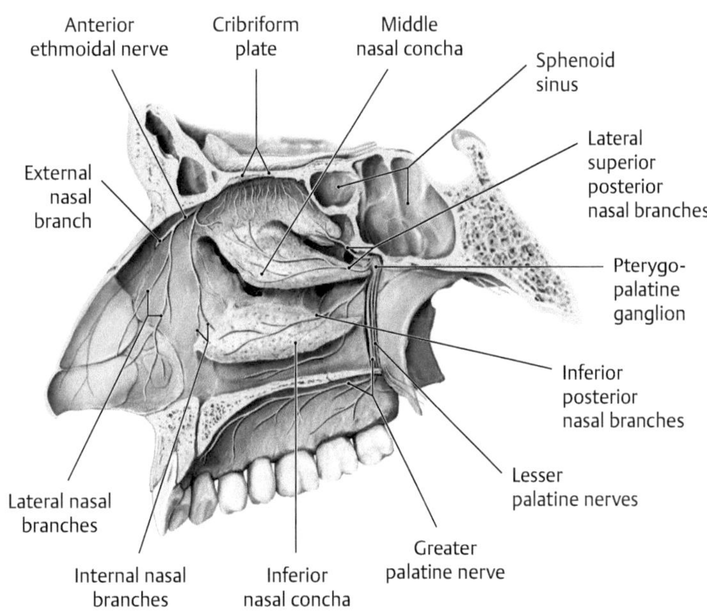

Fig. 7.72 Nerves of the nasal septum and right lateral nasal wall. (From Schuenke M, Schulte E, Schumacher U. THIEME Atlas of Anatomy. Head, Neck, and Neuroanatomy. Illustrations by Voll M and Wesker K. 3rd ed. New York: Thieme Medical Publishers; 2020.)

7.8.2 Nasal Cavity

The **nasal cavity** is divided into a left and right half by the nasal septum. Boundaries of the nasal cavities include:

- Frontal, ethmoid, and sphenoid bones (roof).
- Hard palate (floor).
- Nasal conchae (lateral wall).
- Nasal septum (medial wall) that is formed by the **septal cartilage**, **perpendicular plate of the ethmoid bone**, and the **vomer** (**Fig. 7.74**).

Air enters through the nares, travels through the nasal cavity, and finally exits posteriorly into the nasopharynx through apertures called **choanae**. Nasal mucosa is firmly attached to the perichondrium and periosteum and is continuous with the paranasal sinuses, lacrimal sac, conjunctiva, and nasopharynx. The majority of the mucosa is known as the respiratory area while a specific superior portion is known as the olfactory area. This olfactory area contains the peripheral organ of smell. The nasal conchae (or turbinates) curve inferomedially from the lateral wall and add surface area to the nasal cavities. This surface area is important in heat exchange and humidification of inspired air.

The **superior** and **middle nasal conchae** are parts of the ethmoid bone while the **inferior nasal conchae** are individual bones located bilaterally. When mucosa overlying the conchae is irritated, they become inflamed and cause blockage of the nasal passageways. Below a concha is the recess known as a **nasal meatus** (superior, middle, and inferior) and they are named

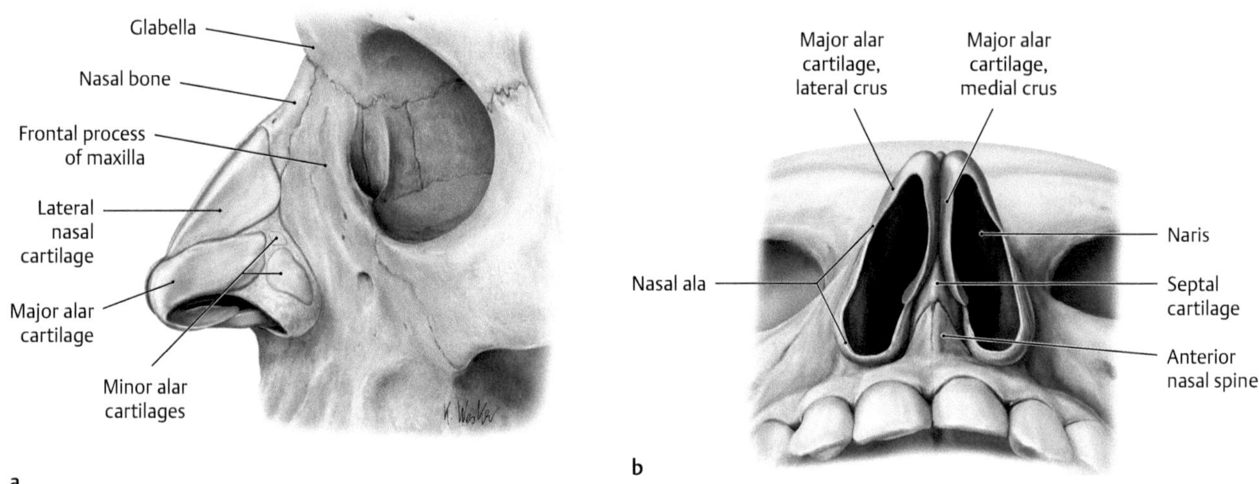

Fig. 7.73 Skeleton and nasal cartilages of the external nose. **(a)** Left lateral view. **(b)** Inferior view. (From Schuenke M, Schulte E, Schumacher U. THIEME Atlas of Anatomy. Head, Neck, and Neuroanatomy. Illustrations by Voll M and Wesker K. 3rd ed. New York: Thieme Medical Publishers; 2020.)

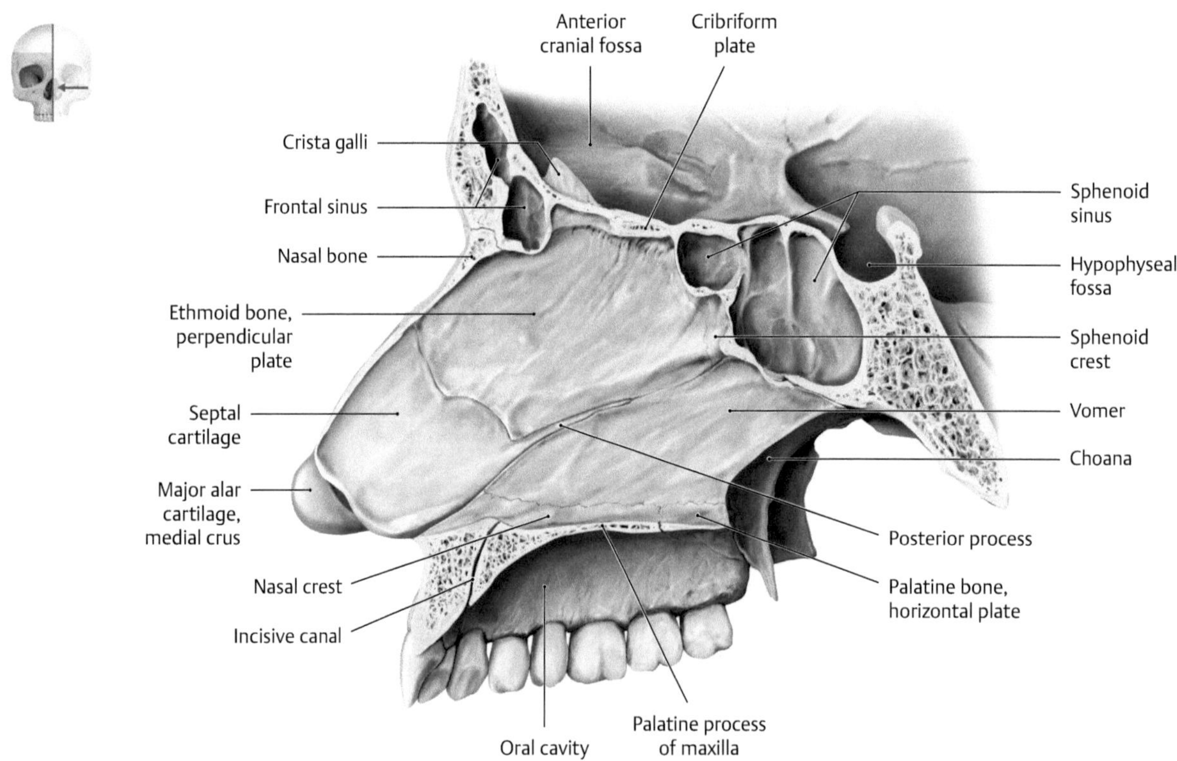

Fig. 7.74 Nasal septum. (From Schuenke M, Schulte E, Schumacher U. THIEME Atlas of Anatomy. Head, Neck, and Neuroanatomy. Illustrations by Voll M and Wesker K. 3rd ed. New York: Thieme Medical Publishers; 2020.)

according to the concha they are located below. Located posterior to the superior concha and anterior to the sphenoid sinus is the **sphenoethmoidal recess (Fig. 7.75)**.

Neurovasculature of the Nasal Cavities and Septum

An oblique line passing from the anterior nasal spine and the sphenoethmoidal recess divides the nasal mucosa into an anterosuperior versus posteroinferior region innervation scheme and includes both the lateral and medial walls of the nasal cavity. Mucosa innervation of the anterosuperior region and both walls is associated with mainly CN V_1 nerves and these include the **anterior** and **posterior ethmoidal nerves**, direct branches of the nasociliary nerve. The **olfactory nerve (CN I)** is responsible for the sense of smell located on both the lateral and medial walls of the anterosuperior portion of the nasal cavity.

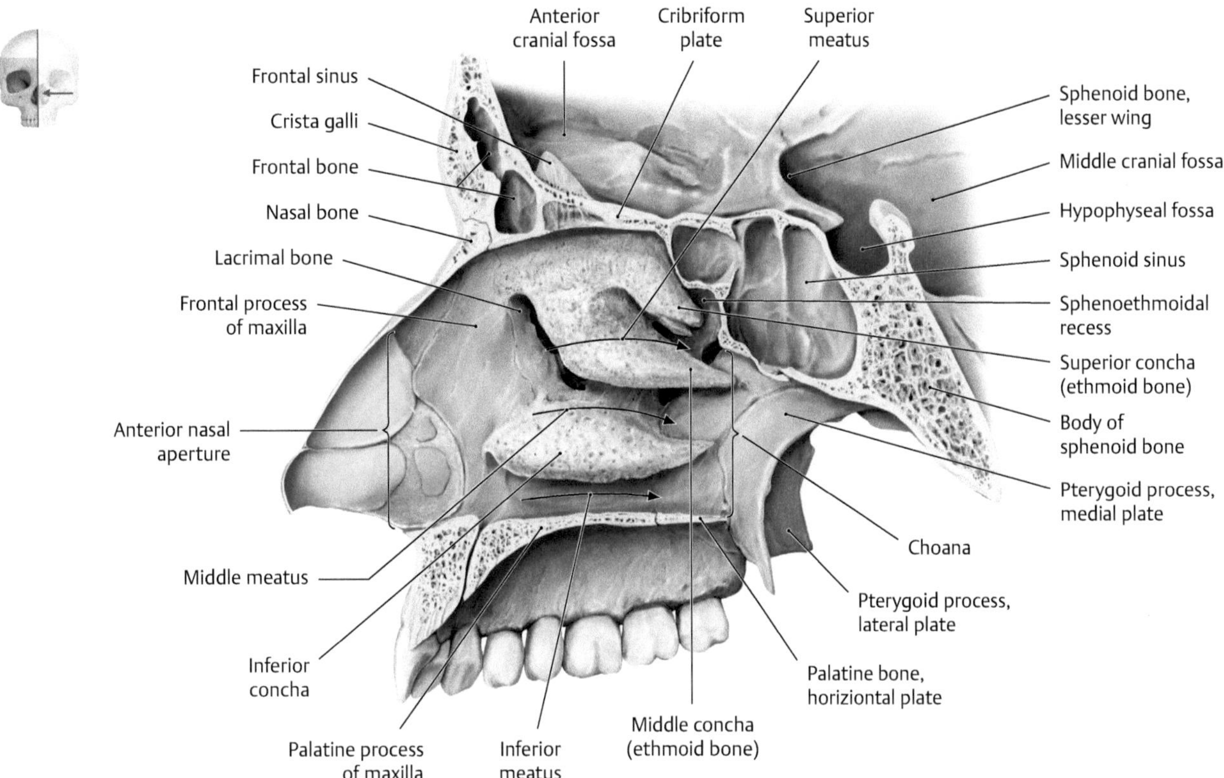

Fig. 7.75 Lateral wall of the right nasal cavity. (From Schuenke M, Schulte E, Schumacher U. THIEME Atlas of Anatomy. Head, Neck, and Neuroanatomy. Illustrations by Voll M and Wesker K. 3rd ed. New York: Thieme Medical Publishers; 2020.)

The **nasopalatine** and **posterior superior lateral/medial nasal** and **posterior inferior lateral/medial nasal nerves** innervate the posteroinferior region of the nasal mucosa. The nasopalatine and posterior superior lateral/medial nasal branches are direct branches of the PPG while the posterior inferior lateral/medial nasal branches come off the greater palatine nerve. However, because the GSA fibers traveling back through these nerves eventually pass through the maxillary nerve, they are commonly referred to as CN V_2 branches. The **external nasal** (anterior ethmoidal br.) and **infratrochlear nerves** (nasociliary br.) supply the dorsum and apex of the external nose while the **nasal branches of the infraorbital nerve** (CN V_2 br.) supply the alae and vestibule of the nose **(Fig. 7.76)**.

Blood supply to the lateral and medial walls of the nasal cavity is from six sources and they can form an anastomosis at many sites. These arteries include the **anterior ethmoidal** (ophthalmic br.), **posterior ethmoidal** (ophthalmic br.), **sphenopalatine** (third part of maxillary br.), **septal branch of superior labial** (facial br.), **lateral nasal** (facial br.), and **greater palatine** (descending palatine br.). All of these vessels contribute to an anastomotic arterial plexus located near the anterior portion of the nasal septum known as *Kiesselbach area*. The anterior ethmoidal, nasal branches of the infraorbital, septal branch of the superior labial and lateral nasal branches of the facial arteries supply the external nose **(Fig. 7.76)**.

Deep to the nasal mucosa, the **submucosal venous plexus** drains venous blood from the nose via the ophthalmic, sphenopalatine, and facial veins. This plexus exchanges heat and warms the air prior to it reaching the lungs and serves as part of the thermoregulatory system of the body. The facial vein through the angular and lateral nasal tributaries receives most of the venous blood from the external nose. This lies within the "danger area" of the face and can communicate with the cavernous sinuses within the skull.

Lymphatic drainage of the external nose and anterior aspect of the nasal cavity is to the **submandibular**, **buccal,** and **parotid lymph nodes.** The posterior aspect of the nasal cavity drains back to the **retropharyngeal** and **superior deep cervical lymph nodes.**

Histology of the Nose and Nasal Cavity

The vestibule consists of *stratified squamous epithelium* just prior to the stereotypical *pseudostratified ciliated columnar epithelium* with abundant goblet cells seen in the nasal cavities **(Fig. 7.77)**. The **olfactory epithelium** located on the superior portions of both the nasal septum and lateral walls of the nasal cavities is made up of special chemoreceptors mixed in with pseudostratified columnar epithelium containing no goblet cells. The **olfactory sensory cells** are bipolar neurons that have dendrite processes with **olfactory vesicles** near the luminal surface. The unmyelinated axons extend in the opposite direction toward the cribriform plate synapse with neurons in the **olfactory bulb (Fig. 7.78)**. Secretions originating from Bowman glands bath the olfactory vesicles and they remove previous ligands to reactivate receptors to pick up additional odors. The olfactory system of a human contains approximately 400 types of scent receptors capable of detecting at least 1 trillion different odors.[3]

7.8.3 Paranasal Sinuses

The **paranasal sinuses** are the air-filled extensions of the respiratory portion of the nasal cavity and are named according to the bones in which they are located (**Fig. 7.79**). They include the

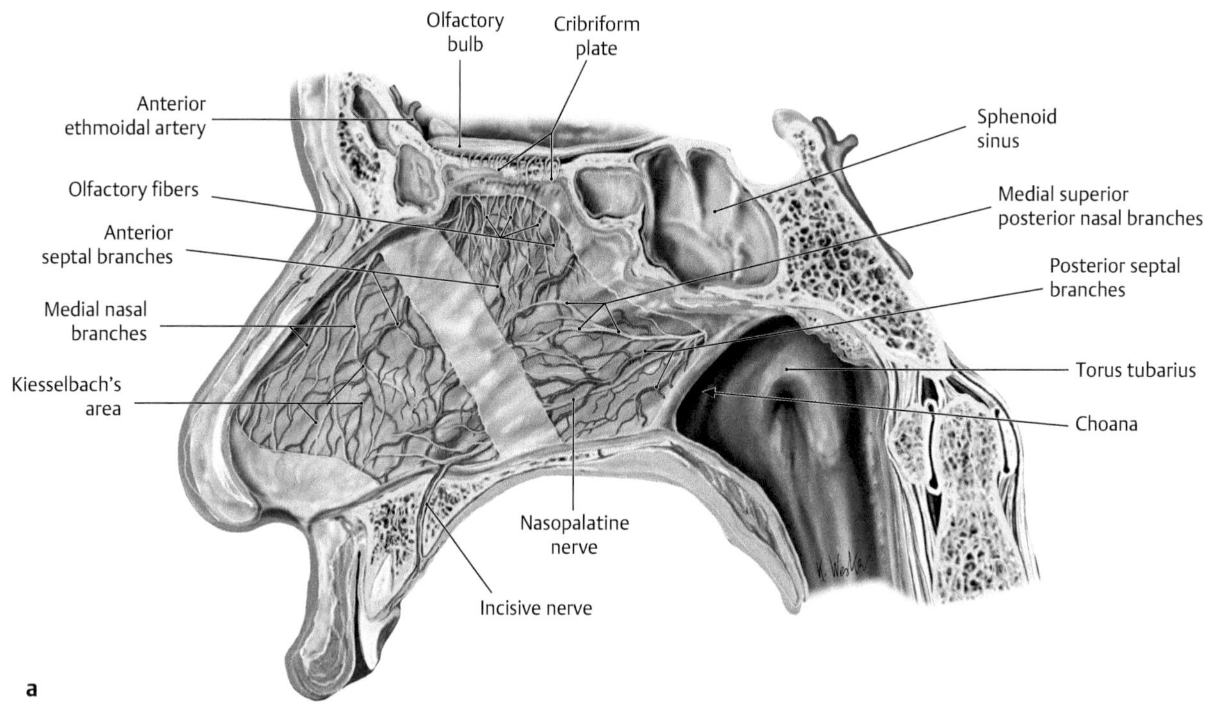

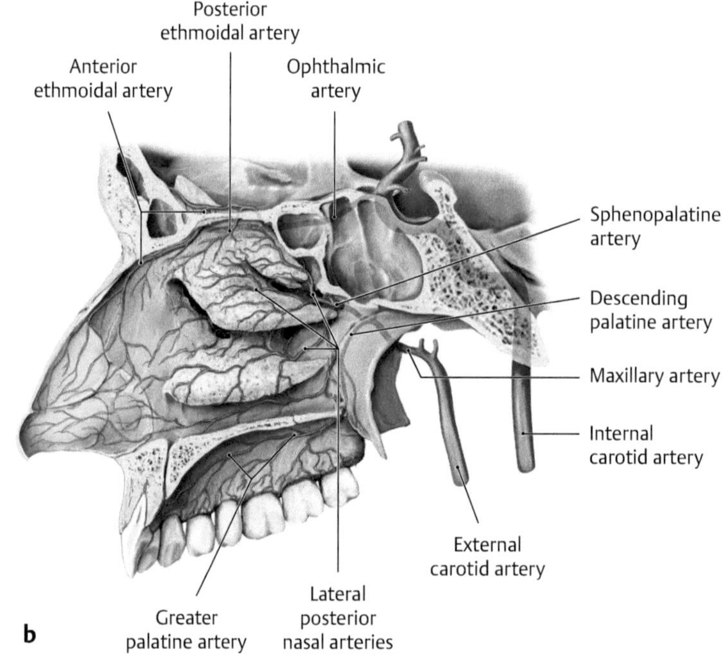

Fig. 7.76 **(a)** Neurovasculature of the nasal septum with the mucosa removed. **(b)** Arteries of the right lateral nasal wall. (From Schuenke M, Schulte E, Schumacher U. THIEME Atlas of Anatomy. Head, Neck, and Neuroanatomy. Illustrations by Voll M and Wesker K. 3rd ed. New York: Thieme Medical Publishers; 2020.)

frontal, ethmoid, sphenoid, and maxillary sinuses. The frontal, sphenoid, and maxillary sinuses continue to develop (pneumatization) and this can extend well into the sixth decade of life as in the case of the maxillary sinuses. The ethmoid sinus is already pneumatized at birth.

- **Frontal sinuses**: are located posterior to the superciliary arches (eyebrow ridge) and root of the nose but in between the external and internal layers of the frontal bone. There is generally a left and right sinus but they are rarely symmetrical and on occasion they may be fused. A small percentage of individuals (<5%) have no frontal sinuses. The frontal sinus drainage initially passes through the **frontonasal duct**, into the **ethmoidal infundibulum** and then **semilunar hiatus** before finally passing to the middle meatus. The mucosa lining these sinuses receives its innervation from the **supraorbital nerves** (GSA) and **orbital branches off the PPG** (para/post

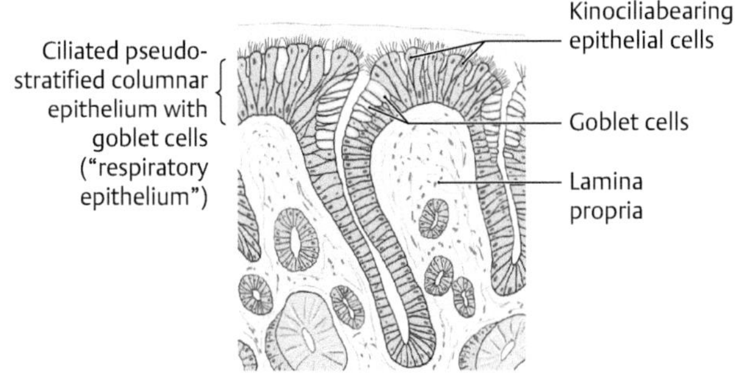

Fig. 7.77 Histology of the nasal mucosa. (From Schuenke M, Schulte E, Schumacher U. THIEME Atlas of Anatomy. Head, Neck, and Neuroanatomy. Illustrations by Voll M and Wesker K. 3rd ed. New York: Thieme Medical Publishers; 2020.)

secretomotor). Blood supply is from the **supraorbital** and **anterior ethmoidal arteries**. Lymph drains to the **submandibular lymph nodes**.

- **Ethmoidal sinuses (air cells)**: are different from other paranasal sinuses because they are formed of multiple thin-walled cavities within the ethmoid bone. The size and number of air cells varies and may not be visible on a radiograph until 2 years of age. There are *anterior, middle,* and *posterior ethmoidal air cells.*
  - **Anterior ethmoidal air cells**: drain directly or indirectly to the *middle meatus* by way of the *ethmoidal infundibulum.*
  - **Middle ethmoidal air cells**: drain directly to the *middle meatus* through the *ethmoid bulla.*
  - **Posterior ethmoidal air cells**: drain directly to the *superior meatus.*

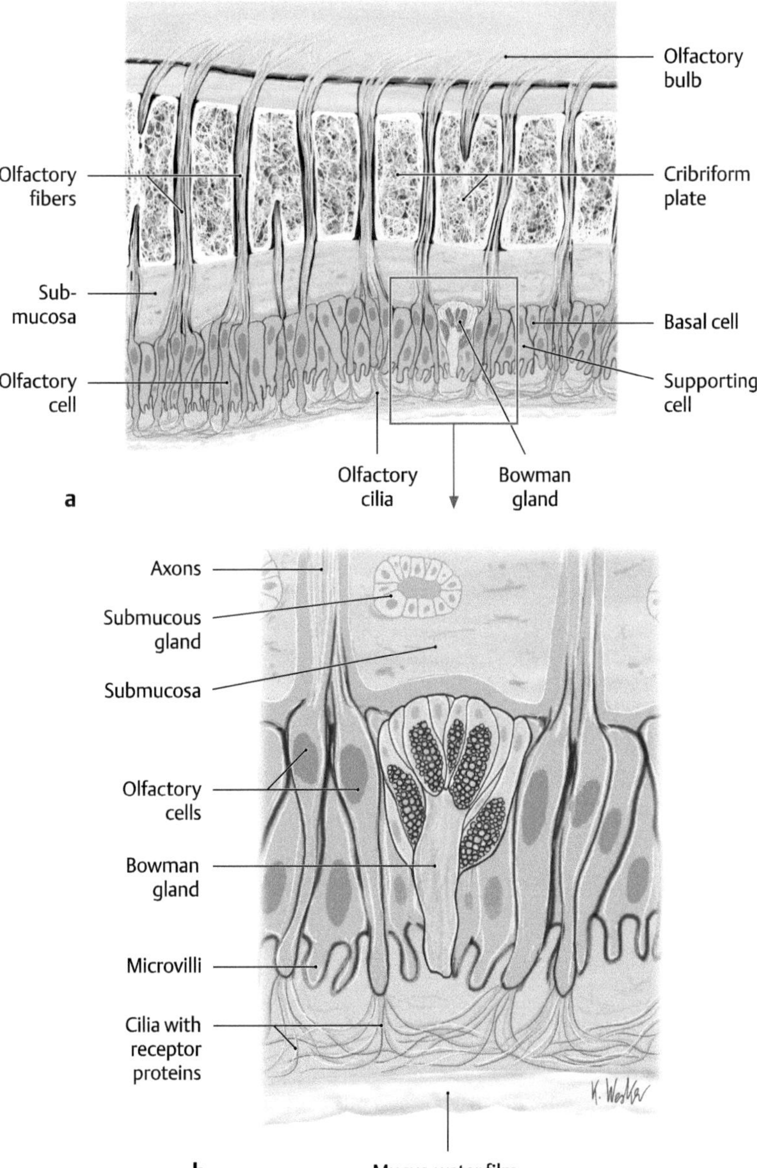

Fig. 7.78 **(a)** The olfactory epithelium at the level of the cribriform plate. **(b)** Close up of the olfactory neuron cell bodies and Bowman glands. (From Schuenke M, Schulte E, Schumacher U. THIEME Atlas of Anatomy. Head, Neck, and Neuroanatomy. Illustrations by Voll M and Wesker K. 3rd ed. New York: Thieme Medical Publishers; 2020.)

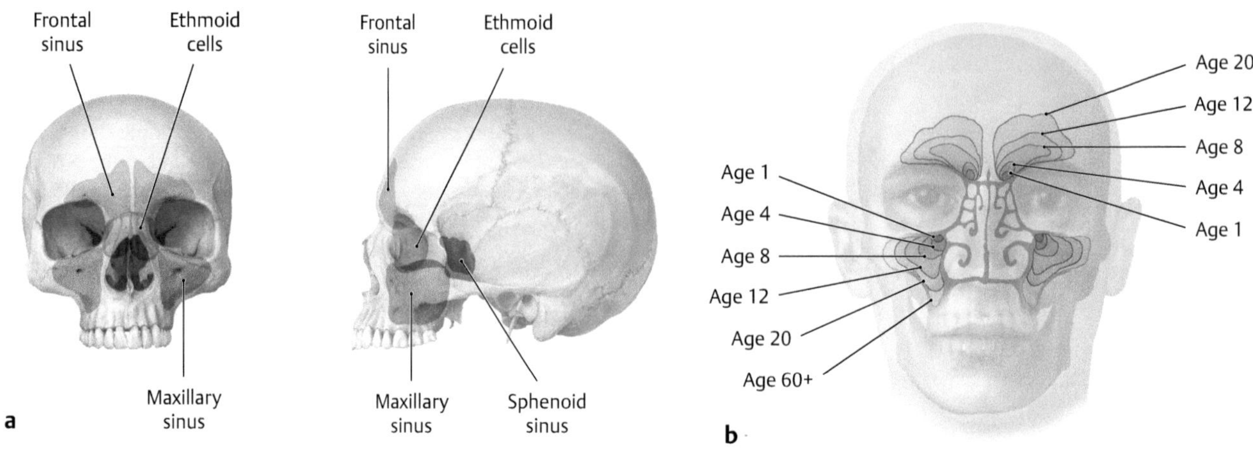

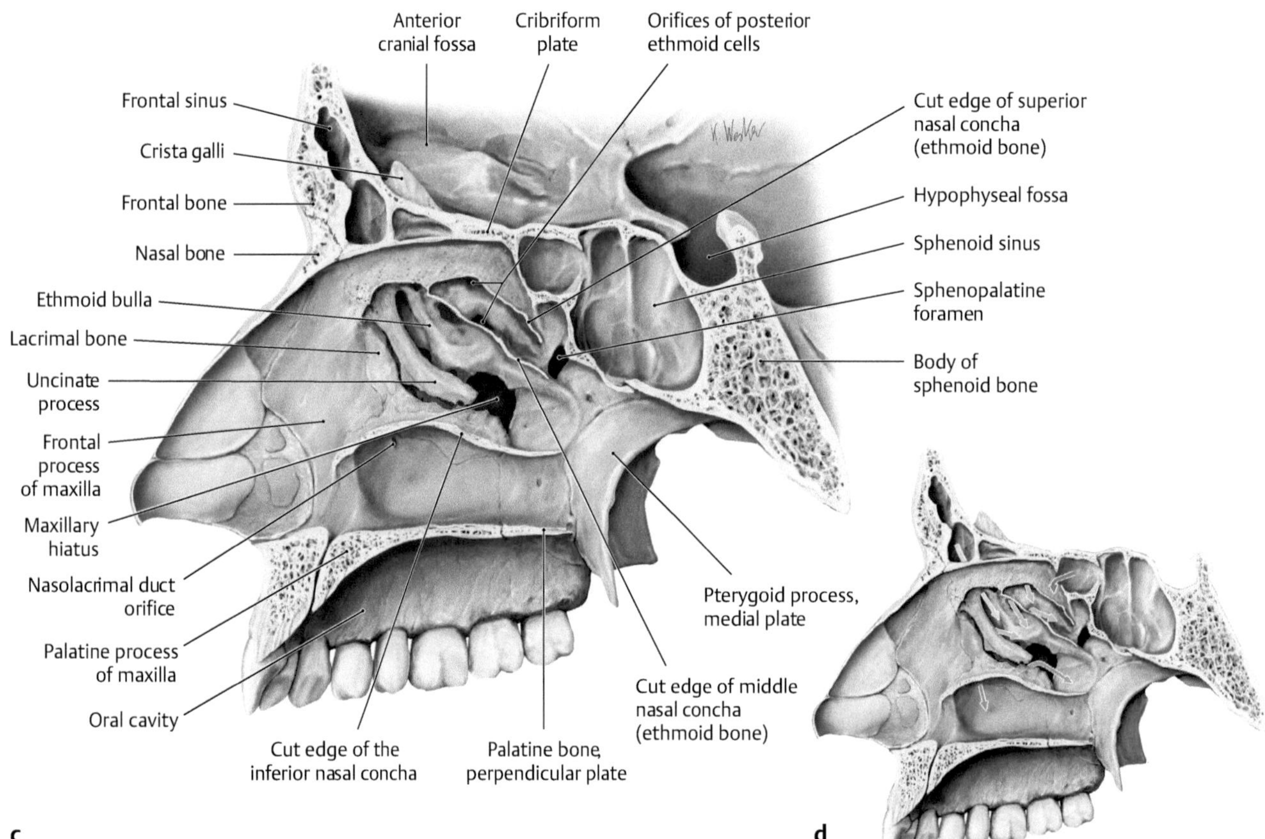

Fig. 7.79 **(a)** Anterior and lateral views of the paranasal sinuses. **(b)** Pneumatization of the frontal and maxillary sinuses. **(c)** Lateral wall of the right nasal cavity. **(d)** Drainage patterns: yellow = frontal sinus; green = ethmoid air cells; blue = sphenoid sinus; red = nasolacrimal duct; orange = maxillary sinus. (From Schuenke M, Schulte E, Schumacher U. THIEME Atlas of Anatomy. Head, Neck, and Neuroanatomy. Illustrations by Voll M and Wesker K. 3rd ed. New York: Thieme Medical Publishers; 2020.)

The mucosal lining receives its innervation from the **anterior** and **posterior ethmoidal nerves** (GSA) and **orbital branches off the PPG** (para/post secretomotor). Blood supply is from the **anterior ethmoidal, posterior ethmoidal,** and **sphenopalatine arteries**. Lymphatic drainage is to the **submandibular** and **retropharyngeal lymph nodes**.

- **Sphenoidal sinuses**: are generally located in the body of the sphenoid but can extend into the pterygoid processes, and the greater and lesser wings. The majority of sphenoid sinus development occurs after puberty. On the anterior wall of these sinuses, a small aperture allows for drainage into the *spheno-ethmoidal recess*. The mucosa lining these sinuses receives its innervation from the **posterior ethmoidal nerves** (GSA) and **orbital branches off the PPG** (para/post secretomotor). Blood supply is from the **posterior ethmoidal** and **sphenopalatine arteries**. Lymph drains to the **retropharyngeal lymph nodes**.

- **Maxillary sinuses**: is the largest of the paranasal sinuses and results in the maxillae being primarily open space. They are pyramidal in shape and can continue to expand into the sixth or seventh decades of life (**Fig. 7.79**). The thinness of the sinuses wall is significant because any tumors originating from these sinuses can easily push through into adjacent regions. The sinuses drain via the **maxillary ostia** located in the *semilunar hiatus*. From here they will drain to the *middle meatus*. Neurovasculature supplying the mucosa of these sinuses is from the **posterior superior alveolar**, **middle superior alveolar**, and **anterior superior alveolar nerves** and **vessels**. The nerves contain both GSA and autonomic fibers. Lymphatic drainage is to the **submandibular lymph nodes**.

7.8.4 Development of the Face, Palate, and Nasal Cavities

Face Development

During the fourth week of development, five facial primordia or prominences begin to appear around the stomodeum. There is one *frontonasal* and two each of the *maxillary* and *mandibular prominences* that consist primarily of neural crest derived mesenchyme. The **frontonasal prominence** surrounds the ventrolateral part of the forebrain. The frontal part of this prominence forms the forehead while the nasal part forms the rostral boundary of the stomodeum and the nose. By the end of the fourth week, bilateral thickenings of surface ectoderm or **nasal placodes** develop on the inferolateral portions of the frontonasal prominence. These placodes invaginate to form the **nasal pits** or precursor to nostrils and the anterior nasal cavity, but this results in the creation of **lateral nasal** and **medial nasal prominences**. Cranial nerve V_1 will become associated with this prominence but it is not a part of the first pharyngeal arch (**Fig. 7.80**).

The **maxillary prominences** give rise to the maxilla (upper jaw), zygomatic bone, squamous portion of the temporal bone, and upper lip. Up till the sixth week, the maxillary prominences continue to grow and their medially driven growth compresses the medial nasal prominences toward the midline. With the medial nasal and maxillary prominences merging, this will result in the continuity of the upper jaw and lip and separation of the nasal pits from the stomodeum. The lower part of the medial nasal prominences becomes deeply positioned and is covered by medial extensions of the maxillary prominences forming the **intermaxillary segment** which helps form the **philtrum**. Cranial nerve V_2 is associated with this part of the first pharyngeal arch. The lateral nasal prominences are separated from the maxillary prominences by the **nasolacrimal groove**. The **nasolacrimal duct** and **lacrimal sac** develop from a solid rodlike thickening of ectoderm in the floor of the nasolacrimal groove that later canalizes (**Fig. 7.80**). The **mandibular prominences** form the mandible and lower lip. These are the first parts of the face to develop. Cranial nerve V_3 is associated with this part of the first pharyngeal arch.

Palate Development

Palatogenesis begins in the 6th week of development but will not be completed until the 12th week. The most critical time period is between weeks 6 and 9. The palate will develop from two primordia known as the *primary* and *secondary palates*. When growth of the *maxillary prominences* causes the two medial nasal prominences to fuse together at the midline this creates the **intermaxillary segment**. This intermaxillary segment will contribute to the **primary palate**, along with the **philtrum of the lip** and the **four incisor teeth**. The primary palate makes up only a small portion of the adult hard palate (**Fig. 7.80; Fig. 7.81**).

Lateral outgrowths from the maxillary prominences are known as **palatine shelves** and they project from each side of the tongue to become the **secondary palate**, with the **palatine raphe** representing the site of fusion. The posterior portions of the palatine shelves do not ossify but will extend in a posterior direction and fuse to form the **soft palate** and **uvula**. This fusion occurs beyond the location of the final nasal septum. The **nasal septum** originated from the medial nasal prominences and continued to develop in a downward direction before fusing with the primary and secondary palates at the level of the palatine raphe. Moving in an anterior to posterior direction, the septum will be complete by the 12th week (**Fig. 7.81**).

Clinical Correlate 7.18

Cleft Palates and Upper Lips

Cleft palates and upper lips can be the result of multifactorial causes such as failed neural crest cell migration, associated with syndromes, or possibly due to the exposure to anticonvulsant and acne medications to name a few. The incisive canal/fossa and papilla are used as reference points to classify these defects (**Fig. 7.82**). **Cleft palates** may or may not include a cleft lip but they generally involve the hard or soft palates and even the uvula.

Cleft lips can present either unilaterally or bilaterally. **Unilateral cleft lips** are the most common congenital malformation of the head and neck regions and affect boys most often. They are the result of the maxillary prominence failing to fuse with the medial nasal prominences of the ipsilateral side. **Bilateral cleft lip** is the failure of maxillary prominences to meet and fuse with the medial nasal prominences. This form of cleft lip results in the intermaxillary segment hanging and projecting anteriorly.

Nasal Cavity Development

The deepening of the **nasal pits** mainly due to the proliferating mesenchyme forming the **medial** and **lateral nasal prominences** results in the formation of **nasal sacs**. The nasal sacs are initially separated from the oral cavity by the **oronasal membrane**. This membrane ruptures around the sixth week, allowing the nasal and oral cavities to communicate with one another. The region of continuity between the nasal and oral cavities is known as the **primitive choanae** and it lies posterior to the primary palate. After the secondary palate develops, the choanae will be located between the nasal cavity and nasopharynx (**Fig. 7.83**).

The **superior**, **middle,** and **inferior nasal conchae** develop from elevations of the lateral nasal cavity walls. Ectodermal epithelium of the roof of the nasal cavities becomes specialized and forms the **olfactory epithelium**. These cells differentiate to form olfactory receptor cells and the axons that extend from these cells constitute the **olfactory nerve** (CN I) that will grow into the olfactory bulb of the brain.

Paranasal sinuses form from outgrowths of the walls of the nasal cavities and become pneumatic (air-filled) extensions of the nasal cavities in the adjacent bones and begin to develop after birth. The original openings of the outgrowths persist as the orifices of the adult sinuses. The **maxillary sinuses**, however, begin to develop during late fetal life and will continue to expand into the sixth or seventh decade of life (**Fig. 7.79**).

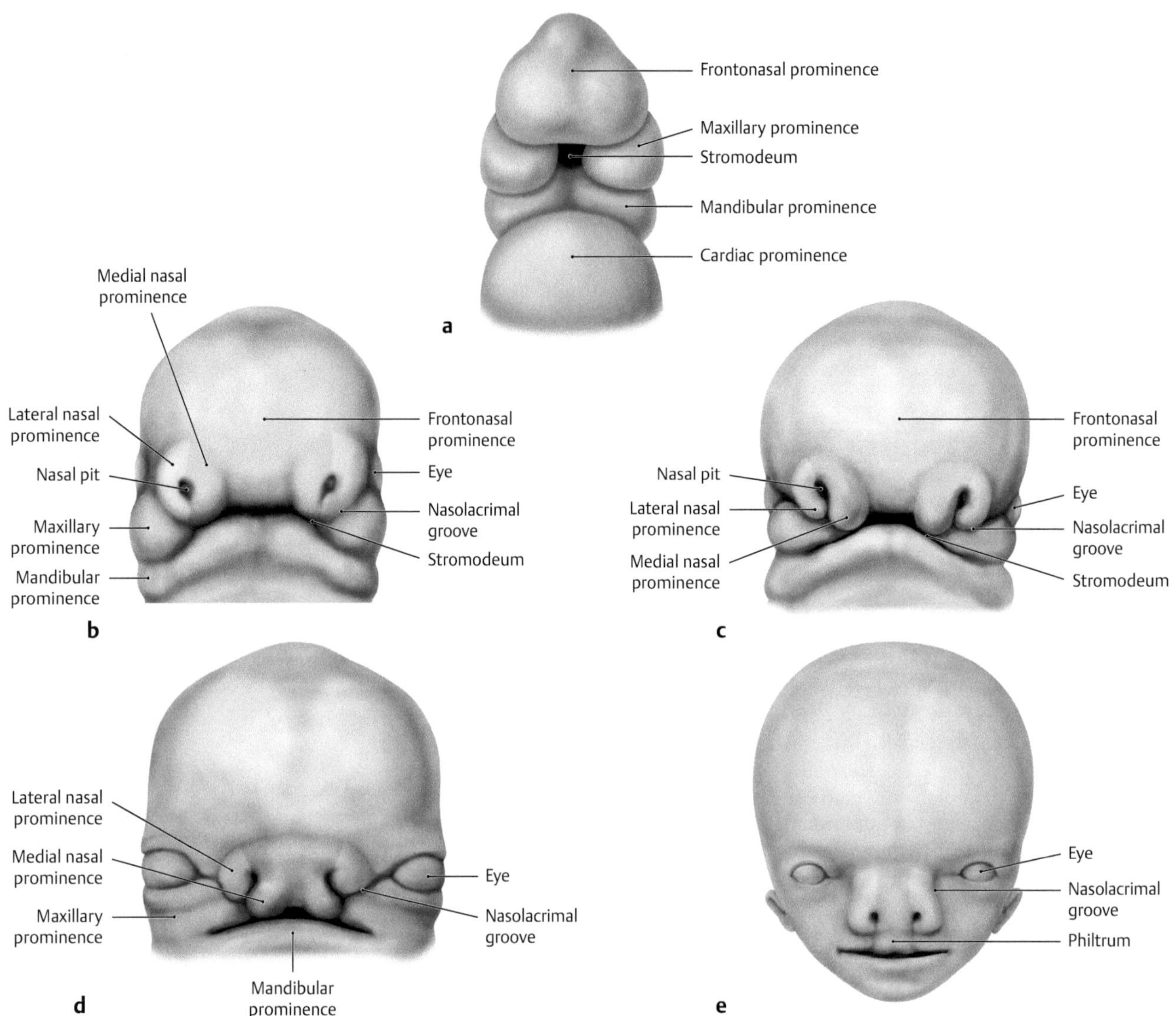

Fig. 7.80 Development of the face. **(a)** Anterior view at 24 days; **(b)** 5 weeks; **(c)** 6 weeks; **(d)** 7 weeks; **(e)** 10 weeks. (From Baker EW. Anatomy for Dental Medicine. 2nd ed. 2015. Based on the work of: Schuenke M, Schulte E, Schumacher U. THIEME Atlas of Anatomy. Illustrations by Voll M and Wesker K.)

7.9 Orbit and Eye

7.9.1 Osteology of the Orbit

The orbit is a cone-shaped, bony cavity in the facial skeleton that protects structures such as the eyeball, lacrimal gland, extraocular muscles, and relevant neurovasculature and ciliary ganglion. The boundaries of the orbit include four *walls* (superior, medial, inferior, and lateral), an *apex* and a *base*. The orbit also includes a *notch/foramen*, two *canals*, a *groove*, two *fossae*, and two *fissures* that allow structures to pass to and from the orbit (**Fig. 7.84**).

- *Superior wall*: formed by the **orbital plate of frontal bone** and **lesser wing of sphenoid bone**. A small depression near the lateral side of this wall represents the **fossa of the lacrimal gland** and where the lacrimal gland resides.
- *Medial wall*: formed by a small portion of the **lesser wing of the sphenoid**, **orbital plate of ethmoid bone, lacrimal bone,** and **frontal process of the maxilla**. The **fossa of the lacrimal sac** along with the **trochlea** of the superior oblique muscle is located on this wall. The **nasolacrimal canal** is located on the anterior aspect of this wall and transmits the *nasolacrimal duct*.
- *Inferior wall*: formed by the **orbital surface of the maxilla, zygomatic bone,** and **orbital process of palatine bone**. The **infraorbital groove** allows for the passage of the infraorbital neurovasculature.
- *Lateral wall*: formed by the **greater wing of the sphenoid** and **frontal process of the zygomatic bone** and is the strongest wall of the orbit. The *inferior orbital fissure* separates the inferior and lateral walls.
- *Apex*: is represented by the **optic canal** that passes through the *lesser wing of the sphenoid bone*. The optic canal allows for only the *optic nerve* and *ophthalmic artery*. The *superior orbital fissure* is located just lateral to the apex.
- *Base*: is represented by the **orbital margin** or outer border of the orbit. The **orbital septum** attaches to the base and is associated with the eyelid.

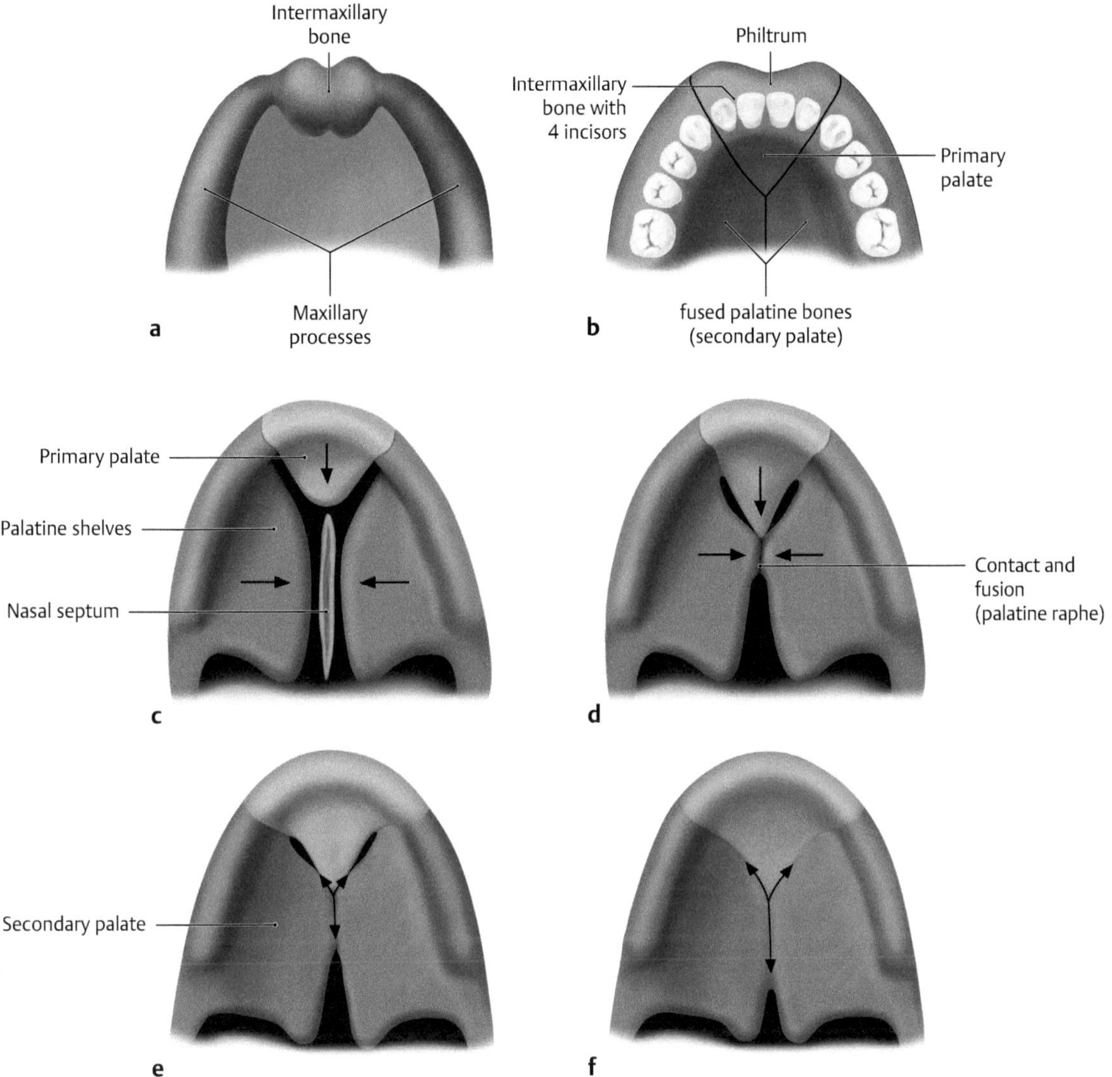

Fig. 7.81 Caudal view of palate. **(a,b)** Formation of the intermaxillary segment and early primary palate. Fusion and merging of the palatine shelves **(c-f)**. Fusion of the palate begins at around 9 weeks **(c)** and is completed posteriorly by week 12 **(f)**. (From Baker EW. Anatomy for Dental Medicine. 2nd ed. 2015. Based on the work of: Schuenke M, Schulte E, Schumacher U. THIEME Atlas of Anatomy. Illustrations by Voll M and Wesker K.)

The bones that form the orbit are lined by a periosteum known as **periorbita**. This periorbita is continuous with the:

- Dura mater (periosteal layer) at the optic canal and superior orbital fissure.
- Periosteum adjacent to the external surface of the cranium (pericranium) at the orbital margins and through the inferior orbital fissure.
- Fascial sheaths of the extraocular muscles.
- Fascial sheath of the eyeball.
- Orbital septa at the orbital margin.

7.9.2 Eyelids

The **eyelids** cover the eyeball anteriorly and protect it from excessive light and injury. The eyelids are movable folds that are covered externally by the skin and internally by palpebral conjunctiva, assist in spreading lacrimal fluid over the cornea to keep it moist, and consist of five layers in order from superficial to deep (1) outer skin; (2) superficial fascia devoid of fat; (3) muscular; (4) tarsofacial; and (5) conjunctiva layers **(Fig. 7.85)**.

The muscular layer contains the *orbicularis oculi* on both the upper and lower eyelids but the *levator palpebrae superioris* is located only with the upper eyelid. A smooth muscle known as the **superior tarsal muscle** extends from the levator palpebrae superioris and onto the superior tarsal plate to assist in elevation of the upper eyelid. The tarsofacial layer contains both the tarsal plates and orbital septum. The **tarsal plates** (superior/inferior) are bands of dense connective tissue and contain **tarsal glands**. The tarsal plates provide support for both eyelids and are attached to a **medial palpebral** and **lateral palpebral ligament**. The **orbital septum** is a fibrous membrane that is also connected to the tarsal plates and extends toward the orbital margins. It functions by containing the orbital fat located posterior to the septum, can limit the spread of an orbital infection, and serves as the posterior fascia of the orbicularis oculi muscle. The tarsal glands produce a lipid

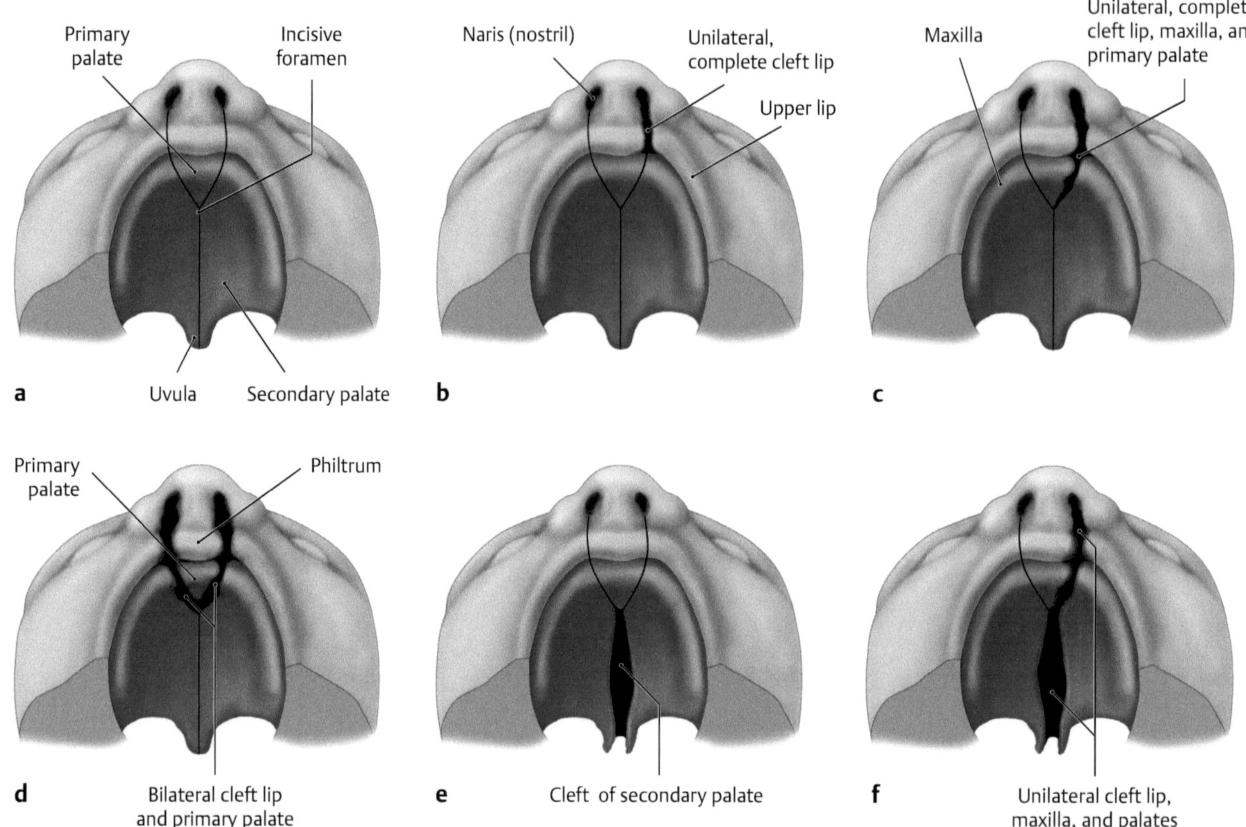

Fig. 7.82 **(a)** Normal lips and palate. **(b)** Unilateral, complete cleft lip (cheiloschisis). **(c)** Unilateral, complete cleft lip, maxilla, and primary palate (cheilognathoschisis). **(d)** Bilateral cleft lip and maxilla. **(e)** Incomplete fusion of the primary and secondary palates (palatoschisis). **(f)** Unilateral, complete cleft lip, maxilla, and palate (cheilognathopalatoschisis). (From Baker EW. Anatomy for Dental Medicine. 2nd ed. 2015. Based on the work of: Schuenke M, Schulte E, Schumacher U. THIEME Atlas of Anatomy. Illustrations by Voll M and Wesker K.)

secretion responsible for lubricating the edges of the eyelids preventing them from sticking to one another when they are closed (**Fig. 7.86**).

The **palpebral conjunctiva** is the transparent mucous membrane located on the internal surface of an eyelid. It is continuous with the **bulbar conjunctiva** that is located on the cornea and a small portion of the sclera. Where these two conjunctivas meet and form deep recesses is known as the **superior** and **inferior fornices (Fig. 7.85)**.

The anterior aperture located between the upper and lower eyelids is called the **palpebral fissure** and the lateral and medial junctions of the eyelids are known as the **lateral palpebral** and **medial palpebral commissures**, respectively. The **eyelashes** are located on the distal margins of the eyelids and are associated with sebaceous glands called **ciliary glands**.

7.9.3 Lacrimal Apparatus

The **lacrimal apparatus** consists of the lacrimal glands, ducts, papilla/punctum, canaliculi, lacrimal sac, and nasolacrimal duct. The lacrimal fluid is responsible for keeping the eyeball moist and contains the bactericidal enzyme lysozyme.

Drainage of tears from the eyeball occurs near the medial angle of the eye. Tears first collect at the **lacrimal lake** and then enter by capillary action through the **lacrimal puncta** of the **lacrimal papillae**. After entering through the puncta, tears drain through the **lacrimal canaliculi** to the **lacrimal sac**. This leads to the **nasolacrimal duct** and finally the inferior nasal meatus of the nasal cavity. A small mound of modified skin tissue can be found in the lacrimal lake and is called the **lacrimal caruncle**. Thus the course of tear drainage is such: (1) lacrimal gland; (2) lacrimal ducts; (3) superior then inferior fornices before reaching the lacrimal lake; (4) lacrimal puncta of the lacrimal papillae; (5) lacrimal canaliculi; (6) lacrimal sac; (7) nasolacrimal duct; (8) and finally the inferior nasal meatus of the nasal cavity (**Fig. 7.87**).

The lacrimal gland is stimulated by parasympathetic impulses that originate from the **superior salivatory nucleus** of the brainstem and pass through the greater petrosal nerve of CN VII. The **greater petrosal** and **deep petrosal nerves** combine to form the **nerve of the pterygoid canal** (Vidian nerve). The nerve of the pterygoid canal and its autonomic fibers empty into the PPG with only the para/pre fibers synapsing. From the PPG, the pathway of para/post fibers to the lacrimal gland is as follows: pterygopalatine ganglion → pterygopalatine nerves → V_2 → zygomatic nerve → zygomaticotemporal nerve (if present) → communicating branch → lacrimal nerve → lacrimal gland (**Fig. 7.94b**).

7.9.4 Muscles of the Eyeball

There are seven extraocular muscles of the orbit and they are involved in the movement of the eyeball and elevating the upper

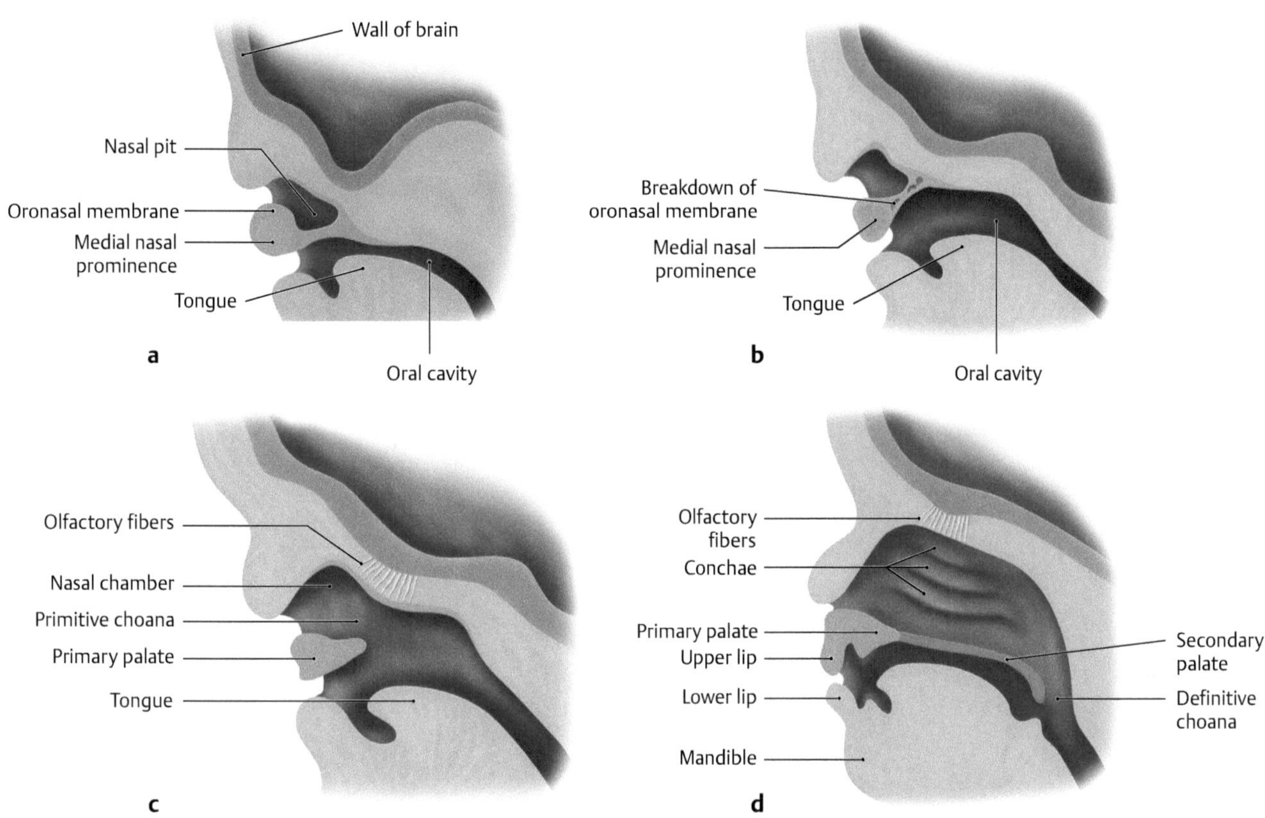

Fig. 7.83 Development of the nasal cavity, midsagittal section from weeks 6-9 **(a-d)**. The nasal septum (not shown) will fuse with the palatine shelves by weeks 9-12. (From Baker EW. Anatomy for Dental Medicine. 2nd ed. 2015. Based on the work of: Schuenke M, Schulte E, Schumacher U. THIEME Atlas of Anatomy. Illustrations by Voll M and Wesker K.)

eyelid. These muscles include the **superior rectus**, **inferior rectus**, **lateral rectus**, **medial rectus**, **superior oblique**, **inferior oblique**, and **levator palpebrae superioris**. These muscles have at least one function and they include elevation of the upper eyelid, abduction, adduction, depression, elevation, lateral rotation (extorsion), and medial rotation (intorsion) of the eyeball.

Movements occur at three different axes of rotation and they are the **anteroposterior** (lateral and medial rotation), **horizontal** (elevation and depression), and **vertical axes** (abduction and adduction), and these movements are described based on the direction the pupil and superior pole deviates from their neutral positions. Movements can occur around one or all three axes simultaneously **(Fig. 7.88; Fig. 7.89)**. Because of this, the optical axis will deviate from the orbital axis by 23 degrees. This results in the point of maximum visual acuity (or *fovea centralis*) being located lateral to the optic disc or "blind spot" of the eye. All of the extraocular muscles are innervated by the oculomotor nerve (CN III), except for the superior oblique (trochlear-CN IV) and lateral rectus (abducent-CN VI) muscles. Muscles of the eyeball are detailed in **Table 7.5**.

In order to direct one's gaze, coordination between functionally paired contralateral extraocular muscles or **yolk muscles** must take place with both eyes. An example would include looking to the left, which involves the left lateral rectus muscle and the right medial rectus muscle.

Clinically, the orientation of the extraocular muscles attaching to the back of the eyeball at an angle must be considered. **Table 7.5** describes all of the functions of a particular eye muscle but further distinction is needed in order to properly identify a defective muscle. *Primary position* of the eyeballs is when the two eyes are looking straight ahead. There are several factors that complicate the understanding of recti and oblique muscle actions. Recall that the *apex* of each orbit, which also represents the *orbital axis*, is located on the medial side of the orbit. This resulted in the *orbital axis* and *optical axis*, the imaginary line that divides the eye into left and right halves, differing by 23 degrees **(Fig. 7.90; Fig. 7.91)**.

Isolating the function of the LR and MR by either abducting or adducting the eyeball, respectively, can clearly demonstrate whether or not those muscles are functioning correctly. An examiner moving his/her finger in an H-pattern can isolate the primary function of the superior/inferior recti and superior/inferior oblique muscles. On a horizontal plane, the patient will be asked to completely abduct or adduct their eyeball **(Fig. 7.92)**.

While in a completely abducted gaze, the only elevator of the eyeball is the SR and the only depressor is the IR. This will test the integrity of the oculomotor nerve (for SR and IR) and the abducent nerve (LR). While in a completely adducted gaze, the only elevator of the eyeball is the IO and the only depressor is the SO. This will test the integrity of the oculomotor nerve (for MR and IO) and the trochlear nerve (SO). The simultaneous and medial movement of both eyes toward one another in order to maintain single binocular vision when viewing an object is known as **convergence**. Thus, this makes the inferior and superior oblique muscles vitally important when an individual is reading up and down the text of a book or other source **(Fig. 7.92)**.

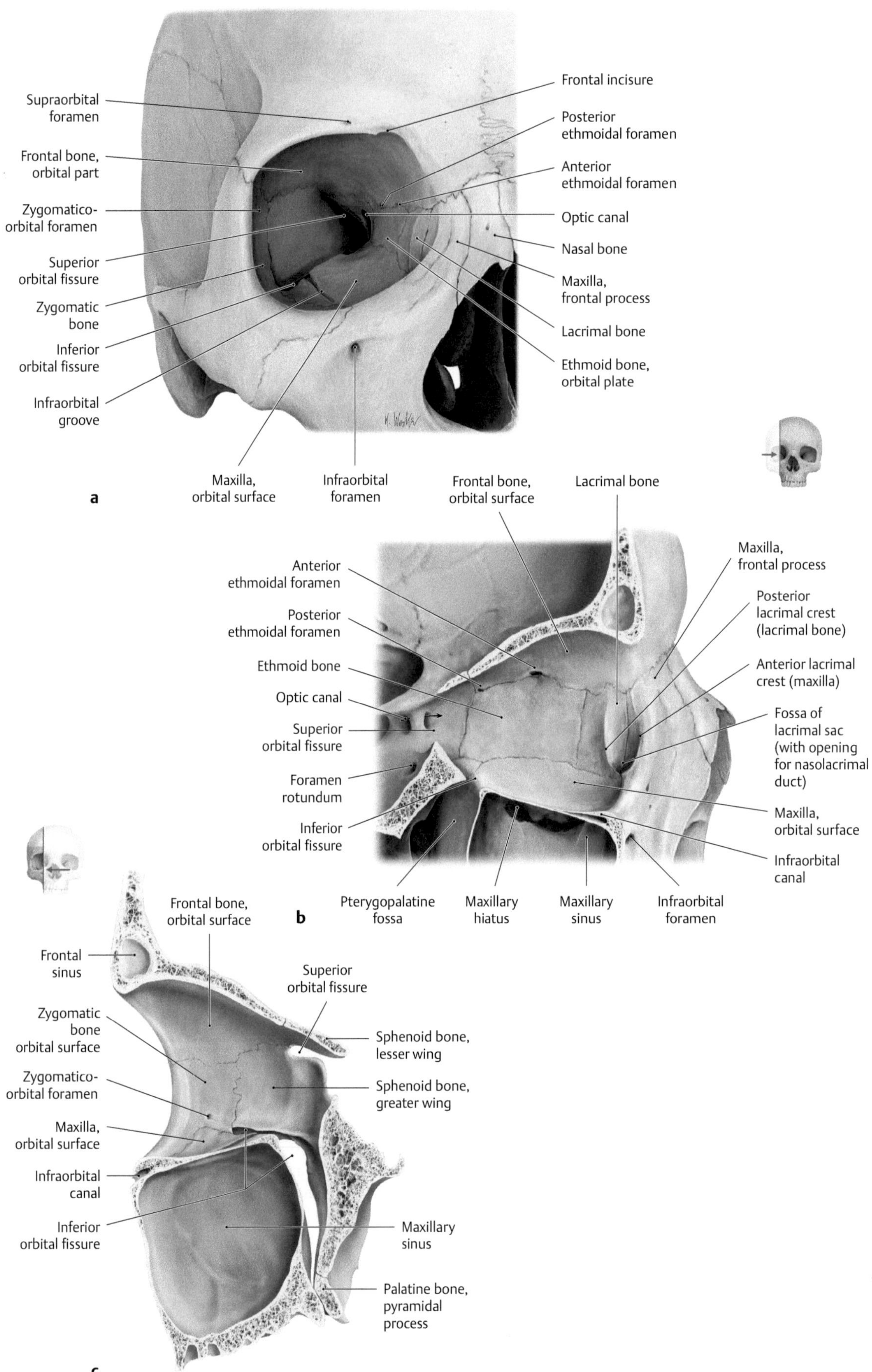

Fig. 7.84 The walls of the right orbit and openings for neurovascular structures. **(a)** Anterior view. **(b)** Medial wall. **(c)** Lateral wall. (From Schuenke M, Schulte E, Schumacher U. THIEME Atlas of Anatomy. Head, Neck, and Neuroanatomy. Illustrations by Voll M and Wesker K. 3rd ed. New York: Thieme Medical Publishers; 2020.)

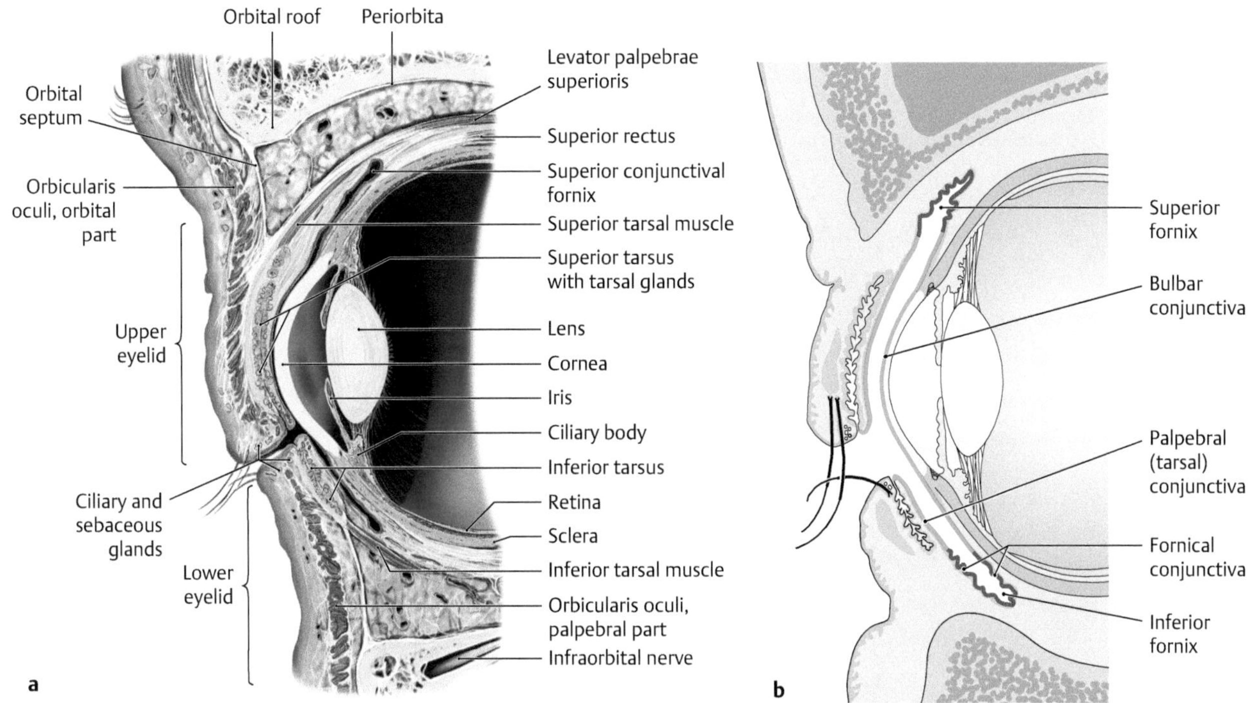

Fig. 7.85 Structure of the eyelids and conjunctiva. **(a)** Sagittal section through anterior orbit cavity. **(b)** Location of the conjunctiva. (From Schuenke M, Schulte E, Schumacher U. THIEME Atlas of Anatomy. Head, Neck, and Neuroanatomy. Illustrations by Voll M and Wesker K. 3rd ed. New York: Thieme Medical Publishers; 2020.)

7.9.5 Neurovasculature of the Orbit and Eyeball

The nerves of the orbit include the **optic (CN II)**, **oculomotor (CN III)**, **trochlear (CN IV)**, **trigeminal-ophthalmic division (CN V_1)**, **abducent (CN VI)**, and their branches. The **optic nerves** are actually a part of the central nervous system formed by secondary neurons that developed originally as paired anterior extensions of the forebrain. These nerves carry only special sensory (SSA) fibers responsible for vision. They begin at the **lamina cribrosa of the sclera** where the unmyelinated fibers pierce the sclera and then become myelinated. After passing posteriorly through the orbit, they exit this space through the optic canal and are paired alongside only with the ophthalmic artery. They are surrounded by extensions of all three cranial meninges and CSF within the subarachnoid space. The **optic nerve sheath** is the intraorbital extensions of cranial dura and arachnoid maters becoming continuous with the *fascial sheath of the eyeball*. Pia mater rests directly on the surface of the optic nerve **(Fig. 7.93)**.

The **oculomotor nerve** enters the orbit through the superior orbital fissure and branches into a superior and inferior division. It innervates most of the extraocular muscles except the superior oblique and lateral rectus. It carries somatic motor (GSE), somatic sensory (GSA), and GVE-para/pre fibers **(Fig. 7.94)**. The para/pre fibers originate from the **Edinger-Westphal nucleus** in the midbrain and will course through the *inferior division of CN III* to reach the **ciliary ganglion**. After synapsing at the ganglion, para/post fibers will continue through the short ciliary nerves to eventually innervate the **ciliary body** and **sphincter (constrictor) pupillae muscles**. Sym/post fibers from the **internal carotid periarterial plexus** course along the *superior division of CN III* in order to reach and innervate the **superior tarsal (*Muller*) muscle**.

The **ophthalmic nerve (CN V_1)** enters the orbit through the superior orbital fissure and divides into three major branches: the **frontal**, **lacrimal**, and **nasociliary nerves**. The frontal nerve divides into the **supraorbital** and **supratrochlear nerves**. The **nasociliary nerve**, which courses from lateral to medial over the optic nerve, gives rise to the **long ciliary**, **posterior ethmoidal**, and **anterior ethmoidal nerves**, and then terminates as the **infratrochlear nerve**. The **lacrimal nerve** is the most lateral of these three initial V_1 branches and courses above the lateral rectus muscle before reaching the lacrimal gland. All ophthalmic nerve branches contain GSA fibers and their cell bodies are located in the **trigeminal ganglion**. The *proximal portion of the nasociliary* and all of the **long ciliary nerve** contain sym/post fibers that are responsible for innervating the **dilator pupillae muscle**. The lacrimal nerve has primarily GSA fibers except for the distal one-half that also contains the para/post fibers destined for the lacrimal gland **(Fig. 7.95)**.

The **trochlear (CN IV)** and **abducent nerves (CN VI)** enter the orbit through the superior orbital fissure and innervate the **superior oblique** and **lateral rectus muscles**, respectively. They both carry GSE and GSA-proprioceptive fibers **(Fig. 7.94; Fig. 7.95)**.

A fibrous cuff known as the **common tendinous ring** is the structure the recti muscles of the orbit originate from. It surrounds the optic canal and divides the superior orbital fissure into a superior, middle, and inferior space/passageways. The trochlear, lacrimal (V_1 br.), and frontal (V_1 br.) nerves along with the superior ophthalmic vein pass through the superior space. Both the superior and inferior divisions of the oculomotor, nasociliary (V_1 br.), and abducent nerves pass through the common tendinous ring and the middle space of the superior orbital fissure created by the ring. If the inferior ophthalmic vein has not joined the superior ophthalmic vein midorbit, then it will pass through the inferior

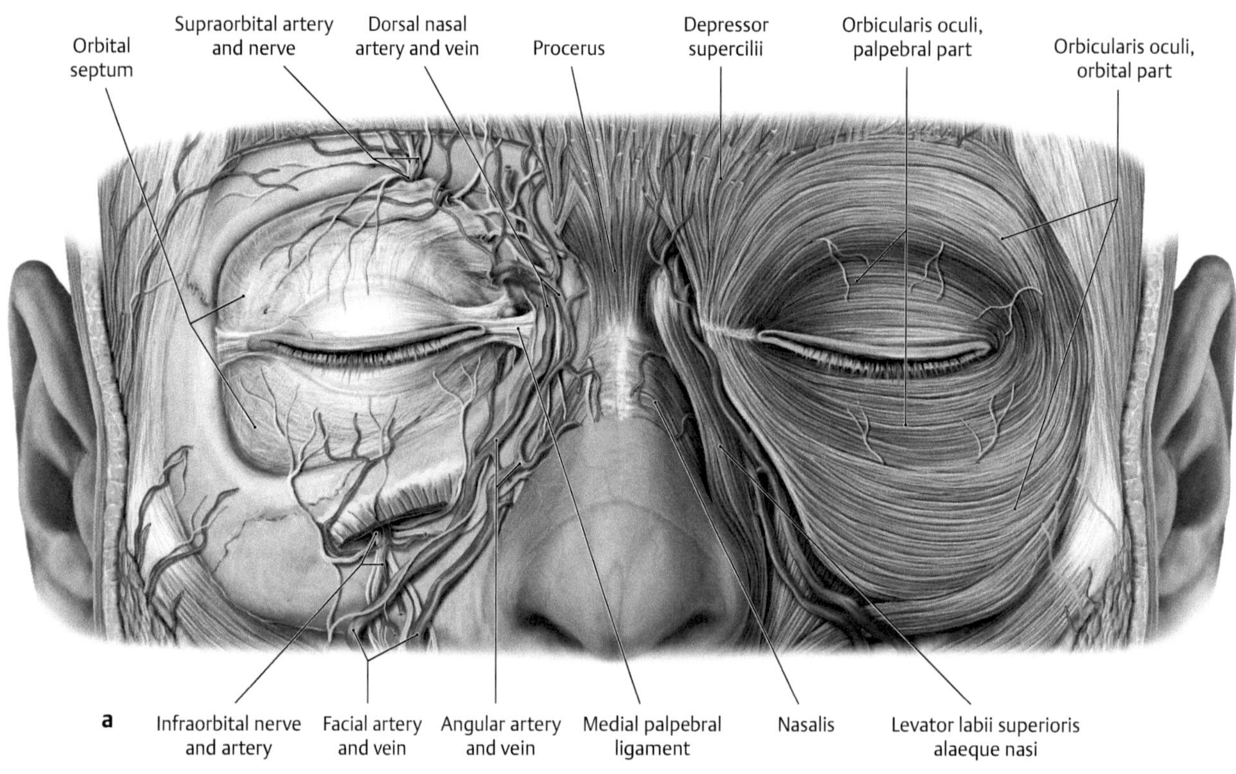

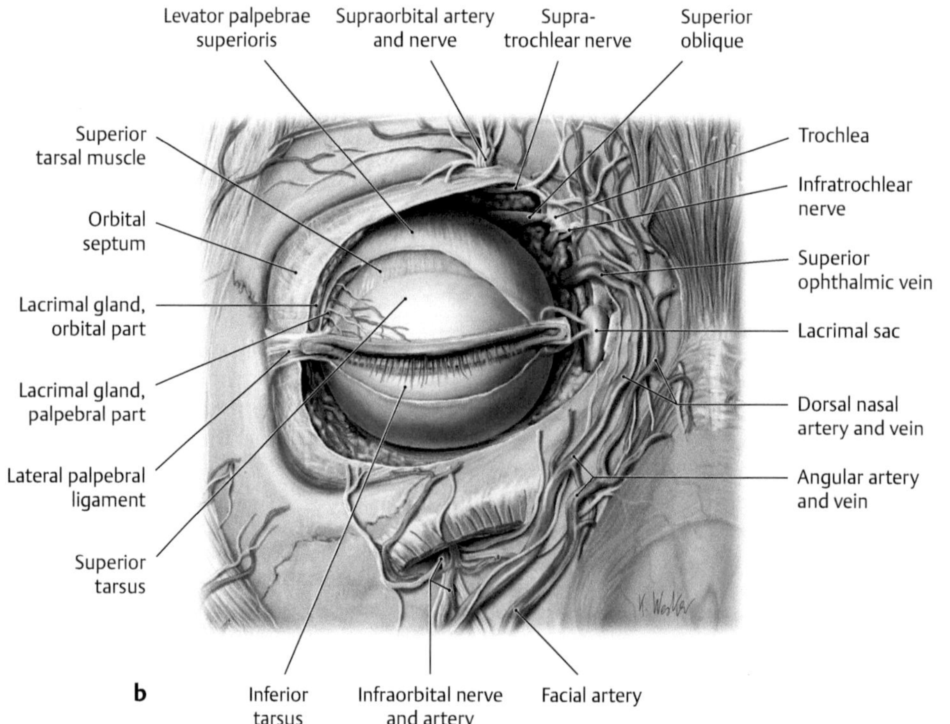

Fig. 7.86 Superficial **(a)** and deep **(b)** structures of the right orbital region. (From Schuenke M, Schulte E, Schumacher U. THIEME Atlas of Anatomy. Head, Neck, and Neuroanatomy. Illustrations by Voll M and Wesker K. 3rd ed. New York: Thieme Medical Publishers; 2020.)

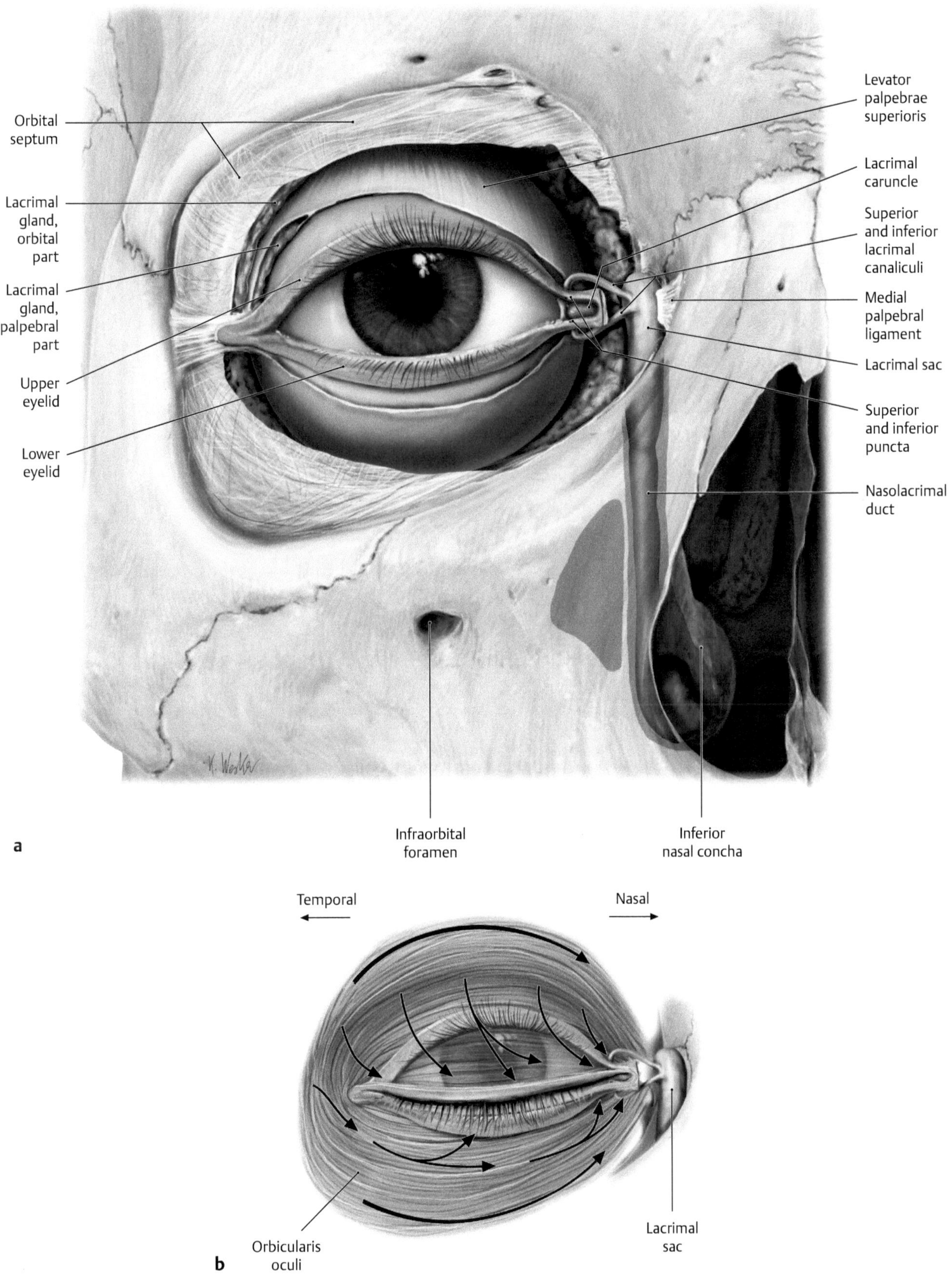

Fig. 7.87 (a) Lacrimal apparatus. Right eye, anterior view. **(b)** Mechanical propulsion of the lacrimal fluid within the right eye. (From Schuenke M, Schulte E, Schumacher U. THIEME Atlas of Anatomy. Head, Neck, and Neuroanatomy. Illustrations by Voll M and Wesker K. 3rd ed. New York: Thieme Medical Publishers; 2020.)

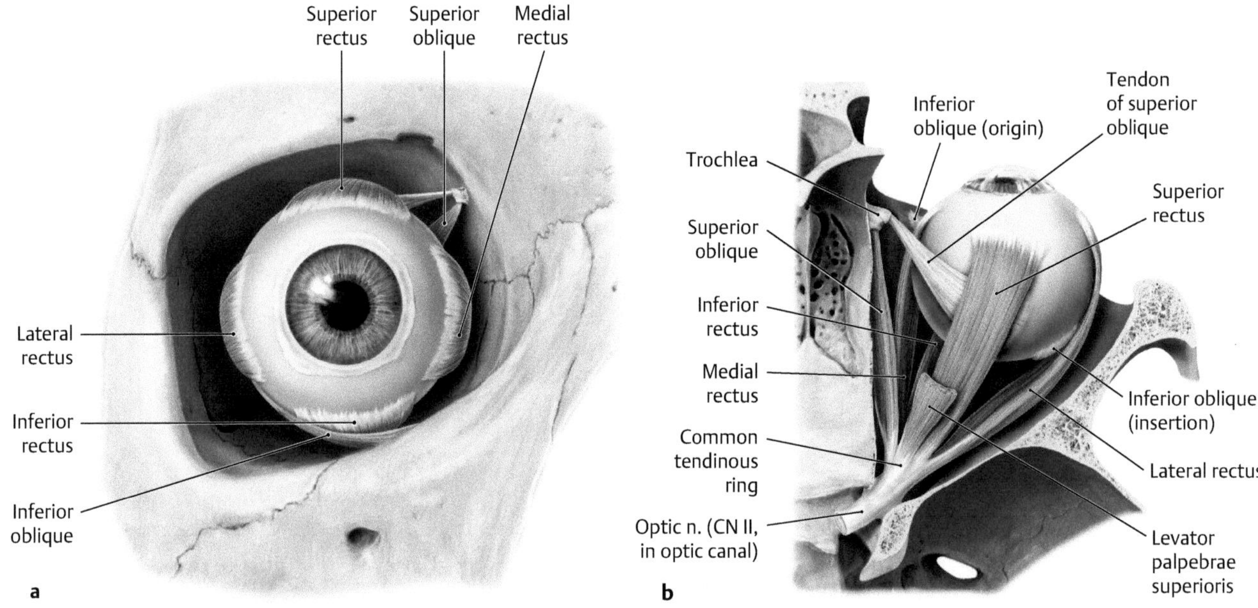

Fig. 7.88 Extraocular muscles. **(a)** Right eye, anterior view. **(b)** Right eye, superior view. (From Schuenke M, Schulte E, Schumacher U. THIEME Atlas of Anatomy. Head, Neck, and Neuroanatomy. Illustrations by Voll M and Wesker K. 3rd ed. New York: Thieme Medical Publishers; 2020.)

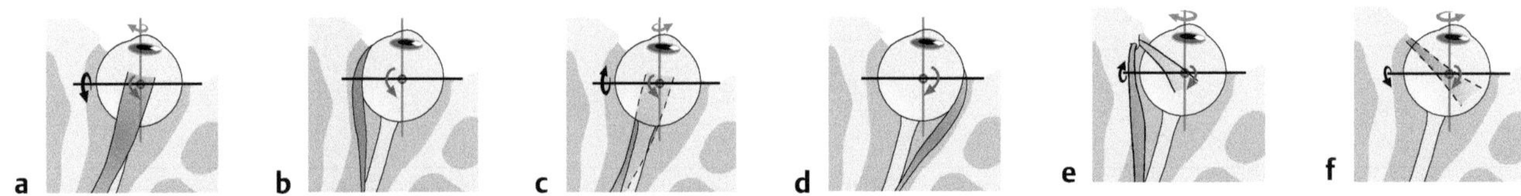

Fig. 7.89 Actions of the extraocular muscles. **(a)** Superior rectus. **(b)** Medial rectus. **(c)** Inferior rectus. **(d)** Lateral rectus. **(e)** Superior oblique. **(f)** Inferior oblique. Vertical axis, red circle; horizontal axis, black line; anteroposterior axis; blue line. (From Schuenke M, Schulte E, Schumacher U. THIEME Atlas of Anatomy. Head, Neck, and Neuroanatomy. Illustrations by Voll M and Wesker K. 3rd ed. New York: Thieme Medical Publishers; 2020.)

Table 7.5 **Muscles of the eyeball**

Muscle	Innervation	Function(s)	Origin	Insertion
Levator palpebrae superioris (LPS)	Oculomotor nerve (CN III-superior division)	Elevates upper eyelid	Lesser wing of sphenoid bone	Superior tarsal plate and upper eyelid
Superior tarsal (smooth muscle)	Sym/post fibers via superior division of CN III	Elevates upper eyelid	Distal portion of LPS muscle	Superior tarsal plate
Superior rectus (SR)	Oculomotor nerve (CN III-superior division)	Elevates, adducts, and medially rotates eyeball	Common tendinous ring (annulus of Zinn)	Superior sclera near corneoscleral junction or limbus
Inferior rectus (IR)	Oculomotor nerve (CN III-inferior division)	Depresses, adducts, and laterally rotates eyeball	Common tendinous ring (annulus of Zinn)	Inferior sclera near corneoscleral junction or limbus
Lateral rectus (LR)	Abducent nerve (CN VI)	Abducts eyeball	Common tendinous ring (annulus of Zinn)	Lateral sclera near corneoscleral junction or limbus
Medial rectus (MR)	Oculomotor nerve (CN III-inferior division)	Adducts eyeball	Common tendinous ring (annulus of Zinn)	Medial sclera near corneoscleral junction or limbus
Superior oblique (SO)	Trochlear nerve (CN IV)	Medially rotates, depresses, and abducts eyeball	Body of sphenoid bone	Superior sclera just deep to the SR
Inferior oblique (IO)	Oculomotor nerve (CN III-inferior division)	Laterally rotates, elevates, and abducts eyeball	Anteromedial portion of orbital floor	Lateral sclera just deep to LR

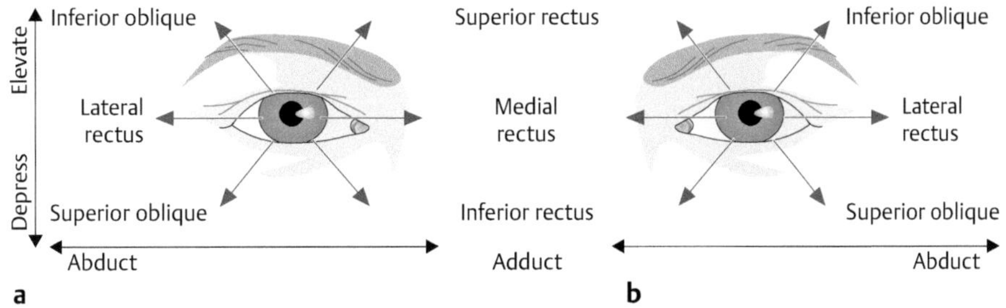

Fig. 7.90 The paired muscles involved in gaze. **(a)** Right eye. **(b)** Left eye. (From Schuenke M, Schulte E, Schumacher U. THIEME Atlas of Anatomy. Head, Neck, and Neuroanatomy. Illustrations by Voll M and Wesker K. 3rd ed. New York: Thieme Medical Publishers; 2020.)

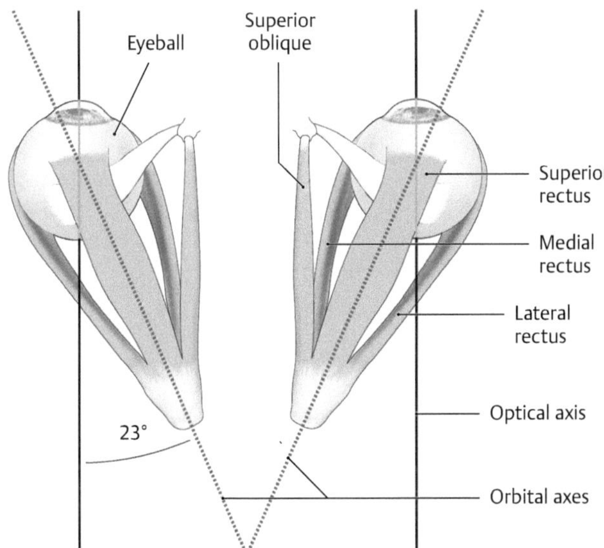

Fig. 7.91 Optical axis and orbital axis. (From Schuenke M, Schulte E, Schumacher U. THIEME Atlas of Anatomy. Head, Neck, and Neuroanatomy. Illustrations by Voll M and Wesker K. 3rd ed. New York: Thieme Medical Publishers; 2020.)

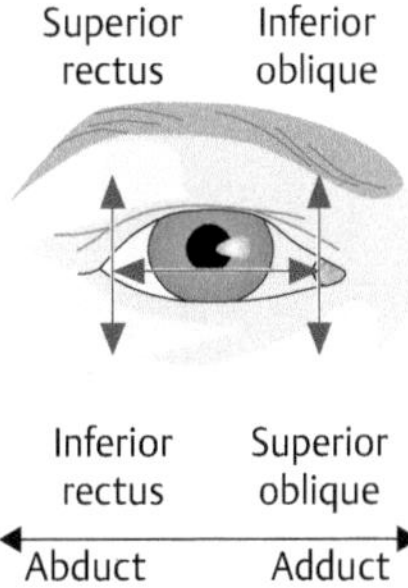

Fig. 7.92 Testing individual extraocular muscles on the right eye. (From Schuenke M, Schulte E, Schumacher U. THIEME Atlas of Anatomy. Head, Neck, and Neuroanatomy. Illustrations by Voll M and Wesker K. 3rd ed. New York: Thieme Medical Publishers; 2020.)

space of the superior orbital fissure created by the common tendinous ring.

The **ophthalmic artery** is the main blood supply to the orbit and it originates off of the ICA. The ophthalmic artery pairs with the optic nerve and enters the orbit through the optic canal where it gives off numerous branches. They include the **central artery of the retina, long/short posterior ciliary, lacrimal, supraorbital, posterior ethmoidal, anterior ethmoidal, dorsal nasal,** and **supratrochlear (Fig. 7.96)**. The **infraorbital artery** is known to contribute some blood to the orbit. The retina receives oxygenated blood from direct and indirect branches of the ophthalmic artery, the *central retinal artery*, and the *ciliary artery* **(Fig. 7.97)**. The *central artery of the retina* pierces the optic nerve and travels to the optic disc of the eyeball where it will branch numerous times over the internal surface of the retina. Terminal branches of the central retinal artery are considered *end arteries* and they provide the only blood supply to the internal retinal surface **(Fig. 7.98)**. End arteries have no anastomosis with other vessels to supply tissue if an occlusion was present.

The external surface of the retina along with the choroid is supplied by multiple **short posterior ciliary arteries** and the **capillary lamina of the choroid**. The "red eye" produced after having a picture taken is caused by the capillary lumina of the choroid. The ophthalmic artery has **muscular branches** that supply the extraocular muscles and these will continue as the **anterior ciliary arteries**. The **long posterior ciliary arteries** travel between the choroid and sclera and will anastomose with the anterior ciliary arteries and together supply the **ciliary plexus**. The **episcleral arteries** are located on the external surface of the sclera and originate from the anterior and posterior ciliary arteries. The common "red eye" brought on by allergies or conjunctivitis causes the episcleral vessels to become engorged with blood when irritated **(Fig. 7.97)**.

Venous drainage of the orbit is primarily associated with the superior and inferior ophthalmic veins. The **supraorbital, supratrochlear,** and **angular veins** form the tributaries that help make up the **superior ophthalmic vein**. The **inferior ophthalmic vein** receives blood from the **angular**, **facial,** and **intraorbital** veins along with the **pterygoid venous plexus** and will generally drain into the superior ophthalmic vein. It is the superior ophthalmic vein that passes through the superior orbital fissure to enter the **cavernous sinus** in most individuals. No lymph nodes are present in the orbit **(Fig. 7.99)**.

The listed arteries above supplying the eyeball all have corresponding veins. The **central vein of the retina** usually drains to the cavernous sinus, and if not it will drain to an ophthalmic vein. The **vorticose veins** (or *vortex veins*) are initially located in the episcleral space between the sclera and fascial sheath of the eyeball and are responsible for draining the vascular *uvea* which consists of the iris, ciliary body, and choroid. There are at least four and as many as eight of these veins present with their

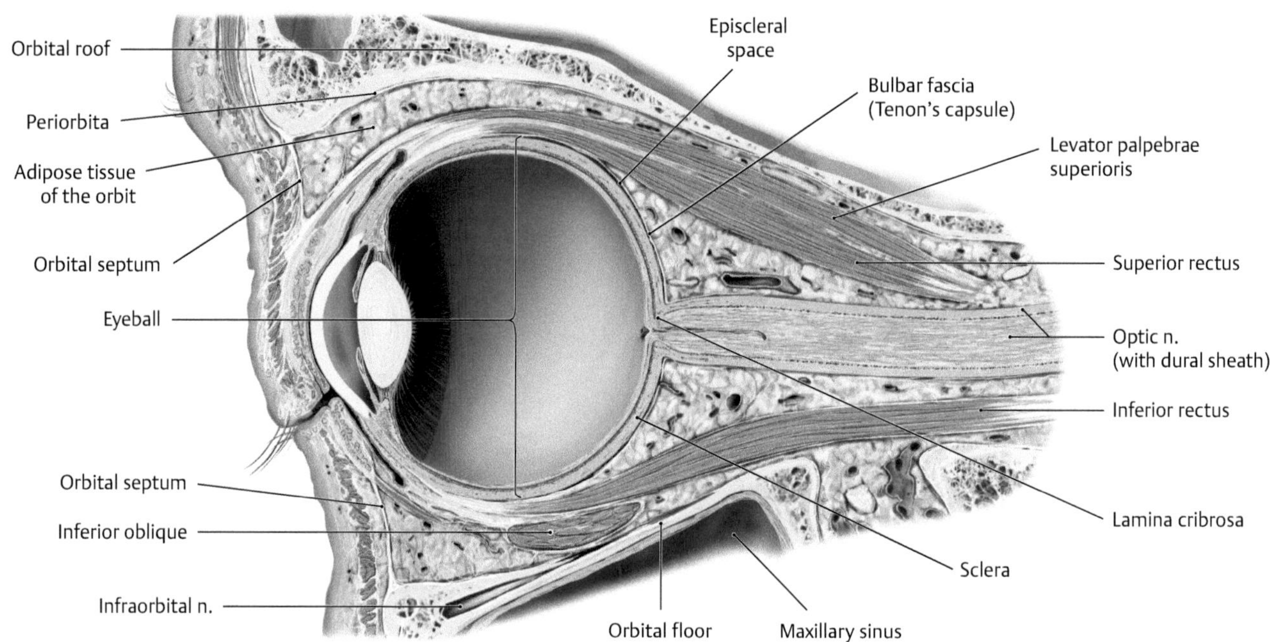

Fig. 7.93 Topography of the orbit: sagittal section through the right orbit, medial view. (From Schuenke M, Schulte E, Schumacher U. THIEME Atlas of Anatomy. Head, Neck, and Neuroanatomy. Illustrations by Voll M and Wesker K. 3rd ed. New York: Thieme Medical Publishers; 2020.)

tributaries including the limbal plexus, anterior/posterior ciliary, and capillary layer of the choroid and episcleral veins. The vorticose veins will drain into the superior or inferior ophthalmic veins **(Fig. 7.97)**.

7.9.6 Ciliary Ganglion

The **ciliary ganglion** is located on the superior and lateral edge of the optic nerve and has a parasympathetic (motor) root, sensory root, and a sympathetic root **(Fig. 7.94)**. The para/pre fibers that coursed through the inferior division of CN III before heading toward the ganglion represent the parasympathetic root. The nasociliary nerve serves as the sensory root. The sym/post fibers from the internal carotid plexus that course along the artery and directly to the ganglion from the ICA or from the ophthalmic artery will serve as the sympathetic root. **Short ciliary nerves** extend from the ganglion and enter the eyeball carrying para/post (innervate ciliary body and sphincter pupillae muscles), GSA (sensory from eyeball), and sym/post (innervate blood vessels) fibers.

7.9.7 Internal Eyeball

The optical apparatus or organ of the visual system is the eyeball. Structures of the eyeball are circular or spherical in nature and it is made up of three layers. These layers include the: fibrous (outer) layer, vascular (middle) layer, and the inner (internal most) layer **(Fig. 7.100)**.

The **fibrous layer** acts as the external skeleton of the eyeball and provides shape and resistance. It is made up of two parts: the *cornea* and *sclera* **(Fig. 7.101)**.

- The **cornea** is transparent, anterior one-sixth of the fibrous layer and is largely responsible for refraction of light entering the eyeball. It is highly sensitive to touch and is innervated by the ophthalmic nerve (CN V_1). It is nourished by aqueous humor and lacrimal fluid.
- The **sclera** is the opaque and dense fibrous tissue that makes of the posterior five-sixth of the fibrous layer. It is pierced posteriorly by the optic nerve at the **lamina cribrosa** and provides the attachment of all the extraocular muscles except for the LPS as well as the intrinsic muscles of the eye. The sclera represents the *"white of the eyes."* It is continuous with the cornea anteriorly and dura mater posteriorly.
- The **corneoscleral junction (limbus)** is where these two layers meet and the location of numerous capillaries.

The **vascular layer** (*uvea* or *uveal tract*) of the eyeball is made up of three parts, the *iris*, *ciliary body*, and *choroid*.

- The **iris** is an anteriorly placed, thin, contractile, and pigmented diaphragm that rests on the lens and has a central aperture known as the **pupil (Fig. 7.102)**. There are two smooth muscles that control the size of the pupil: the **dilator pupillae** increases the size of the pupil and is innervated by *sympathetic fibers* passing through the long ciliary nerve (nasociliary br.) while the **sphincter (constrictor) pupillae** constricts the pupil and is innervated by *parasympathetic fibers* originating from CN III (**Fig. 7.103**). Sympathetic responses are immediate while the parasympathetic response, like in most of the body, is slow and can take many minutes. The iris divides the space between the lens and the cornea into an *anterior* and *posterior chamber.*
- The **ciliary body** is a thickening of the layer posterior to the corneoscleral junction, is made up of a muscular and vascular part, and connects the choroid to the iris. The muscular portion contains circular and longitudinal orientated smooth muscle fibers. **Zonular fibers** (**suspensory ligament of the lens**)

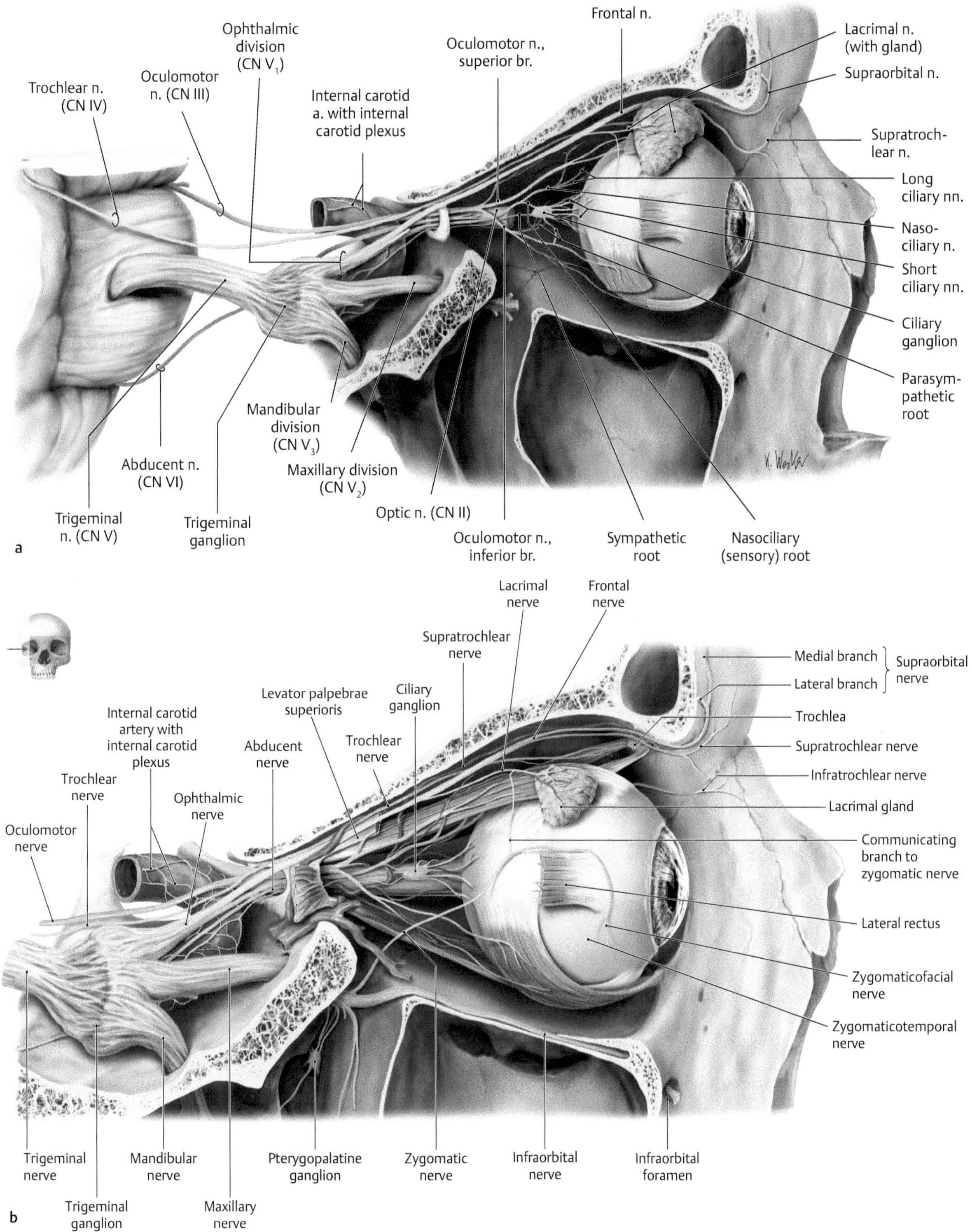

Fig. 7.94 Innervation of the orbit: lateral view of the right orbit with temporal bony wall removed. **(a)** Orbit cranial nerves and the autonomic roots of the ciliary ganglion. **(b)** Addition of extraocular muscles and the nerves related to the lacrimal gland innervation. (From Schuenke M, Schulte E, Schumacher U. THIEME Atlas of Anatomy. Head, Neck, and Neuroanatomy. Illustrations by Voll M and Wesker K. 3rd ed. New York: Thieme Medical Publishers; 2020.)

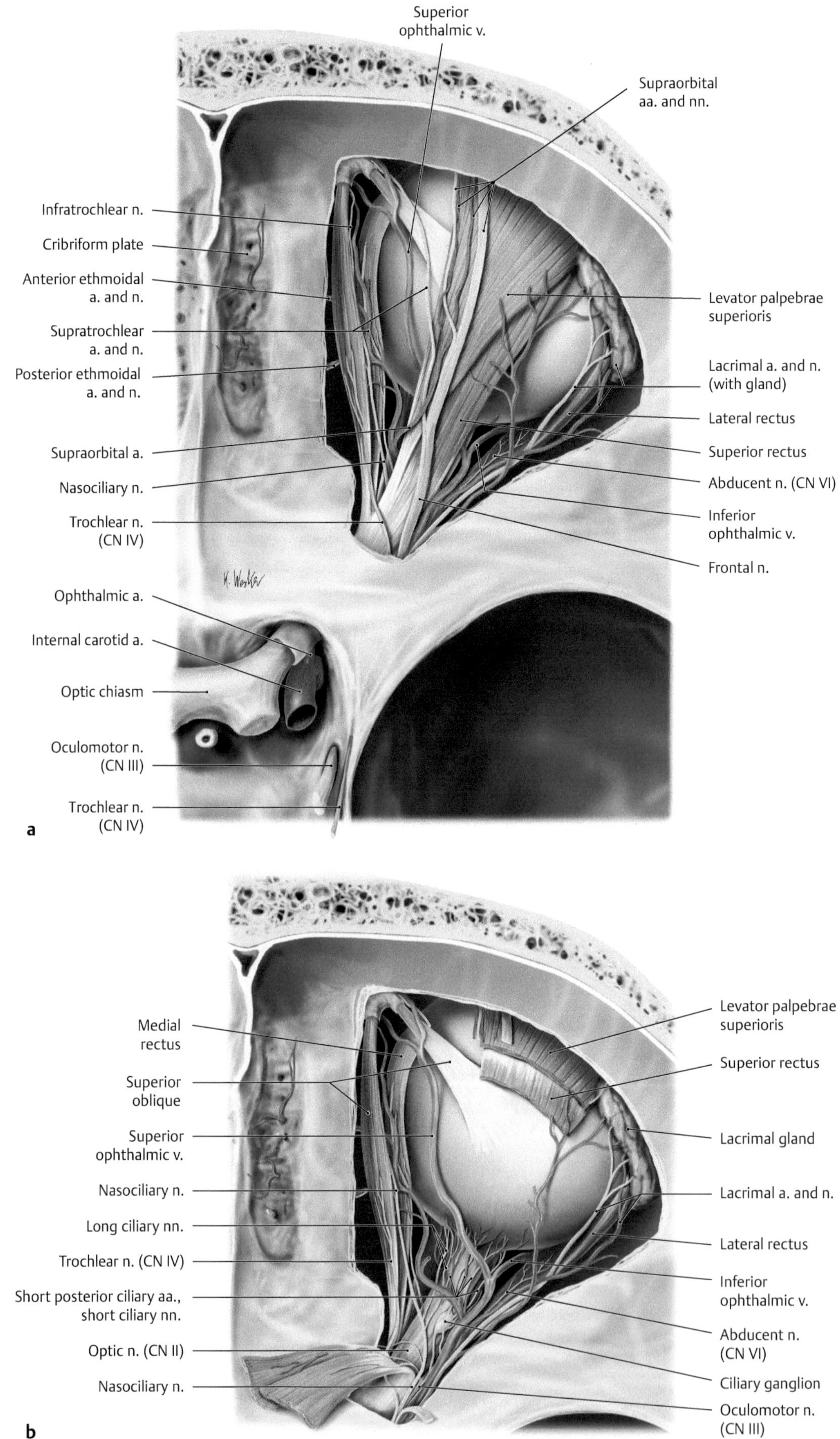

Fig. 7.95 Neurovascular contents of the orbit. **(a)** Upper level of dissection. **(b)** Middle level of dissection. (From Schuenke M, Schulte E, Schumacher U. THIEME Atlas of Anatomy. Head, Neck, and Neuroanatomy. Illustrations by Voll M and Wesker K. 3rd ed. New York: Thieme Medical Publishers; 2020.)

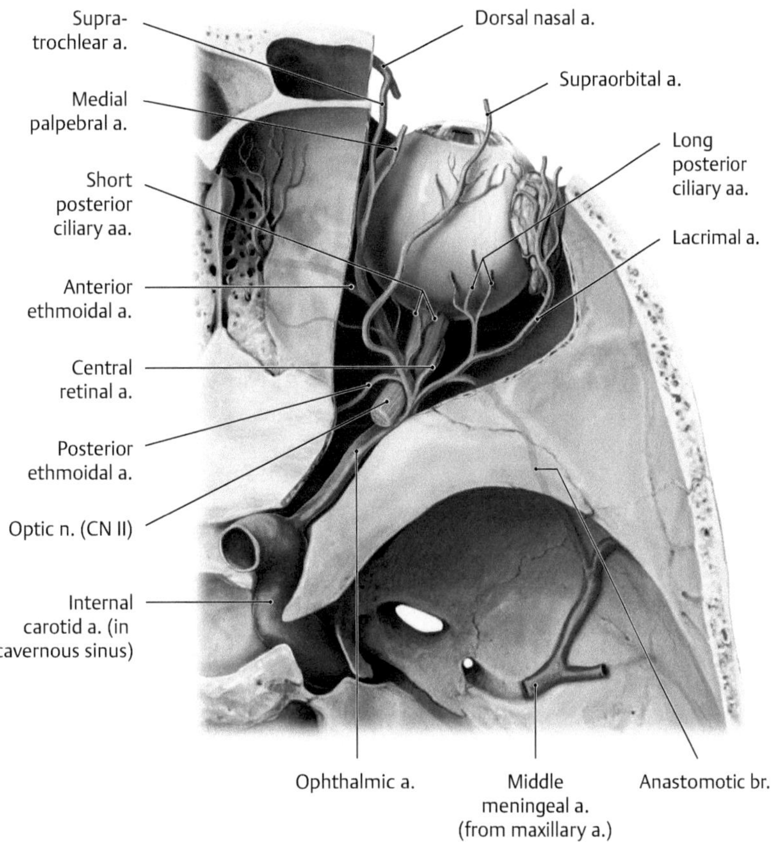

Fig. 7.96 Arteries of the orbit: superior view of the right orbit with the optic canal and orbital roof opened. (From Schuenke M, Schulte E, Schumacher U. THIEME Atlas of Anatomy. Head, Neck, and Neuroanatomy. Illustrations by Voll M and Wesker K. 3rd ed. New York: Thieme Medical Publishers; 2020.)

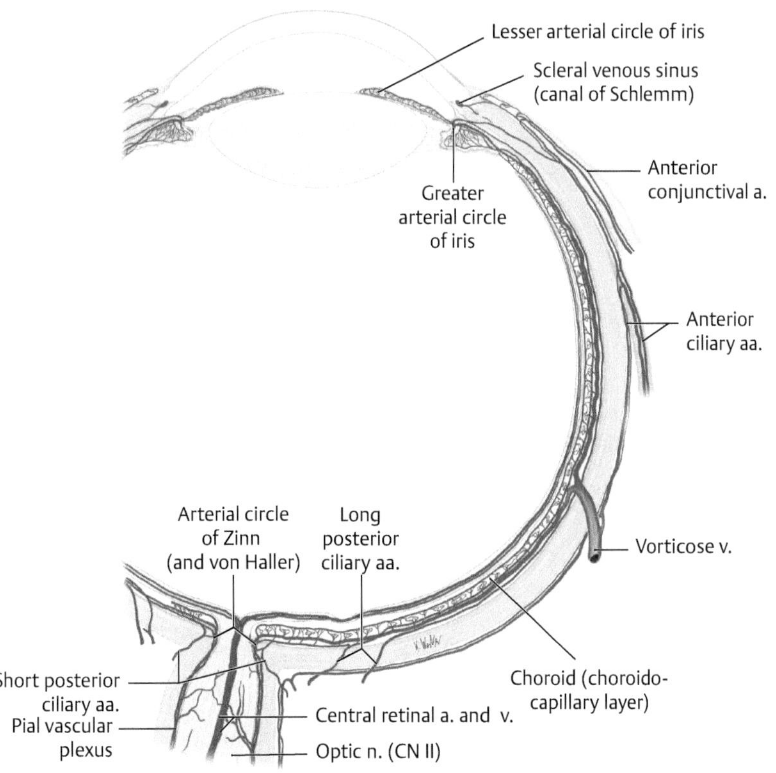

Fig. 7.97 Blood vessels of the eye. (From Schuenke M, Schulte E, Schumacher U. THIEME Atlas of Anatomy. Head, Neck, and Neuroanatomy. Illustrations by Voll M and Wesker K. 3rd ed. New York: Thieme Medical Publishers; 2020.)

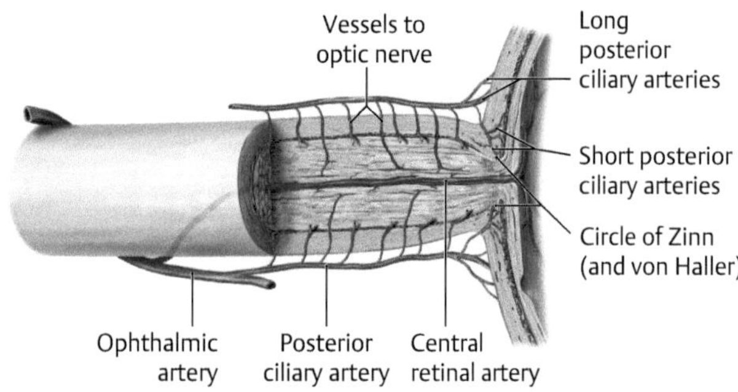

Fig. 7.98 Arterial blood supply of the optic nerve. (From Schuenke M, Schulte E, Schumacher U. THIEME Atlas of Anatomy. Head, Neck, and Neuroanatomy. Illustrations by Voll M and Wesker K. 3rd ed. New York: Thieme Medical Publishers; 2020.)

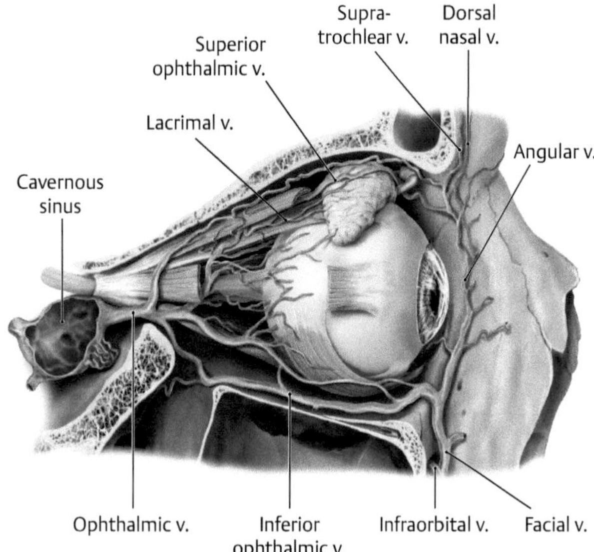

Fig. 7.99 Veins of the orbit, lateral view of the right orbit: lateral orbital wall removed and the maxillary sinus is opened. (From Schuenke M, Schulte E, Schumacher U. THIEME Atlas of Anatomy. Head, Neck, and Neuroanatomy. Illustrations by Voll M and Wesker K. 3rd ed. New York: Thieme Medical Publishers; 2020.)

connect to the lens and ciliary processes of the ciliary body and their tension level affects the shape of the lens (**Fig. 7.104**). Contraction/relaxation of the **ciliary muscle** is what affects the tension level on the zonular fibers. The **ciliary processes** are folds located on the internal surface of the ciliary body and are responsible for secreting the **aqueous humor** that fills the **anterior/posterior chambers of the eyeball**.

- The **choroid** is the reddish-brown layer located between the sclera and retina and is highly vascular. **Bruch membrane** (*lamina vitrea*) is traditionally considered the innermost layer of the choroid and the thin refractive basement membrane that extends from the *ora serrata* to the optic disc. It is continuous from the iris and ciliary body anteriorly to the pia and arachnoid posteriorly. The attachment with the sclera can be easily stripped but the attachment of the choroid to the pigmented layer of the retina is quite firm. The larger vessels are located closer to the sclera while the smallest of vessels or **capillary lamina of the choroid** (*choriocapillaris*) are closest to the avascular portion of the retina. It supplies the light-sensitive region of the retina with oxygen and nutrients. The appearance of "red eye" in photos is due to the engorgement of blood in the capillary lamina vessels.

The **inner layer** of the eyeball is made up of the **retina (Fig. 7.100; Fig. 7.105)**. The retina consists of an *outer pigmented* and *inner neural layer* both of which are part of the **optic part of the retina**. The **pigmented layer** consists of a single layer of cells (simple cuboidal) adjacent to Bruch membrane that reinforces the light absorbing property of the choroid and reduces the scattering of light. The pigmented layer extends anteriorly over the posterior surfaces of both the ciliary body (*ciliary part of retina*) and iris (*iridial part of retina*) at the **ora serrata (Fig. 7.104)**, which defines the border between the *visual* and *nonvisual portions of the retina*. The **neural layer** is light-receptive layer and is composed of three types of neurons: the photoreceptors known as cones and rods, bipolar neurons, and ganglion neurons. It is the axons of the ganglion neurons that form the optic nerve (CN II).

Where the light enters and focuses on the posterior portion of the internal eyeball is called the **fundus**. The retina of this fundus or posterior region has a circular area called the **optic disc** and is where the optic nerve and central retinal vessels are found. There are no photoreceptors located here and it is insensitive to light. This portion of the retina is known as the *"blind spot."* The **macula lutea** (yellow spot) is located lateral to the optic disc and has a small, central depression called the **fovea centralis**. The highest concentrations of the photoreceptor cones are located here and this is the area of most acute or distinct vision. Although this area makes up less than 1% of the total retina, its relayed information takes up over 50% of the visual cortex in the brain **(Fig. 7.106; Fig. 7.107)**.

7.9.8 Histology of the Retina

There are ten histological layers to the retina and they are formed by elements of three neurons. Light will pass through all the inner layers of the retina before reaching the photosensitive elements of the photoreceptors. The transmission of visual sensory information is the opposite of incoming light. The visual pathway involves a connection between these three ordered neurons prior to reaching the *lateral geniculate nucleus* and *superior colliculus*, parts of the thalamus and midbrain, respectively.

First-order neurons are the light-sensitive **photoreceptor cells** known as *cones* and *rods* and they transform light stimuli into electrochemical signals. *Second-order neurons* are the **bipolar cells** that receive the impulses from the cones and rods and relay them to the ganglion cells. *Third-order neurons* are the **ganglion cells** whose axons converge at the optic disc and form the optic nerve. There are retinal glial cells (non-neuronal) called **Müller cells** that span the neural layer and support the surrounding cells, participate in bidirectional communication, and can collect light to channel it to the cones and rods. Other cells include the **horizontal cells** that allow for adjustment to bright and dim light conditions and **amacrine cells** that alternate routes between bipolar and ganglion cells. The 10 layers of the retina in order from excitation to the optic nerve are as follows **(Fig. 7.108)**:

1. *Pigmented epithelium*: a simple cuboidal epithelium with melanin granules adjacent to Bruch membrane.
2. *Processes of photoreceptors cells*: flattened vesicles filled with the visual pigment proteins iodopsin (cones) and rhodopsin (rods). **Cones** function best in bright light and pick up

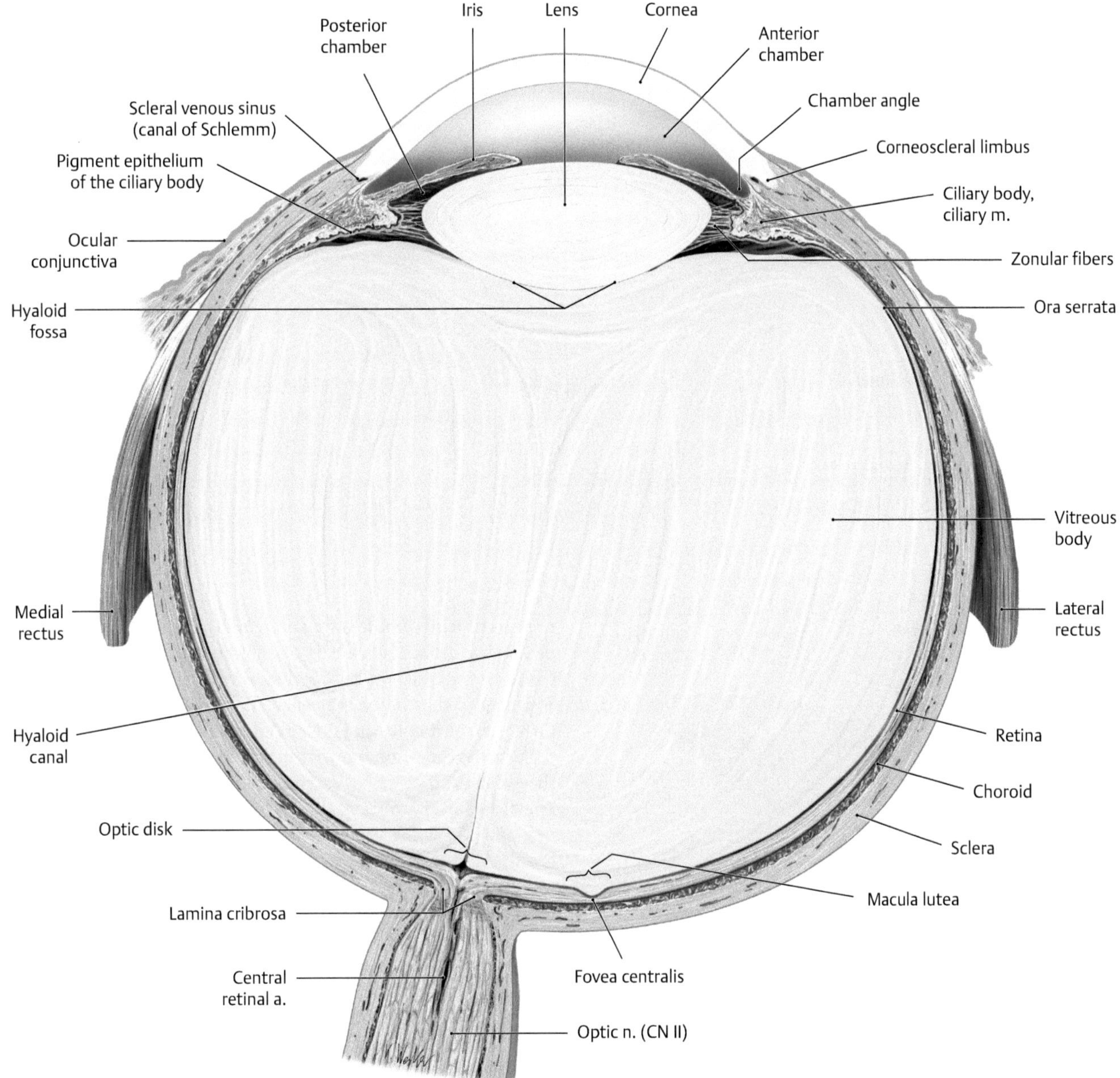

Fig. 7.100 Structure of the eyeball. Transverse section through right eyeball, superior view. (From Schuenke M, Schulte E, Schumacher U. THIEME Atlas of Anatomy. Head, Neck, and Neuroanatomy. Illustrations by Voll M and Wesker K. 3rd ed. New York: Thieme Medical Publishers; 2020.)

wavelengths associated with red, green, and blue color. **Rods** work well in low light and are associated with black, white, and peripheral vision.

3. *Outer limiting membrane*: site of Müller cell processes and dense junctional complexes.
4. *Outer nuclear*: nuclei of photoreceptor cells.
5. *Outer plexiform*: synapses between photoreceptor cell processes and the bipolar and horizontal cells.
6. *Inner nuclear*: contains the nuclei of bipolar, horizontal, amacrine, and Müller cells.
7. *Inner plexiform*: synapses between bipolar, ganglion, and amacrine cells.
8. *Ganglion cell*: large nuclei of ganglion cells.
9. *Nerve fiber*: ganglion cell axons that will form the optic nerve.
10. *Internal limiting membrane*: basement membrane produced by Müller cells.

7.9.9 Compartments and Refractive Media of the Eyeball

The primary refractory medium of the eyeball is the **cornea**. This means it bends light to the greatest degree focusing an inverted image onto the light-sensitive portion of the retina at the fundus of the eyeball. The corneal epithelium facing anteriorly is a

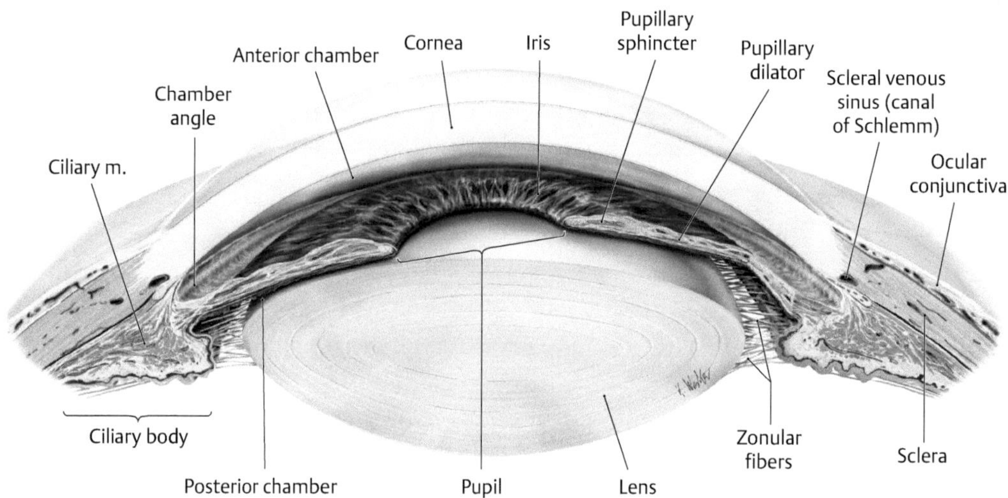

Fig. 7.101 Location of the cornea, iris, lens, and the anterior and posterior chambers. (From Schuenke M, Schulte E, Schumacher U. THIEME Atlas of Anatomy. Head, Neck, and Neuroanatomy. Illustrations by Voll M and Wesker K. 3rd ed. New York: Thieme Medical Publishers; 2020.)

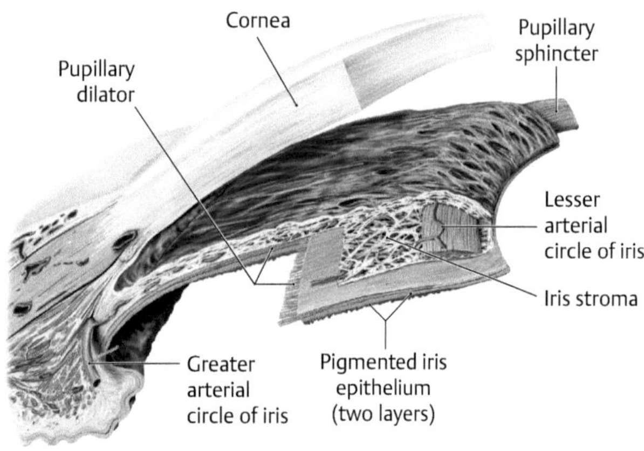

Fig. 7.102 Structure of the iris. (From Schuenke M, Schulte E, Schumacher U. THIEME Atlas of Anatomy. Head, Neck, and Neuroanatomy. Illustrations by Voll M and Wesker K. 3rd ed. New York: Thieme Medical Publishers; 2020.)

nonkeratinizing stratified squamous epithelium while the posteriorly facing surface is made up of a simple squamous/cuboidal epithelium (endothelium) that regulates water content in the cornea. Touching of the cornea may elicit the *corneal reflex* that involves CN V_1 (afferent limb) and CN VII (efferent limb).

The **anterior compartment** makes up the anterior one-fifth of the eyeball and contains two chambers filled with aqueous humor. The **anterior chamber** of the eyeball is located between the cornea and iris while the **posterior chamber** is located between the iris and lens. **Aqueous humor** is a watery-solution similar to plasma produced by the ciliary processes of the ciliary body within the posterior chamber and passes through the pupil to enter the anterior chamber. It then drains at the *iridocorneal angle* into the **scleral venous sinus** (*canal of Schlemm*). It then passes through a network of scleral veins close to the limbus called the **limbal plexus** that ultimately drain to the anterior ciliary and vorticose veins. Obstruction of aqueous humor drainage could lead to increased intraocular pressure or glaucoma, resulting in blindness due to degenerative changes to the retina (**Fig. 7.100; Fig. 7.101**).

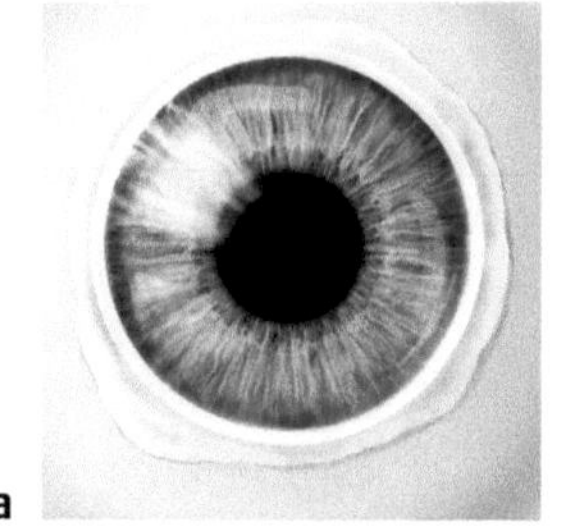

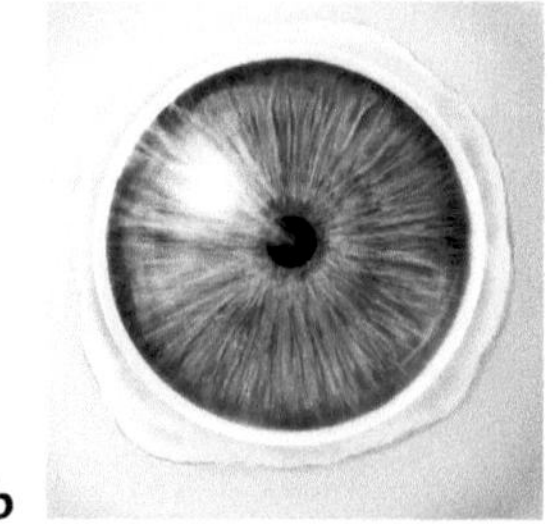

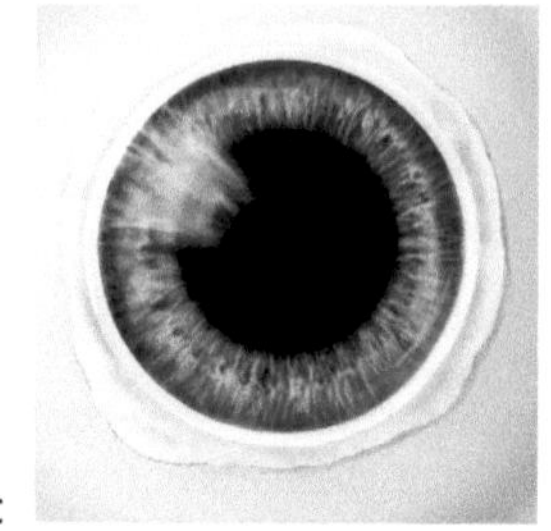

Fig. 7.103 Pupil: pupil size is regulated by two intraocular muscles of the iris—the sphincter pupillae and the dilator pupillae. **(a)** Normal pupil size. **(b)** Maximum constriction (miosis). **(c)** Maximum dilation (mydriasis). (From Schuenke M, Schulte E, Schumacher U. THIEME Atlas of Anatomy. Head, Neck, and Neuroanatomy. Illustrations by Voll M and Wesker K. 3rd ed. New York: Thieme Medical Publishers; 2020.)

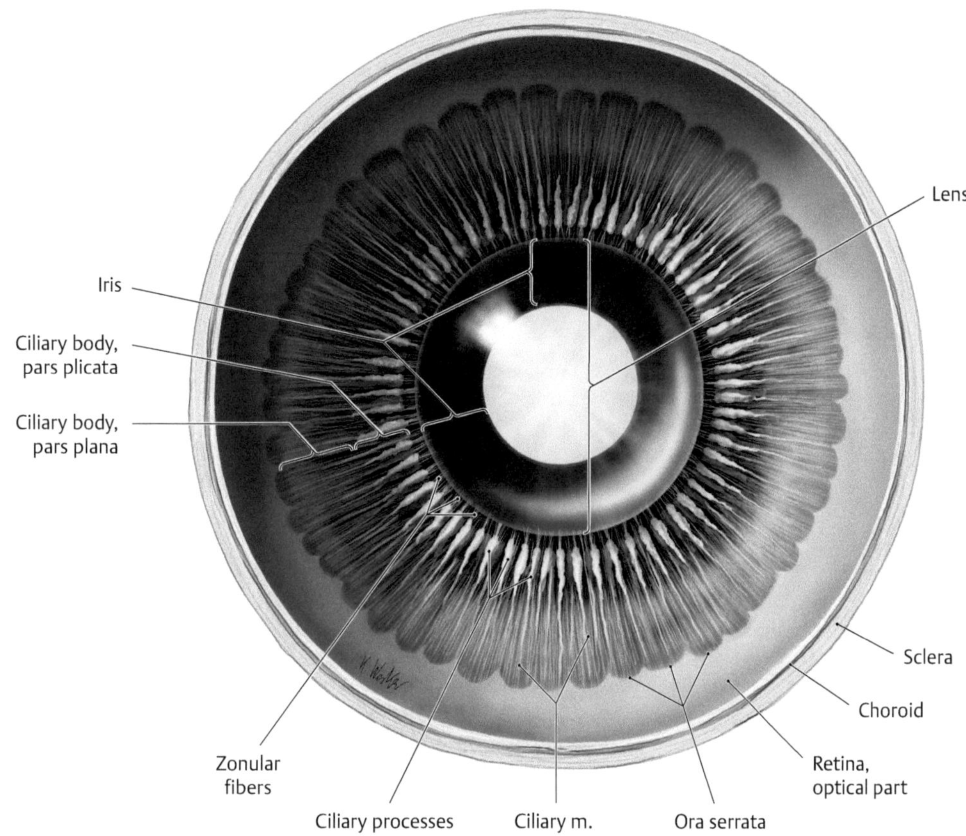

Fig. 7.104 Lens and ciliary body, posterior view. (From Schuenke M, Schulte E, Schumacher U. THIEME Atlas of Anatomy. Head, Neck, and Neuroanatomy. Illustrations by Voll M and Wesker K. 3rd ed. New York: Thieme Medical Publishers; 2020.)

The **lens** is a transparent, biconvex structure enclosed in a capsule, and located posterior to the iris but anterior to the vitreous body. On only the anterior surface just below the capsule, a simple cuboidal epithelium is responsible for producing lens fibers and transporting nutrients. The **capsule**, which is composed primarily of type IV collagen and completely surrounds the lens, is attached to the zonular fibers that are themselves attached to the ciliary processes of the ciliary body. The convexity of the lens constantly fine-tunes the focus of distant or near objects on the retina. The **ciliary muscle** (smooth muscle) of the ciliary body is responsible for changing the shape of the lens. When contracting (via parasympathetic innervation), tension on the **zonular fibers** (collectively the **suspensory ligament of the lens**) is reduced causing the lens to thicken and brings near objects into focus (near vision). **Accommodation** is the active process of changing the shape of the lens for near vision. If the ciliary muscle relaxes, this increases the tension on the zonular fibers causing the lens to stretch and become thinner resulting in the focusing of distant objects (far vision) (**Fig. 7.100; Fig. 7.101; Fig. 7.109**).

The **posterior compartment** (or *vitreous chamber*) makes up the posterior four-fifth of the eyeball and contains the **vitreous body**. The vitreous body is a transparent jellylike substance that contains **vitreous humor** that is made up of primarily water (99%) but also contains hyaluronic acid and collagen. The vitreous body and humor are generally referred together as just the vitreous. It functions in transmitting light, supports the lens, and holds the neural layer of the retina up against the pigmented layer.

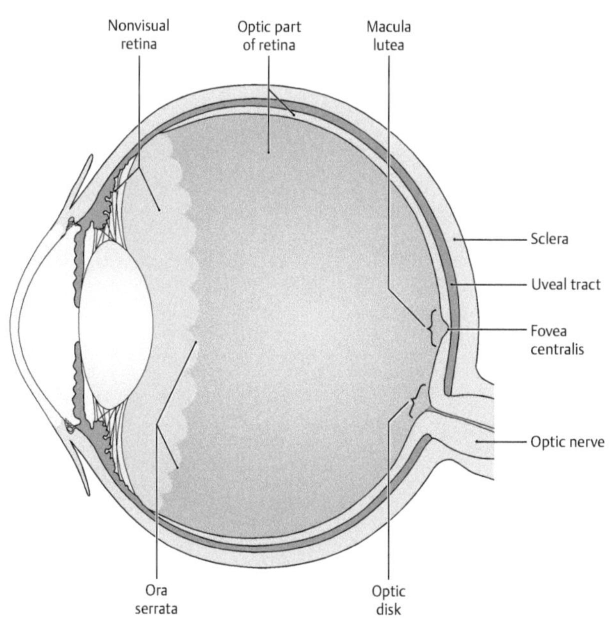

Fig. 7.105 Overview of the retina. The photosensitive optic part and the non-photosensitive nonvisual retina are separated by the ora serrata. (From Schuenke M, Schulte E, Schumacher U. THIEME Atlas of Anatomy. Head, Neck, and Neuroanatomy. Illustrations by Voll M and Wesker K. 3rd ed. New York: Thieme Medical Publishers; 2020.)

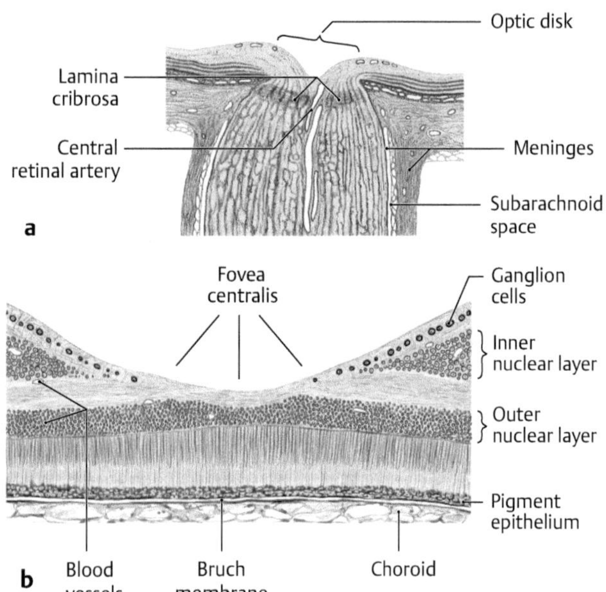

Fig. 7.106 **(a)** Optic disc ("blind spot") and lamina cribrosa. **(b)** Macula lutea and fovea centralis. (From Schuenke M, Schulte E, Schumacher U. THIEME Atlas of Anatomy. Head, Neck, and Neuroanatomy. Illustrations by Voll M and Wesker K. 3rd ed. New York: Thieme Medical Publishers; 2020.)

The **hyaloid canal** is a narrow channel running through the vitreous body from the optic disc to the posterior lens and during development it contained the *hyaloid vessels*, of which the proximal portions of these vessels remain as the central retinal vessels (**Fig. 7.100**).

7.9.10 Fascia of the Eyeball

The **fascial sheath** (bulbar sheath or capsule of Tenon) envelops the eyeball from the optic nerve to the corneoscleral junction (limbus), and forms an actual socket for the eyeball. The fascial sheath is pierced by the tendons of extraocular muscles and is reflected onto each of them as a **tubular (muscle) sheath**. Expansions of the fascial sheath at the lateral and medial rectus muscles are called the **lateral** and **medial check ligaments**. Transverse sections generally describe these ligaments as triangular in shape and they act by preventing the overaction (abduction and adduction) of these muscles. The other extraocular muscles do not have any distinct check ligaments. A blending of the check ligaments with the fascia of the inferior rectus and inferior oblique muscles forms the **suspensory ligament** (*of Lockwood*). This hammock-like sling supports the eyeball and limits depression of the eyeball (**Fig. 7.110**).

7.9.11 Development of the Eye

Eye development begins on day 22 with the formation of a pair of **optic grooves** near the forebrain. As the neural tube closes, the optic grooves evaginate from the walls of the diencephalon and form the hollow **optic vesicles** that consist of neuroectoderm. The optic vesicle will then come into contact with the surface ectoderm, invaginate, and form the double-layered **optic cup** and **optic stalk**. The optic cup consists of an *outer pigmented* and an *inner neural layer* and is the source for the retina, iris, and ciliary body (**Fig. 7.111**).

The **retina** has an outer pigmented and inner neural layer and they originate from the outer pigmented and inner neural layers of the optic cup, respectively. These two layers are originally separated from one another by the **intraretinal space** that is normally obliterated in the adult (**Fig. 7.112**). This space can be opened due

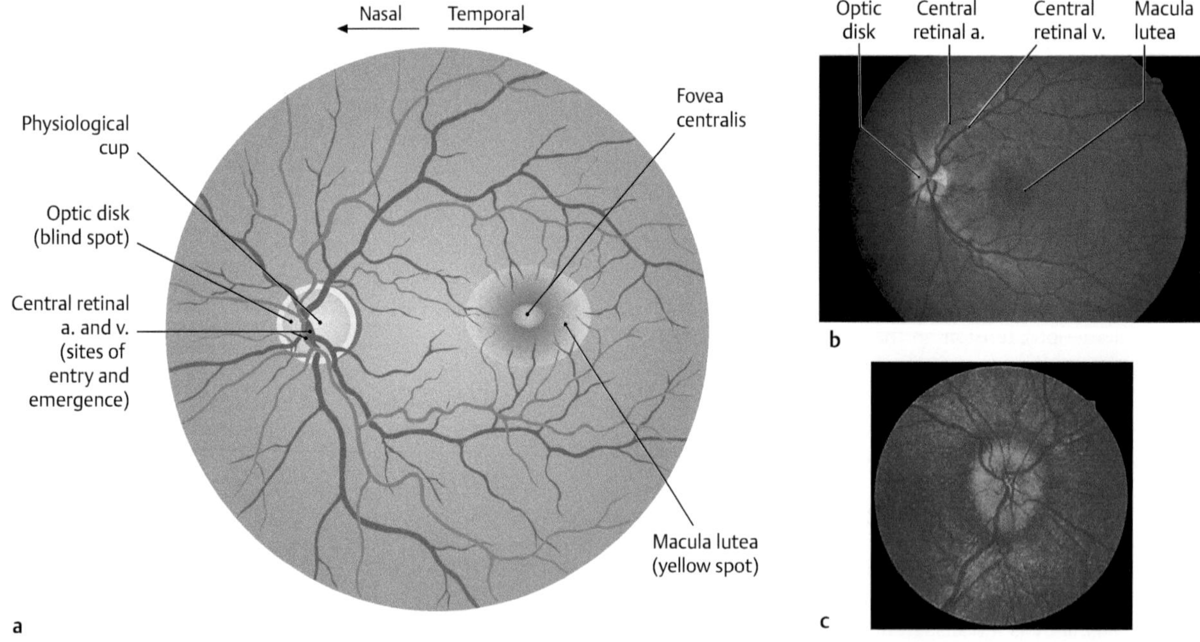

Fig. 7.107 Optic fundus. **(a)** Retina of left eyeball, anterior view, schematic. **(b)** Normal optic fundus in the ophthalmoscopic examination. (c) High intracranial pressure; the edges of the optic disk appear less sharp. (From Schuenke M, Schulte E, Schumacher U. THIEME Atlas of Anatomy. Head, Neck, and Neuroanatomy. Illustrations by Voll M and Wesker K. 3rd ed. New York: Thieme Medical Publishers; 2020.)

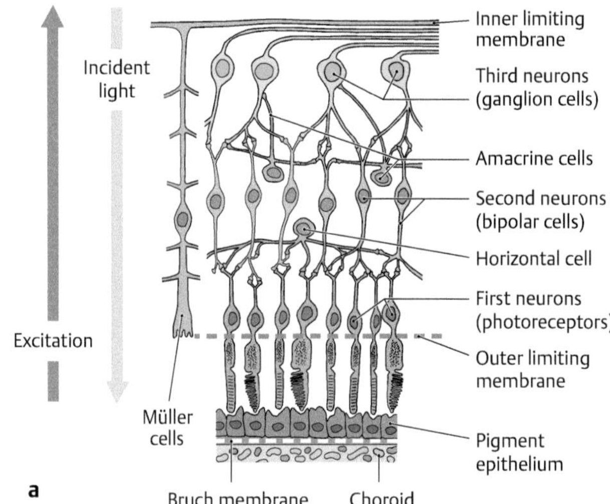

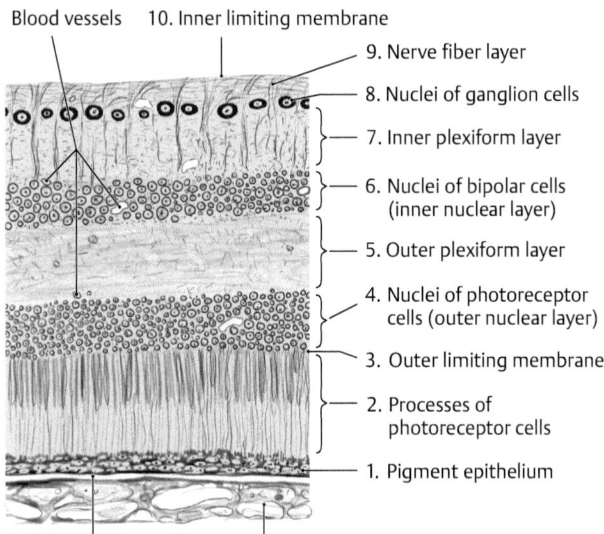

Fig. 7.108 Structure of the retina. **(a)** Schematic diagram of the first three neurons in the visual pathway and their connections. **(b)** The ten anatomical layers of the retina. (From Schuenke M, Schulte E, Schumacher U. THIEME Atlas of Anatomy. Head, Neck, and Neuroanatomy. Illustrations by Voll M and Wesker K. 3rd ed. New York: Thieme Medical Publishers; 2020.)

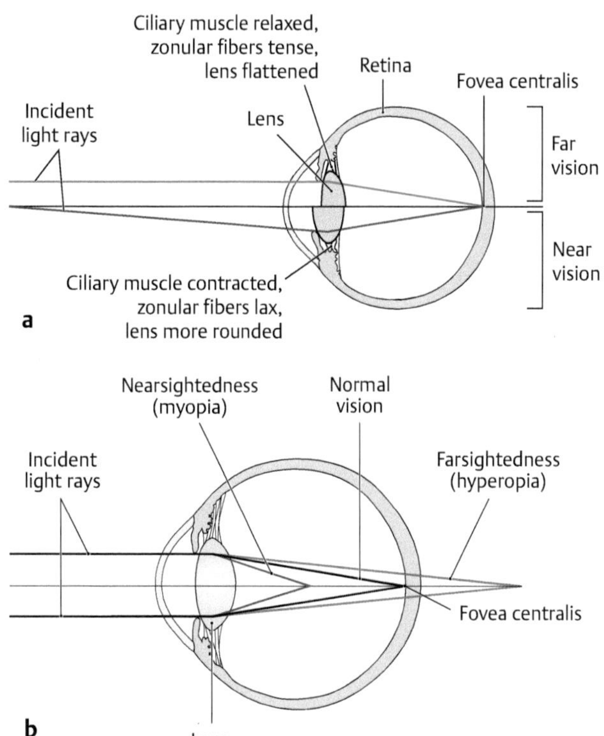

Fig. 7.109 Light refraction and dynamics of the lens. **(a)** Normal dynamics of the lens. **(b)** Abnormal dynamics. In nearsightedness (myopia), the light rays are focused to a point in front of the retina. In farsightedness (hyperopia), the light rays are focused behind the retina. (From Schuenke M, Schulte E, Schumacher U. THIEME Atlas of Anatomy. Head, Neck, and Neuroanatomy. Illustrations by Voll M and Wesker K. 3rd ed. New York: Thieme Medical Publishers; 2020.)

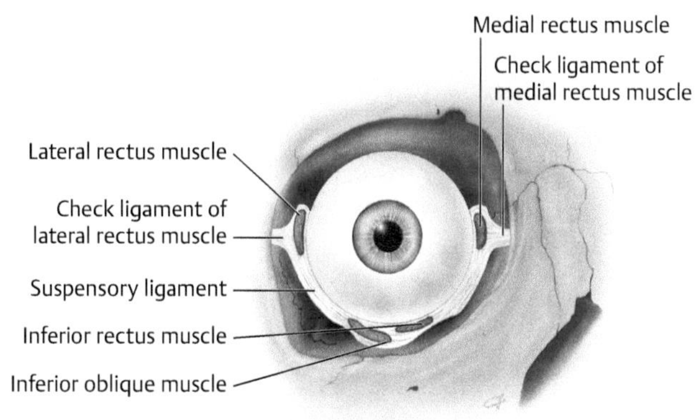

Fig. 7.110 Check and suspensory ligaments of the eyeball. Illustration by Calla Heald.

to leaking of vitreous fluid into it and thus becoming the site for *retinal detachment.* The epithelium of both the **iris** and **ciliary body** develop from the anterior portions of the pigmented and neural layers of the optic cup. The stroma of both these structures originates from the mesoderm that is continuous with the choroid. The *sphincter/constrictor pupillae* and *dilator pupillae* muscles of the iris develop from a transformation of epithelial cells into contractile cells within the epithelium of the optic cups' outer pigment layer. The *ciliary muscle* of the ciliary body develops from mesoderm within the choroid.

The surface ectoderm adjacent to the optic vesicles will thicken and form the **lens placode**, the future **lens** of the eyeball. The placode will then invaginate and sink deep into the surface ectoderm forming a **lens pit**. The edges of this pit will fuse and form the spherical **lens vesicles**. As the lens vesicles develop, the optic vesicles continue their own invagination to form the double-walled optic cups resulting in the enveloping of the early lens. The lens vesicle induces the **cornea** but the cornea will receive contributions from three different sources (**Fig. 7.112**). Surface ectoderm forms the *anterior/external corneal epithelium*; mesoderm contributes to *Bowman membrane*, the *stroma (substantia propria)*, and *Descemet membrane*; neural crest cells form the posteriorly facing *corneal endothelium*.

The outer fibrous **sclera** and inner vascular **choroid** develop from mesoderm that surrounds the optic cup (**Fig. 7.112**). The sclera is continuous with the cornea and dura mater while the choroid is continuous with the iris, ciliary body, and both the arachnoid and pia maters. The **anterior chamber** undergoes vacuolization

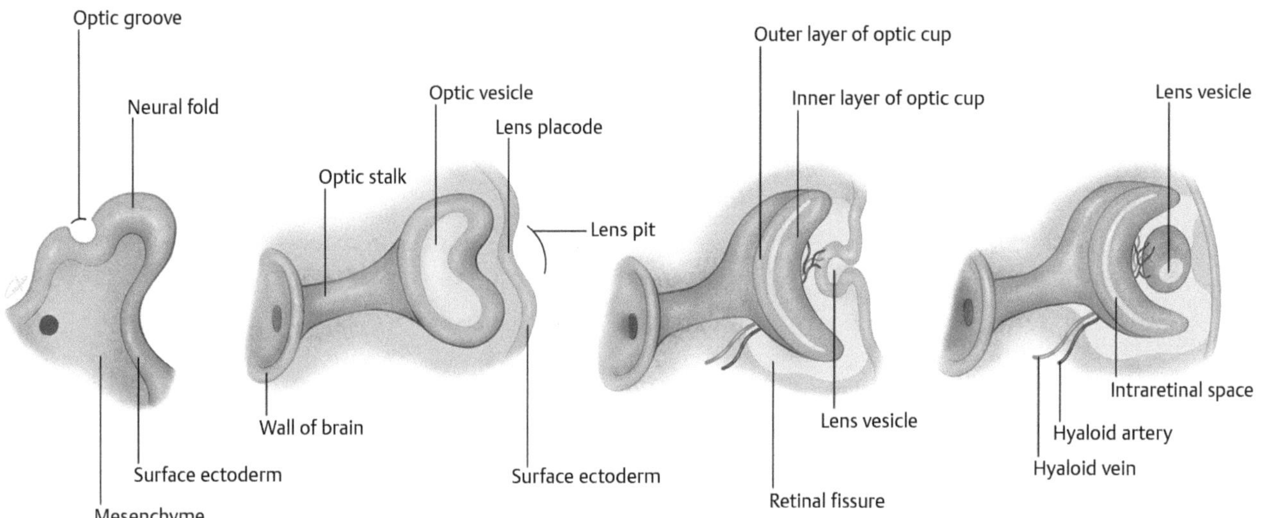

Fig. 7.111 Early stages of eye development. Demonstrated are the successive stages in the development of the optic cup and lens vesicle beginning at approximately 22 days. Illustration by Calla Heald.

Clinical Correlate 7.19

Preseptal (Periorbital) Cellulitis

Preseptal cellulitis is the inflammation due to an infection and is located *anterior* to the orbital septum. A patient may present with a fever and swollen eyelids but there is no limited eye movement or pain associated with that movement, no proptosis (bulging of the eye), and no loss of vision. Blurry vision may be a symptom however. Oral antibiotics may be prescribed and the patient is sent home.

Clinical Correlate 7.20

Orbital Cellulitis

Orbital cellulitis is the inflammation due to an infection located *posterior* to the orbital septum. This is considered a life-threatening condition and the patient should be admitted to a hospital immediately. There may be a sudden loss of vision, pain when moving the eye, proptosis of the eye, or swelling of the eyelid similar to preseptal cellulitis. Prompt administration of intravenous antibiotics in the hospital must be given. If an abscess is located it may have to be removed surgically.

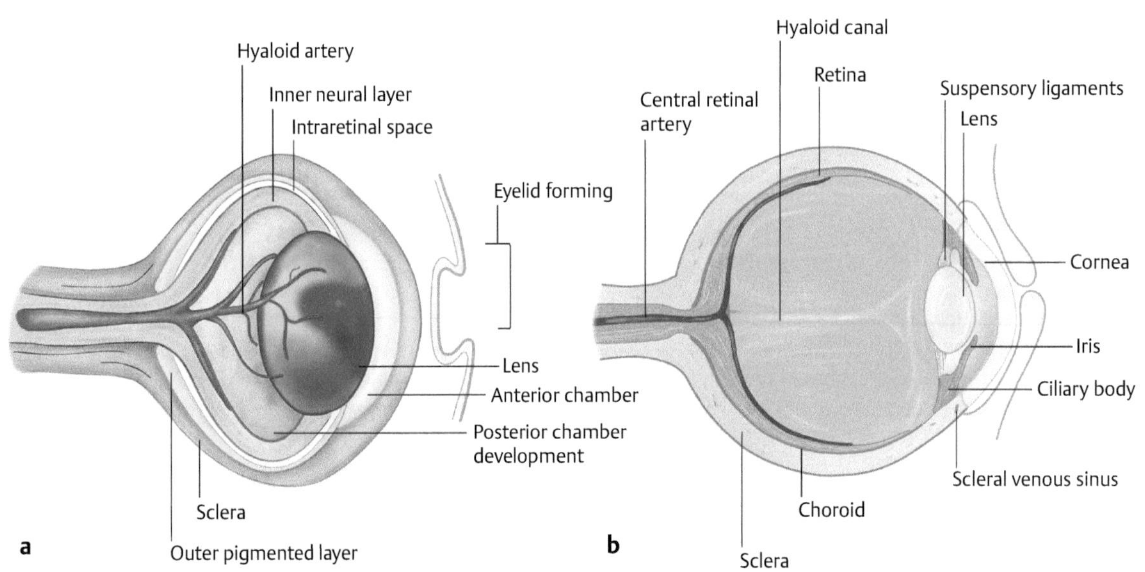

Fig. 7.112 Sagittal section through the eye demonstrating lens, retina, iris, and cornea development. **(a)** 6 weeks. **(b)** Newborn infant. Illustration by Calla Heald.

Clinical Correlate 7.21

Palpebral Gland Inflammation

Glands associated with the eyelids may become inflamed or swollen due to an infection or an obstruction of their ducts. If the ducts of the *tarsal glands* (sebaceous in nature) become inflamed and produce a lesion they are called **tarsal chalazia.** When the *ciliary glands* become obstructed and inflamed, a red pus-producing swelling develops on the eyelid. This is commonly known as having a **"sty."**

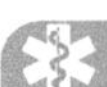

Clinical Correlate 7.22

Detached Retina

A detached retina is the result of fluid drainage into an open space now located between the pigmented cell layer and neural layer. The filling of this potential space through retinal tears can take several days or longer and the first symptoms may be seeing floaters or small moving spots. Flashes of light and darkening of one's peripheral vision is also noted. Treatment must include repair within a couple days or presentation or total blindness in the affected eye could occur. *Laser photocoagulation* or *cryopexy* treatments work best when the detachment is found early. Other procedures to correct for the detachment include *vitrectomy*, *scleral buckle surgery*, and *pneumatic retinopexy*.

Clinical Correlate 7.23

Presbyopia and Cataracts

As individuals age, their lenses will become harder and more flattened. These changes will gradually reduce the focusing power of the lenses, and this condition is known as **presbyopia**. A **cataract** is a clouding of the lens. A common practice has become the combined cataract extraction with an intraocular lens implant. An *extracapsular cataract extraction* involves removing the lens but leaving the capsule of the lens intact to receive a synthetic intraocular lens. An *intracapsular lens extraction* involves removing the lens and lens capsule and then implanting a synthetic intraocular lens into the anterior chamber.

Clinical Correlate 7.24

Glaucoma

The drainage of aqueous humor through the scleral venous sinus and back into the blood circulation must occur at the same rate at which the aqueous humor is produced **(a)**. If there is a reduction in the amount of outflow due to some form of blockage, pressure builds up in the anterior and posterior chambers of the eye, a condition known as **glaucoma**. If there is compression of the retina and the retinal arteries due to the aqueous humor production not being reduced in order to maintain normal intraocular pressure, this will result in blindness. There are two main types of glaucoma.

- ***Chronic*** (*open angle*): the drainage angle formed by the cornea and the iris remains open but the drainage canals in the angle are partially blocked causing the fluid to drain out of the eye too slowly (**b**).
- ***Acute*** (*closed angle*) occurs when the iris bulges anteriorly to narrow or block the drainage angle formed by the cornea and the iris (**c**).

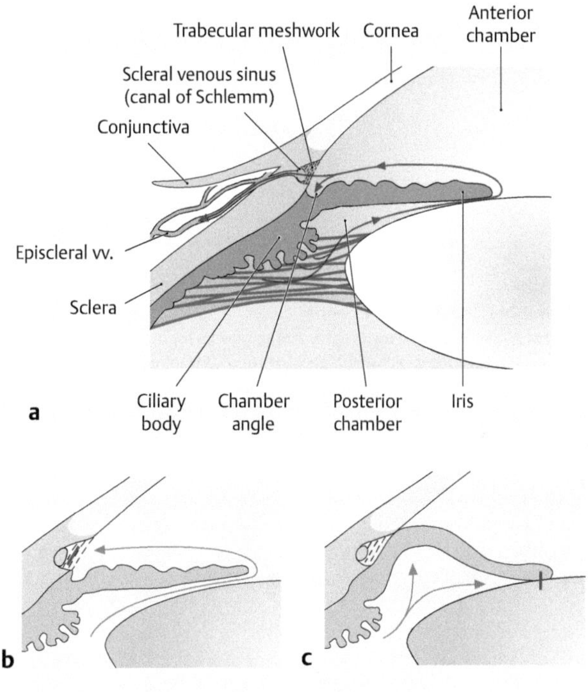

(From Schuenke M, Schulte E, Schumacher U. THIEME Atlas of Anatomy. Head, Neck, and Neuroanatomy. Illustrations by Voll M and Wesker K. 3rd ed. New York: Thieme Medical Publishers; 2020.)

and splits the mesoderm into two layers. Mesoderm located anterior to the chamber contributes to the *stroma* of the cornea and mesoderm posterior to the chamber forms the **iridopupillary membrane**, a membrane normally reabsorbed prior to birth. The anterior and posterior chambers located between the iris are filled with *aqueous humor* produced by the ciliary processes while the transparent and gelatinous *vitreous body*, located between the lens and retina, develops from mesoderm that migrated through the *choroid fissure.*

The optic stalk contains the **choroid (retinal) fissure** and this is the location of the **hyaloid blood vessels**. The hyaloid vessels will become the **central artery/vein of the retina** (**Fig. 7.111; Fig. 7.112**). With closure of the choroid fissure during the seventh week of development, the optic stalk that already contains the axons of ganglion cells forms the **optic nerve (CN II)**, **optic chiasm,** and **optic tracts**. The optic nerve will be invested by the meninges but will not become completely myelinated until approximately three months after birth. **Extraocular muscles** located within the orbit develop from mesoderm that surrounds the optic cup. This mesoderm originates specifically from *somitomeres 1-3 and 5.*

7.10 Ear

The **ear** is divided into an **external**, **middle,** and **internal ear** (**Fig. 7.113**). The *tympanic membrane (eardrum)* will serve as the separation between the external and middle ears. The *pharyngotympanic (auditory or Eustachian) tube* joins the middle ear to the nasopharynx. The external and middle ears are responsible for transferring sound to the internal ear. The internal ear contains the organs responsible for hearing and equilibrium.

The **external ear** has two major components, an auricle and the external acoustic meatus. The **auricle (or pinna)** is an irregularly shaped structure made of an elastic cartilage plate and covered with skin. Features include a deep depression known as

Clinical Correlate 7.25

Oculomotor Nerve (CN III) Palsy

An **oculomotor nerve palsy** can affect the majority of the ocular muscles. The individual will display a "down and out" gaze when looking straight ahead due to the unopposed actions of the lateral rectus and superior oblique muscles. The upper eyelid will display *ptosis* due to the paralysis of the levator palpebrae superioris muscle. There will be no accommodation of the lens (near vision) or constriction of the pupil because of disruption to the parasympathetic fibers affecting the ciliary and sphincter (constrictor) pupillae muscles, respectively.

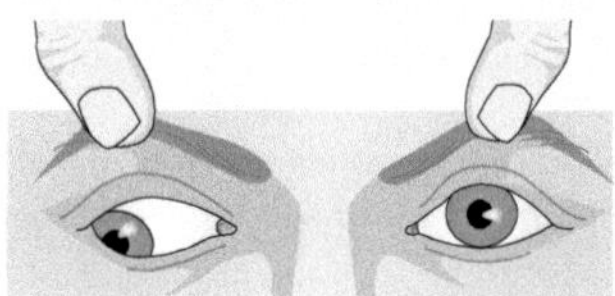

(From Schuenke M, Schulte E, Schumacher U. THIEME Atlas of Anatomy. Head, Neck, and Neuroanatomy. Illustrations by Voll M and Wesker K. 3rd ed. New York: Thieme Medical Publishers; 2020.)

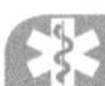

Clinical Correlate 7.26

Trochlear Nerve (CN IV) Palsy

A **trochlear nerve palsy** targets the superior oblique muscle and the individual displays an "up and in" gaze when looking forward. Characteristic to this type of palsy is *diplopia* (double vision) when looking down and this is because the superior oblique normally assists the inferior rectus in depressing the eyeball and is the only one to do so if the eye is adducted. One of the most common causes for *hypertropia*, a type of strabismus where there is a vertical misalignment of the eyes, is a trochlear nerve palsy. To accommodate for a nonfunctioning superior oblique muscle, the individual will tilt their head away from the affected side to correct for extortion and then tuck their chin while looking up to correct for the hypertropia.

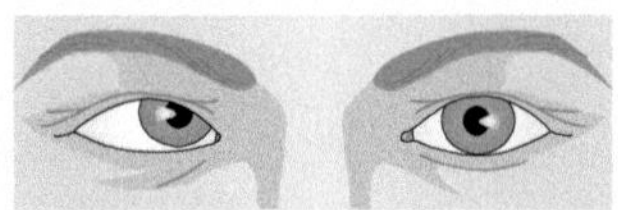

(From Schuenke M, Schulte E, Schumacher U. THIEME Atlas of Anatomy. Head, Neck, and Neuroanatomy. Illustrations by Voll M and Wesker K. 3rd ed. New York: Thieme Medical Publishers; 2020.)

Clinical Correlate 7.27

Abducent Nerve (CN VI) Palsy

An abducent nerve palsy could be the result of a brain tumor and would affect the function of the lateral rectus muscle which is responsible for abducting the eye. There will be adduction of the affected eye when a person looks forward due to the unopposed action of the medial rectus muscle.

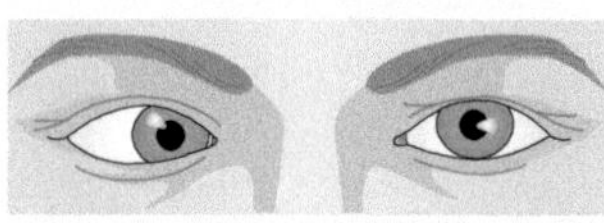

(From Schuenke M, Schulte E, Schumacher U. THIEME Atlas of Anatomy. Head, Neck, and Neuroanatomy. Illustrations by Voll M and Wesker K. 3rd ed. New York: Thieme Medical Publishers; 2020.)

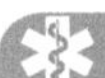

Clinical Correlate 7.28

Corneal Reflex

The **corneal reflex** is evaluated by touching the cornea with a cotton wisp. A bilateral blinking response should result. If this reflex is lost or diminished it may be due to a lesion related to either the ophthalmic nerve (V_1) or the facial nerve (CN VII). The afferent limb is associated with CN V_1 while the efferent limb is related to CN VII.

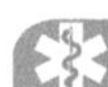

Clinical Correlate 7.29

Pupillary Light Reflex

The **pupillary light reflex** (photopupillary reflex) is responsible for controlling the diameter of the pupil, thus regulating the amount of light entering the eye, and it is tested by using a pen light during a neurological examination. When light is flashed toward one eye, both of the pupils will constrict because each of the retinas send fibers to the optic tracts of both sides. The sphincter (constrictor) pupillae muscle is innervated by parasympathetic fibers coursing through the inferior division of CN III and if there is any disruption of these fibers, this will cause dilation of the pupil because of the unopposed action of the sympathetically innervated dilator pupillae muscle. The first sign of CN III compression is ipsilateral slowness of the pupillary response to light. The afferent limb of the reflex involves the optic nerve (CN II) and the efferent limb is related to the oculomotor nerve (CN III).

the **concha** that is made up of two regions, the *cymba* and *cavity*. Just below the concha is the **lobule**, which is noncartilaginous and is a common site to pierce one's ear. The **tragus** is a posteriorly directed projection that overlaps the external acoustic meatus while the **antitragus** is located just superoposteriorly from the lobule and marks the beginning of the *antihelix*. The **helix** is an outer rim extending from near the scalp and down to the lobule. The **antihelix** is located mainly anterior to the helix and separated only by the **scaphoid fossa**. It extends up from the antitragus before bifurcating into two crura. Located between the antihelix crura is the **triangular fossa (Fig. 7.114)**.

The **external acoustic (auditory) meatus** is a canal that begins at the cavity of the concha and travels through the tympanic portion of the temporal bone before reaching the tympanic membrane. The lateral one-third is cartilaginous and the skin lining it is continuous with the skin of the auricle. Specialized sweat glands known as ceruminous glands along with sebaceous glands in this lateral one-third of the meatus produce **cerumen (earwax)**, which is responsible for lubrication, waterproofing, and trapping foreign particles. The medial two-thirds is bony and the skin in this region is continuous with the outer layer of the tympanic membrane **(Fig. 7.115)**.

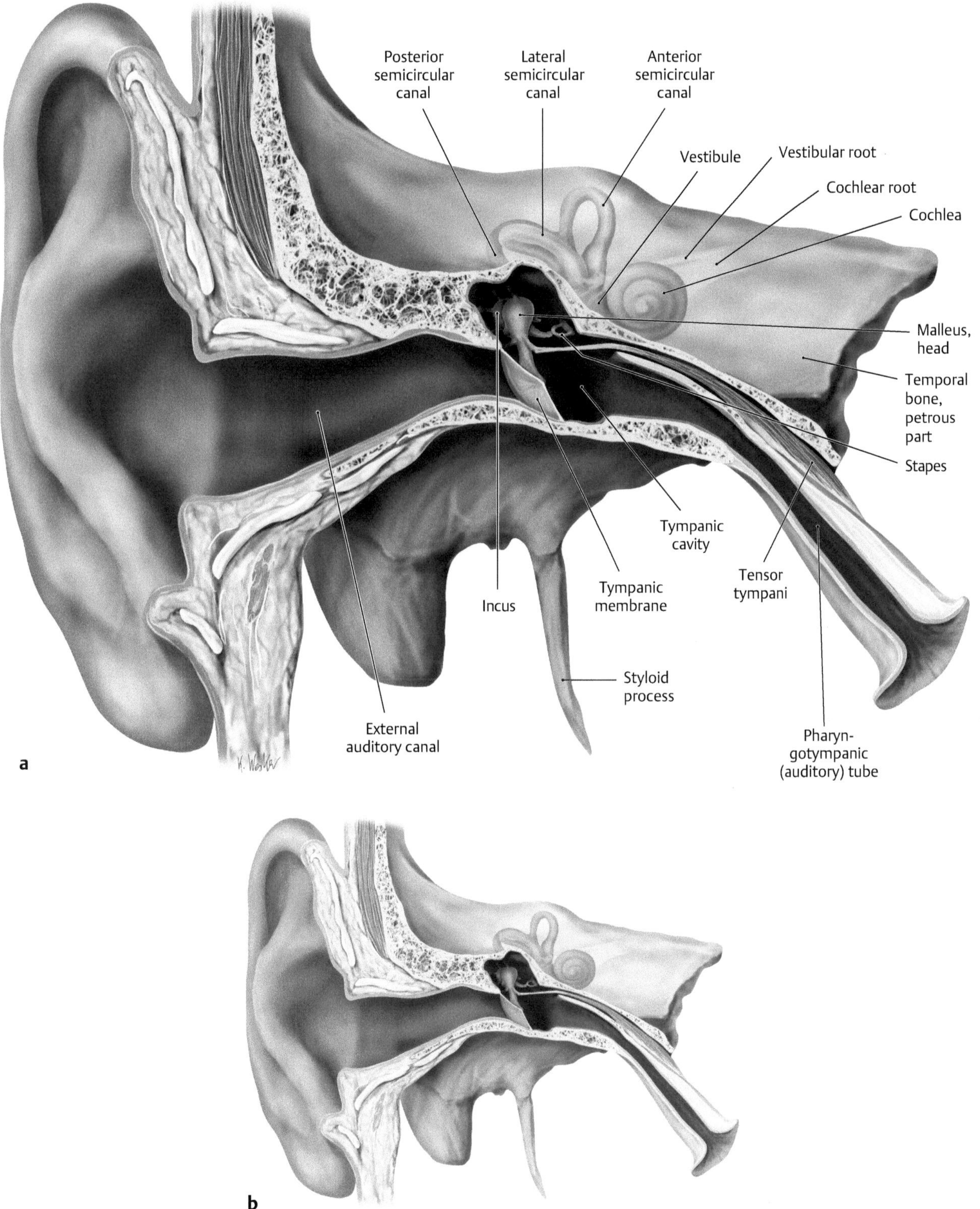

Fig. 7.113 Auditory and vestibular apparatus in situ. **(a)** Coronal section through the right ear, anterior view. **(b)** External ear (*yellow*), middle ear (*blue*), and inner ear (*green*). (From Schuenke M, Schulte E, Schumacher U. THIEME Atlas of Anatomy. Head, Neck, and Neuroanatomy. Illustrations by Voll M and Wesker K. 3rd ed. New York: Thieme Medical Publishers; 2020.)

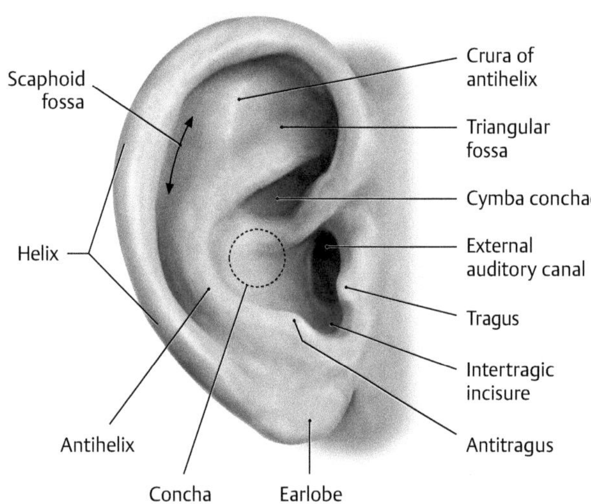

Fig. 7.114 Right auricle. (From Schuenke M, Schulte E, Schumacher U. THIEME Atlas of Anatomy. Head, Neck, and Neuroanatomy. Illustrations by Voll M and Wesker K. 3rd ed. New York: Thieme Medical Publishers; 2020.)

The **tympanic membrane** is a thin, semitransparent, and oval-shaped membrane located at the terminal end of the external acoustic meatus and separates it from the tympanic cavity of the middle ear. Skin is located on the outer surface while the inner surface is lined with a mucous membrane. It is concave toward the external acoustic meatus and has a conelike central depression that peaks forming the **umbo**. It is orientated in such a way to receive signals from the anterior and lateral sides of the head, thus moving in response to air vibrations that push against the membrane. The majority of the tympanic membrane is known as the **pars tensa**, the tense portion of the membrane that extends inferiorly from the anterior and posterior malleolar folds at the level of the lateral process of the malleus. The **pars flaccida** is the smaller flaccid portion of the membrane that is located just superior to the lateral process of the malleus **(Fig. 7.116)**.

7.10.1 Neurovasculature of the External Ear, External Acoustic Meatus, and Tympanic Membrane

The **great auricular nerve** (C2–C3) is responsible for cutaneous innervation to most of the lateral surface of the auricle, including the lobule, helix, and antihelix along with most of the medial (cranial/back of ear) surface. The **lesser occipital nerve** (C2–C3) supplies the superior aspect of the medial (cranial) surface. The **auriculotemporal nerve** (CN V_3) supplies the auricle skin anterior to the external acoustic meatus, superior portions of the external acoustic meatus, and the majority of the outer surface of the tympanic membrane. The **auricular branches of the vagus nerve** (CN X) supply the concha and the remainder of both the external acoustic meatus and outer tympanic membrane. The **facial nerve** (CN VII) will also contribute to the innervation of the concha, outer borders of the auricle, and possibly the medial surface. The **glossopharyngeal nerve** (CN IX) is better known for innervating the internal surface of the tympanic membrane and mucosa of the middle ear cavity (visceral sensory) but it may also contribute to regions of the concha, external acoustic meatus, and medial surface **(Fig. 7.117)**.

Blood supply to these regions is derived from the *perforating branches* of the **posterior auricular**, *auricular branches* of the **superficial temporal**, and *deep auricular branches* of the **maxillary artery (Fig. 7.118)**. Venous drainage would travel back toward the **external jugular**, **retromandibular**, and **maxillary veins**.

Lymphatic drainage is divided into three zones and will eventually drain to the **deep cervical lymph nodes** located adjacent to the IJV before continuing to the thoracic or right lymphatic duct. The *anterior zone*, which includes the majority of the anterior half of the auricle, tragus, and external acoustic meatus, drains first

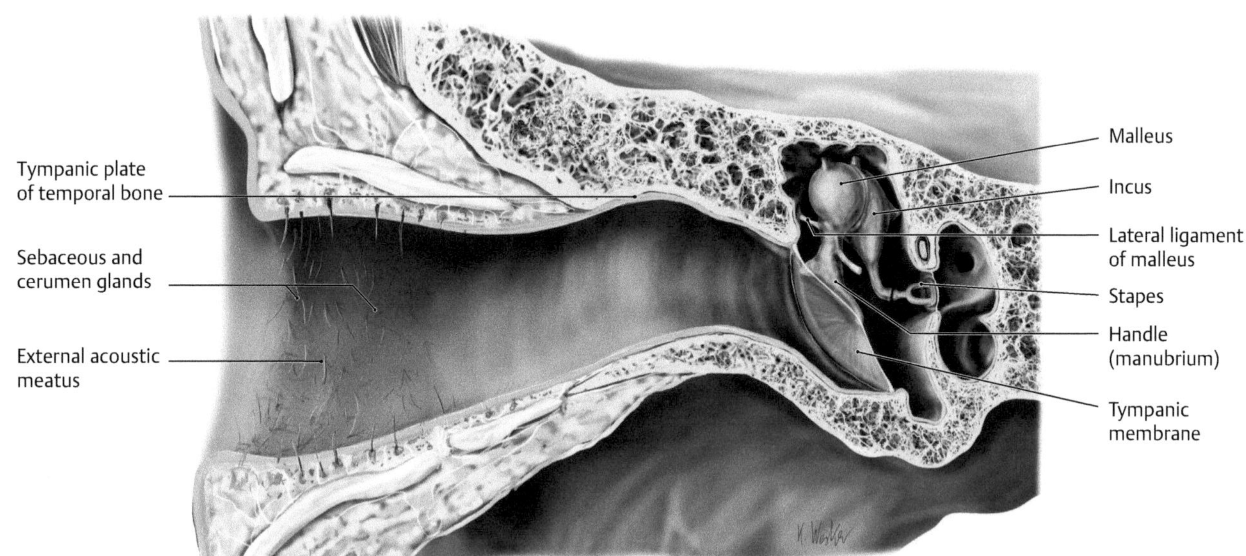

Fig. 7.115 External acoustic (auditory) meatus, tympanic membrane, and tympanic cavity. (From Schuenke M, Schulte E, Schumacher U. THIEME Atlas of Anatomy. Head, Neck, and Neuroanatomy. Illustrations by Voll M and Wesker K. 3rd ed. New York: Thieme Medical Publishers; 2020.)

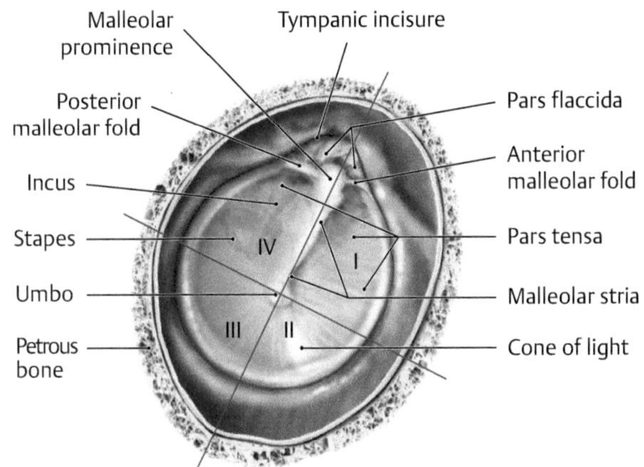

Fig. 7.116 Tympanic membrane. (From Schuenke M, Schulte E, Schumacher U. THIEME Atlas of Anatomy. Head, Neck, and Neuroanatomy. Illustrations by Voll M and Wesker K. 3rd ed. New York: Thieme Medical Publishers; 2020.)

to the **superficial parotid lymph nodes**, then the **deep parotid lymph nodes** before reaching the **deep cervical lymph nodes**. The *posterior zone*, which includes the majority of the posterior half of the auricle, drains initially to the **mastoid (retroauricular) lymph nodes** before reaching the **deep cervical lymph nodes**. The *lower zone* includes the remainder of the auricle and lobule, and drains initially to the **superficial cervical lymph nodes** followed by the **deep cervical lymph nodes**. It may also drain directly to the deep cervical lymph nodes **(Fig. 7.119)**.

7.10.2 Middle Ear (Tympanic Cavity)

The **middle ear (tympanic cavity)** is an air-filled and irregularly shaped space located within the petrous portion of the temporal bone and sandwiched between the tympanic membrane and inner ear. This cavity is connected posterosuperiorly with the *mastoid cells* through the **mastoid antrum** and anteromedially to the nasopharynx by the **pharyngotympanic tube**. The contents of this cavity include the auditory ossicles, tensor tympani muscle, stapedius muscle, tympanic plexus, chorda tympani nerve, and a mucous membrane innervated by the glossopharyngeal nerve. This mucous membrane is continuous with the lining of the mastoid cells, mastoid antrum, and pharyngotympanic tube **(Fig. 7.120a)**.

The tympanic cavity is said to have six borders (**Fig. 7.120b**):

- *Tegmental wall (superior or roof)*: formed by a thin plate of the petrous portion of the temporal bone known as the **tegmen tympani**. It forms a separation between the tympanic cavity and the dura mater lying on the floor of the middle cranial fossa.
- *Labyrinthine wall (medial)*: the **promontory** formed by the cochlea, *oval window*, and *round window* form much of this wall. The **tympanic nerve plexus** (formed by the tympanic br. of CN IX) rests directly on the promontory. This wall separates the tympanic cavity from the internal ear.
- *Jugular wall (or floor)*: formed by a thin layer of the temporal bone. It separates the tympanic cavity from the superior bulb of the IJV.
- *Membranous wall (lateral)*: formed almost entirely by the tympanic membrane. The lateral bony wall of the **epitympanic recess** forms the superior aspect of this lateral wall. The *handle of the malleus* extends into the epitympanic recess.
- *Mastoid wall (posterior)*: the superior portion of this wall has an opening called the **aditus to the mastoid antrum**. It forms the connection from the mastoid cells to the tympanic cavity. The *facial nerve canal* passes between the mastoid antrum and posterior wall.
- *Carotid wall (anterior)*: separates the tympanic cavity from the carotid canal. The *pharyngotympanic tube opening* and the *canal for the tensor tympani muscle* can be located on the superior aspect of this wall.

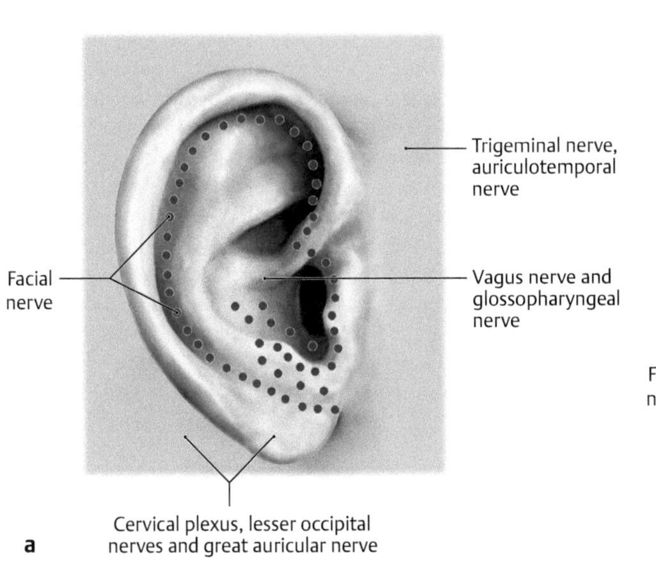

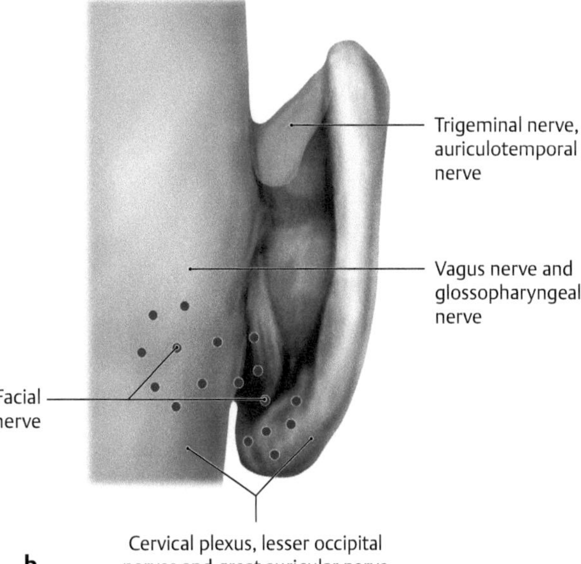

Fig. 7.117 Sensory innervation of the auricle. (From Schuenke M, Schulte E, Schumacher U. THIEME Atlas of Anatomy. Head, Neck, and Neuroanatomy. Illustrations by Voll M and Wesker K. 3rd ed. New York: Thieme Medical Publishers; 2020.)

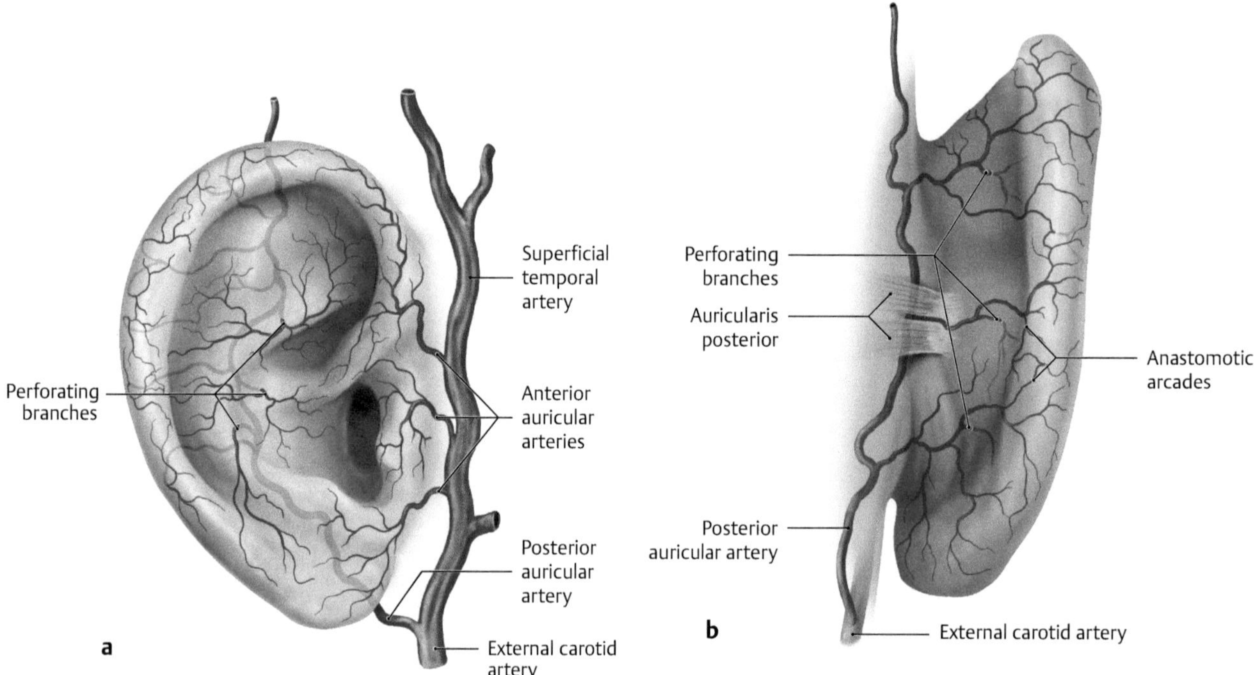

Fig. 7.118 Arterial supply to the auricle. **(a)** Lateral view. **(b)** Posterior view. (From Schuenke M, Schulte E, Schumacher U. THIEME Atlas of Anatomy. Head, Neck, and Neuroanatomy. Illustrations by Voll M and Wesker K. 3rd ed. New York: Thieme Medical Publishers; 2020.)

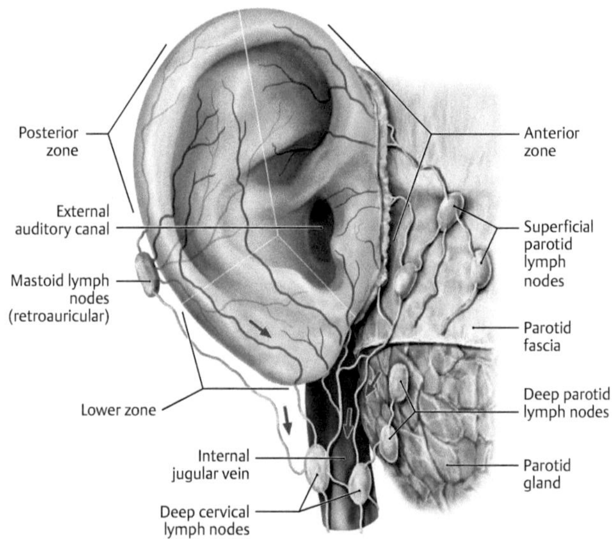

Fig. 7.119 Lymphatic drainage of the auricle and external acoustic (auditory) meatus/canal. (From Schuenke M, Schulte E, Schumacher U. THIEME Atlas of Anatomy. Head, Neck, and Neuroanatomy. Illustrations by Voll M and Wesker K. 3rd ed. New York: Thieme Medical Publishers; 2020.)

7.10.3 Auditory Ossicles

The sequence of small bones located in the middle ear is known as the **auditory ossicles** and they are the first bones to be fully ossified during development. They are known individually as the malleus, incus, and stapes (**Fig. 7.120b**). They connect the tympanic membrane to the *oval window*, an oval opening on the labyrinthine (medial) wall that leads to the *vestibule of the bony labyrinth*. They are covered with a mucous membrane but lack a layer of osteogenic periosteum.

The **malleus** (L. for hammer) has a **handle** portion that is embedded in the tympanic membrane, of which the terminal portion is known as the **umbo**. The **neck** lies against the flaccid portion of the tympanic membrane while the superior portion known as the **head** is located in the epitympanic recess and articulates with the incus (**Fig. 7.121**).

The **incus** (L. for anvil) has a body, long limb, and short limb and is located between the malleus and stapes. Its **body** lies in the epitympanic recess just like the head of the malleus. The **lenticular process** of the **long process** articulates with the stapes while the **short process** is connected to the posterior portion of the epitympanic recess by a ligament (**Fig. 7.121**).

The **stapes** (L. for stirrup) has a head, neck, anterior limb, posterior limb, and base. The **head** articulates with the incus; the tendon of the stapedius muscle attaches to the posterior surface of the **neck**. Both the **anterior crus** and **posterior crus** attach to the base. The **base** (or footplate) is attached to the margin of the oval window by a ring of fibrous tissue constituting the **annular ligament of the stapes** (**Fig. 7.121**). Hardening of the annular ligament is associated with the *otosclerosis*. Vibratory force of the stapes is increased ~10 times over that of the tympanic membrane. This is due to the base being much smaller than the tympanic membrane. Thus, the ossicles increase the force but decrease the amplitude of the vibrations traveling from the tympanic membrane back to the internal ear (**Fig. 7.122**).

7.10.4 Muscles of the Middle Ear

The two muscles of the middle ear are the tensor tympani and stapedius. The **tensor tympani muscle** is innervated by CN V_3. It originates from cartilaginous portion of the pharyngotympanic

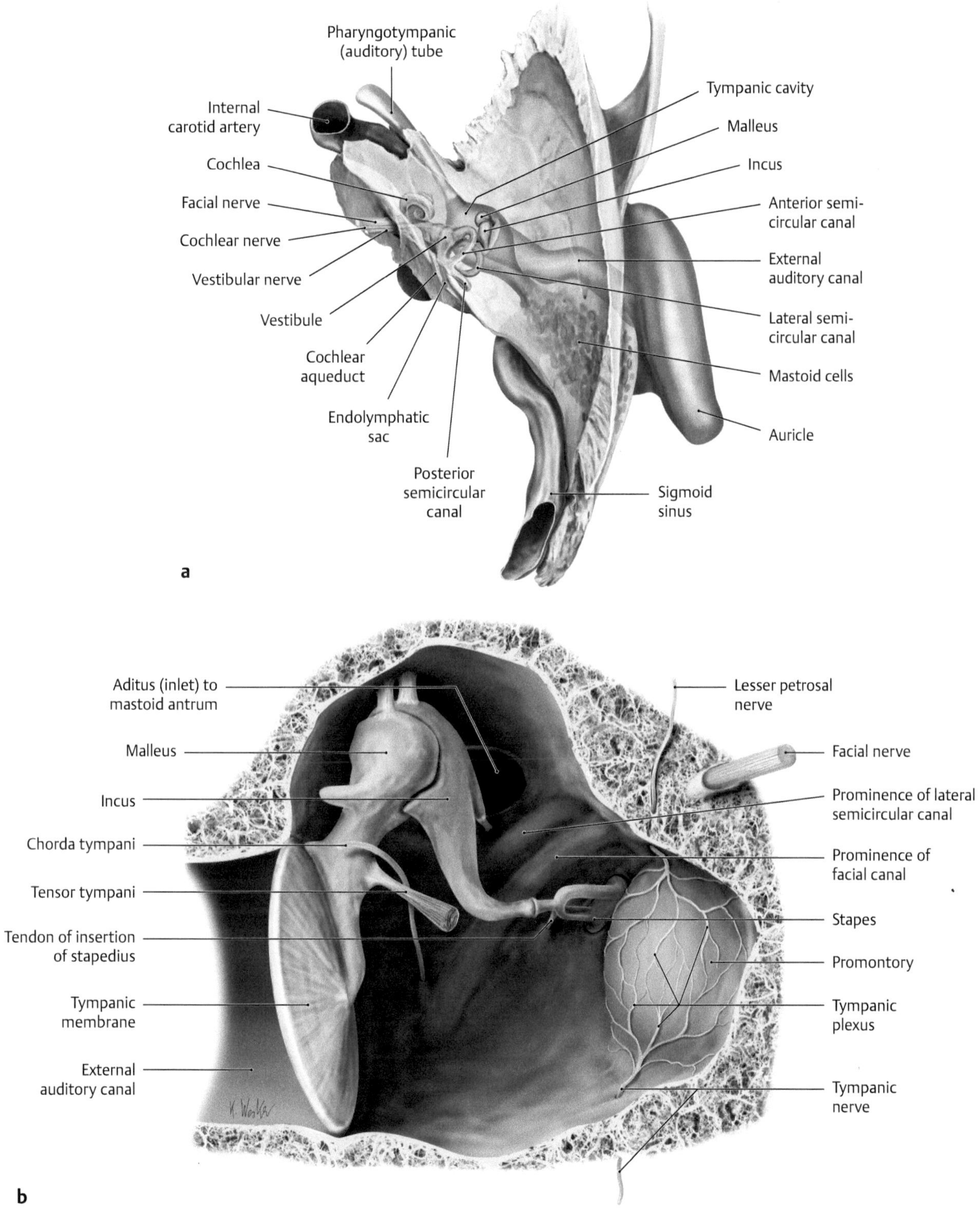

Fig. 7.120 **(a)** The middle ear and associated structures. **(b)** Walls of the tympanic cavity. (From Schuenke M, Schulte E, Schumacher U. THIEME Atlas of Anatomy. Head, Neck, and Neuroanatomy. Illustrations by Voll M and Wesker K. 3rd ed. New York: Thieme Medical Publishers; 2020.)

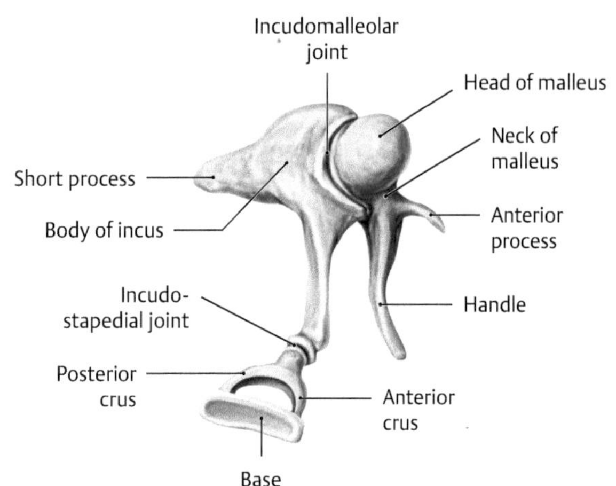

Fig. 7.121 Medial view of the auditory ossicles. (From Schuenke M, Schulte E, Schumacher U. THIEME Atlas of Anatomy. Head, Neck, and Neuroanatomy. Illustrations by Voll M and Wesker K. 3rd ed. New York: Thieme Medical Publishers; 2020.)

tube, petrous portion of the temporal bone, and greater wing of the sphenoid bone before inserting near the neck of the handle of the malleus. It functions by reducing the amplitude of the tympanic membranes' oscillations, thus preventing damage when an individual is exposed to loud sounds. The **stapedius muscle**, which is the smallest skeletal muscle in the body, is innervated by CN VII. It originates from the **pyramidal eminence** located on the mastoid (posterior) wall and inserts onto the neck of the stapes. It functions primarily in limiting movements of the stapes, thus reducing the oscillatory range. These two muscles together function by dampening or reducing the vibrations experienced by the ossicles (**Fig. 7.120b**).

The **acoustic/auditory reflex** occurs just prior to an individual beginning to speak or in response to a high-intensity sound. Protecting the *organ of Corti* from an initial and excessive stimulation is the basis of this reflex. It involves the involuntary contraction of the stapedius muscle in humans but both the stapedius and tensor tympani muscles in all other animals.

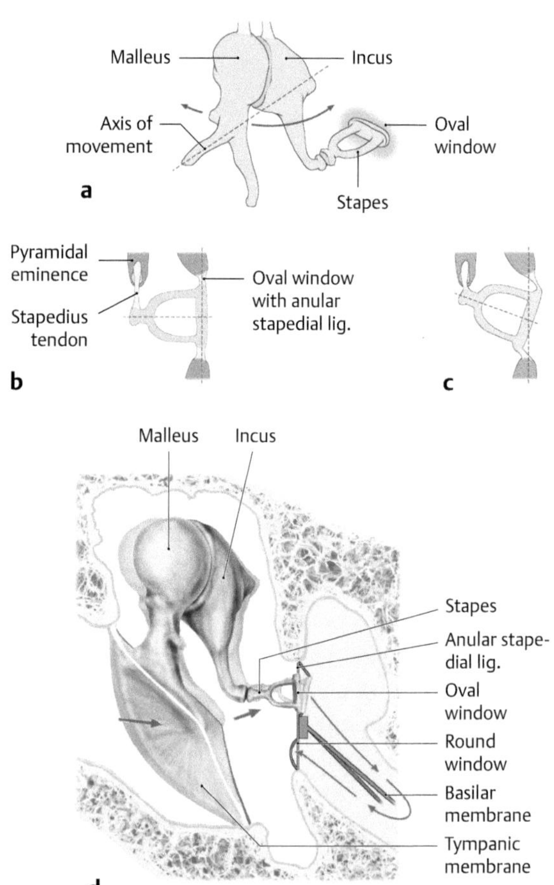

Fig. 7.122 Ossicular chain in hearing. **(a)** Vibration of the tympanic membrane causes a rocking movement in the ossicular chain. **(b)** The stapes in its normal position lies in plane of the oval window. **(c)** Rocking of the ossicular chain causes the stapes to tilt. **(d)** Propagation of sounds waves by the ossicular chain. (From Schuenke M, Schulte E, Schumacher U. THIEME Atlas of Anatomy. Head, Neck, and Neuroanatomy. Illustrations by Voll M and Wesker K. 3rd ed. New York: Thieme Medical Publishers; 2020.)

7.10.5 Pharyngotympanic Tube

The **pharyngotympanic tube** is also known as the *auditory* or *Eustachian tube*. It connects the tympanic cavity to the nasopharynx, just posterior to the inferior nasal meatus. Most of the tube is cartilaginous except for the posterolateral one-third that is bone. The mucous membrane of this tube is continuous with the tympanic cavity and nasopharynx. Its function is to equalize the pressure in the tympanic cavity with that of atmospheric pressure. This thus allows free movement of the tympanic membrane. The tensor veli palatini and levator veli palatini muscles are associated with the soft palate and actively keep this tube opened. Swallowing or yawning is an activity associated with equalizing these pressures (**Fig. 7.123**).

Innervation is autonomic in nature and comes from a combination of the **tympanic plexus** and **pharyngeal nerve branch of the pterygopalatine ganglion**. Blood supply to the pharyngotympanic tube is from the **ascending pharyngeal** (external carotid br.), **middle meningeal** (maxillary br.), and the **artery of the pterygoid canal** (maxillary br.). Venous drainage is mainly to the **pterygoid plexus** of veins in the deep face region. Lymphatic drainage is to the **deep cervical lymph nodes**.

The **tympanic plexus** is made of autonomic fibers and contains no ganglia. It rests upon the promontory of the tympanic cavity and the functional components of this plexus are GVE-para/pre, sym/post, and GVA. The sym/post fibers arise from the **caroticotympanic nerve**, which extends from the periarterial plexus wrapped around the ICA to the tympanic cavity. The para/pre fibers pass through the **tympanic nerve** branch of the glossopharyngeal nerve (CN IX) to reach the plexus. These autonomic fibers continue through the **lesser petrosal nerve** before reaching the **otic ganglion**, at this point the para/pre fibers will synapse and continue as para/post fibers through the *auriculotemporal temporal nerve of CN V_3*. Visceral sensory (GVA) fibers responsible for the innervation of the mucous membrane in the tympanic cavity travel back through the tympanic plexus, followed by the tympanic nerve, and their cell bodies are located in the inferior ganglion of CN IX (**Fig. 7.120**).

7.10.6 Internal Ear

The **internal ear** contains the vestibulocochlear organ, a structure that is responsible for the maintenance of balance and the reception of sound, respectively. It is located in the petrous portion of

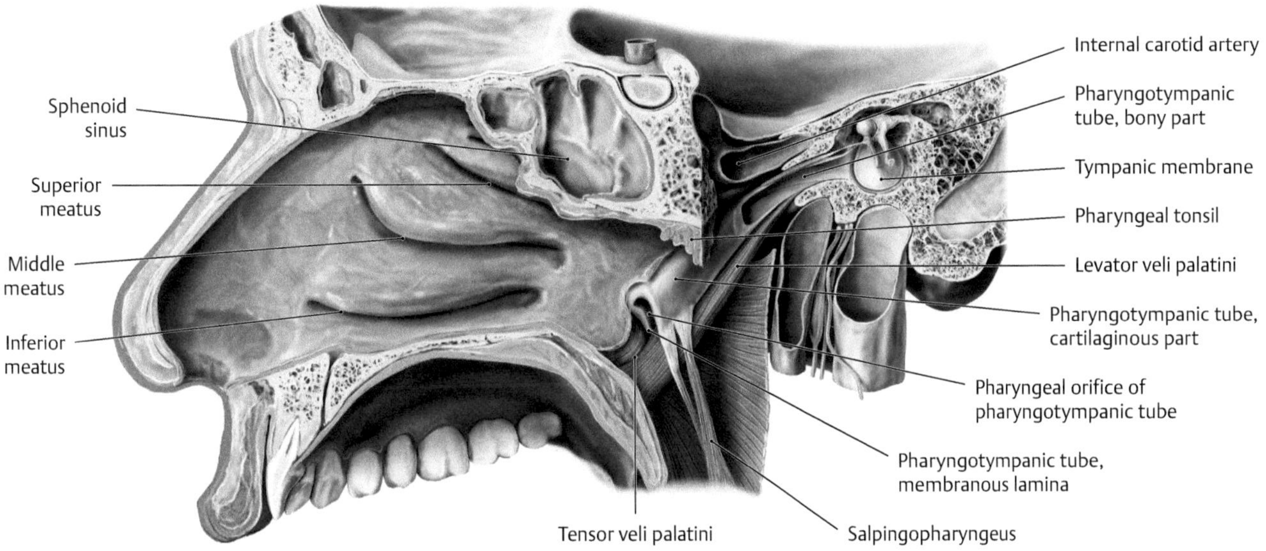

Fig. 7.123 Pharyngotympanic (auditory) tube. (From Schuenke M, Schulte E, Schumacher U. THIEME Atlas of Anatomy. Head, Neck, and Neuroanatomy. Illustrations by Voll M and Wesker K. 3rd ed. New York: Thieme Medical Publishers; 2020.)

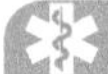 **Clinical Correlate 7.30**

Otitis Media

After upper respiratory infections, **otitis media** or inflammation of the middle ear cavity is the second most common childhood disease but the most common cause of earaches. When air is unable to pass freely through the middle ear it becomes warm and damp resulting in an environment prone to germs. Any allergies, cold virus, sinus infections, or exposure to tobacco smoke and even day care can help lead to otitis media. If it is suspected to be bacterial in nature, amoxicillin is the first choice for an antibiotic unless the child is allergic to it.

the temporal bone and consists of a bony labyrinth and membranous labyrinth.

The **bony labyrinth** is covered by an **otic capsule**, a bony layer denser than the rest of the petrous portion of the temporal bone. The bony labyrinth is made up of a series of three cavities filled with **perilymph**, a fluid similar to extracellular fluid that consists of a high Na+/low K+ ratio. These cavities include the *semicircular canals, vestibule,* and *cochlea*. The bony labyrinth is best described as a cast of the otic capsule after removing the surrounding bone (**Fig. 7.124**).

7.10.7 Semicircular Canals

The **semicircular canals** communicate with the vestibule and consist of three parts, the anterior, posterior, and lateral canals that are set at right angles to one another. The **anterior canal** (or superior) is positioned vertically and is directed approximately anterolaterally from the vestibule at about 45 degrees to the sagittal plane. The **posterior canal** is also positioned vertically, at approximately 45 degrees to the sagittal plane, and thus at about a right angle to the anterior canal. The **lateral canal** lies approximately on a horizontal plane. Each canal generally has two limbs that make up about two-thirds of a full circle. However, there are only five openings into the adjacent vestibule and this is because the anterior and posterior canals form a common limb. At one end of a limb for each canal, a swelling appears and forms a bony **ampulla**. The semicircular ducts are suspended within perilymph of the bony semicircular canals (**Fig. 7.125**).

7.10.8 Vestibule

The **vestibule** is the small, oval, and centrally located chamber that lies between the semicircular canals and cochlea. The vestibule contains the *saccule* and *utricle*, structures associated with balance. On the lateral wall of the vestibule the **oval window** houses the base or footplate of the stapes. The semicircular canals open into the vestibule posteriorly while the cochlea opens into it from the anterior end. The vestibule communicates with the posterior cranial fossa by way of the **vestibular aqueduct**, a structure that contains the *endolymphatic duct* (**Fig. 7.124**).

7.10.9 Cochlea

The shell-shaped portion of the bony labyrinth is known as the **cochlea** and it is made of two chambers that are continuous with one another. The **scala vestibuli** ascends from the vestibule to the cochlear apex known as the **helicotrema**. From the helicotrema, this chamber descends as the **scala tympani** and it will end at the **round window**. Located between these two bony cavities is the **cochlear duct (scala media)**, the structure responsible for hearing. The promontory located on the medial wall of the tympanic cavity is formed by the large basal turn of the cochlea (**Fig. 7.124; Fig. 7.125; Fig. 7.126**). Also near this basal turn, the round window is found closed by the **secondary tympanic membrane** along with the **cochlear aqueduct** that forms a communication between the bony labyrinth and subarachnoid space superior to the jugular foramen. Beginning at the vestibule, the helical cochlea represents approximately 2 ¾ spirals of the bony labyrinth cavity around a centrally located, and cone-shaped bony axis known as the **modiolus** (**Fig. 7.127**). The apex of the modiolus is directed laterally, anteriorly, and inferiorly, much like the axis of the tympanic membrane. The modiolus contains

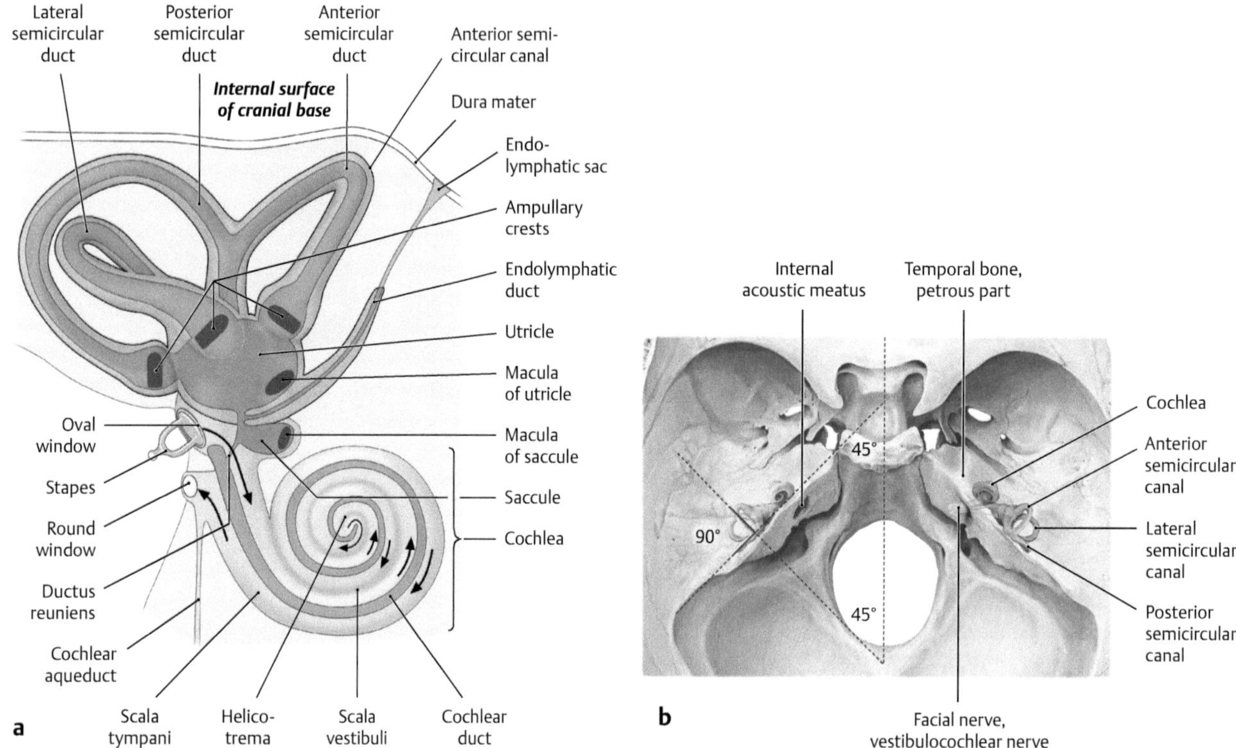

Fig. 7.124 (a) Schematic diagram of the inner ear. **(b)** Projection of the inner ear onto the bony skull (superior view). (From Schuenke M, Schulte E, Schumacher U. THIEME Atlas of Anatomy. Head, Neck, and Neuroanatomy. Illustrations by Voll M and Wesker K. 3rd ed. New York: Thieme Medical Publishers; 2020.)

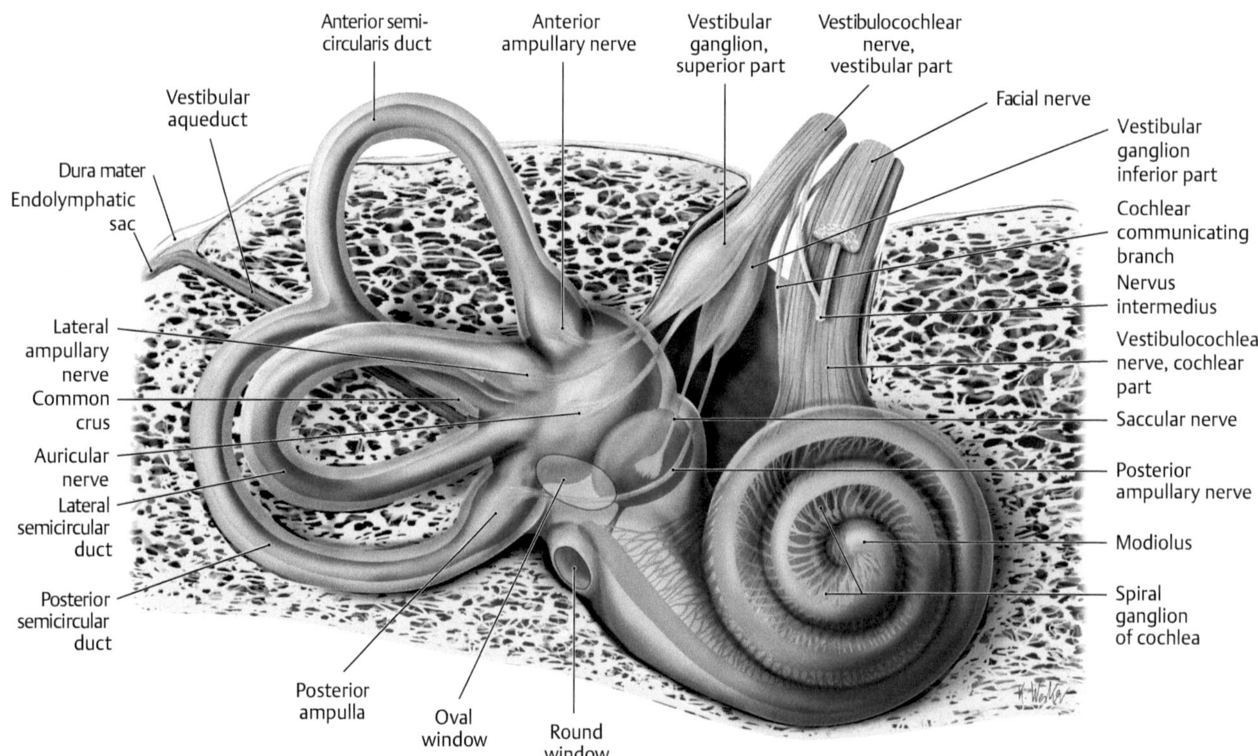

Fig. 7.125 Innervation of the membranous labyrinth. Right ear, anterior view. (From Schuenke M, Schulte E, Schumacher U. THIEME Atlas of Anatomy. Head, Neck, and Neuroanatomy. Illustrations by Voll M and Wesker K. 3rd ed. New York: Thieme Medical Publishers; 2020.)

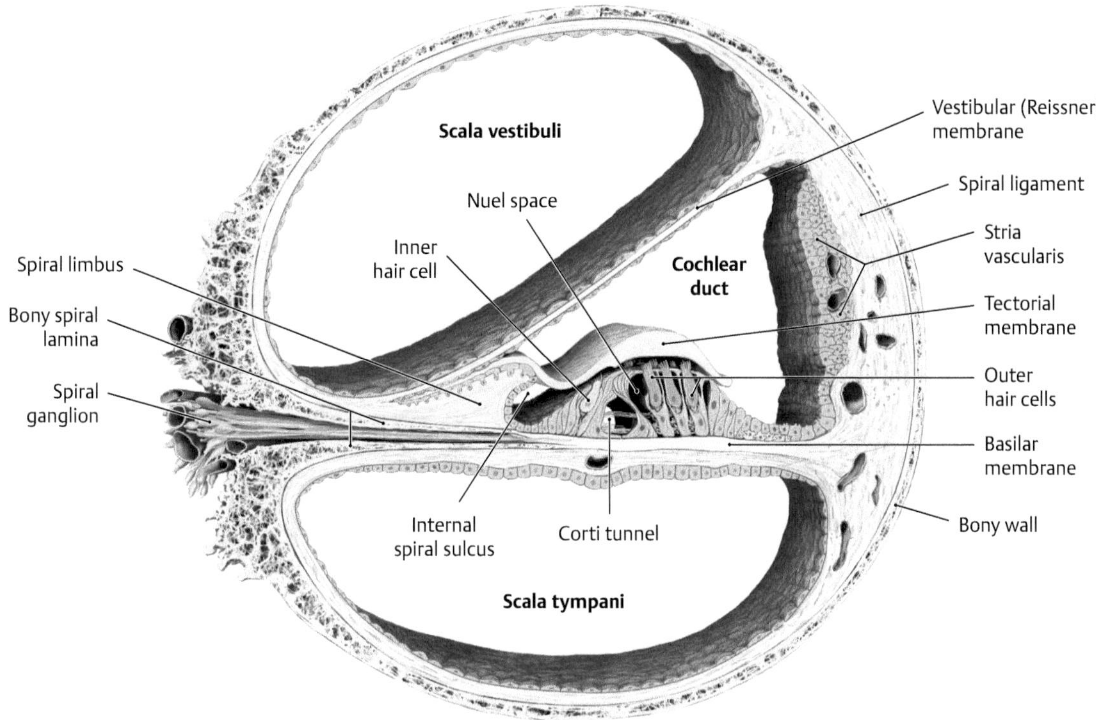

Fig. 7.126 Cochlear turn with sensory apparatus. (From Schuenke M, Schulte E, Schumacher U. THIEME Atlas of Anatomy. Head, Neck, and Neuroanatomy. Illustrations by Voll M and Wesker K. 3rd ed. New York: Thieme Medical Publishers; 2020.)

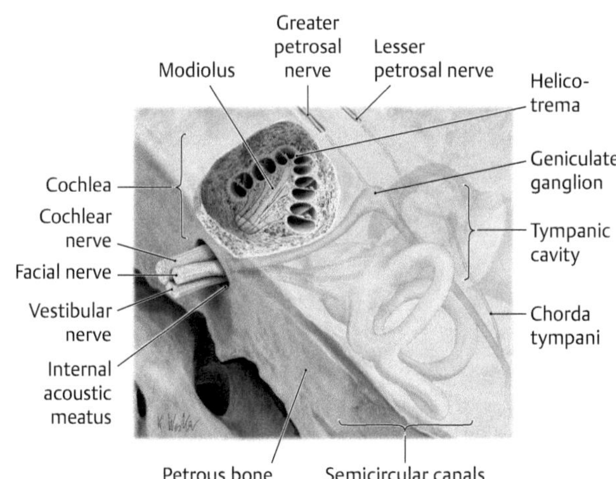

Fig. 7.127 Cross-section through the cochlea in the petrous bone. (From Schuenke M, Schulte E, Schumacher U. THIEME Atlas of Anatomy. Head, Neck, and Neuroanatomy. Illustrations by Voll M and Wesker K. 3rd ed. New York: Thieme Medical Publishers; 2020.)

canals for neurovasculature especially of those of the cochlear nerve branches. Projecting out from the modiolus like a bony shelf or thread of a screw is the **osseous spiral lamina**. It serves to partially separate the scala vestibuli and scala tympani from one another.

The **membranous labyrinth** is a closed network of communicating and epithelial-lined sacs and ducts that are suspended within the bony labyrinth. The membranous labyrinth is filled with **endolymph**, a fluid similar to intracellular fluid that consists of a high K+/low Na+ ratio. The membranous labyrinth includes the *semicircular ducts, utricle, saccule,* and *cochlear duct.*

7.10.10 Semicircular Ducts

The **semicircular ducts** each have a swelling or **ampulla** at one end that contain a sensory organ known as the **ampullary crest**. These crests contain **hair cells** and they are covered by a gelatinous cap or **cupula** that protrudes into the endolymph. Movement of the endolymph pulls on the cupula and this excites the hair cells. The ampullary crests respond to rotational (angular) acceleration and deceleration of the head **(Fig. 7.128)**.

7.10.11 Utricle and Saccule

Located within the vestibule are the **utricle** and **saccule.** The semicircular ducts open into the larger utricle through five openings similar to the way the semicircular canals open into the vestibule. The utricle connects to the saccule by way of the **utriculosaccular duct**. The saccule directly connects to the cochlear duct by way of the **ductus reunions**. The **endolymphatic duct** extends from about the central portion of the utriculosaccular duct and through the vestibular aqueduct before reaching the **endolymphatic sac**, a blind pouch located on the petrous portion of the temporal bone. It can function in the storage of endolymph, is possibly related to the immune system, and may play a role in the development of *Meniere disease.*

Both the utricle and the saccule contain special sensory structures known as **maculae** that are important in responding to linear accelerations and the force of gravity. The **utricular macula** is located on the floor of the utricle and parallel with the base of the cranium while the **saccular macula** is located vertically on the medial wall of the saccule. The maculae are covered with a gelatinous **otolithic membrane** containing **otoliths** (or otoconia). Otoliths are small particles of crystalline calcium carbonate that are overly sensory hair cells. The changes in head position cause

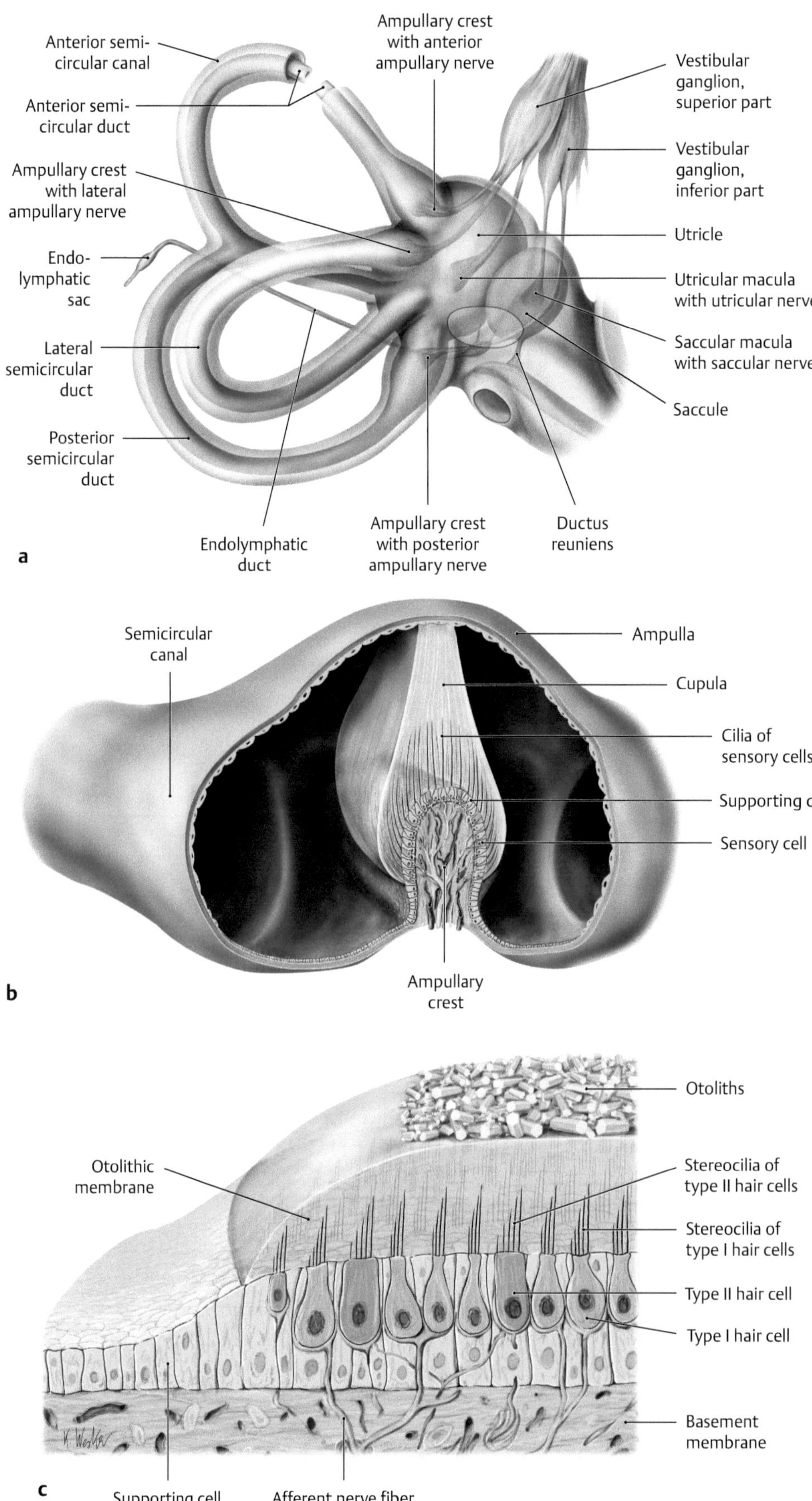

Fig. 7.128 **(a)** Structure of the vestibular apparatus. **(b)** Structure of the ampulla and ampullary crests. **(c)** Structure of the utricular and saccular maculae. (From Schuenke M, Schulte E, Schumacher U. THIEME Atlas of Anatomy. Head, Neck, and Neuroanatomy. Illustrations by Voll M and Wesker K. 3rd ed. New York: Thieme Medical Publishers; 2020.)

the otolithic membrane to bend the *kinocilium* and *sterocilia* of hair cells, thus generating a nerve impulse that is transmitted through the vestibular branch of CN VIII. The utricular macula functions to measure horizontal motion and is maximally stimulated when the head is bent forward or backward. The saccular macula functions to measure vertical motion and is maximally stimulated when the head is bent to the side **(Fig. 7.128)**.

7.10.12 Cochlear Duct

The **cochlear duct** (scala media) is a spiral, blind tube closed at one end near the apex of the cochlea and it is responsible for hearing. It is firmly suspended across the cochlear canal between the **spiral ligament** on the external wall of the cochlear canal and the *osseous spiral lamina*. Sound transmission begins when vibrations picked up by the tympanic membrane are transferred from the ossicles to the oval window. Vibrations at the base (footplate) of the stapes create pressure waves in the perilymph that pass from the vestibule to the scala vestibuli. The endolymph of the cochlear duct thus "receives" these vibrations or pressure waves and they then cause displacement of the **basilar membrane** of the cochlear duct. It is movement of the basilar membrane that bends the hair cells of the **spiral organ of Corti**, the structure responsible for auditory reception **(Fig. 7.126; Fig. 7.129)**. Pressure waves continue up to the helicotrema and back down the scale tympani toward the round window. Remaining pressure waves are dampened by the secondary tympanic membrane of the round window into the air of the middle ear cavity. High-frequency sound waves (20,000 Hz) cause displacement of the basilar membrane closer to the oval window while low-frequency sound waves (20 Hz) are detected closer to the apex and helicotrema. Humans are most sensitive to the frequencies between 2000 and 5000 Hz.[4]

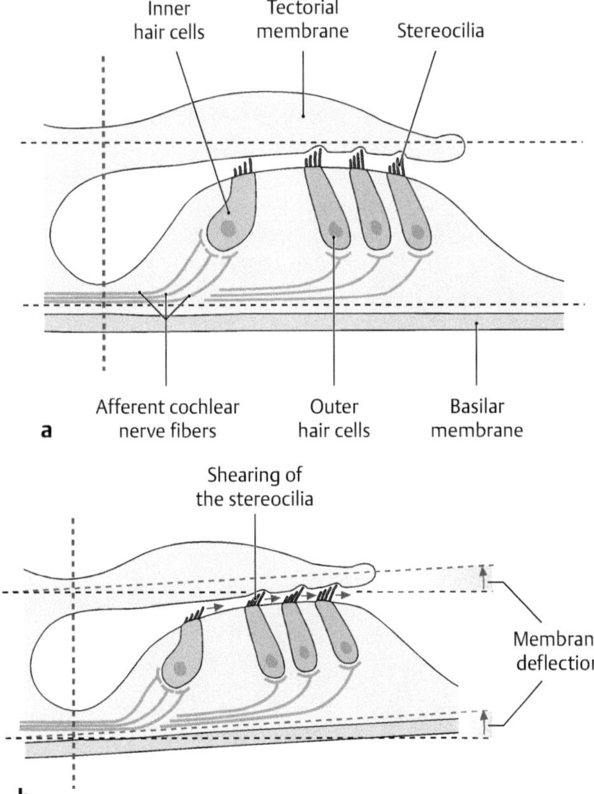

Fig. 7.129 Organ of Corti at rest **(a)** and deflected by a traveling wave **(b)**. (From Schuenke M, Schulte E, Schumacher U. THIEME Atlas of Anatomy. Head, Neck, and Neuroanatomy. Illustrations by Voll M and Wesker K. 3rd ed. New York: Thieme Medical Publishers; 2020.)

7.10.13 Vestibulocochlear Nerve (CN VIII)

The **vestibulocochlear nerve (CN VIII)** is the main cranial nerve associated with the function of the internal ear. It has a vestibular branch that contains special sense (SSA) fibers important for balance and equilibrium and a cochlear branch that contains special sense (SSA) fibers important for hearing. Bipolar neurons are associated with the hair cells of the ampullary crests, maculae, and spiral organ of Corti. The cell bodies of neurons associated with the ampullary crests and maculae are located in the **vestibular ganglion** while the cell bodies of the neurons related to the spiral organ of Corti are located in the **spiral (cochlear) ganglion**. The vestibulocochlear nerve along with the facial nerve (CN VII) and the labyrinthine vessels pass through the **internal acoustic meatus**. This meatus is located in the posteromedial part of the petrous portion of the temporal bone. The lateral end of the internal acoustic meatus is separated from the internal ear by a thin perforated plate, which allows for passage of CN VII, CN VIII, and some small blood vessels **(Fig. 7.125)**.

7.10.14 Histology of the Ear

The auricle of the external ear has a core of elastic and fibrocartilage covered with a "thin" skin composed of *stratified squamous epithelium*. The external acoustic meatus is a tube that has an outer one-third portion formed by elastic cartilage that is continuous with the auricle. The inner two-third of the meatus is formed by the temporal bone. The meatus changes from a *keratinized* to a *nonkeratinized stratified squamous epithelium* as it reaches the tympanic membrane. Although quite thin, the tympanic membrane is made up of three layers. *Nonkeratinized stratified squamous epithelium* makes up the outer covering, the core is made of fibroelastic connective tissue, and the inner covering is covered with a *simple squamous/cuboidal epithelium.*

A *simple squamous/cuboidal epithelium* covers the middle ear cavity and mastoid antrum regions. The ossicles are made of compact bone and linked together by synovial joints. The tensor tympani and stapedius muscles that act on the ossicles by dampening vibrations are skeletal muscles. The pharyngotympanic tube that is connected to the middle ear cavity is mostly a *ciliated, pseudostratified columnar epithelium* with increasing numbers of goblet cells as it approaches the nasopharynx.

The internal ears' bony labyrinth fluid-filled spaces are lined with a *simple squamous epithelium.* The membranous labyrinth is lined with a *simple squamous epithelium* in most areas. A *simple columnar epithelium* is found near hair cells of the sensory areas and a *simple cuboidal/columnar epithelium* is found near fluid production/resorption areas.

The cochlear duct has multiple membranes and the spiral organ of Corti associated with it. The thin **vestibular (Reissner) membrane** forms the roof of the cochlear duct and is made of two apposed layers of *simple squamous epithelium* and their associated basement membranes. The floor is formed by the thicker **basilar membrane** and the outer edge of the osseous spiral lamina. The basilar membrane is connected to the osseous spiral ligament laterally and to the spiral ganglia more centrally. The lateral wall of the cochlear duct attaches to the periosteum of the cochlea and is

Clinical Correlate 7.31

Meniere Syndrome

Meniere syndrome is a disorder involving the inner ear and is not yet completely understood. It is related to excess endolymph production or blockage of the endolymphatic duct. Patients have symptoms ranging from recurring episodes of vertigo (sensation of spinning), tinnitus (ringing ears), hearing loss, migraines, and the feeling of pressure in the affected ear. Individuals should avoid excess salt intake, smoking, caffeine, and alcohol. Treatment may include a diuretic, antivertigo medications, and even surgery but hearing loss may become permanent.

Clinical Correlate 7.32

Conductive and Sensorineural Hearing Loss

Conductive hearing loss occurs when there is a deficiency in the conduction of sound through the external and/or middle ear. There is a reduction in sound level or the ability to hear more faint sounds. Causes could include otitis externa, perforation of the tympanic membrane, otitis media, allergies, and possibly due to a tumor. This type of hearing loss can be corrected surgically or with the use of a hearing aid. **Sensorineural hearing loss** is linked to damage involving the inner ear or pathways that connect the inner ear to the brain. Causes include aging, developmental, or long-term exposure to loud noises to name a few. This may be permanent from birth as in a deaf individual but *cochlear implants* have given the opportunity to people to hear again. A combination of both conductive and sensorineural hearing loss can occur.

covered by the **stria vascularis** (**Fig. 7.126**). The stria vascularis is made up of a *pseudostratified columnar epithelium*, overlies highly vascularized connective tissue, and secretes endolymph. The spiral organ of Corti is supported by the basilar membrane and is composed of inner or outer *neuroepithelial hair cells* and several types of supporting cells known as *pillar, phalangeal, border,* and *Hensen cells.* The apical portion of the hair cell contains around 50 to 100 **stereocilia** that are arranged symmetrically and in a graded fashion. These stereocilia of the outer hair cells are embedded into the **tectorial membrane**, a gelatinous extracellular structure. Vibrations of the basilar membrane create a shearing force against the stationary tectorial membrane, thus causing displacement of the stereocilia and a conversion of mechanical energy into an electrochemical signal (**Fig. 7.126; Fig. 7.129**).

7.10.15 Development of the Ear

Development of the ear first begins with the internal ear. During the fourth week of development, a thickening of the surface ectoderm near the caudal part of the hindbrain on both sides of the embryo will appear and is known as the **otic placode**. The otic placodes invaginate the surface ectoderm and into the underlying mesenchyme to form the **otic pit**. The otic pit edges fuse forming the **otic vesicle**, which then loses its connection to the surface ectoderm (**Fig. 7.130**). A diverticulum extends and grows from the otic vesicle to become the **endolymphatic duct** and **sac** (**Fig. 7.131**).

The two recognizable regions of the otic vesicle include the dorsal *utricular* and ventral *saccular* regions. The **utricular region** has three disk-like diverticula that grow out from it. The central parts of these diverticula will fuse and disappear while the

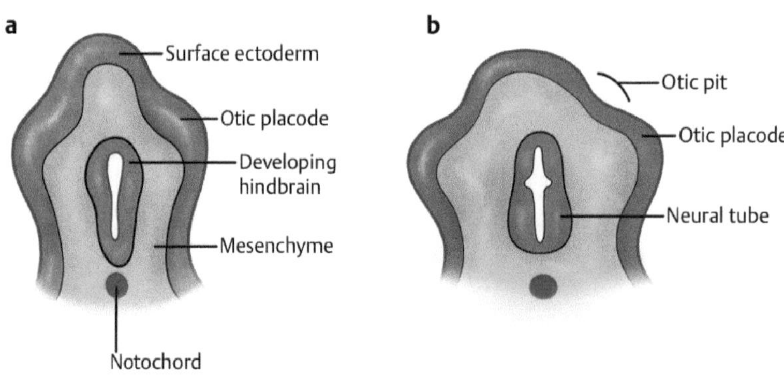

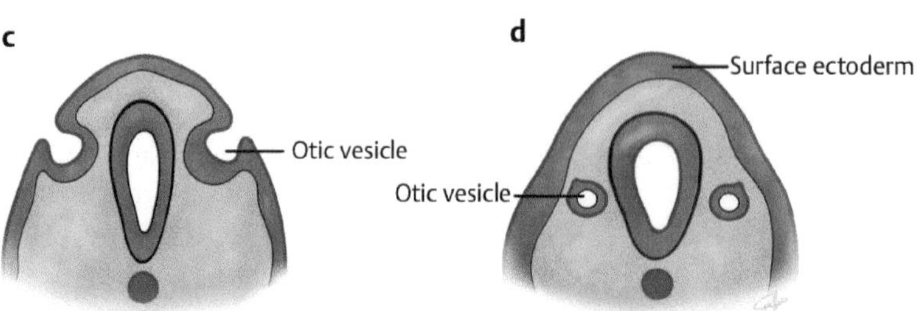

Fig. 7.130 (a-d) Development of the internal ear. Schematic coronal sections showing the development of the otic vesicles beginning at 4 weeks.
Illustration by Calla Heald.

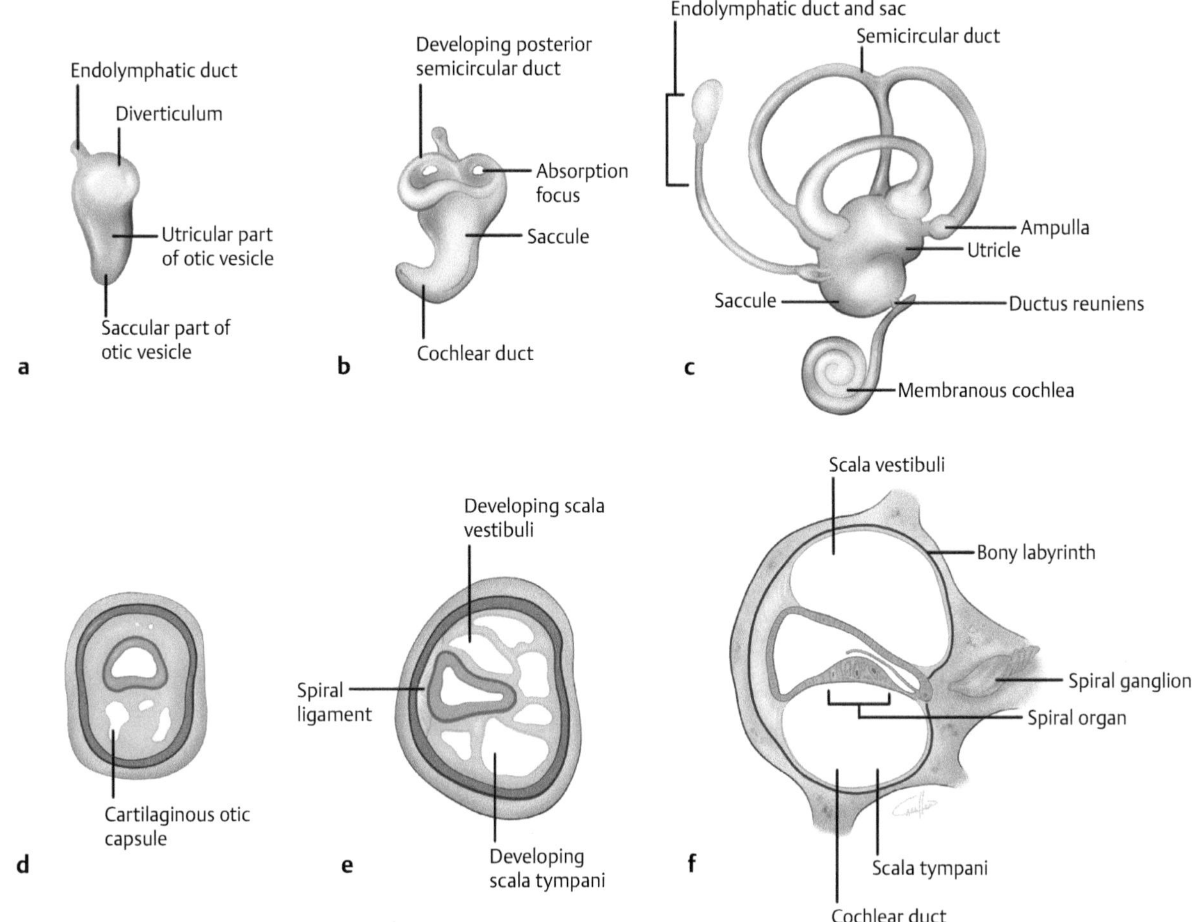

Fig. 7.131 (a-c) Lateral views from the 5th-8th weeks demonstrating the successive stages in the development of the otic vesicle in the membranous labyrinth. **(d-f)** Sections through the early cochlear duct from about the 10th-20th weeks demonstrating successive stages of spiral organ and scala vestibuli and scala tympani development. Illustration by Calla Heald.

unfused peripheral parts become the **semicircular ducts** of the membranous labyrinth. What is left of the utricular region connecting to the semicircular ducts will be known as the utricle. The semicircular ducts are later enclosed by the semicircular canals of the bony labyrinth. The **ampullary crest** sensory organs develop as localized dilations within the ampulla of the semicircular ducts. The **vestibular ganglion** of CN VIII will also develop from the early utricular region and have a final location near the base of the internal acoustic meatus **(Fig. 7.131)**.

The **saccular region** initially has a tubular diverticulum extending out from it and this will become the **cochlear duct** of the membranous labyrinth. Cells from the wall of the cochlear duct differentiate into the **spiral organ (of Corti)**. The **spiral (cochlear) ganglion** of CN VIII also originates from the saccular region. With enlargement of the membranous labyrinth, vacuoles soon appear in the otic capsule and form the scala vestibuli and scala tympani.

The middle ear develops from **pharyngeal pouch 1**. It begins first as the **tubotympanic recess** with the proximal portion becoming the *pharyngotympanic tube* and the distal portion expanding to become the *tympanic cavity*. The malleus and incus ossicles, along with the tensor tympani muscle, develop from **pharyngeal arch 1** while the stapes bone and stapedius muscle develop from **pharyngeal arch 2**. The tympanic membrane develops from **pharyngeal membrane 1** and it consists of endo-, meso-, and ectoderm **(Fig. 7.132)**.

The external acoustic meatus of the external ear originates from **pharyngeal groove 1**. A temporary **meatal plug** proliferates as depth of the meatus is being established; however, it will disappear prior to birth. Surrounding pharyngeal groove 1 are six **auricular hillocks**. These are the basis of development for the auricle, which initially develops near the base of the neck before assuming its normal position **(Fig. 7.133)**.

7.11 The Neck

The **neck** is the portion of the body that connects the head with the trunk and upper limbs. It is divided into two main sections, the anterior and posterior (lateral cervical) triangles **(Fig. 7.134; Fig. 7.139)**. The posterior triangle contains structures that lead down to the upper limb such as the brachial plexus while the remainder of the neck contains extensive neurovasculature, the thyroid and parathyroid glands, larynx, and pharynx **(Fig. 7.135)**.

Just below the outer skin layer, lying just superficial to the investing layer of the deep cervical fascia, the **superficial cervical fascia** consists of a thin layer of subcutaneous connective tissue of

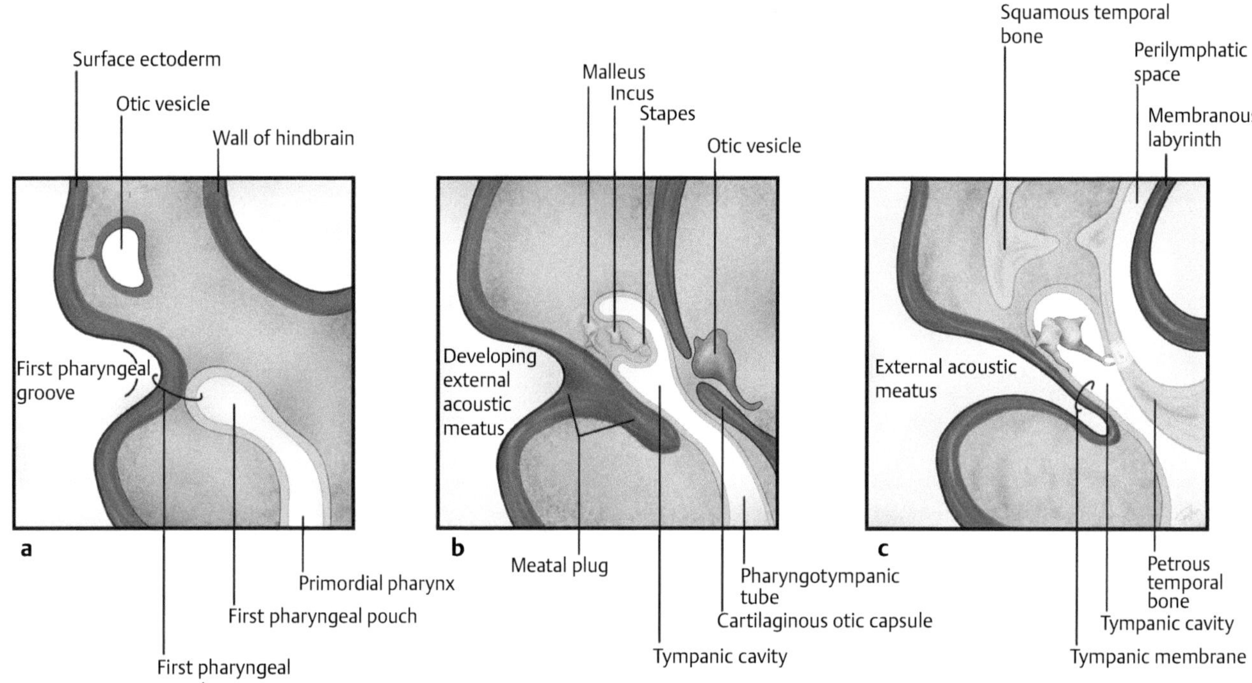

Fig. 7.132 **(a)** At 4 weeks demonstrating the relationship between the otic vesicle and pharyngeal apparatus leading to ear development. **(b)** The tubotympanic recess has formed the tympanic cavity and the ossicles are developing from the 1st and 2nd pharyngeal arches. **(c)** The external acoustic meatus and tympanic membrane have formed. The tympanic cavity has enveloped the ossicles. Illustration by Calla Heald.

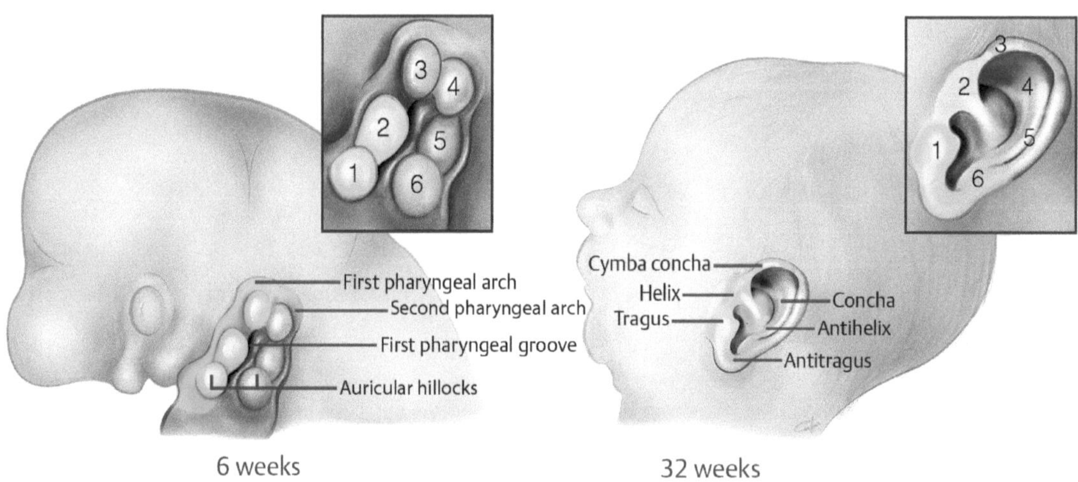

Fig. 7.133 Development of the auricle of the external ear. Illustration by Calla Heald.

which it invests the **platysma muscle**. Just deep to the platysma, deep cervical fascia can be located. The **deep cervical fascia** consists of three layers: *investing, pretracheal,* and the *prevertebral layers*. They support the viscera, neurovasculature, muscles, and deep lymph nodes of the neck (**Fig. 7.136**).

The **investing layer of deep cervical fascia** circles the entirety of the neck. It splits to engulf the sternocleidomastoid and trapezius muscles. Near the level of the mandible it again splits in order to surround the submandibular gland and it forms the fibrous capsule of the parotid gland. The investing layer attaches superiorly to the zygomatic arches, inferior border of the mandible, hyoid bone, mastoid processes, superior nuchal line and spinous processes of the cervical vertebrae. This layer attaches inferiorly at the manubrium, clavicle, acromion and spine of the scapulae, the C7 spinous process periosteum and finally the nuchal ligament (**Fig. 7.136**).

The **pretracheal layer of deep cervical fascia** is located in the anterior half of the neck. It extends from the hyoid bone down to the fibrous pericardium and can be further subdivided into a visceral versus muscular portion. The *visceral portion* surrounds the thyroid and parathyroid glands, trachea, and esophagus while the *muscular portion* surrounds the infrahyoid muscles. The pretracheal layer is continuous posteriorly with the **buccopharyngeal fascia**, a fascia in close proximity to the *pharyngeal nerve plexus* (**Fig. 7.136**).

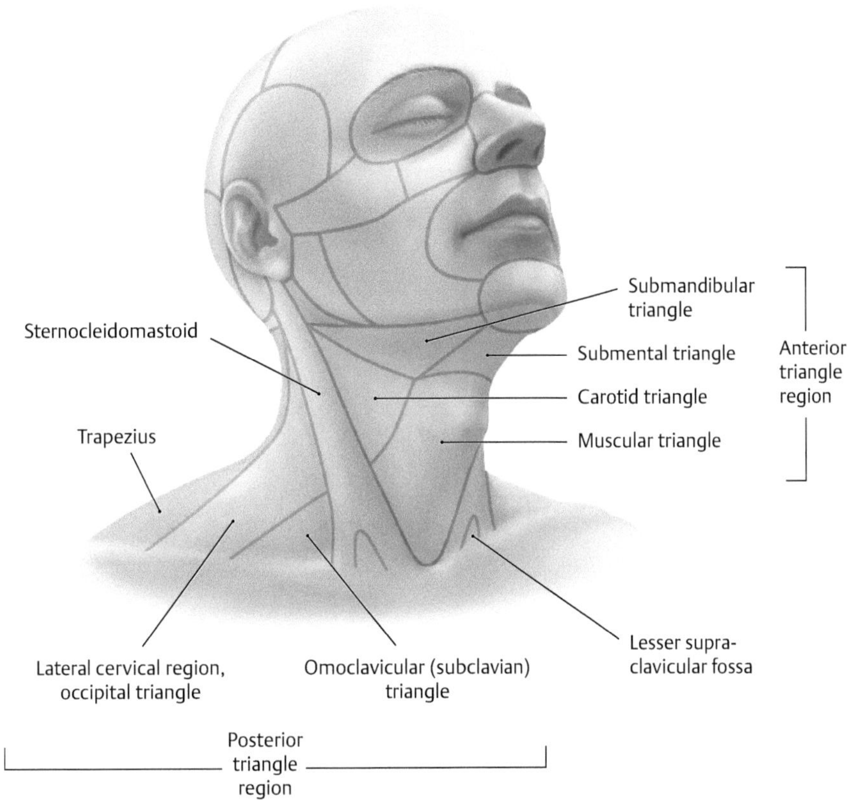

Fig. 7.134 Regions of the neck. (From Schuenke M, Schulte E, Schumacher U. THIEME Atlas of Anatomy. Head, Neck, and Neuroanatomy. Illustrations by Voll M and Wesker K. 3rd ed. New York: Thieme Medical Publishers; 2020.)

Clinical Correlate 7.33

Congenital Muscular Torticollis

Congenital muscular torticollis is a condition involving the sternocleidomastoid muscle which is found to be tight and shortened, resulting in the individuals head to be flexed and tilted toward the nonaffected side. It can also be referred to as *twisted neck* or *wryneck*. This diagnosis is usually made at birth or within the first couple of months of life. The cause is unknown but it may be related to a breeched position or crowding in utero; thus, there is no form of prevention. Standard treatment involves an exercise program that aims to stretch the SCM. Very rarely will surgery be needed to correct a shortened SCM.

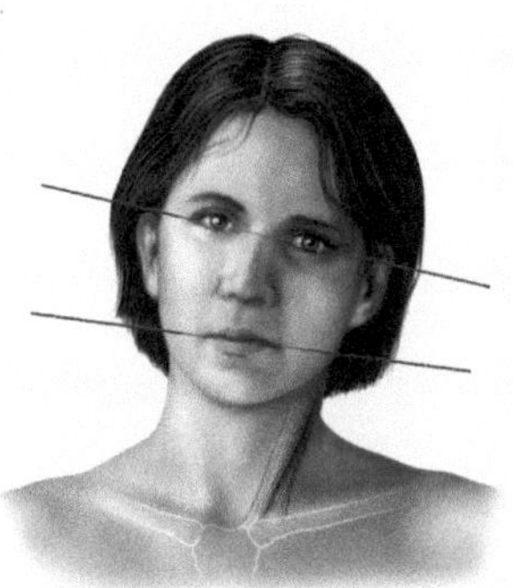

(From Schuenke M, Schulte E, Schumacher U. THIEME Atlas of Anatomy. Head, Neck, and Neuroanatomy. Illustrations by Voll M and Wesker K. 3rd ed. New York: Thieme Medical Publishers; 2020.)

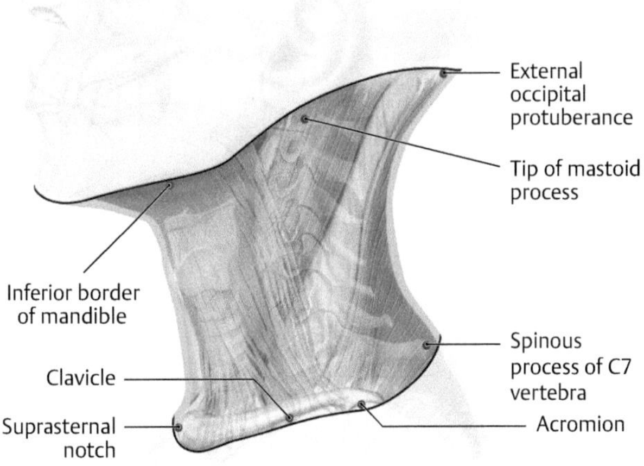

Fig. 7.135 Superior and inferior borders of the neck. (From Schuenke M, Schulte E, Schumacher U. THIEME Atlas of Anatomy. Head, Neck, and Neuroanatomy. Illustrations by Voll M and Wesker K. 3rd ed. New York: Thieme Medical Publishers; 2020.)

The **prevertebral layer of deep cervical fascia** is located in the posterior half of the neck and wraps around the vertebral column but is more superficial to the longus capitis, longus colli, the scalenes, levator scapulae, and deep cervical muscles. The cervical portion of the sympathetic trunk is embedded in this prevertebral layer and it lies adjacent to the carotid sheath. This fascia is fixed

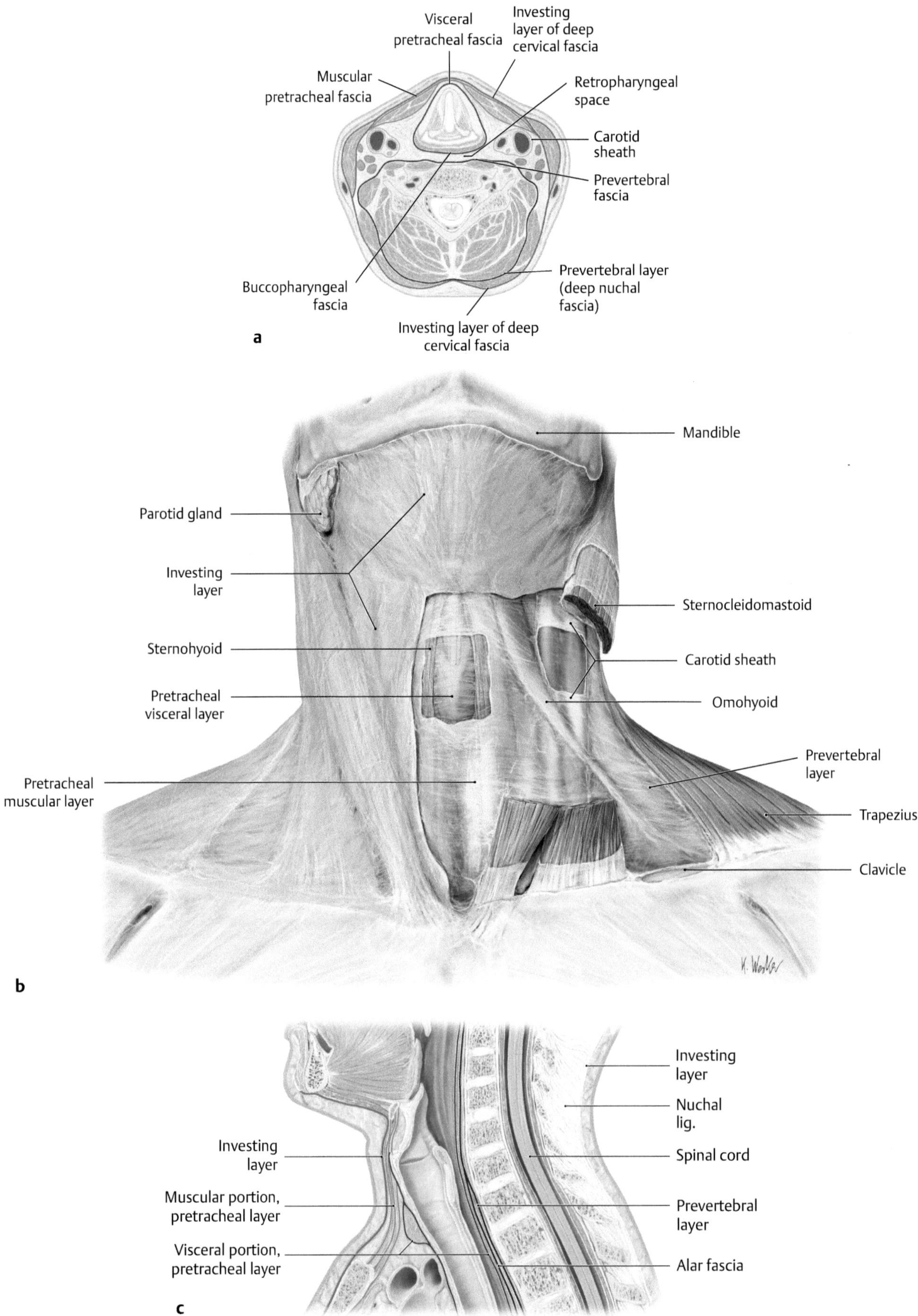

Fig. 7.136 **(a)** Relationships of the deep fascia in the neck, transverse section at the C5 vertebral level. **(b)** Fascial relationships in the neck, anterior view. **(c)** Fascial relationships in the neck, left lateral view. (From Schuenke M, Schulte E, Schumacher U. THIEME Atlas of Anatomy. Head, Neck, and Neuroanatomy. Illustrations by Voll M and Wesker K. 3rd ed. New York: Thieme Medical Publishers; 2020.)

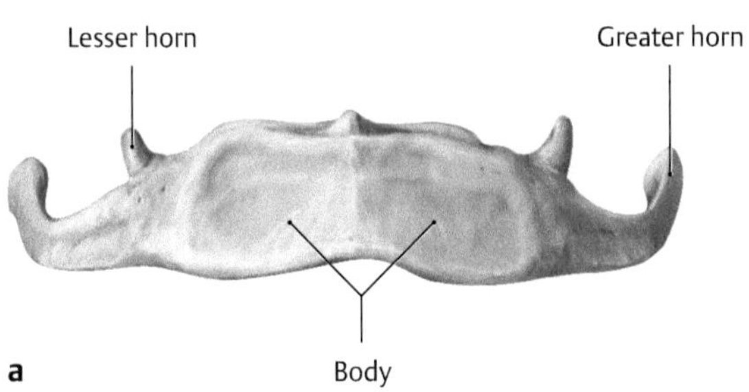

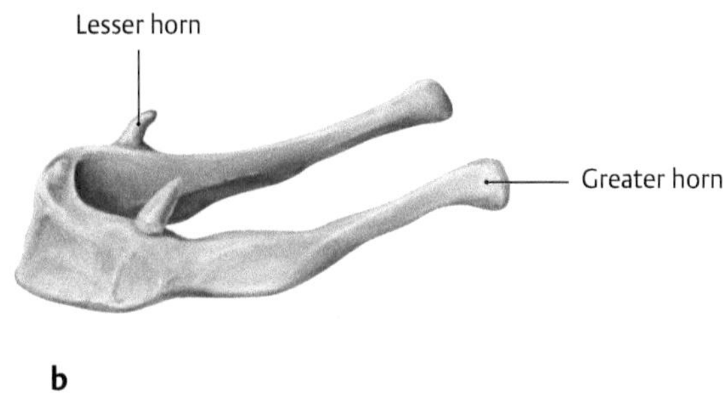

Fig. 7.137 Hyoid bone. **(a)** Anterior view. **(b)** Oblique left lateral view. (From Schuenke M, Schulte E, Schumacher U. THIEME Atlas of Anatomy. Head, Neck, and Neuroanatomy. Illustrations by Voll M and Wesker K. 3rd ed. New York: Thieme Medical Publishers; 2020.)

to the cranial base, fuses with the anterior longitudinal ligament at approximately the T3 vertebra, and continues laterally into the upper limbs as the *axillary sheath* (**Fig. 7.136**).

All three of the deep cervical fascial layers contribute to the **carotid sheath (Fig. 7.136)**, a condensation of fascia that contains multiple structures including the *common* and *internal carotid arteries, internal jugular vein (IJV), vagus nerve, carotid sinus nerve, periarterial plexuses* (sym/post fibers), and *deep cervical lymph nodes*. Structures such as the glossopharyngeal (CN IX), spinal accessory (CN XI), and hypoglossal nerves (CN XII) initially pass through the superior portion of the carotid sheath before reaching their final destinations. The superior and inferior roots of ansa cervicalis are found embedded within the anterior aspect of this sheath. The carotid sheath extends from the cranial base to the root of the neck. It communicates with the cranial cavity and mediastinum, thus representing a potential pathway for extravasation of fluids or blood and the spread of an infection.

The orientation of deep cervical fascial layers leads to the development of a couple of clinically significant spaces in the neck. Located between the buccopharyngeal fascia and the prevertebral fascia and blending with the carotid sheath is the **alar fascia**. The alar fascia creates the retropharyngeal and prevertebral spaces and it also extends from the midline of the buccopharyngeal fascia at the base of the cranium and inferiorly to the C7 vertebra. The anatomical space located between the buccopharyngeal fascia and the alar fascia and leading to the superior mediastinum is known as the **retropharyngeal space**. The anatomical space located between the alar fascia and the prevertebral fascia and leading to the posterior mediastinum is known as the **prevertebral space**, also known as the "danger space." Clinically, the terms "retropharyngeal space" and "danger space" are used synonymously (**Fig. 7.136**).

Much of the skeleton of the neck centers on the seven cervical vertebrae that were described in Chapter 1. The clavicles and manubrium form a border of the neck and can serve as attachment sites for muscles located in the neck region. One other bony structure in this region is the hyoid bone. The **hyoid bone** is located on the anterior side of the neck and at vertebral level C3. It serves as the attachment point for the thyrohyoid ligament associated with the larynx, most of the infrahyoid muscles important for speaking and swallowing, and it does not articulate with any other bone (**Fig. 7.137**).

The first three superficial muscles initially encountered when discussing the neck are the platysma, sternocleidomastoid, and trapezius. The **platysma** is a facial expression muscle best seen when an individual displays the expression of sadness or fright. The **sternocleidomastoid** serves as the border for the anterior and posterior triangles of the neck. It is a two-headed muscle seen on the anterior neck attaching to the temporal bone, manubrium, and clavicle and is responsible for producing movements at the atlanto-occipital joints, cervical vertebrae, and even the manubrium and clavicle during forced/deep respiration. The **trapezius** is seen on the more posterior aspect of the neck and functions in both scapular and neck movements (**Fig. 7.138**). Muscles of the superficial neck are detailed in **Table 7.6**.

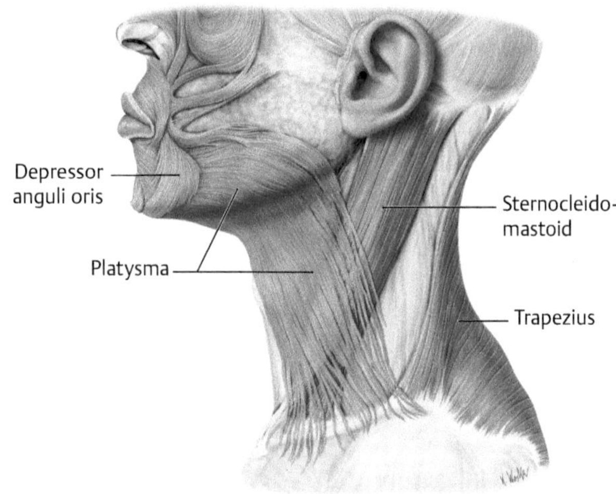

Fig. 7.138 Superficial muscles of the neck. (From Schuenke M, Schulte E, Schumacher U. THIEME Atlas of Anatomy. Head, Neck, and Neuroanatomy. Illustrations by Voll M and Wesker K. 3rd ed. New York: Thieme Medical Publishers; 2020.)

7.12 Anterior Triangle of the Neck

There is a superior, anterior, and posterior boundary along with a roof, floor, and apex that help define the anterior triangle. This triangle is defined by (**Fig. 7.139**):

- Inferior border of mandible (superior boundary).
- Midline of the neck (anterior boundary).
- Sternocleidomastoid muscle (posterior boundary).
- Subcutaneous tissue enveloping the platysma muscle (roof).
- Larynx, thyroid gland, and pharynx (floor).
- Jugular notch of the manubrium (apex).

This larger anterior triangle is subdivided into four smaller triangles on each side of the neck by the **anterior/posterior bellies**

Table 7.6 **Superficial muscles of the neck**

Muscle	Innervation	Function(s)	Origin	Insertion
Platysma	Cervical branch of facial nerve (CN VII)	Depress the angle of the mouth and draw the skin of the neck superiorly as in facial expressions of anxiety, fright, or sadness	Fascia overlying the superclavicular and infraclavicular regions near the pectoralis major and deltoid	Mandible (inferior border); skin of lower lip, angle of the mouth and cheek
Sternocleidomastoid	Spinal accessory nerve (CN XI); ventral rami of C2–C4 (pain and proprioception)	*Unilateral action*: lateral flexion of neck toward the ipsilateral shoulder and simultaneously rotates the head so the face is turned superiorly toward the contralateral side; *Bilateral contraction*: flexes head and cervical vertebrae of neck	*Sternal head*: upper part of anterior surface of the manubrium; *clavicular head*: upper part and anterior surface of medial one-third of clavicle	Mastoid process of temporal bone and superior nuchal line
Trapezius	Spinal accessory nerve (CN XI); ventral rami of C2–C4 (pain and proprioception)	With shoulders fixed, *unilateral contraction* does lateral flexion to ipsilateral shoulder and *bilateral contraction* extends neck; elevates, retracts, and depresses scapula; descending and ascending fibers together superiorly rotate scapula	Superior nuchal line, external occipital protuberance, nuchal ligament, and spinous processes of C7–T12	Lateral one-third of clavicle, acromion, and spine of scapula

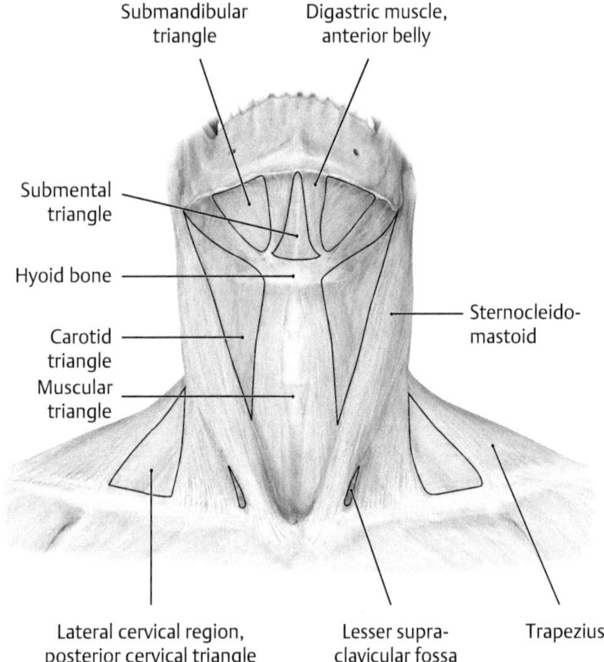

Fig. 7.139 Anterior triangle of the neck. (From Schuenke M, Schulte E, Schumacher U. THIEME Atlas of Anatomy. Head, Neck, and Neuroanatomy. Illustrations by Voll M and Wesker K. 3rd ed. New York: Thieme Medical Publishers; 2020.)

of digastric and **omohyoid muscles** along with the **hyoid bone.** The **stylohyoid muscle** lies just superior to the posterior belly of digastric and thus may be considered a boundary along with it. These four smaller triangles are called the *submental, submandibular, muscular,* and *carotid triangles.*

The **submental triangles** are bounded inferiorly by the body of the *hyoid bone*, laterally by the *anterior bellies of digastric muscle*, and it has a floor formed by the *mylohyoid muscle*. The contents are minimal and include the **submental lymph nodes, mylohyoid muscle**, distal portion of the **mylohyoid nerve** (CN V_3 br.), and the smaller venous tributaries that unite to form the **anterior jugular veins (Fig. 7.139; Fig. 7.140).**

The **submandibular triangles** are bounded by both the *anterior* and *posterior bellies of digastric muscles* and the inferior border of the *mandible*. The floor of these triangles is formed by the **mylohyoid, hyoglossus,** and **middle pharyngeal constrictor muscles**. The contents include the **submandibular gland** and **lymph nodes, facial vessels**, and proximal portions of the **mylohyoid** and **hypoglossal nerves** (CN XII) **(Fig. 7.139; Fig. 7.140; Fig. 7.141; Fig. 7.142).**

The **muscular triangles** are bounded by the *midline of the neck* and *sternocleidomastoid* and *omohyoid muscles* (superior belly). The contents include the **infrahyoid muscles, anterior jugular veins, recurrent laryngeal nerves** (CN X br.), **thyroid** and **parathyroid glands, larynx,** and **trachea**. The last two structures will be discussed in detail later in this chapter **(Fig. 7.139; Fig. 7.140; Fig. 7.143; Fig. 7.144; Fig. 7.145).**

The **infrahyoid muscles** (or "strap muscles") consist of four total muscles that are divided equally into a superficial and deep layer. The superficial layer includes the **omohyoid** and **sternohyoid muscles** while the deep layer includes the **thyrohyoid** and **sternothyroid muscles.** The sternothyroid muscle covers the lateral surface of the thyroid gland. These muscles as a group anchor the *hyoid bone, sternum, clavicle,* and *scapula* and function to depress the hyoid bone and larynx during speaking and swallowing movements. The thyrohyoid also functions in elevating the larynx. These muscles work with the *suprahyoid muscles* to provide a firm base for the tongue by steadying the hyoid bone. Refer to **Table 7.7** and **Table 7.8** for a summary of the suprahyoid and infrahyoid muscles (**Fig. 7.140; Fig. 7.141**).

The **anterior jugular veins** arise near the hyoid bone from the confluence of superficial submandibular veins before descending through the muscular triangle and passing posterior to the sternocleidomastoid muscle, ultimately draining into either the external jugular or subclavian vein **(Fig. 7.143).**

The **left recurrent laryngeal nerve** wraps around the arch of the aorta while the **right recurrent laryngeal nerve** wraps around the proximal right subclavian artery prior to entering the neck. The left recurrent laryngeal ascends vertically while the right recurrent laryngeal is more angled initially before reaching the

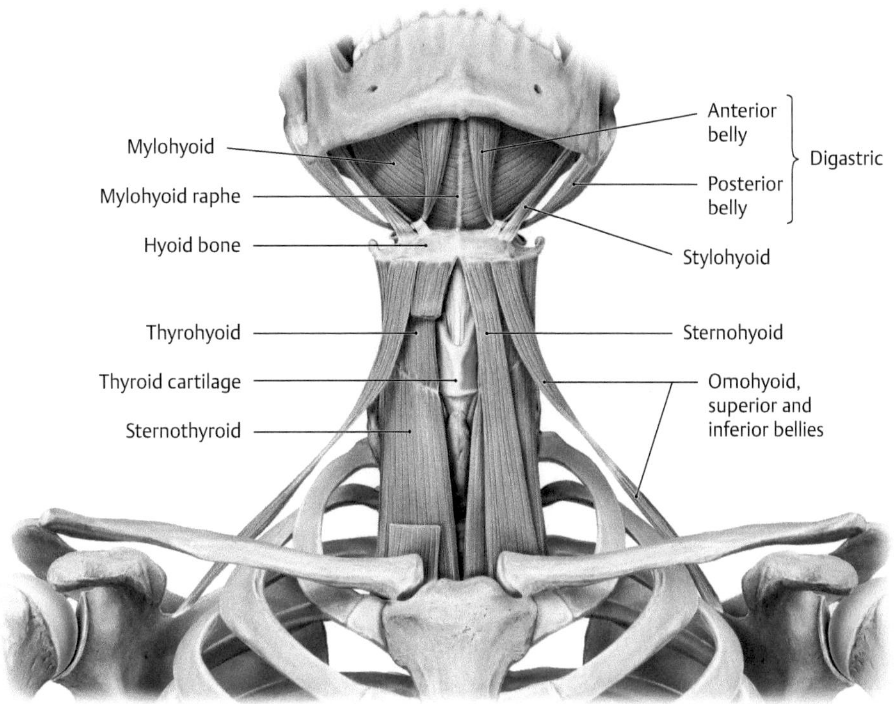

Fig. 7.140 Supra- and infrahyoid muscles, anterior view. The sternohyoid has been cut (right). (From Schuenke M, Schulte E, Schumacher U. THIEME Atlas of Anatomy. Head, Neck, and Neuroanatomy. Illustrations by Voll M and Wesker K. 3rd ed. New York: Thieme Medical Publishers; 2020.)

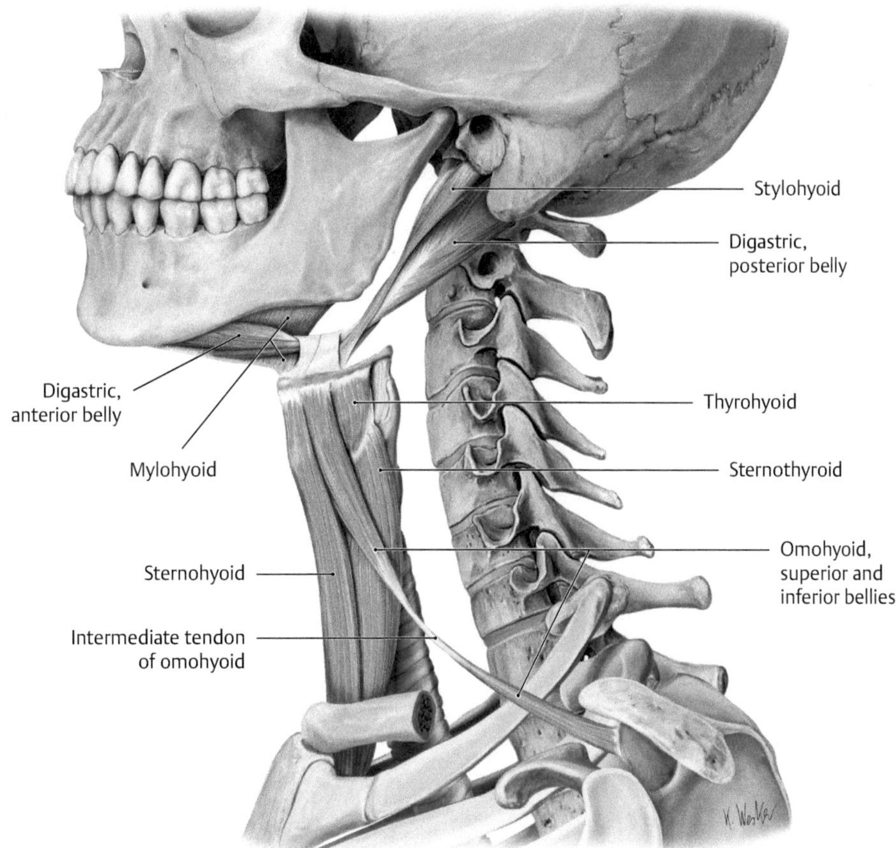

Fig. 7.141 Supra- and infrahyoid muscles, left lateral view. (From Schuenke M, Schulte E, Schumacher U. THIEME Atlas of Anatomy. Head, Neck, and Neuroanatomy. Illustrations by Voll M and Wesker K. 3rd ed. New York: Thieme Medical Publishers; 2020.)

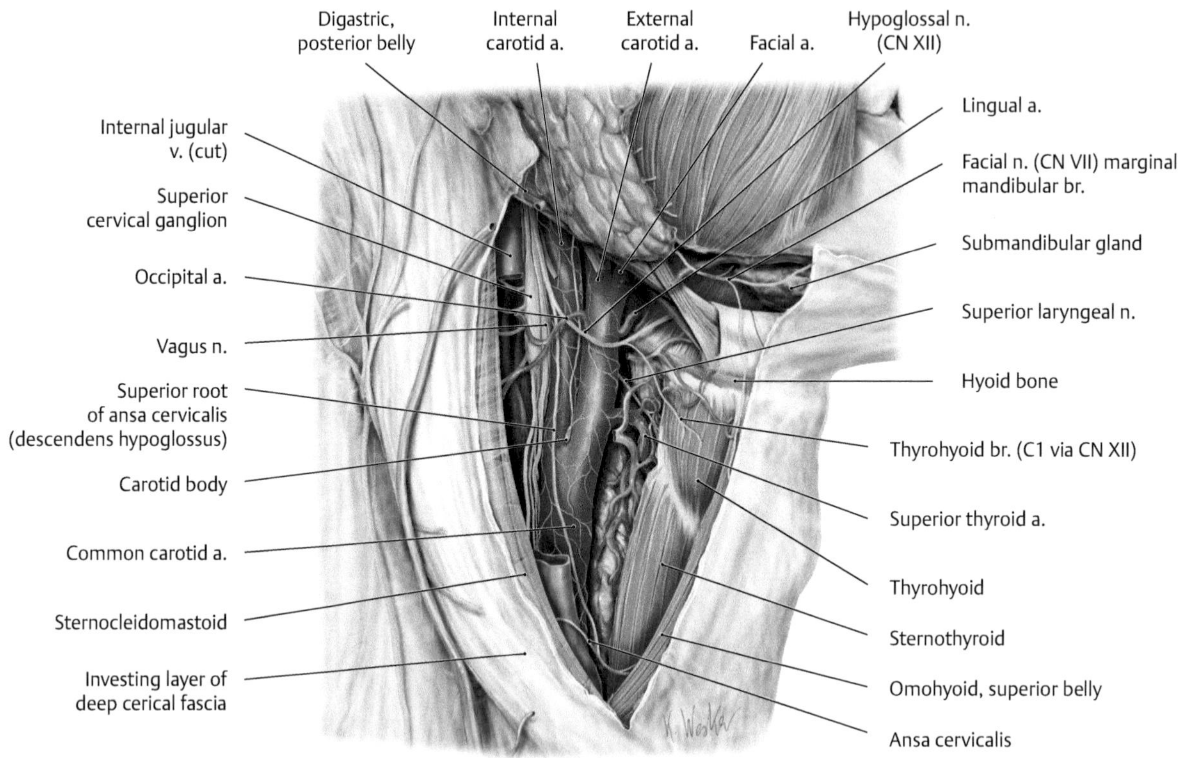

Fig. 7.142 Submandibular and carotid triangles, right lateral view. Internal jugular and facial veins removed. (From Schuenke M, Schulte E, Schumacher U. THIEME Atlas of Anatomy. Head, Neck, and Neuroanatomy. Illustrations by Voll M and Wesker K. 3rd ed. New York: Thieme Medical Publishers; 2020.)

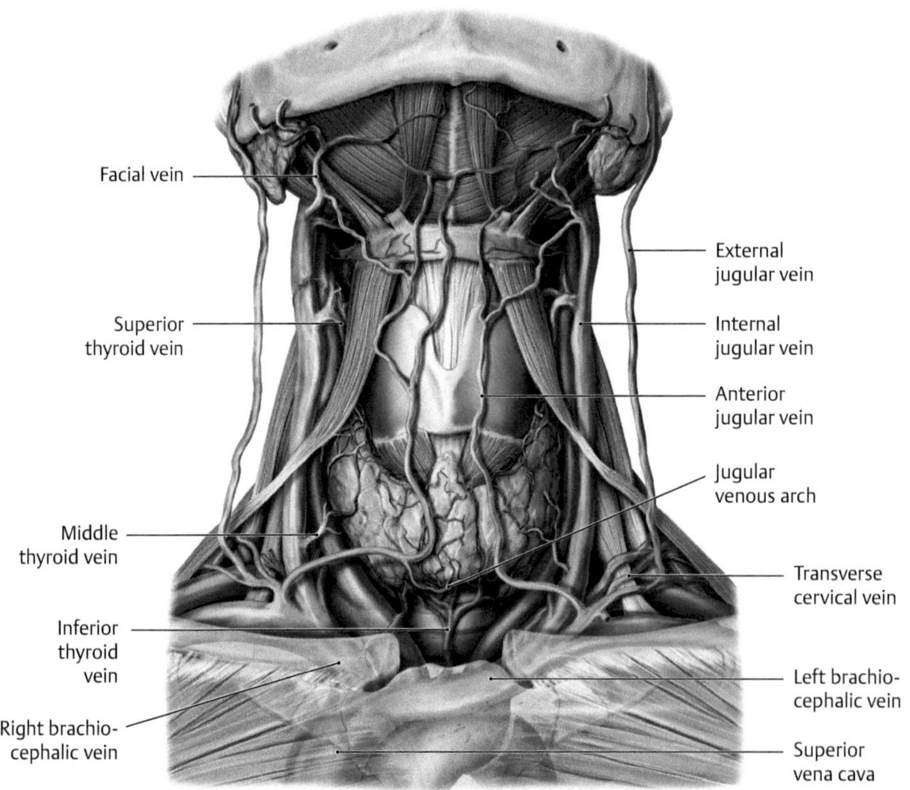

Fig. 7.143 Cervical veins, anterior view. (From Schuenke M, Schulte E, Schumacher U. THIEME Atlas of Anatomy. Head, Neck, and Neuroanatomy. Illustrations by Voll M and Wesker K. 3rd ed. New York: Thieme Medical Publishers; 2020.)

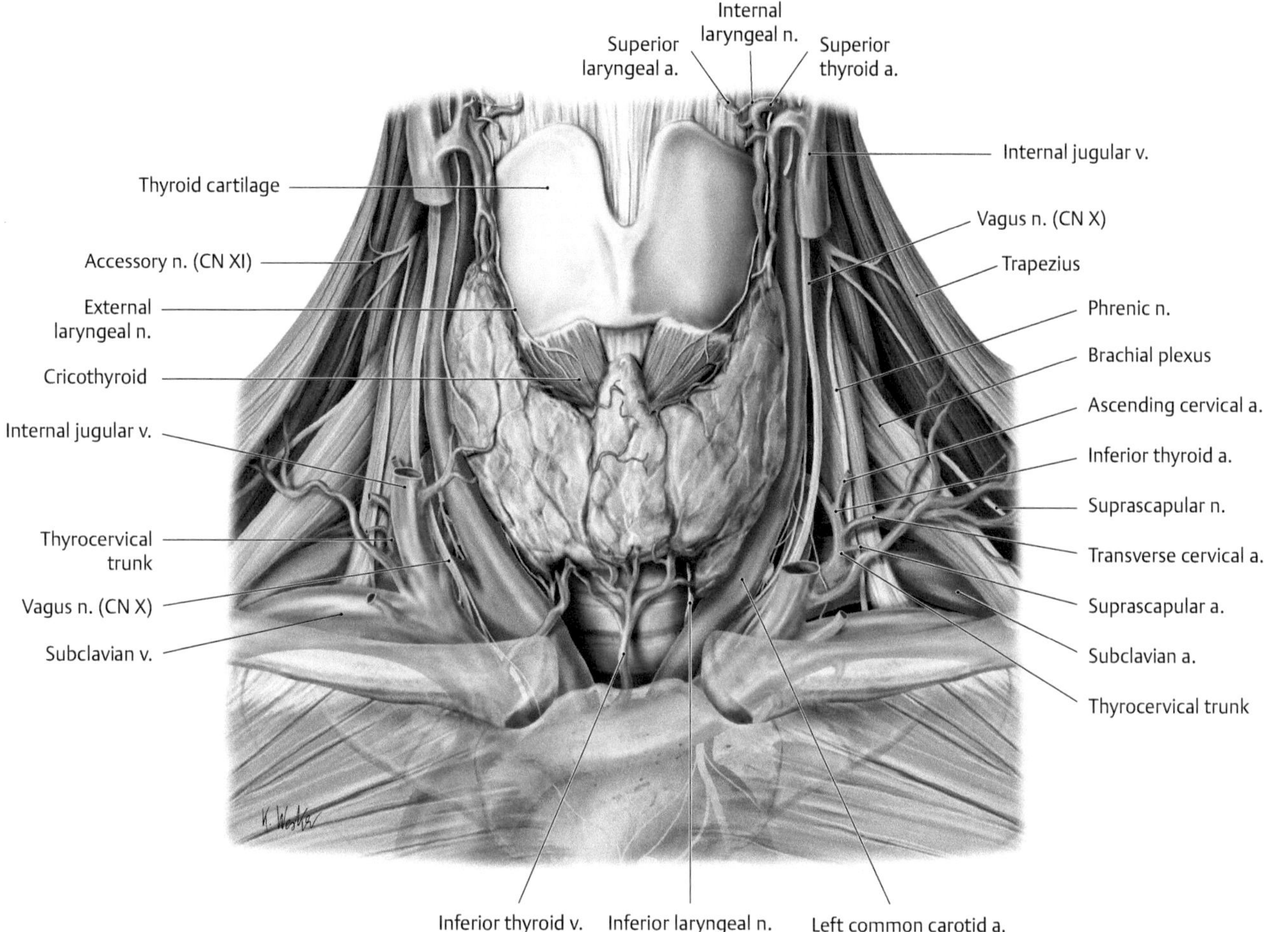

Fig. 7.144 Deep anterior cervical region with the thyroid gland. (From Schuenke M, Schulte E, Schumacher U. THIEME Atlas of Anatomy. Head, Neck, and Neuroanatomy. Illustrations by Voll M and Wesker K. 3rd ed. New York: Thieme Medical Publishers; 2020.)

tracheoesophageal groove. This must be considered if a surgical procedure such as a thyroidectomy is being performed. Recurrent laryngeal nerves terminate near the laryngeal muscles as the **inferior laryngeal nerves** and are responsible for innervating all laryngeal muscles except for the cricothyroid muscle (*external laryngeal nerve*) (**Fig. 7.145**).

7.12.1 Thyroid Gland

The **thyroid gland**, a butterfly-shaped, highly vascularized and brownish-red structure, consists of a **left lobe** and a **right lobe** connected by a centrally located **isthmus**. The **pyramidal (*Lalouette*) lobe** is a vestigial remnant of the *thyroglossal duct* and may only be present in approximately 50% of the population. This lobe extends superiorly and most commonly to the level of the thyroid cartilage. The thyroid gland is found at approximately the C5–T1 vertebral levels and will attain about half the adult size by 2 years of age (**Fig. 7.146**).

The thyroid gland is responsible for how quickly the body burns energy, makes proteins, and controls how sensitive the body should be to other hormones. The primary function is to produce **triiodothyronine (T3)**, **thyroxine (T4),** and **calcitonin**. T3 and T4 are hormones important for regulating metabolism while calcitonin is a hormone that aids in calcium homeostasis by decreasing calcium levels.

7.12.2 Parathyroid Gland

The **parathyroid glands** are small, yellowish-brown, and ovoid structures located on the posterior surface of the thyroid glands. There are generally a total of four in which one each is found on the superior and inferior aspects of the left and right lobes. Parathyroid glands function mainly by maintaining calcium levels but can also have an effect on phosphate, sodium, and potassium levels. **Parathyroid hormone (PTH)** increases blood calcium levels by stimulating osteoclasts to break down bone, thus releasing calcium. It is antagonistic to calcitonin produced by the thyroid gland (**Fig. 7.146**).

7.12.3 Neurovasculature of the Thyroid and Parathyroid Glands

The thyroid and parathyroid glands are mostly hormonally regulated. The thyroid gland responds to thyroid-stimulating hormone produced by the anterior pituitary and blood calcium levels. The parathyroid glands respond mostly to lower levels of serum calcium by secreting PTH, thus increasing calcium. Sympathetic innervation is related to the vasculature supplying these organs and does not serve a secretomotor function.

Blood supply to the thyroid and parathyroid glands is similar to one another. These glands' arterial supply comes from the

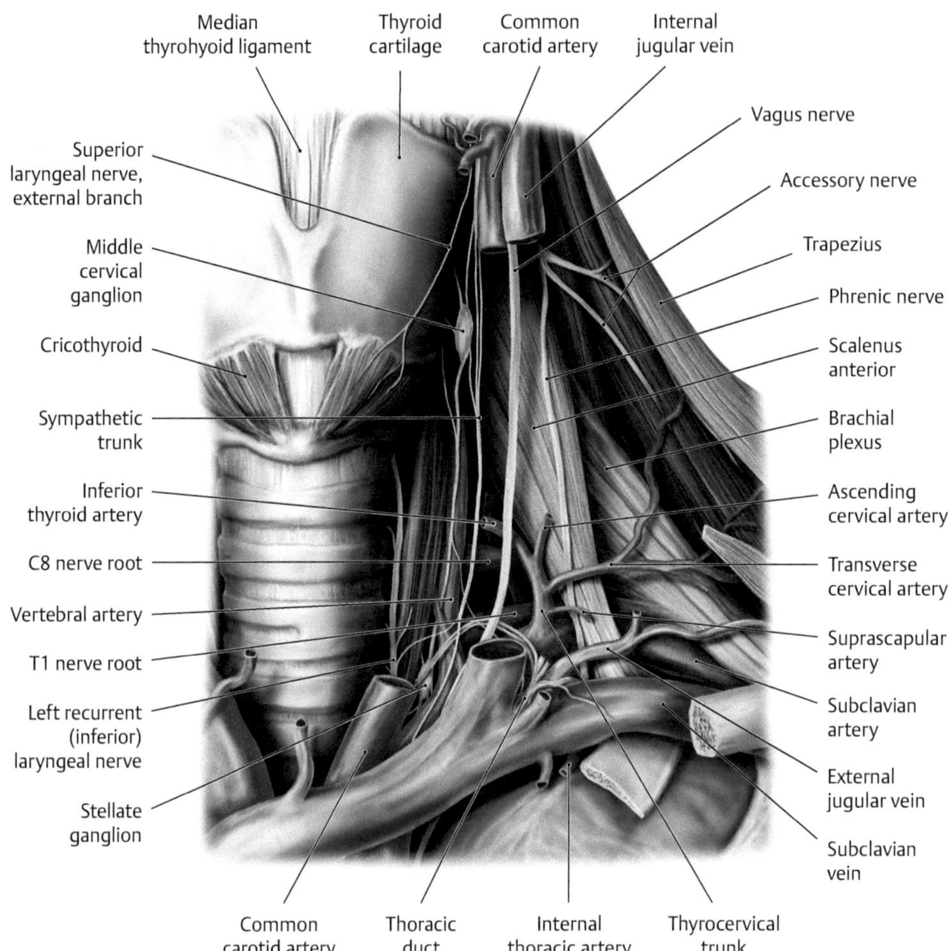

Fig. 7.145 Base of neck and thoracic inlet on the left side. (From Schuenke M, Schulte E, Schumacher U. THIEME Atlas of Anatomy. Head, Neck, and Neuroanatomy. Illustrations by Voll M and Wesker K. 3rd ed. New York: Thieme Medical Publishers; 2020.)

superior thyroid (external carotid br.) and **inferior thyroid arteries** (thyrocervical trunk br.). An unpaired **thyroid ima artery** may be present in approximately 10% of the population. It generally branches from the brachiocephalic trunk and extends superiorly and parallel to the trachea. Understanding this possible arterial anomaly is important when performing a tracheostomy **(Fig. 7.147)**.

Venous drainage of the thyroid and parathyroid glands is to the **superior**, **middle,** and **inferior thyroid veins**. Lymph drainage of the thyroid and parathyroid glands is primarily to the **prelaryngeal**, **paratracheal,** and **pretracheal lymph nodes**. The prelaryngeal nodes drain to the **superior deep cervical lymph nodes** while paratracheal and pretracheal lymph nodes drain to the **inferior deep cervical lymph nodes**.

7.12.4 Histology of the Thyroid and Parathyroid Glands

A **capsule** covers the thyroid gland and the septa of this capsule help divide the parenchyma into lobules. This is unique for an endocrine gland because the cells are arranged into spherical structures called **follicles** and they serve as the basic structural units of this gland. The **follicular cells**, which are generally *simple cuboidal* in nature, surround the follicle and synthesize and release colloid into the lumen of the follicle. **Colloid** is composed of an iodinated glycoprotein called **thyroglobulin** and it is the inactive form of thyroid hormones (TH) **(Fig. 7.148)**.

A low level of TH in circulating blood stimulates the production of **thyroid-stimulating hormone** (TSH) from the anterior pituitary. In response to TSH, the follicular cells begin to take up **iodide** from the surrounding capillaries and then oxidize it to form iodine. **Iodine** is then released into the lumen of the follicle and combines with the amino acid tyrosine to form iodinated thyroglobulin. The hormones **T3** and **T4** are the principal products of iodinated thyroglobulin.

The inactive forms of T3 and T4 remain bound to iodinated thyroglobulin until TSH stimulates its release. Follicular cells by pinocytosis take up iodinated thyroglobulin from the colloid and through proteolytic hydrolysis of iodinated thyroglobulin, yield T3 and T4. T3 and T4 are released into the general circulation and will be responsible for accelerating the metabolic rate of the body, increasing cell, fat, protein, and carbohydrate metabolism, and can be involved in neurologic development in the fetus. T3 accounts for only 10 to 20% of the total secretion while T4 is closer to 80 to 90%, but T3 is more potent.

The **parafollicular cells** are located along the edge of the follicular epithelium as a single cell or clusters of cells in between the follicles but are not in contact with the colloid. These cells synthesize and secrete the hormone **calcitonin** into the surrounding capillaries. The function of calcitonin is to lower blood calcium levels by reducing the number of osteoclasts in bones. Calcitonin will also increase the excretion of calcium and phosphate ions from the kidneys into the urine (**Fig. 7.148**).

A **capsule** surrounds each parathyroid gland and has delicate septa that help separate the secretory cells into clusters. The parenchyma consists of two different cell types, chief and oxyphil cells. The **chief (principal) cells** form the bulk of the cells and are responsible for the secretion of **parathyroid hormone (PTH)**. PTH induces the release of osteoclast-stimulating factor, thus stimulating the proliferation and increased activity of osteoclasts in bones. This results in an increase in blood calcium levels. PTH also influences the proximal convoluted tubule of the nephron to produce the hormone **calcitriol**, the active form of vitamin D, and this results in increased calcium absorption by way of the gastrointestinal tract into the bloodstream. The **oxyphil cells** are less numerous but increase with age and are quite rare before puberty. They are larger than the chief cells but their function is unknown (**Fig. 7.149**).

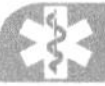

Clinical Correlate 7.34

Hyperthyroidism
When the thyroid gland becomes overactive it begins to secrete excessive amounts of thyroid hormones. The most common cause of hyperthyroidism is *Grave disease*, an autoimmune disorder that produces an antibody resembling thyroid-stimulating hormone, thus overriding normal regulation of the thyroid gland. This can result in the enlargement of the thyroid gland now known as a **goiter**. Ocular protrusion (exophthalmos or bulging eyes), irregular heartbeat, weight loss, anxiety, and irritability can all be symptoms associated with Grave disease.

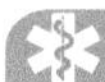

Clinical Correlate 7.35

Hypothyroidism
An underactive thyroid gland does not produce enough thyroid hormone. The most common cause of hypothyroidism is *Hashimoto thyroiditis*, an autoimmune disorder where the body produces antibodies that attack and destroy the thyroid gland. Iodine deficiency in an individual's diet can lead to thyroid hormone impairment and this can also produce a goiter. Other causes of hypothyroidism include surgical removal of the thyroid gland and radiation therapy in the neck region. After giving birth, women may have hypothyroidism due to an inflamed thyroid; however, the reason for this is still unclear and this issue generally reverses itself. Congenital hypothyroidism results in **cretinism**, a condition characterized by mental and growth retardation.

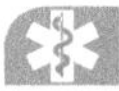

Clinical Correlate 7.36

Hyperparathyroidism
When the parathyroid glands become overactive they secrete too much parathyroid hormone. Two types of hyperparathyroidism exist. *Primary hyperparathyroidism* is the result of hyperactivity due most often to a parathyroid adenoma. Patients may present with multiple issues such as having kidney stones, hypercalcemia, peptic ulcers, constipation, and even depression. Patients undergoing lithium treatments for bipolar disorder are at a greater risk of developing hyperparathyroidism. *Secondary hyperparathyroidism* is the result of PTH being secreted in response to hypocalcemia, which is generally due to vitamin D deficiency or chronic kidney failure. Reduced calcium absorption by the intestinal walls will lead to hypocalcemia, thus increasing PTH. Bones and joints become weak due to the overstimulation of osteoclasts.

Clinical Correlate 7.37

Hypoparathyroidism
When the parathyroid glands have lost much of their function, they fail to secrete enough PTH. Hypocalcemia can interfere with normal nerve conduction and muscle contraction leading to seizures or cardiac arrhythmias. Causes could include the surgical removal of the parathyroids, magnesium deficiency, or congenital absence of the parathyroid glands seen in *DiGeorge syndrome*.

Clinical Correlate 7.38

Thyroglossal Duct Cysts
If there is a remnant of the thyroglossal duct it is known as a **thyroglossal duct cyst**. They are the most common congenital neck cysts and the majority of these patients present before the age of 10. They are located anywhere along the migration pattern of the thyroid gland but are most commonly found near the body of the hyoid bone or just inferior to it. They can also be found near the base of the tongue or near the thyroid cartilage. On occasion, the cyst is connected to the outside surface by a canal and this is called a **thyroglossal fistula**. Treatment involves performing the *Sistrunk procedure*, which removes as one complete specimen, the cyst, middle third of the hyoid bone, and any other tissue leading to the base of the tongue.

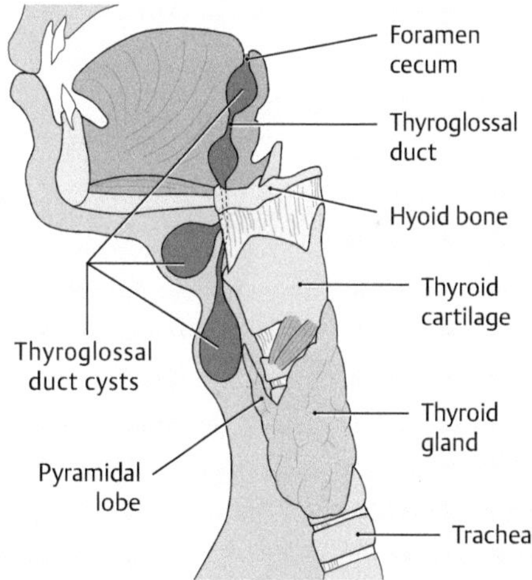

(From Schuenke M, Schulte E, Schumacher U. THIEME Atlas of Anatomy. Head, Neck, and Neuroanatomy. Illustrations by Voll M and Wesker K. 3rd ed. New York: Thieme Medical Publishers; 2020.)

7.12.5 Development of the Thyroid Gland

The **thyroid gland** begins to form at approximately the 24th day of development and it is also the first endocrine gland to develop.

Table 7.7 **Suprahyoid muscles**

Muscle	Innervation	Function(s)	Origin	Insertion
Geniohyoid	C1 via hypoglossal nerve (CN XII)	Elevates and draws hyoid anteriorly; retracts and depresses mandible when hyoid is fixed; shortens floor of mouth; widens pharynx	Mandible (inferior mental spines)	Hyoid (body)
Mylohyoid	Mylohyoid nerve branch of inferior alveolar nerve (CN V_3 br.)	Elevates hyoid, floor of mouth, and tongue during speaking and swallowing	Mandible (mylohyoid line)	Mylohyoid raphe and hyoid (body)
Anterior belly of digastric	Mylohyoid nerve branch of inferior alveolar nerve (CN V_3 br.)	Steadies and elevates hyoid during speaking and swallowing; depresses mandible when hyoid is fixed	Mandible (digastric fossa)	The intermediate tendon is attached to the body of the hyoid via "digastric sling"
Posterior belly of digastric	Facial nerve (CN VII)	Steadies and elevates hyoid during speaking and swallowing; depresses mandible when hyoid is fixed	Mastoid notch of temporal bone	The intermediate tendon is attached to the body of the hyoid via "digastric sling"
Stylohyoid	Facial nerve (CN VII)	Elevate and retract hyoid	Styloid process of temporal bone	Hyoid (body)

Table 7.8 **Infrahyoid muscles**

Muscle	Innervation	Function(s)	Origin	Insertion
Omohyoid	Ansa cervicalis	Steady, depress, and retract hyoid	Superior border of scapula near suprascapular notch	Inferior border of hyoid
Sternohyoid	Ansa cervicalis	Steady and depress hyoid	Manubrium and clavicle (medial end)	Body of hyoid
Thyrohyoid	C1 via hypoglossal nerve (CN XII)	Elevate larynx; steady and depress hyoid	Thyroid cartilage (oblique line)	Greater horn and body (inferior border) of hyoid
Sternothyroid	Ansa cervicalis	Depress hyoid and larynx	Manubrium (posterior surface)	Thyroid cartilage (oblique line)

In the midline of the floor of the early pharynx between the *tuberculum impar* and *copula* near the foramen cecum, the endoderm thickens to form an outpouching known as the **thyroid primordium**. The thyroid migrates caudally, passing ventral to the hyoid bone and laryngeal cartilages. While the thyroid migrates, it remains connected to the tongue by the **thyroglossal duct**, which will become obliterated around the seventh week. The thyroid gland also assumes its definitive shape and final location in the neck by the seventh week **(Fig. 7.150)**.

The small, proximal opening of the thyroglossal duct persists as a blind pit known as the **foramen cecum** of the tongue. If there is a remnant of the thyroglossal duct, this is known as a *thyroglossal cyst*. Near the end of the third month of development, the thyroid becomes functional with iodine thyroid hormones synthesis. Parathyroid gland development is discussed at the end of the chapter and involves the pharyngeal pouches.

The **carotid triangles** are bounded by the *sternocleidomastoid*, *omohyoid* (superior belly), and the *posterior belly of digastric muscles*. Contents include the **structures isolated by the carotid sheath**, proximal **external carotid artery** and limited branches, **carotid body** and **carotid sinus**, **superior**, **external** and **internal laryngeal nerves**, **spinal accessory** (CN XI) and **hypoglossal nerves** (CN XII), and the **ansa cervicalis (Fig. 7.145)**.

The **carotid sheath (Fig. 7.146c)** is the condensation of all three layers of the deep cervical fascia and contains multiple structures of which the larger ones include the **common carotid** and **internal carotid arteries, internal jugular vein, vagus nerve,** and **deep cervical lymph nodes**. While bundled in the carotid sheath, the common carotid artery is located medially, the IJV laterally, and the vagus nerve posteriorly. The most common location (~65%) for the bifurcation of the common carotid arteries into an internal and external carotid artery is at vertebral level C4.

The common carotid arteries originate from different locations. The **left common carotid** branches from the arch of the aorta between the brachiocephalic trunk and left subclavian artery while the **right common carotid** is one of two branches of the brachiocephalic trunk, the other being the right subclavian artery. The *carotid pulse* is taken by placing the second and third digits near the anterior border of the sternocleidomastoid muscle and near the level of the superior border of the thyroid cartilage. Palpation should be done below the level of the common carotid bifurcation to avoid undue pressure being applied to the carotid sinus, which could result in a reflex drop in blood pressure.

The **internal carotid artery** (ICA) continues superiorly from the common carotid artery bifurcation (cervical portion) and then enters the cranium through the carotid canal of the petrous portion of the temporal bone. The ICA supplies the majority of the blood to the brain and is devoid of any branches while in the neck. It is divided into a *cervical, petrous, cavernous,* and *cerebral part.* Branches of this artery do not exist until after reaching the cranium **(Fig. 7.151)**.

The **external carotid artery** (ECA) exits the carotid sheath immediately and begins to branch into multiple distal arteries. These branches supply regions such as the neck viscera, superficial face, deep face, oral cavity, and scalp. The ECA has six direct and two terminal branches. The direct branches include the *superior thyroid, ascending pharyngeal, lingual, facial, occipital,* and *posterior auricular* arteries. The two terminal branches include the

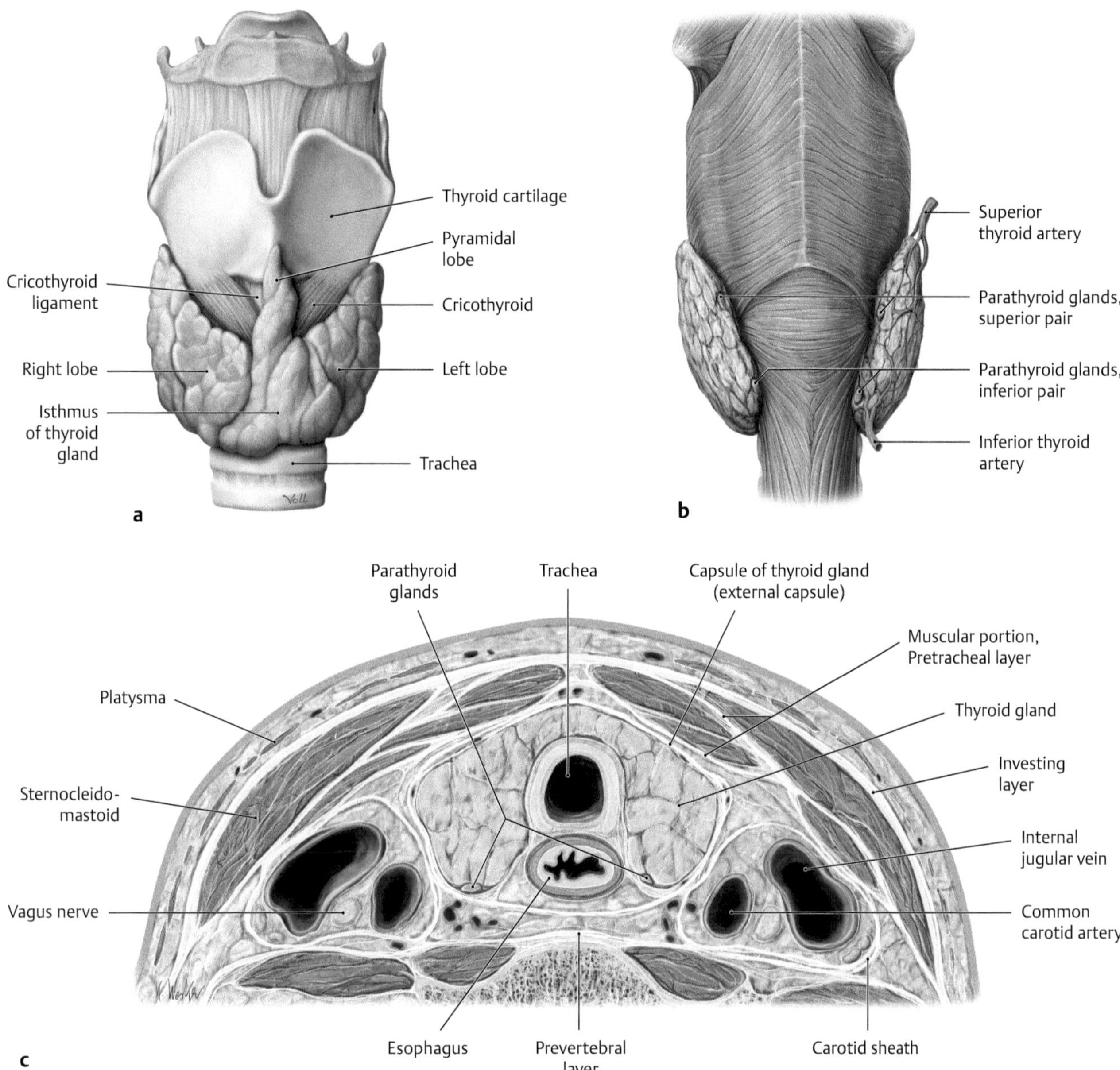

Fig. 7.146 **(a)** Thyroid gland, anterior view. **(b)** Thyroid and parathyroid glands, posterior view. **(c)** Relationship of the thyroid and parathyroid glands to the trachea and neurovascular structures. (From Schuenke M, Schulte E, Schumacher U. THIEME Atlas of Anatomy. Head, Neck, and Neuroanatomy. Illustrations by Voll M and Wesker K. 3rd ed. New York: Thieme Medical Publishers; 2020.)

maxillary and *superficial temporal* arteries. Of all these branches, generally the superior thyroid, lingual, ascending pharyngeal, and occipital arteries are the only ones located in the carotid triangle. The list below represents the most common order of branching from the external carotid artery (**Fig. 7.152**).

- **Superior thyroid artery**: this is the first branch of the ECA and the only one that extends inferiorly toward its target structures, the thyroid and parathyroid glands. The **superior laryngeal artery** branches from it and supplies blood to the superior half of the larynx.
- **Ascending pharyngeal artery**: this is the smallest of ECA branches and ascends superiorly between the pharynx and medial side of the ICA up to the base of the cranium. Smaller branches from it help supply the pharynx, prevertebral muscles, middle ear cavity, and cranial meninges.
- **Lingual artery**: is the chief blood supply to the tongue and floor of the mouth. It extends anteriorly adjacent to the middle pharyngeal constrictor muscle but medial to the hypoglossal nerve. It continues to course medial to the hyoglossus muscle before bifurcating into the **sublingual** and **deep lingual arteries**.
- **Occipital artery**: this artery extends posteriorly from the ECA and is initially hooked by the hypoglossal nerve posteriorly and laterally. It continues along the posteromedial border of the posterior belly of digastric muscle and on the lateral side of the ICA, cranial nerves IX, X, and XI, before coursing through the

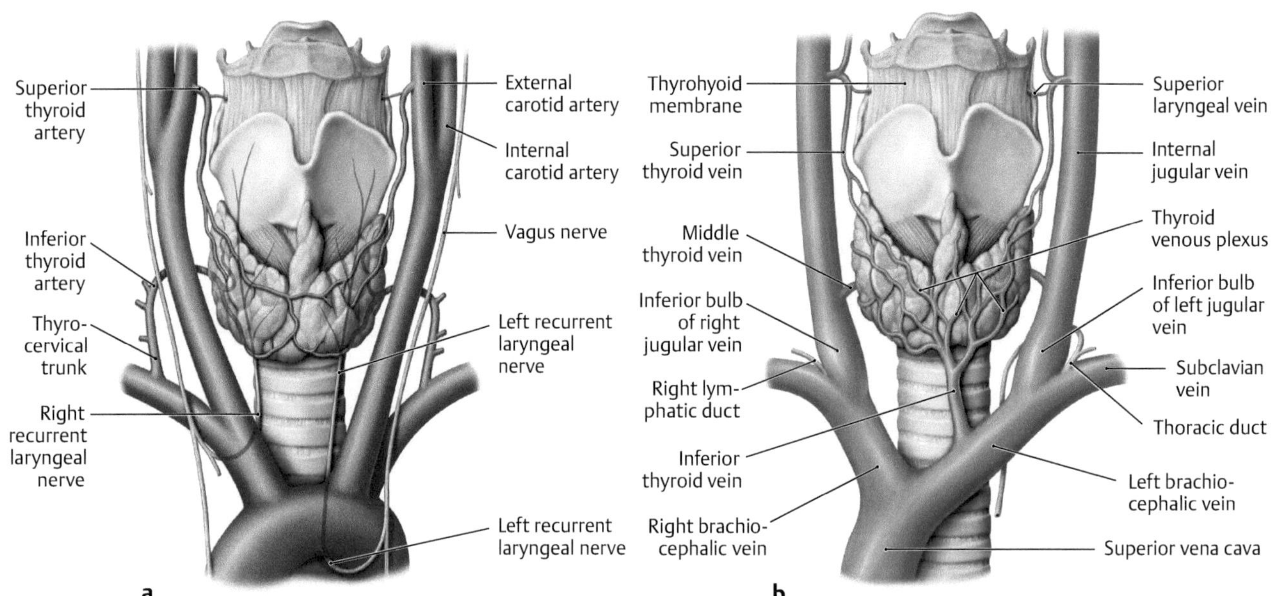

Fig. 7.147 (a, b) Arterial supply and venous drainage of the thyroid and parathyroid glands, anterior view. (From Schuenke M, Schulte E, Schumacher U. THIEME Atlas of Anatomy. Head, Neck, and Neuroanatomy. Illustrations by Voll M and Wesker K. 3rd ed. New York: Thieme Medical Publishers; 2020.)

occipital groove of the temporal bone. It supplies the posterior scalp, ear, and head regions.

- **Facial artery**: this artery branches anteriorly just opposite the occipital, superior to the lingual, or from a common trunk with the lingual artery. It is quite torturous and it initially passes medial to the posterior belly of digastric and stylohyoid muscles. Near the mandibular ramus it arches back around the superior aspects of these muscles to rest near the submandibular gland, lateral mandibular surface, and masseter muscle before continuing onto the superficial surface of the face. In the neck, it gives rise to the **ascending palatine**, **tonsillar**, **glandular branches** to the submandibular gland and the **submental artery**. This artery supplies blood to the palate, palatine tonsil, submandibular gland, floor of the mouth, and other aspects of the face described in the "Scalp and Superficial Face" section of this chapter.
- **Posterior auricular artery**: this is generally the last of the direct branches of the ECA and it ascends posteriorly just above the stylohyoid and posterior belly of digastric muscles and between the mastoid process and external acoustic meatus. It supplies blood to the nearby muscles, parotid gland, auricle, mastoid antrum, some scalp, and the facial nerve.
- **Maxillary artery**: is a terminal branch of the ECA and is responsible primarily for supplying blood to the *"Infratemporal Fossa."*
- **Superficial temporal artery**: is the other terminal branch of the ECA and it divides into a *frontal* and *parietal* branch. It primarily supplies blood to the scalp as described in the "Scalp and Superficial Face" section of this chapter.

Back at the bifurcation of the common carotid artery, a *carotid body* and *carotid sinus* can be found. The **carotid body** is small mass of specialized tissue that lies at the bifurcation of the common carotid artery. It is the most vascularized tissue in the human body and functions as a *chemoreceptor* responsible mainly for detecting the level of oxygen (O_2), carbon dioxide (CO_2), and pH in the blood. When there is a decrease in the partial pressure of oxygen (pO2 (subscript 2)), an increase in partial pressure of carbon dioxide (pCO2 (subscript 2)) or a decrease in pH in arterial blood, a signal is sent to the dorsal inspiratory center of the medulla oblongata to increase the rate and volume of breathing. The carotid body is made up of two different *glomus cells* that are structurally similar to neurons. It is innervated mainly by GVA fibers of the **carotid sinus nerve** (CN IX br.) with a smaller contribution from CN X **(Fig. 7.153)**.

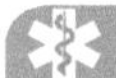

Clinical Correlate 7.39

Carotid Endarterectomy

The main objective of a **carotid endarterectomy** (CEA) is to prevent strokes by removing a plaque buildup causing stenosis of a carotid artery. The stenosis may be creating symptoms such as transient ischemic attacks (TIAs) and may have been the reason the patient made a visit to the clinic in the first place. However, patients are not always symptomatic and these individuals are still at a greater risk of stroke than the general population. Patients that demonstrate a 50% or more stenosis, generally detected with ultrasound and symptoms, are recommended to undergo this procedure within a few weeks of detection. An asymptomatic patient may be best to wait until the stenosis has progressed to 70% or more to avoid any complication due to the surgical procedure.

The **carotid sinus** is a slight dilation at the proximal end of the ICA. It is a *baroreceptor* and reacts to changes in arterial blood pressure. Much like the carotid body, the carotid sinus is innervated by GVA fibers of the **carotid sinus nerve** (CN IX br.) with a smaller contribution from CN X. Note that CN X also has a carotid sinus nerve branch but it is a smaller contributor to the carotid body and sinus innervation. The CN IX versus CN X contribution to these two structures varies among multiple authors **(Fig. 7.153)**.

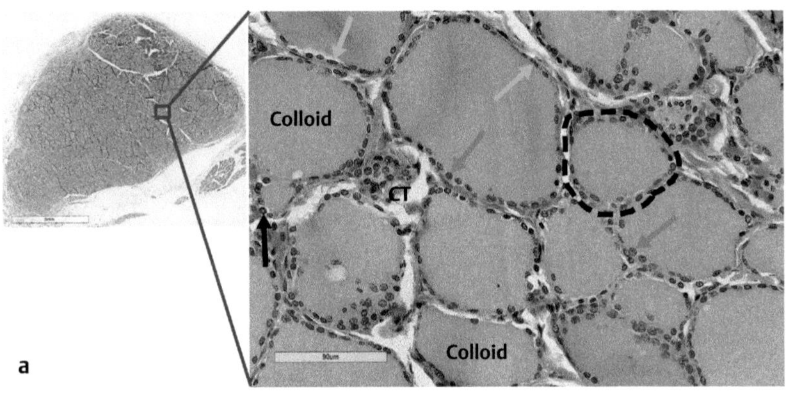

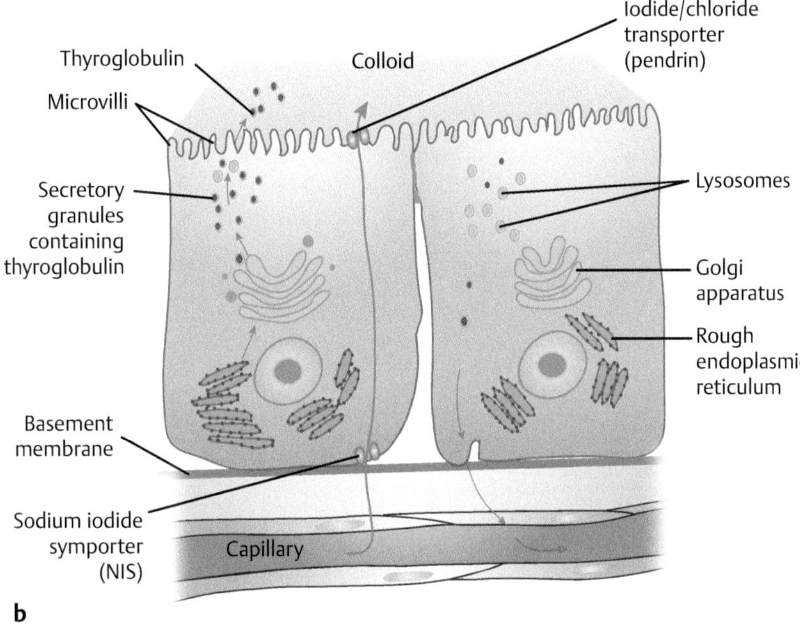

Fig. 7.148 Histology of the thyroid gland. **(a)** Follicles are (*black outline*) filled with colloid. Loose connective tissue (CT) and parafollicular cells are located between the follicles. Follicular cells may be cuboidal (*blue arrows*) or squamous (*green arrows*). Clear cells may also be present (*black arrow*). **(b)** Production of thyroid hormone. (From Lowrie DJ. Histology: An Essential Textbook. New York: Thieme Medical Publishers; 2020.)

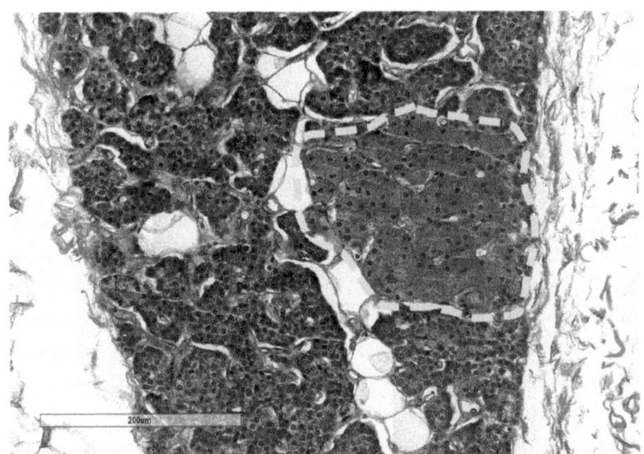

Fig. 7.149 Histology of the parathyroid gland: medium magnification, oxyphil cells (*yellow outline*) and chief (principal) cells (all other cells). (From Lowrie DJ. Histology: An Essential Textbook. New York: Thieme Medical Publishers; 2020.)

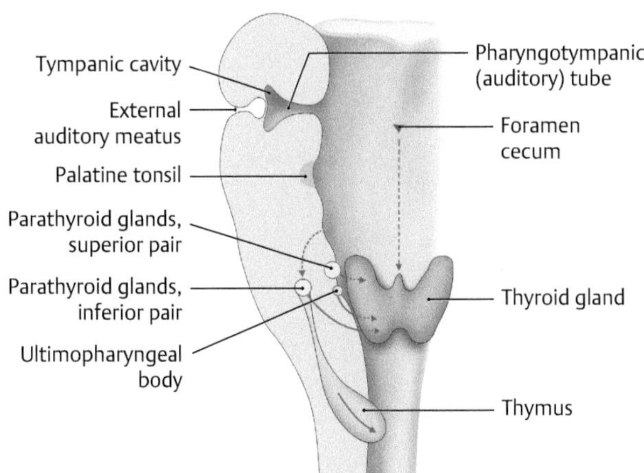

Fig. 7.150 Development of the thyroid gland. (From Baker EW. Anatomy for Dental Medicine. 2nd ed. 2015. Based on the work of: Schuenke M, Schulte E, Schumacher U. THIEME Atlas of Anatomy. Illustrations by Voll M and Wesker K.)

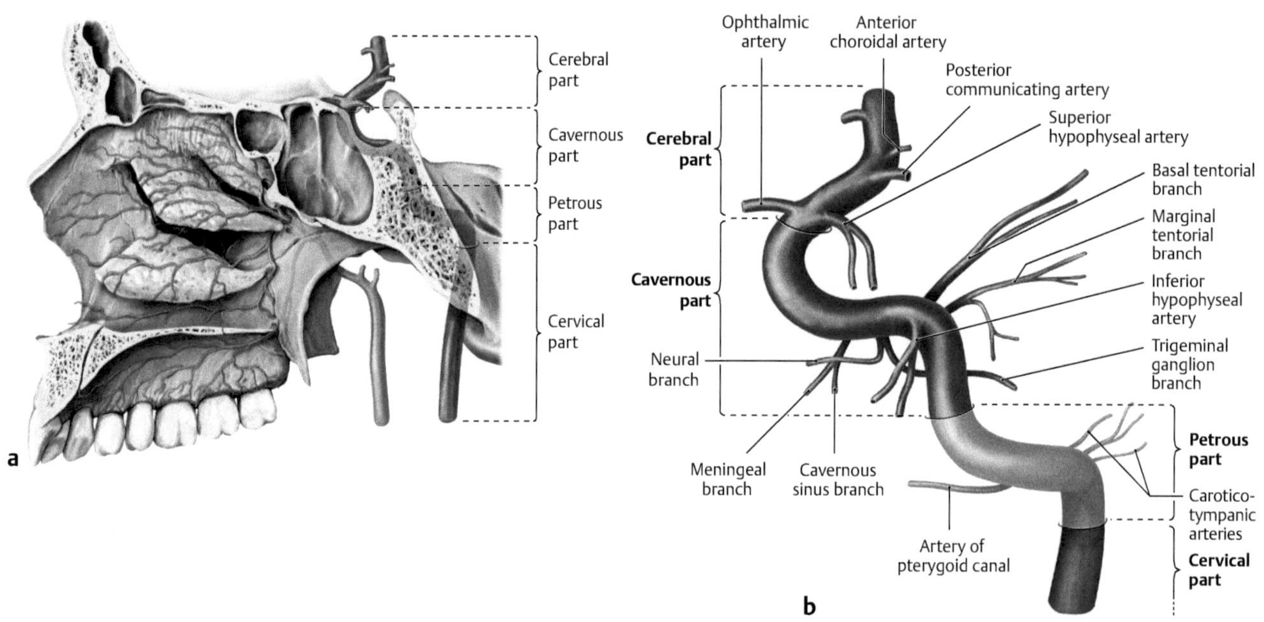

Fig. 7.151 Subdivisions of the internal carotid artery and its four parts. **(a)** Medial view of the right internal carotid artery as it passes through the skull. **(b)** Segments and branches of the internal carotid artery. (From Schuenke M, Schulte E, Schumacher U. THIEME Atlas of Anatomy. Head, Neck, and Neuroanatomy. Illustrations by Voll M and Wesker K. 3rd ed. New York: Thieme Medical Publishers; 2020.)

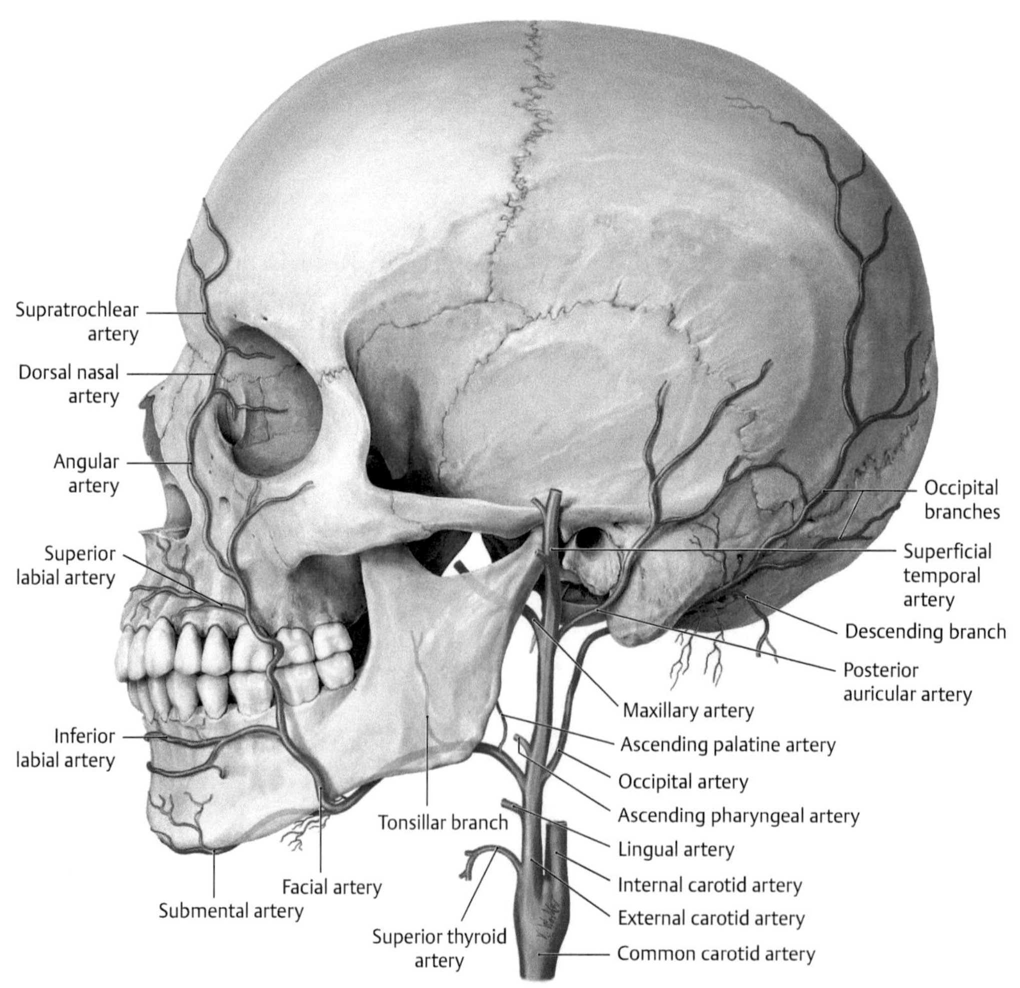

Fig. 7.152 External carotid artery and its branches. (From Schuenke M, Schulte E, Schumacher U. THIEME Atlas of Anatomy. Head, Neck, and Neuroanatomy. Illustrations by Voll M and Wesker K. 3rd ed. New York: Thieme Medical Publishers; 2020.)

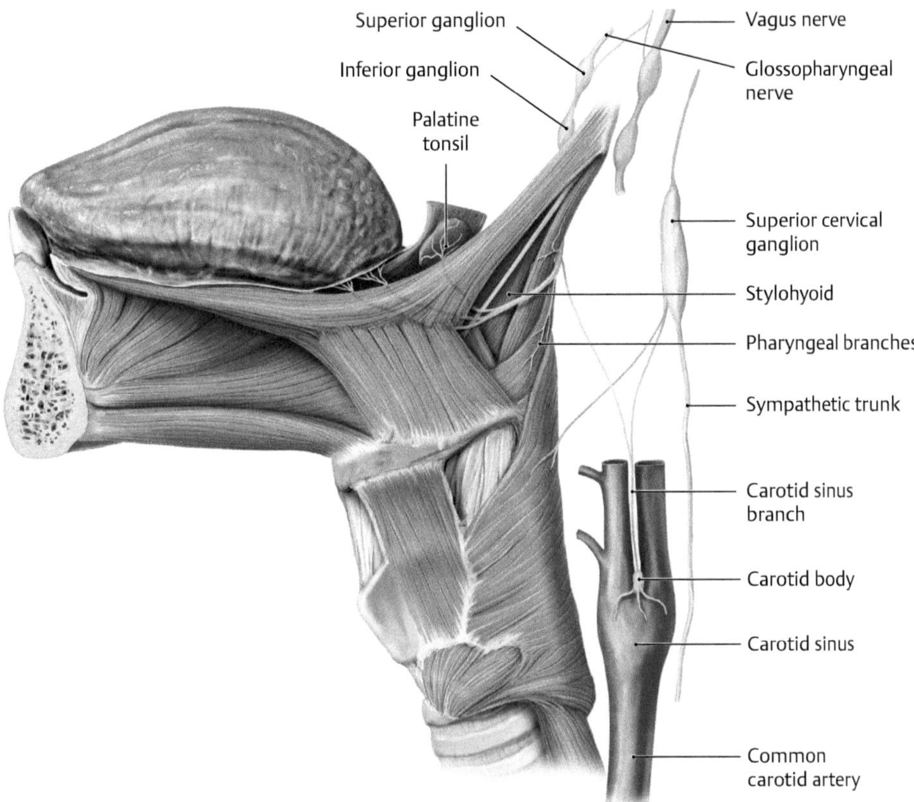

Fig. 7.153 Carotid body and sinus. (From Schuenke M, Schulte E, Schumacher U. THIEME Atlas of Anatomy. Head, Neck, and Neuroanatomy. Illustrations by Voll M and Wesker K. 3rd ed. New York: Thieme Medical Publishers; 2020.)

The procedure while under local or general anesthesia involves making an incision near the anterior border of the sternocleidomastoid muscle that can extend from the angle of the mandible down to the level of the laryngeal prominence (Adam's apple) or lower. Exposure of the internal, external, and common carotid arteries is crucial so that they may be controlled with vessels loops and clamped. The lumen of the carotid artery is exposed, the plaque is removed, and then the artery is sutured closed. Minimally invasive procedures may involve a catheter being routed up from the femoral artery to the carotid artery before inflating a balloon with a wire-mesh stent. This is similar to coronary artery angioplasty.

The **superior laryngeal nerve** branches from the vagus nerve near the jugular foramen and has two branches **(Fig. 7.154)**. The **internal laryngeal nerve** supplies visceral sensory (GVA) and autonomic GVE-para/pre fibers for innervation of the laryngeal mucosal membrane *above* the level of the vocal folds along with GVA and special sensory (SVA-taste) fibers from the anterior epiglottis. The internal laryngeal nerve is paired with the superior laryngeal vessels as they pass through a foramen in the thyrohyoid membrane. The **external laryngeal nerve** is an isolated structure that supplies SVE/BM and GSA fibers to the **cricothyroid muscle**.

The **spinal accessory nerve** (CN XI) exits the jugular foramen and courses through the carotid triangle containing GSE fibers for innervation to the **trapezius** and **sternocleidomastoid muscles**. The GSA fibers related to proprioception course back through the ventral rami of C2–C4 **(Fig. 7.155)**.

The **hypoglossal nerve** (CN XII) exits the hypoglossal canal containing GSE and GSA fibers and it will pass through both the submandibular and carotid triangles on its way to innervating all the muscles of the tongue except the palatoglossus muscle. Attached to CN XII and following the initial contours of this nerve is a C1 ventral ramus nerve branch. After "hitching a ride" with CN XII, these C1 nerves will leave at three different locations. The first C1 nerves to leave contribute to the superior root of ansa cervicalis while the next two branches leave to supply the thyrohyoid and geniohyoid muscles, respectively **(Fig. 7.156)**.

Ansa cervicalis is formed by the ventral rami of C1–C3 of the cervical plexus. It has a **superior root** made up solely of C1 and an **inferior root** consisting of C2–C3 ventral rami branches. The roots of ansa cervicalis are initially located embedded within the carotid sheath but after they are dissected the combined roots will have the appearance of it resting on the IJV. The functional components of all ansa cervicalis branches are GSE, GSA, and GVE-sym/post. Ansa cervicalis is responsible for the innervation of all the infrahyoid muscles except the thyrohyoid muscle **(Fig. 7.156)**.

7.13 Posterior (Lateral Cervical) Triangle of the Neck

There is an anterior, posterior, and inferior boundary along with a roof, floor, and apex that help define the posterior triangle. This particular triangle of the neck is defined by:

- Sternocleidomastoid muscle (anterior boundary).
- Trapezius muscle (posterior boundary).
- Middle one-third of clavicle between the SCM and trapezius muscles (inferior boundary).
- Investing fascia (roof).

- Prevertebral fascia (floor).
- Where the SCM and trapezius muscles meet superiorly (apex).

The posterior triangle is subdivided into two additional triangles by the **inferior belly of the omohyoid muscle**. These two triangles are known as the **occipital** and **omoclavicular triangles (Fig. 7.157)**.

The larger **occipital triangle** will be the location for the bulk of the structures associated with the posterior triangle. These include the *cervical plexus*, *spinal accessory nerve (CN XI)*, origin of the *brachial plexus*, *phrenic nerve*, *dorsal scapular nerve*, *suprascapular nerve*, *nerve to subclavius*, *occipital artery*, *transverse cervical artery* and *suprascapular artery*, and the *mid-portion of the external jugular vein*.

The **cervical plexus (Fig. 7.158)** is made up of the ventral rami of C1–C4 spinal nerves and supplies select neck muscles and the diaphragm, along with a large section of the head and neck skin. The plexus is located anteromedial to the middle scalene and levator scapulae muscles but deep to the sternocleidomastoid muscle. This plexus consists of each ramus, except for the first, dividing into both an ascending and descending branch that unites to form a communicating loop. Superficial branches of this plexus are cutaneous in nature and mostly pass in a posterior fashion. The deep branches are considered the motor fibers and pass through the neck mostly in an anteromedial fashion. The dorsal rami of cervical nerves are not associated with the cervical plexus but contribute to mixed motor and sensory innervation of the posterior head and neck region. A select few of these dorsal rami have specific names, suboccipital nerve (C1), greater occipital (C2), and the third occipital (C3) while the rest just refer to where they originate.

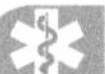

Clinical Correlate 7.40

Cervical Nerve Plexus Block

The **nerve point of the neck (Fig. 7.157)**, also known as *Erb's point* or the *punctum nervosum*, is the site for a **cervical nerve plexus block**. It is used in surgical procedures whereas anesthesia is needed to target the ipsilateral skin over the anterolateral neck. All four of the major cutaneous nerves (lesser occipital, great auricular, transverse cervical, and supraclavicular) of the cervical plexus exit near the midpoint of the posterior border of the SCM. Hence targeting only this central region allows the physician to anesthetize the entire anterolateral neck.

The **cutaneous branches of the cervical plexus** consist of four nerves **(Fig. 7.158)**. The **lesser occipital nerve** originates primarily from C2 and supplies skin over the neck and scalp posterosuperior to the auricle. The **great auricular** and **transverse cervical nerves** both come from C2 and C3. The great auricular nerve innervates the skin over a portion of the parotid gland and

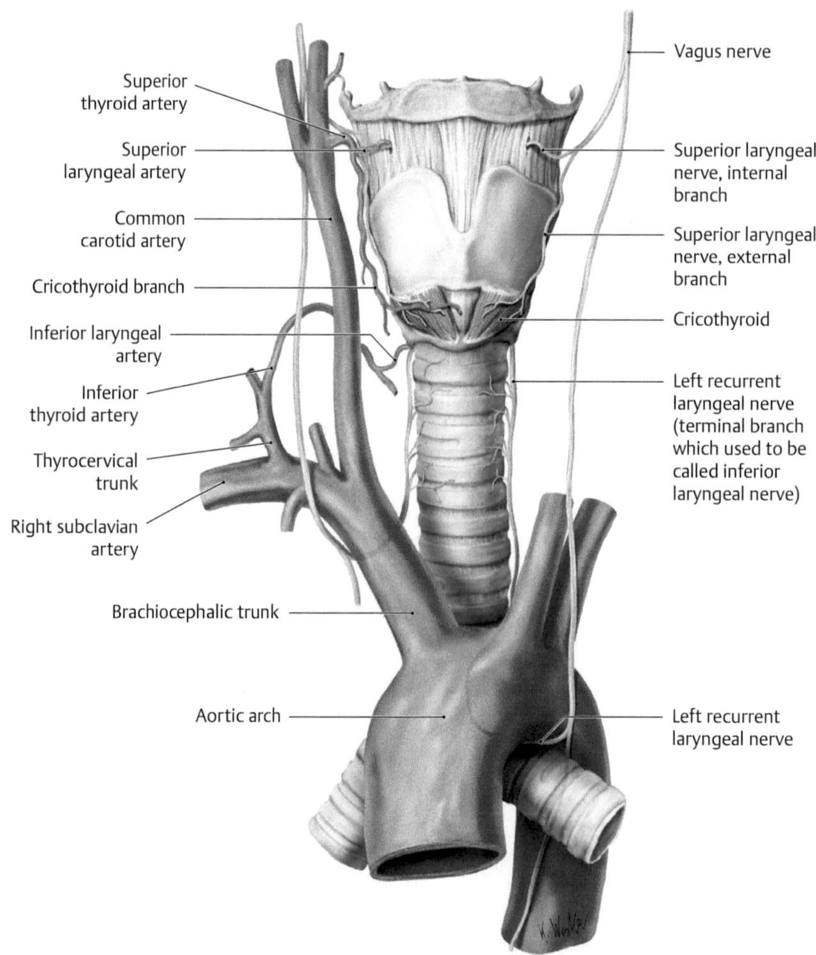

Fig. 7.154 Laryngeal nerves branches of the vagus nerve. (From Schuenke M, Schulte E, Schumacher U. THIEME Atlas of Anatomy. Head, Neck, and Neuroanatomy. Illustrations by Voll M and Wesker K. 3rd ed. New York: Thieme Medical Publishers; 2020.)

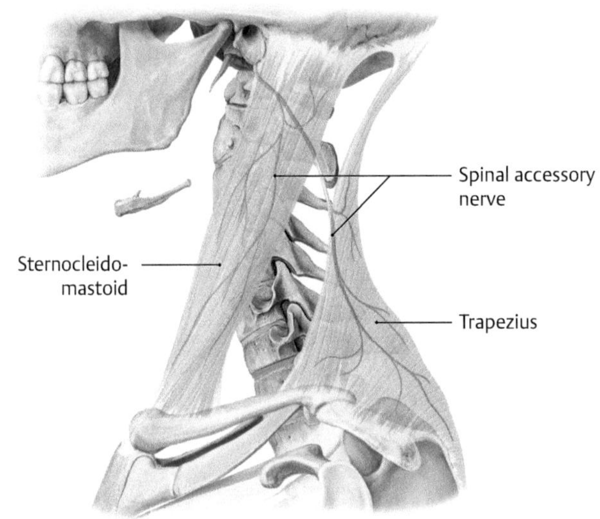

Fig. 7.155 Spinal accessory nerve in neck. (From Schuenke M, Schulte E, Schumacher U. THIEME Atlas of Anatomy. Head, Neck, and Neuroanatomy. Illustrations by Voll M and Wesker K. 3rd ed. New York: Thieme Medical Publishers; 2020.)

its sheath, posterior aspect of the auricle on both sides, and an area extending from the angle of the mandible to the mastoid process. The transverse cervical nerve passes anteriorly over the sternocleidomastoid muscle to supply a good portion of the skin related to the anterior triangle. The **supraclavicular nerves** originate from C3 and C4, and will generally form a common trunk before branching into an individual anterior, middle, and posterior branch. This nerve supplies the skin over the inferior neck, clavicle, and unto the shoulder. The **muscular branches of the cervical plexus** help contribute to the ansa cervicalis and phrenic nerves along with some of the individual segmental branches that innervate the anterior and middle scalene muscles.

The **spinal accessory nerve (CN XI)** while in the occipital triangle will pass from the superoposterior border of the sternocleidomastoid muscle and extend posteroinferiorly over the levator scapulae muscle before reaching the anterior aspect of the trapezius muscle. Once it reaches the trapezius it will slide underneath the muscle and pair with the superficial cervical vessels. Initially, there are two branches of CN XI, and the more anterior branch not seen in either the anterior or posterior triangle will be responsible for innervating the sternocleidomastoid muscle **(Fig. 7.155)**.

The **brachial plexus** was described in great detail in Chapter 6 but in the posterior triangle the roots and trunks of this plexus are best seen here. The ventral rami of C5–T1 form the *roots of the*

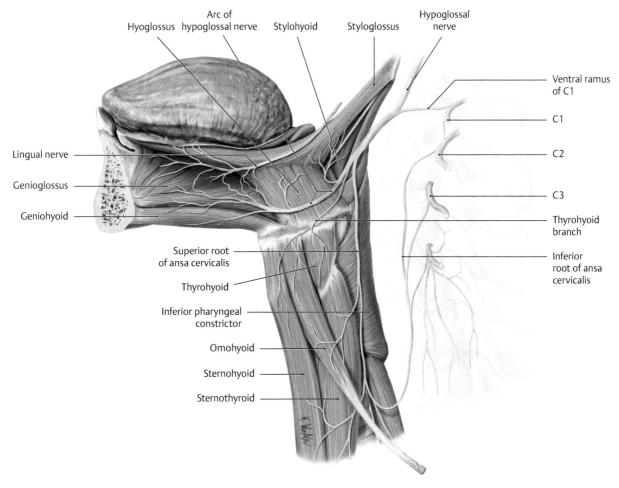

Fig. 7.156 Hypoglossal nerve and ansa cervicalis. (From Schuenke M, Schulte E, Schumacher U. THIEME Atlas of Anatomy. Head, Neck, and Neuroanatomy. Illustrations by Voll M and Wesker K. 3rd ed. New York: Thieme Medical Publishers; 2020.)

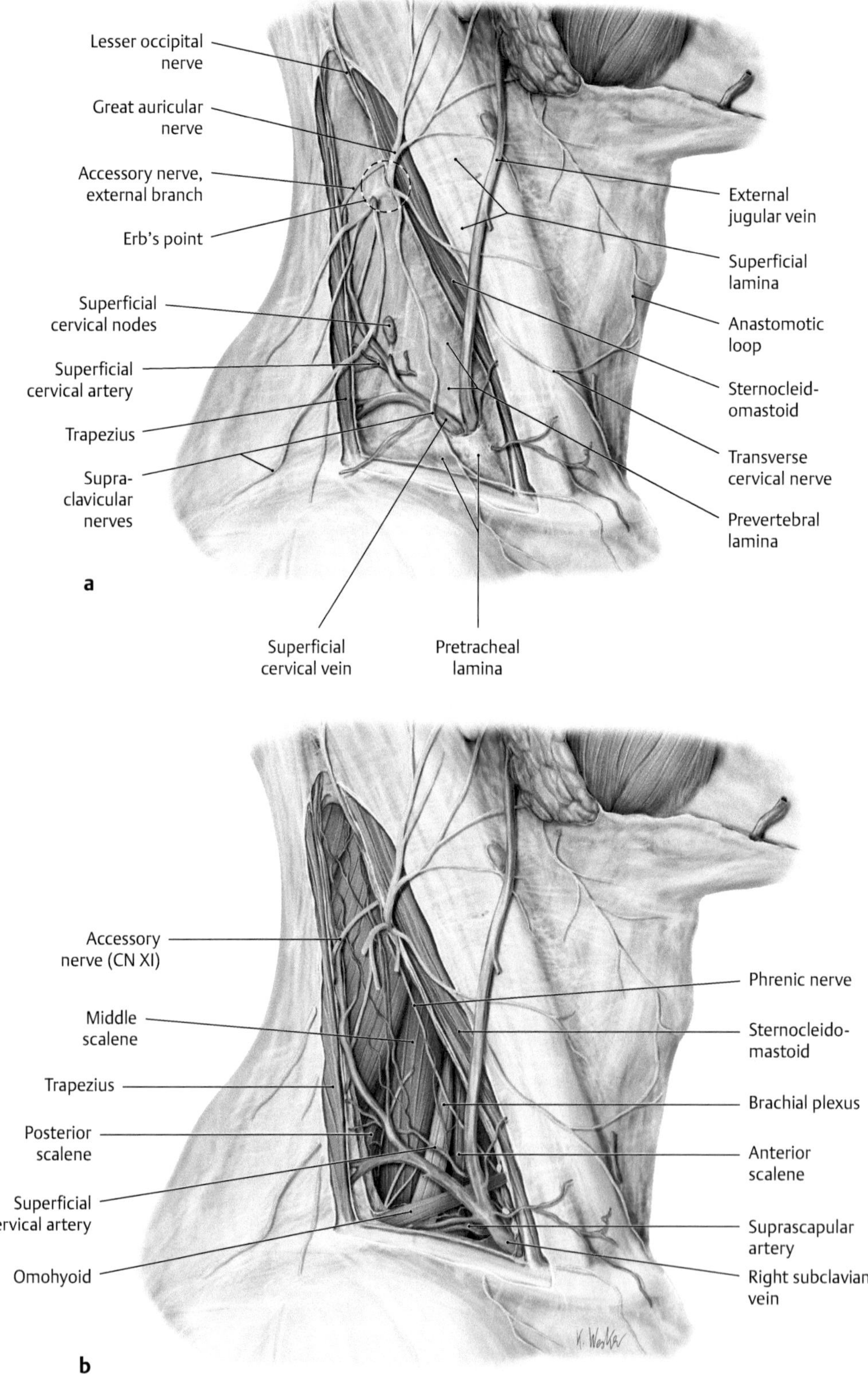

Fig. 7.157 Posterior triangle of the neck. **(a)** Deep layer with the pretracheal layer of deep cervical fascia removed. **(b)** Deepest layer with the prevertebral layer of deep cervical fascia removed. (From Schuenke M, Schulte E, Schumacher U. THIEME Atlas of Anatomy. Head, Neck, and Neuroanatomy. Illustrations by Voll M and Wesker K. 3rd ed. New York: Thieme Medical Publishers; 2020.)

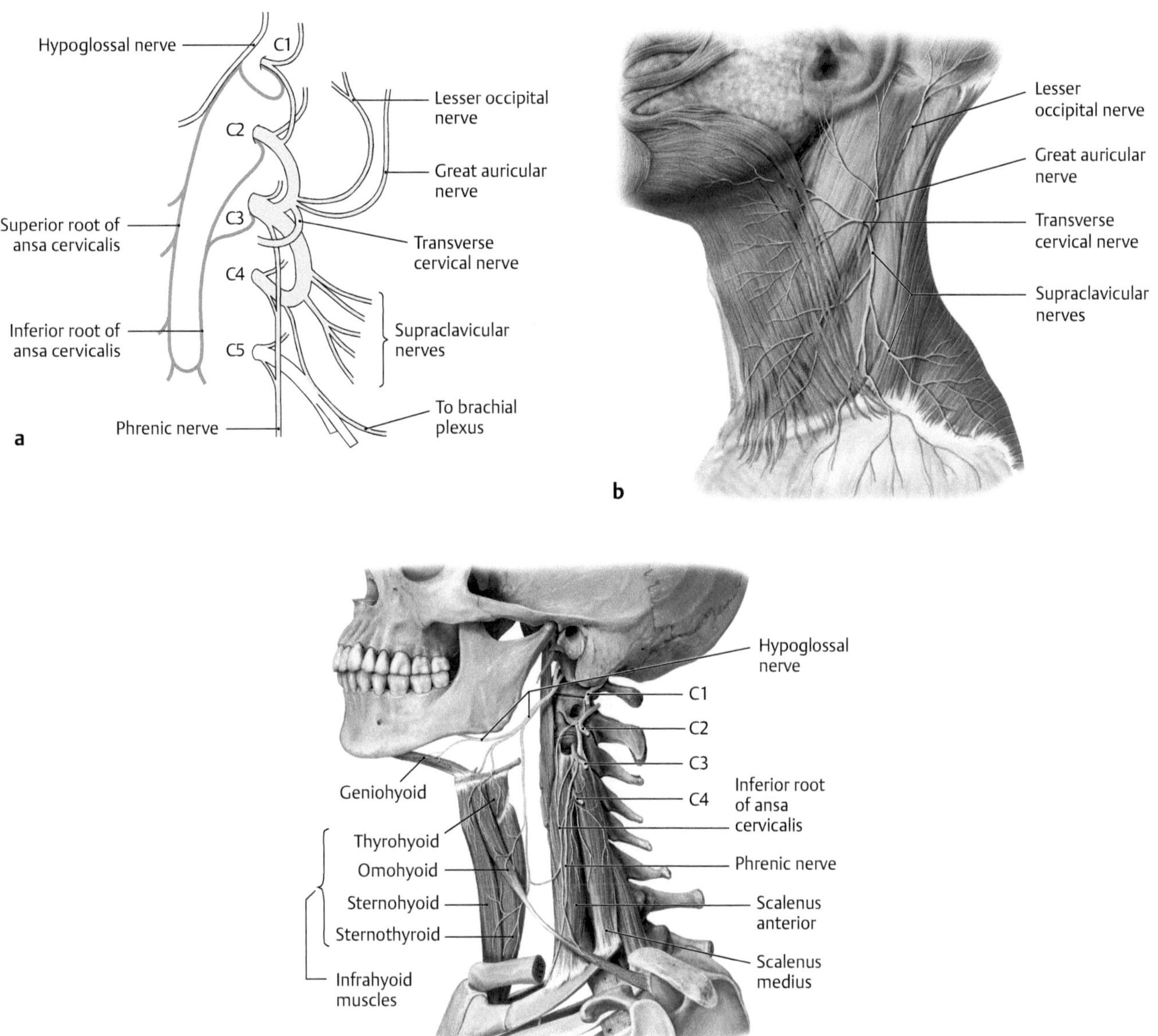

Fig. 7.158 **(a)** Branching pattern of the cervical plexus. **(b)** Sensory branches of the cervical plexus. **(c)** Motor branches of the cervical plexus. (From Schuenke M, Schulte E, Schumacher U. THIEME Atlas of Anatomy. Head, Neck, and Neuroanatomy. Illustrations by Voll M and Wesker K. 3rd ed. New York: Thieme Medical Publishers; 2020.)

brachial plexus. The C5 and C6 roots combine to form the *superior trunk*; C7 forms the *middle trunk*; and finally C8 and T1 form the *inferior trunk*. The roots are located between the anterior and middle scalene muscles while the trunks extend inferolaterally between the clavicle, first rib, and superior border of the scapula before reaching the axilla (**Fig. 7.157**).

The **dorsal scapular nerve** originates from the ventral ramus of C5 and generally pierces the middle scalene muscle before passing posterior to the levator scapulae and pairing with the dorsal scapular vessels (**Fig. 7.157**). It innervates the levator scapulae and rhomboid muscles. The **suprascapular nerve** comes from the superior trunk of the brachial plexus and thus contains the ventral rami of C5 and C6 spinal nerves (**Fig. 7.144**). It passes posterolaterally before pairing with the suprascapular vessels near the clavicle and it innervates the supraspinatus and infraspinatus muscles.

The **nerve to subclavius** originates from the superior trunk but it descends anterior to the brachial plexus and the third part of the subclavian artery before passing above the subclavian vein to innervate the subclavius muscle.

The **phrenic nerves** were detailed during Chapter 2 but to recap, the phrenic nerve is the sole motor supply to the diaphragm and the functional components are GSE, GSA, and GVE-sym/post. The phrenic nerves originate from the ventral rami of C3–C5 with its largest contribution coming from C4. They descend across the superficial surface of the anterior scalene muscles just posterior to the transverse cervical and suprascapular arteries and lie just deep to the prevertebral layer of deep cervical fascia. On its way to the thorax, the left phrenic will pass anterior to the first part of the subclavian artery while the right phrenic passes anterior to the second part of the subclavian artery. Both phrenic nerves pass posterior to

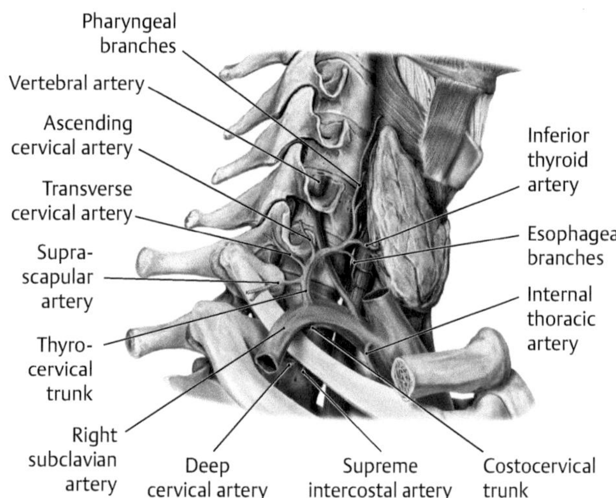

Fig. 7.159 The thyrocervical trunk and costocervical trunk and their branches. (From Schuenke M, Schulte E, Schumacher U. THIEME Atlas of Anatomy. Head, Neck, and Neuroanatomy. Illustrations by Voll M and Wesker K. 3rd ed. New York: Thieme Medical Publishers; 2020.)

the subclavian vein and anterior to the internal thoracic artery upon entering the thorax (**Fig. 7.145; Fig. 7.158**). An **accessory phrenic nerve** may exist and is frequently a branch of the *nerve to the subclavius*. The C5 contribution to the phrenic nerve may be derived from the accessory phrenic nerve. If present, it will lie lateral to the phrenic nerve and pass either posterior or anterior to the subclavian vein before joining the phrenic nerve at the root of the neck or in the thorax.

The main blood vessels of this triangle include the **occipital artery** located near the apex of the posterior triangle (**Fig. 7.152**). The **transverse cervical** and **suprascapular arteries** are both branches of the *thyrocervical trunk* that originated off the *first part of the subclavian artery*. The external jugular vein is most prominent in the occipital triangle but its inferior bulb will be located in the omoclavicular triangle (**Fig. 7.159**).

The smaller **omoclavicular** (subclavian or supraclavicular) **triangle** is located between the inferior belly of omohyoid and the clavicle. This is the location where the terminal portion or inferior bulb of the EJV, and after receiving the **transverse cervical, suprascapular,** and **anterior jugular veins**, drains into the subclavian vein. The third part of the subclavian artery and vein reside in this triangle.

7.14 Prevertebral Region and Root of the Neck

The **prevertebral region** is located anterolateral to the vertebral column and posterior to the cervical viscera and consists of the **prevertebral muscles** (**Fig. 7.160; Fig. 7.161**). The prevertebral muscles are divided into anterior and lateral muscle groups. The **anterior group** is made up of the **rectus capitis anterior, longus capitis, longus colli**, and **anterior scalene muscles** (**Table 7.9**). This group is found mainly posterior to the prevertebral fascia and the prevertebral space. The lateral group consists of the **rectus capitis lateralis, splenius capitis, middle scalene,** and **posterior scalene** (**Table 7.10**). These muscles can be located posterior to the prevertebral fascia and the neurovascular plane of the cervical and brachial plexus along with the subclavian artery. The **levator scapulae** are considered part of the lateral group; however, because their functions are not similar to the rest of the prevertebral muscles it will not be discussed in this section. The anterior and lateral muscle groups have functions that include head and cervical vertebrae flexion in either the anterior or lateral direction, and during forced inspiration, some of these muscles elevate the first or second ribs (**Fig. 7.160**). Refer to **Table 7.9** and **Table 7.10** for a summary of the anterior and lateral prevertebral muscles.

7.14.1 Nerves of the Root

The junction between the neck and the thorax and at the level of the superior thoracic aperture is the **root of the neck.** It will serve as the conduit for all the structures that pass to and from the neck and thorax regions. Nerves that pass through the root include the *phrenic, vagus (CN X), recurrent laryngeal,* and the *sympathetic trunks*. All others have been described except for the sympathetic trunk and their ganglion.

Lying just anterolateral to the cervical vertebrae and extending from the root of the neck to the cranial base is the **cervical portion of the sympathetic trunk**. Sympathetic preganglionic nerve fibers that ascend through the neck region originate mostly from the T1–T4 lateral horns of the spinal cord. Along this portion of the sympathetic trunk there is a superior, middle, and inferior cervical sympathetic ganglion.

The **superior cervical ganglion** is the largest sympathetic ganglion and it is located at the level of the C1 and C2 vertebrae; the **middle cervical ganglion** is inconstant but if present it rests on the anterior aspect of the inferior thyroid artery at the level of the transverse process of the C6 vertebra; and finally the **inferior cervical ganglion**, which in a large percentage of the population fuses with the first thoracic ganglion forming a **cervicothoracic (stellate) ganglion**, and it is generally located anterior to the transverse process of the C7 vertebra, posterior to the origin of the vertebral artery and just superior to the neck of the first rib (**Fig. 7.145**). The **ansa subclavia** originates from the inferior cervical ganglion and will loop around the subclavian artery before connecting to the middle cervical ganglion.

Sympathetic preganglionic fibers pass through the cervical sympathetic trunk before synapsing at one of these ganglions. After they synapse and become postganglionic, there are three options for which these sympathetic postganglionic fibers will travel.

1. Pass through a gray rami communicantes before continuing with a ventral or dorsal cervical rami nerve branch.
2. Extend directly off the ganglion and onto an artery, thus forming a **periarterial nerve plexus**. These plexuses are prominent around the common carotid, external/internal carotid, and vertebral arteries and continue distally to supply the head and

Clinical Correlate 7.41

Cervicothoracic (Stellate) Ganglion Block

The stellate ganglion is part of the sympathetic nervous system and is commonly formed by the fusion of the last cervical and first thoracic sympathetic ganglions. This type of nerve block is used to diagnose or treat circulation problems or nerve injuries that can include *herpes zoster infection* (shingles), *reflex sympathetic dystrophy, phantom limb pain, causalgia*, or *complex regional pain syndromes*. After a local anesthetic is injected near the root of the neck, a second needle will be guided by either ultrasound or fluoroscopy to target the stellate ganglion where anesthetic will again be injected to block activity from this ganglion.

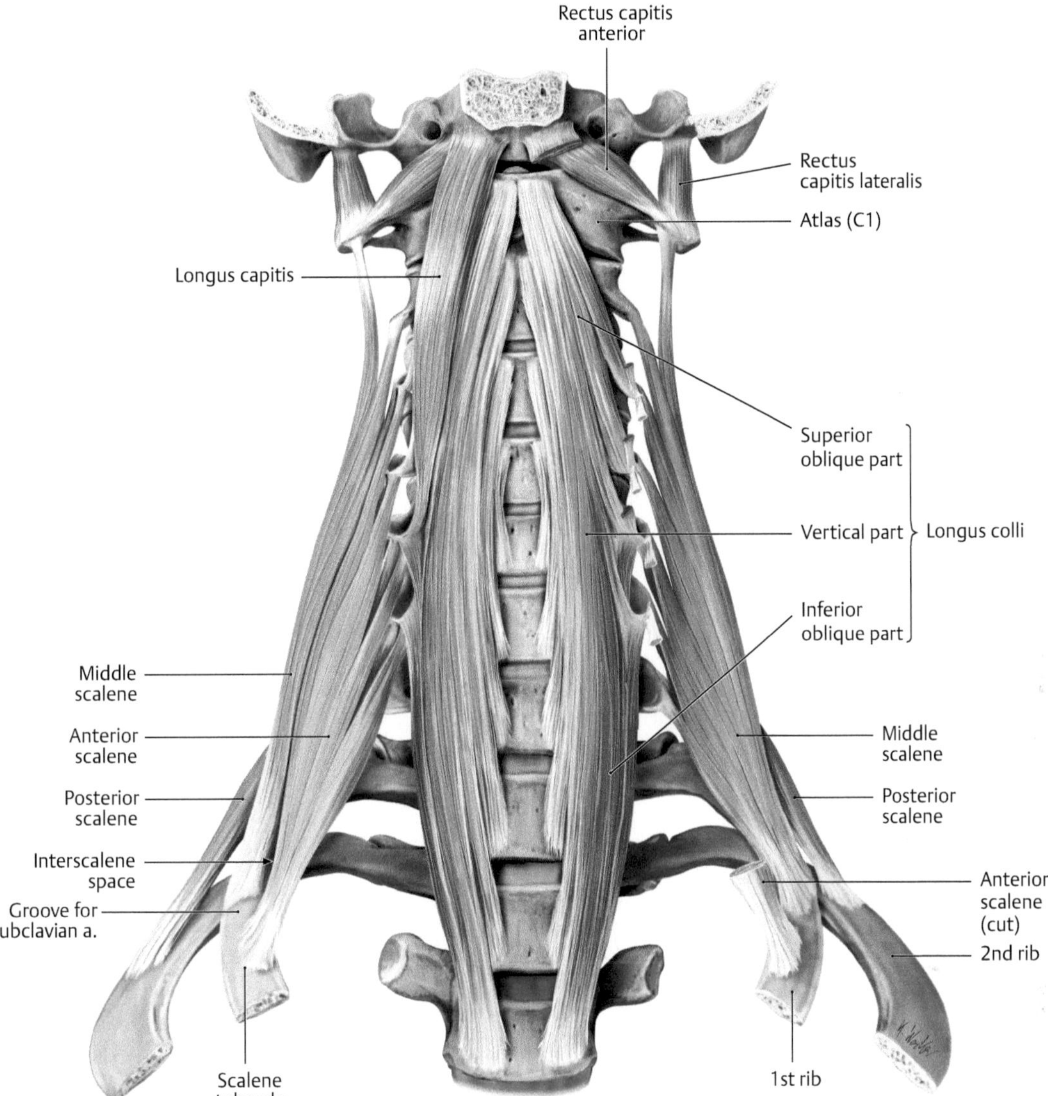

Fig. 7.160 Prevertebral and scalene muscles, anterior view. (From Schuenke M, Schulte E, Schumacher U. THIEME Atlas of Anatomy. Head, Neck, and Neuroanatomy. Illustrations by Voll M and Wesker K. 3rd ed. New York: Thieme Medical Publishers; 2020.)

neck viscera or skin. A periarterial plexus in the head and neck region only contains sympathetic postganglionic autonomics unlike the abdominal and pelvic regions where periarterial plexuses contain sympathetic postganglionic and parasympathetic preganglionic autonomics.

3. The **superior**, **middle,** and **inferior cardiopulmonary splanchnic nerves** extend inferiorly from their equivalent named ganglion to contribute additional sympathetic postganglionic fibers to the *cardiac* and *pulmonary visceral nerve plexuses* supplying the heart and lungs.

7.14.2 Arteries of the Root

The root is associated with the *brachiocephalic trunk, common carotids*, and the *subclavian arteries* and their subsequent branches (**Fig. 7.161**). The **brachiocephalic (innominate) trunk** bifurcates into the *right subclavian* and *right common carotid arteries* near the border of the root of the neck and thorax. These are generally the only branches of the brachiocephalic trunk, but rarely the anatomical variation known as the *thyroid ima artery* may originate from this trunk.

The **subclavian arteries** rest upon the subclavian artery grooves of the first rib and are posterior to the anterior scalene muscle after originating from either the brachiocephalic trunk on the right or the arch of the aorta on the left. Both subclavian arteries are divided into three parts and this is based on their relationship to the anterior scalene muscle.

- The *first part of the subclavian artery* is medial to the anterior scalene and has three branches. From medial to lateral these branches include the *vertebral, internal thoracic,* and *thyrocervical trunk.*
  - The **vertebral artery** is divided into four parts (**Fig. 7.161; Fig. 7.162**).

    1. The **cervical part** comes directly off the subclavian and passes through the *pyramidal space* located

Clinical Correlate 7.42

Horner Syndrome

If there is a disturbance in the sympathetic pathway usually due to a lesion of the cervical portion of the sympathetic trunk, this is called **Horner syndrome**. Other causes can include dissecting carotid aneurysms, proximal brachial plexus injuries, and even brainstem damage resulting from a tumor or stroke. This syndrome is characterized by drooping of the upper eyelid (*ptosis*) caused by paralysis of the superior tarsal muscle; contraction of the pupil (*miosis*) caused by paralysis of the dilator pupillae muscle; excessive vasodilation given the appearance of flushed skin (*hyperemia*) and the absence of sweating on the face and neck (*anhydrosis*), both of which are caused by no innervation by sympathetics to the blood vessels or sweat glands, respectively; and finally the appearance of the eyeball sinking (*enophthalmos*) but this is generally thought to be an illusion due to the already present ptosis. Some believe a paralyzed *orbitalis muscle* could cause it, but this particular smooth muscle is a vestigial structure and not always present. When present it is also known as Muller muscle, not to be confused with the already present superior tarsal (Muller) muscle.

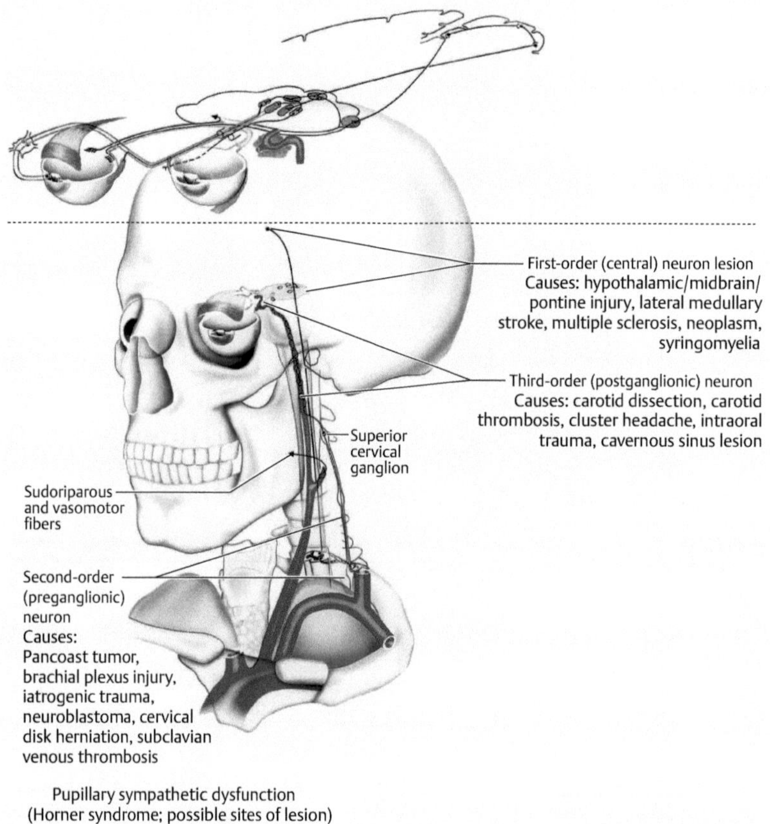

Pupillary sympathetic dysfunction (Horner syndrome; possible sites of lesion)

(From Rohkamm, Color Atlas of Neurology, 2nd ed. Stuttgart: Thieme Medical Publishers, 2014.)

Table 7.9 **Prevertebral muscles—anterior group**

Muscle	Innervation	Function(s)	Origin	Insertion
Rectus capitis anterior	Ventral rami of C1–C2	Anterior and lateral flexion at atlanto-occipital joint	Lateral mass of atlas (C1)	Basilar part of occipital bone
Longus capitis	Ventral rami of C1–C3	Flex head; tilts and rotates head to ipsilateral side	Anterior tubercles of transverse processes of C3–C6 vertebrae	Basilar part of occipital bone
Longus colli	Ventral rami of C2–C6	Flex neck; tilts and rotates neck to ipsilateral side	Anterior tubercles of transverse processes of C3–C5 vertebrae; anterior sides of C5–T3 vertebral bodies	Anterior tubercles of atlas; anterior tubercles of transverse processes of C5–C6 vertebrae; anterior sides of C2–C4 vertebrae
Anterior scalene	Ventral rami of C4–C6	Elevate the first rib; anterior and lateral flexion of neck; assists in forced respiration	Anterior tubercles of transverse processes of C3–C6 vertebrae	Scalene tubercle of the first rib

Table 7.10 **Prevertebral muscles—lateral group**

Muscle	Innervation	Function(s)	Origin	Insertion
Rectus capitis lateralis	Ventral rami of C1–C2	Anterior and lateral flexion at atlanto-occipital joint	Transverse process of atlas (C1)	Basilar part of occipital bone (lateral to occipital condyles)
Splenius capitis	Dorsal rami of middle cervical nerves	Extends head and neck; flexes and rotates head to ipsilateral side	Spinous processes of C3–T3 vertebrae	Lateral part of superior nuchal line; mastoid process
Middle scalene	Ventral rami of C3–C8	Elevate the first rib; anterior and lateral flexion of neck; assists in forced respiration	Posterior tubercles of transverse processes of C2–C7 vertebrae	First rib and posterior to subclavian artery groove
Posterior scalene	Ventral rami of C7–C8	Elevate the second rib; anterior and lateral flexion of neck; assists in forced respiration	Posterior tubercles of transverse processes of C5–C7 vertebrae	Outer surface of the second rib

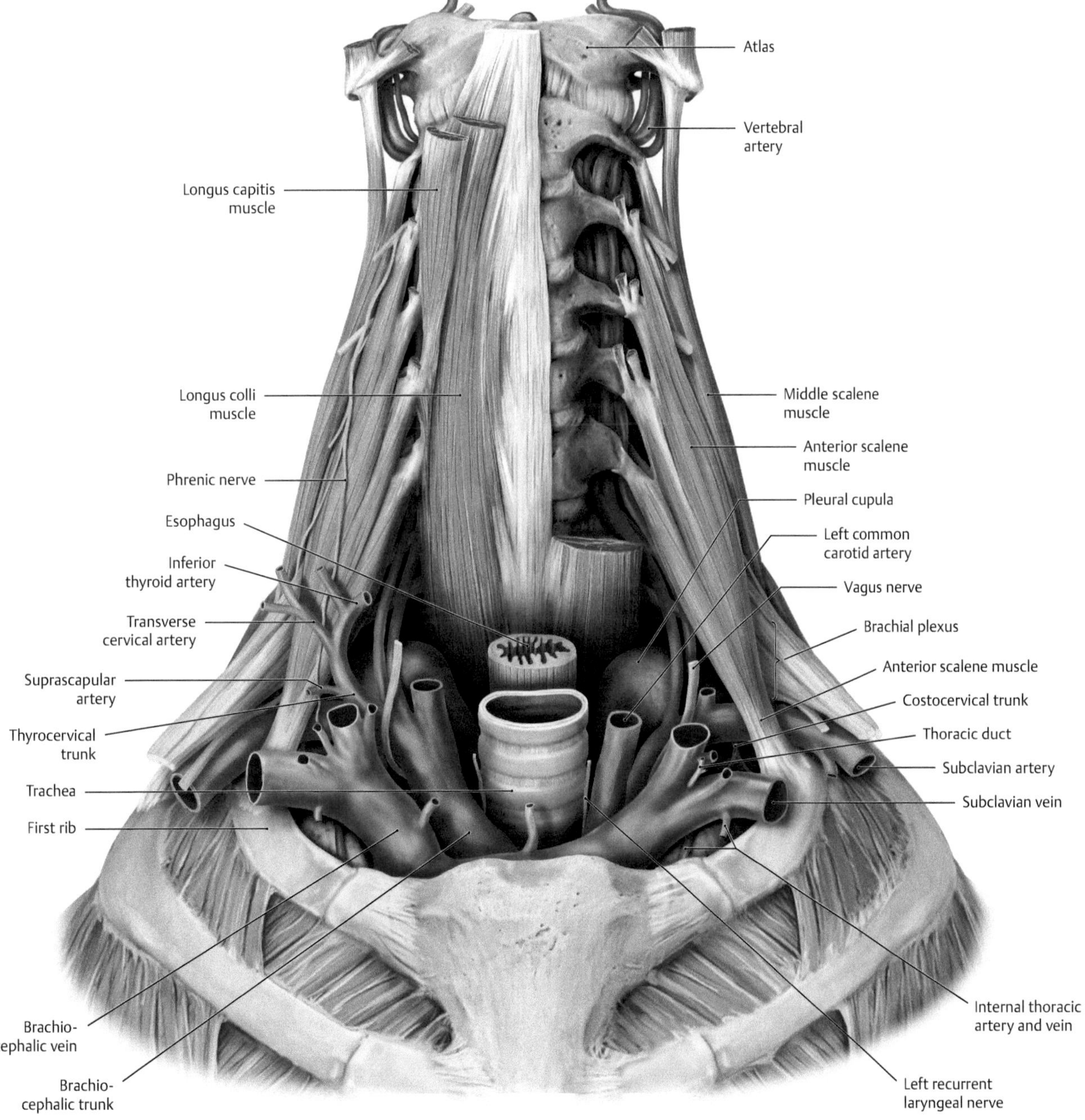

Fig. 7.161 Neurovasculature and muscles at the root of the neck. (From Schuenke M, Schulte E, Schumacher U. THIEME Atlas of Anatomy. Head, Neck, and Neuroanatomy. Illustrations by Voll M and Wesker K. 3rd ed. New York: Thieme Medical Publishers; 2020.)

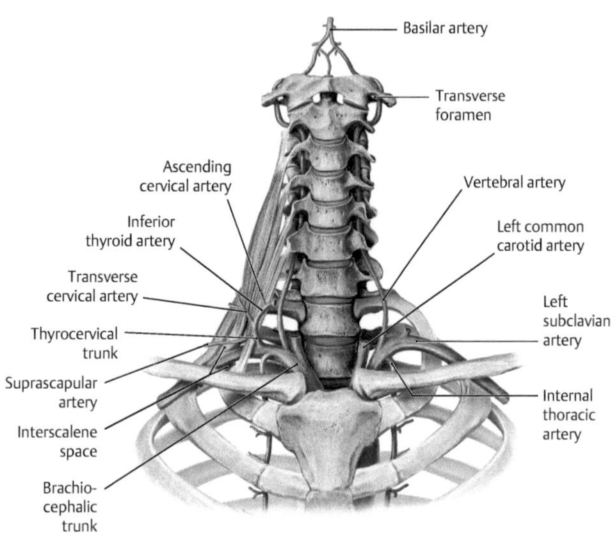

Fig. 7.162 Subclavian artery and its branches. (From Schuenke M, Schulte E, Schumacher U. THIEME Atlas of Anatomy. Head, Neck, and Neuroanatomy. Illustrations by Voll M and Wesker K. 3rd ed. New York: Thieme Medical Publishers; 2020.)

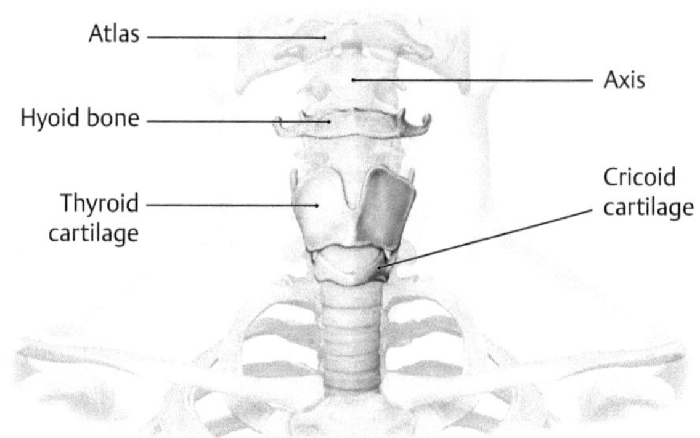

Fig. 7.163 Location of the larynx in the neck. (From Schuenke M, Schulte E, Schumacher U. THIEME Atlas of Anatomy. Head, Neck, and Neuroanatomy. Illustrations by Voll M and Wesker K. 3rd ed. New York: Thieme Medical Publishers; 2020.)

between the longus colli and anterior scalene muscles where its apex is near the *carotid tubercle* of the C6 vertebra.

2. The **vertebral part** passes deep near the pyramidal space apex to then course through the *transverse foramina* of the C1–C6 vertebrae.
3. After passing through the transverse foramina of the C1 vertebra, the **suboccipital part** of this artery rests on a groove located on the posterior arch of the C1 vertebra.
4. After passing through the foramen magnum it becomes the **cranial part**. These parts fuse superiorly to become the *basilar artery*.

- The **internal thoracic artery (Fig. 7.161; Fig. 7.162)** passes inferiorly through the thorax before lying on the parasternal edge of the anterior rig cage. It will bifurcate near the xiphoid process into the *musculophrenic* and *superior epigastric artery*.
- The **thyrocervical trunk** arises as a superior extension just above the internal thoracic artery and near the medial border of the anterior scalene muscle. It has three main branches **(Fig. 7.161; Fig. 7.162)**:

1. **Inferior thyroid artery**: the **ascending cervical artery** is normally a branch of the inferior thyroid but it is occasionally referred to as the fourth branch of the thyrocervical trunk.
2. **Suprascapular artery**: extends back into the posterior triangle of the neck and into the shoulder region.
3. **Transverse cervical artery**: supplies posterior triangle of the neck region. It has two of its own branches, the *superficial cervical* and *dorsal scapular*.

- The *second part of the subclavian artery* is located posterior to the anterior scalene and it has only one branch. The **costocervical trunk (Fig. 7.159)** bifurcates superiorly into the *deep cervical artery* and inferiorly as the *supreme intercostal artery*.
- The *third part of the subclavian artery* is located lateral to the anterior scalene and at the lateral border of the first rib becomes the axillary artery. This portion of the subclavian generally doesn't have any branches but in approximately 30% of the population, the *dorsal scapular artery* originates from here instead of the transverse cervical artery.

7.14.3 Veins of the Root

The *subclavian, external jugular (EJV), internal jugular (IJV),* and *anterior jugular veins* are the major veins of the root region. The **subclavian vein** is the continuation of the *axillary vein* and it begins at the lateral border of the first rib and will terminate after it unites with the IJV. Both the **EJV** and **IJV** drain into the subclavian vein. Where the subclavian and IJV meet, this is referred to as the **venous angle**. The left venous angle generally receives the *thoracic duct* while on the right it would receive the *right lymphatic trunk*. The **anterior jugular veins** arise near the hyoid bone and descend before passing posterior to the sternocleidomastoid muscle at the level of the root. They may drain either into the EJV or subclavian vein. Where both sides of the anterior jugular veins meet near the root is called the **jugular venous arch (Fig. 7.143; Fig. 7.161)**.

7.15 Larynx and Trachea

The **larynx** is an organ responsible for the protection of the airway and the production of sound (phonation). It is located anterior to the pharynx and between the C3–C6 vertebral levels. At vertebral level C6 the larynx continues as the **trachea (Fig. 7.163)**.

7.15.1 Laryngeal Skeleton

The outer shell of the larynx is known as the **laryngeal skeleton** and it is not made of bone but nine cartilages. The larger unpaired cartilages include the *thyroid, cricoid,* and *epiglottic cartilages* and the smaller paired cartilages include the *arytenoid, corniculate,* and *cuneiform cartilages* **(Fig. 7.164)**.

The **thyroid cartilage** is the largest of the laryngeal cartilages and functions mainly to protect the airway and also serves as the attachment sites for certain muscles (**Fig. 7.164**). It is actually a double, square-like laminae made of hyaline cartilage that is fused anteriorly. The anterior projection, which is most prominent in males, is known as the **laryngeal prominence** or *Adam's*

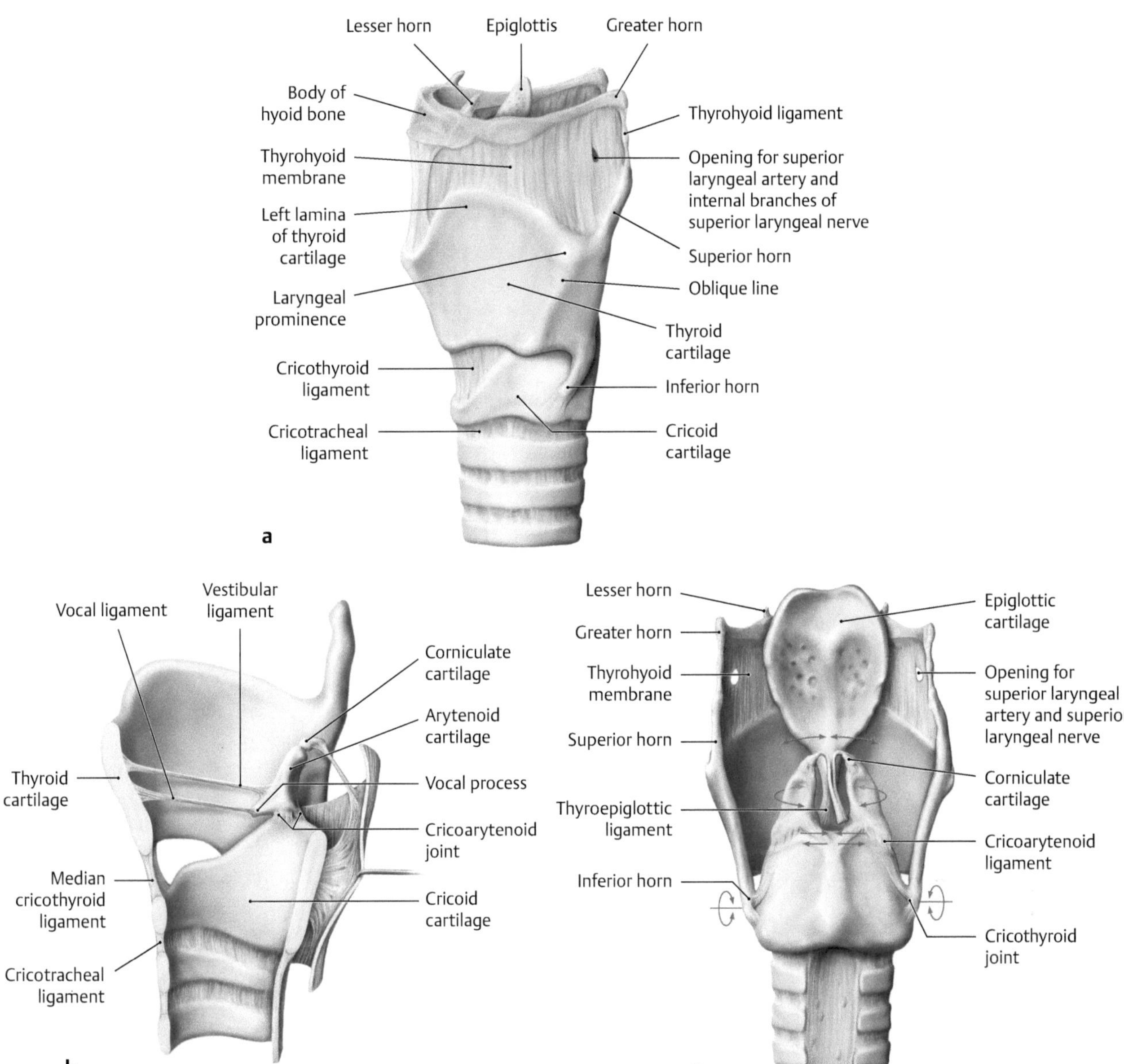

Fig. 7.164 Structure of the larynx. **(a)** Left anterior oblique view. **(b)** Sagittal section, viewed from the left medial aspect. **(c)** Posterior view. Arrows indicate the directions of movement in the various joints. (From Schuenke M, Schulte E, Schumacher U. THIEME Atlas of Anatomy. Head, Neck, and Neuroanatomy. Illustrations by Voll M and Wesker K. 3rd ed. New York: Thieme Medical Publishers; 2020.)

apple. Just above the laryngeal prominence is the V-shaped **superior thyroid notch**. The **oblique lines** are located on the lateral sides of the thyroid cartilage and serve as an attachment point for the *thyrohyoid*, *sternothyroid*, and *inferior constrictor muscles*. **Superior horns** and **inferior horns** are located on the posterior aspect of this cartilage. The superior horns are related to a smaller and not always present *triticeal cartilage* located near the tip of the greater horn of the hyoid bone. The inferior horn articulates with the cricoid cartilage and forms the **cricothyroid joint**. This is a synovial joint that allows for anteroposterior sliding and rotation movements that change the tension put on the *vocal ligaments* of the vocal folds.

The **cricoid cartilage** is a signet ring-shaped structure made of hyaline cartilage and it is the only laryngeal cartilage to encircle the entire airway. There is a steep incline from anterior to posterior and this leaves a space that is filled in with the *cricothyroid membrane*. This cartilage attaches to the thyroid cartilage by way of the **median cricothyroid ligament (cricothyroid membrane)**. It also attaches to the first tracheal ring by way of the **cricotracheal ligament (Fig. 7.164)**.

The **epiglottic cartilage** or just **epiglottis** is leaf-shaped and made of elastic cartilage (**Fig. 7.164**). It is situated anterior to the **laryngeal inlet** but posterior to the root of the tongue. The space or depressions located between the anterior epiglottis and root of the tongue are known as the **valleculae**. The **median** and **lateral glossoepiglottic folds** help delineate these depressions. The **hyoepiglottic ligament** attaches the hyoid bone to the anterior surface of the epiglottis. The inferior end of the epiglottis tapers off to form the *stalk of the epiglottis* and it attaches to the thyroid cartilage superior to the vocal ligament by way of the **thyroepiglottic**

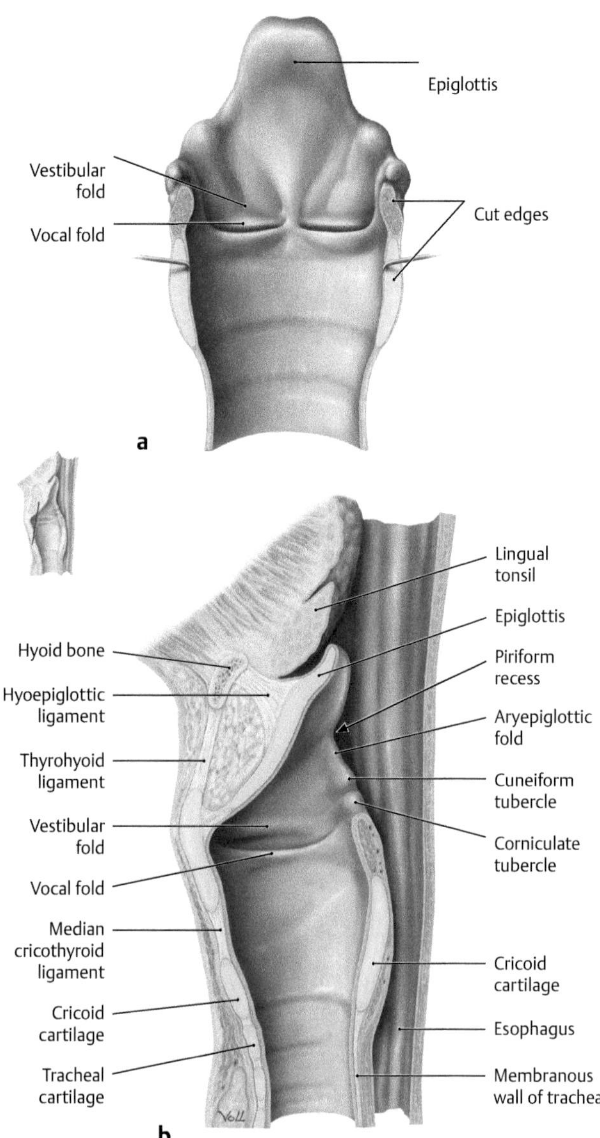

Fig. 7.165 Cavity of the larynx: mucosal surface anatomy and division into levels. **(a)** Posterior view. **(b)** Midsagittal section viewed from the left side. (From Schuenke M, Schulte E, Schumacher U. THIEME Atlas of Anatomy. Head, Neck, and Neuroanatomy. Illustrations by Voll M and Wesker K. 3rd ed. New York: Thieme Medical Publishers; 2020.)

ligament. The epiglottis functions primarily by folding down during swallowing, forcing food to enter the esophagus instead of the trachea.

The **arytenoid cartilages** (**Fig. 7.165; Fig. 7.166**) are pyramidal-shaped and made of hyaline cartilage. They consist of an *apex* superiorly, a *vocal process* anteriorly, and a *muscular process* laterally. The apex articulates with the corniculate cartilages while the vocal process articulates with the vocal ligament. An elastic **vocal ligament** is covered by mucosa and together constitutes the **vocal fold** or *true vocal cord* (**Fig. 7.165; Fig. 7.166; Fig. 7.167; Fig. 7.168**). The ligament spans from the vocal processes of the arytenoid cartilage to the internal surface of the thyroid cartilage approximately in the middle of the laryngeal prominence and inferior border of the thyroid cartilage. The arytenoids articulate with the posterior aspect of the cricoid cartilage forming the synovial **cricoarytenoid joint**. This joint allows for side-to-side sliding, rotation, and anterior/posterior tilting of the arytenoids, thus affecting the orientation of the vocal ligaments.

The smaller **corniculate (Fig. 7.166)** and **cuneiform cartilages** are both made of elastic cartilage. The corniculates are located at the apex of the arytenoids while the cuneiforms are located just lateral and superior to the corniculates within the aryepiglottic folds (**Fig. 7.165; Fig. 7.169**). Their functions are mostly structural support for the airway.

Located between these cartilages are membranes or fibroelastic tissue that add support to the overall structure of the larynx. These include the *thyrohyoid membrane*, *quadrangular membrane*, and the *conus elasticus*.

- **Thyrohyoid membrane**: will bind the inferior edges of the hyoid bone to the superior edges of the thyroid cartilage. The internal laryngeal nerve and superior laryngeal vessels penetrate it (**Fig. 7.164**).
- **Quadrangular membrane**: extends from the epiglottis to the arytenoid cartilages. The superior margin of this membrane forms the **aryepiglottic ligament** while the inferior margin constitutes the **vestibular ligament**. This ligament is covered with mucosa and combine to form the **vestibular fold** or *false vocal cords* (**Fig. 7.168**). There is minimal phonation produced by these ligaments, hence the term "false vocal cords." The vestibular folds are located just superior to the vocal folds.
- **Conus elasticus**: a combination of both *lateral cricothyroid ligaments* and *vocal ligaments*. The **lateral cricothyroid ligaments** extend superiorly and medially before meeting the vocal ligaments. It is the anterior most portion that attaches to both the thyroid cartilage and median cricothyroid ligament. This structure forms the roof of the infraglottic space (**Fig. 7.166; Fig. 7.167**).

The *internal laryngeal cavity*, which spans from the **laryngeal inlet** to the junction of the larynx and trachea, is divided into three main spaces with another located specifically between the vocal folds. These spaces are (**Fig. 7.167**):

- **Supraglottic space**: located between the laryngeal inlet and the vestibular folds.
- **Transglottic (ventricle) space**: located between the vestibular and vocal folds.
- **Infraglottic space**: located between the vocal folds and inferior border of the larynx.
- **Glottis**: is defined as the *vocal folds* plus the space or **rima glottidis** located between them. Note: the **rima vestibuli** (**Fig. 7.168**) is the space between the vestibular folds.

The **vocal folds** (true vocal cords) control phonation or the production of sound. Sound production is a combination of air passing by the vocal folds causing them to vibrate along with the laryngeal muscles adjusting the tension and length of the vocal ligaments resulting in pitch and quality control. Sounds can also be fine-tuned by the openness of the nasal passages, tongue, lips, and palate and with the onset of puberty especially in a male. The vocal folds lie inferior to the vestibular folds and slightly medial to them. The mucous membrane of the vocal fold overlies the vocal ligaments and these ligaments attach to the arytenoid and thyroid cartilages. The vocal folds also contain the *vocalis* and *thyroarytenoid muscles* (**Fig. 7.168**).

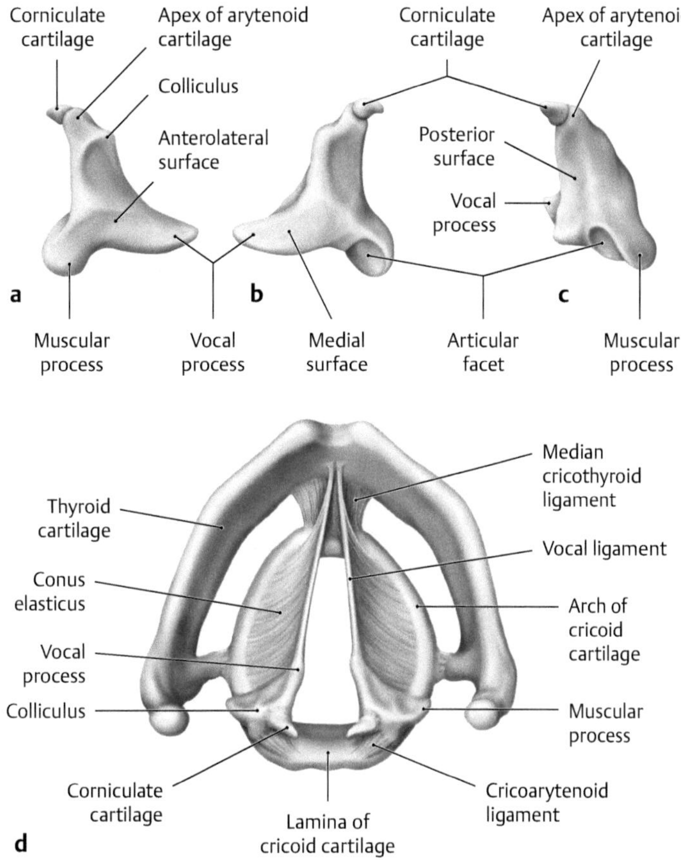

Fig. 7.166 Arytenoid and corniculate cartilages. **(a)** Right lateral view. **(b)** Medial view. **(c)** Posterior view. **(d)** Superior view. (From Schuenke M, Schulte E, Schumacher U. THIEME Atlas of Anatomy. Head, Neck, and Neuroanatomy. Illustrations by Voll M and Wesker K. 3rd ed. New York: Thieme Medical Publishers; 2020.)

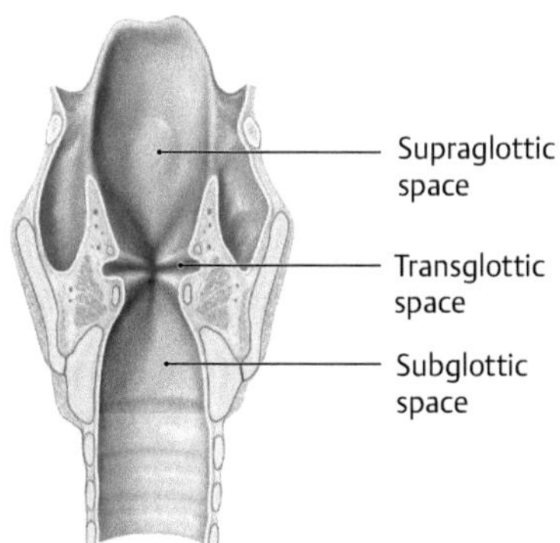

Fig. 7.167 Levels of the larynx and their boundaries, posterior view. (From Schuenke M, Schulte E, Schumacher U. THIEME Atlas of Anatomy. Head, Neck, and Neuroanatomy. Illustrations by Voll M and Wesker K. 3rd ed. New York: Thieme Medical Publishers; 2020.)

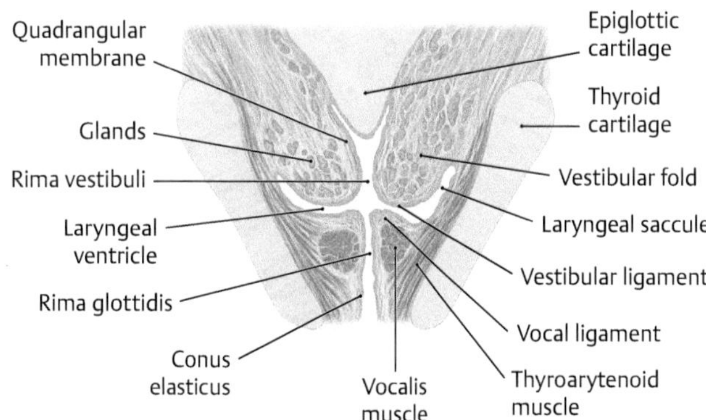

Fig. 7.168 Vestibular folds and vocal folds, coronal section. (From Schuenke M, Schulte E, Schumacher U. THIEME Atlas of Anatomy. Head, Neck, and Neuroanatomy. Illustrations by Voll M and Wesker K. 3rd ed. New York: Thieme Medical Publishers; 2020.)

7.15.2 Laryngeal Muscles

The muscles that act on the larynx are described as being either extrinsic or intrinsic. **Extrinsic laryngeal muscles** move the larynx as a complete structure often during speaking and swallowing. These muscles include the suprahyoid and infrahyoid muscle groups. The **intrinsic laryngeal muscles** (**Table 7.11**) act directly on the vocal folds and size of the rima glottidis. The *inferior laryngeal nerves* innervate all of these muscles except for the cricothyroid, which is innervated by the *external laryngeal nerves* (**Fig. 7.169**).

The **vocalis muscles** are located medial to the **thyroarytenoid muscles** and both serve to primarily relax the vocal ligaments, thus lowering the pitch of the voice. The **cricothyroid muscle** is the only intrinsic muscle located externally and not under a mucosal layer. It functions to tense the vocal ligaments by tilting the laryngeal prominence anteriorly and inferiorly toward the cricoid cartilage to raise the pitch (**Fig. 7.169**).

The **lateral cricoarytenoid**, **oblique arytenoid,** and **transverse arytenoid muscles** function by adducting the vocal ligaments. The

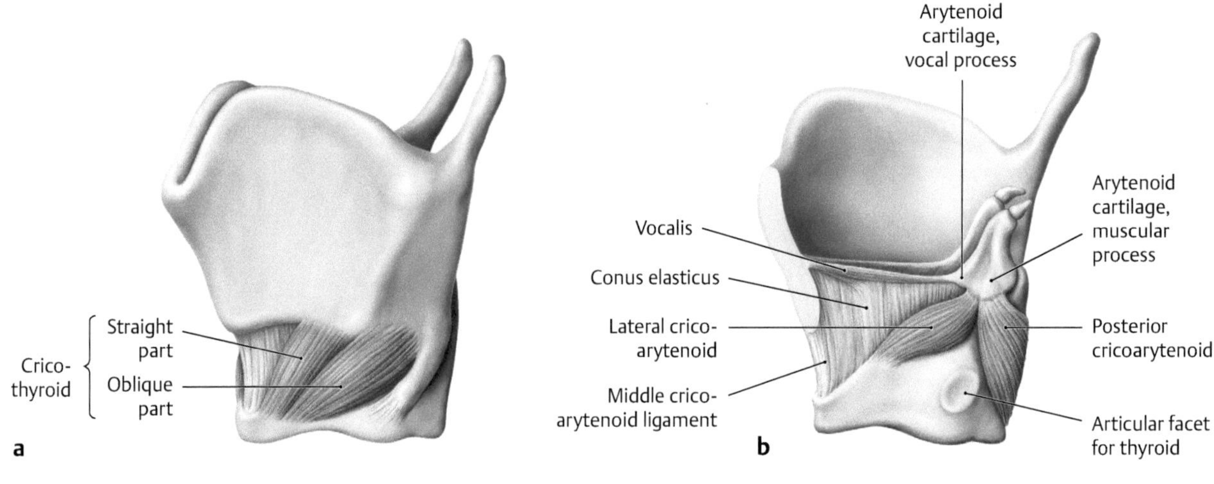

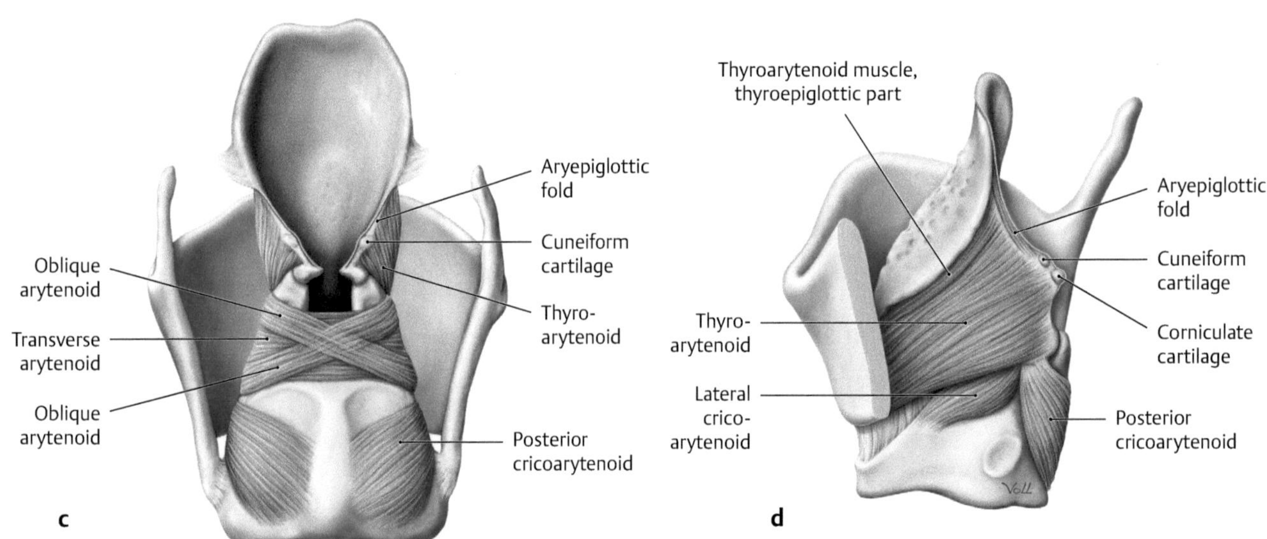

Fig. 7.169 Muscles of the larynx. **(a)** Left lateral oblique view. **(b)** Left lateral view with the epiglottis and left half of the thyroid cartilage removed. **(c)** Posterior view. **(d)** Left lateral view with left half of the thyroid cartilage removed. (From Schuenke M, Schulte E, Schumacher U. THIEME Atlas of Anatomy. Head, Neck, and Neuroanatomy. Illustrations by Voll M and Wesker K. 3rd ed. New York: Thieme Medical Publishers; 2020.)

Table 7.11 **Intrinsic laryngeal muscles**

Muscle	Innervation	Function(s)	Origin	Insertion
Vocalis	Inferior laryngeal nerve	Relax posterior portion of vocal ligament while tensing anterior portion	Lateral surface of vocal process on arytenoid cartilage	Ipsilateral vocal ligament
Thyroarytenoid	Inferior laryngeal nerve	Relax vocal ligament	Posterior aspect of thyroid laminae near the median cricothyroid ligament	Anterolateral surface of the arytenoid cartilage
Cricothyroid	External laryngeal nerve	Tenses vocal ligament	Anterolateral portion of cricoid cartilage	Inferior margin and horn of thyroid cartilage
Lateral cricoarytenoid	Inferior laryngeal nerve	Adduct vocal ligament	Arch of the cricoid cartilage	Vocal processes of the arytenoid cartilages
Oblique and transverse arytenoids	Inferior laryngeal nerve	Adduct vocal ligament	Arytenoid cartilage	Contralateral arytenoid cartilage; oblique bellies will then extend superiorly to form the aryepiglottic muscles
Posterior cricoarytenoid	Inferior laryngeal nerve	Abduct vocal ligament	Posterior surface of cricoid cartilage	Vocal processes of the arytenoid cartilages

lateral cricoarytenoids rotate the arytenoid cartilages medially creating adduction of the vocal ligaments. The oblique and transverse arytenoids adduct the vocal ligaments by sliding the arytenoid cartilages toward the midline. Adducting the vocal ligaments can lead to whispering. The **posterior cricoarytenoid muscles** are the only muscles that abduct the vocal ligaments. They do this by rotating the arytenoid cartilages laterally, leading to abduction of the vocal ligaments and widening of the rima glottidis. This would be seen in forced respiration (**Fig. 7.169; Fig. 7.179**).

The lateral cricoarytenoid, oblique arytenoid, and transverse arytenoid muscles along with the **aryepiglottic muscles** can act as a sphincter in order to close the laryngeal inlet. This sphincter-like action is more reflexive in nature and in response to liquid or food particles in or near the supraglottic space (**Fig. 7.169**). Intrinsic laryngeal muscles are detailed in **Table 7.11**.

7.15.3 Neurovasculature of the Larynx

Innervation of the mucosa can be divided into a superior versus inferior half by way of the vocal folds. The **internal laryngeal nerves** innervate the superior half while the combination of the **recurrent/inferior laryngeal nerves** supply the inferior half. All of these nerves carry GVE-para/pre fibers before synapsing at submucosal ganglion and are paired with GVA fibers.

Innervation to the laryngeal muscles is primarily from the **inferior laryngeal nerves** that are terminal branches of the **recurrent laryngeal nerves**. The **external laryngeal nerve**, a branch of the superior laryngeal nerve, innervates the cricothyroid muscle. After passing through the tracheoesophageal groove the recurrent laryngeal nerves terminate prior to the laryngeal muscles as the inferior laryngeal nerves. The functional components of the recurrent/inferior laryngeal nerves are SVE/BM, GSA, GVE-para/pre, and GVA while the external laryngeal nerve has only SVE/BM and GSA fibers (**Fig. 7.170**).

Blood supply to the larynx is primarily from the **superior laryngeal** (superior thyroid br.) and the **inferior laryngeal arteries** (inferior thyroid br.). The superior laryngeal vessels are paired with the *internal laryngeal nerves* while the inferior laryngeal vessels are paired with the *recurrent laryngeal nerves*. Venous drainage of the superior one-half of the larynx passes first through the **superior laryngeal vein**, followed by the **superior thyroid vein**, before reaching the **IJV**. The venous drainage of the inferior one-half passes first through the **inferior laryngeal vein** before reaching the **inferior thyroid vein**. The inferior thyroid vein will then drain directly into one of the **brachiocephalic veins** (**Fig. 7.170**).

Lymphatic drainage of the superior one-half of the larynx is to the **prelaryngeal lymph nodes** before reaching the **superior deep cervical lymph nodes**. Lymphatic drainage of the inferior one-half is primarily to the **pretracheal** and **paratracheal lymph nodes** before reaching the **inferior deep cervical lymph nodes**. The vocal folds are devoid of lymphatics, and it serves as the demarcation between the superior and inferior halves of the laryngeal lymphatic drainage.

7.15.4 Histology of the Larynx

As mentioned previously the thyroid, cricoid, and arytenoid cartilages of the larynx are made of *hyaline cartilage*. The corniculate, cuneiform, and epiglottic cartilages are made of *elastic cartilage*. The mucosa of the larynx is mostly covered with the typical respiratory epithelium or *pseudostratified ciliated columnar epithelium* with a few exceptions. The anterior portion of the epiglottis facing the oral cavity and the vocal folds (true vocal cords) are lined with a *stratified squamous epithelium* (**Fig. 7.171**).

Clinical Correlate 7.43

Laryngitis

Inflammation and swelling of the larynx is called laryngitis. It may occur due to an allergic, bacterial, viral, or chemical reaction. The most common causes are a generalized upper respiratory tract infection and exposure to environmental toxins such as cigarette smoke. Although the infection generally resolves itself without medical treatment, the disorder may cause airway obstruction in infants and children. Examination of the airway may reveal edema and erythema of the vocal folds and irregularities on the surfaces of the vocal folds.

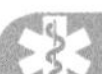

Clinical Correlate 7.44

Vocal Fold/Cord Nodules

Vocal fold/cord nodules or polyps are chronic lesions or masses of tissue that grow on the vocal folds. These lesions typically appear as symmetrical swellings on both sides of the vocal cords near the point of maximum contact that is at the border of the anterior one-third and posterior two-thirds of the vocal ligament. Vocal fold nodules are most commonly seen in individuals who have poor singing techniques ("singer's nodes") or in heavy smokers. Initially the trauma may only include subepithelial hemorrhaging or bruising but later become more pathological in nature.

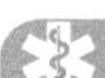

Clinical Correlate 7.45

Laryngoscopy

The interior of the larynx can be viewed through a procedure known as **laryngoscopy**. There are two different versions, an indirect or direct approach. **Indirect laryngoscopy** uses a laryngeal mirror to view the larynx (**Fig. 7.173; Fig. 7.174**). The tongue is generally protracted in order to minimize the blocked view of the epiglottis and laryngeal inlet by the posterior tongue. **Direct laryngoscopy** involves the use of a **laryngoscope**, a flexible fiber optic endoscope equipped with lighting for examining or operating on the internal larynx. Both the vestibular and vocal folds are visible during laryngoscopy primarily because the rima vestibuli between the vestibular folds is naturally larger allowing for a clearer view of the vocal folds. The vestibular folds normally appear pink while the vocal folds have a more white-like appearance.

7.15.5 Histology of the Trachea

The **trachea** is a fibrocartilaginous tube that begins at vertebral level C6 and is connected to the larynx. It will descend into the thorax before bifurcating at vertebral level T4/T5 to become the left and right main bronchi. It primarily functions as the conduit for air traveling to and from the lungs. There are 16 to 20 C-shaped rings made of hyaline cartilage that support and maintain a patent airway leading to the lungs. The posterior portion of the trachea is the area displaying a gap in tracheal ring positioning. These gaps contain the smooth muscle known as the **trachealis muscle**. The epithelium is made of a *pseudostratified ciliated columnar epithelium* containing goblet cells (**Fig. 7.172**).

Clinical Correlate 7.46

Tracheostomy and Cricothyrotomy

In the case of respiratory failure or an upper airway obstruction, a **tracheostomy** can provide an air passage to help an individual breathe when the usual route is obstructed or impaired. A tracheostomy is often needed when health problems require long-term use of a ventilator machine to help a person breathe or in an emergency situation that involves trauma especially to the neck if the airway is suddenly blocked. A **tracheotomy** is the surgical procedure used to create the opening or tracheostomy. After a midline incision is made between the laryngeal prominence (Adam's apple) and near the sternal notch, the infrahyoid muscles are retracted and the thyroid gland is divided in half allowing full access to the trachea. An opening generally between the first and second tracheal rings is formed and a tracheostomy tube is then inserted.

A **cricothyrotomy** establishes an airway generally in an emergency situation. A midline incision is made just below the level of the laryngeal prominence and eventually through the cricothyroid membrane before a tracheostomy or endotracheal tube is inserted. These are meant to be short term before they are replaced with a tracheotomy.

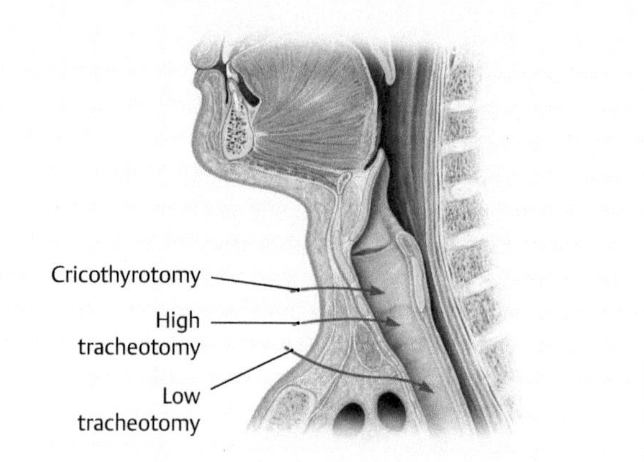

(From Schuenke M, Schulte E, Schumacher U. THIEME Atlas of Anatomy. Head, Neck, and Neuroanatomy. Illustrations by Voll M and Wesker K. 3rd ed. New York: Thieme Medical Publishers; 2020.)

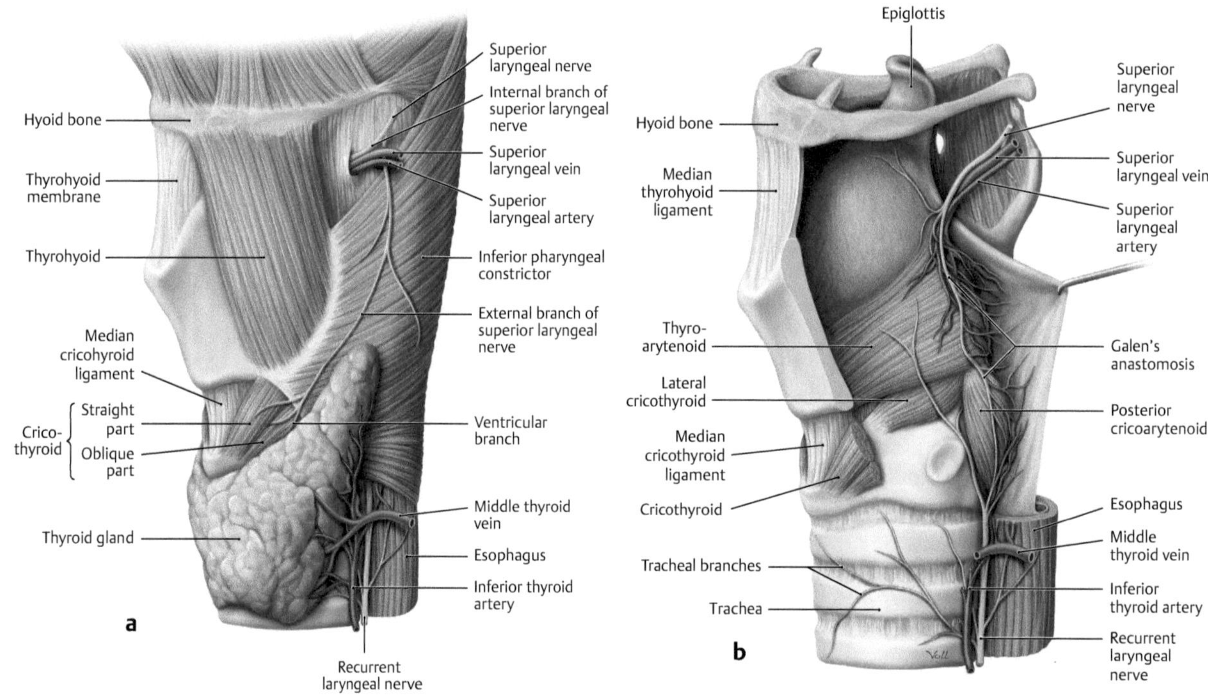

Fig. 7.170 Neurovasculature of the larynx, left lateral view. **(a)** Superficial layer. **(b)** Deep layer. (From Schuenke M, Schulte E, Schumacher U. THIEME Atlas of Anatomy. Head, Neck, and Neuroanatomy. Illustrations by Voll M and Wesker K. 3rd ed. New York: Thieme Medical Publishers; 2020.)

7.16 Pharynx and the Cervical Region of the Esophagus

The region located posterior to both the nasal and oral cavities is known as the pharynx. It is one of the earliest portions of the GI tract that will continue posterior to the larynx before becoming the cervical portion of the esophagus at vertebral level C6. It allows for the passage of both air and food and is divided into three parts: the *nasopharynx*, *oropharynx*, and *laryngopharynx* (**Fig. 7.175**).

- **Nasopharynx**: this part is located posterior to the **choanae**, paired openings that lead from the nasal cavity to the nasopharynx, and superior to the level of the soft palate. It serves as the posterior extension of the nasal cavity and this is evident due to its respiratory-like *pseudostratified columnar epithelium*. The opening of the *pharyngotympanic (auditory or Eustachian) tube* is evident and has a superior border formed by the *torus tubarius*. The **salpingopharyngeal fold** extends inferiorly from the pharyngotympanic tube and contains the *salpingopharyngeus muscle*. The **pharyngeal tonsils** are found in the

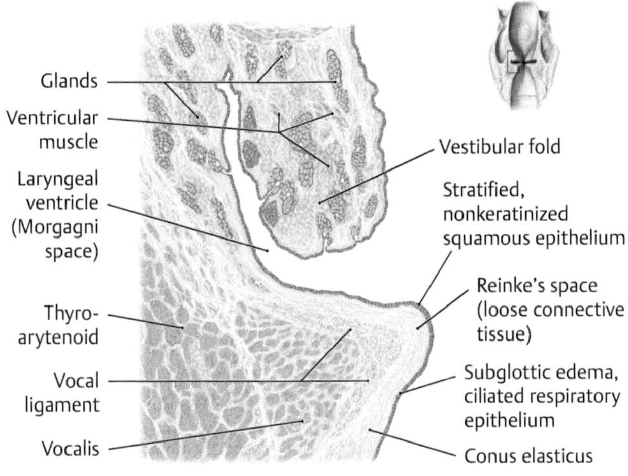

Fig. 7.171 Schematic coronal histological section of the vocal fold, posterior view. (From Schuenke M, Schulte E, Schumacher U. THIEME Atlas of Anatomy. Head, Neck, and Neuroanatomy. Illustrations by Voll M and Wesker K. 3rd ed. New York: Thieme Medical Publishers; 2020.)

mucosa superior and posterior to the opening of the pharyngotympanic tube and the **tubal tonsils** are located on the torus tubarius (**Fig. 7.176**).

- **Oropharynx**: this part is located posterior to the oral cavity and extends from the border of the soft palate to the superior border of the epiglottis. The epithelium must deal with abrasive food boluses passing against it and thus made up of *stratified squamous epithelium*. The **palatine tonsil** lies within the *tonsillar sinus* positioned between the **palatoglossal** and **palatopharyngeal arches** on both the left and right side of the oropharynx (**Fig. 7.177**).
- **Laryngopharynx** (hypopharynx): this part is located from the superior border of the epiglottis to the C6 vertebral level where the pharynx ends and the esophagus begins. It rests posterior to the larynx and serves as the conduit for a food bolus to travel toward the esophagus. For reasons similar to the oropharynx, this mucosa is made up of *stratified squamous epithelium*. The *laryngeal inlet* represents the communication between the larynx and laryngopharynx while the small depression located between the laryngopharynx and the lateral portion of the larynx is known as the **piriform recess**.

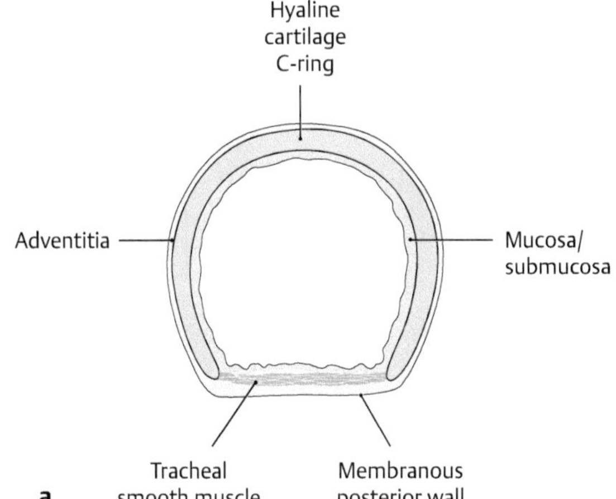

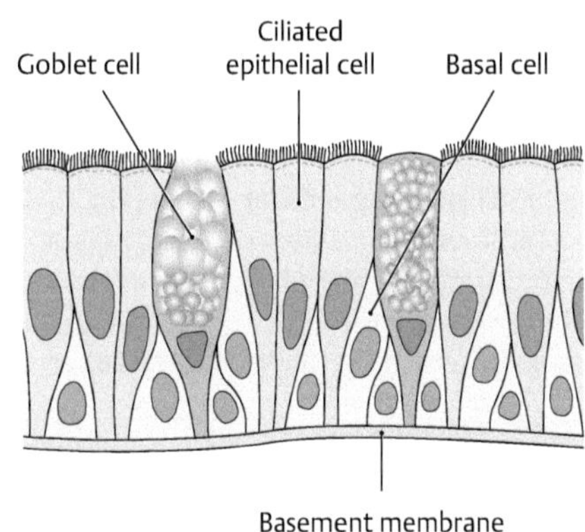

Fig. 7.172 **(a)** Histological organization of the wall of the trachea. **(b)** Tracheal epithelium. (From Schuenke M, Schulte E, Schumacher U. THIEME Atlas of Anatomy. Internal Organs. Illustrations by Voll M and Wesker K. 3rd ed. New York: Thieme Medical Publishers; 2020.)

Clinical Correlate 7.47

Laryngeal Nerve Blocks and Injury

When an endotracheal intubation in a conscious person must be done, a **superior laryngeal nerve block** can be employed. If the needle is inserted halfway between the hyoid bone and thyroid cartilage and anterior to the posterior tip of the greater horn of the hyoid, this nerve block technically targets the **internal laryngeal nerve branch** of the larger superior laryngeal nerve. The anesthesia will block the innervation of the mucosa above the vocal folds, posterior tongue, and near the epiglottis. A **recurrent laryngeal nerve block** can anesthetize the laryngeal mucosa below the vocal folds. The procedure is done (translaryngeal) by inserting a needle through the cricothyroid membrane until air is aspirated. After withdrawing the needle a catheter is left in its place. Coughing is induced after the anesthetic is injected, thus further scattering it and only affecting sensory innervation. No motor innervation of the laryngeal muscles is effected. Generally, these nerve blocks are done together since multiple nerves innervate the mucosa of the larynx. On occasion, the glossopharyngeal nerve may also be blocked near the palatoglossal arch.

Injury to the recurrent laryngeal nerves can occur during neck surgery and more often when the procedure takes place near the thyroid gland. The left recurrent laryngeal is more vertical unlike the right recurrent laryngeal nerve that extends back up toward the larynx at an angle after wrapping around the right subclavian artery. It is closely related to the inferior thyroid artery so ligation of the artery prior to reaching the level of the nerve may be done to preserve the nerve. Abduction movements of the vocal folds and thus having continuously opened airway were thought at one time to be the most greatly affected by injury to a recurrent laryngeal nerve but the axons destined for the intrinsic laryngeal muscles are randomly distributed. Unilateral injury usually results in a hoarse sounding voice that may return to normal over time. Difficulty with phonation or voice production (aphonia) including laryngeal spasms can occur.

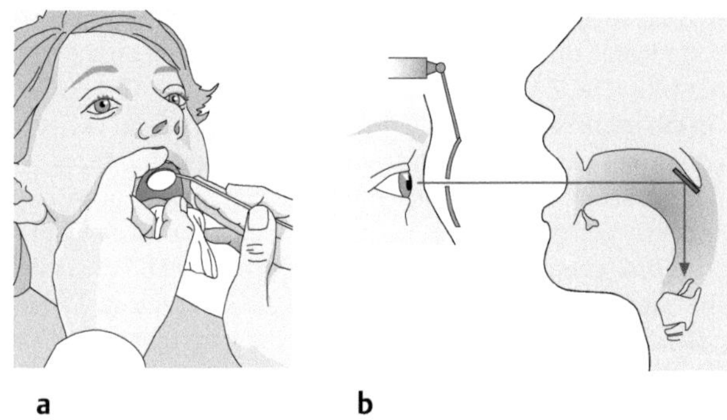

Fig. 7.173 Indirect laryngoscopy. **(a)** Mirror examination of the larynx. **(b)** Optical path. (From Schuenke M, Schulte E, Schumacher U. THIEME Atlas of Anatomy. Head, Neck, and Neuroanatomy. Illustrations by Voll M and Wesker K. 3rd ed. New York: Thieme Medical Publishers; 2020.)

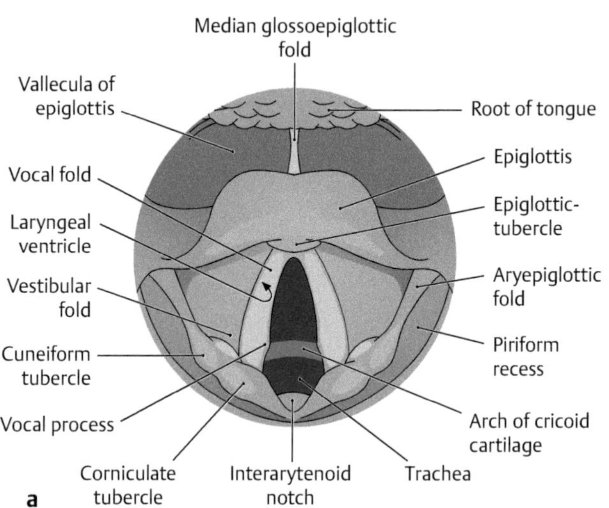

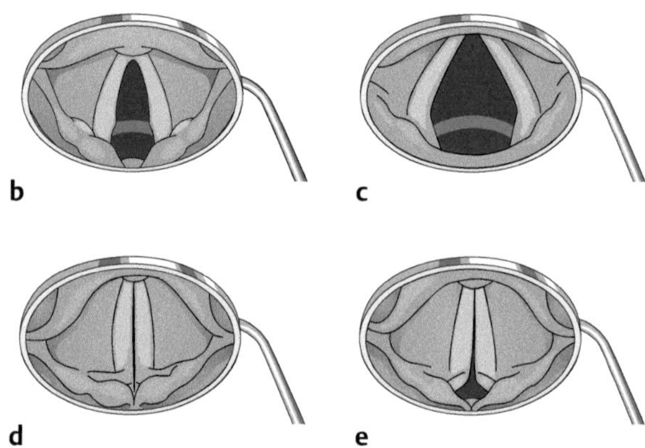

Fig. 7.174 Appearance of the larynx on indirect laryngoscopy. **(a)** Depiction of the laryngoscopic mirror image. **(b)** Rima glottidis during normal respiration. **(c)** Rima glottidis during vigorous respiration. **(d)** Vocal folds completely adducted. **(e)** Slightly abducted vocal folds during whispered speech. (From Schuenke M, Schulte E, Schumacher U. THIEME Atlas of Anatomy. Head, Neck, and Neuroanatomy. Illustrations by Voll M and Wesker K. 3rd ed. New York: Thieme Medical Publishers; 2020.)

7.16.1 Muscles of the Pharynx

The pharynx is made up of skeletal muscles orientated in either a circular or longitudinal fashion. The circular layer is external to the more internal longitudinal layer of musculature. The circular layer consists of the **superior**, **middle**, and **inferior pharyngeal constrictor muscles.** The longitudinal layer is made up of the **palatopharyngeus, salpingopharyngeus**, and **stylopharyngeus muscles (Fig. 7.177; Fig. 7.178; Fig. 7.179)**. Muscles of the pharynx are detailed in **Table 7.12**.

The pharyngeal muscles are lined by supporting fascia consisting of a strong internal **pharyngobasilar fascia (Fig. 7.178)** just deep to the mucosal layer and a thinner externally placed **buccopharyngeal fascia** containing the **pharyngeal nervous plexus.** The orientation of the constrictor muscles creates four gaps that allow for the passage of certain structures **(Fig. 7.178)**.

- Gap #1: located between the cranium and superior constrictor muscle, the ascending palatine artery, levator veli palatini muscle, and pharyngotympanic tube pass through this gap. This gap is primarily filled by the pharyngobasilar fascia that helps form the pharyngeal recess.
- Gap #2: located between the superior and middle constrictor muscles and allows for the passage of the glossopharyngeal nerve, stylopharyngeus muscle, and stylohyoid ligament.
- Gap #3: located between middle and inferior constrictor muscles and allows for the passage of the internal laryngeal nerve and superior laryngeal vessels.
- Gap #4: located inferior to the inferior constrictor muscles and allows for the passage of the recurrent laryngeal nerve and inferior laryngeal vessels.

7.16.2 Neurovasculature of Pharynx

The **pharyngeal plexus** is made up of the pharyngeal branches of both the glossopharyngeal and vagus nerves along with sympathetic postganglionic fibers originating from the superior cervical ganglion. The plexus lies within the buccopharyngeal fascia primarily at the level of the middle pharyngeal constrictor muscle. The plexus supplies most of the soft palate and pharynx muscles. The exceptions include the tensor veli palatini muscle (supplied by CN V_3) of the soft palate and the stylopharyngeus muscle (supplied by CN IX) of the pharynx. In addition, this plexus supplies all of the pharyngeal mucosa except for the anterosuperior portion of the nasopharynx **(Fig. 7.180)**.

Sympathetic fibers supply the blood vessels whereas the parasympathetic fibers associated with the vagus nerve innervate the mucosal glands. The branchiomotor (BM) fibers that pass through the vagus nerve technically innervate the majority of the soft palate and pharynx muscles. Somatic sensory information from the inferior portion of the nasopharynx along with all of the oropharynx passes back through the glossopharyngeal nerve. It is visceral sensory information that comes from the laryngopharynx but it passes back through with the vagus nerve. Note there is considerable overlap between the somatic and visceral sensory innervation of the pharyngeal mucosa. The mucosa of the anterosuperior portion of the nasopharynx receives autonomic fibers that originally passed through the pterygopalatine ganglion. The parasympathetic fibers are associated with the facial nerve while the sympathetic fibers originated from the deep petrosal nerve. The sensory innervation to this portion of the nasopharynx is somatic in nature and passes back through the maxillary nerve (V_2) **(Fig. 7.181)**.

The **swallowing pattern generator (SPG)** is located in the brainstem and is responsible for the timing of striated muscle

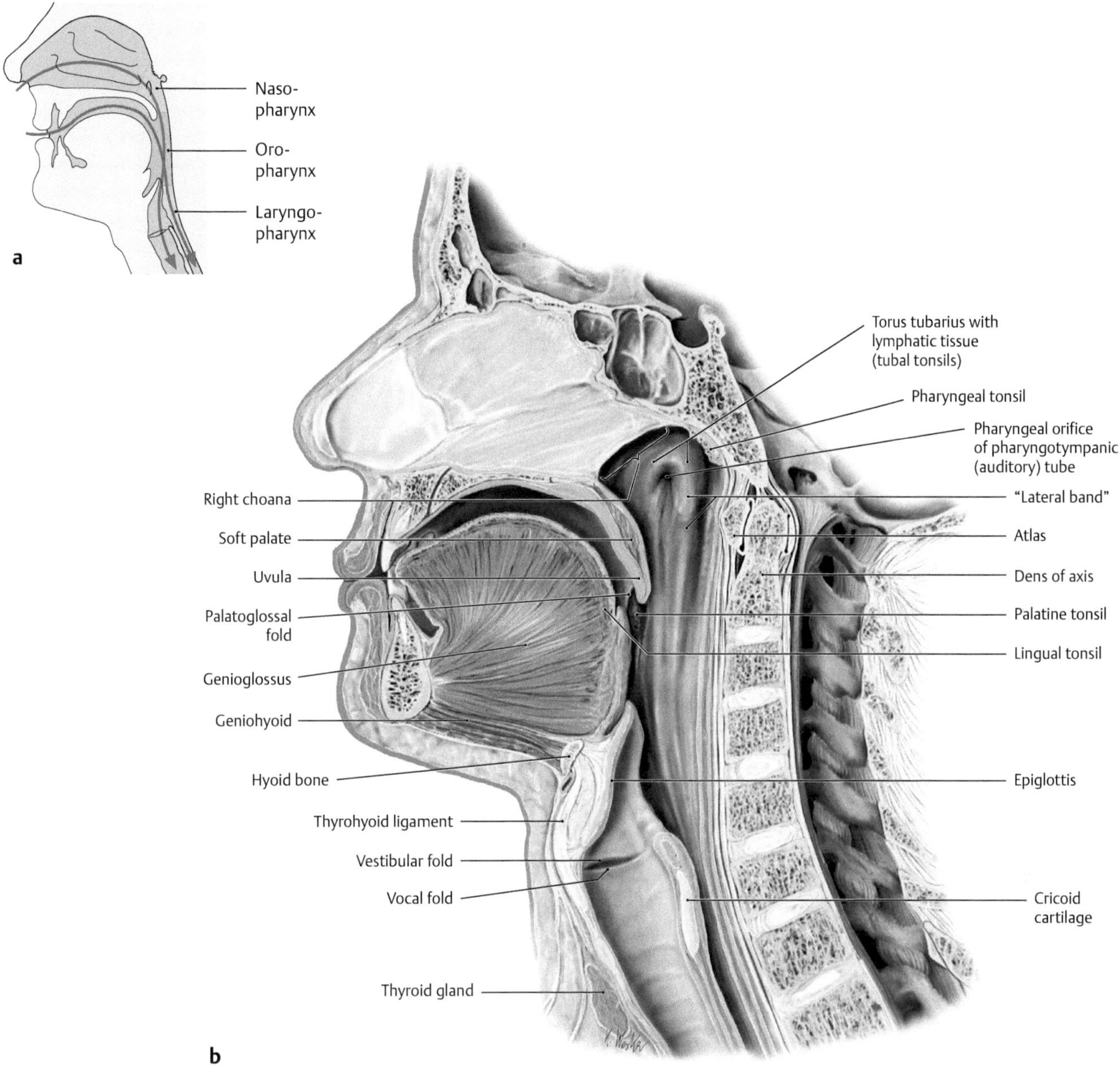

Fig. 7.175 Topographical anatomy of the pharynx. **(a)** Organization of the pharynx. **(b)** Midsagittal section, left lateral view. (From Schuenke M, Schulte E, Schumacher U. THIEME Atlas of Anatomy. Head, Neck, and Neuroanatomy. Illustrations by Voll M and Wesker K. 3rd ed. New York: Thieme Medical Publishers; 2020.)

contraction during swallowing. The SPG is made up of several brainstem nuclei and two different groups of interneurons located in the dorsal and ventral parts of the medulla known as the dorsal (DSG) and ventral swallowing groups (VSG), respectively. The DSG contains neurons responsible for generating the swallowing pattern while the VSG contains neurons that distribute swallowing activation to motor neurons in the trigeminal, facial, nucleus ambiguus, and hypoglossal brainstem nuclei **(Fig. 7.182)**.

Blood supply is from the **ascending pharyngeal** (external carotid br.), **ascending palatine** (facial br.), and smaller branches of the **lingual** (external carotid br.) and **pharyngeal artery branches** (inferior thyroid br.) **(Fig. 7.180)**.

Venous drainage follows the **pterygoid venous plexus**, **facial**, and **internal jugular veins**. Lymphatic drainage can involve the **retropharyngeal** and **paratracheal lymph nodes** before reaching the **superior deep cervical lymph nodes** or they may just drain directly to the **superior deep cervical lymph nodes**.

7.16.3 Histology of the Pharynx

Due to the pharynx connecting to two different regions, the nasal and oral cavities, the epithelium differs. The nasopharynx is lined by a *pseudostratified ciliated columnar epithelium containing goblet cells* of which the pharyngeal and tubal tonsils located in this region are also lined with this epithelium. The oropharynx and laryngopharynx along with the palatine tonsils are lined by a *stratified squamous epithelium*. The lamina propria and connective tissue will be surrounded by circular and longitudinally orientated skeletal muscle.

7.16.4 Cervical Region of the Esophagus

The **cervical region of the esophagus** begins posterior to the inferior border of the cricoid cartilage at vertebral level C6. This is also the location of the **cricopharyngeus muscle** that serves

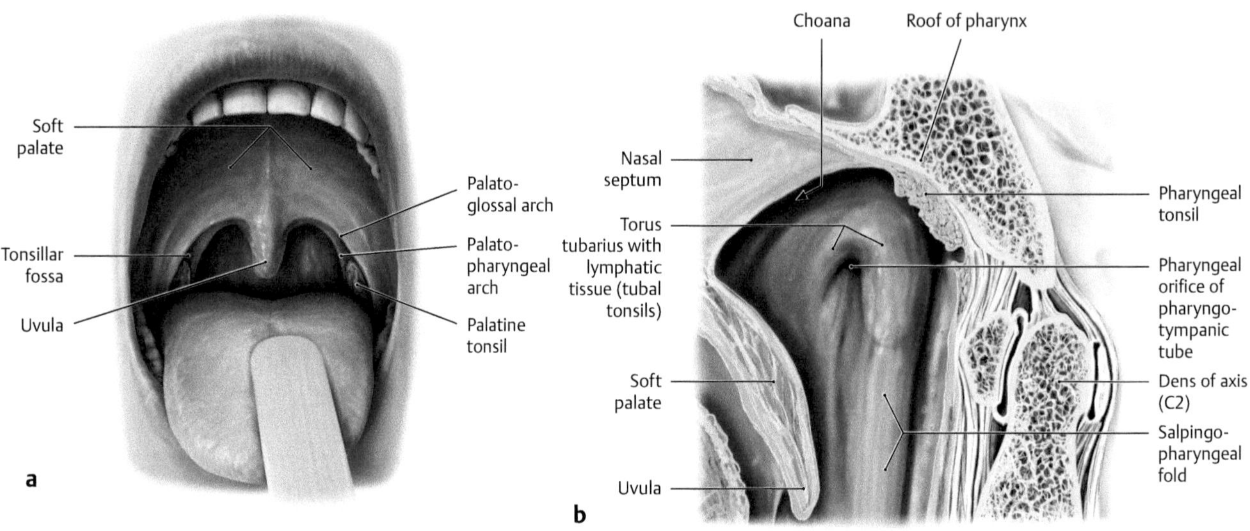

Fig. 7.176 **(a)** Anterior view of the oral cavity. **(b)** Sagittal section through the nasopharynx. (From Schuenke M, Schulte E, Schumacher U. THIEME Atlas of Anatomy. Head, Neck, and Neuroanatomy. Illustrations by Voll M and Wesker K. 3rd ed. New York: Thieme Medical Publishers; 2020.)

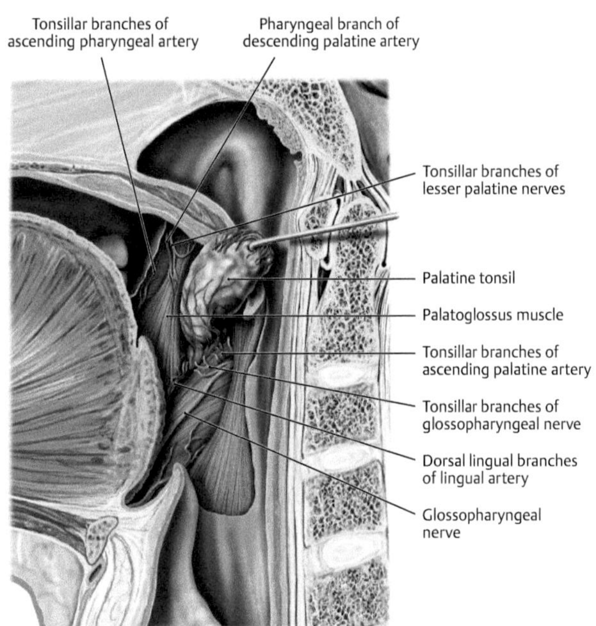

Fig. 7.177 Vascular and nerve supply of the palatine tonsil within the oropharynx. (From Schuenke M, Schulte E, Schumacher U. THIEME Atlas of Anatomy. Head, Neck, and Neuroanatomy. Illustrations by Voll M and Wesker K. 3rd ed. New York: Thieme Medical Publishers; 2020.)

as the upper esophageal sphincter (UES) and relaxes during swallowing but contracts when there is no swallowing taking place **(Fig. 7.183)**. The cervical region, much like the rest of the esophagus, has a ***stratified squamous epithelium*** but the muscularis externa layer is primarily made of skeletal muscle unlike the rest of the esophagus.

7.16.5 Neurovasculature of the Cervical Esophagus

Branchiomotor fibers (BM) passing through the recurrent laryngeal nerves innervate the skeletal muscle while the smooth muscle is innervated by parasympathetic fibers originating from the vagus nerve. Sympathetic fibers then innervate the blood vessels. Blood supply and venous drainage are associated with the **inferior thyroid vessels**. Lymphatic drainage is to the **paratracheal** and **deep cervical lymph nodes**.

7.17 The Process of Deglutition (Swallowing)

Deglutition is a complex but mainly involuntary process involving the transfer of a food/liquid bolus from the mouth to the stomach and it involves three stages (**Fig. 7.184**).

Clinical Correlate 7.48

Pharyngeal (Gag) Reflex

The gag reflex is triggered when an unusually large food bolus or object reaches the back of the mouth. It results in a quick elevation of the soft palate to close off the upper airway, closure of the glottis to seal off the lower airway, and bilateral contraction of the pharyngeal muscles to expel any object causing the reflex when the more sensitive areas such as the palatoglossal arches are stimulated. However, nearly 40% of the general population may not even have a functional gag reflex and that there is little relationship between this reflex and a person's ability to swallow normally. The afferent limb of the gag reflex is mediated by the glossopharyngeal nerve while the efferent limb is controlled by the vagus nerve.

Table 7.12 **Pharynx muscles**

Muscle	Innervation	Function(s)	Origin	Insertion
Superior pharyngeal constrictor	Pharyngeal branch of vagus nerve (CN X) and pharyngeal plexus	Constrict the walls of the pharynx and induce peristaltic waves during swallowing	Pterygoid hamulus of sphenoid bone; pterygomandibular raphe; mylohyoid line of mandible	Pharyngeal tubercle of occipital bone; pharyngeal raphe
Middle pharyngeal constrictor	Pharyngeal branch of vagus nerve (CN X) and pharyngeal plexus	Constrict the walls of the pharynx and induce peristaltic waves during swallowing	Greater and lesser horns of hyoid bone	Pharyngeal raphe
Inferior pharyngeal constrictor	Pharyngeal branch of vagus nerve (CN X) and pharyngeal plexus	Constrict the walls of the pharynx and induce peristaltic waves during swallowing	Oblique line of thyroid cartilage; lateral aspect of cricoid cartilage	Pharyngeal raphe; cricopharyngeal part wraps around pharyngoesophageal junction with no formation of a raphe
Palatopharyngeus	Pharyngeal branch of vagus nerve (CN X) and pharyngeal plexus	Elevate the pharynx and larynx during swallowing or speaking	Posterior border of hard palate; palatine aponeurosis	Posterior border of thyroid cartilage; lateral wall of pharynx
Salpingopharyngeus	Pharyngeal branch of vagus nerve (CN X) and pharyngeal plexus	Elevate the pharynx and larynx during swallowing or speaking	Cartilaginous part of the pharyngotympanic tube	Fuses with palatopharyngeus fibers on lateral pharyngeal wall
Stylopharyngeus	Glossopharyngeal nerve (CN IX)	Elevate the pharynx and larynx during swallowing or speaking	Styloid process of the temporal bone	Posterolateral borders of thyroid cartilage; lateral wall of pharynx between superior and middle constrictors

- **Stage 1** or **Oral Preparatory/Transfer Stage**: a voluntary action where the food is first placed in the mouth and reduced or grinded down by the action of the muscles of mastication while simultaneously being mixed with saliva. Food remains in contact with the teeth by the action of the buccinator muscle in the cheek region and closure of the lips by the orbicularis oris muscles. The continuous cycling of food over the anterior and posterior surfaces of the tongue forms a food bolus. This stage ends after the food bolus passes through the palatoglossal and palatopharyngeal arches of the soft palate and into the oropharynx. This occurs with the combined movements of the tongue and soft palate muscles.
- **Stage 2** or **Pharyngeal Stage**: an involuntary action and the most critical stage of swallowing that involves the pharynx changing from an exclusive air channel to a now food channel. Delivery of the food bolus into the oropharynx triggers the pharyngeal stage. This stage involves the nasopharynx being sealed off from the remainder of the pharynx by the elevation of the soft palate and contraction of the superior pharyngeal constrictor muscle. As the suprahyoid and longitudinal pharyngeal muscles contract, thus elevating the larynx, the pharynx shortens and widens to receive the bolus and helps relax the UES. Total time from initiation of the pharyngeal stage to the re-establishment of the airway is approximately one second.
- **Stage 3** or **Esophageal Stage**: an involuntary action much like stage 2 but can last up to 20 seconds. It begins after the relaxation of the UES and involves the sequential contraction of the pharyngeal constrictor muscles that propel the bolus inferiorly into the esophagus and ultimately into the stomach. The epiglottis serves to deflect the bolus from entering the trachea but does not completely close the laryngeal inlet during swallowing.

7.18 Venous Drainage of the Neck

The larger veins located in the neck region are the external and internal jugular veins. As discussed earlier in the chapter, the *superficial temporal* and *maxillary veins* meet and form the **retromandibular vein (Fig. 7.47)**. This vein is generally found coursing through the substance of the parotid gland and posterior to the mandibular ramus but continues as an anterior and posterior tributary. The *posterior auricular vein* and the **posterior tributary of the retromandibular vein** form the **external jugular vein (EJV)**. The *occipital vein* can also contribute to the formation of the EJV (**Fig. 7.143; Fig. 7.157**). The EJV descends inferiorly and superficial to the sternocleidomastoid muscle before joining the subclavian vein. A valve does exist near the junction with the subclavian vein but it does not prevent regurgitation of blood. The EJV is responsible for draining blood mainly from the face and scalp (**Fig. 7.143**).

The **internal jugular vein (IJV)** is continuous with the termination of the sigmoid sinus at the level of the jugular foramen. It actually begins as the **superior bulb of IJV** before descending through the carotid sheath and finally terminating as the **inferior bulb of IJV** at the subclavian vein. The inferior bulb contains a bicuspid valve that allows blood to pass to the heart and prevents regurgitation. It is the IJV and subclavian veins that form the brachiocephalic veins. The majority of smaller veins located in the neck region are tributaries of the internal pageantry jugular vein. These tributaries include the inferior petrosal sinus, pharyngeal,

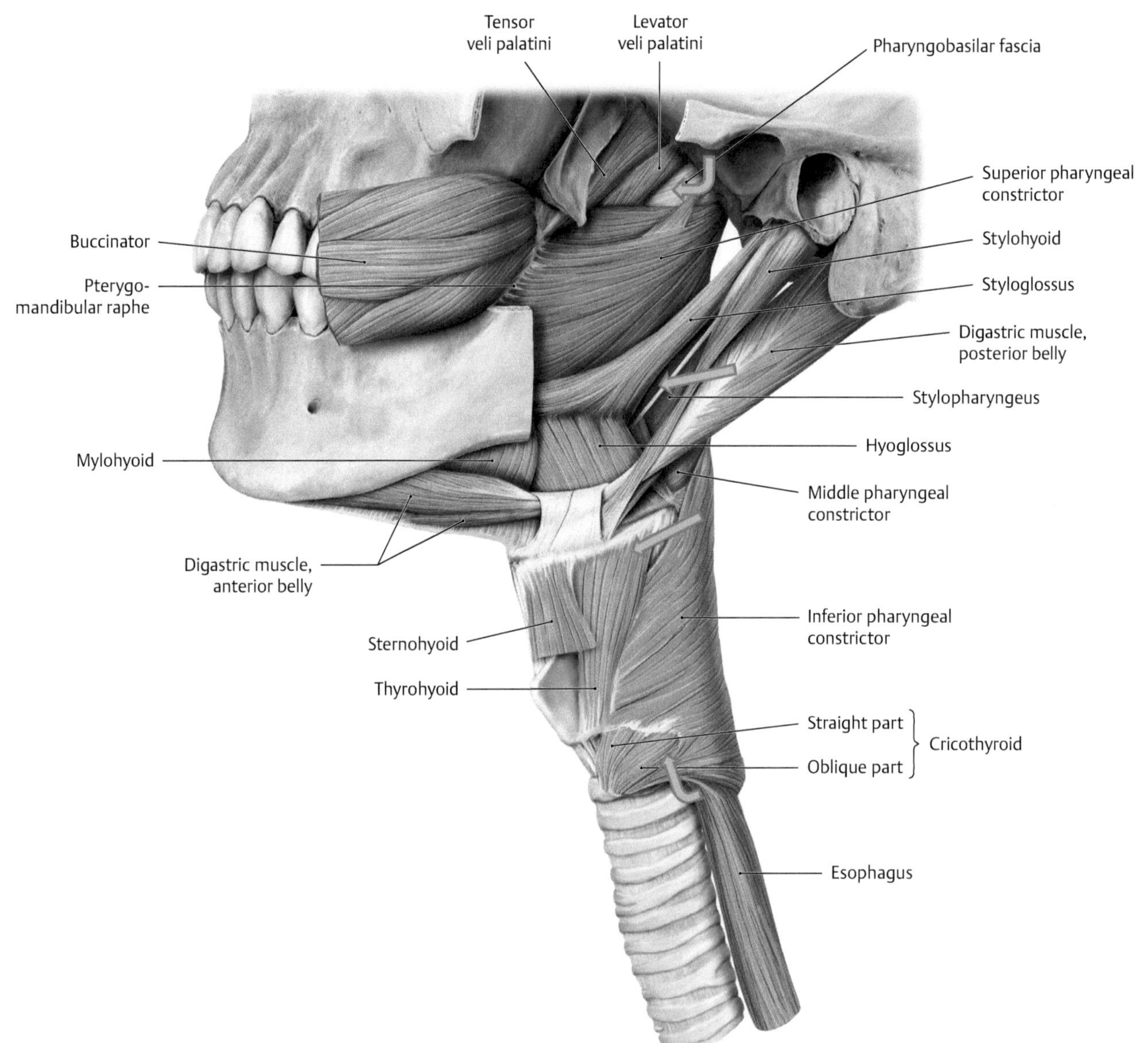

Fig. 7.178 Muscles and pharyngeal wall gaps of the pharynx, left lateral view. (From Schuenke M, Schulte E, Schumacher U. THIEME Atlas of Anatomy. Head, Neck, and Neuroanatomy. Illustrations by Voll M and Wesker K. 3rd ed. New York: Thieme Medical Publishers; 2020.)

facial, lingual, superior thyroid, middle thyroid, and occasionally the occipital vein (**Fig. 7.143; Fig. 7.144; Fig. 7.145**).

7.19 Lymphatic Drainage of the Neck

As mentioned earlier in the chapter there is general principle with lymphatics of the scalp, face, and neck. Lymph will drain from a superior to inferior and superficial to deep direction, eventually reaching the *deep cervical lymph nodes* located near the IJV. Lymph from the scalp and face can drain to the **submental, submandibular, buccal, superficial/deep parotid, mastoid (retroauricular)**, or **occipital lymph nodes**, known collectively as the *superficial ring/pericervical collar of lymph nodes* (**Fig. 7.38**).

These lymph nodes along with the superficial tissues of the neck will drain toward the **superficial cervical lymph nodes** that are adjacent to the external jugular and anterior jugular veins. Lymph then will drain toward the **deep cervical (superior/inferior) lymph nodes** that are located mainly near the IJV. Other deep cervical lymph nodes include the **retropharyngeal, jugulodigastric, jugulo-omohyoid, infrahyoid, prelaryngeal, pretracheal, paratracheal**, and **supraclavicular lymph nodes**. From the deep cervical lymph nodes, lymph will pass through **jugular lymphatic trunks** and from the upper limb lymph will pass through the **subclavian lymphatic trunks**. These trunks connect to the **thoracic duct** on the left side and help form the **right lymphatic duct** on the right side. The thoracic and right lymphatic ducts drain into the **left/right venous angles**, respectively, located at the junction of the internal jugular and subclavian veins. The right lymphatic duct generally has a direct route to the right venous angle. However, the

Clinical Correlate 7.49

Waldeyer Tonsillar Ring

The incomplete ring of lymphoid tissue situated between the nasopharynx, soft palate, oropharynx, and posterior tongue is collectively known as the **Waldeyer tonsillar ring**. Named after the German anatomist Heinrich Wilhelm Gottfried von Waldeyer-Hartz, this tonsillar ring includes the pharyngeal, tubal, palatine, and lingual tonsils. It acts as a first-line defense against incoming microbes.

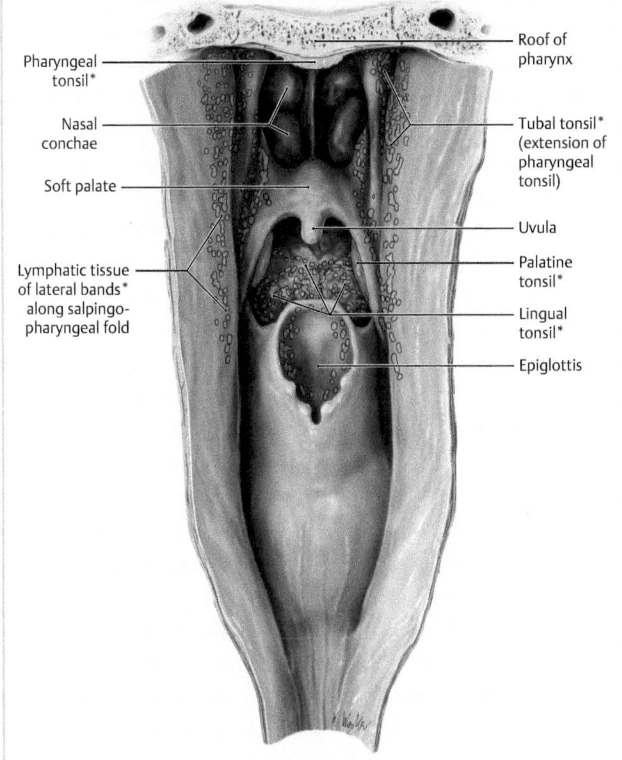

(From Schuenke M, Schulte E, Schumacher U. THIEME Atlas of Anatomy. Head, Neck, and Neuroanatomy. Illustrations by Voll M and Wesker K. 3rd ed. New York: Thieme Medical Publishers; 2020.)

Clinical Correlate 7.50

Adenoiditis and Tonsillitis

When the pharyngeal tonsils become inflamed, an individual has **adenoids** or **adenoiditis**. Adenoids can be caused by bacterial or viral infections and may obstruct the pharyngotympanic tubes and airway between the nasal cavity and nasopharynx. Surgical removal may be necessary and this is called an *adenoidectomy*.

Inflammation of the palatine tonsils is known as **tonsillitis**. This may also be caused by a bacterial or viral infection but it is more commonly the result of streptococcus (strep) bacteria. The removal of the palatine tonsils is known as a *tonsillectomy* and the glossopharyngeal nerve is at risk of being damaged.

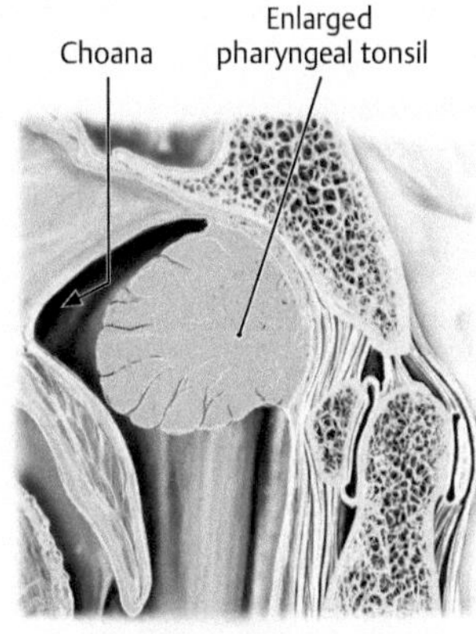

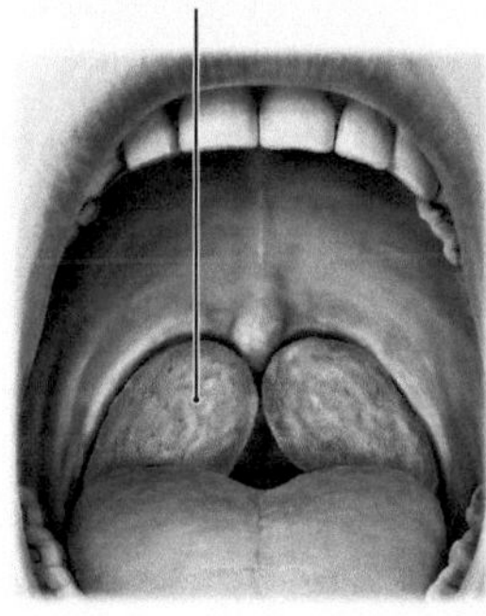

(From Schuenke M, Schulte E, Schumacher U. THIEME Atlas of Anatomy. Head, Neck, and Neuroanatomy. Illustrations by Voll M and Wesker K. 3rd ed. New York: Thieme Medical Publishers; 2020.)

thoracic duct must pass superiorly through the superior thoracic aperture near the left border of the esophagus; arch laterally in the root of the neck; and then pass posterior to the IJV before reaching the left venous angle. The final insertion point of both the thoracic duct and right lymphatic duct is variable.

7.20 Neck and Remaining Viscera Development

Much of the development involving head and neck structures have already been discussed. This section focuses on the development of the **pharyngeal (branchial) apparatus** that is first observed in week 4 of development. The pharyngeal apparatus consists of **pharyngeal arches**, **pharyngeal pouches**, **pharyngeal grooves**, and **pharyngeal membrane (Fig. 7.185; Fig. 7.186)**. After regression of multiple portions of this larger apparatus, namely the fifth pharyngeal arch and pouch there will be a total of five arches numbered 1-4 and 6, four pouches (1-4), one groove, and one membrane.

The pharyngeal arches consist of *neural crest cells* and *somitomeric mesoderm* and have a *cranial nerve* and *pharyngeal arch artery* associated with it. The first two arches also have a specific cartilaginous rod incorporated into it that helps contribute to bone and cartilage. The neural crest cells differentiate into bone and connective tissue while the mesoderm contributes primarily to muscle but also to the vessels. The pharyngeal pouches are evaginations of *endoderm* that line the foregut while the remaining pharyngeal groove is an invagination of *ectoderm* located between the first two pharyngeal arches. The only surviving pharyngeal

Clinical Correlate 7.51

Central Venous Catheters of the Neck

A **central venous catheter** done in the neck region involves either the subclavian or internal jugular veins but rarely the external jugular vein. Also known as a *central line*, it is used to deliver concentrated nutritional solutions or medications, permits monitoring of venous pressures, and can be used over short and longer durations.

A *subclavian vein approach* **(a)** involves placing a thumb of one hand on the middle portion of the clavicle and the index finger on the jugular notch of the manubrium. After the needle punctures the skin near the thumb, some advocate hitting the clavicle with the needle before "walking" the needle medially along the clavicle and toward the jugular notch until the subclavian vein is punctured. This is to help reduce the possibility of causing a pneumothorax. Once venous access is obtained (presence of a "flash"), the needle is stabilized and the syringe is removed. The J-tipped end of a guide wire is inserted into the needle and after reaching its terminal position the needle will then be removed leaving only the wire in place. An introducer and dilator assembly is then inserted over the wire, and after reaching the skin with the introducer, the dilator and wire are removed together. Final suturing and dressing is done to secure the central line.

An *IJV approach* **(b)** can be done anteriorly, centrally, or posteriorly based on the needle insertion to the SCM with the central approach being the most common. After rotating the patient's head opposite the side the needle will be inserted, the apex of the bifurcating bellies of the SCM is the target of the practitioner's needle and it is inserted at a 30-degree angle while aiming toward the ipsilateral nipple. After the vein has been accessed, the continuation of the central line procedure is similar to that of the subclavian approach. The right IJV is preferred because it is straighter and slightly larger than the left IJV.

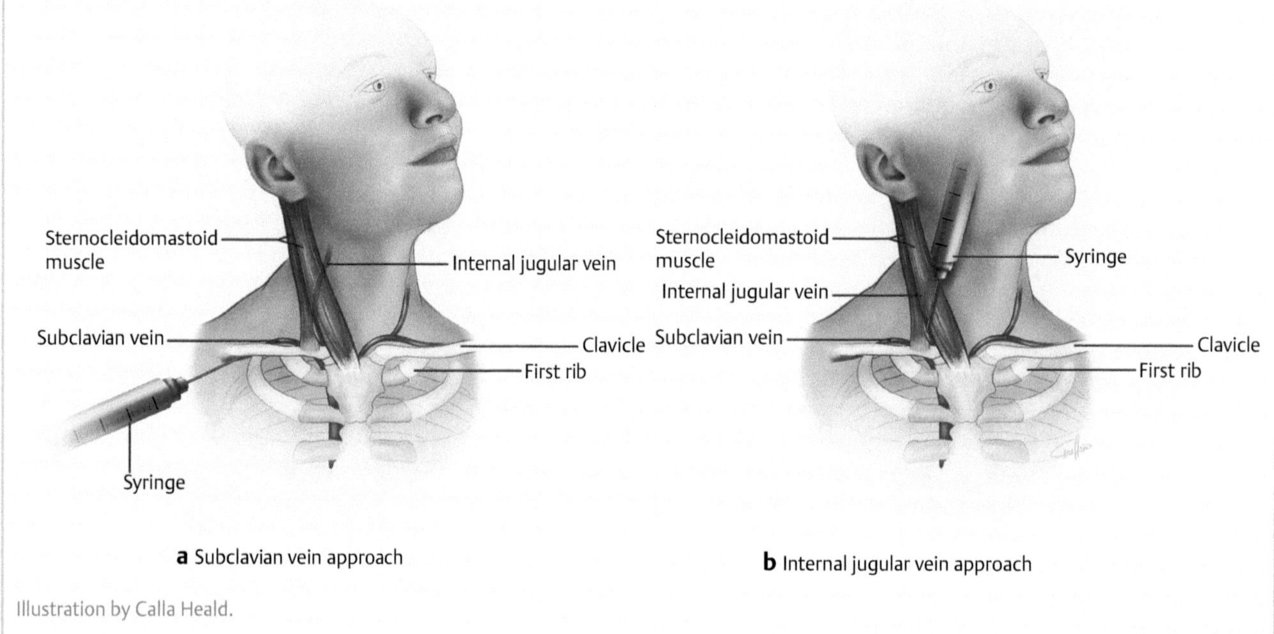

a Subclavian vein approach

b Internal jugular vein approach

Illustration by Calla Heald.

Clinical Correlate 7.52

External Jugular Vein Prominence and Severance

The external jugular vein may be easily visible near the posterior border of the SCM. It becomes more prominent and even displays the look of engorgement when venous pressure rises as in congestive heart failure or pulmonary hypertension for example; thus, the EJV can be used as an early diagnostic sign for such conditions. If the EJV is cut or severed, firm pressure to the damaged vein needs to be applied. This is because the lumen of the vein will be held open by the investing layer of deep cervical fascia. Then due to the negative intrathoracic pressure, air will be sucked into the vein and this will produce *cyanosis* (bluish discoloration of skin due to inadequate oxygenation of the blood) and a churning noise in the thorax. If an air embolism forms, it will produce a froth that fills the right side of the heart altering blood flow and resulting in *dyspnea* (shortness of breath).

membrane is also located between the first two arches and consists of an outer ectoderm, middle mesoderm, and inner endoderm layer (**Fig. 7.187**).

Pharyngeal arch 1 is made up of a *dorsal* and *ventral process* and is termed the "mandibular arch"; however, this is not entirely correct because the dorsal process contributes to maxillofacial, middle ear, and palatopharyngeal structures. The embryonic cartilaginous rod is also known as *Meckel cartilage* (**Fig. 7.187**). **Pharyngeal arch 2** is commonly referred to as the "hyoid arch" although it is both the second and third arches that contribute

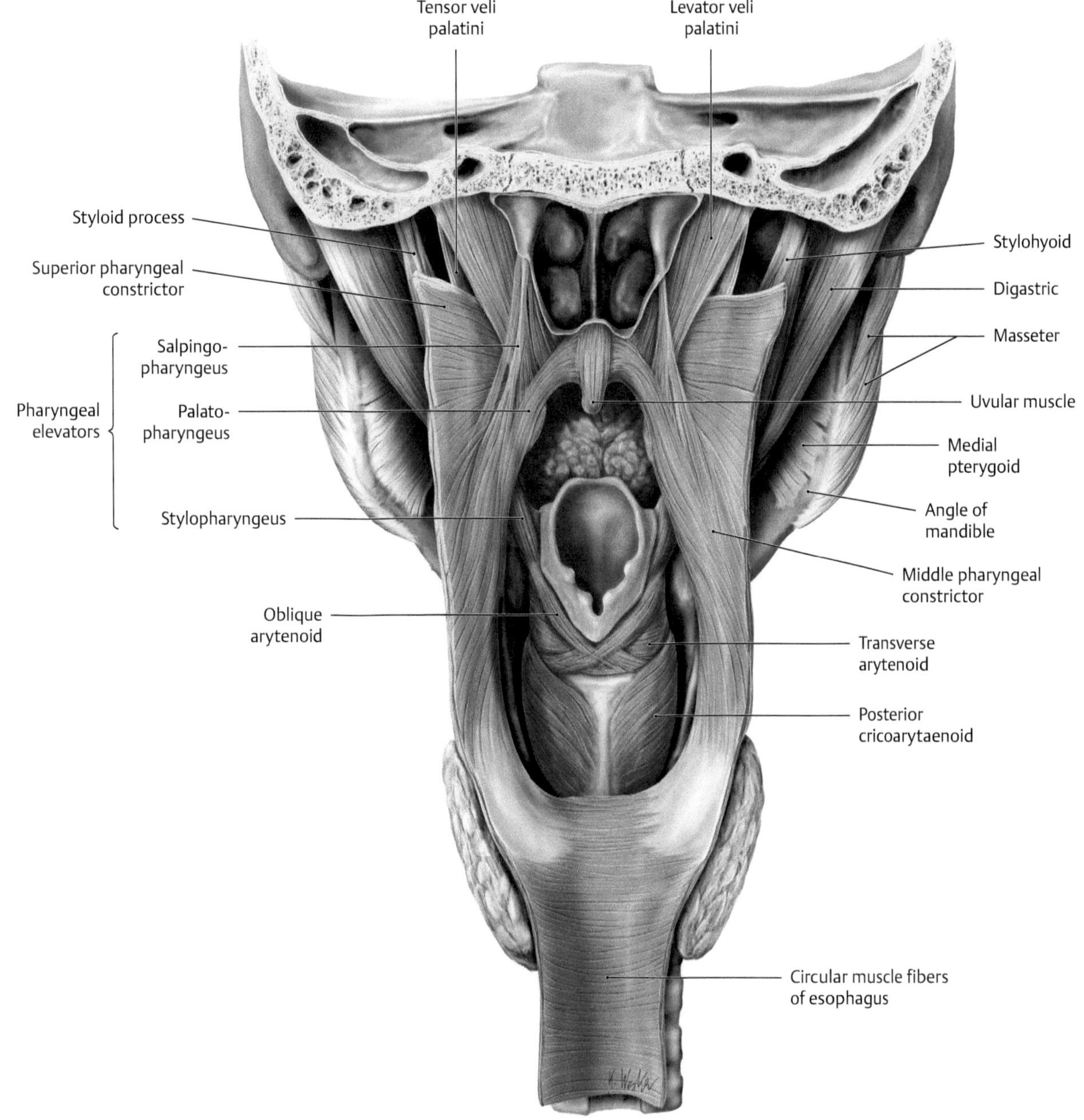

Fig. 7.179 Pharyngeal and laryngeal musculature, posterior view. Posterior pharynx has been opened. (From Schuenke M, Schulte E, Schumacher U. THIEME Atlas of Anatomy. Head, Neck, and Neuroanatomy. Illustrations by Voll M and Wesker K. 3rd ed. New York: Thieme Medical Publishers; 2020.)

to the overall development of the hyoid bone. The cartilaginous rod in this arch is known as *Reichert cartilage* (**Fig. 7.187**). All laryngeal cartilages are associated with pharyngeal arch development. However, the epiglottis develops from the mesenchyme of the *hypopharyngeal eminence* of the third and fourth pharyngeal arches. Refer to **Table 7.13** for a summary of all structures that originate from the pharyngeal arches.

Pharyngeal pouch 1 gives rise to the **tubotympanic recess.** This recess gives rise to the epithelial lining of the **tympanic cavity** and **mastoid antrum** and **mastoid air cells.** The connection of the tubotympanic recess with the pharynx forms the **pharyngotympanic tube**. **Pharyngeal pouch 2** forms the **palatine tonsil** and a portion of this pouch will remain as the **tonsillar sinus/fossa. Pharyngeal pouch 3** expands into dorsal and ventral portions

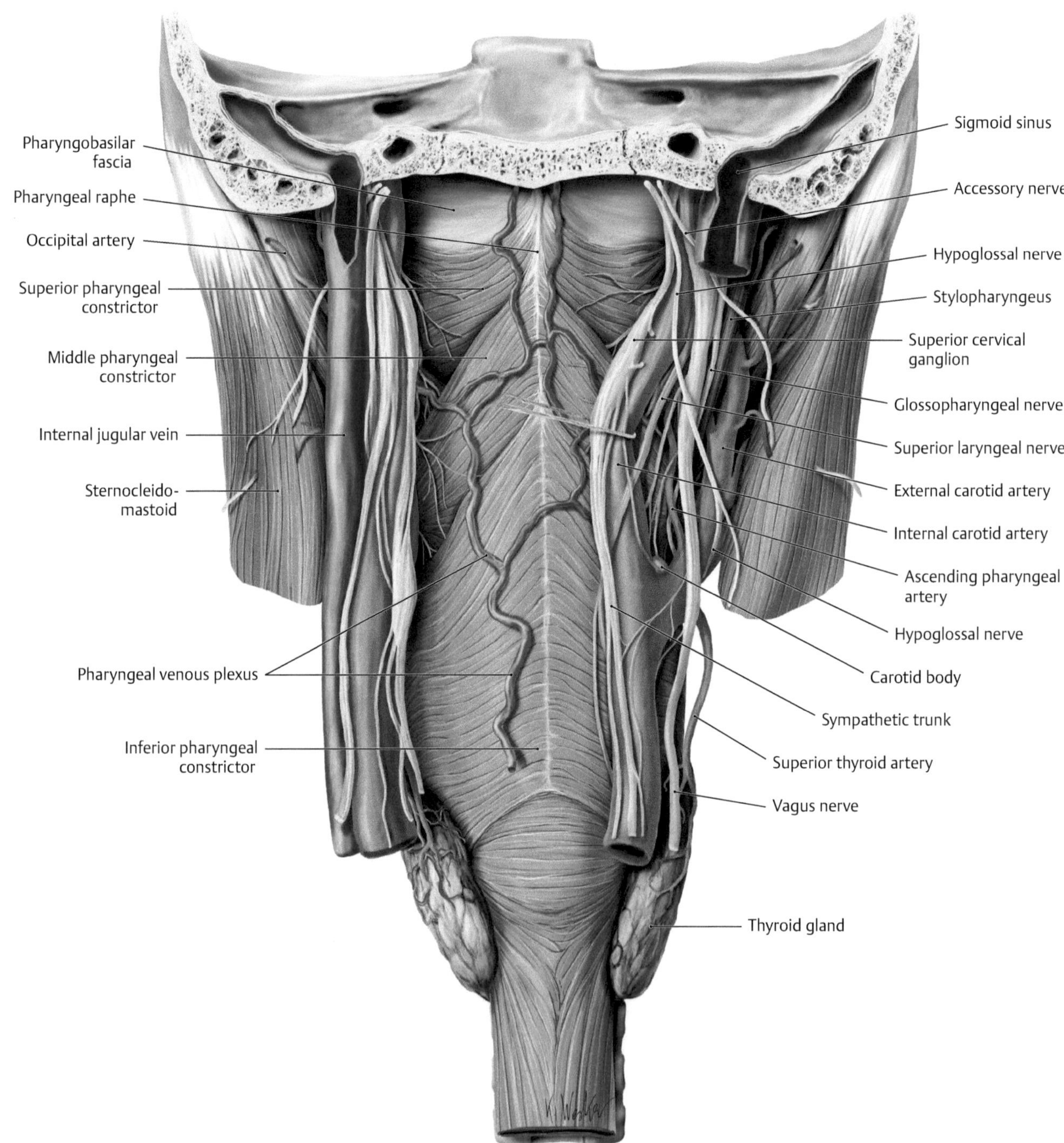

Fig. 7.180 Neurovasculature of the posterior pharynx. (From Schuenke M, Schulte E, Schumacher U. THIEME Atlas of Anatomy. Head, Neck, and Neuroanatomy. Illustrations by Voll M and Wesker K. 3rd ed. New York: Thieme Medical Publishers; 2020.)

Corticonuclear tract
Principal sensory (pontine) nucleus of trigeminal nerve
Principal sensory nucleus of trigeminal nerve
Sensation (pain, temperature, touch)
From the ear (tympanic nerve)
Sensation
Taste
To thalamus and cortex (medial lemniscus)
Solitary nucleus
Nucleus ambiguus
Superior ganglion
Inferior ganglion
IX
X
Spinal nucleus of trigeminal nerve
Stylo-pharyngeus
Pharyngeal constrictor
Motor
Somatic sensory
Visceral sensory

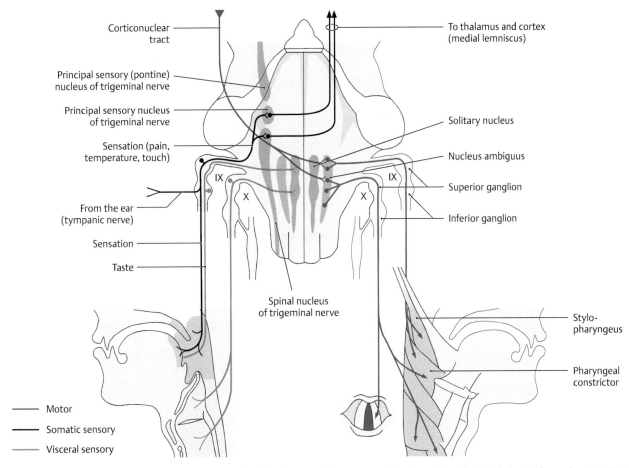

Fig. 7.181 Glossopharyngeal and vagus nerve: their peripheral distribution and brainstem nuclei. (From Schuenke M, Schulte E, Schumacher U. THIEME Atlas of Anatomy. Head, Neck, and Neuroanatomy. Illustrations by Voll M and Wesker K. 3rd ed. New York: Thieme Medical Publishers; 2020.)

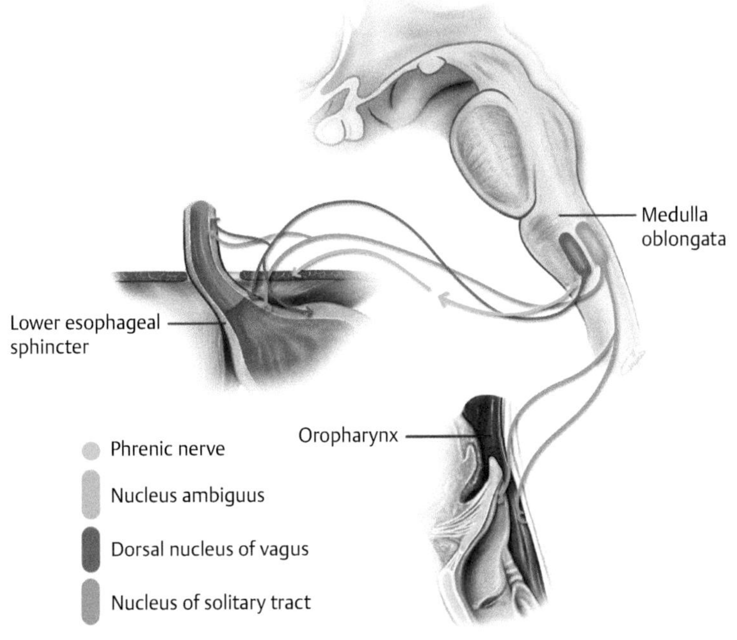

Fig. 7.182 Swallowing pattern generator (SPG). The SPG is located in and around the reticular formation of the nucleus ambiguus and nucleus of solitary tract of the brainstem. It receives all descending motor drives and peripheral inputs. The cerebral cortex and some subcortical structures connect the SPG to corticobulbar tracts. Corticobulbar tracts are composed of upper motor neurons that synapse on the motor nuclei of cranial nerves. The SPG involves motor nuclei of CN V, VII, IX, X, & XII in the brainstem along with two groups of interneurons known as the dorsal swallowing group (DSG) located in the nucleus of solitary tract and the ventral swallowing group (VSG) located above the nucleus ambiguus. Illustration by Calla Heald.

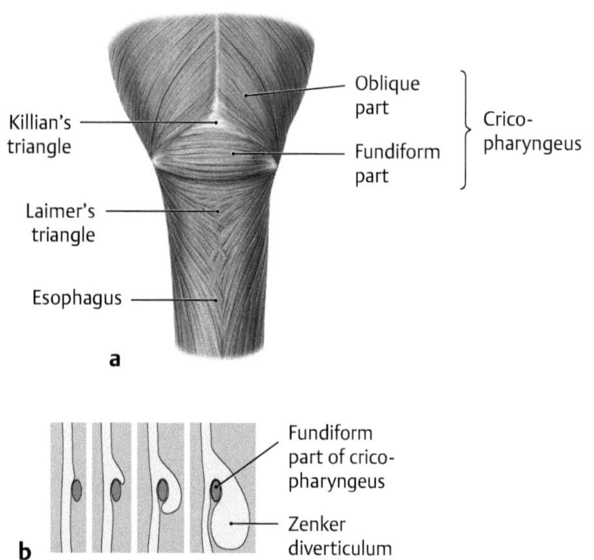

Fig. 7.183 **(a)** Junction of the pharyngeal and esophageal musculature, posterior view. **(b)** Development of Zenker diverticula, left lateral view. (From Schuenke M, Schulte E, Schumacher U. THIEME Atlas of Anatomy. Head, Neck, and Neuroanatomy. Illustrations by Voll M and Wesker K. 3rd ed. New York: Thieme Medical Publishers; 2020.)

with the dorsal portions forming the **inferior parathyroid glands** and the ventral portions forming two masses that eventually meet and fuse to form the **thymus gland**. The thymus and inferior parathyroid glands migrate caudally but later the inferior parathyroid glands separate from the thymus and come to lie on the dorsal surface of the thyroid gland. **Pharyngeal pouch 4** also develops into a dorsal and ventral portion. Each dorsal portion develops into a **superior parathyroid gland** whereas the ventral portions develop into the **ultimopharyngeal body**. The ultimopharyngeal body fuses with the thyroid gland and gives rise to **parafollicular cells** (C cells) that are responsible for producing calcitonin **(Fig. 7.188)**.

Pharyngeal groove 1 gives rise to the epithelial lining of the **external acoustic meatus** while the other grooves lie in a slit-like depression known as the **cervical sinus.** As pharyngeal arch 2 grows over the third and fourth arches it will obliterate the cervical sinus. **Pharyngeal membrane 1** becomes the **tympanic membrane**. Refer to **Table 7.14** for a summary of all structures that originate from the pharyngeal pouches, groove, and membrane.

All voluntary musculature of the head and neck regions are derived from paraxial mesoderm that develops into somitomeres and somites. Examples include: somitomeres 1-3 and 5 contribute to eye musculature; somitomere 4 contributes to muscles of mastication in pharyngeal arch 1; somitomere 6 contributes to the facial expression muscles in pharyngeal arch 2; somitomere 7 contributes to the stylopharyngeus muscle in pharyngeal arch

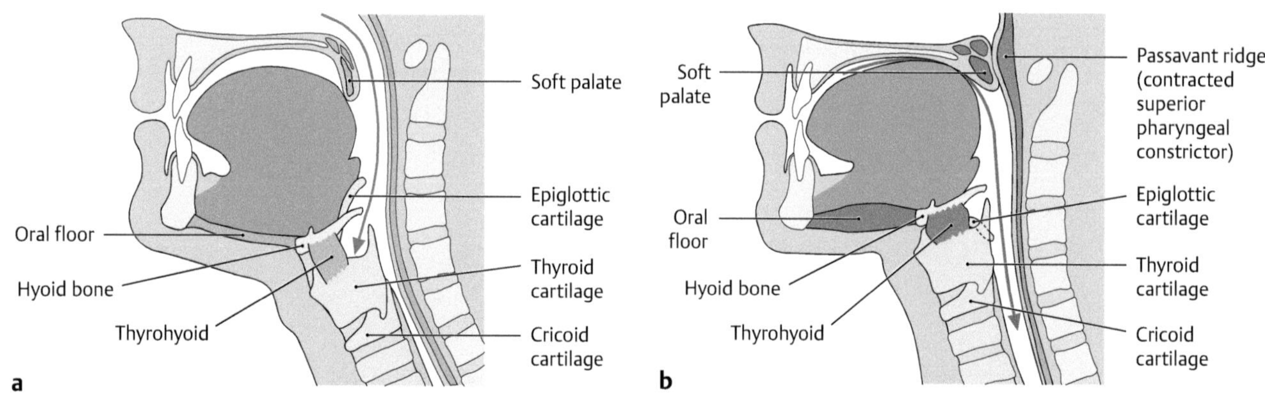

Fig. 7.184 The process of deglutition. **(a)** An open airway prior to swallowing a food bolus. **(b)** Elevation of the soft palate to seal off the nasopharynx; elevation of the larynx shortens and widens the pharynx; and the bolus is propelled toward the esophagus. (From Schuenke M, Schulte E, Schumacher U. THIEME Atlas of Anatomy. Head, Neck, and Neuroanatomy. Illustrations by Voll M and Wesker K. 3rd ed. New York: Thieme Medical Publishers; 2020.)

Clinical Correlate 7.53

Virchow's Node

A left supraclavicular node is specifically known as *Virchow node* (*Troisier sign*). Enlargement of this specific lymph node is a strong indicator of the presence of an abdominal cancer, especially gastric cancer, and may be referred to as a *sentinel node*. Virchow node is the end node of the thoracic duct, which is the lymphatic duct responsible for draining lymph from the majority of the body. Its location can be near the anterior scalene muscle. The German pathologist Rudolf Virchow (1821–1902) first described the specificity of this node and its correlation with gastric cancer.

Clinical Correlate 7.54

Zones of Penetrating and Blunt Neck Trauma

The neck is commonly divided into three distinct zones that serve as clinical guides to the initial assessment and management of neck trauma. *Asymptomatic patients* will be evaluated with diagnostic work-ups initially and if any pathologic findings are observed they will be taken to the operating room for open neck exploration. Symptomatic patients may first have a CT scan done before open exploration in the operating room. This could present the best surgical approach before entering the operating room.

- **Zone 1**: the lower zone and it is located between the level of the clavicle and jugular notch and superiorly to the level of the cricoid cartilage. A vascular injury in this zone could be challenging and mortality is generally high. A sternotomy may be needed to control a hemorrhage in this zone. Structures at risk in this zone include the proximal common carotid arteries, vertebral and subclavian arteries, subclavian, brachiocephalic and terminal jugular veins, recurrent laryngeal and vagus nerves trachea, esophagus, thoracic duct, cervical pleurae, and cervical vertebrae.
- **Zone 2**: the middle zone that is located between the cricoid cartilage and angles of the mandible. Neck explorations after a vertical or horizontal incision in this zone are generally uncomplicated. Structures at risk include the carotid arteries, vertebral and jugular veins, recurrent laryngeal and vagus nerves, larynx, upper trachea, pharynx, and cervical vertebrae.
- **Zone 3**: the upper zone extending from the angles of the mandible to the base of the skull and surgical access is difficult. A craniotomy or mandibulotomy may be needed to gain access to vascular structures. Structures at risk include the internal and external carotid arteries, jugular veins, cranial nerves IX, X, XI, and XII, nasopharynx, oropharynx, oral and nasal cavities, and salivary glands.

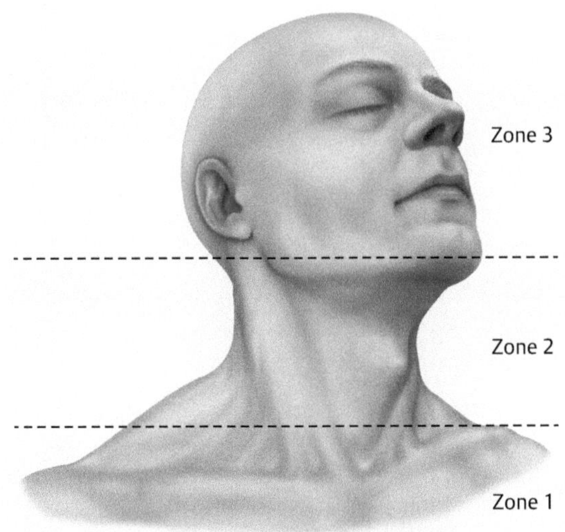

(From Schuenke M, Schulte E, Schumacher U. THIEME Atlas of Anatomy. Head, Neck, and Neuroanatomy. Illustrations by Voll M and Wesker K. 3rd ed. New York: Thieme Medical Publishers; 2020.)

Clinical Correlate 7.55

First Arch Syndromes

First arch syndromes are caused by a lack of neural crest cells migrating into pharyngeal arch 1. The two most well-described first arch syndromes are known as *Treacher Collins syndrome (mandibulofacial dysotstosis)* and *Pierre Robin sequence*. Individuals with **Treacher Collins** have underdeveloped cheek bones, micrognathia (small jaw), and possibly a cleft palate. They often have eyes that slant downward, sparse eyelashes, and a notch in the lower eyelids. Individuals may also demonstrate absent, small, or unusually formed ears and hearing loss occurs in about half of all affected individuals. These individuals usually have normal intelligence. It is the result of mutations in the TCOF1 or POLR1D genes.

Pierre Robin sequence is more of a sequence of malformations than a syndrome like it is usually misrepresented as but it has three main features: micrognathia, cleft palate, and posterior displacement of the tongue (glossoptosis) accompanied by an airway obstruction. There is no known cause for Pierre Robin but may involve multiple chromosomes or environmental factors.

Clinical Correlate 7.56

Pharyngeal Fistula and Cysts

A **pharyngeal fistula** is the result of the second pharyngeal arch failing to grow over the third and fourth arches, thus closing off the entire cervical sinus that was associated with pharyngeal grooves 2-4. There will remain a patent opening that extends to the outer neck and it is generally located along the anterior border of the SCM. A **pharyngeal cyst** is a remnant of the cervical sinus due to these same pharyngeal grooves 2-4 remaining when they are normally obliterated. A pharyngeal cyst is also located on the anterior border of the SCM and may connect to the fistula.

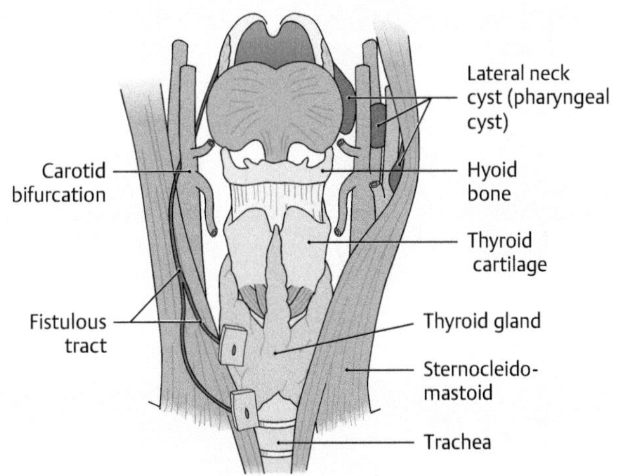

(From Schuenke M, Schulte E, Schumacher U. THIEME Atlas of Anatomy. Head, Neck, and Neuroanatomy. Illustrations by Voll M and Wesker K. 3rd ed. New York: Thieme Medical Publishers; 2020.)

Clinical Correlate 7.57

DiGeorge Syndrome

DiGeorge syndrome is caused by a microdeletion of a region in chromosome 22q11.2 and is a complex of congenital malformations caused by abnormalities of neural crest migration and proliferation occurring during the formation of the third and fourth pharyngeal arches. It is characterized by (1) neonatal hypocalcemia due to hypoplasia of the parathyroid glands; (2) susceptibility to infection due to low levels of T cells caused by hypoplasia of the thymus gland; (3) cardiovascular defects that can include tetralogy of Fallot and truncus arteriosus; and (4) minor craniofacial defects including micrognathia, low set ears, auricular abnormalities, and cleft palate.

3; somites 1 and 2 contribute to the intrinsic laryngeal muscles located in pharyngeal arches 4 and 6; somites 2-5 contribute to tongue musculature; and finally a combination of somites 2-7 help form the sternocleidomastoid and trapezius muscles.

Due to the phylogenetic/embryologic derivation of muscles associated with the pharyngeal arches, these muscles have been historically classified as being innervated by a special visceral motor fiber or a somatic (branchial) motor fiber. In this text the abbreviations are SVE or BM and these fibers will be associated specifically with any muscle originating from the five pharyngeal arches.

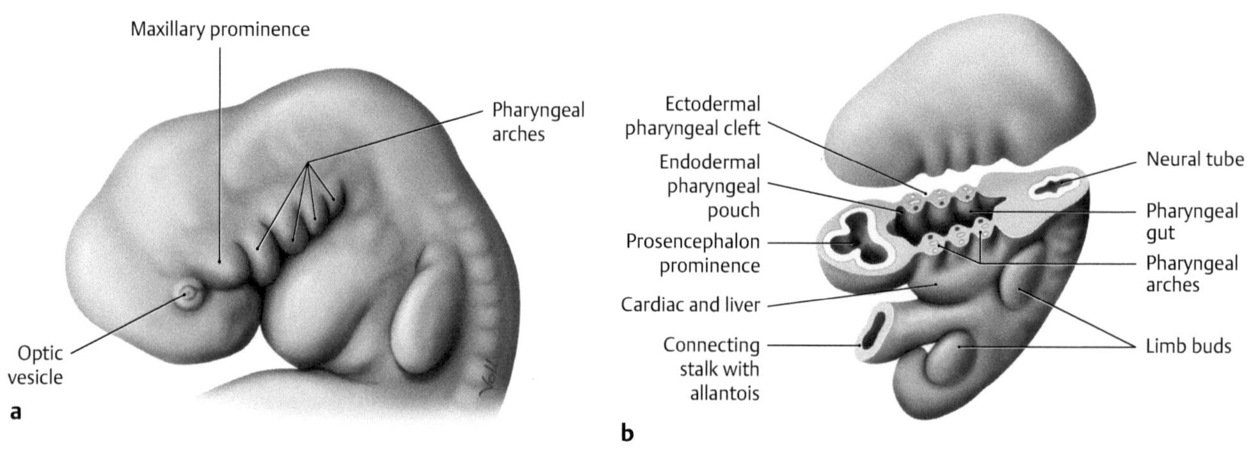

Fig. 7.185 (a) Head and neck region of a 5-week-old embryo displaying the pharyngeal (branchial) arches and grroves. **(b)** Cross-section through an embryo at the level of the pharyngeal gut. (From Baker EW. Anatomy for Dental Medicine. 2nd ed. 2015. Based on the work of: Schuenke M, Schulte E, Schumacher U. THIEME Atlas of Anatomy. Illustrations by Voll M and Wesker K.)

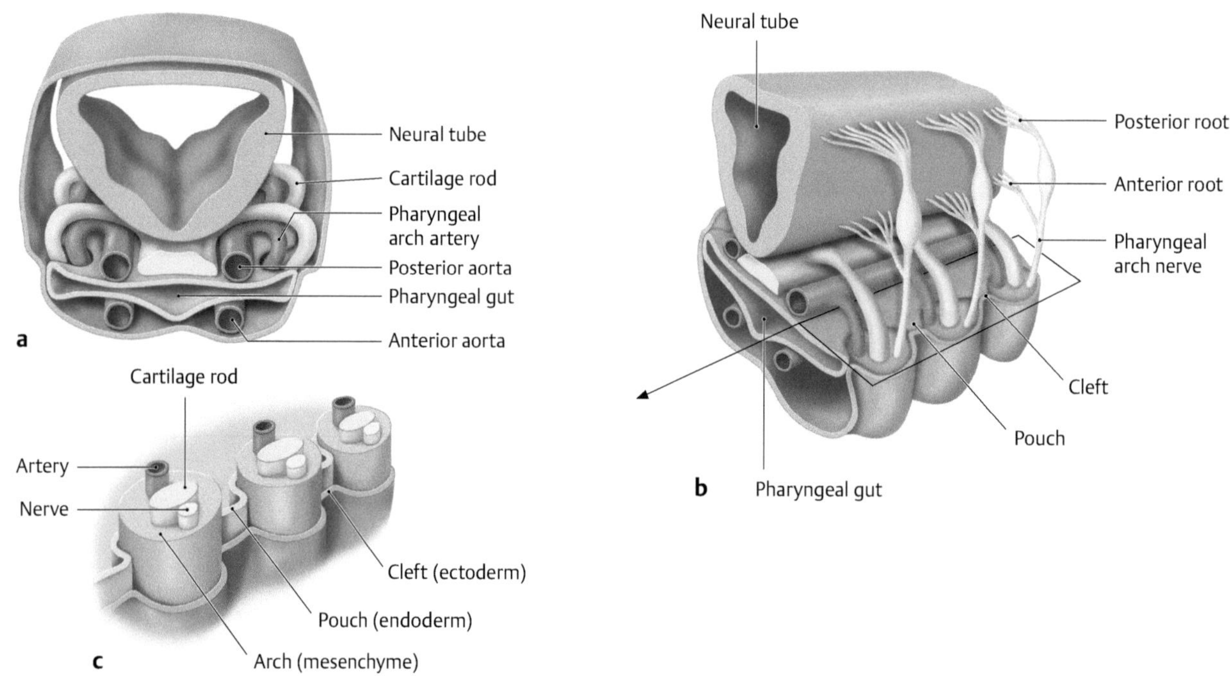

Fig. 7.186 (a) Cross-section through the pharyngeal arch and the neural tube, showing the pharyngeal arch cartilage and artery. **(b)** Oblique section showing the pharyngeal arch nerves. **(c)** Close up of section in **(b)** showing the relationship between the pharyngeal arch cartilage, artery, and nerve in the pharyngeal arches. (From Baker EW. Anatomy for Dental Medicine. 2nd ed. 2015. Based on the work of: Schuenke M, Schulte E, Schumacher U. THIEME Atlas of Anatomy. Illustrations by Voll M and Wesker K.)

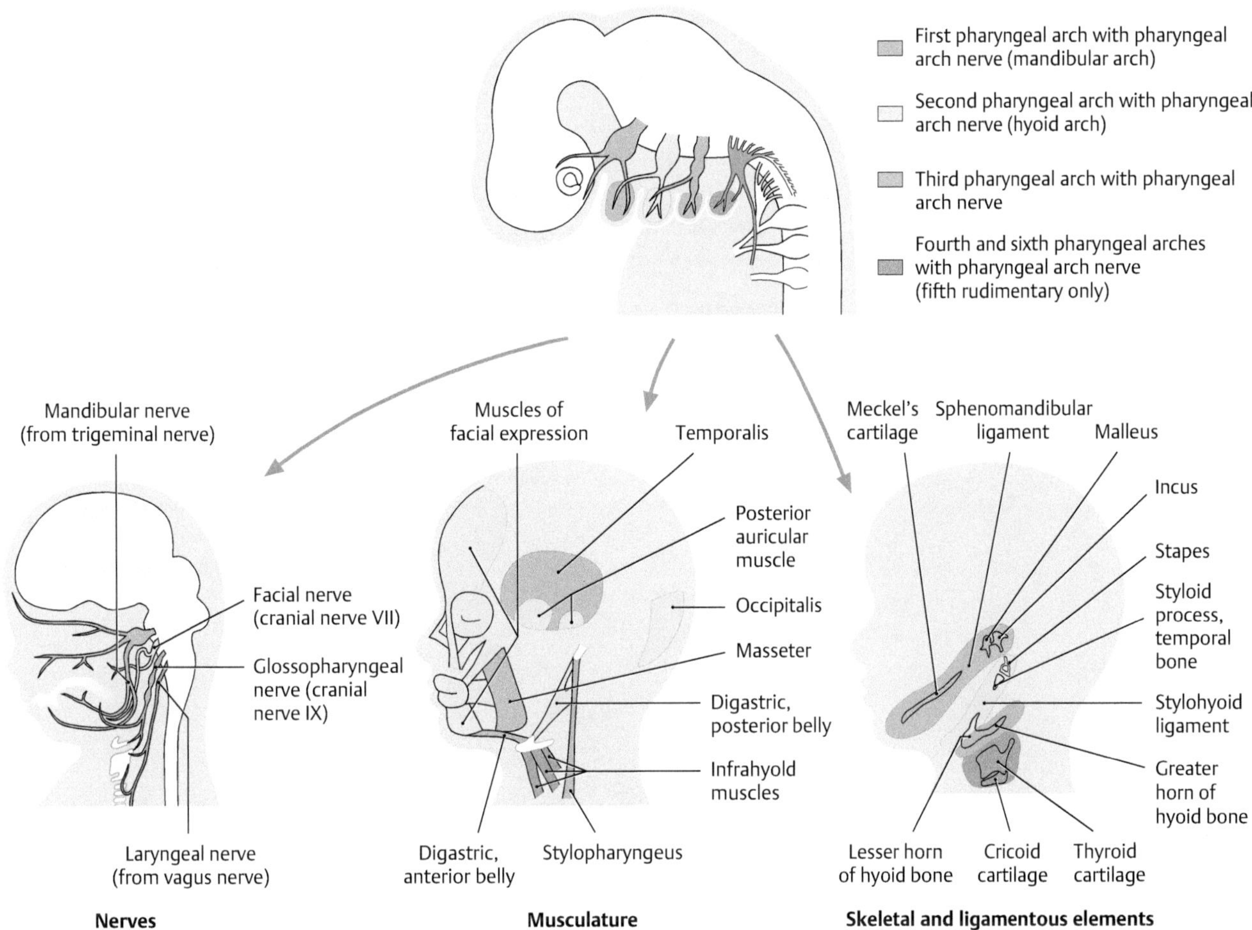

Fig. 7.187 The arrangement and derivatives of the pharyngeal arches. (From Baker EW. Anatomy for Dental Medicine. 2nd ed. 2015. Based on the work of: Schuenke M, Schulte E, Schumacher U. THIEME Atlas of Anatomy. Illustrations by Voll M and Wesker K.)

Table 7.13 **Derivatives of the pharyngeal arches**

Arch	Embryonic cartilage	Cartilage derivative	Cranial nerve	Muscle	Artery
1	Meckel	• Malleus • Incus • Anterior ligament of malleus • Sphenomandibular ligament • Spine of sphenoid • Mental (genial) tubercle of mandible	Trigeminal (V_3)	• Muscles of mastication • Mylohyoid • Anterior belly of digastric • Tensor veli palatini • Tensor tympani	Most first arch arteries regress but some remain to form parts of the maxillary artery
2	Reichert	• Stapes • Stylohyoid ligament • Styloid process of temporal bone • Lesser horn and upper half of hyoid bone body	Facial (VII)	• Facial expression muscles • Stylohyoid • Posterior belly of digastric • Stapedius	Most second arch arteries regress but remnants form the hyoid and stapedial arteries
3		• Greater horn and lower half of hyoid bone body	Glossopharyngeal (IX)	• Stylopharyngeus	Proximal ICA and common carotid arteries
4		• Thyroid cartilage	Vagus (X)—superior laryngeal branch	• Soft palate muscles except tensor veli palatini • Pharynx muscles except stylopharyngeus • Cricothyroid	Arch of aorta between the left common carotid and left subclavian arteries; proximal right subclavian artery
6		• Cricoid cartilage • Arytenoid cartilages • Corniculate cartilages • Cuneiform cartilages	Vagus (X)—recurrent laryngeal branch	• Intrinsic laryngeal muscles except cricothyroid	Proximal left and right pulmonary arteries and ductus arteriosus

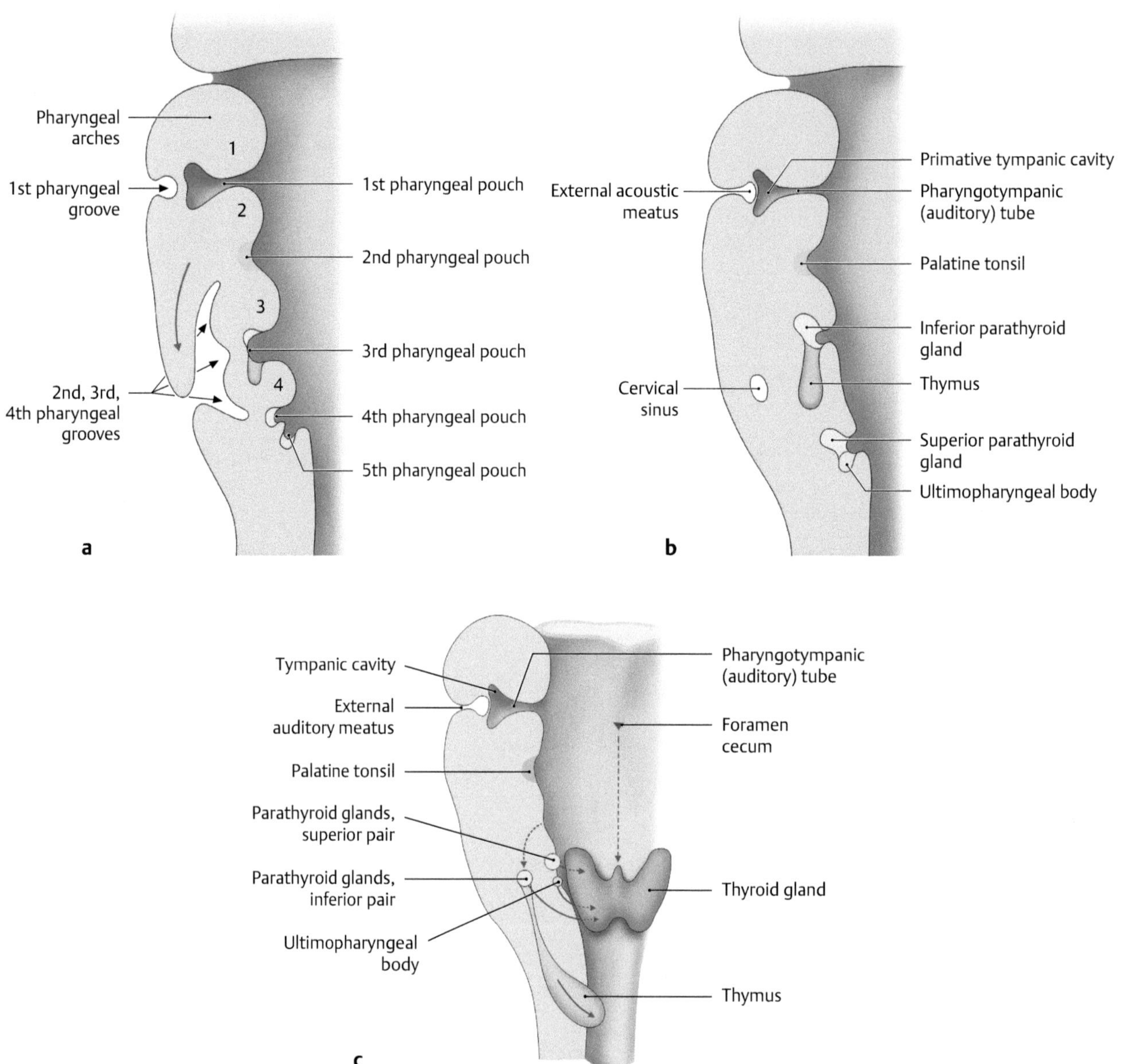

Fig. 7.188 **(a)** Schematic view of developing pharyngeal pouches and grooves. **(b)** Schematic view of adult structures formed by pharyngeal pouches. **(c)** Migration of the pharyngeal arch tissues. (From Baker EW. Anatomy for Dental Medicine. 2nd ed. 2015. Based on the work of: Schuenke M, Schulte E, Schumacher U. THIEME Atlas of Anatomy. Illustrations by Voll M and Wesker K.)

Table 7.14 **Derivatives of the pharyngeal pouches, groove, and membrane**

Pouch	Adult derivative
1	Tympanic cavity, mastoid antrum/air cells and pharyngotympanic tube
2	Palatine tonsil and tonsillar fossa
3	Inferior parathyroid glands and thymus
4	Superior parathyroid glands and ultimopharyngeal body
Groove	
1	External acoustic meatus
Membrane	
1	Tympanic membrane

PRACTICE QUESTIONS

1. An individual has been in an automobile accident and has a major fracture to the skull. The patient presents with a loss of skin sensation over their mandible and anterior to the ear regions. The patient is also complaining that their mouth seems a little dry. The nerves responsible for these innervations originated near which foramen or fissure?
   A. Foramen ovalE.
   B. Petrotympanic fissure.
   C. Greater palatine foramen.
   D. Mental foramen.
   E. Stylomastoid foramen.
2. A 41-year-old woman presents to the clinic with headaches and dizziness. It is found that she has an infection within the dural venous sinus that is located within the posterior margins of the tentorium cerebelli and just lateral to the confluence of sinuses. Which of the following sinuses is the infection located in?
   A. Sigmoid sinus.
   B. Transverse sinus.
   C. Cavernous sinus.
   D. Inferior petrosal sinus.
   E. Straight sinus.
3. An individual has just finished his MMA bout but during the last round, he suffered a posterior dislocation of the mandible resulting in the laceration of the nerve that passes through the petrotympanic fissure. What were the functional components of the nerve that were damaged due to this trauma?
   A. GVE-sym/post, SVA/SS-taste from soft palate.
   B. GVE-para/post, SVA/SS-taste from anterior two-third of tongue.
   C. GVE-para/pre, GSA, SVA/SS-taste from posterior one-third of tonguE.
   D. GSA, SVA/SS-taste from posterior one-third of tongue.
   E. GVE-para/pre, GVA, SVA/SS-taste from anterior two-third of tongue.
4. During a schoolyard brawl, a 17-year-old individual is struck at the pterion on the lateral side of the skull causing an epidural hematoma. Which specific artery is damaged when a blow to the pterion takes place resulting in this epidural hematoma?
   A. Maxillary artery.
   B. Ophthalmic artery.
   C. Accessory meningeal artery.
   D. Anterior branch of the middle meningeal artery.
   E. Posterior branch of the middle meningeal artery.
5. The fontanelles are anatomical soft spots associated with the neurocranium of a newborn and an infant's head. Which of the following fontanelles is the last to close?
   A. Sphenoid.
   B. Anterior.
   C. Posterior.
   D. Mastoid.
6. Which statement about the meningeal layers is INCORRECT?
   A. Large portions of the dura mater are innervated by CN V.
   B. Cerebrospinal fluid passes between the arachnoid and pia maters.
   C. A subarachnoid hemorrhage is venous in nature (a vein ruptures).
   D. The pia mater is not innervated by any nerves.
   E. The subdural space is a potential space between the dura and arachnoid maters.
7. Which combination of cranial foramen and the structure passing through it is INCORRECT?
   A. Superior orbital fissure/Abducent nerve (CN VI).
   B. Foramen rotundum/Maxillary nerve (CN V_2).
   C. Foramen spinosum/Middle meningeal artery.
   D. Jugular foramen/Glossopharyngeal nerve (CN IX).
   E. Inferior orbital fissure/Oculomotor nerve (CN III).
8. Which statement about ansa cervicalis is CORRECT?
   A. It is formed by the dorsal rami of C1–C3.
   B. It has the functional components GSE, GSA, and GVE-para/post.
   C. It innervates all suprahyoid muscles except the hyoglossus muscle.
   D. It innervates all infrahyoid muscles except the thyrohyoid muscle.
   E. Its superior root consists of C1–C2 fibers.
9. A 68-year-old male has a carotid endarterectomy procedure done in order to remove a plaque that is causing stenosis of the common carotid artery near its bifurcation into the internal and external carotid arteries. The procedure can involve making an incision through the carotid sinus of the internal carotid artery thus damaging it. The carotid sinus is innervated mainly by GVA fibers of what cranial nerve?
   A. Trigeminal nerve.
   B. Facial nerve.
   C. Glossopharyngeal nerve.
   D. Vagus nerve.
   E. Hypoglossal nerve.
10. Which structure listed below is not a content of the muscular triangle?
    A. Sternothyroid muscle.
    B. Thyroid gland.
    C. Larynx.
    D. Recurrent laryngeal nerves.
    E. Geniohyoid muscle.
11. An individual suffers a swallow knife wound near the angle of the mandible damaging a facial nerve branch. Which muscle listed below would be affected by damage to the facial nerve?
    A. Hyoglossus.
    B. StylohyoiD.
    C. Middle pharyngeal constrictor.
    D. Anterior belly of digastric.
    E. Mylohyoid.
12. Which layer of the scalp allows free movement of the scalp proper?
    A. Skin layer.
    B. Connective (dense) tissue layer.
    C. Aponeurosis layer.
    D. Loose connective tissue layer.
    E. Pericranium layer.
13. Which statement regarding the "superficial face" is CORRECT?
    A. The zygomatic branch of the facial nerve has SVE/BM and GSA for functional components.
    B. The mental nerve is a V_2 branch.
    C. The posterior auricular vein and the posterior branch of retromandibular vein form the internal jugular vein.
    D. The orbicularis oris muscle is innervated by CN V_3.
    E. Injury to CN V_1 can result in Bell palsy.

14. Which pathway of parasympathetic fibers from CN IX to the parotid gland is CORRECT?
    A. CN IX, tympanic nerve, tympanic plexus, otic ganglion, lesser petrosal nerve, auriculotemporal nerve, parotid gland.
    B. CN IX, tympanic plexus, tympanic nerve, lesser petrosal nerve, otic ganglion, auriculotemporal nerve, parotid gland.
    C. CN IX, tympanic plexus, tympanic nerve, otic ganglion, lesser petrosal nerve, auriculotemporal nerve, parotid gland.
    D. CN IX, tympanic nerve, tympanic plexus, lesser petrosal nerve, otic ganglion, auriculotemporal nerve, parotid gland.
    E. CN IX, lesser petrosal nerve, tympanic plexus, tympanic nerve, otic ganglion, auriculotemporal nerve, parotid gland.
15. What are the functional components of the second portion of the lingual nerve located between the chorda tympani insertion and submandibular ganglion?
    A. SVE/BM, GSA, GVE-sym/post.
    B. GSA, GVE-Para/pre, SVA/SS-taste from soft palate.
    C. SVE/BM, GSA, GVE-Para/pre.
    D. GSA, GVE-Para/post, SVA/SS-taste from anterior two-third of tongue.
    E. GSA, GVE-Para/pre, SVA/SS-taste from anterior two-third of tongue.
16. Which set of functions listed below best describes the actions of the lateral pterygoid muscle, one of four muscles of mastication?
    A. Elevates and protracts the jaw/mandible.
    B. Depresses, retracts, and lateral deviation of the jaw/mandible.
    C. Elevates, protracts, and lateral deviation of the jaw/mandible.
    D. Depresses, protracts, and lateral deviation of the jaw/mandible.
    E. Elevates and retracts the jaw/mandible.
17. An individual suffers a deep penetrating wound cutting the second (pterygoid) part of the maxillary artery. Which artery listed below is not a branch off the second part of the maxillary artery?
    A. Buccal.
    B. Pterygoid.
    C. Accessory meningeal.
    D. Masseteric.
    E. Deep temporal.
18. A 43-year-old patient presents to the emergency department with a deep knife wound to the submandibular triangle of the neck that resulted in damage to the hypoglossal nerve. The following day the patient is asked to protract or stick out their tongue but it deviates toward the side of the knife wound. Which of the muscles of the tongue listed below would not be innervated by the hypoglossal nerve?
    A. Palatoglossus muscle.
    B. Hyoglossus muscle.
    C. Genioglossus muscle.
    D. Superior longitudinal muscle fibers of the tongue.
    E. Styloglossus muscle.
19. A 66-year-old female has made a visit to her primary care physician's office with the chief complaint that she has had trouble tasting food. You recall from your anatomy course that there are multiple lingual papillae connected to our taste buds. Which of the listed lingual papillae does not connect to taste buds?
    A. Fungiform.
    B. Filiform.
    C. Foliate.
    D. Vallate.
    E. All listed papillae connect to taste fibers.
20. A 65-year-old man suffers from a benign tumor affecting the middle of the pterygoid canal. Which of the following nerve fibers could be injured by this condition?
    A. Parasympathetic preganglioniC.
    B. Sympathetic preganglionic.
    C. Taste from the anterior epiglottis.
    D. Parasympathetic postganglionic.
    E. Taste from the anterior two-third of tongue.
21. Which pathway of GVE-para/post fibers from the pterygopalatine ganglion to the lacrimal gland is CORRECT?
    A. PPG, V_2, pterygopalatine nerves, zygomatic nerve, zygomaticofacial nerve, communicating branch, lacrimal nerve.
    B. PPG, pterygopalatine nerves, V_2, communicating branch, zygomatic nerve, zygomaticofacial nerve, lacrimal nerve.
    C. PPG, pterygopalatine nerves, V_2, zygomatic nerve, communicating branch, lacrimal nerve.
    D. PPG, V_2, pterygopalatine nerves, zygomatic nerve, communicating branch, lacrimal nerve.
    E. PPG, pterygopalatine nerves, V_2, zygomatic nerve, communicating branch, zygomaticofacial nerve, lacrimal nerve.
22. What are the functional components of the nerve that supplies the majority of the hard palate?
    A. GSA, GVE-para/post, GVE-sym/post.
    B. GSA, GVE-para/pre, GVE-sym/post.
    C. GVE-para/pre, GVE-sym/pre.
    D. GSA, GVE-para/pre, GVE-sym/post, SVA/SS-taste.
    E. GVE-para/post, GVE-sym/post, SVA/SS-taste.
23. Identify all the muscles involved in abduction of the eyeball?
    A. Medial rectus, inferior rectus, and superior rectus.
    B. Lateral rectus, inferior rectus, and superior rectus.
    C. Lateral rectus, inferior oblique, and superior oblique.
    D. Medial rectus, inferior oblique, and superior oblique.
    E. Medial rectus, levator palpebrae superioris, and lateral rectus.
24. The H-pattern test on a patient's right eye is performed in order to verify the integrity of the extraocular muscles. While the patient's right eye is fully adducted, you ask them to look down and they are unable to. What muscle is impaired?
    A. Inferior rectus.
    B. Superior obliquE.
    C. Lateral rectus.
    D. Inferior oblique.
    E. Medial rectus.
25. If a patient presents with a fully adducted or medially deviated eye while looking straight ahead, this would be consistent with which cranial nerve palsy?
    A. Optic nerve.
    B. Oculomotor nerve.
    C. Trochlear nerve.
    D. Trigeminal nerve.
    E. Abducent nerve.
26. During a neurological exam, a light is flashed at each individual eye to determine the reflex activity of the sphincter (constrictor) pupillae muscle acting on the pupil. The pupillary light reflex involves the afferent and efferent limbs of what cranial nerves?
    A. CN II (afferent) & CN III (efferent).
    B. CN VII (afferent) & CN V_1 (efferent).
    C. CN V_1 (afferent) & CN VII (efferent).
    D. CN II (afferent) & CN V_1 (efferent).
    E. CN III (afferent) & CN VII (efferent).

27. A 56-year-old patient presents with a downward and outward gaze, dilated pupil, and eyelid drooping of the right eye. A CT scan is performed and a space-occupying lesion is identified. Which cranial nerve palsy is present?
  A. Optic nerve.
  B. Oculomotor nerve.
  C. Trochlear nerve.
  D. Trigeminal nerve.
  E. Abducent nerve.

28. A patient is diagnosed with a trochlear nerve (CN IV) injury. Which statement regarding this injury is INCORRECT?
  A. The patient has diplopia (double vision) when looking down.
  B. Head tilt toward the affected eye corrects for extortion (lateral rotation).
  C. The superior oblique muscle is unable to function.
  D. Head tilt away from the affected eye with a chin tuck and then looking up corrects hypertropia.
  E. When looking straight ahead, the affected eye is directed "up and in."

29. The stapedius muscle originates from the pyramidal eminence of what middle ear cavity wall?
  A. Carotid wall.
  B. Mastoid wall.
  C. Labyrinthine wall.
  D. Membranous wall.
  E. Tegmental wall.

30. An individual has otitis media or inflammation of the middle ear cavity. Which cranial nerve listed below is responsible for the sensory innervation (GVA) of the mucosa for the middle ear cavity?
  A. Trigeminal nerve.
  B. Facial nerve.
  C. Vestibulocochlear nerve.
  D. Glossopharyngeal nerve.
  E. Vagus nerve.

31. Which statement about the inner ear is INCORRECT?
  A. The saccule and utricle respond to linear acceleration.
  B. The helicotrema is the communication between the scala vestibuli and scala tympani.
  C. The membranous labyrinth contains perilymph.
  D. The roof of the cochlear duct is formed by the vestibular membrane.
  E. The semicircular ducts respond to rotational head movements.

32. A lesion of the sympathetic trunk in the neck results in Horner syndrome. Which symptom would not be seen in Horner syndrome?
  A. Sinking of the eyeball (enophthalmos).
  B. Flushed skin due to the vasodilation of blood vessels.
  C. Pupillary constriction.
  D. Dropping of the upper eyelid (ptosis).
  E. Profuse sweating on the affected side.

33. An individual has been diagnosed with a left-sided thyroid tumor and it has been decided that they will undergo a left thyroidectomy; however, during the procedure a nerve had been severed. The patient upon coming out of anesthesia is asked to speak and they display a hoarse voice. You suspect the recurrent laryngeal nerve was cut. What muscle acting on the vocal ligaments would not be affected if the recurrent laryngeal nerve were severed?
  A. Posterior cricoarytenoid.
  B. Lateral cricoarytenoid.
  C. Oblique arytenoid.
  D. Vocalis.
  E. Cricothyroid.

34. A 24-year-old presents to the emergency department gasping for air. It is quickly decided that a cricothyrotomy would be performed in order to establish a more complete airway. After a midline incision is made just below the level of the laryngeal prominence, which membrane or ligament is opened to insert an endotracheal tube?
  A. Quadrangular membrane.
  B. Cricothyroid membrane.
  C. Vocal ligament.
  D. Thyrohyoid membrane.
  E. Conus elasticus.

35. A 10-year-old boy has had a tonsillectomy and after the procedure the patient complains of a loss of taste from the posterior one-third of the tongue as well as the general sensation of the same region. Which of the following nerves was most likely damaged?
  A. Lingual branch of CN IX.
  B. Internal laryngeal nerve of CN X.
  C. Lingual nerve of CN V_3.
  D. Chorda tympani of CN VII.
  E. Hypoglossal nerve.

36. Which statement about the "pharynx" is INCORRECT?
  A. Anatomically, the space between the buccopharyngeal and alar fascia is known as the retropharyngeal space.
  B. GSA fibers from CN IX are responsible for sensory innervation of the oropharynx.
  C. The internal laryngeal nerve/superior laryngeal vessels pass through the third pharyngeal wall gap.
  D. SVE/BM fibers from CN IX contribute to the pharyngeal plexus.
  E. Pharyngeal constrictor muscles participate in the third stage of deglutition.

37. Which prevertebral muscle is specifically innervated by the ventral rami of C7–C8?
  A. Longus colli.
  B. Longus capitis.
  C. Anterior scalene.
  D. Middle scalene.
  E. Posterior scalene.

38. From the mucosa, what is the correct order of pharyngeal wall layers?
  A. Mucosa, pharyngobasilar fascia, pharyngeal muscles, submucosa, buccopharyngeal fascia.
  B. Mucosa, submucosa, prevertebral fascia, pharyngobasilar fascia, pharyngeal muscles, buccopharyngeal fascia.
  C. Mucosa, submucosa, pharyngobasilar fascia, pharyngeal muscles, buccopharyngeal fascia.
  D. Mucosa, submucosa, alar fascia, pharyngeal muscles, pharyngobasilar fascia, buccopharyngeal fascia.
  E. Mucosa, submucosa, pharyngeal muscles, pharyngobasilar fascia, buccopharyngeal fascia.

39. Which statement about the pharyngeal arches is CORRECT?
    A. The stapedius muscle develops from the first pharyngeal arch.
    B. Inferior parathyroid glands develop from the third pharyngeal pouch.
    C. Treacher-Collins syndrome involves the malformation of the fourth pharyngeal arch.
    D. Soft palate muscles develop from the second pharyngeal arch.
    E. The lens of the eye develops from the optic vesicle.

40. DiGeorge syndrome is a complex of congenital malformations caused by abnormalities of neural crest migration and proliferation. This occurs during the formation of what pharyngeal arch or arches?
    A. First pharyngeal arch.
    B. Fourth pharyngeal arch.
    C. Sixth pharyngeal arch.
    D. First & second pharyngeal arches.
    E. Third & fourth pharyngeal arches.

ANSWERS

1. **A.** With the patient presenting with a loss of sensation over the mandible and anterior ear along with a sudden dry mouth, structures passing through the foramen ovale would have to be considered. These structures include the lesser petrosal nerve that carries parasympathetic fibers destined to innervate the parotid gland after synapsing at the otic ganglion along with the numerous branches of the mandibular nerve (CN V_3), which represents the facial dermatome located adjacent to the mandible, anterior ear, and posterior temporal region.
2. **B.** The transverse sinus traverses laterally from the confluence of sinuses and until it meets the superior petrosal sinus to form the sigmoid sinus.
3. **E.** The chorda tympani nerve can be damaged during a posterior dislocation of the mandible and the functional components passing through this nerve are GVE-para/pre and SVA/SS-taste from the anterior two-third of the tongue.
4. **D.** The anterior branch of the middle meningeal artery passes just deep to the pterion and is the damaged artery related to an epidural hematoma.
5. **B.** The anterior fontanelle is the last fontanelle to normally close and this occurs between 18 and 36 months of age.
   A. The sphenoid fontanelles close at around 6 months of age.
   C. The posterior fontanelle is generally the first to close at around 1 to 3 months of age.
   D. The mastoid fontanelles close between 6 and 18 months of age.
6. **C.** A subarachnoid hemorrhage is arterial in nature and generally involves the rupture of a saccular/berry aneurysm of a cerebral artery.
7. **E.** The oculomotor nerve (CN III) passes through the superior orbital fissure.
8. **D.** The ansa cervicalis innervates all infrahyoid muscles except for the thyrohyoid muscle.
   A. The ansa cervicalis is formed by ventral rami of C1–C3.
   B. The functional components of ansa cervicalis are GSE, GSA, and GVE-sym/post.
   C. Ansa cervicalis does not innervate any suprahyoid muscles including the hyoglossus muscle.
   E. The superior root only consists of C1 fibers.
9. **C.** Although GVA fibers from both the glossopharyngeal and vagus nerves innervate the carotid sinus, it is believed the GVA fibers passing through the glossopharyngeal nerve play a larger role.
10. **E.** All structures listed above can be found in the muscular triangle of the larger anterior triangle of the neck except for the geniohyoid muscle.
11. **B.** The stylohyoid muscle is innervated by the facial nerve (CN VII).
    A. Hyoglossus—CN XII.
    C. Middle pharyngeal constrictor—CN X.
    D. Anterior belly of digastric—mylohyoid nerve of CN V_3.
    E. Mylohyoid—mylohyoid nerve of CN V_3.
12. **D.** The loose connective tissue of the scalp is the layer that allows free movement of the scalp proper.
13. **A.** The functional components of the zygomatic branch of the facial nerve are SVE/BM and GSA.
    B. The mental nerve is a V_3 branch.
    C. The posterior auricular vein and the posterior branch of retromandibular vein form the external jugular vein and not the internal jugular vein.
    D. The orbicularis oris muscle is innervated by CN VII and not CN V_3.
    E. Bell palsy is related to CN VII and not CN V_1.
14. **D.** The correct pathway for parasympathetic fibers to reach the parotid gland from CN IX is as follows: CN IX, tympanic nerve, tympanic plexus, lesser petrosal nerve, otic ganglion, auriculotemporal nerve, parotid gland.
15. **E.** GSA, GVE-Para/pre, and SVA/SS-taste from anterior two-third of tongue are the functional components of the second portion of the lingual nerve.
16. **D.** The lateral pterygoid muscle will function in depression, protraction, and lateral deviation of the jaw/mandible.
17. **C.** The accessory meningeal artery is a branch of the first (mandibular) part of the maxillary artery.
18. **A.** All of tongue muscles are innervated by the hypoglossal nerve except for the palatoglossus muscle, which is innervated by the vagus nerve (CN X).
19. **B.** The filiform papillae are long and conical projections located on the majority of the dorsal tongue surface and contain afferent nerve endings but no taste buds.
20. **A.** The nerve that passes through the pterygoid canal is called the nerve of the pterygoid canal or Vidian nerve. This nerve is formed with the fusion of the greater petrosal and deep petrosal nerves. The functional components passing through the nerve of the pterygoid canal are GVE-parasympathetic preganglionic, sympathetic postganglionic, and SVA/SS taste from the soft palate. Thus, A is the only answer.
21. **C.** The correct pathway for GVE-para/post fibers to travel from after originating from the pterygopalatine ganglion (PPG) would be as follows: PPG, pterygopalatine nerves, V_2, zygomatic nerve, communicating branch, and then the lacrimal nerve.
22. **A.** The greater palatine nerve innervates the majority of the hard palate mucosa. It carries GSA, GVE-para/post, and sym/post fibers.
23. **C.** The lateral rectus, inferior oblique, and superior oblique have the ability to abduct the eyeball.

24. **B.** With the eye fully adducted, the superior oblique muscle is the primary muscle that allows the eye to move downward. Thus, if a patient is unable to look down, the superior oblique muscle itself or the trochlear nerve that innervates it has been damaged.
25. **E.** While looking straight ahead, if a patient has a fully adducted or medially deviated eye, the patient is presenting with an abducent nerve palsy.
26. **A.** The pupillary reflex has an afferent limb involving CN II and an efferent limb involving CN III. The efferent limb is more focused on the parasympathetics fibers that course through the inferior division of CN III before synapsing at the ciliary ganglion and continuing to the sphincter (constrictor) pupillae muscle.
27. **B.** An oculomotor nerve (CN III) palsy would be the reason a patient presents with a downward and outward gaze, dilated pupil, and the eyelid drooping.
28. **B.** Head tilt away from the affected eye corrects for extortion (lateral rotation). This can be combined with answer E where an individual does a chin tuck and then looks up to correct hypertropia.
29. **B.** The stapedius muscle originates from the pyramidal eminence located on the mastoid (posterior) wall.
30. **D.** The middle ear cavity mucosa is innervated by GVA fibers that pass through.
31. **C.** All statements are correct except C. The membranous labyrinth would contain endolymph and not perilymph.
32. **E.** If the sympathetic fibers were damaged, sweating would be reduced, not increased on the affected side.
33. **E.** The cricothyroid muscle is innervated by the external laryngeal nerve.
34. **B.** The cricothyroid membrane is opened to allow passage of an endotracheal tube during a cricothyrotomy.
35. **A.** The lingual branch of the glossopharyngeal nerve (CN IX) passes just deep to the tonsils and is at risk of being damaged during a tonsillectomy.
36. **D.** The SVE/BM fibers from CN IX that ultimately innervate the stylopharyngeus muscle do not contribute to the pharyngeal plexus.
37. **E.** The posterior scalene is innervated by the ventral rami of C7–C8.
    A. The longus colli is innervated by the ventral rami of C2–C6.
    B. The longus capitis is innervated by the ventral rami of C1–C3.
    C. The anterior scalene is innervated by the ventral rami of C4–C6.
    D. The middle scalene is innervated by the ventral rami of C3–C8.
38. **C.** The correct order from the internal mucosal layer to the outer pharyngeal wall is as follows: mucosa, submucosa, pharyngobasilar fascia, pharyngeal muscles, and then the buccopharyngeal fascia.
39. **B.** The inferior parathyroid glands develop from the third pharyngeal pouches.
    A. The stapedius muscle develops from the second pharyngeal arch.
    C. Treacher-Collins syndrome involves the malformation of the first pharyngeal arch.
    D. Soft palate muscles develop from the fourth pharyngeal arch.
    E. The lens of the eye develops from the lens placode.
40. **E.** Congenital malformations related to DiGeorge syndrome can be traced back to abnormalities of neural crest cell migration and proliferation to the third and fourth pharyngeal arches.

References

1. Ernest A, Herzog M, Seidl RO. Head and Neck Trauma: An Interdisciplinary Approach. New York: Thieme; 2006
2. Hardt N., Kuttenberger J. Anatomy of the Craniofacial Region. In: Hardt N., Kuttenberger J. (eds) Craniofacial Trauma. Berlin, Heidelberg: Springer; 2010
3. Bushdid C, Magnasco MO, Vosshall LB, Keller A. Humans can discriminate more than 1 trillion olfactory stimuli. Science. 2014;343(6177):1370–1372
4. Gelfand S. Essentials of Audiology. New York: Thieme; 2011

8 Introductory Concepts of the Nervous System

LEARNING OBJECTIVES

- To understand the general structure of the nervous system.
- To describe neurons and how they are classified by the number of neurites, axonal length or function.
- To describe an action potential.
- Know the difference between a myelinated and unmyelinated nerve fiber. Describe multiple motor and sensory nerve fibers and their functions.
- To understand where a synapse occurs and the different types of synapses.
- To describe the specific neuroglia of the nervous system.
- To describe clinical correlates such as transneuronal degeneration, multiple sclerosis and gliomas.

The cells (neurons) of the nervous system communicate by way of electrical signals that produce almost immediate responses. As described previously in the Introductory Concepts chapter, the nervous system is divided into structural and functional components.

- The **central nervous system (CNS)** and **peripheral nervous system (PNS)** make up the structural portion of this system. The CNS is made up of the brain and spinal cord and they are the main centers where integration and correlation of nervous information occurs. The PNS consists of most cranial nerves and all of the spinal nerves, which are made up of bundles of axons or nerve fibers responsible for carrying information to and from the CNS (**Fig. 8.1**).
- The **somatic nervous system (SNS)** and the **autonomic nervous system (ANS)** make up the functional portion of this system. Somatic motor and sensory fibers supply the skeletal muscles and sensation from the skin and joints. The ANS is motor only to visceral organs, smooth muscle and glands and is made up of either *parasympathetic* or *sympathetic* fibers. Visceral sensory fibers can pair with the visceral motor fibers but they by definition are not part of the ANS (**Fig. 8.2**).

8.1 Neurons

The parenchymal cell of the nervous system is known as the **neuron**. A neuron itself refers to a nerve cell and all of its processes. They can be located in the brain, spinal cord and ganglia. These specialized excitable cells serve two functions: to receive stimuli and to conduct nerve impulses. The shape and size of neurons varies considerably and mature neurons mostly lose the ability to undergo division and replication like other cells in the body. There are as many as 100 million neurons in the nervous system, each having contact with more than 1,000 other individual neurons.

Each neuron possesses a **cell body** of which there are one or more surface projections called **neurites** (processes). Neurites that receive information are called **dendrites** and can they can form an extensive *dendritic arborization* or branching density. The longer individual neurite conducting impulses is called the **axon**. The axon arises from a small conical elevation on the cell body called the **axon hillock** and this area is devoid of *Nissl substance*. The impulses are amplified or increased when **myelin** or the **myelin sheath** is present around these axons. Myelin does not form a continuous layer because it is interrupted at regular intervals called **nodes of Ranvier**. The distance between two nodes is called an **internode** and represents the distance covered by a single *oligodendroglia* or *Schwann cell*. Depolarization occurs at the nodes and demonstrates a salutatory (or leaping) conduction; thus the myelin serves to increase the velocity of conduction of the nerve impulse. The term **nerve fiber** can refer to either the dendrite or axon. Neurons can be classified by the number of neurites (processes), axonal length and their functions (**Fig. 8.3**).

8.1.1 Classifying Neurons Based on the Number of Neurites

- **Multipolar**: numerous dendrites and a single axon extending out from the cell body. These are the most abundant type of neuron in the CNS and are found in both the brain and spinal cord. They include motor neurons, interneurons, pyramidal cells of the cerebral cortex, and the Purkinje cells of the cerebellar cortex (**Fig. 8.4a,b**).
- **Pseudounipolar**: a short single process extending down from the cell body that divides the axon into a peripheral process extending from a sensory receptor and a central process that connects to the CNS. These neurons relay sensory information from a peripheral receptor to the CNS without modifying the signal. They are primarily sensory afferent neurons in spinal or cranial nerves of the PNS and their cell bodies are located in a dorsal root or cranial nerve ganglia (**Fig. 8.4f**).
- **Bipolar**: elongated cell body that is connected on one side by either the axon or a single main dendrite. These types of neurons are related to special senses and are commonly found in the retina, olfactory epithelium and the vestibular and cochlear ganglia (**Fig. 8.4e**).

8.1.2 Classifying Neurons Based on Axonal Length

- **Golgi Type I**: have a long axon and are the neurons that form the long fiber tracts of the brain and spinal cord and fibers of the peripheral nervous system. Examples include pyramidal cells of the cerebral cortex, Purkinje cells of the cerebellar cortex, and the motor neurons of the spinal cord (**Fig. 8.4a,c,d**).
- **Golgi Type II**: may have a short axon or none at all. They greatly outnumber Golgi type I neurons. They are numerous in both the cerebral and cerebellar cortexes. An example would be interneurons (**Fig. 8.4b**).

8.1.3 Classifying Neurons Based on Function

- **Motor (efferent)**: these multipolar neurons have their cell bodies mostly located in the ventral horn of the spinal cord and make up the motor division of the PNS. The notable exception

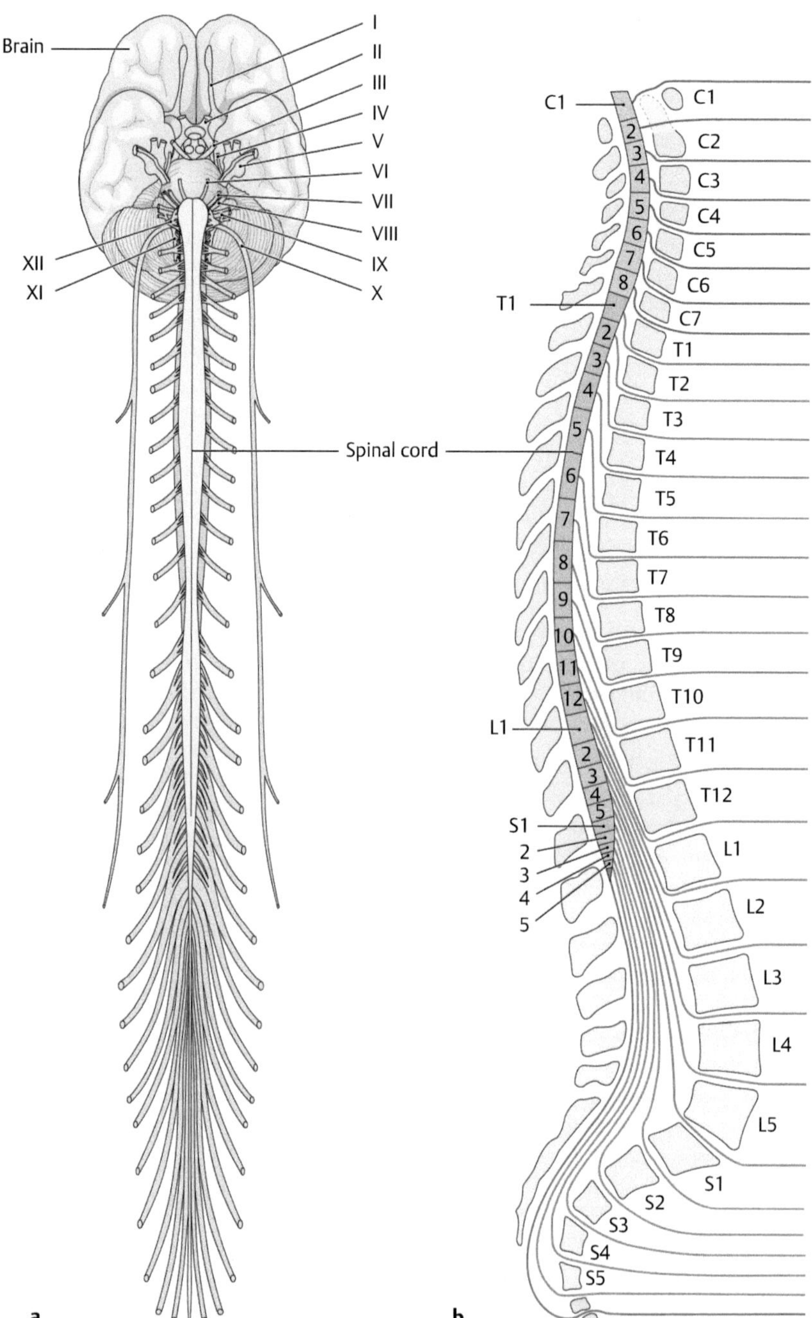

Fig. 8.1 **(a)** Central and peripheral nervous system. **(b)** Spinal segments of the spinal cord and spinal nerves. (From Schuenke M, Schulte E, Schumacher U. THIEME Atlas of Anatomy. General Anatomy and Musculoskeletal System. Illustrations by Voll M and Wesker K. 3rd ed. New York: Thieme Medical Publishers; 2020.)

to cell body location would be the postganglionic fibers of the ANS. These neurons conduct impulses away from the CNS to effector organs such as skeletal muscle, glands and smooth muscle of blood vessels.

- **Sensory (afferent)**: these are almost entirely pseudounipolar neurons that have cell bodies located in a dorsal root or cranial nerve ganglia. These neurons conduct impulses from sensory receptors back towards the CNS and make up the sensory division of the PNS.
- **Interneuron (association)**: these multipolar neurons link together motor and sensory neurons to form complex neuronal pathways. They make up over 99.9% of all neurons in the body but are confined to the CNS.

8.2 Nerve Cell Body and Action Potentials

The nerve cell body is similar to other cells, in which a nucleus is embedded within the cytoplasm. The nucleus is generally centrally located and round. There is a single nucleolus that functions

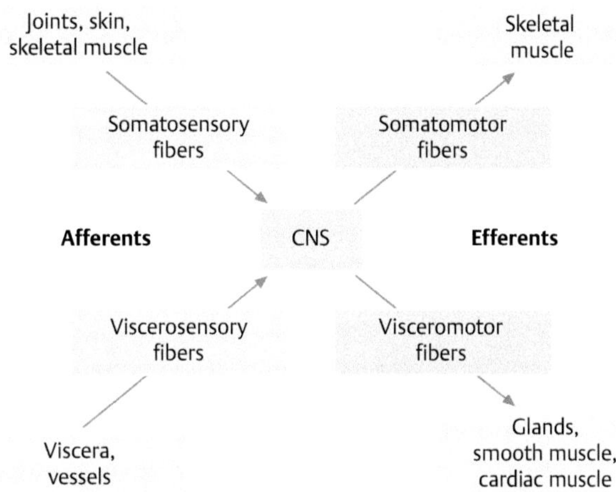

Fig. 8.2 Schematic representation of information flow in the nervous system. (From Schuenke M, Schulte E, Schumacher U. THIEME Atlas of Anatomy. General Anatomy and Musculoskeletal System. Illustrations by Voll M and Wesker K. 3rd ed. New York: Thieme Medical Publishers; 2020.)

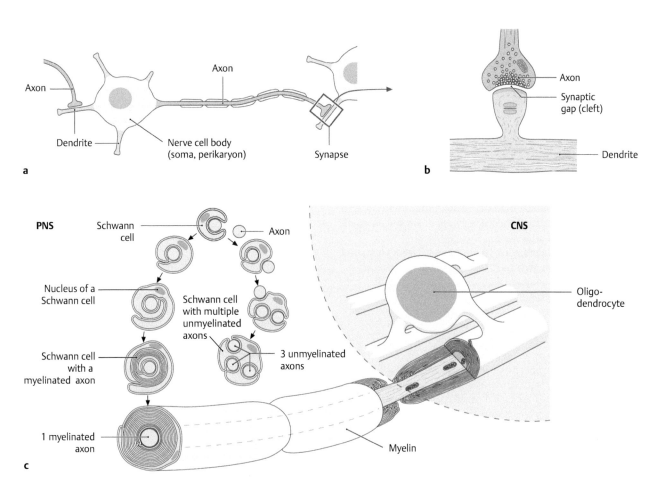

Fig. 8.3 **(a,b)** Nerve cell body and action potentials. **(c)** Myelination differences in the PNS and CNS. (From Schuenke M, Schulte E, Schumacher U. THIEME Atlas of Anatomy. Head, Neck, and Neuroanatomy. Illustrations by Voll M and Wesker K. 2nd ed. New York: Thieme Medical Publishers; 2016.)

in ribosomal ribonucleic acid (rRNA) synthesis and ribosome subunit assembly. The cytoplasm has an abundant amount of both granular and agranular endoplasmic reticulum along with organelles located in other cells. **Nissl substance** has an important role in protein synthesis. It is characteristic to nerve cells and is found in the cytoplasm and dendrites but not at the axon hillock or axon. The **Golgi complexes** appear near the nucleus and receive proteins produced by the Nissl substance. The Golgi complex may help produce lysosomes and synthesize cell membranes particular to synaptic vesicles located at the axon terminals. **Lysosomes** are

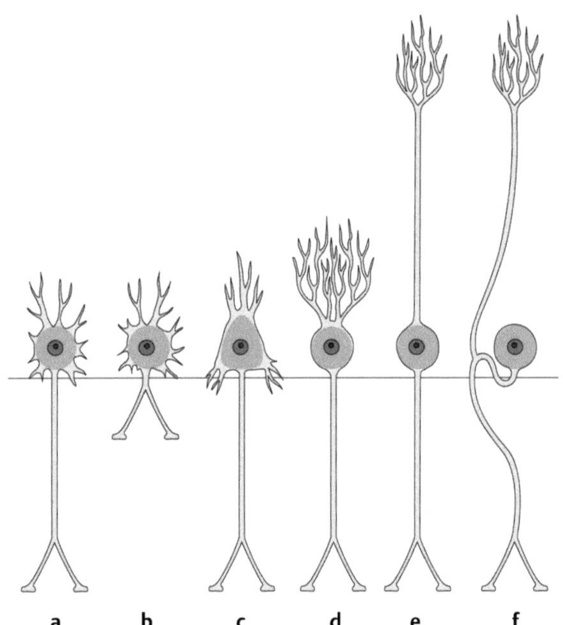

Fig. 8.4 Basic forms of the neuron and its functionally adapted variants. (a) Multipolar neuron with a long axon. (b) Multipolar neuron with a short axon. (c) Pyramidal cell. (d) Purkinje cell. (e) Bipolar neuron. (f) Pseudounipolar neuron. (From Schuenke M, Schulte E, Schumacher U. THIEME Atlas of Anatomy. Head, Neck, and Neuroanatomy. Illustrations by Voll M and Wesker K. 2nd ed. New York: Thieme Medical Publishers; 2016.)

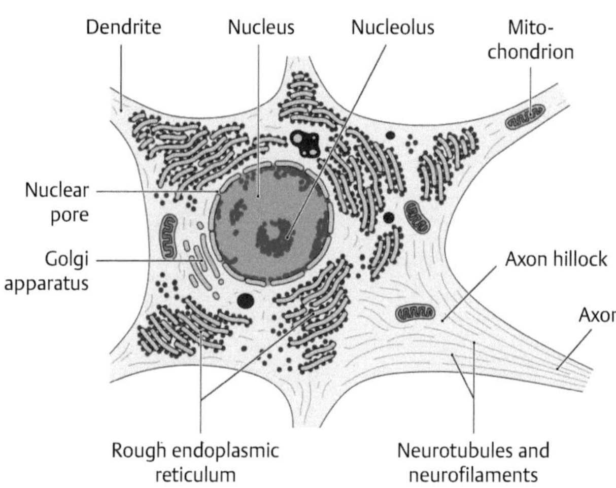

Fig. 8.5 Electron microscopy of the neuron. (From Schuenke M, Schulte E, Schumacher U. THIEME Atlas of Anatomy. Head, Neck, and Neuroanatomy. Illustrations by Voll M and Wesker K. 2nd ed. New York: Thieme Medical Publishers; 2016.)

membrane-bound vesicles that contain hydrolytic enzymes and are involved in intracellular digestion. **Mitochondria** are located throughout the cytoplasm of the cell body, dendrites and axon and produce energy **(Fig. 8.5)**.

The **cytoskeleton** is the internal supportive network composed of filamentous protein structures. **Microtubules** are the largest and located in the cell body and neurites. They are arranged in parallel, pointing to and from the cell body. Their function is in intracellular transportation and the development and maintenance of cell shape. **Neurofilaments** form the main component of the cytoskeleton and are located in the cell body and neurites. They have a role in developing and regenerating nerve fibers. However, when they begin to degenerate they form **neurofibrillary tangles** and this is associated with Alzheimer's disease. The smallest of these protein structures are called **microfilaments** are they are composed of actin. They are concentrated at the periphery of the cytoplasm near the plasma membrane and at the tips of growing axons. They assist the microtubules with the formation of new and the retraction of old cell processes in addition to facilitating axon transport **(Fig. 8.5)**.

The **dendrites** are short neurites that arise from the cell body and can branch profusely **(Fig. 8.3)**. The finer branches may contain **dendritic spines**, small projections that are involved in synaptic strength and transmission of electrical signals toward the cell body. Dendrites increase the surface area to which axons from other neurons can attach. The cytoplasm is consistent with that of the cell body but dendrites do not contain Golgi complexes. They essentially receive a synaptic impulse and transmit it to the cell body.

The **axon (Fig. 8.3)** is a tubular structure with a uniform diameter and is either myelinated or unmyelinated. Larger diameter axons conduct impulses more rapidly while smaller diameter axons have slower impulses. Collateral branches can occur along the length of an axon but generally not near the cell body. There is profuse branching at the axon's most distal end and these branches are referred to as **axon terminals**. A series of swellings occur at these terminal ends and are called **varicosities**. The axon cytoplasm, known as **axoplasm**, lacks Nissl granules and Golgi complexes that are normally found in the cell body cytoplasm. This means protein production is not possible and axon survival is dependent on the transportation of substances from the cell body. Movement of these substances is done through **axoplasmic (axonal) transport**, a cellular process responsible for distributing secretory proteins, lipids, organelles and cytoskeletal structures back and forth between the cell body and axon of a neuron. Movement may be described as either fast or slow and in an anterograde (away from the cell body) or retrograde (back to the cell body) direction.

- **Fast anterograde**: movement of newly formed synaptic vesicles and precursor of neurotransmitters. This process is mediated by microtubules and the protein *kinesin*. The rate of transport is ~100-400 mm/day.
- **Slow anterograde**: involves the movement of neurofilaments, microtubules and additional cytoskeletal elements. The rate of transport is ~0.1-5 mm/day.
- **Fast retrograde**: used materials from the axon terminal are sent back to the cell body to be recycled and broken down. The process is mediated by microtubules and the protein *dynein* and proceeds at a rate of 100-200 mm/day. This is the common pathogen invasion pathway of the herpes simplex, polio and rabies viruses, along with the tetanus toxin.
- **Fast mitochondrial**: transport of mitochondria in either direction, which proceeds at a rate of ~75 mm/day.

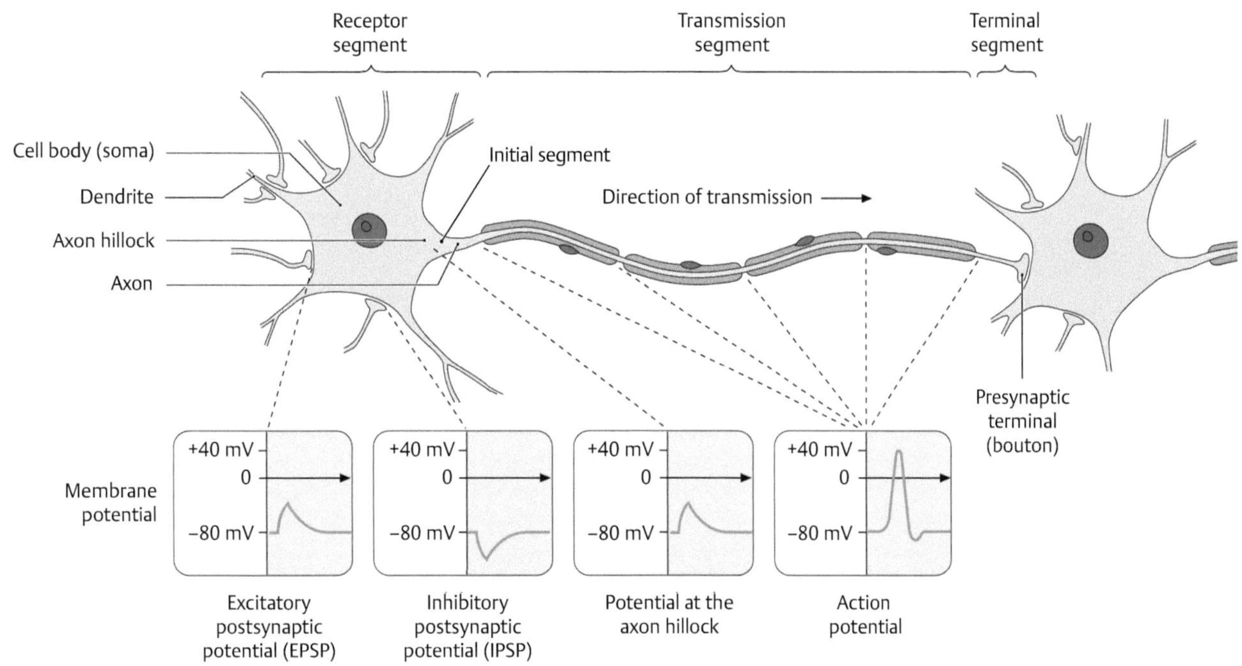

Fig. 8.6 The nerve cell (neuron): The receptor segment corresponds to the cell body and the dendrites. The transmission segment (axon) carries the information to the target cell. The terminal segment is responsible for relaying the information to the target cell. (From Schuenke M, Schulte E, Schumacher U. THIEME Atlas of Anatomy. Head, Neck, and Neuroanatomy. Illustrations by Voll M and Wesker K. 2nd ed. New York: Thieme Medical Publishers; 2016.)

Clinical Correlate 8.1

Transneuronal Degeneration

With the central nervous system, if one group of neurons is injured, then a second group of neurons further along the pathway and serving the same function can also show signs of degeneration. This is a form of *anterograde* **transneuronal degeneration.** Alzheimer's and Huntington's disease have been linked to this degeneration. A form of *retrograde* transneuronal degeneration would include amyotropic lateral sclerosis (ALS) or Lou Gehrig's disease.

The most excitable part of the axon is the **initial segment**, the portion of the axon just distal to the axon hillock of the cell body. This is where an *action potential* originates. Axons generally conduct impulses away from the cell body except for sensory neurons, where impulses head back toward the cell body (**Fig. 8.6**).

An **action potential** or *nerve impulse* occurs when there is a rapid change in membrane permeability to Na^+ ions. The Na^+ ions move into the axon through Na^+ channels, causing depolarization. An action potential is approximately +40 mV and lasts about 2-5 milliseconds. The increased membrane permeability for the Na^+ ions quickly dissipates while permeability for K^+ ions increases, thus K^+ ions begin to flow from the cell cytoplasm and return the localized area of the cell to the resting state (-80 mV). A nerve cell can be stimulated by chemical, electrical or mechanical means (**Fig. 8.6**).

Action potentials spread over the plasma membrane and away from the site of initiation. The impulse is self-propagated and its size and frequency does not alter. After an impulse has occurred over a portion of the plasma membrane, an additional action potential cannot be elicited immediately. This non-excitable state is known as the **refractory period** and it has control over the maximum frequency of the action potentials. The greater the strength of the initial stimulus or excitation, the more widely the initial depolarization is spread into the surrounding areas of the plasma membrane. If multiple stimuli are applied to the surface of a neuron there is a cumulative effect.

Additional axons of other neurons form synapses with the target neuron and at these synapses there can be either an excitatory or inhibitory release of neurotransmitters. These neurotransmitters bind to receptors at the cell membrane of the target neuron and create either a local increase or decrease in the membrane potential. This is known as an excitatory postsynaptic potential (EPSP) or inhibitory postsynaptic potential (IPSP) respectively (**Fig. 8.6**).

8.3 Nerve Fibers

The general **nerve fiber** is defined primarily as the axon of a nerve cell. Some authors include the dendrites as part of a nerve fiber. Bundles of nerve fibers represent nerve tracts in the CNS while bundles of nerve fibers in the PNS are referred to as peripheral nerves. A nerve fiber in either the CNS or PNS can be either myelinated or unmyelinated. The myelin sheath is not part of the neuron but of a supporting cell. The supporting cell in the CNS is known as the **oligodendrocyte** while in the PNS it is known as the **Schwann cell.** The oligodendrocyte may form and maintain myelin sheaths of up to 60 individual axons. There is only one Schwann cell for each segment of one nerve fiber. The myelin sheath is segmented

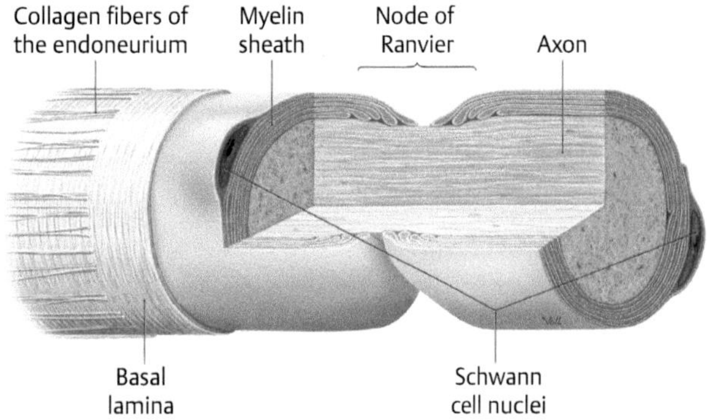

Fig. 8.7 (a) Myelinated axon in the PNS. (From Schuenke M, Schulte E, Schumacher U. THIEME Atlas of Anatomy. Head, Neck, and Neuroanatomy. Illustrations by Voll M and Wesker K. 2nd ed. New York: Thieme Medical Publishers; 2016.)

Clinical Correlate 8.2

Multiple Sclerosis

The most common autoimmune disorder affecting the central nervous system is multiple sclerosis (MS). It is a demyelinating disease wherein the myelin surrounding neurons slowly becomes disrupted or damaged and lesions within the white matter are apparent. This creates communication problems between the brain and the rest of the body. There may be trouble with motor, sensory, vision, mental, or autonomic problems. The first symptoms may begin between 20-40 years of age and generally include blurred vision. Most MS patients have some form of muscle weakness in their extremities and have difficulty with coordination and balance. There is no known cure but treatments attempt to improve overall function. MS may range from fairly benign to disabling.

and interrupted at regular intervals by the **nodes of Ranvier** (**Fig. 8.7**).

Nerve fiber **conduction velocity** is proportional to the cross-sectional area of the axon, thus the thicker diameter nerve fibers conduct an impulse more quickly than those of a smaller diameter. Conduction velocities can be as high as 120 m/sec in an alpha fiber or as low as 0.5 m/sec in an unmyelinated nerve fiber. The myelin sheath acts as an insulator, increasing the speed at which action potentials propagate along an axon. A myelinated fiber is only stimulated at the nodes of Ranvier, where the axon allows ions to pass freely through the plasma membrane. Action potentials ultimately jump from one node to the next and this creates a current in the surrounding tissue fluid that quickly becomes depolarized at the next node. This leaping effect is referred to as **saltatory conduction**. The action potential through an unmyelinated fiber passes continuously through the axon progressively exciting adjacent areas of the membrane, like a wave.

Axons can be classified into A, B and C groups based on their contribution to a compound action potential in a mixed nerve. Group A is further subdivided into alpha (α), beta (β), delta (δ) and gamma (γ) subgroups, where alpha is the fastest- and gamma is the slowest-conducting axon. Somatic alpha motor neurons are large, whereas gamma motor neurons are smaller. Both are myelinated and part of the A group axons. Sensory fibers may be classified on the basis of axon diameter and myelin thickness into groups I, II, III and IV. Group I axons are large and heavily myelinated and each successive group is gradually smaller and less myelinated, with group IV being unmyelinated. The B group axons are isolated to preganglionic autonomic fibers. The C group axons are associated with either postganglionic autonomics or slow pain and temperature fibers. These axons are also the most sensitive to local anesthetics, with group A axons being the least sensitive. Descriptions of different nerve fibers are found in **Table 8.1**.

Table 8.1 **Nerve fibers: motor fibers vs sensory fibers**

Fiber Type	Conduction Velocity (m/s)	Fiber Diameter (mm)	Function
Motor axons			
Alpha (Aα)	70-120	12-20	Alpha motor neurons that innervate the extrafusal fibers of skeletal muscle
Gamma (Aγ)	10-50	2-8	Gamma motor neurons that innervate the intrafusal fibers of skeletal muscle
Preganglionic autonomics (B)	3-15	1-3	Myelinated preganglionic autonomic fibers
Postganglionic autonomics (C)	0.5-2	0.2-1.2	Unmyelinated postganglionic autonomic fibers
Sensory axons			
Ia (Aα)	70-120	12-20	Proprioception from muscle spindles
Ib (Aα)	70-120	12-20	Proprioception from Golgi tendon organs and Ruffini corpuscles
II (Aβ)	30-80	5-15	Touch, pressure, vibration and joint receptors
III (Aδ)	10-30	2-5	Free nerve endings for fast pain and temperature; hair follicles
IV (C)	0.5-2	0.2-1.2	Free nerve endings for slow pain and temperature

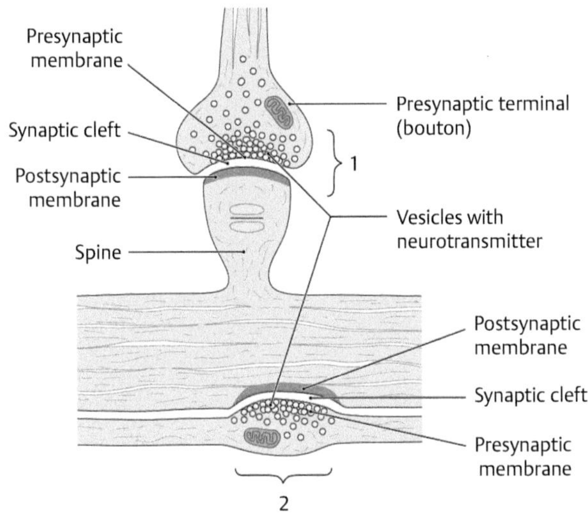

Fig. 8.8 Synapses. A synapse with a dendritic spine (1). A side-by-side synapse called a parallel contact or *bouton en passage* (2). (From Schuenke M, Schulte E, Schumacher U. THIEME Atlas of Anatomy. Head, Neck, and Neuroanatomy. Illustrations by Voll M and Wesker K. 2nd ed. New York: Thieme Medical Publishers; 2016.)

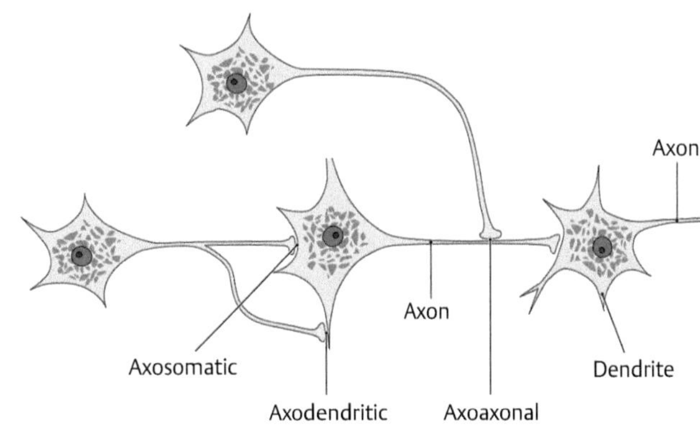

Fig. 8.9 Types of synapses. (From Schuenke M, Schulte E, Schumacher U. THIEME Atlas of Anatomy. Head, Neck, and Neuroanatomy. Illustrations by Voll M and Wesker K. 2nd ed. New York: Thieme Medical Publishers; 2016.)

8.4 Synapses

The nervous system is made up of neurons that are linked together to form functional conducting pathways and the site of communication between two neurons, an effector cell, or sensory receptor cell is referred to as a **synapse (Fig. 8.8)**. This physiological communication occurs in one direction only. A synapse is made up of a **presynaptic membrane**, **synaptic cleft** and **postsynaptic membrane.** On the presynaptic side there are membrane-bound sacs called **synaptic vesicles** filled with neurotransmitters. The axon terminal has an abundant amount of mitochondria because neurotransmitter secretion uses a great deal of energy. An impulse stimulates the vesicles to discharge neurotransmitters into the synaptic cleft. They then bind to receptors located on the plasma membrane of the postsynaptic membrane.

8.4.1 Types of Synapses

- **Axodendritic**: between an axon and dendrite and they are the most common synapses in the CNS. The dendritic arborization pattern allows for thousands of axodendritic synapses to occur, leading to the generation of an electrical signal or action potential **(Fig. 8.9)**.
- **Axosomatic**: between an axon and a cell body. A much more powerful signal for a new action potential because the synapse is near the axon hillock but it is less common in the CNS.
- **Axoaxonic**: between an axon and another axon. These synapses are also near or on the axon hillock leading to either a powerful action potential or inhibition of an action potential.

A particular synapse can be classified as either chemical or electrical in nature.

- **Chemical**: these are the vast majority of all synapses and involve neurotransmitters. Acetylcholine (ACh), norepinephrine (NE), epinephrine, gamma-aminobutyric acid (GABA), dopamine, serotonin, glycine, substance P, glutamic acid and enkephalins are all considered neurotransmitters and some are either excitatory or inhibitory.
- **Electrical**: consist of presynaptic and postsynaptic membranes connected by gap junctions that allow ions to pass from one cell to the other.

8.5 Neuroglia

The supportive/stromal cells of nervous system are called **neuroglia**. The neuroglia (glial) cells provide structural and metabolic support and outnumber neurons as much as 50:1. They are non-neuronal and non-excitable and vary depending on if they are found in the CNS or PNS. There are six different types of neuroglia and the CNS contains *astrocytes*, *oligodendroglia*, *microglia* and *ependymal cells* while the PNS contains *Schwann* and *satellite cells*.

1. **Astrocytes**: the largest of the neuroglia and the most common cell type of the nervous system. A few of the functions include; helping regulate the transmission of electrical impulses within the brain; neurotransmitter uptake; providing nutrition to neurons, andhelping form the blood-brain barrier. They proliferate and form scar tissue following injury to neurons. There are two types:
   - **Fibrous astrocytes**: found mainly in white matter and their processes pass between nerve fibers **(Fig. 8.10)**.
   - **Protoplasmic astrocytes**: found mainly in gray matter and their processes pass between nerve cell bodies **(Fig. 8.10)**.

   Astrocyte processes end as expansions or **astrocyte end feet** and they can line the blood vessels (perivascular feet) in the brain and contribute to the blood-brain barrier. These end feet can also contribute to the outer and inner glial limiting membranes. The **outer glial limiting membrane** is located below the pia mater. The **inner glial limiting membrane** is located beneath the ependyma lining the ventricles of the brain and central canal of the spinal cord.
2. **Oligodendroglia**: also known as oligodendrocytes, these are smaller than astrocytes and myelinate up to 60 neuronal axons at one time to increase impulse speed **(Fig. 8.7)**.

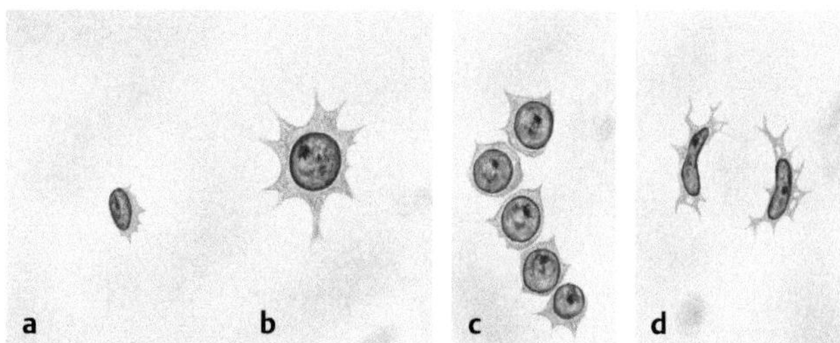

Fig. 8.10 Types of neuroglia with cell nuclei demonstrated with a basic stain. **(a)** Fibrous astrocyte. **(b)** Protoplasmic astrocyte. **(c)** Oligodendrocytes. **(d)** Microglia. (From Schuenke M, Schulte E, Schumacher U. THIEME Atlas of Anatomy. Head, Neck, and Neuroanatomy. Illustrations by Voll M and Wesker K. 2nd ed. New York: Thieme Medical Publishers; 2016.)

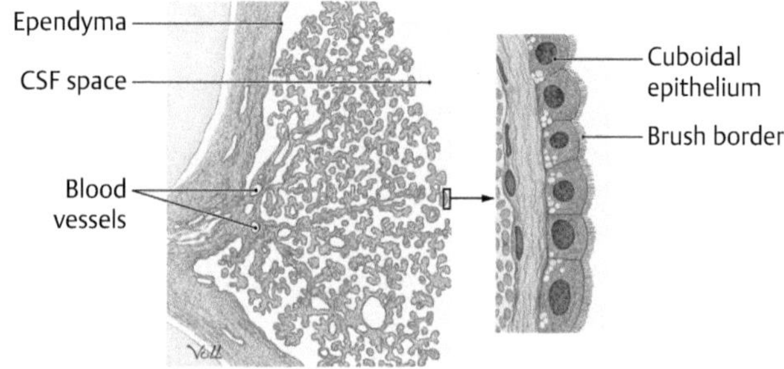

Fig. 8.11 Ependyma of the choroid plexus. (From Schuenke M, Schulte E, Schumacher U. THIEME Atlas of Anatomy. Head, Neck, and Neuroanatomy. Illustrations by Voll M and Wesker K. 2nd ed. New York: Thieme Medical Publishers; 2016.)

3. **Microglia**: they are resident macrophages and appear after an injury. They continuously scavenge for infectious agents, plaques or damaged neurons. They arise from monocytes that have entered the CNS from the blood **(Fig. 8.10)**.
4. **Ependymal**: these mainly *cuboidal cells* are found lining the ventricles and central canal of the spinal cord. They form a single layer and their microvilli and cilia help circulate cerebrospinal fluid (CSF). Ependymal cells are divided into three groups **(Fig. 8.11)**:
   - **Ependymocytes**: the cells in contact with CSF and that line the brain ventricles and central canal of the spinal cord.
   - **Choroidal epithelial cells**: these cells cover the choroid plexus and produce and absorb CSF. Tight junctions between these cells prevent leakage of CSF into underlying tissues.
   - **Tanycytes**: these cells mainly line the floor of the third ventricle and help form a blood-CSF barrier overlying the median eminence of the hypothalamus.
5. **Schwann**: the PNS equivalent of oligodendroglia and encloses the axons of the PNS. These cells only insulate one axon at a time and aid in the regeneration of peripheral nerves **(Fig. 8.7)**.
6. **Satellite**: provide support for the cell bodies of sensory, parasympathetic and sympathetic ganglia in the PNS.

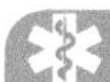

Clinical Correlate 8.3

Gliomas

Gliomas are named according to the specific cell type they are derived from and this will include astrocytes, oligodendrocytes or ependymocytes. They may be classified based on their location above (supratentorial) or below (infratentorial) the tentorium cerebelli. Low-grade gliomas may initially begin benign but have the potential to reach high-grade status and become malignant. The exact causes of gliomas are unknown but the most common primary brain tumor among adults is an astrocytoma.

PRACTICE QUESTIONS

1. Which part of an axon is the most excitable?
   A. Terminal segment.
   B. Initial segment.
   C. Transmission segment.
   D. Axon terminals.
   E. Node of Ranvier.
2. Which statement regarding specific nerve fibers is INCORRECT?
   A. Preganglionic autonomic (B) motor axons are myelinated fibers with a conduction velocity of 3-15 m/s.
   B. Ib (Aα) sensory axons receive proprioceptive information from Golgi tendon organs and Ruffini corpuscles.
   C. III (Aδ) sensory axons are free nerve endings that receive fast pain and temperature information.
   D. Alpha (Aα) motor axons have a conduction velocity of 70-120 m/s.
   E. Gamma (Aγ) motor axons function as unmyelinated postganglionic autonomic fibers.
3. These type of neuroglia are the resident macrophages and appear after an injury or continuously scavenge for infectious agents, plaques or damaged neurons.
   A. Microglia.
   B. Oligodendroglia.
   C. Astrocyte.
   D. Ependymal.
   E. Schwann.
4. Which statement regarding a neuron is INCORRECT?
   A. Pseudounipolar neurons have a short single process extending from the cell body and both a central and peripheral axon process.
   B. Bipolar neurons are related to the special senses.
   C. Sensory or afferent neurons are multipolar and have cell bodies located in the dorsal root ganglion or cranial nerve ganglia.
   D. Multipolar neurons have numerous dendrites and a single axon extending out from the cell body.
   E. Golgi type I cells form the long fiber tracts of the brain, spinal cord, and peripheral nervous system.

ANSWERS

1. **B.** The initial segment of the axon is the most excitable part of an axon.
2. **E.** Gamma (Aγ) motor axons innervate the intrafusal fibers of skeletal muscle.
3. **A.** Microglia.
4. **C.** Sensory or afferent neurons are almost exclusively pseudounipolar and have their cell bodies located in the dorsal root ganglion or cranial nerve ganglia.

9 Central Nervous System

LEARNING OBJECTIVES

- To understand the general structure of gray and white matter, the meningeal layers, and ventricular system of the central nervous system.
- To describe the feature differences between the gray and white matter of the spinal cord.
- To describe the different parts of the brainstem and the role of the reticular formation. Clinical correlates of the brainstem include lateral medullary, dorsal medullary, medial medullary, caudal basal pontine, tegmental pontine, rostral basal pontine, tegmental pontine, Weber, Parinaud, and Benedikt syndromes.
- To describe the gross structure, peduncles, histology, and nuclei of the cerebellum. Clinical correlates include ataxia, hypotonia, cerebellar nystagmus, and the anterior vermis, posterior vermis, and cerebellar hemispheric syndromes.
- To describe the specific nuclei and functions of the thalamus and hypothalamus.
- To describe the gross structure, histology, hormone functions, and the hypophyseal portal circulation of the pituitary gland.
- To understand the subthalamus, epithalamus, and the function of the pineal gland.
- To describe the structure, nuclei, connections, and neurotransmitters of the basal ganglia. Clinical correlates include dyskinesias, dystonias, hypokinesia, Parkinson disease, and ballism.
- To describe the structure, function, connections, and Papez circuit of the limbic system.
- Describe the structure and the fiber tracts that pass through the internal capsule.
- To describe the individual lobes, Brodmann areas, histology, white matter fibers, blood supply, and cerebral dominance of the cerebral hemispheres and cortex. Clinical correlates include split-brain syndrome, epilepsy, and sleep.
- To understand all ascending sensory and descending motor pathways. Clinical correlates include upper versus lower motor neuron lesions, subacute combined degeneration, syringomyelia, poliomyelitis, amyotropic lateral sclerosis, and the central cord, Brown-Séquard, anterior cord, posterior cord, conus medullaris, cauda equina, and corticospinal tract syndromes.
- To distinguish between monosynaptic and polysynaptic reflexes.
- To describe the structures, pathways, and specific lesions related to the olfactory, visual, auditory, vestibular, and gustatory systems.
- To understand the blood supply and venous drainage related to the cerebral hemispheres, brainstem, cerebellum, and spinal cord. Clinical correlates include subclavian steal syndrome, stroke, transient ischemic attacks, and cerebral artery occlusions.
- To understand the central nervous system development. Clinical correlates include craniopharyngioma, anencephaly, and hydrocephalus.

9.1 Structure of the Central Nervous System

Made up of the brain and spinal cord, the central nervous system (CNS) has the role of integrating and coordinating incoming and outgoing neuron signals. These signals may continue through the peripheral nervous system by way of cranial and spinal nerves. It is also involved in carrying out higher mental functions such as learning and memory. The brain and spinal cord are made up of gray matter and white matter.

The **gray matter** has a gray color appearance and contains numerous collections of cell bodies (or a **nucleus**), supporting neuroglia, and relatively few myelinated axons. The **white matter** is white in appearance due to lipid material located in the myelin sheaths and is composed of bundles of myelinated axons that connect to various gray matter locations along with supporting neuroglia (**Fig. 9.1**).

A bundle of axons (nerve fibers) within the CNS that connects nuclei of the cerebral cortex are known as **tracts**. The CNS is protected by cranial bones and the vertebral column and by system of membranes known as the meninges. The CNS is suspended by cerebrospinal fluid that is situated between two of the three meninges.

9.2 Meninges of the Brain and Spinal Cord

The external surface of the CNS is covered by the meninges and there are three of these membranes. They are called the dura, arachnoid, and pia maters. The meninges have multiple functions that include protecting the brain, forming a structural framework for blood vessels and the dural venous sinuses, and creating a fluid-filled subarachnoid space that cushions the CNS.

The **dura mater** (**Fig. 9.2; Fig. 9.3**) is composed of a tough, fibrous, and elastic tissue, and it is the furthest from the brain and spinal cord but closest to the surrounding bone. There are two layers in the cranium adjacent to the brain. The cranial dura is divided into an external **periosteal layer** and an internal **meningeal layer**. When these two layers split from each other, they form dural venous sinuses and dural reflections. Specifics regarding both dural venous sinuses and dural reflections were presented in Chapter 7. The primary innervation of the cranial dura is from the meningeal branches of all three trigeminal nerves. Additional innervation comes from the C2 and C3 spinal nerves. These may be direct branches or they may be distributed by CN X and CN XII. Blood supply to the dura originates from multiple sources. These include the anterior and posterior branches of the middle meningeal, accessory meningeal, or small meningeal branches of the anterior ethmoidal, ophthalmic, internal carotid, ascending meningeal, occipital, and vertebral arteries.

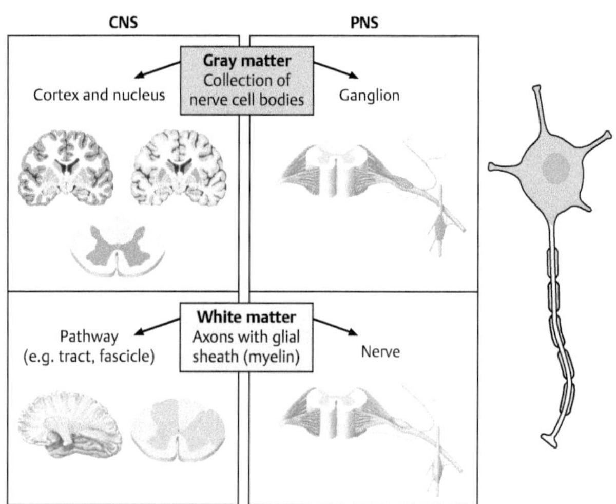

Fig. 9.1 Structural classification of the nervous system: gray and white matter. (From Schuenke M, Schulte E, Schumacher U. THIEME Atlas of Anatomy. Head, Neck, and Neuroanatomy. Illustrations by Voll M and Wesker K. 3rd ed. New York: Thieme Medical Publishers; 2020.)

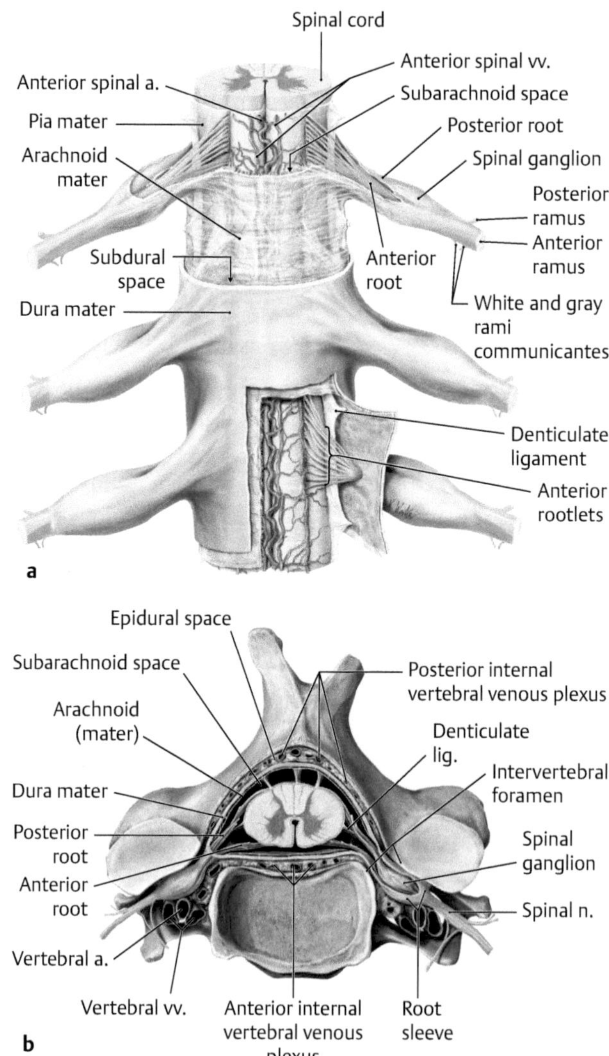

Fig. 9.2 **(a)** Spinal cord and its meningeal layers; posterior view with the dura mater opened and the arachnoid is sectioned. **(b)** Transverse section of the spinal cord at the C4 vertebral level; superior view. (From Schuenke M, Schulte E, Schumacher U. THIEME Atlas of Anatomy. Head, Neck, and Neuroanatomy. Illustrations by Voll M and Wesker K. 3rd ed. New York: Thieme Medical Publishers; 2020.)

The dura mater at the level of the spinal cord (**Fig. 9.2; Fig. 9.3**) consists of only one layer, and it is the outermost meningeal layer of the spinal cord composed of a tough, fibrous, and elastic tissue. The dura mater forms the **dural sac**, a long tubular sheath within the vertebral canal structure that extends from the junction of the cranial dura mater located at the foramen magnum and inferiorly to about the S2 vertebral level. The dural sac extends into the intervertebral foramina and along the ventral and dorsal nerve roots distal to the dorsal root ganglia to form the **dural root sheaths**. The dural root sheaths are continuous with the outer epineurium of the spinal nerves.

The space located between the vertebrae and the dura mater is called the **epidural space**. This space runs the entire length of the vertebral canal beginning at the level of the foramen magnum and inferiorly to the level of the sacral hiatus being sealed off by the *sacrococcygeal ligament*. It extends laterally at the intervertebral foramina just as the dura mater adheres to the periosteum surrounding each opening. In addition to a thin layer of **epidural fat**, the **internal vertebral venous plexus** fills the epidural space.

The **arachnoid mater** (**Fig. 9.2; Fig. 9.3**) is the thin, avascular intermediate meningeal layer that is composed of fibrous and elastic tissue and lies adjacent to the spinal dura layer or the meningeal layer of dura in the cranium. Pressure from the **cerebrospinal fluid (CSF)** located in the **subarachnoid space**, a space located between the arachnoid and pia maters, is the reason the arachnoid is pressed against the dura. The subarachnoid space is present in both the vertebral canal and cranium. Spanning the subarachnoid space are very delicate strands of connective tissue called the **arachnoid trabeculae** and they connect the arachnoid to the pia mater (**Fig. 9.3**).

There is a potential space between arachnoid and dura mater layers and it is called the *subdural space*. A trauma situation is generally the cause of bleeding, which results in the creation of this space. The lack of CSF passing through the subarachnoid space in a cadaver naturally opens the subdural space that is not normally present in living individuals.

The **pia mater** (**Fig. 9.2; Fig. 9.3**) is the innermost layer of the meninges consisting of flattened cells with long and equally flattened processes that follow the surface of the CNS. The **filum terminale** while passing through the lumbar cistern of the subarachnoid space is made of condensed pia mater. The filum terminale along with the **denticulate ligaments** help suspend the spinal cord within the spinal dural sac but both have a limited role in preventing unwanted motion of the spinal cord. Denticulate ligaments are tooth-like extensions or sheets of pia mater passing between a ventral and dorsal nerve root before anchoring itself into the dura mater. There are approximately 20 to 22 of them, and they are located from the craniovertebral junction down to T12–L1 nerve root (**Fig. 9.2**).

9.3 The Ventricular System

Within the brain, there are four fluid-filled cavities known as the ventricles. There are two laterals, a third and fourth ventricle. The **lateral ventricles** are C-shaped, and their **central part** occupies the parietal lobe. The **anterior**, **posterior**, and **inferior horns**

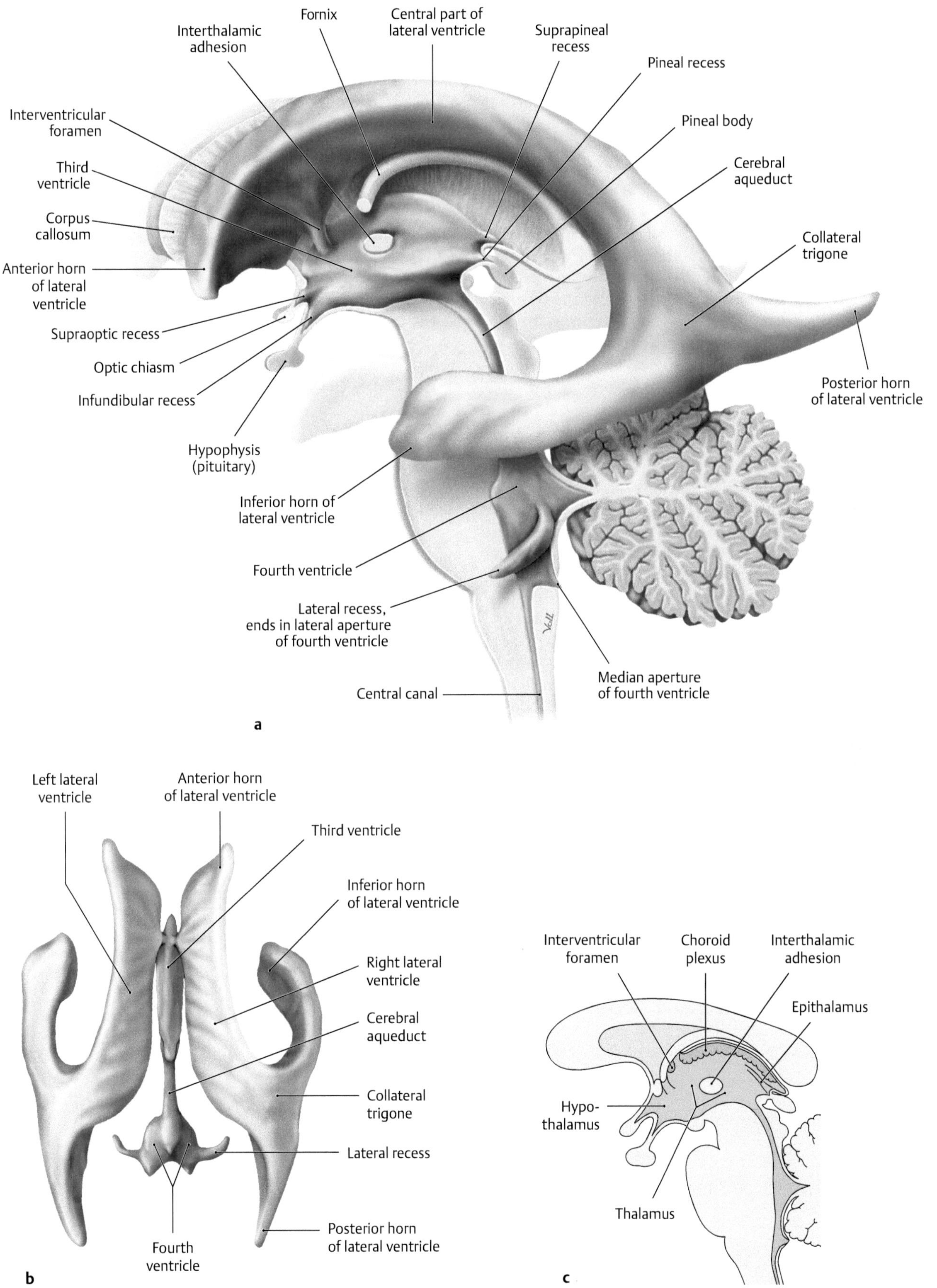

Fornix
Central part of lateral ventricle
Interthalamic adhesion
Suprapineal recess
Pineal recess
Interventricular foramen
Pineal body
Third ventricle
Cerebral aqueduct
Corpus callosum
Collateral trigone
Anterior horn of lateral ventricle
Supraoptic recess
Optic chiasm
Infundibular recess
Posterior horn of lateral ventricle
Hypophysis (pituitary)
Inferior horn of lateral ventricle
Fourth ventricle
Lateral recess, ends in lateral aperture of fourth ventricle
Median aperture of fourth ventricle
Central canal
a

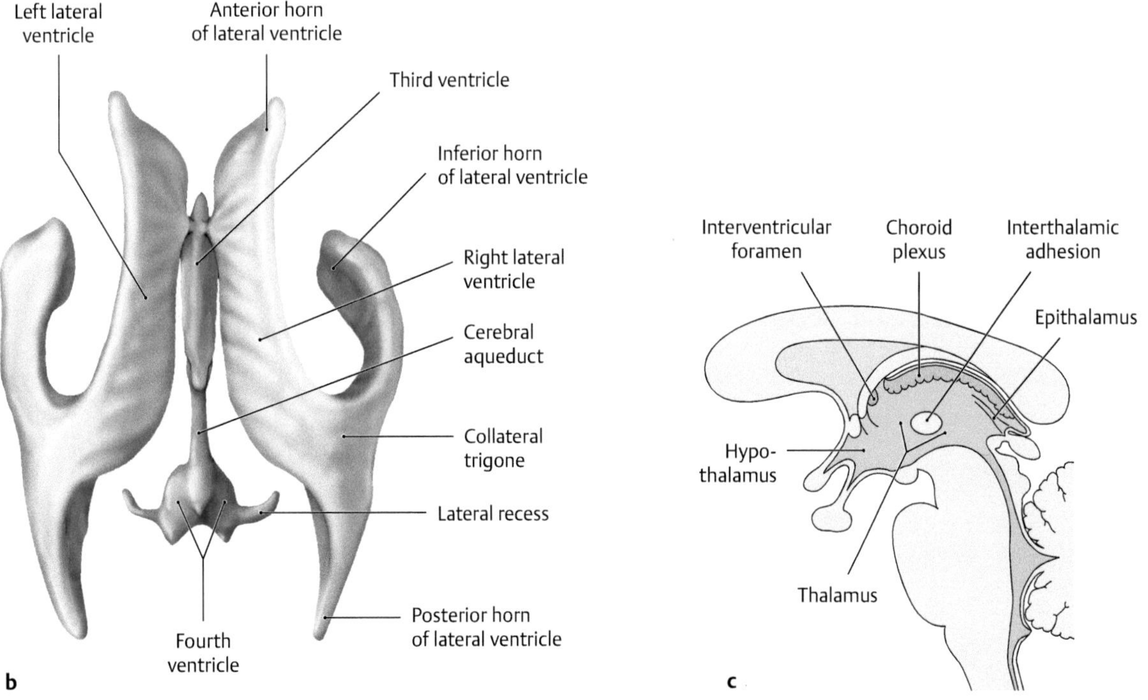

Fig. 9.3 **(a)** Overview of the ventricular system and neighboring structures. **(b)** Cast of the ventricular system, superior view. **(c)** Lateral wall of the third ventricle. (From Schuenke M, Schulte E, Schumacher U. THIEME Atlas of Anatomy. Head, Neck, and Neuroanatomy. Illustrations by Voll M and Wesker K. 3rd ed. New York: Thieme Medical Publishers; 2020.)

occupy the frontal, occipital, and temporal lobes, respectively. The two lateral ventricles communicate with the third ventricle by way of the **interventricular foramen** (of ***Monro***) (**Fig. 9.3**).

The **third ventricle** is located between the two thalami. Near the center of this ventricle, the **interthalamic adhesion** passes through it and connects the paired thalami. The anteroinferior wall extends out to form the **supraoptic** and **infundibular recesses**. Posteriorly, this ventricle extends out to form the **suprapineal** and **pineal recesses**. The **cerebral aqueduct** (of ***Sylvius***) connects the third ventricle with the fourth ventricle.

The **fourth ventricle** is located anterior to the cerebellum but posterior to the pons and superior portion of the medulla oblongata. It is continuous caudally with the **central canal** of the spinal cord and this canal ends as a small dilation called the **terminal ventricle**. The fourth ventricle also communicates with the subarachnoid space by way of the **median aperture** (of ***Magendie***) and **lateral apertures** (of ***Luschka***) (**Fig. 9.3a, b**).

9.3.1 Tela Choroidea and the Choroid Plexus

The **tela choroidea** is a thin but highly vascularized two-layered fold of pia mater that gives rise to the choroid plexus. It can be thought of as the lamina propria of the ependyma. It lies along the **choroidal fissure** in the medial wall of the lateral ventricles and the roof of both the third and fourth ventricles. The **choroid plexus** is essentially the irregular lateral edge of the tela choroidea. They are located along the roof of the inferior horns and floor of the central part along with the roofs of both the third and fourth ventricles. Histologically the choroid plexus is lined by *ependyma*, a cuboidal-shaped epithelium. The lines of attachment on the ventricles for the tela choroidea are referred to as the **taenia choroidea** (**Fig. 9.4**).

Blood supply to the choroid plexuses of the lateral ventricles and third ventricle come from **choroidal branches of the internal carotid** and **basilar arteries**. The choroid plexus of the fourth ventricle receives blood from branches of the **posterior inferior cerebellar arteries**.

The function of the choroid plexuses is to produce CSF. The CSF serves as a cushion and shock absorber for the CNS, circulates nutrients and chemicals filtered from the blood, and removes waste products from the brain. It is produced by ependymal cells of the choroid plexuses and reabsorbed by the **arachnoid granulations**, small protrusions of the arachnoid mater that are most notably found at the level of the superior sagittal dural venous sinus (**Fig. 9.5**). CSF circulates from the lateral ventricles and through the third and fourth ventricles before passing through the central canal and subarachnoid space. Approximately 150 mL of CSF are present at one time but it is replaced two to four times daily; thus, about 500 mL is produced each day. If there are any obstructions to CSF drainage, it causes an increase in intracranial pressure.

9.4 Spinal Cord

The major bundle of nervous tissue that begins at the *medulla oblongata* at the level of the foramen magnum and terminates inferiorly at the L1 vertebral level represents the **spinal cord** and it passes within the vertebral canal of the vertebral column. The tapering off end of the spinal cord is called the **conus medullaris** and in newborns may extend down to the L3 vertebral level or even lower. The spinal cord is made up of **spinal segments** of which each has a paired ventral and dorsal root that will fuse to become a spinal nerve. There are 31 total and specifically 8 cervical, 12 thoracic, 5 lumbar, 5 sacral, and 1 coccygeal spinal

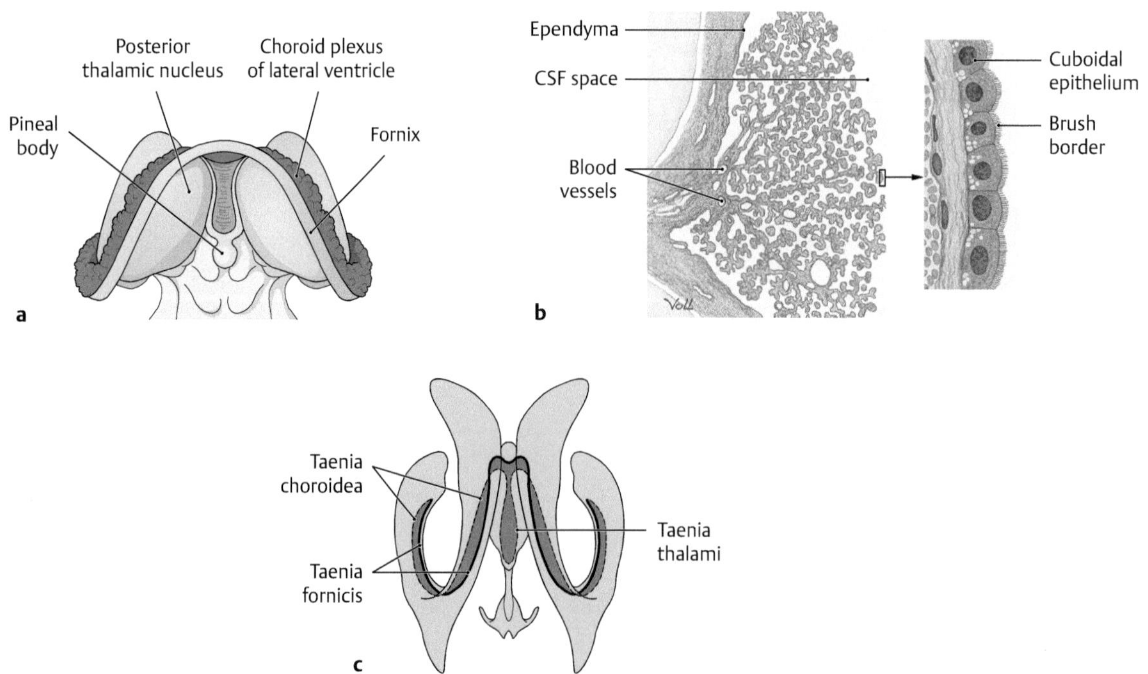

Fig. 9.4 **(a)** Choroid plexus in the lateral ventricles. **(b)** Histological section of the choroid plexus. **(c)** Taeniae of the choroid plexus. (From Schuenke M, Schulte E, Schumacher U. THIEME Atlas of Anatomy. Head, Neck, and Neuroanatomy. Illustrations by Voll M and Wesker K. 3rd ed. New York: Thieme Medical Publishers; 2020.)

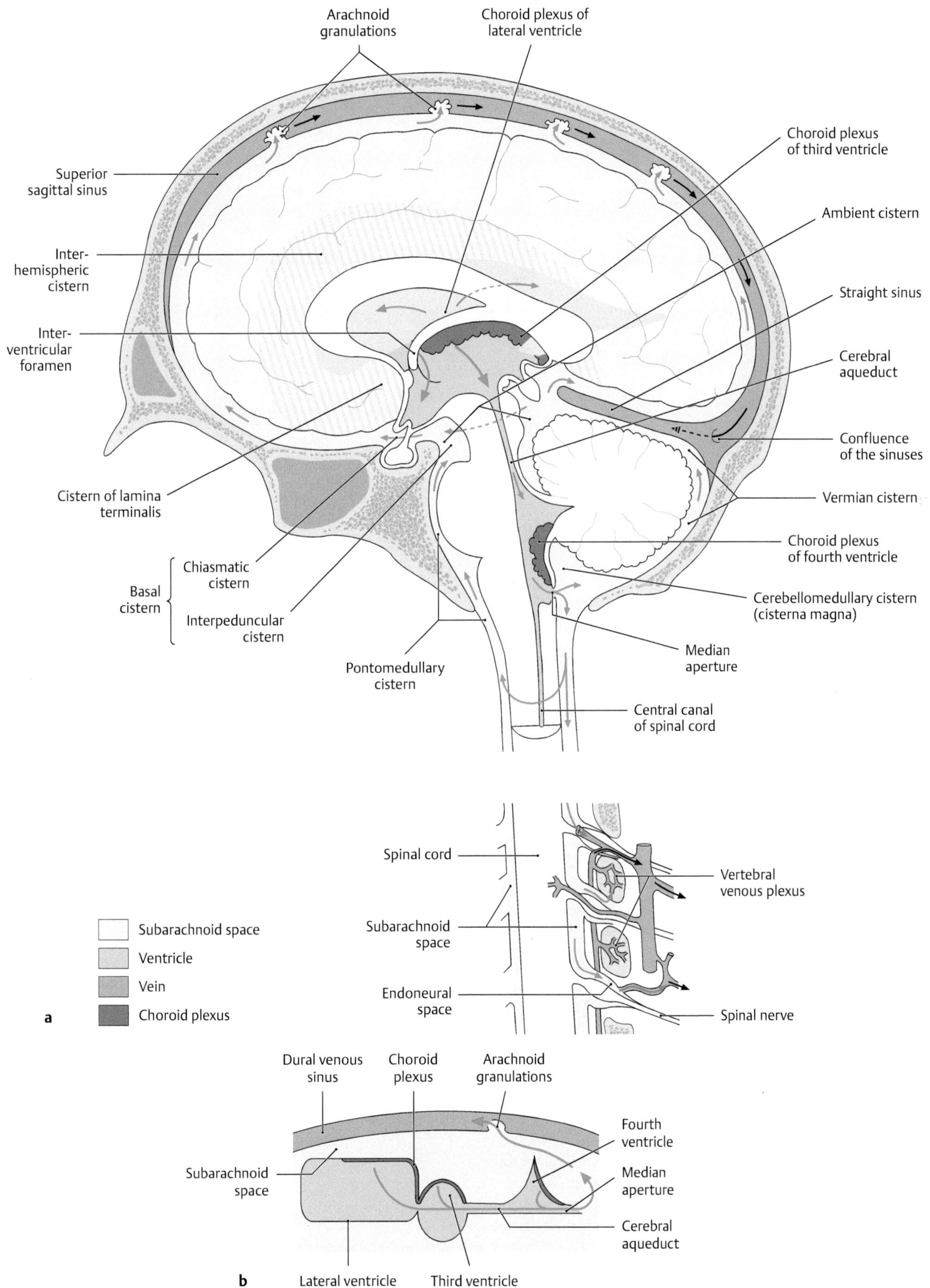

Fig. 9.5 (a) Cerebrospinal fluid circulation and the cisterns. **(b)** Schematic diagram of cerebrospinal fluid circulation. (From Schuenke M, Schulte E, Schumacher U. THIEME Atlas of Anatomy. Head, Neck, and Neuroanatomy. Illustrations by Voll M and Wesker K. 3rd ed. New York: Thieme Medical Publishers; 2020.)

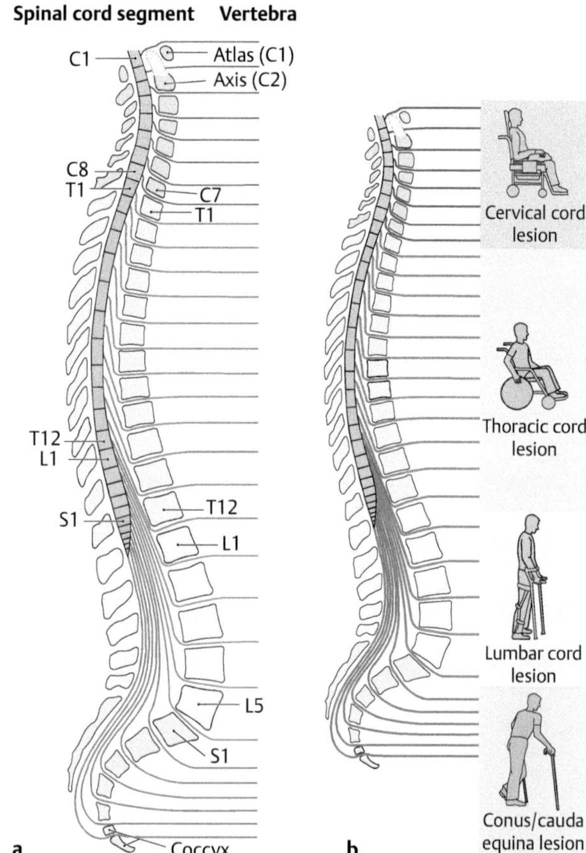

Fig. 9.6 **(a)** Spinal cord segments. **(b)** Effects of spinal cord lesions. (From Schuenke M, Schulte E, Schumacher U. THIEME Atlas of Anatomy. Head, Neck, and Neuroanatomy. Illustrations by Voll M and Wesker K. 1st ed. New York: Thieme Medical Publishers; 2010.)

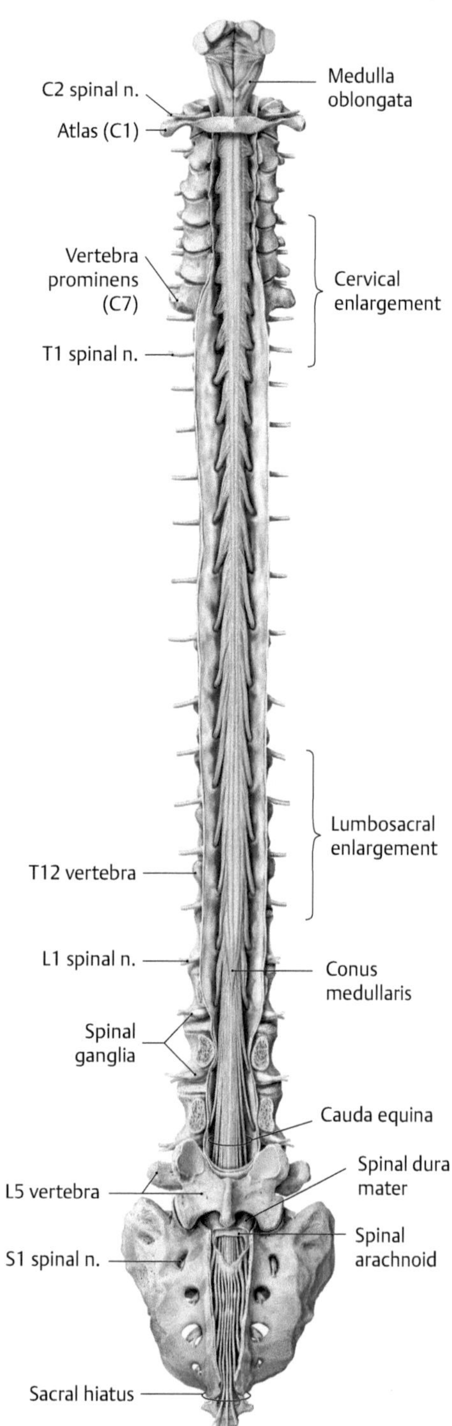

Fig. 9.7 Spinal cord in situ; posterior view with vertebral canal windowed. (From Schuenke M, Schulte E, Schumacher U. THIEME Atlas of Anatomy. Head, Neck, and Neuroanatomy. Illustrations by Voll M and Wesker K. 1st ed. New York: Thieme Medical Publishers; 2010.)

segments (**Fig. 9.6a; Fig. 9.7**). The effects of spinal cord lesions are shown in **Fig. 9.6b**.

Two enlargements of the spinal cord are associated with the innervation to the limbs. The **cervical enlargement** is made up of the C4–T1 spinal segments, and the ventral rami that are associated with these spinal segments form the *brachial plexuses* that are responsible for innervating the upper limbs. The **lumbosacral enlargement** is made up of the L1–S3 spinal segments (between the T9 and T12 vertebral levels) and the ventral rami that are associated with them form the *lumbar* and *sacral plexuses* that are responsible for innervating the lower limbs (**Fig. 9.7**).

Extending out from the spinal cord is a set of ventral and dorsal rootlets and roots, of which the dorsal root contains a dorsal root ganglion (DRG), before fusing to become the spinal nerve. The C1 dorsal roots are absent in about 50% of the general population. The T1–Co1 nerves bear the same alphanumeric name as the vertebra forming the superior margin of their intervertebral foramen; thus, the T6 spinal nerve passes between the T6 and T7 vertebrae. Due to the cervical nerves having eight pairs and there only being seven pairs of cervical vertebrae, the C1–C7 spinal nerves pass above their same alphanumeric vertebra but the C8 spinal nerve passes between the C7 and T1 vertebrae.

The spinal cord in adults is shorter than the vertebral column so there will be a progressive increase in length of both the ventral and dorsal rootlet/roots before they reach the corresponding intervertebral foramen and become a spinal nerve. The lumbar and sacral rootlet/roots are the longest and any of these located inferior to the conus medullaris are known collectively as the **cauda equina**. The cauda equina is located in a particular portion of the subarachnoid space called the **lumbar cistern** and is a clinically relevant location when doing *spinal taps*. Also passing through this region is an isolated extension from the conus medullaris called the **filum terminale** and it acts as an anchor for the spinal cord and spinal meninges (**Fig. 9.7; Fig. 9.8**).

On the anterior surface and in the midline, there is a deep and longitudinal groove called the **anterior median fissure**. Where the ventral rootlets emerge, it is called the **anterolateral sulcus**. The posterior surface has a much shallower furrow called the **posterior median sulcus**. The dorsal rootlets enter the spinal cord at the **posterolateral sulcus**. The shallow groove located between the posterior median and posterolateral sulci is called the **posterior intermediate sulcus** (**Fig. 9.9**).

9.4.1 Gray Matter

The spinal cord in cross-section has an embedded inner core of **gray matter** that is surrounded by an outer covering of white matter. The H-shaped gray matter has an **anterior (ventral) horn** associated with *efferent (motor) neurons*; a **posterior (dorsal) horn** associated with *afferent (sensory) neurons*; and in specific regions, a **lateral horn** that is the site for *preganglionic autonomic neurons*. These horns are also referred to as columns (**Fig. 9.10**). The **gray matter** is described as containing prominent nuclei and being divided into multiple layers called **Rexed laminae**.

The distribution of cells and fibers within the gray matter exhibits a pattern of lamination or layering. The cellular pattern of each lamina is composed of various sizes or shapes of neurons (or cytoarchitecture) and it is based on a total of ten laminae. This classification is useful since it is related more accurately to function versus major nuclear groups. In general, laminae I–IV are concerned with exteroceptive sensation and comprise the posterior horn. Laminae V and VI are concerned primarily with proprioceptive sensations and are still a part of the posterior horn. Lamina VII is the equivalent to the lateral horn or intermediate zone and can extend into the ventral horn depending on its location in the spinal cord. This region is concerned with the autonomic nervous system, receives information from lamina II and VI, visceral afferents, and muscle and tendon afferents, and contains numerous interneurons called **Renshaw cells**. Renshaw cells regulate the output of alpha motor neurons. When an alpha motor neuron is excited, it activates Renshaw cells via excitatory axon collaterals that extend from it. In turn, the Renshaw cells inhibit the activity of the same alpha motor neuron (**Fig. 9.11**). Laminae VIII–IX comprise the ventral horn and contain alpha and gamma motor neurons. The axons of these neurons innervate mainly skeletal muscle. Lamina X surrounds the central canal and allows for axon decussating.

The prominent nuclei of the gray matter that can be located in certain laminae include the posteromarginal nucleus, substantia gelatinosa, nucleus proprius, and posterior thoracic nucleus of the posterior horn; the intermediolateral nucleus of the lateral horn and the intermediomedial nucleus in the intermediate zone just anterior to the posterior thoracic nucleus; and finally the spinal accessory nuclei, phrenic nuclei, nucleus of Onuf, and multiple lateral and medial motor nuclei in the ventral horn (**Fig. 9.12**).

- Posterior (dorsal) horn
  - **Posteromarginal nucleus**: located in Rexed lamina I and at all spinal cord levels. It is associated with pain, temperature, and light touch of the anterolateral system.
  - **Substantia gelatinosa**: located in Rexed lamina II and at all spinal cord levels. It is associated with pain, temperature, and light touch of the anterolateral system, and it is homologous with the spinal trigeminal nucleus.
  - **Nucleus proprius**: located in Rexed laminae III and IV and at all spinal cord levels. It is associated with pain, temperature, and light touch of the anterolateral system.
  - **Posterior thoracic nucleus (dorsal nucleus of Clarke)**: located in Rexed lamina VII and between the C8 and L2 spinal cord segments. It accepts unconscious proprioception from muscle spindles and Golgi tendon organs and is the origin of the posterior spinocerebellar tract. It is homologous with the accessory cuneate nucleus of the medulla.
- Lateral horn
  - **Intermediolateral nucleus/column**: located in Rexed lamina VII and between the T1 and L2 spinal cord segments. This is the location of sympathetic preganglionic neurons. At the S2–S4 spinal segments there is a less conspicuous intermediolateral nucleus (or sacral autonomic nucleus) that is the location for parasympathetic preganglionic neurons targeting the hindgut and pelvic structures. Extending from C8 to T2, the **ciliospinal center** (of ***Budge***) is associated with the sympathetic innervation to the dilator pupillae muscle of the eye.
  - **Intermediomedial nucleus/column**: located in Rexed lamina VII and at all spinal cord levels. Autonomic afferents, in particular pain afferents, are received here and they are joined through interneurons to the visceral motor neurons for visceral responses.
- Anterior (ventral) horn
  - **Spinal accessory nucleus**: located in Rexed lamina IX and between the C1 and C6 spinal cord segments. It is responsible for innervating both the sternocleidomastoid and trapezius muscles.
  - **Phrenic nucleus**: located in Rexed lamina IX and between the C3 and C5 spinal cord segments. It is responsible for innervating the diaphragm.
  - **Lateral motor nuclei**: located in Rexed lamina IX and at all spinal cord levels. These nuclei can be subdivided into anterior, posterior, and retroposterior groups. Innervation is to the appendicular muscles and they receive input from the corticospinal and rubrospinal tracts.
  - **Medial motor nuclei**: located in Rexed lamina IX and at all spinal cord levels. These nuclei can be divided into anterior and posterior subgroups. Innervation is to the axial muscles and they receive input from the vestibulospinal and reticulospinal tracts.
  - **Nucleus of Onuf**: located in Rexed lamina IX and between the S1 and S3 spinal cord segments. It is responsible for innervation to the external urethral sphincter but it has also been cited for pelvic muscle innervation during orgasm, innervation of the external anal sphincter muscles, and the maintenance of micturition and defecation continence.

9.4.2 White Matter

The white matter is divided bilaterally into an anterior, lateral, and posterior column or funiculus (**Fig. 9.13**). White matter surrounds the H-shaped gray matter and consists of myelinated nerve fiber bundles, neuroglia, and blood vessels. The ascending and descending fiber pathways that travel through it are known as tracts.

- **Anterior funiculus**: located between the anterior median fissure and anterior lateral sulcus. It contains the **anterior**

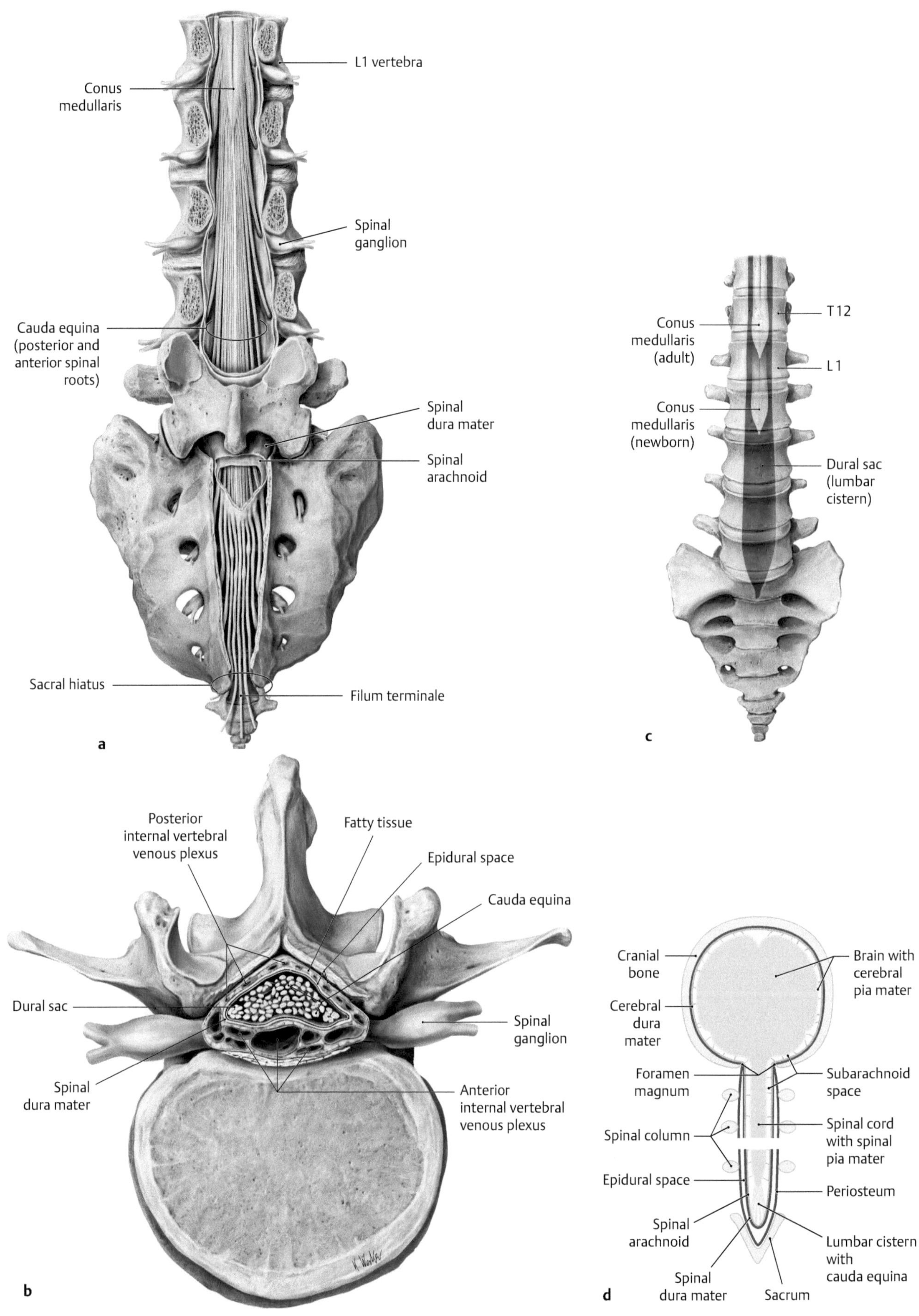

Fig. 9.8 **(a)** Cauda equina in the vertebral canal: posterior view. **(b)** Cauda equina in situ: transverse section. Superior view at level of L2 vertebra. **(c)** The spinal cord, dural sac, and vertebral column at different stages: anterior view. **(d)** Meninges in the cranial cavity and spinal canal. (From Schuenke M, Schulte E, Schumacher U. THIEME Atlas of Anatomy. Head, Neck, and Neuroanatomy. Illustrations by Voll M and Wesker K. 1st ed. New York: Thieme Medical Publishers; 2010.)

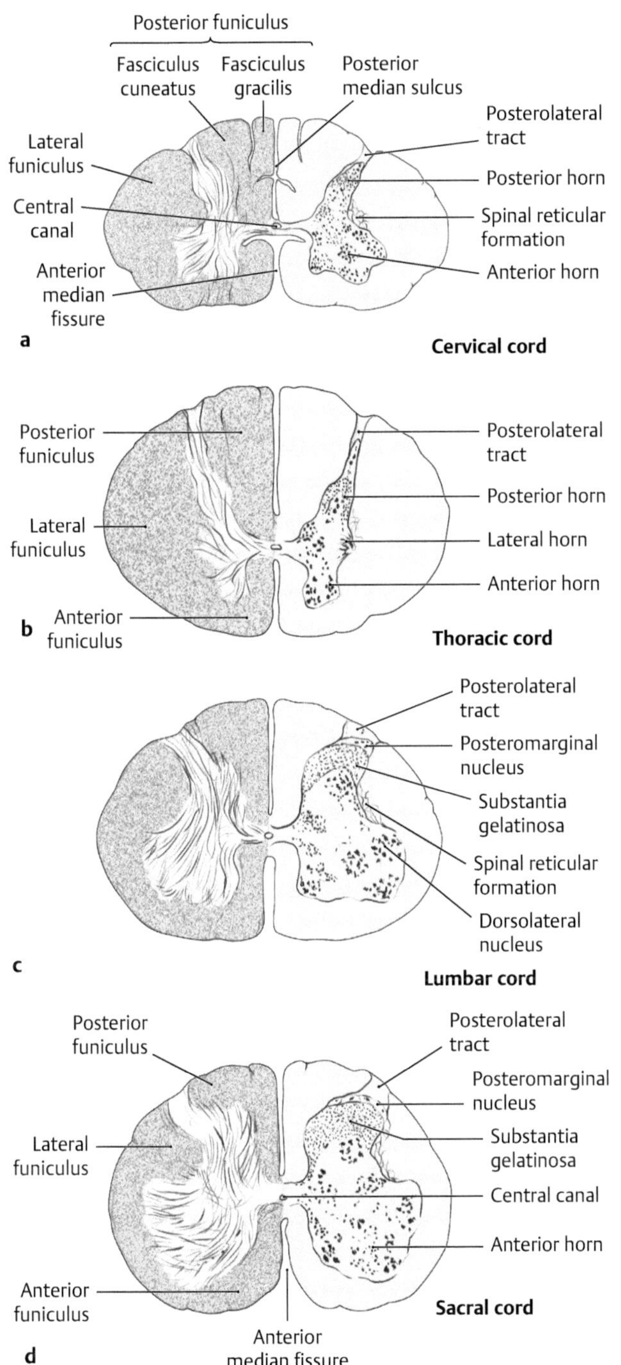

Fig. 9.9 Transverse sections of the cervical **(a)**, thoracic **(b)**, lumbar **(c)**, and sacral **(d)** spinal cord. (From Schuenke M, Schulte E, Schumacher U. THIEME Atlas of Anatomy. Head, Neck, and Neuroanatomy. Illustrations by Voll M and Wesker K. 3rd ed. New York: Thieme Medical Publishers; 2020.)

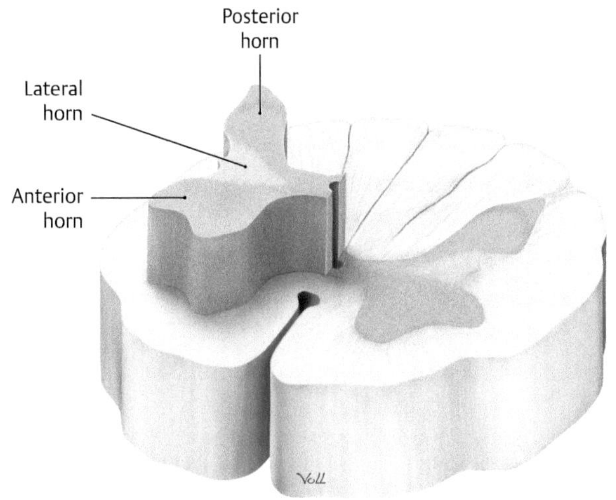

Fig. 9.10 Gray matter of spinal cord. (From Schuenke M, Schulte E, Schumacher U. THIEME Atlas of Anatomy. Head, Neck, and Neuroanatomy. Illustrations by Voll M and Wesker K. 3rd ed. New York: Thieme Medical Publishers; 2020.)

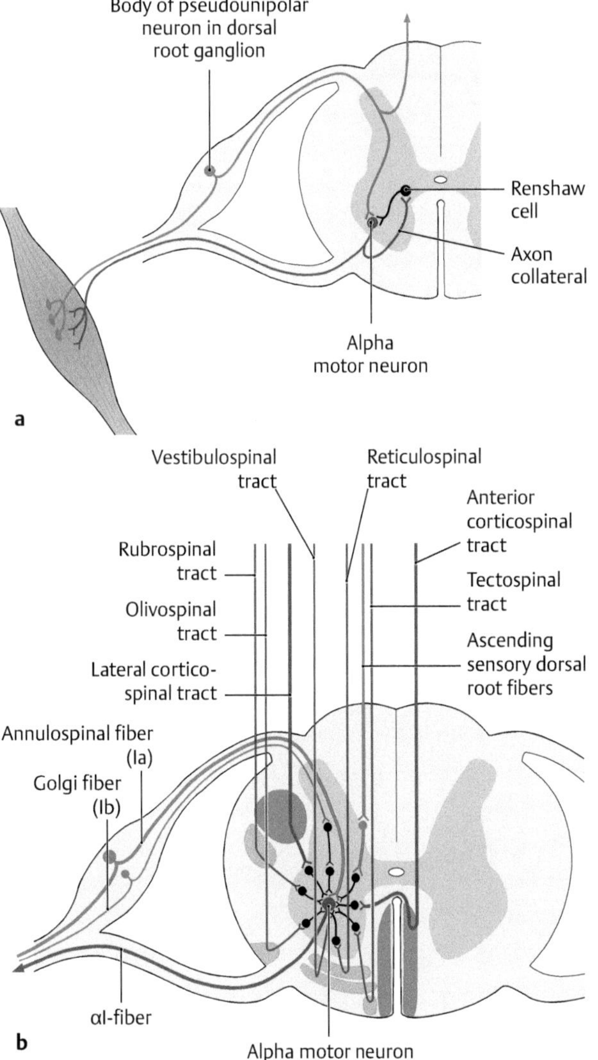

Fig. 9.11 **(a)** Effects of the Renshaw cell on the alpha motor neuron. **(b)** Effects of long tracts on the alpha motor neuron. (From Schuenke M, Schulte E, Schumacher U. THIEME Atlas of Anatomy. Head, Neck, and Neuroanatomy. Illustrations by Voll M and Wesker K. 3rd ed. New York: Thieme Medical Publishers; 2020.)

white commissure, the site of decussating spinothalamic fibers.

- **Lateral funiculus**: located between the anterior lateral and posterior lateral sulci.
- **Posterior funiculus**: as a whole it is located between the posterior lateral and posterior median sulci. Above the T6 spinal level, it is divided into a fasciculus gracilis and cuneatus.
  - **Fasciculus gracilis**: located at all spinal cord levels and between the posterior intermediate sulcus and septum and

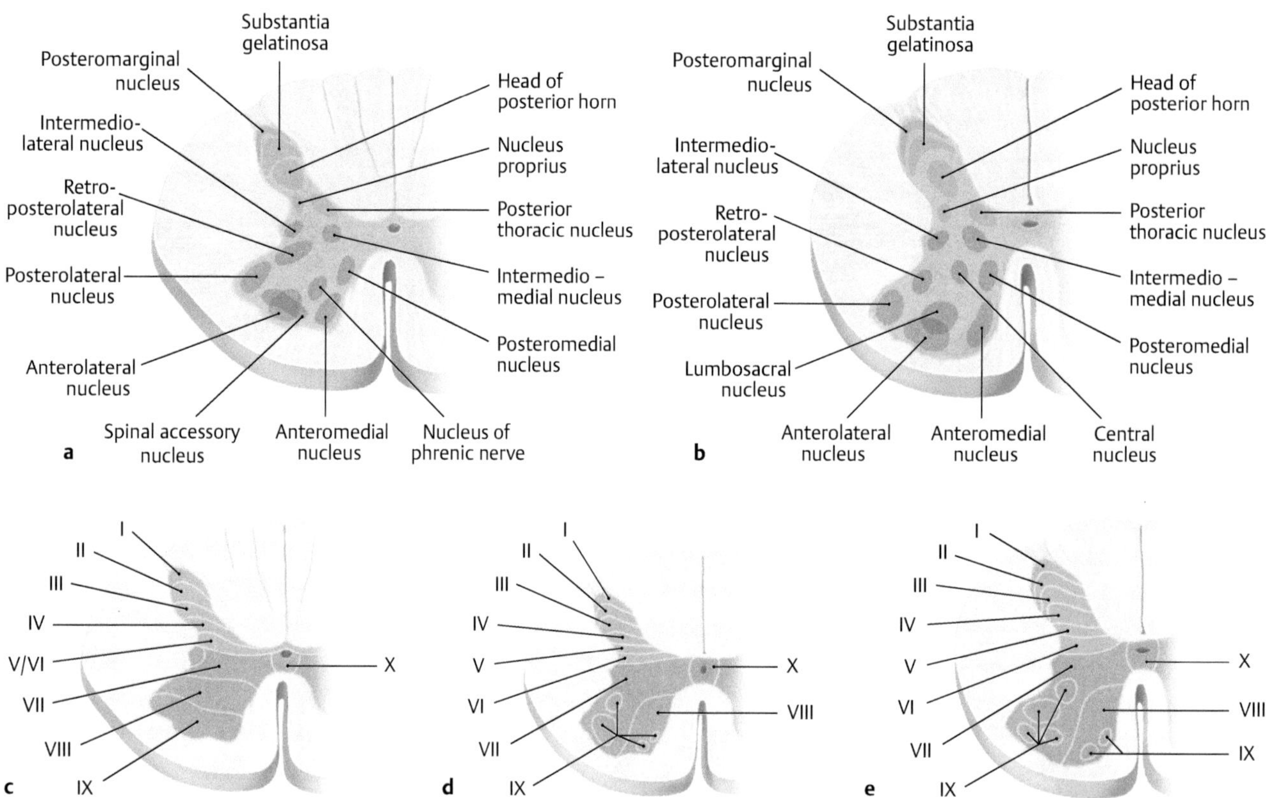

Fig. 9.12 Cell groups in the gray matter of the spinal cord: **(a)** Cervical cord. **(b)** Lumbar cord. Synaptic layers in the gray matter: **(c)** Cervical cord. **(d)** Thoracic cord. **(e)** Lumbar cord. (From Schuenke M, Schulte E, Schumacher U. THIEME Atlas of Anatomy. Head, Neck, and Neuroanatomy. Illustrations by Voll M and Wesker K. 3rd ed. New York: Thieme Medical Publishers; 2020.)

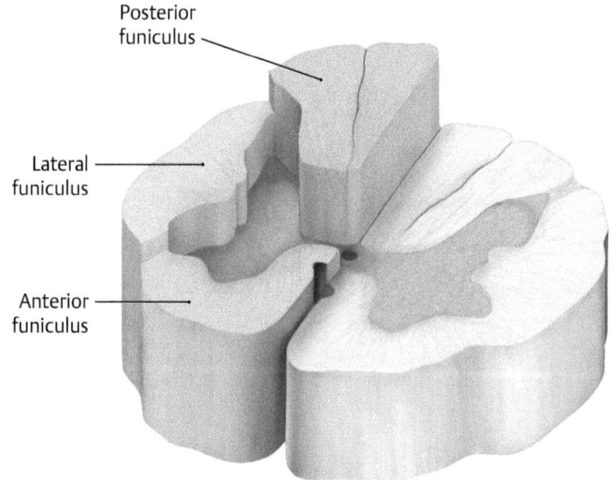

Fig. 9.13 White matter of the spinal cord. (From Schuenke M, Schulte E, Schumacher U. THIEME Atlas of Anatomy. Head, Neck, and Neuroanatomy. Illustrations by Voll M and Wesker K. 3rd ed. New York: Thieme Medical Publishers; 2020.)

the posterior median sulcus. Long ascending fibers from the sacral, lumbar, and lower six thoracic spinal nerves pass through it.

- **Fasciculus cuneatus**: located between the C1 and T6 spinal cord levels and between the posterior intermediate sulcus and septum and the posterior lateral sulcus. Long ascending fibers from the upper six thoracic and all of the cervical spinal nerves pass through it.

9.5 Brainstem

9.5.1 Gross Anatomy of the Brainstem

The brainstem consists of three main parts: an inferiorly located medulla, middle pons, and superiorly placed midbrain. The medulla connects directly to the spinal cord. The medulla and pons form a connection to the cerebellum through cerebellar peduncles. The midbrain is found between the pons and forebrain. Coursing through the brainstem are multiple ascending or descending tracts that travel between the spinal cord and brain. In addition, there are numerous nuclei that contribute to motor, sensory, and autonomic fibers (**Fig. 9.14; Fig. 9.15**). A common feature of the entire brainstem is the dorsally situated tegmentum and reticular formation. The **tegmentum** is the phylogenetically older part of the brainstem that contains nuclei. The tegmentum is covered by the **tectum** at only the level of the midbrain. The cerebellum forms a covering over the pons and medulla portion. Ventral to the tegmentum is the region of the brainstem that consists of ascending and descending tracts. This region is known as the pyramids for the medulla, basilar part for the pons, and finally the cerebral peduncle (crus cerebri) for the midbrain (**Fig. 9.16**).

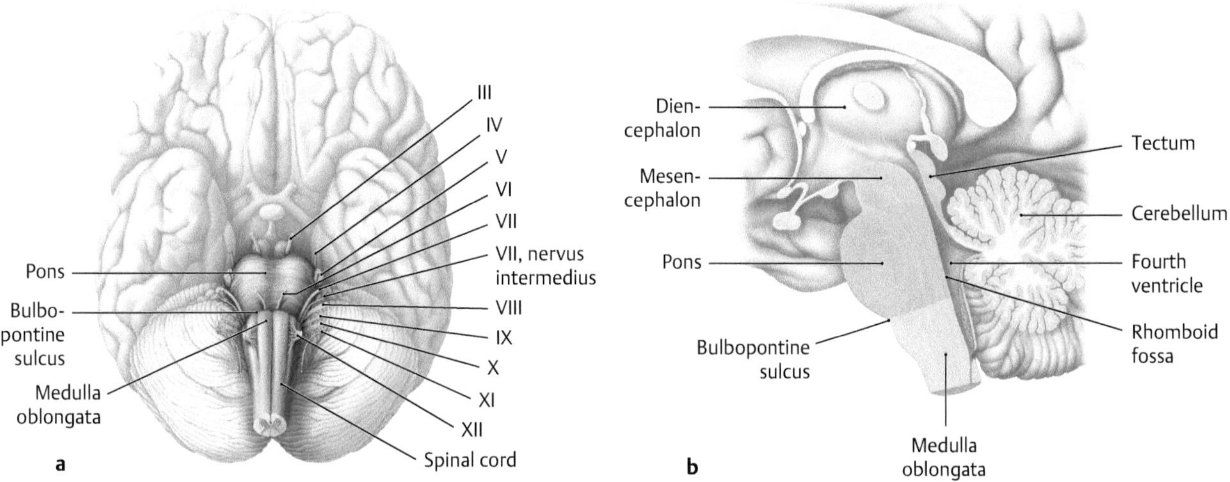

Fig. 9.14 Brainstem. **(a)** View of intact brain from below. **(b)** Midsagittal section, left lateral view. (From Schuenke M, Schulte E, Schumacher U. THIEME Atlas of Anatomy. Head, Neck, and Neuroanatomy. Illustrations by Voll M and Wesker K. 3rd ed. New York: Thieme Medical Publishers; 2020.)

9.5.2 Reticular Formation

The **reticular formation (RF)** is a morphologically ill-defined collection of numerous small nuclei located throughout the brainstem tegmentum (**Fig. 9.17a, b**). The nuclei are divided into three longitudinal zones (**Fig. 9.17b**):

- **Lateral zone (parvocellular nuclei)**: contain small-cell nuclei, which receive and process afferent fibers from regions of the neighboring brainstem along with the spinal cord through the spinoreticular tract. These neurons project to the medial zone in order to balance motor function.
- **Medial zone (magnocellular nuclei)**: contain large-cell nuclei, which primarily give rise to efferent fibers involved in motor output and tone.
- **Median zone (raphe nuclei)**: a collection of serotonergic neurons involved in the modulation of moods and feelings. They project to a wide range of areas such as the thalamus, prefrontal cortex, basal ganglia, and cranial nerve nuclei.

Neurotransmitters such as *dopamine, norwepinephrine*, and *serotonin* play a large role in the RF. Within the rostral midbrain, dopaminergic neurons are located in two distinct areas called the substantia nigra and ventral tegmental area. The **substantia nigra** (**Fig. 9.16a; Fig. 9.18; Fig. 9.21a**) projects to the caudate nucleus and putamen and plays an important role in the modulation of movements. The **ventral tegmental area** (**Fig. 9.16a**) projects to regions of the limbic system such as the amygdala, cingulate gyrus, and hippocampus, along with the nucleus accumbens, olfactory bulb, and prefrontal cortex. It plays a role in emotional learning and memory, motivation and reward. Clinically, the connection between the ventral tegmental area and the nucleus accumbens has been implicated in drug-seeking behaviors.

The **locus coeruleus** (**Fig. 9.17b; Fig. 9.21b**) is located in the pons adjacent to the fourth ventricle. This structure uses norepinephrine as its principal neurotransmitter and projects to structures such as the amygdala, hippocampus, hypothalamus, thalamus, cerebellum, and spinal cord. It functions in arousal and wakefulness, attention, pain, panic, and stress. Destruction of this structure has been linked to *Alzheimer's disease*.

The raphe nuclei of the RF release serotonin and project to areas such as the thalamus, prefrontal cortex, basal ganglia, cranial nerve nuclei, and spinal cord. The number of individually named raphe nuclei differs in the literature but they can include the *nucleus raphe dorsalis, nucleus raphe pontis*, and *nucleus raphe pallidus*. They function in memory and learning, appetite, mood, wakefulness, and the modulation of pain. Clinically, these serotonin-releasing neurons are related to depression and anxiety disorders and are the targets of antidepressants such as selective serotonin reuptake inhibitors (SSRIs).

The larger functions of the RF include (**Fig. 9.17c**):

- *Somatic motor control*: the RF can receive axons from motor neurons that give rise to the reticulospinal tract, a tract that plays a large role in maintaining posture and balance during movements. Motor nuclei include gaze centers that enable the eyes to track and fixate on certain objects. Nuclei known as the central pattern generators produce rhythmic signals to muscles involved in breathing and swallowing. Motor coordination can be integrated with visual, auditory, and vestibular stimuli back to the cerebellum by the RF.
- *Sleep and consciousness*: the RF plays a central role in states of sleep and alertness. Projections to the thalamus, hypothalamus, and cerebral cortex from the RF can exert some control over which sensory signals reach the cerebrum. The regulation of sleep–wake transitions and an individual's level of alertness are referred to as the **ascending reticular activating system (ARAS)**.
- *Control of the autonomic nervous system*: the RF can regulate both sympathetic and parasympathetic outflow through the reticulospinal and reticulobulbar tracts.
- *Control of the vital functions*: individual nuclear regions of the RF have influence on functional centers such as the vasomotor center important in regulating blood pressure, inspiration and expiration centers involved in breathing, swallowing, or micturition. Some of the functional centers may be more protective in nature such as controlling the gagging and vomiting reflexes.
- *Pain modulation*: how pain signals from the lower body reach the cerebral cortex. Descending analgesic pathways do exist

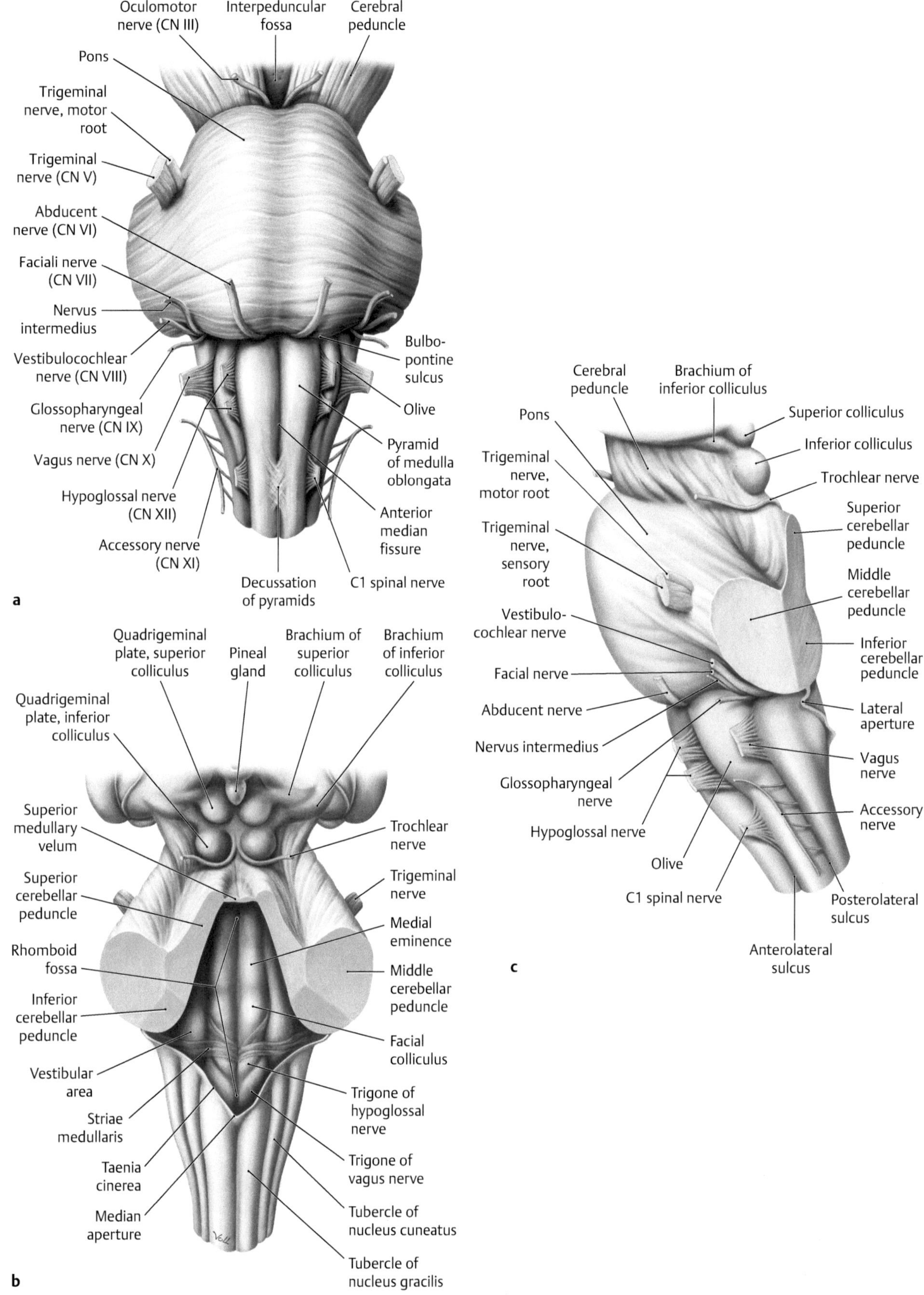

Fig. 9.15 Brainstem: external structures. **(a)** Ventral view. **(b)** Dorsal view. **(c)** Lateral view from left. (From Schuenke M, Schulte E, Schumacher U. THIEME Atlas of Anatomy. Head, Neck, and Neuroanatomy. Illustrations by Voll M and Wesker K. 3rd ed. New York: Thieme Medical Publishers; 2020.)

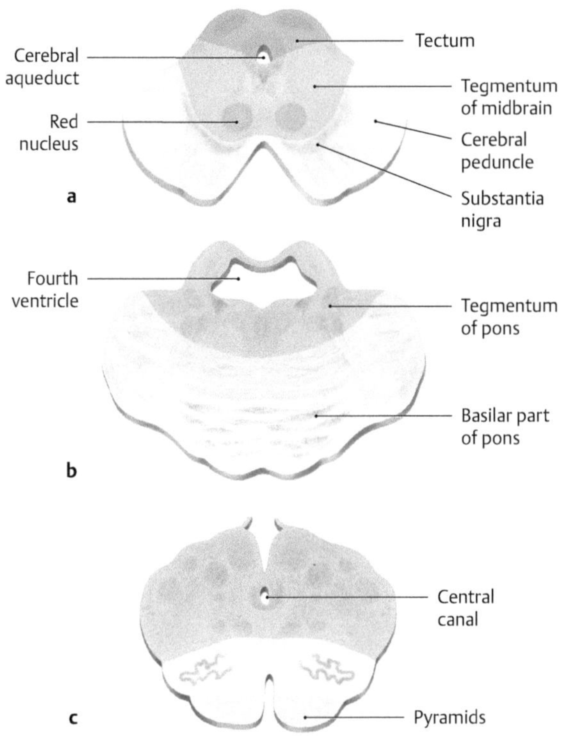

Fig. 9.16 Cross-sectional structure of the brainstem at different levels. **(a)** Midbrain. **(b)** Pons. **(c)** Medulla oblongata. (From Schuenke M, Schulte E, Schumacher U. THIEME Atlas of Anatomy. Head, Neck, and Neuroanatomy. Illustrations by Voll M and Wesker K. 3rd ed. New York: Thieme Medical Publishers; 2020.)

and can act in the spinal cord to block pain transmission back to the brain.

- *Habituation*: a process whereby the brain has learned to ignore repetitive and inconsequential stimuli while remaining more sensitive to other stimuli.

9.5.3 Medulla

The **medulla oblongata** (or just medulla), or **myelencephalon**, has a caudal end attached to the spinal cord and a rostral end continuous with the pons. The caudal portion displays the position of the **fasciculus cuneatus** and **gracilis**, structures that ascend from the spinal cord. Their locations can be isolated externally as two swellings, the **tuberculum cuneatus** and **gracilis**, respectively. The termination of these swellings helps identify the location of the **nucleus cuneatus** and **gracilis.** The fasciculi and nuclei mediate conscious proprioception, vibratory sensation, and tactile impulses are destined for higher regions of the brain (**Fig. 9.19c, d**).

The **pyramid** is located on the ventral surface and is composed of numerous nerve fibers that arise from the precentral, postcentral, and premotor regions of the cerebral cortex. These nerve fibers belong to the corticospinal and corticobulbar tracts. The pyramid near the caudal portion of the medulla and just rostral to the spinal cord is the location where approximately 90% of the corticospinal tract crosses to the contralateral side. This is called the **decussation** of the pyramids. Nerve fibers that decussate are known as the lateral corticospinal tract while the fibers that do not are known as the anterior corticospinal tract (**Fig. 9.19c, d**). Still externally and lying just laterally to the pyramids are the **olives.** The olives contain the **inferior olivary nucleus** (**Fig. 9.19a-c**), a relay station for mainly proprioceptive sensory information originating from the spinal cord that ultimately travels to the cerebellum. Connecting the medulla to the cerebellum are the **inferior cerebellar peduncles**, structures that contain both motor and sensory tracts (**Fig. 9.19a**).

There are numerous nuclei located in the medulla. Specific functions for most nuclei will be discussed in appropriate sections of this chapter. The nucleus cuneatus, nucleus gracilis, and inferior olivary nucleus have already been mentioned but others include the **accessory cuneate**, **superior**, **inferior**, **lateral**, and **medial vestibular nuclei** (**Fig. 9.103c**). The **anterior** and **posterior cochlear nuclei** are found near the medullopontine junction (**Fig. 9.20**). The **spinal nucleus of the trigeminal nerve (CN V)** helps mediate somatosensory information from the head region and thalamus. The **nucleus ambiguus** is where the branchiomotor fibers of cranial nerve IX and X reside. The **dorsal vagal nucleus** is the origin of parasympathetic preganglionic fibers that course through the vagus nerve (CN X). The **hypoglossal nuclei** are where somatic motor fibers of most tongue muscles originate (**Fig. 9.19a, b; Fig. 9.21a, b**).

In addition to the larger ascending and descending tracts, there is the **medial lemniscus** (**Fig. 9.19a–c**), a large ascending myelinated set of axons that decussate in the medulla. It is formed by the **internal arcuate fibers**, which are composed of axons originating from the nucleus cuneatus and gracilis and associated with the PCMLS sensory pathway. The function of the medial lemniscus is to transmit information associated primarily with conscious proprioception and vibratory stimuli to the thalamus. The **medial longitudinal fasciculus (MLF)** is situated near the midline of the brainstem and is made up of both ascending and descending axons (**Fig. 9.19a–d**). Ascending axons arise from the **superior**, **lateral**, and **medial vestibular nuclei** and project to the pons and midbrain. They provide information about the position of the head in space to cranial nerve nuclei that coordinate movements and position of the eyes such as cranial nerves III, IV, and VI. The descending axons arise from the medial vestibular nucleus and extend down to the cervical levels of the spinal cord. This is commonly known as the **medial vestibulospinal tract** and it serves to adjust changes in the position of the head in response to changes in vestibular inputs. The **solitary tract and nucleus** are located in the medulla and pons, and these are associated with both taste and visceral sensory information (**Fig. 9.19a–d; Fig. 9.21a, b**).

9.5.4 Pons

The **pons** serves as a bridge between the medulla and midbrain. Anatomically, the pons can be divided into a ventral **basilar pons** and a dorsal **tegmentum** (**Fig. 9.16b**). The tegmentum is continuous with both the medulla and midbrain tegmentums. The basilar pons is broken into two different groups of neurons and fibers. One massive group of fibers runs in a transverse direction across the pons and is called the **transverse pontine (pontocerebellar) fibers.** These fibers arise from the neurons of deep pontine nuclei scattered throughout the basilar pons. The second group of fibers consists of the corticobulbar and corticospinal fibers.

The basilar artery forms a groove called the **basilar sulcus** along the midline of the basilar pons. Lateral to this is the large **middle cerebellar peduncle** fiber bundle that is a continuation of the transverse pontine fibers. This peduncle passes posterolaterally into the cerebellum. The floor of the fourth ventricle and roof of the pons are located at the dorsal aspect of the tegmentum. The lateral walls of the fourth ventricle are formed by the superior cerebellar peduncles that originate primarily from the cerebellum

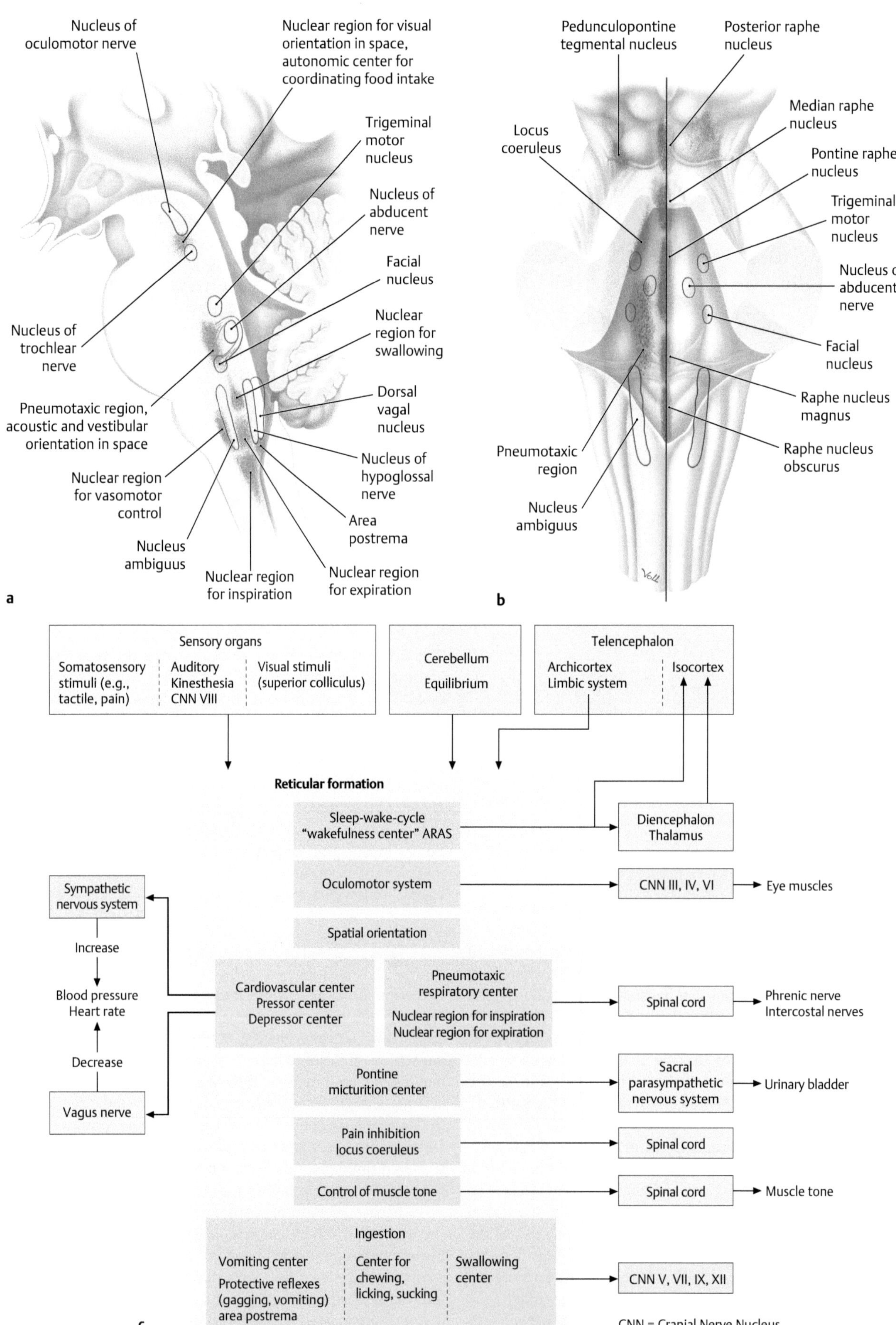

Fig. 9.17 (a) Functional centers of the reticular formation and cranial nerve nuclei, left lateral view. **(b)** Three longitudinal zones of the reticular formation, posterior view. **(c)** Overview of the functions of the reticular formation. (From Schuenke M, Schulte E, Schumacher U. THIEME Atlas of Anatomy. Head, Neck, and Neuroanatomy. Illustrations by Voll M and Wesker K. 3rd ed. New York: Thieme Medical Publishers; 2020.)

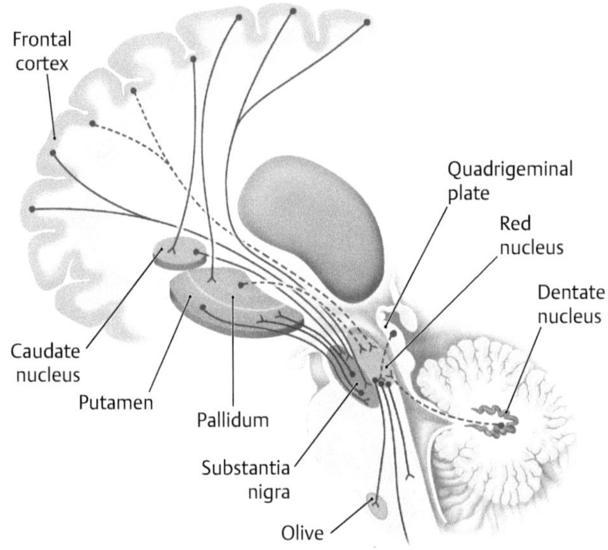

Fig. 9.18 Afferent (*blue*) and efferent (*red*) connections of the red nucleus and substantia nigra. (From Schuenke M, Schulte E, Schumacher U. THIEME Atlas of Anatomy. Head, Neck, and Neuroanatomy. Illustrations by Voll M and Wesker K. 3rd ed. New York: Thieme Medical Publishers; 2020.)

before entering the brainstem from a posterolateral position at the level of the rostral pons. A bulge called the **facial colliculus** can be identified on the floor of the fourth ventricle, and it is formed by the fibers of the facial nerve that pass over the dorsal aspect of the abducent motor nucleus (**Fig. 9.22d**).

The tegmentum of the pons is the location of both nuclei and fiber pathways. The **abducent nucleus**, **facial nucleus**, **superior salivatory nucleus**, **superior** and **lateral vestibular nuclei**, **trapezoid body** (with nucleus), **superior olivary nucleus**, **lateral lemniscus**, and **reticular formation nuclei** and fibers are present in the caudal half of the tegmentum (**Fig. 9.21a, b; Fig. 9.22b-d**). The abducent and facial nuclei are motor to those corresponding cranial nerve skeletal muscles. The superior salivatory nucleus is where parasympathetic preganglionic fibers originate from and are motor to the lacrimal, submandibular, sublingual, nasal cavity, and palate glands. The superior and lateral vestibular nuclei receive direct information from the vestibular apparatus and supply fibers to the MLF. The lateral vestibular nuclei specifically are where the lateral vestibulospinal tract originates. Auditory inputs from the cochlear nuclei are received by the nucleus of the trapezoid body and superior olivary nucleus and then they are sent to higher centers of the brainstem. The lateral lemniscus is made up of fibers extending from both the cochlear nuclei and superior olivary nucleus to the inferior colliculus. The reticular formation related to the pons is divided into three different regions: a midline region containing **raphe nuclei** that produce serotonin, a medial two-thirds region containing larger cells giving rise to ascending and descending fibers related to the central tegmental tract, and a lateral region containing small cells that create additional inputs to the reticular formation.

The rostral half of the tegmentum is the site of the **mesencephalic, main (principal)** and **motor nucleus of the trigeminal nerve**, **locus coeruleus**, and the **superior cerebellar peduncle** (**Fig. 9.21a, b; Fig. 9.22b, c**). Portions of the trigeminal nerve are described extensively in Chapter 12 but the locus coeruleus consists of norepinephrine-containing neurons that project to different cell groups in the cerebellum, brainstem, and cerebral cortex. The superior cerebellar peduncle contains the majority of cerebellar efferent fibers to the midbrain and thalamus in addition to forming the lateral walls of the fourth ventricle. Superior cerebellar peduncle fibers cross at the caudal midbrain to the contralateral side.

Most of the same pathways coursing through the medulla are also present in the pons. The two most prominent ascending tracts would be the **medial lemniscus** and **medial longitudinal fasciculus**. Others include the **lateral spinothalamic** and **trigeminothalamic pathways** responsible for mediating somatosensory information from the body and head region to the ventral posterolateral and ventral posteromedial nuclei of the thalamus, respectively, which are located on the more lateral portion of the tegmentum (**Fig. 9.22b-d**). These two pathways are situated between the medial lemniscus and the **lateral lemniscus** (auditory relay circuit). Descending pathways include the **corticobulbar**, **corticospinal**, **rubrospinal**, and **tectospinal tracts**. The **central tegmental tract**, a combination of ascending and descending fibers, courses through the pons (**Fig. 9.22b-d**).

9.5.5 Midbrain

The midbrain is located between the pons and forebrain. It is divided into three parts: a ventral **crus cerebri**, a central **tegmentum**, and a dorsal **tectum** also referred to as the **corpora quadrigemina** (**Fig. 9.16a**). The **crus cerebri** include large bundles of descending fibers to pass from the cerebral cortex to the brainstem and spinal cord. The **tegmentum** is continuous with that of the pons. The **substantia nigra** (**Fig. 9.22a**) cell group separates the crus cerebri from the tegmentum. The tegmentum is separated from the tectum by the **periaqueductal gray** (**Fig. 9.22a**) that surrounds the cerebral aqueduct. The **tectum/corpora**

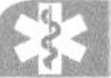
Clinical Correlate 9.1

Lateral Medullary Syndrome

Lateral medullary (Wallenberg, PICA) syndrome is the result of a vascular lesion associated with the vertebral artery or its posterior inferior cerebellar artery (PICA) branches. Structures affected and their deficits include:

- *Spinothalamic tracts*: contralateral loss of pain and temperature of the trunk and limbs.
- *Sensory nucleus of trigeminal nerve*: ipsilateral loss of pain and temperature from face.
- *Vestibular (inferior and medial) nuclei*: vertigo, nausea, vomiting, and nystagmus.
- *Glossopharyngeal nerve*: loss of afferent limb of gag reflex.
- *Vagus nerve*: loss of efferent limb of gag reflex.
- *Nucleus ambiguus of CN IX and X*: ipsilateral loss of palatal, laryngeal, and pharyngeal muscle activity resulting in hoarseness (dysphonia) and difficulty swallowing (dysphagia).
- *Inferior cerebellar peduncles*: ipsilateral limbs and gait ataxia.
- *Central sympathetic tract*: ipsilateral Horner syndrome.

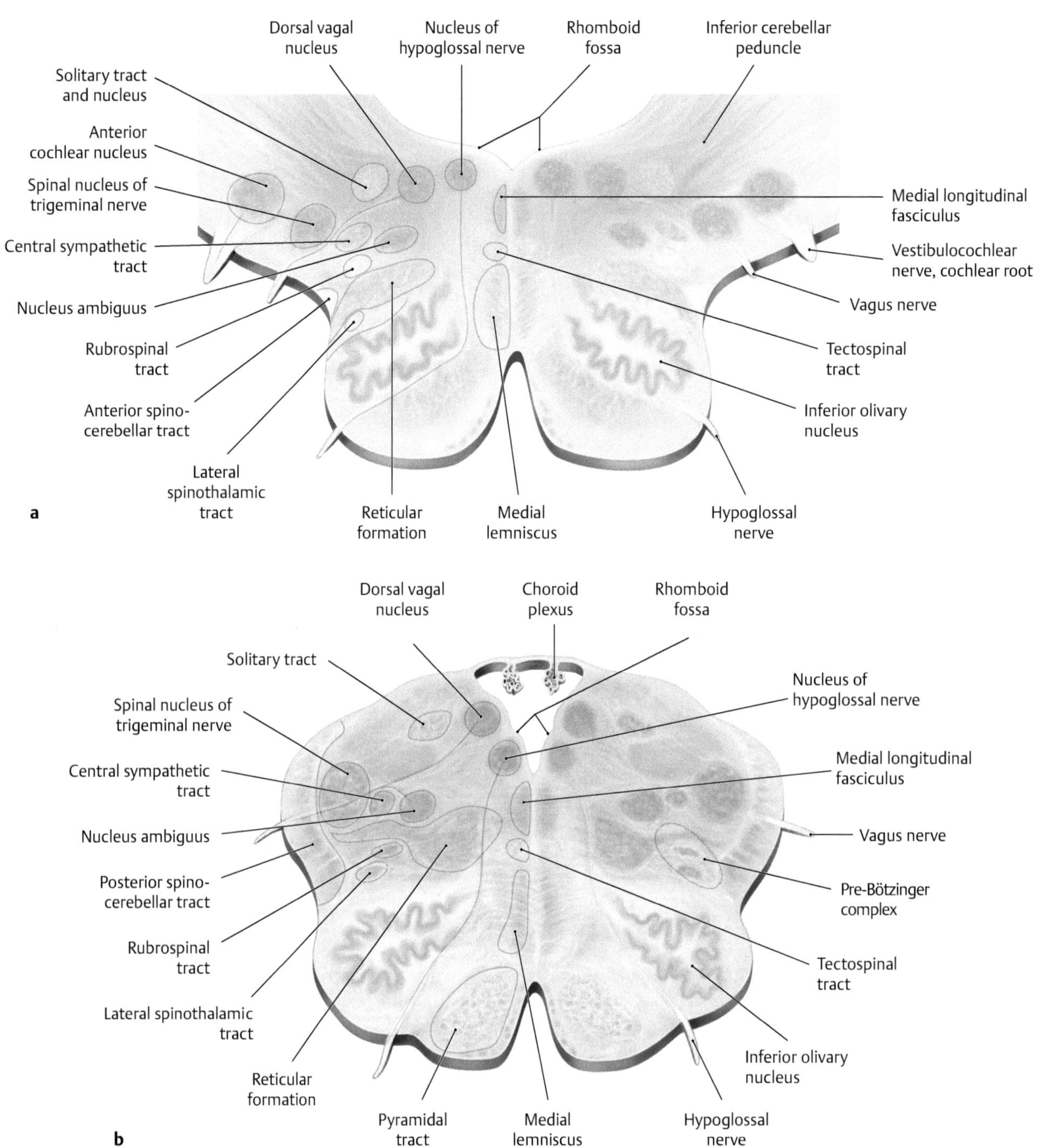

Fig. 9.19 Medulla oblongata; transverse sections. **(a)** Upper medulla. **(b)** Just above the middle of the medulla oblongata. (*continued*) (From Schuenke M, Schulte E, Schumacher U. THIEME Atlas of Anatomy. Head, Neck, and Neuroanatomy. Illustrations by Voll M and Wesker K. 3rd ed. New York: Thieme Medical Publishers; 2020.)

quadrigemina consists of four bodies and these are collectively the **superior** and **inferior colliculi** (**Fig. 9.15b, c**). Additional nuclei in this region include **red nucleus**, and the **oculomotor**, **trochlear**, and **Edinger-Westphal motor nuclei** associated with eye muscles (**Fig. 9.21a, b; Fig. 9.22a**).

The **inferior colliculus** is located in the tectum. It receives ascending inputs from auditory relay nuclei of the medulla and pons, which includes the cochlear and superior olivary nuclei along with the nucleus of the trapezoid body. These neurons supplied the inferior colliculus via the **lateral lemniscus pathway**. The inferior colliculus then projects fibers through a bundle called the brachium of the inferior colliculus to the medial geniculate nucleus of the thalamus. At the level of the inferior colliculus but in the tegmentum is the **periaqueductal gray (PAG)**, a structure important in the regulation of autonomic activities and emotional processes, and in the control of pain impulses. The PAG contains high concentrations of a neurotransmitter peptide called *enkephalin*. Axons arising from the forebrain and PAG ascend through different levels of the PAG to terminate within the PAG or at lower parts of the brainstem. The MLF lies just beneath the trochlear

Nucleus cuneatus
Nucleus gracilis
Solitary tract
Accessory cuneate nucleus
Spinal nucleus of trigeminal nerve
Central canal
Posterior spino-cerebellar tract
Nucleus of accessory nerve
Reticular formation
Medial longitudinal fasciculus
Central sympathetic tract
Accessory nerve
Rubrospinal tract
Nucleus of hypoglossal nerve
Lateral spinothalamic tract
Hypoglossal nerve
Pyramidal tract
Tectospinal tract
Medial lemniscus
c

Nucleus gracilis
Fasciculus gracilis
Nucleus cuneatus
Fasciculus cuneatus
Substantia gelatinosa
Solitary tract
Spinal nucleus of trigeminal nerve
Nucleus of accessory nerve
Reticular formation
Central canal
Central sympathetic tract
Decussation of pyramids
Posterior spino-cerebellar tract
Lateral corticospinal tract
Rubrospinal tract
Medial longitudinal fasciculus
Lateral spinothalamic tract
Tectospinal tract
Anterior corticospinal tract
d

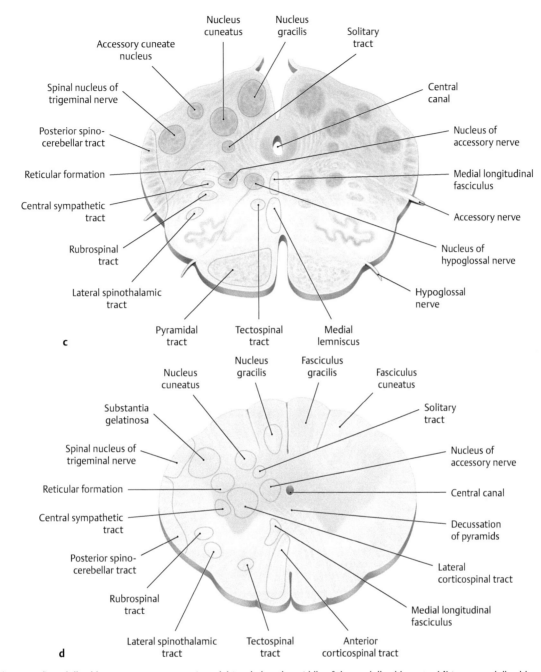

Fig. 9.19 (*continued*) Medulla oblongata; transverse sections. **(c)** Just below the middle of the medulla oblongata. **(d)** Lower medulla oblongata. (From Schuenke M, Schulte E, Schumacher U. THIEME Atlas of Anatomy. Head, Neck, and Neuroanatomy. Illustrations by Voll M and Wesker K. 3rd ed. New York: Thieme Medical Publishers; 2020.)

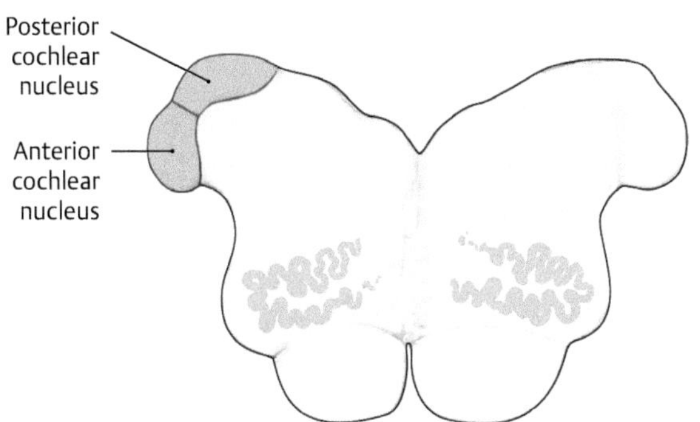

Fig. 9.20 Cochlear nuclei. (From Schuenke M, Schulte E, Schumacher U. THIEME Atlas of Anatomy. Head, Neck, and Neuroanatomy. Illustrations by Voll M and Wesker K. 3rd ed. New York: Thieme Medical Publishers; 2020.)

motor nucleus and is an afferent source to this nucleus. The **central tegmental area** is located at this level as well.

The **crus cerebri** has a particular pattern of fibers that pass through it. Fibers passing through the lateral fifth originate from the parietal, occipital, and temporal neocortices and terminate at the deep pontine nuclei. Within the middle three-fifths there is the passage of the corticospinal and corticobulbar fibers. The organization is set up so that the fibers associated with the trunk and limbs are located laterally while the fibers associated with the head region are more medial. Within the medial fifth, fibers arise from the frontal lobe but also terminate at the deep pontine nuclei.

The **substantia nigra** (**Fig. 9.16a; Fig. 9.18; Fig. 9.22a**) contains two groups of cells: the lateral group, which is called the pars reticulata, and the medial group, which is called the pars compacta. **Pars reticulata** neurons project to the thalamus using the

Clinical Correlate 9.2

Dorsal Medullary Syndrome

Dorsal medullary syndrome is related to lateral medullary syndrome to some degree. It is due to a vascular lesion involving the medial branch of the PICA. Structures affected and their deficits include:

- *Inferior cerebellar peduncles*: ipsilateral limbs and gait ataxia.
- *Vestibular nuclei*: vertigo, nausea, vomiting, and nystagmus.
- *Nucleus prepositus hypoglossi (NPH)*: direction changing gaze-evoked nystagmus. NPH is a structure located adjacent to the MLF in the medullopontine junction and serves as a key constituent of a vestibular-cerebellar-brainstem neural network. It ensures that the eyes are held steady in all positions of gaze.

Clinical Correlate 9.3

Medial Medullary Syndrome

Medial medullary (Dejerine) syndrome is the result of a vascular lesion involving the anterior spinal or paramedian branches of the vertebral arteries. Structures affected and their deficits include:

- *Hypoglossal nerve*: ipsilateral paralysis of the tongue with deviation of the tongue while protruding to the side of the lesion.
- *Corticospinal tract*: contralateral weakness of the trunk and limbs.
- *Medial longitudinal fasciculus*: ipsilateral internuclear ophthalmopegia.
- *Medial lemniscus*: contralateral loss of proprioception, discriminative tactile, and vibration sensation from trunk and limbs.

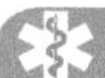

Clinical Correlate 9.4

Lateral Superior Pontine Syndrome

Lateral superior pontine syndrome is due to a vascular lesion involving the long circumferential or superior cerebellar arteries of the basilar artery. Structures affected and their deficits include:

- *Superior and middle cerebellar peduncles*: ipsilateral trunk and limb dystaxia.
- *Dentate nucleus of cerebellum*: lack of muscle coordination (dystaxia), intention tremors, and inability to estimate distance with muscle actions (dysmetria).
- *Central sympathetic tract*: ipsilateral Horner syndrome.
- *Sensory nucleus of trigeminal nerve*: ipsilateral loss of pain and temperature from face.
- *Spinothalamic tracts*: contralateral loss of pain and temperature of the trunk and limbs.
- *Medial lemniscus*: contralateral loss of proprioception, discriminative tactile and vibration sensation of the trunk and lower limbs.

neurotransmitter gamma-aminobutyric acid (GABA). The **pars compacta** is associated with the neurotransmitter dopamine and is released onto neurons of the neostratium. The loss of dopamine production from these neurons of the substantia nigra results in Parkinson disease.

At the level of the superior colliculus, there are a few other structures associated with the midbrain. The **superior colliculus** (**Fig. 9.22a**) itself receives input from the retina and its projections via the tectospinal tract to the cervical spinal cord and serves to produce reflex movements of the head and neck in response to sensory inputs. The periaqueductal gray is still present at this

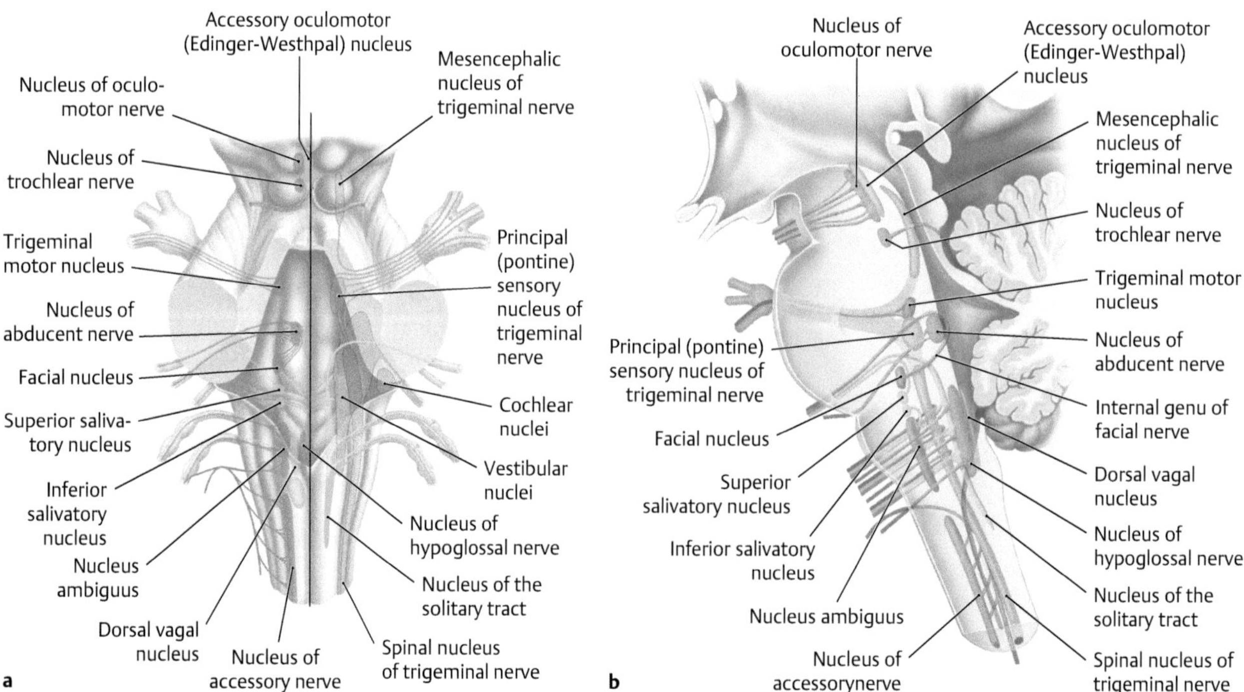

Fig. 9.21 Cranial nerve nuclei in the brainstem. **(a)** Posterior view with the cerebellum removed, exposing the rhomboid fossa. **(b)** Midsagittal section of the right half of the brainstem viewed from the left side. Note: vestibular and cochlear nuclei are not shown. (From Schuenke M, Schulte E, Schumacher U. THIEME Atlas of Anatomy. Head, Neck, and Neuroanatomy. Illustrations by Voll M and Wesker K. 3rd ed. New York: Thieme Medical Publishers; 2020.)

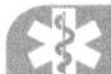 Clinical Correlate 9.5

Lateral Mid-Pontine Syndrome
Lateral mid-pontine syndrome is due to a vascular lesion involving mainly the short circumferential arteries of the basilar artery. Structures affected and their deficits include:

- *Trigeminal sensory and motor nuclei and nerve root*: ipsilateral muscle of mastication paralysis, jaw deviation to weak side, and touch, proprioception, pain, and temperature loss on face.
- *Middle cerebellar peduncle*: ipsilateral limb and gait dystaxia.
- Ipsilateral loss of corneal reflex.

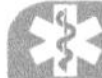 Clinical Correlate 9.6

Lateral Inferior Pontine Syndrome
Lateral inferior pontine (AICA) syndrome is due to a vascular lesion involving the long circumferential arteries or generally the anterior inferior cerebellar artery (AICA) of the basilar artery. Structures affected and their deficits include:

- *Middle and inferior cerebellar peduncles*: ipsilateral limb and gait ataxia.
- *Sensory nucleus of trigeminal nerve*: ipsilateral loss of pain and temperature from face.
- *Facial motor nucleus*: ipsilateral facial nerve paralysis, loss of stapedial and corneal reflexes, and loss of taste (anterior two-thirds of tongue).
- *Vestibular nuclei*: vertigo, nausea, vomiting, and nystagmus.
- *Cochlear nuclei*: unilateral central nerve deafness.
- *Central sympathetic tract*: ipsilateral Horner syndrome.
- *Spinothalamic tracts*: contralateral loss of pain and temperature of the trunk and limbs.

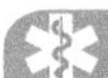 Clinical Correlate 9.7

Medial Pontine Syndrome
Medial pontine syndrome is due to a vascular lesion involving the paramedian branches of the basilar artery. Structures affected and their deficits include:

- *Middle cerebellar peduncle*: ipsilateral limb and gait ataxia.
- *Corticospinal tract*: contralateral weakness of the trunk and limbs.
- *Corticobulbar tract*: contralateral weakness of the lower face.
- *Abducent nerve*: ipsilateral lateral rectus paralysis.
- *Medial longitudinal fasciculus*: ipsilateral internuclear ophthalmopegia.
- *Medial lemniscus*: contralateral loss of proprioception, discriminative tactile and vibration sensation from trunk and limbs.

Clinical Correlate 9.8

Ventral Pontine Syndrome
Ventral pontine (locked-in) syndrome is due to a vascular lesion involving the basilar artery at the base of the pons and the effect is bilateral. Structures affected and their deficits include:

- *Corticospinal tract*: bilaterally affected; thus, the individual is a quadriplegic.
- *Corticobulbar tract*: bilaterally affecting lower cranial nerves; thus, weakness is seen on both sides of the face and there is an inability to speak (aphonia).
- *Reticular formation*: generally spared, so the patient is awake but communication occurs by blinking or moving the eyes vertically.

level, but the superior cerebellar peduncles begin to be replaced by the **red nucleus** (**Fig. 9.16a; Fig. 9.18, 9.22a**). The red nucleus supplies all levels of the spinal cord and aids in the discharge of flexor motor neurons along with influencing cerebellar activity by sending axons to the inferior olivary nucleus, which helps supply the contralateral cerebellar cortex. The **ventral tegmental area** is located near the pars compacta and produces dopamine that is responsible for supplying both the striatum and forebrain.

The **crus cerebri** at the level of the superior colliculus has the same orientation as before. However, the superior colliculus begins to be replaced by a mass of cells called the **pretectal region**, which is related to the *pupillary light reflex*. The **posterior commissure** is located just dorsal to the periaqueductal gray, and it contains fibers that originate from multiple nuclei that include the pretectal region and synapse with the cranial nerve nuclei related to eye movements in order to coordinate their total movements. There are three thalamic nuclei that lie adjacent to the upper portion of the midbrain and these include the **lateral geniculate**, **medial geniculate**, and **pulvinar**.

9.5.6 Brainstem Lemnisci Summary

Coursing through all parts of the brainstem are the lemnisci. These ribbon-like structures pertain to a portion of one of four specific afferent pathways. The specific names are based on (1) their location relative to each other, (2) their origin in the spinal cord, or (3) their origin from the trigeminal nerve nucleus (**Fig. 9.23**).

- **Medial lemniscus:** serves as the continuation of the fasciculus gracilis or cuneatus. This entire lemniscus is formed by fibers that cross in the decussation of the medial lemnisci and terminates in the ventral posterolateral nucleus of the thalamus. It is related to the posterior column-medial lemniscus (PCML) sensory pathway.
- **Lateral spinothalamic (spinal) lemniscus**: serves as the continuation of the anterior and lateral spinothalamic tracts or the larger anterolateral sensory system (ALS). Second-order neuron cell bodies are located in the posterior horn of the spinal cord and their axons decussate while still in the spinal cord. This lemniscus thus receives information from the contralateral side and ascends until reaching the ipsilateral ventral posterolateral nucleus of the thalamus.
- **Trigeminal lemniscus:** originates from the spinal and main (principal) sensory nuclei related to the trigeminal nerve (CN V). It carries both anterior (crossed) and posterior (uncrossed) trigeminothalamic tract fibers that convey light touch, pressure, pain, and temperature input related to the head (except the posterior portion).
- **Lateral lemniscus**: associated with the organs of hearing and the auditory pathway. Second-order neurons mainly from the anterior cochlear nucleus can pass through the superior olivary nucleus or trapezoid body prior to ascending contralaterally or ipsilaterally. The lateral lemniscus conveys third-order neurons to the nucleus of the inferior colliculus. This lemniscus contains its own nuclei that serve as relay stations for the auditory pathway. Neurons from the inferior colliculus ascend and terminate at the medical geniculate body.

9.6 Cerebellum

The **cerebellum** plays a major role in the integration of motor functions. It is situated in the posterior cranial fossa and separated from the occipital lobes of the cerebral hemispheres by the tentorium cerebelli. It lies adjacent to the fourth ventricle

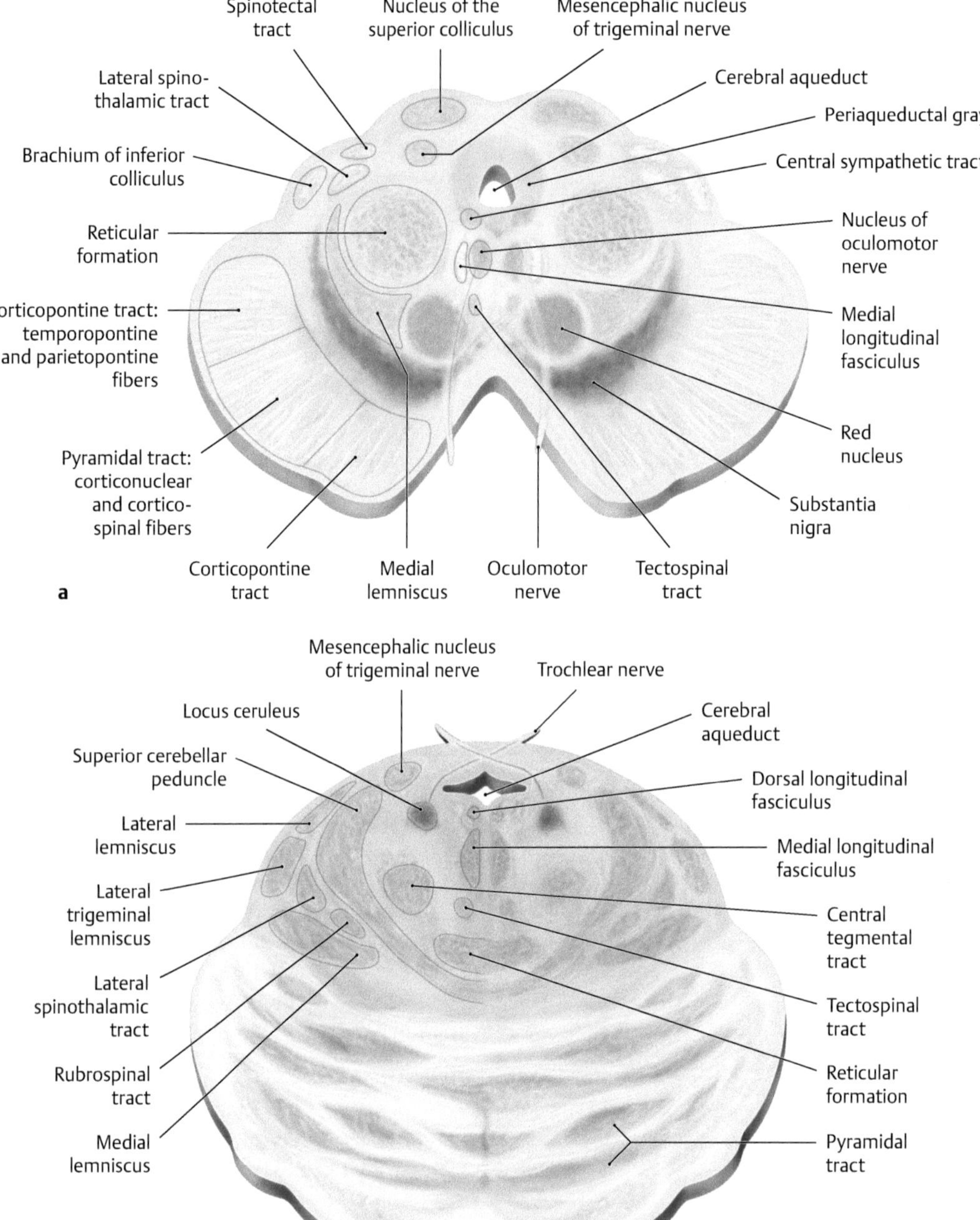

Fig. 9.22 Midbrain and pons; transverse sections. **(a)** Midbrain. **(b)** Upper pons. (*continued*) (From Schuenke M, Schulte E, Schumacher U. THIEME Atlas of Anatomy. Head, Neck, and Neuroanatomy. Illustrations by Voll M and Wesker K. 3rd ed. New York: Thieme Medical Publishers; 2020.)

Clinical Correlate 9.9

Medial Midbrain Syndrome

Medial midbrain (Weber) syndrome is the result of a vascular lesion involving posterior choroidal or posterior communicating branches of the posterior cerebral artery and it affects the medial portion of the cerebral peduncle at the level of the superior colliculus and root of the oculomotor nerve (CN III). Structures affected and their deficits include:

- *Oculomotor nucleus:* an ipsilateral oculomotor paralysis in conjunction with a contralateral upper motor neuron paralysis. A dropping eyelid (ptosis) is present and there is a dilated, unresponsive pupil (complete internal ophthalmoplegia).
- *Corticospinal tract:* contralateral weakness of the trunk and limbs.
- *Corticobulbar tract:* contralateral weakness of the lower face (CN VII), palate (CN X), and tongue (CN XII).

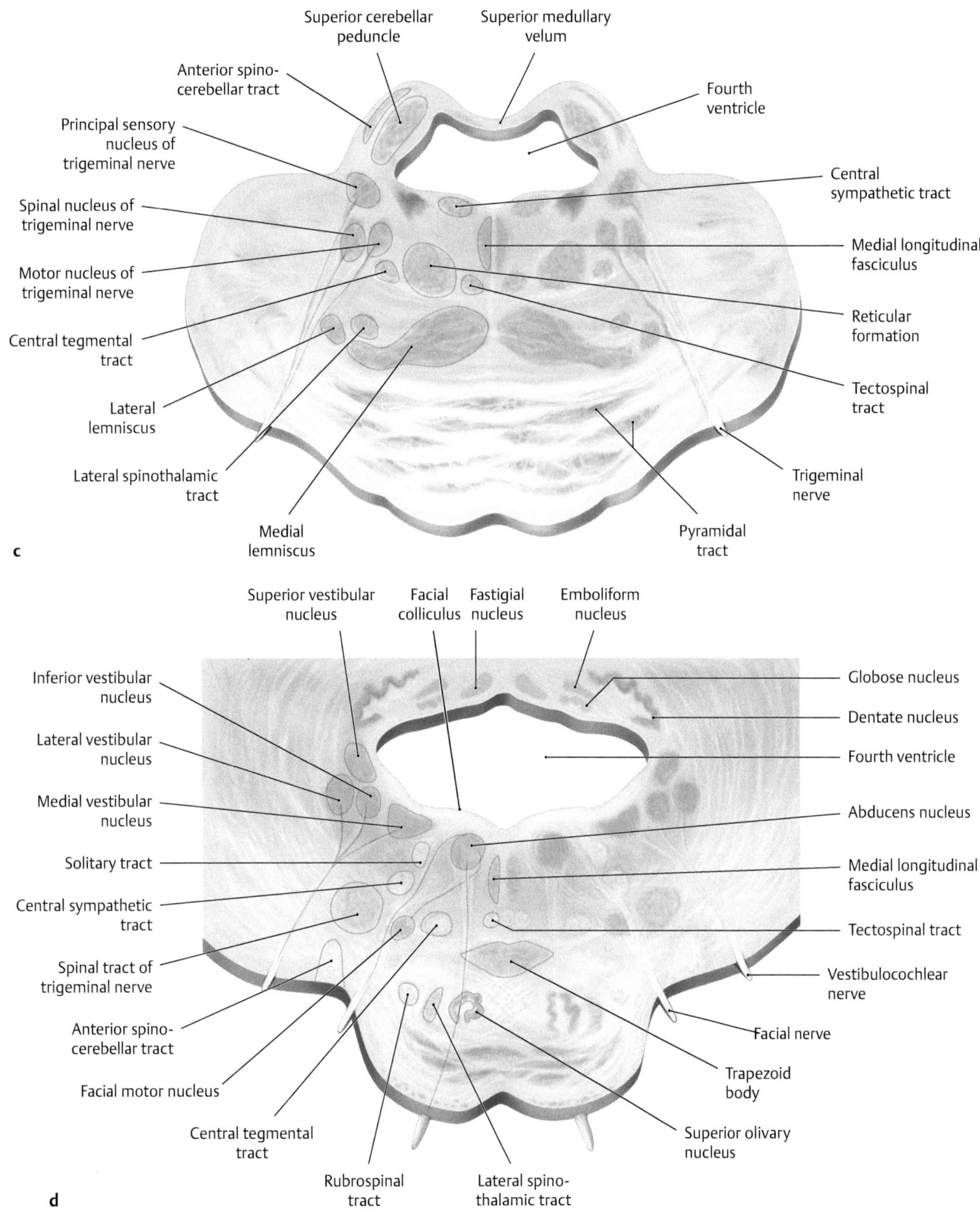

Fig. 9.22 (*continued*) Midbrain and pons; transverse sections. **(c)** Midportion of the pons. **(d)** Lower pons. (From Schuenke M, Schulte E, Schumacher U. THIEME Atlas of Anatomy. Head, Neck, and Neuroanatomy. Illustrations by Voll M and Wesker K. 3rd ed. New York: Thieme Medical Publishers; 2020.)

and attaches to the brainstem by way of the superior, middle, and inferior cerebellar peduncles. The cerebellum receives input from all levels of the CNS and its output projections are focused on almost all components of the skeletal motor system, which indirectly influence the activity of lower motor neurons. The cerebellum is able to integrate sensory input in order to shape motor output. This leads to smooth and coordinated movements and the maintenance of stable posture. Damage to it could cause unstable balance, lack of coordination of muscles, and reduced muscle tone and tremors.

Clinical Correlate 9.10

Paramedian Midbrain Syndrome

Paramedian (Benedikt) syndrome is the result of a vascular lesion of the posterior communicating branches of the posterior cerebral artery. Structures affected and their deficits include:

- *Oculomotor nucleus:* an ipsilateral oculomotor paralysis in conjunction with a contralateral upper motor neuron paralysis. A dropping eyelid (ptosis) is present and there is a dilated, unresponsive pupil (complete internal ophthalmoplegia).
- *Red nucleus and superior cerebellar peduncle:* the dentatorubrothalamic tract is damaged, resulting in contralateral cerebellar dystaxia and an intention tremor. The tremors are related to the damage to the superior cerebellar peduncle or fibers of the basal ganglia that pass near the red nucleus.
- *Spinothalamic tracts:* contralateral loss of pain and temperature of the trunk and limbs.
- *Medial lemniscus:* contralateral loss of proprioception, discriminative tactile and vibration sensation from trunk and limbs.

Clinical Correlate 9.11

Dorsal Midbrain Syndrome

Dorsal midbrain (Parinaud) syndrome is the result of a vascular lesion involving the posterior cerebral artery or a pineal gland tumor. Structures affected and their deficits include:

- *Superior colliculus and pretectal area:* an ipsilateral oculomotor paralysis in conjunction with a contralateral upper motor neuron paralysis. A dropping eyelid (ptosis) is present and there is a dilated, unresponsive pupil (complete internal ophthalmoplegia). Deficits can also include a vertical gaze paralysis, possible nystagmus with a downward gaze, and an accommodation paralysis.
- *Cerebral aqueduct:* noncommunicating hydrocephalus.

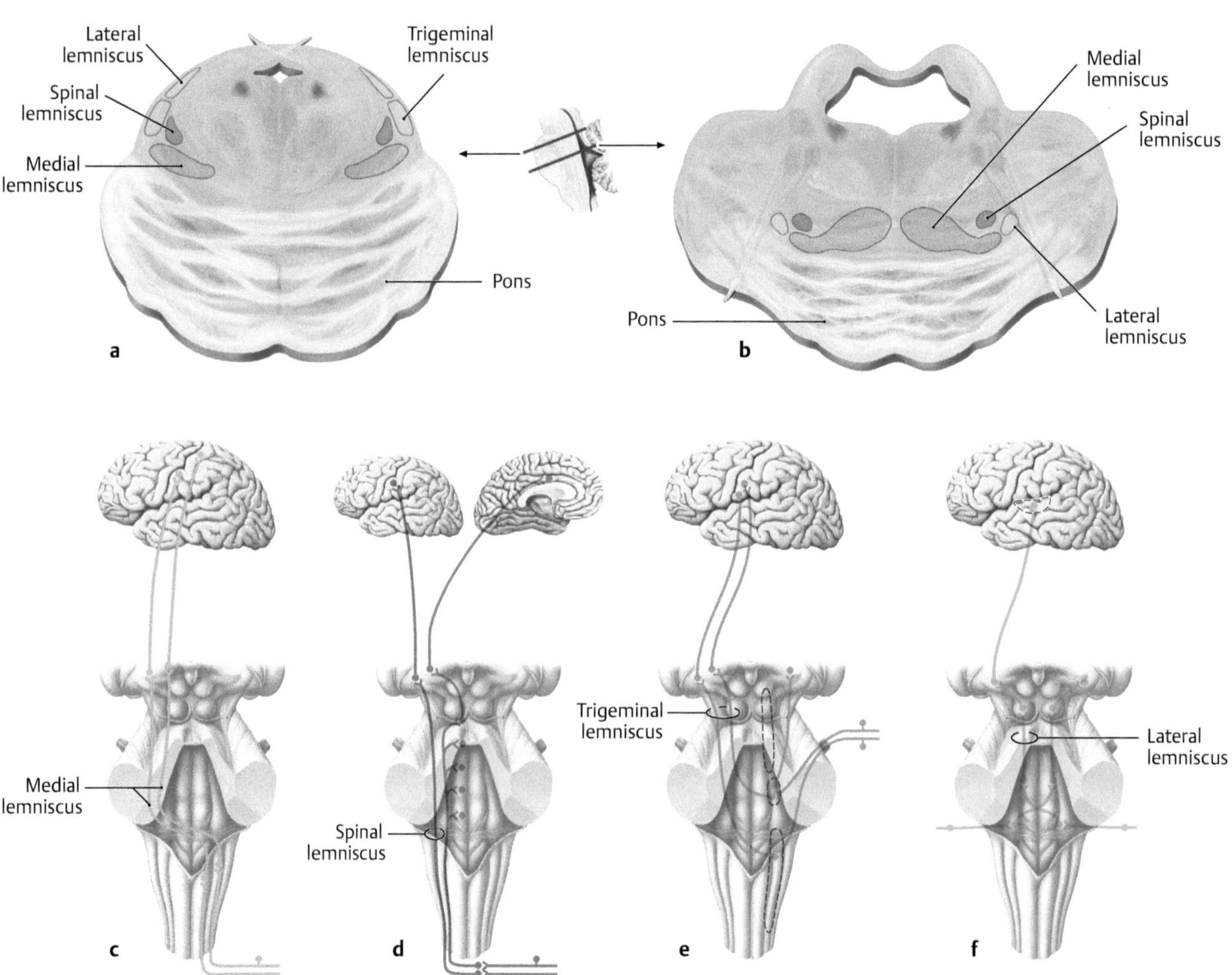

Fig. 9.23 The four lemnisci in the brainstem: **(a)** Cross-section through the upper pons. **(b)** Cross-section through the midportion of the pons. Schematic representation of the medial lemniscus **(c)**; spinal lemniscus **(d)**; trigeminal lemniscus **(e)**; lateral lemniscus **(f)**. (From Schuenke M, Schulte E, Schumacher U. THIEME Atlas of Anatomy. Head, Neck, and Neuroanatomy. Illustrations by Voll M and Wesker K. 3rd ed. New York: Thieme Medical Publishers; 2020.)

It is made up of two hemispheres that are continuous with a median vermal region. The hemispheres are divided into an anterior, posterior, and flocculonodular lobe. The **anterior lobe** occupies the majority of the superior surface of the cerebellum and the **primary fissure** separates it from the posterior lobe. The anterior lobe and the adjacent vermal region of the posterior lobe receive inputs from the spinal cord and are also referred to functionally as the **spinocerebellum**. It plays a significant role in the maintenance of muscle tone. The **posterior lobe** fills the remainder of the superior surface and the majority of the inferior surface of the cerebellum. It is the largest lobe with a link to the cerebral cortex. It is functionally referred to as the **pontocerebellum (cerebrocerebellum)** and is essential for the coordination of skilled movements. The **flocculonodular lobe** is the smallest and most inferior portion of the cerebellum separated from the posterior lobe by the **posterolateral fissure**. It receives inputs from the vestibular system and thus is also referred to functionally as the **vestibulocerebellum**. This lobe functions in the control of equilibrium and posture. The **horizontal fissure** is the largest and deepest of the cerebellar fissures and it separates the cerebellum into an upper and lower portion (**Fig. 9.24**).

There are three longitudinal and functional zones to the cerebellum, with each zone having an association with specific deep cerebellar nuclei and pathways. The **median (vermal) zone** contains the vermal cortex and projects to the *fastigial nucleus*. The **paramedian (paravermal) zone** contains the paravermal cortex and projects to the *globose* and *emboliform nuclei*. The **lateral zone** contains the hemispheric cortex and projects to the *dentate nucleus* (**Fig. 9.24a-c**).

The cerebellum has a highly convoluted outer **cortex** that receives and processes information from multiple sources. **White matter** underlies the cortex and consists of intrinsic, afferent, and efferent axons. It has a tree-like appearance and thus is referred to as the **arbor vitae** (**Fig. 9.25a, b**). The white matter helps make up the cerebellar peduncles. Embedded within the white matter are **deep cerebellar nuclei**, these gray matter structures serve as output centers for the cerebellum (**Fig. 9.25b**).

9.6.1 Cerebellar Peduncles

The cerebellar peduncle white matter is formed by axons passing to and from the cerebellum. There are superior, middle, and inferior cerebellar peduncles (**Fig. 9.24c; Fig. 9.26**).

- **Superior cerebellar peduncles (brachium conjunctivum)** connect the cerebellum with the midbrain and are made up of nearly all cerebellar efferent fibers except for the afferent fibers of the anterior spinocerebellar tract.
- **Middle cerebellar peduncles (brachium pontis)** connect to the lateral aspect of the pons and contain mainly afferent fibers that originate from the contralateral cerebral cortex (*pontocerebellar tract*) before projecting mainly to the neocerebellum. The bulk of all afferent fibers traveling to the cerebellum are through these peduncles.
- **Inferior cerebellar peduncles (restiform body)** are attached to the dorsolateral portion of the upper medulla and contain both afferent and efferent fibers. The largest component of these peduncles is the *olivocerebellar tract* fibers that arise from the contralateral inferior olive. Also included are the *posterior spinocerebellar tract* fibers originating from cells in the ipsilateral Clarke column in the spinal cord and the *cuneocerebellar tract* fibers that arise from the ipsilateral accessory cuneate nucleus. Lastly, the *vestibulocerebellar tract* fibers originating from cells of both the vestibular ganglion and the vestibular nuclei pass through this peduncle to reach the cerebellum.

9.6.2 Cerebellum Histology

The gray matter orientation is consistent throughout the cerebellar cortex. It forms folds or folia that are arranged transversely within the long axis of the hemisphere. White matter is located deep into the gray matter and contains both the afferent and efferent axons of the cerebellar cortex. The cerebellar cortex consists of three layers (**Fig. 9.27a**):

- **Molecular cell layer**: the most superficial or outer layer. It contains the dendrites of Purkinje cells, parallel axons of granule cells, stellate and basket cells.
- **Purkinje cell layer**: the middle layer. It contains only Purkinje cells. The cell body is flask-shaped and the neck ascends vertically toward the molecular layer.
- **Granular cell layer**: the innermost layer. It contains primarily granule cells. These cells have three to five dendrites and receive mossy fiber cerebellar afferents. This layer also contains Golgi cells.

The ultimate destination for fibers entering the cerebellum is the **Purkinje cells**. Their extensive dendritic trees reach through the molecular layer and to the cortical surface. The axons of Purkinje cells project primarily to cerebellar nuclei. They are *inhibitory neurons* and use GABA to inhibit the deep cerebellar nuclei. The **granule cells** are the only *excitatory neurons* of the cerebellar cortex. Their axons ascend through the Purkinje layer and into the molecular layer before bifurcating and each of these branches become an unmyelinated **parallel fiber**. These parallel fibers travel parallel to the long axis of the folia before making *excitatory* connections with numerous Purkinje cells. A single Purkinje cell can receive contact from a couple hundred thousand parallel fibers. The **Golgi cells** inhibit the granule cells while the **stellate cells** and **basket cells** serve to inhibit the Purkinje cells (**Fig. 9.27a**).

The axons that enter the cerebellum by way of the cerebellar peduncles belong to either a climbing fiber or a mossy fiber. These fibers are the two main lines of input to the cerebellar cortex and are both excitatory to the Purkinje cells. They both send collateral branches to deep cerebellar nuclei.

- **Climbing fibers** have a slow-firing rate and are related more to the muscle learning that has already occurred with activities such as throwing a ball or signing your signature. The input of a climbing fiber to that of a Purkinje fiber is one of the strongest excitatory connections in the CNS. The climbing fibers are the terminal fibers of the olivocerebellar tract that emanate from the contralateral inferior olive. They branch into a dozen or so collaterals as they approach the cerebellar cortex and each of these collaterals ascends to the molecular layer before synapsing with the dendrites of the Purkinje cell. A single Purkinje cell receives only one climbing fiber collateral; however, one climbing fiber can synapse with as many as 10 Purkinje cells (**Fig. 9.27b**).
- **Mossy fibers** have a fast-firing rate due to the rapid adjustments necessary for ongoing muscle activity. They are the terminal fibers of all other cerebellar afferent tracts and have multiple branches that exert a much more diffuse effect as they can stimulate thousands of Purkinje cells via the granule cells (**Fig. 9.27b**).

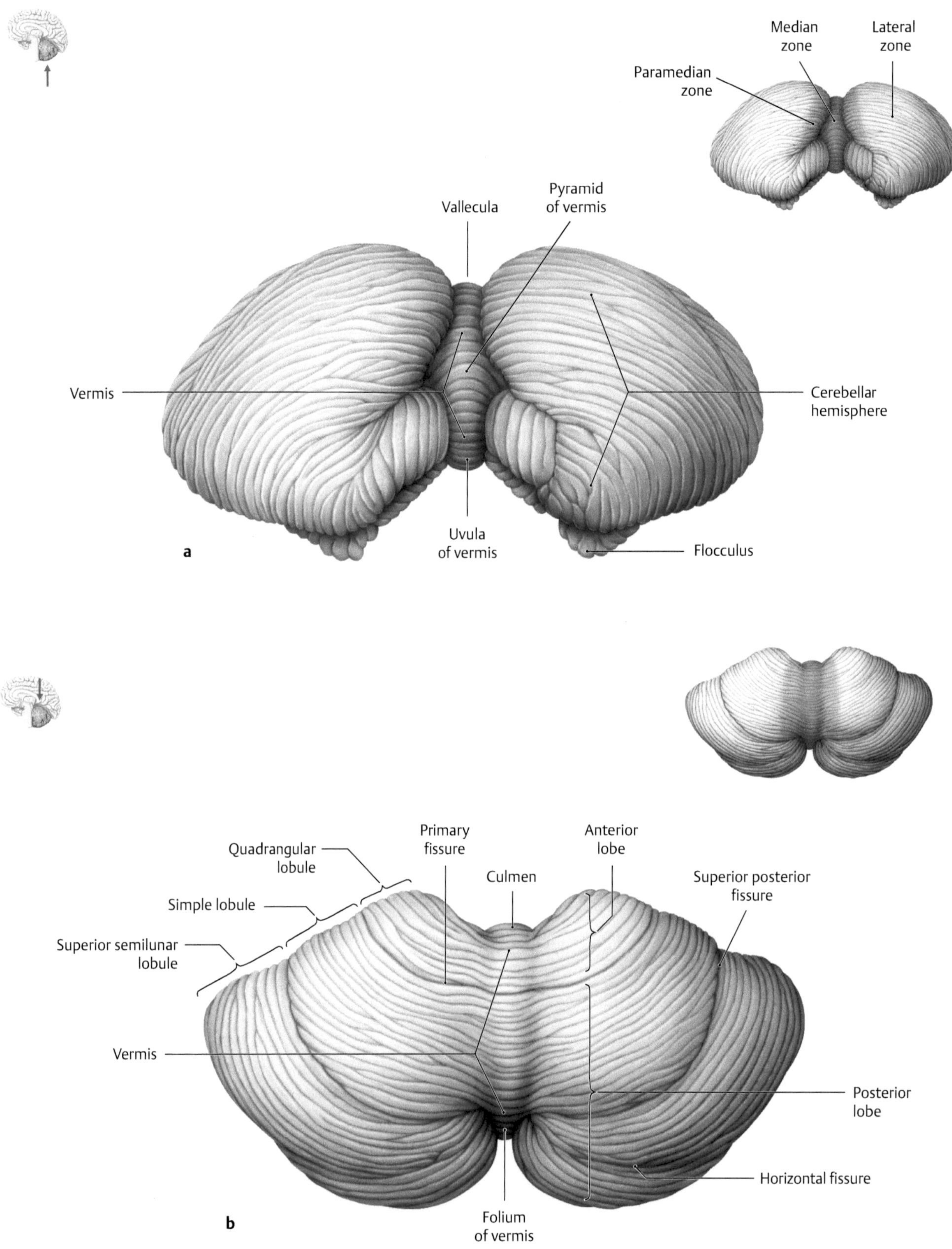

Fig. 9.24 Isolated cerebellum. **(a)** Inferior view. **(b)** Superior view. (*continued*) (From Schuenke M, Schulte E, Schumacher U. THIEME Atlas of Anatomy. Head, Neck, and Neuroanatomy. Illustrations by Voll M and Wesker K. 3rd ed. New York: Thieme Medical Publishers; 2020.)

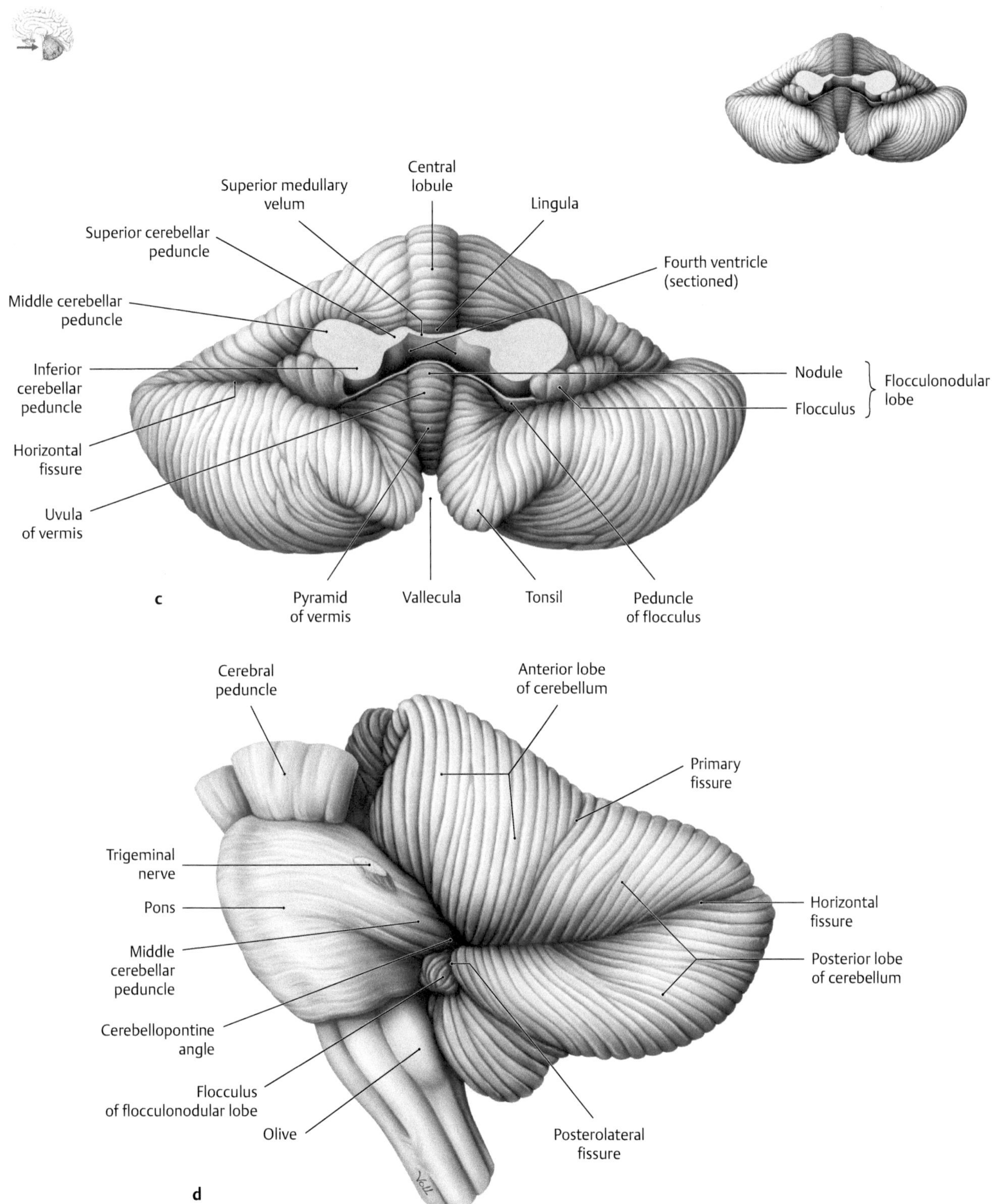

Fig. 9.24 *(continued)* Isolated cerebellum. **(c)** Anterior view. **(d)** Cerebellum on the brainstem, left lateral view. (From Schuenke M, Schulte E, Schumacher U. THIEME Atlas of Anatomy. Head, Neck, and Neuroanatomy. Illustrations by Voll M and Wesker K. 3rd ed. New York: Thieme Medical Publishers; 2020.)

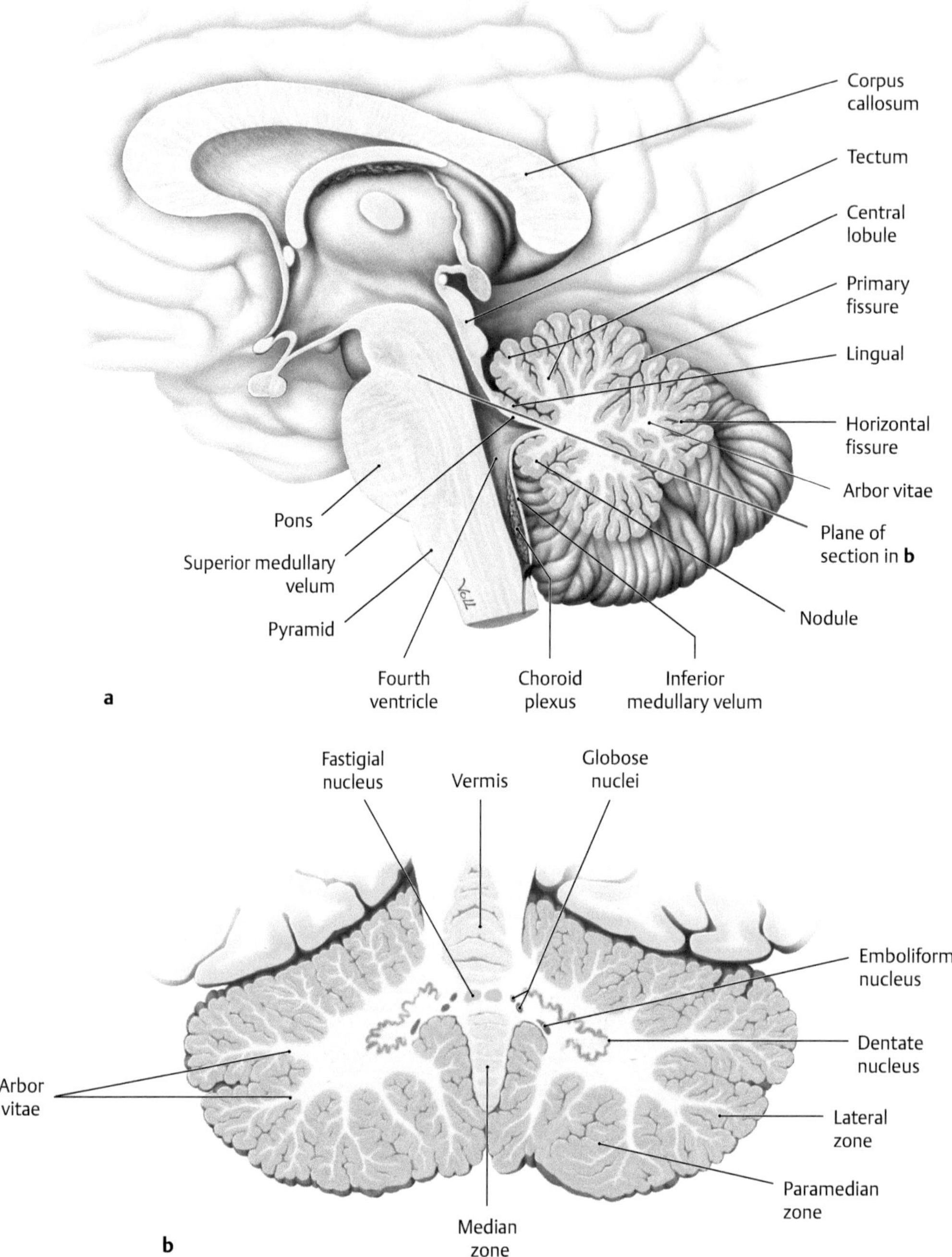

Fig. 9.25 Cerebellum, internal surface. **(a)** Cerebellum: positional relationship and cut surface. Midsagittal section, left lateral view. **(b)** Nuclei of the cerebellum. Section through the superior cerebellar peduncles (plane of section in **a**). (From Schuenke M, Schulte E, Schumacher U. THIEME Atlas of Anatomy. Head, Neck, and Neuroanatomy. Illustrations by Voll M and Wesker K. 3rd ed. New York: Thieme Medical Publishers; 2020.)

9.6.3 Cerebellar Nuclei

There are four pairs of cerebellar nuclei embedded within the white matter which are the principal source of efferent fibers originating from the cerebellum. Moving from medial to lateral, beginning near the midline, the nuclei are arranged as the fastigial, globose, emboliform, and the dentate. The Purkinje cells are responsible for inhibiting these nuclei (**Fig. 9.25b**).

- **Fastigial nucleus**: serves as the chief output nucleus for the vestibulocerebellum and assists with the spinocerebellum. This nucleus projects to multiple locations including the vestibular nuclei via the inferior cerebellar peduncle. Projections from the vestibular nuclei then pass to the ventral horn cells of the spinal cord via the lateral and medial vestibulospinal tracts and to the motor nuclei of CN III, IV, and VI by way of rostral projections through the MLF. These nuclei can also project

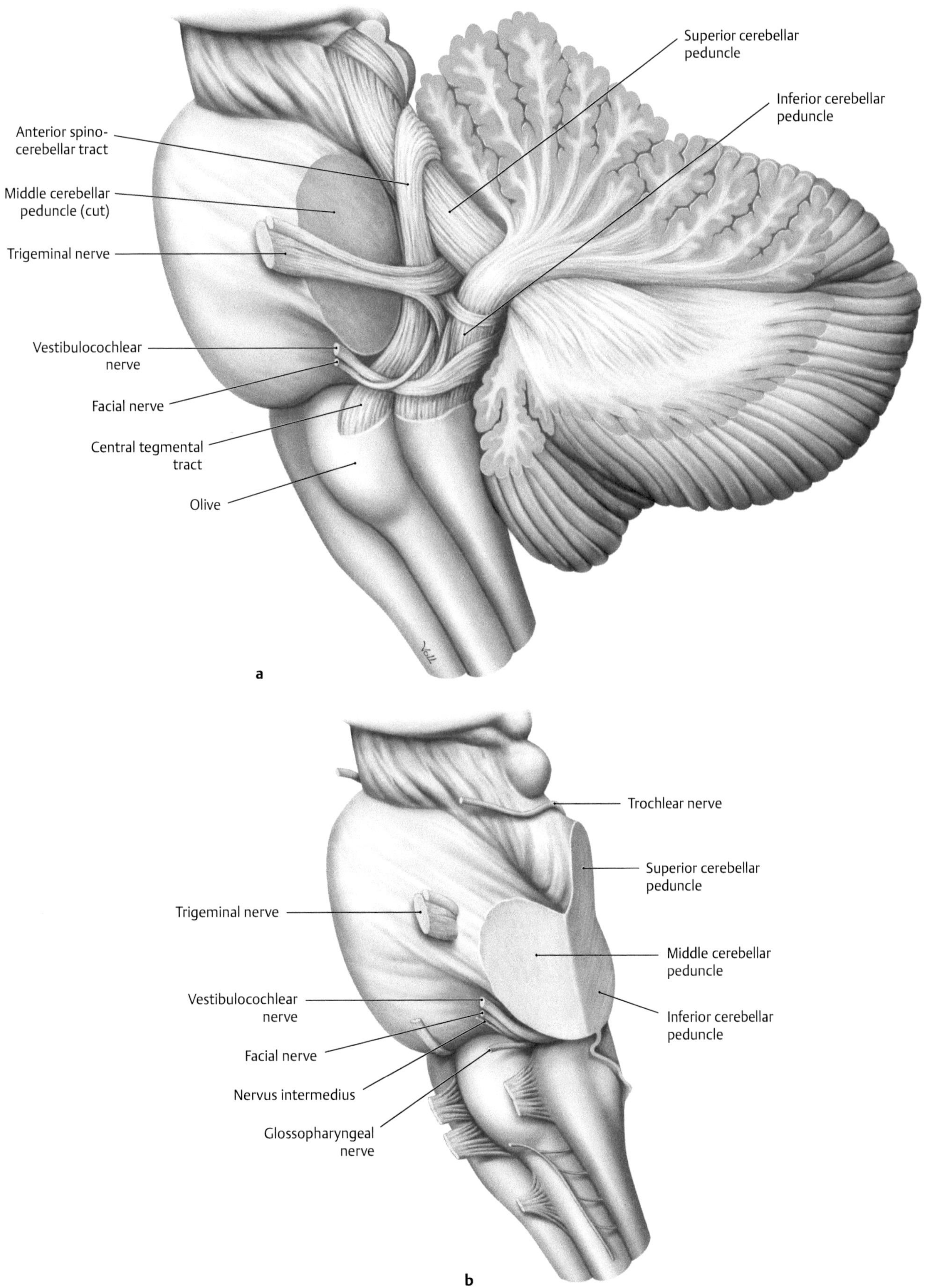

Fig. 9.26 Cerebellar peduncles. **(a)** Left lateral view with the upper portion of the cerebellum and lateral portions of the pons removed. **(b)** Left lateral view with the cerebellum detached and demonstrating the surface of the peduncles. (From Schuenke M, Schulte E, Schumacher U. THIEME Atlas of Anatomy. Head, Neck, and Neuroanatomy. Illustrations by Voll M and Wesker K. 3rd ed. New York: Thieme Medical Publishers; 2020.)

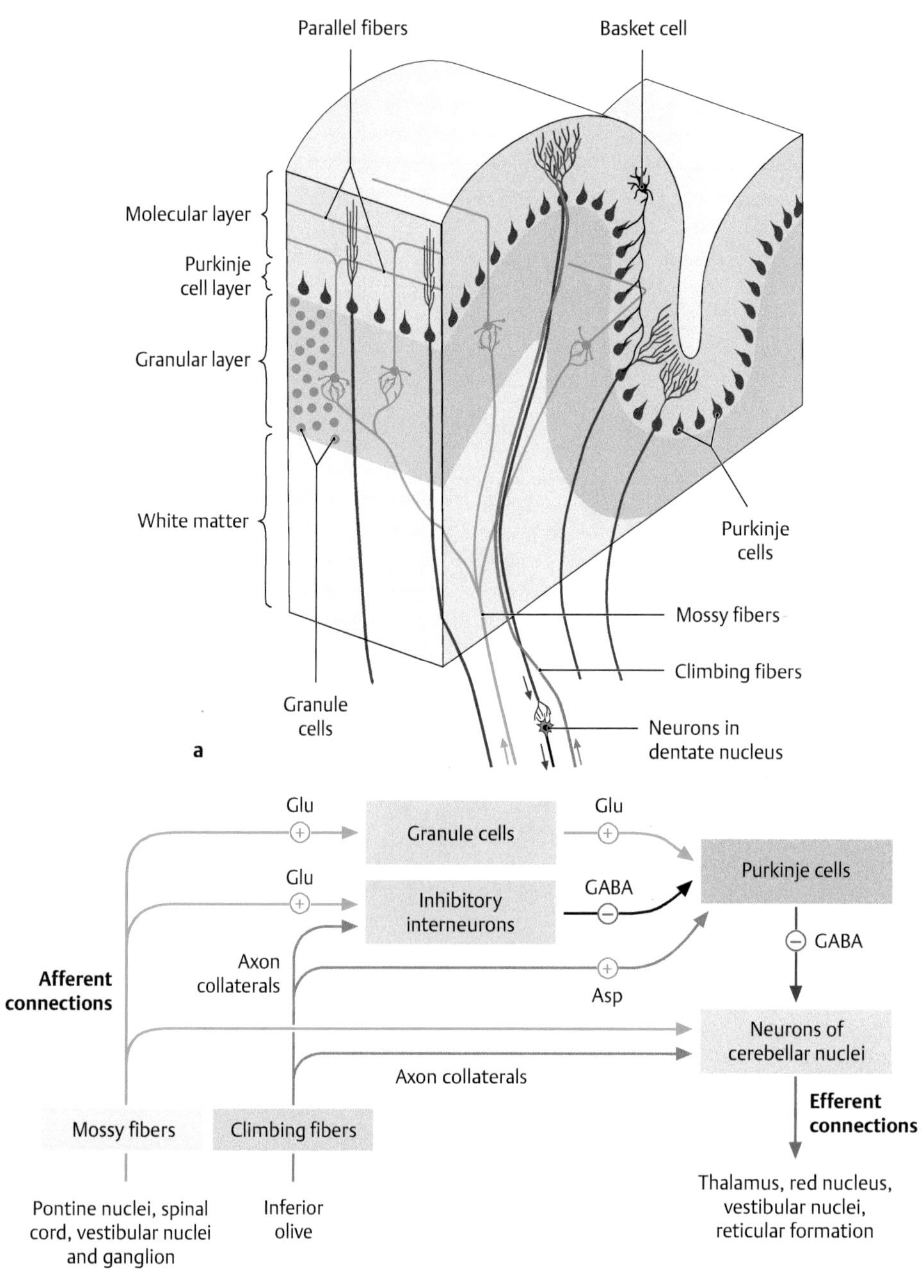

Fig. 9.27 (a) Cerebellar cortex. **(b)** Synaptic circuitry of the cerebellum. (From Schuenke M, Schulte E, Schumacher U. THIEME Atlas of Anatomy. Head, Neck, and Neuroanatomy. Illustrations by Voll M and Wesker K. 3rd ed. New York: Thieme Medical Publishers; 2020.)

via the superior cerebellar peduncles to the reticular formation in the brainstem in order to influence the reticulospinal tracts that are important in mediating posture and autonomic functions.

- **Globose** and **emboliform nuclei**: together these two nuclei are known as the **interposed nuclei**. They are the chief output nuclei for the spinocerebellum. These nuclei extend through the superior cerebellar peduncles to the contralateral red nucleus (magnocellular part) and to the contralateral ventral lateral nucleus of the thalamus. Projections to the red nucleus are related to the rubrospinal tract, while the projections through the ventral lateral nuclei of the thalamus are associated with the corticospinal tract. Both of these tracts are important in the innervation of distal musculature.
- **Dentate nuclei**: the only output nucleus for the neocerebellum. These nuclei extend through the superior cerebellar peduncles to the contralateral ventral lateral nuclei of the thalamus before continuing to the motor cortex areas. The dentate nuclei also project to the contralateral red nucleus (parvocellular part) and from here the fibers can extend to the ipsilateral inferior olivary nucleus via the central tegmental tract or to the ventral lateral nucleus of the thalamus.

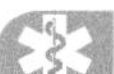

Clinical Correlate 9.12

Ataxia

Ataxia can be described as a lack of muscle control or coordination of voluntary movements. This lack of muscle coordination can affect activities such as walking, eye movements, swallowing, and speech. Cerebellar lesions are known to create **asynergy** or the loss of coordination. **Dysmetria** is a type of ataxia that involves overshooting (hypermetria) or undershooting (hypometria) the intended position of the hand or leg for example. **Dysdiadochokinesia** is the inability to make rapid and alternating rotational movements. It may be caused by the inability to switch on and off antagonizing muscle groups in a coordinated fashion due to poor muscle tone (hypotonia). If an individual voluntarily attempts to move their limb and displays a tremor, this is called an intention tremor and is common among individuals with multiple sclerosis. These disorders are most frequently the result of lesions affecting the cerebellar hemispheres.

Gait ataxia presents with an individual walking with a very wide and slow gait and they have a tendency to fall toward the side of the lesion. The lesion is generally located in the flocculonodular lobe or the vermal regions of the anterior or posterior lobes. Feedback circuits are disrupted and these include the vestibulocerebellum and/or spinocerebellum and their connections to the fastigial nucleus along with its own output to the vestibular nuclei, reticular formation, and eventually the spinal cord.

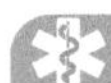

Clinical Correlate 9.13

Hypotonia

Low muscle tone or **hypotonia** is generally associated with damage to the cerebellar cortex. Hypotonia is a resistance to passive movement whereas muscle weakness is the result of impaired active movement. It is not a specific medical disorder but more of a manifestation of different diseases. Lesions may involve the paravermal region or posterior lobe. It may manifest due to a disruption of afferent information from stretch receptors and/or a loss of excitatory output to the spinal cord motor neurons.

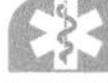

Clinical Correlate 9.14

Cerebellar Nystagmus

A **cerebellar nystagmus** may be the result of a lesion targeting the fastigial nucleus or vermal region of the cerebellar cortex. The disruption of inputs into the MLF from the vestibular nuclei seems to be a likely result of the lesion.

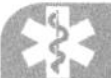

Clinical Correlate 9.15

Anterior Vermis Syndrome

Chronic alcohol abuse can affect the lower limb region of the anterior lobe of the cerebellum and lead to atrophy of the rostral vermis. This is called **anterior vermis syndrome** and it results in the **dystaxia** or lack of muscle coordination with the trunk and leg muscles and the individual would present with an unsteady gait.

Clinical Correlate 9.16

Posterior Vermis Syndrome

Posterior vermis syndrome is generally caused by a medulloblastoma or ependymoma located in the cerebellum of young children. It involves the flocculonodular lobe and results in truncal dystaxia.

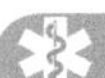

Clinical Correlate 9.17

Cerebellar Hemispheric Syndrome

Cerebellar hemispheric syndrome usually involves only one cerebellar hemisphere and is the result of a brain tumor or abscess. It produces dystaxia of the ipsilateral upper limb, lower limb, and trunk musculature and leads to an unstable gait.

Clinical Correlate 9.18

Functional Anatomy and Lesions of the Cerebellum

See Fig. 9.28.

(a) Simplified functional anatomy of the cerebellum Two-dimensional representation of the cerebellum. The left side illustrates the afferent information from the periphery, which the cerebellum involved in voluntary motor movement requires; and cerebellar functions divided based on the origin of its afferents (spinocerebellum, pontocerebellum, and vestibulocerebellum). The afferents are not segregated by externally visible anatomical boundaries. After the afferent information has been processed, the cerebellar cortex sends efferent impulses to the cerebellar nuclei, the eventual cerebellar efferents (shown on the right side).

- The fastigial nucleus and lateral vestibular nucleus coordinate the activity of skeletal muscles and thus movement via the medial descending systems (lateral vestibulospinal, reticulospinal, and tectospinal tracts); emboliform and globose nuclei via the lateral descending systems (lateral corticospinal and rubrospinal tracts).
- The dentate nucleus projects to the cerebral cortex and thus exerts influences on the planning and programming of movements.
- Efferents from the vestibulocerebellum control balance and oculomotor functions.
- Note: visual inputs have not been considered here.

(b) Synopsis of cerebellar classifications and their relationships to motor deficits.

(c-f) Cerebellar lesions. Cerebellar lesions may remain clinically silent for some time because other brain regions can functionally compensate for them with reasonable effectiveness. Exceptions are direct lesions of the efferent cerebellar nulcei, which cannot be clinically compensated.

9.7 Cerebrum

The forebrain or **cerebrum** is the structure that makes up any of the brain rostral to the midbrain. The structures of the forebrain include the diencephalon, basal ganglia, limbic system, internal capsule, anterior commissure, and cerebral cortex. The diencephalon includes the thalamus, hypothalamus, subthalamus, and epithalamus.

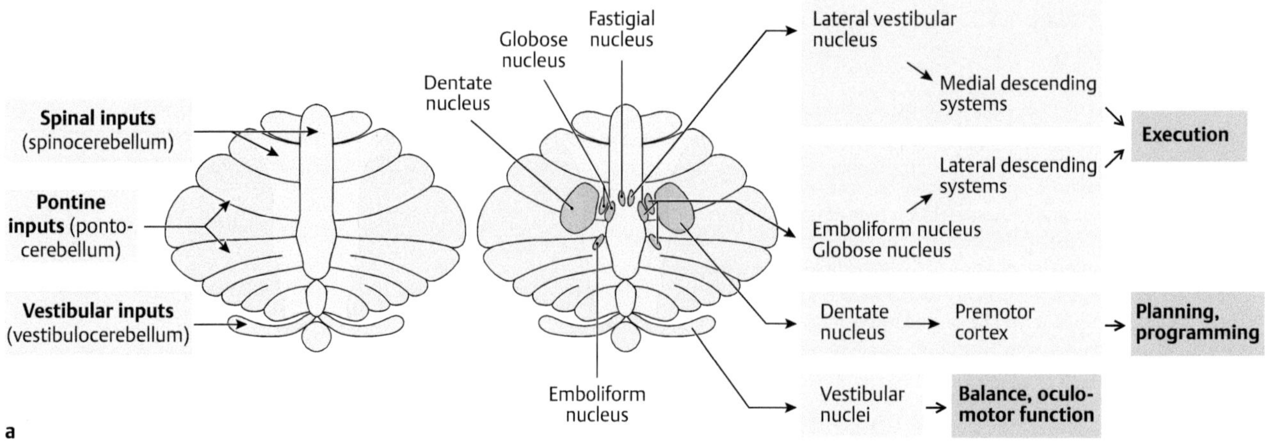

Functional classification	Anatomical classification	Deficit symptoms
• Vestibulocerebellum	• Flocculonodular lobe	• Truncal, stance, and gait ataxia • Vertigo • Nystagmus • Vomiting
• Spinocerebellum	• Anterior lobe, parts of vermis; Posterior lobe, medial parts	• Ataxia, chiefly affecting the lower limb • Oculomotor dysfunction • Speech disorder (asynergy of speech muscles)
• Pontocerebellum (= cerebrocerebellum)	• Posterior lobe, hemispheres	• Dysmetria and hypermetria (positive rebound) • Intention tremor • Nystagmus • Decreased muscle tone

b

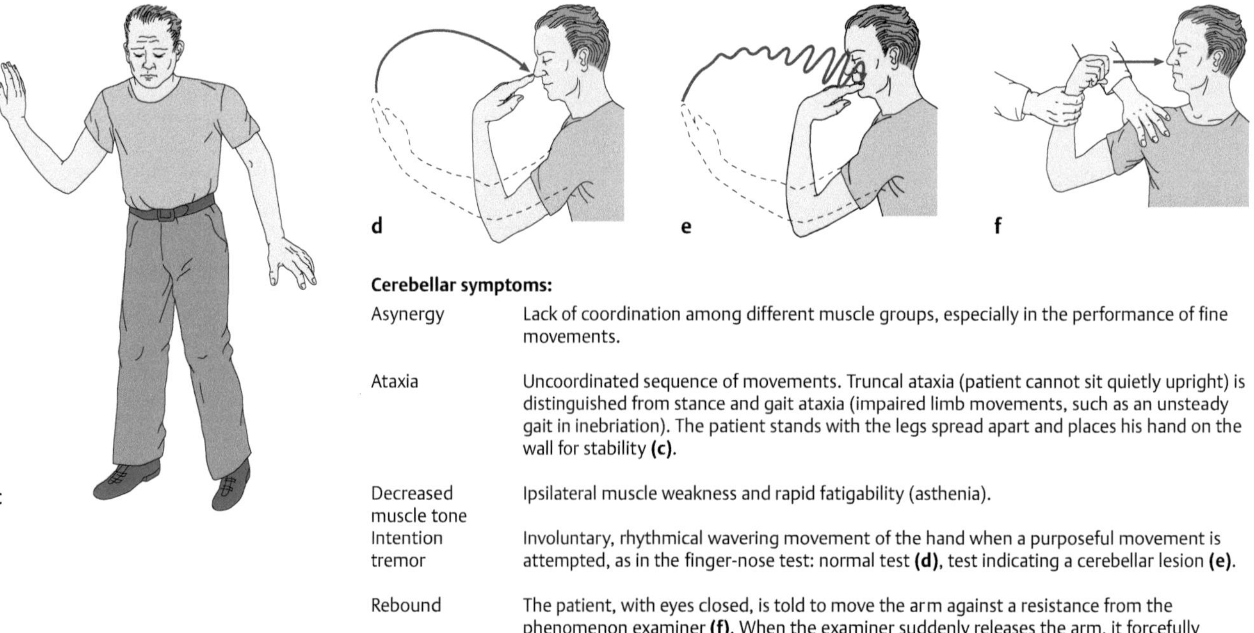

Cerebellar symptoms:

Asynergy	Lack of coordination among different muscle groups, especially in the performance of fine movements.
Ataxia	Uncoordinated sequence of movements. Truncal ataxia (patient cannot sit quietly upright) is distinguished from stance and gait ataxia (impaired limb movements, such as an unsteady gait in inebriation). The patient stands with the legs spread apart and places his hand on the wall for stability **(c)**.
Decreased muscle tone	Ipsilateral muscle weakness and rapid fatigability (asthenia).
Intention tremor	Involuntary, rhythmical wavering movement of the hand when a purposeful movement is attempted, as in the finger-nose test: normal test **(d)**, test indicating a cerebellar lesion **(e)**.
Rebound phenomenon	The patient, with eyes closed, is told to move the arm against a resistance from the examiner **(f)**. When the examiner suddenly releases the arm, it forcefully "rebounds" toward the patient (hypermetria).

Fig. 9.28 (a-f) Cerebellum, simplified functional anatomy and lesions. (From Schuenke M, Schulte E, Schumacher U. THIEME Atlas of Anatomy. Head, Neck, and Neuroanatomy. Illustrations by Voll M and Wesker K. 3rd ed. New York: Thieme Medical Publishers; 2020.)

9.8 Thalamus

The **thalamus** is located on the rostral end of the brainstem and serves as a relay and integration center for information passing to the cerebral cortex, brainstem, basal ganglia, and hypothalamus (**Fig. 9.29**).

Sensory information of all types concentrates on the thalamus and is integrated through interconnections between different thalamic nuclei. The sense of smell may first be integrated at lower levels, along with the sense of taste, before being relayed to the thalamus from the multiple nuclei of the amygdaloid complex and the hippocampus via the mammillothalamic tract. The thalamus and cerebral cortex are anatomically and functionally linked. If a portion of the cerebral cortex is surgically removed, the thalamus is able to still comprehend crude sensations due to the fiber connections between the two structures. The cerebral cortex, however, would be required to interpret these sensations based on past experiences. Neurons of the thalamus are 75 to 80% projection neurons while the rest are inhibitory interneurons.

The thalamus can be divided into specific and nonspecific nuclei. Specific nuclei and their fibers have direct connections with the cerebral cortex and nonspecific nuclei and their fibers do not. All thalamic nuclei are specific except for the intralaminar and central thalamic (midline) nuclei.

This egg-shaped “gatekeeper” is a mass of gray matter that is found bilaterally and forms the majority of the diencephalon. A band of gray matter called the **interthalamic adhesion** connects the two sides. The anterior end of the thalamus forms the posterior boundary of the interventricular foramen while the posterior end expands and forms the **pulvinar**. The medial surface contributes to the lateral wall of the third ventricle while the inferior surface is continuous with the midbrain tegmentum. A thin layer of white matter covers the superior and lateral surfaces of the thalamus. The superior surface is covered by the **stratum zonale** and the lateral surface by the **external medullary lamina**. A vertical sheet of white matter called the **internal medullary lamina**, which itself is a sheet of myelinated axons consisting of thalamic interconnections, divides the thalamus into three unequal parts or groups of nuclei. In addition, there are the surrounding reticular, intralaminar, and midline nuclei (**Fig. 9.30; Fig. 9.31; Fig. 9.32; Fig. 9.33**).

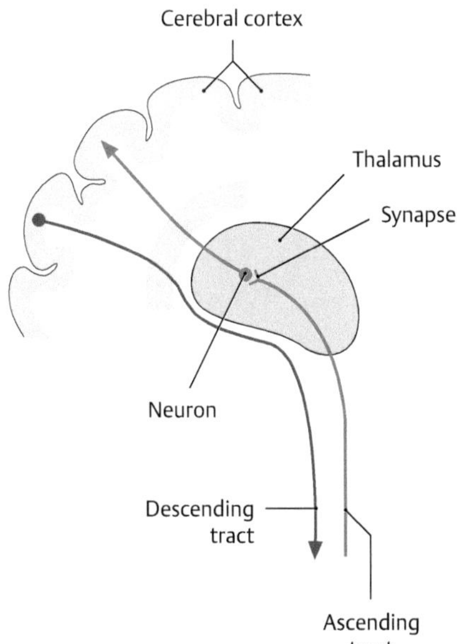

Fig. 9.29 Functional organization of the thalamus. (From Schuenke M, Schulte E, Schumacher U. THIEME Atlas of Anatomy. Head, Neck, and Neuroanatomy. Illustrations by Voll M and Wesker K. 3rd ed. New York: Thieme Medical Publishers; 2020.)

- **Anterior group**: represented only by the **anterior nucleus**. This nucleus receives input from the mammillary bodies (via the mammillothalamic tract) and the hippocampus (via the fornix). It projects to the cingulate gyrus and is part of the *Papez circuit* of the limbic system related to emotion and memory formation (**Fig. 9.30a, b; Fig. 9.31**).
- **Medial group**: represented only by the **dorsomedial** (or **mediodorsal) nucleus** (DM). This nucleus has a reciprocal connection with the prefrontal cortex; a region involved in abstract thinking, long-term goal-directed behavior, and it is also related to emotions and memory formation. There are numerous connections with the intralaminar nuclei. Principal input originates from the amygdala, basal ganglia, olfactory, and entorhinal cortices (**Fig. 9.30a; Fig. 9.32**).
- **Lateral group**: this group of nuclei is broken up into a dorsal or ventral tier.
  - **Dorsal tier**: nuclei related to association areas of the cerebral cortex (**Fig. 9.30a; Fig. 9.32**).
    - **Lateral dorsal nucleus**: considered a caudal extension of the anterior nuclei group. It is functionally related to the anterior nucleus. It has reciprocal connections with the limbic system. It receives input via the mammillothalamic tract and projects to the cingulate and parietal cortices. It plays a role in memory consolidation, motivation, and attention to a specific stimulus.
    - **Lateral posterior nucleus**: has reciprocal connections with areas 5 and 7 of the superior parietal lobule. It is functionally related to the pulvinar.
    - **Pulvinar**: the largest thalamic nucleus. The pulvinar has reciprocal connections with the visual and auditory association cortices, frontal, parietal, temporal, and occipital lobe areas. It receives input from the superior colliculus, lateral geniculate, and medial geniculate bodies and is concerned primarily with the integration of visual, auditory, and somatosensory input.
  - **Ventral tier** (**Fig. 9.30a, c; Fig. 9.33**)
    - **Ventral anterior nucleus**: receives input from the globus pallidus and substantia nigra. It projects to the premotor cortex (area 6) and diffusely to both the prefrontal and orbital cortices. It functions during movements by providing feedback for the outputs of the basal ganglia.
    - **Ventral lateral nucleus**: receives input from the globus pallidus, substantia nigra, and the dentate nucleus of the cerebellum. It projects to the primary motor cortex (area 4) and the supplementary motor cortex (area 6). It functions in coordination and planning of movements. The VA and VL form the motor relay nuclei of the thalamus.
    - **Ventral posterior nucleus**: divided into three parts and serves as a portion of the sensory relay nuclei of the thalamus. This larger nucleus is responsible for receiving general sensory (i.e., pain and temperature) and special visceral (taste) information.
      - **Ventral posterolateral nucleus**: receives input from the posterior column-medial lemniscus (PCML) and

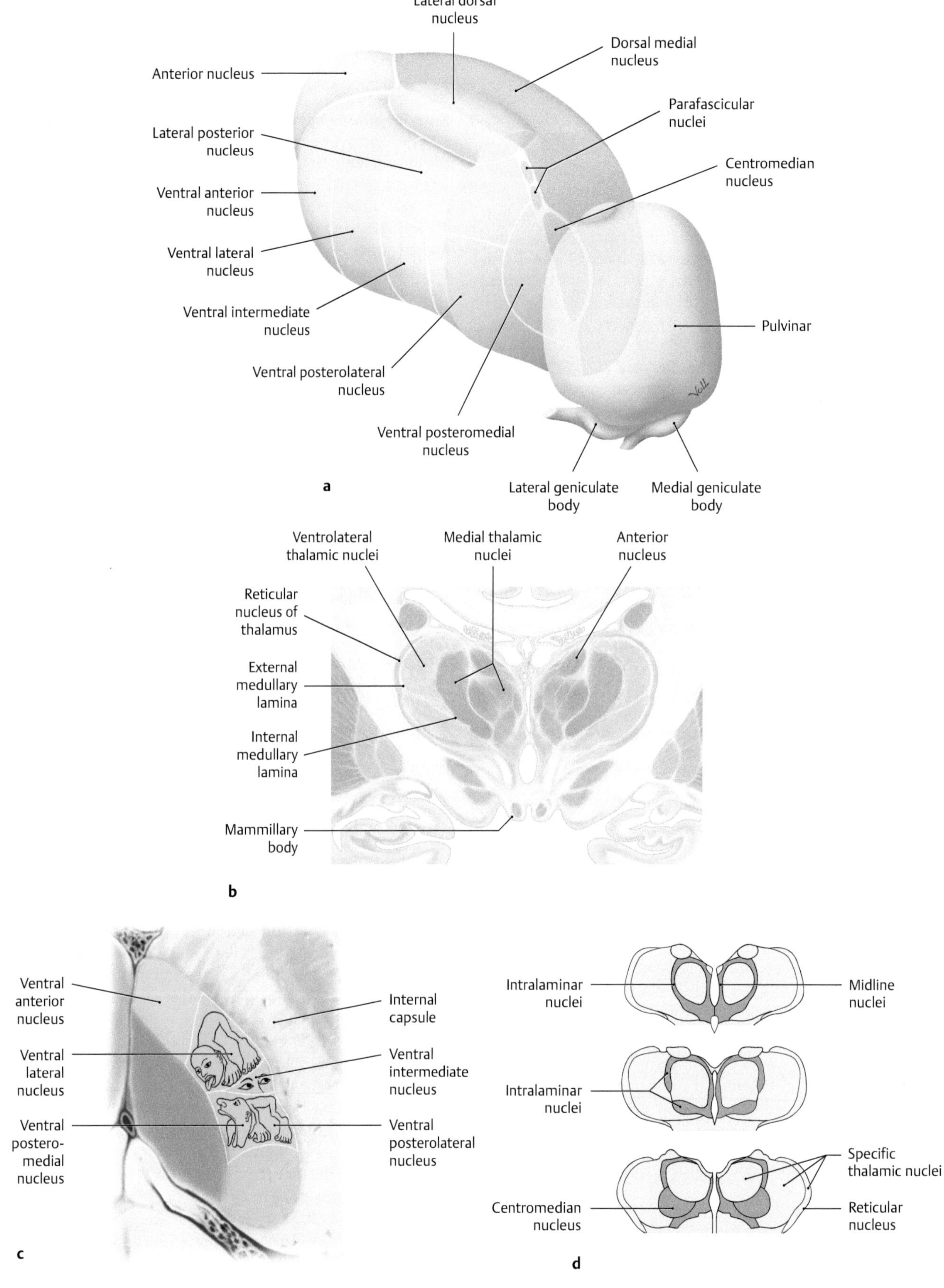

Fig. 9.30 **(a)** Spatial arrangement of the thalamic nuclei. **(b)** Division of the thalamic nuclei by the medullary laminae. **(c)** Somatotopic organization of specific thalamic nuclei. **(d)** Nonspecific thalamic nuclei. (From Schuenke M, Schulte E, Schumacher U. THIEME Atlas of Anatomy. Head, Neck, and Neuroanatomy. Illustrations by Voll M and Wesker K. 3rd ed. New York: Thieme Medical Publishers; 2020.)

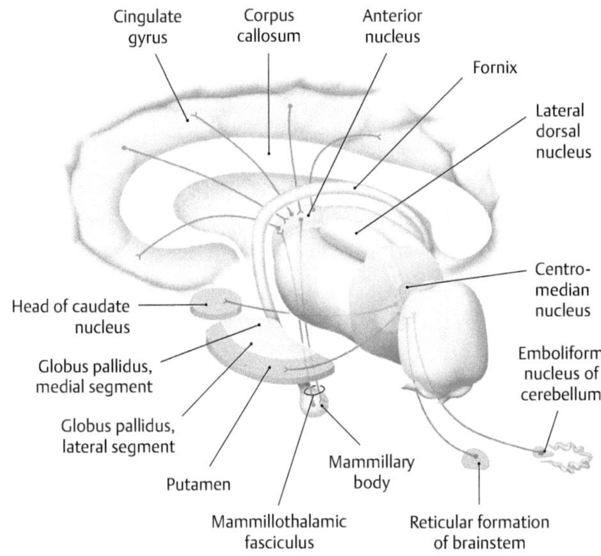

Fig. 9.31 Anterior nucleus and centromedian nucleus: afferent and efferent connections. (From Schuenke M, Schulte E, Schumacher U. THIEME Atlas of Anatomy. Head, Neck, and Neuroanatomy. Illustrations by Voll M and Wesker K. 3rd ed. New York: Thieme Medical Publishers; 2020.)

anterolateral system (ALS) pathways. It projects to the primary somatosensory cortex (areas 3, 1, and 2). Lesions result in the contralateral loss of pain and temperature sensation and tactile discrimination of the trunk and extremities.

- **Ventral posteromedial nucleus**: receives input from both trigeminothalamic tracts along with taste information from the solitary nucleus and the parabrachial nucleus located near the border of the pons and midbrain. It projects to the primary somatosensory cortex (areas 3, 1, and 2). Lesions result in the contralateral loss of pain and temperature sensation and tactile discrimination in the head region along with the ipsilateral loss of taste.
- **Ventral intermediate (posteroinferior) nucleus**: receives input from the vestibular nuclei related to the coordination of gaze toward the ipsilateral side. It projects to the ill-defined vestibular regions of the cortex near the temporoparietal junction and posterior insula.

- **Lateral geniculate body**: receives retinal input from both eyes by way of the optic tract. It projects to the primary visual cortex (area 17) and association cortices (areas 18 and 19) in the occipital lobe by way of the optic radiation (**Fig. 9.30a; Fig. 9.32**).

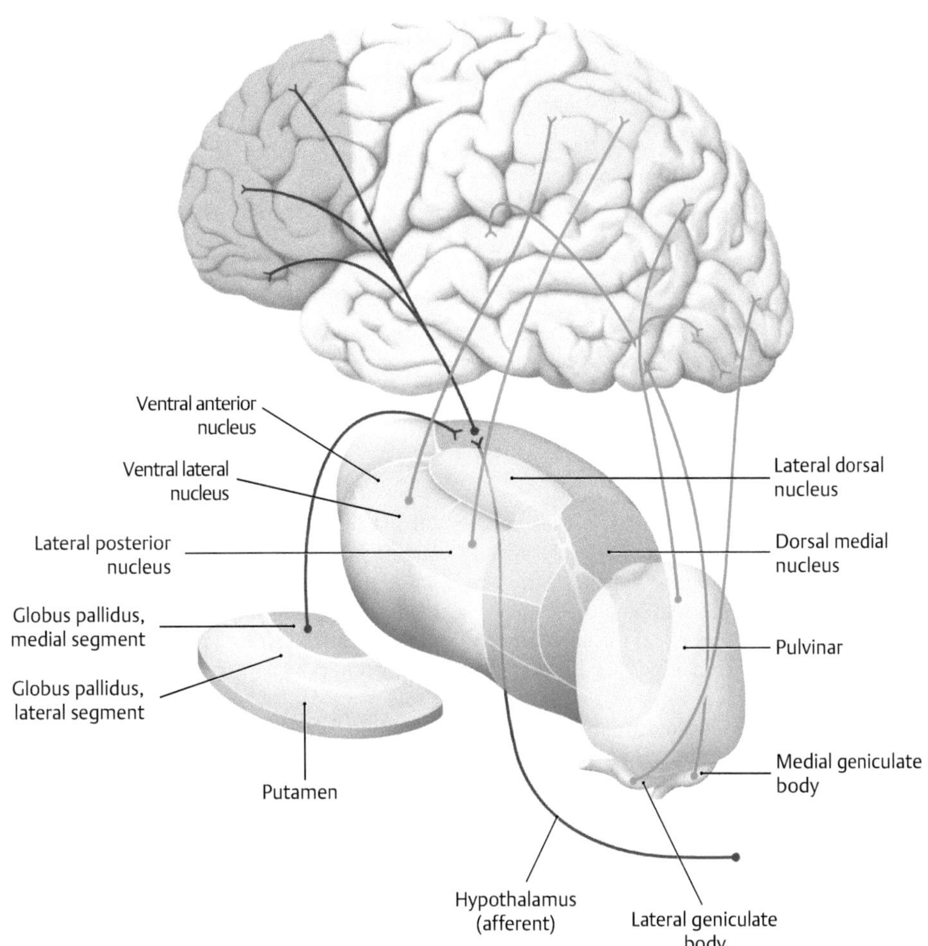

Fig. 9.32 Medial, posterior, and lateral thalamic nuclei: afferent and efferent connections. (From Schuenke M, Schulte E, Schumacher U. THIEME Atlas of Anatomy. Head, Neck, and Neuroanatomy. Illustrations by Voll M and Wesker K. 3rd ed. New York: Thieme Medical Publishers; 2020.)

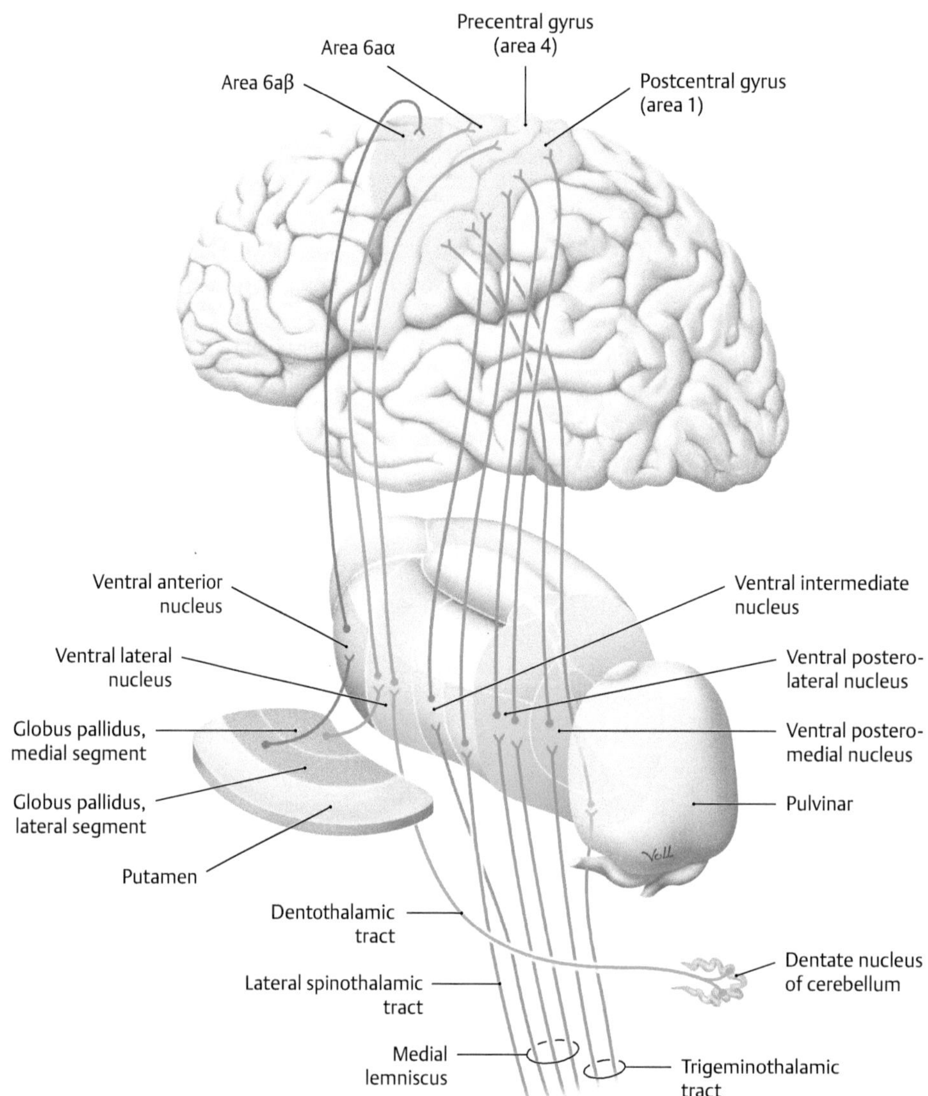

Fig. 9.33 Ventrolateral thalamic nuclei: afferent and efferent connections. (From Schuenke M, Schulte E, Schumacher U. THIEME Atlas of Anatomy. Head, Neck, and Neuroanatomy. Illustrations by Voll M and Wesker K. 3rd ed. New York: Thieme Medical Publishers; 2020.)

- **Medial geniculate body**: receives auditory input from the inferior colliculus via the inferior brachium. This auditory information comes from both ears but mostly from the opposite ear. From the medial geniculate body, the information projects to the primary auditory cortex (areas 41 and 42) of the superior temporal gyrus by way of the auditory radiation (**Fig. 9.30a; Fig. 9.32**).
- **Reticular nucleus**: shaped like a shield located around the anterior and lateral aspects of the thalamus, and separated by the external medullary lamina. Connections between the thalamus and cortex are reciprocal. These thalamocortical and corticothalamic projections send collateral branches to the reticular nucleus and in turn they project back to the exact location of the thalamus the input originated from. This nucleus plays a large role in selective attention and possibly in consciousness because it controls access to the cortex. It is the source of the electrical impulses recorded in an electroencephalogram (EEG) (**Fig. 9.30b, d**).
- **Intralaminar nuclei**: considered nonspecific thalamic nuclei and lie within the internal medullary lamina. They receive input from the reticular formation, spinothalamic and trigeminothalamic tracts, and other thalamic nuclei. They can project to the corpus striatum or indirectly to the cerebral cortex by way of other thalamic nuclei. The intralaminar nuclei may play a role in arousal and goal-orientated behaviors. There are two main nuclei (**Fig. 9.30a, b, d; Fig. 9.31**):
  - **Centromedian nucleus**: receives input from the globus pallidus and projects to the corpus striatum and diffusely to the cerebral cortex. It is reciprocally connected to the primary motor cortex (area 4).
  - **Parafascicular nucleus**: projects to the premotor cortex (area 6) and the corpus striatum.
- **Midline nuclei**: the **central thalamic (midline) nuclei** are small groups of cells adjacent to the wall of the third ventricle and are considered nonspecific thalamic nuclei much like the intralaminar nuclei. These nuclei are not fully understood but

they do receive afferent fibers from the reticular formation (**Fig. 9.30d**).

9.8.1 Blood Supply to the Thalamus

The chief blood supply to the thalamus is by way of the small end-arteries called the **posterior choroidal** and **posterior thalamoperforating arteries** that originate from the **posterior cerebral arteries.** Additional blood comes from the **anterior thalamoperforating arteries** that originate from the **posterior communicating arteries.** The **anterior choroidal artery** supplies the lateral geniculate body.

9.9 Hypothalamus

The hypothalamus is located just below the thalamus and anatomically is part of the diencephalon but functionally it is part of the limbic system. It is the main visceral control center of the body, regulating many activities of the visceral organs. It helps form the inferolateral walls of the third ventricle and projects inferiorly as the pituitary gland. It has multiple nuclei that have multiple functions:

- To control emotional responses, motivational behaviors, the autonomic nervous system, and the endocrine system through the pituitary gland.
- To form memories.
- To regulate body temperature, the sleep–wake cycle, sensations of hunger and thirst.

The functional zones or regions of the hypothalamic nuclei are divided along a lateral/medial axis and an anterior/posterior axis. The connection between the columns of the fornix and mammillary bodies divides the hypothalamus into either a lateral or medial zone. The **lateral zone** is made up of scattered or diffuse neurons distributed among major fiber bundles. The **medial zone** consists of the bulk of functionally important hypothalamic nuclei. There are three functional regions that pass along the anterior-to-posterior axis. The **anterior region** lies above the optic chiasm and contains the preoptic, suprachiasmatic, paraventricular, anterior and supraoptic nuclei. The **middle/tuberal region** includes the dorsomedial, ventromedial, and arcuate (infundibular) nuclei. The **posterior region** is located at the level of the mammillary bodies, which along with the posterior nucleus make up the nuclei of this region.

- **Lateral zone nuclei:** promotes eating and digestive functions, and wakefulness, and reduces pain perception. Lesions of this zone may lead to eating disorders such as anorexia, motility disorders, and narcolepsy (**Fig. 9.34**).
- Anterior region (**Fig. 9.34**):
  - **Preoptic nuclei**: there are up to four different specific preoptic nuclei (median, medial, ventrolateral/intermediate, and periventricular), and they function in thermoregulation, generating thirst, regulating the release of gonadotropic hormones from the adenophysis, and mediating the onset of non-REM sleep. The medial preoptic nucleus is sexually dimorphic.
  - **Suprachiasmatic nucleus**: plays a role in circadian rhythm and receives direct input from the retina.
  - **Paraventricular nucleus**: regulates water balance and releases oxytocin, antidiuretic hormone (ADH), and corticotropin-releasing hormone (CRH). A lesion here could lead to *diabetes insipidus*.
  - **Anterior nucleus**: stimulates the parasympathetic nervous system and plays a role in temperature regulation. A lesion here could lead to hyperthermia.
  - **Supraoptic nucleus**: releases ADH and oxytocin.

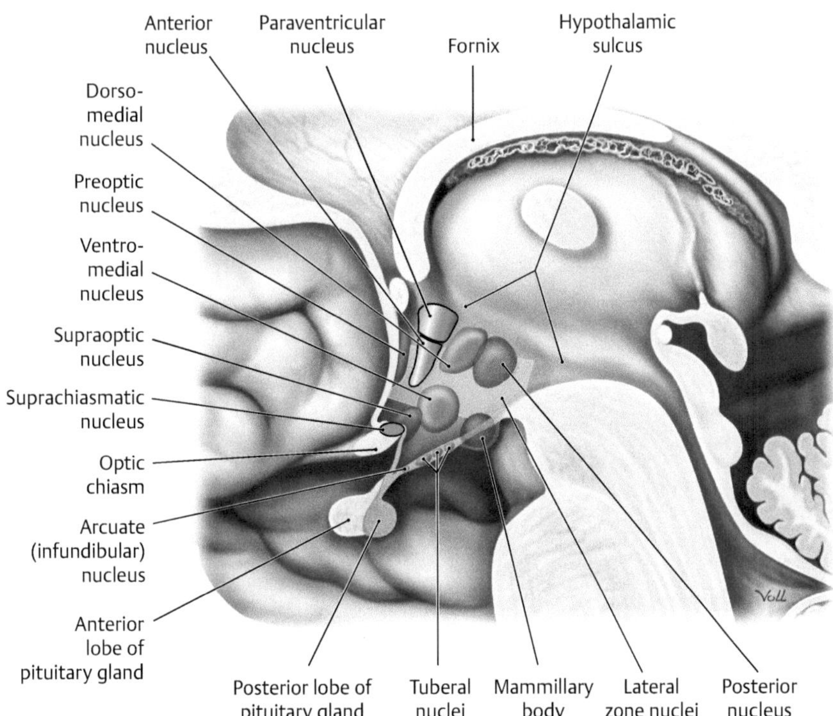

Fig. 9.34 Nuclei of the hypothalamus: midsagittal section of the right hemisphere viewed from the medial side. (From Schuenke M, Schulte E, Schumacher U. THIEME Atlas of Anatomy. Head, Neck, and Neuroanatomy. Illustrations by Voll M and Wesker K. 3rd ed. New York: Thieme Medical Publishers; 2020.)

- Middle/tuberal region (**Fig. 9.34**):
  - **Dorsomedial nucleus**: plays a role in drinking, body weight and feeding, emotional behavior, and the circadian rhythm.
  - **Ventromedial nucleus**: serves as the satiety center and when stimulated it inhibits drinking and eating.
  - **Arcuate (infundibular) nucleus**: contains neurons that control the endocrine functions of the adenohypophysis and produces hypothalamic releasing factors that enter the hypophyseal portal system.
- Posterior region:
  - **Posterior nucleus**: stimulates the sympathetic nervous system and plays a role in both thermoregulation and arousal or wakefulness.
  - **Mammillary bodies**: made up of lateral and medial mammillary nuclei that receive information from the hippocampus via the fornix and function in consolidation of memories.

9.9.1 Afferent and Efferent Connections of the Hypothalamus

In order to maintain homeostasis, the hypothalamus has multiple afferent and efferent connections or tracts that act on the autonomic nervous system, and endocrine and limbic systems. Most of these tracts are reciprocal, with the majority of information passing through the medial forebrain bundle and the dorsal longitudinal fasciculus. The **medial forebrain bundle** passes through the lateral hypothalamus and connects it to the forebrain, reticular formation of the midbrain, and rostral pons. The **dorsal longitudinal fasciculus** also connects the hypothalamus with the reticular formation through the caudal medulla.

- The **afferent connections** include (Note: not all pathways are shown) (**Fig. 9.35**):
  - From the primary olfactory cortex to the preoptic nuclei via the medial forebrain bundle.
  - From the amygdala via the stria terminalis and ventral amygdalofugal pathway.
  - From the hippocampus via the fornix.
  - From erogenous zones to the mammillary bodies via the peduncle of the mammillary body.
  - From the frontal lobe to the lateral nuclei via the corticohypothalamic tract.
  - From the retina to the suprachiasmatic nucleus via the retinohypothalamic tract.
  - From the dorsomedial nucleus of the thalamus and to mostly the lateral nuclei via the thalamohypothalamic tract (or inferior thalamic peduncle).
  - General somatic, visceral, and gustatory information passing through the spinal cord or brainstem can reach the hypothalamus through collateral branches of the anterolateral system, medial lemniscus, or solitary tract by way of the reticular formation.
- The **efferent connections** include (Note: not all pathways are shown) (**Fig. 9.36**):
  - To the neurohypophysis from the paraventricular and supraoptic nuclei via the hypothalamic-hypophyseal (supraoticohypophyseal) tract (**Fig. 9.37**).
  - To the adenohypophysis and hypophyseal portal system from the arcuate nucleus via the tuberohypophyseal tract.
  - To the tegmentum of the midbrain from the mammillary bodies via the mammilotegmental tract.
  - To the anterior thalamic nucleus from the mammillary bodies via the mammilothalamic tract/fasciculus.
  - To the dorsomedial nucleus of the thalamus from the lateral zone nuclei via the inferior thalamic peduncle.
  - To the septal area of the frontal lobe via the medial forebrain bundle.
  - To the amygdala via the stria terminalis and ventral amygdalofugal pathway.
  - To the parasympathetic brainstem nuclei and spinal cord via the medial forebrain bundle and dorsal longitudinal fasciculus.

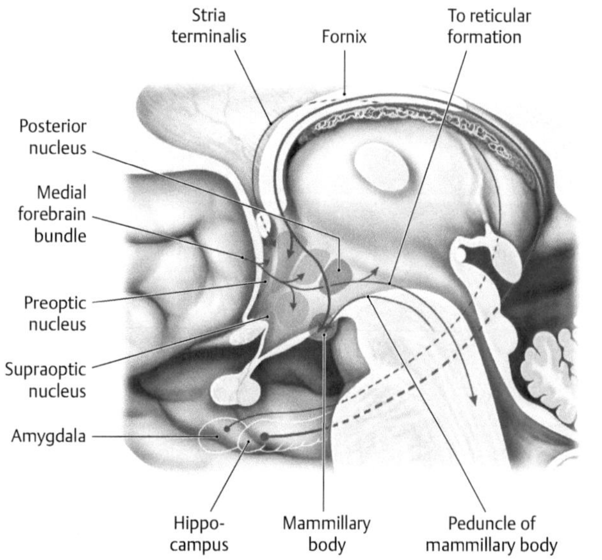

Fig. 9.35 Afferent connections to the hypothalamus. (From Schuenke M, Schulte E, Schumacher U. THIEME Atlas of Anatomy. Head, Neck, and Neuroanatomy. Illustrations by Voll M and Wesker K. 3rd ed. New York: Thieme Medical Publishers; 2020.)

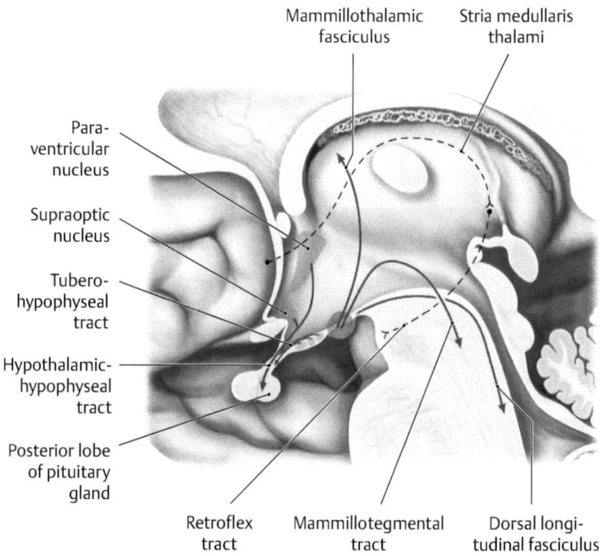

Fig. 9.36 Efferent connections to the hypothalamus. (From Schuenke M, Schulte E, Schumacher U. THIEME Atlas of Anatomy. Head, Neck, and Neuroanatomy. Illustrations by Voll M and Wesker K. 3rd ed. New York: Thieme Medical Publishers; 2020.)

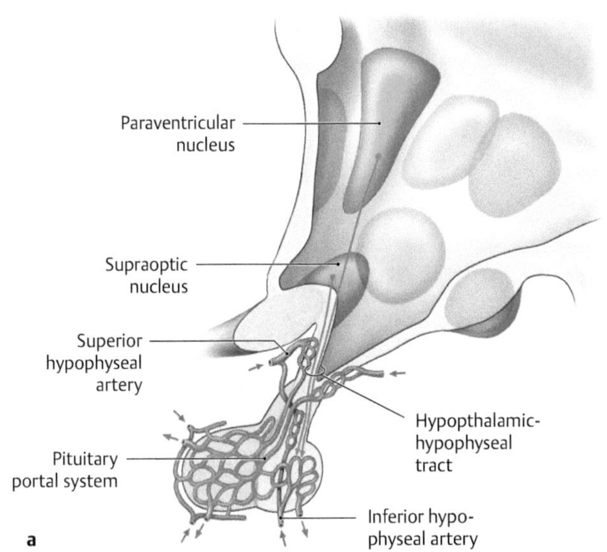

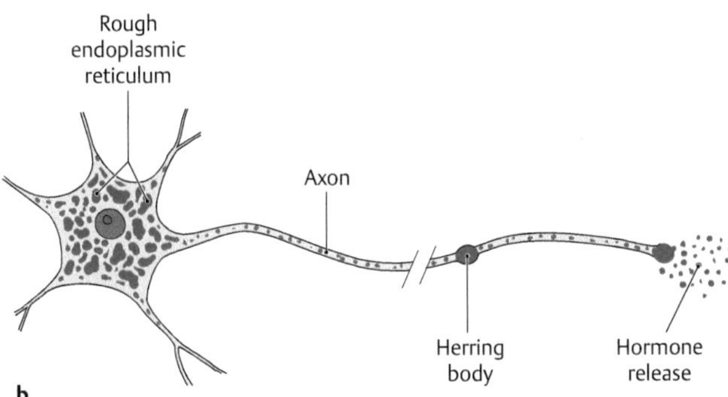

Fig. 9.37 **(a)** Connections of the hypothalamic nuclei to the posterior lobe of the pituitary gland. **(b)** Neurosecretory neuron in the hypothalamic nucleus. (From Schuenke M, Schulte E, Schumacher U. THIEME Atlas of Anatomy. Head, Neck, and Neuroanatomy. Illustrations by Voll M and Wesker K. 3rd ed. New York: Thieme Medical Publishers; 2020.)

9.10 Pituitary Gland

The **pituitary gland** (**Fig. 9.38**) is a small bean-shaped structure that lies in the hypophyseal fossa of the sphenoid bone. The gland is a coalition of secretory cells regulated by hypothalamic-releasing factors. It is made up of an anterior and posterior lobe. The **anterior lobe (adenohypophysis)** makes up about 80% of the pituitary gland and functions in both producing and secreting hormones. It originates from an evagination of oral ectoderm called ***Rathke pouch***. Remnants of *Rathke pouch* remain as colloid-filled cysts. The adenohypophysis is subdivided into the **pars tuberalis**, **pars distalis**, and **pars intermedia**.

The **posterior lobe (neurohypophysis)** makes up 20% of the pituitary gland and is the hormone-releasing part for hormones produced in the hypothalamus. It originates as an extension of neuroectoderm related to the diencephalon. The neurohypophysis is made up of the **pars nervosa** and **infundibulum** (or pituitary stalk) (**Fig. 9.38**).

9.10.1 Histology of Pituitary Gland

The adenohypophysis is arranged as cords and includes chromophobes (~50% of the cell population), acidophils (~40%), and basophils (~10%). **Chromophobes** may be actively secreting or precursor cells, thus having the appearance of a clear cytoplasm. **Acidophils** produce growth hormone (GH) or prolactin. **Basophils** produce follicle-stimulating hormone (FSH), luteinizing hormone (LH), thyroid-stimulating hormone (TSH), adrenocorticotrophic hormone (ACTH), and melanocyte-stimulating hormone (MSH) (**Fig. 9.39a, b**).

The pars nervosa of the neurohypophysis contains unmyelinated axons and axon terminals of secretory hypothalamic neurons, modified astrocytes called pituicytes, and neurosecretory granules called Herring bodies (**Fig. 9.39a, c**). **Pituicytes** assist in the storage and release of hormones in the neurohypophysis. **Herring bodies** store **oxytocin** and **antidiuretic hormone (ADH)** also known as *vasopressin*. Oxytocin and ADH are synthesized in the paraventricular and supraoptic nuclei of the hypothalamus, respectively, and migrate down into the Herring bodies by way of axoplasmic transport through the hypothalamic-hypophyseal

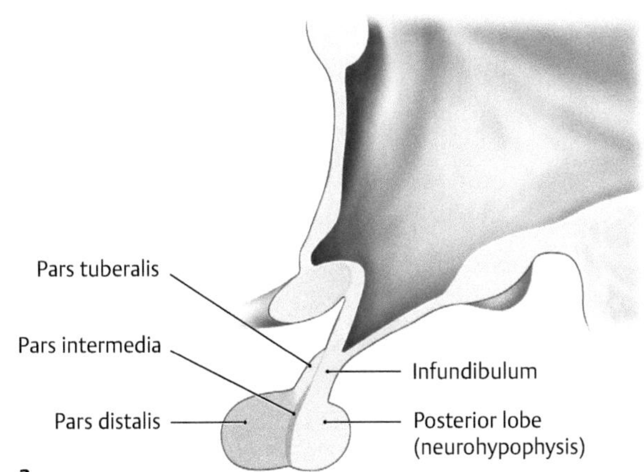

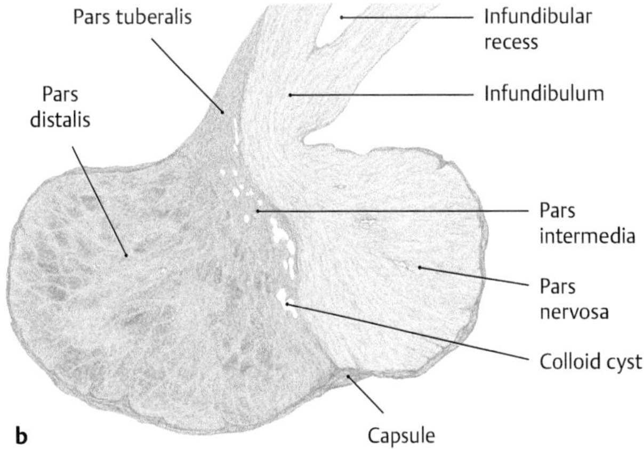

Fig. 9.38 Divisions of the pituitary gland, midsagittal sections. **(a)** Schematic representation. **(b)** Histological appearance. (From Schuenke M, Schulte E, Schumacher U. THIEME Atlas of Anatomy. Head, Neck, and Neuroanatomy. Illustrations by Voll M and Wesker K. 3rd ed. New York: Thieme Medical Publishers; 2020.)

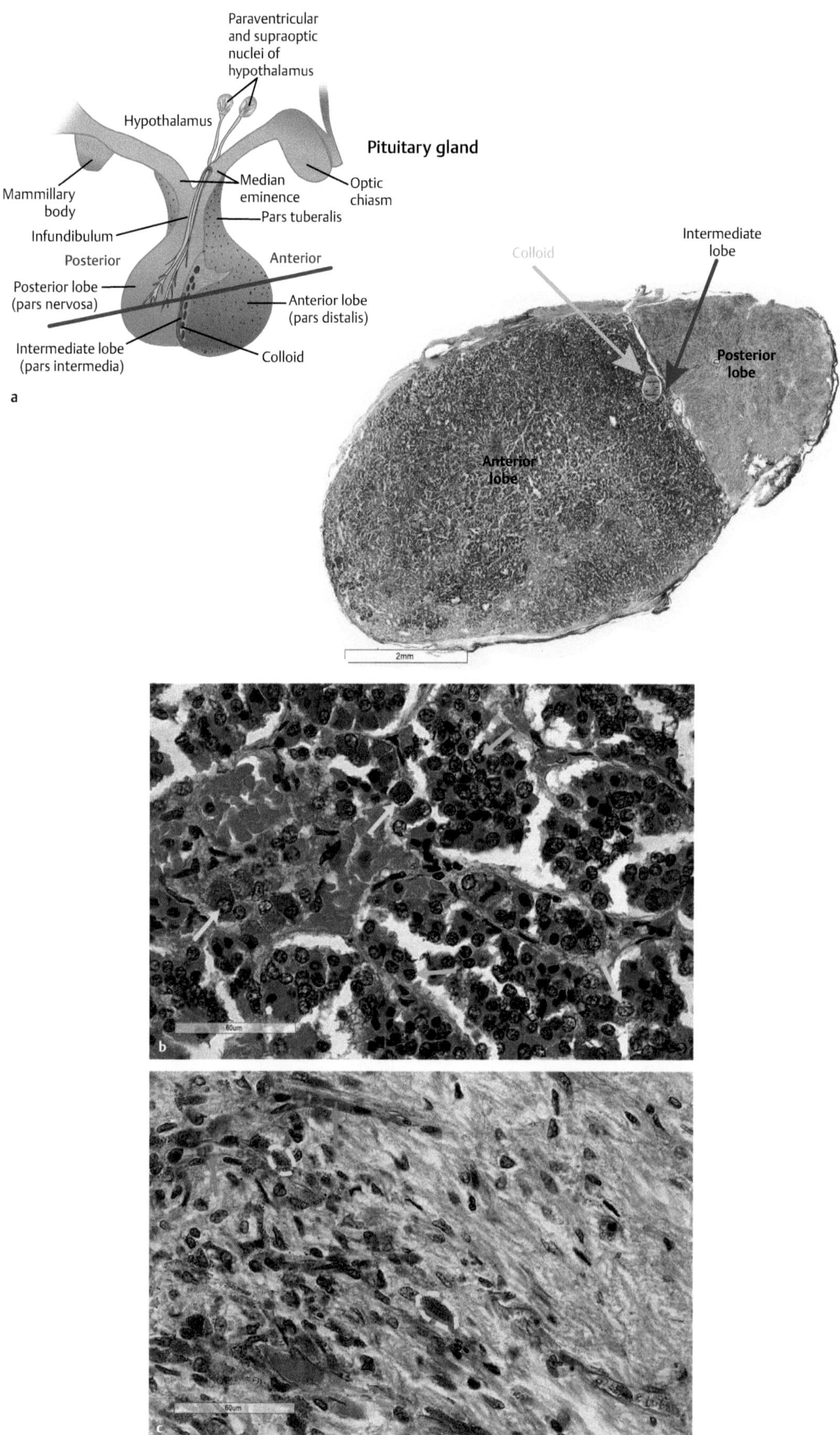

Fig. 9.39 Histology of the pituitary gland. **(a)** Scanning view of the pituitary gland with Mallory stain. Note that the anterior-posterior orientation of the histological section is reversed from the drawing. **(b)** Anterior lobe, high magnification, H&E stain, showing basophils (*yellow arrows*), acidophils (*blue arrows*), and chromophobes (*green arrows*). **(c)** Posterior lobe, PAS and orange G stain, showing synaptic termini (Herring bodies, outlined) and blood vessels (*blue arrows*). (From Lowrie DJ. Histology: An Essential Textbook. New York: Thieme Medical Publishers; 2020.)

Table 9.1 **Adenohypophysis and neurohypophysis hormones**

Hormone	Function
Growth hormone (GH)	Promotes body growth and protein synthesis
Prolactin	Promotes breast development during pregnancy and stimulates milk production and secretion in the breast tissue
Follicle-stimulating hormone (FSH)	Stimulates follicular development and estrogen in the ovaries; stimulates sperm maturation in the Sertoli cells of the testes
Luteinizing hormone (LH)	Stimulates ovulation, corpus luteum formation, progesterone and estrogen synthesis from the ovaries; stimulates Leydig cells in the testes to produce testosterone
Thyroid-stimulating hormone (TSH)	Promotes synthesis and secretion of thyroid gland hormones
Adrenocorticotropic hormone (ACTH)	Promotes synthesis and secretion of suprarenal cortical hormones such as cortisol, androgens, and aldosterone
Melanocyte-stimulating hormone (MSH)	Stimulates melanin synthesis
Oxytocin	Stimulates milk ejection from the breasts and contractions of the uterus
Antidiuretic hormone (ADH)	Stimulates water reabsorption in the collecting ducts of the kidneys

tract. The hormones are released from the Herring bodies upon neural stimulation (**Fig. 9.37b**). Hormones of the pituitary gland are listed in **Table 9.1**.

9.10.2 Hypophyseal Portal Circulation

The **superior hypophyseal arteries** (internal carotid artery br.) form a vascular plexus around the infundibulum. Axons from hypothalamic nuclei terminate at this plexus and secrete hormones that have been produced in smaller (parvocellular) neurons of the hypothalamus. These secreted hormones are of two types:

- Releasing factors that stimulate hormone release from cells of the adenohypophysis.
- Inhibiting factors that inhibit hormonal release from these cells.

The hormones are ushered by the **hypophyseal portal venous system** to capillaries located in the adenohypophysis. This establishes a communication between the hypothalamus and endocrine cells of the adenohypophysis (**Fig. 9.40**).

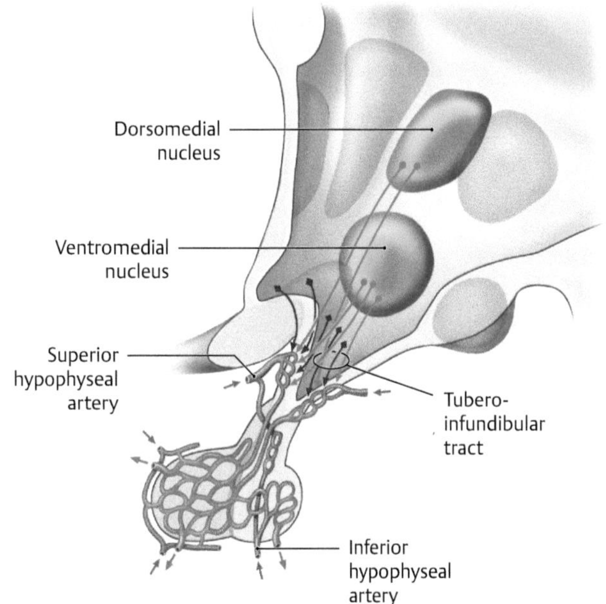

Fig. 9.40 Hypophyseal portal circulation and connections of the hypothalamic nuclei to the anterior pituitary gland. (From Schuenke M, Schulte E, Schumacher U. THIEME Atlas of Anatomy. Head, Neck, and Neuroanatomy. Illustrations by Voll M and Wesker K. 3rd ed. New York: Thieme Medical Publishers; 2020.)

9.11 Subthalamus

The **subthalamus** consists of several nuclei and fiber pathways that relate to motor functions associated with the basal ganglia. The **subthalamic nucleus** lies near the internal capsule and maintains complementary connections with the globus pallidus. The **zona incerta** is formed by thin bands of cells separating the lenticular fasciculus from the thalamic fasciculus but its function is unclear (**Fig. 9.41a,b**).

9.12 Epithalamus

The **epithalamus** (**Fig. 9.41a**) helps form the roof of the diencephalon and includes the habenular complex, stria medullaris, and pineal gland. There are two sets of lateral and medial nuclei that connect anatomically on each side by the **habenular commissure** (**Fig. 9.42a**). The **stria medullaris** contains largely habenular afferent fibers. It links the **habenular nuclei** to the anterior perforated substance, septal nuclei (medial olfactory area), and preoptic nuclei of the hypothalamus. Afferents from the amygdala reach the habenular nuclei via the **stria terminalis**. Efferent connections include the *habenulotectal*, *habenulotegmental*, and *habenulointerpeduncular tracts* (**Fig. 9.43**).

The **pineal gland** (**Fig. 9.42**) is a small cone-shaped structure attached to the roof of the posterior aspect of the third ventricle. It is covered by pia mater and receives inputs from the sympathetic nervous system via the superior cervical ganglia. It displays a circadian rhythm to light due to the release of several hormones. An indirect pathway may be involved in this and it is likely due to the

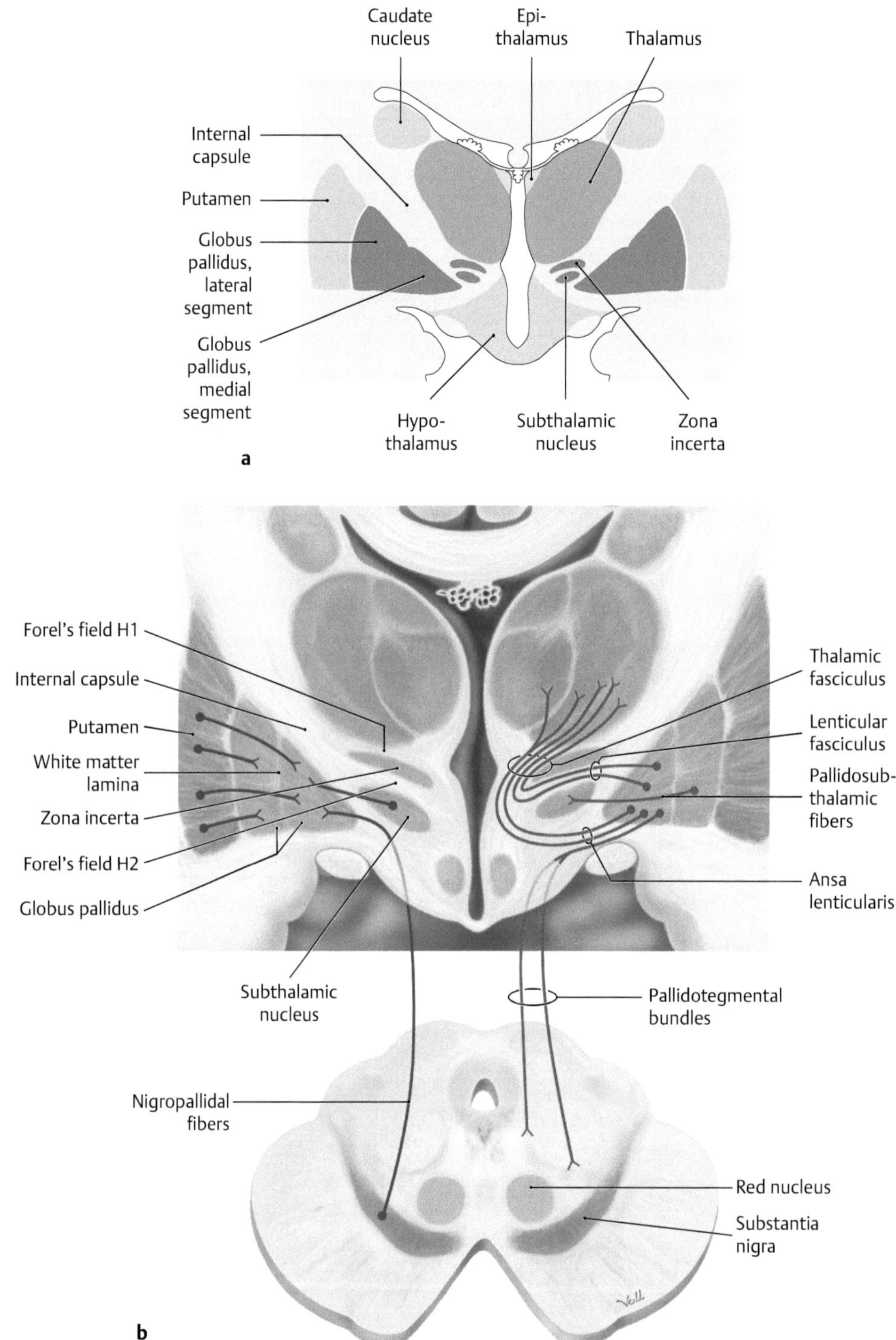

Fig. 9.41 (a) Location of the epithalamus and subthalamus. **(b)** Subthalamic nuclei with their afferent (*blue*) and efferent (*red*) connections. (From Schuenke M, Schulte E, Schumacher U. THIEME Atlas of Anatomy. Head, Neck, and Neuroanatomy. Illustrations by Voll M and Wesker K. 3rd ed. New York: Thieme Medical Publishers; 2020.)

light cycle information extending to the **suprachiasmatic nucleus** of the hypothalamus from the retina.

The pineal gland contains cells called **pinealocytes** (~95% of the gland) that are involved in the secretion of primarily *melatonin*, but also serotonin and norepinephrine. The pineal gland affects the CNS through hormones being released into the general circulation and into the brain through the blood–brain barrier because there are no direct CNS connections with it. Secretory activity is stimulated by darkness and inhibited by exposure to light. **Astrocytes** (5%) make up the remainder of cells. Present among the pineal gland cells are **corpora arenacea** or "*brain sand*," calcium-containing concretions that increase in size and numbers as an individual ages.

9.13 Basal Ganglia

The **basal ganglia** have a role in regulating motor functions. The major components or nuclei consist of the caudate nucleus, putamen, and globus pallidus. These structures together have also been termed the **corpus striatum**. The caudate and putamen are referred together as the **striatum**. There are some additional terms related to the basal ganglia. The **lenticular nucleus** equals the putamen and globus pallidus. The **deep telencephalic nuclei** equal the caudate nucleus plus the lenticular nucleus. The neostriatum is the primary receiving area for input into while the globus pallidus is the primary region for the outflow of information from the basal ganglia. Because of the functional and anatomical relationships shared with these three structures, the **substantia nigra** and **subthalamic nucleus** are considered a part of the basal ganglia (**Fig. 9.41**).

The **caudate nucleus** is C-shaped, consists of a head, body, and tail, and follows the lateral ventricle for its entire length. The internal capsule forms the lateral and ventral borders while the dorsal border is formed by the corpus callosum. The **putamen** lies between the globus pallidus and the external capsule. Along with the globus pallidus, the putamen lies lateral to the internal capsule. The **globus pallidus** lies medial to the putamen and consists of two parts: a lateral and medial segment separated by white matter called the **medial medullary lamina**. The globus pallidus and the putamen are separated by white matter called the **lateral medullary lamina** (**Fig. 9.44**).

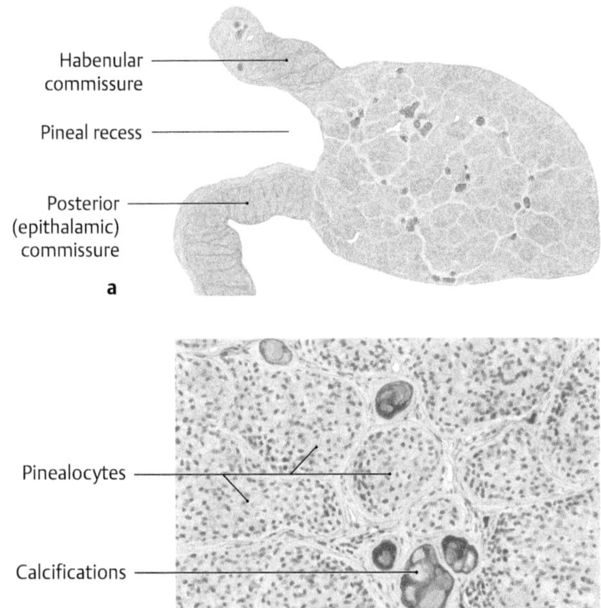

Fig. 9.42 Structure of the pineal gland. **(a)** Gross midsagittal tissue section. **(b)** Histological section. (From Schuenke M, Schulte E, Schumacher U. THIEME Atlas of Anatomy. Head, Neck, and Neuroanatomy. Illustrations by Voll M and Wesker K. 3rd ed. New York: Thieme Medical Publishers; 2020.)

9.13.1 Basal Ganglia Connections

The basal ganglia are connected in such a way that it has the appearance of loops. These loops are the way the basal ganglia are able to modulate the activity of the motor and premotor cortices before finally the lower motor neuron. The loop is essentially set up in this order: (1) neocortex, (2) caudate and putamen, (3) globus pallidus, (4) ventral anterior (VA) and ventral lateral (VL) nuclei of the thalamus, and (5) motor and premotor cortices. **Corticostriatal fibers** involve the internal capsule and they are an organized projection system originating mainly from association areas of much of the neocortex but they can come from the motor and sensory cortex as well. Projections to the caudate and putamen are excitatory and utilize the neurotransmitter **glutamate** (**Fig. 9.45**).

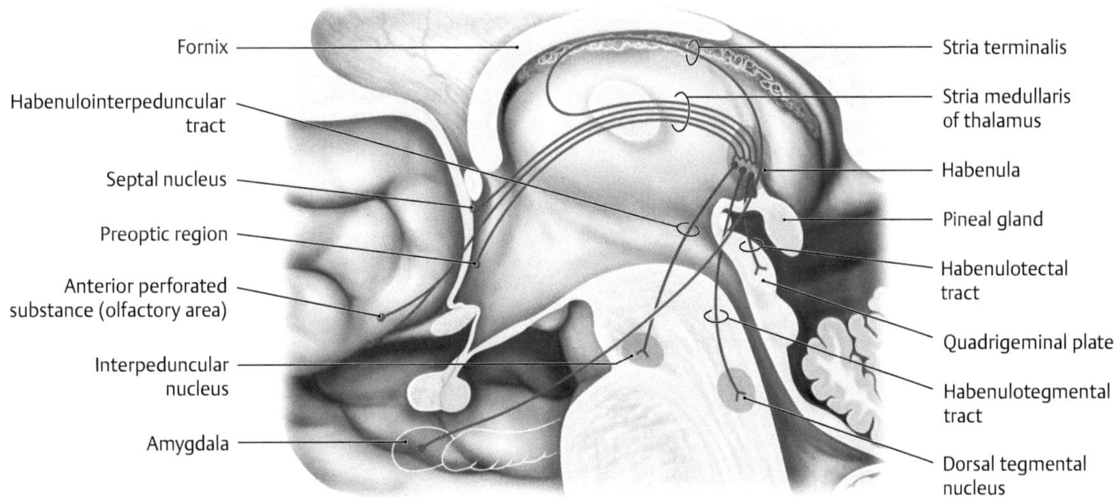

Fig. 9.43 Habenular nuclei and their fiber connections. Afferent connections (blue): afferent impulses from the anterior perforated substance (olfactory area), septal nuclei, and preoptic region are transmitted by the stria medulaaris to the habenular nuclei. These nuclei also recieve impulses from the amygdala via the stria terminalis. Efferent connections (red): efferent fibers from the habenular nuclei are projected to the midbrain along three tracts: (1) **Habenulotectal tract:** terminates at the quadrigeminal plate supplying it with olfactory impulses; (2) **Habenulotegmental tract:** terminates in the dorsal tegmental nulceus to establish connections with the dorsal longitudinal fasciculus and with the salivatory and motor cranial nerve nuclei; (3) **Habenulointerpeduncular tract:** terminates in the interpeduncular nucleus before connecting with the reticular formation. (From Schuenke M, Schulte E, Schumacher U. THIEME Atlas of Anatomy. Head, Neck, and Neuroanatomy. Illustrations by Voll M and Wesker K. 3rd ed. New York: Thieme Medical Publishers; 2020.)

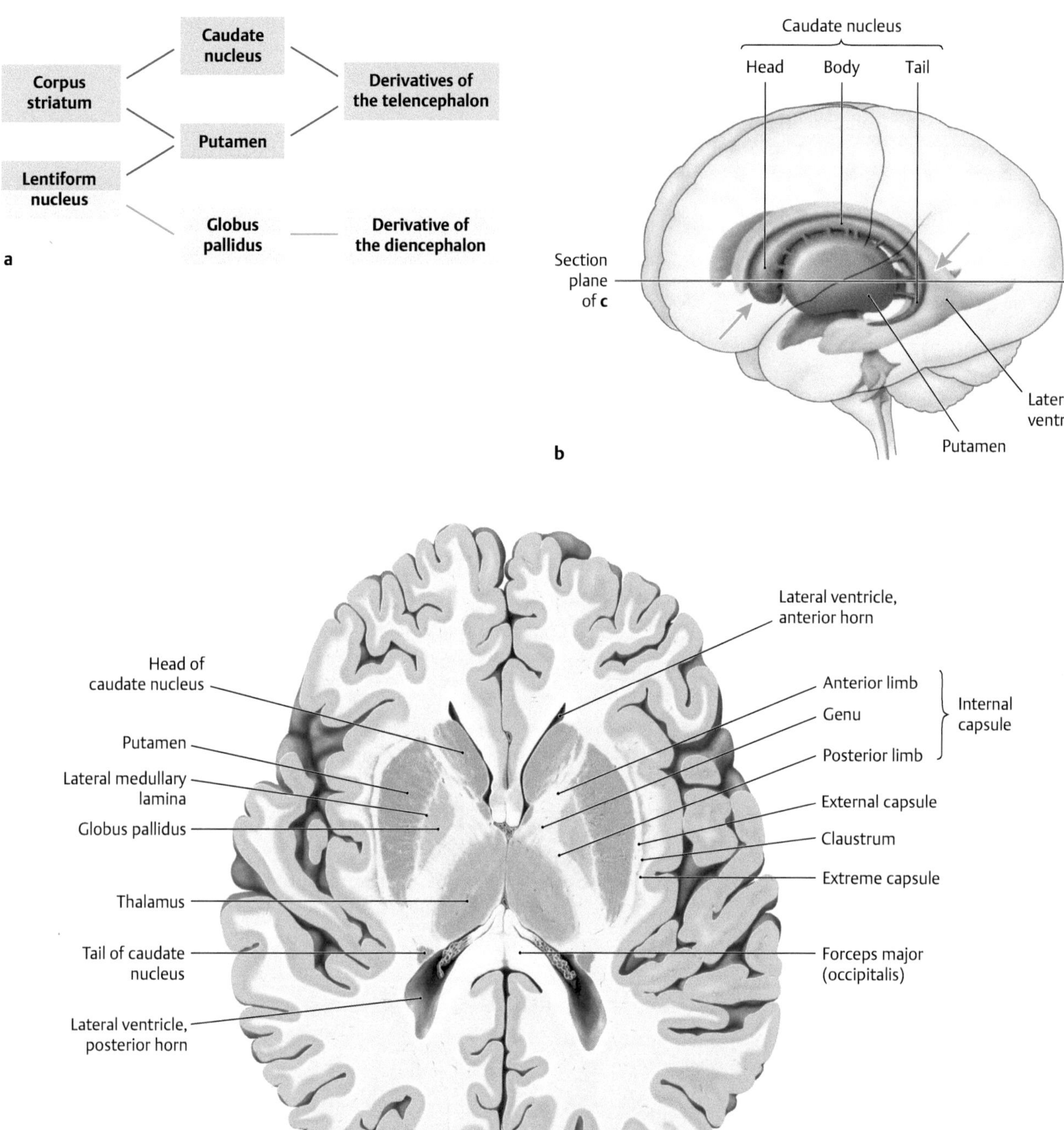

Fig. 9.44 **(a)** Definition and classification of basal ganglia. **(b)** Location and projection of basal ganglia. **(c)** Horizontal section through brain at the telencephalon-diencephalon border, superior view. (*continued*) (From Schuenke M, Schulte E, Schumacher U. THIEME Atlas of Anatomy. Head, Neck, and Neuroanatomy. Illustrations by Voll M and Wesker K. 3rd ed. New York: Thieme Medical Publishers; 2020.)

9.13.2 Striatum (Caudate and Putamen) Projections (Direct vs Indirect)

- *Direct pathway*: output from the striatum extends to the *internal segment* of the globus pallidus using the inhibitory neurotransmitter **GABA**. The internal segment of the globus pallidus contains GABAergic neurons that extend primarily to the VA of the thalamus. The VA nucleus then sends excitatory projections to areas 4 and 6 of the cerebral cortex using **glutamate**. Ultimately this pathway increases the activity of the VA nucleus and excites the motor areas of the cerebral cortex.
- *Indirect pathway*: GABAergic neurons of the striatum project to the *external segment* of the globus pallidus and from here GABAergic extensions to the **subthalamic nucleus**. Neurons from the subthalamic nucleus project to the internal segment

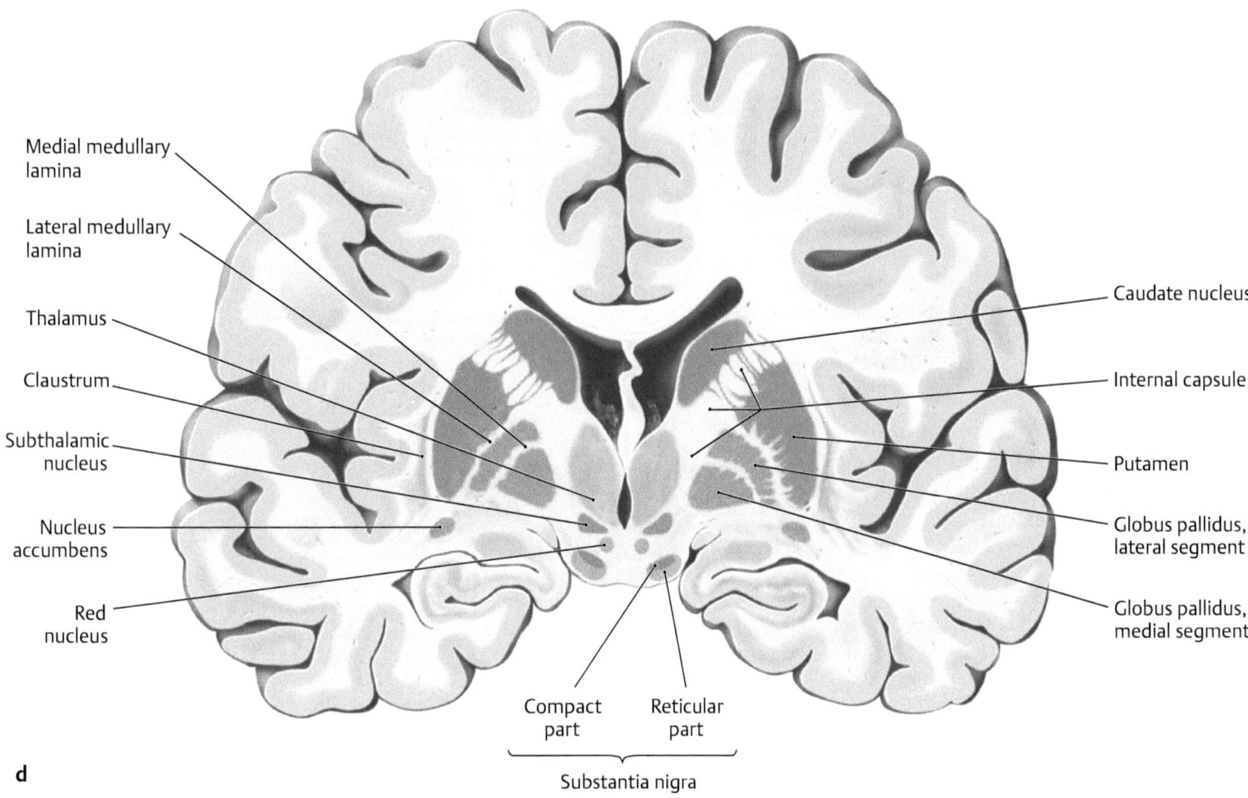

Fig. 9.44 (*continued*) **(d)** Coronal section through the brain showing the basal ganglia. (From Schuenke M, Schulte E, Schumacher U. THIEME Atlas of Anatomy. Head, Neck, and Neuroanatomy. Illustrations by Voll M and Wesker K. 3rd ed. New York: Thieme Medical Publishers; 2020.)

of the globus pallidus using **glutamate**. The internal segment then sends its inhibitory extensions to the VA nucleus, which then sends excitatory projections to areas 4 and 6. Ultimately this pathway decreases the activity of the VA nucleus and excites the motor areas of the cerebral cortex (**Fig. 9.45**).

9.13.3 Additional Basal Ganglia Circuitry

- The pars compacta of the substantia nigra has neurons that produce dopamine and they can project to the striatum. They are mainly modulatory to the striatum. The pars reticulata is functionally similar to the internal segment of the globus pallidus.
- Local neurons of the striatum contain the neurotransmitter acetylcholine (ACh). The striatum output neurons receive two distinct but opposite modulatory inputs: dopamine from the substantia nigra and ACh from its own local neurons.
- Dopamine plays a critical role in the ability of the striatum to initiate and block the initiation of individual motor impulses. This helps balance the activity between the direct and indirect pathways. Dopamine is excitatory on striatal neurons that project directly to the internal segment of the globus pallidus. If the direct pathway is activated, activation of the VA nucleus occurs and a selected motor impulse is permitted to advance. Dopamine at the same time inhibits the indirect loop, enhancing the effect of the VA nucleus on the cerebral cortex.
- Dopamine is inhibitory on striatal neurons that project to the external segment of the globus pallidus. If the indirect pathway is activated, inhibition of the VA nucleus is strengthened; thus, reduced VA nucleus activity does not allow for the completion of a motor impulse to occur, or slows it down.

9.13.4 Additional Fiber Bundles

- **Lenticular fasciculus:** fibers exit from the *dorsal portion* of the internal segment of globus pallidus and pass through the posterior limb of the internal capsule before passing medially above the subthalamic nucleus. This fasciculus then becomes part of the thalamic fasciculus (**Fig. 9.41b**).

Clinical Correlate 9.19

Basal Ganglia Disorders

Lesions of the basal ganglia produce motor deficits. Movement disorders are known as **dyskinesias** while disturbances of muscle tone are called **dystonias. Hypokinesia** is a partial or complete loss of muscle movement and is frequently accompanied by rigidity. Hypokinesia, rigidity, postural instability, and tremors at rest are consistent with **Parkinson disease**. Parkinson is a degenerative disorder centered on damage to the pars compacta of the substantia nigra.

Ballism is the abnormal flailing of the extremities and is usually the result of a stroke affecting the subthalamic nucleus, with symptoms occurring on the contralateral side. These movements are typical of Huntington disease and it is due to the profound loss of neurons in the caudate nucleus and throughout the cerebral cortex. Cells of the caudate nucleus that are lost are specifically GABAergic neurons.

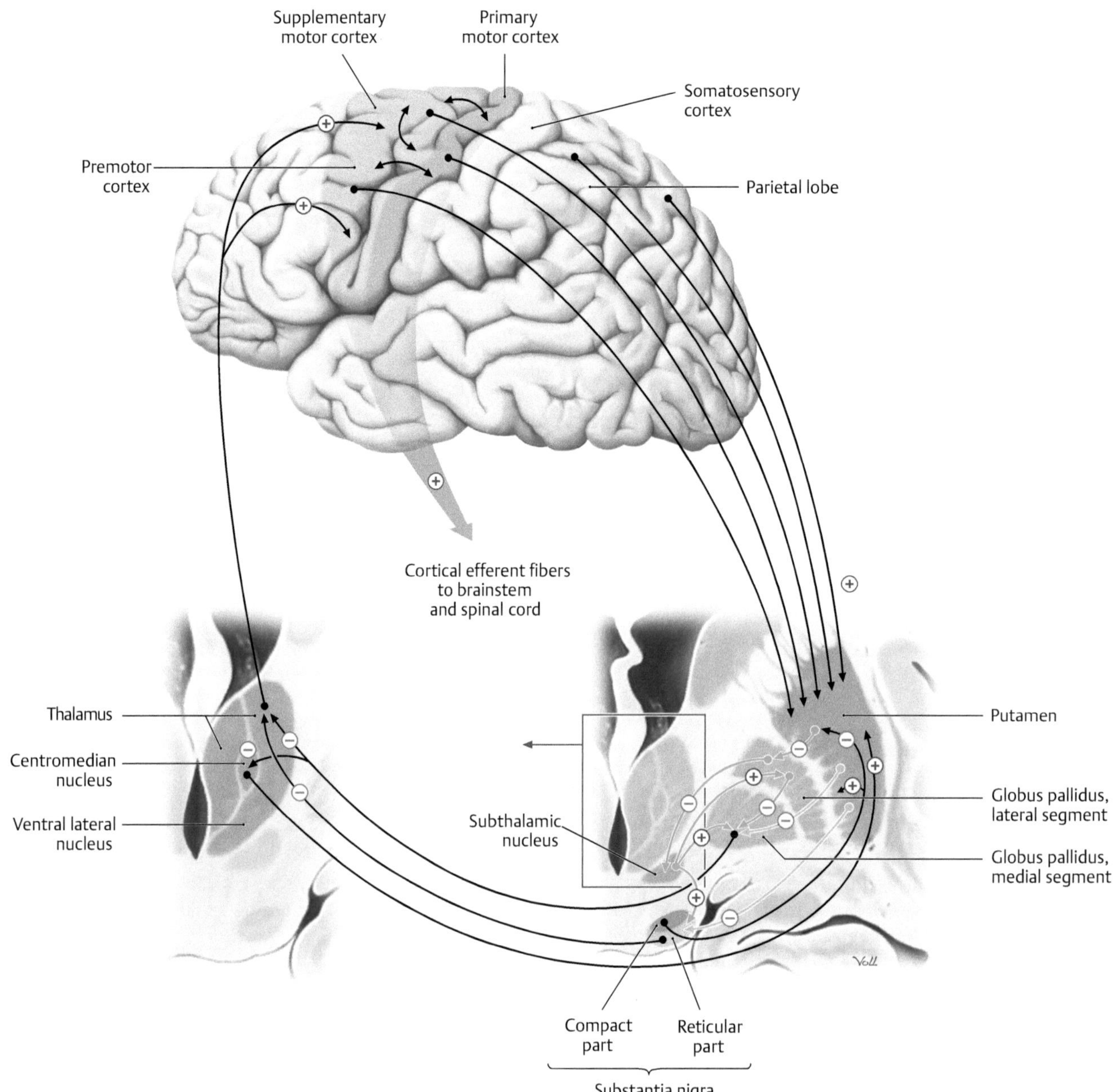

Fig. 9.45 Flow of information between motor cortical areas and basal ganglia: motor loop. (From Schuenke M, Schulte E, Schumacher U. THIEME Atlas of Anatomy. Head, Neck, and Neuroanatomy. Illustrations by Voll M and Wesker K. 3rd ed. New York: Thieme Medical Publishers; 2020.)

- **Ansa lenticularis:** fibers exit the *ventral portion* of the internal segment of globus pallidus and loop below the posterior limb of the internal capsule before turning dorsally and joining the thalamic fasciculus (**Fig. 9.41a,b**).
- **Thalamic fasciculus:** fibers of the lenticular fasciculus and ansa lenticularis, in addition to fibers from the dentate (rubro) thalamic tract (dentate nucleus to VL nucleus), enter the VA and VL nuclei from below.

9.14 Limbic System

The **limbic lobe** is not a true lobe; rather, it comprises a ring of cerebral cortex on the medial surface of the brain and includes parts of the frontal, parietal, and temporal lobes. Structures that make up the limbic lobe include the cingulate gyrus, parahippocampal gyrus, and subcallosal gyrus, and they are related to the limbic system. The **limbic system** is a ring of structures that lie between the neocortex and diencephalon and are involved in behaviors essential for self-preservation and preservation of the species such as feeding and mating, respectively. It is a collection of interconnected neurons in the telencephalon and diencephalon (**Fig. 9.46; Fig. 9.47**).

The telencephalic portion includes the **cingulate gyrus**, **parahippocampal gyrus**, **hippocampal formation**, **amygdala**, and **septal area**. Some authors also include the ventral portions of the **putamen** and **globus pallidus**, and the **prefrontal cortex**. The diencephalon contribution comes from **anterior thalamic nuclear group**, **dorsomedial (DM) thalamic nucleus**, **hypothalamus**, **mammillary bodies**, **nucleus accumbens**, and the **habenulae**. The **cingulum** connects these cortical and subcortical regions.

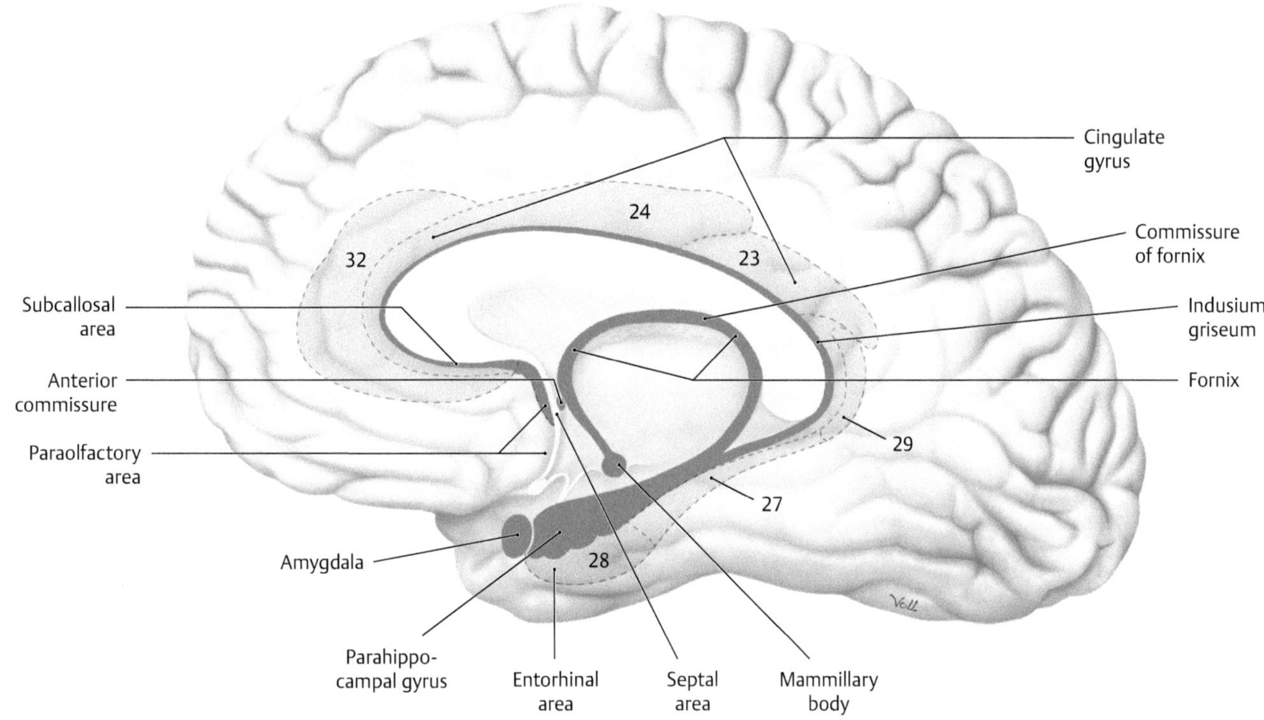

Fig. 9.46 Limbic system viewed through the partially transparent cortex. (From Schuenke M, Schulte E, Schumacher U. THIEME Atlas of Anatomy. Head, Neck, and Neuroanatomy. Illustrations by Voll M and Wesker K. 3rd ed. New York: Thieme Medical Publishers; 2020.)

9.14.1 Cingulate and Parahippocampal Gyrus

The **cingulate** and **parahippocampal gyri** are part of the cortical components of the limbic system termed the "limbic association cortex," and they receive information from higher-order sensory cortices such as the prefrontal cortex and areas 18 and 19 for vision. This information is then sent to the amygdala and hippocampal formation. The anterior portion of the parahippocampal gyrus is called the **entorhinal cortex**. It receives input from the cortical association areas, which include the prefrontal region, somatosensory, visual, auditory, and taste areas. A lesion of the cingulate gyrus results in a lack of emotion or interest (apathy), unable to speak physically or psychologically (mutism), or having an indifference to pain (**Fig. 9.46; Fig. 9.47**).

9.14.2 Hippocampal Formation

The **hippocampal formation** lies deep within the parahippocampal gyrus of the temporal lobe and floor of the third ventricle. It has three main parts: the **hippocampus** (hippocampal proper or Ammon horn), **dentate gyrus**, and **subiculum** (**Fig. 9.47**).

The **hippocampus** has an important role in the mediation of learning and the formation of memories and can be viewed as a primitive form of three-layered cortical tissue. Its primary cell type is the pyramidal cell with basal dendrites that extend toward the ventricular surface and apical dendrites that extend toward the dentate gyrus. The axons of these pyramidal cells pass into the superficial layer of the hippocampus also known as the **alveus** before ultimately reaching the fimbria-fornix or entorhinal cortex. The pyramidal cells are arranged into a C-shaped orientation that is interlocked with another C-shaped appearance of the dentate gyrus. There are four distinct sectors or fields classified as CA1, CA2, CA3, and CA4. The pyramidal cells located closest to the subiculum are CA1. The CA1 field is referred to as *Sommer's sector* and is susceptible to anoxia especially during periods of temporal lobe epilepsy. It receives collateral axons from CA3 pyramidal cells known as *Schaffer collaterals*. The CA4 field is located within the hilus of the dentate gyrus. The CA2 and CA3 fields are situated between CA1 and CA4 (**Fig. 9.47; Fig. 9.48**).

The hippocampus is connected to other regions of the brain through the fornix and perforant pathway. The alveus fibers converge to form the **fimbria** near the medial border of the hippocampus. The fimbria leaves the hippocampus as the **crus of the fornix**. The crus curves posteriorly and superiorly beneath the splenium of the corpus callosum and around the posterior surface of the thalamus. The two crura converge to form the **body of the fornix**. The two crura are connected by the **commissure of the fornix**. Anteriorly, the body of the fornix is connected to the undersurface of the corpus callosum by the septum pellucidum before continuing and splitting into two **columns of the fornix**. The **fornix** interconnects the hippocampal formation with the septal area and with the mammillary bodies of the hypothalamus. The **perforant pathway** is mostly an inflow tract for the hippocampal formation and receives fibers from the entorhinal cortex of the parahippocampal gyrus and other parts of the temporal lobe. The entorhinal cortex is considered the gateway to the hippocampus. It contributes to memory, autonomic and hormonal regulation, motivation, and the central regulation of emotional behavior. Bilateral lesions result in the inability to form long-term memories (**Fig. 9.47; Fig. 9.48b; Fig. 9.49**).

The **dentate gyrus** is a tooth-like band of gray matter that lies between the fimbria and the parahippocampal gyrus. It can also be thought of as a primitive three-layered cortical structure. Its

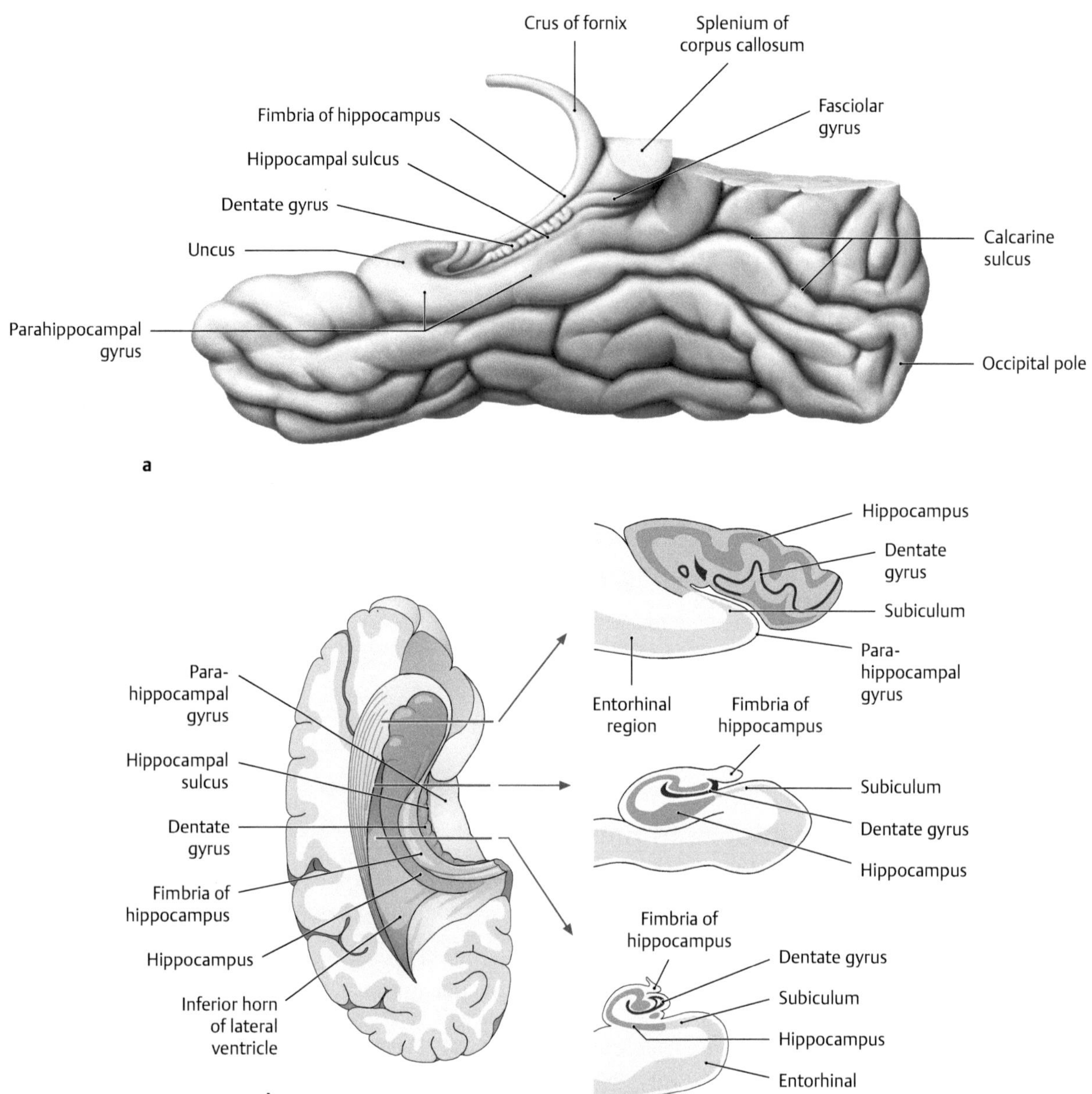

Fig. 9.47 **(a)** Right hippocampal formation and the caudal part of the fornix. Left temporal lobe with the inferior horn of the lateral ventricle exposed. **(b)** Transverse section, posterior view of the hippocampus on the floor of the inferior (temporal) horn. **(c)** Coronal sections through the left hippocampus. (From Schuenke M, Schulte E, Schumacher U. THIEME Atlas of Anatomy. Head, Neck, and Neuroanatomy. Illustrations by Voll M and Wesker K. 3rd ed. New York: Thieme Medical Publishers; 2020.)

principal cell is the granule cell. The axon of the granule cell is called a mossy fiber and it makes synaptic contact with pyramidal cells in the CA3 field. The granule cells of the dentate gyrus along with the olfactory bulb are one of the few regions of the adult brain where neurogenesis takes place. They are thought to play a role in the formation of new memories and possibly adjusting to symptoms of stress and depression (**Fig. 9.47; Fig 9.48; Fig. 9.49b**).

The dentate gyrus accompanies the fimbria almost to the splenium of the corpus callosum before becoming continuous with the **indusium griseum** (**Fig. 9.46; Fig. 9.49a**). The indusium griseum is a thin, vestigial layer of gray matter that covers the superior surface of the corpus callosum and is flanked by the **lateral** and **medial longitudinal striae** (**Fig. 9.49a**). Its function in humans is unclear, but a recent study has shown that it is a glial membrane with no neuronal content or obvious connections to the hippocampus[1]

The **subiculum** serves as a transition zone of cortex and is continuous with the hippocampus on one side and with the parahippocampal gyrus on the other side. It has a considerably thicker pyramidal cell layer than the hippocampus (**Fig. 9.47b, c; Fig. 9.48**).

9.14.3 Afferent Connections to the Hippocampus

- Fibers from the opposite hippocampus pass through the commissure of the fornix.
- Fibers from cingulate, parahippocampal, and dentate gyri.

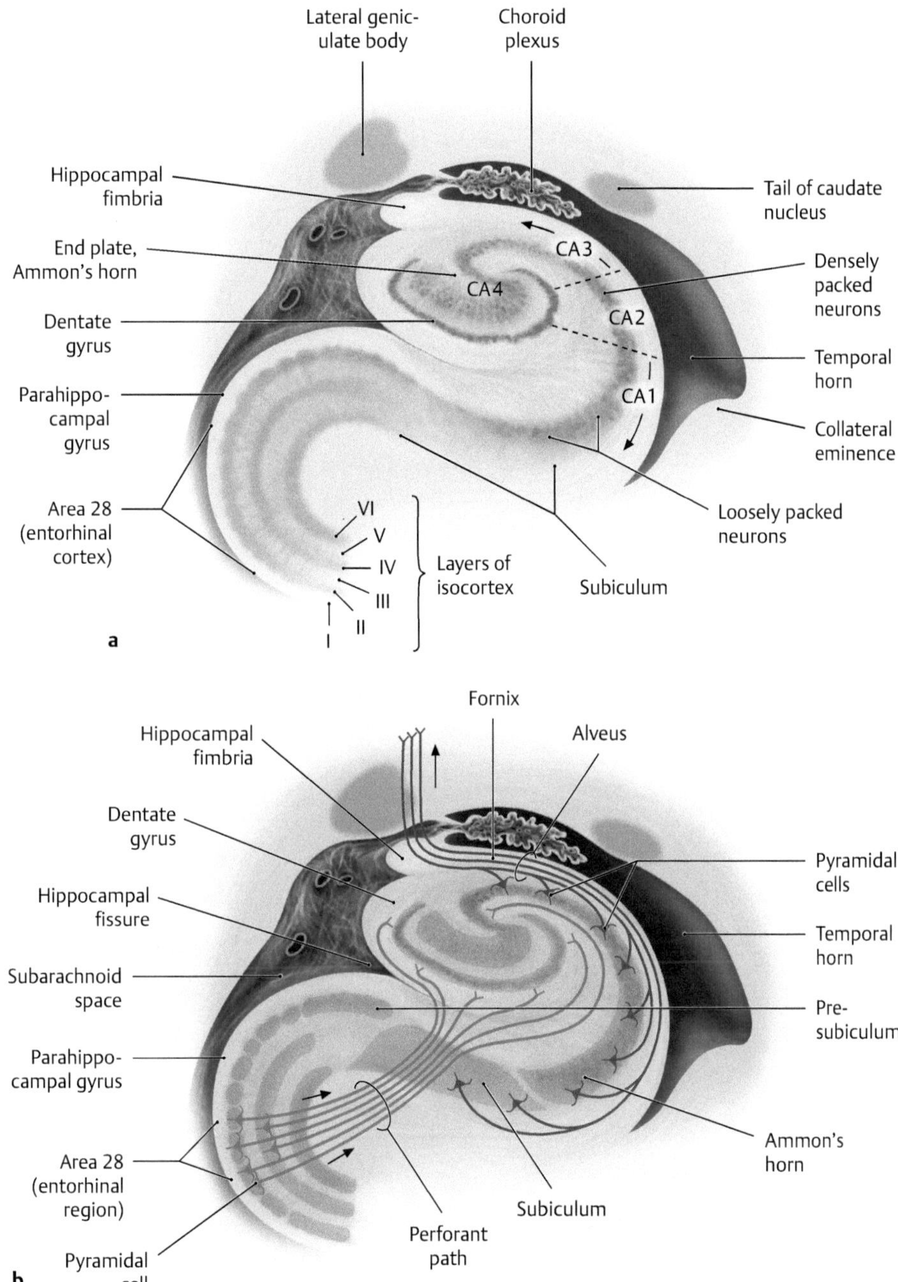

Fig. 9.48 (a) Cytoarchitecture of the hippocampal formation. **(b)** Connections of the hippocampus. (From Schuenke M, Schulte E, Schumacher U. THIEME Atlas of Anatomy. Head, Neck, and Neuroanatomy. Illustrations by Voll M and Wesker K. 3rd ed. New York: Thieme Medical Publishers; 2020.)

- Fibers from the entorhinal cortex or olfactory-associated cortex.
- Fibers from the septal nuclei pass posteriorly through the fornix before reaching the hippocampus.
- Fibers from the indusium griseum pass posteriorly through the longitudinal striae (unclear).

9.14.4 Efferent Connections to the Hippocampus (via the Fornix)

- Fibers pass to the medial nucleus of the mammillary body.
- Fibers pass to the anterior nuclei of the thalamus.
- Fibers pass to the midbrain tegmentum.
- Fibers pass to the lateral preoptic area, septal nuclei, and the anterior part of the hypothalamus.
- Fibers follow the stria medullaris thalami before reaching the habenular nuclei.

9.14.5 Amygdala

The amygdala is an almond-shaped structure that lies deep within the temporal lobe near the anterior limit of the hippocampal formation. Bilateral lesions result in a loss of fear, rage, and aggression or being serenely quiet or undisturbed (placidity).

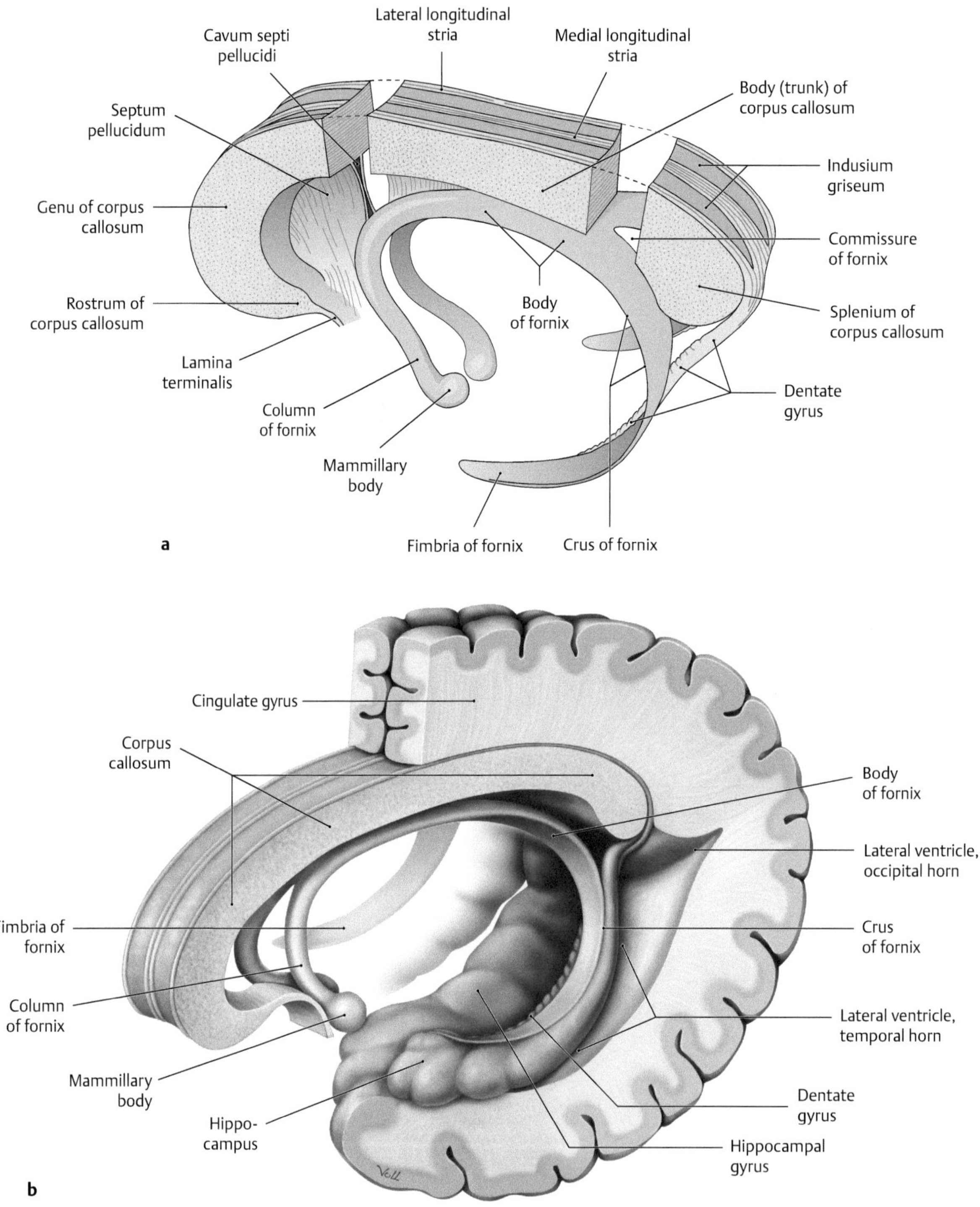

Fig. 9.49 Topography of the fornix, corpus callosum, septum pellucidum, and hippocampus. **(a)** Occipital view from upper left. **(b)** Viewed from the upper left and anterior aspect. (From Schuenke M, Schulte E, Schumacher U. THIEME Atlas of Anatomy. Head, Neck, and Neuroanatomy. Illustrations by Voll M and Wesker K. 3rd ed. New York: Thieme Medical Publishers; 2020.)

It has been described as an amygdaloid nuclear complex consisting of basolateral, central, and corticomedial nuclei (**Fig. 9.46; Fig. 9.50**).

- **Basolateral nuclei**: these nuclei are the largest of the amygdala and are well developed in humans. They play a role in attaching emotional significance to a particular stimulus. They receive highly processed sensory information from the sensory association cortices and are connected with the limbic lobe cortex (cingulate and parahippocampal gyrus), orbitofrontal cortex, medial prefrontal cortex, and the DM nucleus of the thalamus. This nucleus primarily uses the **ventral amygdalofugal fibers** to reach the DM nucleus of the thalamus, basal forebrain structures like the septal area, ventral basal ganglia, and the basal nucleus *of Meynert*. The basal nucleus *of Meynert* may be related to **Alzheimer's disease**.

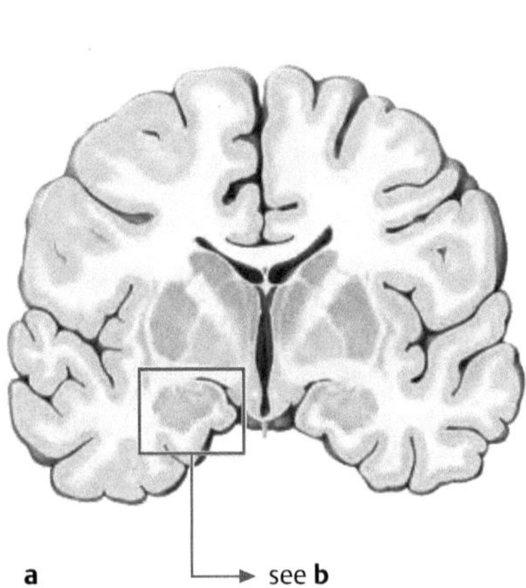

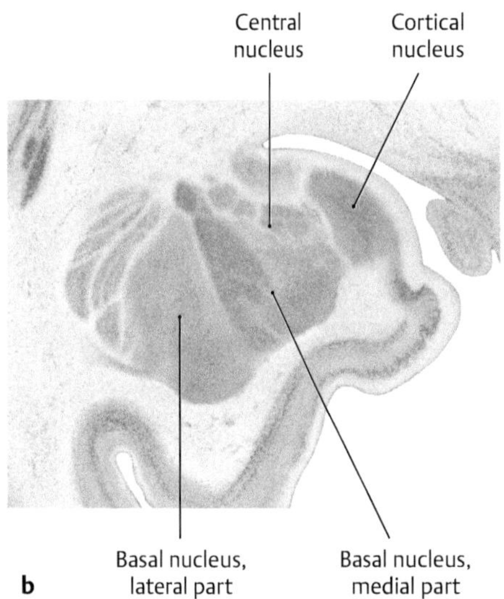

Fig. 9.50 Amygdala. **(a)** Coronal section at the level of the interventricular foramen. **(b)** Detail showing the three groups of nuclei in the amygdala. (From Schuenke M, Schulte E, Schumacher U. THIEME Atlas of Anatomy. Head, Neck, and Neuroanatomy. Illustrations by Voll M and Wesker K. 3rd ed. New York: Thieme Medical Publishers; 2020.)

- **Central nuclei**: these nuclei mediate general emotional responses. They receive input from the basolateral nucleus and have reciprocal connections with visceral nuclei of the spinal cord and brainstem. The ventral amygdalofugal fibers originate from both the central and basolateral nuclei and terminate in the hypothalamus and septal area. They can also project to prefrontal, frontal, cingulate, and inferior temporal cortices along with the ventral striatum.
- **Corticomedial nuclei**: these nuclei are not well defined in humans but are interconnected with the olfactory bulb and the primary olfactory cortex. This part of the amygdala can regulate the activity of the autonomic nervous system and the neurons of the hypothalamus that help control the pituitary gland. It connects to the hypothalamus by way of the **stria terminalis**. The stria terminalis is a small tract originating primarily from the centromedial nuclei, and it projects to the hypothalamus, septal area, and ventral striatum.

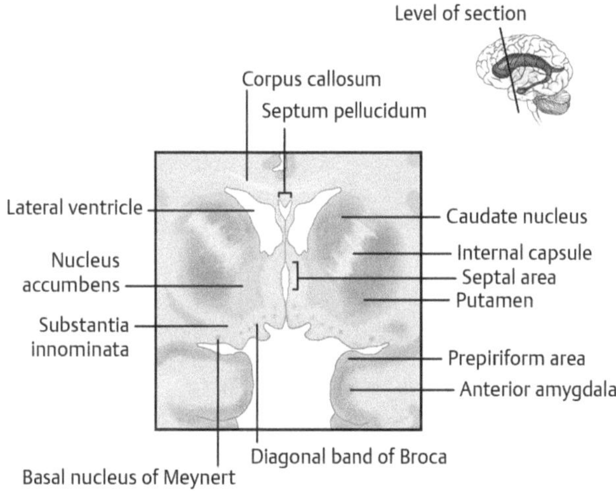

Fig. 9.51 The substantia innominata, diagonal band of Broca, and the basal nucleus of Meynert. The plane of section passes through the body of the caudate nucleus. Illustration by Calla Heald.

9.14.6 Septal Area

The **septal area** is a small group of nuclei located in the medial wall of the frontal lobe and rostral to the anterior commissure, near the anterior horn of the lateral ventricle. These nuclei have reciprocal connections with the hippocampus, the amygdala, and the olfactory bulb. It serves as a relay nucleus of the hippocampal formation to the lateral and medial hypothalamus. It is a primary receiving area for fibers contained within the precommissural fornix that arise from the hippocampal formation. It may be seen as a functional extension of the hippocampal formation (**Fig. 9.46; Fig. 9.51**).

9.14.7 Nucleus Accumbens

The **nucleus accumbens** is located near the head of the caudate nucleus, putamen, septal area, and substantia innominate. It is believed to process rewarding stimuli and reinforce those rewarding behaviors. It receives a larger dopaminergic projection from the brainstem and other areas such as the amygdala and hippocampal formation. It then sends axons to the substantia nigra, substantia innominate, and ventral tegmental area (**Fig. 9.45; Fig. 9.51**).

9.14.8 Substantia Innominata

The **substantia innominata** is located at the level of the septal nuclei and immediately below the striatum. Its medial border is the **diagonal band of Broca** and preoptic region. It is sometimes identified as an extension of the amygdala. It extends laterally where it appears to merge with that of the **prepiriform area**, which is located near the olfactory trigone. The substantia innominata shares connections with the amygdala and projects its axons to the lateral hypothalamus (**Fig. 9.51**).

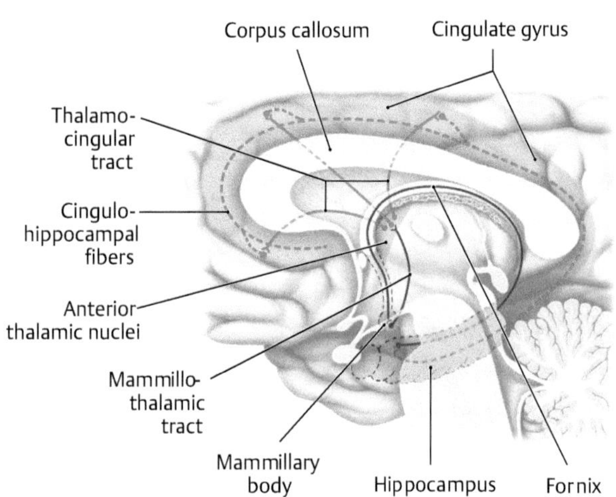

Fig. 9.52 Papez circuit. (From Schuenke M, Schulte E, Schumacher U. THIEME Atlas of Anatomy. Head, Neck, and Neuroanatomy. Illustrations by Voll M and Wesker K. 3rd ed. New York: Thieme Medical Publishers; 2020.)

9.14.9 Papez Circuit

The **Papez Circuit** is a "closed loop" of connections within the limbic system involved in learning and memory, emotion, and social behavior. The overly simplified circuitry of the Papez circuit is as follows: hippocampus → fornix → mammillary body → mammillothalamic tract → anterior thalamic nucleus → thalamocingular tract → cingulate gyrus → cingulum (cingulohippocampal fibers) → entorhinal cortex → perforant pathway → hippocampus (**Fig. 9.46; Fig. 9.48b; Fig. 9.52**).

9.14.10 Additional Pathways of the Limbic System

- **Stria medullaris thalami**: connects the septal nuclei to the **habenula.** It is situated along the point of attachment of the roof of the third ventricle.
- **Habenulointerpeduncular fibers**: connect the habenula to the **interpeduncular nucleus.** The fibers extending from the interpeduncular nucleus descend to the reticular formation of the brainstem and ultimately parasympathetic nuclei including both the salivary nuclei and dorsal motor nucleus of vagus.
- **Cingulum**: the primary interconnections between the areas of the cingulate and parahippocampal gyri.
- **Uncinate fasciculus**: the interconnections between the amygdala and orbital surface of the frontal lobe.

9.14.11 Pathology of the Limbic System

The hypothalamus energizes visceral reactions through its connections with the brainstem reticular formation and autonomic centers located in both the brainstem and spinal cord. It does this in response to input received from the limbic system. Overlap and duplication is prevalent within the limbic system and it is not possible to pinpoint a single symptom on a single element. Lesions of the limbic system may produce a large range of issues such as memory loss, autonomic dysfunction, olfactory abnormalities, or bizarre behavioral patterns. The mechanism of memory seems to still be processed in the hippocampus. Incoming stimuli going to all neocortical primary sensory and association areas must be copied to the hippocampus. Here a memory of ongoing events or short-term memory is laid down. What will be processed as long-term memory is then moved to other cortical association areas and does not remain in the hippocampus.

9.15 Internal Capsule

The **internal capsule**, when viewed horizontally, has three parts: the anterior limb, genu, and posterior limb. It contains both descending fibers from the cerebral cortex that course down to the brainstem and spinal cord along with ascending fibers that pass from the thalamus to the cerebral cortex.

- The **anterior limb** has the *frontopontine (corticopontine) tracts* that connect the frontal lobe to the pons and serve to coordinate planned motor functions with the contralateral cerebellum. Also present are the *anterior thalamic peduncle (thalamocortical) fibers* that primarily consist of fibers connecting the dorsomedial and anterior thalamic nuclei to the prefrontal cortex.
- The **genu** contains the *corticobulbar (corticonuclear) fibers*, which carry impulses from the lower portion of the precentral and premotor cortices to the motor nuclei of cranial nerves.
- The **posterior limb** has multiple components. The *corticospinal tract* is the motor pathway, starting primarily in the motor cortices of the cerebral cortex and terminating on lower motor neurons and interneurons in the spinal cord. It functions in controlling movements of the limbs and is somatotopically organized with control of the arms closest to the genu and the legs nearest the posterior aspect of this limb. The *temporopontine (corticopontine) tract* connects the temporal lobe with the pontine nuclei. The *posterior thalamic peduncle (thalamocortical) tracts* are composed of fibers that extend back from the ventral anterior, ventral lateral, and ventral posterior thalamic nuclei before reaching motor or sensory cortices. Optic radiations are also found passing through this peduncle (**Fig. 9.53**).

9.16 Cerebral Hemispheres and Cortex

The largest part of the brain is the cerebral hemispheres and they are separated into a left and right portion by the deep **longitudinal cerebral fissure.** The **falx cerebri**, a dural infolding, along with the **anterior cerebral arteries**, are located within this cerebral fissure. The deepest portion of the fissure is the location of the **corpus callosum**, the largest commissural fibers responsible for connecting the two hemispheres. The **tentorium cerebelli** is another dural infolding but it separates the cerebral hemispheres from the cerebellum (**Fig. 9.54**).

The cerebral hemispheres are divided into six major lobes bilaterally and some are named according to the cranial bones they rest against, the **frontal, parietal, temporal**, and **occipital lobes**, while the **insula** and **limbic lobe** are located deep or medial to the other lobes. The surface area of the cerebral cortex is increased by the appearance of **gyri** or folds, which are separated from each other by a **sulcus** or **fissure.** The **central sulcus** separates the precentral and postcentral gyri, the portions of the cortex related to the primary motor and primary sensory areas, respectively. The **lateral sulcus** is a deep ridge located on the lateral surfaces of the cerebral hemispheres. It extends at three locations to form the **anterior**

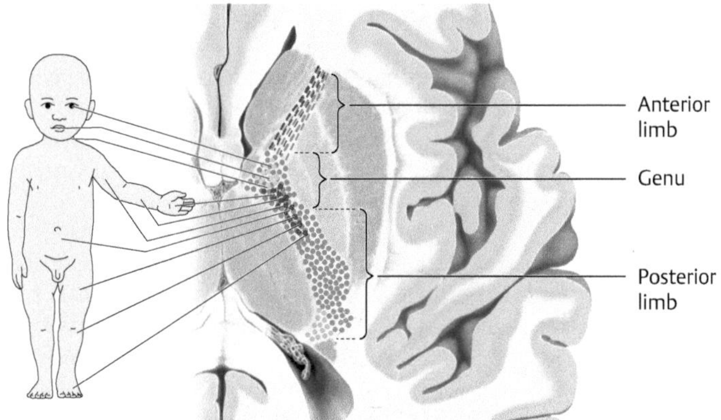

Fig. 9.53 Somatotopic organization of the internal capsule. Frontopontine tracts (*red dashes*); anterior thalamic peduncle (*blue dashes*); corticonuclear fibers (*yellow dots*); corticospinal fibers (*red dots*); posterior thalamic peduncle (*blue dots*); temporopontine tract (*orange dots*); posterior thalamic peduncle (*light blue dots*). (From Schuenke M, Schulte E, Schumacher U. THIEME Atlas of Anatomy. Head and Neuroanatomy. Illustrations by Voll M and Wesker K. 1st ed. New York: Thieme Medical Publishers; 2010.)

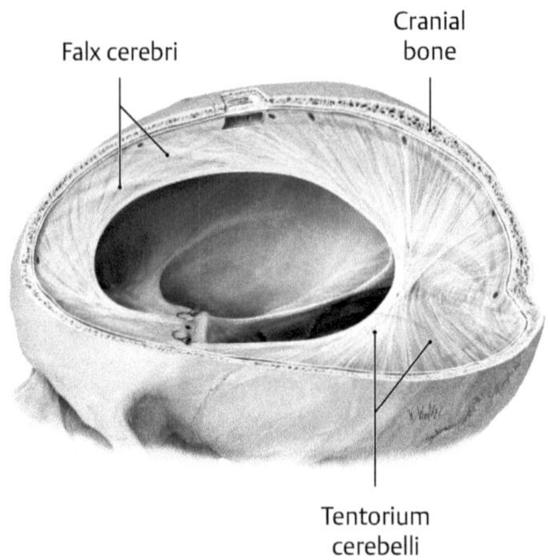

Fig. 9.54 Dural infoldings. (From Schuenke M, Schulte E, Schumacher U. THIEME Atlas of Anatomy. Head, Neck, and Neuroanatomy. Illustrations by Voll M and Wesker K. 3rd ed. New York: Thieme Medical Publishers; 2020.)

horizontal, **anterior ascending**, and **posterior rami**. The **insula** is part of the cortex that lies just deep to the lateral sulcus. The **parieto-occipital sulcus** is orientated on the superomedial margin of the hemisphere approximately 4 to 5 cm anterior to the occipital lobe. It extends anteriorly and inferiorly on the medial surface before reaching the calcarine sulcus. The **calcarine sulcus** is located on the medial surface of the cerebral hemispheres near the occipital lobe (**Fig 9.55**).

The cerebral cortex is divided into **Brodmann areas** based on its cytoarchitecture. These areas were originally described by the German anatomist Korbinian Brodmann, who originally described 52 distinct regions of the cerebral cortex with many of these areas correlating to specific cortical functions (**Fig. 9.56**).

9.16.1 Frontal Lobe

The **frontal lobe** is located anterior to the central sulcus and superior to the lateral sulcus. The surface of this lobe is divided into four gyri by three individual sulci (**Fig. 9.55 a-c**). The **precentral gyrus** is located between the central and **precentral sulcus**. The superior frontal and inferior frontal sulci extend anteriorly from the precentral sulcus. The **superior frontal gyrus** is found superior to the superior frontal sulcus. The **middle frontal gyrus** is located between the superior frontal and inferior frontal sulci, while the **inferior frontal gyrus** rests inferior to the inferior frontal sulcus. On the inferior surface of this lobe, the olfactory bulb and tract overlie the **olfactory sulcus**. Medial to this sulcus is the **straight (rectus) gyrus** and lateral to it are numerous **orbital gyri** (**Fig. 9.55b**). Special features of the cortex of this lobe include:

- **Primary motor cortex**: located in the precentral gyrus and anterior portion of the paracentral lobule. It corresponds with **Brodmann area 4** and contributes to the corticospinal tract. The giant pyramidal cells *of Betz* are located here and activity at this location results in contralateral motion of voluntary muscles especially the distal limb muscles. A lesion at this area results in contralateral upper motor neuron paralysis. If there is a bilateral lesion targeting the paracentral lobule region, this could cause urinary incontinence (**Fig. 9.56a, b**).
- **Premotor cortex**: located just anterior to the precentral gyrus and corresponds to **area 6**. Much of this cortex is associated with the superior frontal gyrus and it functions in motor movement planning involving head, trunk, and limb flexion and extension. The **supplementary motor cortex** is also a part of **area 6**, but it is located more on the medial side and anterior to the paracentral lobule. It involves planning complex motor sequences and bilateral movements. Both cortices contribute to the corticospinal tract. Lesions of the premotor cortex create the inability to perform movements in the correct sequence (apraxia). If a lesion targets the supplementary motor cortex, this leads to speech deficits (aphasia) or hypertonus of flexor muscles if the lesion is bilateral (**Fig. 9.56a, b**).
- **Frontal eye field**: found anterior to the premotor cortex (area 6) and on the posterior part of the middle frontal gyrus. This cortex corresponds with **area 8** and plays a role in contralateral conjugate eye movements. Studies have shown that this cortex is also involved in motor, language, memory, attention, and executive functions. Lesions here result in contralateral horizontal conjugate gaze palsy (**Fig. 9.56a, b**).
- **Prefrontal cortex**: includes **areas 9–12** and **area 46** and serves as the highest cortical region responsible for motor planning, organization, and regulation. Areas 9 and 10 have a strong connection with memory encoding and memory retrieval

along with working memory. A lesion to the prefrontal cortex could lead to problems that affect executive memory, concentration, social judgment and behavior, abstract thinking, and problem solving. **Area 11** is also referred to as the orbitofrontal area, and a lesion of this region can cause personality changes and disinhibited behavior. Examples include the inability to empathize, compulsive drug use or gambling, and hypersexuality (**Fig. 9.56a, b**).

- **Broca speech area**: located in the posterior part of the inferior frontal gyrus of the dominant hemisphere and corresponds with **areas 44** and **45**. The arcuate fasciculus connects it with *Wernicke's speech area* (**Fig. 9.56b**).

9.16.2 Parietal Lobe

The **parietal lobe** is found posterior to the central sulcus and superior to the lateral sulcus and it extends as far posteriorly as the parieto-occipital sulcus (**Fig. 9.55a, c**). The **intraparietal sulcus** extends from the postcentral sulcus to the parieto-occipital sulcus. The **superior parietal** and **inferior parietal lobules** are located superior and inferior to the intraparietal sulcus, respectively. Located inferior to the more anterior half of the intraparietal lobule and adjacent to the posterior most portion of the lateral sulcus is the **supramarginal gyrus**. The **angular gyrus** lies between the superomarginal gyrus, inferior parietal lobule, temporal lobe, and occipital lobe. On the medial surface, the **paracentral lobule** is continuous anteriorly with the precentral gyrus and posteriorly with the postcentral gyrus. The paracentral lobule may be separated from the **precuneus** by the **marginal sulcus**, a posterosuperior extension of the cingulate sulcus (**Fig. 9.55c**). Special features of the cortex of this lobe include:

- **Primary somatosensory cortex**: located in the postcentral gyrus and posterior portion of the paracentral gyrus. This cortex is related to areas **3, 1,** and **2** and contributes to the corticospinal tract. Information is sent to it by the ventral posterior nucleus of the thalamus, and it is somatotopically organized into the sensory homunculus. Damage to this region of the cortex results in a contralateral loss of tactile discrimination and the inability to localize sensation (**Fig. 9.56a, b**).
- **Secondary somatosensory cortex**: just anterior to the primary somatosensory region along the superior border of the lateral sulcus. This cortex includes portions of **area 40**. This region may be involved in remembering the differences between tactile shapes and textures (**Fig. 9.56a**).
- **Somatosensory association cortex** comprises the superior parietal lobule and/or **areas 5** and **7**, the supramarginal gyrus or **area 40**, and the angular gyrus that is related to **area 39**. Areas 39 and 40 can be considered part of *Wernicke's speech area*. The superior parietal lobule portion receives input from

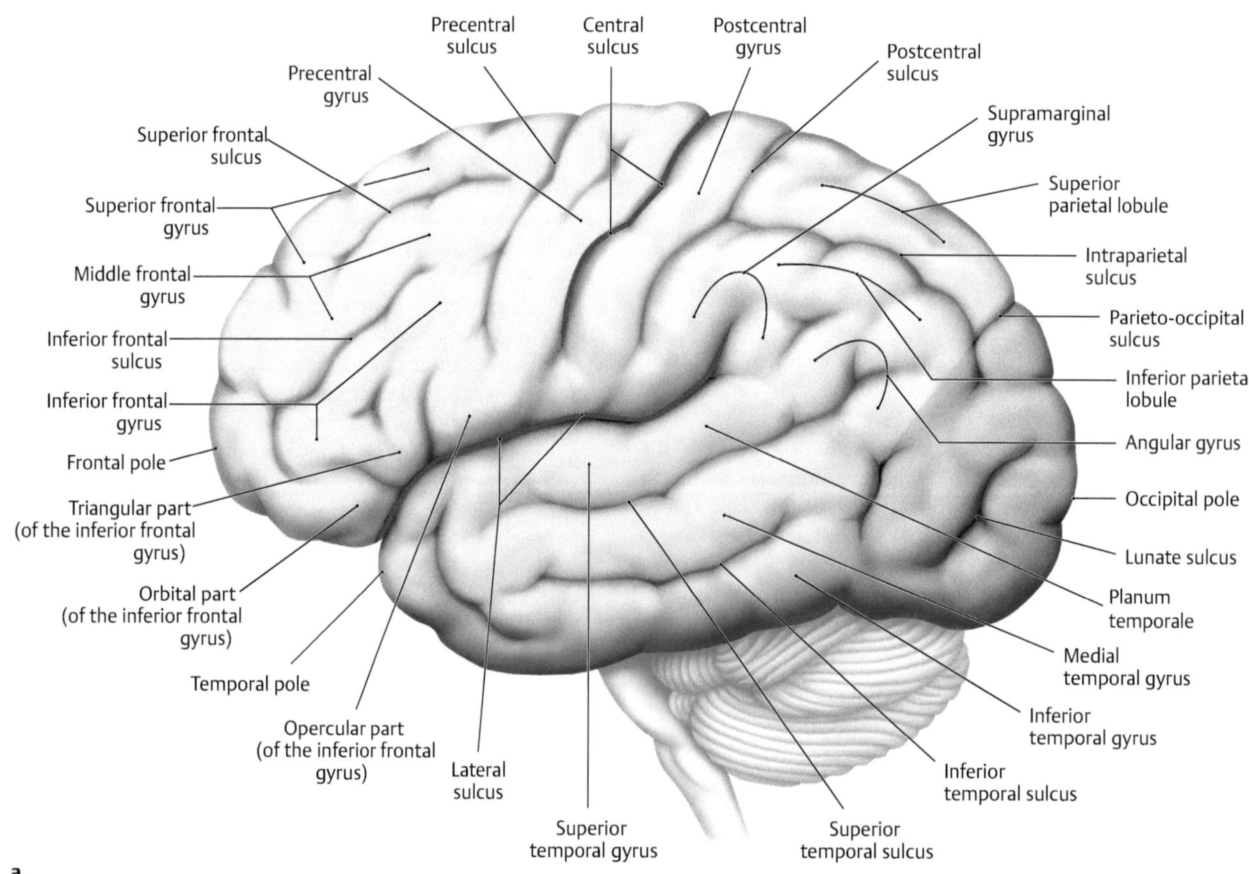

Fig. 9.55 (a) Gyri and sulci of the convex surface. (*continued*) (From Schuenke M, Schulte E, Schumacher U. THIEME Atlas of Anatomy. Head, Neck, and Neuroanatomy. Illustrations by Voll M and Wesker K. 3rd ed. New York: Thieme Medical Publishers; 2020.)

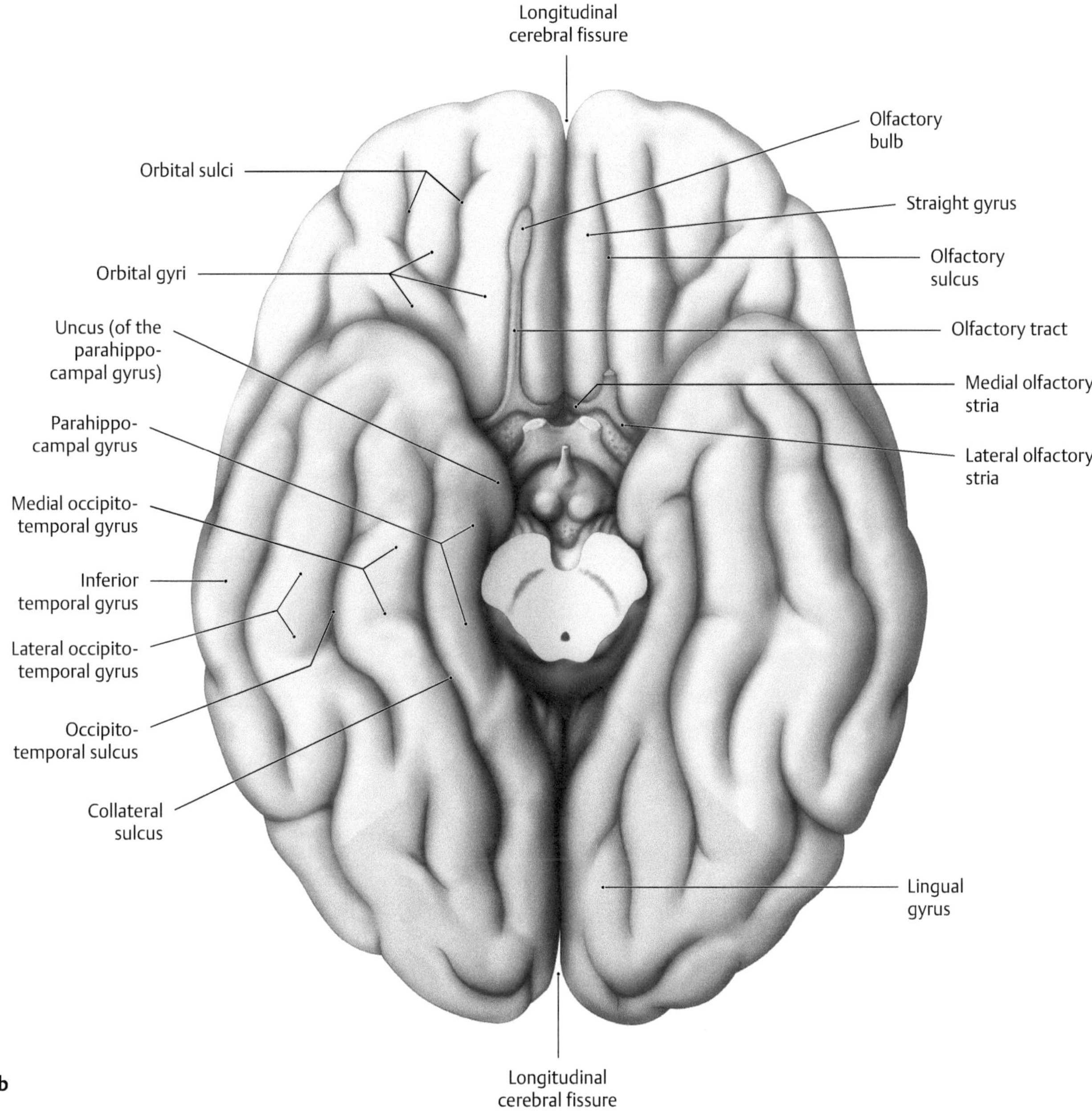

Fig. 9.55 *(continued)* **(b)** Gyri and sulci at the base of the brain. *(continued)* (From Schuenke M, Schulte E, Schumacher U. THIEME Atlas of Anatomy. Head, Neck, and Neuroanatomy. Illustrations by Voll M and Wesker K. 3rd ed. New York: Thieme Medical Publishers; 2020.)

areas 3, 1, and 2 but area 7 also receives visual information from area 19. Damage to this region results in contralateral losses of tactile discrimination, loss of the ability to recognize the position of body parts in space (statognosis), and loss of the ability to recognize form (stereognosis). The supramarginal gyrus portion incorporates somatosensory, visual, and auditory information. Damage to this specific region could lead to both motor and sensory apraxia (**Fig. 9.56a, b**).

- **Primary gustatory cortex**: also known as **area 43**, this cortex is located in the parietal operculum and parainsular cortex. Little is known about its exact function but it does receive taste information from the ventral posteromedial nucleus of the thalamus. Lesions of this region would ultimately have an effect on taste sensation (**Fig. 9.56b**).

9.16.3 Temporal Lobe

The **temporal lobe** is located inferior to the lateral sulcus and consists of three gyri separated by two sulci. The **superior temporal** and **middle temporal gyri** are separated by the **superior temporal sulcus**. The **inferior temporal** and **middle temporal gyri** are separated by the **inferior temporal sulcus**. The inferior temporal gyrus continues onto the inferior surface of the cerebral hemisphere. On the inferior surface of the temporal lobe, the **lateral occipitotemporal (fusiform) gyrus** is separated from the **medial occipitotemporal gyrus** by the **occipitotemporal sulcus**. The **parahippocampal gyrus** is continuous posteriorly with the lingual gyrus of the occipital lobe but is separated from the medial occipitotemporal gyrus by the **collateral sulcus**. Anteriorly it

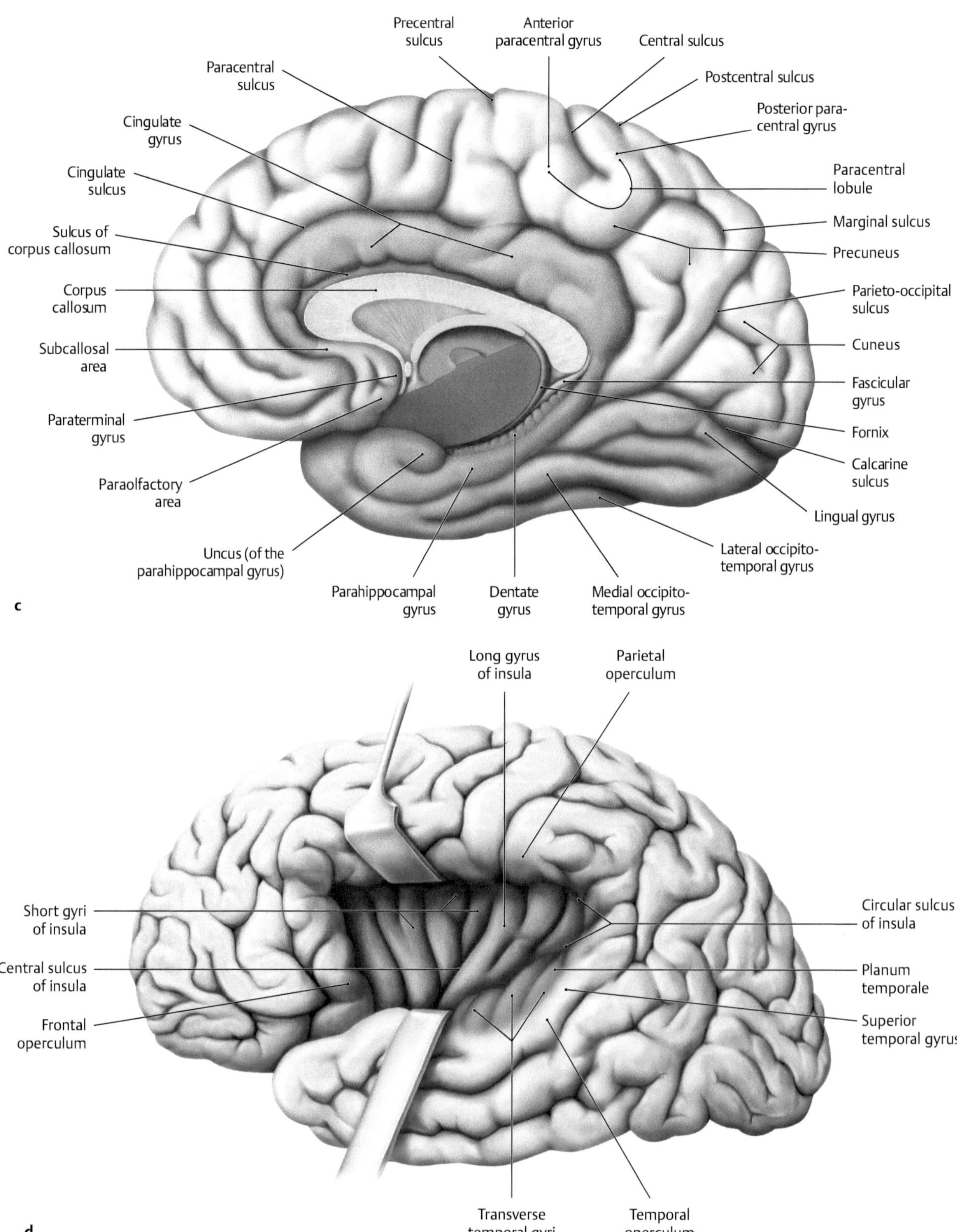

Fig. 9.55 *(continued)* **(c)** Gyri and sulci of the medial surface. **(d)** Gyri and sulci of the insula. (From Schuenke M, Schulte E, Schumacher U. THIEME Atlas of Anatomy. Head, Neck, and Neuroanatomy. Illustrations by Voll M and Wesker K. 3rd ed. New York: Thieme Medical Publishers; 2020.)

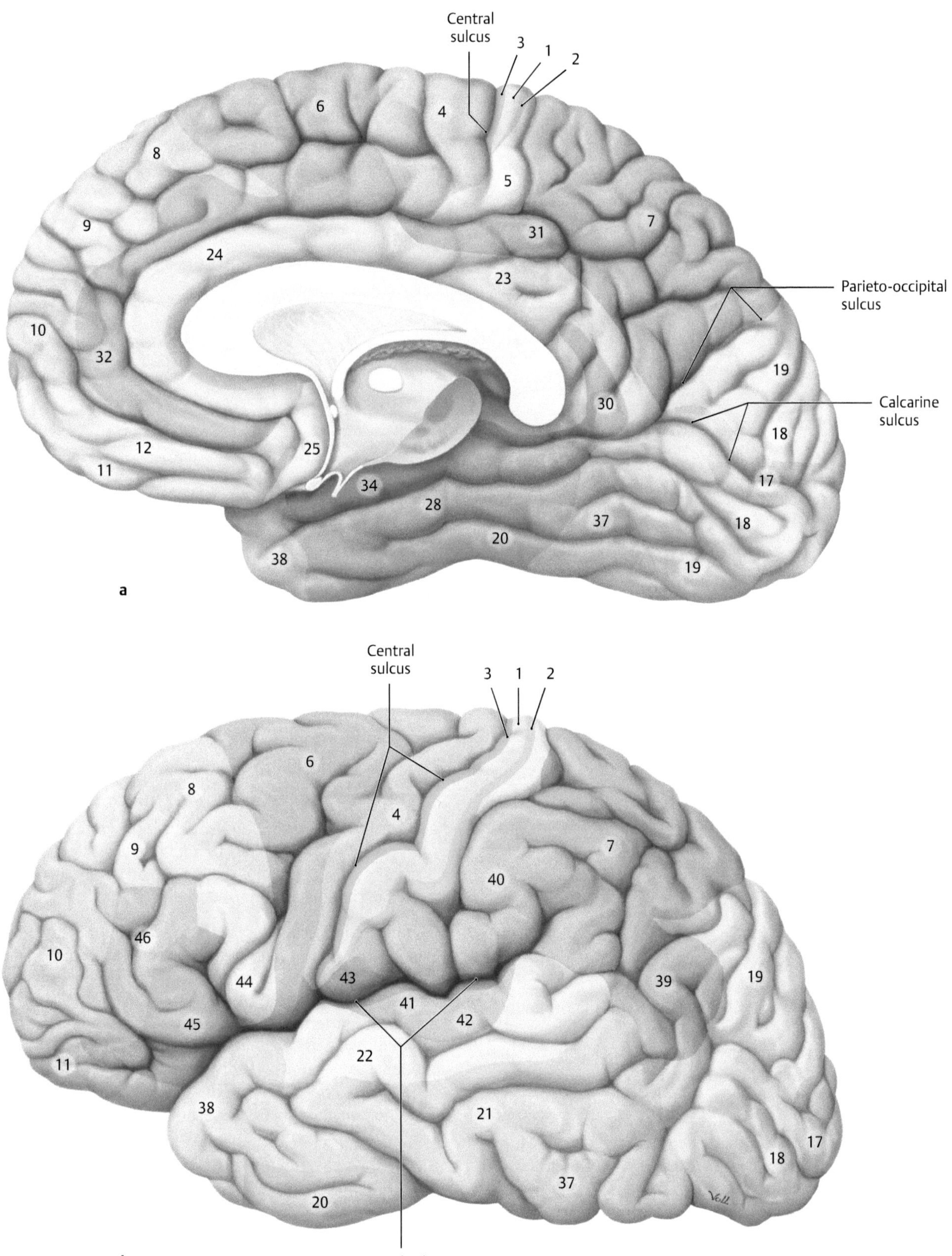

Fig. 9.56 Neocortex, cortical areas. **(a)** Brodmann areas in a midsagittal section of the right cerebral hemisphere, viewed from the left side. **(b)** Brodmann areas seen from the lateral view of the left cerebral hemisphere. (*continued*) (From Schuenke M, Schulte E, Schumacher U. THIEME Atlas of Anatomy. Head, Neck, and Neuroanatomy. Illustrations by Voll M and Wesker K. 3rd ed. New York: Thieme Medical Publishers; 2020.)

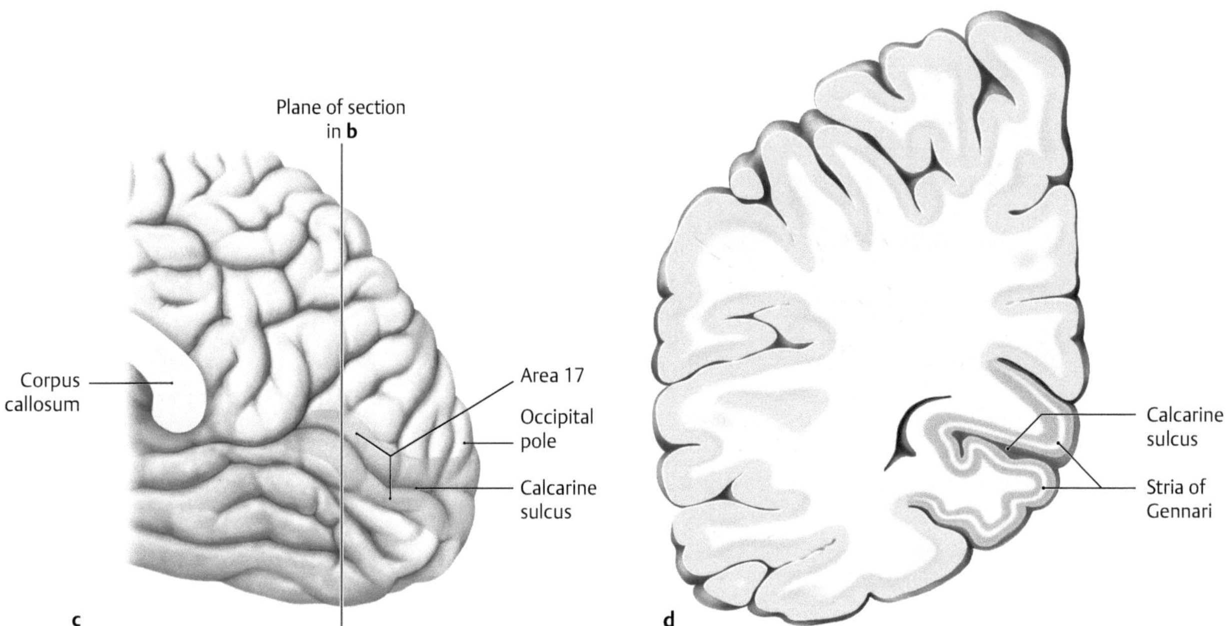

Fig. 9.56 *(continued)* **(c)** The visual cortex on the medial aspect of the right hemisphere viewed from the left side; **(d)** The visual cortex through a coronal section, anterior view. (From Schuenke M, Schulte E, Schumacher U. THIEME Atlas of Anatomy. Head, Neck, and Neuroanatomy. Illustrations by Voll M and Wesker K. 3rd ed. New York: Thieme Medical Publishers; 2020.)

terminates as a hook-like structure called the **uncus**. The **transverse temporal gyri** (*of Heschl*) are buried within the lateral sulcus and close to the insula. Special features of the cortex of this lobe include (**Fig. 9.55**):

- **Primary auditory cortex**: located in the superior temporal gyrus and the transverse temporal gyri (*of Heschl*) and receives information from the medial geniculate body. It corresponds to **areas 41** and **42** and a unilateral lesion of damage to it would result in only partial deafness due to bilateral cochlear input. A bilateral lesion would result in cortical deafness (**Fig. 9.56b**).
- **Auditory association cortex**: located in the posterior portion of the superior temporal gyrus, corresponds to **area 22**, and includes ***Wernicke's speech area***. The **planum temporale** (**Fig. 9.55a**) is located within Wernicke's area and is most prominent on the left cerebral hemisphere. It is important in auditory processing and language. Wernicke's area is connected to *Broca's speech area* by the arcuate fasciculus. Lesions or damage to the dominant hemisphere results in *Wernicke sensory aphasia* while damage to the nondominant hemisphere creates an inability to perceive the pitch or rhythm of speech (sensory dysprosody). The middle temporal gyrus (**area 21**) and inferior temporal gyrus (**area 20**) are part of the auditory association cortex (**Fig. 9.56b**).
- **Primary olfactory cortex**: related to the entorhinal region or **area 34** of the parahippocampal gyrus. A lesion here results in ipsilateral loss of smell (anosmia). The uncal region of the parahippocampal gyrus is related to **area 28** and a lesion here could lead to both olfactory and gustatory hallucinations (**Fig. 9.56a**).
- The **occipitotemporal (fusiform) gyri** are related to **area 37** and are involved in processing color information and recognizing faces, numbers, and words. Lesions of this region cause difficulties with word retrieval and word generation (**Fig. 9.56a, b**).

9.16.4 Occipital Lobe

The **occipital lobe** is the most posterior part of the cerebral hemispheres but the orientation of gyri and sulci on the lateral surface is quite variable. There may or may not be **superior**, **middle**, and **inferior occipital gyri**, which are divided by the lateral occipital (if present) and **lunate sulci**. The medial surface is more consistent. Adjacent to the **parieto-occipital sulcus** is the **cuneus**. Inferior to the cuneus is the **calcarine sulcus** and this sulcus lies adjacent to the **lingual gyrus** (**Fig. 9.55a–c; Fig. 9.56c, d**). Special features of the cortex of this lobe include:

- **Primary visual cortex**: located in the calcarine sulcus and corresponds with **area 17**. It receives information from the lateral geniculate body and damage to the region leads to visual field defects (**Fig. 9.56**).
- **Visual association cortices**: related to **areas 18** and **19** and damage to these areas could lead to visual hallucinations. An additional association cortex is located at the angular gyrus of the temporal lobe. Damage to this region could lead to contralateral homonymous hemianopia or inferior quadrantanopia along with *Gerstmann syndrome*, which involves the inability to express thoughts in writing (agraphia), inability to recognize your own fingers (finger agnosia), difficulty in learning and comprehending mathematics (dyscalculia), and left-right confusion disorientation (**Fig. 9.56**).

9.16.5 Limbic Lobe

The **limbic lobe** is seen on the medial side and is represented by the **cingulate gyrus**. This gyrus is bordered superiorly by the **cingulate sulcus** and inferiorly by the **corpus callosum**. The sulcus that separates the cingulate gyrus and corpus callosum can be

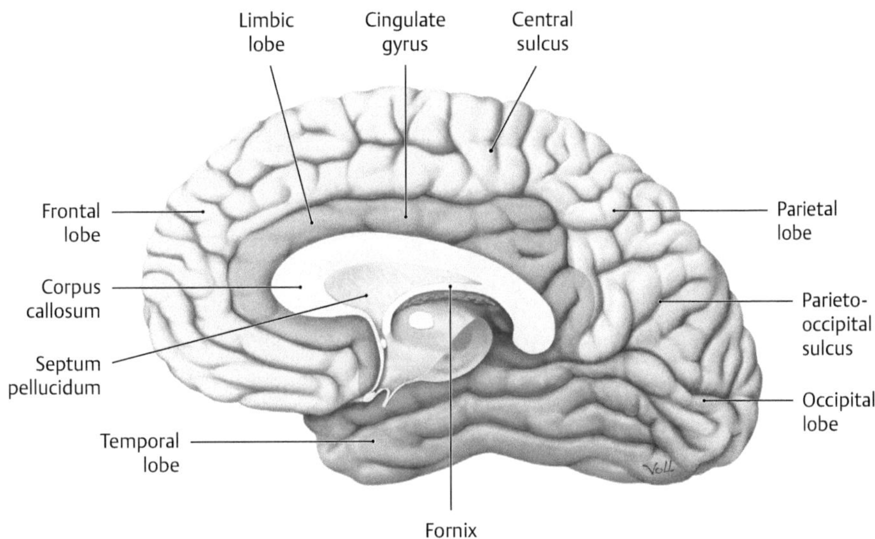

Fig. 9.57 Division of the cerebral hemispheres into lobes; medial view of the right hemisphere. (From Schuenke M, Schulte E, Schumacher U. THIEME Atlas of Anatomy. Head, Neck, and Neuroanatomy. Illustrations by Voll M and Wesker K. 3rd ed. New York: Thieme Medical Publishers; 2020.)

simply referred to as the **sulcus of the corpus callosum (callosal sulcus)** (**Fig. 9.55c; Fig. 9.57**).

The **insula** can be seen after the lateral sulcus is retracted. Anterior to the **central sulcus of insula**, there are a number of **short gyri** and posterior to it there is the **long gyrus of insula**. Retraction of the lateral sulcus also helps expose certain areas that are unrelated to the insula. The **frontal operculum** is a part of the frontal lobe and is associated with *Broca's area*, a region referred to as the motor speech center. The **parietal operculum** is part of the parietal lobe and it covers the superior surface of the insula while the **temporal operculum** is part of the temporal lobe and covers the inferior surface of the insula. The transverse temporal gyri (*of Heschl*) are separated from the insular gyri by the **circular sulcus of insula** (**Fig. 9.55d**).

9.16.6 Cortical Homunculus

A somatotopic organization exists depicting both sensory and motor innervation. The **cortical homunculus** is a pictorial representation of the anatomical divisions of the primary somatosensory and motor cortices, the particular parts of the brain responsible for the exchange of sensory and motor information traveling from and to parts of the body. The primary somatosensory cortex is concerned with the signals within the postcentral gyrus coming from the thalamus (**Fig. 9.58**), while the primary motor cortex pertains to impulses within the precentral gyrus from the premotor area of the frontal lobes (**Fig. 9.59**).

The homunculus demonstrates an upside-down sensory or motor map of the contralateral side of the body. For example, structures related to the face are represented closer to the lateral sulcus whereas the toes and feet are near the longitudinal fissure. The distorted appearance is due to the amount of total cerebral tissue devoted to a particular body region.

9.16.7 Histology of the Cerebral Cortex

The cerebral cortex is composed of gray matter and forms a complete outer covering of the cerebral hemispheres. The surface area is increased with the creation of gyri. The cortex is thickest over the crest of a gyrus and thinnest deep within a sulcus. There is a mixture of nerve cells, nerve fibers, neuroglia, and the blood vessels that supply the region. The cerebral cortex is divided into six layers and the cells that are present in the cortex include the pyramidal cells, stellate cells, horizontal cells *of Cajal*, cells *of Martinotti*, and the fusiform cells.

- **Pyramidal cells**: have pyramid-shaped cell bodies with the dendrites originating from the apex and the axons from the base. The largest pyramidal cells are called ***Betz cells*** and they are located in the motor precentral gyrus of the frontal lobe. The apical dendrites have **dendritic spines** and are the preferential site for synapses. Most of these cells have long axons that either extend to deeper cortical layers or enter the white matter as a commissural, association, or projection fiber. They serve as the principal output cells.
- **Stellate cells (or granule cell)**: typically small multipolar neurons that have multiple branching dendrites and a short axon that terminates on a nearby neuron. These cells serve as the principal interneurons of the cortex.
- **Horizontal cells of Cajal**: small and horizontally placed within the most superficial layer of the cortex. There is a dendrite and an axon that runs horizontally before making contact with pyramidal cell dendrites.
- **Cells of Martinotti**: small multipolar neurons that traverse all layers of the cortex. They have short dendrites and their axons are directed toward the pial surface. There may be a few collateral branches that extend from the axon.
- **Fusiform cells**: spindle-shaped and concentrated in the deepest layers of the cortex with a function similar to that of the pyramidal cells. The dendrites extend from each end of the cell body and branch within the same cellular layer while the more superior dendrites ascend toward the more superficial cortex layers. The axon originates from the inferior portion of the cell body and enters the white matter as a commissural, association or projection fiber.

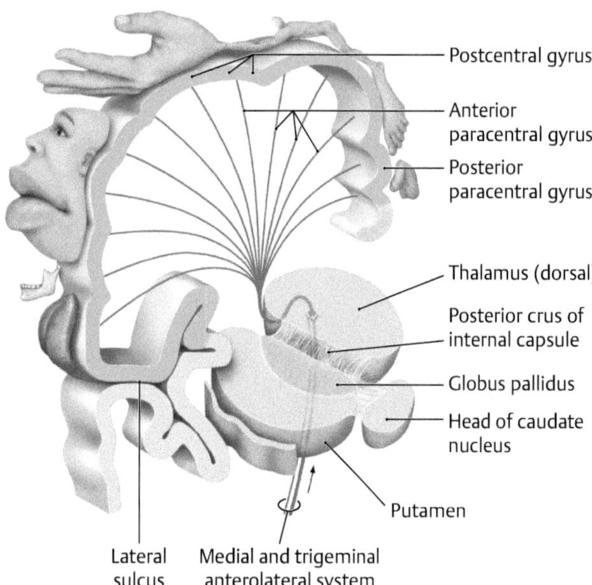

Fig. 9.58 Somatotopic organization of the somatosensory cortex: the sensory homunculus. (From Schuenke M, Schulte E, Schumacher U. THIEME Atlas of Anatomy. Head, Neck, and Neuroanatomy. Illustrations by Voll M and Wesker K. 3rd ed. New York: Thieme Medical Publishers; 2020.)

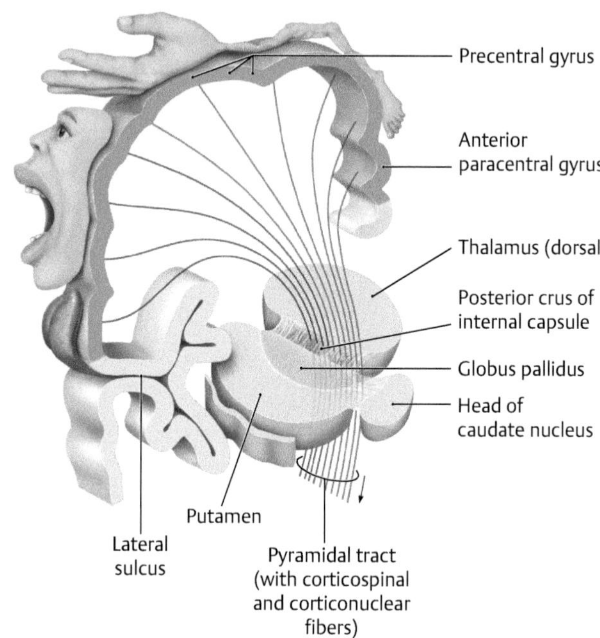

Fig. 9.59 Somatotopic organization of the somatomotor cortex: the motor homunculus. (From Schuenke M, Schulte E, Schumacher U. THIEME Atlas of Anatomy. Head, Neck, and Neuroanatomy. Illustrations by Voll M and Wesker K. 3rd ed. New York: Thieme Medical Publishers; 2020.)

Layers of the cortex are described from the most superficial to the deepest (**Fig. 9.60**).

- **Molecular (plexiform) layer**: the most superficial layer, just deep to the pia mater. A large number of synapses occur here. This layer consists primarily of a dense network of tangentially orientated nerve fibers. These nerve fibers originate from the apical dendrites of both fusiform and pyramidal cells and the axons of the cells *of Martinotti* and stellate cells.
- **External granular layer**: contains small pyramidal cells and numerous stellate cells. Dendrites of these cells terminate in the molecular layer. Axons terminate in deeper cortex layers or enter the white matter.
- **External pyramidal layer**: contains slightly larger pyramidal cells whose dendrites travel to the molecular layer and whose axons pass through the white matter as a commissural, association, or projection fiber.
- **Internal granular layer**: tightly packed stellate cells make up this layer. It receives thalamocortical fibers from the ventrolateral group of the thalamus such as the ventral posterolateral and ventral posteromedial nuclei. Higher concentrations of these fibers are horizontally arranged and are referred to as the **external band *of Baillarger***. In area 17 this external band is called the **stria *of Gennari*** (**Fig. 9.56d**).
- **Internal pyramidal layer**: much larger pyramidal cells are located in this layer with the largest ones known as the giant pyramidal cells *of Betz*. The *Betz* cells are located only in the motor cortex (area 4) and the anterior portion of the paracentral lobule. This layer gives rise to the corticospinal, corticobulbar, and corticostriatal fibers. Stellate cells and cells *of Martinotti* are scattered among the pyramidal cells and there is a large number of cells that are horizontally arranged to form the **internal band *of Baillarger***.
- **Multiform layer**: most cells of this layer are fusiform cells, with the remaining being modified pyramidal cells. The cells *of Martinotti* are clearly visible in this layer. This layer is the major source of corticothalamic fibers and also gives rise to commissural, association, and projection fibers.

Not all regions of the cerebral cortex have six layers. The regions that do have the recognizable six layers are referred to as a **homotypical cortex**. In regions of the cortex where the six layers are not recognizable this is referred to as **heterotypical cortex**. There are two heterotypical areas and they are described as either a granular or agranular type of cortex.

The **granular type** of cortex consists of granular layers that are well pronounced and contain densely packed stellate cells that receive afferent impulses. This would mean layers II and IV are well developed with layers III and V being less developed. Thus layers II-V merge into a single layer of predominately granular cells and are known for receiving thalamocortical fibers. The granular cortices are located in regions such as the postcentral, superior temporal, and parts of the hippocampal gyri. Areas related to primary sensory regions like the somatosensory, auditory, and visual cortices (**Fig. 9.61a**). The **agranular type** of cortex is defined by tightly packed pyramidal cells in layers III and V but poorly developed in layers II and IV. The agranular cortices give rise to mainly efferent motor fibers and can be found in the precentral gyrus and other regions of the frontal lobe. Areas that give rise to corticospinal and corticobulbar projections (**Fig. 9.61b**).

9.16.8 White Matter of the Cerebral Hemispheres

Myelinated nerve fibers of different diameters make up the white matter of the cerebral hemispheres. They are classified into three

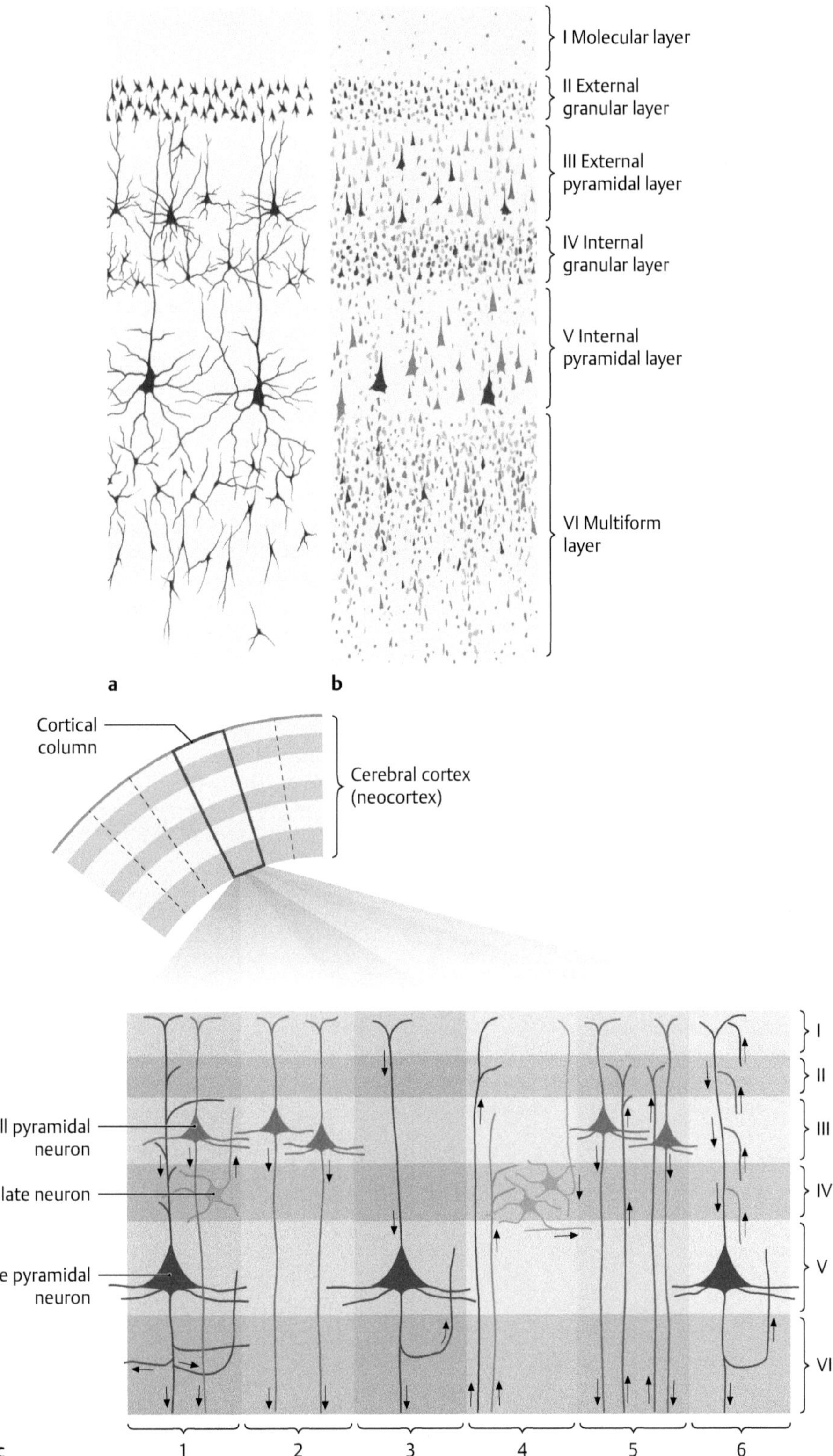

Fig. 9.60 Cerebral cortex, histological structure, and function. **(a)** Histology of the cerebral cortex (silver impregnation). **(b)** Histology of the cerebral cortex (Nissl staining). **(c)** Columnar organization of the cortex. Panels 1-3 show the principal types of cells particpating in a cortical column. Panels 4-6 contain axons projecting into the cerebral cortex. (1) Several thousand stellate neurons of various subtypes and one hundred or so large and small pyramid neurons. (2) The isolation of small pyramidal cells whose axons tend to terminate within the cortex itself. (3) The deeper, large pyramidal neurons have axons that generally project to subcortical structures. The larger cells are responsible for tracts of corticospinal and corticobulbar motor axons, which project to the spinal cord and brainstem respectively. (4) Isolation of thalamocortical projections that enter from the thalamus and synapse mostly on the stellate neurons of layer IV. (5) Association fibers of the neighboring cortex and commissural fibers from the contralateral hemisphere often terminate on the dendrites of the small pyramidal neurons. (6) Large pyramidal neurons whose apical dendrites stretch from layer V to I. (From Schuenke M, Schulte E, Schumacher U. THIEME Atlas of Anatomy. Head, Neck, and Neuroanatomy. Illustrations by Voll M and Wesker K. 3rd ed. New York: Thieme Medical Publishers; 2020.)

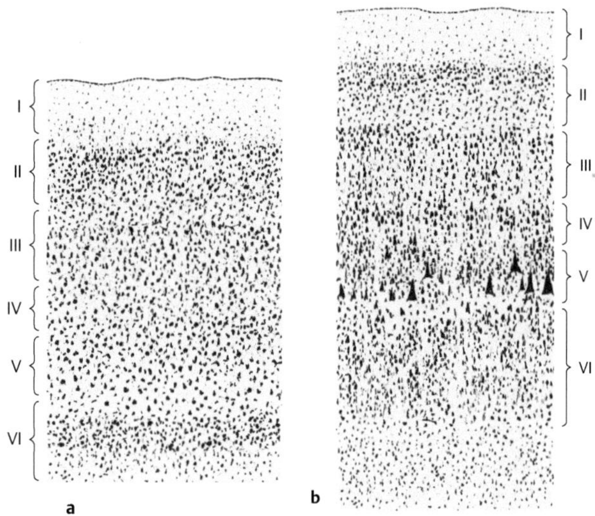

Fig. 9.61 (a) Granular cortex. **(b)** Agranular cortex. (From Schuenke M, Schulte E, Schumacher U. THIEME Atlas of Anatomy. Head, Neck, and Neuroanatomy. Illustrations by Voll M and Wesker K. 3rd ed. New York: Thieme Medical Publishers; 2020.)

groups: commissural fibers, association fibers, and projection fibers.

- **Commissural fibers**: connect corresponding regions of the two cerebral hemispheres.
  - **Corpus callosum**: connects the two cerebral hemispheres and is the largest commissure of the brain. It is located at the most inferior aspect of the longitudinal fissure and is divided into a rostrum, genu, body, and splenium. The **rostrum** is the thinner anterior portion that becomes continuous with the lamina terminalis. The curved anterior portion is the **genu** and fibers from here curve anteriorly into the frontal lobe to form the **forceps minor**. The **body** arches posteriorly and fibers from this region that extend laterally are called the **radiation of the corpus callosum**. These laterally passing fibers intersect with other association and projection fibers and are related to the posterior and lateral horns of the lateral ventricle of which these fibers are called the **tapetum**. The body terminates as the **splenium** and fibers that extend posteriorly toward the occipital lobe form the **forceps major** (**Fig. 9.62**).
  - **Anterior commissure**: a small bundle of fibers that cross the midline in the **lamina terminalis**, a structure that

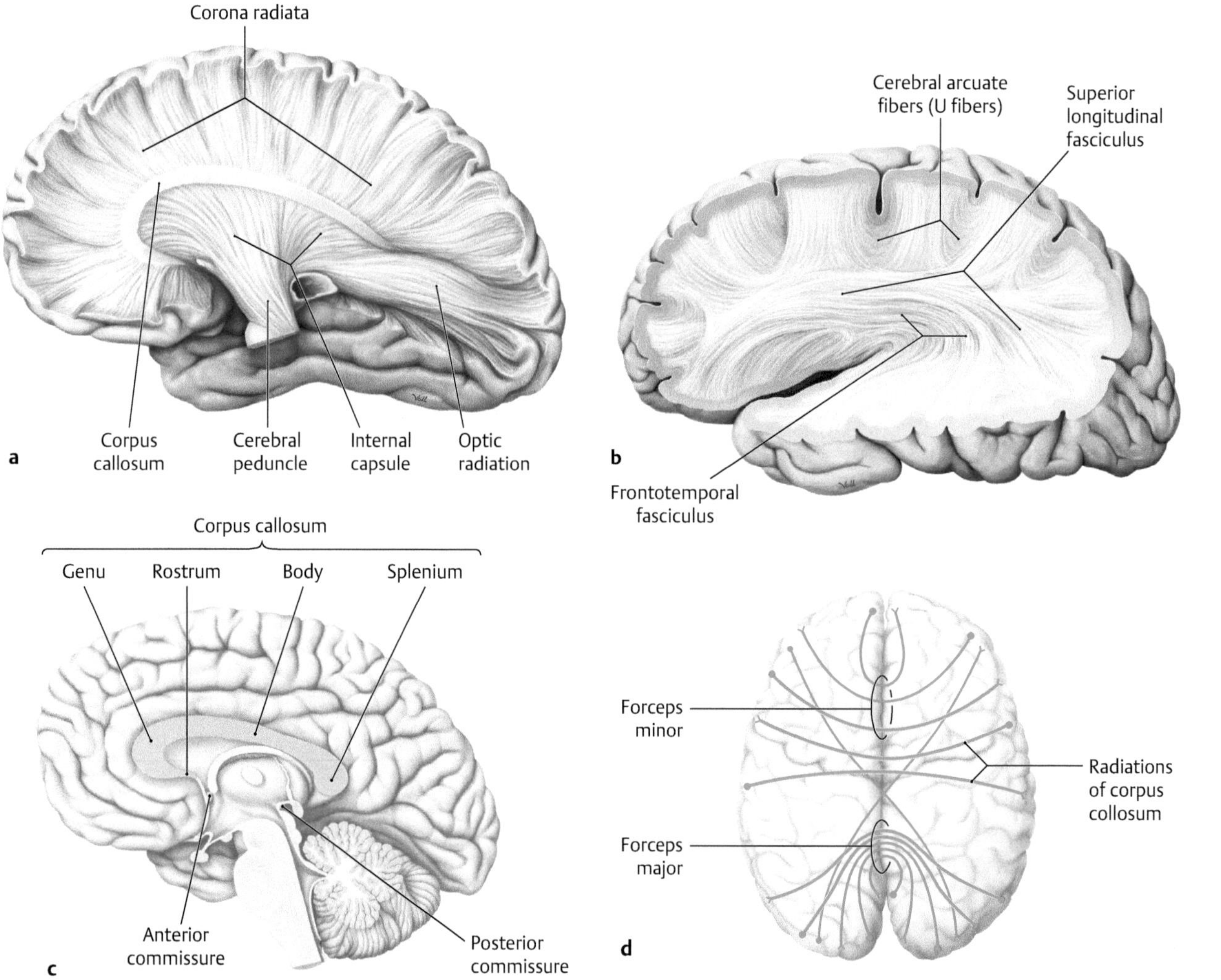

Corona radiata
a
Corpus callosum
Cerebral peduncle
Internal capsule
Optic radiation

b
Cerebral arcuate fibers (U fibers)
Superior longitudinal fasciculus
Frontotemporal fasciculus

c
Corpus callosum
Genu
Rostrum
Body
Splenium
Anterior commissure
Posterior commissure

d
Forceps minor
Forceps major
Radiations of corpus collosum

Fig. 9.62 (a) Midsagittal view of the right hemisphere viewed from the left. **(b)** Parasagittal view of the left hemisphere viewed from the left, a fiber dissection specimen. **(c)** Commissural fibers, medial view. **(d)** Commissural fibers, superior view of the transparent brain. (From Schuenke M, Schulte E, Schumacher U. THIEME Atlas of Anatomy. Head, Neck, and Neuroanatomy. Illustrations by Voll M and Wesker K. 3rd ed. New York: Thieme Medical Publishers; 2020.)

helps form the anterior wall of the third ventricle. Fibers extend anteriorly toward the olfactory tract and anterior perforated substance. Fibers can also pass posteriorly near the inferior surface of the lentiform nucleus before reaching the temporal lobes (**Fig. 9.62c**).

- **Posterior commissure**: a bundle of fibers that cross the midline just above the opening of the cerebral aqueduct into the third ventricle. These fibers are related to the inferior portion of the stalk of the pineal gland (**Fig. 9.62c**).
- **Fornix**: fibers that establish the efferent system of the hippocampus that passes to the mammillary bodies of the hypothalamus. These fibers first form the **alveus**, a thin layer of white matter covering the ventricular surface of the hippocampus before forming the **fimbria**. As they reach the posterior end of the hippocampus, the fimbria arches anteriorly above the thalamus and below the corpus callosum to form the **posterior columns**. These columns continue as the **crura** before meeting near the midline to form the **body of the fornix**. The region between the crura and body is connected by the **commissure of the fornix**. The body splits into two **anterior columns** before reaching the **mammillary bodies** (**Fig. 9.49a**).
- **Habenular commissure**: a smaller set of fibers that cross the midline near the pineal stalk. This commissure is related to the **habenular nuclei** of the **habenula**. These nuclei receive afferents from the anterior perforated substance, septal nuclei, preoptic region, amygdala, and hippocampus, of which these fibers pass to the habenular nuclei by way of the **stria medullaris of thalamus** or **stria terminalis** (**Fig. 9.42a; Fig. 9.43**).

- **Association fibers**: these types of fibers connect various cortical regions within the same hemisphere and are divided into short and long association groups.
  - **Short association**: located beneath the cortex and connect adjacent gyri (**Fig. 9.63c**).
  - **Long association**: named bundle groups that connect the more widely separated gyri. The major examples are included (**Fig. 9.62b; Fig. 9.63a, b**).
    - **Superior longitudinal fasciculus**: the largest of these types of fibers. They connect the anterior portion of the frontal lobe to the temporal and occipital lobes.
    - **Inferior longitudinal fasciculus**: passes anteriorly from the occipital lobe and continues lateral to the optic radiations before reaching the temporal lobe.
    - **Uncinate fasciculus**: connects the anterior temporal lobe with the medial and lateral orbitofrontal cortex. Function is unknown but it is considered a part of the limbic system and may be involved in the formation and retrieval of episodic memories.
    - **Cingulum**: lies within the cingulate gyrus and connects the frontal and parietal lobes with the parahippocampal gyrus and uncus of the temporal lobe. It is associated with the spinothalamic tract.
    - **Occipitofrontal fasciculus**: located deep within the cerebral hemisphere near the lateral border of the caudate nucleus (superior) or putamen (inferior). It connects the frontal lobe to the temporal and occipital lobes. There is strong evidence for the inferior occipitofrontal fasciculus but not so much for a superior version.
- **Projection fibers**: the afferent and efferent fibers that connect the cerebral cortex with the brainstem and spinal cord. Most of these types of fibers rest medial to the association fibers but can converge with the anterior commissure and corpus callosum. Projection fibers produce the **internal capsule**, which consists of an **anterior limb**, **genu**, and **posterior limb**. The most posterior portion of the posterior limb contributes to the **optic radiation**, a structure that connects to the primary visual

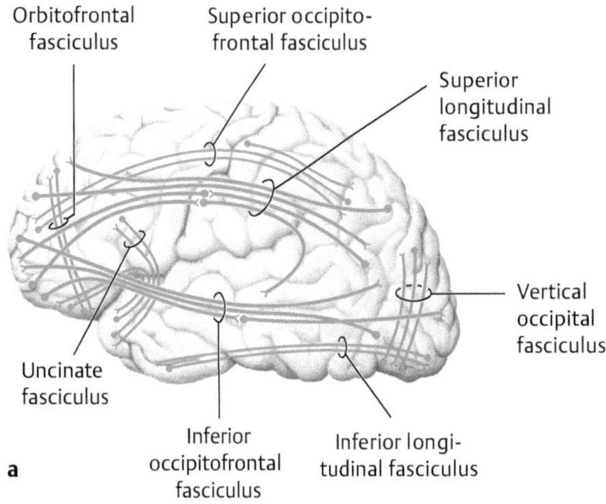

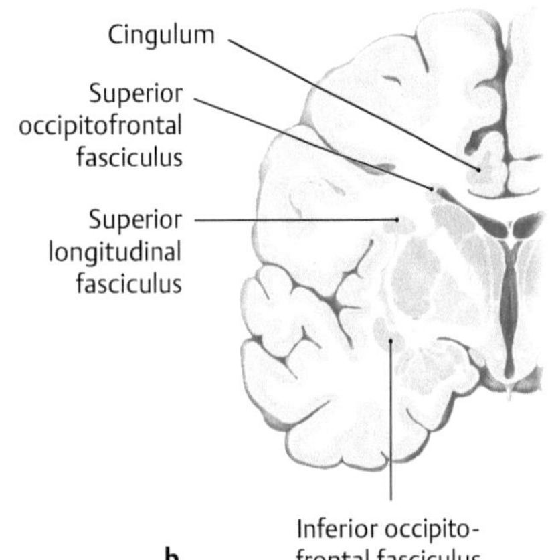

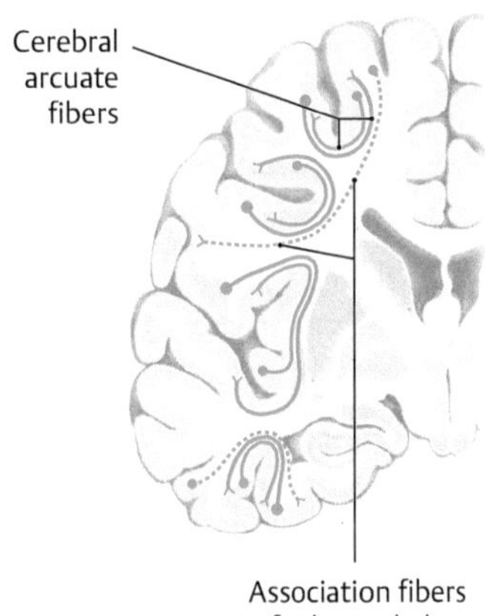

Fig. 9.63 Association fibers. **(a)** Lateral view of the left hemisphere. **(b)** Anterior view of coronal section of the right hemisphere. **(c)** Anterior view of short association fibers. (From Schuenke M, Schulte E, Schumacher U. THIEME Atlas of Anatomy. Head, Neck, and Neuroanatomy. Illustrations by Voll M and Wesker K. 3rd ed. New York: Thieme Medical Publishers; 2020.)

cortex. When the internal capsule fibers continue superiorly, they extend in all directions to the cerebral cortex. These projecting fibers are called the **corona radiata** (**Fig. 9.62a**).

9.16.9 Cerebral Dominance

Certain nervous activity is predominately performed by one of the two cerebral hemispheres. The left hemisphere is the dominant side in over 90% of the population. The dominant hemisphere controls the perception of language, speech, calculation, and handedness. Studies have determined that the hemispheres are equal in their capabilities in a newborn, but that during childhood one hemisphere becomes more dominant than the other and by the age of 10 the dominant hemisphere has been clearly established. The nondominant hemisphere becomes responsible for three-dimensional perception, musicality, and nonverbal formation of ideas and sound.

9.16.10 Blood Supply of the Cerebral Hemispheres

The **anterior cerebral arteries** are branches of the internal carotid arteries and help form a portion of the circle of Willis. The **anterior communicating artery** connects these two vessels near the longitudinal fissure. Together the anterior cerebral arteries and their branches contribute blood to the medial aspect of the cerebral hemispheres, specifically the midline and superior portions of the frontal lobe, olfactory cortex, the superomedial part of the parietal lobe, cingulate gyrus of the limbic lobe, and all of the corpus callosum except the splenium portion. Occlusion of these arteries could result in contralateral somatosensory loss and weakness and hyperflexia in the lower extremity. It may also involve a partial loss of coordinated movements (dyspraxia) or tactile agnosia (**Fig. 9.64**).

The **middle cerebral arteries** originate from the internal carotid arteries and they continue into the lateral sulcus before giving off branches responsible for supplying blood to the majority of the lateral surfaces of the cerebral hemispheres including Broca's and Wernicke's areas. Occlusions could result in contralateral facial and upper extremity weakness, altered judgment, mood issues, conjugate deviation of the eyes to the affected side, Broca's and/or Wernicke's aphasia, auditory hallucinations, loss of sensory discrimination, Gerstmann syndrome, and topographic memory loss among other symptoms (**Fig. 9.64**).

The **posterior cerebral arteries** originate between the junction of the basilar and posterior communicating arteries. They supply the occipital lobe, posteromedial portion of the temporal lobe, and the splenium of the corpus callosum. Occlusions of this artery could result in contralateral homonymous hemianopia with macular sparing and the inability to create and store long-term memories. If the occlusion was bilateral it could result in cortical blindness, the inability to identify a familiar face (prosopagnosia), and color blindness (achromatopsia) (**Fig. 9.64**).

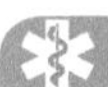

Clinical Correlate 9.20

Split-Brain Syndrome

For patients suffering from a kind of epilepsy that results in chronic and reoccurring seizures, a surgical procedure known as a *corpus callosotomy* is done and involves transecting the corpus callosum. The result of this surgery is **split-brain syndrome**. Assuming left hemisphere dominance, there would be an inability to see words (alexia) from the left visual fields because the right visual cortex has no connection with the language centers in the left hemisphere. If the patient is blindfolded they are unable to match an object held in one hand with that of an object held in the opposite hand. There is also the inability to match an object seen in the right half of the visual field with one seen in the left half. Olfaction would be perceived on the same side while hearing would be predominately on the opposite hemisphere.

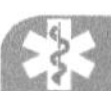

Clinical Correlate 9.21

Epilepsy

Epilepsy is a neurological disorder characterized by epileptic seizures. These seizures can be brief or progress over a longer period. They can be nearly undetectable or involve intense shaking. The cause of epilepsy is unknown but could be the result of a stroke, brain injury, brain tumor, or a birth defect. Epileptic seizures are generally the result of abnormal and excessive nerve cell activity in the cortex of the brain. Epilepsy may be confirmed with an electroencephalogram (EEG) and the seizures associated with it can be controlled for the majority of patients with anticonvulsant medications.

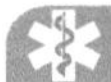

Clinical Correlate 9.22

Sleep

Sleep is the naturally occurring condition of rest the body and mind undertake for several hours every night. It involves the eyes being closed, the nervous system becoming relatively inactive, relaxation of the muscles, and suspension of an individual's consciousness. Structures related to sleep include the suprachiasmatic nucleus of the hypothalamus, pineal gland, thalamus, brainstem, and amygdala. Sleep is described as either rapid eye movement (REM) or non-REM sleep (three total stages). A sleeper cycles through all stages of REM and non-REM sleep multiple times each night. The cycles become increasingly longer and deeper during a typical night of sleep.

Stage 1 non-REM is moving from wakefulness to sleep and may only last a few minutes. A person's breathing, heartbeat, and eye movements slow with occasional muscle twitches. **Stage 2 non-REM** is a period of light sleep before entering deeper sleep. An individual's heart rate, breathing, and brain activity slow but there will be brief bursts of electrical brain activity. The body temperature drops and the muscles become more relaxed. Most sleep takes place in stage 2. **Stage 3 non-REM** is deep sleep and it occurs in longer periods during the first half of a normal sleep pattern. It is the sleep that allows a person to wake up feeling refreshed in the morning. The heart and breathing rates are at the lowest during this stage. Brain waves are even slower and it is often difficult to awaken someone during this stage of sleep. **REM sleep** first begins approximately 90 minutes after falling asleep. The eyes move rapidly and brain activity is similar to when a person is nearing waking up. Heart, blood pressure, and breathing rates all increase but muscles are temporarily paralyzed. This stage is when most dreams take place and may be the time when memory consolidation occurs. Older people spend a smaller proportion of time in REM sleep.

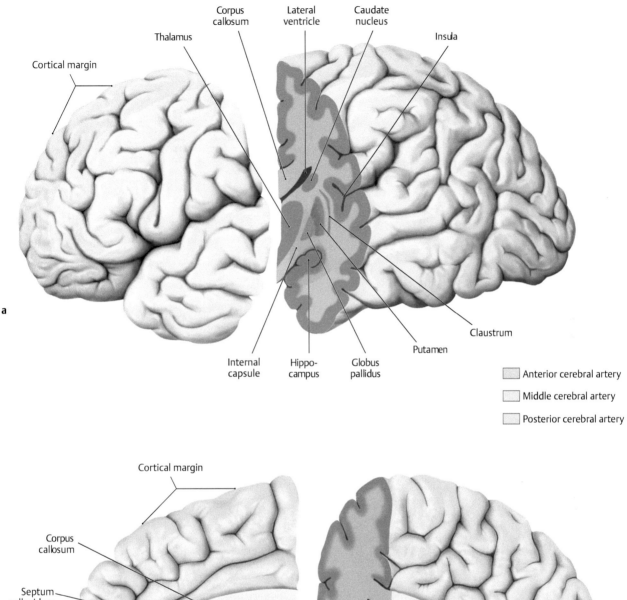

Cortical margin
Thalamus
Corpus callosum
Lateral ventricle
Caudate nucleus
Insula
Claustrum
Putamen
Internal capsule
Hippo-campus
Globus pallidus

a

Anterior cerebral artery
Middle cerebral artery
Posterior cerebral artery

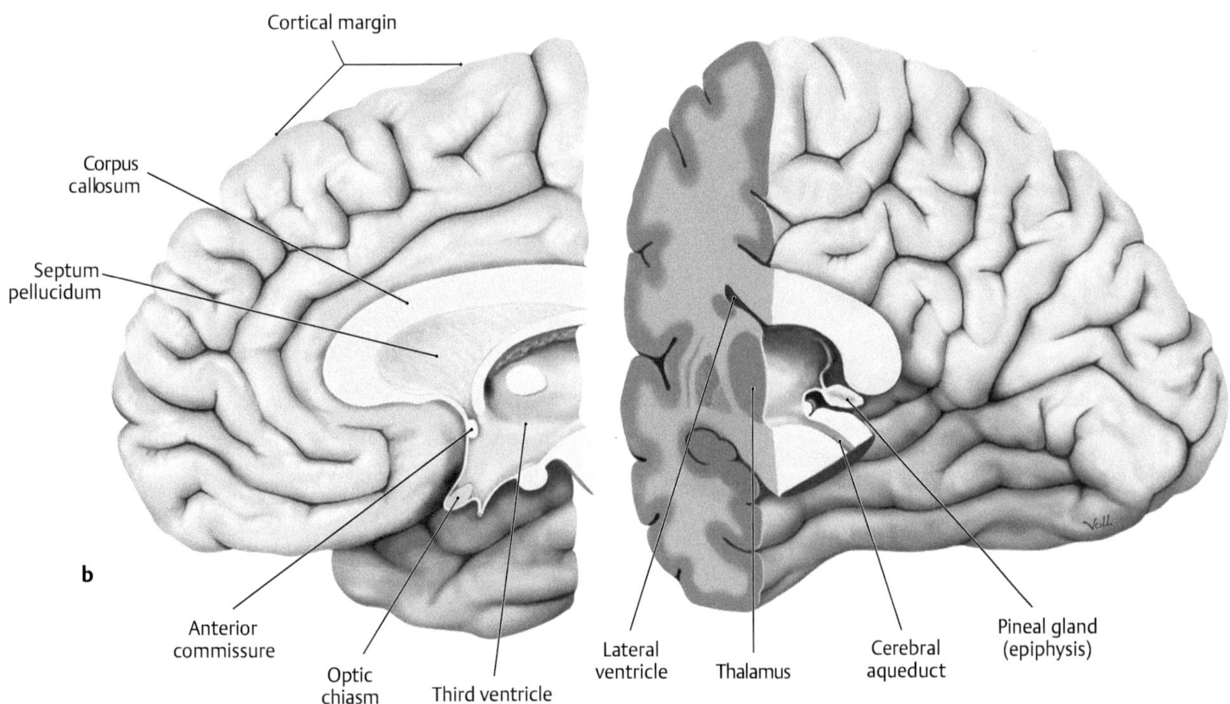

Fig. 9.64 Distribution areas of the main cerebral arteries. **(a)** Lateral view of the left cerebral hemisphere. **(b)** Medial view of the right cerebral hemisphere. (*continued*) (From Schuenke M, Schulte E, Schumacher U. THIEME Atlas of Anatomy. Head, Neck, and Neuroanatomy. Illustrations by Voll M and Wesker K. 3rd ed. New York: Thieme Medical Publishers; 2020.)

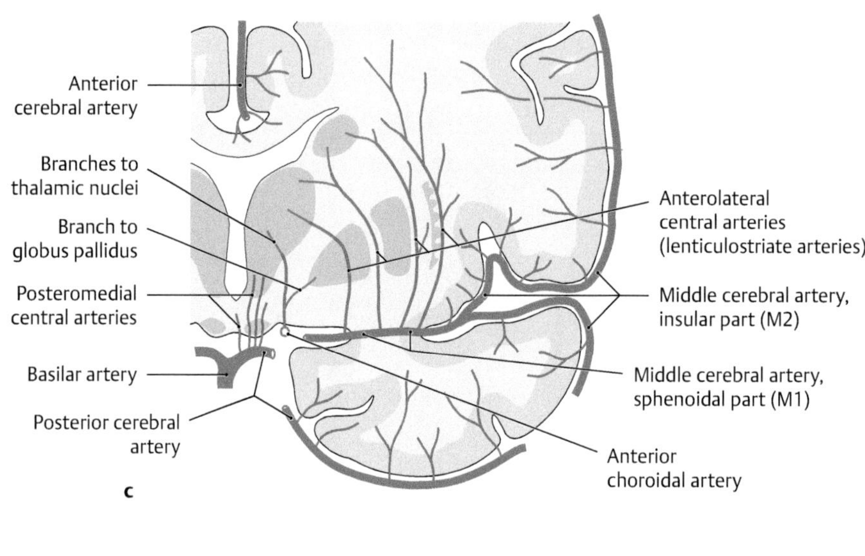

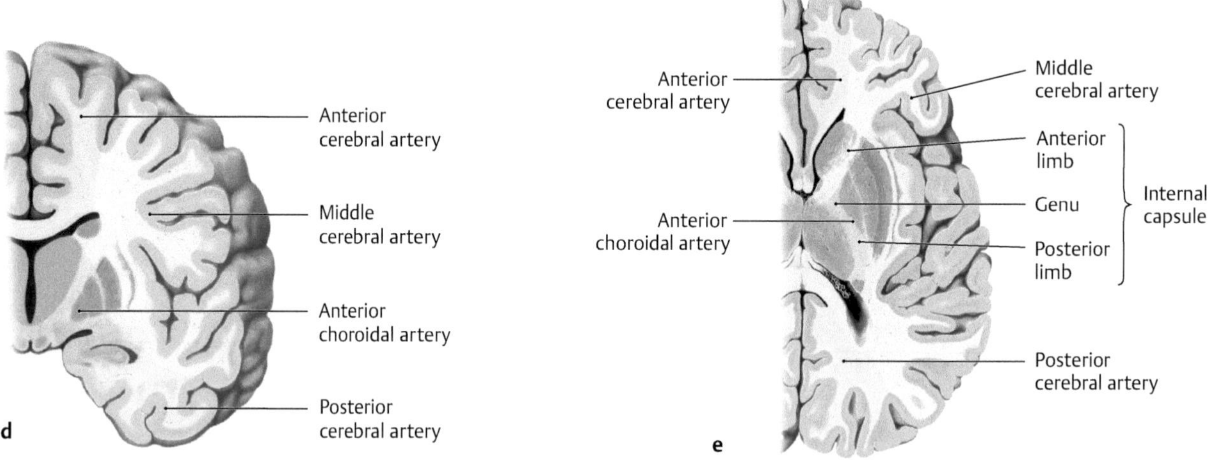

Fig. 9.64 *(continued)* Distribution areas of the main cerebral arteries. **(c, d)** Coronal sections at the level of the mammillary bodies. **(e)** Transverse section at the level of the internal capsule. (From Schuenke M, Schulte E, Schumacher U. THIEME Atlas of Anatomy. Head, Neck, and Neuroanatomy. Illustrations by Voll M and Wesker K. 3rd ed. New York: Thieme Medical Publishers; 2020.)

9.17 Ascending Sensory Pathways

The ascending sensory pathways or tracts serve as functional pathways that are responsible for conveying sensory information from the periphery to higher brain levels (**Fig. 9.65**). There is usually an organized group of first-, second-, and third-order neurons. The first-order neuron has its cell body located in the dorsal root ganglion. Upon the axon's central processes entering a spinal cord segment, they decussate or cross to the contralateral side of the spinal cord. From here the axons ascend, before reaching their final destination. The many collateral branches given off by these ascending axons serve local spinal reflex arcs.

9.18 Posterior Column-Medial Lemniscus Pathway

The **posterior column-medial lemniscus (PCML) pathway** is a somatotopically organized pathway that mediates fine touch, proprioception, and vibratory senses. Input is received from Meissner, Pacinian, and Ruffini corpuscles, hair follicles, muscle spindles, joint receptors, and Golgi tendon organs passing through A-β group II (Meissner, Pacinian, and Ruffini corpuscles and hair follicles), A-α group Ia (nuclear bag and chain fibers), and A-α group Ib fibers (Golgi tendon organs). Collateral branches can contribute to local spinal reflexes. Lesions of this tract result in the ipsilateral loss of fine discriminative touch, proprioception, and vibratory senses. A patient demonstrates a positive Romberg sign, meaning they sway or become unsteady when standing and when their eyes are closed. If their eyes are open, the visual system can help compensate for the interruption in proprioceptive input (**Fig. 9.66**).

1. 1. First-order neurons:
   1. Cell bodies are located in the **dorsal root ganglion** at all levels.
   2. Give rise to the **fasciculus gracilis** from the lower extremity and the **fasciculus cuneatus** from the upper extremity.
   3. Axons immediately ascend through the posterior columns before synapsing at the **nucleus gracilis** and **nucleus cuneatus** of the medulla, respectively.

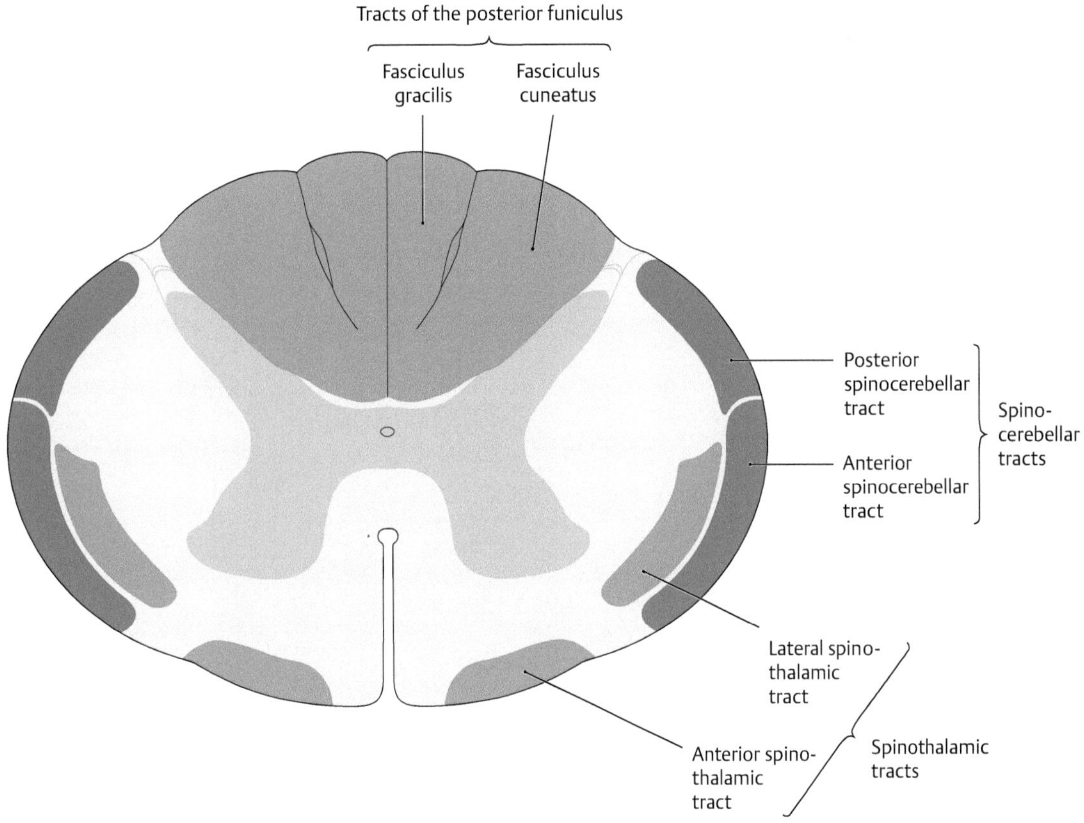

Fig. 9.65 Ascending tracts in the spinal cord. (From Schuenke M, Schulte E, Schumacher U. THIEME Atlas of Anatomy. Head, Neck, and Neuroanatomy. Illustrations by Voll M and Wesker K. 3rd ed. New York: Thieme Medical Publishers; 2020.)

4. 2. Second-order neurons:
   1. Cell bodies are located in the **nucleus gracilis** and **nucleus cuneatus**.
   2. A decussation of axons at the medulla called the **internal arcuate fibers** occurs and forms the contralateral **medial lemniscus** fiber bundle.
   3. Axons of the medial lemniscus ascend through the brainstem before terminating at the **ventral posterolateral (VPL) nucleus** of the thalamus.
4. 3. Third-order neurons:
   1. Cell bodies are located in the **VPL** of the thalamus.
   2. Axons project via the **posterior limb of the internal capsule** to the somatosensory cortex areas 3, 1, and 2 of the **postcentral gyrus**.

9.19 Anterolateral System

The **anterolateral system (ALS)** is comprised of two main functionally distinct sets of fibers called the *anterior* and *lateral spinothalamic tracts.* However, these tracts run alongside each other and can be considered a single direct pathway. Input is received from free-nerve endings and thermal receptors passing through A-δ (well-localized pain and temperature) and C fibers (itch and poorly localized dull pain, chemonociception, and temperature). The ascending and descending axons help form the **posterolateral tract** (of ***Lissauer***). The ALS originates primarily from the nucleus proprius of Rexed laminae III and IV.

Collateral branches from the direct pathway can project by way of multiple indirect pathways that are involved in the motor, autonomic, endocrine, and arousal components of pain, temperature, and nondiscriminative touch and pressure. These indirect pathways include the *spinoreticular, spinomesencephalic, spinotectal,* and *spinohypothalamic tracts.*

9.19.1 Direct Pathways

Anterior spinothalamic tract: this tract transmits nondiscriminative light (crude) touch and pressure. Input is received from free-nerve endings and Merkel disks. Lesions of this tract result in the contralateral loss of crude touch sensation starting three to four segments below the lesion (**Fig 9.67a, b; Fig. 9.68**).

1. First-order neurons:
   - Cell bodies are located in the **dorsal root ganglion** at all levels.
   - The central processes of these axons enter the spinal cord and either remain, ascend, or descend through the posterior horn of the gray matter. The entering axons generally ascend or descend multiple spinal segments before synapsing at a neuron in the posterior horn somewhere in laminae I–IV.

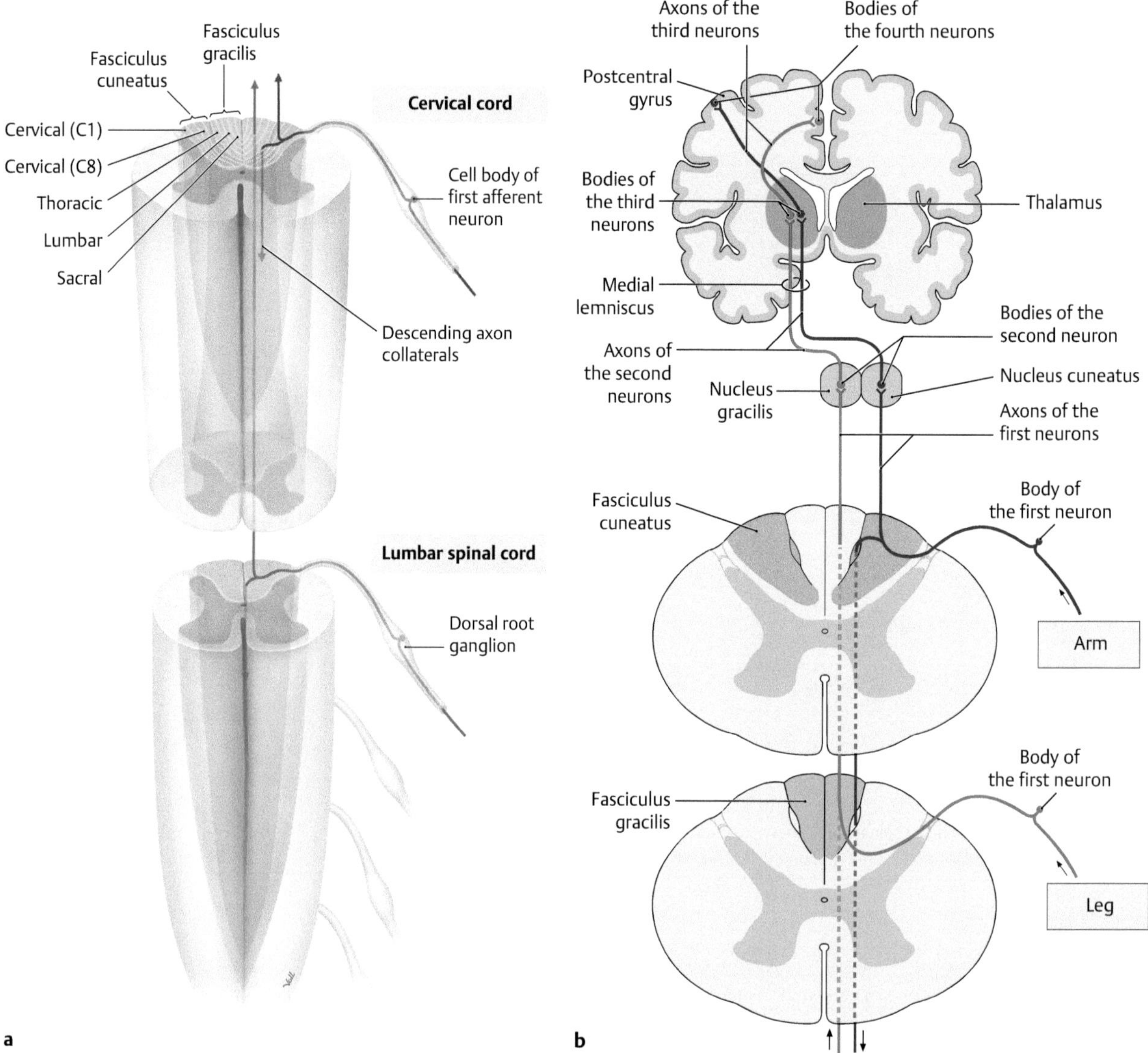

Fig. 9.66 **(a)** Ascending axons in the fasciculus gracilis and fasciculus cuneatus of the posterior column-medial lemniscus pathway. **(b)** Central connections of the posterior column-medial lemniscus pathway. (From Schuenke M, Schulte E, Schumacher U. THIEME Atlas of Anatomy. Head, Neck, and Neuroanatomy. Illustrations by Voll M and Wesker K. 3rd ed. New York: Thieme Medical Publishers; 2020.)

2. Second-order neurons:
   - Cell bodies are located in the **posterior horn.**
- Their axons decussate at the **anterior white commissure** before reaching the contralateral anterior spinothalamic tract.
   - These axons continue and ascend to the brainstem before terminating at the **VPL nucleus** of the thalamus.
3. Third-order neurons:
   - Cell bodies are located in the **VPL nucleus** of the thalamus.
   - Axons project via the **posterior limb of the internal capsule** and **corona radiata** to the somatosensory cortex areas 3, 1, and 2 of the **postcentral gyrus.**

Lateral spinothalamic tract: this tract is a somatotopically organized pathway that mediates pain, temperature, and itch sensations. Input is received from free-nerve endings and thermal receptors. Lesions of this tract result in the contralateral loss of pain, temperature, and itch sensations starting one segment below the lesion (**Fig 9.67a, c; Fig. 9.68**).

1. First-order neurons:
   - Cell bodies are located in the **dorsal root ganglion** at all levels.
   - The central processes of these axons enter the spinal cord and synapse at the posterior horn generally at the same level but possibly one to two segments above or below.
2. Second-order neurons:
   - Cell bodies are located in the **posterior horn.**
   - Their axons decussate at the **anterior white commissure** before reaching the contralateral lateral spinothalamic tract.
   - These axons continue and ascend to the brainstem before terminating at the contralateral **VPL nucleus** and bilaterally at the intralaminar nuclei of the thalamus.
3. Third-order neurons:
   - Cell bodies are located in the **VPL nucleus** of the thalamus and **intralaminar nuclei.**

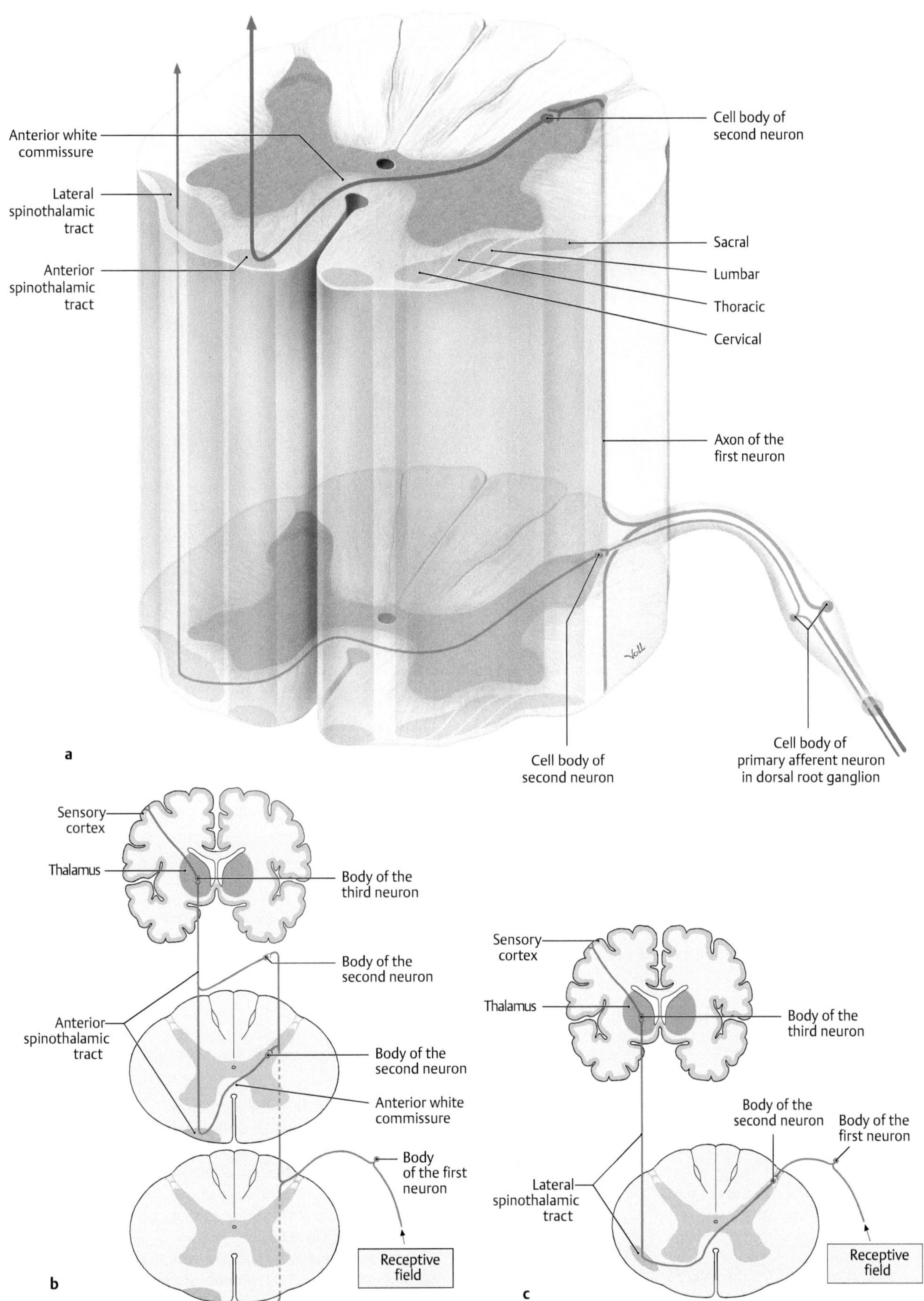

Fig. 9.67 (a) Course of the anterior and lateral spinothalamic tracts in a transverse section of the spinal cord. **(b)** Central connections of the anterior spinothalamic tract. **(c)** Central connections of the lateral spinothalamic tract. (From Schuenke M, Schulte E, Schumacher U. THIEME Atlas of Anatomy. Head, Neck, and Neuroanatomy. Illustrations by Voll M and Wesker K. 3rd ed. New York: Thieme Medical Publishers; 2020.)

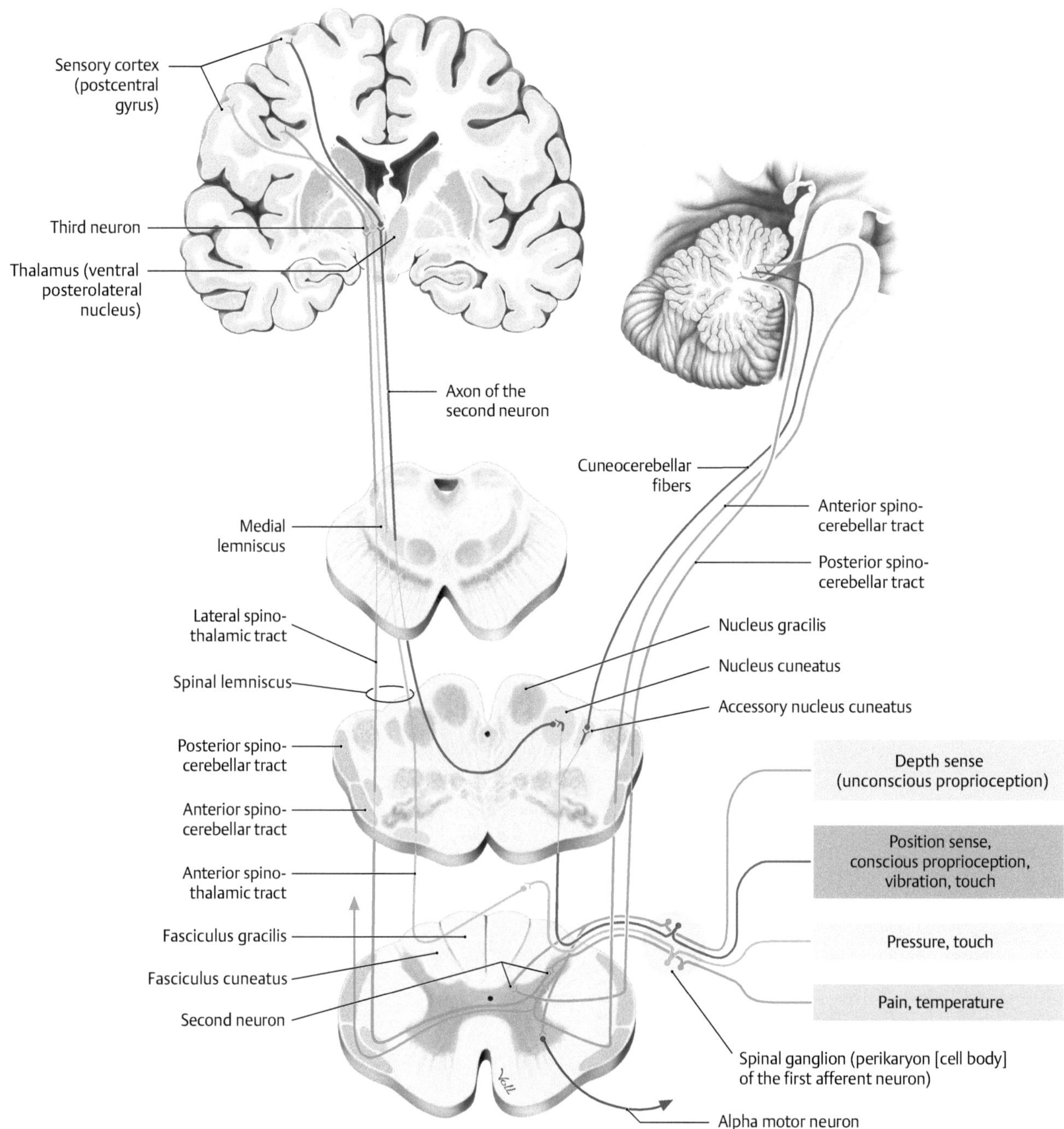

Fig. 9.68 Simplified diagram of the somatosensory pathways of the spinal cord. (From Schuenke M, Schulte E, Schumacher U. THIEME Atlas of Anatomy. Head, Neck, and Neuroanatomy. Illustrations by Voll M and Wesker K. 3rd ed. New York: Thieme Medical Publishers; 2020.)

- Axons project via the **posterior limb of the internal capsule** to the somatosensory cortex areas 3, 1, and 2 of the **postcentral gyrus**.
- Axons also project by way of intralaminar neurons to the caudatoputamen and to the frontal and parietal lobes of the cerebral cortex.

9.19.2 Indirect Pathways

- **Spinoreticular tract**: fibers convey information to the **brainstem reticular formation**, an area responsible for arousal and wakefulness. From the reticular formation, impulses are sent to the **intralaminar nuclei of the thalamus**. Both the reticular formation and the intralaminar nuclei of the thalamus are components of the **reticular-activating system (RAS)**, which functions in the activation of an individual's entire nervous system in order to elicit responses that enable them to evade painful stimuli (**Fig. 9.69**).
- **Spinomesencephalic tract**: fibers terminate in the **periaqueductal gray matter** and the **midbrain raphe nuclei**, structures that give rise to additional fibers that modulate nociceptive transmission through the *descending pain inhibiting system*.

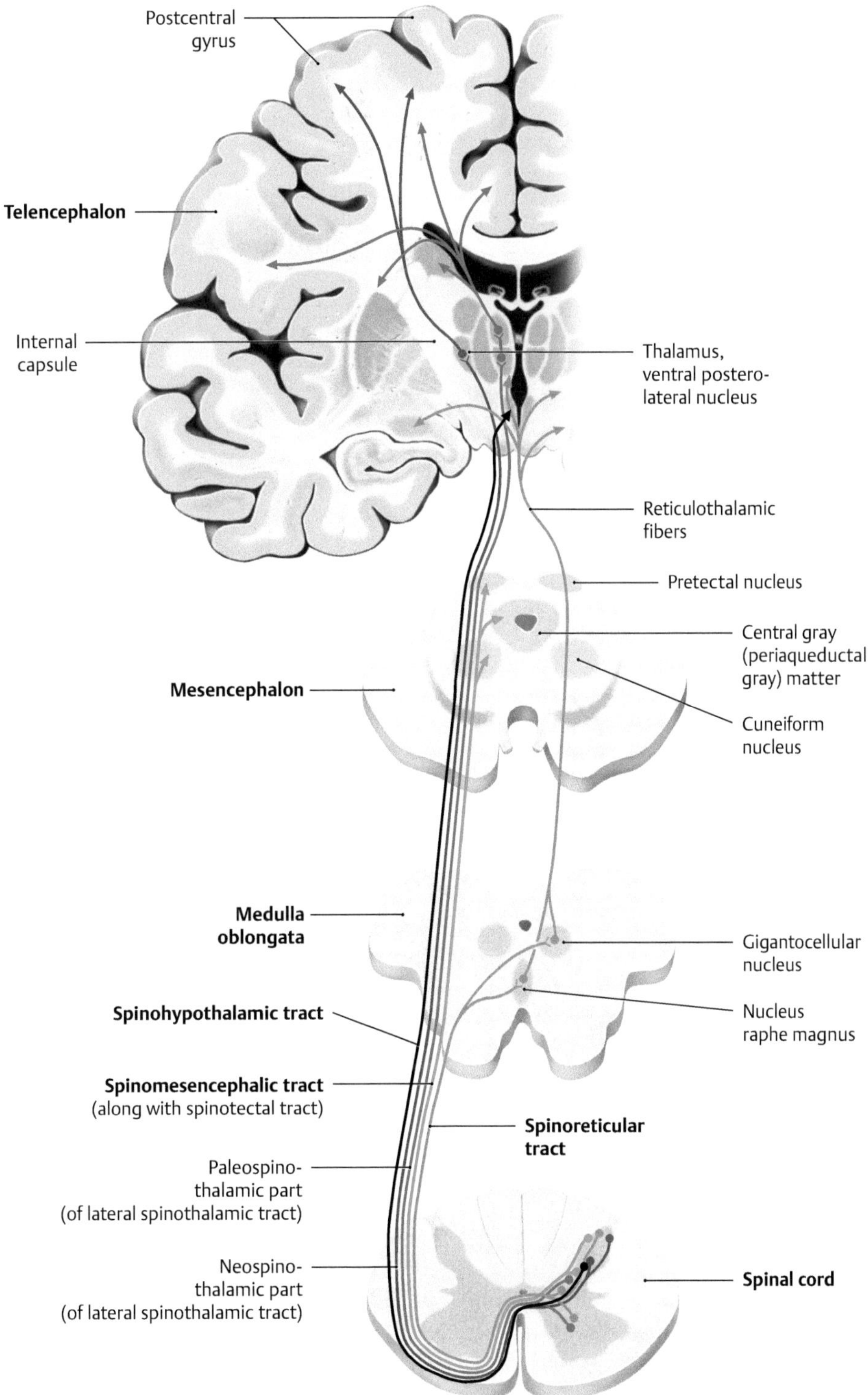

Fig. 9.69 Indirect pathways related to the anterolateral system. (From Schuenke M, Schulte E, Schumacher U. THIEME Atlas of Anatomy. Head, Neck, and Neuroanatomy. Illustrations by Voll M and Wesker K. 3rd ed. New York: Thieme Medical Publishers; 2020.)

Additional fibers of this main tract can terminate at the **parabrachial nucleus**, which sends information to the amygdala and plays a role in the emotional response to pain (**Fig. 9.69**).

- **Spinotectal tract**: fibers terminate primarily in the deep layers of the **superior colliculus** and have a reflex action to turn the upper body, head, and eyes in the direction of a painful stimulus.
- **Spinohypothalamic tract**: fibers terminate in the **hypothalamus** and are associated with autonomic reflex responses to nociception (**Fig. 9.69**).

9.20 Cerebellar Tracts

Posterior spinocerebellar tract: this tract transmits unconscious proprioceptive information back to the cerebellum. It is concerned with maintaining posture and coordinating movements of the lower extremity and ipsilateral trunk muscles. Input is received from muscle spindles, Golgi tendon organs, and pressure receptors. Fibers of this tract do not decussate. Lesions of this individual tract are rare, but if present there would include an ipsilateral lack of muscle coordination (dystaxia) of the lower limb (**Fig. 9.68; Fig. 9.70a, c**).

1. First-order neurons:
   - Cell bodies are located in the **dorsal root ganglion** from C8 to S3.
   - The axons from spinal segments C8–L2 synapse directly at the ipsilateral posterior thoracic nucleus (dorsal nucleus of Clarke).
   - The axons from below the L2 spinal segment must ascend through the fasciculus gracilis before synapsing at the caudal portion of the posterior thoracic nucleus.
2. Second-order neurons:
   - Cell bodies are located in the **posterior thoracic nucleus (dorsal nucleus of Clarke)**.
   - The axons of the second-order neurons ascend ipsilaterally in the lateral funiculus before continuing through the **restiform body** of the **inferior cerebellar peduncle**.
   - After passing through the inferior cerebellar peduncle, the axons terminate ipsilaterally as **mossy fibers** into the caudal **vermis** of the cerebellum.

Cuneocerebellar tract: transmits unconscious proprioceptive information back to the cerebellum from the neck, upper limb, and upper half of the trunk. It is the upper extremity equivalent of the posterior spinocerebellar tract. Input is received from muscle spindles and Golgi tendon organs (**Fig. 9.68**):

1. First-order neurons:
   - Cell bodies are located in the **dorsal root ganglion** and their central processes enter spinal segments C2–T5.
   - Axons ascend through the fasciculus cuneatus before synapsing at the **accessory cuneate nucleus** of the medulla.
2. Second-order neurons:
   - Cell bodies are located in the **accessory cuneate nucleus**.
   - The axons of the second-order neurons project ipsilaterally through the **restiform body** of the **inferior cerebellar peduncle** before entering the **anterior lobe** of the cerebellum.

Anterior spinocerebellar tract: transmits unconscious proprioceptive information back to the cerebellum. It is concerned with maintaining posture and coordinating movements of the lower extremity and ipsilateral trunk muscles. Input is received from muscle spindles, Golgi tendon organs, and pressure receptors. Fibers of this tract decussate. Much like the posterior spinocerebellar tract, lesions of this individual tract are rare; however, if one were present there would be a contralateral lack of muscle coordination (dystaxia) of the lower limb (**Fig. 9.68; Fig. 9.70a, b**).

1. First-order neurons:
   - Cell bodies are located in the **dorsal root ganglion** from L1 to S2.
   - Axons from these spinal segments synapse directly at the spinal border cells.
2. Second-order neurons:
   - Cell bodies are located in the **spinal border cells**.
   - Their axons decussate at the **anterior white commissure** and ascend through the lateral funiculus before continuing through the **superior cerebellar peduncle (brachium conjunctivum)**.
   - After passing through the superior cerebellar peduncle, the axons decussate again and terminate as **mossy fibers** into the rostral **vermis** of the cerebellum.

Rostral spinocerebellar tract: the head and upper limb equivalent to the anterior spinocerebellar tract but has not been well described in humans. Input is received from muscle spindles and Golgi tendon organs. Originates from cells rostral to Clarke's column and sends uncrossed axons through the lateral funiculus to the cerebellum. It reaches the cerebellum partly through the brachium conjunctivum and partly through the restiform body, terminating bilaterally in the anterior lobe of the cerebellum (not shown).

1. First-order neurons:
   - Cell bodies are located in the **dorsal root ganglion** from C4 to C8.
   - Axons from these spinal segments synapse with cell bodies located rostral to the posterior thoracic nucleus in Rexed lamina VII.
2. Second-order neurons:
   - Cell bodies of **Rexed lamina VII**.
   - Their axons ascend ipsilaterally through the lateral funiculus before continuing through both the **superior** and **inferior cerebellar peduncles**.
   - After passing through a combination of both peduncles, the axons terminate in the **anterior lobe** of the cerebellum.

Lesions of the ascending sensory pathways and those of the spinal cord and peripheral nerves are summarized in **Fig. 9.71**.

9.21 Descending Motor Pathways

The descending motor pathways or tracts originate in the brain and are responsible for initiating or modifying motor activity. The motor signals sent from the brain target lower motor neurons. The lower motor neurons then directly innervate muscles to produce movement (**Fig. 9.72**). Somatic motor activity is not an isolated action but rather an action that works along with reflex connections. Activities such as chewing, walking, and respiration operate in a reflex mode unless the action is modulated or adjusted. Motor neurons maintain a minimal basal firing rate and this represents the neurological basis of **muscle tone**. In general, the CNS transmits motor commands in response to sensory information.

The somatic nervous system includes neurons located in the cerebral cortex, brainstem, and spinal cord that serve to regulate and/or modulate the activity of the motor neurons and their interneuron pools. Motor neurons are located in Rexed lamina IX and consist of **alpha** and **gamma motor neurons**. The alpha neurons innervate extrafusal fibers or the principal contractile elements of a skeletal muscle while the gamma neurons innervate the intrafusal fibers of a muscle spindle. Motor neurons that innervate the flexor musculature are located on the posterior half of the ventral horn and the neurons that innervate the extensor musculature are on the anterior half of the ventral horn.

Interneurons are located in Rexed laminae VII and VIII, are topographically organized, and supply much of the input to lower motor neurons. Laterally located interneurons of the anterior horn are associated with lower motor neurons innervating more distal

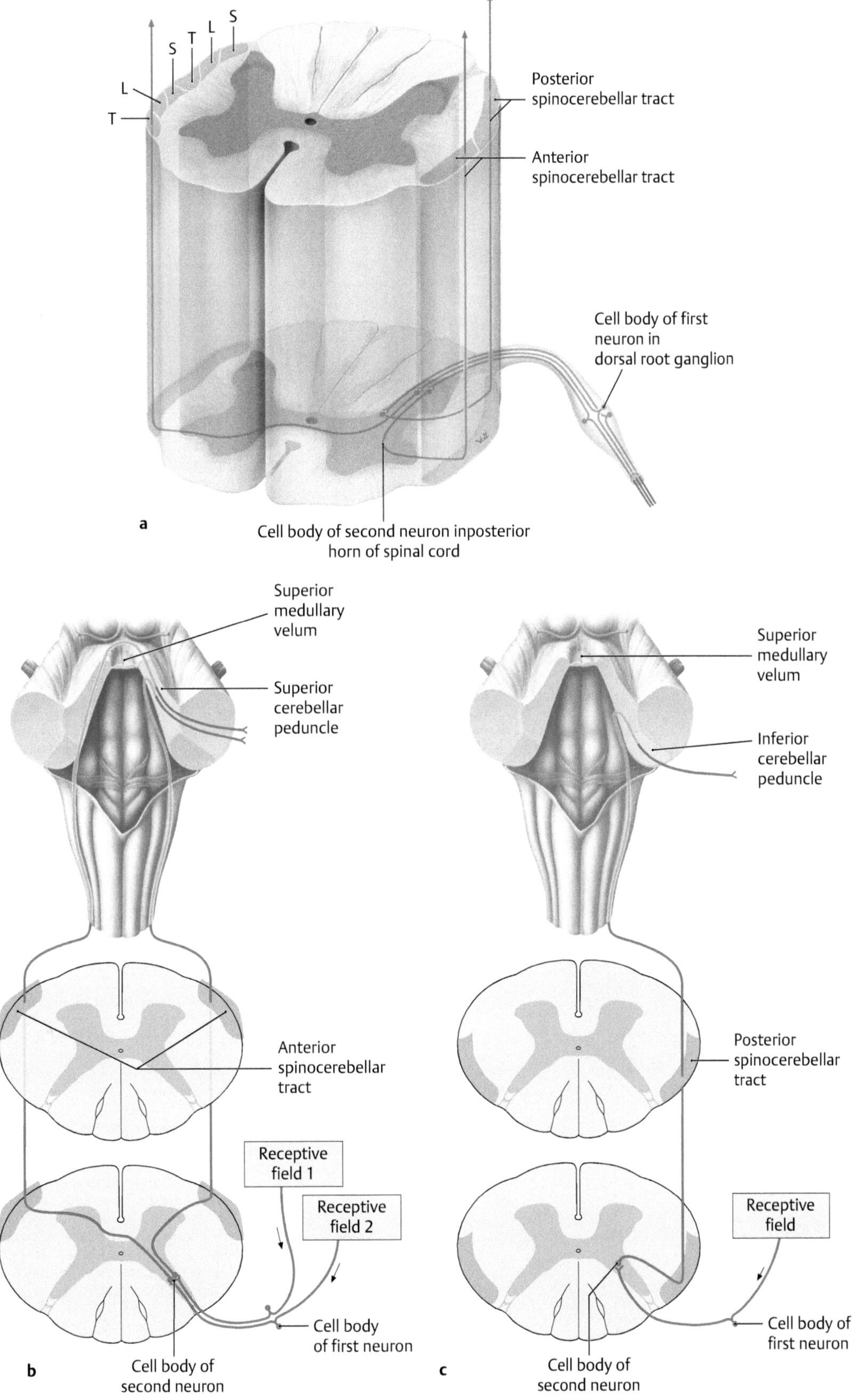

Fig. 9.70 **(a)** Course of the anterior and posterior spinocerebellar tracts in a transverse section of the spinal cord. **(b)** Central connections of the anterior spinocerebellar tract. **(c)** Central connections of the posterior spinocerebellar tract. (From Schuenke M, Schulte E, Schumacher U. THIEME Atlas of Anatomy. Head, Neck, and Neuroanatomy. Illustrations by Voll M and Wesker K. 3rd ed. New York: Thieme Medical Publishers; 2020.)

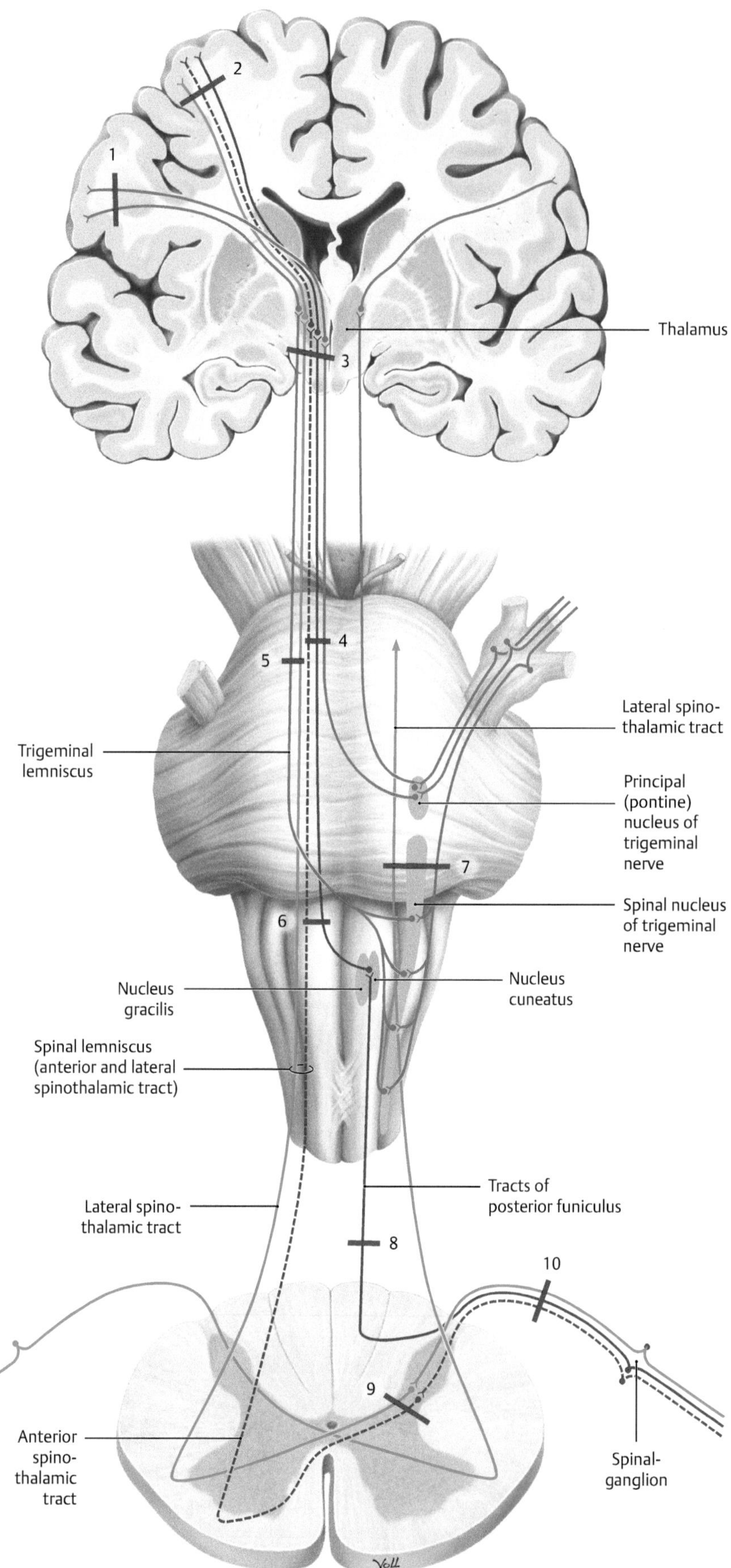

Sites of occurrence of lesions in the somatosensory pathways (after Bähr and Frotscher): The central portions of the somatosensory pathways may be damaged at various sites from the spinal root to the somatosensory cortex as a result of trauma, tumor mass effect, hemorrhage, or infarction. The signs and symptoms are helpful in determining the location of the lesion. This unit deals strictly with lesions in conscious pathways. The innervation of the trunk and limbs is mediated by the spinal erves. The innervation of the head is mediated by the trigeminal nerve, which has its own nuclei (see below).

Cortical or subcortical lesion (1, 2): A lesion at this level is manifested by paresthesia (tingling) and numbness in the corresponding regions of the trunk and limbs on the *opposite* side of the body. The symptoms may be most pronounced distally because of the large receptive fields on the fingers and the relatively small receptive fields on the trunk (see previous unit). The motor and somatosensory cortex are closely interlinked because fibers in the sensory tracts from the thalamus also terminate in the motor cortex, and because the cortical areas are adjacent (pre- and postcentral gyrus).

Lesions caudal to the thalamus (3): All sensation is abolished in the *contralateral* half of the body (thalamus = "gateway to consciousness"). A partial lesion that spares the pain and temperature pathways **(4)** is characterized by hypesthesia (decreased tactile sensation) on the *contralateral* face and body. Pain and temperature sensation are unaffected.

Lesion of the trigeminal lemniscus and lateral spinothalamic tract (5): Damage to these pathways in the brainstem causes a loss of pain and temperature sensation in the *contralateral* half of the face and body. Other sensory modalities are unaffected.

Lesion of the medial lemniscus and anterior spinothalamic tract (6): All sensory modalities on the *opposite* side of the body are abolished except for pain and temperature. The medial lemniscus transmits the axons of the second neurons of the anterior spinothalamic tract and both tracts of the posterior funiculus.

Lesion of the trigeminal nucleus, spinal tract of the trigeminal nerve, and lateral spinothalamic tract (7): Pain and temperature sensation is abolished on the *ipsilateral* side of the face (uncrossed axons of the first neuron from the trigeminal ganglion) and on the *contralateral* side of the body (axons of the crossed second neuron in the lateral spinothalamic tract).

Lesion of the posterior funiculi (8): This lesion causes an *ipsilateral* loss of position sense, vibration sense, and two-point discrimination. Because coordinated motor function relies on sensory input that operates in a feedback loop, the lack of sensory input leads to ipsilateral sensory ataxia.

Posterior horn lesion (9): A circumscribed lesion involving one or a few segments causes an *ipsilateral* loss of pain and temperature sensation in the affected segment(s), because pain and temperature sensation are relayed to the second neuron within the posterior horn. Other sensory modalities including crude touch are transmitted in the posterior funiculus and relayed to the dorsal column nuclei; hence they are unaffected. The effects of a posterior horn lesion are called a "dissociated sensory deficit."

Dorsal root lesion (10): This lesion causes *ipsilateral*, radicular sensory disturbances that may range from pain in the corresponding dermatome to a complete loss of sensation. Concomitant involvement of the ventral root leads to segmental weakness. This clinical situation may be caused by a herniated intervertebral disk. Lesions of *unconscious* cerebellar tracts that lead to sensorimotor deficits are not considered here.

Fig. 9.71 Lesions of the somatosensory system. (From Schuenke M, Schulte E, Schumacher U. THIEME Atlas of Anatomy. Head, Neck, and Neuroanatomy. Illustrations by Voll M and Wesker K. 3rd ed. New York: Thieme Medical Publishers; 2020.)

(appendicular) musculature, have shorter axons, and have collateral branches that remain mostly ipsilateral and can only extend several spinal segments. The more medially located interneurons are related to the proximal (axial) musculature, have longer axons, and have collateral branches capable of decussating to the opposite side and to many spinal segments. Due to the more restricted nature of the laterally placed interneurons, they affect muscles that participate in finer and more delicate movements. The medially placed interneurons control muscles that play a larger role in posture control (**Fig. 9.73**).

An **upper motor neuron** is a neuron that can descend from the cerebral cortex to the brainstem or spinal cord. It can also include a neuron that descends from the brainstem to the spinal cord and synapses with a lower motor neuron. The neurons can be thought of as corticospinal or corticobulbar neurons. A **lower motor neuron** is a neuron whose cell body is located in the CNS but its axon innervates muscles. These neurons are generally the ones that course through multiple cranial nerves and all 31 pairs of spinal nerves (**Fig. 9.74**).

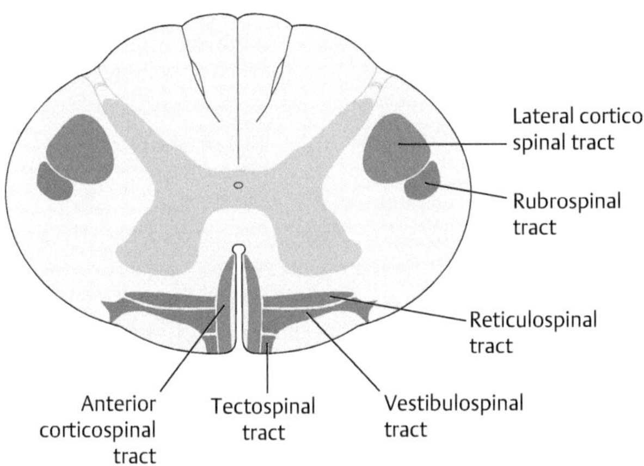

Fig. 9.72 Descending tracts in the spinal cord. (From Schuenke M, Schulte E, Schumacher U. THIEME Atlas of Anatomy. Head, Neck, and Neuroanatomy. Illustrations by Voll M and Wesker K. 3rd ed. New York: Thieme Medical Publishers; 2020.)

9.21.1 Upper Motor Neuron versus Lower Motor Neuron Lesions

A lesion located on any part of a lower motor neuron results in hypoactive muscle stretch reflexes and reduced muscle tone (hypotonicity). This is due to the fact that lower motor neurons form the motor component of the reflex. The early signs of a lower motor neuron lesion are muscle fasciculations or contractions of groups of muscles that may produce visible twitches seen on the skin. Fibrillations, which are invisible potentials seen with electromyography, soon follow muscle fasciculations. Muscle wasting and atrophy occur with lower motor neuron lesions. Ultimately with lower motor neuron lesions, there is a **flaccid paralysis**, which is the combination of muscle weakness (paresis) with suppressed or absent reflexes, fasciculations, and wasting or atrophy of the muscles. The flaccid paralysis of lower motor neuron lesions is seen ipsilateral and at the level of the lesion.

Upper motor neuron lesions have an inhibitory effect on muscle stretch reflexes. This type of lesion combines skeletal muscle weakness with either hyperactive or hypertonic muscle stretch or deep tendon reflexes. Hypertonia can be seen as *decorticate rigidity* (postural flexion of the upper limbs and extension of the lower limbs) or *decerebrate rigidity* (postural extension of both upper and lower limbs) depending on the site of the lesion. Lesions above the midbrain lead to *decorticate rigidity* and lesions below the midbrain lead to *decerebrate rigidity*. Muscle atrophy due to an upper motor neuron lesion is the result of only inactivity because muscles can still be contracted by stimulating muscle

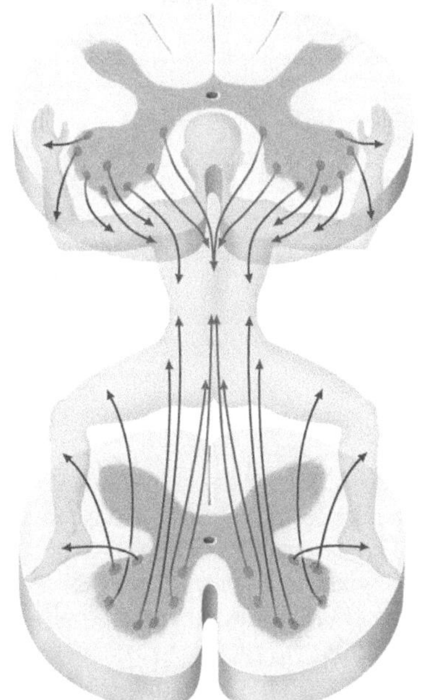

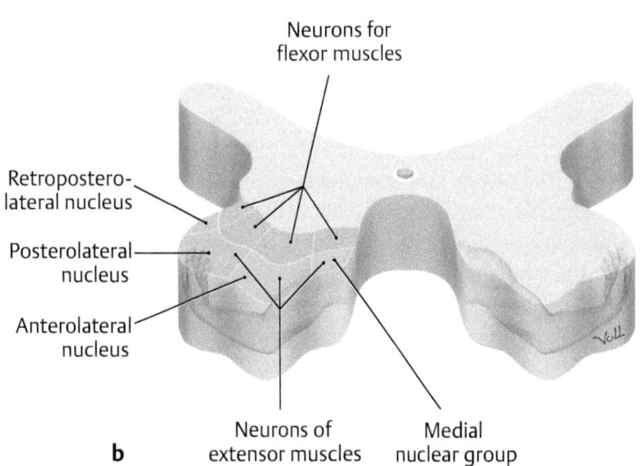

Fig. 9.73 **(a)** Somatotopic organization of nuclear columns of the anterior horns. **(b)** Enlargement of the cervical cord demonstrating medial-to-lateral and anterior-to-posterior organization of motor nuclei. (From Schuenke M, Schulte E, Schumacher U. THIEME Atlas of Anatomy. Head, Neck, and Neuroanatomy. Illustrations by Voll M and Wesker K. 3rd ed. New York: Thieme Medical Publishers; 2020.)

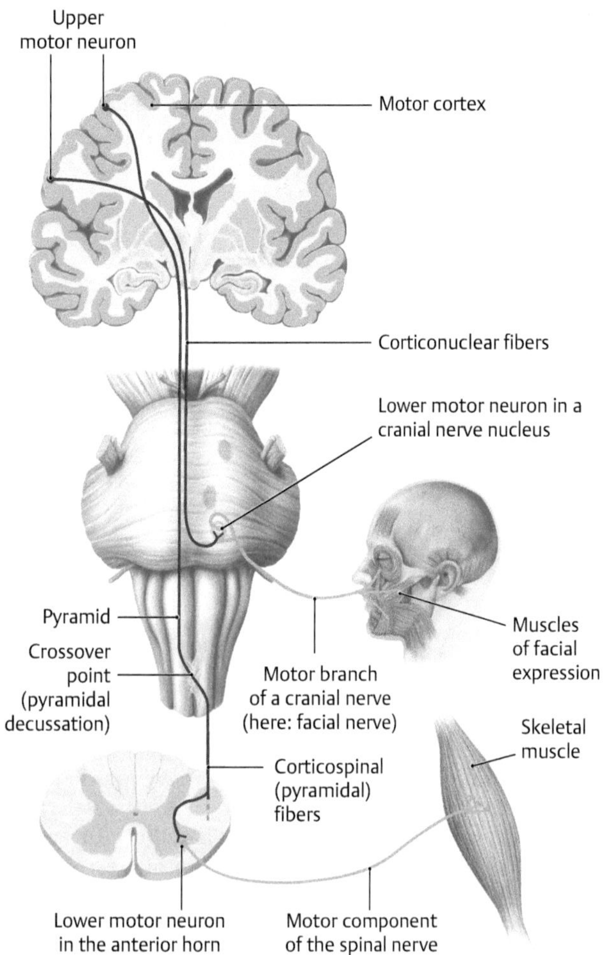

Fig. 9.74 Upper motor neuron versus lower motor neuron. (From Schuenke M, Schulte E, Schumacher U. THIEME Atlas of Anatomy. Head, Neck, and Neuroanatomy. Illustrations by Voll M and Wesker K. 3rd ed. New York: Thieme Medical Publishers; 2020.)

stretch reflexes. In addition, these lesions are accompanied by the reversal of cutaneous reflexes that normally yield a flexor motor response most notably the ***Babinski sign.*** After stroking the sole of the foot, the normal response would be plantar flexion of the toes. If there were a lesion, a Babinski sign would be apparent due to the extension of the big toe and fanning out of the other digits.

Ultimately with upper motor neuron lesions there is a **spastic paresis**, which is the combination of muscle weakness with hyperactive reflexes, atrophy of the muscles, and a reversal of cutaneous reflexes. If the upper motor neuron lesion is located between the cerebral cortex and the pyramidal decussation, it results in a contralateral spastic paresis below the level of the lesion. If this type of lesion occurs anywhere in the spinal cord, it results in an ipsilateral spastic paresis below the level of the lesion.

9.22 Corticospinal Tract

The **corticospinal** (or **pyramidal**) **tract** is vital for the expression of precise and voluntary movements. It arises from lamina V of the cerebral cortex and three specific regions of the cortex. About 30% of the fibers arise from the **primary motor cortex (M1, area 4)** and is located in the **precentral gyrus**. Less than 5% of the axons of this particular region belong to the **giant pyramidal cells** (of ***Betz***) and this region is thought to be involved in the actual execution of a movement. Another 30% of the fibers arise from the **premotor cortex (PMC)** and **supplemental motor area (SMA)** located on the lateral and medial surfaces of **area 6**, respectively. These regions, especially the SMA, are thought to be involved in the planning and initiation of motor movements. The remaining 40% of these fibers originate from the **primary somatosensory cortex (S1, areas 3, 1,** and **2)** located in the **postcentral gyrus** and with **area 5** and **area 7** of the **posterior parietal cortex**. These regions form a connection through association fibers with areas 4 and 6 and provide cortical representation of space, which is important in eye movements and precision grasping movements (**Fig. 9.75; Fig. 9.76**).

The tract descends first through the **corona radiata** and then to the **posterior limb of the internal capsule**. It continues through the middle three-fifths of the **cerebral peduncle (crus cerebri)** of the midbrain followed by the **basilar part** of the pons (pontine enlargement). While in the pons, the fibers are broken into smaller axon bundles. The fibers become grouped together to form the **pyramids** of the medulla before continuing through the spinal cord. At the level of the pyramids, 90% of the tract fibers decussate and descend through the posterior portion of the contralateral lateral funiculus of the spinal cord as the **lateral corticospinal tract**. The fibers from this tract descend through all levels of the spinal cord, with the axons finally terminating on interneurons located on the lateral aspect of laminae IV–VII. A smaller percentage of these fibers synapse with alpha and gamma motor neurons in lamina IX. The lateral tract functions to primarily control limb musculature (**Fig. 9.75; Fig. 9.76**).

The remaining 10% of tract fibers do not decussate in the medulla but instead through the spinal cord as the **anterior corticospinal tract**. At their levels of termination, the axons decussate in the **anterior white commissure** of the spinal cord before synapsing with interneurons of the contralateral spinal cord. The anterior tract functions to control axial and postural musculature (**Fig. 9.75; Fig. 9.76**).

If a lesion is located above the pyramidal decussation, there is muscle weakness on the contralateral side of the body. Muscle weakness on the ipsilateral side of the body would be due to a lesion located below the decussation.

9.23 Corticobulbar Tract

The **corticobulbar** (or **corticonuclear**) **tract** fibers arise from the part of **area 4** just above the lateral fissure on the lateral surface of the hemisphere and this area is related to the head of the motor homunculus (**Fig. 9.75b; Fig. 9.76a, b**). The axons of this tract accompany those of the corticospinal tract until the level of the pons. Here the axons begin to travel dorsally through the brainstem tegmentum before reaching the motor nuclei of the trigeminal (CN V), facial (CN VII), glossopharyngeal (CN IX), vagus (CN X), spinal accessory (CN XI), and hypoglossal (CN XII) nerves. The corticobulbar fibers are located in the genu of the internal capsule and are the most medial of all cortically arising upper motor neurons in the cerebral peduncle. This tract innervates the cranial nerve lower motor neurons ***bilaterally*** and for most cases the muscles are unable to be contracted voluntarily on one side only. The facial (only facial muscles below the eye) and hypoglossal nuclei receive the majority of their innervation from the *contralateral* cerebral cortex.

Generally not considered part of the corticobulbar tract system would be the motor innervation to the oculomotor (CN III), trochlear (CN IV), and abducent (CN VI) motor nuclei. They instead receive direct input from **area 8** (frontal eye fields) and not from

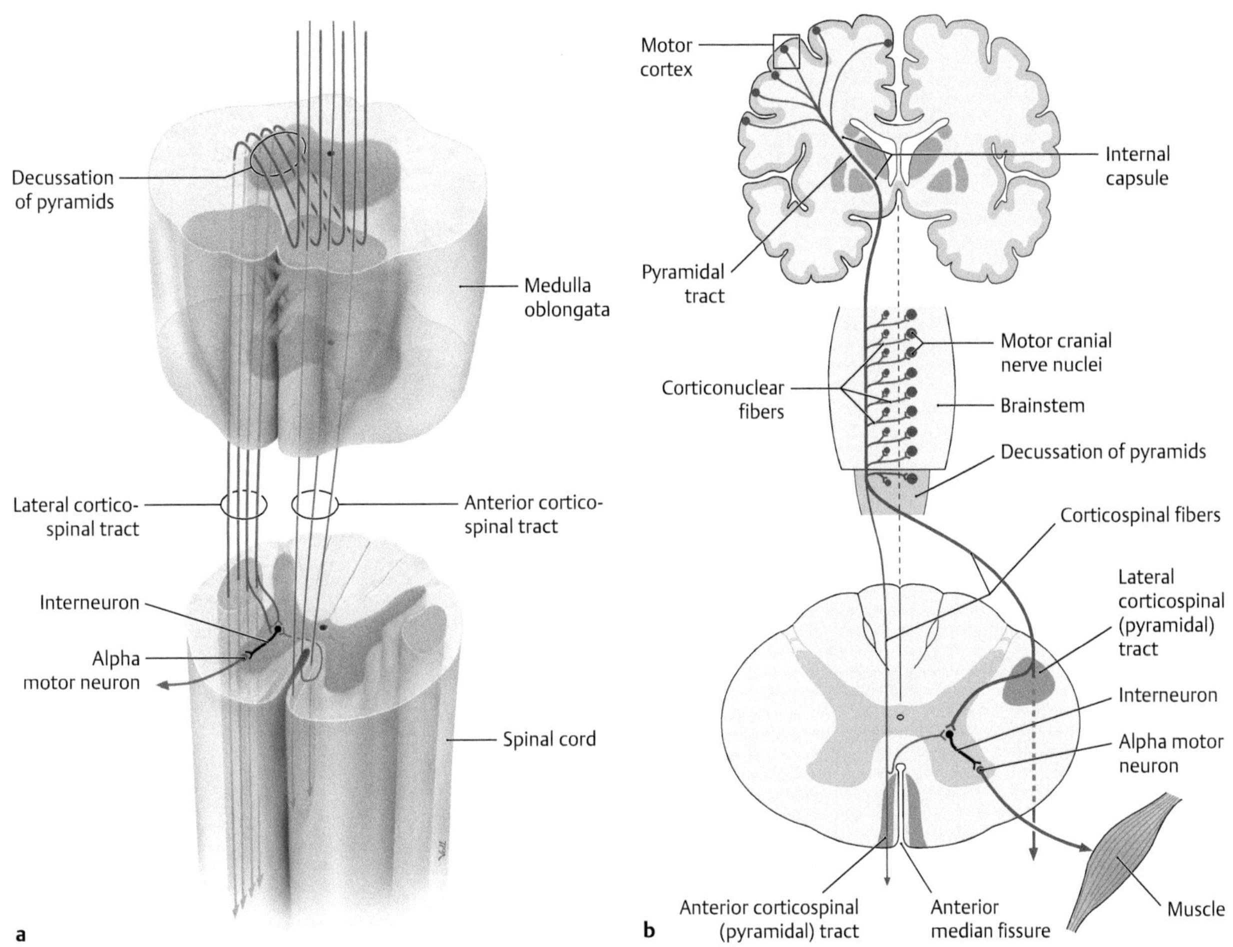

Fig. 9.75 (a) Course of the anterior and lateral corticospinal tracts (pyramidal tract) in the lower medulla and spinal cord. **(b)** Course of the corticospinal (pyramidal) tract. (From Schuenke M, Schulte E, Schumacher U. THIEME Atlas of Anatomy. Head, Neck, and Neuroanatomy. Illustrations by Voll M and Wesker K. 3rd ed. New York: Thieme Medical Publishers; 2020.)

area 4. Area 8 input is not direct but instead passes through gaze centers located in the reticular formation.

9.24 Rubrospinal Tract

The **rubrospinal tract** is located just anterior to the lateral corticospinal tract (**Fig. 9.77**). It arises from the **red nucleus**, a structure located in tegmentum of the midbrain and at the level of the superior colliculus. Axons decussate immediately through the ventral midbrain tegmentum and its tract fibers synapse in the intermediate and lateral portions of laminae VII and VIII. The tract terminates primarily in the cervical and upper thoracic segments but can extend throughout the spinal cord, suggesting that it functions mostly in upper limb control. Activation of this tract causes excitation of flexor muscles and tone along with inhibition of extensor muscles.

9.25 Tectospinal Tract

The **tectospinal tract** originates in the **superior colliculus** and the axons decussate soon after to the contralateral side through the dorsal midbrain tegmentum (near the level of the rubrospinal tract decussation) and descend through the brainstem near the MLF (**Fig. 9.77**). This tract descends through the anterior funiculus of the spinal cord near the anterior median fissure and its tract fibers synapse in laminae VII and VIII of the cervical segments of the spinal cord. This is in relationship to motor neurons that are concerned with musculature of the neck and shoulder regions and reflex movements in response to visual stimuli. Activation of this tract causes excitation of flexor muscles and tone along with inhibition of extensor muscles.

9.26 Vestibulospinal Tract

Originating from the vestibular nuclei are the **lateral** and **medial vestibulospinal tracts** (**Fig. 9.77**). The vestibular nuclei are located in the brainstem at the level of the medulla and pons near the floor of the fourth ventricle. The vestibular nuclei are not influenced by the cerebral cortex but instead serve as an important integration center for information originating from the contralateral vestibular nuclei, the vestibular apparatus, and the cerebellum and visual system.

The **lateral vestibulospinal tract** is important in maintaining balance in response to vestibular stimuli, for example, postural adjustments in response to head turning or for the body position relative to gravity. The highest level of activity passing through this tract is from the excitatory input to extensor musculature of

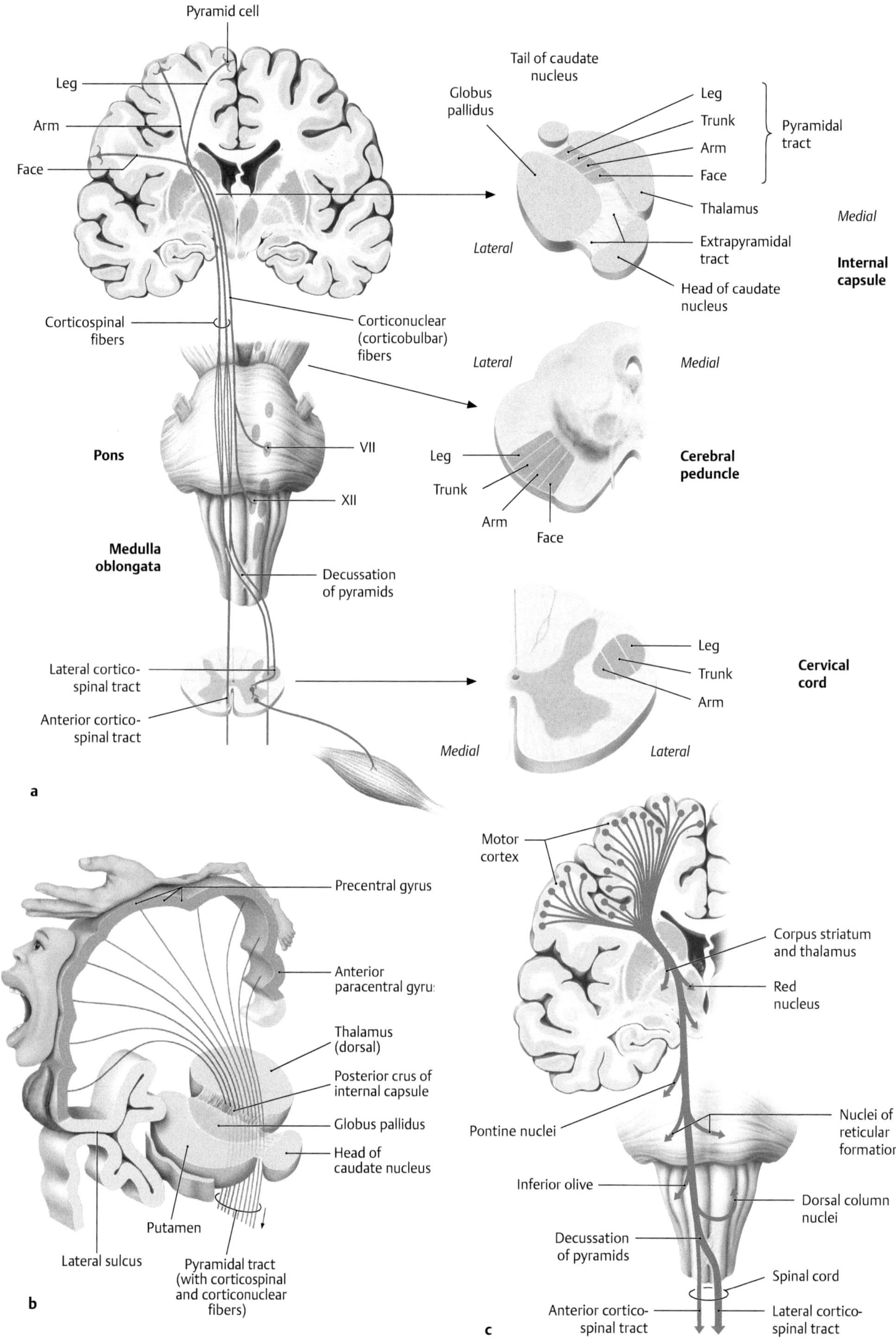

Fig. 9.76 **(a)** Course of the corticospinal and corticobulbar tracts. **(b)** Somatotopic representation of the skeletal muscle in the precentral gyrus (motor homunculus). **(c)** Variety of cortical efferent fibers. (From Schuenke M, Schulte E, Schumacher U. THIEME Atlas of Anatomy. Head, Neck, and Neuroanatomy. Illustrations by Voll M and Wesker K. 3rd ed. New York: Thieme Medical Publishers; 2020.)

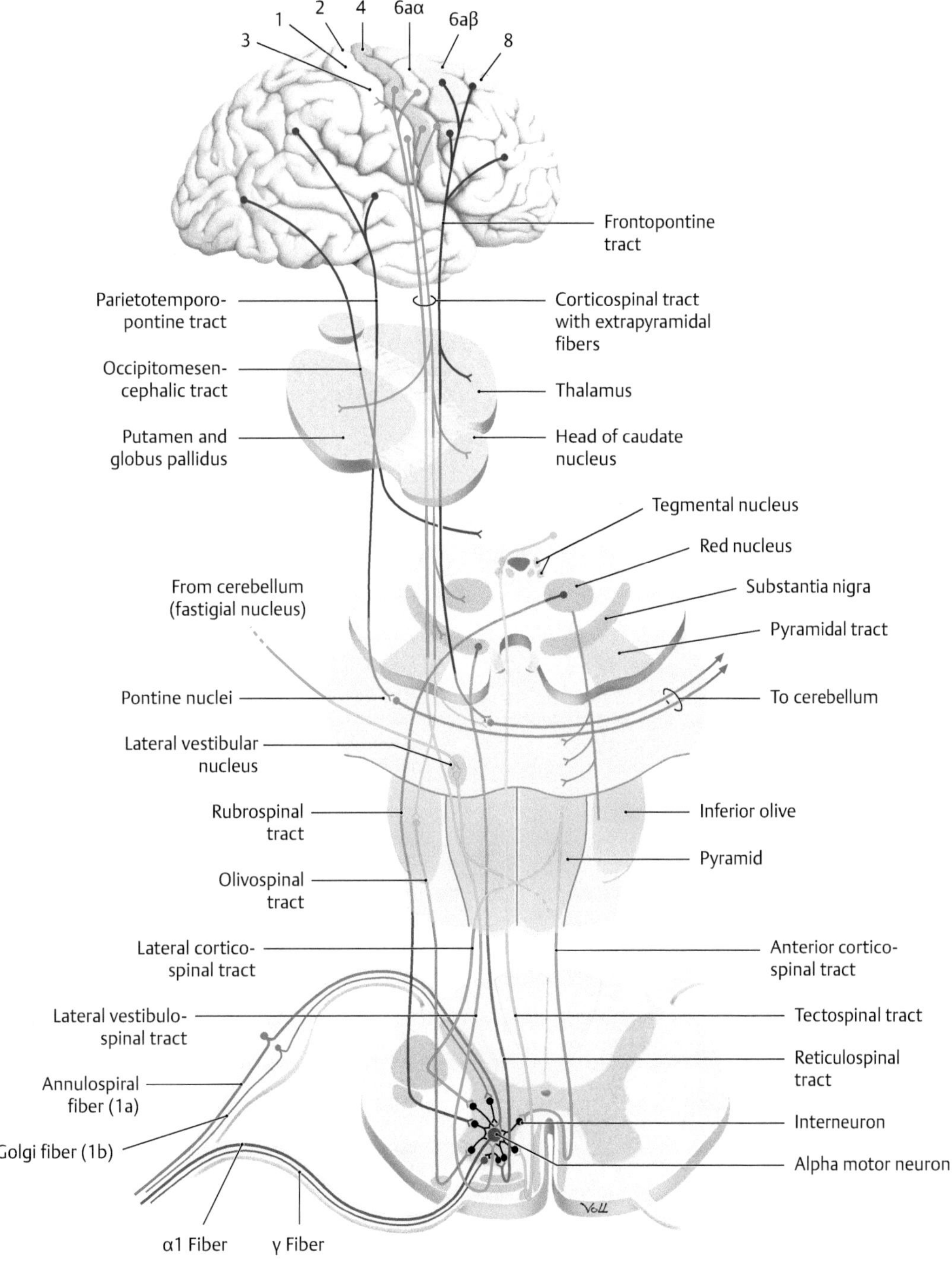

Fig. 9.77 Descending tracts of the extrapyramidal motor system. (From Schuenke M, Schulte E, Schumacher U. THIEME Atlas of Anatomy. Head, Neck, and Neuroanatomy. Illustrations by Voll M and Wesker K. 3rd ed. New York: Thieme Medical Publishers; 2020.)

the neck, back, and limbs. This tract also evokes a reciprocal inhibition in the flexor musculature. This tract begins in the lateral vestibular nucleus and descends *ipsilaterally* through the medial portion of the anterior funiculus before terminating at laminae VII and VIII of all spinal cord levels.

The **medial vestibulospinal tract** impacts the activity in lower motor neurons of the neck and upper back regions only because it does not descend into the lumbar and sacral regions of the spinal cord. Fibers from this tract originate primarily from the medial vestibular nucleus and descend *bilaterally* through the anterior funiculus before reaching laminae VII and VIII of the cervical and thoracic spinal cord levels.

9.27 Recticulospinal Tract

The **reticulospinal tracts** (**Fig. 9.77**) center on the complicated network of neurons and circuits called the reticular formation. Functions of the reticular formation vary greatly and include the regulation and modification of states of consciousness, the

Clinical Correlate 9.23

Types of Spinal Cord Lesions or Syndromes

- **Central Cord Syndrome**: seen most often with hyperextension injuries of the cervical spine and in individuals over the age of 50. The pneumonic is MUD because there are greater motor versus sensory deficits, involves the upper extremities more than the lower extremities, and finally muscle weakness is seen most often with the distal musculature versus proximal musculature (**Fig. 9.79**).
- **Brown-Séquard Syndrome**: due to a penetrating injury that has hemisected one side of the spinal cord but incomplete lesions are the most common. There will be a loss of ipsilateral proprioception, light touch, and motor function, in addition to the loss of contralateral pain and temperature sensations two to three segments below the lesion (**Fig. 9.80**).
- **Anterior Cord Syndrome**: the most common form of spinal cord infarction that involves the anterior spinal artery. It affects the majority of the spinal cord except for the posterior column. Due to this, light touch, vibratory sensation, and proprioception are preserved but there is a bilateral loss of both motor function and any pain and temperature sensations below the level of the lesion. Autonomic control may be lost, resulting in sexual, bowel, and/or bladder dysfunctions (**Fig. 9.81**).
- **Posterior Cord Syndrome**: very rare and the result of a tumor or infarction of the posterior spinal artery. This artery helps supply the posterior columns of the spinal cord. Proprioception, tactile recognition (stereognosis), two-point discrimination, and the ability to recognize writing on the skin by touch (graphesthesia) are lost below the level of the lesion. Tabes dorsalis is a form of neurosyphilis that slowly degenerates the neural tracts of the posterior column and thus presents similar to posterior cord syndrome (**Fig. 9.82**).
- **Subacute Combined Degeneration**: seen most commonly in cases of vitamin B_{12} deficiency, which is sometimes associated with pernicious anemia. It, most commonly, affects the lower cervical and upper thoracic spinal cord segments. It is characterized as patchy losses of myelin in the posterior columns and lateral corticospinal tracts. The result is a bilateral spastic paralysis and a bilateral loss of touch, vibration, and pressure sensations below the lesion level (**Fig. 9.83**).
- **Syringomyelia**: a slowly developing disease resulting in a progressive cavitation of the central canal. This lesion is usually isolated to the middle to lower parts of the cervical and upper thoracic spinal cord segments. Early on, there is a bilateral loss of pain and temperature sensation in the hands and forearms due to the destruction of spinothalamic fibers that cross the anterior white commissure. With continued cavitation, lower motor neurons of the ventral horns are compressed and result in bilateral flaccid paralysis of the upper limb muscles. Later manifestations could result in Horner syndrome because descending hypothalamic fibers that target preganglionic sympathetic neurons located in the lateral horn are compressed (**Fig. 9.84**).
- **Conus Medullaris Syndrome**: involves the lumbar and sacral nerve roots and causes loss of bowel control; areflexic bladder; ankle jerk reflex is absent but the knee jerk reflex is preserved; signs similar to cauda equina syndrome but effects are more likely to be bilateral (**Fig. 9.85**).
- **Cauda Equina Syndrome**: results in a lower motor neuron lesion involving the nerve roots and not the spinal cord itself and is generally below the L1 vertebral level. This type of lesion tends to be incomplete, and regeneration of the peripheral nerves is possible. There is a decrease in bladder and bowel control reflexes (areflexia); and there is a decreased level of sensation at the affected dermatome level and muscle weakness (flaccidity) (**Fig. 9.86**).
- **Poliomyelitis**: an infectious disease caused by the poliovirus. It results in the relatively selective destruction of lower motor neurons found in the ventral horn of the spinal cord and most commonly in the lumbar region. The virus is usually spread from person to person through the ingestion of food or water containing infected fecal matter. There is a vaccine and it has been in use since 1955. The disease causes muscle weakness or flaccidity along with both the accompanying reduced reflexes (hyporeflexia) and muscle tone (hypotonicity) (**Fig. 9.87**).
- **Amyotropic Lateral Sclerosis**: ALS, or *Lou Gerhig disease*, is primarily a motor system disease that affects both upper and lower motor neurons. This disease typically begins at the cervical region of the spinal cord before progressing either superior or inferior through the rest of the cord. Men are affected twice as much as women and it usually occurs between the ages of 50 and 70. Patients present with bilateral spastic paralysis in the lower limbs and bilateral flaccid weakness in the upper limbs (**Fig. 9.88**).
- **Corticospinal Tract Syndrome**: characterized by a progressive degeneration of the cortical neurons in the motor cortex with increasing failure of the corticospinal tracts, meaning there is axonal degeneration of the first motor neuron. The course of the disease involves a progressive spastic paralysis in the lower limbs before reaching the upper limbs (**Fig. 9.89**).

location of cardiovascular and respiratory centers, and eye movement organization, to name a few. There is a **lateral** and **medial reticulospinal tract** and these are similar to the vestibulospinal tracts, in that their axons terminate at the medial portions of the ventral horn gray matter. At this location, they have a primary influence on the local circuits that coordinate both axial and proximal limb movements but they are largely inhibitory to interneurons, alpha, and gamma motor neurons in the spinal cord.

The **lateral reticulospinal tract** originates from neurons in the reticular formation of the medulla. It projects *bilaterally* to laminae VII and VIII of all spinal cord levels. The axon terminals generally branch and both ascend and descend multiple segments before terminating at several adjacent spinal segments. This specific tract may act as upper motor neurons for the autonomic lower motor neurons located at the lateral horns of the thoracic and upper lumbar spinal segments. This would be in conjunction with the sympathetic nervous system.

The **medial reticulospinal tract** originates from the reticular formation of the pons. The tract remains mostly *uncrossed* and projects to laminae VII and VIII in a similar fashion to how the lateral reticulospinal axon terminals terminate.

9.28 Olivospinal Tract

The **olivospinal tract** (**Fig. 9.77**) and its existence have been questioned for some time. If present, it may function by modulating reflex movements and facilitating muscle tone. However, the tract has been described as arising from the inferior olivary nucleus and descending within the ipsilateral anterolateral portion of the white matter funiculus before terminating on ventral horn cells in the cervical spinal cord region only.

Lesions of the descending motor pathways and those of the spinal cord and peripheral nerves are summarized in **Fig. 9.78.**

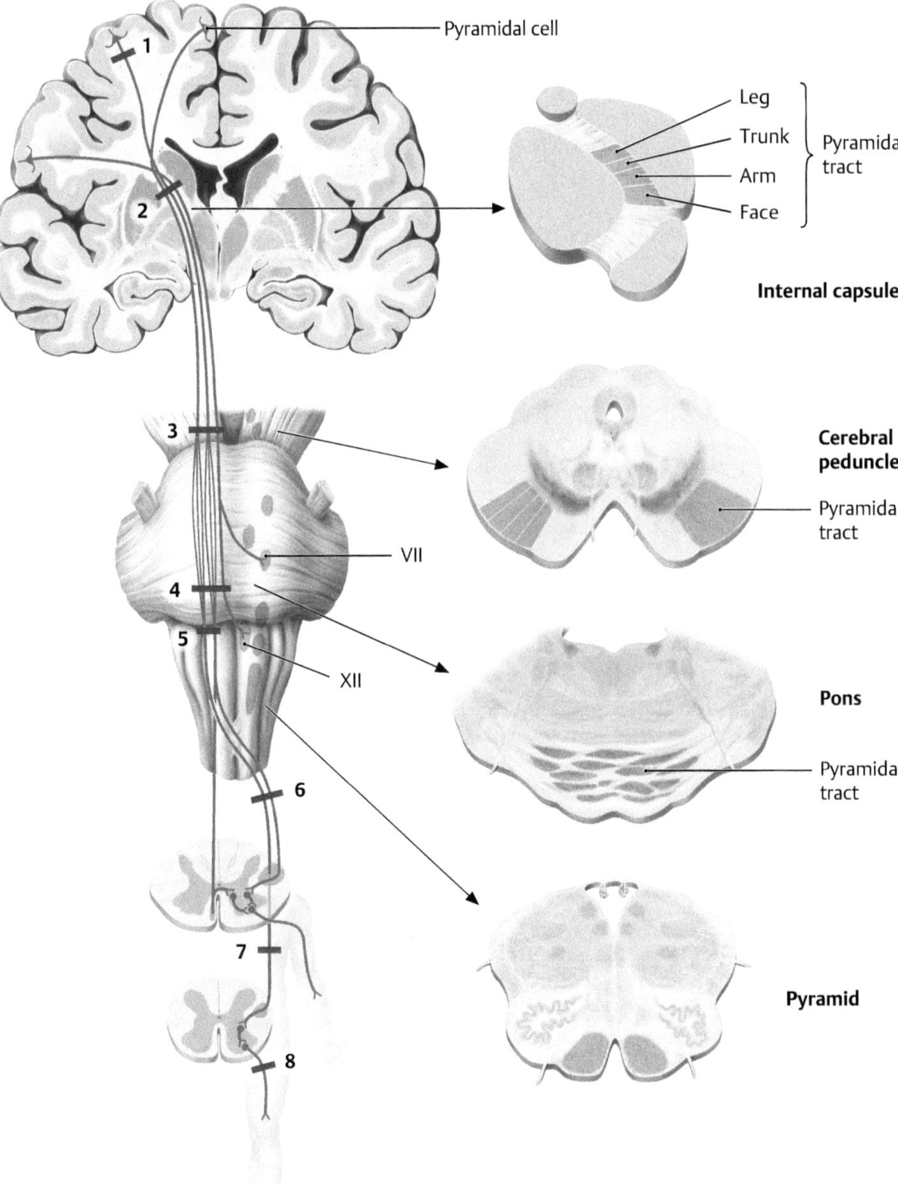

Lesion near the cortex (1): Paralysis of the muscles innervated by the damaged cortical area. Because the face and hand are represented by particularly large areas in the motor cortex, paralysis often affects primarily the arm and face ("brachiofacial" paralysis). The paralysis invariably affects the side opposite the lesion (due to decussation of the pyramids) and is flaccid and partial (*paresis*) rather than complete because the extrapyramidal fibers are not damaged. If the extrapyramidal fibers were also damaged, the result would be contralateral *complete* spastic *paralysis*.

Lesion at the level of the internal capsule (2): This leads to chronic, contralateral, spastic hemi*plegia* (complete paralysis) because the lesion affects both the extrapyramidal motor pathways, which mix with pyramidal tract fibers in front of the internal capsule. Stroke is a frequent cause of lesions at this level.

Lesion at the level of the cerebral peduncle (crus cerebri) (3): Contralateral spastic hemi*paresis*.

Lesion at the pons (4): Contralateral hemiparesis or bilateral paresis, depending on the size of the lesion. Because the fibers of the pyramidal tract occupy a larger cross-sectional area in the pons than in the internal capsule, not all of the fibers are damaged in many cases. For example, the fibers for the facial nerve and hypoglossal nerve are usually unaffected because of their dorsal location. Damage to the abducens nucleus may cause ipsilateral damage to the trigeminal nucleus (not shown).

Lesion at the level of the pyramid (5): Flaccid contralateral paresis occurs because the fibers of the extrapyramidal motor pathways (e.g., the rubrospinal and tectospinal tracts) are more dorsal than the pyramidal tract fibers and are therefore unaffected by an isolated lesion of the pyramid.

Lesion at the level of the spinal cord (6,7): A lesion at the level of the cervical cord (6) leads to ipsilateral spastic hemiplegia because the fibers of the pyramidal and extrapyramidal system are closely interwoven at this level and have already crossed to the opposite side. A lesion at the level of the thoracic cord (7) leads to spastic paralysis of the ipsilateral leg.

Lesion at the level of the peripheral nerve (8): This lesion damages the axon of the alpha motor neuron, resulting in flaccid paralysis.

Fig. 9.78 Lesions of the central motor pathways and their effects. (From Schuenke M, Schulte E, Schumacher U. THIEME Atlas of Anatomy. Head, Neck, and Neuroanatomy. Illustrations by Voll M and Wesker K. 3rd ed. New York: Thieme Medical Publishers; 2020.)

9.29 Spinal Reflexes

A **reflex** can be defined as an efferent motor neuron discharge that automatically follows a sufficient afferent stimulation, bringing about a stereotypical and generally specific activity in an effector structure. A reflex can act independently of supraspinal (i.e., corticospinal tract) control, and if the supraspinal effect is cut off, the reflex activity is generally exaggerated.

A reflex arc involves a minimal number of neurons that when stimulated lead to a simple reflex behavior. Reflexes are unlearned and involuntary responses that can be related to either somatic or visceral structures. There are five components to a reflex arc:

1. **Receptor**: located at the terminal end of the peripheral processes of an axon and this is where the stimulus occurs.
2. **Sensory neuron**: afferent impulses are transmitted to the CNS.
3. **Integration center**: the gray matter of the CNS where one or more synapses occur.
4. **Motor neuron**: the structure that carries an efferent impulse to an effector organ.
5. **Effector**: the muscle or gland that responds to an efferent impulse.

A **monosynaptic reflex** (**Fig. 9.90a**) is the simplest of all reflexes where there is no interneuron between the sensory and motor neuron. These one synapse reflexes include among others the bicep or knee-jerk reflexes. There are many skeletal muscles that an upright posture and equilibrium. These are the fastest of all reflexes.

A **polysynaptic reflex** (**Fig. 9.90a**) is much more common than a monosynaptic reflex and there are one or more interneurons that make up the reflex pathway. With just one interneuron present, there are at least two synapses. Withdrawal reflexes such as the flexor (withdrawal) reflex and the crossed extensor reflex are both examples of a polysynaptic reflex.

The **flexor withdrawal reflex** is the combined ipsilateral flexor excitation and extensor inhibition of a limb. Flexion of a limb due to a nociceptive or painful stimulus serves as a protective mechanism. The afferents involved are usually exteroceptive (external) and the axons are relatively small. A strong noxious stimulation would result in a greater excitation of the ipsilateral flexor motor neurons and inhibition of the ipsilateral extensor motor neurons. The **crossed extensor reflex** usually occurs simultaneously with the flexor withdrawal reflex when the afferent stimulus is intense enough. The afferents send collaterals across to the contralateral dorsal horn and synapse with interneurons that are eventually excitatory to the relevant extensor motor neurons in their half of the spinal cord and inhibitory to the appropriate flexor motor neurons in their half of the spinal cord.

9.30 The Olfactory System

The **olfactory receptor cells** are bipolar neurons located about a square inch in size in the epithelium of the nasal cavity. The central processes of the axons pass through the cribriform plate of the ethmoid bone and penetrate the dura and arachnoid maters

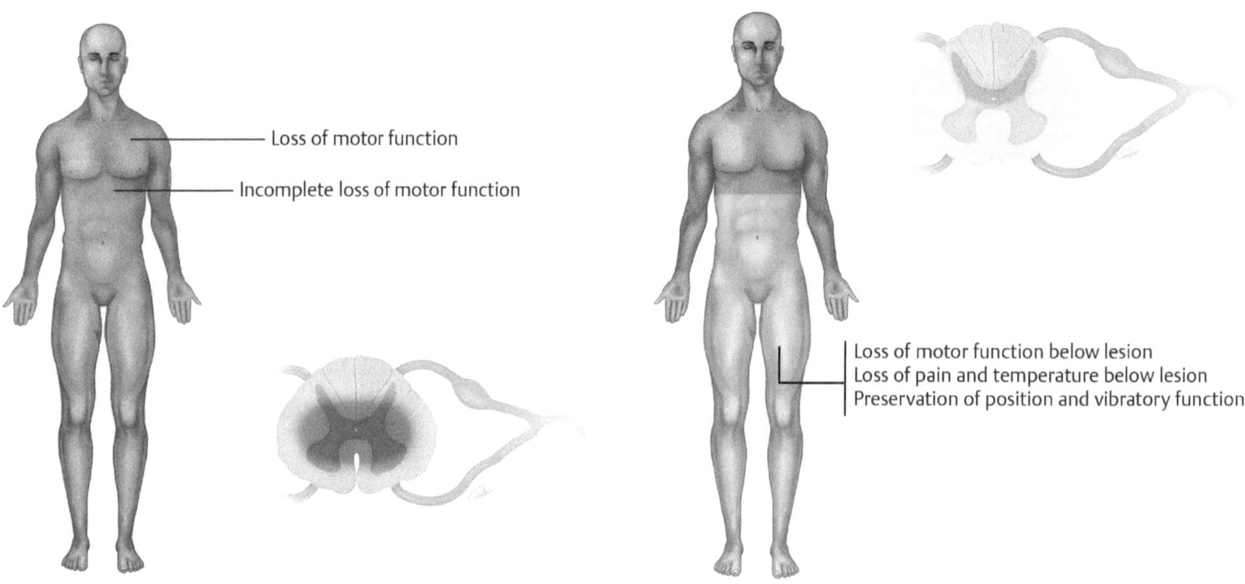

Fig. 9.79 Central cord syndrome. Illustration by Calla Heald.

Fig. 9.81 Anterior cord syndrome. Illustration by Calla Heald.

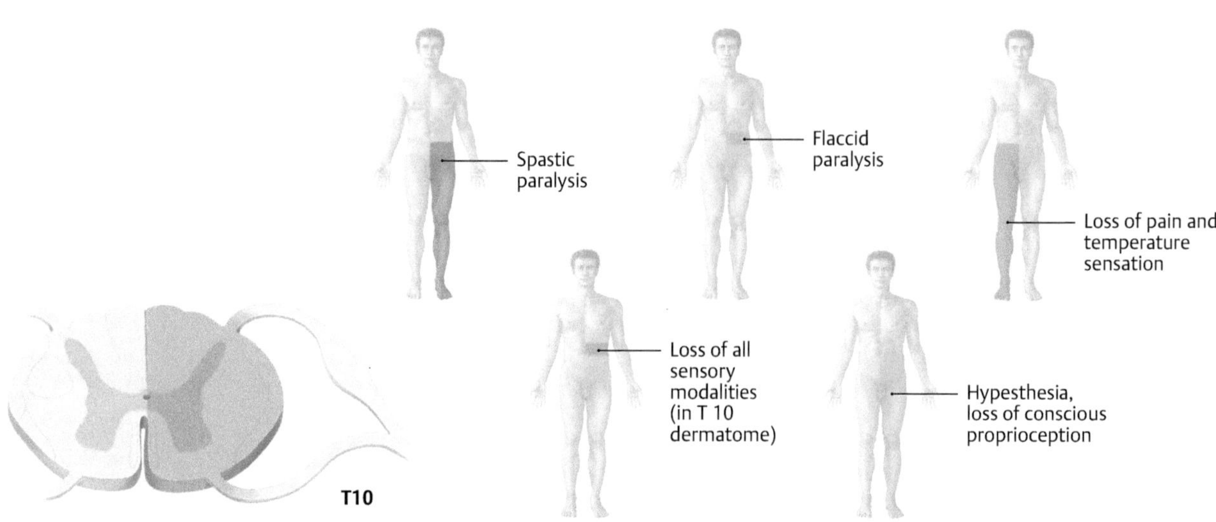

Fig. 9.80 Brown-Sequard syndrome. (From Schuenke M, Schulte E, Schumacher U. THIEME Atlas of Anatomy. Head, Neck, and Neuroanatomy. Illustrations by Voll M and Wesker K. 3rd ed. New York: Thieme Medical Publishers; 2020.)

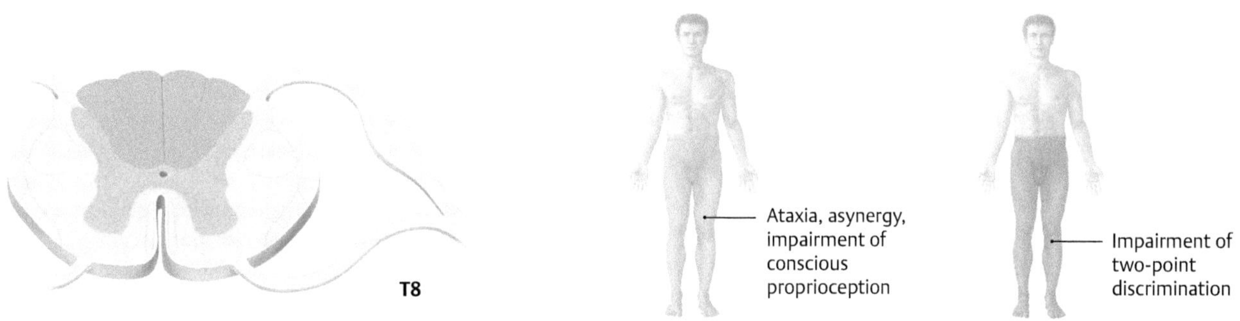

Fig. 9.82 Posterior cord syndrome. (From Schuenke M, Schulte E, Schumacher U. THIEME Atlas of Anatomy. Head, Neck, and Neuroanatomy. Illustrations by Voll M and Wesker K. 3rd ed. New York: Thieme Medical Publishers; 2020.)

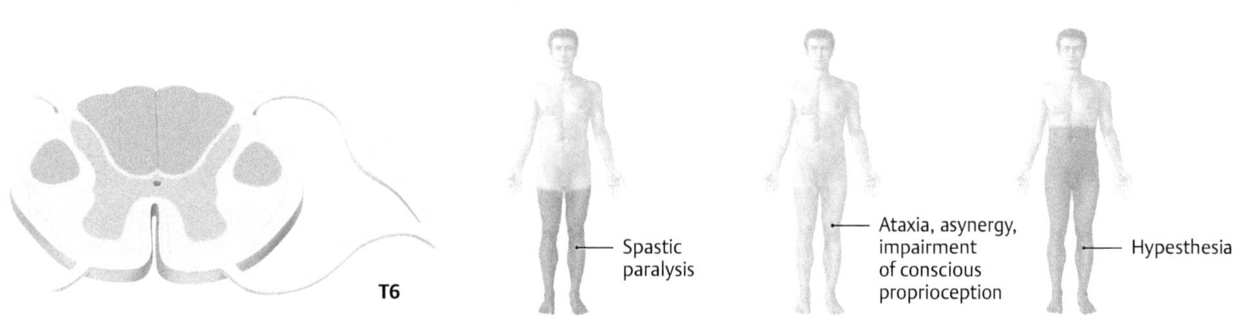

Fig. 9.83 Subacute combined degeneration. (From Schuenke M, Schulte E, Schumacher U. THIEME Atlas of Anatomy. Head, Neck, and Neuroanatomy. Illustrations by Voll M and Wesker K. 3rd ed. New York: Thieme Medical Publishers; 2020.)

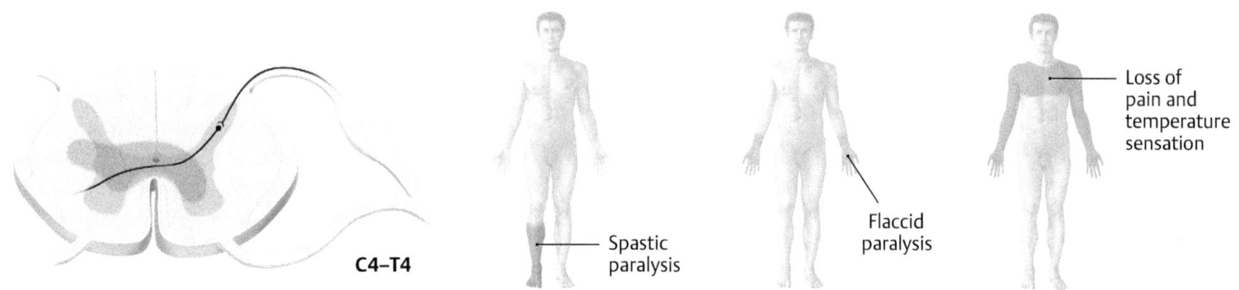

Fig. 9.84 Syringomyelia. (From Schuenke M, Schulte E, Schumacher U. THIEME Atlas of Anatomy. Head, Neck, and Neuroanatomy. Illustrations by Voll M and Wesker K. 3rd ed. New York: Thieme Medical Publishers; 2020.)

before reaching the **olfactory bulb**. A synapse in the olfactory bulb occurs with the **olfactory mitral cells**. The olfactory tract is formed by the axons of the mitral cells and it runs caudally on the basal surface of the frontal lobe before reaching the **anterior perforated substance**. At the rostral end of the anterior perforated substance is the olfactory trigone, which is formed by the division of the flattened olfactory tract into lateral and medial olfactory striae (**Fig. 9.91**).

The **lateral olfactory stria** passes caudally at the lateral edge of the anterior perforated substance before curling into the **uncus** of the temporal lobe (**Fig. 9.91d, e**). Olfactory fibers terminate in the cortex at the lateral edge of the anterior perforated substance, cortex of the uncus, and in a portion of the amygdala. These areas of synapse make up the **olfactory cortex**. The association cortex responsible for processing olfactory information received in the primary olfactory cortex forms the bulk of the anteromedial **parahippocampal gyrus**. This parahippocampal gyrus cortex is also called the **entorhinal cortex**. This cortex projects heavily onto the hippocampal formation and may be involved in remembering certain smells. The olfactory and entorhinal cortices, or the entire olfactory area, are often referred to as the prepiriform area (**Fig. 9.91 d, e**).

The **medial olfactory stria** contains olfactory tract fibers that end in the cortex of the olfactory trigone (**Fig. 9.91 d,e**). Other fibers connect the olfactory areas of the left and right hemispheres via the anterior commissure, as some of these fibers passing through the medial olfactory stria terminate bilaterally in the septal area and **subcallosal area** (**Fig. 9.46**).

Olfactory information projects bilaterally. It reaches its own primary cortex along with direct projections to the amygdala and subcallosal area of the limbic system, and the septal area. The primary olfactory cortex has an indirect thalamocortical connection to the neocortex by way of the dorsomedial (DM) nucleus of the thalamus, which then projects from the DM nucleus to the orbitofrontal cortex.

Bowman glands secrete a watery mucus that protects and moistens the olfactory epithelium (**Fig. 9.91a, b**). The existence of the **vomeronasal (Jacobson's) organ** in humans is debated but some evidence has it located bilaterally on the anterior portion of the nasal septum. Its central connections in humans are unknown but in other mammals it is used to detect pheromones.

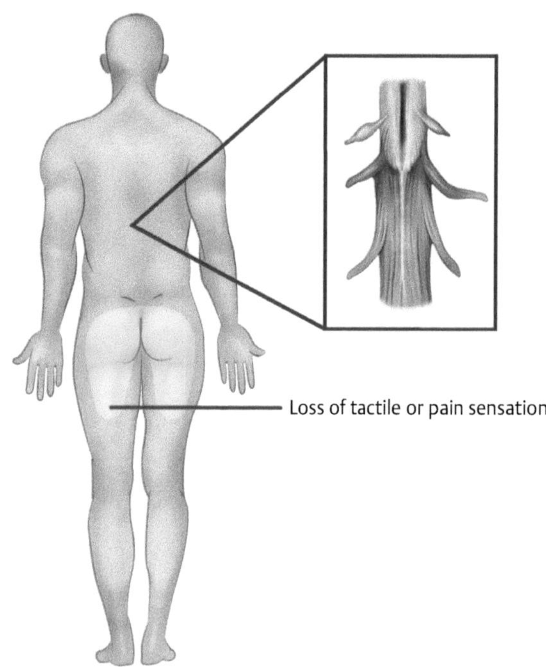

Fig. 9.85 Conus medullaris syndrome. Illustration by Calla Heald.

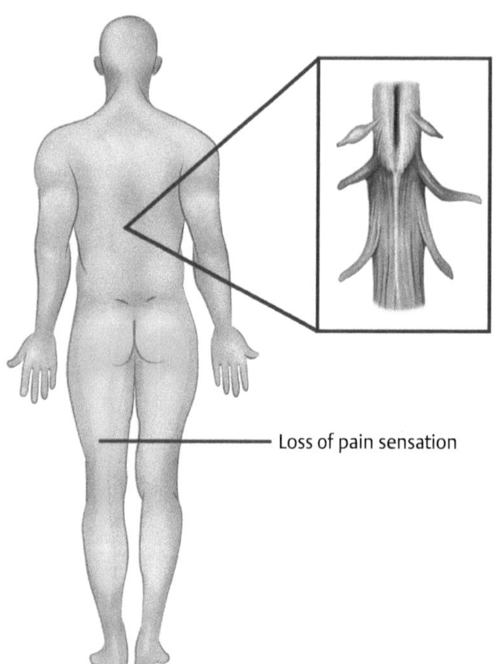

Fig. 9.86 Cauda equina syndrome. Illustration by Calla Heald.

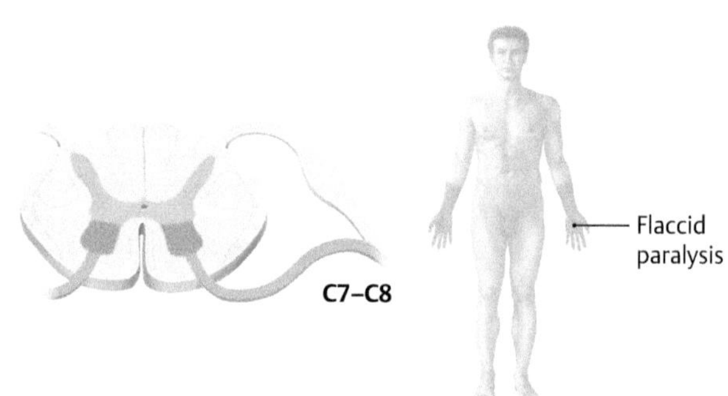

Fig. 9.87 Poliomyelitis. (From Schuenke M, Schulte E, Schumacher U. THIEME Atlas of Anatomy. Head, Neck, and Neuroanatomy. Illustrations by Voll M and Wesker K. 3rd ed. New York: Thieme Medical Publishers; 2020.)

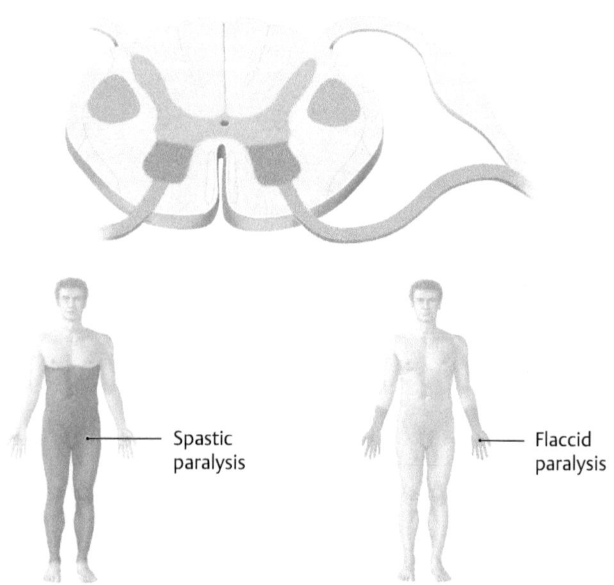

Fig. 9.88 Amyotropic lateral sclerosis. (From Schuenke M, Schulte E, Schumacher U. THIEME Atlas of Anatomy. Head, Neck, and Neuroanatomy. Illustrations by Voll M and Wesker K. 3rd ed. New York: Thieme Medical Publishers; 2020.)

9.31 The Visual System

The **visual system** (**Fig. 9.92a**) is responsible for the special sense of vision. The eyeball or oculus is the peripheral organ of vision and the retina specifically serves as the main information-processing structure. The structures of the eyeball including the histology of the retina were described in Chapter 7. For discussion purposes, we will begin at the photoreceptors of the retina.

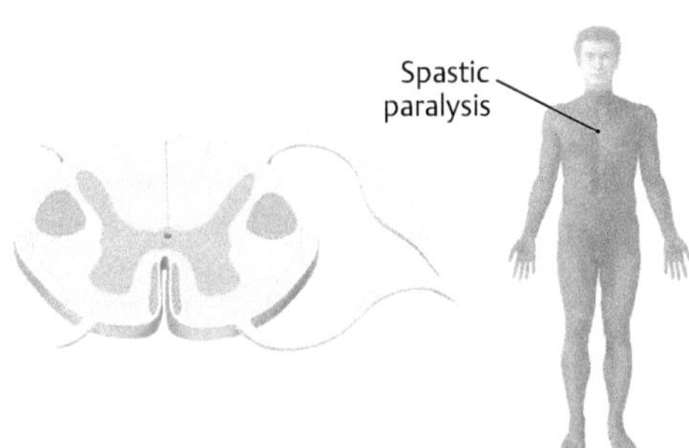

Fig. 9.89 Corticospinal tract syndrome. (From Schuenke M, Schulte E, Schumacher U. THIEME Atlas of Anatomy. Head, Neck, and Neuroanatomy. Illustrations by Voll M and Wesker K. 3rd ed. New York: Thieme Medical Publishers; 2020.)

The photoreceptor cells are known as the cones and rods (**Fig. 9.92b**). **Cones** (~7 million) are responsible for sharp visual definition and color discrimination. They are relatively insensitive to light but they have a higher threshold of excitability than rods. **Rods** (~100 million) are detectors of motion and are best suited for detecting low levels of light and serve an individual in night vision. They are not involved in color vision and do not provide good resolution. Most visual input that reaches the brain originates from the **fovea centralis** and it is populated only by cones (**Fig. 9.93**). The concentration of cones increases while the concentration of rods decreases as these cells near the fovea centralis. The **macula lutea** of the fovea is the area for most acute vision and the eyes fix themselves in such a way that the perceived image or object is always focused on the maculae (**Fig. 9.93**). The remainder of the retina is more concerned with peripheral vision. The loss of cone function makes an individual legally blind whereas the loss of rod function results in a person having night blindness.

These first-order photoreceptor neurons transform light stimuli to electrochemical signals and pass this to the second-order bipolar neurons. The signal then passes from the bipolar cells to the third-order ganglion cells whose axons become the **optic nerves**. The optic nerves leave the eyeball at the optic disc and meet each other at the **optic chiasm**. The optic chiasm is the location where ganglion cell axons may or may not decussate. The ganglion cell axons of the *nasal half* of each retina decussate to the contralateral

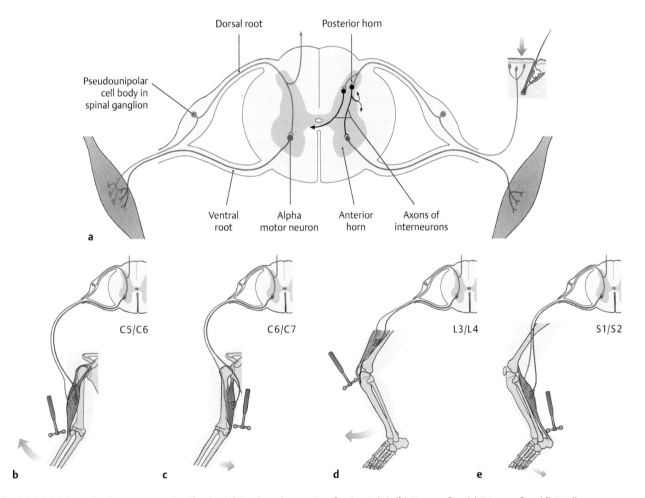

Fig. 9.90 **(a)** Schematic of a monosynaptic reflex (on left) and a polysynaptic reflex (on right). **(b)** Biceps reflex. **(c)** Triceps reflex. **(d)** Patellar (quadriceps) reflex. **(e)** Achilles tendon reflex. (From Schuenke M, Schulte E, Schumacher U. THIEME Atlas of Anatomy. Head, Neck, and Neuroanatomy. Illustrations by Voll M and Wesker K. 3rd ed. New York: Thieme Medical Publishers; 2020.)

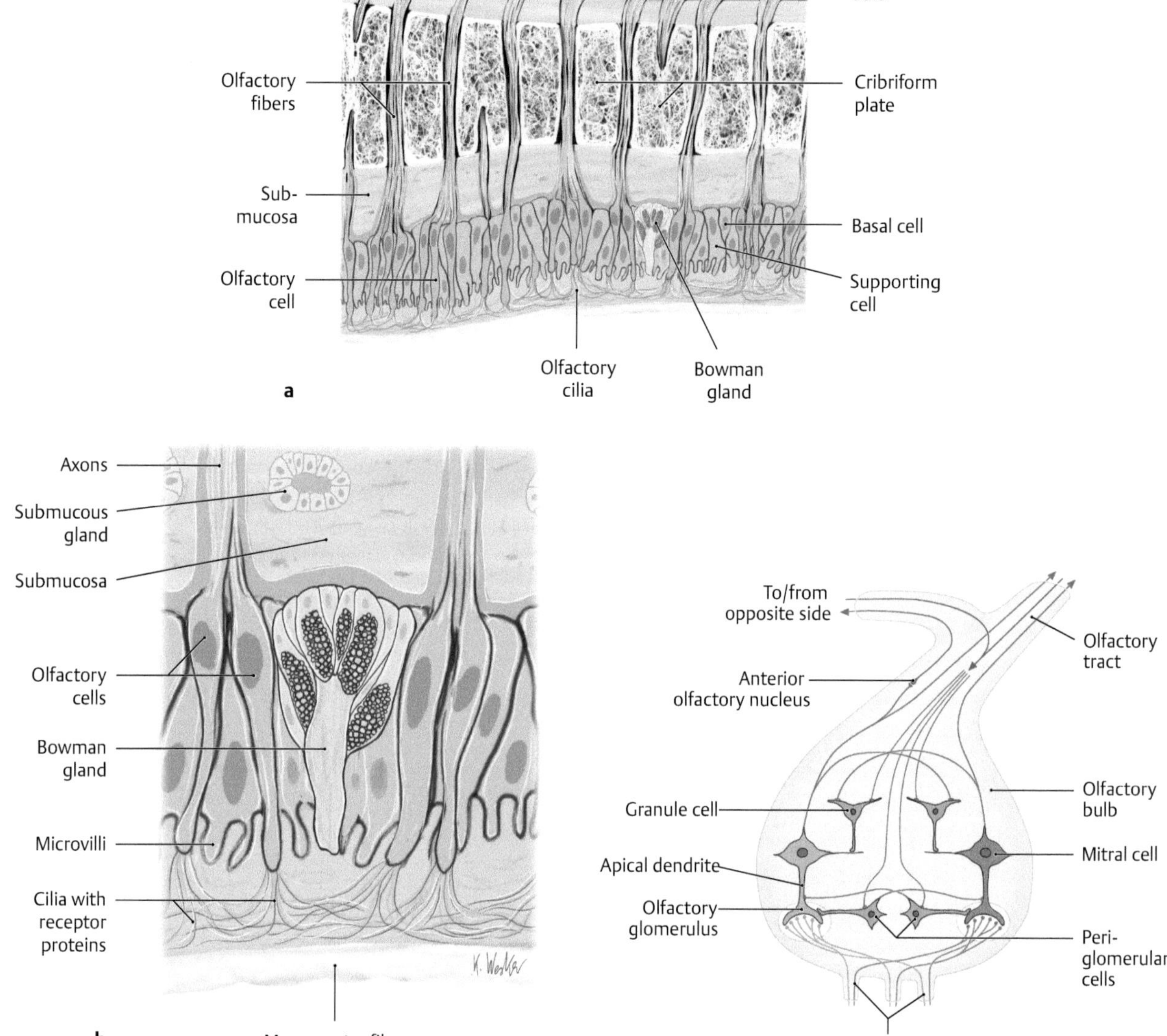

Fig. 9.91 Olfactory system. **(a, b)** Olfactory mucosa. **(c)** Synaptic patterns in an olfactory bulb. (*continued*) (From Schuenke M, Schulte E, Schumacher U. THIEME Atlas of Anatomy. Head, Neck, and Neuroanatomy. Illustrations by Voll M and Wesker K. 3rd ed. New York: Thieme Medical Publishers; 2020.)

optic tract but the axons from the *temporal half* of the retina remain on the ipsilateral side. This means the visual information from one-half of the visual field is carried within the contralateral optic tract and processed at the adjoining **lateral geniculate body** before continuing via the optic radiations to the occipital lobe of the cerebral cortex. The **retinogeniculate pathway** represents the pathway from the retina to the lateral geniculate body (**Fig. 9.92b, c; Fig. 9.93**).

While the majority of fibers passing through the optic tract terminate in the lateral geniculate body (~90%), some fibers bypass it as the **brachium of the superior colliculus** and terminate at the **superior colliculus**. The superior colliculus functions in orientating the head and eyes to both visual and auditory stimuli from the external environment. Additional fibers that have bypassed or are collateral branches that terminated in the lateral geniculate body can terminate at the **pretectal area**, an area that serves as the afferent limb of the light reflex. There are additional optic tract axons that target the **suprachiasmatic nucleus of the hypothalamus** and are sensitive to circadian rhythms. These nongeniculate parts of the visual pathway are described in **Fig. 9.94**.

The lateral geniculate bodies are made up of six layers and all of these layers process information from the contralateral visual field. Each of the layers processes information exclusively from only one retina and from either cones or rods. This segregation of information from the retinae is preserved in the **optic radiations (geniculocalcarine pathway)** that span the lateral geniculate bodies to

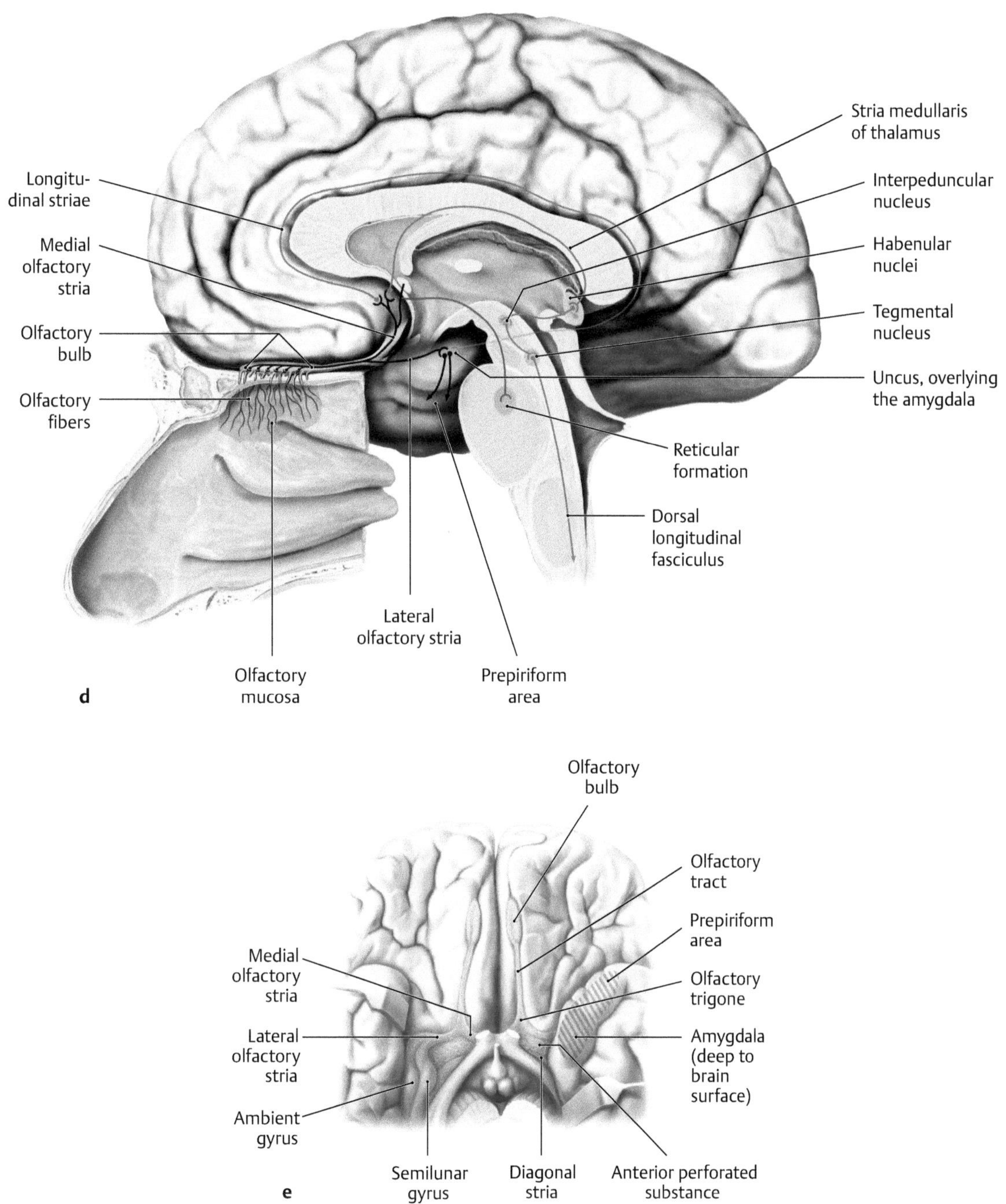

Fig. 9.91 (*continued*) Olfactory system. **(d, e)** Central connections of the olfactory system. (From Schuenke M, Schulte E, Schumacher U. THIEME Atlas of Anatomy. Head, Neck, and Neuroanatomy. Illustrations by Voll M and Wesker K. 3rd ed. New York: Thieme Medical Publishers; 2020.)

the **primary visual cortex (area 17** or **striate cortex)** located just above and below the **calcarine fissure** on the medial surface of the occipital lobe (**Fig. 9.56a, c, d; Fig. 9.92a, b; Fig. 9.93).** The primary visual cortex is the only location where information from both retinae can converge upon a single cortical cell. The projection neurons from all six layers transmit their axons to the primary visual cortex. The optic radiations form the retrolenticular portion of the internal capsule. As these radiations pass just anterior to the most vertical portion of the lateral ventricle, they form a loop that extends forward into the temporal lobe. These looping fibers that originate from the contralateral temporal superior visual field represent fibers of the contralateral inferior nasal retinal quadrant. This loop is called **Meyer's loop** (**Fig. 9.92a**).

The primary visual cortex is thicker in layer 4 and it is marked by a dense plexus of myelinated axons that are actually axon collaterals of the primary visual cortex and referred to as the *stripe of Gennari* (**Fig. 9.56d**). The visual association areas are located in **area 18** and **area 19**. These two areas contain at least a partial representation of the retinal fields and receive input directly from area 17. The visual cortex demonstrates a precise localization pattern

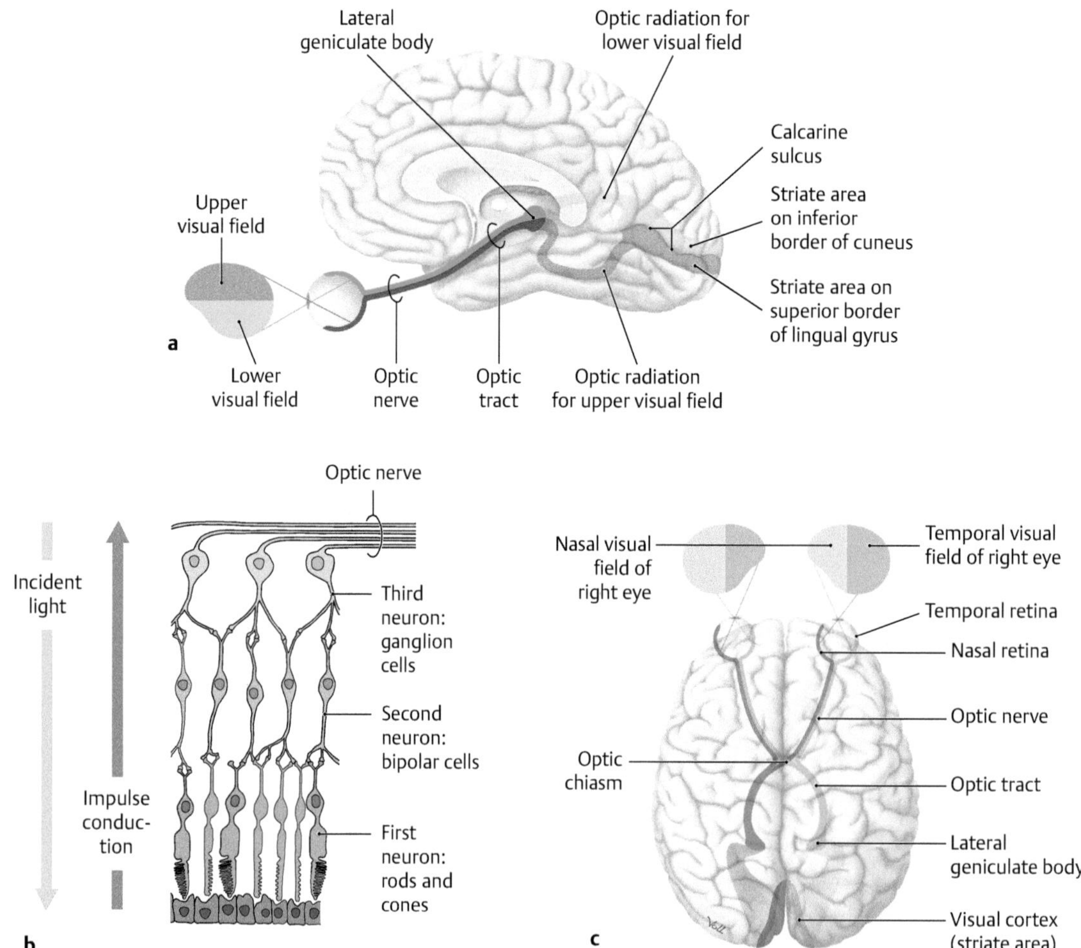

Fig. 9.92 **(a)** Overview of the visual system. **(b)** The retina and the first three neurons of the visual pathway. **(c)** Representation of each visual field in the contralateral visual cortex. (From Schuenke M, Schulte E, Schumacher U. THIEME Atlas of Anatomy. Head, Neck, and Neuroanatomy. Illustrations by Voll M and Wesker K. 3rd ed. New York: Thieme Medical Publishers; 2020.)

with the macular portion of the retina representing a much larger cortical area than the peripheral parts of the retina. This translates to the central 10 degrees of visual space occupying around 50% of the visual cortex. The **macular area** of the retina is a small region that surrounds the fovea centralis, which serves central vision and contains cones. This area projects to the most posterior portion of the visual cortex. The **paramacular (parafoveal) area** of the retina is a larger area that surrounds the macular portion and contains mostly rods. This area projects to the visual cortex anterior to that of the macular portrayal. The **monocular area** represents the peripheral retinal field and projects to the visual cortex just anterior to the paramacular portrayal.

The flow of information that originates from the cones and is represented by smaller axons in the retinogeniculate pathway before terminating in the lateral geniculate body (parvocellular layer) is involved with recognition of form, shape, and color of the stimulus and proceeds by way of a multisynaptic course to area 37 of the middle temporal cortex. The flow of information that originates from rods, is represented by larger axons in the retinogeniculate pathway, and terminates in the lateral geniculate body (magnocellular layer) is used to determine where relevant visual stimuli are located and whether they are moving. This information was relayed to area 17 but can proceed to area 7a of the posterior parietal cortex through multisynaptic pathways. Areas 18 and 19 and the previously listed temporal and parietal cortices are essential for visual fixation and other reflexes in addition to the aforementioned recognition of form, shape, color, and movement functions. The pulvinar can send inputs to areas 18 and 19 and adjacent cortices. The pulvinar and/or lateral posterior nucleus of the thalamus may receive neurons from the superior colliculus before projecting to areas 18 and 19 and the association areas of the parietal, occipital, and temporal lobes. This information may be related to evaluating the importance of the visual stimulus, its speed, and the direction of eye movements.

Visual defects and lesions are described relative to a visual field defect and are from the perspective of the patient. The term **anopia** means absence of vision in a visual field while the term **scotoma** refers to a partial defect within the field of vision (**Fig. 9.95**).

1. **Monocular blindness** of the left eye is caused by a lesion of the ipsilateral left optic nerve.
2. **Bitemporal hemianopia** is caused by a lesion of the optic chiasm. This type of lesion interrupts the fibers from the nasal portions of the retina that themselves represent the temporal

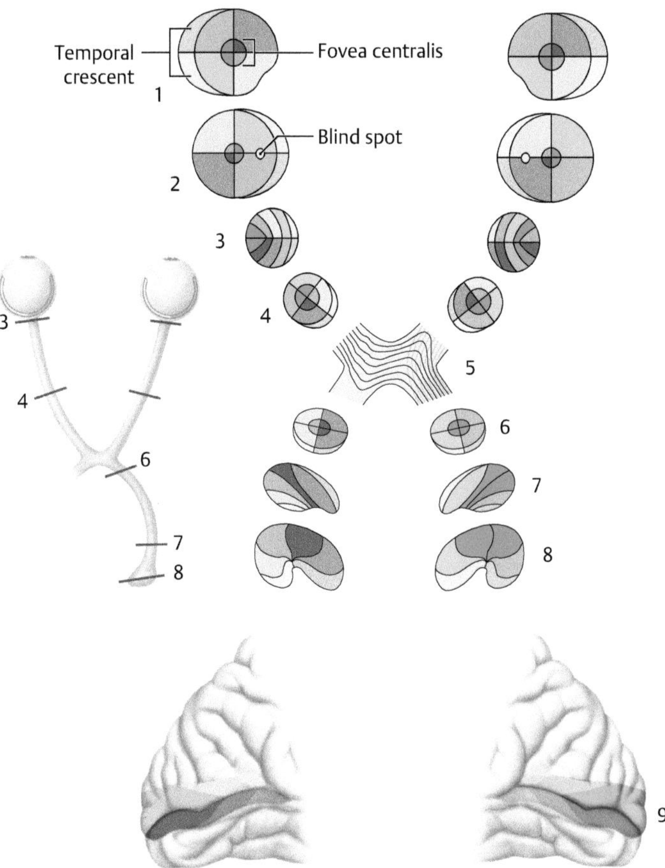

The fovea centralis, the point of maximum visual acuity on the retina, has a high receptor density. Accordingly, a great many axons pass centrally from its receptors, and so the fovea centralis is represented by an exceptionally large area in the visual cortex. Other, more peripheral portions of the retina contain fewer receptors and therefore fewer axons, resulting in a smaller representational area in the visual cortex. Note: Only the left half of the complete visual field is shown. It is subdivided into four quadrants (clockwise from top left in 1): upper temporal, upper nasal, lower nasal, and lower temporal. The representation of this subdivision is continued into the visual cortex.

1 The three zones that make up a particular visual hemifield (left, in this case) are each indicated by color shading of decreasing intensity: The smallest and darkest zone is at the center of the fovea centralis; it corresponds to the central visual field. The largest zone is the macular visual field, which also contains the "blind spot" (= optic disk, see **2**). The "temporal crescent" represents the temporal, monocular part of the visual field. Note that the lower nasal quadrant of each visual field is indented by the nose (small medial depression).

2 Because all light that reaches the retina must first pass through the narrow pupil (which is like the aperture of a camera), up/down and temporal/nasal are exactly reversed when the image is projected onto the **retina**.

3, 4 In the initial part of the optic nerve, the fibers that represent the macular visual field first occupy a lateral position (**3**) and then move increasingly toward the center of the nerve (**4**).

5 In traversing the **optic chiasm**, the nasal fibers of the optic nerve cross the midline to the opposite side.

6 At the **start of the optic tract**, the fibers from the corresponding halves of the retinae unite—the right halves of the retinae in the right tract, the left halves in the left tract. The impulses from the right visual field finally terminate in the left striate area. Initially the macular fibers continue to occupy a central position in the optic tract.

7 At the **end of the optic tract**, just before it enters the lateral geniculate body, the fibers are collected to form a wedge.

8 In the **lateral geniculate body**, the wedge shape is preserved, the macular fibers occupying almost half the wedge. These fibers synapse with the fourth neurons, which project to the posterior end of the occipital pole (**visual cortex**).

9 This figure shows that the central part of the visual field is represented by the largest area in the visual cortex compared with other portions of the field. This is due to the large number of axons that run to the optic nerve from the fovea centralis. This large proportion of axons is continued into the visual cortex, establishing a point-to-point (retinotopic) correlation between the fovea centralis and the visual cortex. The other parts of the visual field also show a point-to-point correlation but have fewer axons. The central lower half of the visual field is represented by a large area on the occipital pole above the calcarine sulcus, while the central upper half of the visual field is represented below the sulcus. The region of central vision also occupies the largest area within the lateral geniculate body (see **8**).

Fig. 9.93 Topographic organization of the geniculate part of the visual pathway. (From Schuenke M, Schulte E, Schumacher U. THIEME Atlas of Anatomy. Head, Neck, and Neuroanatomy. Illustrations by Voll M and Wesker K. 3rd ed. New York: Thieme Medical Publishers; 2020.)

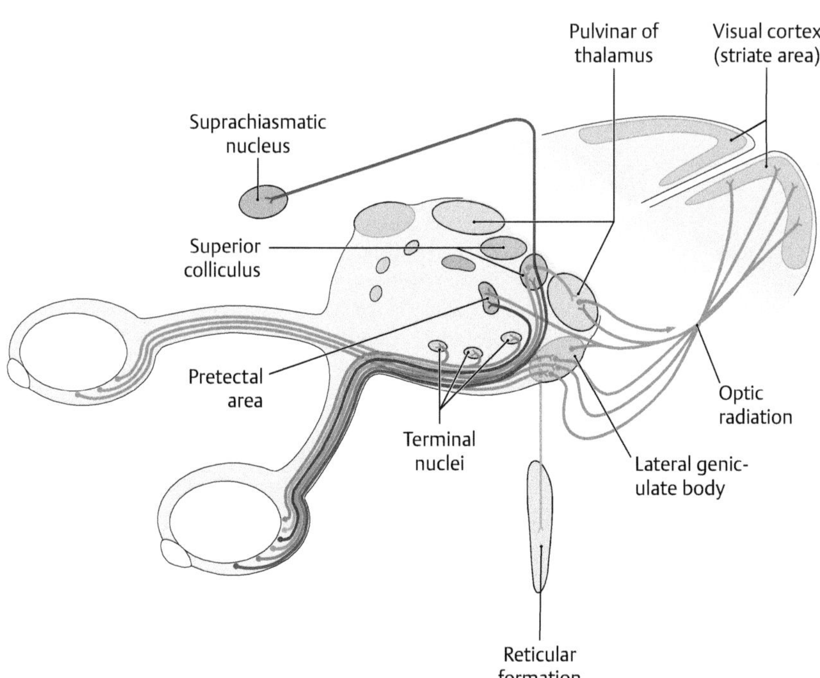

Approximately 10% of the axons of the optic nerve do not terminate on neurons in the lateral geniculate body. These axons will continue along the medial root of the optic tract and form the nongeniculate part of the visual pathway. The information from these fibers plays an important role in unconscious regulation of various vision-related processes and in visually mediated reflexes (e.g., the afferent limb of the pupillary light reflex). Axons from the nongeniculate part of the visual pathway terminate in the following regions:

- Superior colliculus: will transmit kinetic information that is necessary for tracking moving objects by unconscious eye and head movements (retinotectal system).
- Pretectal area: afferents for pupillary responses and accommodation reflexes (retinopretectal system).
- Suprachiasmatic nucleus of the hypothalamus: will influence circadian rhythms.
- Thalamic nuclei (optic tract) in the tegmentum of the midbrain and to the vestibular nuclei: afferent fibers for optokinetic nystagmus (jerky, physiological eye movements during the tracking of fast-moving objects). This has been called the "accessory visual system."
- Pulvinar of the thalamus: visual association cortex for oculomotor function (neurons are relayed in the superior colliculus).
- Parvocellular nucleus of the reticular formation: arousal function.

Fig. 9.94 Nongeniculate part of the visual pathway. (From Schuenke M, Schulte E, Schumacher U. THIEME Atlas of Anatomy. Head, Neck, and Neuroanatomy. Illustrations by Voll M and Wesker K. 3rd ed. New York: Thieme Medical Publishers; 2020.)

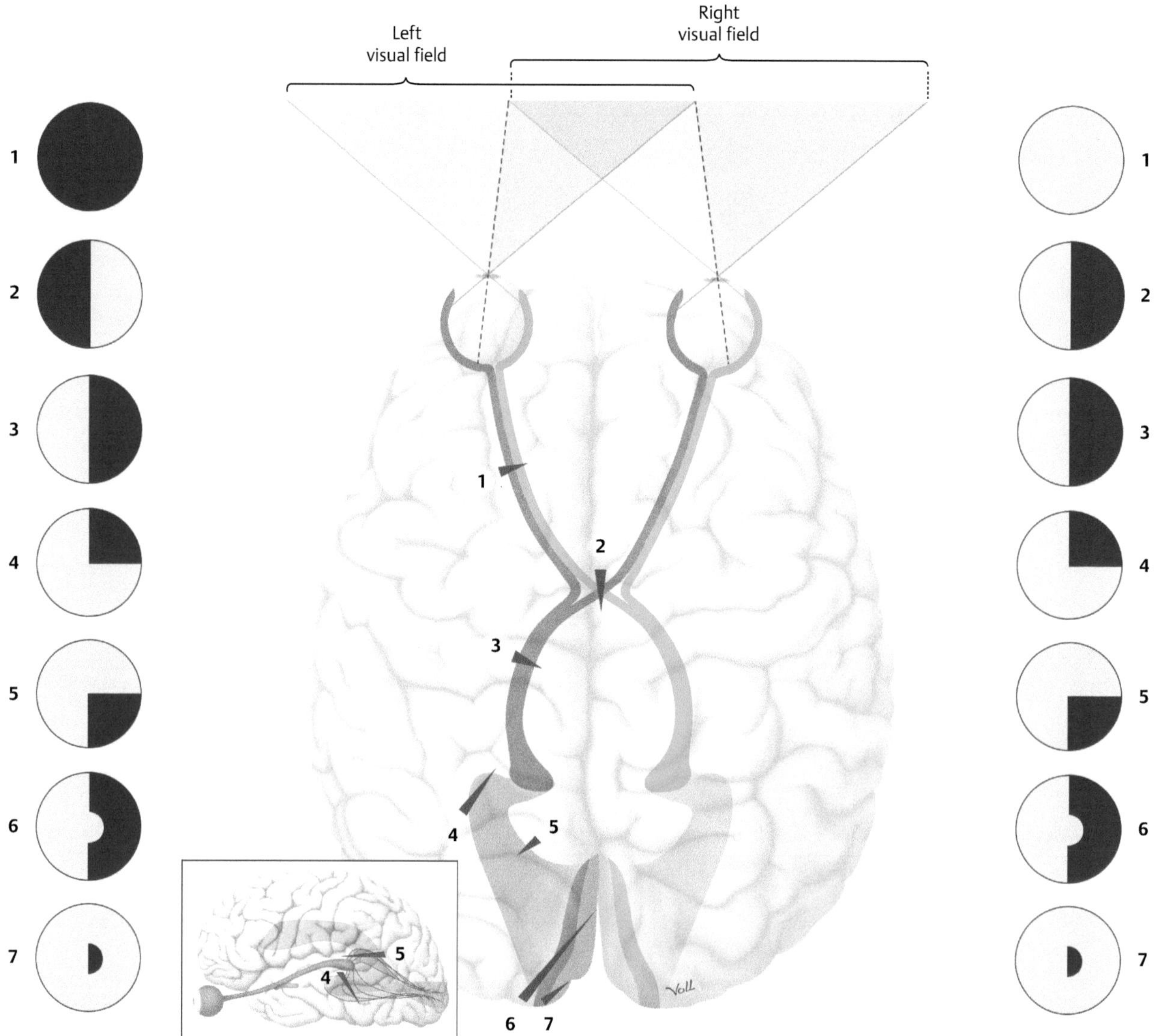

Fig. 9.95 Visual field defects (scotomata) and their location along the visual pathway. (From Schuenke M, Schulte E, Schumacher U. THIEME Atlas of Anatomy. Head, Neck, and Neuroanatomy. Illustrations by Voll M and Wesker K. 3rd ed. New York: Thieme Medical Publishers; 2020.)

visual fields. These fibers were the only ones that cross at the optic chiasm. The individual will describe having tunnel vision.

3. **Right homonymous hemianopia** is due to a lesion of the optic tract. In the figure, the left optic tract is damaged and interrupts fibers from the temporal portions of the retina on the ipsilateral side and the nasal portions on the contralateral side. The right or left half of the visual field is affected in each eye.
4. **Right superior homonymous quadrantanopia** is caused by a unilateral lesion of optic radiations specifically referred to as *Meyer's loop* located in the anterior temporal lobe. This is also referred to as a "pie-in-the-sky" deficit. The affected fibers rap around the inferior horn of the lateral ventricle in the temporal lobe before heading back to the visual cortex.
5. **Right inferior homonymous quadrantanopia** is caused by a unilateral lesion of the optic radiations not associated with *Meyer's loop* and closer to the parietal lobe. This type of lesion is rare.
6. **Right homonymous hemianopia with macular sparing** is the result of a lesion affecting the occipital lobe. They are most commonly the result of intracerebral hemorrhages. Macular sparing occurs because the optic radiations fan out before entering the visual cortex and there is an anastomotic blood supply related to that part of the visual cortex. A bilateral lesion targeting the same area results in *peripheral anopia* or "keyhole vision."
7. **Right homonymous macular hemianopia** is the result of a lesion targeting the cortical areas of the occipital lobe specific to the macula. A bilateral lesion targeting the same area results in *macular anopia*.

9.31.1 Pupillary Light Reflex

The **pupillary light reflex** (**Fig. 9.96**) enables the eye to adapt to multiple intensities of brightness. It is comprised of an afferent limb (CN II) and an efferent limb (CN III). With large amounts of light entering the eye, the pupil must constrict in order to protect

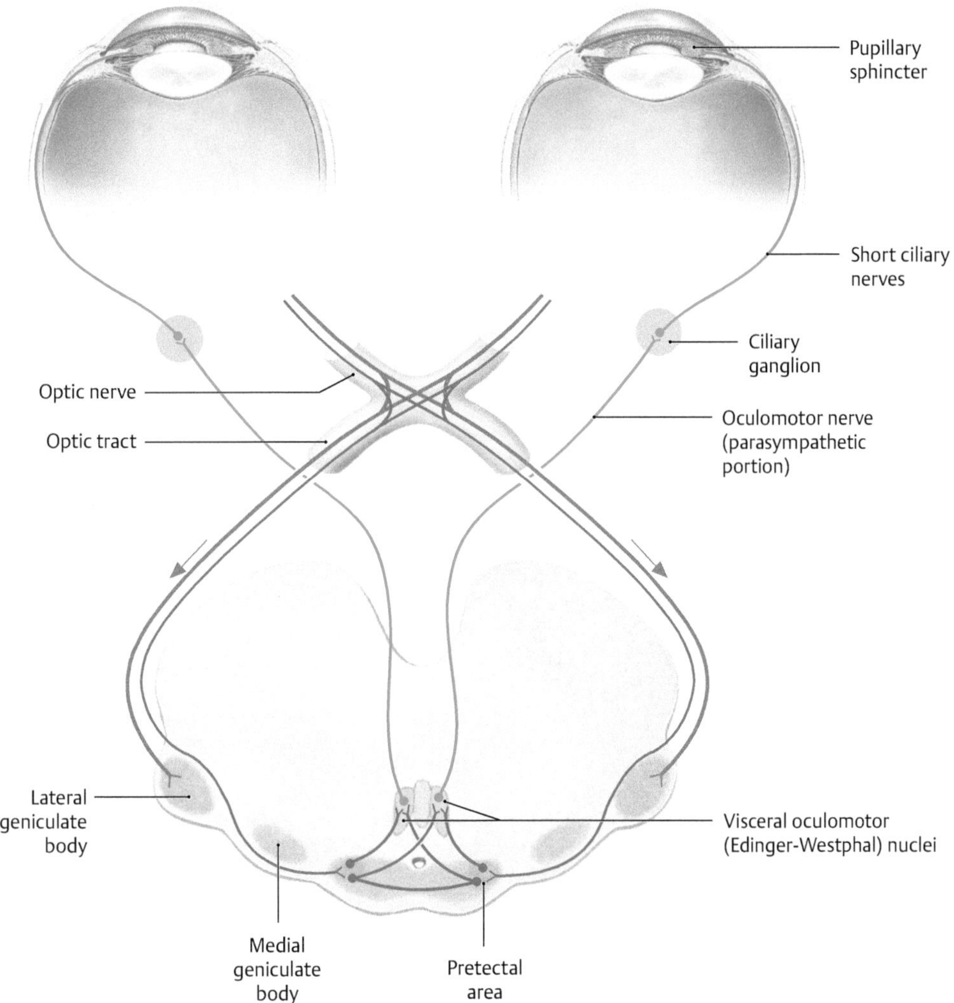

Fig. 9.96 Pupillary light reflex. (From Schuenke M, Schulte E, Schumacher U. THIEME Atlas of Anatomy. Head, Neck, and Neuroanatomy. Illustrations by Voll M and Wesker K. 3rd ed. New York: Thieme Medical Publishers; 2020.)

the photoreceptors of the retina. The pupil then dilates when the intensity of the light has decreased. The afferent limb begins in the retina and fibers related to the reflex (blue) pass to the **pretectal area/nucleus**. After the synapse in the pretectal area occurs, the axons pass bilaterally to the **Edinger-Westphal nuclei** of the oculomotor nerve (CN III). The efferent limb begins at the Edinger-Westphal nuclei (*parasympathetic preganglionic fibers*) and their axons project to the ipsilateral **ciliary ganglion** and synapse. From the ciliary ganglion, *parasympathetic postganglionic fibers* travel through the **short ciliary nerves** before innervating the **sphincter pupillae muscles** forcing constriction of the pupils.

To test the **direct light response**, the individual must be conscious and have both of their eyes covered. The patient then uncovers one eye, exposing it to light and after a short period the pupil should contract. For testing the **indirect (consensual) light response**, the medical professional places their hand on the bridge of the patient's nose, thus shading one of the eyes from the beam of a flashlight while they shine it into the other eye. If there is no defect, both pupils still constrict, even though one of the eyes is shaded from the light. If there is a unilateral optic nerve lesion, there is no direct response when light is shone into the affected eye. The indirect light response on the opposite side is also lost because of the impairment of the afferent limb of the light response on the affected side. If light is applied to the unaffected side, as expected there is pupillary constriction in that eye. The indirect light response is also present because of the afferent signals related to this reflex are mediated by the unaffected side while the efferent signals are not mediated by the optic nerve. If there is a lesion involving the Edinger-Westphal nucleus or even the ciliary ganglion, the efferent limb is lost. In both cases there are no direct or indirect light responses.

9.31.2 Convergence and Accommodation

When an object moves closer to the head, the visual axes of the eyes must move closer together, and this is called **convergence**. Simultaneously, **accommodation** occurs and this is when the eye lenses adjust their focal length (**Fig. 9.97**). The combination of these two processes is important to maintain a sharp and three-dimensional visual image. Convergence is important to keep an image of the approaching object on the fovea centralis, and contracting both medial recti muscles inward does this. During accommodation, the ciliary muscle relaxes but this increases the

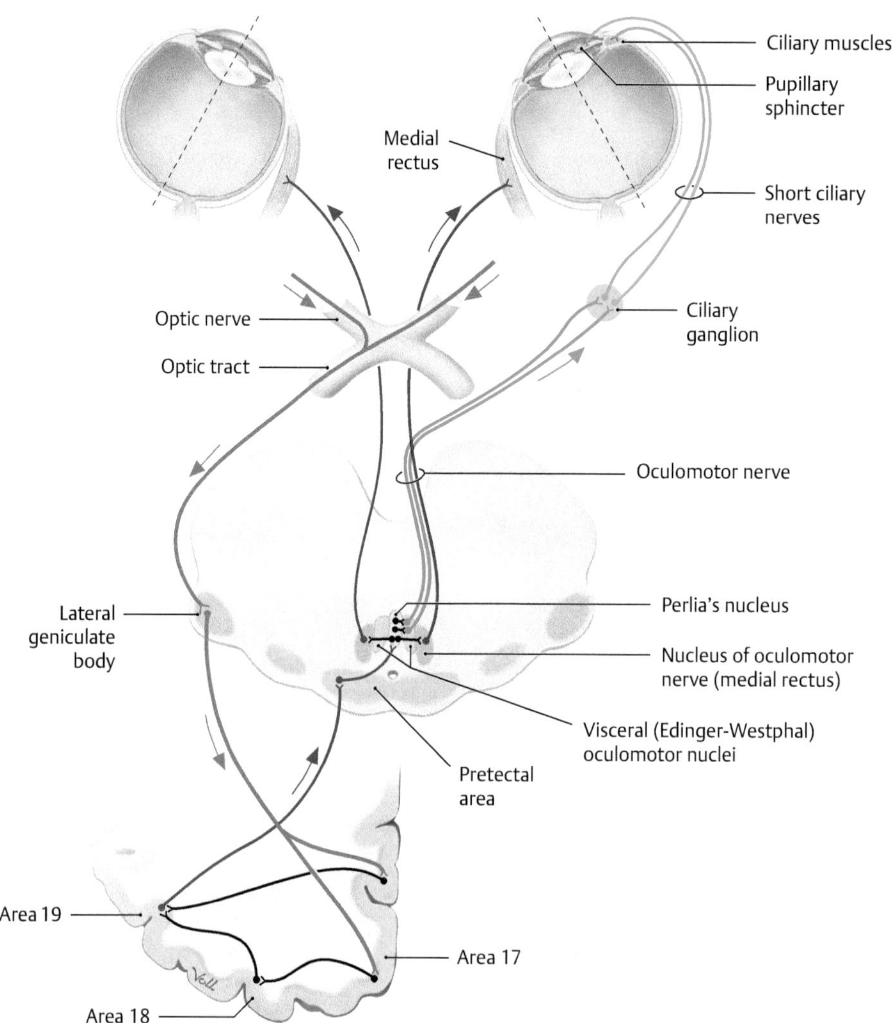

Fig. 9.97 Pathways for convergence and accommodation. (From Schuenke M, Schulte E, Schumacher U. THIEME Atlas of Anatomy. Head, Neck, and Neuroanatomy. Illustrations by Voll M and Wesker K. 3rd ed. New York: Thieme Medical Publishers; 2020.)

tension on the zonular fibers. This causes the lens to stretch and the image remains sharply focused on the retina. In addition to convergence and accommodation, the visual acuity increases with constriction of the pupil by the sphincter pupillae.

Both of these processes can occur while conscious, as in fixing the gaze onto a nearby object, or unconscious, when fixing ones gaze on an approaching object such as an automobile. After fibers of the visual pathway reach the lateral geniculate body, they are relayed to the primary visual cortex (area 17). Fibers that originate from the visual association areas 18 and 19 reach the pretectal area by way of synaptic relays and interneurons. Another relay targets **Perlia's nucleus**, which lies between the Edinger-Westphal nuclei. From Perlia's nucleus, one group of neurons related to convergence synapses on the oculomotor nucleus whose axons then pass directly to the medial rectus muscle. The other group related to accommodation and pupillary constriction projects relay neurons to the Edinger-Westphal nucleus.

9.31.3 Coordination of Eye Movements

The cerebellum and several portions of the brainstem are involved in the coordination of eye movements (**Fig. 9.98; Fig. 9.99**).

- **Nuclei of CN III, IV, and VI**: the extraocular muscles are yoked in pairs so that eyes move conjugately with one another. This includes both direction and speed of movements. The principle of equal innervation of paired extraocular muscles is called *Hering's Law.*
- **Paramedian pontine reticular formation (PPRF)**: referred to as the horizontal gaze center. It relies on the structure of the MLF to mediate horizontal conjugate eye movements.
- **Rostral interstitial nucleus of the medial longitudinal fasciculus (riMLF)**: referred to as the vertical gaze center. It relies on the connections related to the oculomotor and trochlear motor nuclei.
- **Superior colliculi**: the superior colliculi can project to the gaze centers and can receive either direct or indirect visual input. It contains an orderly visual map and the activation of visually related neurons in the superior colliculus by a visual stimulus can lead to the production of fast eye movements sufficient enough to align the foveas with the visual stimulus. It can receive auditory information from the inferior colliculus that helps in the localization of sounds and mediates reflex adjustments with the position of the eyes and head in response to an auditory stimulus. It receives cortical projections from areas 8 and 19.

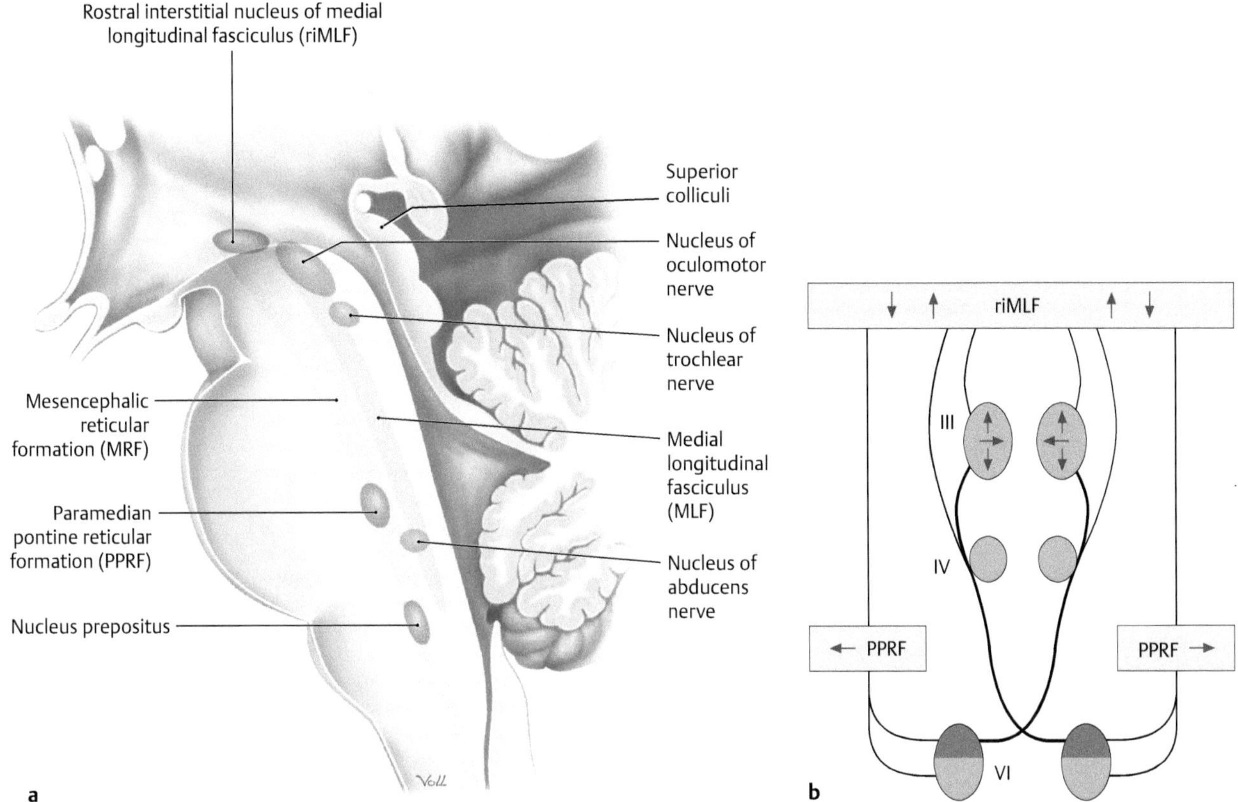

Fig. 9.98 Oculomotor nerve nuclei and their higher connections in the brainstem. **(a)** Midsagittal section viewed from the left side. **(b)** Circuit diagram showing the supranuclear organization of eye movements. When we shift our gaze to a new object, we swiftly move the axis of vision of our eyes toward the intended target. These rapid, precise, "ballistic" eye movements are called saccades. They are preprogrammed and, once initiated, cannot be altered until the end of the saccadic movement. The nuclei of all the nerves that supply the eye muscles (nuclei of cranial nerves III, IV, and VI, shaded red) are involved in carrying out these movements. They are interconnected for this purpose by the *medial longitudinal fasciculus* (shaded blue; see **Fig. 9.99a** for its location). Because these complex movements essentially involve all of the extraocular muscles and the nerves supplying them, the activity of the nuclei must be coordinated at a higher or *supranuclear level*. This means, for example, that when we gaze to the right with the *right* eye, the right lateral rectus muscle (CN VI, abducens nucleus activated) must contract while the right medial rectus muscle (CN III, oculomotor nucleus inhibited) must relax. For the left eye, the left lateral rectus (CN VI) must relax while the left medial rectus (CN III) must contract. Movements of this kind that involve both eyes are called *conjugate eye movements*. These movements are coordinated by several centers (premotor nuclei, shaded purple). Horizontal gaze movements are programmed in the nuclear region of the paramedian pontine reticular formation (PPRF), while vertical gaze movements are programmed in the rostral interstitial nucleus of the medial longitudinal fasciculus (riMLF). Both gaze centers establish bilateral connections with the nuclei of cranial nerves III, IV, and VI. The tonic signals for maintaining the new eye position originate from the nucleus prepositus (see **a**). (From Schuenke M, Schulte E, Schumacher U. THIEME Atlas of Anatomy. Head, Neck, and Neuroanatomy. Illustrations by Voll M and Wesker K. 3rd ed. New York: Thieme Medical Publishers; 2020.)

- **Cortical eye fields**: area 8 in the frontal lobe and area 19 of the parieto-occipital cortex. The frontal eye field (area 8) can project to the gaze centers and receive both direct and indirect visual input much like the superior colliculus. Area 8 contains the cortical upper motor neurons for innervation of the lower motor neurons of CN III, IV, and VI. Stimulation of area 8 results in conjugate deviation of the eyes to the opposite side of the initial stimulation. Area 8 projects both to the horizontal gaze center and superior colliculus. Area 19 receives direct input from area 17 before projecting to area 8 and the superior colliculi.
- Vestibular nuclei and their connections via the MLF and the abducent nucleus.

9.31.4 Saccades

Saccadic eye movements or **saccades** are defined as rapid conjugate eye movements. These are eye movements that quickly bring an image to the fovea and establish visual fixation. These movements can be *voluntary* and in response to a command or a remembered target. The control of voluntary saccades is dependent on frontal eye fields projecting to the horizontal or vertical gaze centers. A *reflexive* saccade would be in response to a visual, auditory, or somatosensory input. The control of a reflexive saccade depends on the superior colliculi projecting to a horizontal or vertical gaze centers.

Saccadic movements involve neuronal activity from the cerebral cortex streaming downward to the contralateral PPRF. Voluntary saccades are related to impulses from the frontal eye fields that travel directly to the PPRF. A reflexive saccade is related to an impulse originating from the parietal eye fields and traveling first to the superior colliculus before continuing to the PPRF. Signals for horizontal saccades activate the PPRF, which in turn activates both motor neurons and interneurons in the abducent motor nucleus. Then by way of the MLF, signals are sent to the contralateral oculomotor nucleus. Vertical saccades use the same pathway to the

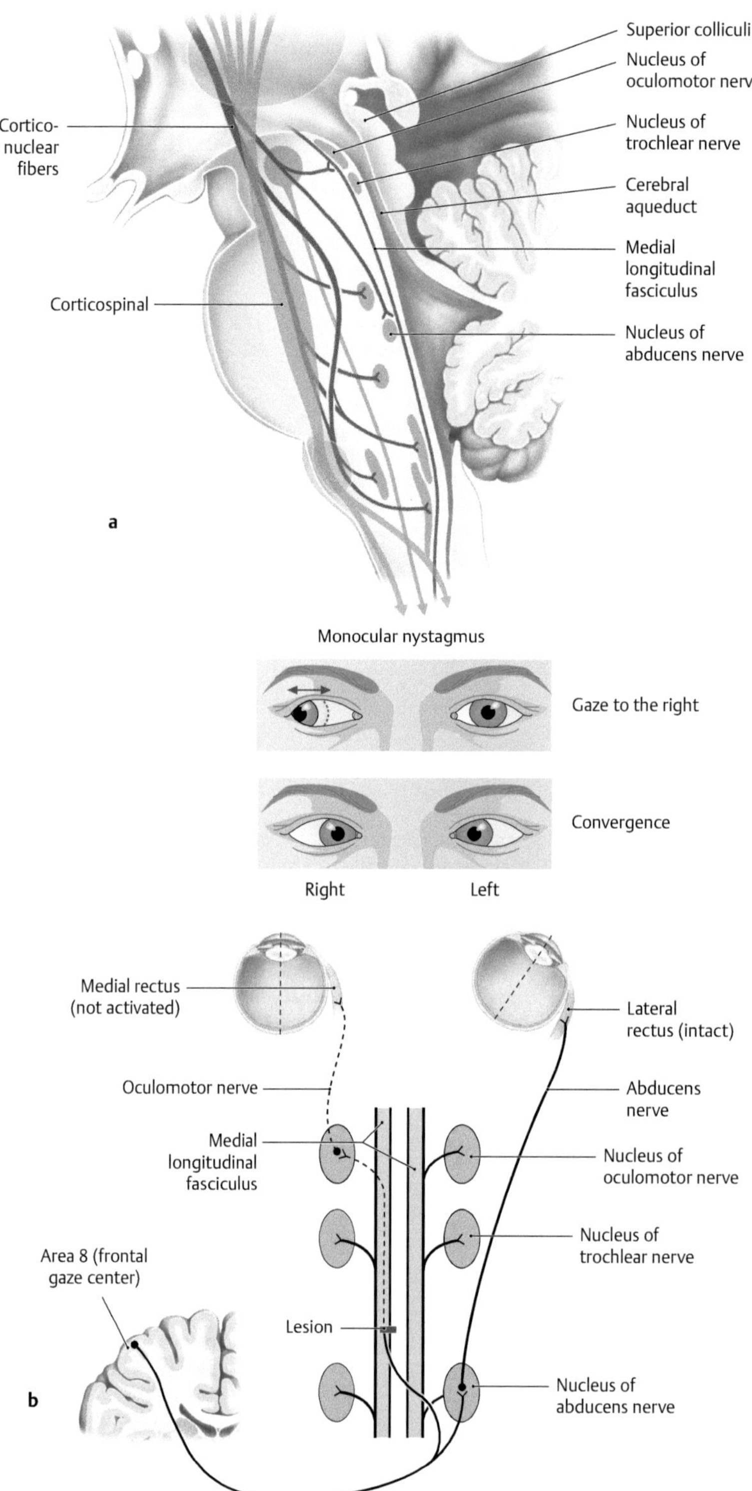

Fig. 9.99 **(a)** Course of the medial longitudinal fasciculus in the brainstem; midsagittal section viewed from the left side. **(b)** Lesion of the medial longitudinal fasciculus and internuclear ophthalmoplegia. The medial longitudinal fasciculus runs anterior to the cerebral aqueduct on both sides and continues from the mesencephalon to the cervical spinal cord. It transmits fibers for the coordination of conjugate eye movements. A lesion of the MLF results in internuclear ophthalmoplegia (see **b**). The medial longitudinal fasciculus interconnects the oculomotor nuclei and also connects them with the opposite side. When this "information highway" is interrupted, internuclear ophthalmoplegia develops. This type of lesion most commonly occurs between the abducens nucleus and the oculomotor nucleus. It may be unilateral or bilateral. Typical causes are multiple sclerosis and diminished blood flow. The lesion is manifested by the loss of conjugate eye movements. With a lesion of the left medial longitudinal fasciculus, as shown here, the left medial rectus muscle is no longer activated during gaze to the right. The eye cannot be moved inward on the side of the lesion (loss of the medial rectus), and the opposite eye goes into an abducting nystagmus (lateral rectus is intact and innervated by the abducent nerve). Reflex movements such as convergence are not impaired because there is no peripheral or nuclear lesion and this reaction is not mediated by the medial longitudinal fasciculus. (From Schuenke M, Schulte E, Schumacher U. THIEME Atlas of Anatomy. Head, Neck, and Neuroanatomy. Illustrations by Voll M and Wesker K. 3rd ed. New York: Thieme Medical Publishers; 2020.)

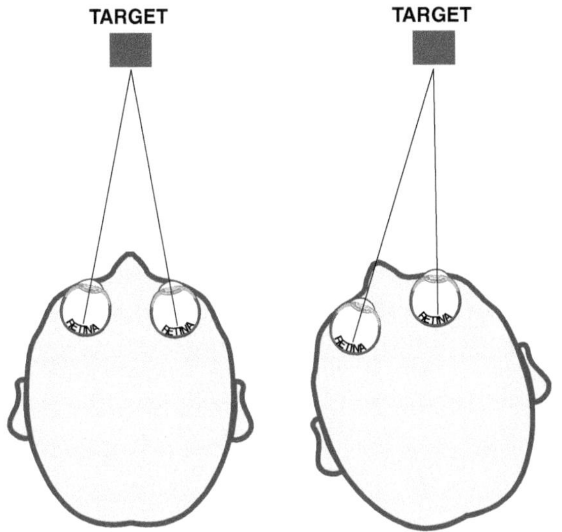

Fig. 9.100 Vestibulo-ocular reflex. (From Albertstone CD et al. Anatomic Basis of Neurologic Diagnosis. New York: Thieme Medical Publishers; 2009.)

PPRF but the impulses from the PPRF cells travel to the riMLF and nearby interstitial nucleus *of Cajal* located near the oculomotor nuclei.

9.31.5 Vestibulo-ocular Reflex

The **vestibulo-ocular reflex (VOR)** is responsible for maintaining an image on the foveae during brief head rotations. This reflex serves as a stabilizing mechanism responsible for keeping the eyes directed at a target when external stimuli are present. Without the VOR, images of the visual world would move from the foveae with every head movement and our vision would be blurry. Stationary objects would actually appear to be moving every time the head turned. The receptors for this reflex are located in the semicircular ducts and neural activity is integrated by the vestibular nuclei. The VOR involves a conjugate eye movement equal in magnitude but is in the direction opposite to that of the head movement perceived by the vestibular apparatus (**Fig. 9.100**).

9.31.6 Optokinetic Eye Movements

Optokineitc eye movements are a way to compensate for prolonged and continuous velocity movements such as staring out of a window while traveling on a highway. To compensate, an individual's eyes automatically move to stabilize images on the retina, which is previously described as VOR. After a prolonged period of continuous velocity movement, VOR fades because vestibular apparatus stimulation reaches equilibrium with the movement of the head. At this time, however, compensatory eye movements begin to occur in order to find another visual target. This normal reflex adjustment of the eyes is called **optokinetic nystagmus**. The phenomenon known as a **nystagmus** is related to a sequence of slow eye movements in one direction followed by quick movements back in the opposite direction.

9.32 The Auditory System

The **auditory system** (**Fig. 9.101**) is responsible for the special sense of hearing. The external and middle ears were described in detail in Chapter 7. For discussion purposes, we begin at the inner ear to review the auditory system pathway. The inner ear is housed in the petrous portion of the temporal bone and it contains two parts: the **bony** and **membranous labyrinth**. The bony labyrinth is filled with perilymph and the membranous labyrinth is filled with endolymph.

The **cochlea** is the auditory portion of the bony labyrinth and it is connected to the open vestibule. The cochlea is a spiral-shaped canal that winds 2 ½ times around a central bony axis known as the **modiolus**. The **spiral (cochlear) ganglion** spirals around the inner margin of the cochlea and within the modiolus. The peripheral processes of these bipolar neurons innervate the receptors of the cochlear duct while the central processes enter the core of the modiolus and become the **cochlear nerve of the vestibulocochlear nerve (CN VIII)**.

The **cochlear duct (scala media)** is the endolymph-filled membranous labyrinth of the cochlea and the auditory apparatus responsible for hearing. The portions of the bony labyrinth that surround the cochlear duct are called the scala vestibuli and scala tympani, and these two structures are continuous with each other at the apex of the cochlea called the **helicotrema**. The **scala vestibuli** is positioned above the cochlear duct and communicates with the oval window. The **scala tympani** is positioned below the cochlear duct and ends at the round window. The scala vestibuli begins at the oval window and waves of hydraulic pressure created by vibrations of the stapes spiral upward within it toward the helicotrema. At the helicotrema these pressure waves spiral down through the scala tympani and end at the round window.

The cochlear duct is made up of three walls. The outer and highly vascularized wall is called the **stria vascularis**. The roof is located between the scala vestibuli and cochlear duct and is called the **vestibular (*Reissner's*) membrane**. The floor is located between the cochlear duct and the scala tympani and is called the **basilar membrane**. Residing on this membrane would be the wave-sensitive **hair cells** of the **spiral organ (of *Corti*)** and these hair cells are embedded in the **tectorial membrane**. The terminal ends of the peripheral processes of the cochlear nerve are connected to these hair cells. The stereocilia of the hair cells are exposed to shearing forces of the tectorial membrane that are produced due to vibrations at the basilar membrane. Movement of the hair cells transduces mechanical energy produced by pressure waves into electrochemical energy that travels as a nerve impulse through the cochlear nerve of CN VIII. The basilar membrane is the most sensitive to higher tones (faster frequency and shorter wavelengths) at the base of the cochlea and to lower tones (slower frequency and longer wavelengths) at the apex. The basilar membrane is narrowest at the base and widest at the apex and it is said to be *tonotopically organized*. Frequencies are measured in *Hertz* and frequency determines the pitch of sound. Amplitude of a sound wave is related to the loudness of a sound and this is measured in *decibels*. The human ear can detect sound frequencies between 20 and 20,000 Hertz and loudness between 1 and 120 decibels (discussed in Chapter 7).

Hearing information travels through the cochlear nerve and continues through the internal auditory meatus before reaching the pontomedullary junction of the brainstem. The cochlear nerve fibers of CN VIII pass over the surface of the inferior cerebellar peduncle and finally terminate in the **anterior** and **posterior cochlear nuclei**. These are the only auditory nuclei that do not receive binaural input. The ascending pathways of this system create a bilateral and multisynaptic system with a number of relay nuclei (**Fig. 9.101**).

All of the first-order cochlear nerve fibers enter the **anterior cochlear nucleus** but the axon terminal bifurcates and one axon terminal continues to the **posterior cochlear nucleus**. Second-order neurons from the cochlear nuclei ascend ipsilaterally or cross to the contralateral side chiefly in the **trapezoid body**. Much of the secondary auditory fibers both crossed and uncrossed terminate at the **superior olivary nucleus**. This nucleus plays a role in the localization of sound. From the superior olivary nucleus, third-order neurons ascend through the **lateral lemniscus** before terminating at the **inferior colliculus nuclei**. The inferior colliculus serves as an auditory relay and information station, with the fibers projecting from it creating the **brachium of the inferior colliculus** and finally terminating at the **nucleus of the medial geniculate body**. Fibers projecting from the medial geniculate body enter the **posterior limb (sublenticular part) of the internal capsule** and project to the **primary auditory cortex** on the superior temporal gyrus—a location also referred to as the **transverse gyri (of *Heschl*)** or **area 41**. The primary auditory cortex connects to the **secondary auditory cortex (area 42)** and **Wernicke's (area 22)**. These two connections are important for the interpretation of spoken word. Area 41 can project to additional cortical regions including the contralateral area 41 via the corpus callosum. Central lesions involving the auditory pathway and located only on the ipsilateral side have a minimal effect on hearing. This is because auditory stimuli project bilaterally in the brainstem (**Fig. 9.101**).

Information from one ear only (monaural) is routed primarily to the contralateral side of the brain whereas information from both ears (binaural) involves bilateral auditory pathways. Arising from the superior olivary nucleus is the **olivocochlear tract/bundle**, an uncrossed efferent tract that plays a role in suppressing auditory nerve activity and selective tuning of the hair cells to focus on specific auditory stimuli (**Fig. 9.102a**).

The **stapedius reflex** (**Fig. 9.102b**) is a reflex mechanism present to protect the inner ear from high intensity sounds; however, it is not effective for higher frequencies. It most likely serves to reduce the number of acoustic stimuli reaching the brainstem when the ambient level of sound is greater.

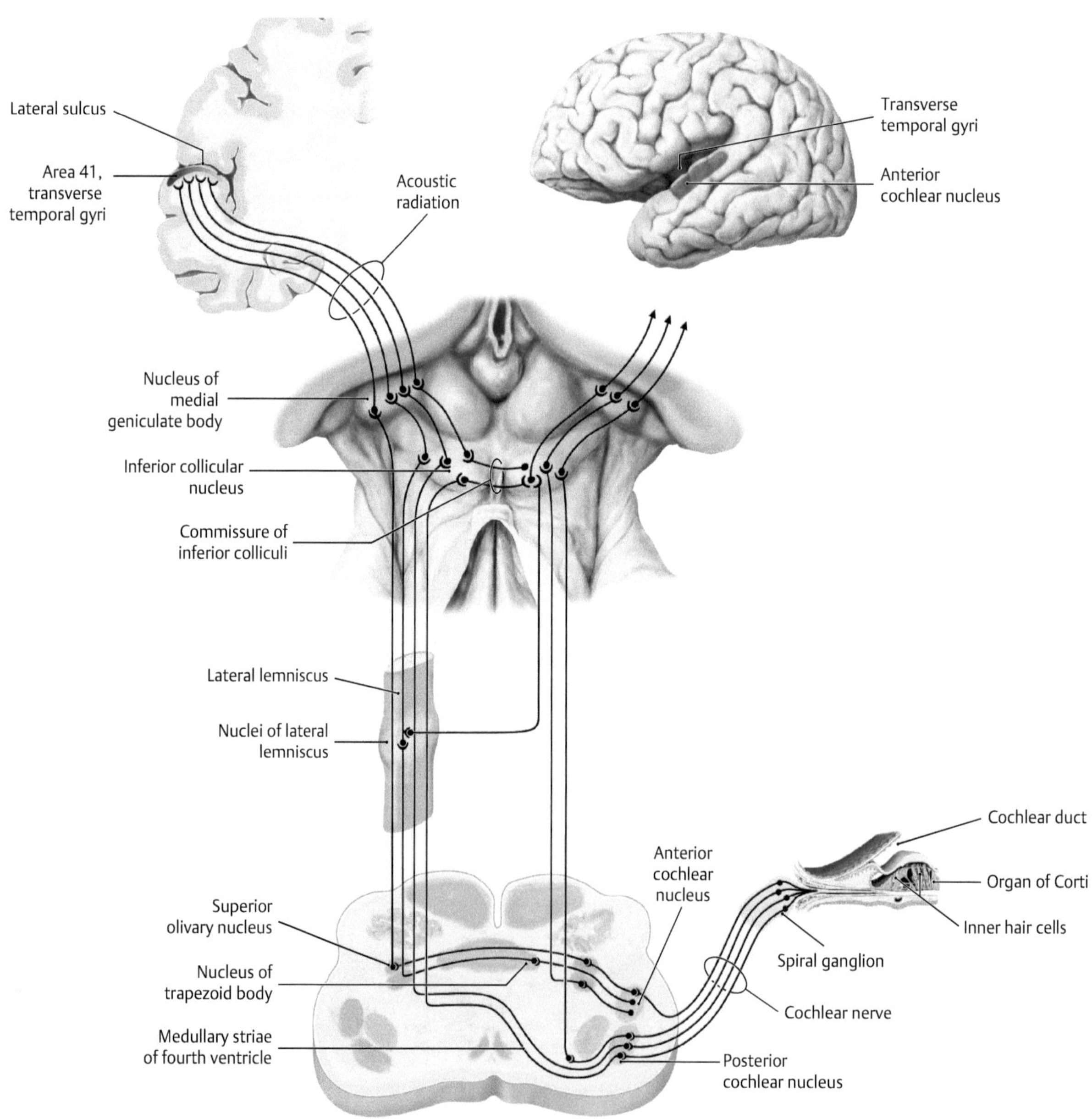

Fig. 9.101 Auditory system: afferent auditory pathway of the left ear. (From Schuenke M, Schulte E, Schumacher U. THIEME Atlas of Anatomy. Head, Neck, and Neuroanatomy. Illustrations by Voll M and Wesker K. 3rd ed. New York: Thieme Medical Publishers; 2020.)

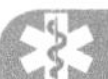 *Clinical Correlate 9.24*

Conductive and Sensorineural Hearing Loss
Both conductive hearing loss and sensorineural hearing loss were discussed in Chapter 7. Briefly, **conductive hearing loss** is the reduction in sound level or the ability to hear more faint sounds because of a deficiency in the conduction of sound (i.e., cerumen "ear wax" buildup) through the external and/or middle ear. Causes could include otitis media, tympanic membrane perforation, allergies, or a tumor. Surgery or the use of a hearing aid can correct this. **Sensorineural hearing loss** involves damage to the inner ear or pathways that connect the inner ear to the brain. Monaural hearing loss may be the result of lesions involving the cochlear duct (auditory apparatus), cochlear division of CN VIII, or the cochlear nuclei. *Cochlear implants* provide an opportunity for the severely hard of hearing or deaf to finally hear.

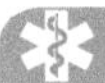 *Clinical Correlate 9.25*

Presbycusis
The loss of hearing occurring over normal aging is called **presbycusis** and it is the most common cause of hearing loss. Degenerative disease affecting the organ of *Corti* is the result of this condition.

 *Clinical Correlate 9.26*

Acoustic Neuroma
A peripheral nerve tumor of the vestibulocochlear nerve is called an **acoustic neuroma**. These are located generally in the internal acoustic meatus or in the posterior cranial fossa at the level of the cerebellopontine angle. Symptoms can include monaural hearing loss and tinnitus.

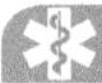 *Clinical Correlate 9.27*

Testing for Hearing Loss
Certain tests can be done to help distinguish between conduction and sensorineural hearing loss. They may also distinguish between air and bone conduction issues. These tests can include the Weber, Rinne, and Schwabach test.

- **Weber test**: a vibrating tuning fork is placed on the vertex of the skull. A normal result would mean a person is able to hear equally from both sides. If there is unilateral sensorineural hearing loss, the vibration is louder on the unaffected side, whereas if there is unilateral conduction hearing loss, the vibration is louder on the affected side.
- **Rinne test**: this test compares air and bone conduction issues. This test is performed by placing a vibrating tuning fork on the mastoid process of the temporal bone until it is no longer heard and then it is held in front of the ear. A normal patient hears vibrations in the air after the bone conduction is gone. A patient having unilateral sensorineural hearing loss hears vibrations in the air after bone conduction is gone, whereas a patient with unilateral conduction hearing loss fails to hear vibrations in the air after bone conduction is gone.
- **Schwabach test**: compares bone conduction of a patient to that of the examiner. This test assumes the examiner has normal hearing. If the patient stops hearing before the examiner, it suggests a sensorineural hearing loss. If the patient hears it longer than the examiner, it suggests a conductive hearing loss.

9.33 The Vestibular System

The **vestibular system** (**Fig. 9.103**) functions to maintain the balance of the body, coordination of eye, head, and body movements during the maintenance of equilibrium, and permits the eyes to remain fixed on a target as the head changes position. The bony vestibular labyrinth is made up of the vestibule and three semicircular canals. The semicircular canals communicate with the vestibule at both ends but at one end has a slight swelling. The membranous vestibular labyrinth is filled with endolymph and consists of the semicircular ducts, utricle, and saccule, and these structures make up the vestibular apparatus. The **semicircular ducts** are located in the semicircular canals and they communicate with the utricle directly. The swelling at one end of the semicircular duct is called the **ampulla**, and the sensory receptors called ampullary crests are located in this ampulla. The **ampullary crests** contain **hair cells** that project into a gelatinous **cupola** and they respond to rotational (angular) acceleration and deceleration of the head. The **utricle** and **saccule** are located in the vestibule and both have sensory receptors called maculae. The **maculae** are small and are covered with a gelatinous **otolithic membrane** containing **otoliths** (or otoconia). These receptors respond to linear acceleration and the force of gravity. The cilia of the **hair cells** project into either the cupula of the ampullary crest or the otolithic membrane of the utricle and saccule (discussed in Chapter 7).

When the head undergoes angular acceleration or deceleration (i.e., spinning or turning), the endolymph lags behind from inertia in the semicircular ducts and this pushes on the cupulae in the ampullae. This creates a receptor potential in the hair cells of the ampullary crests activating the peripheral processes of the vestibular ganglion cells. The otolithic membranes move the hair cells of the maculae if the head is tilted or if the head is stationary and there is a linear acceleration or deceleration. This movement induces changes in the membrane potential of the peripheral processes of the vestibular ganglion cells.

The **superior**, **lateral**, **medial**, and **inferior vestibular nuclei** are located dorsally and laterally in the brainstem tegmentum in the floor of the fourth ventricle throughout the rostral medullary and caudal pontine regions (**Fig. 9.103c**). The vestibular nuclei as a whole are important centers of integration of information in the CNS. They receive information from other ipsilateral or contralateral vestibular nuclei, send and receive information from the cerebellum, and receive information from the visual system and somatic sensory systems. Vestibular nuclei give rise to second-order neurons that project to the (1) spinal cord, (2) specific cranial nerve nuclei, (3) specific parts of the cerebellum, and/or (4) higher levels of the neuraxis.

- **Projections to spinal cord**: projections to the spinal cord are for postural adjustments. The **lateral vestibular nucleus** receives input primarily from the maculae. The **lateral vestibulospinal tract** arises from the lateral vestibular nucleus and descends ipsilaterally to the cervical through lumbar levels of the spinal cord. This facilitates the motor neurons that innervate extensor (antigravity) musculature to maintain posture, especially with the axial and proximal extensor musculature. The **medial vestibular nucleus** receives input primarily from the ampullary crests. The **medial vestibulospinal tract** constitutes the descending (crossed or uncrossed) fibers that originate from the medial vestibular nucleus and passes through the **medial longitudinal fasciculus (MLF)** before reaching the cervical levels of the spinal

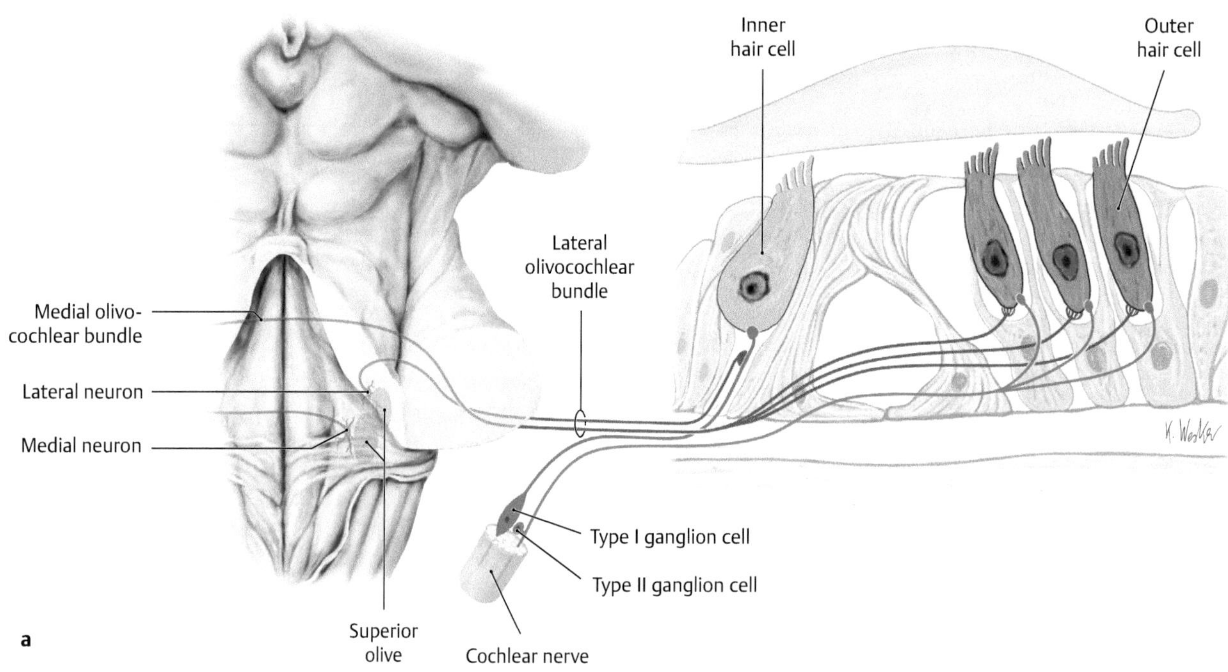

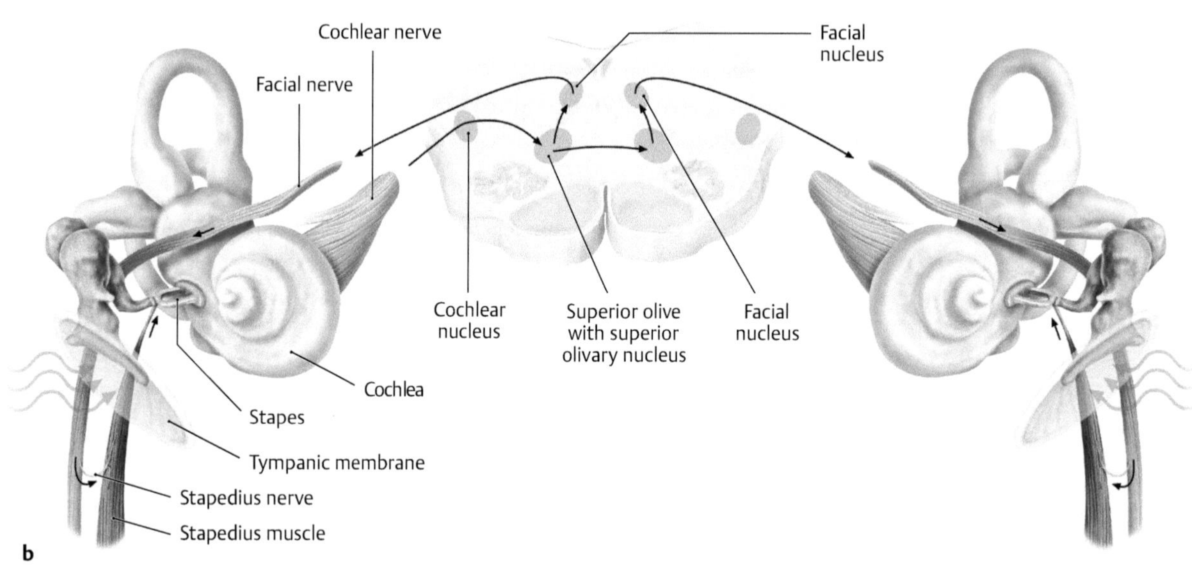

Fig. 9.102 (a) Efferent fibers from the olive to the organ of Corti. **(b)** The stapedius reflex. (From Schuenke M, Schulte E, Schumacher U. THIEME Atlas of Anatomy. Head, Neck, and Neuroanatomy. Illustrations by Voll M and Wesker K. 3rd ed. New York: Thieme Medical Publishers; 2020.)

cord. Here they synapse with interneurons that influence lower motor neurons that innervate neck and shoulder musculature (**Fig. 9.103a, c**).

- **Projections to specific cranial nerve nuclei**: crossed and uncrossed ascending fibers passing through the MLF originate from vestibular nuclei and project to the motor nuclei of CN III, IV, and VI (**Fig. 9.103a–c**). The **vestibulo-ocular reflex (VOR)** represents the mechanism for producing eye movements that counter head movements. It tends to keep the eyes on a horizontal plane and to allow an object in the visual field to remain on a fixed point on the retina. An example would include the increased activity of the right horizontal semicircular duct caused by turning the head to the right results in an increased input to the right vestibular nuclei. Originating from the right vestibular nuclei, excitatory projections cross the midline and terminate in the contralateral (left) abducent motor nucleus, which has two excitatory outputs: one to the left lateral rectus muscle via CN VI and the other from the abducent internuclear neurons, the axons of which cross the midline and project to the contralateral (right) oculomotor motor nucleus in the right MLF for innervation of the right medial rectus muscle. Hence, the horizontal conjugate movement of the eyes to the left occurs in response to turning the head to the right.

- **Projections to the cerebellum**: primary vestibular afferent fibers originating from all four vestibular nuclei project to the cortex of the **flocculonodular lobe** of the cerebellum via the **juxtarestiform body** of the inferior cerebellar peduncle. Purkinje cells from the cortex of the flocculonodular lobe send signals to the **nucleus fastigius**. Complementary connections between the vestibular system and the cerebellum act to regulate eye movements, head and neck movements, and postural adjustments (**Fig. 9.103a–c**).
- **Projections to the cerebral cortex**: these projections are important for conscious recognition of the position of the body in space. There are bilateral ascending projections that originate from the vestibular nuclei and are believed to pass through the ventral intermediate nucleus of the thalamus. There is no specific primary vestibular cortex in humans but from the thalamus, ascending fibers reach the regions of the temporoparietal junction and posterior insula (**Fig. 9.103a, b**).

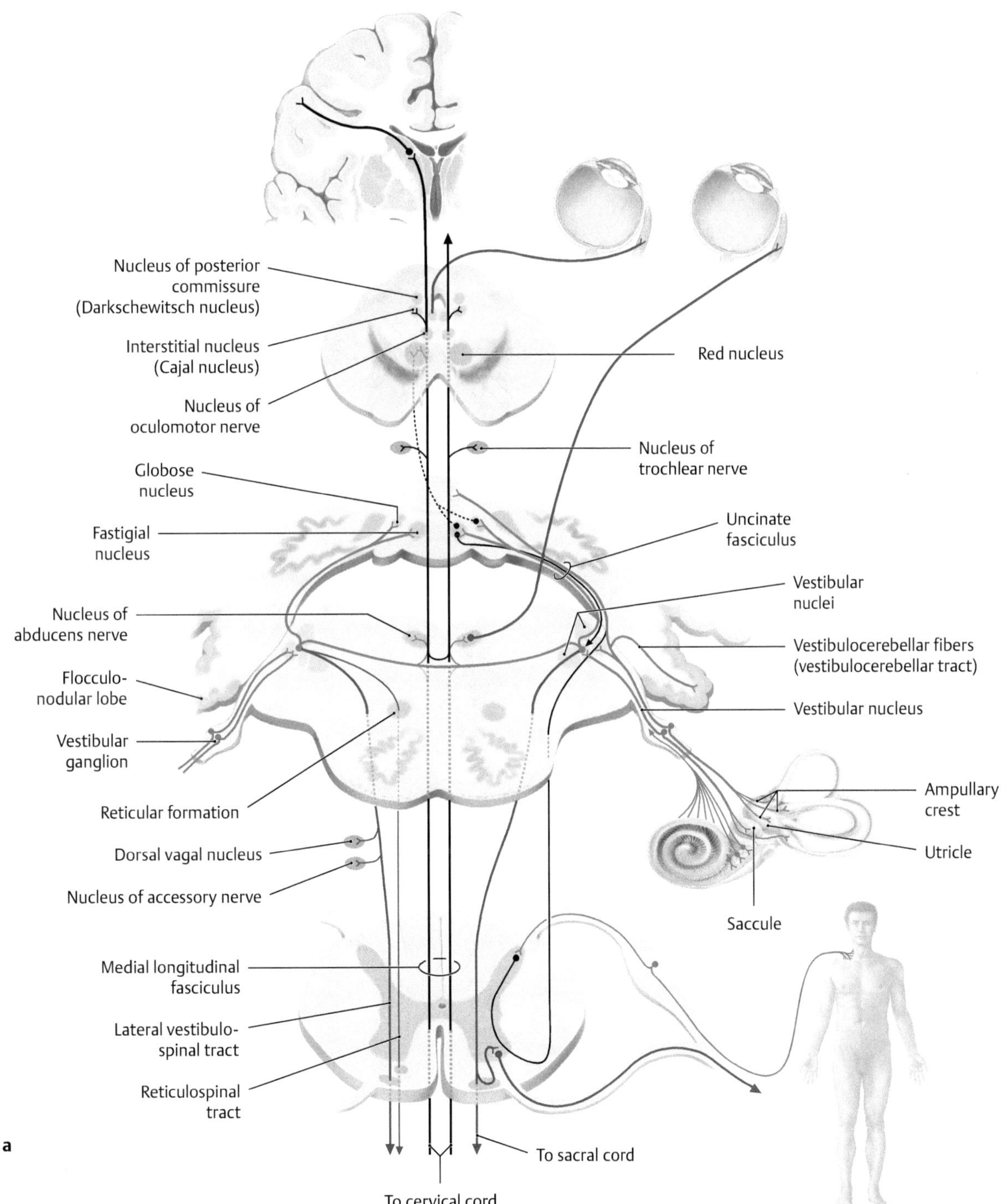

Fig. 9.103 (a) Central connections of the vestibular nerve. (*continued*) (From Schuenke M, Schulte E, Schumacher U. THIEME Atlas of Anatomy. Head, Neck, and Neuroanatomy. Illustrations by Voll M and Wesker K. 3rd ed. New York: Thieme Medical Publishers; 2020.)

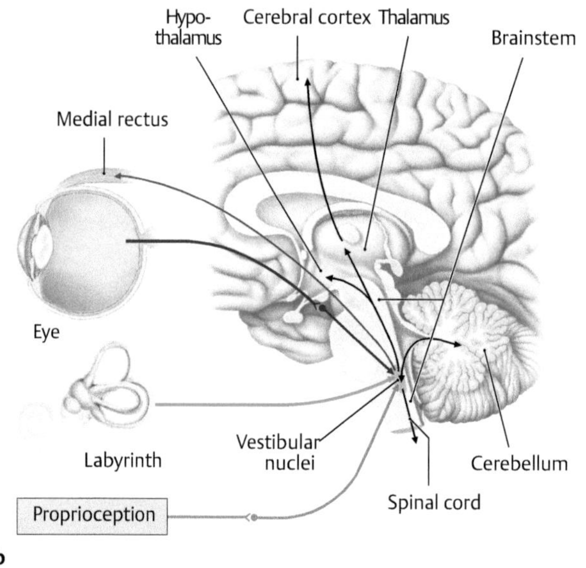

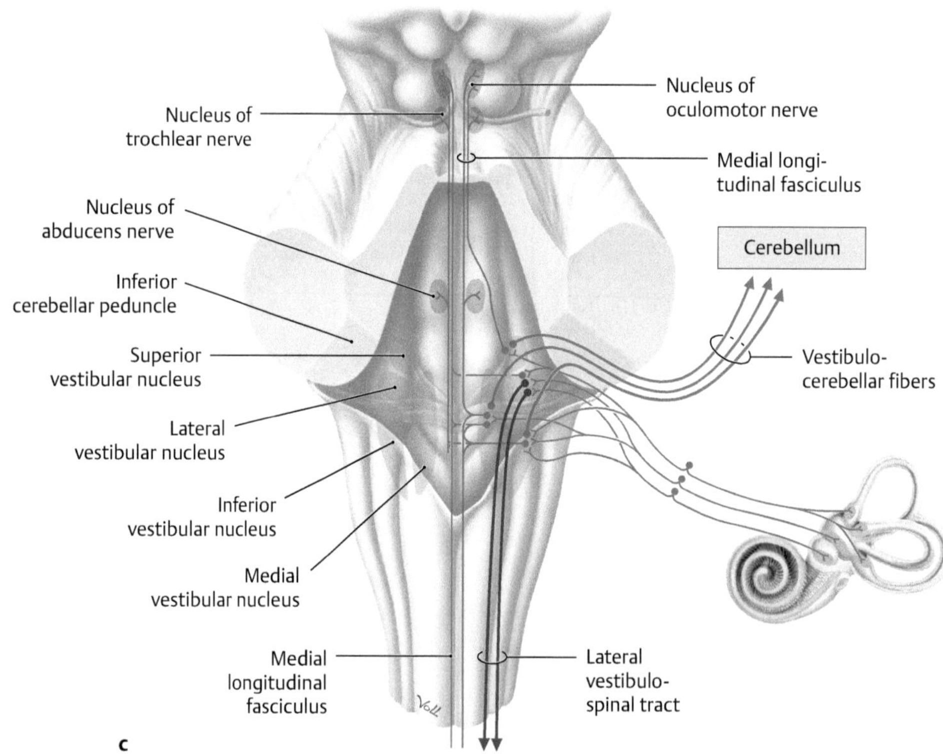

Fig. 9.103 *(continued)* **(b)** Central role of the vestibular nuclei in the maintenance of balance. **(c)** Vestibular nuclei: topographic organization and central connections. (From Schuenke M, Schulte E, Schumacher U. THIEME Atlas of Anatomy. Head, Neck, and Neuroanatomy. Illustrations by Voll M and Wesker K. 3rd ed. New York: Thieme Medical Publishers; 2020.)

9.34 The Gustatory System

The **gustatory system** (**Fig. 9.104**) is related to the sense of taste. The main taste buds are located mainly on the tongue but can also be picked up from the anterior epiglottic and soft palate regions. Peripheral processes of pseudounipolar neurons associated with the **facial (CN VII)**, **glossopharyngeal (CN IX)**, and **vagus nerves (CN X)** terminate on taste buds. The anterior two-thirds of the tongue and the soft palate are associated with the facial nerve. The posterior one-third of the tongue is paired with the glossopharyngeal nerve. The anterior epiglottic region is associated with the vagus nerve.

The **geniculate** (CN VII) and **inferior ganglions** (CN IX and X) are the locations of these pseudounipolar neuron cell bodies. The central processes of these first-order neurons send their information to the most rostral portion of the **nucleus of the solitary tract**. Second-order neurons project ipsilaterally via the **central tegmental tract** to the **ventral posteromedial (VPM) nucleus**. From the VPM, third-order neurons project to the **gustatory**

Clinical Correlate 9.28

Oculocephalic Reflex

The **oculocephalic (doll's eye) reflex** is tested by turning a patient's head from side to side. Absence of a fracture to the cervical spine must be ruled out before testing this reflex. When this reflex is present, the eyes do not turn with the head and it appears the patient is able to maintain fixation on a single point in space (positive doll's eye). Movements can be performed in the horizontal or vertical planes to test the reflex. The eyes are thus moving relative to the head in the direction opposite to the head movement. This is a normal finding in comatose patients but the reflex can be suppressed in conscious patients and is therefore not generally tested in them. Absence or asymmetry of this reflex in a comatose patient indicates possible dysfunction in the reflex pathway and multiple points for this do exist. A lesion could be in the afferent limb (vestibular nerve and neck proprioceptors), the efferent limb (CN III and VI and the muscles they innervate), or the pathways bridging the two limbs in the pons and medulla.

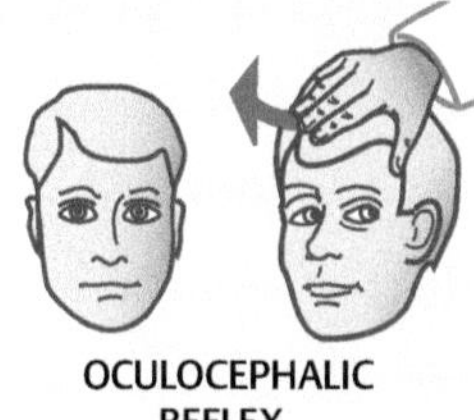

(From Albertstone CD et al. Anatomic Basis of Neurologic Diagnosis. New York: Thieme Medical Publishers; 2009.)

Clinical Correlate 9.29

Caloric Reflex Test

The caloric reflex or caloric nystagmus test is used to test the vestibulo-ocular reflex (VOR). Nystagmus is the condition where the eyes move rapidly and uncontrollably. To begin, the individual is left sitting erect or they may lie down before the head is tilted back 60°. This aligns the lateral/horizontal semicircular ducts in a plane best for easy observation. Cold or warm water is then irrigated through the external auditory meatus, producing a convective current in the endolymph of the lateral semicircular duct.

- *If cold water is used*: the endolymph falls within the ipsilateral lateral semicircular duct and decreases the rate of vestibular afferent stimulation. This emulates a person turning their head to the ipsilateral side. The eyes then turn toward the ear that was injected with water and horizontal nystagmus would be seen moving toward the opposite ear.
- *If warm water is used*: the endolymph rises within the ipsilateral lateral semicircular duct and increases the rate of vestibular afferent stimulation. This emulates a person turning their head to the contralateral side. The eyes turn away from the ear injected with water and horizontal nystagmus would be seen moving toward the ipsilateral ear.
- The common mnemonic is COWS: Cold Opposite, Warm Same. Thus this translates to a nystagmus to the side contralateral of the cold water-filled ear or a nystagmus to the side ipsilateral of the warm water-filled ear.

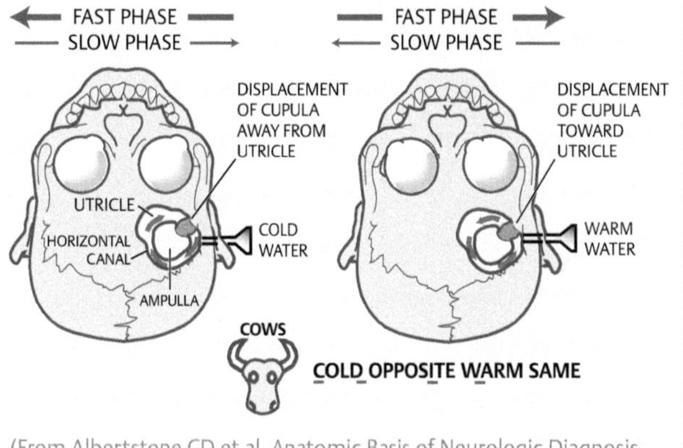

(From Albertstone CD et al. Anatomic Basis of Neurologic Diagnosis. New York: Thieme Medical Publishers; 2009.)

cortex located near the **postcentral gyrus** and the **insular cortex**. Some second-order neurons can travel to the **medial parabrachial nucleus**, which then project as third-order neurons to the VPM and then finally as fourth-order neurons to the postcentral gyrus and insular cortex. The medial parabrachial nucleus can send taste information to the hypothalamus and amygdala.

9.35 Blood Supply and Venous Drainage of the Brain and Spinal Cord

9.35.1 Blood Supply to the Brain

Blood flow to the brain centers on two main arteries and those being the **internal carotid** (*anterior* or *carotid circulation*) and **vertebral arteries** (*posterior* or *vertebral-basilar circulation*). The cerebral hemispheres receive blood from both the anterior and posterior circulations while the brainstem receives blood from only the posterior circulation. The spinal cord in contrast is supplied primarily by the systematic circulation and with only a limited amount originating from the vertebral arteries.

The anterior and posterior circulations are not independent of each other but are connected by networks of arteries on the ventral surface of the diencephalon and midbrain and on the cortical surface. These arteries and the numerous branches that originate from them deliver oxygen, glucose, and other nutrients to support nervous tissue. The cerebral arteries, which directly supply the brain tissue, can anastomose at the circle of Willis and near the surface of the cerebral hemispheres. Once they enter the brain substance, there are no anastomoses.

A local increase in blood flow can be induced by an increase in neuronal activity. Arterial blood pressure is the most important factor in forcing blood through parts of the brain. Cerebral blood flow is notably constant despite changes in the general blood pressure. This constant physiological state of the circulation is accomplished by a compensatory lowering of the cerebral vascular resistance when the arterial pressure is decreased and a raising of the vascular resistance when the arterial pressure is increased. The diameter of cerebral blood vessels is the main factor contributing to the cerebrovascular resistance. Sympathetic innervation to these blood vessels plays a minimal part in the control of cerebrovascular resistance. Instead, the most powerful vasodilator is an increase in carbon dioxide or hydrogen ions along with a reduction in oxygen concentrations.

9.35.2 Internal Carotid Artery

The common carotid artery bifurcates into an external and **internal carotid artery (ICA)** at approximately the C4 vertebral level. The ICA begins initially as a slight dilation called the **carotid sinus**,

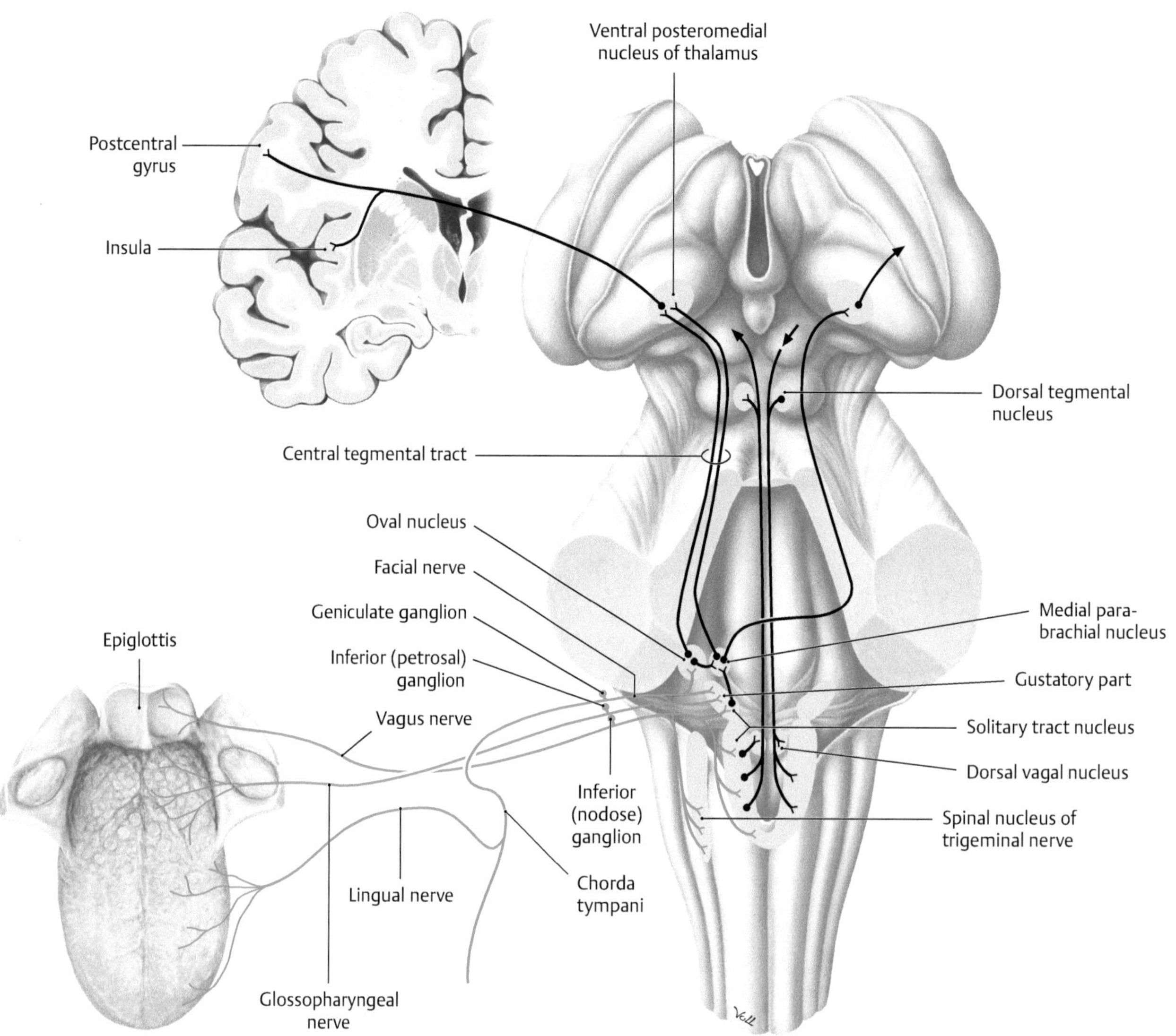

Fig. 9.104 Gustatory system. (From Schuenke M, Schulte E, Schumacher U. THIEME Atlas of Anatomy. Head, Neck, and Neuroanatomy. Illustrations by Voll M and Wesker K. 3rd ed. New York: Thieme Medical Publishers; 2020.)

a baroreceptor that monitors blood pressure, before ascending through the neck and perforating the base of the skull through the carotid canal of the temporal bone. The artery courses through this canal anteromedially, and ascends toward and then through the cavernous sinus before emerging on the medial side of the anterior clinoid process by perforating the dura mater. After piercing the arachnoid mater to enter the subarachnoid space, the ICA extends posteriorly to near the medial end of the lateral cerebral sulcus and divides into the **anterior** and **middle cerebral arteries** (**Fig. 9.64; Fig. 9.106**).

The artery is divided into four anatomical sections: cervical, petrous, cavernous, and cerebral part. The cervical part generally has no branches. Clinically, the intracranial parts that include the cerebral and cavernous parts are referred to as C1–C5. Collectively, the C2–C4 portions are called the **carotid siphon**. The major branches of the internal carotid artery are noted in **Table 9.2** (**Fig 9.64; Fig. 9.105; Fig. 9.106**).

9.35.3 Vertebral Artery

The **vertebral arteries** (**Fig. 9.106a; Fig. 9.107**) originate from the first part of the subclavian artery. As they ascend the neck they pass bilaterally through the upper six transverse foramina of the cervical vertebrae. The vertebral artery generally skips the transverse foramina of the seventh cervical vertebra. Both enter the foramen magnum and pass along the ventral surface of the medulla before uniting to form the **basilar artery** near the border of the medulla and pons. A summary of the blood supply to the brainstem and cerebellum that originates from branches of both the vertebral and basilar arteries is provided

Clinical Correlate 9.30

Subclavian Steal Syndrome

Stenosis of the left subclavian artery located proximal to the origin of the vertebral artery can lead to **subclavian steal syndrome**. Blood in a sense is stolen from the vertebral artery and shunted to the subclavian artery. A muscular effort of the upper limbs may produce a deficiency in blood flow originally destined for the brain because it is now being diverted to the upper limb musculature. The individual may complain of lightheadedness because of insufficient blood flow to the brain.

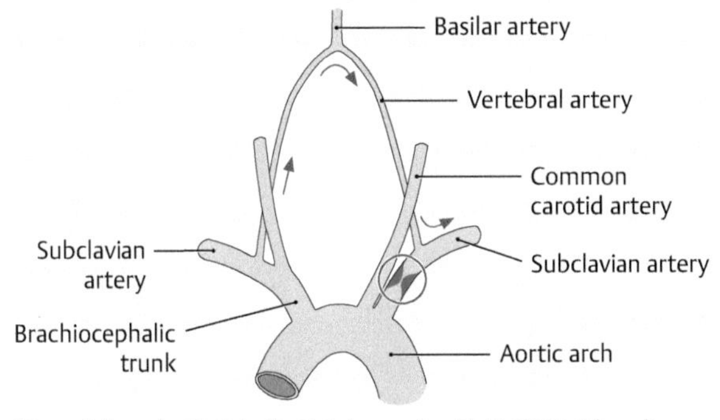

(From Schuenke M, Schulte E, Schumacher U. THIEME Atlas of Anatomy. Head, Neck, and Neuroanatomy. Illustrations by Voll M and Wesker K. 3rd ed. New York: Thieme Medical Publishers; 2020.)

in **Fig. 9.108**. The major branches of the vertebral arteries are noted in **Table 9.3**.

9.35.4 Basilar Artery

The **basilar artery** (**Fig. 9.106a; Fig. 9.107**) is formed inferiorly by the fusion of the two vertebral arteries and terminates superiorly as the posterior cerebral arteries. The major branches of the basilar artery are noted in **Table 9.4**.

9.35.5 Circle of Willis

An arterial anastomosis known as the **circle *of Willis*** (**Fig. 9.109**) is found within an area at the base of the brain called the interpeduncular fossa. It is both the internal carotid and vertebral arteries that provide the bulk of the blood to this anastomosis. However, the vertebral artery is an indirect supplier of blood as it is the basilar artery that directly feeds it. The function is to create a redundancy of blood flow in order to prevent ischemia of any brain tissue. Reduction of blood flow could be due to stenosis (narrowing) or a blocked vessel.

The arteries that directly form the anastomosis include the *anterior cerebral, anterior communicating, internal carotid, posterior communicating,* and the *posterior cerebral.* The middle cerebral arteries are not considered part of the circle. This circle displays multiple variations that can include the absence of certain vessels. The arteries of the circle have **cortical branches** named according to the areas they supply and **central branches** that are responsible for blood flow internal to the circle, namely the interpeduncular fossa region.

9.35.6 Venous Drainage of the Brain

The venous drainage of the brain does not parallel that of the arterial supply. Venous drainage originates from the surface, base, and interior of the brain. **Cerebral veins** are divided into superficial and deep veins. These veins are thin walled and possess no valves. After emerging from the brain, they move into the subarachnoid space. After piercing the arachnoid and meningeal layer of the dura mater, these veins drain into the dural venous sinuses.

The superficial veins drain blood from the cerebral cortex and white matter to the dural venous sinuses, which were discussed in Chapter 7. Superficial veins can include the **superior cerebral, anterior cerebral**, **superficial middle cerebral**, **deep middle cerebral**, and **basilar veins**. The basilar veins form a venous circle analogous to the arterial *circle of Willis*. The deep veins can include the **internal cerebral**, **thalamostriate**, **basal**, and **great cerebral** (of ***Galen***) (**Fig. 9.111; Fig. 9.112; Fig. 9.113**).

The veins that drain the brainstem are ones that form a continuation with the basal veins of the cerebral hemispheres and those of the spinal cord. These veins are more consistent with a venous plexus system. Together the veins of the medulla, pons, and cerebellum make up the *infratentorial venous system* (below the tentorium cerebelli) (**Fig. 9.114**).

The cerebellar veins are similar to those of the cerebral hemispheres where they are distributed independently of the cerebral arteries. A *medial group* of cerebellar veins focus on the venous drainage of the vermis and adjacent parts of the cerebellar hemispheres. A *lateral group* drains the remainder of the two cerebellar hemispheres. Either group of veins has a connection with the dural venous sinuses (**Fig. 9.113b**).

9.35.7 Blood Supply to the Spinal Cord

There is a single anterior spinal and a set of posterior spinal arteries that supply blood to the spinal cord. These arteries extend the entire length of the spinal cord and terminate as a plexus near the conus medullaris. The **anterior spinal artery** supplies the anterior two-thirds of the spinal cord, namely the anterior and lateral funiculi and the pyramids, medial lemniscus, and a part of the hypoglossal nerve at the level of the medulla. The **posterior spinal artery** supplies blood to the posterior one-third of the spinal cord, namely the posterior horns and columns and the cuneate and gracile fasciculi and nuclei of the medulla (**Fig. 9.115**).

There are numerous *segmental medullary* vessels that reinforce the spinal cord blood supply because the spinal arteries are fairly small. Segmental medullary arteries originate from the spinal branches that themselves originate from regional arteries such as the vertebral, posterior intercostal, and lumbar arteries. These arteries do not arise from every spinal branch but instead extend from alternating spinal branches. There are on average 8 **anterior segmental medullary** and 12 **posterior segmental medullary arteries**. These arteries enter the intervertebral foramen and supply primarily the cervical and lumbosacral enlargements. An isolated segmental vessel known as the **great anterior segmental medullary artery** (*of* ***Adamkiewicz***) mostly arises from the left side and from any spinal branch generally between T7 and L4, with most originating at T12 or L1. This artery plays a large role in supplementing the blood supply to the inferior two-thirds of the spinal cord and the lumbosacral enlargement specifically.

Table 9.2 **Major branches of the internal carotid artery**

Major branches	Sub-branches	Major structures supplied
Ophthalmic		Retina, orbital structures, ethmoid and frontal sinuses, anterior scalp, dorsum of the nose, and cranial dura
Posterior communicating		Pituitary (hypophysis) gland, infundibulum, anterior part of the ventral portion of the thalamus, hypothalamus, subthalamus, mammillary bodies, a portion of the red nucleus, substantia nigra, and the optic chiasm and tract
Anterior choroidal		Choroid plexus of lateral ventricles, optic tract, lateral geniculate body, hippocampus, amygdala, globus pallidus, genu and posterior limb of the internal capsule, and lateral portions of thalamus
Anterior cerebral		Medial aspect of cerebral hemisphere, including frontal and parietal lobes, postcentral gyrus, precentral gyrus, and the corpus callosum
	Anterior communicating	Connects the anterior cerebral arteries on both sides
	Medial striate artery (recurrent artery of *Heubner*)	Anterior limb of the internal capsule, anteromedial part of head of caudate nucleus, putamen, and septal area (nuclei)
	Orbital branches	Orbital and medial surfaces of frontal lobe
	Polar frontal branches	Medial portions of the frontal lobe and lateral parts of the convexity of the hemisphere
	Callosomarginal	Paracentral lobule and portions of the cingulate gyrus
	Pericallosal artery	Precuneus (portion of parietal lobe caudal to paracentral lobule and proximal to occipital cortex)
Middle cerebral		Lateral surface of the cerebral hemisphere, which includes parts of the temporal, frontal, parietal, and occipital lobes; *Broca's* area, prefrontal cortex, and primary and association auditory cortices including *Wernicke's* area, and supramarginal and angular gyri (association cortex)
	Lenticulostriate branches	Posterior limb of internal capsule, and parts of the caudate nucleus and putamen
	Lateral frontobasal (orbitofrontal)	Portions of the frontal lobe specifically the inferior frontal gyrus
	Precentral (pre-*Rolandic*) and central sulcus (*Rolandic*) branches	Primary sensory and motor cortices
	Anterior and posterior parietal branches	Portions of the parietal lobe
	Angular gyral branch	Angular gyrus
	Anterior, middle, and posterior temporal branches	Portions of the temporal lobe and lateral portions of the occipital lobe

Additional arteries arising from the spinal branches include the **anterior** and **posterior radicular arteries**. These vessels target the ventral and dorsal nerve roots but generally do not connect to the spinal arteries. They, however, communicate with the outer **vasocorona**.

9.35.8 Venous Drainage of the Spinal Cord

There are as many as three **anterior** and **posterior spinal veins** each and approximately 12 **anterior** and **posterior medullary veins** along with numerous **radicular veins** (**Fig. 9.116**). These veins are tributaries to the **internal** (***Batson's***) and the **external vertebral venous plexuses**, **vertebral**, **spinal**, **intercostal**, and **ascending lumbar veins** among others.

9.36 Development of the Nervous System

The process of **neurulation** refers to the formation and closure of the **neural tube**. The **notochord** induces the overlying ectoderm to differentiate into **neuroectoderm** and form the **neural plate**, from which the CNS originates, and all these initially begin during the third week of development. The notochord goes on to become the nucleus pulposus of the intervertebral disk in the adult. The peripheral and autonomic nervous systems are derived primarily form neural crest cells (**Fig. 9.117; Fig. 9.118**).

The **neuroectodermal cells** of the neural tube give rise to neuroblasts and glioblasts. The **neuroblasts** form all the neurons of the CNS. The **glioblasts** form supporting cells of the CNS such as astrocytes, oligodendrocytes, and ependymocytes. **Neural**

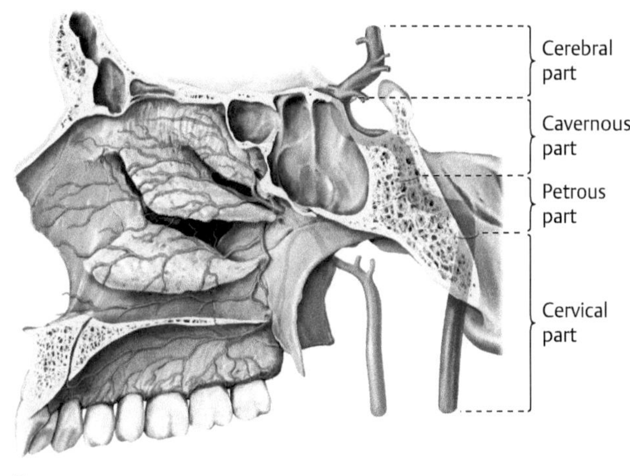

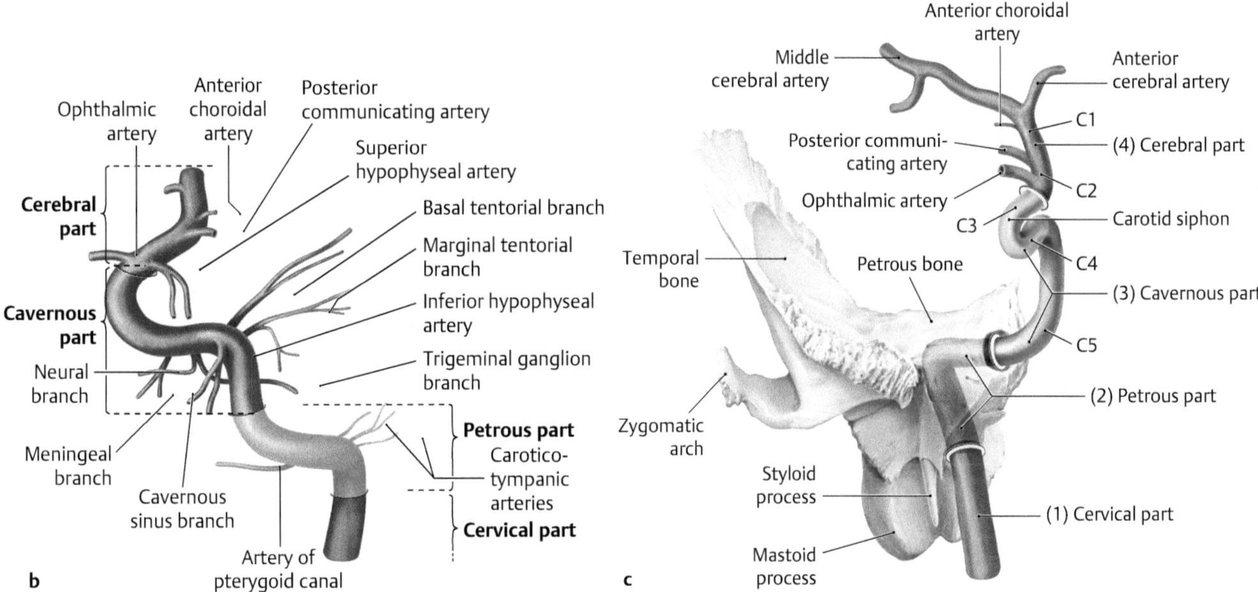

Fig. 9.105 The four anatomical divisions of the internal carotid artery and branches that supply extracerebral structures of the head. **(a)** Medial view of the right internal carotid artery. **(b)** Anatomical segments of the internal carotid artery and their branches. **(c)** Anterior view of the left internal carotid artery. (From Schuenke M, Schulte E, Schumacher U. THIEME Atlas of Anatomy. Head, Neck, and Neuroanatomy. Illustrations by Voll M and Wesker K. 3rd ed. New York: Thieme Medical Publishers; 2020.)

crest cells differentiate from cells of the neural plate and migrate throughout the embryo to form multiple adult cells and structures (**Fig. 9.117**). Neural crest from the *cranial region* migrates from the rhombencephalon to the pharyngeal arches and contributes to muscles and connective tissue. Additional structures formed include the bones of the neurocranium; sensory ganglia of CN V, CN VII, CN IX, and CN X; parasympathetic ganglia of CN III, CN VII, and CN IX; parafollicular cells of thyroid gland; arachnoid and pia maters; odontoblasts; and the hearts aorticopulmonary septum and parts of the outflow tract. The *trunk region* neural crest differentiates into melanocytes, Schwann cells, dorsal root ganglia, paravertebral (chain) and prevertebral sympathetic ganglia, enteric, abdominal, and pelvic parasympathetic ganglia, and chromaffin cells of the suprarenal gland.

The lateral edges of the neural plate begin to elevate forming the **neural folds.** The neural folds continue to elevate and shortly approach one another until they fuse to form the **neural tube**. Fusion of the neural tube begins in the cervical region but proceeds in both a cephalic and caudal direction. Fusion of the neural folds creates an opening at both the cranial and caudal ends called the **cranial (anterior)** and **caudal (posterior) neuropores** and these communicate with the overlying amniotic cavity. The cranial and caudal neuropores close on the 25th and 28th days after fertilization, respectively, and the process of neurulation is now complete. The lumen of the neural tube gives rise to the ventricular system (**Fig. 9.118; Fig. 9.119**). The lumen adjacent to the cerebral hemispheres becomes the *lateral ventricles*; near the diencephalon would be the *third ventricle*; and finally the cavity near the rhombencephalon becomes the *fourth ventricle*. The cranial end of the neural tube is associated with brain development and the caudal end (caudal to the fourth pair of somites) is related to the spinal cord.

The cranial portion of the neural tube demonstrates three dilations or **primary brain vesicles** and two **flexures** during the fourth week of development. The primary brain vesicles consist of the **prosencephalon (forebrain), mesencephalon (midbrain),**

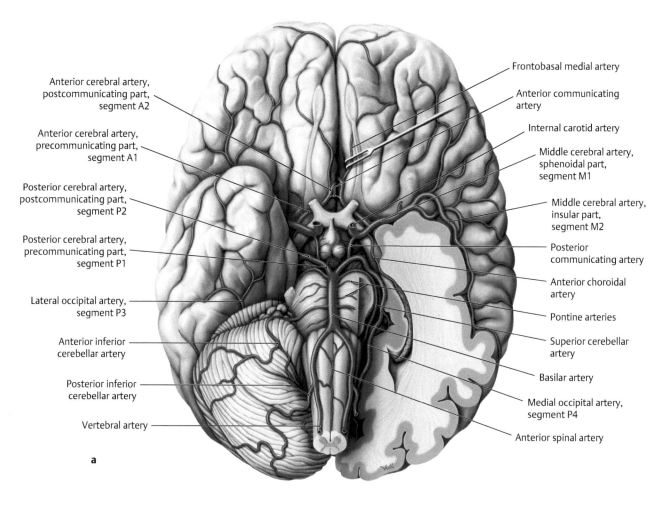

Anterior cerebral artery, postcommunicating part, segment A2
Anterior cerebral artery, precommunicating part, segment A1
Posterior cerebral artery, postcommunicating part, segment P2
Posterior cerebral artery, precommunicating part, segment P1
Lateral occipital artery, segment P3
Anterior inferior cerebellar artery
Posterior inferior cerebellar artery
Vertebral artery
Frontobasal medial artery
Anterior communicating artery
Internal carotid artery
Middle cerebral artery, sphenoidal part, segment M1
Middle cerebral artery, insular part, segment M2
Posterior communicating artery
Anterior choroidal artery
Pontine arteries
Superior cerebellar artery
Basilar artery
Medial occipital artery, segment P4
Anterior spinal artery
a

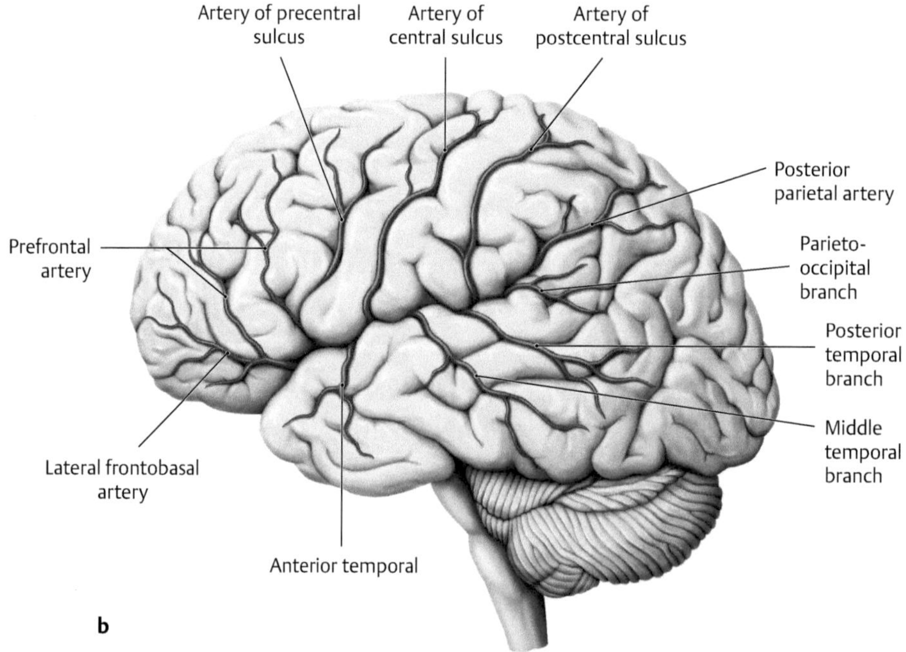

Fig. 9.106 (a) Arteries at the base of the brain. **(b)** Terminal branches of the middle cerebral artery on the lateral cerebral hemisphere, left lateral view. (*continued*) (From Schuenke M, Schulte E, Schumacher U. THIEME Atlas of Anatomy. Head, Neck, and Neuroanatomy. Illustrations by Voll M and Wesker K. 3rd ed. New York: Thieme Medical Publishers; 2020.)

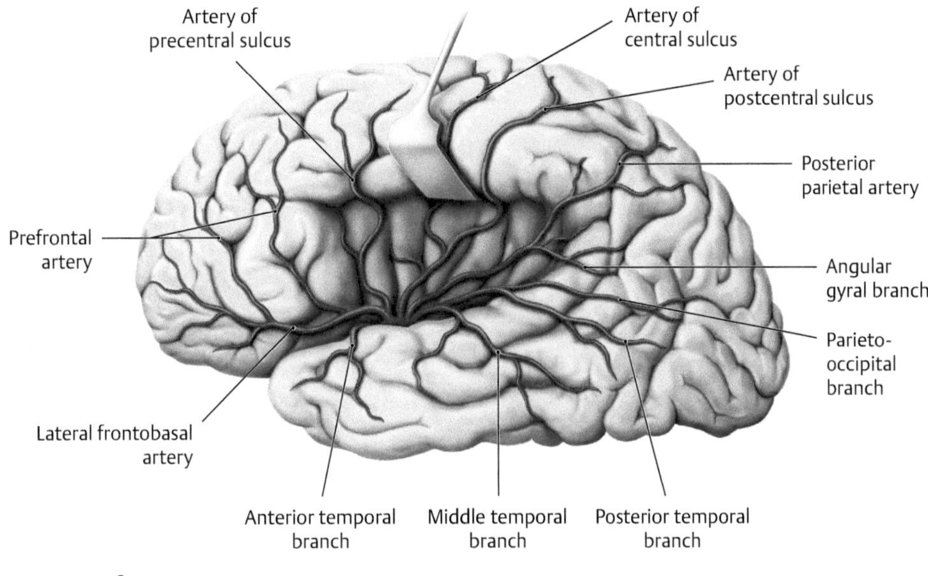

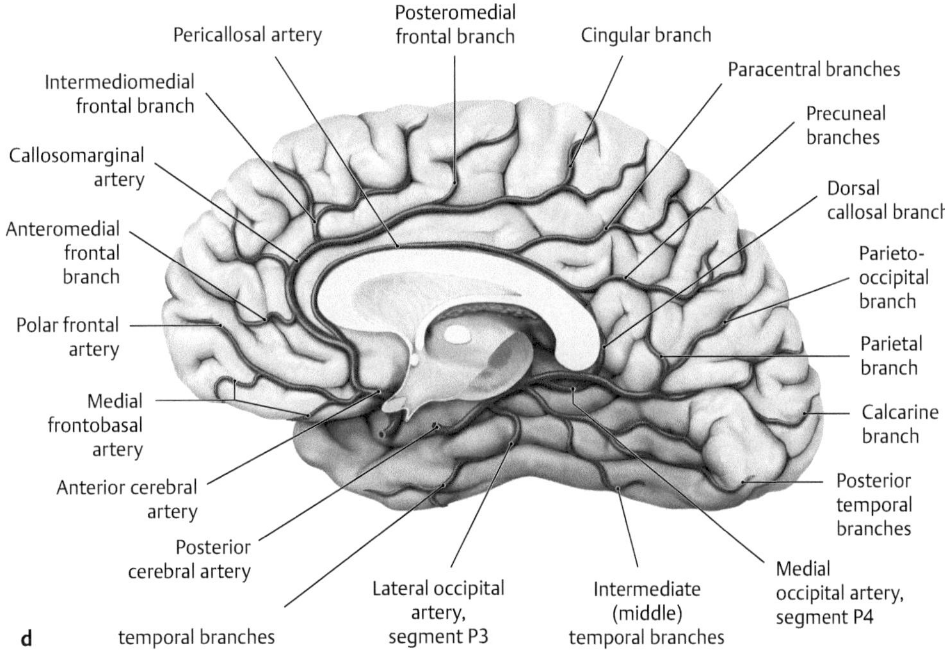

Fig. 9.106 (*continued*) **(c)** Course of the middle cerebral artery in the interior of the lateral sulcus, left lateral view. **(d)** Branches of the anterior and posterior cerebral arteries on the medial surface of the cerebrum. (From Schuenke M, Schulte E, Schumacher U. THIEME Atlas of Anatomy. Head, Neck, and Neuroanatomy. Illustrations by Voll M and Wesker K. 3rd ed. New York: Thieme Medical Publishers; 2020.)

and **rhombencephalon (hindbrain)**. The **mesencephalic flexure** is located between the prosencephalon and the rhombencephalon. The **cervical flexure** is located between the rhombencephalon and developing spinal cord. The **secondary brain vesicles** or regions arise from the primary vesicles during the sixth week and are as follows: the prosencephalon gives rise to the **telencephalon** and **diencephalon**; the mesencephalon is unchanged; and the rhombencephalon becomes the **metencephalon** and **myelencephalon** (**Fig. 9.119; Fig. 9.120**). Adult derivatives of brain vesicles or regions are found in **Table 9.5**.

The neural tube is made up of three layers or zones: the inner *ventricular zone*, the *intermediate zone*, and the outer *marginal zone* (**Fig. 9.117**). The **ventricular zone** contains neuroectoderm which give rise to neuroblasts and glioblasts and that later migrate to the intermediate zone. The neuroectoderm that remains differentiates into ependymocytes and is related to the ventricular system. The **intermediate zone** contains neuroblasts and glioblasts. The neuroblasts differentiate into neurons that have both axons and dendrites. The glioblasts form astrocytes and oligodendrocytes. The **gray matter** of the CNS originates from this zone and

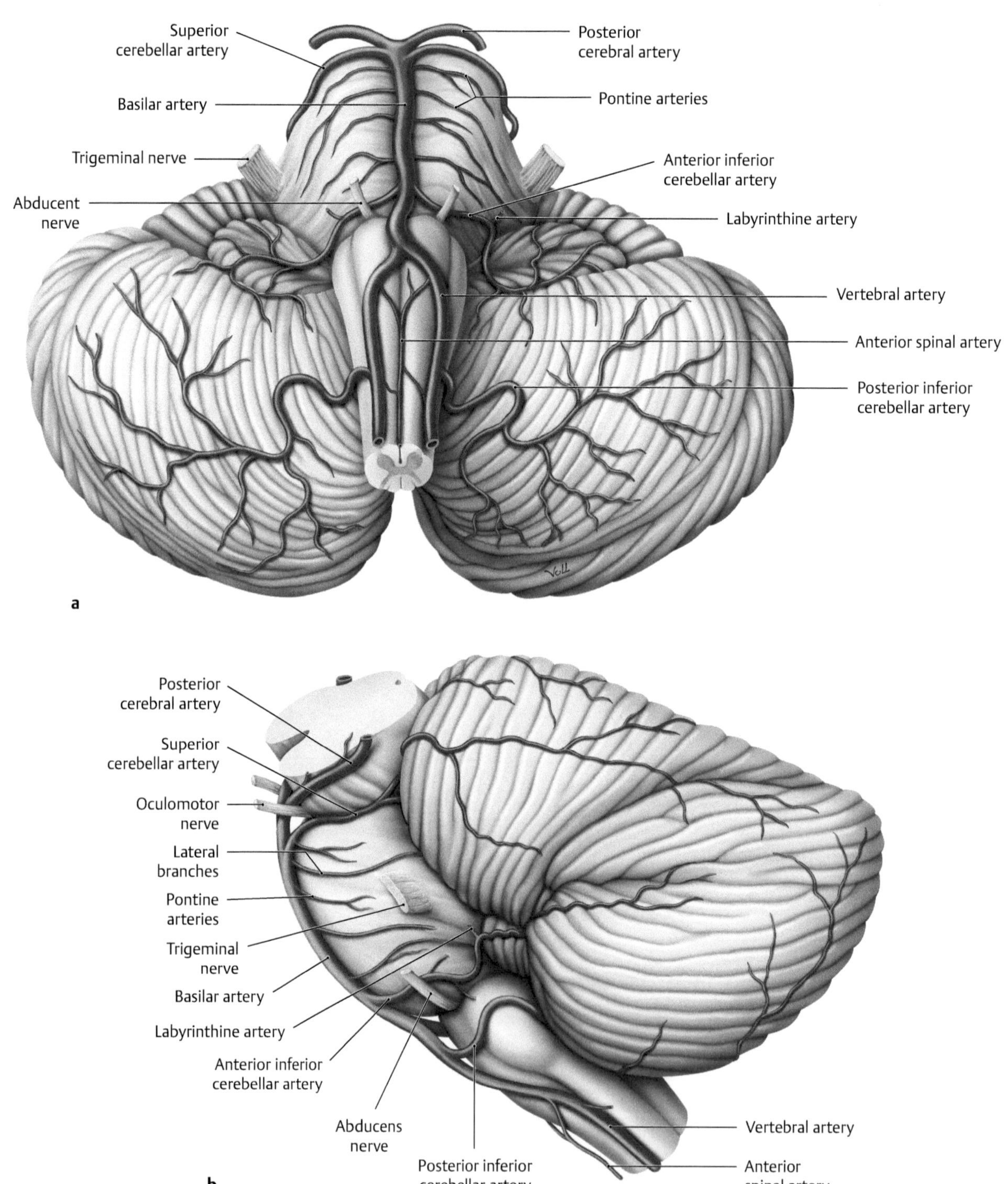

Fig. 9.107 Arteries of the brainstem and cerebellum. **(a)** Basal view. **(b)** Left lateral view. (From Schuenke M, Schulte E, Schumacher U. THIEME Atlas of Anatomy. Head, Neck, and Neuroanatomy. Illustrations by Voll M and Wesker K. 3rd ed. New York: Thieme Medical Publishers; 2020.)

is also divided into an **alar plate** (sensory/afferent functions) and a **basal plate** (motor/efferent functions). The **marginal zone** contains axons that originate from the intermediate zone. Glioblasts are located in this zone and they differentiate into astrocytes and oligodendrocytes. The **white matter** of the CNS originates from this zone.

The **sulcus limitans** is a longitudinal groove in the lateral wall of the neural tube that marks the boundary between the alar and basal plates. It extends from the rostral midbrain and down through the spinal cord during development but it is only present in the adult in the rhomboid fossa of the brainstem. The **roof** and **floor plates** are located on the dorsal and ventral surfaces of the neural tube, respectively. They do not contain any neuroblasts and serve as pathways for nerve fibers to cross. The floor plate is where the anterior white commissure can be located.

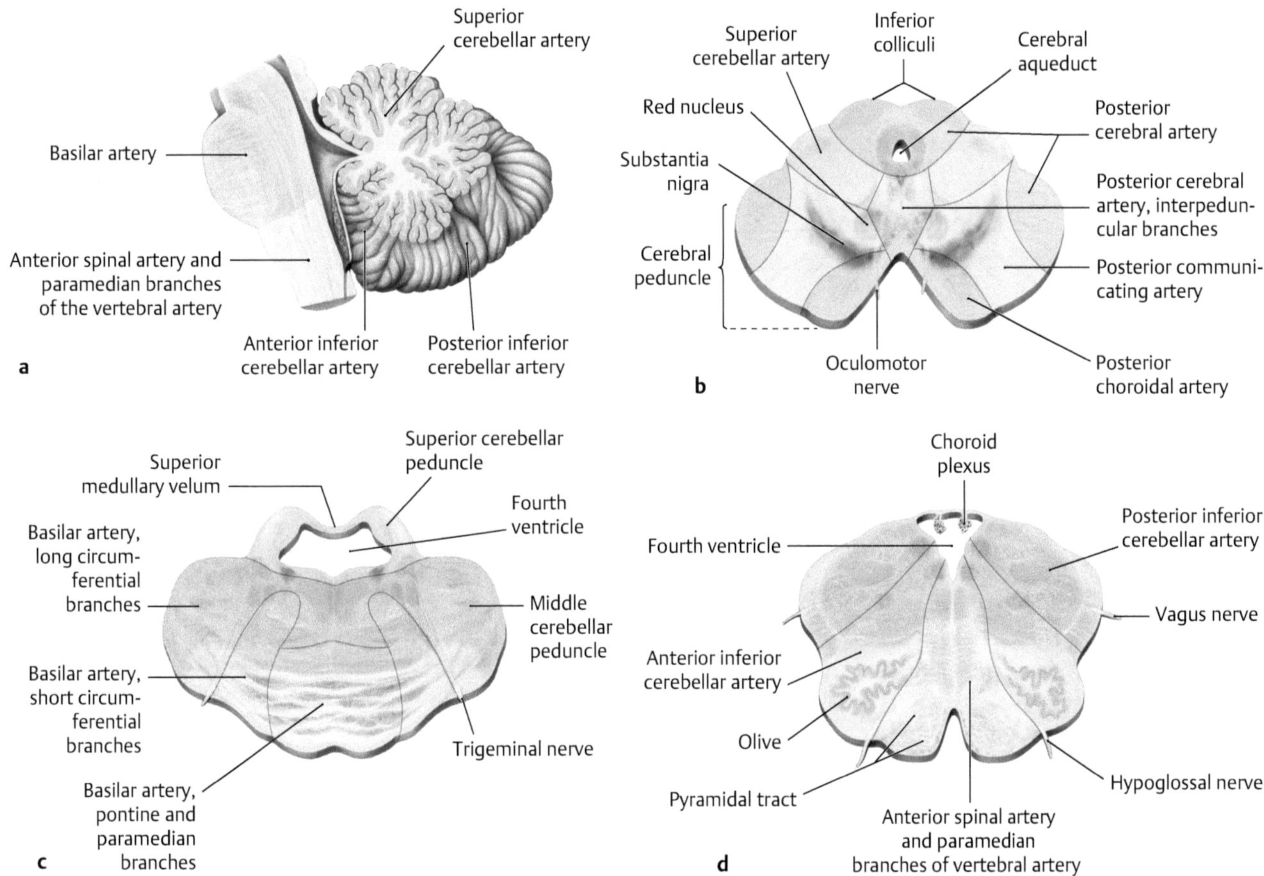

Fig. 9.108 **(a)** Distribution of the arteries of the brainstem and cerebellum in midsagittal section. **(b)** Distribution of the arteries of the midbrain in transverse section. **(c)** Distribution of the arteries of the pons in transverse section. **(d)** Distribution of the arteries of the medulla oblongata in transverse section. (From Schuenke M, Schulte E, Schumacher U. THIEME Atlas of Anatomy. Head, Neck, and Neuroanatomy. Illustrations by Voll M and Wesker K. 3rd ed. New York: Thieme Medical Publishers; 2020.)

Table 9.3 **Major branches of the vertebral artery**

Major branches	Major structures supplied
Anterior spinal	Anterior two-thirds of the spinal cord, medial structures of medulla including pyramids, medial lemniscus, tectospinal tract, medial longitudinal fasciculus, and hypoglossal nucleus
Posterior spinal	Posterior one-third of spinal cord, caudal medulla: fasciculus gracilis and cuneatus, gracile and cuneate nuclei, spinal trigeminal nucleus, dorsal and caudal portions of inferior cerebellar peduncle, portions of the solitary tract, and dorsal motor nucleus (CN X)
Posterior inferior cerebellar	Choroid plexus of fourth ventricle, central nuclei and inferior surface of cerebellum, inferior surface of vermis, inferior cerebellar peduncles, and inferior and medial vestibular nuclei. Of the posterolateral medulla: spinothalamic tract, anterior and posterior spinocerebellar tracts, hypothalamospinal tract, spinal trigeminal nucleus and tract (CN V), portions of CN IX and dorsal motor nucleus (CN X), nucleus ambiguus (CN IX and X), and solitary tract

Regional Development of the Neural Tube

9.36.1 Spinal Cord Development

- The **alar plate** of the developing spinal cord becomes the **posterior horn**. It gives rise to the **sensory neuroblasts** of the posterior horn and receives the axons of GSA and GVA fibers from the dorsal root ganglia that become the dorsal sensory roots of the spinal cord (**Fig. 9.121**).
- The **basal plate** becomes the **anterior horn** of the spinal cord. It gives rise to the **motor neuroblasts** of the anterior (GSE) and lateral horns (GVE) (**Fig. 9.121**). Motor neuroblasts project from the basal plate and become the ventral motor roots of the spinal cord. Located between the alar and basal plates is the intermediate region or lateral horn that contains neurons of the preganglionic sympathetic nervous system situated specifically at the T1–L2 spinal segments. This region also gives rise to the preganglionic parasympathetic fibers located between the S2 and S4 spinal segments. The basal

Table 9.4 **Major branches of the basilar artery**

Major branches	Sub-branches	Major structures supplied
Anterior inferior cerebellar		Anteroinferior surface of cerebellum and flocculus, inferolateral portions of the pons including facial motor nucleus (CN VII) and vestibular and cochlear nuclei (CN VIII), inferior and middle cerebellar peduncle, and spinothalamic tract, hypothalamospinal tract, spinal trigeminal nucleus and tract (CN V), and inferior olivary nucleus of medulla
Labyrinthine (internal auditory)		Vestibular apparatus and cochlea
Pontine arteries		
	Paramedian branches	Medial portion of lower and upper pons: pontine nuclei, corticopontine fibers, corticospinal and corticobulbar tracts, and portions of ventral pontine tegmentum and medial lemniscus
	Short circumferential branches	A wedge-shaped area in the ventrolateral pons
	Long circumferential branches	Most of tegmentum of the rostral and caudal pons, lateral portions of midbrain tegmentum, and middle cerebellar peduncle
Superior cerebellar		Superior surface of the cerebellum and cerebellar nuclei, superior medullary velum, superior and middle cerebral peduncles, caudal part of midbrain, rostral level of pons, medial and lateral lemniscus, part of spinal trigeminal nucleus and tract (CN V), and spinothalamic tract
Posterior cerebral		Most of midbrain, thalamus, and subthalamic nucleus
	Anterior, intermediate, and posterior temporal; parieto-occipital	Medial surfaces of temporal lobes and the medial and inferior surfaces of the occipital lobe
	Calcarine	Primary visual cortex
	Posterior choroidal branches	Choroid plexuses of lateral and third ventricles
	Central branches	Parts of the thalamus and lentiform nucleus, most of the midbrain, medial geniculate bodies, and pineal gland

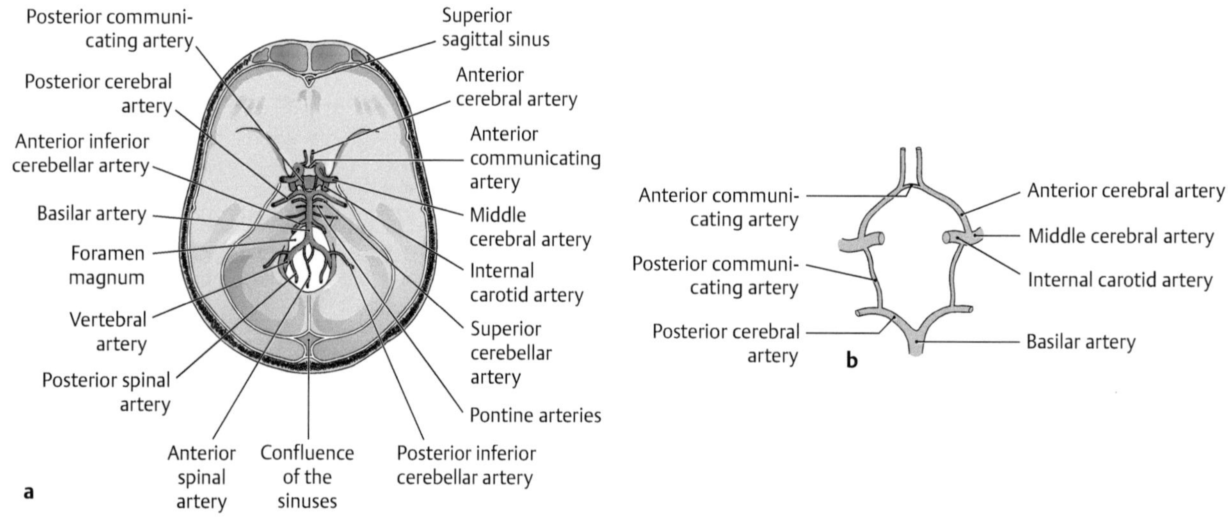

Fig. 9.109 **(a)** Projection of the circle of Willis onto the base of the skull. **(b)** General orientation of the circle of Willis. (From Schuenke M, Schulte E, Schumacher U. THIEME Atlas of Anatomy. Head, Neck, and Neuroanatomy. Illustrations by Voll M and Wesker K. 3rd ed. New York: Thieme Medical Publishers; 2020.)

plate specifically of the C1–C6 spinal segments contributes to the development of the **spinal accessory nerve** (CN XI) motor nuclei.

- Myelination of the spinal cord begins in the fourth month and targets the motor axons first. Oligodendrocytes and Schwann cells myelinate the CNS and PNS, respectively. Corticospinal tracts are not completely myelinated until around the second year of age. The spinal cord courses through the entire vertebral canal but at birth the terminal portion or conus medullaris is located at the L3 vertebral level. In the adult, the conus medullaris is located at approximately L1.

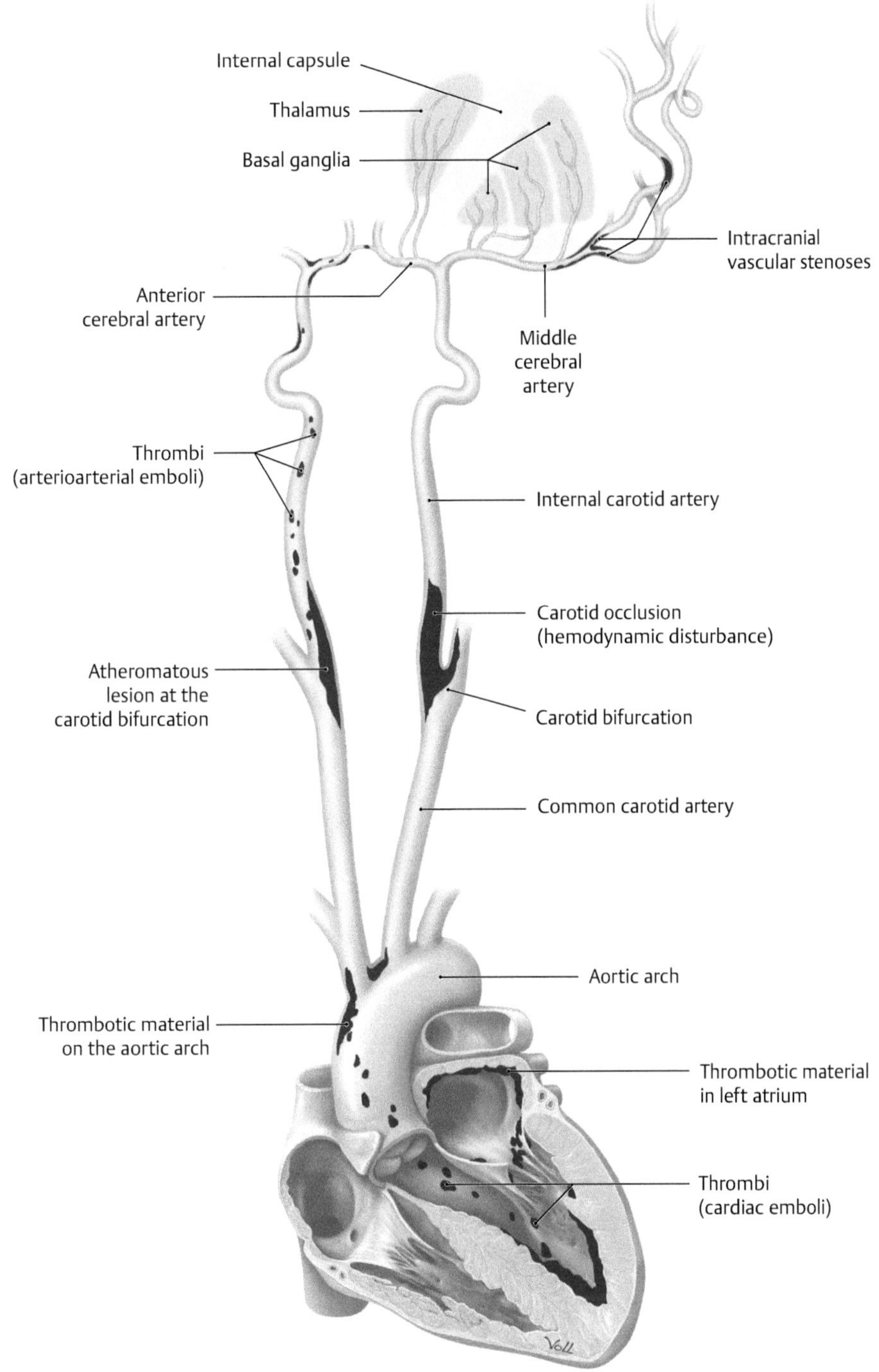

Fig. 9.110 Frequent causes of cerebrovascular disease. (From Schuenke M, Schulte E, Schumacher U. THIEME Atlas of Anatomy. Head, Neck, and Neuroanatomy. Illustrations by Voll M and Wesker K. 3rd ed. New York: Thieme Medical Publishers; 2020.)

9.36.2 Myelencephalon Development

- The **myelencephalon** becomes the medulla of the brainstem.
- The sensory neuroblasts of the **alar plate** give rise to the **inferior olivary nuclei**, **cuneate** and **gracile nuclei**, **cochlear** and **vestibular nuclei** (SSA), **spinal trigeminal nucleus** (GSA), and the **solitary nucleus** (SVA and GVA).
- The motor neuroblasts of the **basal plate** give rise to the **inferior salivatory nucleus of CN IX** (SVE), **dorsal motor nucleus of vagus nerve** (SVE), **nucleus ambiguus** (SVE of CN IX and X); and the **hypoglossal motor nucleus** (GSE).
- The roof plate, or **tela choroidea** in this region, contributes to the roof of the fourth ventricle and is penetrated by pial blood vessels to form the **choroid plexus**.

Clinical Correlate 9.31

Stroke

Ischemia is the result of an inadequate blood supply to a particular tissue. This typically occurs when an artery becomes occluded or when systematic blood pressure drops substantially, such as during a myocardial infarction (heart attack). Occlusions are generally due to an acute blockade, for example, an embolus or gradual narrowing (stenosis) of the arterial lumen as seen in atherosclerosis (**Fig. 9.110**). A **transient ischemic attack (TIA)** is the result of a brief reduction in blood flow lasting only a few minutes, but the individual during this time displays transient or short-term neurological deficits. If this ischemia persists and is uncorrected, it may lead to an **infarction** or localized tissue death. An infarction causes more permanent impairments and describes an **ischemic stroke** and can be termed *thrombotic* (diseased or damaged cerebral artery) or *embolic strokes* (clot forms somewhere other than the brain itself).

A **hemorrhagic stroke** occurs when an artery ruptures, thereby releasing blood into the surrounding tissue. A common cause of this type of stroke is when an **aneurysm** of an artery due to weakening of the muscular wall ruptures. A hemorrhagic stroke not only produces a loss of downstream blood flow but also damages brain tissue at the rupture site because of the blood volume now occupying and compressing that region outside the vessel.

Clinical Correlate 9.32

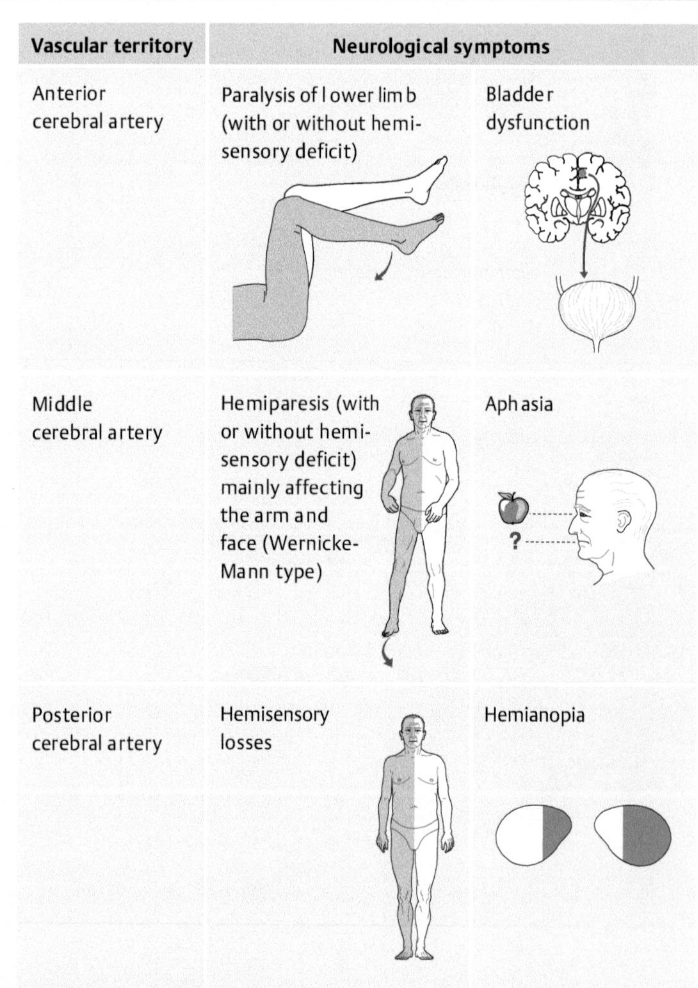

Vascular territory	Neurological symptoms	
Anterior cerebral artery	Paralysis of lower limb (with or without hemisensory deficit)	Bladder dysfunction
Middle cerebral artery	Hemiparesis (with or without hemisensory deficit) mainly affecting the arm and face (Wernicke-Mann type)	Aphasia
Posterior cerebral artery	Hemisensory losses	Hemianopia

(From Schuenke M, Schulte E, Schumacher U. THIEME Atlas of Anatomy. Head, Neck, and Neuroanatomy. Illustrations by Voll M and Wesker K. 3rd ed. New York: Thieme Medical Publishers; 2020.)

The Cardinal Symptoms related to an Anterior, Middle, and Posterior Cerebral Artery Occlusion

- Vesicula urinaria weakness (cortical bladder center) and paralysis of the lower limb (with or without hemisensory deficit, predominately affecting the leg) on the side opposite the occlusion indicates an infarction in the territory of the **anterior cerebral artery**.
- Contralateral hemiplegia affecting the arm and face more than the leg indicates an infarction in the territory of the **middle cerebral artery**. If the dominant hemispherium is affected, aphasia (individual cannot name objects) also occurs. Middle cerebral artery occlusions are the most common because they are a direct continuation of the internal carotid artery.
- Visual disturbances affecting the contralateral visual field (contralateral homonymous hemianopsia) may signify an infarction in the territory of the **posterior cerebral artery** because this artery supplies the visual cortex in the calcarine sulcus of the occipital lobe. Branches of this artery help supply the thalamus and the patient may exhibit a contralateral hemisensory deficit because the afferent fibers have already decussated below the thalamus.

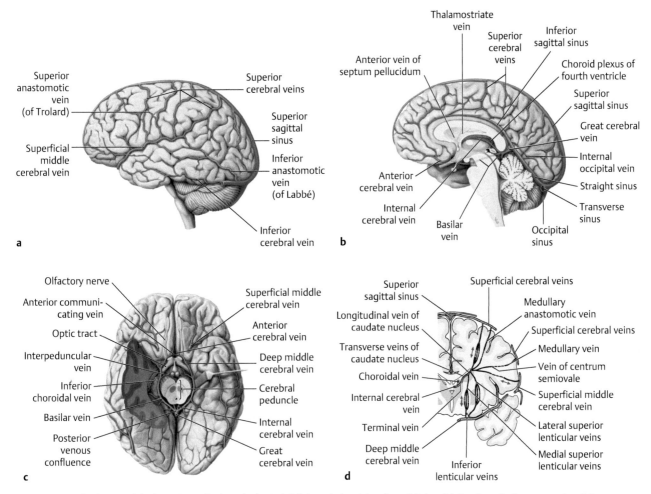

Fig. 9.111 Superficial veins of the brain (superficial cerebral veins), left lateral view **(a)** and medial view **(b)**. Basal cerebral venous system **(c)**. Anastomoses between the superficial and deep cerebral veins **(d)**. (From Schuenke M, Schulte E, Schumacher U. THIEME Atlas of Anatomy. Head, Neck, and Neuroanatomy. Illustrations by Voll M and Wesker K. 3rd ed. New York: Thieme Medical Publishers; 2020.)

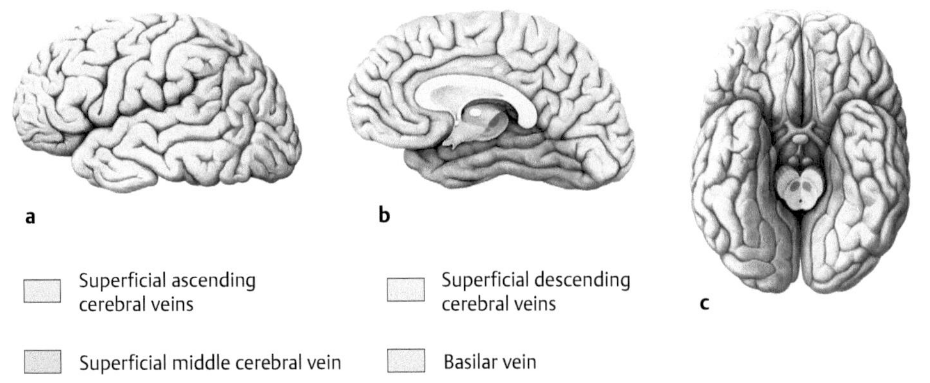

Fig. 9.112 Regions drained by the superficial cerebral veins. **(a)** Left lateral view. **(b)** View of the medial surface of the right hemisphere. **(c)** Basal view. (From Schuenke M, Schulte E, Schumacher U. THIEME Atlas of Anatomy. Head, Neck, and Neuroanatomy. Illustrations by Voll M and Wesker K. 3rd ed. New York: Thieme Medical Publishers; 2020.)

9.36.3 Metencephalon Development

- The **metencephalon** becomes the pons of the brainstem and the cerebellum.
- **Pons**:
  - The sensory neuroblasts of the **alar plate** give rise to the **pontine nuclei**, **cochlear** and **vestibular nuclei** (SSA), **spinal** and **main (principal) trigeminal nuclei** (GSA), and the **solitary nucleus** (SVA and GVA).
  - The motor neuroblasts of the **basal plate** give rise to the **trigeminal motor nucleus** (GSE of CN V), **abducent motor nucleus** (GSE of CN VI), **facial motor nucleus** (SVE of CN VII), and the **superior salivatory nucleus** (GVE of CN VII).
- **Cerebellum**:
  - Cerebellum development begins with two dorsolateral swellings of the alar plate called **rhombic lips**. The rhombic lips have neuroectoderm organized in the same fashion or zones as the neural tube but they thicken to form the **cerebellar plate**, which is separated into a cranial and caudal section.
  - The cranial section gives rise to the **cerebellar hemispheres** and the **vermis**.
  - The caudal section forms the most primitive part of the cerebellum, the **flocculonodular lobe**.
  - Neuroectoderm in the ventricular zone forms the **internal germinal layer**, a layer responsible for producing the **deep cerebellar nuclei** (dentate, globose, emboliform, and fastigial nuclei), **Golgi cells**, **Purkinje cells**, **astrocytes**, and **oligodendrocytes**.
  - The **external germinal layer** forms after neuroectoderm cells of the internal germinal layer migrate to the marginal zone. This layer produces **granule**, **stellate** and **basket cells** along with **astrocytes**, and **oligodendrocytes**.

9.36.4 Mesencephalon Development

- The **mesencephalon** becomes the midbrain of the brainstem.
- The sensory neuroblasts of the **alar plate** give rise to the **superior** and **inferior colliculi**.
- The motor neuroblasts of the **basal plate** give rise to the **oculomotor nucleus** (GSE of CN III), **trochlear motor nucleus** (GSE of CN IV), **Edinger-Westphal nucleus** (GVE of CN III), **red nucleus**, and the **substantia nigra**.

9.36.5 Diencephalon Development

- The **diencephalon** gives rise to the thalamus, hypothalamus, epithalamus, subthalamus, and the posterior lobe of the

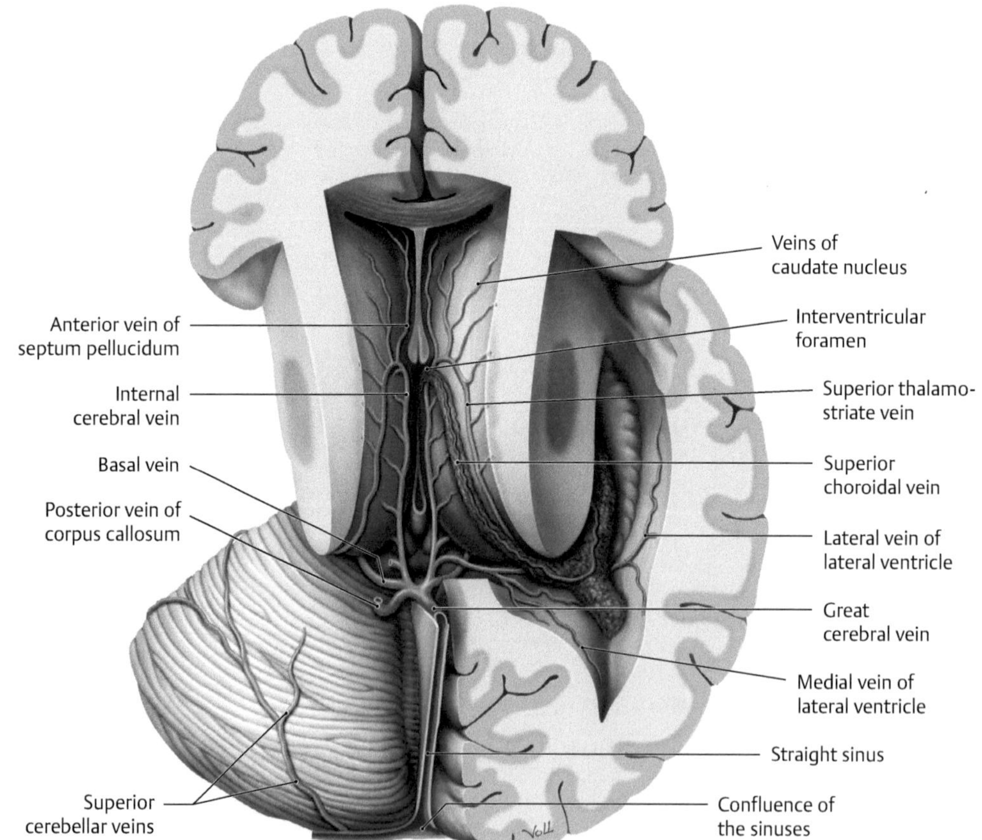

Fig. 9.113 **(a)** Deep cerebral veins. (*continued*) (From Schuenke M, Schulte E, Schumacher U. THIEME Atlas of Anatomy. Head, Neck, and Neuroanatomy. Illustrations by Voll M and Wesker K. 3rd ed. New York: Thieme Medical Publishers; 2020.)

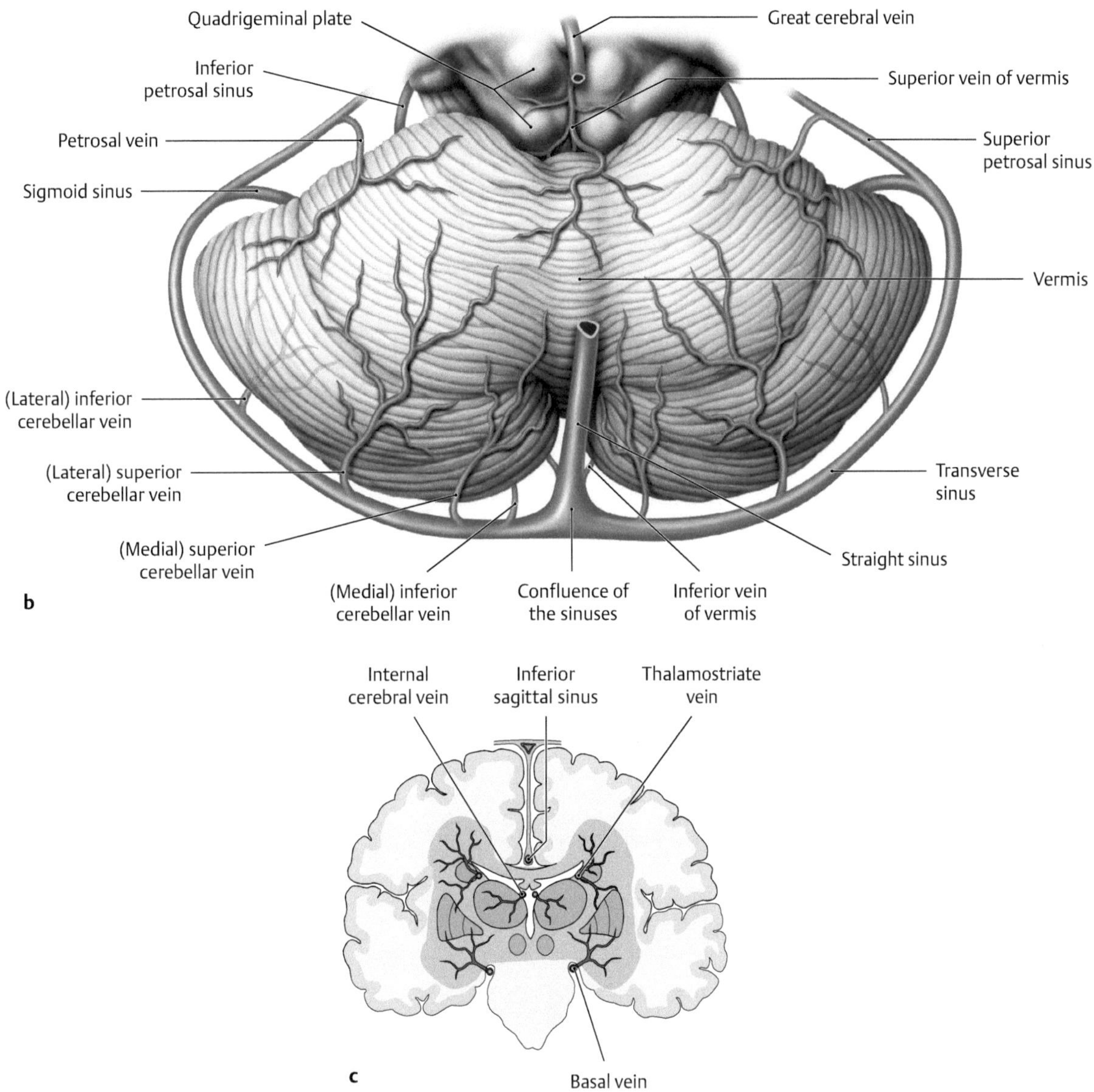

Fig. 9.113 *(continued)* **(b)** Cerebellar veins. **(c)** Regions drained by the deep cerebral veins. (From Schuenke M, Schulte E, Schumacher U. THIEME Atlas of Anatomy. Head, Neck, and Neuroanatomy. Illustrations by Voll M and Wesker K. 3rd ed. New York: Thieme Medical Publishers; 2020.)

pituitary gland (neurohypophysis) among other structures. The choroid plexus of this region develops from the roof plate of the diencephalon. The optic vesicles, cups, and stalks related to eye and retina development originate from derivatives of the diencephalon.

- **Thalamus**: originates from the alar plate and gives rise to the multiple **thalamic nuclei**, and **lateral** and **medial geniculate bodies.**
- **Hypothalamus**: originates from both the alar and floor plates inferior to the *hypothalamic sulcus*. It gives rise to the multiple **hypothalamic nuclei, mammillary bodies,** and **posterior lobe of the pituitary gland.**
- **Epithalamus**: develops from the dorsal portions of the alar plate along with the roof plate. It gives rise to the **tela choroidea** and **choroid plexus** of the third ventricle, **pineal gland, habenular nuclei** and **commissure**, and the **posterior commissure.**
- **Subthalamus**: originates from the alar plate and has a number of neuroblasts that migrate into the white matter of the telencephalon to form the **globus pallidus.**
- **Pituitary gland (hypophysis)**: the pituitary gland attaches to the hypothalamus and has an anterior and posterior lobe. The **anterior lobe (adenohypophysis)** develops from an ectodermal extension (***Rathke pouch***) of the early oral cavity or *stomodeum*. The **posterior lobe (neurohypophysis)** develops from a ventrally located neuroectodermal evagination of the hypothalamus called the **infundibulum.**
- **Eye structures**: detailed in Chapter 7.

9.36.6 Telencephalon Development

The **telencephalon** gives rise to structures such as the cerebral hemispheres and cortex, caudate, putamen, claustrum, amygdala, hippocampus, and commissure fibers. The choroid plexus of the

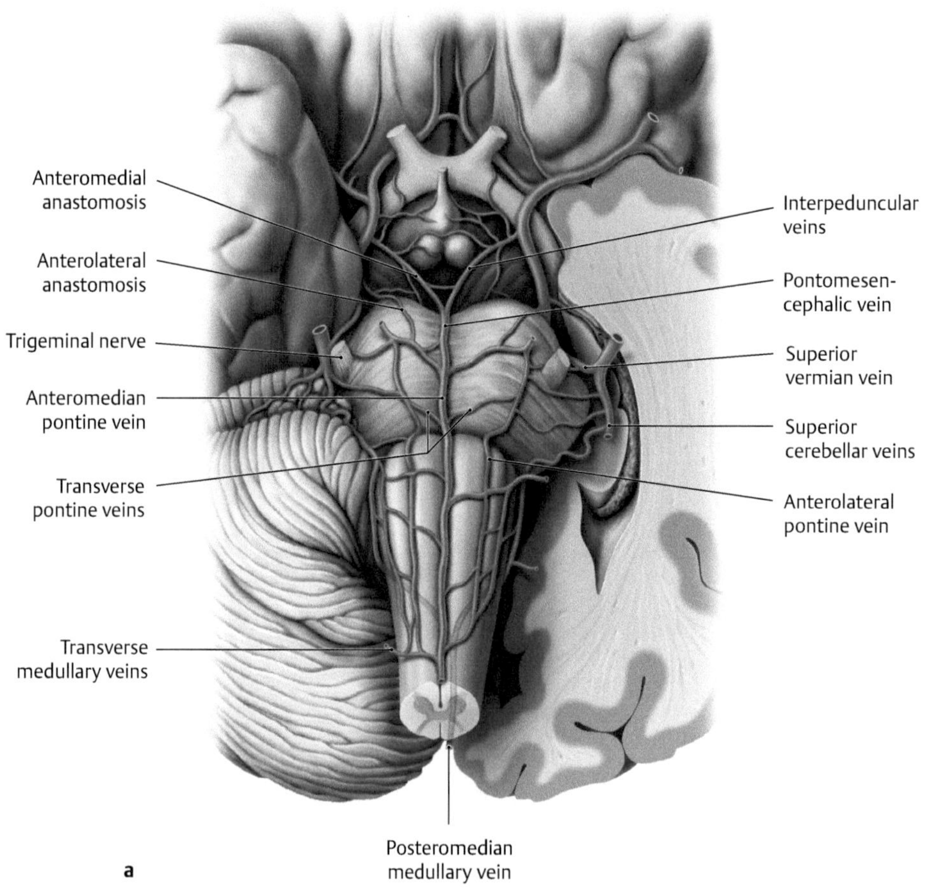

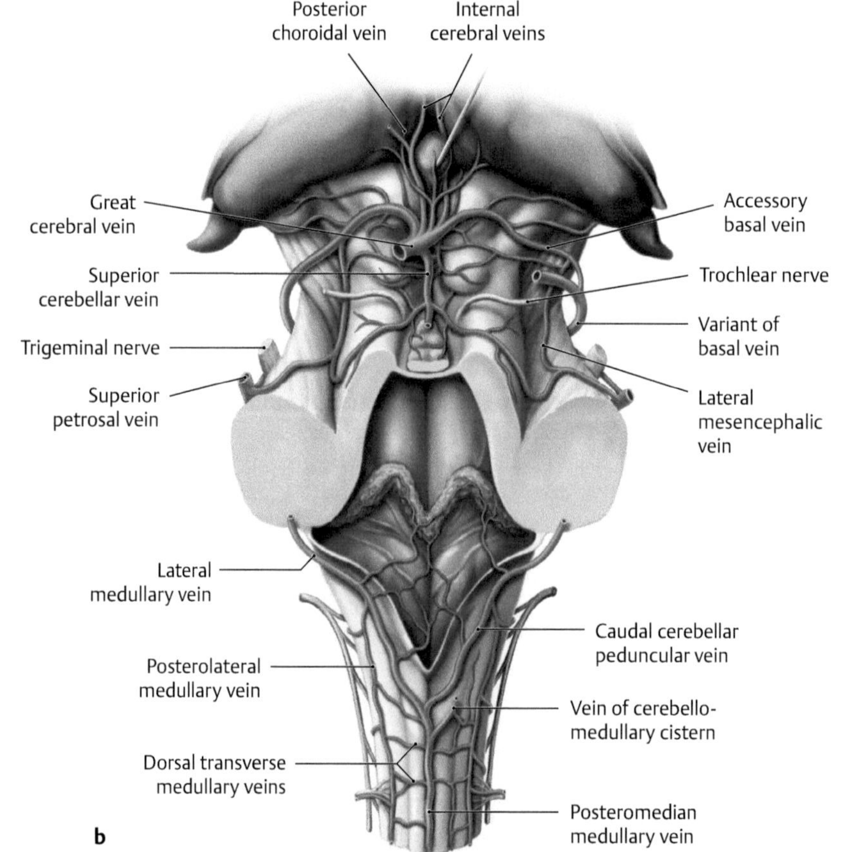

Fig. 9.114 Veins of the brainstem. **(a)** Anterior view of the brainstem in situ (the cerebellum and part of the occipital lobe have been removed on the left side). **(b)** Posterior view of the isolated brainstem with the cerebellum removed. (From Schuenke M, Schulte E, Schumacher U. THIEME Atlas of Anatomy. Head, Neck, and Neuroanatomy. Illustrations by Voll M and Wesker K. 3rd ed. New York: Thieme Medical Publishers; 2020.)

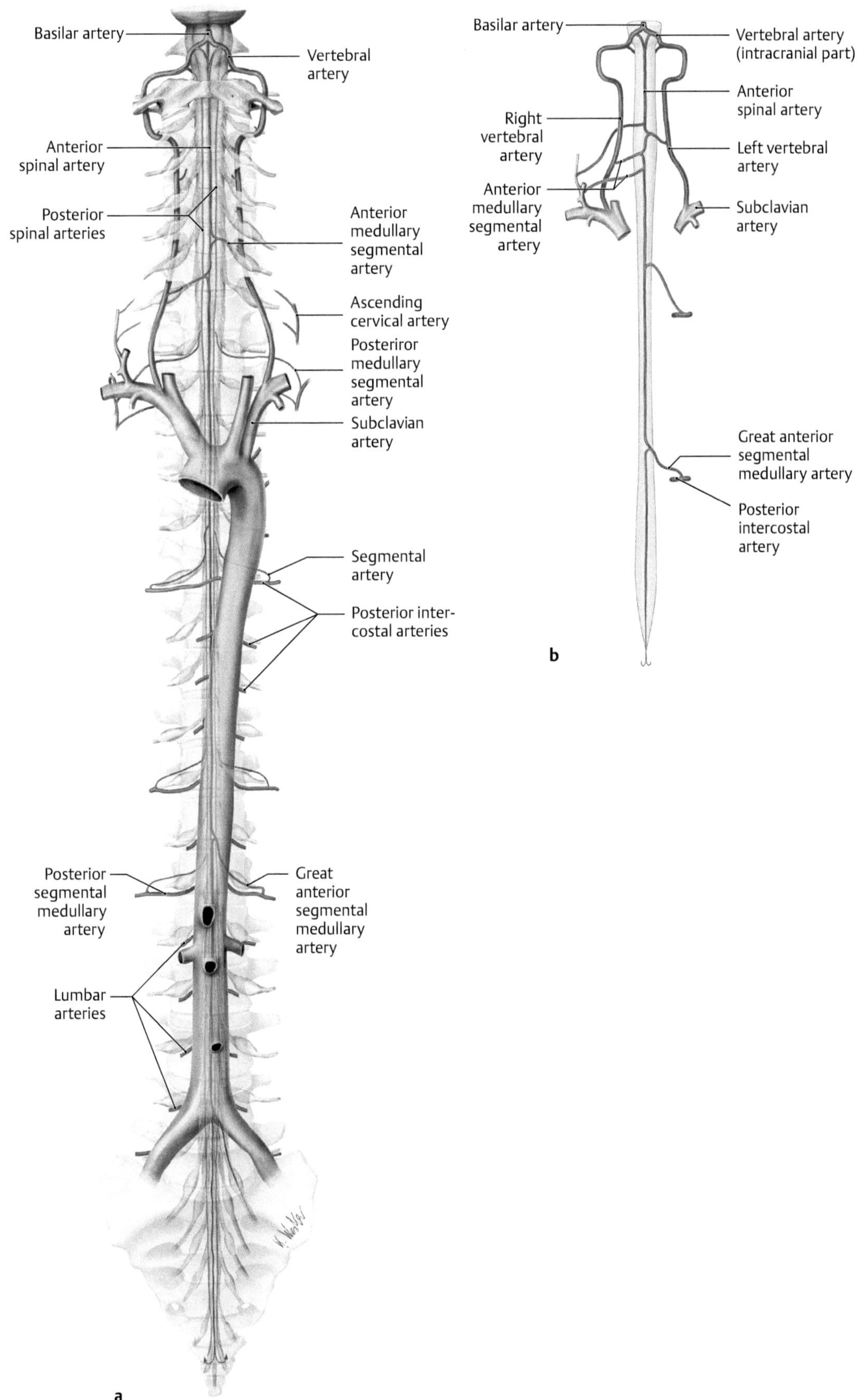

Fig. 9.115 Arterial blood supply to the spinal cord, anterior view. **(a)** Overview of the arterial supply system. **(b)** Vessels supplying the vertical system. *(continued)* (From Schuenke M, Schulte E, Schumacher U. THIEME Atlas of Anatomy. Head, Neck, and Neuroanatomy. Illustrations by Voll M and Wesker K. 3rd ed. New York: Thieme Medical Publishers; 2020.)

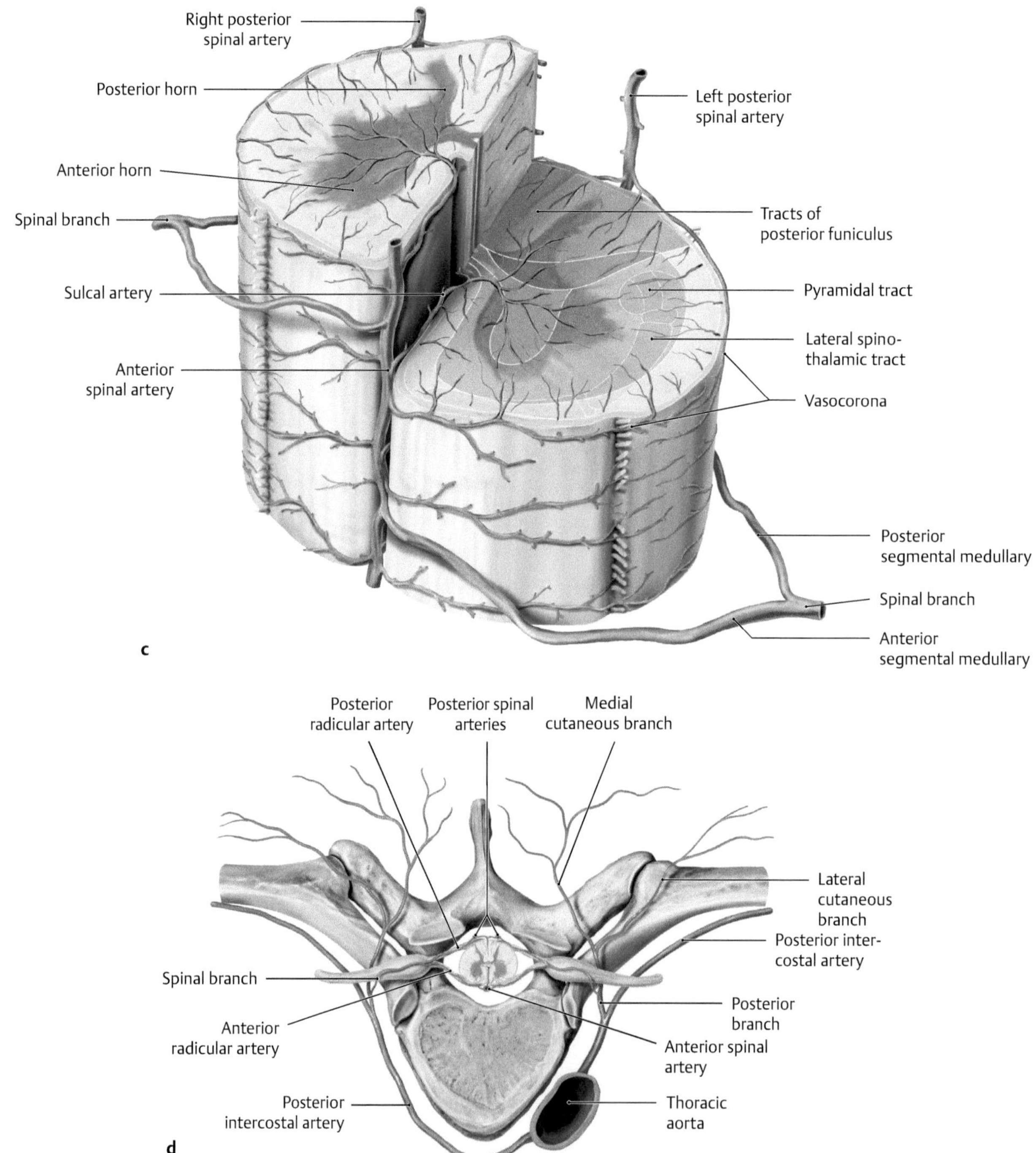

Fig. 9.115 (*continued*) Arterial blood supply to the spinal cord, anterior view. **(c)** Blood supply to the spinal cord segments. **(d)** Blood vessels supplying the spinal cord. (From Schuenke M, Schulte E, Schumacher U. THIEME Atlas of Anatomy. Head, Neck, and Neuroanatomy. Illustrations by Voll M and Wesker K. 3rd ed. New York: Thieme Medical Publishers; 2020.)

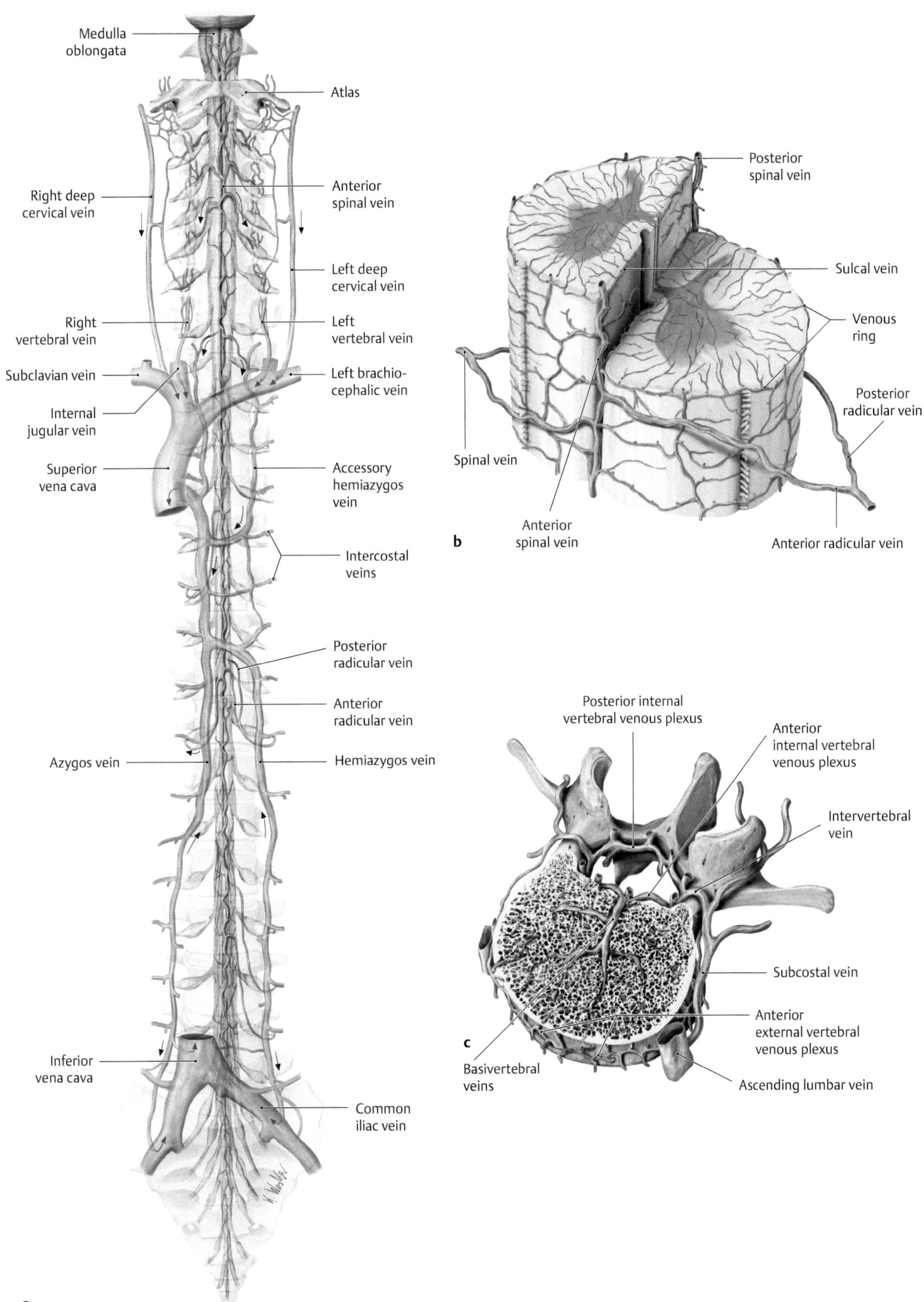

Fig. 9.116 **(a)** Venous drainage of the spinal cord, anterior view. **(b)** Venous drainage of a spinal cord segment. **(c)** Vertebral venous plexus.
(From Schuenke M, Schulte E, Schumacher U. THIEME Atlas of Anatomy, Head, Neck, and Neuroanatomy. Illustrations by Voll M and Wesker K. 3rd ed. New York: Thieme Medical Publishers; 2020.)

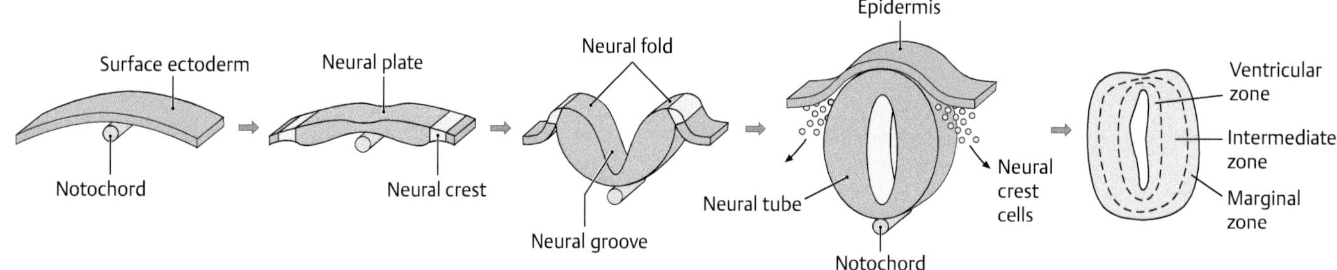

Fig. 9.117 Development of the neural tube, neural crest, and their derivatives. (From Schuenke M, Schulte E, Schumacher U. THIEME Atlas of Anatomy. Head, Neck, and Neuroanatomy. Illustrations by Voll M and Wesker K. 3rd ed. New York: Thieme Medical Publishers; 2020.)

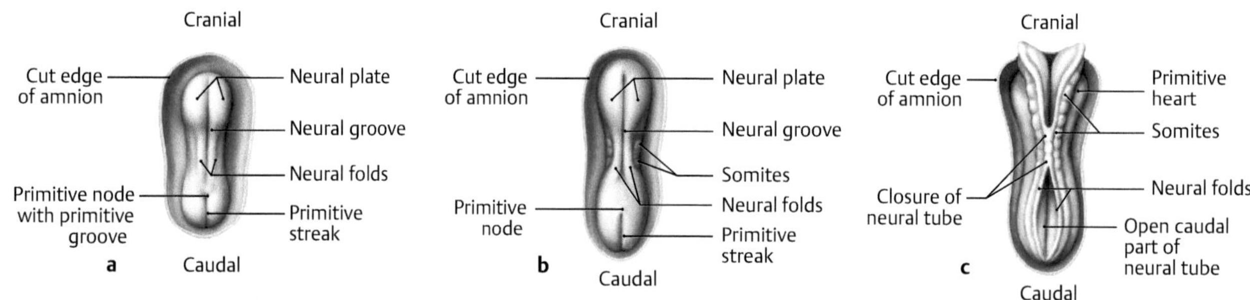

Fig. 9.118 Neurulation during early human development. **(a–c)** Dorsal view after removal of the amnion. (From Schuenke M, Schulte E, Schumacher U. THIEME Atlas of Anatomy. Head, Neck, and Neuroanatomy. Illustrations by Voll M and Wesker K. 3rd ed. New York: Thieme Medical Publishers; 2020.)

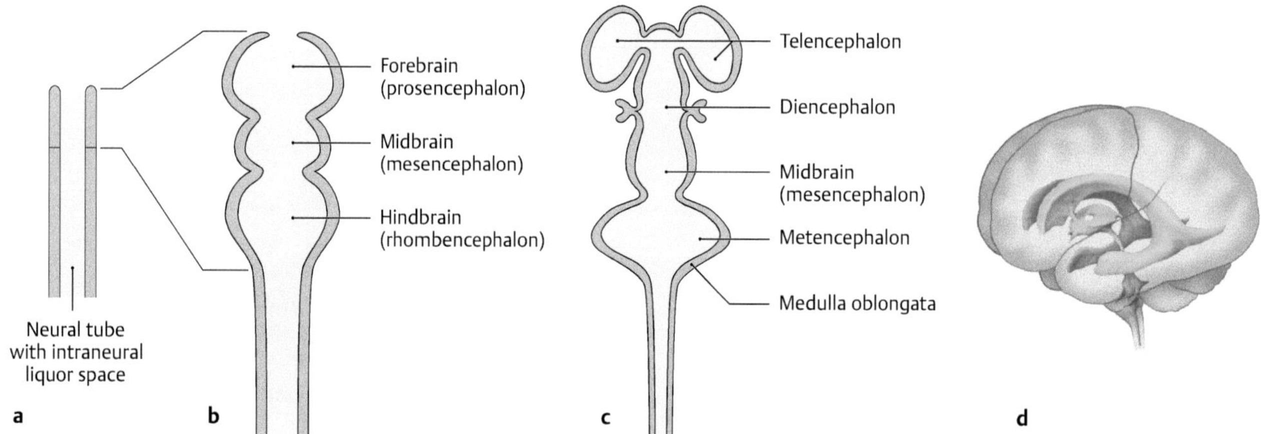

Fig. 9.119 Neural tube and its derivatives; dorsal view. **(a-c)** The neural tube is cut open. **(d)** Mature brain with subarachnoid spaces in situ. (From Schuenke M, Schulte E, Schumacher U. THIEME Atlas of Anatomy. Head, Neck, and Neuroanatomy. Illustrations by Voll M and Wesker K. 3rd ed. New York: Thieme Medical Publishers; 2020.)

Table 9.5 **Adult derivatives of the brain vesicles**

Primary vesicle	Secondary vesicle/region	Adult derivative
Prosencephalon	Telencephalon	Cerebral cortex and hemispheres, olfactory bulbs, caudate, putamen, claustrum, amygdala, hippocampus, lamina terminalis
	Diencephalon	Thalamus, hypothalamus, epithalamus, subthalamus, globus pallidus, posterior lobe of pituitary gland, mammillary bodies, pineal gland, optic tract, optic nerve, retina, iris, and ciliary body
Mesencephalon	Mesencephalon	Tectum, tegmentum, and cerebral peduncles of midbrain
Rhombencephalon	Metencephalon	Fiber tracts and nuclei of pons; cerebellar cortex, nuclei and peduncles of cerebellum
	Myelencephalon	Fiber tracts and nuclei of medulla

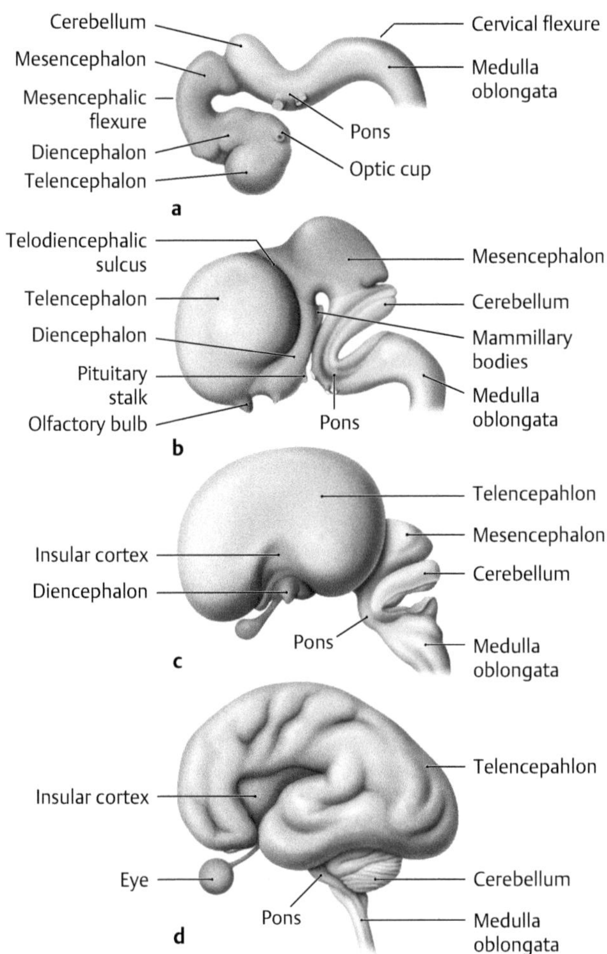

Fig. 9.120 Development of the brain from the neural tube. **(a)** Second month of pregnancy. **(b)** Third month of pregnancy. **(c)** Fourth month of pregnancy. **(d)** Sixth month of pregnancy. (From Schuenke M, Schulte E, Schumacher U. THIEME Atlas of Anatomy. Head, Neck, and Neuroanatomy. Illustrations by Voll M and Wesker K. 3rd ed. New York: Thieme Medical Publishers; 2020.)

lateral ventricles originates from within the choroid fissure of the telencephalon.

- **Cerebral hemispheres**: develop from the bilateral evaginations of the lateral walls of the prosencephalon. Continued growth creates the individual frontal, parietal, temporal, and occipital lobes. The hemispheres contain the cerebral cortex, lateral ventricles, white matter, and basal ganglia. The anterior commissure, hippocampal commissure, and corpus callosum serve as connections between the hemispheres. Near the *choroidal fissure* the hemispheres thicken to form the **hippocampus**, a structure responsible for processing long-term memory and emotional responses.
- **Cerebral cortex**: known as the **pallium** during development. Neuroblasts from the ventricular and intermediate zones migrate to form a **cortical plate.** Additional neuroblasts from the ventricular zone proliferate and form the **subventricular zone.** From the subventricular zone, neuroblasts migrate peripherally to form the **subplate zone.** The intermediate zone eventually becomes devoid of neuroblasts and this constitutes the **white matter** of the cerebral hemispheres. The **molecular layer** of the cortex originates from the marginal zone. The cortical and subplate zones together represent the **cerebral cortex.**
- The cerebral cortex is broken down into a **neocortex (neopallium)** and allocortex. The **neocortex (neopallium)** has six layers, represents 90% of the cerebral cortex, and is located between the paleocortex and the hippocampus. The **allocortex** has three layers and makes up only 10% of the cortex. It is subdivided into a **paleocortex (paleopallium)** and **archicortex (archipallium).** The paleopallium is related to the olfactory and piriform cortices. The archipallium is related to the hippocampus and dentate gyrus.
- **Corpus striatum**: the corpus striatum is the rapidly growing region near the basal part of the cerebral hemispheres. It bulges into the lumen of the lateral ventricles and onto the floor of the interventricular foramen (of *Monro*). It gives rise to basal ganglia such as the **caudate** and **lentiform nucleus** (putamen and globus pallidus). Note the globus pallidus originates initially from the subthalamus. In addition, it gives rise to the **amygdala** and **claustrum.** The amygdala is part of the limbic system and is responsible for the response and memory of emotions, especially fear, while the claustrum may function in communication between the hemispheres.
- **Commissure fibers**: the **lamina terminalis** forms the anterior wall of the third ventricle and it is related to the first bundle of crossing nerve fibers to form the **anterior commissure**, and this structure connects the olfactory system to the middle and inferior temporal gyri. The **hippocampal (fornix) commissure** begins in the hippocampus, and the fibers meet on the lamina terminalis. From here the fibers arch toward the **mammillary body** and hypothalamus. The **corpus callosum** is the largest but third commissure to form. It connects the homologous left and right cerebral hemispheres. The **posterior commissure** connects the pretectal nuclei and helps mediate the pupillary light reflex. The **habenular commissure** connects the habenular nuclei, structures involved in the sleep–wake cycle, stress responses, and reproductive behaviors, to name a few. The **optic chiasma** is related to the optic nerve (CN II).
- **Olfactory system**: develops in two different regions. The **olfactory bulbs** are associated with the telencephalon while the **olfactory nerves (CN I)** are related to the nasal placode and olfactory epithelium. Axons of the olfactory nerves eventually make contact with secondary neurons in the olfactory bulbs.

9.36.7 Peripheral Nervous System Development

- During the 4th week of development, the motor nerve fibers originate from the basal plates of the spinal cord. They condense to form the ventral nerve roots.
- Initially, neural crest cells migrate and give rise to the dorsal root ganglion. The central nerve processes originating from the ganglion form bundles that migrate toward the alar plates of the spinal cord while the peripheral processes extend out toward the ventral root. The central and peripheral processes create the dorsal sensory root which forms mostly during the fifth week of development.
- The neural crest–derived Schwann cells are responsible for the myelination of peripheral nerves and each cell only myelinates a single axon. Myelin begins to be deposited during the fourth month of fetal development (**Fig. 9.122**).

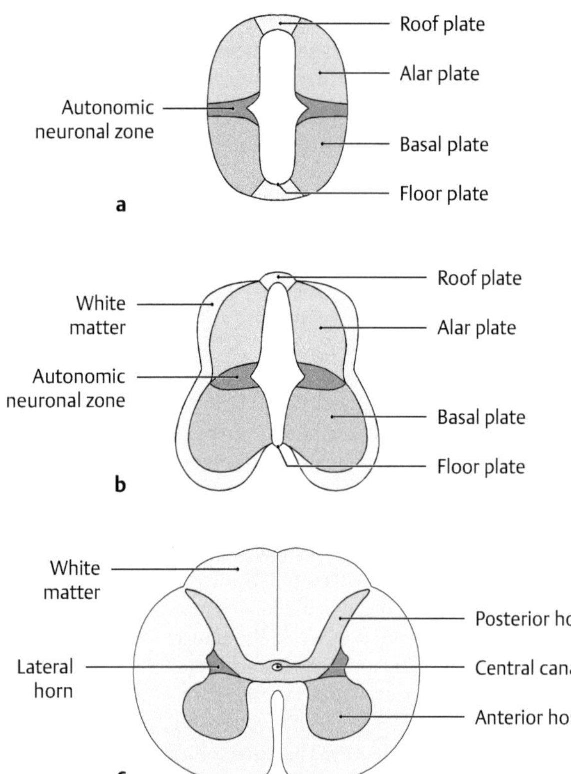

Fig. 9.121 Differentiation of the neural tube in the spinal cord region during embryonic development; cross section, cranial view. **(a)** Early neural tube development. **(b)** Intermediate stage. **(c)** Adult spinal cord. (From Schuenke M, Schulte E, Schumacher U. THIEME Atlas of Anatomy. Head, Neck, and Neuroanatomy. Illustrations by Voll M and Wesker K. 3rd ed. New York: Thieme Medical Publishers; 2020.)

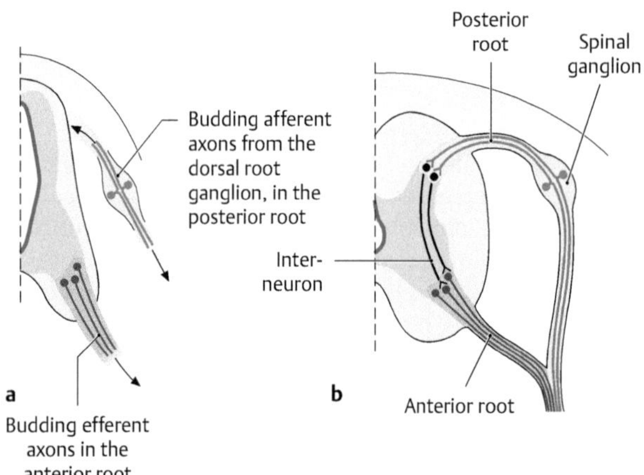

Fig. 9.122 (a, b) Development of a spinal nerve. (From Schuenke M, Schulte E, Schumacher U. THIEME Atlas of Anatomy. Head, Neck, and Neuroanatomy. Illustrations by Voll M and Wesker K. 3rd ed. New York: Thieme Medical Publishers; 2020.)

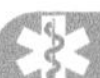

Clinical Correlate 9.33

Craniopharyngioma

A **craniopharyngioma** is a rare and generally benign type of brain tumor. They are derived from the ectoderm related to Rathke pouch or the embryonic tissue involved in the development of the anterior lobe of the pituitary gland. These tumors are most common in children ages 5 to 10 but can occur in adults as well. Early symptoms could include pressure on the optic nerve or optic chiasm affecting vision and a disruption of hormone production related to the pituitary gland. Increased pressure of the brain due to hydrocephalus could also result in frequent headaches and vomiting. The most common treatment is surgery but radiation therapy may accompany this option.

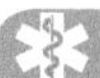

Clinical Correlate 9.34

Anencephaly

Anencephaly is a rare birth defect that is due to the cranial portion of the neural tube failing to close. Prenatal tests and ultrasound can be used to diagnose anencephaly while the fetus is in utero. A low intake of folic acid prior to and during pregnancy has shown to increase the risk of neural tube defects including caudal versions such as spina bifida discussed in Chapter 1. The newborn will be missing much of the brain and portions of the brainstem. There are no treatments and the baby will generally die shortly after birth.

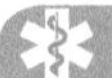

Clinical Correlate 9.35

Hydrocephalus

The abnormal accumulation of cerebrospinal fluid (CSF) within the ventricular system is called **hydrocephalus.** This can occur in both infants and adults but if it occurs during development there could be an enlargement of the skull. Hydrocephalus in a newborn is normally due to an obstruction of the cerebral aqueduct (of *Sylvius*) preventing CSF to pass from both the lateral and third ventricles and into the fourth ventricle. The accumulation of CSF in the lateral ventricles especially causes the brain to be compressed and can enlarge the skull. Treatment most often involves surgically inserting a shunt that allows for proper CSF drainage.

9.36.8 Autonomic Nervous System Development

- **Parasympathetics**: the **basal plates** of the neural tube related to the developing brainstem give rise to the **preganglionic parasympathetic neurons** that pass through **CN III, CN VII, CN IX**, and **CN X.** The **basal plate** of the neural tube related to **spinal cord segments S2–S4** also gives rise to preganglionic neurons that originate from an area similar to the lateral (intermediolateral) horns of T1–L2. **Postganglionic neurons** located within the **ciliary** (CN III), **submandibular** (CN VII), **pterygopalatine** (CN VII), and **otic ganglia** (CN IX), along with the **enteric ganglia** of the GI tract (CN X, *Auerbach* and *Meissner plexuses*) and the **pelvic ganglia**, develop from **neural crest cells.**
- **Sympathetics**: the **basal plates** of the neural tube related to **spinal cord segments T1–L2** give rise to **preganglionic sympathetic neurons.** These neurons are located specifically in an area known as the lateral (intermediolateral) horns. **Postganglionic neurons** located within the **sympathetic chain (paravertebral)** and **preaortic (prevertebral) ganglia**, along with the **chromaffin cells** located in the medulla of the suprarenal gland, all develop from **neural crest cells.**

PRACTICE QUESTIONS

1. On average there are approximately 500 mL of cerebrospinal fluid (CSF) produced daily by the choroid plexuses, but at what location is CSF reabsorbed into the venous circulation?
   A. Central canal.
   B. Median aperture (of *Magendie*).
   C. Arachnoid granulations.
   D. Lateral apertures (of *Luschka*).
   E. Cerebral aqueduct.
2. A 65-year-old man is demonstrating progressive memory loss, sleeplessness, and the inability to recognize family members. Multiple tests are performed and the individual is diagnosed with Alzheimer's disease. Destruction of what structure located in the brainstem has been linked to Alzheimer's disease?
   A. Substantia nigra.
   B. Locus coeruleus.
   C. Inferior olivary nucleus.
   D. Red nucleus.
   E. Ventral tegmental area.
3. All of the following statements regarding the gray matter of the spinal cord are correct EXCEPT?
   A. The phrenic nucleus is responsible for innervating the diaphragm.
   B. The nucleus of *Onuf* is responsible for innervation of the external urethral sphincter and the maintenance of micturition and defecation continence.
   C. The lateral motor nuclei are responsible for appendicular muscle innervation.
   D. The posteromarginal nucleus, substantia gelatinosa, and nucleus proprius are associated with the anterolateral system or spinothalamic tract.
   E. The posterior thoracic nucleus is the location of sympathetic preganglionic neurons.
4. All of the following arteries directly form the circle of Willis EXCEPT:
   A. Posterior communicating.
   B. Middle cerebral.
   C. Anterior communicating.
   D. Anterior cerebral.
   E. Posterior cerebral.
5. All of the following statements regarding the nuclei of the hypothalamus are correct EXCEPT:
   A. The suprachiasmatic nucleus plays a role in circadian rhythm and receives direct input from the retina.
   B. The anterior nucleus stimulates the parasympathetic nervous system.
   C. The mammillary bodies function in the consolidation of memories.
   D. The preoptic nuclei serve as the satiety center and inhibit drinking and eating when stimulated.
   E. The arcuate nucleus controls the endocrine functions of the adenohypophysis and produces hypothalamic-releasing factors that enter the hypophyseal portal system.
6. A unilateral lesion has developed on the left optic tract. In this case, what clinical condition would a patient present with?
   A. Bitemporal hemianopia.
   B. Monocular blindness.
   C. Homonymous macular hemianopia.
   D. Superior quadrantanopia.
   E. Homonymous hemianopia.
7. An occlusion of the left posterior inferior cerebellar artery (branch of the vertebral artery) has occurred and it affects the posterolateral portion of the caudal medulla. This leads to what is known as lateral medullary or Wallenberg syndrome. All listed symptoms would occur EXCEPT:
   A. Loss of gag reflex (efferent limb) on ipsilateral side.
   B. Contralateral loss of pain and temperature sensation from the trunk and extremities.
   C. Contralateral loss of proprioception, discriminative tactile sensation, and vibrations from the trunk and extremities.
   D. Ipsilateral lack of muscle coordination (dystaxia).
   E. Ipsilateral loss of pain and temperature sensation from the face.
8. A 73-year-old woman is visiting with family when she loses consciousness. After regaining consciousness she complains of double vision, ptosis is noted on the left eye, and there is a significant tremor involving her left upper limb. While at the hospital, an angiogram is performed and there is evidence of a posterior cerebral artery rupture. Further examination demonstrates a contralateral lack of muscle coordination (dystaxia) and a contralateral loss of proprioception, discriminative tactile sensation, and vibration senses from the trunk and limbs. Her symptoms are consistent with what syndrome?
   A. Dorsal medullary syndrome.
   B. Benedikt syndrome.
   C. Caudal basal pontine syndrome.
   D. Weber syndrome.
   E. Parinaud syndrome.
9. There is a spinal cord infarction involving the anterior spinal artery and this is known as anterior cord syndrome. All structures and tracts would be affected EXCEPT:
   A. Lateral corticospinal tract.
   B. Anterior (ventral) horn.
   C. Lateral spinothalamic tract.
   D. Posterior funiculus.
   E. Anterior white commissure.
10. What type of cerebellar cortex neuron is excitatory?
    A. Basket cells.
    B. Granule cells.
    C. Purkinje cells.
    D. Golgi cells.
    E. Stellate cells.
11. The adenohypophysis of the pituitary gland has three different types of cells, the chromophobes, acidophils, and basophils. All of the following hormones are secreted by basophils EXCEPT:
    A. Thyroid-stimulating hormone (TSH).
    B. Melanocyte-stimulating hormone (MSH).
    C. Growth hormone (GH).
    D. Luteinizing hormone (LH).
    E. Adrenocorticotropic hormone (ACTH).
12. An individual has been in an automobile accident and sustained damage to their spinal cord. An MRI has revealed a left hemisection of the spinal cord at T10. This is known as Brown-Séquard syndrome. All symptoms would be seen in this patient EXCEPT:
    A. Contralateral loss of crude touch and sensation starting three to four segments below the lesion.
    B. Ipsilateral loss of fine discriminative touch, proprioception, and vibratory senses below the lesion.

C. Ipsilateral flaccid paralysis at the level of the lesion and spastic muscle weakness (paresis) below the level of the lesion with a Babinski sign.
D. Contralateral loss of pain, temperature, and itch sensations starting one segment below the lesion.
E. Ipsilateral loss of lower extremity muscle coordination (dystaxia).

13. All of the following pairings between the cerebral cortices and Brodmann areas are correct EXCEPT:
A. Primary motor cortex/Area 6.
B. Broca speech area/Areas 44 and 45.
C. Primary olfactory cortex/Area 34.
D. Visual association cortices/Areas 18 and 19.
E. Primary somatosensory cortex/Areas 3, 1, and 2.

14. A 52-year-old office worker has noticed over the past few years that there is an involuntary shaking or tremor involving his hands, especially near his thumb and pointer finger. His limbs seem very rigid or tight and after standing up and taking a few steps his balance seems to be a little off. After a battery of tests, which included blood work, an MRI, and PET scans, and even a dopamine transporter (DAT) scan, a diagnosis of Parkinson disease is made. Parkinson's is a degenerative disorder involving the substantia nigra. What combination of thalamic nuclei function during motor movements by providing feedback for the outputs of the basal ganglia before projecting to cerebral motor cortices?
A. Lateral dorsal and lateral posterior.
B. Ventral posterolateral and ventral posteromedial.
C. Centromedian and parafascicular.
D. Ventral anterior and ventral lateral.
E. Lateral geniculate and medial geniculate.

15. The frontal lobe contains all the following structures or cortices EXCEPT:
A. Straight gyrus.
B. Orbital sulci.
C. Postcentral gyrus.
D. Broca speech area.
E. Premotor cortex.

16. An individual has just been diagnosed with a stroke. If the vascular lesion seen on an MRI was focused on Broca's area, what particular artery was occluded to allow this to happen?
A. Superior cerebellar.
B. Anterior cerebral.
C. Posterior cerebral.
D. Middle cerebral.
E. Basilar.

17. Basilar membrane deflection causes shearing forces on the stereocilia attached to the hair cells resulting in an action potential. From the hair cells, what would be the correct order of structures regarding the auditory system neuropathway before reaching the primary auditory cortex?
A. Hair cells, cochlear nuclei, inferior colliculi, lateral lemniscus, superior olivary nuclei, medial geniculate body, primary auditory cortex.
B. Hair cells, superior olivary nuclei, cochlear nuclei, lateral lemniscus, inferior colliculi, medial geniculate body, primary auditory cortex.
C. Hair cells, superior olivary nuclei, cochlear nuclei, lateral lemniscus, medial geniculate body, inferior colliculi, primary auditory cortex.
D. Hair cells, cochlear nuclei, superior olivary nuclei, lateral lemniscus, inferior colliculi, medial geniculate body, primary auditory cortex.
E. Hair cells, cochlear nuclei, lateral lemniscus, superior olivary nuclei, inferior colliculi, medial geniculate body, primary auditory cortex.

18. Which structure listed below is NOT directly related to the Papez circuit, a closed loop of connections within the limbic system that is involved in learning and memory, emotion, and social behavior?
A. Cingulate gyrus.
B. Basolateral nuclei of amygdala.
C. Hippocampus.
D. Mammillothalamic tract.
E. Anterior thalamic nucleus.

19. The central processes of first-order neurons that contain taste information from the tongue send that information to the nucleus of the solitary tract. What thalamic nucleus receives taste information from the second-order neuron?
A. Ventral posterolateral nucleus.
B. Ventral intermediate nucleus.
C. Pulvinar.
D. Ventral posteromedial nucleus.
E. Dorsomedial nucleus.

20. A 55 year-old male has noticed he has been having difficulty in walking and seems to be short of breath. He has also noticed some slurred speech along with twitching in his hands. All of these symptoms seem to be getting progressively worse. After a battery of tests including blood and urine samples, electromyogram, MRI, and a spinal tap it is confirmed the patient has amyotropic lateral sclerosis (ALS) or *Lou Gehrig's disease*. Where could damage of the spinal cord be seen if an individual was diagnosed with ALS?
A. Lateral corticospinal tract and ventral horns of gray matter.
B. Posterior spinocerebellar tract and posterior horns of gray matter.
C. Tectospinal tract and rubrospinal tract.
D. Anterior corticospinal tract and lateral horns of gray matter.
E. Posterior column-medial lemniscus pathway and anterior spinocerebellar tract.

ANSWERS

1. **C.** CSF is reabsorbed into the venous circulation at the arachnoid granulations primarily located at the superior sagittal sinus.
2. **B.** Recently, scientists have shown that the locus coeruleus located in the pons of the brainstem has been linked to Alzheimer's disease.
3. **E.** The posterior thoracic nucleus (or dorsal nucleus of *Clarke*) is located in Rexed lamina VII and between the C8 and L2 spinal cord segments. It accepts unconscious proprioception from muscle spindles and Golgi tendon organs and is the origin of the posterior spinocerebellar tract. It is homologous with the accessory cuneate nucleus of the medulla. Sympathetic preganglionic neurons would originate from the lateral horn of the gray matter of the spinal cord and specifically at the intermediolateral nucleus/column of Rexed lamina VII between the T1 and L2 spinal cord segments.
4. **B.** The middle cerebral arteries are branches of the internal carotid arteries and do not contribute to the circle of Willis. The internal carotid arteries help form the circle of Willis along with the other four answers.
5. **D.** The preoptic nuclei function in thermoregulation, generation of thirst, regulates the release of gonadotropic hormones from the adenophysis, mediates the onset of non-REM sleep, and the medial preoptic nucleus is sexually dimorphic. The ventromedial nucleus of the middle/tuberal region of the hypothalamus serves as the satiety center and inhibits drinking and eating.
6. **E.** If the lesion were present on the left optic tract, this would be known as a right homonymous hemianopia. With the left optic tract damaged, it interrupts fibers from the temporal portions of the retina on the ipsilateral side and the nasal portions on the contralateral side. The left and right half of the visual field is affected in each eye. Bitemporal hemianopia (A) would have occurred at the optic chiasm; monocular blindness (B) at the optic nerve; homonymous macular hemianopia (C) at cortical areas of the occipital lobe specific to the macula; and superior quadrantanopia (D) at Meyer's loop.
7. **C.** The deficit seen here would involve the medial lemniscus, a structure located closer to the midline of the current medullary location and a structure affected by medial medullary (Dejerine) syndrome. In this situation, Wallenberg syndrome would affect the nucleus ambiguus (A), spinothalamic tracts (B), inferior cerebellar peduncle (D), and spinal trigeminal nucleus and tract (E). This syndrome also has an effect on multiple vestibular nuclei and descending sympathetic tracts.
8. **B.** Benedikt syndrome. Benedikt, Weber, and Parinaud syndromes all involve the rupture of the posterior cerebral artery (PCA) or a direct branch off this artery. More specifically, Benedikt syndrome involves the paramedian branches of the PCA, and the midbrain structures affected include the oculomotor nerve roots, red nucleus, and medial lemniscus. The oculomotor nerve involvement would explain the double vision and ptosis. The red nucleus would be the reason behind the dystaxia while the medial lemniscus pathway involves proprioception, tactile, and vibration sensations from the trunk and limbs.
9. **D.** Posterior funiculus. Anterior cord syndrome generally preserves fine touch, proprioception, and vibratory senses because these are related to the PCML pathway that passes through the posterior funiculus of the spinal cord. Blood supply to this region is from the posterior spinal artery.
10. **B.** The only cells in the cerebellar cortex that are excitatory are granule cells.
11. **C.** Growth hormone along with prolactin is produced by acidophils.
12. **E.** There would be both an ipsilateral (posterior cerebellar tract) and contralateral (anterior spinocerebellar tract) loss of lower extremity muscle coordination.
13. **A.** The primary motor cortex located in the frontal lobe corresponds with Brodmann area 4.
14. **D.** The ventral anterior (VA) and ventral lateral (VL) thalamic nuclei receive input from parts of the basal ganglia (VA and VL) along with the cerebellum (VL) before projecting to cortical area 4 (VL) and area 6 (VA and VL).
15. **C.** The postcentral gyrus is part of the parietal lobe and related to both the primary and secondary somatosensory cortices.
16. **D.** Broca's speech area is located in the posterior part of the inferior frontal gyrus of the dominant hemisphere and is supplied by the middle cerebral artery.
17. **D.** The auditory pathway progress in this order: hair cells, cochlear nuclei, superior olivary nuclei, lateral lemniscus, inferior colliculi, medial geniculate body, primary auditory cortex.
18. **B.** The basolateral nuclei of the amygdala play a role in attaching emotional significance to a particular stimulus. They receive highly processed sensory information from the sensory association cortices and are connected with the limbic lobe cortex, among other areas, but they are not part of the Papez circuit. The Papez circuit is as follows: hippocampus ® fornix ® mammillary body ® mammillothalamic tract ® anterior thalamic nucleus ® thalamocingular tract ® cingulate gyrus ® cingulum (cingulohippocampal fibers) ® entorhinal cortex ® perforant pathway ® hippocampus.
19. **D.** Most second-order neurons from the nucleus of the solitary tract ascend through the brainstem and synapse at the ventral posteromedial nucleus (VPM) of the thalamus. Historically, the tract that delivers the second-order neurons to the VPM is the central tegmental tract but they may also involve the trigeminothalamic tracts. A limited amount of second-order neurons may travel first to the medial parabrachial nucleus near the junction of the midbrain and pons before sending third-order neurons to the VPM.
20. **A.** The progressive degeneration of motor neurons with someone having ALS would be seen in a combination of the corticospinal tracts and ventral horn gray matter.

Reference

1. Tubbs RS, Prekupec M, Loukas M, Hattab EM, Cohen-Gadol AA. The Indusium Griseum: Anatomic Study with Potential Application to Callosotomy. *Neurosurgery*. 2013;73(2):312–316

10 Peripheral Nervous System

LEARNING OBJECTIVES

- To describe the basic structure and function of the peripheral nervous system.
- To describe the different sensory receptors based on their location, stimulus detected, and anatomical structure
- To understand a motor unit and the neuromuscular junction.
- To understand dermatomes and myotomes.
- To describe the somatic peripheral nerve plexuses and the main branches that originate from the cervical, brachial, lumbar, sacral, and coccygeal plexuses.
- To describe nerve regeneration, rhizotomy, nerve transplantation and transfers, phantom limbs, peripheral nerve tumors, polyneuropathy, and herpes zoster.

10.1 Structure of the Peripheral Nervous System

All of the nerve fibers and cell bodies located outside of the CNS that conduct impulses to or away from the CNS are part of the peripheral nervous system (PNS). It is organized into nerves that connect the CNS with peripheral structures.

Structures of the PNS include:

- **Nerves**: bundle of nerve fibers located outside the CNS. Nerves that contain both sensory and motor fibers are known as mixed nerves.
- **Ganglia**: a collection of cell bodies that may or may not involve a synapse. A synapse will occur at an autonomic ganglion. Sympathetic ganglia can include the sympathetic chain and pre-aortic ganglia while parasympathetic autonomic ganglia are located in the head or adjacent to various viscera. Sensory ganglia do not involve synapses and are located on the dorsal roots of each spinal nerve along with specific sensory ganglia of cranial nerves V, VII, VIII, IX, and X.
- **Sensory receptors**: pick up stimuli from both inside and outside the body and send this information back to the CNS.
- **Motor endings**: the axon terminals of motor neurons that innervate effector organs, muscles or glands.

A **nerve** contains the following characteristics: (1) a bundle of nerve fibers outside the CNS or fascicles that are a bundle of bundled fibers, (2) connective tissue that surrounds and binds nerve fibers and fascicles together, and (3) is nourished by blood vessels known as *vasa nervorum*. The connective tissues of the nerve fibers are as follows **(Fig. 10.1)**:

- **Endoneurium**: surrounds the neurolemma of myelinated and unmyelinated nerve fibers.
- **Perineurium**: a dense connective tissue layer that encloses a fascicle and prevents penetration of most foreign substances.
- **Epineurium**: the outermost layer of a nerve and is a thick, dense connective tissue sheath that wraps around multiple bundles of fascicles. Blood vessels and lymphatics can also be found near this layer.

The **nerve fiber** is defined as consisting of an *axon*, a *neurolemma*, and its surrounding *endoneurium*. The **neurolemma** is the outermost nucleated cytoplasmic layer of the Schwann cells that surround the axon of the neuron and separate it from other axons. It takes two forms in the PNS **(Fig. 10.2)**:

1. With myelinated nerve fibers, the neurolemma consists of Schwann cells specific to an individual axon that is organized into a continuous series of segmented myelin sheathes separated by **nodes of Ranvier**.
2. With unmyelinated nerve fibers, the neurolemma, still composed of Schwann cells, does not produce myelin but instead embeds multiple axons in a **mesaxon** within its cytoplasm. There are no nodes of Ranvier.

Types of nerves associated with the PNS include the cranial and spinal nerves. The 12 pairs of cranial nerves are discussed extensively in Chapter 7 and exclusively in Chapter 12. They are peripheral nerves that arise from the brain or spinal cord with the exception of the optic nerve (CN II) that is more of an extension of the diencephalon. Originating from the spinal cord are 31 pairs of spinal nerves that correspond to either the cervical (8), thoracic

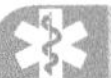
Clinical Correlate 10.1

Nerve Regeneration

Nerve regeneration can occur in the peripheral nervous system unlike the central nervous system. **Wallerian (anterograde) degeneration** is a process that results after a nerve fiber has been damaged or cut and involves the part of the axon distal to the initial injury. The distal axon stumps are still electrically excitable but show signs of degeneration within 2-3 days after the initial injury. In the event axons are damaged and the cell bodies are still intact the regeneration of motor, sensory and autonomic axons is possible and is dependent on the special properties of the Schwann cells and the presence of the endoneurium forming endoneurial tubes. Initially with a nerve injury, the axon becomes fragmented and eventually macrophages will begin to remove portions of the axon distal to the injury. Axon sprouts (or filaments) originating from the proximal portion of the nerve stump move towards the more distal stump through regeneration tubes formed by the Schwann cells. The multiple sprouts or filaments condense to form a single but enlarging axon that will eventually be wrapped by a new myelin sheath. The mechanisms thought to be involved allowing axon regeneration are as follows: (1) axons are attracted to chemotropic factors originating from the Schwann cells of the distal stump; (2) the distal stump may have growth-stimulating factors; and (3) the perineurium has inhibitory factors that prevent the axons from leaving the nerve.

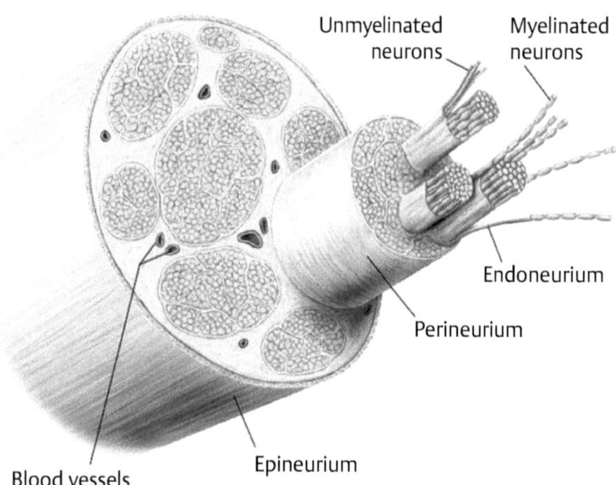

Fig. 10.1 Peripheral nerve. (From Schuenke M, Schulte E, Schumacher U. THIEME Atlas of Anatomy. Head and Neuroanatomy. Illustrations by Voll M and Wesker K. 1st ed. New York: Thieme Medical Publishers; 2010.)

(12), lumbar (5), sacral (5) or coccygeal (1) spinal segments of the spinal cord **(Fig. 10.3)**.

The architecture extending out from the spinal cord is as such: **ventral/dorsal rootlets**, **ventral/dorsal roots**, and the **spinal nerve**, which bifurcates into a **ventral** and **dorsal ramus** branch just distal to the intervertebral foramen. The dorsal root contains a **dorsal root ganglion**. The ventral rami branches of spinal nerves make up the majority of named nerves, can form plexuses, and innervate the anterior and lateral body walls along with the upper and lower limbs. The dorsal rami branches of spinal nerves are smaller contributors than their ventral counterparts and target the deep muscles of the back, the overlying skin of the back, and the synovial joints of the vertebral column **(Fig. 10.4)**.

The **ventral rootlet** and **roots** contain only **efferent (motor) fibers**. These are always somatic motor in nature but there are visceral motor fibers traveling through the T1-L2 and S2-S4 ventral rootlets and roots. The visceral motor fibers are part of the autonomic nervous system, which is further divided into sympathetic and parasympathetic components. The fibers passing through T1-L2 are sympathetic while those passing through S2-S4 they are parasympathetic. The **dorsal rootlets** and **roots** contain only **afferent (sensory) fibers**. They will include both somatic and visceral sensory fibers with their cell bodies both located in the **dorsal root ganglion**.

Motor and sensory fibers will not mix until reaching the **spinal nerve**. The **ventral** and **dorsal rami** branches of the spinal nerve are both considered mixed nerves. Each contains a combination of somatic motor (GSE), somatic sensory (GSA), visceral motor (GVE-sym/post) and in some locations visceral sensory (GVA) fibers that briefly pass back through with a ventral rami branch **(Fig. 10.5)**.

10.2 Sensory Receptors

Sensory receptors of the PNS fit into two categories; (1) **free nerve endings** or (2) specialized **receptor cells**. Most types of general sensory information that includes proprioception, touch, pressure, pain and temperature are monitored by free nerve endings. Specialized receptor cells monitor special sensory information such as vision and hearing. Sensory receptors can be classified by their location, by what stimulus they detect, or by their anatomical structure.

10.2.1 Sensory Receptors Based on Location

- **Exteroceptors**: located at or near the superficial surface of the body and these receptors are sensitive to the stimuli from outside the body. These receptors respond to touch, pressure, pain and temperature in the skin as well as most special sense organs.
- **Interoceptors (visceroreceptors)**: receive stimuli originating from the internal viscera. These stimuli may include chemical secretions, temperature and tissue stretching.
- **Proprioceptors**: located in skeletal muscle, tendons, ligaments and joints. Respond to the degree of stretch and send input regarding body movements back to the CNS.

10.2.2 Sensory Receptors Based on Stimulus Detected

- **Mechanoreceptors**: respond to mechanical deformation.
- **Thermoreceptors**: respond to temperature changes. Some receptors are specific to heat or cold.
- **Chemoreceptors**: respond to chemical changes associated with oxygen and carbon dioxide concentrations in the blood as well as smell and taste.
- **Nociceptors**: respond to a stimulus that results in pain.
- **Photoreceptors**: rods and cones of the retina that respond to light intensity and wavelength.

10.2.3 Sensory Receptors Based on Anatomical Structure

From a structural standpoint, sensory receptors are divided into two groups: (1) nonencapsulated and (2) encapsulated where nerve endings are surrounded with a capsule of connective tissue. Both groups are mechanoreceptors and respond to some form of mechanical deformation.

- *Nonencapsulated Receptors* **(Fig. 10.6)**
  - **Free nerve endings**: widely distributed throughout the body but densest in connective tissues (i.e. dermis, fascia, ligaments, joint capsules, tendons, muscles or periosteum) and between the epithelia of the skin, GI tract and cornea. They detect pain, temperature, light (crude) touch, pressure and tickle sensations and can be fast, intermediate or slowly adapting.

Clinical Correlate 10.2

Rhizotomy

A **rhizotomy** is a neurological procedure that will selectively destroy nerve roots in order to relieve the symptoms of neuromuscular conditions such as *spastic cerebral palsy*. As described in the introductory chapter, these individuals generally present with hypertonic or very tight muscle groups that are continuously contracting. Weakness is seen in the antagonistic muscle group resulting in abnormal positioning of the patients joints. Spasticity originates from the sensory roots thus the electrical activity of the dorsal roots are isolated using electromyographic (EMG) stimulation. The specific roots responsible for producing spasticity are then destroyed with tiny electrical pulses.

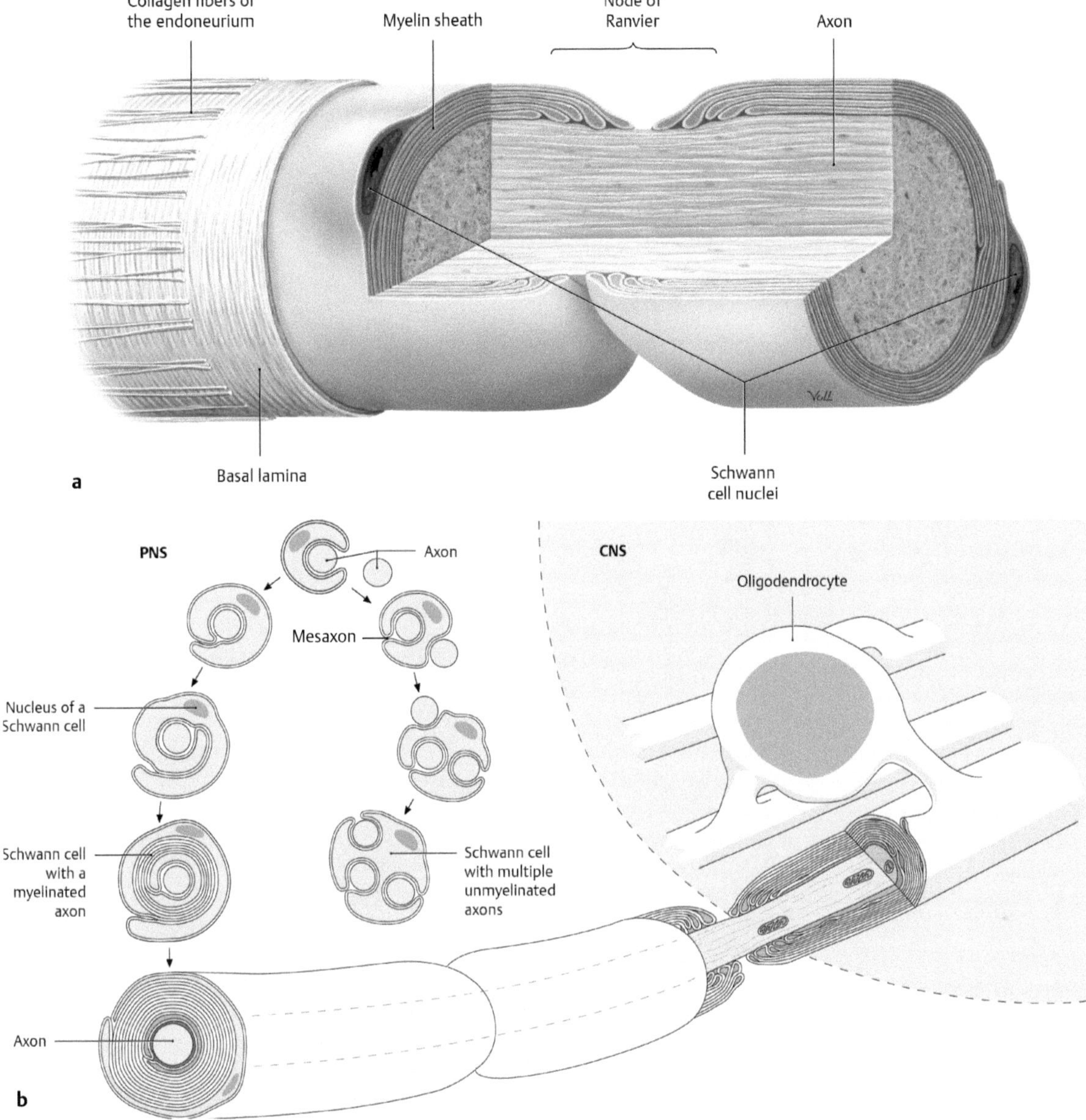

Fig. 10.2 **(a)** Myelinated axon in the PNS. **(b)** Myelination differences in the PNS and CNS. (From Schuenke M, Schulte E, Schumacher U. THIEME Atlas of Anatomy. Head, Neck, and Neuroanatomy. Illustrations by Voll M and Wesker K. 2nd ed. New York: Thieme Medical Publishers; 2016.)

- **Merkel disks**: found in the basal layer of the epidermis of hairless skin. They mediate light touch and are slowly adapting.
- **Hair follicle receptors**: located wrapped around the hair follicle in its outer connective tissue sheath. These receptors are stimulated when the hair bends and they rapidly adapt.

• *Encapsulated Receptors* **(Fig. 10.6)**
- **Pacinian (Vater-Pacini) corpuscles**: widely distributed throughout the body but abundant in the nipples, external genitalia, dermis, subcutaneous tissue, pleura, peritoneum, ligaments, joint capsules and periosteum. They detect pressure and vibration sensations and are rapidly adapting.
- **Meissner's corpuscles**: located in the dermal papillae of skin and especially near the palm of the hand and sole of the foot. Additionally, the external genitalia and nipples have these receptors. They mediate fine discriminative touch and are rapidly adapting. They allow a person to distinguish between two pointed structures when placed together on the skin.
- **Ruffini corpuscles**: are located in the dermis of hairy skin. They respond to stretch and are slowly adapting receptors.
- **Muscle spindles** (proprioceptor): are innervated by both motor and sensory neurons and will respond to changes in length of skeletal muscle fibers and to rates of change in length. There are 50-100 muscle spindles per muscle

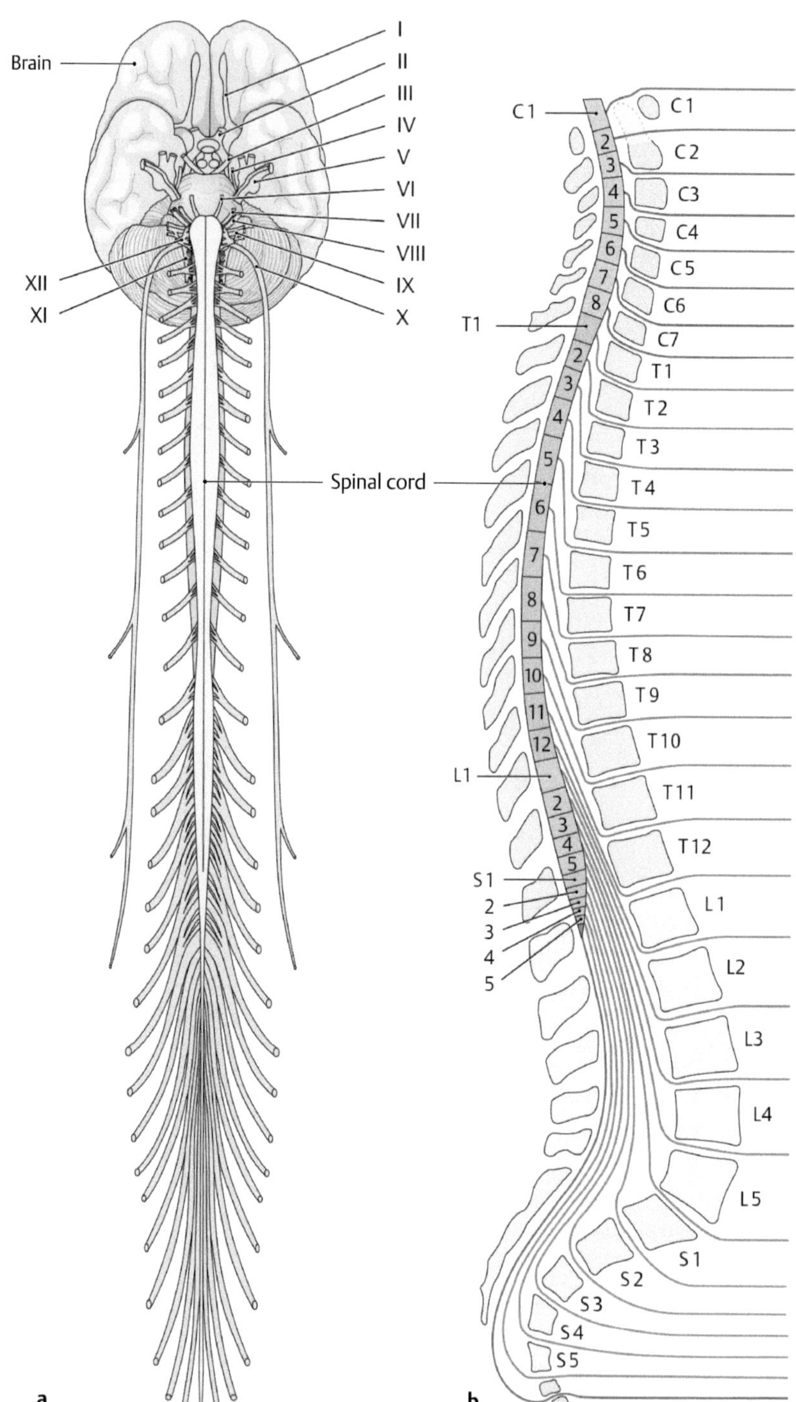

Fig. 10.3 (a) Central and peripheral nervous systems. **(b)** Spinal segments of the spinal cord and spinal nerves. (From Schuenke M, Schulte E, Schumacher U. THIEME Atlas of Anatomy. General Anatomy and Musculoskeletal System. Illustrations by Voll M and Wesker K. 3rd ed. New York: Thieme Medical Publishers; 2020.)

and they consist of on average 7-10 **intrafusal nerve fibers** that are specialized muscle cells within a collagen sheath anchored to the endomysium and perimysium. There are two types of intrafusal fibers: (1) **nuclear bag fibers** that receive type Ia primary afferent fibers (annulospiral endings) and respond primarily to the rate of change of muscle length; (2) **nuclear chain fibers** that receive type Ia primary and Type II secondary afferent fibers (flower spray endings) and respond primarily to muscle length.

When the muscle stretches, the sensory nerve fibers send feedback to the brain and spinal cord before the CNS activates spinal motor neurons called **alpha efferent neurons**. These neurons innervate the **extrafusal nerve fibers**, of which most of the muscle is made up of, and results in the muscle contracting and resisting any further stretching. Additional motor neurons called **gamma efferent neurons** innervate the intrafusal nerve fibers and preset the sensitivity of the muscle spindle to stretch. The *simple reflex arc reaction* is the result of muscle spindles being suddenly stretched.

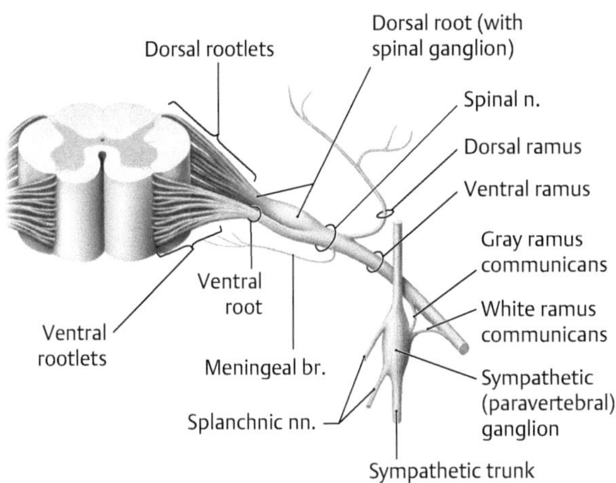

Fig. 10.4 Structure of a spinal cord segment. (From Schuenke M, Schulte E, Schumacher U. THIEME Atlas of Anatomy. Head and Neuroanatomy. Illustrations by Voll M and Wesker K. 1st ed. New York: Thieme Medical Publishers; 2010.)

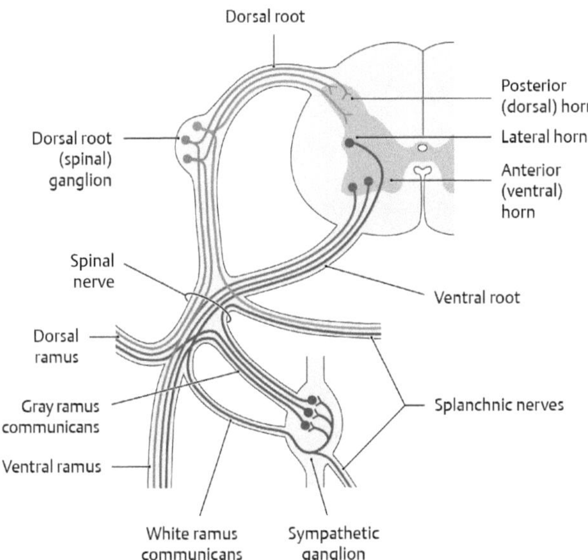

Fig. 10.5 Topographical and functional organization of a spinal cord segment. (From Schuenke M, Schulte E, Schumacher U. THIEME Atlas of Anatomy. General Anatomy and Musculoskeletal System. Illustrations by Voll M and Wesker K. 3rd ed. New York: Thieme Medical Publishers; 2020.)

- **Golgi tendon organs** (proprioceptor): respond to total muscle tension during muscle stretch and contraction and not the length or rate. They are also sensitive to the velocity of tension development. They are located at the muscle-tendon junction, are innervated by type Ib afferent fibers, and are responsible for protecting the tendons from excessive muscle contraction.
- **Joint receptors** (proprioceptor): monitor stretch in synovial joints and body movements and they will send this information back to the cerebellum and cerebrum. Each joint capsule includes free nerve endings, Pacinian corpuscles, Ruffini corpuscles and receptors that resemble Golgi tendon organs.

Clinical Correlate 10.3

Nerve Transplantation and Transfers

Nerve transplantation or grafts have been used to restore muscle activity generally after some form of trauma or surgical removal of a tumor that resulted in heavy tissue loss. The sural nerve located on the posterior leg has been used to bridge nerves while addressing brachial plexus, facial nerve and sciatic nerve injuries. A **nerve transfer** will involve taking a nerve that has a less important role or one that has multiple branches performing a redundant function and then transfer them to restore function to an area that has seen damage to its native nerve.

10.3 Motor Endings

One or more nerves may innervate skeletal muscle. Single innervation may include muscles of the head and neck or even the limbs whereas large sheet like muscles such as the abdominal muscles will receive innervation from multiple nerves. A nerve to a muscle contains three types of motor fibers: (1) large type A-alpha myelinated fibers that target extrafusal fibers; (2) small type A-gamma myelinated fibers that target intrafusal fibers; and (3) thin type C unmyelinated fibers that are generally sympathetic postganglionic and target smooth muscle of blood vessels, arrector pili and sweat glands. The nerve responsible for innervating a muscle contains both motor and sensory fibers of which the sensory fibers and receptors were listed previously.

A **motor unit** can be defined as the single alpha motor neuron and the muscle fibers that it innervates. The muscle fibers of a single motor unit will be found scattered throughout the muscle. Fine precision movements seen in small hand and extraocular muscles are possible because they will have motor units that occupy only a few muscle fibers. A large bulky muscle such as the gastrocnemius will have a motor unit that innervates hundreds of muscle fibers.

The type A-alpha myelinated nerve fibers originating from the ventral horns of the spinal cord or motor nuclei of cranial nerves will enter a skeletal muscle and branch many times. A single branch will then terminate on a muscle fiber at a site called the **neuromuscular junction** (or **motor end plate**). After reaching the muscle fiber, the nerve will lose its myelin sheath and branch into a number of fine branches. A nerve impulse will stimulate the release of the neurotransmitter acetylcholine (ACh) from the **axon terminal** and into the **synaptic cleft**. The synaptic cleft serves as a separation between the axon terminal and **sarcolemma** (plasma membrane of muscle cells) and is approximately 40 nm wide. Only a single contraction is allowed after the release of ACh because enzymes located in the synaptic cleft will immediately break it down to prevent any additional and undesirable contractions (**Fig. 10.7**). Even at rest, every skeletal muscle is in a partial state of contraction and this is known as **muscle tone**.

10.4 Dermatomes

The area of skin that is mainly supplied by the sensory neurons of a single spinal nerve of the ipsilateral (same) side is called a **dermatome**. There is overlap from one dermatome to the next so if a lesion of a specific spinal nerve was to occur; there is still some sensory input to the affected dermatome (**Fig. 10.8**). For example, if there was compression or a lesion of the fourth spinal nerve

Clinical Correlate 10.4

Phantom Limb Syndrome

If a patient has undergone an amputation they may experience the phenomenon known as **phantom limb**. In this situation, the patient is experiencing pain due to the pressure that is applied to nerve fibers at the end of the limb stump. For some patients the symptoms will resolve on their own over time. For others, chronic pain may have to be controlled by analgesics (from aspirin to narcotics), antidepressants, and anticonvulsants or even with the help of electroconvulsive therapy.

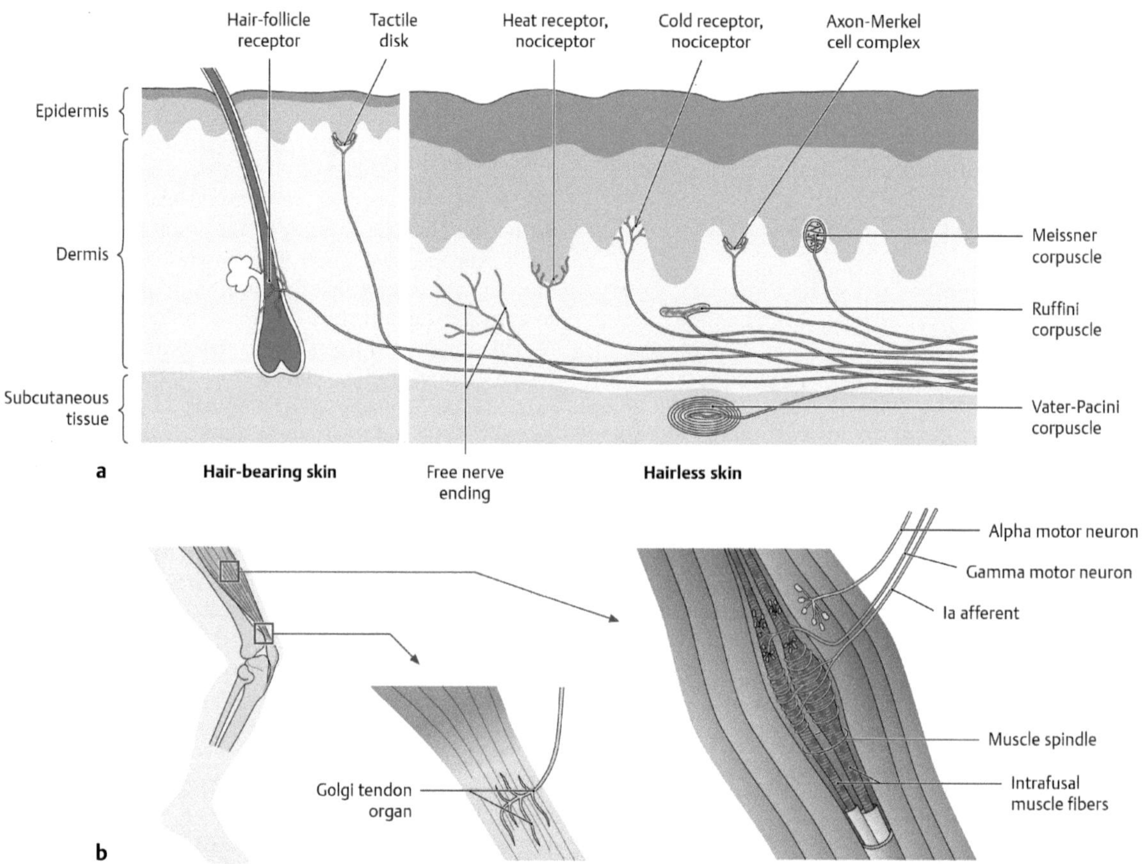

Fig. 10.6 Nonencapsulated and encapsulated receptors. **(a)** Skin receptors. **(b)** Joint receptors. (From Schuenke M, Schulte E, Schumacher U. THIEME Atlas of Anatomy. Head, Neck, and Neuroanatomy. Illustrations by Voll M and Wesker K. 2nd ed. New York: Thieme Medical Publishers; 2016.)

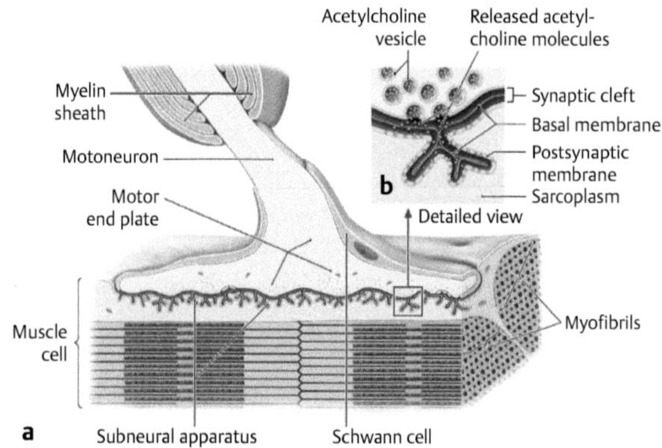

Fig. 10.7 (a, b) Neuromuscular junction. (From Schuenke M, Schulte E, Schumacher U. THIEME Atlas of Anatomy. Head, Neck, and Neuroanatomy. Illustrations by Voll M and Wesker K. 2nd ed. New York: Thieme Medical Publishers; 2016.)

of which it corresponds to the dermatome the nipple is located in, fibers of the adjacent third and fifth spinal nerves overlap the fourth dermatome and thus provide a double or redundant coverage. At least three contiguous or adjacent spinal nerves would have to be blocked in order to eliminate the sensation to a particular dermatome. The degree of overlap of fibers carrying pain and temperature information is much more extensive than fibers carrying tactile sensation thus the area of tactile sensation loss is always greater than the area of pain and temperature sensations.

It is important to distinguish the fibers carried by an individual spinal nerve that contributes to a segmental innervation such as a dermatome and the fibers carried by a named cutaneous nerve that can originate from a plexus of peripheral nerves and thus innervates a peripheral region not defined by dermatomes **(Fig. 10.9)**. A cutaneous nerve supplies an area of the skin that is related to a peripheral nerve. This cutaneous nerve may contain fibers from several individual spinal nerves and therefore

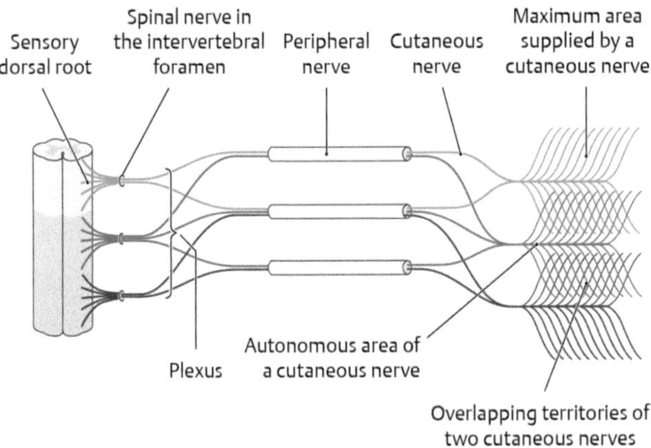

Fig. 10.8 Course of sensory fibers from the dorsal root to the dermatome. (From Schuenke M, Schulte E, Schumacher U. THIEME Atlas of Anatomy. General Anatomy and Musculoskeletal System. Illustrations by Voll M and Wesker K. 3rd ed. New York: Thieme Medical Publishers; 2020.)

the peripheral cutaneous nerve and dermatome mapped regions will show much overlapping. A cutaneous nerve area is generally broader and wider than an area or segment defined as a single dermatome. Overlap is seen with individual cutaneous nerves much like that of an individual spinal nerve overlapping another defined dermatome. The details listed above are the reason a dermatome map differs from that of a peripheral cutaneous nerve map (**Fig. 10.10**).

The concept of **referred pain** is the perception of somatic pain at a particular location but in reality it is pain from a visceral organ and travels back with the visceral sensory (GVA) fibers associated with the sympathetic nervous system. It may be located in an area corresponding to multiple dermatomes but referred pain in itself is not associated with a specific dermatome.

10.5 Myotomes

A **myotome** represents a group of muscles that a single spinal nerve innervates. Most of the muscles located in the upper and lower limbs receive innervation from one or more spinal nerves that collectively form a "nerve" and are therefore comprised of multiple myotomes. In order to paralyze a muscle completely, it would be necessary to section multiple spinal nerves or several segments of the spinal cord. When spinal nerves become compressed or irritated by trauma, disc herniation, bones spurs or even reduced blood supply due to diabetes for example, it leads to what is known as *radiculopathy*. This results in pain, numbness, or even muscle weakness with it most commonly occurring at the level of the cervical and lumbar regions (**Fig. 10.11**).

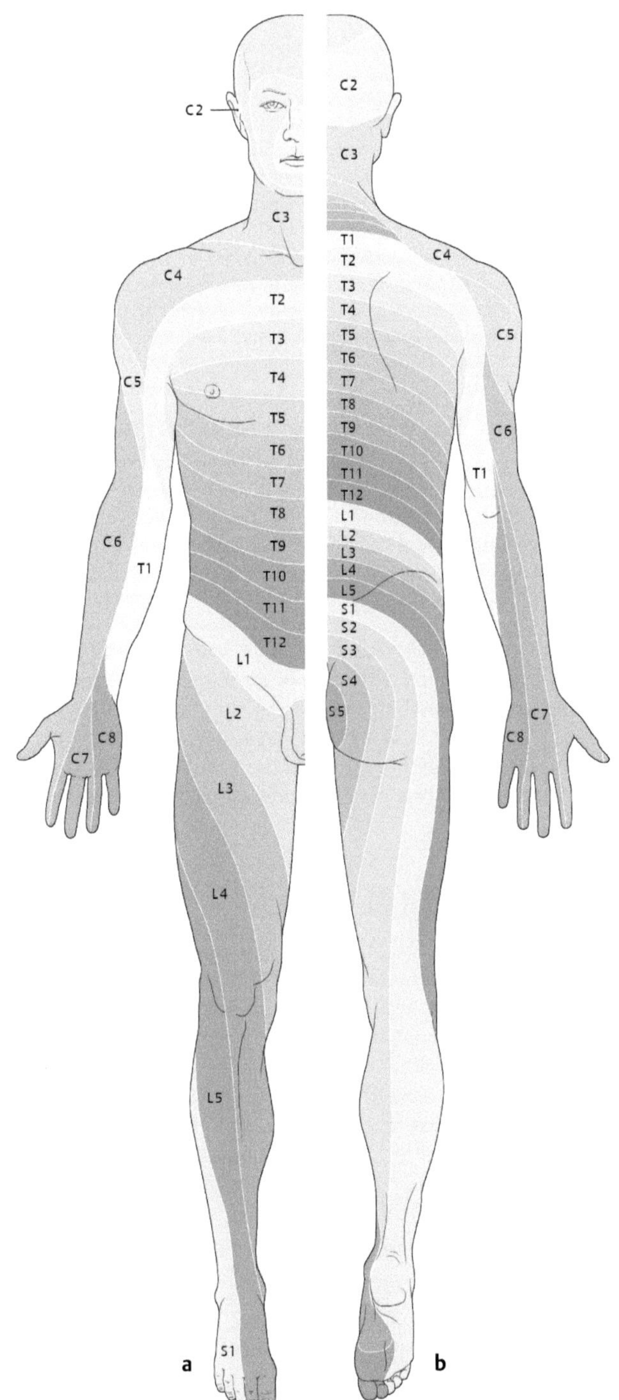

Fig. 10.9 Dermatome map. **(a)** Anterior view. **(b)** Posterior view. (From Schuenke M, Schulte E, Schumacher U. THIEME Atlas of Anatomy. General Anatomy and Musculoskeletal System. Illustrations by Voll M and Wesker K. 3rd ed. New York: Thieme Medical Publishers; 2020.)

10.6 Peripheral Nerve Plexuses

Peripheral nerves are composed of bundles of nerve fibers but along their course they may divide into branches that join nearby peripheral nerves. The formation of a network of nerves occurs and this is known as a **nerve plexus**. A nerve plexus allows for individual nerve fibers to pass from one peripheral nerve to another. Ultimately, a plexus permits the redistribution of nerve fibers within the different peripheral nerves. A nerve plexus is solely made of ventral rami of the spinal nerves.

10.6.1 Cervical Plexus

The **cervical plexus** is made up of the ventral rami of C1-C4 spinal nerves and supplies select neck muscles and the diaphragm, along with a large section of the head and neck skin. The plexus is located anteromedial to the middle scalene and levator scapulae muscles but deep to the sternocleidomastoid muscle. This plexus consists of each ramus, except for the first, dividing into both an ascending and descending branch that unites to form a

Clinical Correlate 10.5

Peripheral Nerve Tumors

The majority of peripheral nerve tumors are benign with primary tumors of the axons being quite rare. These tumors can affect the function of the nerve and result in pain or some form of disability. *Schwannomas* are commonly caused by *schwannomatosis* and are a slowly growing tumor consisting of only Schwann cells. These tumors are generally held within a capsule and can be surgically removed. The vestibulocochlear nerve (CN VIII) is the most susceptible to Schwannomas. *Neurofibromas* are benign nerve sheath tumors that are generally stand-alone tumors. A minority of these cases are due to *neurofibromatosis type I*. They arise from Schwann cells but incorporate additional cell types. *Dermal neurofibromas* originate from nerves in the skin while *plexiform neurofibromas* can also originate from nerves of the skin or internal nerve plexuses. Plexiform neurofibromas can manifest themselves into *malignant peripheral nerve sheath tumors*, very aggressive tumors classified as a sarcoma of the connective tissue surrounding nerves. Surgical resection along with both chemotherapy and radiation may be prescribed for the patient. Most originate from larger nerve plexuses such as the brachial plexus and nearly half of all cases are diagnosed with individuals who have neurofibromatosis.

communicating loop. Superficial branches of this plexus are cutaneous in nature and mostly pass in a posterior fashion. The deep branches are considered the motor fibers and pass through the neck mostly in an anteromedial fashion. Like all somatic nerve plexuses the functional components of their nerves contain GSE, GSA and GVE-sym/post fibers unless it is a cutaneous nerve and it only has GSA and GVE-sym/post fibers.

- The *muscular branches* contribute to the **ansa cervicalis** and **phrenic nerve** along with some of the individual segmental branches that contribute to the innervation of multiple muscles of the prevertebral region **(Fig. 10.12).**
- The *cutaneous branches* consist of the **lesser occipital**, **great auricular**, **transverse cervical** and **supraclavicular nerves (Fig. 10.12).**

10.6.2 Brachial Plexus

The nerves that innervate the upper extremity originate from the **brachial plexus** (ventral rami of C5-T1) located mainly in the posterior triangle of the neck and axilla regions. This somatic nerve plexus enters the shoulder region and down into the rest of the upper extremity to provide (1) motor innervation to the muscles; (2) sensory innervation from the skin, muscles and joints; and (3) sympathetic innervation to the blood vessels, sweat glands and arrector pili muscles. The brachial plexus itself is made up of *roots, trunks, divisions, cords* and *terminal branches*. The individual branches that directly originate from these structures or serve as the main terminal branches from this plexus are listed below **(Fig. 10.13).**

- Roots
  - **Dorsal scapular** (C5) and **long thoracic** (C5-C7).
- Upper Trunk
  - **Suprascapular** (C5-C6) and **nerve to subclavius** (C5-C6).
- Lateral Cord
  - **Lateral pectoral** (C5-C7), **musculocutaneous** (C5-C7), and **lateral root of median nerve.**
- Medial Cord
  - **Medial pectoral** (C8-T1), **medial brachial cutaneous** (C8-T1), **medical antebrachial cutaneous** (C8-T1), **ulnar** (C8-T1), and **medial root of median nerve.**
- Posterior Cord
  - **Upper subscapular** (C5-C6), **thoracodorsal** (C6-C8), **lower subscapular** (C5-C6), **axillary** (C5-C6), and **radial nerve** (C5-T1).
- Terminal Branches
  - Although previously described, the musculocutaneous, median (C5-T1), ulnar, axillary and radial nerves are considered the terminal branches.

10.6.3 Lumbar and Sacral Plexuses

The nerves that innervate the lower extremity originate from both the **lumbar plexus** (ventral rami of L1-L4) located in the abdomen and the **sacral plexus** (ventral rami of L4-S4) found in the pelvic region. These somatic nerve plexuses are commonly referred together as the *lumbosacral plexus* and they will provide the lower extremity and perineum with (1) motor innervation to the muscles; (2) sensory innervation from the skin, muscles and joints; and (3) sympathetic innervation to the blood vessels, sweat glands and arrector pili muscles.

The **lumbar plexus** is made up of the **iliohypogastric** (L1), **ilioinguinal** (L1), **lateral femoral cutaneous** (L2-L3), **femoral** (L2-L4), **genitofemoral** (L1-L2), and the **obturator nerves** (L2-L4). In addition, there are direct muscular branches originating from L1-L4 that contribute to the innervation of select posterior abdominal wall muscles **(Fig. 10.14).**

The **sacral plexus** is made up of the **lumbosacral trunk** (L4-L5), **superior gluteal** (L4-S1), **nerve to quadratus femoris** (L4-S1), **nerve to piriformis** (S1-S2), **inferior gluteal nerve** (L5-S2), **nerve to obturator internus** (L5-S2), **posterior femoral cutaneous** (S1-S3), **sciatic** (L4-S3), and both of its **tibial** (L4-S3) and **common fibular (peroneal)** (L4-S2) divisions, the **superficial fibular** (L4-S1) and **deep fibular nerves** (L5-S2) of the superficial fibular and finally the **pudendal nerve** (S2-S4). The pelvic splanchnic nerves arise from the S2-S4 ventral rami but carry parasympathetic preganglionic fibers destined for the pelvic and hindgut organs **(Fig. 10.14).**

10.6.4 Coccygeal Plexus

The ventral rami of S4-Co1 contribute to the much smaller **coccygeal plexus**. This somatic nerve plexus is quite limited and may

Clinical Correlate 10.6

Polyneuropathy

The simultaneous impairment of multiple peripheral nerves is known as **polyneuropathy**. Both motor and sensory functions can be affected and degeneration can involve either the axon or cell body. Interrupted function of the distal axons of peripheral nerves or *distal axonopathy* is the most common response due to a metabolic disorder or exposure to toxic materials. The loss of myelin or *myelinopathy* reduces the rate of conduction of action potentials through the axon. Causes of polyneuropathy can include diabetes, heavy metal poisoning, vitamin B_1 and B_{12} deficiency and Guillain-Barré syndrome but mild conditions have been reversible.

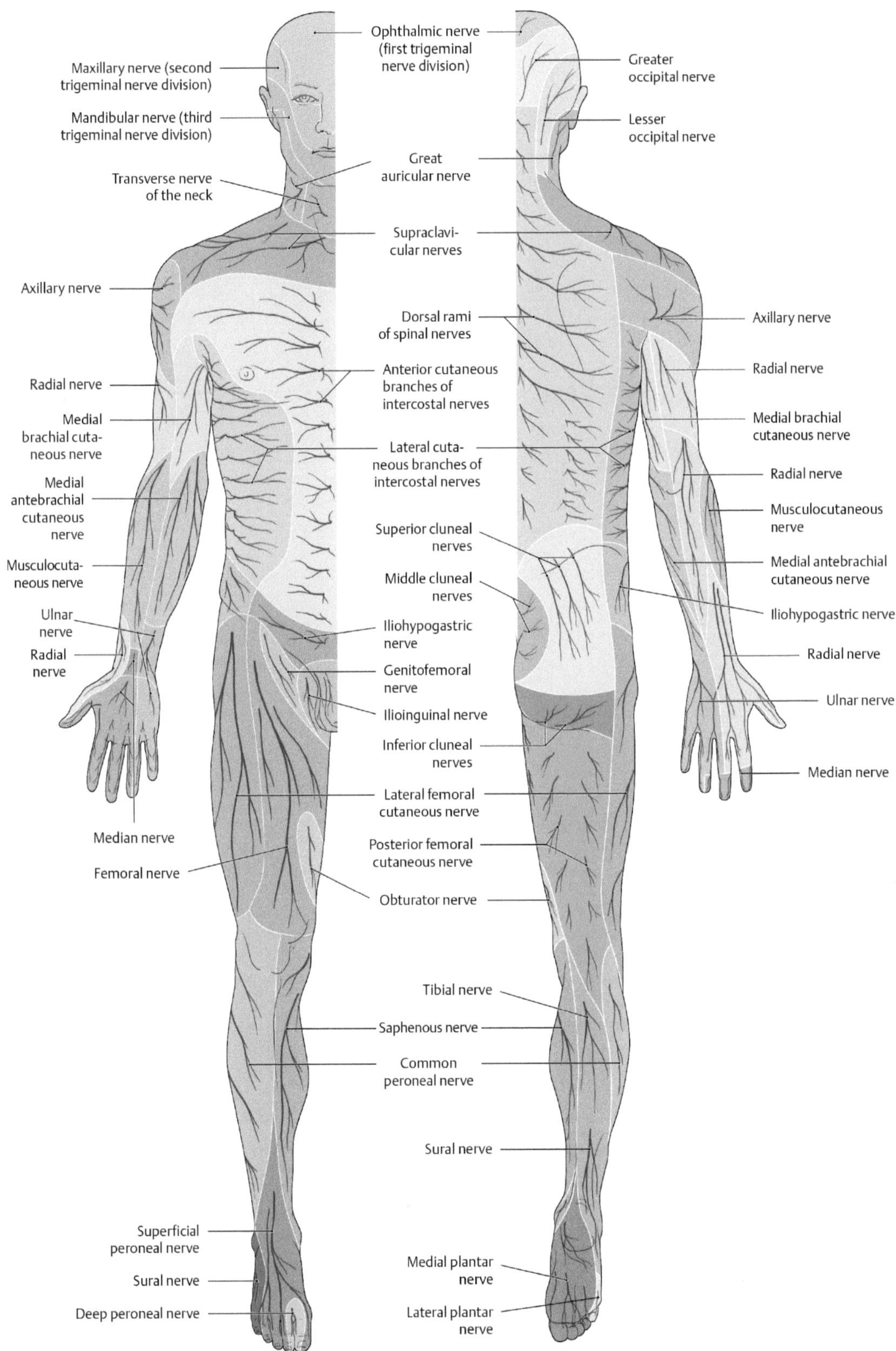

Fig. 10.10 Peripheral cutaneous nerve map. (From Schuenke M, Schulte E, Schumacher U. THIEME Atlas of Anatomy. General Anatomy and Musculoskeletal System. Illustrations by Voll M and Wesker K. 3rd ed. New York: Thieme Medical Publishers; 2020.)

be considered part of the sacral plexus but it supplies the levator ani, coccygeus and external anal sphincter muscles, along with the sacrococcygeal joint and a small area of skin between the tip of the coccyx and the anus. The individual nerves of this plexus include the **nerve to levator ani**, **nerve to coccygeus** and **anococcygeal nerve (Fig. 10.14)**.

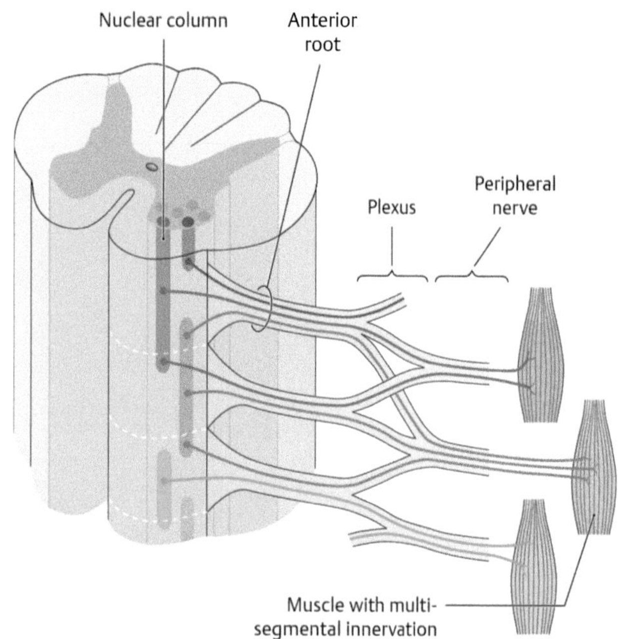

Fig. 10.11 Organizational principles of the anterior column of the spinal cord. (From Schuenke M, Schulte E, Schumacher U. THIEME Atlas of Anatomy. Head, Neck, and Neuroanatomy. Illustrations by Voll M and Wesker K. 3rd ed. New York: Thieme Medical Publishers; 2020.)

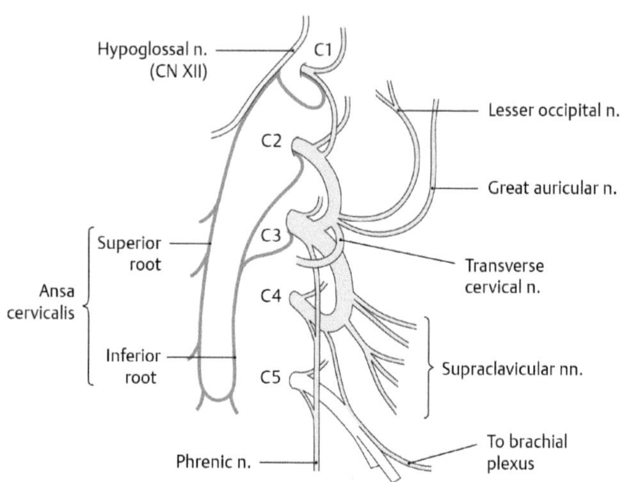

Fig. 10.12 Muscular and cutaneous branches of the cervical plexus. (From Schuenke M, Schulte E, Schumacher U. THIEME Atlas of Anatomy. Head, Neck, and Neuroanatomy. Illustrations by Voll M and Wesker K. 3rd ed. New York: Thieme Medical Publishers; 2020.)

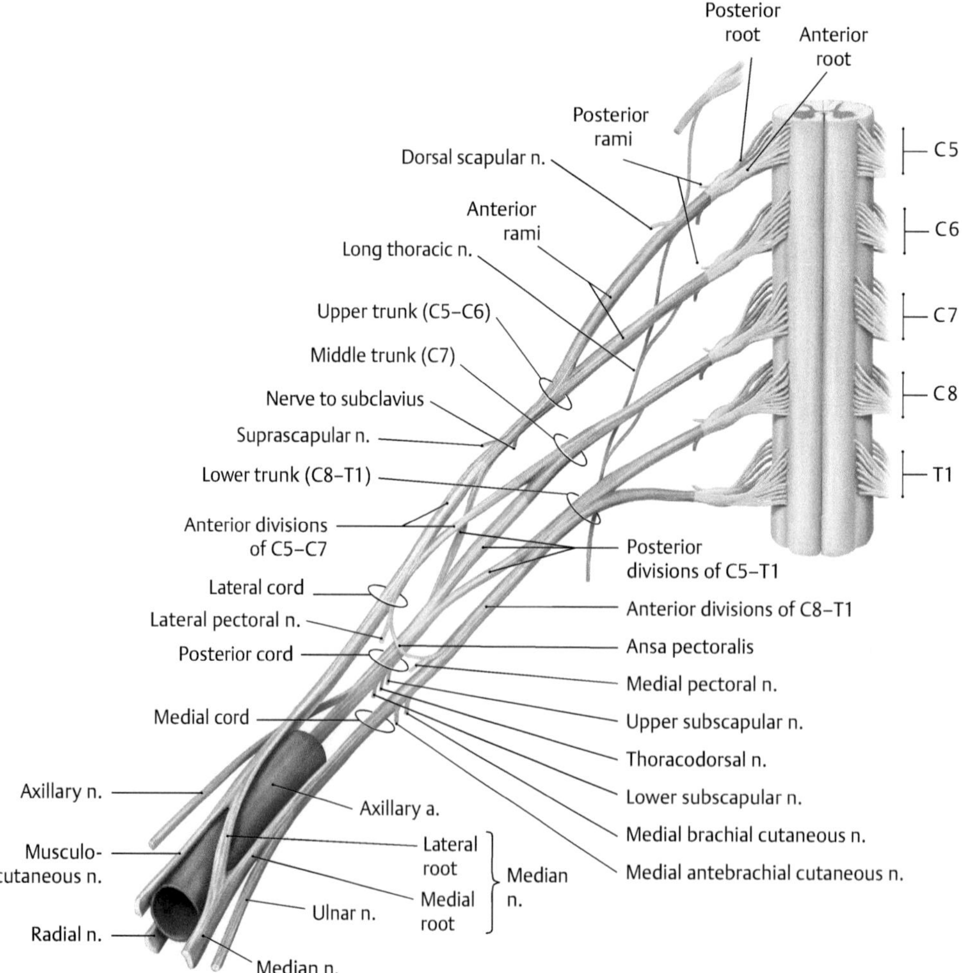

Fig. 10.13 Brachial plexus. (From Gilroy AM et al. Atlas of Anatomy. 4th ed. New York: Thieme Medical Publishers 2020. Based on Schuenke M, Schulte E, Schumacher U. THIEME Atlas of Anatomy. Head, Neck, and Neuroanatomy. Illustrations by Voll M and Wesker K. 3rd ed. New York: Thieme Medical Publishers; 2020)

Clinical Correlate 10.7

Herpes Zoster

The relatively common condition known as **Herpes zoster** or *shingles* is the result of the reactivation of the latent varicella-zoster virus in a patient who has previously had chickenpox. The virus remains dormant in any dorsal root ganglion or trigeminal ganglion. Herpes zoster is only possible if a person had the chickenpox most likely as a child. When the virus becomes active again it will travel down the nerve to the endings in the skin and produce inflammation and blisters. It will follow the dermatome pattern that corresponds with the sensory neuron it originated from. First symptoms may include fever and malaise but then be followed by itching and burning pain. Rashes develop and later become small blisters filled with a serous exudate. It is most common in people over 50 years of age and may typically take up to 3-5 weeks to resolve itself.

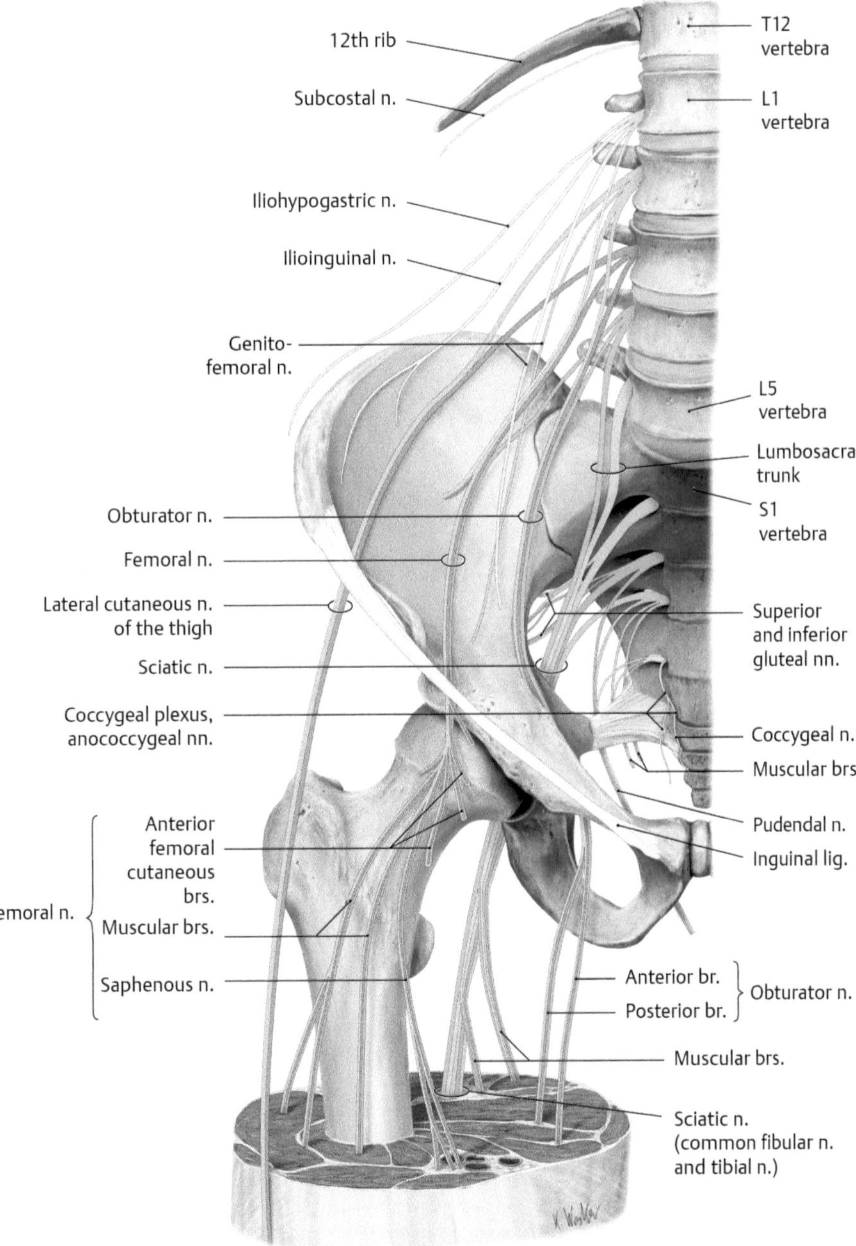

Fig. 10.14 Lumbar, sacral and coccygeal plexuses. (From Gilroy AM et al. Atlas of Anatomy. 4th ed. New York: Thieme Medical Publishers 2020. Based on Schuenke M, Schulte E, Schumacher U. THIEME Atlas of Anatomy. Head, Neck, and Neuroanatomy. Illustrations by Voll M and Wesker K. 3rd ed. New York: Thieme Medical Publishers; 2020.)

PRACTICE QUESTIONS

1. What type of sensory receptor responds to the degree of stretch and sends input regarding body movements back to the central nervous system?
   A. Proprioceptors.
   B. Interoceptors.
   C. Nociceptors.
   D. Exteroceptors.
   E. Chemoreceptors.
2. What type of receptor mediates fine discriminative touch, rapidly adapts, and allows a person to distinguish between two pointed structures when placed together on the skin?
   A. Pacinian corpuscles.
   B. Merkel disks.
   C. Meissner's corpuscles.
   D. Ruffini corpuscles.
   E. Free nerve endings.
3. Which statement about motor endings is INCORRECT?
   A. Small type A-gamma myelinated fibers target intrafusal fibers.
   B. The neurotransmitter acetylcholine is released from the axon terminal and into the synaptic cleft.
   C. A motor unit is a single alpha motor neuron and the muscle fibers that it innervates.
   D. Multiple contractions are allowed after the release of acetylcholine.
   E. Large type A-alpha myelinated fibers target extrafusal fibers.
4. All of the listed nerves are cutaneous branches of the cervical plexus EXCEPT?
   A. Great auricular.
   B. Ansa cervicalis.
   C. Transverse cervical.
   D. Supraclavicular.
   E. Lesser occipital.
5. The brachial plexus is made up of the nerves responsible for upper extremity innervation. From the spinal cord, what is the correct order of the components that make up the brachial plexus?
   A. Roots, cords, trunks, divisions, and terminal branches.
   B. Trunks, cords, roots, terminal branches, and divisions.
   C. Roots, trunks, divisions, cords, and terminal branches.
   D. Terminal branches, cords, divisions, trunks, and roots.
   E. Cords, roots, divisions, trunks, and terminal branches.
6. Which combination of spinal nerves makes up the inferior gluteal nerve of the sacral plexus?
   A. S1-S2.
   B. L4-S1.
   C. S2-S4.
   D. L4-S3.
   E. L5-S2.

ANSWERS

1. **A.** Proprioceptors.
2. **C.** Meissner's corpuscles.
3. **D.** Only a single contraction is allowed after the release of acetylcholine because enzymes located in the synaptic cleft will immediately break it down to prevent additional or undesirable contractions.
4. **B.** The ansa cervicalis is a muscular branch of the cervical plexus and innervates most of the infrahyoid muscles located in the anterior neck.
5. **C.** The correct order extending distally from the spinal cord is roots, trunks, divisions, cords, and terminal branches.
6. **E.** The combination of L5-S2 spinal nerves contribute to the inferior gluteal nerve.

11 Autonomic Nervous System

LEARNING OBJECTIVES

- To understand the structural differences between the parasympathetic and sympathetic divisions of the autonomic nervous system (ANS).
- To describe the effects of the parasympathetic and sympathetic divisions on individual organs.
- To describe the cell body locations and pathways of both the parasympathetic and sympathetic divisions of the ANS.
- To understand the visceral sensory fibers that are paired with both divisions of the ANS and the make-up of a visceral nerve plexus.
- To describe the neurotransmitters released at the preganglionic and postganglionic axon terminals for both the parasympathetic and sympathetic divisions of the ANS.
- To describe how agonists and antagonists act on neurotransmitter receptor sites.
- To understand how the central nervous system can have an effect on the activity of the ANS.
- To describe Horner's syndrome, autonomic dysreflexia, Raynaud's disease, gustatory sweating, and Hirschsprung's disease.

The **autonomic nervous system (ANS)** is defined as the visceral motor fibers that innervate visceral organs and these include vital organs, smooth muscle or glandular tissues **(Fig. 11.1)**. The ANS is comprised of two divisions: the sympathetic and parasympathetic divisions. The **sympathetic division** is concerned with the "fight or flight" response (the response of a person under threat) while the **parasympathetic division** is concerned with homeostasis and can be referred to as the "calming, digesting and resting" response.

These **general visceral efferent (GVE)** motor fibers consist of a two-neuron motor system that differs from the entire somatic nervous system that only has one neuron involved. The cell body of the first **preganglionic (presynaptic) neuron** is located in the gray matter of the CNS. After traveling through the nerve fiber, a synapse will occur on the cell body of the **postganglionic (postsynaptic) neuron** that is located in *autonomic ganglion* outside the CNS. The postganglionic fibers will then terminate on a target organ that could include cardiac muscle, smooth muscle or glandular tissue **(Fig. 11.2)**.

Nerve impulses move much slower through the ANS than through the somatic nervous system due to the fact that the

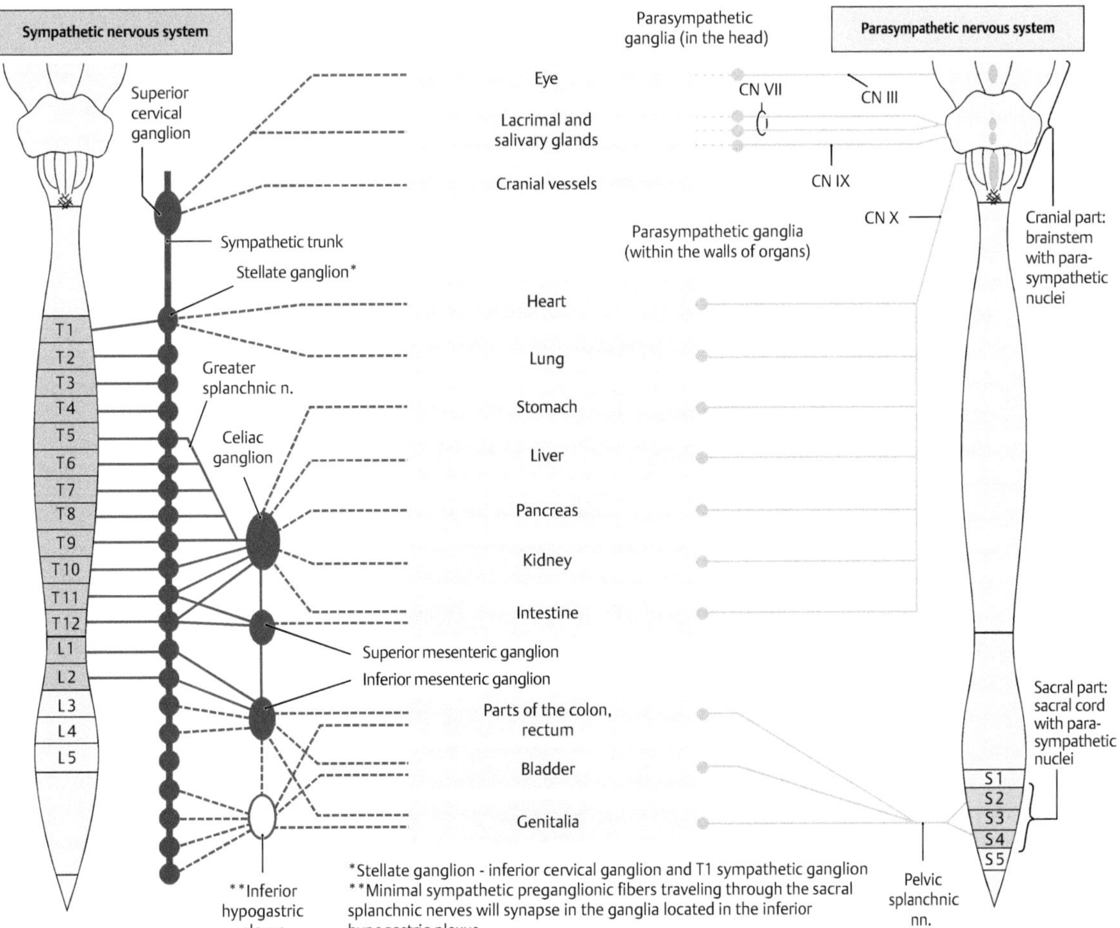

Fig. 11.1 Organization of the sympathetic and parasympathetic nervous systems. (From Gilroy AM et al. Atlas of Anatomy. Illustrations by Voll M and Wesker K. 4th ed. New York. Thieme Medical Publishers 2020.)

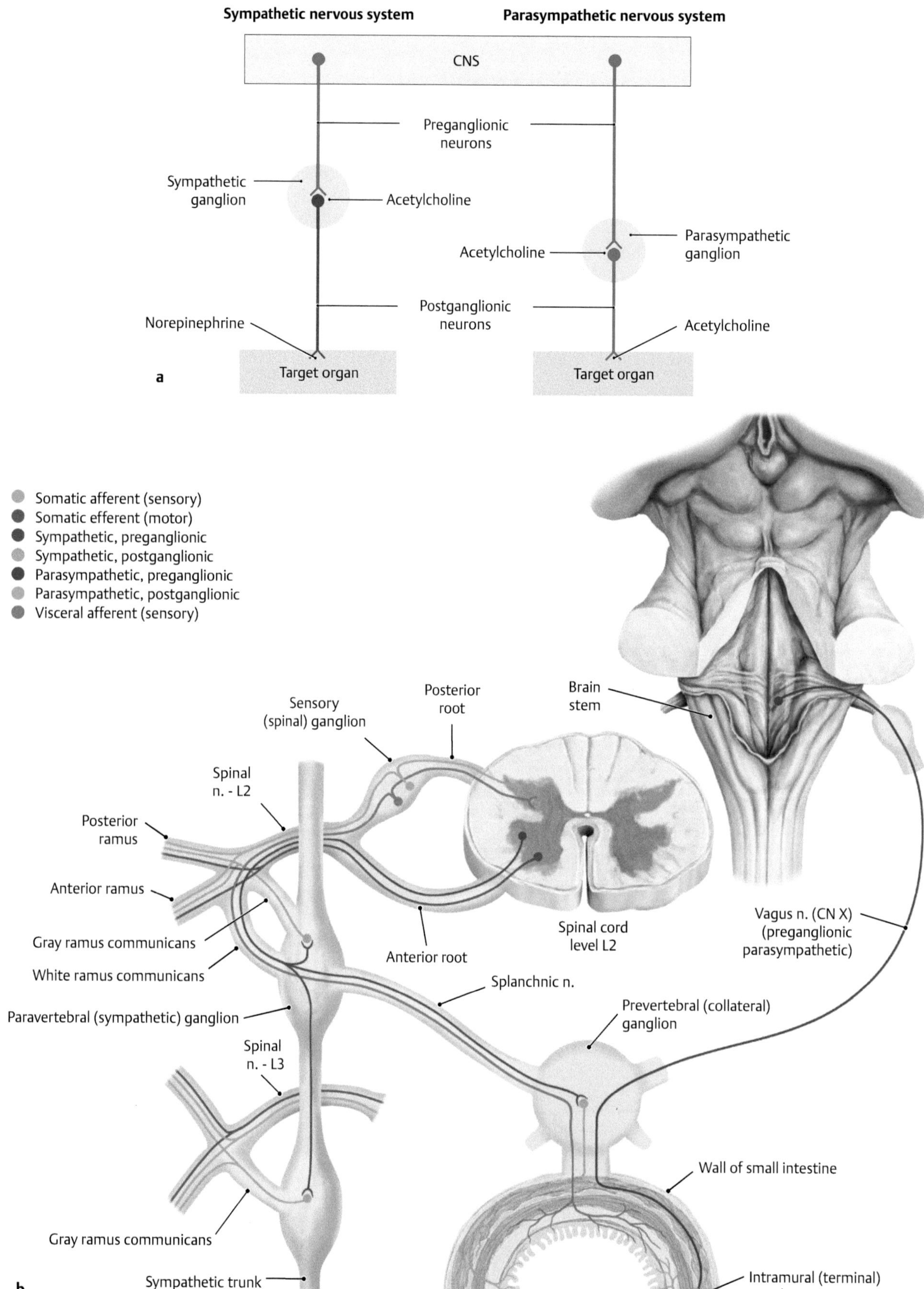

Fig. 11.2 (a) Circuit diagram of the autonomic nervous system. (From Schuenke M, Schulte E, Schumacher U. THIEME Atlas of Anatomy. Head, Neck, and Neuroanatomy. Illustrations by Voll M and Wesker K. 2nd ed. New York: Thieme Medical Publishers; 2016.) **(b)** Synaptic organization of the autonomic nervous system. (From Gilroy AM et al. Atlas of Anatomy. 4th ed. New York: Thieme Medical Publishers 2020. Based on Schuenke M, Schulte E, Schumacher U. THIEME Atlas of Anatomy. Head, Neck, and Neuroanatomy. Illustrations by Voll M and Wesker K. 3rd ed. New York: Thieme Medical Publishers; 2020)

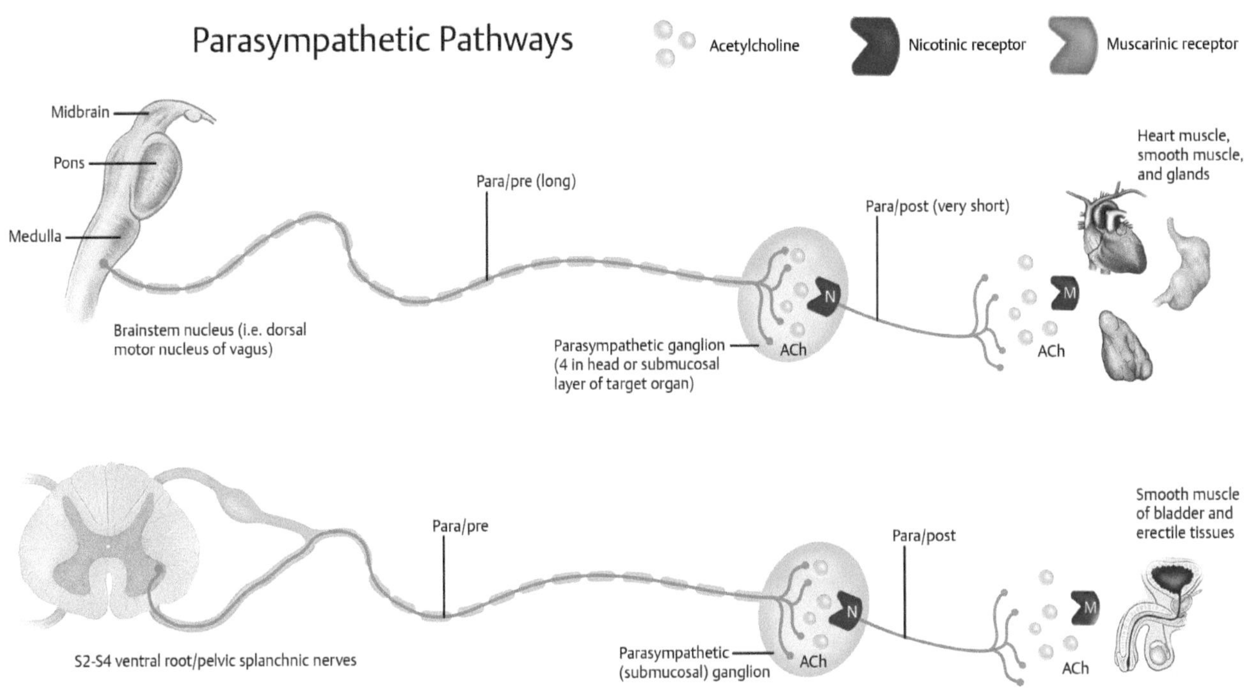

Fig. 11.3 Parasympathetic division pathways. Illustration by Calla Heald.

somatic motor axons are thick and heavily myelinated, they conduct nerve impulses rapidly, and there is only one synapse. **Preganglionic axons** of the ANS are thin and lightly myelinated whereas the **postganglionic axons** are thinner and unmyelinated but ultimately there are two synapses.

11.1 Parasympathetic Division

The parasympathetic division of the ANS is a *homeostatic system* or energy conserving system concerned with the calming, resting or digestive actions of the body **(Fig. 11.3)**. This division is also known as the *craniosacral division* because it originates from the brainstem or sacral regions of the spinal cord. Specific organ functions are listed in **Table 11.1**.

11.1.1 Parasympathetic Division Pathways

1. **Preganglionic cell body**: located in the **Edinger-Westphal**, **superior salivatory**, **inferior salivatory** and the **dorsal motor nucleus of vagus** brainstem nuclei associated with the oculomotor (III), facial (VII), glossopharyngeal (IX), and vagus (X) cranial nerves respectively **(Fig. 11.4)**. Cell bodies will also be found in the spinal cord gray matter between the S2-S4 spinal cord segments similar in location to the lateral (intermediolateral) horns of the T1-L2 spinal cord segments **(Fig. 11.5)**.
2. **Preganglionic axon (fiber)**: generally very long. The para/pre axons from the S2-S4 spinal segments travel through the ventral roots of spinal nerves S2-S4, ventral rami of S2-S4, and the pelvic splanchnic nerves that arise from the S2-S4 ventral rami. From the pelvic splanchnic nerves, para/pre fibers travel through visceral nerve plexuses to hindgut and pelvic structures before synapsing on para/post cell bodies.
3. **Postganglionic cell body**: located in the **ciliary**, **pterygopalatine**, **submandibular** and **otic ganglion** of the head or the **submucosal ganglion** of a target organ such as the heart, lungs, esophagus and most of the gastrointestinal tract. The ganglia of the head are associated with cranial nerves III, VII and IX while the submucosal ganglia are associated with cranial nerve X and the preganglionic axons originating from the sacral region of the spinal cord **(Fig. 11.4)**.
4. **Postganglionic axon (fiber)**: very short. The para/post axons that extend out from the four head ganglia will normally travel on one of the three branches of the trigeminal nerve (CN V) before reaching their target organ. Submucosal ganglia lie adjacent to the target organ already so the para/post axons have a very short course before acting.
   - **Parasympathetics to the thorax**: after originating from the brainstem, the vagus nerve (CN X) travels through the neck and delivers para/pre fibers into the thorax. These para/pre fibers then join visceral nerve plexuses of various organs. These include the cardiac, pulmonary and esophageal plexuses. The para/pre fibers then pierce the wall of the organ and travel to the submucosa before synapsing with the para/post cell bodies.
   - **Parasympathetics to the abdomen and pelvis**: the anterior and posterior vagal trunks of the vagus nerve deliver para/pre fibers to foregut and midgut structures respectively. Para/pre fibers originating from S2-S4 and via the pelvic splanchnic nerves supply the hindgut and pelvic structures. The para/pre fibers reach their target organs by passing through peri-arterial plexuses originating from arteries of the aorta with regards to gut innervation or through extensions of the inferior hypogastric plexus for pelvic structures.

Table 11.1 **Effects of the ANS on various organs**

Organ		Parasympathetic effects	Sympathetic effects
Systematic arteries			
	Skin		Constricts
	Skeletal		Dilates (β_2); constricts (α_1)
	Abdominal		Constricts
Arrector pili muscles			Contracts
Adipose			Lipolysis
Glands			
	Sweat		Stimulates sweating
	Lacrimal, parotid, submandibular, sublingual and nasal	Stimulates secretion	Reduces secretion
Eye			
	Pupil	Constrict	Dilate
	Ciliary muscle	Contract	
Heart			
	Cardiac muscle	Decrease force of contraction	Increases force of contraction
	Coronary arteries (mainly effected by metabolic factors)	Constrict	Dilate
Lungs		Constrict bronchioles; dilate arteries; increased secretions	Dilate bronchioles; constrict arteries; decreased secretions
GI tract			
	Peristalsis activity	Increase	Decrease
	Sphincters	Relax	Contract
	Glands	Increases secretions	Decreases secretions
	Liver		Glycogenolysis
	Gallbladder	Contract	Relax
Adrenal gland			
	Cortex		Stimulates release of cortex hormones
	Medulla		Stimulates release of epinephrine and norepinephrine
Kidney			Constricts arteries to reduce urine output
Urinary Bladder		Contracts detrusor muscle; relaxes urethral sphincter	Relaxes detrusor muscle; contracts urethral sphincter
Male genitalia		Causes an erection	Ejaculation
Uterus (mainly under hormonal control)		Relaxes smooth muscle; dilates arteries	Contracts smooth muscle; constricts arteries
Vagina			Contracts smooth muscle

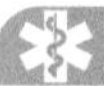

Clinical Correlate 11.1

Hirschsprung's Disease

Hirschsprung's disease or *megacolon* is a congenital condition in which the myenteric (Auerbach) plexus fails to develop in the distal portions of the colon. Peristalsis is absent because this part of the colon possess no parasympathetic ganglion cells. This effectively prevents the passage of feces and results in distension of the colon that can be corrected surgically.

11.2 Sympathetic Division

The sympathetic division of the ANS is a *catabolic system* or energy-expending system concerned with the "fight or flight" response **(Fig. 11.6)**. This division is also known as the *thoraco-lumbar division* because it originates from the thoracic and upper lumbar regions of the spinal cord. Specific organ functions are listed in **Table 11.1**.

The sympathetic pathway is a connection between the spinal cord with the **sympathetic trunk** (or **chain**), **sympathetic chain** (or **paravertebral) ganglion**, **pre-aortic (prevertebral** or

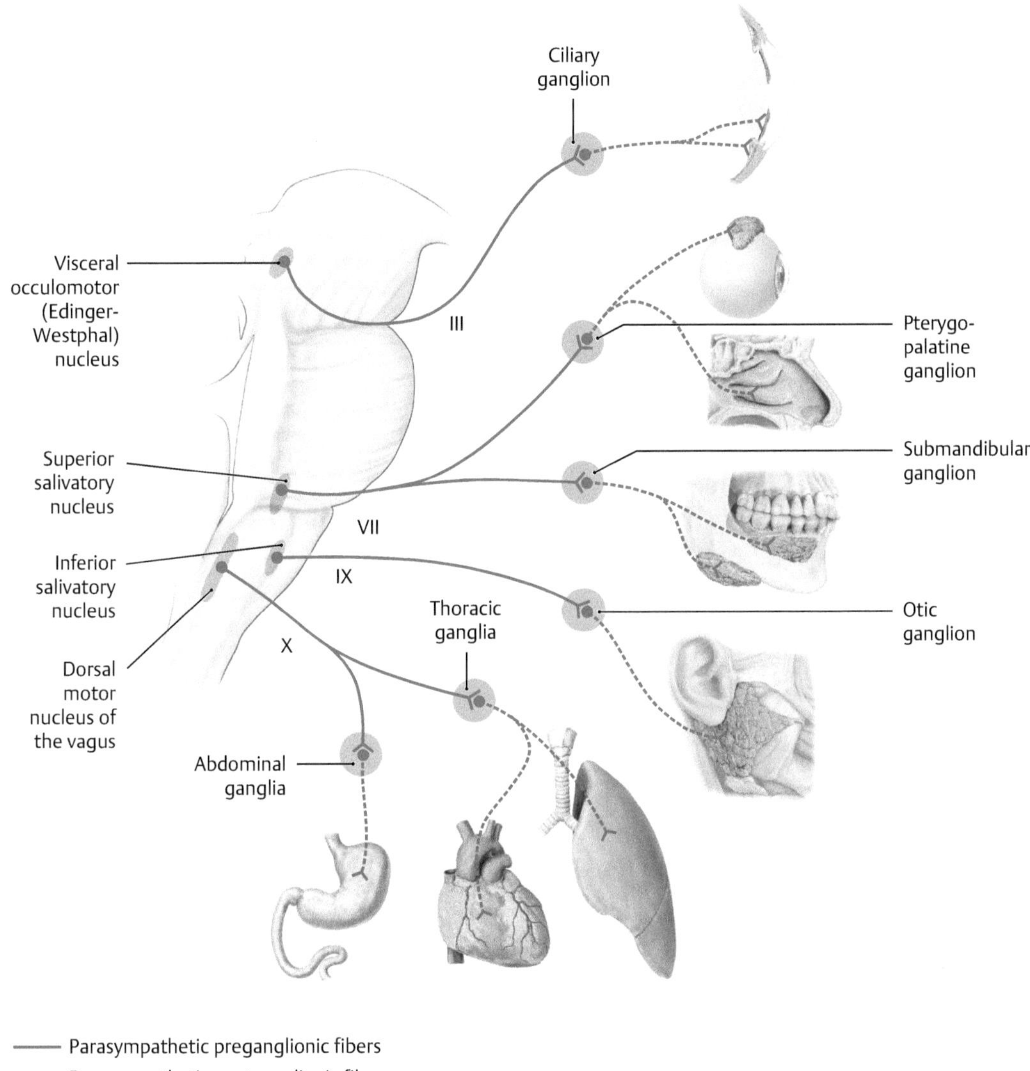

Fig. 11.4 Overview: parasympathetic nervous system (cranial part). (From Gilroy AM et al. Atlas of Anatomy. Illustrations by Voll M and Wesker K. 4th ed. New York: Thieme Medical Publishers 2020.)

collateral) ganglion and in a special case with the **suprarenal gland**. The sympathetic trunk extends from the upper cervical region near the base of the skull down to the coccyx. The ganglia associated with the trunk are bilateral and in conjunction with the region they are located in. There are **cervical**, **thoracic**, **lumbar**, **sacral** and **coccygeal ganglia** with the last set of ganglia near the coccyx being fused and known as the **ganglion impar**.

11.2.1 Sympathetic Division Pathways

1. **Preganglionic cell body**: located in the lateral horns (intermediolateral columns) between T1-L2 spinal cord segments **(Fig. 11.7)**.
2. **Preganglionic axon (fiber)**: can vary in length depending on where the axon originates and where it ultimately travels before synapsing. These sym/pre axons leave the spinal cord in order through the ventral rootlets, ventral root, spinal nerve, and very briefly through the ventral rami before entering the sympathetic trunk through the **white rami communicantes**. White rami communicantes are only connected to the T1-L2 proximal ventral rami and lateral to the **gray rami communicantes** (**Fig. 11.2; Fig. 11.7**).

   Once in the sympathetic trunk these sym/pre axons can:
   a) *Synapse immediately* at a sympathetic chain ganglion.
   b) *Ascend* or *descend* through the trunk before finally synapsing at a sympathetic chain ganglion.
   c) *Continue through a splanchnic nerve* before synapsing at a pre-aortic ganglion of the aortic plexus.
   d) *Innervate the suprarenal gland* by first passing through a splanchnic nerve and then bypassing the pre-aortic ganglion of the aortic plexus before synapsing on chromaffin cells of the suprarenal gland medulla.
3. **Postganglionic cell body**: located in the sympathetic chain ganglia or pre-aortic ganglia (i.e. celiac, superior mesenteric, aorticorenal and inferior mesenteric ganglion). A limited amount of cell bodies are located in the inferior hypogastric

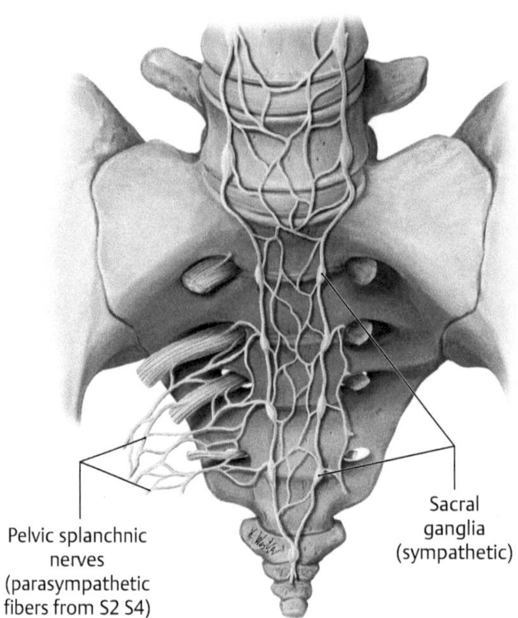

Fig. 11.5 Overview: parasympathetic nervous system (lumbosacral part). (From Schuenke M, Schulte E, Schumacher U. THIEME Atlas of Anatomy. Head, Neck, and Neuroanatomy. Illustrations by Voll M and Wesker K. 2nd ed. New York: Thieme Medical Publishers; 2016.)

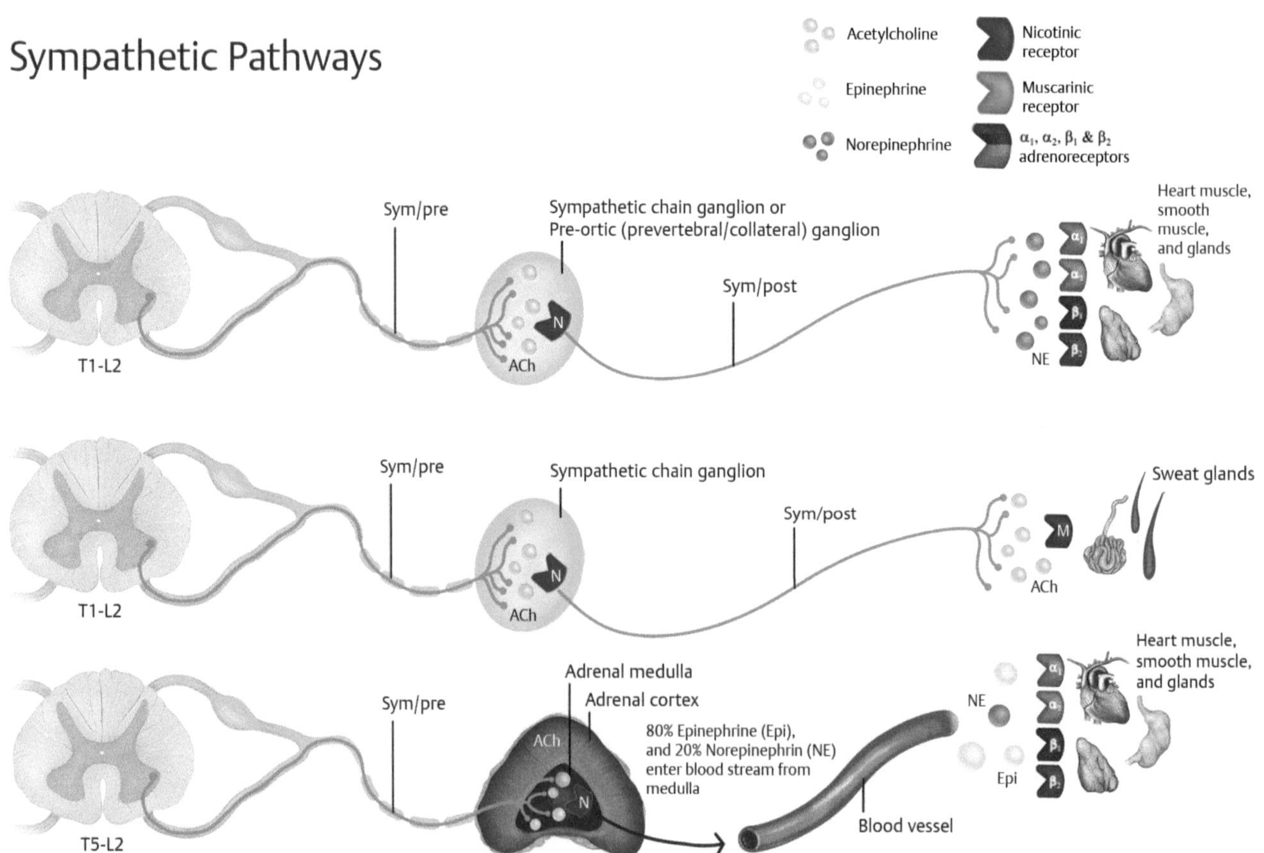

Fig. 11.6 Sympathetic division pathway. Illustration by Calla Heald.

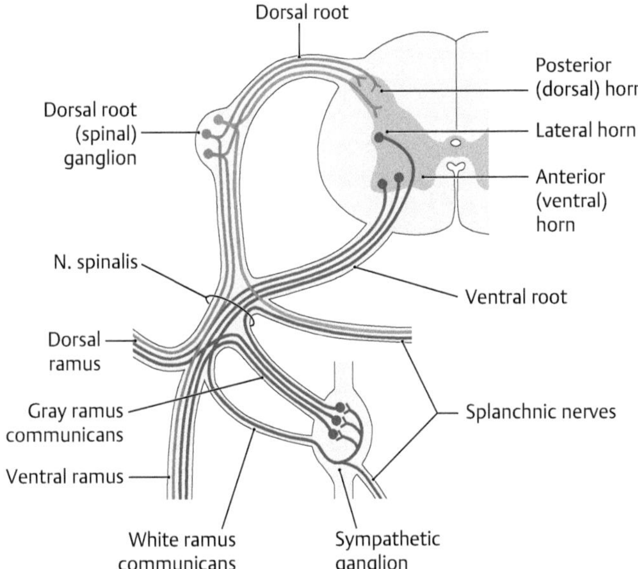

Fig. 11.7 Topographical and functional organization of a spinal cord segment. (From Schuenke M, Schulte E, Schumacher U. THIEME Atlas of Anatomy. General Anatomy and Musculoskeletal System. Illustrations by Voll M and Wesker K. 1st ed. New York: Thieme Medical Publishers; 2010.)

plexuses located in the pelvis. The **chromaffin cells** located in the medulla of the suprarenal gland are structurally similar to sympathetic postganglionic neurons and when stimulated by the sym/pre axons, they release epinephrine and norepinephrine directly into the systematic circulation. **(Fig. 11.6).**

4. **Postganglionic axon (fiber)**: can be relatively long. After the sym/pre axons have synapsed at a sympathetic chain ganglion, the sym/post axons must pass through **gray rami communicantes** attached to one of the 31 spinal nerves before continuing through either a ventral or dorsal rami branch. Sym/post fibers traveling through this route are destined to innervate the blood vessels, arrector pili muscles and sweat glands of the head, neck, trunk or limb regions. The sym/post axons leaving the pre-aortic ganglion pass through the aortic plexus and onto a blood vessel (via a periarterial plexus) or down into the pelvic region and innervate blood vessels or certain sphincters of the abdominal and pelvic organs.

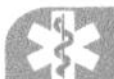

Clinical Correlate 11.2

Horner's Syndrome

If there is a disturbance in the sympathetic pathway, usually due to a lesion of the cervical portion of the sympathetic trunk, this is called **Horner's syndrome.** Other causes can include dissecting carotid aneurysms, proximal brachial plexus injuries and even brainstem damage from a tumor or stroke. This was described in Chapter 7, but to summarize, this syndrome is characterized by (1) drooping of the upper eyelid (*ptosis*); (2) contraction of the pupil (*miosis*); (3) excessive vasodilation given the appearance of flushed skin (*hyperemia*); (4) the absence of sweating on the face and neck (*anhydrosis*), and (5) the appearance of a sinking eyeball (*enophthalmos*) generally thought to be more of an illusion due to the already present ptosis.

Clinical Correlate 11.3

Raynaud's Disease

More commonly seen in the elderly, **Raynaud's disease** is an exaggerated and sympathetic response provoked by exposure to a cold environment or strong emotion resulting in the vasoconstriction of blood vessels. These tend to be intermittent and painful attacks of the digits making them appear blue and pale. Treatment may require the administration of drugs that inhibit vasoconstriction.

The cardiopulmonary splanchnic nerves originating from the neck region have sym/post axons that continue to and pass through the cardiac and pulmonary plexuses. The esophageal plexus may receive its sym/post axons directly from the sympathetic trunk by way of splanchnic nerve-like branches.

11.3 Visceral Sensory

The **general visceral afferent (GVA)** fibers transmit reflex or pain impulses from the blood vessels or visceral organs such as the heart, lungs and gastrointestinal tract back to the CNS. Although these fibers pass along with the parasympathetic and sympathetic motor fibers, they are not considered part of the ANS. The information that passes through them can help alter blood pressure, blood chemistry and digestion activity. Visceral sensation that reaches a conscious level is generally perceived as poorly localized pain related possibly to hunger, cramps or nausea. Visceral reflex arcs are associated with urination (micturition), defecation, baroreceptors, chemoreceptors and the enteric nervous system.

- **GVA pain fibers**: from all locations travel back primarily with sympathetic fibers and their cell bodies are located in a dorsal root ganglion. Visceral pain is not felt if the viscera is cut or scrapped but is felt when there is chemical irritation or inflammation, smooth muscle spasms (cramping) or excessive stretching of the visceral organ. This pain will be perceived as somatic but is a phenomenon known as **referred pain** and is closely associated with the sympathetic nervous system **(Fig. 11.8)**.
- **GVA reflex fibers** from the thorax, foregut and midgut travel back through the vagus nerve (CN X) and their cell bodies are located in the inferior sensory ganglion of CN X. The GVA reflex fibers originating from the hindgut or pelvis travel back through the pelvis splanchnic nerves and their cell bodies are located in the S2-S4 dorsal root ganglions **(Fig. 11.9)**.
- A **visceral nerve plexus** is located near a visceral organ and is generally named according to the specific organ or region it rests upon. Examples include the cardiopulmonary, aortic or inferior hypogastric plexuses. The plexuses will be composed of both general visceral efferent (GVE) motor and general visceral afferent (GVA) sensory fibers. The GVE fibers that pass through these plexuses consist of sympathetic postganglionic (sym/post) and parasympathetic preganglionic (para/pre) fibers and they are accompanied by either visceral pain or reflex fibers. Thus, for the bulk of visceral nerve plexuses the functional components are GVE-sym/post, GVE-para/pre, and GVA (pain and reflexes) **(Fig. 11.10)**.

There are generally no ganglia located in a visceral nerve plexus except for that of the larger aortic plexus. The inferior hypogastric

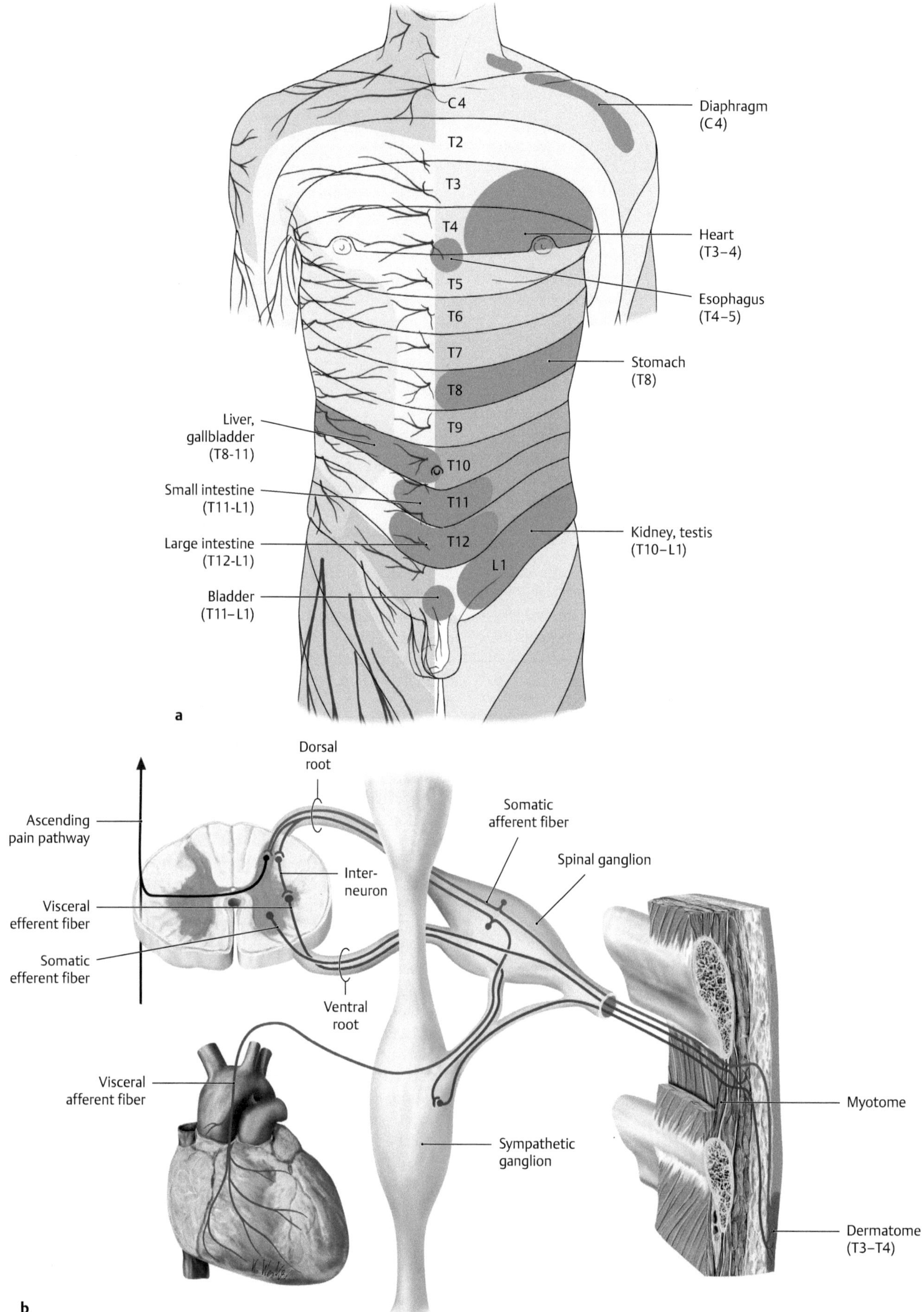

Fig. 11.8 Referred pain. **(a)** Pain impulses from a particular internal organ are consistently projected to the same well-defined skin area. **(b)** The convergence of somatic and visceral afferent pain. (From Schuenke M, Schulte E, Schumacher U. THIEME Atlas of Anatomy. Head, Neck, and Neuroanatomy. Illustrations by Voll M and Wesker K. 2nd ed. New York: Thieme Medical Publishers; 2016.)

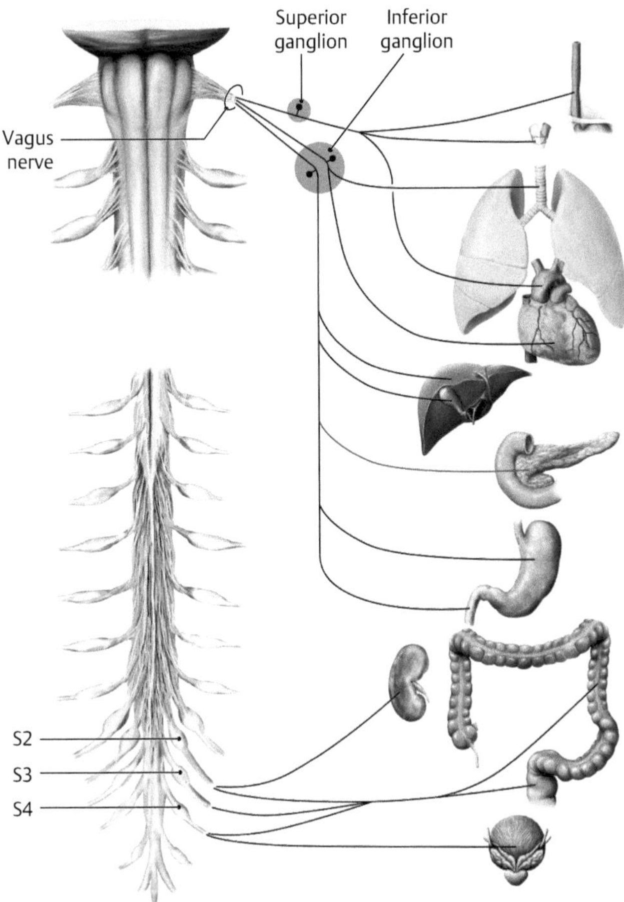

Fig. 11.9 General visceral afferent reflex fibers. (From Schuenke M, Schulte E, Schumacher U. THIEME Atlas of Anatomy. Head, Neck, and Neuroanatomy. Illustrations by Voll M and Wesker K. 2nd ed. New York: Thieme Medical Publishers; 2016.)

(pelvic) plexus is known to have a minimal amount of ganglion-like cells that represent sym/post cell bodies while the cardiac plexus contains a limited amount of isolated ganglia that consist of para/post cell bodies.

11.4 Preganglionic Neurotransmitters

Both the parasympathetic and sympathetic **preganglionic axon terminals** are known as *cholinergic*, meaning they release the neurotransmitter **acetylcholine** (ACh). There are two types of ACh receptors, known as either the **nicotinic** or **muscarinic receptors**. ACh binds initially with the nicotinic receptor located on the outside of the cell membrane of the postganglionic neurons **(Fig. 11.3; Fig. 11.6)**.

11.5 Postganglionic Neurotransmitters

The parasympathetic **postganglionic axon terminals** are also *cholinergic* because they release ACh. ACh from this axon terminal will bind to the **muscarinic receptor** located on an effector organ such as the heart, smooth muscle or glands. The sympathetic **postganglionic axon terminals** are known as *adrenergic* because they release norepinephrine (NE). However, sympathetic postganglionic axon terminals that innervate sweat glands and blood vessels in skeletal muscle of the periphery are cholinergic. The NE binds to **alpha** and **beta receptors** on the effector organs, both of which consist of subgroups (alpha-1 and alpha-2 or beta-1 and beta-2). Alpha receptor sites are associated mostly with excitatory functions of the sympathetic division whereas the beta receptors are mostly inhibitory in nature. NE has its greatest effect on the alpha receptors **(Fig. 11.3; Fig. 11.6), (Table 11.2)**.

11.6 Central Nervous System Control over the ANS

The ANS helps maintain homeostasis, with the hypothalamus and other portions of the CNS having an effect on it. Stimulation of the anterior nucleus of the hypothalamus can influence the parasympathetic division while stimulation of the posterior nucleus can have an effect on the sympathetic division. There are direct connections between these preganglionic neurons and the hypothalamic nuclei that pass through the reticular formation and periaqueductal gray matter of the brainstem. The reticular formation found primarily in the medulla oblongata has a cardiac center that regulates heart rate, a respiratory center that regulates the rate and rhythm of breathing, and a vasomotor center that helps regulate blood pressure. There are additional centers that have an effect on swallowing, sneezing and coughing.

Certain thoughts originating from the cerebral cortex have been known to influence the ANS. The amygdala, which is part of the limbic system, can increase sympathetic activity through previously learned, fear-related behavior. The spinal cord is involved in spinal visceral reflexes such as defecation and urination (micturition).

Clinical Correlate 11.4

Autonomic Dysreflexia

Autonomic dysreflexia develops in individuals who have had a spinal cord injury at or above the T6 spinal segment. This type of injury results in an imbalanced sympathetic reflex discharge that leads to potentially life-threatening hypertension. A noxious stimulus, most often from bladder or bowel distension, causes a peripheral sympathetic response through spinal reflexes resulting in vasoconstriction below the level of the initial injury. Baroreceptors located in the aortic arch and carotid sinus that normally respond to this perceived hypertension can only signal as far as the spinal cord injury. Therefore the hypertension will remain uncontrolled. When spinal cord injuries first occur, there are no reflexes, but they return later and are exaggerated due to the lack of inhibitory signals from the brain.

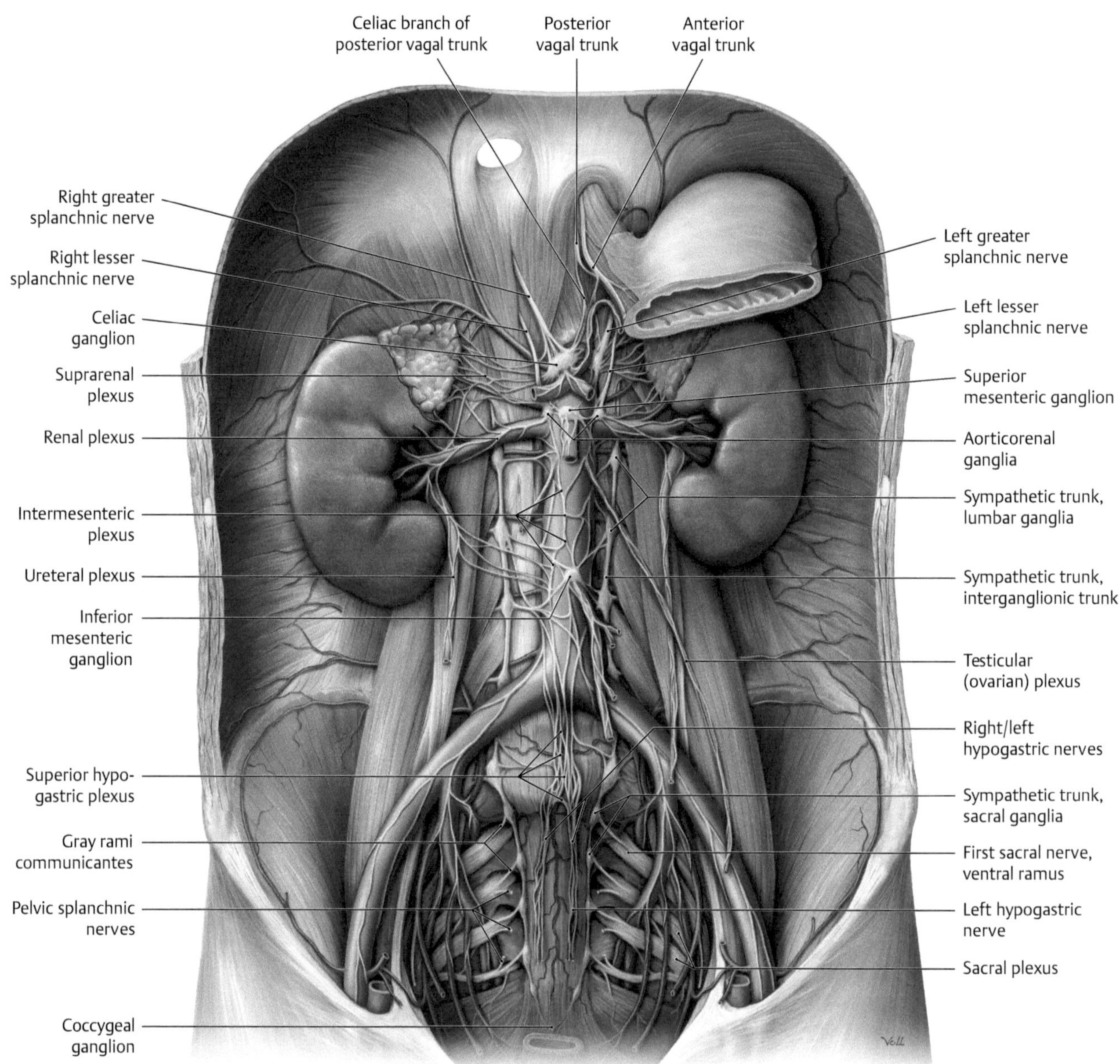

Fig. 11.10 Aortic plexus. An example of a visceral nerve plexus. (From Schuenke M, Schulte E, Schumacher U. THIEME Atlas of Anatomy. Head, Neck, and Neuroanatomy. Illustrations by Voll M and Wesker K. 2nd ed. New York: Thieme Medical Publishers; 2016.)

Table 11.2 **Receptor agonist versus antagonists**

Receptor	Target tissue	Agonists	Antagonists
Cholinergic			
Nicotinic	Motor end plate of skeletal muscle; postganglionic neurons of both parasympathetic and sympathetic nervous systems; adrenal medulla	Acetylcholine Carbachol Nicotine	Atracurium Curare Trimethaphan
Muscarinic	All effector organs (parasympathetics) and sweat glands (sympathetics)	Acetylcholine Bethanechol Carbachol Muscarine Pilocarpine	Atropine Glycopyrrolate Ipratropium Scopolamine
Adrenergic			
Alpha-1	Vascular smooth muscle of skin, skeletal muscle and visceral organs; sphincters of bladder and GI tract; dilator muscle of iris	Cirazoline Midodrine Norepinephrine Phenylephrine Xylometazoline	Acepromazine Doxazosin Phenoxybenzamine Phentolamine Prazosin
Alpha-2	Presynaptic adrenergic nerve terminals; smooth muscle walls of GI tract; platelets	Agmatine Clonidine Dexmedetomidine Lefexidine Xylazine	Atipamezole Phentolamine Trazodone Yohimbine
Beta-1	Prominent in SA node, AV node and ventricular muscle of heart; kidney; adipose; salivary glands	Dobutamine Isoproterenol Norepinephrine	Bisoprolol Metoprolol Propranolol Timolol Vortioxetine
Beta-2	Vascular smooth muscle of skeletal muscle; smooth muscle of bronchioles, bladder and GI tract	Albuterol Epinephrine Isoproterenol Levosalbutamol Terbutaline	Butoxamine Propranolol Timolol

PRACTICE QUESTIONS

1. Which statement regarding the architecture of the autonomic nervous system is CORRECT?
   A. The axon terminals of the parasympathetic preganglionic and parasympathetic postganglionic neurons release acetylcholine (ACh) and norepinephrine (NE) respectively.
   B. Parasympathetic preganglionic cell bodies of CN III, VII, IX and X are located in submucosal (intramural) ganglion.
   C. Sympathetic preganglionic axons must always enter a white rami communicans in order to reach the sympathetic trunk.
   D. Sympathetic postganglionic axons course through a thoracic splanchnic nerve.
   E. For either sympathetics or parasympathetics, preganglionic ACh always binds to the muscarinic receptor located on the cell body of the postganglionic neuron.
2. A five-year-old girl was recently treated for an asthma attack and is prescribed albuterol.Albuterol belongs to a category of medications called bronchodilators that relax the bronchial smooth muscle fibers and allow more air to pass through when an individual is having difficulty breathing. Albuterol acts as an agonist to what type of receptor?
   A. Alpha-1.
   B. Alpha-2.
   C. Beta-1.
   D. Beta-2.
   E. Muscarinic.
3. Which statement regarding the autonomic nervous system of the head and neck specifically is INCORRECT?
   A. Parasympathetic fibers destined for the constrictor pupillae muscle originated from the oculomotor nucleus.
   B. Parasympathetic postganglionic cell bodies associated with the lacrimal gland are found in the pterygopalatine ganglion.
   C. The middle cervical sympathetic ganglion is located at vertebral level C6.
   D. Sympathetic preganglionic fibers pass through the white rami communicantes before entering the sympathetic trunk.
   E. Sympathetic postganglionic fibers pass through gray rami communicantes to reach cervical spinal nerves.
4. Which statement regarding the autonomic nervous system of the head and neck specifically is INCORRECT?
   A. Sympathetic preganglionic fibers destined to reach the head and neck region originate from the lateral horns of the T1-T4 spinal cord.
   B. Parasympathetic pre- and postganglionic axon terminals release acetylcholine (ACh).
   C. Parasympathetic preganglionic fibers that synapse at the otic ganglion are associated with CN IX.
   D. Parasympathetic preganglionic fibers associated with CN X will synapse at both the pterygopalatine and submandibular ganglia.
   E. Sympathetic postganglionic fibers destined to reach the dilator pupillae muscle pass through both the nasociliary and long ciliary nerves.

5. A 28-year-old male presents to the emergency department with a deep laceration near the root of the neck. This deep cut has extended all the way down to the sympathetic trunk and the subsequent damage has resulted in Horner's syndrome. All symptoms can manifest in Horner's syndrome EXCEPT?
   A. Sinking of the eyeball (enophthalomos).
   B. Flushed skin due to the vasodilation of blood vessels.
   C. Pupillary constriction.
   D. Dropping of the upper eyelid (ptosis).
   E. Profuse sweating on the affected side.
6. A 72 year-old woman walks out to grab a package located on her porch in the middle of winter when the temperature is near freezing. Although she has done this numeroustimes it seems that it takes longer for her fingers to warm up or turn back to their normal color. This is a result of vasospasm or a sudden constriction of the vessels supplying blood to her digits. These symptoms are associated with what clinical correlate?
   A. Horner's syndrome.
   B. Raynaud's disease.
   C. Hirschsprung's disease.
   D. Autonomic dysreflexia.

ANSWERS

1. **C.** In order for sympathetic preganglionic axons to reach the sympathetic trunk they must first pass through white rami communicans attached somewhere between the T1-L2 ventral rami.
2. **D.** Smooth muscle of the bronchioles have the Beta-2 receptor.
3. **A.** Parasympathetic fibers destined to innervate the constrictor pupillae and ciliary muscles originate from the Edinger-Westphal nucleus located in the midbrain of the brainstem.
4. **D.** Parasympathetic preganglionic fibers traveling through CN X will synapse at the submucosal (intramural) ganglion adjacent to organs found in the head and neck, thorax, and most of the abdomen.
5. **E.** Sympathetic innervation controls sweating and since the sympathetic trunk has been damaged, there would be no sweating on the affected side.
6. **B.** Raynaud's disease.

12 Cranial Nerves

LEARNING OBJECTIVES

- To understand the different functional components that pass through each cranial nerve.
- To describe the cranial nuclei and their locations.
- To describe the individual branches of the cranial nerves and the foramen they may pass through.
- To describe any clinical correlates associated with each cranial nerve.

There are 12 pairs of cranial nerves originating mostly from the brainstem of the brain. They continue through the skull foramina, canals or fissures before exiting and innervating specific structures mainly of the head and neck region. The vagus nerve (CN X) in particular can extend all the way into the abdominal cavity. Roman numerals are used to number the cranial nerves sequentially in order of which they arise from the brain. The sequence proceeds from rostral to caudal (**Fig. 12.1**).

All of the cranial nerves are considered part of the peripheral nervous system except for the optic nerve (CN II) because this nerve is really an outgrowth of the brain that emerges from the prosencephalon. The spinal accessory nerve has an odd course in that it arises from the cervical spinal cord before passing through the foramen magnum and later the jugular foramen, continuing to the sternocleidomastoid and trapezius muscles in the neck.

Cranial nerves are described as having functional components passing through them. Terms to follow would be *efferent*, a motor output that can be *somatic* (skeletal muscle), *visceral* (smooth muscle) or *special* (striated muscle that develops from branchial arches). Sensory input nerves are referred to as *afferent*. The term *general* refers to those functional components that are carried by either a cranial or spinal nerve and the term *special* refers to functional components carried only by cranial nerves. The functional component categories are described below (**Fig. 12.2**).

- **General Somatic Efferent (GSE)**: fibers that provide general motor innervation to the skeletal muscles derived by somites. These fibers pass through the oculomotor, trochlear, abducent and hypoglossal nerves.
- **General Somatic Afferent (GSA)**: fibers that carry general sensation (touch, pain, pressure and temperature) from the skin and mucous membranes. General proprioception (GP) from somatic structures including muscles, tendons and joints of the head and neck are also classified under this category.
- **General Visceral Efferent (GVE)**: fibers that provide motor innervation to the viscera. The parasympathetic preganglionic fibers initially pass through the oculomotor, facial, glossopharyngeal and vagus nerves. The parasympathetic postganglionic fibers related to the oculomotor, facial and glossopharyngeal nerves remain in the head but course along with branches of the trigeminal nerve.
- **General Visceral Afferent (GVA)**: general sensation originating from the viscera and mucosa-lined structures such as the middle ear cavity, pharynx and larynx.
- **Special Somatic Afferent (SSA)**: the special sensory fibers that convey the special sense of vision/sight and the sense of equilibrium and hearing. Input derived from the retina will travel through the optic nerve while equilibrium and hearing are related to the vestibulocochlear nerve.
- **Special Visceral Efferent (SVE)**: fibers that provide motor innervation to muscles originating from the pharyngeal (branchial) arches. They are commonly referred to as branchiomotor fibers and they pass through the trigeminal, facial, glossopharyngeal and vagus nerves.
- **Special Visceral Afferent (SVA)**: the special sensory fibers from the viscera that convey the special sense of smell and taste. The sense of smell is related to the olfactory nerve while the sense of taste is associated with the facial, glossopharyngeal and vagus nerves.

12.1 Olfactory Nerve

The **olfactory nerves** (CN I) convey the special sense of smell back to the brain and only contain functional component SVA (**Fig. 12.2**). The olfactory epithelium lines the midline and lateral portions of the upper nasal cavities. The bipolar **olfactory receptor neurons** (first order) and their cell bodies are located within this olfactory epithelium. The axons of the olfactory neurons are assembled into bundles and form approximately 20 olfactory nerves on each side. These fibers pass through **olfactory foramina** of the cribriform plate of the ethmoid bone and are surrounded by sleeves of dura and arachnoid maters before entering the **olfactory bulb** of the anterior cranial fossa (**Fig. 12.3**).

The olfactory nerve fibers synapse with second-order **mitral** and **tufted cells** along with interneurons of the olfactory bulb. It is the axons of the mitral and tufted cells that form the olfactory tract and carry the olfaction information from the olfactory bulb to the central nervous system. The olfactory bulbs and tracts are often mistaken as part of CN I but they are truly just extensions of the forebrain.

Clinical Correlate 12.1

Anosmia

A decrease or loss of olfaction is known as anosmia. Natural aging decreases an individual's sense of smell, but this is generally accompanied with a reduction in the sense of taste and the dysfunction is primarily associated with the olfactory system. Acute anosmia can be the result of sinus infections and allergic or non-allergic rhinitis. Chronic anosmia could be the result of trauma to the cribriform plate, nasal polyps that block the flow of air through the nasal cavities, or, less commonly, by damage due to a brain tumor, Alzheimer's disease, diabetes, multiple sclerosis or radiation therapy. Psychiatric disorders such as schizophrenia can distort smells or produce smells when they are not present in the environment.

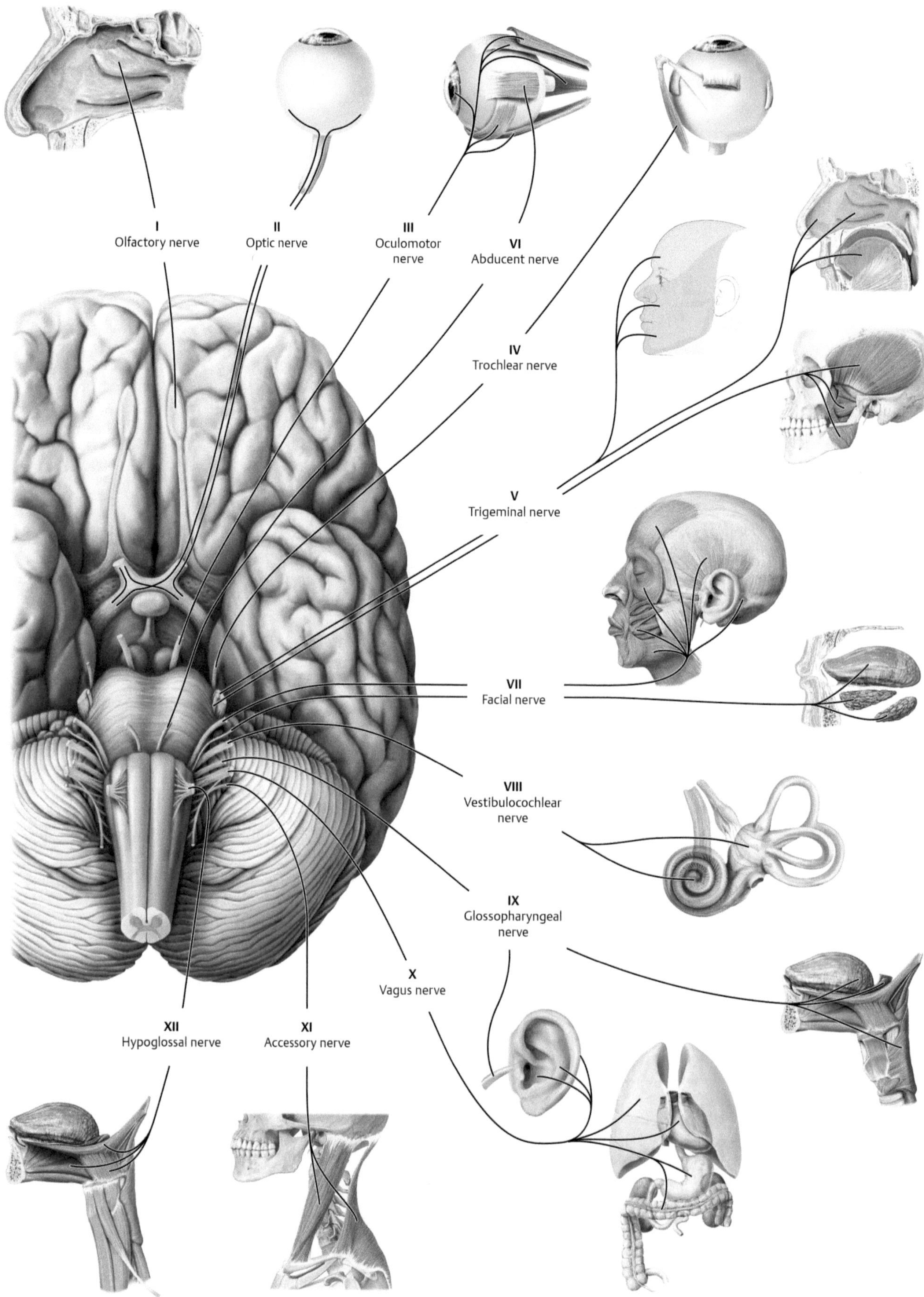

Fig. 12.1 Overview of the cranial nerves. (From Schuenke M, Schulte E, Schumacher U. THIEME Atlas of Anatomy. Head, Neck, and Neuroanatomy. Illustrations by Voll M and Wesker K. 3rd ed. New York: Thieme Medical Publishers; 2020.)

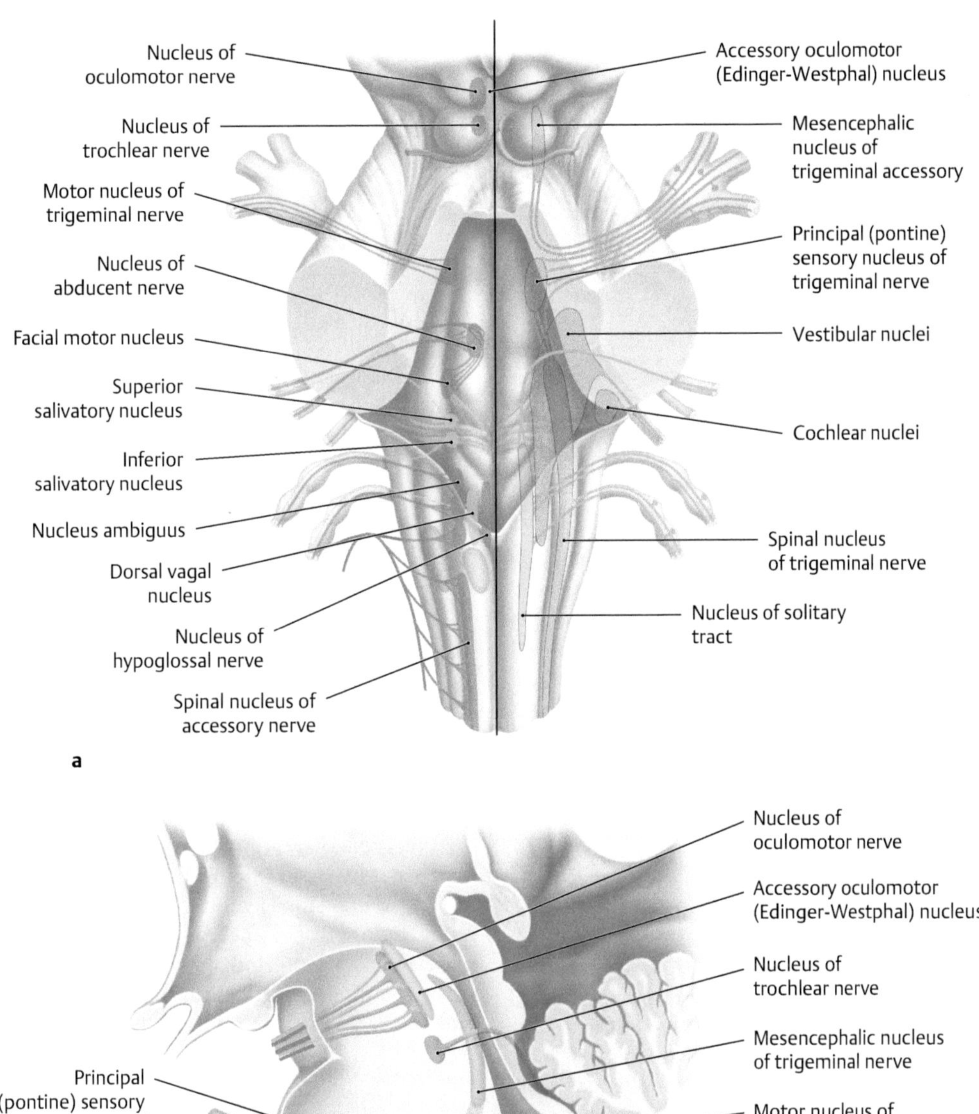

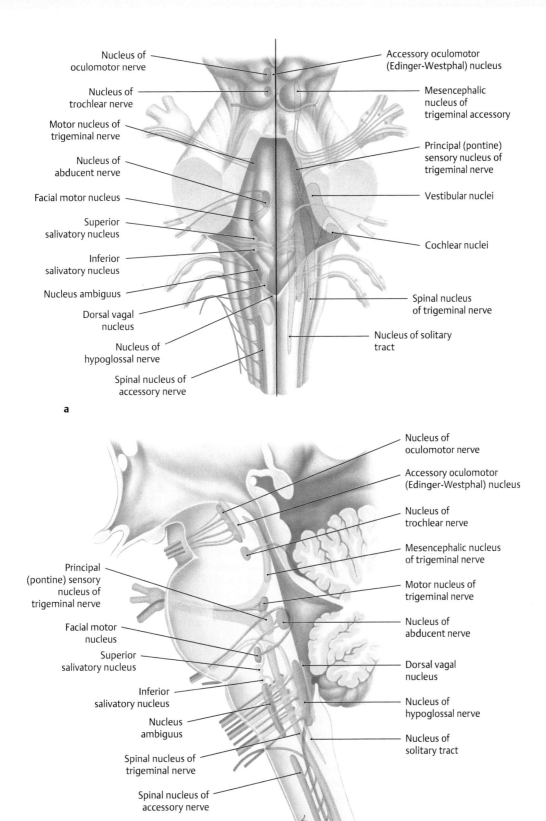

Fig. 12.2 Location of cranial nerves III-VII in the brainstem. **(a)** Posterior view (with cerebellum removed). **(b)** midsagittal section, left lateral view. (From Schuenke M, Schulte E, Schumacher U. THIEME Atlas of Anatomy. Head, Neck, and Neuroanatomy. Illustrations by Voll M and Wesker K. 3rd ed. New York: Thieme Medical Publishers; 2020.)

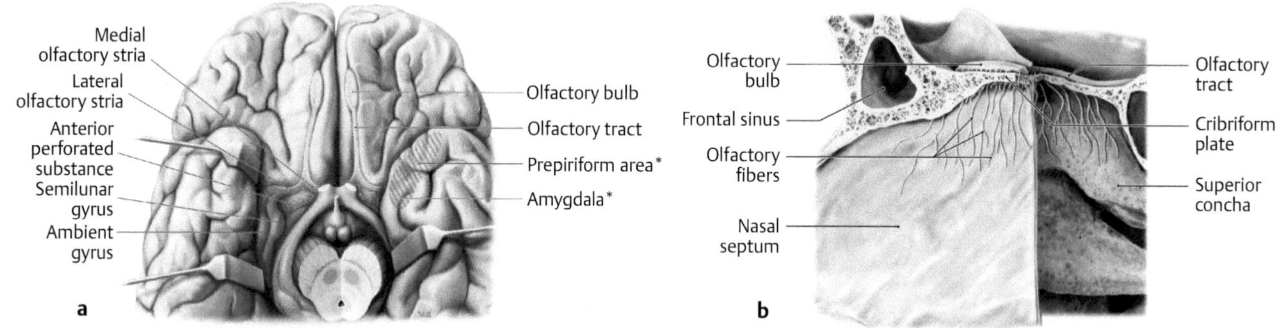

Fig. 12.3 (a) Olfactory bulb and olfactory tract on the basal surface of the frontal lobes of the brain. **(b)** Extent of the olfactory mucosa (olfactory region) * The shaded structures are deep to the basal surface of the brain. (From Schuenke M, Schulte E, Schumacher U. THIEME Atlas of Anatomy. Head, Neck, and Neuroanatomy. Illustrations by Voll M and Wesker K. 3rd ed. New York: Thieme Medical Publishers; 2020.)

12.2 Optic Nerve

The **optic nerve** (CN II) conveys the special sense of vision/sight and contains only the functional component SSA **(Fig. 12.4)**. Light penetrates the retina of the eye and activates the photoreceptors called **cones** and **rods.** Electrical signals generated by the cones and rods are processed and integrated by additional cells located in the retina. The cones and rods will synapse and transmit information to the **bipolar cells** (first order) before these signals reach the **ganglion cells** (second order). The ganglion cells give rise to unmyelinated axons that converge at the optic disk and traverse the lamina cribrosa of the sclera before emerging from the back of the eye and at this point obtain a myelin sheath and form the optic nerve. The signal of a particular synapse can be influenced and refined horizontally by the **horizontal** and **amacrine cells** located in the retina.

The optic nerve is not a true peripheral nerve but an extension of the diencephalon. It exits the orbit through the **optic canal** before reaching the middle cranial fossa. The left and right optic nerves join each other and form the **optic chiasma**. At this location, all of the ganglion cell axons originating from the *nasal half* of the retina will decussate, or cross to the contralateral side of the opposite optic tract. All of the ganglion cell axons arising from the *temporal half* of the retina pass through the optic chiasma but continue through the ipsilateral or same side optic tract.

The **optic tracts** are continuations of the ganglion cell axons that curve around the cerebral peduncle of the mesencephalon before mostly terminating at the thalamic relay station for vision called the **lateral geniculate nucleus.** Other fibers of the optic tract will bypass the lateral geniculate ganglion and terminate at either the **superior colliculus, pretectal area** or **suprachiasmatic nucleus of the hypothalamus.** The optic tract fibers that primarily target the lateral geniculate nucleus will project to the primary visual cortex via **optic radiations** while maintaining their *retinotopic organization*, details of which were discussed in Chapter 9.

Clinical Correlate 12.2

Optic Neuritis

Optic neuritis may be caused by an autoimmune response to a person's own myelin covering the optic nerve, resulting in inflammation of the nerve. Multiple sclerosis, bacterial and viral infections, lupus, certain drugs, and antibiotics have been linked to optic neuritis. Symptoms include pain behind the affected eye, loss of color vision and visual field defects. Certain visual field defects were discussed in Chapter 9. Complications include permanent damage to the optic nerve and decreased visual acuity. Optic neuritis can lead to optic neuropathy.

12.3 Oculomotor Nerve

The **oculomotor nerve** (CN III) provides innervation to five of the seven extraocular muscles that control movements of the upper eyelid and eye **(Fig. 12.5)**. The functional components of this nerve are GSE, GSA and GVE. As it emerges from the brainstem it will extend anteriorly within the lateral border of the cavernous sinus before entering the orbit through the **superior orbital fissure**. CN III passes through the **superior orbital fissure** before dividing into a **superior division** that is responsible for innervating the **levator palpebrae superioris** and **superior rectus muscles** and an **inferior division** that is responsible for innervating the **medial rectus, inferior rectus** and **inferior oblique muscles.**

- GSE: the cell bodies originate from the **oculomotor nucleus** located in the midbrain.
- GSA: general proprioceptive input from these muscles is transmitted back by pseudounipolar neurons that have their cell bodies located in the **mesencephalic nucleus of the trigeminal nerve.**
- GVE: the visceral motor fibers are both parasympathetic and sympathetic.
  - The **para/pre** fibers originate from the **Edinger-Westphal nucleus** of the midbrain and course with the inferior division before synapsing at the **ciliary ganglion.** From this ganglion, **para/post** fibers travel with the **short ciliary nerves** before reaching and innervating the **ciliary** and **sphincter (constrictor) pupillae muscles.** Contraction of the ciliary muscle releases the tension of the zonular fibers attached to the lens leading to accommodation for near vision. Contraction of the sphincter pupillae causes pupil constriction.
  - The **sym/post** fibers may originate from either the periarterial plexus of the internal carotid or ophthalmic arteries. If these fibers course along the superior division they will innervate the **superior tarsal (Müller's) muscle**, an extension of smooth muscle adjacent to the levator palpebrae superioris that assists in elevating the upper eyelid. If these fibers course along the inferior division, they contribute to the sympathetic root of the ciliary ganglion and go on to be a vasomotor to the blood vessels supplying the eye.

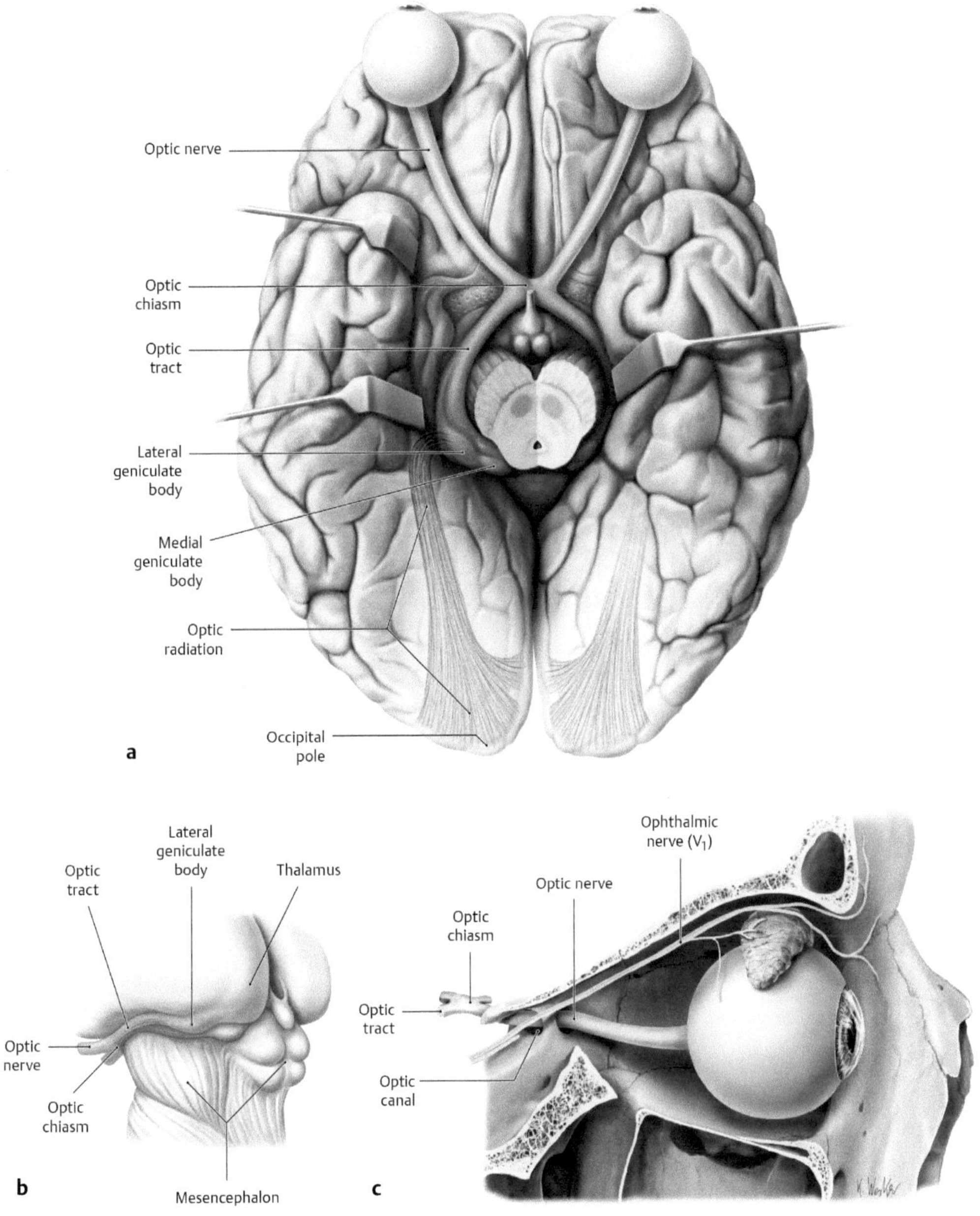

Fig. 12.4 (a) View of the eye, optic nerve, optic chiasm, and optic tract from the base of the brain. **(b)** Posterolateral view of the left side of the brainstem. **(c)** Course of the optic nerve in the right orbit. (From Schuenke M, Schulte E, Schumacher U. THIEME Atlas of Anatomy. Head, Neck, and Neuroanatomy. Illustrations by Voll M and Wesker K. 3rd ed. New York: Thieme Medical Publishers; 2020.)

12.4 Trochlear Nerve

The **trochlear nerve** (CN IV) provides motor innervation to just the **superior oblique muscle** of the eye (**Fig. 12.5**). The superior oblique muscle *depresses, abducts* and *medially rotates* the eye. The functional components of this nerve are GSE and GSA. The cell bodies of the motor fibers are located in the **trochlear nucleus** which itself is located near the midline in the tegmentum of the caudal midbrain. The general proprioceptive input of this muscle is transmitted back with pseudounipolar neurons that have their cell bodies located in the **mesencephalic nucleus of the trigeminal nerve**.

The trochlear nerve is both the thinnest and longest of all cranial nerves. It is also the only cranial nerve whose fibers originate from a contralateral nucleus. As it emerges from the brainstem it curves around the cerebral peduncles and extends anteriorly within the lateral border of the cavernous sinus before entering the orbit through the **superior orbital fissure**.

12.5 Trigeminal Nerve

The largest of all the cranial nerves is the **trigeminal nerve** (CN V) and it is most comparable to the ventral and dorsal roots of a spinal nerve (**Fig. 12.6**). This nerve is associated with the first pharyngeal arch of development and consists of an **ophthalmic** (CN V_1), **maxillary** (CN V_2) and **mandibular** (CN V_3) **division (Fig. 12.7)**. Both the motor and sensory roots pass near the ventrolateral aspect of the pons before they seem to expand at the trigeminal ganglion. The ophthalmic division passes back through the **superior orbital fissure**; the maxillary division traverses the **foramen rotundum**;

Clinical Correlate 12.3

Oculomotor Nerve Palsies

Damage to the oculomotor nerve affects the ipsilateral eye. There is a "down and out" appearance when a person looks straight ahead. The unopposed action of the lateral rectus muscle forces the eye to deviate laterally (*lateral strabismus*) and because the superior oblique muscle still functions to depress the eyeball this forces the "down and out" appearance. There is a loss of function to the levator palpebrae superioris as well, causing drooping of the upper eyelid (*ptosis*). Any damage to the somatic motor fibers would be referred to as *external ophthalmoplegia* and involves the loss of most extraocular muscle functions.

A partial CN III palsy could be the result of a rapid increase in intracranial pressure possibly due to an acute epidural or subdural hematoma, which will often compress CN III against the petrous portion of the temporal bone. Aneurysms involving the posterior cerebral or superior cerebellar arteries have been known to compress CN III because it passes between these two arteries. Due to the parasympathetic fibers being located on the superficial surface of the nerve, they are affected first and may be the first clinical sign demonstrating damage to this nerve because there would be no constriction of the pupil and no accommodation for near vision. The *pupillary light reflex* is lost because the affected eye cannot constrict the pupil in response to a bright light.

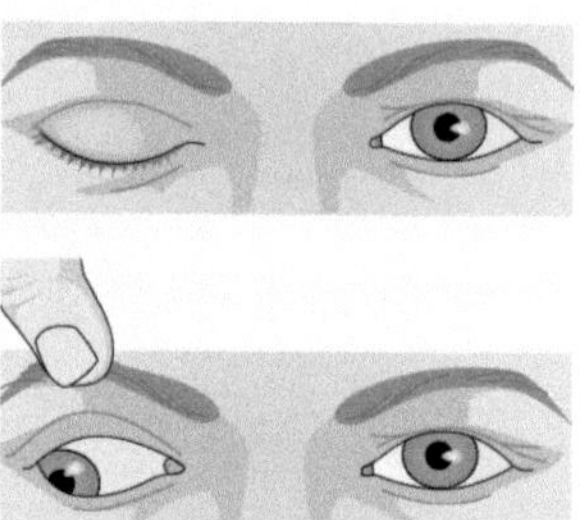

(From Schuenke M, Schulte E, Schumacher U. THIEME Atlas of Anatomy. Head, Neck, and Neuroanatomy. Illustrations by Voll M and Wesker K. 3rd ed. New York: Thieme Medical Publishers; 2020.)

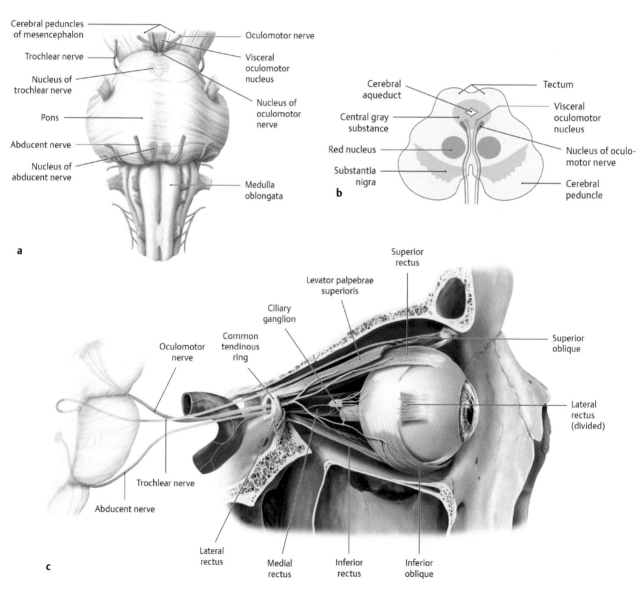

Fig. 12.5 **(a)** Emergence of the nerves from the brainstem. **(b)** Topography of the oculomotor nucleus. **(c)** Course of the nerves supplying the ocular muscles in right orbit, lateral view. (*continued*) (From Schuenke M, Schulte E, Schumacher U. THIEME Atlas of Anatomy. Head, Neck, and Neuroanatomy. Illustrations by Voll M and Wesker K. 3rd ed. New York: Thieme Medical Publishers; 2020.)

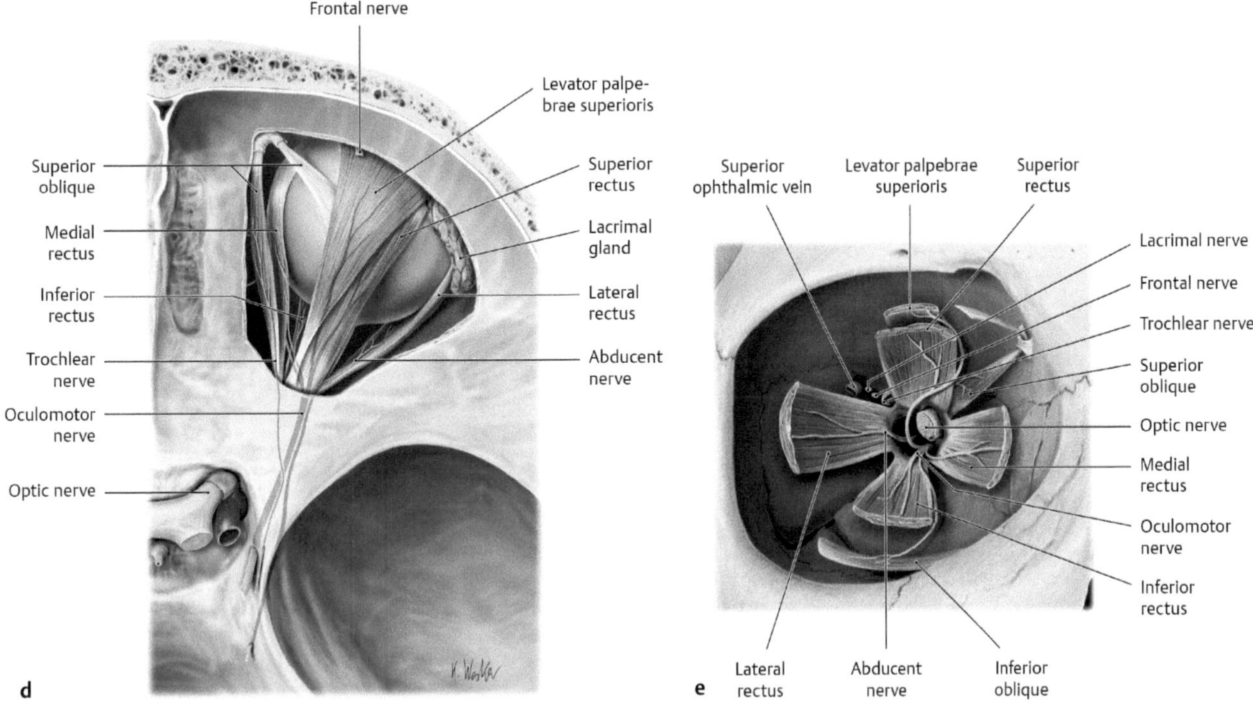

Fig. 12.5 *(continued)* Course of the nerves supplying the ocular muscles: **(d)** Superior view. **(e)** Anterior view. (From Schuenke M, Schulte E, Schumacher U. THIEME Atlas of Anatomy. Head, Neck, and Neuroanatomy. Illustrations by Voll M and Wesker K. 3rd ed. New York: Thieme Medical Publishers; 2020.)

Clinical Correlate 12.4

Trochlear Nerve Palsies

Damage to the trochlear nerve results in paralysis of the ipsilateral eye while damage to the trochlear nucleus affects the contralateral eye. There is an "up and in" appearance when a person looks straight ahead. A characteristic sign of a trochlear nerve injury is vertical diplopia (or double vision) and this is amplified when a person is looking down and in as in reading a book or walking down a flight of stairs. This is due to the fact that the superior oblique muscle normally assists the inferior rectus in depressing the pupil and it is the only muscle to do so when the pupil is adducted. There are many causes of vertical strabismus or vertical misalignment of the eyes called *hypertropia* but one of the most common causes is a trochlear nerve palsy. If a patient has a trochlear nerve palsy they will tilt their head away from the affected side to correct for extorsion or external rotation of the eye which is not usually visible to the examiner. In addition, there is a chin tuck while looking upward to correct for hypertropia.

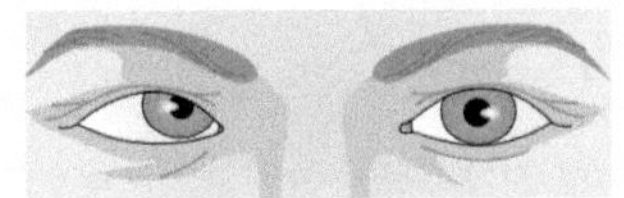

(From Schuenke M, Schulte E, Schumacher U. THIEME Atlas of Anatomy. Head, Neck, and Neuroanatomy. Illustrations by Voll M and Wesker K. 3rd ed. New York: Thieme Medical Publishers; 2020.)

and the mandibular division extends back through the **foramen ovale** before merging with the trigeminal ganglion. The functional components of this nerve are SVE and GSA.

The smaller **motor root** carries SVE branchiomotor fibers responsible for innervating the **muscles of mastication**, **tensor tympani**, **tensor veli palatini**, **mylohyoid** and **anterior belly of digastric muscles**. It joins the mandibular nerve (CN V_3) just outside the skull. The **motor nucleus** is located in the mid-pons region of the brainstem and anterolateral to the edge of the fourth ventricle.

The much larger **sensory root** carries GSA fibers responsible for the touch, pressure, temperature and pain (nociception) sensation of the anterior half of the scalp and face, cornea and conjunctiva, lacrimal gland, anterior two-thirds of the tongue, mucosa of nasal and oral cavities, and innervation of the upper and lower teeth. This trigeminal sensory pathway consists of a first, second and third-order neuron sequence that extends from the periphery to the cerebral cortex respectively. The first-order pseudounipolar neurons have their cell bodies located in the **trigeminal ganglion**. The peripheral processes contribute to the formation of the individual V_1, V_2, and V_3 branches while the central processes enter the pons and join the spinal tract of the trigeminal nerve before terminating in the trigeminal nuclei where they establish contacts with the second-order neurons also located in these nuclei.

Second-order neurons and interneurons are found in the trigeminal nuclei except in the mesencephalic nucleus. These second-order neurons give rise to fibers that decussate in the brainstem before joining the *anterior trigeminothalamic tract* or fibers that do not decussate and follow the *posterior trigeminothalamic tract*. The fibers from both of these tracts will then synapse on third-order neurons located in the *VPM nucleus of the thalamus*. Third-order neurons then relay the sensory information to the postcentral gyrus of the cerebral cortex (**Fig. 12.8**).

The sensory nuclei are arranged into a nearly complete vertical cylinder extending from the mesencephalon to the uppermost cervical spinal cord levels. The mesencephalic nucleus is the most superior structure, followed by the main (principal) sensory nucleus and the spinal nucleus, which is the longest of the three sensory nuclei (**Fig. 12.6a**).

- **Mesencephalic nucleus**: found at the level of the mesencephalon or midbrain. Located here are the cell bodies of first-order

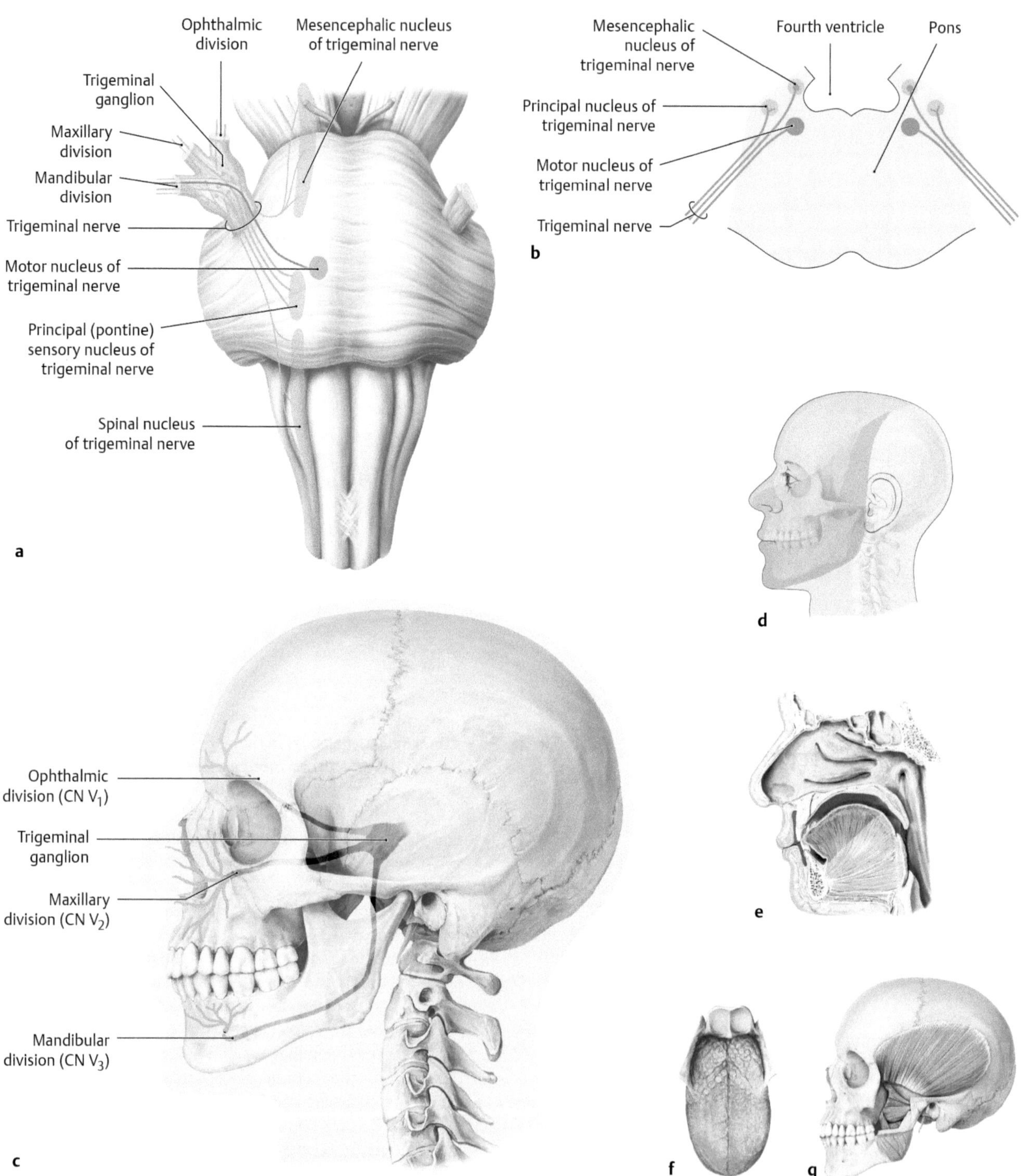

Fig. 12.6 **(a)** Trigeminal nerve nuclei locations. **(b)** Course and distribution of the trigeminal nerve. **(c)** Left lateral view of the three divisions. **(d)** Nerve supply to the skin of the face. **(e)** Mucosa of the nasal cavity and nasopharynx. **(f)** Touch, pain and thermal sensation of the anterior two-thirds of the tongue. **(g)** Motor innervation to the muscles of mastication. (From Schuenke M, Schulte E, Schumacher U. THIEME Atlas of Anatomy. Head, Neck, and Neuroanatomy. Illustrations by Voll M and Wesker K. 3rd ed. New York: Thieme Medical Publishers; 2020.)

pseudounipolar neurons and there are no synapses that occur at this nucleus. This is not a true nucleus but instead a sensory ganglion, much like others that contain cells that are both structurally and functionally ganglion cells. The neurons associated with this nucleus are related to the general proprioceptive input confirmed to be traveling back from the extraocular muscles (CN III, IV and VI), the muscles of mastication (CN V), and the periodontal ligaments (CN V). Proprioceptive input from skeletal muscles related to CN VII, IX, X, and XII may also travel back to this nucleus. However, this has yet to be confirmed.

- **Main (principal) nucleus**: found at the level of the mid-pons or metencephalon. The transmission of mechanoreceptor information for discriminatory (fine) tactile and pressure sense is related to this nucleus. Synapses involving a first-order pseudounipolar neuron whose cell bodies are located in the trigeminal ganglion occur at this nucleus. It is homologous to

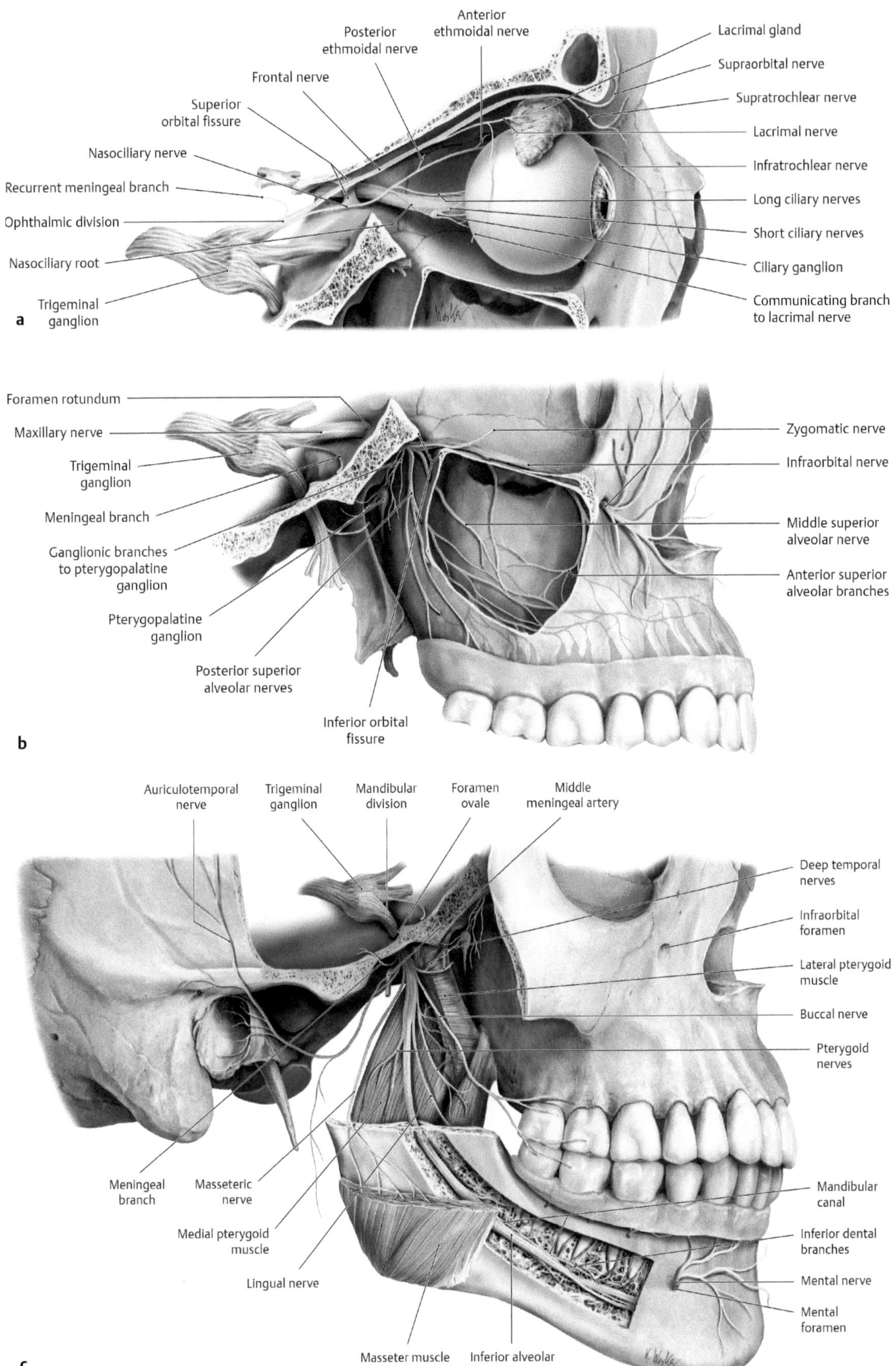

Fig. 12.7 **(a)** Branches of the ophthalmic division. **(b)** Branches of the maxillary division. **(c)** Branches of the mandibular division. (From Schuenke M, Schulte E, Schumacher U. THIEME Atlas of Anatomy. Head, Neck, and Neuroanatomy. Illustrations by Voll M and Wesker K. 3rd ed. New York: Thieme Medical Publishers; 2020.)

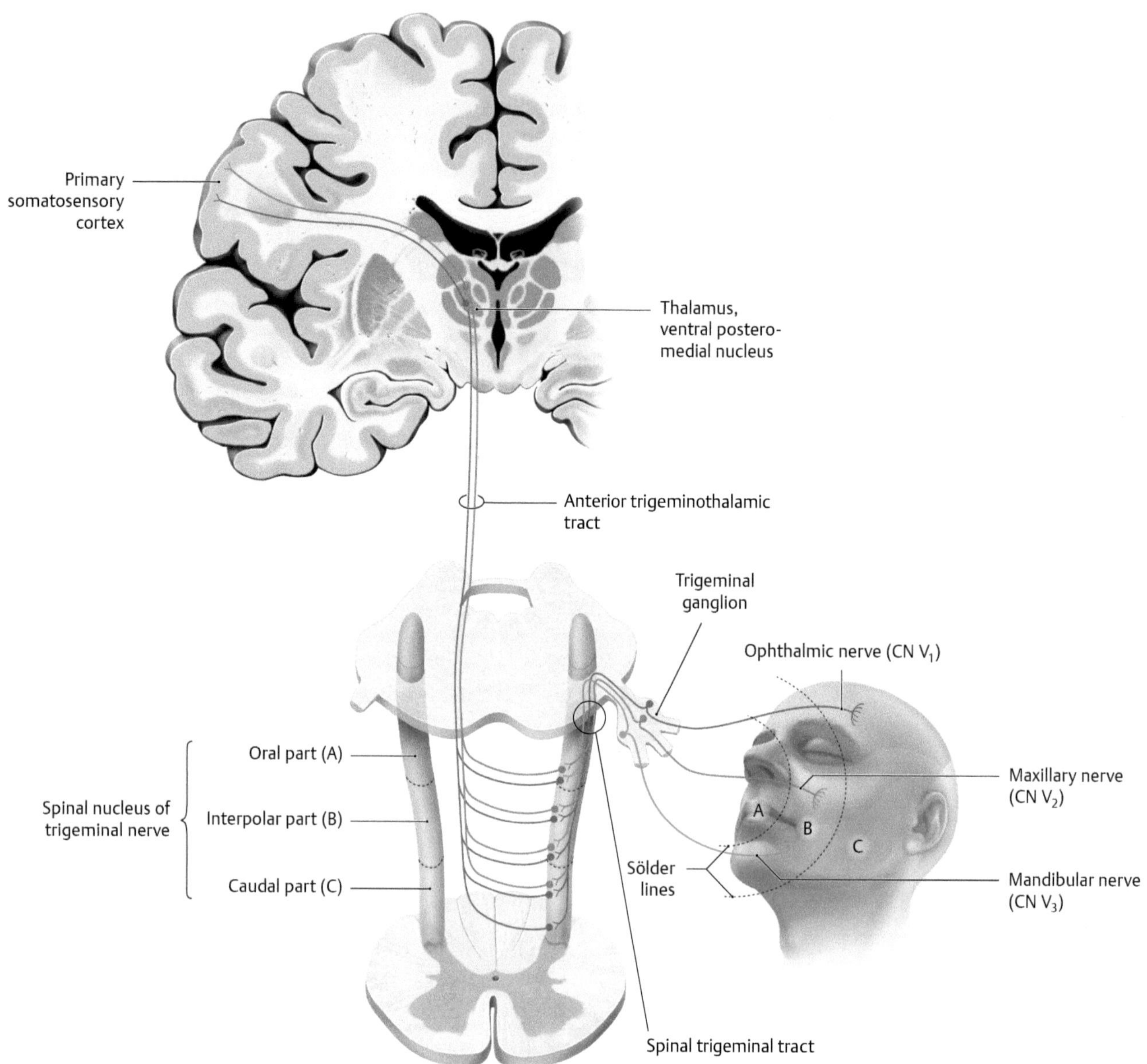

Fig. 12.8 Trigeminal tracts. Posterior trigeminothalamic tract not shown. (From Schuenke M, Schulte E, Schumacher U. THIEME Atlas of Anatomy. Head, Neck, and Neuroanatomy. Illustrations by Voll M and Wesker K. 3rd ed. New York: Thieme Medical Publishers; 2020.)

Clinical Correlate 12.5

Trigeminal Nerve Damage and Trigeminal Neuralgia

Trigeminal nerve damage due to trauma, meningeal infections, aneurysms or tumors may lead to a loss of general sensation to the face or mucous membranes of the nasal and oral cavities; flaccid paralysis of the muscles of mastication; deviation of jaw to the weak side due to the unopposed contraction of the opposite lateral pterygoid muscle; partial deafness to low-pitched sounds (hypacusis) due to tensor tympani muscle paralysis; and the loss of the afferent limb of the corneal reflex.

Trigeminal neuralgia (or tic douloureux), previously discussed in Chapter 7, is a neuropathic disorder associated with the sensory root of CN V and characterized by episodes of sudden, sharp and excruciating pain involving the face. This pain may last for a few seconds or several minutes. The most affected part is V_2, followed by V_3. Compression of the sensory root by an aberrant artery or demyelination of sensory axons may be a cause. Symptoms generally do not begin until middle age and can be triggered by many stimuli, some as gentle as wind blowing on the face. Treatment may begin with anticonvulsant medications. If episodes persist, surgical intervention is inevitable. There is a high rate of suicide associated with this diagnosis because the individuals live in constant pain.

Clinical Correlate 12.6

Jaw Jerk Reflex

The **jaw jerk reflex** is a monosynaptic myotatic reflex similar to spinal stretch reflexes. The gentle tapping of a hammer on the chin will cause the intrafusal muscle fibers within muscle spindles of the masseter muscles to stretch, thus stimulating the sensory nerve fibers innervating them. The afferent limb of the reflex is CN V_3 and the ipsilateral pseudounipolar neurons have their peripheral processes located in the muscle spindles, cell bodies in the mesencephalic nucleus, and their central processes synapse bilaterally at the motor nucleus of CN V. The efferent limb is made up of the multipolar motor neurons traveling through CN V_3 that innervate the masseter muscle. The presence of a pronounced jaw jerk reflex is abnormal and is a sign of hyperreflexia associated with lesions of upper motor neuron pathways projecting to the trigeminal motor nucleus.

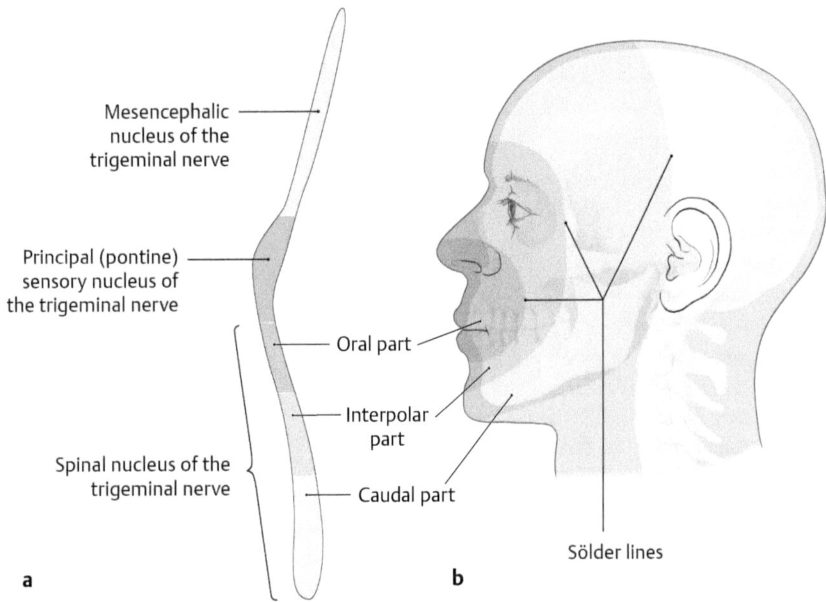

Fig. 12.9 Somatotopic organization of the spinal nucleus of the trigeminal nerve **(a)** and facial zones **(b)** in which sensory deficits arise. (From Schuenke M, Schulte E, Schumacher U. THIEME Atlas of Anatomy. Head, Neck, and Neuroanatomy. Illustrations by Voll M and Wesker K. 3rd ed. New York: Thieme Medical Publishers; 2020.)

the *nucleus cuneatus* and *nucleus gracilis* located in the dorsal portion of the caudal medulla.

- **Spinal nucleus**: extends from the level of the mid-pons and to about C3 of the spinal cord. This nucleus is primarily concerned with the transmission of temperature and pain sensations from the oral and facial regions, but it will also process discriminative tactile sense and itch information. Inferiorly, it is continuous with the substantia gelatinosa of the dorsal horn of the spinal cord. Synapses involving a first-order pseudounipolar neuron whose cell bodies are located in the trigeminal ganglion occur at this nucleus. This nucleus displays a somatotopic organization defined by *Sölder lines* (**Fig. 12.9**) and it is divided into three subnuclei from rostral to caudal: the **subnucleus oralis (oral part)**, **subnucleus interpolaris (interpolar part)**, and the **subnucleus caudalis (caudal part)**, a homologue of the substantia gelatinosa.

12.5.1 Trigeminal Tracts

The majority of somatosensory information from the craniofacial structures including the nasal and oral cavities is transmitted to the brainstem by way of the trigeminal nerve (**Fig. 12.8**). The central processes of the first-order pseudounipolar neurons whose cell bodies are located in the trigeminal ganglion bifurcate into ascending and descending branches before terminating on the second-order neurons of the main sensory nucleus (ascending branches) and spinal nucleus (descending branches). The trigeminal system consists of three tracts: the *spinal trigeminal tract, anterior trigeminothalamic tract* and *posterior trigeminothalamic tract.*

- **Spinal trigeminal tract**: this tract receives GSA temperature, light touch and pain input from the ipsilateral face, palate, anterior 2/3 of the tongue and the teeth. The tract is made up of ipsilateral first-order sensory fibers whose cell bodies are located in the trigeminal ganglion. These fibers descend lateral to the spinal nucleus before synapsing at various levels of this same nucleus. This tract will also carry light touch, temperature and pain input from the ear, larynx, pharynx and upper esophagus in first-order neurons associated with the facial, glossopharyngeal and vagus nerves. The cell bodies of these first-order neurons are located in the geniculate ganglion of CN VII and both of the superior ganglia of CN IX and CN X.
- **Anterior trigeminothalamic tract**: this tract conveys GSA light touch, temperature and pain input from the face, dura mater and oral cavity to the thalamus. First-order neurons with cell bodies from the trigeminal ganglion will synapse at the spinal nucleus. Second-order neurons from the spinal nucleus will decussate and travel superiorly to the ventral posterior medial (VPM) nucleus of the thalamus. Third-order neurons

from the VPM project through the posterior limb of the internal capsule before reaching the postcentral gyrus (3, 1, and 2) of the cerebral cortex.

- **Posterior trigeminothalamic tract**: this tract conveys GSA discriminative (fine) tactile and pressure sensation originating from the face and oral cavity. First-order neurons with cell bodies from the trigeminal ganglion will synapse at the main (principal) nucleus. Second-order neurons from the main (principal) nucleus will remain ipsilateral as they travel superiorly to the ventral posterior medial (VPM) nucleus of the thalamus. Third-order neurons from the VPM project through the posterior limb of the internal capsule before reaching the postcentral gyrus (3, 1, and 2) of the cerebral cortex.

12.6 Abducent Nerve

The **abducent nerve** (CN VI) is responsible for innervating only one of the extraocular muscles, the **lateral rectus muscle** (**Fig. 12.5**). The lateral rectus muscle *abducts* the eye. The functional components of this nerve are GSE and GSA. The general proprioceptive input of this muscle is transmitted back with pseudounipolar neurons that have their cell bodies located in the **mesencephalic nucleus of the trigeminal nerve**.

This nerve will exit the brainstem at the pontomedullary junction and course ventrally before traversing the cavernous sinus just lateral to the internal carotid artery. Upon leaving the cavernous sinus, it will pass through the **superior orbital fissure** and into the orbit before innervating the ipsilateral lateral rectus. During horizontal gaze, there is a simultaneous contraction of both the lateral rectus and medial rectus muscles. If looking to the right, the lateral rectus of the right eye would contract along with the contralateral medial rectus of the left eye.

The **abducent nucleus** contains motor nerve cell bodies that have axons that course ventrally through the pontine tegmentum before exiting at the pontomedullary junction (~70%) and innervate the ipsilateral lateral rectus or interneurons (~30%) that decussate and project via the **medial longitudinal fasciculus** (MLF) to the contralateral oculomotor motor nucleus. From here, neurons go on to innervate the medial rectus. This means the abducent motor nucleus negotiates horizontal eye movements and allows for the two muscles to move in unison.

Clinical Correlate 12.7

Lesion of the Abducent Nerve or Nucleus

A lesion of the abducent nerve distal to the motor nucleus results in paralysis of the lateral rectus and forces the eye to deviate towards the midline because of the unopposed action of the medial rectus. This type of paralysis results in a *medial strabismus* and the individual experiences *horizontal diplopia* (double vision). Diplopia can be reduced if the individual turns their head towards the affected side when looking forward.

If the lesion is located at the abducent motor nucleus, the deficiency is similar to damage involving the individual nerve, but in addition there is the inability to provide excitatory input to the contralateral oculomotor nucleus and its neurons responsible for medial rectus innervation. This is called *lateral gaze paralysis*.

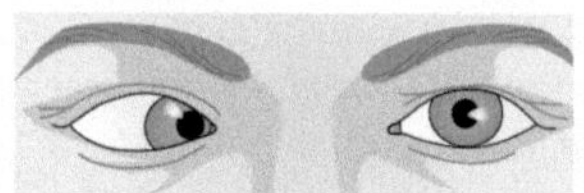

(From Schuenke M, Schulte E, Schumacher U. THIEME Atlas of Anatomy. Head, Neck, and Neuroanatomy. Illustrations by Voll M and Wesker K. 3rd ed. New York: Thieme Medical Publishers; 2020.)

12.7 Facial Nerve

The **facial nerve** (CN VII) is associated with the second pharyngeal arch of development and it consists of two initial roots, a **facial nerve proper** (or **motor root**) and an **intermediate nerve** (or **sensory root**), both of which emerge from the brainstem at the cerebellopontine angle. Both roots continue through the **internal acoustic meatus** alongside the vestibulocochlear nerve and labyrinthine vessels. While in the **facial canal** of the temporal bone, the facial nerve will give rise to three branches: the *greater petrosal nerve* (adjacent to the *geniculate ganglion*), the *nerve to stapedius*, and the *chorda tympani nerve*. The motor root continues through the facial canal before exiting the **stylomastoid foramen** and its SVE fibers will target mimetic muscles. The smaller intermediate nerve carries GSA, GVE, GVA and SVA fibers and their cell bodies are located in the **geniculate ganglion** (**Fig. 12.10**).

- SVE: the cell bodies originate from the **facial nucleus** located in the caudal pons. These fibers loop around the ipsilateral abducent nucleus before continuing through the motor root. Prior to exiting the stylomastoid foramen the SVE fibers innervate the **stapedius muscle** of the middle ear. After passing through the foramen, the SVE fibers are responsible for innervating the muscles of facial expression, scalp and auricular region, the stylohyoid and posterior belly of digastric muscles. These fibers pass through the **posterior auricular**, **temporal**, **zygomatic**, **buccal**, **marginal mandibular** and **cervical branches.**
- GSA: these pseudounipolar neurons convey temperature, touch and pain input and have peripheral processes terminating at specific parts of the external ear such as the concha, helix, antihelix and scaphoid fossa. Their cell bodies are found in the geniculate ganglion with the central processes passing through the intermediate nerve before joining the ipsilateral **spinal trigeminal tract** and finally synapsing at the **spinal nucleus of CN V.**
- GVE: the **para/pre** cell bodies originate from the **superior salivatory nucleus** and their axons may travel through the **greater petrosal nerve**, followed by the **nerve of the pterygoid canal** (*Vidian nerve*), before ultimately synapsing at the **pterygopalatine ganglion.** Individual nerves that directly or indirectly branch from this ganglion distribute the para/post fibers to the mucous membranes of the nasal and oral cavities or the lacrimal gland in the orbit. Additional **para/pre** fibers travel through the **chorda tympani nerve**, which passes through the **petrotympanic fissure** before continuing via the **lingual nerve of** V_3, before synapsing at the **submandibular ganglion.** The **para/post** fibers from this ganglion are distributed to the submandibular and sublingual glands.
- GVA: a limited amount of GVA sensation originates from the mucosa of the soft palate and adjacent pharyngeal wall but there is no known clinical significance. This pathway follows that of SVA taste fibers from the soft palate. The cell bodies of these neurons are located in the geniculate ganglion and their central processes will synapse at the ipsilateral **solitary nucleus of the solitary tract.**

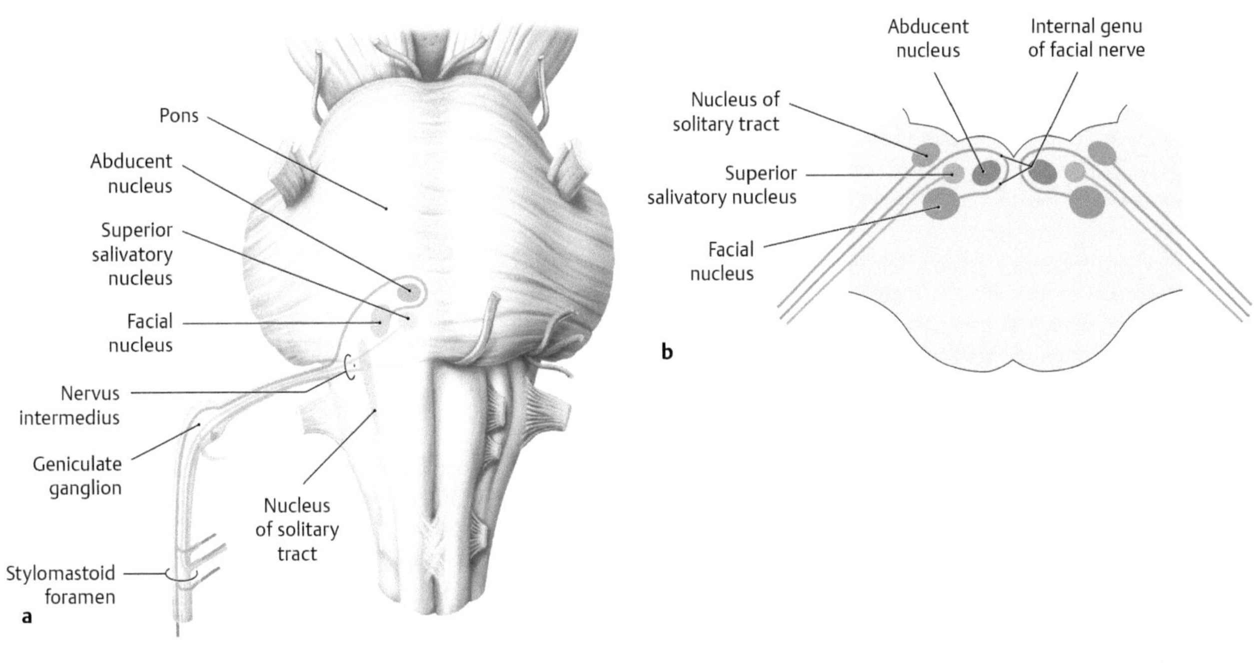

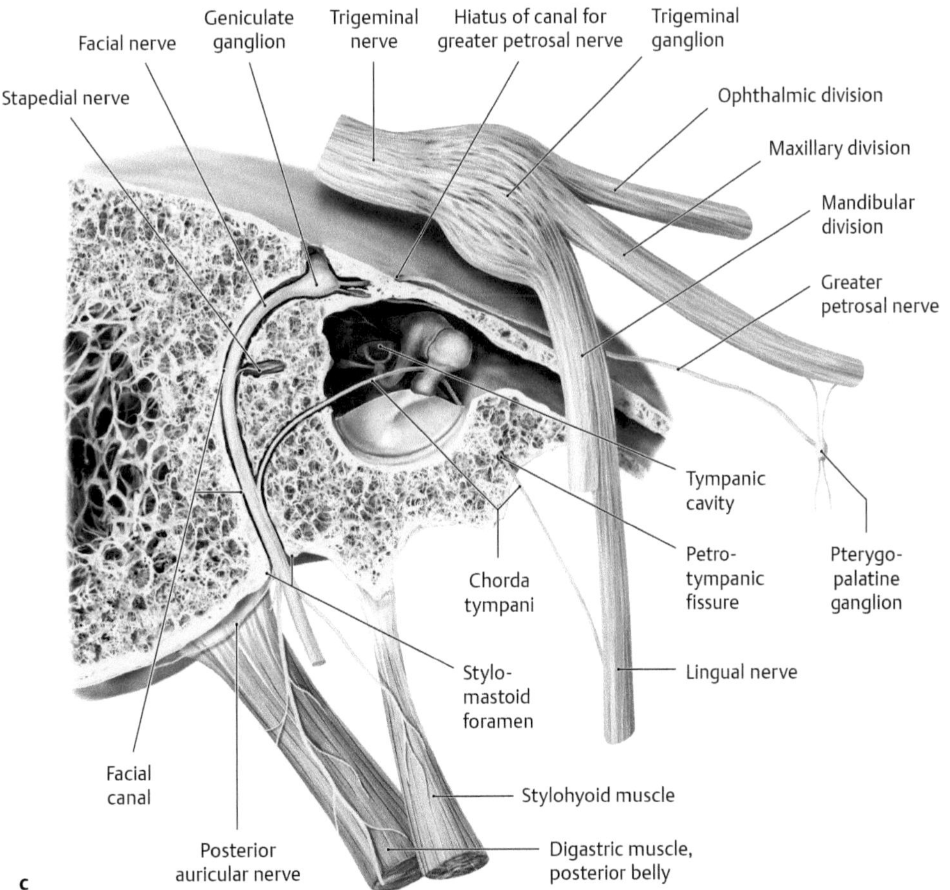

Fig. 12.10 (a) Nuclei locations and principal branches of the facial nerve. **(b)** Facial nerve branches for the muscles of facial expression. **(c)** Facial nerve branches in the temporal bone. (*continued*) (From Schuenke M, Schulte E, Schumacher U. THIEME Atlas of Anatomy. Head, Neck, and Neuroanatomy. Illustrations by Voll M and Wesker K. 3rd ed. New York: Thieme Medical Publishers; 2020.)

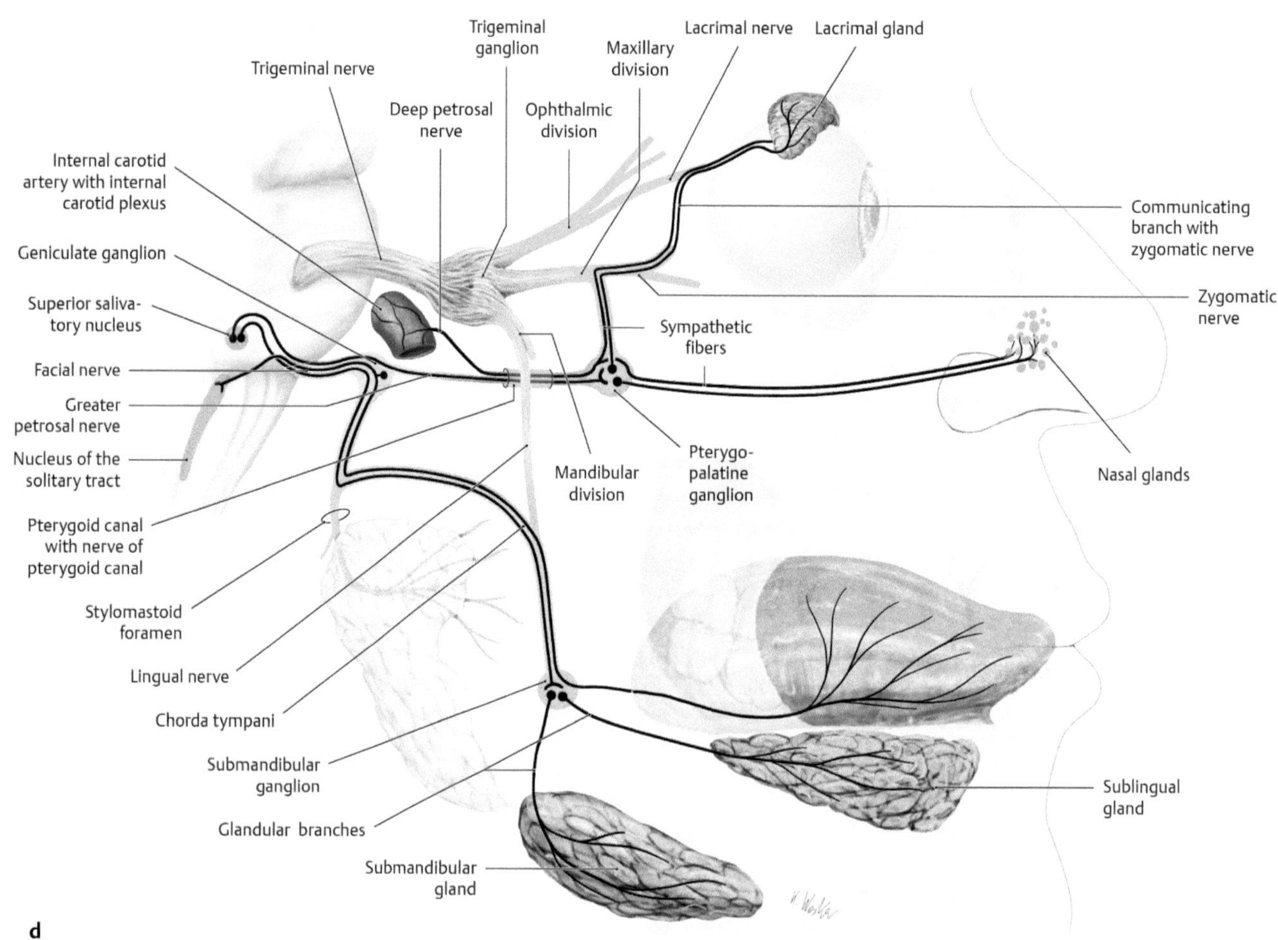

Fig. 12.10 (*continued*) **(d)** Parasympathetic and taste fibers of the facial nerve. (From Schuenke M, Schulte E, Schumacher U. THIEME Atlas of Anatomy. Head, Neck, and Neuroanatomy. Illustrations by Voll M and Wesker K. 3rd ed. New York: Thieme Medical Publishers; 2020.)

- SVA: the peripheral processes of taste sensation fibers from the anterior two-thirds of the tongue travel back through the **lingual nerve of V_3**, continue through the chorda tympani, and have their cell bodies located in the geniculate ganglion. A minimal amount of taste originates from the soft palate and follows the **lesser palatine nerve** back to the pterygopalatine ganglion. The fibers pass through the nerve of the pterygoid canal before continuing through the greater petrosal nerve, and have their cell bodies located in the geniculate ganglion. The central processes of both pathways pass through the intermediate nerve before synapsing at the ipsilateral **solitary nucleus of the solitary tract**.

12.8 Vestibulocochlear Nerve

The **vestibulocochlear nerve** (CN VIII) consists of two distinct and separate nerves that are enclosed within a single sheath (**Fig. 12.11**). The **vestibular nerve** is associated with equilibrium and balance while the **cochlear nerve** is concerned with hearing. The functional component of both nerves is SSA.

The peripheral processes of bipolar neurons of the vestibular nerve are connected to a special receptor called an **ampullary crest** (crista ampullaries) located in each ampulla of the semicircular ducts and the **maculae** found in both the utricle and saccule. The central processes of these neurons extend back from the vestibular ganglion to the **superior**, **inferior**, **lateral**, and **medial vestibular nuclei** located near the rhomboid fossa of the medulla oblongata (**Fig. 12.11b**). Central processes may also pass directly via the **juxtarestiform body** of the inferior cerebellar peduncle to the **flocculonodular lobe** of the cerebellum. The vestibular pathway was discussed in Chapter 9. It eventually projects to the region that corresponds with areas 2v and 3a of the primary vestibular cortex of the parietal lobe.

The peripheral processes of the cochlear nerve originate from the hair cells of the **organ of Corti**, a special receptor that transduces sounds waves into electrical impulses. The cell bodies of the first-order bipolar neurons are located in the **spiral (cochlear) ganglion** and along with the organ of Corti, these two structures are located within the cochlea of the inner ear. Central processes of these neurons synapse with second-order neurons located in the **anterior** and **posterior cochlear nuclei** of the medullopontine junction of the brainstem (**Fig. 12.11c**). The auditory pathway was discussed in Chapter 9. It eventually reaches the **transverse temporal gyri of Heschl** of the superior temporal gyrus. This is a region that corresponds with areas 41 and 42 of the primary auditory cortex of the temporal lobe.

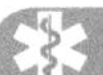

Clinical Correlate 12.8

Facial Nerve Damage

Upper motor neurons from the primary somatomotor cortex (precentral gyrus) have axons that pass through the corticonuclear (corticobulbar) tract before reaching the facial motor nucleus. The facial motor nucleus is broken up into an upper/posterior part and supplies muscles of the forehead and eyes while the lower/anterior part supplies muscles of the lower half of the face. The upper part receives bilateral innervation while the lower part receives only contralateral innervation from upper motor neurons (**a**).

- Central (supranuclear) paralysis: **(b)** involves a loss or lesion of the upper motor neurons. It presents with paralysis of the contralateral facial expression muscles in the lower half of the face while the contralateral forehead and eyelid region remain functional.
- Peripheral (infranuclear) paralysis: **(c)** involves a loss or lesion of the lower motor neurons. It presents with a compete paralysis of the ipsilateral facial expression muscles. This is representative of Bell's palsy, which was discussed in Chapter 7.
- Crocodile tears syndrome: involves a facial nerve lesion proximal to the geniculate ganglion. Lacrimation occurs while eating because select regenerating parasympathetic preganglionic fibers that originate from the superior salivatory nucleus and are destined to reach the submandibular ganglion are misdirected to the pterygopalatine ganglion. The inappropriate synaptic contacts increase tear production when they would have normally increased saliva production.

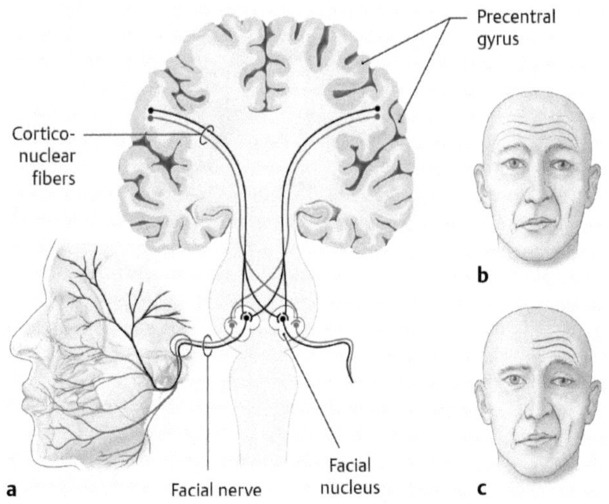

(From Schuenke M, Schulte E, Schumacher U. THIEME Atlas of Anatomy. Head, Neck, and Neuroanatomy. Illustrations by Voll M and Wesker K. 3rd ed. New York: Thieme Medical Publishers; 2020.)

Clinical Correlate 12.9

Lesions of the Vestibulocochlear Nerve

Lesions of the vestibular nerve may result in an abnormal sensation of motion (vertigo), involuntary eye movements (nystagmus), or the sensation of an impending fall (disequilibrium). Lesions of the cochlear nerve lead to ringing in the ears (tinnitus). Tinnitus could also be the result of sensorineural deafness, which is damage located somewhere between the inner ear and pathways back to the brain.

Clinical Correlate 12.10

Acoustic Neuromas

Acoustic neuromas are rare, benign tumors of the neurolemma of Schwann cells and present unilaterally over 90% of the time. These tumors generally begin in the vestibular nerve while it is still in the internal acoustic meatus and are known not to metastasize. Further tumor growth may begin to compress the cerebellum and brainstem. Symptoms include one-sided hearing loss, tinnitus and vertigo. Treatment may include radiation or surgical removal.

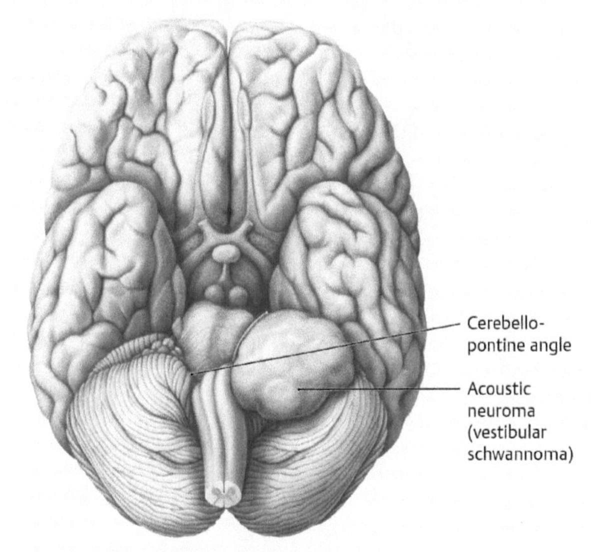

(From Schuenke M, Schulte E, Schumacher U. THIEME Atlas of Anatomy. Head, Neck, and Neuroanatomy. Illustrations by Voll M and Wesker K. 3rd ed. New York: Thieme Medical Publishers; 2020.)

12.9 Glossopharyngeal Nerve

The **glossopharyngeal nerve** (CN IX) is associated with the third pharyngeal arch of development and has the functional components SVE, GSA, GVE, GVA, and SVA. As it emerges from the brainstem as a group of rootlets posterior to the olive of the medulla oblongata it will merge to form a main trunk (**Fig. 12.12**). It will shortly exit the cranial vault via the **jugular foramen** paired with the vagus and spinal accessory nerves. Near the jugular foramen it will form two ganglia. The **superior ganglion** is intracranial and contains cell bodies of GSA first-order pseudounipolar neurons while the **inferior ganglion** is extracranial and consists of the cell bodies of both SVA and GVA first-order pseudounipolar neurons. Major branches of CN IX include the *nerve to stylopharyngeus, tympanic, lingual, tonsillar, pharyngeal* and the *carotid sinus nerves* **(Fig. 12.13).**

- SVE: the cell bodies originate from the **nucleus ambiguus** located primarily in the medulla oblongata. After exiting the jugular foramen along with the rest of CN IX, these fibers pass through the **nerve to stylopharyngeus** before innervating the ipsilateral **stylopharyngeus muscle** of the pharynx.
- GSA: these pseudounipolar neurons convey temperature, touch and pain input and have peripheral processes terminating at the concha, external acoustic meatus and skin located medial to the posterior aspect of the external ear. These fibers pass

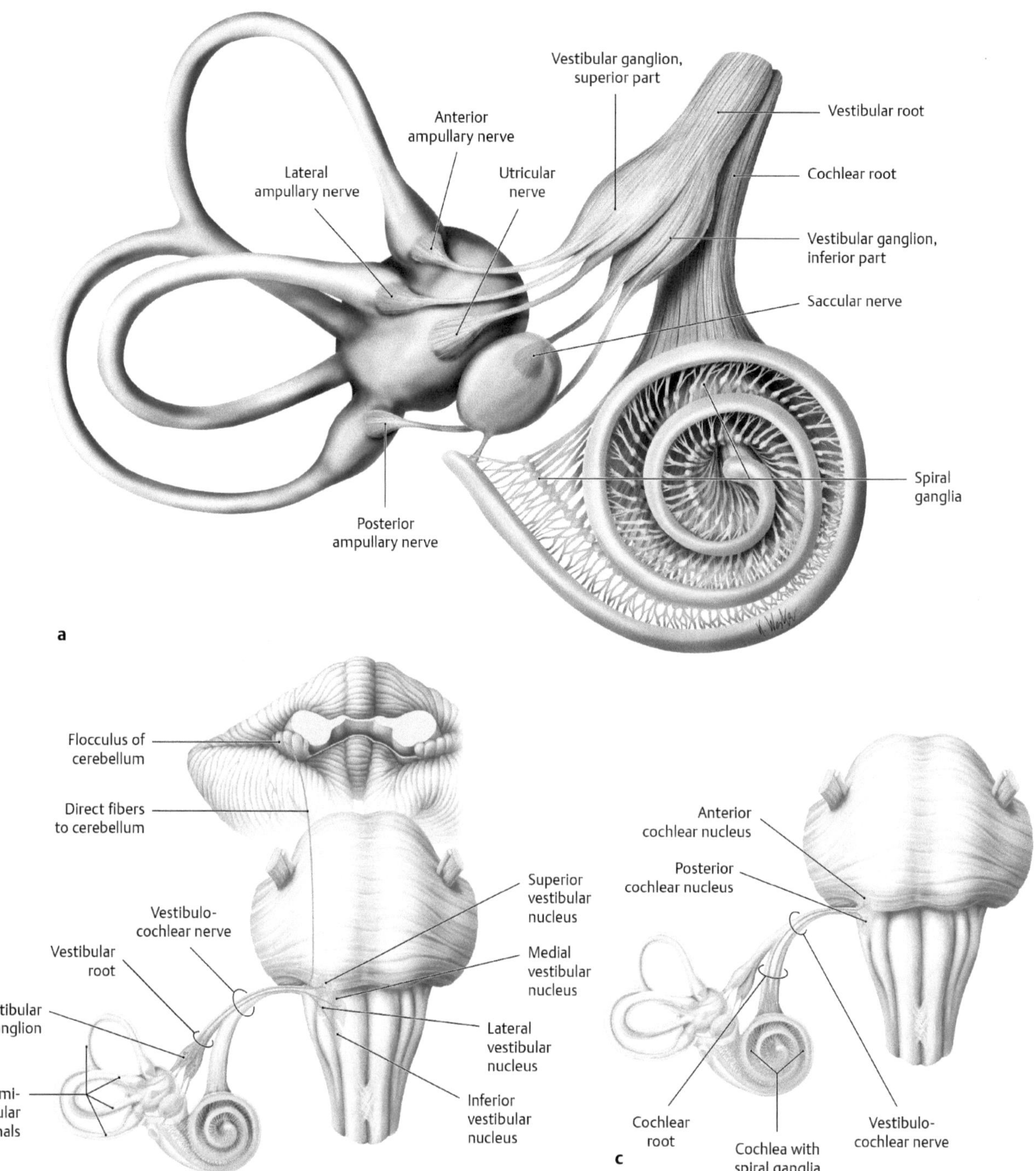

12.11 (a) Vestibular and cochlear ganglia. **(b)** Vestibular nuclei of the vestibulocochlear nerve. **(c)** Cochlear nuclei of the vestibulocochlear nerve. (From Schuenke M, Schulte E, Schumacher U. THIEME Atlas of Anatomy. Head, Neck, and Neuroanatomy. Illustrations by Voll M and Wesker K. 3rd ed. New York: Thieme Medical Publishers; 2020.)

along a *communicating branch* to the auricular nerve of CN X. In addition, peripheral processes extend to the mucosa of the middle ear cavity and pharyngotympanic tube (via the **tympanic nerve**), posterior one-third of the tongue (via **lingual nerve br.**), tonsils (via **tonsillar nerve br.**), and the soft palate, lower portion of the nasopharynx and the entire oropharynx (via **pharyngeal branches of the pharyngeal plexus**). The soft palate innervation overlaps with that of the lesser palatine nerve associated with CN V_2. The central processes join the ipsilateral **spinal trigeminal tract** before synapsing at the **spinal nucleus of CN V.**

- GVE: the **para/pre** cell bodies originate from the **inferior salivatory nucleus** and their axons travel in order through the **tympanic nerve**, the **tympanic plexus** (of the middle ear cavity), and then the **lesser petrosal nerve** before passing through the **foramen ovale** to synapse at the **otic ganglion.** The **para/post** fibers from this ganglion are distributed to the parotid gland via the **auriculotemporal nerve of V_3 (Fig. 12.14).**
- GVA: these fibers convey changes in arterial blood pressure from the **carotid sinus** (a baroreceptor) and the level of certain gases such as oxygen from the **carotid body** (a chemoreceptor).

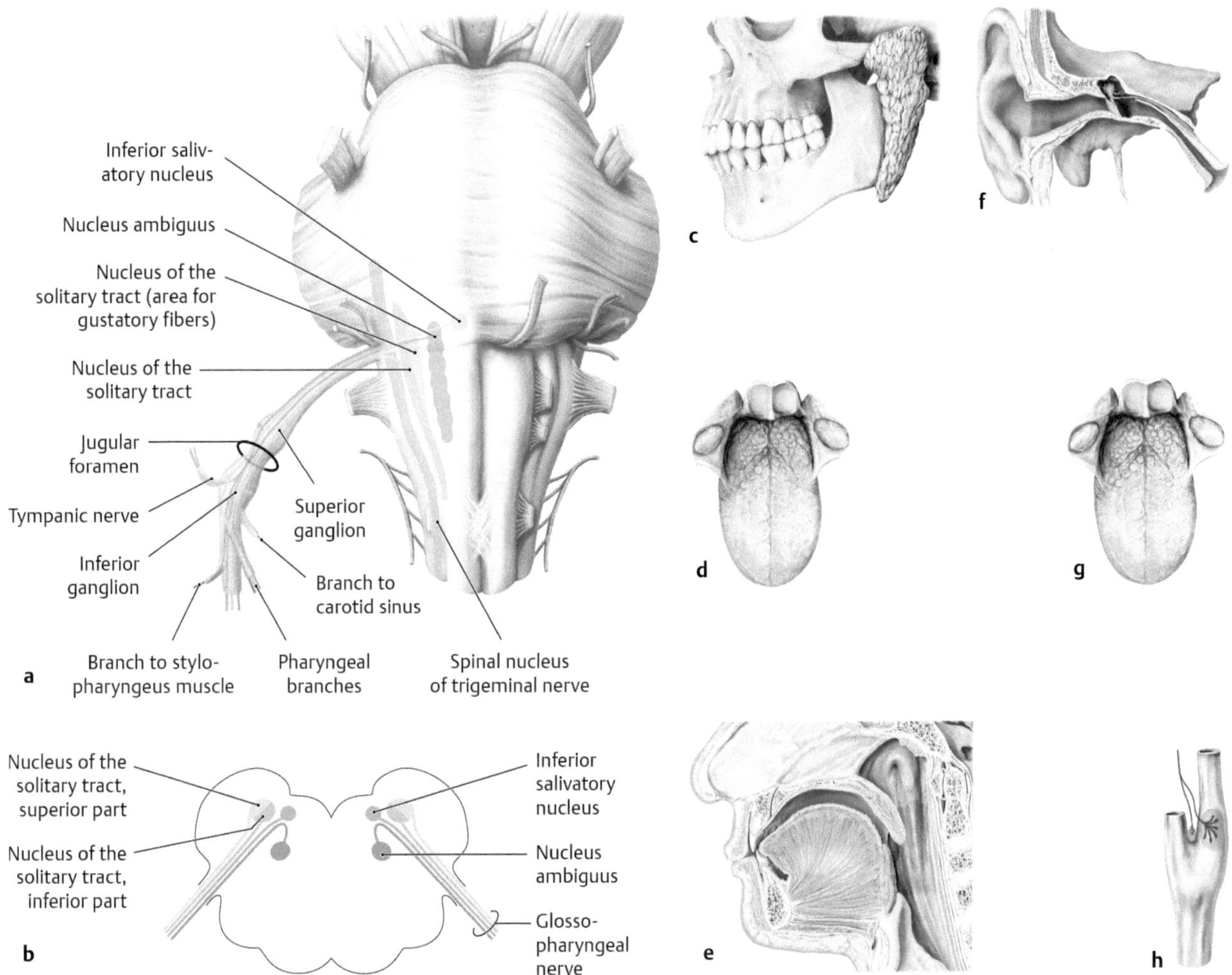

Fig. 12.12 **(a)** Nuclei of the glossopharyngeal nerve, anterior view. **(b)** Cross-section through the medulla oblongata (for clarity, the trigeminal nerve nuclei are not shown). **(c)** Parasympathetic innervation to the parotid gland. **(d, g)** Somatic sensory and taste innervation to the posterior one-third of the tongue. **(e)** Somatic sensory innervation of the mucosa over the posterior one-third of the tongue, soft palate, parts of the nasopharynx and oropharynx, and tonsils. **(f)** Sensory innervation of the mucosa of the tympanic cavity and pharyngotympanic tube. **(h)** Visceral sensory innervation of the carotid body and carotid sinus. (From Schuenke M, Schulte E, Schumacher U. THIEME Atlas of Anatomy. Head, Neck, and Neuroanatomy. Illustrations by Voll M and Wesker K. 3rd ed. New York: Thieme Medical Publishers; 2020.)

Most information originating from the carotid sinus and body pass via the **carotid sinus nerve of CN IX**, however, limited information will pass via the carotid sinus nerve of CN X. The central processes enter the brainstem and synapse at the ipsilateral **solitary nucleus of the solitary tract**.

- SVA: the peripheral processes of taste sensation fibers from the posterior one-third of the tongue travel back through the **lingual nerve of CN IX**. The central processes will synapse at the ipsilateral **solitary nucleus of the solitary tract**.

12.10 Vagus Nerve

The **vagus nerve** (CN X) is associated with the fourth and sixth pharyngeal arches of development and has the functional components SVE, GSA, GVE, GVA, and SVA (**Fig. 12.15**). As it emerges from the brainstem as a group of rootlets just inferior to CN IX and posterior to the olive of the medulla oblongata, it merges to form a main trunk. It exits the cranial vault via the **jugular foramen** paired with the glossopharyngeal and spinal accessory nerves. It has two ganglia similar to CN IX. The **superior ganglion** is located at the level of the jugular foramen and contains cell bodies of GSA first-order pseudounipolar neurons while the **inferior ganglion** is extracranial and consists of the cell bodies of both SVA and GVA first-order pseudounipolar neurons. Major branches of CN X include the *auricular, superior laryngeal, internal laryngeal, external laryngeal, recurrent laryngeal, pharyngeal, carotid sinus,* and the *vagal trunks* (**Fig. 12.16**).

- SVE: the cell bodies originate from the **nucleus ambiguus.** These fibers pass through the **superior laryngeal, external laryngeal**, and **recurrent laryngeal nerves** to innervate the laryngeal muscles. They also pass through the **pharyngeal branches of the pharyngeal plexus** to innervate the soft palate (except tensor veli palatini) and pharyngeal muscles (except stylopharyngeus).
- GSA: these pseudounipolar neurons convey temperature, touch and pain input and have peripheral processes originating from the concha, external acoustic meatus, outer tympanic membrane and skin located medial to the posterior aspect of the

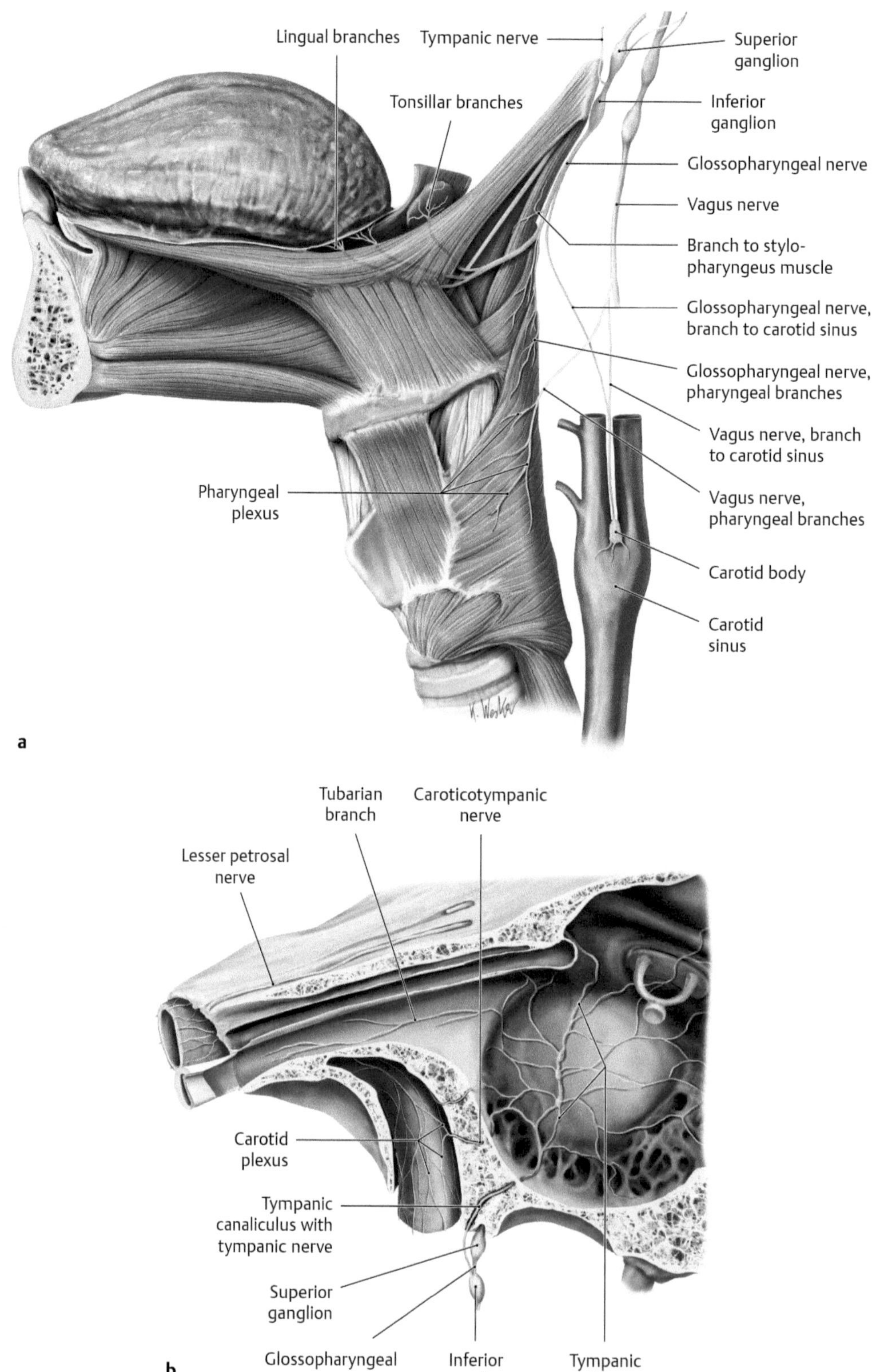

Fig. 12.13 **(a)** Branches of the glossopharyngeal nerve beyond the skull base. **(b)** Branches of the glossopharyngeal nerve in the tympanic cavity. (From Schuenke M, Schulte E, Schumacher U. THIEME Atlas of Anatomy. Head, Neck, and Neuroanatomy. Illustrations by Voll M and Wesker K. 3rd ed. New York: Thieme Medical Publishers; 2020.)

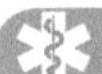

Clinical Correlate 12.11

Glossopharyngeal Neuralgia

Specific lesions involving the glossopharyngeal nerve are rare but when this nerve is involved, the lesion is most likely affecting multiple cranial nerves such as the vagus and spinal accessory nerve all at once (**jugular foramen syndrome**). **Glossopharyngeal neuralgia** may be the result of an abnormally positioned artery and rarely is it due to a tumor. The brief or intermittent attacks of pain that may be present are similar to those of *trigeminal neuralgia*. It is rare, but symptoms can include excruciating pain when chewing or swallowing, bradycardia and swallow syncope. Swallow syncope is when a person loses consciousness during or immediately after swallowing even if there is no pain present. Treatments have included anticonvulsant drugs, nerve resection or microvascular decompressions surgery.

CN IX serves as the afferent limb of the **gag reflex** while CN X serves as its efferent limb. If the gag reflex is absent it will be on the side of the lesion. Only about 60% of the population has a functioning gag reflex and the loss of it does not mean the act of swallowing is affected because they have been shown to be independent of each other (Davies et al., 1995; Lancet 345 (8948): 487-488).

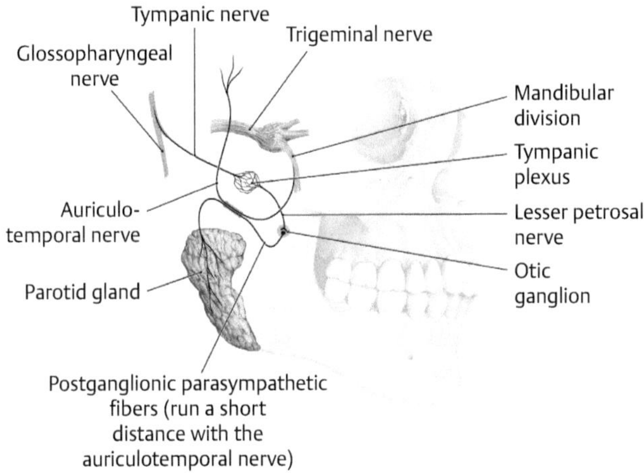

Fig. 12.14 Parasympathetic fibers of the glossopharyngeal nerve. (From Schuenke M, Schulte E, Schumacher U. THIEME Atlas of Anatomy. Head, Neck, and Neuroanatomy. Illustrations by Voll M and Wesker K. 3rd ed. New York: Thieme Medical Publishers; 2020.)

external ear (via the **auricular nerve**). The central processes join the ipsilateral **spinal trigeminal tract** before synapsing at the **spinal nucleus of CN V**.

- GVE: the **para/pre** cell bodies originate from the **dorsal motor nucleus of vagus** and their axons will travel through the **superior laryngeal**, **internal laryngeal**, **recurrent laryngeal**, and **pharyngeal nerve branches of the pharyngeal plexus**, along with the **vagal trunks** that extend inferiorly all the way to the foregut and midgut. The **para/post** fibers extend from ganglia located near or within the viscera (i.e., submucosal ganglion) and are quite short in length.
- GVA: these fibers make up the bulk of the vagus nerve. The peripheral processes are located in the mucous membranes of the soft palate, oropharynx (overlap the CN IX GSA innervation), laryngopharynx, esophagus, larynx and trachea. GVA fibers also travel back from the carotid sinus and carotid body via the **carotid sinus nerve of CN X**. The central processes enter the brainstem and synapse at the ipsilateral **solitary nucleus of the solitary tract**.
- SVA: the peripheral processes of taste sensation fibers originating from a limited area of the anterior epiglottis travel back through the **internal laryngeal** and **superior laryngeal nerves**. The central processes will synapse at the ipsilateral **solitary nucleus of the solitary tract**.

Clinical Correlate 12.12

Lesions of the Vagus Nerve

Much like the glossopharyngeal nerve, isolated lesions of the vagus nerve are rare. If a lesion was on the recurrent laryngeal nerve, this could cause difficulty speaking (dysphonia) or hoarseness because of the paralysis of the vocal cords. Lesions involving the pharyngeal nerve branches could lead to difficulty swallowing (dysphagia). If the soft palate or anterior pharynx is stimulated and a lesion of the vagus nerve is suspected, the uvula and palate will deviate away from the lesion.

12.11 Spinal Accessory Nerve

The **spinal accessory nerve** (CN XI) provides motor innervation to both the **sternocleidomastoid** and **trapezius muscles**. The functional components of this nerve are GSE (**Fig. 12.17**). The cell bodies of the motor fibers are located in the **spinal accessory nucleus**, which is found in the posterolateral aspect of the ventral horns of cervical spinal cord levels C1-C5 (or C6). Thin rootlets extend from between the lateral funiculus of the spinal cord and continue superiorly through the **foramen magnum** before passing through the **jugular foramen** to reach the muscles. This nerve was formally described as having a *cranial* and *spinal root*, however, the cranial root has recently been shown to be more associated with the vagus nerve and originates from the nucleus ambiguus just superior to the spinal accessory nucleus.

The general proprioceptive input from these muscles is transmitted back with branches of the cervical plexus conveying sensory fibers from spinal nerves C2, C3, and C4. These pseudounipolar neurons have their cell bodies located in the dorsal root ganglion.

12.12 Hypoglossal Nerve

The **hypoglossal nerve** (CN XII) is responsible for innervating all of the intrinsic and the majority of the extrinsic tongue muscles with the exception of the palatoglossus muscle (**Fig. 12.18**). The functional components of this nerve are GSE and GSA. There is debate as to where the general proprioceptive input of these muscles transmits. It is thought that pseudounipolar neurons either course through the main nerve and their cell bodies are located in the **mesencephalic nucleus** of the trigeminal nerve, or in a similar fashion to the spinal accessory nerve, where the pseudounipolar neurons pass back with the first couple of cervical spinal nerves and have their cell bodies located in the dorsal root ganglion.

The GSE motor fibers have their cell bodies in the **hypoglossal nucleus**. The nucleus appears as a column located anterior to

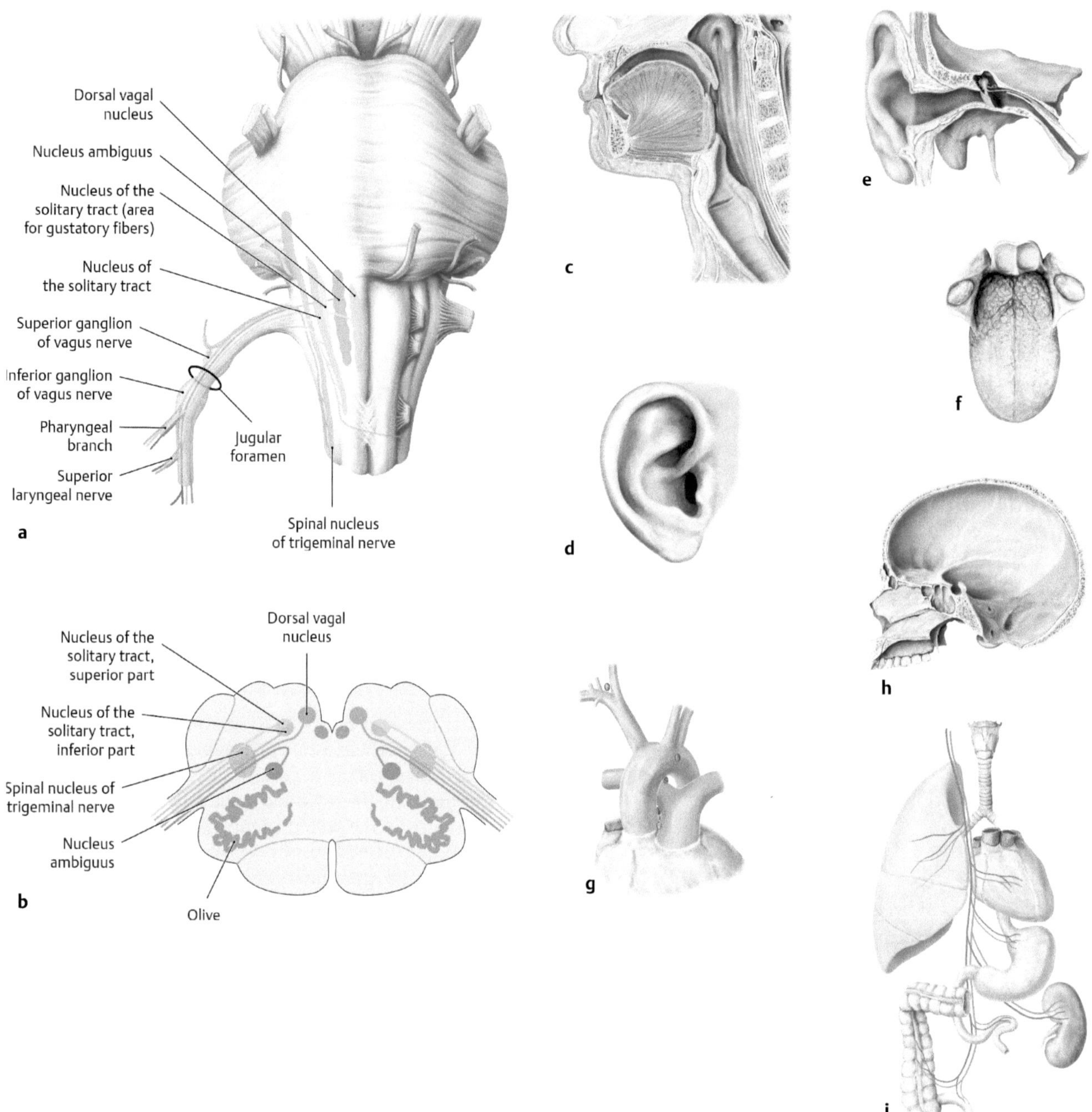

Fig. 12.15 **(a)** Nuclei of the vagus nerve, anterior view. **(b)** Cross-section through the medulla oblongata at the level of the superior olive. **(c)** Visceral sensory innervation of the mucosa of the lower pharynx and larynx. **(d,e)** Somatic sensory innervation of the concha and external acoustic meatus. **(f)** Visceral sensory and taste of the anterior epiglottic region. **(g)** Pressure and chemoreceptors near the aortic arch. **(h)** Dura of the posterior cranial fossa. **(i)** Thoracic and abdominal viscera through the midgut. (From Schuenke M, Schulte E, Schumacher U. THIEME Atlas of Anatomy. Head, Neck, and Neuroanatomy. Illustrations by Voll M and Wesker K. 3rd ed. New York: Thieme Medical Publishers; 2020.)

the floor of the fourth ventricle near the midline of the medulla. This forms a triangular elevation referred to as the **hypoglossal trigone**. The hypoglossal nerve originates anteriorly from the medulla as a series of rootlets in the sulcus separating the pyramid and olive. The rootlets condense to form an isolated nerve that exits the cranial vault through the **hypoglossal canal** and targets the ipsilateral tongue musculature.

There are C1 fibers that course along with the hypoglossal nerve but do not exchange fibers with it. However, these C1 fibers separate at different locations from this nerve and contribute in order to the superior root of ansa cervicalis, the innervation to the thyrohyoid muscle, and finally the innervation to the geniohyoid muscle.

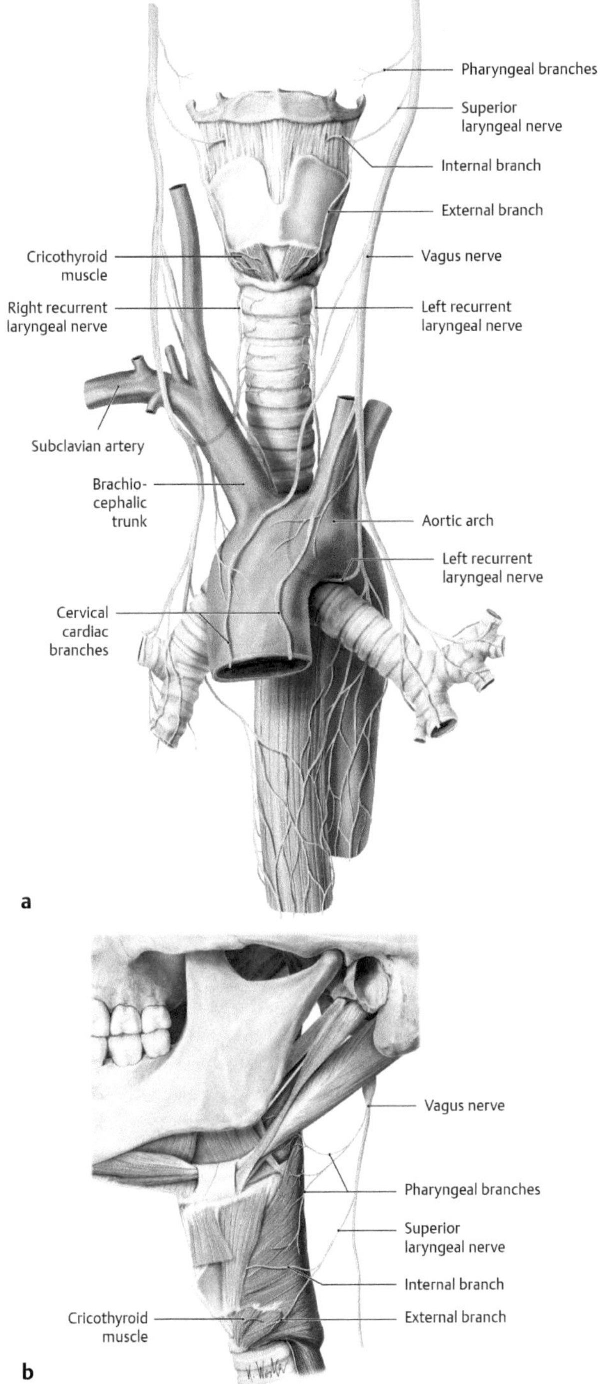

Fig. 12.16 Branches of the vagus nerve in the neck. **(a)** Anterior view. **(b)** Left lateral view. (From Schuenke M, Schulte E, Schumacher U. THIEME Atlas of Anatomy. Head, Neck, and Neuroanatomy. Illustrations by Voll M and Wesker K. 3rd ed. New York: Thieme Medical Publishers; 2020.)

Clinical Correlate 12.13

Damage or Lesions of the Spinal Accessory Nerve

On its way toward the trapezius muscle, CN XI lies superficial to the levator scapulae muscle, making it susceptible to injury during surgical procedures such as a carotid endarterectomy or lymph node biopsy. Lesions of CN XI will produce dropping of the shoulder due to weakness and atrophy of the trapezius muscle **(a)**. Impairment of the sternocleidomastoid muscle would result in a deficiency of rotary movements of the neck towards the opposite side against a resistance **(b)**.

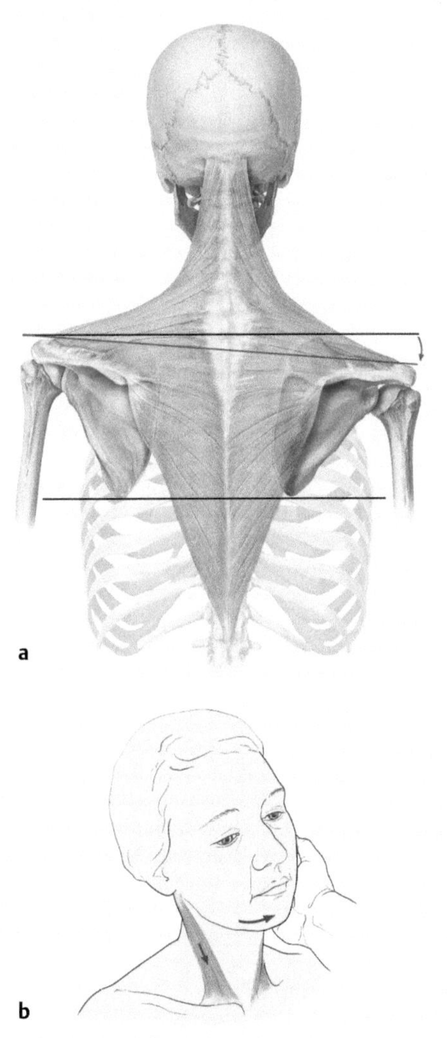

(From Schuenke M, Schulte E, Schumacher U. THIEME Atlas of Anatomy. Head, Neck, and Neuroanatomy. Illustrations by Voll M and Wesker K. 3rd ed. New York: Thieme Medical Publishers; 2020.)

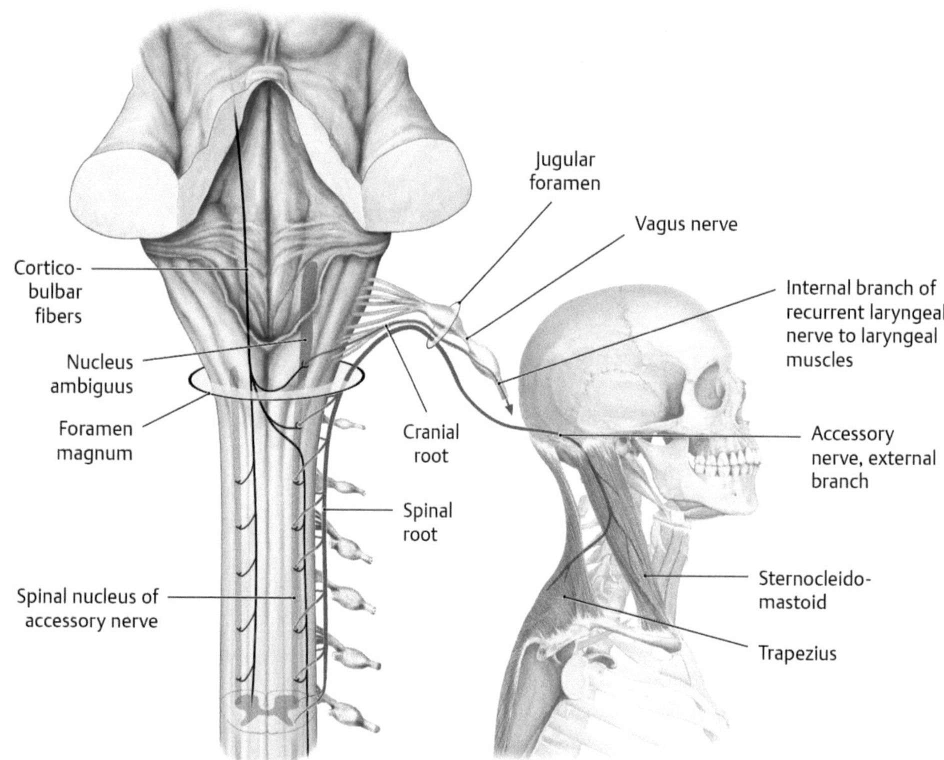

Fig. 12.17 Nucleus and course of the spinal accessory nerve. (From Schuenke M, Schulte E, Schumacher U. THIEME Atlas of Anatomy. Head, Neck, and Neuroanatomy. Illustrations by Voll M and Wesker K. 3rd ed. New York: Thieme Medical Publishers; 2020.)

Clinical Correlate 12.14

Lesions of the Hypoglossal Nerve

A hypoglossal motor nucleus is innervated by upper motor neurons associated with corticobulbar tract fibers that decussate at the medulla oblongata and target the contralateral hypoglossal nucleus. The lower motor neuron then targets the ipsilateral tongue musculature except for the palatoglossus muscle.

An **upper motor neuron lesion** occurring before the decussation causes the tongue to *deviate away* from the side of the lesion. A **lower motor neuron lesion** occurring after the decussation causes the tongue to *deviate to the same side* as the lesion. When protruding the tongue, its apex deviates toward the paralyzed side because of the unopposed action of the genioglossus muscle on the normal side of the tongue.

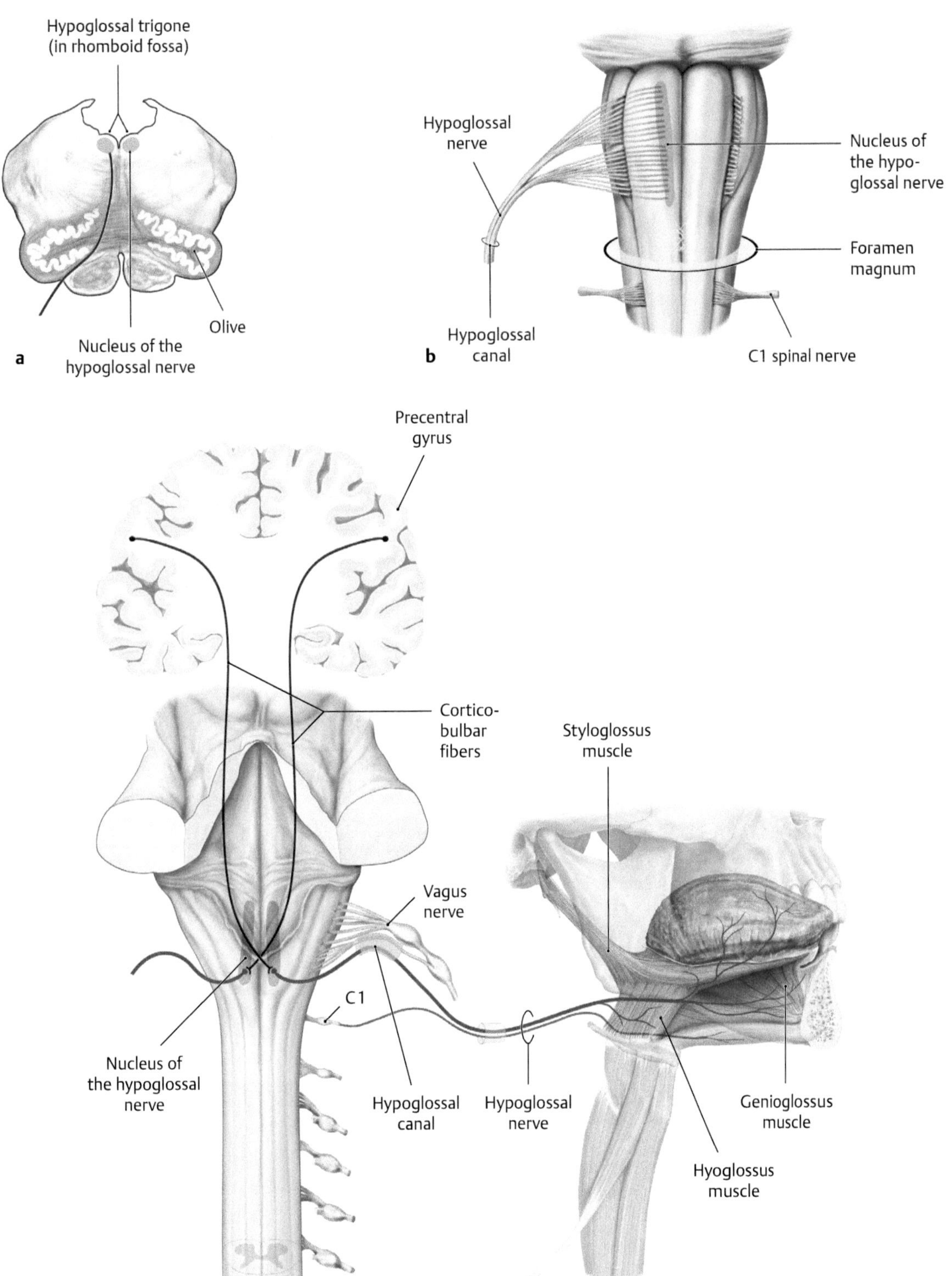

Fig. 12.18 **(a)** Nuclei of the hypoglossal nerve, cross-section through the medulla oblongata at the level of the olive. **(b)** Anterior view of the medulla oblongata. **(c)** Central and peripheral distribution of the hypoglossal nerve. (From Schuenke M, Schulte E, Schumacher U. THIEME Atlas of Anatomy. Head, Neck, and Neuroanatomy. Illustrations by Voll M and Wesker K. 3rd ed. New York: Thieme Medical Publishers; 2020.)

PRACTICE QUESTIONS

1. Which statement regarding cranial nerves is INCORRECT?
   A. V_1 has 3 major initial GSA branches (lacrimal, frontal and nasociliary).
   B. CN IX is responsible for innervating the stylohyoid muscle.
   C. The cell bodies of GSA fibers associated with CN V are located in the trigeminal ganglion.
   D. Parasympathetic preganglionic fibers of CN III course through its inferior division before reaching the ciliary ganglion.
   E. CN XI passes through the jugular foramen before innervating the trapezius muscle.
2. A patient has suffered a stroke and the artery involved helps supply blood to parts of the nucleus ambiguus. SVE (branchiomotor) fibers that originate from this brainstem nucleus will course through which combination of cranial nerves?
   A. CN III, CN IV and CN VI.
   B. CN V3 and CN VII.
   C. CN VII and CN IX.
   D. CN IX and CN X.
   E. CN X and CN XII.
3. Which statement regarding the facial nerve (CN VII) is INCORRECT?
   A. Parasympathetic preganglionic cell bodies of CN VII are located in the inferior salivatory nucleus.
   B. It is associated with Bell's palsy.
   C. It innervates the buccinator muscle.
   D. The cell bodies of GSA, GVA and SSA fibers are located in the geniculate ganglion.
   E. The SVE (branchiomotor) fibers originate from the facial nucleus.
4. A patient presents with a downward and outward gaze, dilated pupil, and eyelid drooping of the right eye when asked to look straight ahead during an eye exam. Which cranial nerve palsy is present?
   A. Optic nerve.
   B. Oculomotor nerve.
   C. Trochlear nerve.
   D. Trigeminal nerve.
   E. Abducent nerve.
5. A patient makes an appointment to see their primary care physician because they have noticed some difficulty swallowing over the past few months. Upon examination, thephysician notices that the palate and pharynx deviate to the right side when the gag reflex is elicited. This is referred to as a "curtain call." An MRI is ordered and a radiodense lesion is noted in the brainstem. Where do you predict the lesion to be located?
   A. Left side of posterior midbrain.
   B. Right side of the paramedian midbrain.
   C. Left side of the anteromedial pons.
   D. Left side of the posterolateral medulla.
   E. Right side of the posterolateral medulla.
6. Which statement regarding the trigeminal nerve (CN V) is INCORRECT?
   A. SVE (branchiomotor) fibers pass only through V3.
   B. The spinal trigeminal tract receives GSA temperature, light touch, and pain input from the ipsilateral face, palate, anterior 2/3 of the tongue, and the teeth.
   C. The posterior trigeminothalamic tract receives GSA discriminative (fine) tactile and pressure input from the face and oral cavity and it will decussate to the contralateral VPM.
   D. The mesencephalic nucleus is associated with GSA proprioceptive input traveling back from CN III, IV, V and VI.
   E. The spinal nucleus is associated with temperature and pain sensation from the oral and facial regions as well as discriminative (fine) tactile sense and itch information.
7. An individual has suffered trauma and the damage has occurred just distal to the geniculate ganglion related to CN VII. All functions would be lost EXCEPT which?
   A. Innervation to the lacrimal gland.
   B. Taste from the anterior 2/3 of the tongue.
   C. Innervation of facial expression muscles.
   D. Innervation to the stapedius muscle.
   E. Innervation to the submandibular and sublingual glands.
8. Which statement regarding the glossopharyngeal nerve (CN IX) is INCORRECT?
   A. The inferior ganglion consists of SVA and GVA first order pseudounipolar neurons.
   B. The SVE (branchiomotor) fibers innervate the stylopharyngeus muscle.
   C. Taste sensation fibers from the posterior 1/3 of the tongue pass back to the contralateral solitary nucleus and tract.
   D. Parasympathetic fibers that target the parotid gland originate from the inferior salivatory nucleus.
   E. Parasympathetic postganglionic cell bodies are located in the otic ganglion.
9. Which cranial nerve is related to the clinical correlate known as anosmia?
   A. Olfactory nerve.
   B. Optic nerve.
   C. Trigeminal nerve.
   D. Abducent nerve.
   E. Hypoglossal nerve.
10. Which cranial nerve is related to the clinical correlate known as crocodile tears syndrome?
    A. Trigeminal nerve.
    B. Facial nerve.
    C. Vestibulocochlear nerve.
    D. Glossopharyngeal nerve.
    E. Vagus nerve.

ANSWERS

1. **B.** CN IX will only innervate the stylopharyngeus muscle associated with the pharynx.
2. **D.** SVE fibers that originate from the nucleus ambiguous course through CN IX and CN X.
3. **A.** Parasympathetic preganglionic cell bodies of CN VII are located in the superior salivatory nucleus.
4. **B.** Oculomotor nerve (CN III).
5. **D.** A left-sided lesion located near the posterolateral medulla would include structures such as the inferior cerebellar peduncle, spinal trigeminal tract and nucleus, anterior spinocerebellar tract, and the nucleus ambiguus among others. With the nucleus ambiguus specifically damaged this would be considered a lower motor neuron injury and the ipsilateral muscles related to the gag reflex would be unable to contract. This results in the palate and pharynx muscles still functioning on the right side thus when the muscles contract they lean toward the side opposite the lesion.

6. **C.** The posterior trigeminothalamic tract receives all of the information as stated, however, after first-order neurons from the trigeminal ganglion synapse at the main (principal) nucleus, second order neurons from the main (principal) nucleus will remain ipsilateral and travel superiorly to the VPM. Ultimately, third order neurons from the VPM will reach the postcentral gyrus (3, 1 and 2) of the cerebral cortex after passing through the internal capsule.
7. **A.** Parasympathetic fibers responsible for innervating the lacrimal gland pass through the greater petrosal nerve that directly branches off the geniculate ganglion thus these fibers would not be affected by damage distal to the ganglion.
8. **C.** Taste sensation from the posterior 1/3 of the tongue does not decussate and travels back to the ipsilateral solitary nucleus and tract.
9. **A.** Anosmia is the decrease or loss of olfaction or smell and is thus related to the olfactory nerve (CN I).
10. **B.** Crocodile tears syndrome involves a facial nerve lesion proximal to the geniculate ganglion. There is an increase in lacrimation or tear production while eating because select regenerating parasympathetic preganglionic fibers that originated from the superior salivatory nucleus and destined to synapse at the submandibular ganglion are misdirected to the pterygopalatine ganglion.

Index

A

B

C

M

N

T

V

W

X

Z